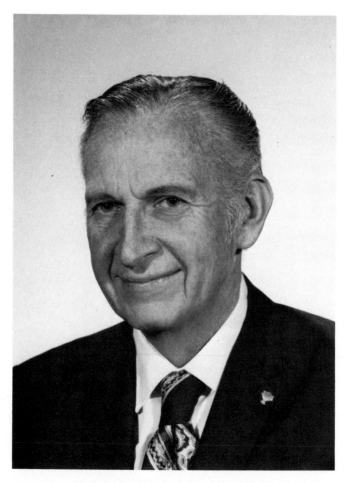

ROBERT H. WILLIAMS

Head of the Division of Endocrinology and Metabolism, University Hospital; Professor of Medicine, School of Medicine, University of Washington, Seattle

Textbook of Endocrinology

Fifth Edition

Edited by
ROBERT H. WILLIAMS, M.D.

With Contributions by Thirty-eight Authorities

W. B. SAUNDERS COMPANY Philadelphia · London · Toronto

W. B. Saunders Company: West Washington Square
                           Philadelphia, Pa. 19105

                           12 Dyott Street
                           London, WC1A 1DB

                           833 Oxford Street
                           Toronto, Ontario M8Z 5T9, Canada

Listed here is the latest translated edition of this
book together with the language of the translation
and the publisher.

Polish (*3rd Edition*) — Lekarskich, Warsaw, Poland

Spanish (*4th Edition*) — Salvat Editores, Barcelona,
                           Spain

French (*4th Edition*) — Flammarion, Paris, France

Italian (*4th Edition*) — Piccin Editore, Padova, Italy

Japanese (*4th Edition*) — Dainihon Seiyaku, Ltd.,
                           Osaka, Japan

Serbo-Croat (*4th Edition*) — Medicinska Knjiga,
                              Belgrade, Yugoslavia

Textbook of Endocrinology   SBN   0-7216-9397-0

Print No.:   9   8   7   6   5   4

DEDICATED

TO

Contributors of the past, who as investigators, educators, and authors have evolved the knowledge summarized in this book,

AND TO

Contributors of the future, who extensively dedicate their activities toward providing universally better health and more happiness, sharing their knowledge readily and collaborating freely in attaining these goals.

CONTRIBUTORS

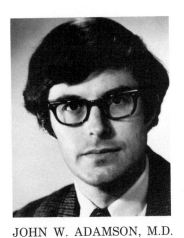

JOHN W. ADAMSON, M.D.

Associate Professor of Medicine, University of Washington School of Medicine, and Chief of Hematology Section, Veterans Administration Hospital, Seattle.

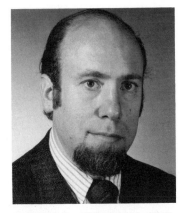

EDWIN L. BIERMAN, M.D.

Professor of Medicine and Head of Division of Metabolism and Gerontology, University of Washington School of Medicine, Seattle.

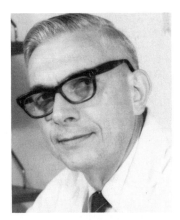

ROBERT M. BLIZZARD, M.D.

Professor of Pediatrics and Chief of Division of Pediatric Endocrinology, Johns Hopkins University School of Medicine, Baltimore.

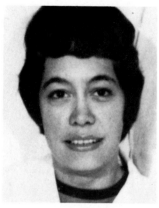

JO ANNE BRASEL, M.D.

Associate Professor of Pediatrics and Chief of the Division of Growth and Development of the Institute of Human Nutrition, Columbia University College of Physicians and Surgeons, New York.

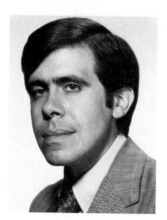

DANIEL P. CARDINALI, M.D.

Research Member of Carrera del Investigador, Comision Nacional de Estudios Geo-Helifisicos, Argentina.

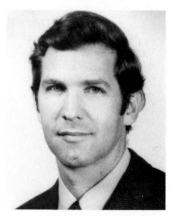

CECIL H. COGGINS, M.D.

Assistant Professor of Medicine, Harvard Medical School, and Acting Chief of Renal Unit, Massachusetts General Hospital, Boston.

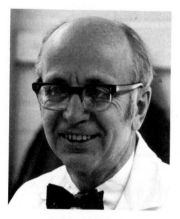

WILLIAM H. DAUGHADAY, M.D.

Professor of Medicine and Director of Metabolism Division, Washington University School of Medicine; Associate Physician at Barnes Hospital, St. Louis.

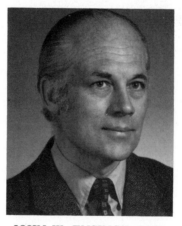

JOHN W. ENSINCK, M.D.

Professor of Medicine, University of Washington School of Medicine, and Director of Clinical Research Center, University Hospital, Seattle.

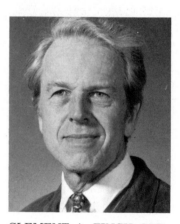

CLEMENT A. FINCH, M.D.

Professor of Medicine and Head of Division of Hematology, University of Washington School of Medicine, Seattle.

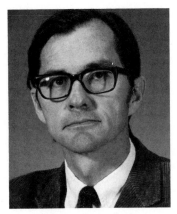

JOHN ASBJÖRN
GLOMSET, M.D.

Professor of Medicine, University of Washington School of Medicine, Seattle.

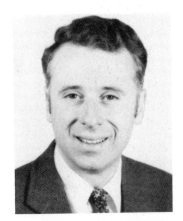

JOSEPH L. GOLDSTEIN,
M.D.

Assistant Professor of Internal Medicine and Head of Division of Medical Genetics, University of Texas Southwestern Medical School, Dallas.

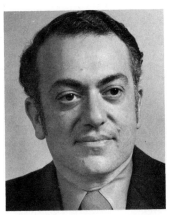

ROBERT I. GREGERMAN,
M.D.

Associate Professor of Medicine, Johns Hopkins University School of Medicine, Baltimore; Chief of Endocrinology Section (Clinical Physiology Branch) of Gerontology Research Center, NIH, Baltimore City Hospitals, Baltimore.

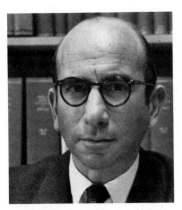

MELVIN M. GRUMBACH,
M.D.

Professor and Chairman of Department of Pediatrics and Director of Pediatric Services, University of California Medical Center, San Francisco.

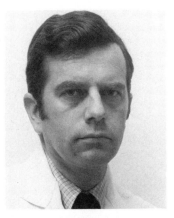

JOEL G. HARDMAN, Ph.D.

Professor of Physiology, Vanderbilt University Medical School, Nashville.

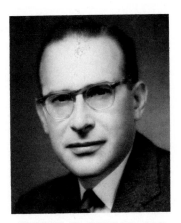

SIDNEY H. INGBAR, M.D.

Professor of Medicine, University of California, and Chief of Section of Endocrinology, Veterans Administration Hospital, San Francisco.

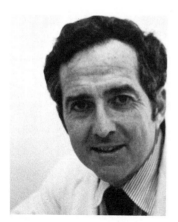

JOHN H. LARAGH, M.D.

Professor of Clinical Medicine, Columbia University, and Attending Physician, Presbyterian Hospital, New York.

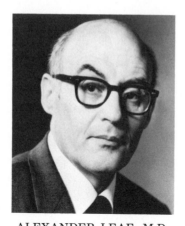

ALEXANDER LEAF, M.D.

Jackson Professor of Clinical Medicine, Harvard Medical School, and Chief of Medical Services, Massachusetts General Hospital, Boston.

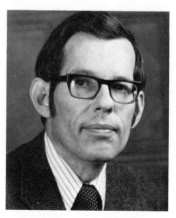

JAMES B. LEE, M.D.

Professor of Medicine, University of Buffalo School of Medicine, and Director of Division of Endocrinology, Buffalo General Hospital, Buffalo.

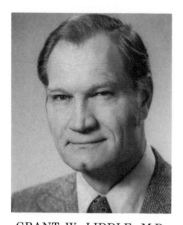

GRANT W. LIDDLE, M.D.

Professor of Medicine, Vanderbilt University School of Medicine; Physician-in-Chief and Director of Endocrinology, Vanderbilt University Hospital, Nashville.

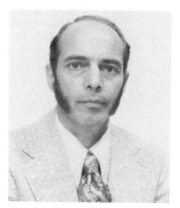

MORTIMER B. LIPSETT, M.D.

Associate Scientific Director of National Institute of Child Health and Human Development, NIH, Bethesda.

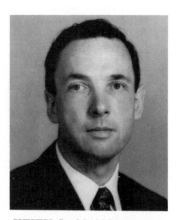

KEITH L. MANCHESTER, Ph.D.

Professor of Biochemistry, University of the Witwatersrand, Johannesburg, South Africa.

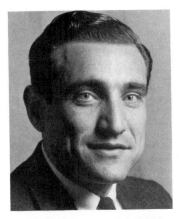

KENNETH L. MELMON,
M.D.

Professor of Medicine and
Pharmacology, University of
California School of Medicine,
and Attending Physician in
H. C. Moffitt Hospital, San
Francisco.

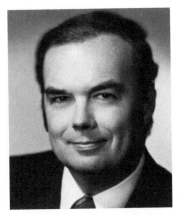

JAMES E. McGUIGAN,
M.D.

Professor of Medicine and
Chief of Division of Gastro-
enterology, University of
Florida College of Medicine,
Gainesville.

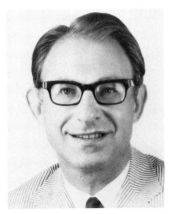

ARNO G. MOTULSKY,
M.D.

Professor of Medicine and
Genetics and Head of Division
of Medical Genetics, Uni-
versity of Washington School
of Medicine, Seattle.

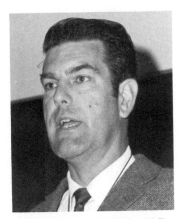

WILLIAM D. ODELL, M.D.,
Ph.D.

Professor of Medicine and
Physiology, UCLA School of
Medicine, and Chairman of
Department of Medicine, Har-
bor General Hospital Campus,
Torrance.

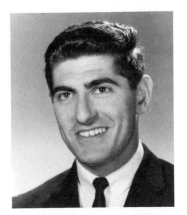

FRANK PARKER, M.D.

Clinical Professor of Medicine,
University of Washington
School of Medicine, Seattle.

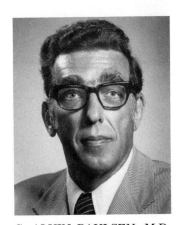

C. ALVIN PAULSEN, M.D.

Professor of Medicine, University of Washington School
of Medicine, and Chief of
Endocrinology, USPHS Hos-
pital, Seattle.

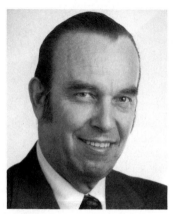

CARL M. PEARSON, M.D.

Professor of Medicine and Director of Division of Rheumatology, UCLA Medical Center, Los Angeles.

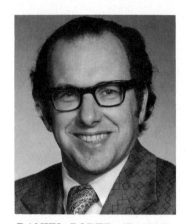

DANIEL PORTE, JR., M.D.

Professor of Medicine, University of Washington School of Medicine, and Associate Chief of Staff for Research, Veterans Administration Hospital, Seattle.

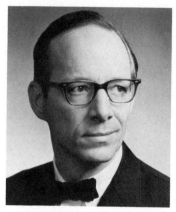

HOWARD RASMUSSEN, M.D., Ph.D.

Benjamin Rush Professor of Biochemistry and Professor of Medicine, University of Pennsylvania School of Medicine; Senior Physician, The Children's Hospital of Philadelphia, Philadelphia.

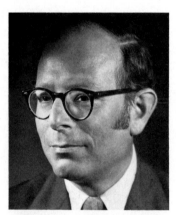

SEYMOUR REICHLIN, M.D., Ph.D.

Professor of Medicine, Tufts University School of Medicine, and Head of Endocrinology Division, Tufts-New England Medical Center, Boston.

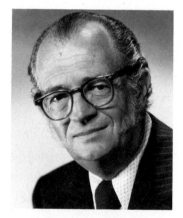

GRIFF T. ROSS, M.D., Ph.D.

Clinical Director of National Institute of Child Health and Human Development; Assistant Chief, Reproduction Research Branch of National Institute of Child Health and Human Development, Bethesda.

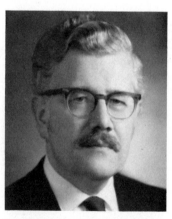

PAUL P. VAN ARSDEL, JR., M.D.

Professor of Medicine and Head of Division of Allergy, University of Washington School of Medicine, Seattle.

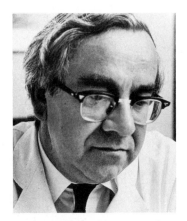

RAYMOND L. VANDE
WIELE, M.D.

Willard C. Rappleye Professor and Chairman of Department of Obstetrics and Gynecology, College of Physicians and Surgeons, Columbia University; Director of Obstetrical and Gynecological Service, Presbyterian Hospital, New York.

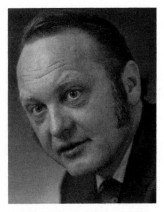

JUDSON J. VAN WYK,
M.D.

Professor of Pediatrics and Chief of Division of Pediatric Endocrinology and Metabolism, University of North Carolina School of Medicine, Chapel Hill.

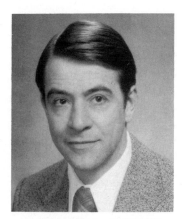

KENNETH A. WOEBER,
M.D.

Professor of Medicine, University of Texas; Chief of Division of Endocrinology and Metabolism, University of Texas Health Science Center, San Antonio.

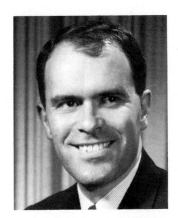

RICHARD J. WURTMAN,
M.D.

Professor of Endocrinology and Metabolism, Department of Nutrition and Food Sciences, Massachusetts Institute of Technology, Cambridge; Clinical Assistant in Medicine, Massachusetts General Hospital, Boston.

PREFACE TO THE FIFTH EDITION

Vast amounts of information are accumulating rapidly concerning metabolic processes involved in the formation, maturation, and function of body tissues and in the pathogenesis of many diseases, including atherosclerosis, heart disease, hypertension, cancer, mental disorders, and genetic abnormalities, among others. Indeed, every illness is associated with metabolic changes. Furthermore, in all body cells hormones influence the metabolism of nucleotides, proteins, lipids, carbohydrates, vitamins, water, and electrolytes. Therefore, knowledge of endocrinology and metabolism is important in every branch of medicine.

The contributors to this book have previously demonstrated excellence as investigators, teachers, and authors. Most of them are engaged in both basic and clinical investigations and teaching. They are adept in the practical application of basic knowledge to clinical problems and use this approach in discussing pathogenesis, diagnosis, and therapy. They have been encouraged to indicate where controversy exists, but to submit tentative conclusions based on available data.

Great efforts were made to restrict the length of each chapter; several chapters are about the same length as in the fourth edition or shorter. A small amount of repetition in different chapters has been permitted and encouraged for emphasis, and because many hormone activities are interrelated.

The authors were asked to use many figures, tables, and prominent headings to aid in clarification and rapid reference. Special attention was devoted to diagnostic tests and treatment, and emphasis given to measures that are most helpful.

The authors were urged to make their references selective and, especially, to include a number of recent reviews. They were told not to attempt to document each statement; sometimes one paragraph includes the results of many investigations.

This is predominantly a new book. Twenty-one of the 38 authors are new, and 12 chapters with new content have been added. In seven other chapters, there are one or more new authors. All of the chapters have been extensively rewritten.

The new chapters discuss (a) hormone actions on skin, on skeletal muscle, on blood elements, on allergic and immunologic reactions, and on cancer; (b) the pineal organ, gastrointestinal hormones, angiotensin-aldosterone system, and prostaglandins; and (c) the interrelationships of hormone secretion and action with cyclic nucleotide metabolism, protein metabolism, and aging.

Chapter 1 deals with major principles, especially with key regulatory and coordinating processes. It considers functions of the cell membrane and reciprocal communications and actions between it, the nucleus, and other intracellular organelles. This chapter also discusses the mechanisms for coordination of metabolic activities in large organisms. The endocrine system and the autonomic nervous system together form a single neuroendocrine unit, with the main endocrine and metabolic coordinative center in the hypothalamus. As discussed particularly in Chapter 12, specific areas in the hypothalamus are inhibited or stimulated by hormones or other constituents in plasma and by neurotransmitters. In turn, individual areas of the hypothalamus respond by releasing specific hormones that are transmitted either directly to the pituitary, or through the autonomic nervous system. The hypophysiotropic hormones consist of those that release ACTH, TSH, GH, FSH, LH, prolactin, and MSH and of those that inhibit the release of GH, prolactin, and MSH. Several chapters emphasize that the site and amount of action by a hormone depend upon its binding to its own specific receptor. From the hormone-receptor complex, messages are transmitted to other cell sites. As discussed particularly in Chapter 16, cyclic nucleotides act as intracellular messengers.

Chapter 25 emphasizes the extensive role of genetics in growth, maturation, aging, and other events, and Chapter 8 details genetic abnormalities in sex differentiation and development.

The special roles of vasopressin, aldosterone, glucosteroids, and angiotensin in water and electrolyte metabolism and in the maintenance of plasma volume and blood pressure are discussed in Chapters 3, 5, 19, and 20.

Hormonal interrelationships between the gastrointestinal tract, pancreas, and liver are presented in Chapters 9, 10, and 14. The roles of gastrin, secretin, pancreozymin, proinsulin, insulin, glucagon, enterogastrone, and serotonin are emphasized.

There are discussions of the latest developments regarding calcitonin, vitamin D metabolites, somatomedin (NSILA), chorionic somatomammotropin, catecholamines, prostaglandins, erythropoietin, thymic hormones, pherhormones, and hormones from ectopic sites.

Newer methods are mentioned for measuring many hormones: melatonin, hypothalamic hormones, vasopressin, oxytocin, anterior pituitary hormones, triiodothyronine, thyroxine, calcitonin, glucagon, glucagon-like hormone, gastrin, secretin, angiotensin, aldosterone, testosterone, estrone, estradiol, progesterone, placental hormones, proinsulin and its connecting peptide, prostaglandins, and erythropoietin. There are discussions of the diagnostic use of hypophysiotropic hormones, ^{131}I-cholesterol, and technetium. Several chapters contain tables listing the order of preference of tests for many clinical disorders.

There are descriptions of the therapeutic uses of calcitonin, mithramycin, o,p'-DDD, propranolol, clomiphene, streptozotocin, diazoxide, monocomponent insulin, clofibrate, cholestyramine, lithium, parachlorophenylalanine, methysergide, vitamin D derivatives, L-dopa, antifertility drugs, and other compounds.

The editor is grateful for the splendid cooperation and superb contributions of the authors, the great assistance given by Alison Ross and other manuscript editors, the excellent secretarial activities of Sharon Kemp, and the many contributions of the members of the W. B. Saunders Company.

ROBERT H. WILLIAMS, M.D.

CONTENTS

Chapter 26

THE INFLUENCE OF THE ENDOCRINE GLANDS UPON GROWTH

By Jo Anne Brasel and Robert M. Blizzard

Chapter 27

By Robert I. Gregerman and Edwin L. Bierman

Chapter 28

By Mortimer B. Lipsett

CHAPTER 1

Organization and Control of Endocrine Systems

By Howard Rasmussen

Claude Bernard was the first to appreciate that the composition of the fluids bathing the cells of multicellular organisms must be controlled. He proposed that the stability of this internal environment, which he termed the *milieu organique interieur,* gave the body a degree of functional freedom from the variability of the external one, the *milieu cosmique ambiant.* Since Bernard, it has become evident that such stability is attained by the coordinated activities of two major systems: the endocrine system and the autonomic nervous system.

At first glance, these two regulatory systems appear rather distinct. Information is carried by neural impulses in the autonomic system, and by the blood in the endocrine system. In general, autonomic responses are more localized and more rapid than hormonal ones. Closer scrutiny, however, reveals that this classification is indistinct. The nerve endings release chemical transmitters, acetylcholine and norepinephrine, which under some circumstances circulate in the plasma and can be

considered endocrine gland products or hormones. There is a gradation from what might be termed a purely neural response through intermediate responses to a purely endocrine one.

The first response can be illustrated by the release of norepinephrine from sympathetic nerve endings in the smooth muscle of the wall of an arteriole; the second by the release of norepinephrine from the adrenal medulla; and the third by the release of parathyroid hormone from the parathyroid gland. Each response is elicited by an afferent stimulus which is neural in the first two instances and humoral in the third. The efferent response in the first is primarily neural, the norepinephrine acting primarily at the site of its release. In the second, the efferent response is initially neural (preganglionic fibers to adrenal medulla) but soon becomes endocrine because the norepinephrine is disseminated by the circulation and acts at widely different sites within the organism. The efferent response in the third is completely endocrine, the hormone being released directly under the influence of the chemical afferent stimulus.

The unique interrelationships between the two systems are even more apparent in the hypothalamus. This portion of the central nervous system is the highest integrative center of both the autonomic and endocrine systems, as well as the major site at which the activities of the two systems merge. In addition to its classic nervous functions, it is the site of synthesis of several polypeptide hormones. Hence in the largest sense the autonomic nervous system and the various endocrine glands represent a single neuroendocrine system that has evolved to integrate and coordinate the metabolic activities of the organism. Although this book deals primarily with the endocrine aspects of this larger system, references to the autonomic system are made, particularly to those aspects most clearly related to endocrine activity.

1

Before a discussion of the general aspects of endocrine organization is undertaken, another facet of the concept of the *milieu intérieur* remains to be considered.

As defined by Bernard, the *milieu intérieur* consists of the plasma and extracellular fluids bathing the cells of a multicellular organism. Yet, from all indications, life developed in a pre-Cambrian sea rich in magnesium and potassium, a milieu differing considerably from that of Bernard's *milieu intérieur* but strikingly similar in composition to the intracellular fluids of present-day animal forms. It is within this milieu that cellular metabolism operates. In reality the intracellular fluids of many simple organisms, such as yeast, as well as those of higher forms, are contained not in a single cellular compartment but in multiple membrane-bounded compartments, each with its own distinct composition. These intracellular fluid compartments are in fact the true chemical environment of life, the *milieu de la vie*.

Each cell of a multicellular organism has inherited a complex system of homeostatic controls with which to regulate and coordinate the activities of its several components. Much of modern biology is concerned with the elucidation and study of these cellular control systems. Considerable unity already has been discovered. For example, it is apparent that the mechanism for transporting glucose into a muscle cell is basically similar to that employed by a bacterial cell and that the intracellular hormone, cyclic AMP ($3',5'$-AMP or C-AMP), was involved in regulating cell metabolism in lower forms long before it became an aspect of hormone action in the rat liver cell.

It is becoming increasingly clear that an understanding of these basic cellular control systems is necessary to define the basis of hormonal action and that the control of the composition of Bernard's *milieu intérieur* is achieved by adaptations to later needs of these ancient but highly sophisticated intracellular systems. In other words, extracellular homeostasis is but an evolutionary extension of intracellular homeostasis. Much of the present chapter is concerned with a discussion of these intracellular control systems and their relationship to hormones and to hormone action.

THE ENDOCRINE SYSTEM

Organization

Basic Concepts

In order to describe how endocrine systems are organized, it is necessary first to introduce certain concepts that have been borrowed from the field of systems analysis and servomechanisms. Basic to an understanding of these concepts are the definitions of systems and a consideration of whether these systems are open or closed. A system for the purpose of our discussion is an organized unit of activity from an enzyme or multienzyme complex to

an entire organism or even a population of organisms. In viewing any one of these systems we can consider them in one of two fashions: either as open or as closed loop systems. The distinction between the two is simple yet consequentially profound. In an open loop system, a cause or input alters the effect or output, but the converse is not true. In a closed loop system, output influences the behavior of the system and its response to an input. In such systems it becomes meaningless to consider simple cause and effect. Not only are responses determined by the nature and strength of the stimuli, but the stimuli depend upon the responses according to the present organization and environment of the system in question.

The paradox of modern endocrinologic research has been that, at the physiologic level of analysis, it has been recognized and generally accepted that the endocrine system and its various subcomponents are organized in a hierarchy of closed loop systems. However, at the biochemical or cellular level of organization, nearly all considerations of the mode of action of hormones have been cast in the mold of open systems, cause and effect relationships in which the hormone acts upon the cell to cause a variety of effects but in which the cell does not in turn act upon the original stimulus.

This paradox has more than merely philosophic interest. The models of cellular organization that we build in innocence and enthusiasm today become the dogma of tomorrow and hence shape the intellect's quest for further understanding. It thus becomes imperative to state explicitly that the mammalian organism and its organized subcomponents, e.g., cells or metabolic pathways, all operate as closed loops. The entire system is a metabolic net. Homeostasis at the level of cell and organism depends fundamentally upon communication between the components. Stimulus (input) leads to response, but response (output), to be meaningful, must in turn influence the stimulus. Disease and dysfunction result when communication in either direction fails.

The most important general concept is that of *feedback control,* and particularly *negative feedback.* The simplest situation to consider is that of two variables, A and B. If A = f(B) and B = f(A), then a feedback relationship exists between the two (Fig. 1–1). If the concentration or effect of A is increased when B increases, then *positive feedback* exists, whereas if A decreases when B increases, *negative feedback* exists. These concepts are illustrated in Figure 1–1 by solid and broken arrows respectively.

The concept of feedback is derived from the operation of electrical networks. As it operates in biochemical or endocrine systems, however, it differs considerably in operational properties from electrical systems. Since much confusion exists on this point, and since many models of biochemical feedback have been constructed as analogues of electrical models, this difference is stressed below.

The most important feature of feedback in a physiologic or biochemical sense is that the *input* to the system is usually a concentration, and the

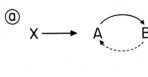

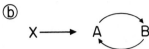

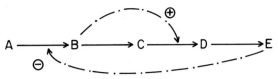

Figure 1–2. A hypothetical metabolic pathway in which positive feed-forward activation operates in an overall system in which negative feedback control exists.

Figure 1–1. Feedback relationships between two variables, A and B. A solid arrow means that when the independent variable changes the dependent variable changes in the same direction. A broken arrow means that when the independent variable changes the dependent variable changes in the opposite direction. (a) Negative feedback. When X increases A increases, leading to an increase in B, but an increase in B leads to a decrease in A. (b) Positive feedback.

output is a rate of change of concentration. Hence the most satisfactory way to analyze biochemical systems is in terms of the mass law equations of the system.

In addition to *feedback* loops in control systems, it is possible to have *feed-forward* loops, which also may be either positive or negative. Feed-forward loops are common in endocrine and metabolic control systems, but a distinctive feature of such loops is their inherent instability. Positive feed-forward signals may increse the flux through a metabolic sequence in an uncontrolled fashion. In order to achieve stability of control (homeostasis), positive feed-forward loops in control systems are nearly always a subcomponent of a larger control system within which negative feedback controls operate to maintain stability (Fig. 1–2).

A question then arises as to the value of positive feed-forward and positive feedback loops in biologic control systems. Their most obvious value is in an anticipatory sense. Such a change in the concentration of a particular intermediate is the signal of a sudden demand upon the pathway. In endocrine systems an extremely important example of this type of feed-forward loop is the release of insulin by the beta cells of the pancreas in response to an increase in intestinal glucose concentration (or rate of transport). By such a feed-forward loop, insulin is mobilized and acts to stimulate the uptake of glucose by the liver. Hence this positive sig-

nal has a very important directive effect in determining the major pathway of glucose disposal (hepatic versus peripheral tissue disposal). Other possible advantages of feed-forward loops may be their role in coordinating activities in divergent pathways (Fig. 1–3) and the possibility that, by activating a late step in a biochemical sequence, the concentrations of intermediates between the initial and final steps in the pathway may be maintained at very low levels in spite of marked increases in overall flux through the pathway.

Two examples in which positive loops exist are blood clotting and glycogenolysis. Both systems are characterized by nearly total inactivity in their resting states; both are activated extremely rapidly because of positive feed-forward and feedback signals and have a *cascade* type of organization (Fig. 1–4), resulting in a marked amplification of the initial signal. A feature of both is their self-limited nature, i.e., there is a relatively fixed amount of either glycogen or fibrinogen (or other clotting factors) available at any given moment. In addition, there are negative feedback loops in both control systems which operate to limit response. In both there is a necessity to go from a state of inactivity to marked activity in a brief period of time. Positive control loops are an effective means of achieving rapid amplification of the initial message or stimulus.

Feed-forward control is also a feature of oscillatory behavior in biologic systems. It has become increasingly evident that time-dependent changes in metabolic and endocrine function are of fundamental homeostatic importance. Periodicities on the order of minutes, hours, days, weeks, and months all have been recognized in human metabolic phenomena. One of the most striking recent findings

Figure 1–3. A hypothetical illustration of divergent metabolic pathways in which the rate of flux through the initial steps of the pathway can, by positive feed-forward control of one branch of the pathway, determine which of the two branches will predominate. In the example given, when the flux from A → B is low, the major product is E, but when it is high, the major products are Z_1 and Z_2.

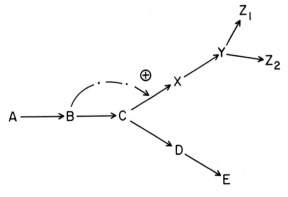

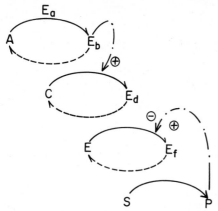

Figure 1–4. A schematic representation of an enzyme cascade such as the ones that operate in blood clotting and glycogenolysis. Here E_a to E_f represents successive enzymes in the cascade, and A, C, and E represent inactive enzymes. The basic sequence depends upon the fact that the successive inactive enzymes, A, C, and E, act as substrates, respectively, for E_a, E_b, and E_d. Hence once the conversion of A to E_b is initiated, there is a successive amplification of response with E_f, the final enzyme catalyzing the first biochemical reaction of glycogenolysis. The dashed arrows (———) represent the conversion of active enzymes back to inactive enzymes, which also must take place for effective control; the broken arrows (— · — · —) represent feedforward or feedback controls within the cascade.

was the discovery of a marked periodicity of growth hormone secretion with a peak of secretion hours after the onset of sleep. These biologic rhythms are of importance to health. A much clearer definition of the various endocrine rhythms other than the menstrual cycle is necessary, however, before this knowledge can be put to diagnostic and therapeutic use. Clearly the day will come when a major aim of therapy, particularly endocrine therapy, will be directed toward restoration of deranged endocrine rhythms.

Information Transfer in Endocrine Systems

Feedback and feed-forward controls in biochemical and endocrine systems represent transfers of information. The chemical messengers indicate to one part of the cell or organism the state of activity of another part of the cell or organism. In order to have the proper flow of this information, there must exist specific receivers or receptors, as well as transmitters. In the endocrine system, this means specific hormonal receptors either upon or within particular cells. These receptors possess sufficient uniqueness of structure to discriminate between the many similar messages that are constantly coming to them. The only known biologic macromolecules that possess sufficient structural plasticity to serve this discriminant function are proteins. It is our present belief that all hormonal receptors are unique proteins or lipoproteins, even though the chemical nature of hormones themselves varies considerably (Table 1–1).

Once the hormone or first chemical messenger has interacted with its receptor, there follows a

transduction of this information into *second* or intracellular messengers. In turn, there exist intracellular targets or receptors to which these second messengers bind and bring about a transduction of information into cellular response. Finally, as a consequence of these changes in cell function, a flow of information in the opposite direction ensues, i.e., specialized receptors in the original gland exist that recognize one or more products of the target cells. Recognition also implies response—a change in hormone output. A bidirectional flow of information is a prerequisite for proper homeostasis.

The Basis of Control

Whether one considers control of biologic processes at the level of populations of organisms, individual organisms, organs, cells, or enzymes, there are fundamentally two means of control: control of unit activity and control of the number of units.

At the physiologic level of organization in the endocrine system, the control units are cells. Hormones act to change the activity of cells, the number of responsive cells, or both. There is a unique feature (in the informational and operational sense) of these biologic control systems, however, that does not have its exact counterpart in the usual electrical analogue. There are qualitative differences in the chemical messengers in biologic systems. These qualitative differences exist in informational content, as well as in chemical structure and type of receptor cell responding. Such differences bring about a plasticity of response that is difficult to duplicate in classical electronic analogues. In addition, there is a very significant historical or unidirectional time sense in the operation of biologic systems. The underlying biologic processes are growth, differentiation, and aging.

The basis of the aging process is not known, but its importance is evident. There is a progressive change with time in the responsiveness of cells existing in an organized framework—an organ. Thus the liver cells of an 80-year-old man respond differently than those of an eight-year-old boy to a standard dose of a particular hormonal agent. In some cases, such differences can be quite dramatic (e.g., effects of calcitonin upon bone), and in other cases small (e.g., the action of insulin upon muscle).

The basis of the processes of differentiation and controlled growth also is not well understood. Nonetheless, differentiation, and particularly the coordinated differentiations underlying embryogenesis, are directional in quality. Their interest to endocrinology lies in the discovery that differentiation of an increasing number of organs requires the presence of specific hormones at some critical time in embryonic life in order for normal organogenesis to occur. The classic example is the testosterone-dependent development of the male genitalia. These hormonally controlled processes

TABLE 1-1. DATES OF DISCOVERY, PURIFICATION, AND DETERMINATION OF STRUCTURE OF MAMMALIAN HORMONES*

Hormone	Source	Discovered	Purified	Structure
Polypeptide				
FSH	AP	1926	1931	—
LH	AP	1926	1940	—
LTH	AP	1929	1933	—
GH	AP	1921	1948	—
TSH	AP	1922	1948	—
ACTH	AP	1924	1948	1956
MSH	IP	1922	1950	1956
Vasopressin	PP or HT	1895	1954	1954
Oxytocin	PP or HT	1901	1954	1954
Insulin	P-β	1889	1926	1953
Proinsulin	P-β	1967	1967	1968
Glucagon	P-α	1930	1953	1957
PTH	PT	1925	1959	1968
ProPTH	PT	1971	1971	—
CT	T	1964	1965	1966
Relaxin	CL	1929	—	—
Erythropoietin	Kid	1906	1959	—
Secretin	Gut	1902	1961	1964
Cholecystokinin	Gut	1928	1962	—
Gastrin	Stom	1902	1964	1964
Progastrin	Stom	1967	1968	—
Angiotensin	Liver plasma	1939	1955	1956
Polypeptide releasing factors				
CRF	HT	1958	1959	—
GHRF	HT	1959	1965	—
TRF	HT	1962	1962	1969
LRF	HT	1960	1961	1971
PRF	HT	1969	—	—
FSHRF	HT	1964	1966	—
MRF	HT	1965	1966	—
GIF	HT	1968	1970	—
PIF	HT	1963	—	—
MIF	HT	1966	1966	1971
Steroids and sterols				
Aldosterone	Ad	1934	1952	1954
Glucocorticoids	Ad	1935	1938	1940
Testosterone	Ts	1889	1931	1935
Estrogen	O	1925	1929	1931
Progesterone	CL	1925	1934	1934
Ad androgen	Ad	1935	1939	1942
Cholecalciferol	Skin	1920	1930	1933
25-Hydroxycholecalciferol	Liver	1967	1968	1968
1,25-Dihydroxycholecalciferol	Kid	1967	1971	1971
Amine				
Acetylcholine	ANS	1921	1868	1867
Thyroxine	T	1895	1915	1926
Triiodothyronine	T	1951	1952	1953
Epinephrine	Ad M	1895	1897	1901
Norepinephrine	Ad M	1948	1904	1904
Melatonin	PP or HT	1954	1958	1958

*Abbreviations: AP, anterior pituitary; IP, intermediate lobe of pituitary; PP, posterior pituitary; HT, hypothalamus; P-β, beta cells of pancreas; P-α, alpha cells of pancreas; PT, parathyroid gland; T, thyroid; CL, corpus luteum; Kid, kidney; Stom, Stomach; Ad, adrenal cortex; O, ovary; Ts, testes; ANS, autonomic nervous system; Ad M, adrenal medulla; FSH, follicle stimulating hormone; LH, luteinizing hormone; LTH, prolactin; GH, growth hormone; TSH, thyroid stimulating hormone; ACTH, adrenal corticotropin; MSH, melanocyte stimulating hormone; PTH, parathyroid hormone; ProPTH, proparathyroid hormone; CT, calcitonin; CRF, corticotropin releasing factor; GHRF, growth hormone releasing factor; TRF, thyrotropin releasing factor; LRF, LH releasing factor; PRF, prolactin releasing factor; FSHRF, FSH releasing factor; MRF, melanocyte stimulating hormone releasing factor; GIF, growth hormone release inhibiting factor; PIF, prolactin release inhibiting factor; MIF, melanocyte stimulating hormone release inhibiting factor.

differ in a qualitative sense from the reversible and recurrent estrogen-induced growth of endometrium and myometrium in the mature female. It is better to talk of these latter processes as hormonally induced modulations of differentiated cells. This type of modulatory process often includes mitosis of the modulated cells. Thus the number of hormone-responsive cells is increased by a shift of a precursor (nonactive) pool of cells to an active pool of cells, cell division, or both, leading to a further increase in the size of the active cell pool.

In summary, hormones can act at the physiologic level of organization to (1) enhance or inhibit an activity of an already differentiated cell, a modulated cell, or both; (2) increase the number of responsive cells by inducing the differentiation or the modulation of precursor cells, or both; or (3) increase cell number by stimulating mitosis of either active or precursor cells; or (4) all of these.

In many instances, the same hormone has all three types of effects on a given organ. For example, adrenocorticotropin (ACTH) not only stimulates steroid hormone production from the adrenal cortex but also causes both hypertrophy and hyperplasia in this gland.

Evolution of Hormonal Control Systems

As emphasized in the introduction, the endocrine system is of major importance in integrating the activities of separate organs in higher organisms. It is concerned with intercellular communication. Obviously throughout evolutionary history, with an increasing complexity of organs and cell types, there developed an increasing complexity of extracellular controls. Just as the paleontologist has come to recognize the phenomenon of homology of structure, so the endocrinologist has come to recognize that new control systems and their extracellular messengers did not simply arise on demand. They evolved from what was already present by a process of gradual change. This ultimately means that extracellular control systems represent an adaptation and extension of the more ancient intracellular control systems.

There is a unique set of features, attributes, capabilities, and limits that all cells share in common. There is a range of temperature, salinity, pH, pressure, oxygen tension, nutrient supply, and so on in which each can function. Free-living forms exhibit a wide range of environmental adaptations, but in a multicellular organism, a degree of freedom has been lost — its cells can function properly only in a restricted extracellular environment. A major prerequisite for their life is the maintenance of this environment.

Solutions of particular evolutionary problems are unique and irrevocable. Oxidative phosphorylation and the Krebs cycle span the biologic ages from yeast to man. So, too, does insulin span the eons of time from fish to man. But the constancy of the basic structural features of insulin overlook an inconstancy of insulin function. In the toadfish, insulin is concerned mainly with the metabolism of amino acids, in the cow with the metabolism of short-chain fatty acids, and in man with the metabolism of glucose. Nonetheless, in man the chemical memory of the fish persists — insulin does alter amino acid and protein metabolism. Adaptation of this chemical, extracellular control system has evolved to fit the nutritional uniqueness of each of these species. In each, insulin serves as a storage hormone in the sense of increasing the conversion of foodstuff into some form of readily mobilizable, energy-yielding substrate. In this sense, the physiologic function of insulin did not change, only the means of fulfilling that function.

Not unique but general solutions have been the evolutionary rule. The importance of this statement lies in its implication for our consideration of the mechanisms of hormone action. Our question is, does each hormone have a unique mode of action, or are there general patterns — a few basic systems by which hormones exert their effects?

A second important question with which endocrinologists have just begun to deal concerns homology of hormone and receptor structure. How, for example, did the receptor site for arginine vasopressin in the rat kidney evolve to become so highly selective for this pituitary hormone, which had in turn evolved from its ancestral form, arginine vasotocin? How were the structural changes in these proteins occurring in two widely separated organs coordinated in evolution? No answer is yet completely acceptable, but present interest lies in the possible impact of gene duplication upon structural change in the two separate organs. The dimension that is so difficult to grasp in our approach to an understanding of this problem is that of time. Dealing as we do with minutes, hours, and days in our experimental approach to endocrine systems, we do not yet comprehend the meaning of billions of years.

A final feature of the extracellular control systems which deserves comment is that of specificity. There appear to be highly specific receptor sites for each hormone on or within the cells of particular target tissues. Careful examination, however, reveals that this biologic specificity is not absolute. Higher than physiologic concentrations of many hormones often affect the function of organs other than those classically assumed to be their target tissues. From the theoretical point of view, this means that there are potential low-affinity receptor sites for a particular hormone in many target tissues. Of particular interest are observations that neoplastic transformation of cells may lead to the appearance of "new" receptor sites of high affinity for a hormone which is not normally considered a prime activation of the cell type in question. These observations indicate that the necessary conditions for an evolutionary change in receptor site location exist within highly differentiated cell types.

The lack of complete specificity at the tissue level of biologic organization is of practical significance. At every level of biologic organization, a similar lack of absolute specificity is the rule. For example, the activity of isolated enzymes can be influenced by adding many different potential effectors in sufficiently high concentration. Clearly, not all of these effectors are of physiologic significance. The problem for the investigator is to deal with this redundancy of experimental information (derived at any given level of biologic organization) and to determine the restricted set of facts that is of physiologic significance at the next higher level of organization.

Organization of Endocrine Control Systems

As can be anticipated, organization within the endocrine system varies greatly. It can be discussed conveniently in order of increasing complexity. Even though this ordering is useful, it must be borne in mind that even the simplest systems do not operate in isolation. Indeed, a most important general rule is that the activity of the entire endocrine system is a highly integrated network. Hence a perturbation, such as removal or malfunction of one gland, leads to changes in the function of many of the other glands, a change in the expression of the activities of other hormones upon target cells, or both. Equally important is the fact that all target cells (cells responsive to hormones) have built-in autoregulatory mechanisms that function in the absence of specific hormones; e.g., the thyroid cells alter their function in response to changes in plasma iodide concentrations in a similar fashion whether pituitary thyroid stimulating hormone (TSH) is present or not. The only difference concerns the magnitude and rapidity of the particular response.

The various types of endocrine control systems that have been recognized are diagrammed schematically in Figures 1–5 to 1–9. The simplest appears to be a system in which the hormone acts on specific cells, thereby promoting a change in the controlled variable in the extracellular fluid, which in turn regulates the output of hormone by the gland (Fig. 1–5). While this negative feedback system operates as a closed loop, its particular setting can be changed by endocrine and neural action exerted either upon the gland itself or upon the hormonally responsive effector cells. Systems of this type appear to operate in the case of insulin-plasma glucose, glucagon-plasma glucose, parathyroid hormone (PTH)-plasma calcium, thyrocalcitonin-plasma calcium, and aldosterone-plasma sodium, although in many of these cases additional mechanisms are operative. A cardinal feature of this type of system is the absence of direct hypothalamic or pituitary control, although pituitary factors may, by altering the general hormonal balance, influence the activity of any one of these systems. For example, excessive growth hormone secretion, by modifying both phosphate and carbohydrate metabolism, alters the homeostatic systems regulating both calcium and glucose homeostasis.

The simple model depicted in Figure 1–5 does not completely represent the complexity and elegance with which these simple feedback systems may operate. For example, in the case of insulin release, factors other than glucose, e.g., glucagon,

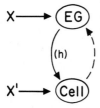

Figure 1–5. Simplest type of endocrine control. Hormone (h) released from endocrine gland (EG) acts upon target cell to release a substance which by negative feedback (——→) decreases the rate of release of h. X and X' represent other factors operating independently of feedback loop and influencing, respectively, the activity of EG and cell. This type of relationship exists between insulin and blood sugar, glucagon and blood sugar, PTH and plasma calcium, calcitonin and plasma calcium, and, to some extent, aldosterone and plasma sodium.

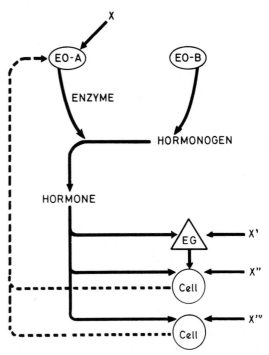

Figure 1–6. Endocrine control by release of a hormone precursor, hormonogen, from one endocrine organ, EO-B, and its activation by an enzyme release from another organ, EO-A. The hormone released acts as a tropic hormone on an endocrine gland, EG, with the release of a hormone which acts on peripheral cells. This type of system exists for angiotensinogen → angiotensin → aldosterone.

parasympathetic activity, and amino acids, can enhance the glucose-induced release of insulin. Of greater physiologic importance, there are glucoreceptors in the intestine that bring about the release of insulin from the beta cells of the pancreas either by hormonal or neural means. Both the hormonal and neural signals induce an increase in insulin release. The magnitude of these signals is related to the amount of glucose in the diet and its rate of transepithelial transport in the intestine. These entero-beta cell control loops are of great importance. They serve an anticipatory function in the sense of alerting the organism (man) to the influx of glucose. As a consequence of their normal operation, over two thirds of a normal glucose load is metabolized by the liver. These controls represent an example of positive feed-forward loops in this homeostatic system. Such loops are common at all levels of biologic organization.

A somewhat more complex system operates in the case of the control of aldosterone secretion by the adrenal cortex (Fig. 1–6). In this case a *hormonogen*, angiotensinogen, is secreted into the bloodstream by one organ, the liver, is acted upon in the blood by an enzyme, renin, from another organ, the kidney, and is converted to a *tropic hormone*, angiotensin, which stimulates the production of aldosterone by the adrenal cortex. This last hormone, acting on the kidney, alters electrolyte excretion. This in turn leads to a decrease in enzyme production by the kidney. The unusual fea-

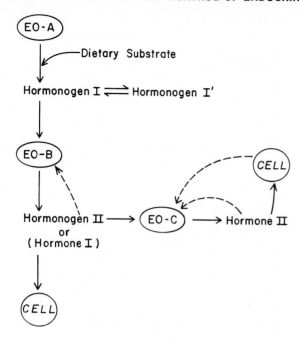

Figure 1–7. Endocrine control by successive conversion of a hormonogen into hormone products in different organs in the body. This type of system operates in the conversion of cholecalciferol to 25-hydroxy- and 1,25-dihydroxycholecalciferol.

ture of this system is the liberation of *hormonogen* into the bloodstream and its conversion to an active substance therein.

The next order of complexity is illustrated in Figure 1–7. In this case the hormonal precursor can be derived from the diet or synthesized within the organism. It goes through successive transformations in several additional organs before becoming a biologically active substance. In some cases, however, it is clear that one of the intermediate hormonogens has biologic activity, i.e., it is, in its own right, a hormone. The clearest example of this type of system is vitamin D metabolism. Vitamin D_3 can be either synthesized in the skin from 7-dehydrocholesterol or ingested in the diet. It then undergoes successive hydroxylations in liver and kidney to form $1,25(OH)_2D_3$. It is also evident, however, that the adrenal glucocorticoids, which classically have been considered end products in terms of hormonal action, undergo further biochemical transformation in the liver into steroids, which exert new hormonal effects. These hepatic steroid hormone metabolites do not fulfill the strict definition of a hormone because they probably act only in the liver to control hemin synthesis. Nonetheless, this situation is clearly distinct from one in which the steroid hormone acts upon its target tissue without conversion. For example, in the case of progesterone upon the hen oviduct, or estradiol in the mammalian uterus, the biologically active steroid is that which reaches and is taken up by the tissue. Thus our present classification of steroid hormones (Table 1–1) is, in a sense, inadequate, and will remain so until the total number of such metabolites with distinct biologic activities has been identified.

The organization of a hormonal control system of a similar order of complexity is shown in Figure 1–8. In this type of system, the activity of the en-

docrine gland is under the control of the hypothalamus. The control of secretion of growth hormone by the anterior pituitary, of epinephrine by the adrenal medulla, and of vasopressin by the posterior pituitary are examples. A differentiating feature of this type of system is that feedback control is exerted not on the endocrine gland directly but upon hypothalamic function, which in turn regulates gland function. The feedback effector appears to be one or more plasma constituents.

In the highest order of complexity, the activity of the final endocrine effector organ is controlled by

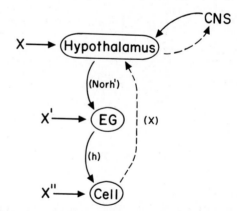

Figure 1–8. Endocrine control achieved by hypothalamus → endocrine gland → target cell hierarchy. The initial afferent signal from hypothalamus may be either neural (N) or hormonal (h′). The release of hormone (h) leads to a change (x) in a plasma constituent that regulates hypothalamic activity rather than the gland itself. X, X′, and X″ represent additional factors that modulate, respectively, the activity of the hypothalamus, endocrine gland, and cell. This type of system is observed in the case of posterior pituitary → vasopressin → kidney → and plasma H_2O; the adrenal medulla → epinephrine; and anterior pituitary → growth hormone. In the former two cases, the signal from hypothalamus to endocrine gland is neural; in the latter, hormonal, growth hormone releasing factor.

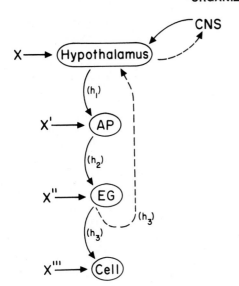

Figure 1–9. Endocrine control achieved by hypothalamus → anterior pituitary (AP) → endocrine gland (EG) → target cell hierarchy. Note that feedback control is exerted primarily at level of hypothalamus, and usually by final endocrine gland product, although there is evidence that some feedback control is exerted at level of anterior pituitary. Each step between hypothalamus to final endocrine gland and return is hormonal (h_1, h_2, h_3). X, X', X'', and X''' are factors regulating respectively and independently the activities of the hypothalamus, anterior pituitary, endocrine gland, and cell. The hypothalamic control of thyroxine and cortisol secretions are examples of this type. The regulation of the secretion of gonadal hormones is similar but has, in addition, positive feed-back loops that serve to coordinate the sequential release of the pituitary and sex hormone.

the anterior pituitary gland, the activity of which is regulated in turn by the hypothalamus (Fig. 1–9). The regulation of thyroid activity by TSH and of adrenal cortical function by ACTH are examples of this type. They are characterized by two important features. First, the final endocrine product is the feedback effector rather than some substance produced as a result of its action on target cells. Second, the site of feedback control is at the hypothalamic level, not at the pituitary gland.

This basic type of organization is also apparent in the regulation of gonadal function, but in the female, it has been elaborated considerably to coordinate the cyclic activity of both gonadal and uterine function. In this development, the final endocrine products, estradiol and progesterone, act as both negative and positive feedback effectors to coordinate the sequential secretion of the hypothalamic and pituitary factors.

As illustrated, all of these systems are closed. In each case, however, the activity of the separate components can be altered by signals arising external to the closed loop, and thus the final balance of the system can be altered. This is best illustrated by the cyclic variations in the rates of secretion of many hormones, even though the essential feedback relationships remain intact.

Prohormones

As discussed above, there is increasing evidence that sterol and steroid hormones secreted by one organ may undergo further metabolic transformation in another with a resultant change in structure, which may lead simply to an increase or decrease in biologic potency or to a qualitative change in biologic activity. The only important difference is that many organs, particularly liver and kidney and some other specific target tissues, do, by controlling sterol and steroid hormone metabolism, function as integral parts of these hormone control systems, not merely as disposal organs for steroid metabolism.

It had been generally thought that peptide hormone metabolism did not exhibit this same diversity of chemical modification following secretion. The possibility cannot yet be completely ruled out, however. It is clear, for example, that for several peptide hormones a precursor molecule or prohormone exists. The example of angiotensin cited above is one in which successive transformations take place in the blood plasma, catalyzed by specific enzymes secreted by other tissues.

A second example of a different type is that of insulin. The synthesis of insulin involves the initial synthesis of proinsulin, a single, long polypeptide chain, which then is folded into a precise three-dimensional structure stabilized by intrachain disulfide bonds. A segment of the proinsulin molecule is then removed by enzymatic hydrolysis of specific peptide bonds, resulting in the formation of the insulin molecule. This conversion normally takes place prior to the secretion of insulin into the bloodstream, i.e., within the cells in which the proinsulin is made. Under abnormal circumstances, however, proinsulin may be secreted into the plasma. Under such circumstances some of it, at least, may be converted into "insulin" by peripheral tissues.

A third example is PTH, in which three distinct species of hormone normally circulate in the blood. The three vary in size. It seems possible, but not yet completely established, that the larger form is secreted by the gland and then undergoes conversion in peripheral organs to the smaller forms, which may be the most important from the point of view of biologic activity.

Larger forms (prohormones) have also been described for ACTH and gastrin. Therefore, these examples would appear to be more than a mere curiosity. They are, in fact, indicators of our increasing awareness of the complexity of the control systems involving peptide hormones. In the case of peptide as well as steroid hormones, peripheral metabolism is an important feature of the overall process. Diseases resulting from dysfunction of peripheral peptide hormone metabolism will probably soon be recognized.

Tissue Hormones

The classical concept of a hormone first proposed by Bayliss and Starling was that of a substance produced in one organ, which, after being transported by the blood, acted upon a distant organ to alter the function of this latter organ. Additional agents have been discovered, however, which may not meet this definition. Among these are various kinins and prostaglandins. Clearly, in the case of some of these substances, although secreted into the bloodstream by one organ, they are rapidly inactivated by another so that they do not normally circulate in the blood in the same sense as does thyroxine. For example, prostaglandin E_2 is released in significant amounts by the spleen but is nearly totally removed from the venous blood in its passage through the pulmonary circulation so that little of this material appears in the arterial blood. The exact hormonal function of many of these agents is yet to be established. In certain cases, they may represent tissue hormones in the sense that they are produced by one cell type in a multicellular tissue and act upon other cell types within the same tissue. These would fulfill the original concept, if not the strict definition, of hormones, being secreted by one cell type and acting upon another, but the extent of transport would be limited to diffusion from cell to cell. This is an attractive concept because, just as the classical endocrine systems and their hormones serve an integrative function within the organism by coordinating the activities of widely separate organs, so these tissue hormones would serve an integrative function at the level of an individual tissue coordinating the activities of the several cell types that go to make up that tissue.

Although many lines of evidence support this integrative action of tissue hormones, the concept is not completely established. In addition, some of the evidence strongly suggests that some of the prostaglandins may serve other functions. In many tissues in which hormone-sensitive adenyl cyclases are activated by specific amine or peptide hormones, one or more prostaglandins have been found to inhibit adenyl cyclase activation. It is possible that in these cases the synthesis of the prostaglandins is stimulated by the particular hormone and acts as a feedback modulator of adenyl cyclase activation.

The problem is complicated by the fact that some prostaglandins in some tissues, such as the fat pad, mimic the effects of the hormones, i.e., activate adenyl cyclase, and it has been proposed that in some of these cases the sequence of events is hormone-receptor interaction, stimulation of prostaglandin formation, and increased prostaglandin-stimulating adenyl cyclase activity. These data serve to emphasize that the effects of prostaglandins are not only diverse but also intimately involved in endocrine regulation. They contribute to both the complexity and plasticity of cellular response. The prostaglandins probably represent hormones that serve an important integrative function at the tissue level of biologic organization.

Blood Cells as Target Cells

Traditionally, fixed tissue cells have been the only recognized target tissues for circulating hormone; however, platelets and white and red blood cells respond to changes in hormone concentrations in blood plasma. In the case of white cells,

these responses are similar to those seen in fixed tissue cells, at least as far as regulation of carbohydrate metabolism is concerned. Platelet responses are specifically related to platelet function, and hormones, such as epinephrine and prostaglandin, control platelet aggregation. The most recently discovered, and potentially most unusual, responses are the hormonal controls of red cell deformability. The importance of this property of deformability is that red cells, in order to pass through many of the smaller capillaries, must undergo reversible changes of shape. By changing the deformability of these cells, hormones may thus alter the relative rates of the capillary blood flow in a given organ or the relative rates of perfusion of different organs within the organism. Several different types of hormonal controls are recognizable. Red cells respond rapidly to tissue hormones, such as prostaglandin E_2, with a decrease in deformability. Red cells respond to catecholamines similarly, and their deformability is also altered by changes in steroid hormone levels. Taken in conjunction with the fact that all these hormone classes alter the properties of capillary beds in one or more organs, the hormonal control of microcirculatory dynamics is based upon the control of both the blood vessel walls and the formed elements, the red blood cells, passing along these walls. The uniqueness of the hormonal controls of red cell deformability lies in the fact that the modified cell itself, rather than a chemical messenger, acts as a circulating messenger that serves to integrate the activities of the various organs of the organism.

Integrative Actions of Endocrine Systems

The preceding discussion of the hierarchy of function can be considered a vertical view of the endocrine system. Endocrine organization can also be viewed in a horizontal fashion by focusing attention upon a particular controlled variable such as blood sugar or plasma calcium (Fig. 1–10). In each of these instances, the concentration of the controlled substance is constant in spite of wide fluctuations in intake, utilization, and excretion. This constancy is achieved by a dual feedback system in which one or more hormones is produced in response to an elevation in the concentration of the controlled substance. This increase in hormone concentration acts to restore the concentration of the controlled chemical toward normal. Conversely, one or more hormones is produced in response to a fall in concentration and acts to restore it toward normal.

When the response to a metabolic perturbation leads to increased activity of two complementary hormones, they often have different time courses of action, one acting quickly but briefly, with a limited capacity for sustained response, the other slowly but with a greater capacity for sustained action. The interplay of these two types of mechanisms provides a finer and more sustained control than either alone can give.

A second aspect of this horizontal view of the en-

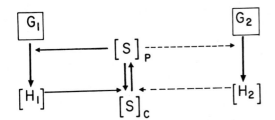

Figure 1-10. A horizontal view of an endocrine control system responsible for controlling the concentration of a metabolite, S (e.g., glucose), in the blood plasma. The figure illustrates the regulation of the concentration of intermediate $[S]_p$ by two endocrine glands, G_1 and G_2, and by the plasma concentrations of their respective hormones $[H_1]$ and $[H_2]$. A heavy solid arrow ($\rightarrow$) represents an increase of flow of intermediate from plasma to cell ($[S]_c$ is the concentration of the intermediate within cells) or vice versa, and an increase in the rate of hormone production. The thin arrows ($\rightarrow$) represent a positive effect of the hormone or intermediate, and the dashed arrows ($\dashrightarrow$) represent a negative effect upon hormone release or intermediate uptake or release by the cell. An increase in uptake of S by the cell leads to a fall in $[S]_p$. This fall leads to a decreased release of H_1 and an increase in release of H_2. The fall in $[H_1]$ leads to a decrease in rate of uptake of S into the cell, and the rise in $[H_2]$ causes an increase in rate of release of S from cell into plasma, thereby restoring S_p toward its original value. Hence, a pulse of S into the plasma or removal of S from plasma will be immediately compensated for by the reciprocal activities of these two control systems.

docrine system is that a single hormone may alter the concentration of more than one plasma constituent; thus insulin alters glucose and nonesterified fatty acid (NEFA) concentrations. The alteration in concentration of one of these constituents may affect the rate of change of the other.

A corollary of these facts is that seldom, if ever, are the two hormones complete antagonists. For example, although calcitonin lowers plasma calcium concentration and PTH raises it, they both cause a fall in plasma phosphate concentration. Furthermore, the major effect of calcitonin is exerted upon one organ, bone, whereas that of PTH is upon another, the kidney. Finally, at the cellular level, PTH activates adenyl cyclase, but calcitonin does not inhibit this action. Thus there is a plasticity of response in the endocrine system similar to the plasticity that Sherrington attributed to the reflex arcs in the nervous system.

The analogy with the nervous system can be made clearer by considering the coordinated reflexes necessary to maintain control of the knee joint during walking and at rest. As the extensors contract, the flexors must relax, but when full extension is to be maintained, as in standing, both muscle systems maintain some degree of contraction. The absence of walking does not bring the activities of the two systems to zero. A dynamic balance is maintained both at rest and when walking. A similar dynamic balance is maintained in the control of plasma calcium, sodium, glucose, and many other bodily constituents. Thus an organism in which both plasma calcitonin and plasma PTH are high, which nonetheless has a normal plasma calcium concentration, is in a different metabolic state than a similar organism with very low

plasma concentrations of these hormones which also has a normal plasma calcium concentration.

None of the preceding discussion has sufficiently emphasized the integrative actions of the endocrine system nor how the basic organization of these control systems is the same at the cellular and supracellular level of biologic organization. In order to establish the prime significance of this integrative aspect of endocrine function, two further features of endocrine control need to be illustrated.

An example of the first is the mode of action of hormones at the level of the organism. For example, testosterone in the male has its most striking effects upon the seminal vesicles and prostate. However, this hormone also exerts effects upon skeletal muscle and brain. It promotes muscular development. Its effects on the brain are related to the psychological problem of gender identity and are critically important to the development of the male personality. Looked at in broader perspective, the hormone acts upon a large number of organs, exerting upon each a distinct effect. The sum total of these effects is integrated into the composite response of the organism. Testosterone has prepared not only the genitalia but the entire organism for its specific sexual function.

A similar kind of integrative action occurs at the cellular level. When a hormone acts, it nearly always has multiple effects upon cell function, all of which are integrated into the cellular response. For example, when ACTH acts upon the adrenal cortex, there is an increase in both the rate of steroid hormone secretion and the capacity to sustain hormone secretion. Both are aspects of the total response of these cells to hormonal stimulation, and both depend upon the integration of the activities of diverse metabolic pathways.

At the supracellular level of organization, the principal role of the endocrine system, or components thereof, is to integrate the metabolic activities of the various tissues and organs that make up the organism. Its integrative function complements that of the central and autonomic nervous systems. At the cellular level, hormones act to integrate the various metabolic activities into a concerted cellular response.

The second aspect of the integrative action of the endocrine system is the interrelatedness of the various hormonal systems. The entire endocrine system operates as a net. For example, when plasma cortisol increases, it not only alters carbohydrate, fat, and protein metabolism but also calcium and phosphate metabolism and, thereby, the plasma concentrations and rates of secretion of PTH, calcitonin, and 1,25-dihydroxycholecalciferol. Similarly, growth hormone alters the metabolism of all the major foodstuffs and of all the major ions, which in turn means an alteration in the rates of secretion of many other hormones. The separation of the endocrine system into isolated subsystems, as in this textbook, must be recognized as an artificial one, convenient from the pedagogical point of view but not accurately reflecting the interrelated nature of all these systems.

The Unique Roles of the Anterior Pituitary and Hypothalamus

The anterior pituitary occupies a special place in the endocrine hierarchy and has often been called the "master gland." It regulates the activity of several subsidiary endocrine organs by secreting tropic hormones for specific endocrine organs. These specific tropic hormones characteristically induce hypertrophy and hyperplasia in the target gland, and, conversely, the absence of tropic hormone leads to pronounced atrophy of the target gland. Even in the absence of a tropic hormone, the target gland continues to produce small quantities of hormones. For this reason, primary dysfunction, which is failure of target gland function resulting from an intrinsic defect, as in primary myxedema, is usually associated with a more profound deficiency of the target gland hormone than is secondary deficiency, which results from a diminished level of tropic hormone, as in secondary or pituitary myxedema.

From the relationships diagrammed in Figures 1–8 and 1–9, it is immediately evident that an increase in target gland hormone normally inhibits production of the corresponding tropic hormone. This is the case whether the target hormone is produced by the gland or administered by the biologist. Improper function of the negative feedback loop may lead to an increase in tropic hormone with a resultant increase in target gland hormone. This type of target gland overactivity is termed *secondary* and is distinct from *primary* hyperplasia and overfunction resulting from autonomous hyperactivity of the target gland.

Although the anterior pituitary occupies a dominant place among endocrine glands, discoveries over the past decade indicate that the activity of the anterior pituitary is regulated in turn by the hypothalamus. This portion of the brain manufactures and releases (under appropriate stimuli) polypeptide releasing factors that are transferred via the pituitary portal circulation to the anterior pituitary, where they lead to the release of the particular anterior pituitary hormone. In addition, factors that inhibit the release of specific pituitary hormones have been identified. Thus the hypothalamus serves as a complex endocrine organ secreting at least ten factors that stimulate or inhibit the release of specific hormones from the anterior pituitary. The hypothalamus is the highest integrative center in the endocrine hierarchy and the center in which the activities of the central nervous system and the endocrine system are integrated to maintain neuroendocrine control over bodily function. Hence the concept of the anterior pituitary as the master gland is incorrect; this appellation belongs more correctly to the hypothalamus.

Hormones

Nature and Characteristics of Hormones

Mammalian hormones fall into three main classes: steroid, polypeptide, and amine. Many have been isolated in pure form, and a significant number of new hormones have been identified in the past 15 years. These include such steroid hormones as aldosterone and such polypeptide hormones as the hypothalamic releasing factors and thyrocalcitonin. Table 1–1 lists the known hormones and their sources, natures, and dates of discovery and isolation.

The most characteristic feature of the endocrine system is that the chemical transmitter is released from specialized cells into the bloodstream and is carried to other cells that are responsive to it. This is, in fact, the classic definition of a hormone first proposed by Starling. Just as with enzymes, hormonal specificity ranges over a wide spectrum of individual functions. Some hormones, such as the growth hormone of the anterior pituitary gland or thyroxine, affect the activity of a wide variety of cells, whereas others act upon only a few specific cell types: e.g., oxytocin acts upon uterine muscle and the myoepithelial cells of the lactating mammary gland.

This restriction of some hormonal effects to specific target tissues has led to the concept that there are specific receptor sites for each hormone. While the nature of these receptor sites will be considered later, it is noteworthy that their interactions with hormones are brought into evidence by minute amounts: physiologic effects are evoked by concentrations of hormone between 10^{-7} and 10^{-12} M.

Within the past several decades, the two-dimensional and in some cases three-dimensional structure of a large number of peptide hormones has been determined. One of the striking structural features of these hormones is that only a small percentage of the total amino acids in the molecule are essential for biologic activity. Other amino acids serve only to enhance specific binding. In these cases, amino acids essential for biologic activity have remained constant throughout evolution, but many changes have occurred in the nature of the nonessential amino acids. Thus, sheep and horse insulin have the same essential structural features but do possess differences at a number of specific loci along their polypeptide chains. An additional structural feature is that some hormone molecules possess several different biologic activities that are dependent upon different essential amino acids in their structure, i.e., different parts of the molecule.

Storage, Transport, Inactivation, and Secretion of Hormones

To meet the needs of the organism, the endocrine system must exhibit a high degree of adaptability. This is achieved in part by the type of hierarchical organization outlined above. An important feature of this endocrine system is the considerable diversity of the time constants characterizing change of its components. The half-life of a given hormone in the plasma may vary from a few minutes to several days. Moreover, a physiologically detectable response of a particular target tissue may be immediate or delayed for several hours, and a given hormone may elicit an immediate response in one tissue and a delayed response in another, or both immediate and delayed responses in the same tissue.

Once released into the bloodstream, the hormones vary considerably in their fates. Many hormones have specific carrier proteins that transport them in body fluids. Whether this is true for the polypeptide hormones is not clear, but it is generally true for the steroid hormones and for thyroxine. Inactivation of the hormone may be achieved in the specific target tissues, by other organs, particularly the liver and kidneys, or by both target tissues and other organs. Some hormones, particularly steroids, are selectively concentrated by specific receptor tissues, as, for example, estrogens by the uterus, or 1,25-dihydroxycholecalciferol by the intestinal mucosal cells.

In most instances, the endocrine glands store only a small percentage of the daily needs of the organism. The thyroid gland is a prominent exception, but most glands possess the ability to alter the rate of hormone synthesis and secretion rapidly and in proportion to need. Very often two phases of secretion can be discerned, particularly in the case of peptide and protein hormones: an initial very rapid and short-lived phase, and a second phase that is slow in onset but sustained for as long as the appropriate stimulus is maintained. In both phases, the rate of stimulation is a function of stimulus strength. It seems likely that initial release is based upon release of stored secretory products in quanta and that there is a distribution of the thresholds at which different quanta or packets are released. This threshold distribution hypothesis explains quite well glucose-induced release of insulin from the rat pancreas. As in other control systems, the rate of secretion in these systems is controlled by increasing the number of packets (units) released as the stimulus strength increases and by stimulating the synthesis of new packets and their migration to the cell surface (i.e., an increase in both activity of individual units and in the number of such units). In a control sense, this is completely analogous to the response of a nerve trunk to increasing strength of stimulus. Individual fibers increase their rate of firing, and as the stimulus strength increases, more and more fibers fire, with activation of responding units and recruitment of new units.

Detection of Hormones in Biologic Fluid

Because of their extremely low concentrations, hormones are difficult to detect and measure accurately in biologic fluids. Some can be detected by chemical means because of unique chemical characteristics; for example, protein-bound iodine is a measure of plasma thyroxine. Some are relatively stable in urine, from which they can be extracted, purified, and detected by chromatographic or other means (e.g., steroids and catecholamines). The polypeptide hormones, on the other hand, generally cannot be measured by these methods. Their detection depends upon a specific biologic or im-

munologic assay. The most sensitive of the latter is the competitive binding assay or radioimmunoassay in which the extent of binding of trace amounts of I^{131}-labeled polypeptide to a specific antisera or binding protein is altered by the amount of nonradioactive hormone in the test plasma sample. This technique, developed by Berson and Yalow, has been applied successfully to the measurement of peptide and protein hormones, steroid hormones, various drugs, and even small molecules such as C-AMP. The basic procedure consists either of extracting a natural protein with a very high affinity for the substance to be measured or of preparing antibodies against the substance in question. Most of the protein and peptide hormones serve as antigens when injected into other species because of structural differences in parts of their polypeptide chains. Steroid hormones and small molecules, however, must first be coupled covalently to proteins such as serum albumin. Once an appropriate antibody has been produced, it can be used as a reagent to measure the concentration of the hormone in human plasma. The assay is based upon the competitive inhibition principle.

Labeled Antigen	Specific Antibody		Labeled Antigen-Antibody Complex
Ag* (F)	+	Ab	$\Longleftrightarrow$	Ag*—Ab (B)
		+		
		Ag	Unlabeled Antigen	
		$\Updownarrow$		
		Ag-A$_b$	Unlabeled Antigen-Antibody Complex	

Unlabeled antigen in unknown or standard samples competes with labeled antigen for binding to antibody. As the concentration of unlabeled antigen is increased, less labeled antigen is bound. Once the reactions have been allowed to proceed to equilibrium, or nearly so, it is necessary only to have a method for separating free (F) labeled antigen from labeled antigen bound to antibody (B). This is commonly done by chromatoelectrophoresis, precipitation, or selective absorption.

The usual technique employs serial dilutions of a standard antigen to prepare a standard curve of the B/F ratio versus concentration of standard (unlabeled) antigen (Fig. 1–11). The concentration in a given sample of human plasma is determined by the B/F ratio determined in a simple manner.

This technique has become of great importance as a diagnostic tool in clinical endocrinology, but it has even greater importance in the study of endocrine physiology and the mechanism underlying control of hormone secretion.

Function, Effects, and Action of Hormones

As first pointed out by R. Levine, the response of the organism to the administration of a hormone can be conveniently considered in three different ways: its *function*, its *effect*, and its *action*. The term *function* of the hormone refers to the manner in

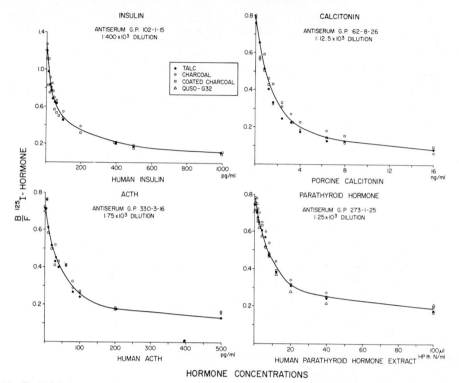

Figure 1–11. Typical dose response patterns obtained in radioimmunoassays of peptide hormones when the bound over free ratio (B/F) of the labeled hormone is plotted against chemical concentration of hormone. [From Yalow, R. S., and Berson, S. A., In *Principles of Competitive Protein-Binding Assays*. Odell, W. O., and Daughaday, W. H. (eds.), Philadelphia, J. B. Lippincott, 1971.]

which we, as endocrinologists, interpret nature's design and purpose. Thus the function of insulin is either to regulate the level of blood glucose or to store energy-yielding substrate in the form of fat or glycogen in times of carbohydrate excess. Which of these one considers to be the function of insulin depends to a considerable extent upon one's point of view. Because of the subjective and imprecise quality of defining hormone responses in terms of function, this appears to be the least helpful way to begin to understand how hormones regulate metabolism.

Hormonal *effects* describe specific measurable and reproducible phenomena that are observed when the hormone is administered *in vivo* or is added to an organ, cell, cell organelle, or enzyme *in vitro*. They represent the body of facts that must be accounted for in any formulation of the precise mechanism of action of the particular hormone in question.

The *mechanism of action* of a hormone is the way the hormone interacts with its specific receptor and the ensuing chain of events that are eventually expressed as the various hormonal effects. It is assumed that the measured response to a hormone is a function of the concentration of hormone-receptor complex, and the latter is the rate-limiting factor in the sequence of reactions from hormone-receptor interaction to physiologic response. A further assumption is that the receptors represent a homogeneous population.

Under these assumptions

$$ap = \frac{\alpha \, (r) \, (h)}{(k_2/k_1) + h} \tag{1}$$

and

$$Ap = \alpha(r) \tag{2}$$

so that

$$ap = \frac{Ap}{[K_h/(h)] + 1} \tag{3}$$

where

(r) = total receptor concentration
(rh) = concentration of complex
(h) = concentration of hormone
k_1 = rate of association of r and h
k_2 = rate of dissociation of rh
α = proportionality constant defined by $ap/(rh)$
ap = physiologic activity, i.e., the measured response
Ap = maximal physiologic activity
K_h = k_2/k_1

This is analogous to the Michaelis-Menten equation, which describes the rate of an enzymatic reaction as a function of substrate and enzyme concentration. Note, however, that in the latter a rate is measured, whereas the equations for hormone-receptor relationships measure an effect, i.e., a change in concentration, not a change in rate.

Equation (3) would predict that the relationship between hormone concentration and effect would follow the pattern depicted in Figure 1–12. Some

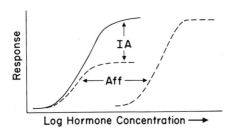

Figure 1–12. Hypothetical plot of physiologic response vs. log of hormone concentration. Solid lines represent response to natural hormone, dashed lines represent change in response pattern when a chemical modification of hormonal molecule leads to a change in affinity (Aff) or intrinsic activity (IA).

hormonal relationships can be reasonably well described by equation (3); however, many others cannot. In many instances, perhaps most, the assumption of direct proportionality between hormonal effect and concentration of hormone receptor is rather unlikely since the physiologic response being measured is usually several steps removed from the initial hormone-receptor interaction. A more general form of equation (3) is that given in equation (4)

$$ap = \frac{Ap}{[K_h/(h)^n] + 1} \qquad (4)$$

where the factor n takes into account the fact that hormone response curves often exhibit a sigmoid character when response is plotted as a function of hormone concentration, suggesting some type of cooperative interaction, i.e., two hormone molecules are bound per receptor. A similar type of kinetics might also be observed if "cascade" effects occur in the sequence of events.

This equation is only a presently useful approximation for describing hormonal effects. It has proved useful in the analysis of hormone-receptor interaction and, in particular, in helping to define the types of functional groups on hormone molecules, most notably on certain polypeptide hormones. In these instances, a large number of synthetic hormone analogues have been prepared with specific alterations or deletions of structure and have been tested in specific hormonally responsive systems. Analysis of the results has clearly indicated that there are two types of amino acids in a hormonal polypeptide chain, those concerned with the binding of hormone to receptor and those concerned with the active site of the hormone molecule. Alterations in the nature of the first type lead to changes in the affinity of hormone for receptor, whereas alterations in those concerned with the second lead to changes in intrinsic activity, or both. These two types of changes lead to different changes in the concentration-response diagram (Fig. 1–12).

There are several alternative mechanisms by which the primary hormone-receptor interaction leads to subsequent biochemical and physiologic changes: (1) the situation in which a single specific hormone-receptor interaction leads to a single initial event, which is in turn responsible for all subsequent events; (2) the situation in which the initial hormone-receptor interaction leads to multiple events; and (3) the situation in which there is more than one specific receptor for the hormone within the cell or organ. Although there is evidence in support of all three models, most consideration has been given to models 1 and 2; however, the study of intracellular control systems indicates that small molecules (e.g., AMP) act at more than one site within a single cell (see below). In this light, model 3 becomes considerably more attractive. This is particularly the case if one views the different cells that respond to a given hormone. It is quite possible that the receptors for a given hormone in different cells differ. Moreover, in the case of steroid hormones (e.g., testosterone), it is clear that some target tissues respond to the parent compound, whereas in others testosterone undergoes reduction to dihydrotestosterone before exerting its biologic effects. Clearly, the physiologic receptors differ in these two tissues.

Another aspect of hormone action is the observation that the action of one hormone upon a cell is often conditioned by the activity of several others. The most dramatic instance of this relationship is the so-called *permissive action* of certain hormones: in the absence of hormone B, A will not exert its usual effects. This relationship is readily explicable in terms of present views of metabolic interrelationships (see below).

HORMONE ACTION: THEORIES

Three general theories of hormone action have been proposed: (1) hormones act upon membranes, (2) hormones act upon enzymes, and (3) hormones act upon genes. These will be discussed in the section on hormonal control mechanisms. To discuss these proposals, however, it is necessary first to consider the organization of the cell. Before doing so, it is worth pointing out that the distinctions between these different modes of action are not always clear; for example, a hormone may alter the activity of a membrane-bound enzyme, or, by acting on a membrane, it may cause the release of an ion.

CELLULAR CONTROL MECHANISMS

Recent investigations in cytology, genetics, and biochemistry have revolutionized our concept of cell structure and function. A highly schematic representation of a typical mammalian cell is given in Figure 1–13.

Membranes and the Ionic Net

The most striking contribution of cytologic investigation is the demonstration of the highly ordered structure within the cell (Fig. 1–13). A large

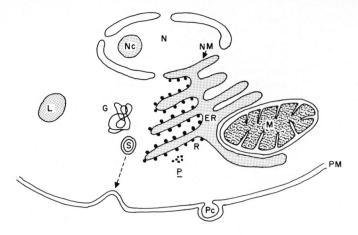

Figure 1–13. A schematic representation of a portion of a mammalian cell. N, nucleus; Nc, nucleolus; G, Golgi; ER, endoplasmic reticulum; M, mitochondria; P, polysomes; Pc, pinocytotic vacuole forming; R, ribosomes; S, secretion vacuole or granule; PM, plasma membrane; L, lysosomes. Note particularly the relationship between nuclear membrane, NM, and endoplasmic reticulum, and the possibility of moving substances into and out of the cell by pinocytosis, Pc, and secretion, S.

variety of organelles have been described, including nucleus, nucleolus, endoplasmic reticulum with attached ribosomes, Golgi apparatus, lysosomes, and mitochondria. The general function of each of these specialized regions of the cell has been defined. A most important property of this highly ordered structure is that of limiting membranes. Each major organelle, as well as the cell itself, is surrounded by one or more limiting membranes. Thus there is not one but several intracellular fluid compartments, each with its unique composition of ions, enzymes, and metabolites.

The Ionic Net

These unique organellar milieu are maintained at the expense of metabolic energy, principally by a number of specific ion pumps in the cellular and subcellular membranes. Just as the entire endocrine system operates as a net at the level of the organism, the various extra- and intracellular ions act as a net at the level of the cell. Of particular interest to the matter of hormone action is the interrelationship between calcium, phosphate, and hydrogen ion (Fig. 1–14). These ions form one of the basic cell buffer systems controlling the extracellular and cytosolic concentrations of H^+, Ca^{2+}, and HPO_4^{2-}. Not shown in Figure 1–14, this basic system is directly coupled to the CO_2/HCO_3^- buffer system by the common ion H^+. It is also coupled to asymmetrical Na^+/K^+ distribution across the plasma membrane of the cell in two ways: (1) $[Ca^{2+}]$ alters the permeability of the plasma membrane to monovalent cations; and (2) the Na^+ gradient and rates of flux of sodium in many cells influence the rate of Ca^{2+} flux and its distribution across the cell membrane. In addition, the Na^+ gradient is a prime regulator of the uptake of many of the major metabolic substrates. This cellular ionic set, only a portion of which is illustrated in Figure 1–14, is one of the principal means of integrating cellular responses. A perturbation in the concentration of any one ionic species leads to a propagated disturbance throughout the cell in the sense that the concentrations of all other ionic species change. These in turn influence the activity of enzymes, transport carriers, and gene expression, and thereby cell function and cell response. In a sense the system acts to amplify the original ionic change.

Organellar Functions and Their Integration

The various membrane-bound cell organelles can be isolated from cellular homogenates by differential centrifugation. The study of the metabolic activities of these isolated organelles has yielded considerable information upon which to base fruitful hypotheses concerning their function in the intact cell. It must be emphasized, however,

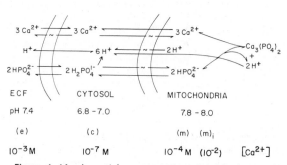

Figure 1–14. A partial representation of the fundamental ionic net within a typical mammalian cell in which there is an asymmetric distribution of calcium, phosphate, and hydrogen ion between extracellular fluids, cell cytosol, and mitochondria. These ionic asymmetries are maintained by the activities of ion pumps in both the cell and mitochondrial membranes. The part of the net represented serves as one of the fundamental cell buffer systems because of the reaction that takes place within the mitochondrial compartment of the cell: $3\ Ca^{2+} + 2\ HPO_4^{2-} \rightleftharpoons 2\ H^+ + Ca_3\ (PO_4)_2$. This means, in turn, that the system depicted is coupled, via the common component H^+, with the HCO_3^-/CO_2 buffer system. Less directly, but no less importantly, the system depicted is coupled to the Na^+/K^+ asymmetry because changes in either extracellular or cytosolic $[Ca^{2+}]$ alter the permeability of the cell membrane to these monovalent cations; moreover, the distribution of Na^+ across the cell membrane influences the flux rates and distribution of Ca^{2+}.

that, by itself, evidence obtained on organelles studied in isolation is not sufficient to provide a complete understanding of the role of the organelle in cell life without confirmation of more integrated systems. Indeed, it is highly probable that the interaction between the various organelles represents a level of functional organization as far above the organization of membrane-bound multienzyme systems as these latter systems are above the level of organization of the individual isolated enzymes.

The study of organellar interaction has barely begun. Nevertheless, there are certain well-defined instances of important membrane-membrane interactions that lead to dramatic changes in membrane properties; e.g., when the portions of the plasma membranes of two cells in an epithelial tissue are apposed, they have a low electrical resistance and a high sodium permeability, but the same areas of the plasma membranes have a high electrical resistance and low sodium permeability when the two cells are separated. There are numerous instances in which cellular and subcellular membranes form closely associated systems, and it is to be expected that the properties of these systems in the living cell differ in a striking fashion from the properties of their components.

Much of the recent attention of endocrinologists has been devoted to an analysis of the cellular actions of hormones. In the case of peptide and protein hormones, a considerable body of evidence has been accumulated in support of the concept that these hormones interact primarily if not exclusively with receptors on the plasma membrane of the cell. This interaction leads to changes in ion transport, enzyme function, and membrane structure, all of which lead to a change in concentration of intracellular messengers, i.e., the plasma membrane talks to the interior of the cell. To date, scant attention has been paid to the fact that, for an integrated and controlled response, it is equally important that the interior of the cell talk to the surface membrane. There must be a number of feedback loops that constantly inform the cell surface of events within the cell, just as there is a constant transmission of the environmental information to the interior of the cell.

The diagram in Figure 1–13 and electron micrographs of cells are only partial and momentary views of the active life of a cell. Such visualization may lead to a static view of cell structure and cellular membranes when in fact these are dynamic structures. Evidence obtained by serial electron micrographs, time-lapse cinematography, or biochemical criteria such as phospholipid turnover indicates that membranes undergo constant changes, that they interact, and that the transport of substances into and out of the cell is often achieved by enclosing them in membrane-limited systems.

Several distinct mechanisms for the regulation of metabolite flow across membranes have been identified:

1. Specific *carrier-mediated transport* across a membrane is considered to take place across the membrane without involving a marked change in membrane structure, although in some instances it is associated with an increase in phospholipid turnover. This type of mechanism is termed *facilitated* when the movement is with the electrochemical gradient of the substrate being transported and *active* when it is against an apparent electrochemical gradient. In some instances a specific permease is associated with the carrier system. This is a protein that specifically allows for the transport of a specific substrate, e.g., β-galactoside. Carrier-mediated mechanisms are most important in moving ions and small molecules across membranes.

2. *Phagocytosis,* the ingestion of particulate matter by a cell, is a process in which the plasma membrane surrounds the particle and then anneals itself to form a membrane-lined vesicle that eventually becomes detached from the plasma membrane and appears as a new intracellular organelle.

3. *Pinocytosis* is similar to phagocytosis, but only the fluid surrounding the cell is taken up in vacuoles.

4. *Micropinocytosis* is a process in which specific extracellular macromolecules are taken up into the cell by the pinching off of small vesicles from the plasma membrane. Thus only specific proteins from a solution containing a variety of proteins are taken up.

5. *Secretion granules* are vesicles containing proteins that are formed in the Golgi apparatus and migrate to the cell surface. There they combine with the plasma membrane and open to discharge their contents.

6. *Vesicles from the smooth-surfaced endoplasmic reticulum* are formed, migrate to the surface, and discharge their contents. Vesicles of this kind are formed when fats are absorbed in the intestine, and they are involved in the movement of triglyceride out of the cell.

The process of secretion is of particular importance in the endocrine system. In addition to the vesicles (described above), the process involves calcium ions, a calcium-activated ATPase, and both microtubules and microfilaments. It has many of the properties of a contractile system.

The general significance of these many modes of transport into and out of cells is that many substances that would react with other cellular components are prevented from doing so by being sequestered or compartmented in specialized membrane-bound structures. Hence this compartmentation of function is an extremely important mechanism for sustained integrated cellular activity. In general, endocrinologists have paid scant attention to these mechanisms when studying hormone action, and a wide gap continues to exist between those who view cells by cytologic means and those who view them by chemical means.

Several orders of control within the cell can be defined and discussed: (1) the regulation of the flow of cofactors and metabolites across membranes; (2) the regulation of the activity of individual enzymes; (3) the organization of individual enzymes into multienzyme complexes; (4) the association of multienzyme systems with membranes, and the control achieved by compartmentation; and (5) the

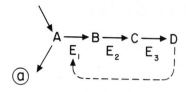

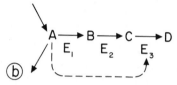

Figure 1–15. End-product inhibition (a) or precursor activation (b). The control of the activity of one enzyme by the product or substrate of a distant enzyme in a metabolic sequence. In (a) the product D interacts with an allosteric site on enzyme E_1 and leads to a decrease in activity of E_1. In (b) the precursor A interacts with an allosteric site of enzyme E_3 and leads to an increase in the activity of E_3.

regulation of enzyme concentration by the regulation of the activity of specific genes (Fig. 1–15).

Control of Individual Enzymes

Just as the cell is the principal unit of physiologic function, the enzyme or protein molecule is the principal unit of biochemical function. Changes in cell function depend upon a change in protein function. Protein functions may be of three basic types: enzymatic catalysis; membrane carrier; or free carrier or binding protein, which may serve to transport a substance from one cell compartment to another or from one metabolic pathway to another. Some proteins may serve purely a structural role.

These functions can be changed either by an alteration in the activity of individual units (proteins) or by an alteration in the concentration of such units. Alteration of protein function is basically of three types. Function may be altered because (1) the multisubunits of the protein undergo association or dissociation; (2) one or several molecules bind to sites other than the catalytic site of the protein and induce a conformational change; or (3) the covalent structure of the protein may be modified by the action of another enzyme, e.g., phosphorylation or adenylation of the protein.

Just as information transfer at the supracellular level involves communication between one cell organ and another, information transfer at the cellular level is necessary between one region of the cell and another. This requires both transmission and reception of information. The ultimate receptors, in a sense, are the individual protein molecules, which may serve as enzymes, membrane carriers, or bulk fluid carriers. Only this class of molecules has sufficient structural plasticity to serve in this capacity. It is the so-called allosteric sites, or noncatalytic sites, on these molecules that are the receptors. Following the binding of a specific ligand to such a site, a structural change in

the protein molecule takes place. In the informational sense, this is a transduction of the messenger. This structural change may lead to a dissociation or association of subunits of the protein molecule, to conformational changes in one subunit that are transmitted via a change in the nature of the interactions between dissimilar subunits, or to a conformational change within the same subunit. Regardless of type, this structural change is eventually expressed as a change in protein activity or function, e.g., an increase or decrease in catalytic activity. In the informational sense, this is the new message or output of the transduction process. As pointed out above, eventually this change in catalytic activity leads to a change in the rate of one or more metabolic pathways, the product or products of which eventually interact with initial elements in the cell metabolic net to indicate the response. Information passes in both directions.

The most important factors controlling the activity of an isolated enzyme are the concentrations of substrates, products, cofactors, and metal ions. The availability of substrate or metal ion may be controlled by the activity of other enzymes, by other cells producing or utilizing the same substrate, or by the activity of transport systems in cellular or subcellular membranes. Each of these is a possible site of hormonal control, and each has been proposed as the mechanism of action of a hormone.

Not only the substrate but also the product has an important regulatory function. The most common effect of the product is that of inhibiting the activity of the enzyme, *product inhibition.* In certain cases (e.g., phosphofructokinase), however, the product activates the enzyme, *product activation,* through an allosteric effect. This is an example of positive feedback in a biochemical system.

Control of Multienzyme Sequences

The activity of an enzyme may be regulated not individually but as part of a sequence involved in the biosynthesis of a specific compound or in the degradation of a particular substrate. An important feature of these systems is that they exhibit end-product inhibition or precursor activation.

In the first, the end-product of a particular sequence of reactions inhibits the activity of the first specific enzyme in the sequence (Fig. 1–15(a)). ("Specific" in this context means the first enzyme that is solely a portion of the sequence.) By regulating the activity of a key enzyme or branch-point in metabolism, the product regulates the flow of metabolites through a sequence of enzymatic reactions. An important feature of this control is that the inhibitor is structurally different from the substrate or product of the controlled enzyme so that it interacts with the enzyme at a site other than the active or catalytic site. The presumption is that this allosteric site is a unique receptor site for the inhibitor. The interaction of inhibitor with this allosteric site leads to a conformational change,

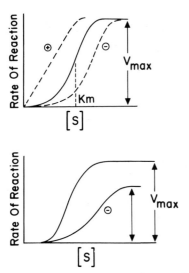

Figure 1–16. The rate of enzyme reaction as a function of substrate concentration. ⊖ is the effect of a negative allosteric interaction, and ⊕ is the effect of a positive allosteric interaction. The top portion of the figure represents the situation in which the allosteric modifier alters the K_m but not the V_{max} of the reaction, and the lower, the case in which a change in V_{max} is produced.

i.e., a change in shape, in the enzyme protein, which in turn alters the conformation of its active or catalytic site. In most cases, the interaction of a regulator with the allosteric site leads to change in the K_m rather than in the V_{max} of the enzymatic reaction (Fig. 1–16), i.e., there ensues a change in the affinity of substrate for enzyme; however, allosteric interactions have been described that lead to a change in V_{max} (note similarity with changes in affinity and intrinsic activity of hormones with receptor).

Allosteric control of enzymatic activity is not confined to end-product inhibition. Precursor activation is also quite common (Fig. 1–15(b)) — a situation in which a molecule of precursor for a metabolic sequence combines with an allosteric, rather than catalytic, site on the enzyme, which catalyzes the first unique step in that sequence, and leads to an activation of the enzyme.

Most important from the point of view of integrated cellular activity, allosteric control is exerted by substances other than precursors, substrates, or end-products, and one enzyme often possesses several allosteric sites. It is possible for intermediates or products of several metabolic sequences to influence the activity of one or more enzymes in a second sequence.

Isozymes and Duplicate Pathways

Metabolic control can be achieved by the presence of *isozymes,* enzymes that, though distinct in structure, catalyze the same reaction, have different kinetic properties, and are controlled by different factors. This is particularly the case when the product of one reaction is a common precursor for two divergent metabolic pathways.

A more general and nearly universal situation is that in which either separate enzymes occur at particular steps in a given reaction sequence or completely different metabolic pathways exist for the synthesis and degradation of both simple molecules and macromolecules. Thus the pathways for glycogen synthesis and degradation involve completely different sets of enzymes as do those involved in fatty acid synthesis and oxidation. On the other hand, the pathways of glycolysis and gluconeogenesis share a number of common enzymes, but at key points separate enzymes exist to catalyze the forward and reverse reaction; e.g., the step from F-6-P to fructose diphosphate (FDP) is catalyzed in the forward direction by the enzyme phosphofructokinase and in the reverse by fructose diphosphate (FDPase).

Two aspects of this general duality of metabolic pathways are worthy of note. The first is that both pathways are thermodynamically feasible and unidirectional under *in vivo* conditions. The second is that, as a consequence of this situation, major controls are kinetic rather than thermodynamic, i.e., by mass action. Thus, for example, under ordinary conditions of metabolism, both the pathway for glycolysis and that for gluconeogenesis are thermodynamically favorable in the directions of pyruvate and glucose, respectively. This means that if the mass action characteristics determined metabolic flux there would be a continual cycling of carbon from glucose to pyruvate to glucose with the expenditure of metabolic energy.

Such futile cycling would represent a serious drain upon metabolism. In order to prevent or minimize such futile cycles, kinetic control of particular steps in each sequence is the rule. This regulation is coordinate in the sense that a given control agent, e.g., AMP, has opposite effects upon steps in the forward and reverse directions, e.g., activation of phosphofructokinase and inhibition of FDPase. Coordinate control is not completely antithetical, however. There are factors that regulate phosphofructokinase but not FDPase and vice versa, which means that under some special circumstances both enzymes are active. In fact, there is a capability for a plasticity of response at all levels of metabolism and metabolic control.

These pairs of oppositely directed unidirectional metabolic sequences are one of the most fundamental features of cellular metabolism. They permit flexibility of response, i.e., they are the basis of homeostasis. It would be wrong, however, to consider them as completely separate. They are not. They are coupled one with the other and with other major pathways by stoichiometric coupling agents. The most universal of these are the adenine and pyridine nucleotides. In a more restricted sense, coenzyme A serves a similar function. The distinctive feature of all such coupling agents is that they exist in rather fixed total amounts (generally), and they exist in one of two (or occasionally three) states. Thus the pyridine nucleotides can be either oxidized or reduced. Their rates of oxidation and reduction must balance over an extended period if metabolism is to maintain a steady state. As a consequence, they couple the oxidative with the reductive systems in the cell. Likewise, the adenine nucleotides can exist in three states, ATP, ADP, or AMP, and their ratios determine the energy charge of the cell—the balance between the synthesis and utilization of phosphate bond energy for osmotic, mechanical, chemical, and electrical work. As such, the coupling between utilization and synthesis must be maintained. It is the basic requirement for continued cell function. In view of this need, it is not surprising that, in addition to serving as coupling agents, the adenine nucleotides serve as basic messengers for exerting kinetic control upon key enzymes in the energy-producing pathways and in some of the energy-utilizing pathways. Additional selective controls are superimposed upon these basic ones. Eventually, in the hierarchical organization, these additional controls are extracellular (hormonal) in nature.

Enzymes, Membranes, and Compartmentation

A most important feature of the organization of some multienzyme sequences is their high degree of structural organization, as illustrated by the reactions of oxidative phosphorylation. All the enzymes involved in electron transport and oxidative phosphorylation are in a highly ordered, membrane-bound sequence within a specific cellular compartment, the mitochondria. The kinetics of the overall process of electron transport indicate that the sequence is shielded from the media on either side of the membrane, and the electron carriers are arranged in a contiguous, highly ordered sequence.

The mitochondria exhibit several important control features. The substrates for the electron transport chain are hydroxybutyrate, succinate, and NADH, all products of fatty acid oxidation or Krebs cycle activity; these cycle enzymes are all located within the mitochondria. The NADH formed by their activity is inaccessible to the enzymes in the cytoplasm; hence this organization confers an important directional component to metabolism. All the NADH generated by the citric acid cycle is reoxidized either by the electron transport chain or by an energy-linked transhydrogenase

$$NADH + NADP^+ \rightleftharpoons NAD^+ + NADPH$$

The latter enzyme is also intramitochondrial and is another site of proposed hormone action. The unique importance of NADPH lies in the fact that it is a crucial cofactor for reductive biosynthesis of fats, steroids, and other compounds.

This compartmentation of the cells into several separate functional units, each with its unique ionic and enzymatic composition, conveys specialization in the same sense as the organization of the multicellular organism into specific cells (such as liver, kidney, and brain). Its importance for the control of metabolism is only dimly perceived, al-

though it is beginning to be apparent. For example, ATP and its products, AMP, P_i, and ADP, play critical roles in the regulation of energy metabolism. An important feature of oxidative phosphorylation is that the reaction

$$ADP^{2-} + HPO_4^{3-} \rightleftharpoons ATP^{2-} + OH^-$$

takes place within the mitochondrion. The substrates, ADP and phosphate, enter this organelle by specific membrane carriers. The product, ATP, leaves in a similar fashion. Hence the nucleotide pool can vary in several cellular compartments, and its balance can be altered by the distribution of metal ions or change in the activity of specific metabolic pathways. Similarly, the processes of gluconeogenesis and fatty acid synthesis are cytoplasmic (extramitochondrial) activities that derive their substrates from mitochondrial intermediates.

Regulation of Membrane Function

One of the unique features of all membranes is that the fluids on their two sides differ strikingly in ionic composition. Likewise, membranes bind metal ions, most notably calcium, and membrane function is controlled by this binding. The maintenance of ion gradients across membranes is brought about by anisotropic energy-requiring enzymes. Over 50 per cent of the energy utilized by the resting cell may be expended in this activity. The maintenance of these gradients is extremely important because they confer a vectorial component to other transport systems within the membrane and thereby to metabolism as a whole. If several carrier systems are affected in the same fashion, then it is apparent that a primary change in the ion pump will lead to an altered distribution of other substances that are transported across the membrane by such carrier-mediated mechanisms. Thus every membrane represents an extremely complex system: the membrane by its activities alters its environment, and its environment in turn modulates the activities of the membrane—a feedback loop.

A second type of membrane control that has been discussed but not considered in depth is that of reversible binding of specific enzymes to membranes. For example, in some species hexokinase or phosphoenolpyruvate carboxykinase are bound to mitochondria, whereas in others they are apparently located in the cytosol. It has been postulated but not established that metabolism might be controlled by a change in enzyme binding to a membrane with a subsequent change in enzyme activity.

A third type of membrane control is that of altering membrane structure and function by influencing membrane turnover. Recent biochemical evidence presents a rather paradoxical view of cell membranes. On the one hand, the phospholipid and protein components of these membranes turn over rapidly and independently, and there appears to be a considerable fluidity of structure. On the other, there is a remarkable stability of structure when viewed in terms of properties such as enzymatic activities, e.g., adenyl cyclase, membrane potential, or glucose transport. It has been known that the turnover of the phosphate group in various phospholipids changes with change in membrane function. Recently it has been discovered, however, that the fatty acid composition of the membrane phospholipids turns over more rapidly than the glycerol backbones of these same phospholipids. This cycle of deacylation and reacylation of membrane phospholipids, particularly in the 2 or beta position of the glycerol, is rapid and, at least in one case (the action of aldosterone), is changed by hormonal action. It is possible that this is a primary effect of the hormone and that the change in fatty acid composition changes the environment of the enzymes and carriers in the membrane sufficiently to change their function. Alternately, the change in lipid composition may be a reflection of a primary change in protein structure with a resultant accommodation of lipid structure to this change.

Regulation of Enzyme Concentration

The overall rate of a particular enzyme-catalyzed reaction depends upon several factors, including enzyme concentration. The concentrations of many enzymes in the cell vary widely in response to environmental change. Hence mechanisms have evolved for increasing or decreasing the rate of synthesis of specific protein molecules and of selectively degrading them. In addition, there are a number of instances in which enzymes are interconvertible from an active to an inactive form; for example:

$$\text{phosphorylase } a \rightleftharpoons \text{phosphorylase } b$$

the different forms having different affinities for substrates and for allosteric modifiers. This conversion from active to inactive form or vice versa is usually regulated by the activity of other enzymes which control the conversion by means of changing the covalent structure of the controlled enzyme. The two most common structural changes involve either adenylation or phosphorylation, both of which use ATP as substrate. In the case of phosphorylase, one enzyme, phosphorylase b kinase, catalyzes the phosphorylation of phosphorylase b, and another, a phosphatase, catalyzes its dephosphorylation.

The ability of cells to control their enzymatic profile is a useful one because it augments the control of metabolism by end-product inhibition, substrate activation, and allosteric regulation of enzymatic activity. In functional terms it means a considerable conservation; enzyme molecules are made or activated during times of need, and their synthesis and activity are suppressed in times of surfeit. Moreover, it represents a second order of control: the time course of the biosynthetic response is sluggish and often less sensitive than end-product inhibition; i.e., a greater accumulation of end product seems required to bring about cessation of enzyme synthesis than to bring about end-product inhibition. This last point, however, is not completely established.

The most widely accepted model of how this type of control is achieved is that of Jacob and Monod. In this model (Fig. 1–17), derived primarily from genetic and biochemical analysis of bacterial systems, a structural gene exists that dictates the primary structure of specific proteins. The information necessary to direct the synthesis of these specific proteins is contained as a triplet code of bases in the nucleotide sequence making up the DNA molecules of the gene. This information is

Figure 1–17. The possible factors regulating the activity of an enzyme E_1. These include regulation by (1) substrate availability or product accumulation across either the plasma membrane, PM, or mitochondrial membrane, MM; (2) availability of metal ions (M^+ or M^{2+}) or cofactor; (3) end-product inhibition, EPI; (4) precursor activation, PA; (5) conversion of enzyme from inactive to active form; and (6) regulation of total enzyme concentration by regulating protein biosynthesis by controlling the translation of the message in mRNA, messenger RNA, to amino acid sequence on individual ribosomes, R, of a polysome, P. In addition to mRNA and R, activated amino acids on specific tRNA, transfer RNA, are necessary (7); amino acid activation is achieved by specific amino acid activating enzymes (8). Translation is blocked by puromycin (9). The availability of mRNA is controlled by the rate of transcription of nucleotide sequence in DNA of structural gene, S_1, by RNA polymerase (10) in the nucleus, N. Regulation of transcription is achieved by the activity of regulator genes, R_1 and R_2. The substrates or products alter the activity of these genes and bring about induction, In (11), or repression, Rp (12). Control of activity of gene S is achieved by regulating activity of operator, O (13). Transcription is blocked by actinomycin D (14). (From Jacob, F., and Monod, J.: *J. Molec. Biol.* 3:318, 1961.)

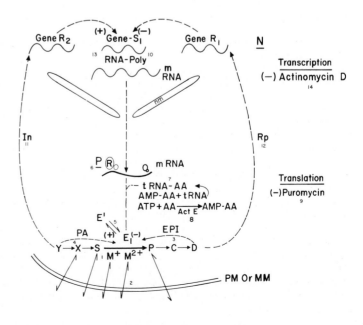

first transcribed to an RNA code in the nucleus by a DNA-dependent RNA polymerase (transcription). The product messenger RNA (mRNA) carries the code in its base sequence, which is complementary to that of the DNA directing its synthesis. The mRNA is presumed to be short-lived and to carry its specific message from its site of synthesis to the site of protein synthesis, the polysome. Polysomes are located in the cytoplasm of the cell and in higher organisms are often bound to the endoplasmic reticulum. On the polysome, the triplet code of mRNA is translated into the specific amino acid sequence of the proteins. The process requires guanosine 5′-triphosphate (GTP), cations, mRNA, transfer RNA (tRNA) — amino acid complexes, and the ribosomes of the polysome. Each ribosome is composed of two subunits, each of which is made up of proteins and larger molecular weight RNA, (ribosomal) rRNA. Specificity resides in the fact that the tRNA-amino acid complexes are formed by enzymes specific for each activated amino acid and for each tRNA, and that the tRNA is also specific in its interaction with the mRNA-polysome complex. The mechanism whereby mRNA directs the synthesis of the protein molecule is known in considerable detail, but it is not yet clear how prosthetic groups are added. All evidence suggests that they are added after the primary sequence of the polypeptide has been completed. It is certain, however, that the primary sequence of the protein molecule is sufficient to determine the secondary and tertiary structure of the molecule once it is released from the ribosome. Synthesis is initiated at the N-terminal end of the polypeptide chain. It is equally clear that attachment of mRNA to the ribosome and the subsequent translation or readout of its message to form a particular protein molecule can vary independently.

The Jacob-Monod model proposes that the major site of control is at the level of transcription, i.e., the synthesis of mRNA by RNA polymerase. Two types of control have been proposed, induction and repression. Induction is the stimulation of the synthesis of one or more specific enzymes in a metabolic sequence when the substrate of the first enzyme in the sequence is added to the bacteria, and repression is the cessation of the synthesis of one or more enzymes in a sequence by the addition of the end-product of that sequence, often a biosynthetic sequence. These two types of effects represent opposites in the same sense as do precursor activation and end-product inhibition.

Genetic evidence indicates that a site upon the chromosome (the regulator gene) distinct from the site specifying the structure of the enzyme (the structural gene) is involved in this regulation. The product of the regulator gene is a protein (the repressor substance) which interacts with another site upon the chromosome (the operator, located near the structural gene) and inhibits further transcription of the particular genetic message. Interaction of an inducer with repressor prevents the binding of the repressor to the operator and thus allows transcription to proceed. There is, in addition, considerable evidence from work in mammalian systems that control can be exerted at the level of translation as well as that of transcription. The exact means of achieving translational control has not yet been established.

A number of the aspects of this sequence of events from gene to enzyme in mammalian cells are not yet fully understood. Ribosomal RNA (rRNA) and tRNA as well as mRNA are usually synthesized when induction occurs. One point of view holds that mRNA is actually transported from nucleus to cytoplasm by one of the ribosomal subunits. Likewise, there is evidence of synthesis of both RNA and protein in mitochondria.

In eukaryotic cells, the process of enzyme degradation as well as synthesis goes on constantly. The rate of breakdown appears to be controlled by both general and specific factors. In general, the larger the protein and the more complex its structure (i.e., the greater its number of subunits), the more rapid its breakdown. It has been proposed that this can be simply related to the greater tendency of the larger molecules to undergo dissociation with a resultant increase in susceptibility to proteolysis. In addition to this general relationship, it appears to be a rule that specific substrates, co-factors, and other ligands all have the ability to stabilize enzyme structure and thereby reduce their rate of proteolytic destruction.

Only a very small percentage of the total number of genes on a mammalian chromosome are active in a mature cell such as liver, kidney, or brain; however, these cells contain the entire genetic potential of the species to which they belong. Some of the inactive genes can be readily activated by changes in diet or hormonal status, whereas others are more or less permanently repressed but do become active during malignant change.

The importance of the relationship of induction to precursor activation and of repression to end-product inhibition is that a single small molecule affects two separate events within the cell, the activity of a specific enzyme and the synthesis of that enzyme. Therefore a small molecule, such as a hormone, may have more than one receptor site within a cell. The corollary to this is that different *functional groups* or topochemical regions of the hormone molecule may be responsible for the chemical interactions with different receptors.

HORMONES AND INTRACELLULAR HOMEOSTASIS

There is no doubt that most of the basic mechanisms responsible for maintaining cellular homeostasis in primitive organisms also operate in the cells of the multicellular organism — in other words, that each cell has inherited a highly developed system of homeostatic controls that permits its individual existence. It is these controls that are in large part responsible for maintaining the constancy of the composition of the various intracellular seas. The multicellular organism, however, is more than a colony of individual cells, and new control mechanisms were necessary to coordinate the activities of the individual cells into the activities of the organism as a whole. The question becomes one of determining how the ancient cellular control systems were altered, supplemented, and integrated to achieve organ and organismal function.

The obvious first development was that of the ability of one cell to communicate with another. This was achieved in two ways: first, by the elaboration of specific extracellular substances, hormones; and second, by the direct communication between contiguous cells in a parenchymatous organ.

Individual cells in a normal organ such as the liver are not autonomous units but function as a syncytium; that is, the plasma membrane of the liver cell has greater permeability and lower electrical resistance when normally joined to other liver cells than when it exists as an isolated liver cell. The importance of this type of organization is that the cells respond as a synchronous single macrocellular complex rather than as many individual cellular units. This communication between cells is direct, i.e., no specialized substances are elaborated into the extracellular fluids, and it seems likely that no fundamentally new type of control mechanism is operative. Stated in another fashion, the homeostatic control of organ function is a direct extension of the autoregulatory control systems possessed by its individual cells.

A second purely cellular type of altered behavior is the development of cellular polarity. This phenomenon is most clearly evident in epithelial organs or membranes such as the kidney tubule, for example. Here a vectoral component is added to cellular function and metabolism by the evolution of asymmetric cell surfaces. In the case of the amphibian urinary bladder, for example, the development of an additional component to the mucosal surface of the epithelial cells lining this organ was associated with the loss of two universal properties of cell membranes: loss of the ability to extrude sodium ions and loss of free permeability to water. These two changes have led to a membrane capable of restricting the movement of water and of bringing about the unidirectional transport of sodium ion. This type of change represents cellular specialization by the loss or alteration of a common cellular function.

On the other hand, the development of intercellular communication by means of neural or humoral signals represents a new type of control system which has evolved in response to a new need. Nevertheless, as should be clear from the foregoing, there is a striking similarity between the supracellular and cellular control systems. For example, the control of the rate of synthesis and release of corticotropin-releasing factor (CRF) from the hypothalamus by the concentration of circulating cortisol is basically the same phenomenon as the control of the rate of synthesis of arginine by the concentration of this amino acid in bacterial cultures.

Nearly all of the present data indicate that hormones act primarily by altering the equilibrium or balance of the cell's autoregulatory systems. Thus iodide uptake by the thyroid, for example, continues in the absence of TSH, and the rate of iodide uptake is responsive to the supply of available iodide. The TSH alters the sensitivity, or in a sense the K_m, of the iodide-trapping system, which continues, however, to be responsive to changing levels of circulating iodide. This type of evidence makes it clear that extracellular homeostasis is but an extension of intracellular homeostasis; in fact, the two represent a single integrated metabolic network. Hormones are thus involved in the control of both intra- and extracellular activities. Viewed in this light, the action of a hormone upon a subcellular membrane such as the mitochondrial membrane naturally leads to an alteration in the composition of the extracellular fluids as well as to changes in intracellular activities. Of particular note is the central role that ions appear to play as integrators and regulators of intra- and extracellular activities; for example, calcium is the intracellular coupling factor between excitation and contraction in a muscle cell as well as the extracellular regulator of the rate of secretion of PTH.

The importance of appreciating this unity of biologic control lies in two general areas: (1) the similarity between extracellular, endocrine, and intracellular control systems; and (2) the necessity of studying intracellular events in order fully to understand extracellular homeostasis and the mechanisms whereby hormones act. Intimate knowledge of cellular control systems thus becomes essential in exploring and understanding endocrine control mechanisms.

A particular analogy between endocrine and cellular controls that deserves attention is that of anticipatory responses. Such responses are a part of many servo-systems as well as of physiologic ones. The best physiologic example is that of the release of epinephrine in preparation for flight or fight, as described by Cannon. Similar anticipatory responses undoubtedly exist at the cellular level, although they have not yet been identified. It seems possible that, in some instances, activation of phosphorylase by C-AMP is a cellular anticipatory response to a hormone; i.e., the need for additional energy is anticipated by the breakdown of glycogen. Moreover, the stimulation of the release of insulin by gastrointestinal hormones in response to a glucose load represents an anticipatory response of a similar nature at the supracellular level of organization.

HORMONAL CONTROL MECHANISMS

As noted above, there have been three general theories of hormone action: they act to alter the function of enzymes, genes, or membranes. There is no recent experimental evidence that supports the concept that hormones are direct activators of single enzymes, although one runs into a semantic problem when considering the membrane-bound enzyme, adenyl cyclase, which is activated by a large number of hormones and other extracellular messengers. The nature of this problem will be discussed below. At present, there is increasing evidence that many hormones act in one of two general ways. The first is by interacting with receptor sites upon the plasma membrane or cell surface with the resultant generation of one or several intracellular messengers; the second is by entering the cell and combining within the cell with specific soluble receptor proteins, which upon interaction with their specific hormone undergo a structural transformation and are transported as the modified receptor-hormone complex into the nucleus where they are responsible for specific gene activation.

The first general model holds for many amine, peptide, and protein hormones, the second for many steroid hormones. It is important to note, however, that not all the effects of all members of either class of hormones are easily explained by these respective models. There may yet prove to be greater diversity of action than presently envisioned.

Because of the rather general correspondence between structural class and mode of action of hormones, it is most convenient to discuss the mode of action of amine peptide and protein hormones as one subsection and that of steroid hormones as another. In doing so, it should be noted that present information about the mode of action of thyroxine and triiodothyronine is confusing, contradictory, and not readily accommodated by either general theory.

Mode of Peptide Hormone Action

Peptide hormones range in size from molecular weights of hundreds to thousands and tens of thousands of daltons. They exhibit enormous differences in structural conformation and are highly specific in their effects and in regard to the target tissues upon which they act. The consequences of their actions are quite different, ranging from a change in the water permeability of the cell membrane in the case of the vasopressins to an inhibition of bone resorption in the case of calcitonin. Given this diversity, it was initially assumed that each had a unique mode of action. In the light of the research conducted over the past 15 years, however, this assumption has been largely invalidated. There appear to be only a few general modes by which these hormones regulate cell function.

The Adenyl Cyclase Model

A present major postulate is that many peptide and amine hormones regulate cell function by controlling the activity of the membrane-bound enzyme, adenyl cyclase, which catalyzes the conversion of ATP to C-AMP and pyrophosphate. The discovery in 1958 by Sutherland and Rall of this cyclic nucleotide as an intermediate in the hepatic action of epinephrine was the major impetus to the subsequent identification of this nucleotide as an intermediate in the action of a large number of peptide and amine hormones (Table 1–2). These discoveries led to the proposal by Sutherland and his colleagues of the second messenger hypothesis, which is presented schematically in Figure 1–18. In this hypothesis, the particular hormone, or extracellular (first) messenger, interacts with a receptor site upon the cell surface. This interaction leads to an increase (or decrease) in the activity of the enzyme, adenyl cyclase, a component of the cell membrane, which results in an increase (or decrease) in the concentration of C-AMP, the second messenger, within the cell. This increase in C-AMP was considered responsible for all the hormonally induced changes in cell function. Subsequent work led to the identification of a class of

TABLE 1–2. CELLULAR SYSTEMS IN WHICH A ROLE FOR BOTH Ca^{2+} AND C-AMP IN CELL ACTIVATION HAS BEEN OBSERVED

Cell	Stimulus	Response	Ca^{2+} Required	C-AMP Produced
Synapse	Electrical	Transmitter release	+	+
Neuromuscular junction	Electrical	Transmitter release	+	+
Anterior pituitary	GHRF	Growth hormone release	+	+
Anterior pituitary	LHRF	LH release	+	+
Anterior pituitary	TRF	TSH release	+	+
Posterior pituitary	Electrical	Vasopressin release	+	?
Salivary gland	Epinephrine	Amylase release	+	+
Beta cell, pancreas	Glucose	Insulin release	+	+
Adrenal cortex	ACTH	Steroid release	+	+
Liver	Glucagon	Glucose synthesis and release	?	+
Thyroid	TSH	Thyroxine release	+	+
Corpus luteum	LH	Progesterone release	+	+
Stomach	Histamine	HCl secretion	+	+
Heart	Epinephrine	Glycogenolysis	+	+
Toad bladder	Vasopressin	$Na^+ + H_2O$ transport	?	+
Kidney tubule	PTH	Gluconeogenesis	+	+
Melanocyte	MSH	Melanin dispersion	+	+
Slime mold	?	Aggregation	+	+
Sea urchin egg	Sperm	Fertilization	+	+
Adipocyte	Epinephrine	Lipolysis	+	+
Fly salivary gland	5-Hydroxytryptamine	Secretion	+	+
Red blood cell	Epinephrine	Change in filterability	+	+
Thymocyte	PTH	Increased mitotic rate	+	?

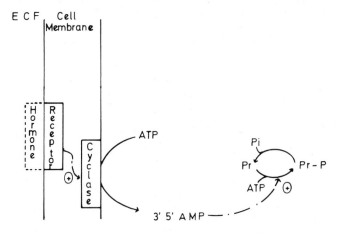

Figure 1–18. The second messenger model of peptide hormone action in which hormone-receptor interaction leads to activation of membrane-bound adenyl cyclase resulting in a rise in the concentration of C-AMP within the cell. The rise in C-AMP concentration leads to the activation of protein kinases (a class of enzyme) that catalyze the phosphorylation of proteins, using ATP as phosphate donor.

enzymes, C-AMP-dependent protein kinases, which have been proposed as the major if not sole site of action of C-AMP within cells.

The specific enzyme, phosphorylase *b* kinase, a protein kinase, has been isolated in highly purified form and has been shown to consist of two dissimilar subunits, a regulatory one and a catalytic one. The mode of action of C-AMP upon this enzyme is that of combining with the regulatory subunit, causing thereby a dissociation of the two subunits (Fig. 1–19). When associated with the regulatory subunit, the activity of the catalytic subunit is inhibited. When free, the catalytic subunit is active and catalyzes the phosphorylation of one or more specific proteins within the particular cell.

There are a number of implications that follow from this hypothesis and a number of questions that it raises, not all of which have been completely answered. It has been proposed that, in order to establish that this model accounts for the mode of action of a particular hormone, the following criteria should be satisfied: (1) the hormone causes an increase (or decrease) in C-AMP within the tissue; (2) C-AMP mimics the effect of the hormone upon the tissue; (3) the effects of submaximal doses of the hormone are enhanced by theophylline or caffeine because these compounds block the activity of the enzyme(s) phosphodiesterase, which

catalyzes the breakdown of C-AMP to 5'-AMP; (4) the hormone causes the activation of particulate adenyl cyclase prepared from a homogenate of the cell (presumably a fraction of the cell membrane); (5) there are present in the tissue one or more C-AMP-dependent protein kinases; (6) specific substrates for these kinases can be identified, and their effects can be related to the physiologic response of the cell; and (7) it should be possible to demonstrate specific activation of the protein kinase *in situ*.

Some of the most important implications of this model are: (1) all peptide hormones act in this way; (2) all the effects of these hormones can be accounted for by the single change, i.e., an increase in C-AMP within the cell; (3) the only important receptors for peptide hormones are upon the plasma membrane, i.e., peptide hormones do not enter cells and interact with subcellular organelles, enzyme complexes, or individual enzymes; (4) C-AMP has only a single universal message, which is expressed by binding to the regulatory subunits of protein and perhaps other kinases; (5) either protein kinases (the catalytic units) in different cells have different specificities in terms of the proteins that will serve as their substrates or there are multiple C-AMP-dependent protein kinases; and (6) the hormone receptor site on the cell surface is an allosteric site on the enzyme adenyl cyclase.

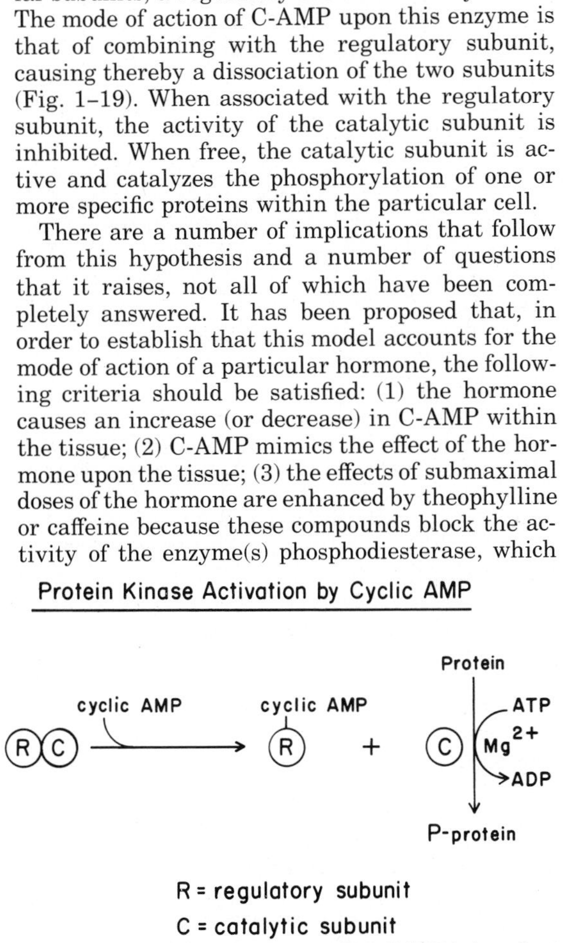

Protein Kinase Activation by Cyclic AMP

$$R\,C \xrightarrow{\text{cyclic AMP}} \quad \text{cyclic AMP} \quad \boxed{R} \;+\; C$$

Protein
ATP
Mg^{2+}
ADP
P-protein

R = regulatory subunit

C = catalytic subunit

Figure 1–19. The mechanism by which C-AMP brings about the activation of protein kinases. The cyclic nucleotide binds to the regulatory subunit of the inactive enzyme causing a dissociation of regulatory from catalytic subunits. The dissociated catalytic subunit is catalytically competent, whereas it is not competent when associated with the regulatory subunit.

Other Models

It is clear that, even though many peptide hormones may act in this fashion, not all do. Insulin is a notable exception. Even though there is evidence that insulin inhibits adenyl cyclase activity in several different target tissues, not all of its effects can be explained by this single action. It has the following additional independent effects upon the function of the cell membrane: (1) increasing glucose transport; (2) altering ionic permeabilities and thereby membrane potential; (3) increasing amino acid transport; and (4) altering the activity of the membrane-bound enzyme, lipoprotein lipase. In the case of insulin, an adequate model to account for these multiple effects is one in which the insulin-receptor interaction leads to a widespread change in membrane structure with a resultant change in multiple membrane functions. In a sense, then, there are multiple second messengers following insulin-receptor interaction. A logical alternative would be a model in which each of these functions is controlled by a unique insulin receptor on the membrane; i.e., multiple insulin receptors exist on each cell type, each coupled directly to a unique membrane functional unit. There is at present no evidence to support this view.

Calcium–C-AMP Relationship: A Modification of the Adenyl Cyclase Model

In the case of many other cellular systems in which C-AMP has been implicated as a second messenger, there is also evidence that other second messengers exist. In particular, in many of these systems calcium also serves as second messenger (Table 1–2). In many of these cases, in the absence of calcium neither the specific hormone nor exogenous C-AMP will initiate a cellular response. Moreover, in most cases, both hormone and exogenous C-AMP will induce radiocalcium efflux from prelabeled cells, but only the hormone will stimulate calcium entry. Finally, an increase in intracellular [Ca^{2+}] leads to an inhibition of hormone-stimulated adenyl cyclase. These facts can be explained by a model (Fig. 1–20), in which hormone-receptor interaction leads to an increase in calcium entry and an activation of adenyl cyclase. The resulting increase in intracellular C-AMP leads to an activation of one or more protein kinases and to an increase in calcium efflux from the major intracellular calcium pool, the mitochondrial calcium pool (Fig. 1–20), into the cell cytosol.

The combined effect of the hormone upon calcium entry at the cell membrane and C-AMP upon the mitochondrial membrane leads to an increase in the concentration of Ca^{2+} in the cell cytosol. The Ca^{2+} activates or inhibits enzymes, some of which are the phosphoprotein products of the C-AMP-dependent protein kinase reactions. It inhibits adenyl cyclase, a negative feedback loop in this intracellular control system, and it alters the permeability of the plasma membrane to monovalent cations. On the basis of the ionic interrelationships depicted in Figure 1–14 and the model in Figure 1–20, it is clear that the final cellular response can be modified by changes in pH and phosphate ion concentration as well as a number of other factors. Moreover, during the adaptation of this kind of control mechanism to the control of function of a specific cell type, one or the other of these two components (or second messengers) may become of greater importance. Thus in the case of insulin release from pancreatic beta cells, for example, the primary messenger appears to be Ca^{2+}, with C-AMP serving only to modify the effects of calcium by controlling its intracellular metabolism. On the other hand, in the liver, the major regulator of glucagon-induced gluconeogenesis appears to be C-AMP. Finally, in other cells, such as those of the renal tubules, both messengers have a primary

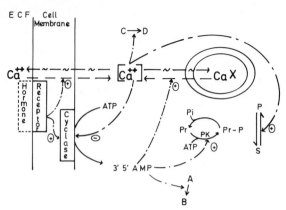

Figure 1–20. A model of peptide hormone action in which hormone receptor-interaction leads to at least two effects: (1) an activation of adenyl cyclase; and (2) an increase in the calcium permeability of the cell membrane. The rise in intracellular 3′,5′-AMP increases calcium efflux from the mitochondria and activates protein kinases. Both Ca^{2+} and C-AMP serve as intracellular messengers, and Ca^{2+} serves as a feedback inhibitor of adenyl cyclase. The Ca^{2+} activates or inhibits the activities of enzymatic reactions (C → D), some of which (S ⇌ P) may be catalyzed by the phosphoprotein products of C-AMP–dependent protein kinases.

function in the integrated cellular response to hormonal stimulation.

An examination of the model depicted in Figure 1–20 shows that it is an augmented and modified version of the original second messenger model (Fig. 1–18). As such, it still probably does not represent a complete description of the second messengers that play a role in the action of many peptide hormones. It is likely that other factors, e.g., other ions and membrane-bound enzymes, will be found to serve this function as well.

A major drawback of the original second messenger hypothesis was its failure to emphasize the need for a feedback of information from cell interior to cell surface. In the model depicted in Figure 1–20, one of the functions of Ca^{2+} is that of acting as a feedback signal. Again, however, it is quite likely that other ions, metabolites, or macromolecules will eventually be found to play a similar role in the transfer of information from inside the cell to the cell surface.

A second drawback of the original model (Fig. 1–18) is that, in the control sense, there was no room for a plasticity of response. When additional second messengers such as Ca^{2+} are incorporated into this cellular control system, however, then the feature of plasticity appears. Obviously, the more numerous the second messengers following a given hormone receptor interaction, the greater the variety of final responses possible, depending upon the state of cell function and its environment at the time of hormonal stimulation.

A difficult question that has yet to be fully answered is whether all peptide and amine hormones act solely at the cell surface. Although the weight of present opinion favors this point of view, the evidence in its support is not completely satisfactory. For example, epinephrine has been shown to activate an adenyl cyclase on the cardiac sarcoplasmic reticulum. If a similar activation takes place when this hormone acts upon the intact heart, it can occur only after epinephrine has entered the cell. Moreover, it has been found that many peptide hormones exhibit highly specific effects upon the function of one or more isolated subcellular organelles. It is difficult, however, to demonstrate that the same changes take place when intact cells are treated with the same hormone. An alternative approach has been to bind small hormone molecules to large molecules (e.g., Sepharose), and then study the effects of these large conjugates upon cell function, assuming that if they exhibit hormonal effects they do so by acting on the cell surface. More data with a large number of peptide hormones are needed before the value of this approach can be fully assessed.

The matter of C-AMP action within the cell is still not completely settled. There do exist, in nearly every cell, C-AMP-dependent protein kinases, most of which are activated by C-AMP in the range of 10^{-7} to 10^{-8} M. The problem is that of establishing that these are the sole sites of action of this nucleotide. The problem is complicated by the fact that these kinases appear to have a very broad specificity in terms of those proteins that will serve as their substrates. Moreover, C-AMP in slightly higher concentrations will influence the activity of a large number of other enzymes without protein kinase activity, another example of the redundancy of information obtained at a single level of investigative analysis. The final validation of the concept that protein kinases are the sole site of C-AMP action requires the demonstration that C-AMP acts only upon these kinases *in situ* and that *in situ* the kinases catalyze the phosphorylation of specific enzymes whose altered function can account for the hormonal effects. This has yet to be accomplished, except in the case of the control of cardiac glycogenolysis by epinephrine. On the other hand, the presence of membrane-bound protein kinases that respond to C-AMP has been discovered. It is difficult at present to see how these enzymes can dissociate in the sense depicted in Figure 1–19; hence C-AMP must be acting to alter enzyme function in a different manner in these cases.

Time Course of Peptide Hormone Action

A major difference between the actions of peptide and steroid hormones concerns the time course of their actions. In general, peptide hormones act rapidly (within seconds to minutes), whereas steroid hormones usually act more slowly (hours). Important as this difference is in the physiologic sense, it is clear that neither characteristic is completely correct. In addition to immediate effects, nearly all peptide hormones have long-term effects. When ACTH acts upon the adrenal cortex, its immediate effects are to increase both steroid synthesis and steroid secretion. In addition, however, it promotes the hypertrophy and hyperplasia of the adrenal cortical cells and thereby the total capacity of the gland to sustain steroid hormone production. Likewise, PTH stimulates the activity of the bone resorbing cells, the osteoclasts, immediately but

also increases the conversion of osteoprogenitor cells to osteoclasts over a much longer period of time. Conversely, steroid hormones have immediate as well as delayed effects. When estrogen acts upon the uterus there are a number of immediate effects, e.g., stimulation of H_2O uptake and phospholipid synthesis, as well as the more delayed effects of stimulating tissue growth. It is not yet clear in the majority of these cases whether the immediate and delayed effects of any given peptide or steroid hormone are mediated by the same second messenger (e.g., do C-AMP and Ca^{2+} regulate cell growth in the adrenal cortex as well as steroid hormone secretion?) or whether there are separate sets of messengers for each of these actions. Available evidence favors the concept that in some cases the same messengers are responsible for both types of effects but that in others this may not be the case.

Any discussion of the time course of action of hormones would be incomplete without a consideration of the phenomenon of hysteresis in biologic systems. This term has been applied to the phenomenon in which, after a particular stimulus has been removed (e.g., the concentration of an allosteric modifier suddenly reduced), there may not be an immediate change in activity (e.g., enzyme function). In isolated enzymes, the function may persist for minutes after the modifier is removed and is thought to represent the time necessary for the enzyme conformation to relax back into its unmodified state. When cellular systems respond to specific hormones, some relax back into the untreated state, but others persist for days or, rarely, even weeks. One of the most dramatic examples of this type of behavior is the action of calcitonin (CT) upon bone resorption. Intermittent therapy of as little as one dose a week is sufficient to suppress bone resorption even though CT acts rapidly (minutes) and, presumably, its primary cellular effects are short-lived. The basis for this type of sustained effect has not been elucidated, but it is of considerable practical significance in therapy.

Mode of Steroid Hormone Action

Estrogen as Prototype

The prototype for the general model of steroid hormone action is the effect of estrogen upon growth and development of the mammalian uterus or hen oviduct. The combined data from these two systems lead to the model of estrogen action depicted in Figure 1–21. The first step is the entry of the active estrogen—estradiol, for example—into the cell cytosol. There it binds to a specific receptor protein. Following this hormone-receptor interaction, the protein undergoes a structural change and is then transported, as the steroid-protein complex, into the nucleus. There it interacts with one or more specific parts of the genome and initiates by this interaction the transcription of specific genes, e.g., the gene for ovalbumin mRNA synthesis in the oviduct.

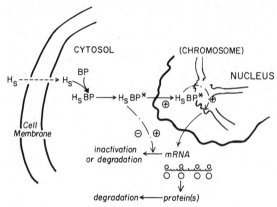

Figure 1–21. A schematic representation of steroid hormone action based upon the action of estradiol upon mammalian uterus and hen oviduct. H_s = steroid hormone; BP = cytosolic binding protein; BP* = altered binding protein; mRNA = messenger RNA.

In addition to these specific gene activations, many hormones also initiate what Tompkins and co-workers have designated as a *pleiotypic response,* consisting of an increase in rRNA and tRNA, a general increase in protein synthesis, and changes in substrate entry, all of which are part of a general growth response. It is not yet clear whether these effects of steroid hormones are mediated by the nuclear steroid-protein complex directly or by some more indirect means. The situation is complex because protein hormones such as insulin induce a similar pleiotypic response in mammalian cells grown in tissue culture. If, as has been postulated, insulin acts only at the level of the plasma membrane of the cell, then some second messenger must be responsible for these generalized and coordinated effects of insulin.

Although the model depicted in Figure 1–21 accounts for many of the known effects of estrogens upon target tissues, it does not explain all of them, and it remains a distinct possibility that the hormone-receptor complex or complexes may have additional, more immediate, direct effects upon cell function. Likewise, when this model is extended to a consideration of the action of other steroid hormones, present evidence indicates that many steroid hormones do have specific intracellular protein receptors. It is not established, however, that they all exert their effects by controlling nuclear gene transcription. In the case of the action of cortisol upon mammalian liver cell function, the available evidence favors the view that the hormone controls specific protein synthesis at the translational rather than the transcriptional level. Moreover, in this tissue and many others, the adrenal hormones exert marked effects upon membrane structure and function. These effects are of such a general nature that they imply a significant change in membrane structure. The nature of this change remains to be elucidated as does the means by which it is regulated. It is possible that the hormones bring about these changes either by being incorporated into the membranes or by altering the specific lipid composition of them. In either case, the distinct possibility exists that the steroid hormone-receptor protein complex or complexes

act not only in the nucleus to control gene function but also in the cell cytosol to regulate mRNA translation (protein synthesis), specific enzyme function, or both. It also remains possible that membrane receptor sites exist for many of these hormones or their mediators.

A final aspect of steroid hormone action concerns so-called permissive action. This term has been applied to define the fact that, in many cases, a specific peptide or amine hormone does not exert its usual physiologic effects in the absence of a particular steroid hormone. Two of the most dramatic of these permissive actions are the role of cortisol in modifying the hepatic response to glucagon and the role of 1,25-dihydroxycholecalciferol in modifying the osseous response to PTH. In both instances, the peptide hormones activate the adenyl cyclase-calcium system, but no physiologic response is observed in the absence of the specific steroid hormone, i.e., the actions of each of the steroids upon the metabolic machinery of each cell type are necessary before the usual second messengers, arising as a consequence of peptide hormone-receptor interaction, can be translated into cellular response. It is assumed that in these instances the steroid hormones control the concentration of key enzymes (or other functional proteins) that are required for expression of C-AMP and calcium action, but the exact enzymes (proteins) have not yet been identified in any of these cases.

Time Course of Hormonal Responses

Just as noted in the case of insulin secretion, many physiologic responses, including those controlled by hormones, are biphasic in nature. In general, there is a sensitive and immediate response that is of limited capacity and a slower less sensitive response of greater magnitude. For example, in the case of blood glucose homeostasis, glycogen mobilization is representative of the first phase and gluconeogenesis of the second. These two phases often correspond, respectively, to the activation of already existing units and to the mobilization of new units of response. At the level of the cell, this means activation of rate-limiting enzymes in one or more metabolic sequences, followed by an increase in the concentration of one or more of these enzymes. The point to be reemphasized is the similarity, in the control or informational sense, of biologic organization at the cellular and supracellular levels. This similarity is based upon the fact that supracellular control systems are adaptations and extensions of the underlying cellular control systems.

Hormones and Energy Metabolism

The addition of hormones to cells or tissues often leads to changes in energy metabolism, e.g., changes in rate of pyridine nucleotide turnover, lactate production, or glucose or oxygen consumption. This is not surprising in view of the fact that hormones alter functions that require energy, such as transport, secretion, movement, and synthesis.

Energy metabolism is regulated by the mechanisms outlined above. For example, the control of energy metabolism in mammalian cells exhibits many of the properties of control systems discussed above: end-product inhibition, precursor activation, negative and positive feedback loops, multiple allosteric sites on key enzymes, isozymes, separate enzymes for the forward and reverse of key reactions in a reversible sequence, and induction and repression. These are illustrated in part in Figure 1–22. Note particularly the complexity of the actual relationships between the enzymes, metabolites, and end products in a small portion of the cell.

In the case of glycolysis, gluconeogenesis, and Krebs cycle-oxidative phosphorylation, the systems are regulated and coupled by the level of the end product, ATP, and its related nucleotides, ADP and AMP. These concentrations are governed by the equilibrium constant

$$(K = [ATP] [AMP]/[ADP]^2)$$

of the adenylate kinase reaction. The activity of this enzyme is usually sufficient to maintain

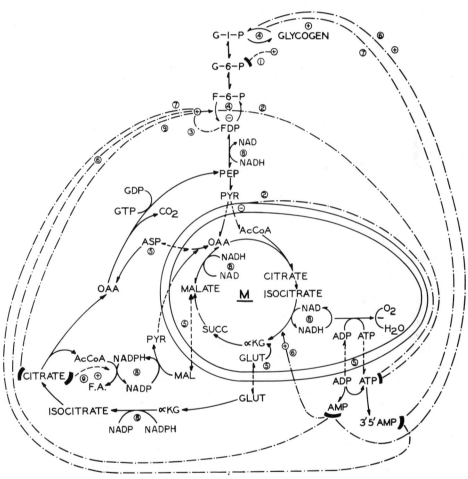

Figure 1–22. The control of energy metabolism in a mammalian cell. Solid arrows ($\rightarrow$) represent biochemical reactions; broken arrows ($- - \rightarrow$), transport steps; alternating arrows ($- \cdot \rightarrow$), allosteric control. $\oplus$ indicates an activation of the particular enzyme, and $\ominus$, inhibition. (indicates a control chemical. The scheme is incomplete, e.g., ADP and ATP participate in several of the steps in glycolysis, and no consideration is given to changes in enzyme concentration or pyridine nucleotide interactions. M represents a mitochondrion enclosed by a double membrane and containing the Krebs cycle enzymes. The following types of control are exhibited: (1) precursor activation of glycogen synthetase by glucose-6-phosphate, G-6-P; (2) end-product inhibition of pyruvate carboxylase and phosphofructokinase by ATP; (3) product activation of phosphofructokinase by fructose diphosphate, FDP; (4) use of two different enzymes (phosphofructokinase-fructose diphosphatase, glycogen synthetase and phosphorylase) to regulate reverse flow of metabolites; (5) compartmentation of adenine nucleotides and various Krebs-cycle intermediates; (6) allosteric control of several key steps by a single allosteric effect, i.e., activation by AMP of phosphorylase, phosphofructokinase, and isocitric dehydrogenase (not shown but equally important, AMP inhibits phosphoenolpyruvate carboxylase and fructose diphosphatase); (7) role of cyclic AMP in regulating both phosphorylase and phosphofructokinase; (8) regulation by pyridine nucleotide availability; (9) activation of one metabolic sequence by intermediate in another, citrate on fatty acid synthesis and on glycolysis; (10) compartmentation of metabolic functions with Krebs cycle activity exclusively within the mitochondria, and fatty acid synthesis in cytoplasm. Abbreviations: G-1-P, glucose-1-phosphate; G-6-P, glucose-6-phosphate; F-6-P, fructose-6-phosphate; FDP, fructose diphosphate; PEP, phosphoenolpyruvate; Pyr, pyruvate; AcCoA, acetyl CoA; αKG, α-ketoglutarate; SUCC, succinate; OAA, oxalacetate; ASP, aspartate; GLUT, glutamate; MAL, malate; AMP, ADP, and ATP, adenosine mono-, di-, and tri-phosphate; GDP and GTP, guanosine di- and tri-phosphate; 3′,5′-AMP, cyclic adenosine monophosphate; and NAD⁺, NADP⁺, NADH, and NADPH, the oxidized and reduced forms of nicotinamide–adenine dinucleotides.

the concentrations of the reactants near equilibrium. Thus a fall in ATP leads to a nearly equivalent rise in AMP. The concentration of the latter is usually 1/10 to 1/100 that of ATP; hence a small fall in ATP concentration leads to a relatively large rise in AMP level. A rise in AMP concentration leads to inhibition of fructose diphosphatase and an activation of phosphofructokinase, i.e., a shift from gluconeogenesis to glycolysis by coordinate control of two enzymes that regulate reverse reactions (Fig. 1–22). The complexity of the possible control is readily apparent when one considers that AMP, ADP, and ATP are not evenly distributed within the various cellular compartments and that their distribution can be altered significantly by alterations in the distribution of the cations, calcium and magnesium.

The other important fact to be derived from the knowledge of the control of energy metabolism is that the overall system exhibits the characteristics of a negative feedback loop in which, however, positive feedback loops have an important directive effect. Because of such arrangements, it is possible to observe oscillations in metabolic systems, particularly of the pulsed or synchronized type. Such systems have considerable relevance to the nature of biologic clocks, including the periodic changes in hormonal secretion rates.

In practical terms, one would expect that the hormonal effects upon energy metabolism result from the hormonal action leading to increased energy demands, i.e., an increased rate of glycolysis and oxidative metabolism. There are, however, certain instances in which it has been postulated that hormones "push" rather than "pull" metabolism by regulating a key early step, such as phosphorylase or glucose-6-dehydrogenase, and thereby drive synthetic reactions. None of these latter instances has been convincingly established.

HORMONES AND CLINICAL MEDICINE

As our knowledge of hormone structure and function has grown, it has become apparent that there are a wide variety of diseases in which either a primary or secondary dysfunction of one or more endocrine glands plays an important pathogenic role. The major endocrinopathies can be classified in a number of ways. The classification presented in Table 1–3 is a functional or etiologic one that defines the cause of the over-, under-, or malfunction of an endocrine organ.

Hormones are widely used in clinical medicine in one of three fashions: (1) as physiologic agents to correct a deficiency, underfunction, or malfunction of a particular endocrine organ or system; (2) as diagnostic aids to determine the adequacy of the function of one or more endocrine or metabolic systems; and (3) as pharmacologic agents that exert effects upon the body, which may be exaggerations of their physiologic actions or entirely new effects not observed when physiologic amounts are employed. The last use is the most common.

Because the use of hormones in this last sense is often complicated by the production of undesirable side effects, much effort is expended in the design and synthesis of hormone analogues that emphasize desirable characteristics and deemphasize undesirable side effects to a greater extent than the natural agent. Conversely, less but increasing attention has been devoted to the development of synthetic or modified natural agents that act as competitive inhibitors of the action of a hormone. Examples of each of these types and their uses will be described in other chapters.

TABLE 1–3.   ENDOCRINOPATHIES

A. Primary dysfunctions
  1. Overproduction
    a. Abnormal gland function
    b. Abnormal tropic stimulus
    c. Change in response to negative feedback signal; change in setpoint
    d. Inappropriate time course of tropic stimuli
  2. Increased target organ sensitivity: normal production but increase in peripheral tissue response
  3. Underproduction
    a. Abnormal gland function
      i. Lack of hydroxylase enzyme in steroid biosynthesis
      ii. Lack of conversion of prohormone to hormone in case of peptide hormone
      iii. Secretion of inactive product which retains immunologic cross-reactivity but not biologic activity
    b. Lack of normal tropic stimulus
    c. Lack of appropriate sequence (in time) of hormonal and neural stimuli
  4. Decreased target organ sensitivity: normal production but decrease in peripheral tissue response
    a. Lack of peripheral tissue receptor
    b. Decrease of peripheral tissue responsiveness due to altered intracellular feedback responses
B. Secondary dysfunctions
  1. Overproduction resulting from sustained normal physiologic stimulus
  2. Underproduction resulting from lack of normal physiologic stimulus

REFERENCES

1. Atkinson, D. E.: Biological feedback control at the molecular level. *Science* 150:851, 1965.
2. Bonner, D. M. (ed.), *Control Mechanisms in Cellular Processes.* New York, The Ronald Press, 1961.
3. Chance, B.: Control characteristics of enzyme systems. *Sympos. Quant. Biol.* 26:289, 1961.
4. Chance, B., Estabrook, R. W., et al. (eds.), *Control of Energy Metabolism.* New York, Academic Press, 1966.
5. Hershko, A., Mamont, P., et al.: Pleiotypic response. *Nature (New Biol.)* 232:206, 1971.
6. Horecker, B. L., and Stadtman, E.: *Current Topics in Cellular Regulation.* Vols. 1–5. New York, Academic Press, 1968-1972.
7. Jacob, F., and Monod, J.: Genetic regulatory mechanisms in the synthesis of proteins. *J. Molec. Biol.* 3:318, 1961.
8. Litwack, G. (ed.), *Biochemical Actions of Hormones.* Vols. I and II. New York, Academic Press, 1971-1972.
9. McCann, S. M., and Porter, J. C.: Hypothalamic pituitary stimulating and inhibiting hormones. *Physiol. Rev.* 49:240, 1969.
10. Monod, J., Changeux, J. P., et al.: Allosteric proteins and cellular control systems. *J. Molec. Biol.* 6:306, 1963.
11. Monod, J., Wyman, J., et al.: On the nature of allosteric transitions. A plausible model. *J. Molec. Biol.* 12:88, 1966.
12. Rasmussen, H., Goodman, D. B. P., et al.: The role of cyclic AMP and calcium in cell activation *CRC Crit. Rev. Biochem.* 1:95, 1972.
13. Robinson, G. A., Butcher, R. W., et al.: *Cyclic AMP.* New York, Academic Press, 1971.
14. Stadtman, E. R.: Enzyme multiplicity and function in the regulation of divergent metabolic pathways. *Bact. Rev.* 27:170, 1963.

CHAPTER 2

The Adenohypophysis

By William H. Daughaday

PITUITARY MORPHOLOGY

Anatomy. The pituitary gland is a complex structure lying in a bony walled cavity, the *sella turcica,* in the sphenoid bone at the base of the skull (Fig. 2–1). The sella turcica is separated superiorly from the cranial cavity by a tough reflection of the dura mater, the *diaphragma sella,* through which the pituitary stalk and its attendant blood vessels reach the main body of the gland. The pituitary is a small organ with normal dimensions of about 10 mm. by 13 mm. by 6 mm. and weighs about 0.5 gm. The anterior lobe consti-

tutes 75 per cent of the total weight of the gland. In women the gland increases in size during pregnancy and may approach 1 gm. in weight. The *pars intermedia,* which is present in the pituitary of most vertebrates, is virtually missing from the human pituitary. The terminology recommended by the International Commission on Anatomical Nomenclature is presented in Table 2–1.

The pituitary is formed early in embryonic life from the fusion of two ectodermal hollow processes of diverse origin. An evagination from the roof of the primitive oral region, Rathke's pouch, extends upward toward the base of the brain and is met by an outpouching of the floor of the third ventricle, destined to become the neurohypophysis. Rathke's pouch undergoes much more extensive proliferation to form the anterior lobe. A pair of lateral buds arises from Rathke's pouch and extends superiorly to invest the neural stalk with cells which later become the *pars tuberalis.* In man the pars tuberalis is a thin cloak of cells on the anterior surface of the stalk; in other species the pars tuberalis forms a complete collar about the neural stalk.

The lumen of Rathke's pouch is nearly obliterated by the proliferation of the anterior and posterior lobes of the hypophysis. It persists in adult human beings as small colloid-filled cysts and clefts at the juncture of the *pars distalis* and the neurohypophysis. The connection of Rathke's pouch with the oral cavity is separated by the developing sphenoid bone. Small remnants of tissue derived from Rathke's pouch, the so-called pharyngeal pituitary, may persist into adult life within or just below the sphenoid bone. These cells contain secretory granules and, at least, growth hormone and prolactin. It is speculated that the pharyngeal pituitary may be of secretory significance after removal of the main body of the pituitary gland.

Secretory granules appear in the fetal pituitary toward the end of the first trimester. At about the same time, several pituitary hormones can be detected by radioimmunoassay. The age at which hormonal secretion is initiated and maintained

31

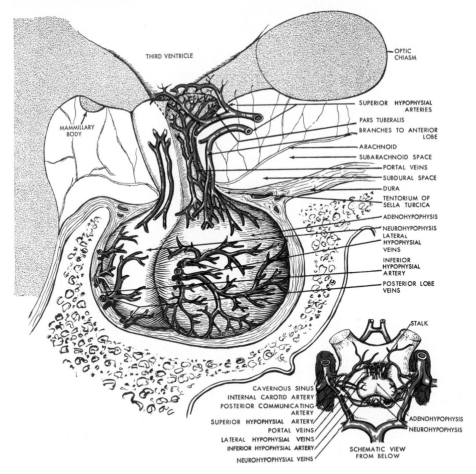

THIRD VENTRICLE

OPTIC CHIASM

MAMMILLARY BODY

SUPERIOR HYPOPHYSIAL ARTERIES
PARS TUBERALIS
BRANCHES TO ANTERIOR LOBE
ARACHNOID
SUBARACHNOID SPACE
PORTAL VEINS
SUBDURAL SPACE
DURA
TENTORIUM OF SELLA TURCICA
ADENOHYPOPHYSIS
NEUROHYPOPHYSIS
LATERAL HYPOPHYSIAL VEINS
INFERIOR HYPOPHYSIAL ARTERY
POSTERIOR LOBE VEINS

STALK

CAVERNOUS SINUS
INTERNAL CAROTID ARTERY
POSTERIOR COMMUNICATING ARTERY
SUPERIOR HYPOPHYSIAL ARTERY
PORTAL VEINS
LATERAL HYPOPHYSIAL VEINS
INFERIOR HYPOPHYSIAL ARTERY
NEUROHYPOPHYSIAL VEINS

ADENOHYPOPHYSIS
NEUROHYPOPHYSIS

SCHEMATIC VIEW FROM BELOW

Figure 2–1. Relationships of pituitary and its blood supply to neighboring structures. (Modified from drawing by Frank Netter. ©Ciba Pharmaceutical Products.)

under feedback control has not been definitely established in man. In the case of corticotropin, this control may be established by the twelfth week. Evidence for this belief has been derived from an analysis of the genital lesions which occur in severe cases of the adrenogenital syndrome. The malformations of the labia and vagina result from excess corticotropin stimulation of defective fetal adrenal and excess androgenic steroid secretion at about the twelfth week of gestation.

The pituitary receives its blood supply from two sources (Fig. 2–1). Arterial blood reaches it from branches of the superior hypophysial artery, a branch of the internal carotid artery. Venous blood enters the pituitary by a physiologically important portal system which originates in specialized vascular structures of the median eminence, the gomitoli, which comprise short straight terminal arterioles with muscular walls surrounded by a dense capillary network. Blood from these capillaries is collected into a series of parallel veins which course down the anterior surface of the pituitary stalk to drain into the sinusoidal capillaries of the anterior lobe. Direct observation in the living animal has confirmed that the direction of blood flow in the portal veins is from the median eminence to the pituitary. These vessels transport neurohumors from the hypothalamus to the adenohypophysis (see Chapter 12).

The detailed vascular organization within the pituitary gland has been clearly recognized only with the help of the electron microscope. The pituitary sinuses are found to be completely lined with endothelium. Between the basement membrane of the sinusoidal endothelium and the parenchymal cells there exists a perisinusoidal space. Scattered cells with cytoplasmic projections, as well as extracellular granules believed to be extruded secretory granules from the pituitary parenchymal cells, are found in the perisinusoidal spaces.

The blood supply to the posterior lobe arises from the inferior hypophysial arteries and is therefore largely separate from the blood supply to the anterior lobe. Venous blood from both pituitary lobes drains into the cavernous sinus by a number of veins.

The nerve supply of the anterior lobe is largely limited to fine nerves derived from the carotid plexus which accompany the arteriolar branches. These nerves appear to have a vasomotor function. A few neural fibers traversing from the posterior lobe to the anterior lobe have been described, but their significance in regulating adenohypophysial function is denied by most authorities.

TABLE 2-1.   DIVISIONS OF PITUITARY GLAND*

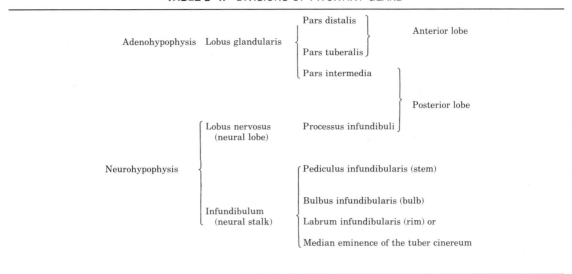

		Pars distalis	Anterior lobe
Adenohypophysis	Lobus glandularis	Pars tuberalis	
		Pars intermedia	Posterior lobe
Neurohypophysis	Lobus nervosus (neural lobe)	Processus infundibuli	
	Infundibulum (neural stalk)	Pediculus infundibularis (stem)	
		Bulbus infundibularis (bulb)	
		Labrum infundibularis (rim) or	
		Median eminence of the tuber cinereum	

*Terminology recommended by the International Commission on Anatomical Nomenclature.

Pituitary Cell Types

The human pituitary is a confederation of several largely independent functional units, each composed of a specific cell type synthesizing and releasing one of the pituitary hormones. The time-honored classification of pituitary cells into acidophil, basophil, and chromophobe types is clearly inadequate to explain the independent secretion of six known hormones and the possible secretion of other hormonal peptides whose physiologic significance remains to be established. In its place there has arisen a jungle of competing classifications based on different histochemical status. The different cell types have been identified by Greek letters or descriptive terms. None of these systems has applicability to all species so that universality cannot be claimed.

Despite the complexities of the cytologic problem, progress has been made by the application of histochemical, immunofluorescent, and electron microscopic techniques. The results of studies of a number of investigators have strengthened the concept that each major hormone is secreted by a distinct cell type. It is logical to classify the pituitary cells on the basis of the hormone secreted.

Somatotropic Cells. The association of acidophilic tumors of the pituitary with acromegaly and gigantism has clearly linked these cells in the normal pituitary with growth hormone secretion. Further confirmation of this conclusion has been obtained by immunofluorescent studies with human pituitary tissue. The human somatotropic cells are easily recognized by numerous large, nearly round, membrane-bound secretory granules measuring 300 to 400 mμ in diameter (Fig. 2-2). These cells

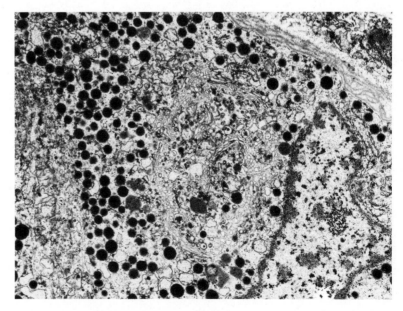

Figure 2-2. Human somatotrope. This cell is characterized by the large, membrane-bound secretory granules. Most granules are uniform in size, shape, and electron density. A large, active Golgi region is characteristic of this cell type. The rough endoplasmic reticulum is often prominent, although it may not be demonstrated because of the plane of section. Note the presence of granule discharge across the plasma membrane (× 14,400). (Courtesy of Dr. D. W. McKeel.)

are predominantly located in the lateral wings of the adenohypophysis.

The process of secretion involves fusion of the granule membranes with the plasma membrane of the cell to a secretory pore and subsequent extrusion of the secretory granule.

Lactotropic Cells. Lactotropic cells, which contain eosinophilic granules, can be distinguished from somatotropic cells by their affinity for erythrosin or carmosin stains. In the lateral "acidophilic wings" of the human pituitary are a limited number of these cells which react with immunofluorescent staining with antisera against ovine prolactin. The lactotropic cells contain large electron-dense granules similar to somatotropic granules but more varied in size and shape (Fig. 2–3).

The relative number of lactotropic cells is increased in fetal pituitaries and during pregnancy. This proliferation of lactotropic cells is the result of the very high concentration of circulating estrogens in human pregnancy.

Thyrotropic Cells. Positive identification of the human thyrotropic cells has been achieved by immunofluorescent staining. Thyrotropic cells, located predominantly in the central "mucoid" wedge of the adenohypophysis, are large and polyhedral. By electron microscopy the granules are small, 50 to 100 mμ in diameter, and of inconstant electron density (Figs. 2–4 and 2–5).

In the thyroprivic state, striking changes occur in pituitary thyrotropic cells. The endoplasmic reticulum becomes greatly enlarged, forming cisternae which occupy most of the cytoplasm. Similar

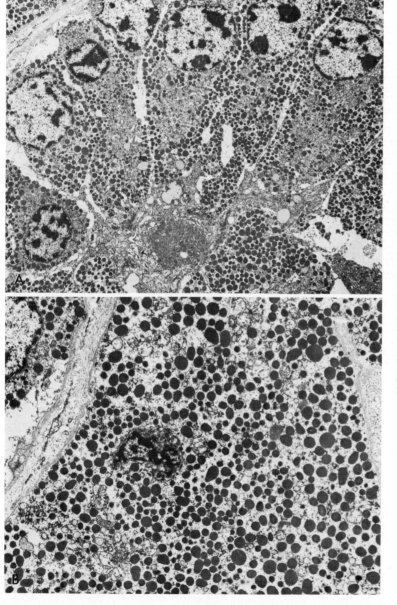

Figure 2–3. *A,* Human lactotrope, autopsy specimen. Electron micrograph of carmosin-positive cells in lateral "acidophil wings" of adenohypophysis of a 17-year-old girl in the third trimester of pregnancy.

On the average, the granules are slightly larger and less regular than human somatotrope granules. The elongated shape of the cells is characteristic, as is the peripheral location of granules in some of the cells. Separation between cells is artifactual due to autolysis. The cells are forming a pseudoacinus around degenerating cells at center, left ($\times$5,040). *B,* Higher magnification to show granule details ($\times$ 10,080). (Courtesy of Dr. D. W. McKeel.)

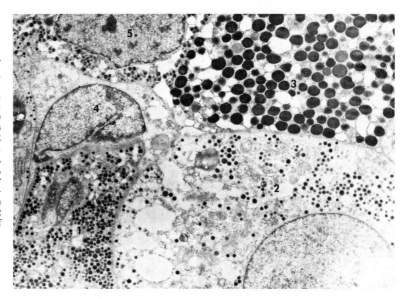

Figure 2–4. Electron micrograph of human adenohypophysis. Cells 1, 2, and 5 are probably thyrotropic cells. Note small granules of varied electron density. Cell 2 is relatively less granulated and may represent a reactive cell depleted by secretion. Cell 3 is probably an ACTH basophil (beta 2-R cell of Phifer, Spicer, and Orth). Variable size and density of granules, vesiculated endoplasmic reticulum, and intracytoplasmic and perinuclear microfilaments (not shown) are characteristic. Cell 4 is a stellate cell with long processes interspersed among other cells (× 11,200). (Courtesy of Dr. D. W. McKeel.)

but less marked hypertrophy of the Golgi apparatus occurs. In addition, secretory granules virtually disappear from the cell, indicating that storage of hormone does not keep pace with secretion. The hypertrophied thyrotropic cells are easily recognized and are called "thyroidectomy cells."

Gonadotropic Cells. The human LH gonadotropic cell is most clearly recognized by immunofluorescent methods employing specific cross-reactive plasma raised against chorionic gonadotropin. These cells are sparsely granulated, usually angular in shape, and distributed singly throughout the pituitary (Fig. 2–5). By staining techniques, they belong to the basophilic subgroup.

The FSH gonadotropic cell is less definitely characterized as separate from the LH gonadotropic cell because of the difficulty of preparing antisera specific for FSH. However, this cell is also believed to be a member of the basophilic subgroup of pituitary cells.

Corticotropic and Melanotropic Cells. Identification of the cells of the human pituitary which secrete corticotropin has been achieved by immunostaining with an antiserum which does not share immunologic determinants with α or β MSH and which, therefore, is specific for corticotropin. Immunoreactive cells are most common in the medial mucoid wedge of the pituitary and relatively infrequent in the lateral, somatotropin-rich areas of the pituitary. Corticotropic cells are also present in the neurohypophysis where it is in apposition to the adenohypophysis. These cells in the neurohypophysis may be the human counterpart to the pars intermedia. Corticotropic cells are also incon-

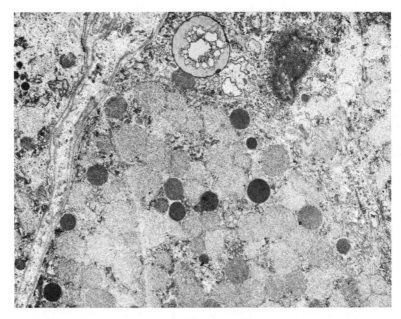

Figure 2–5. Electron micrograph of human pituitary. The cell on the left is one type of gonadotrope. The presence of large granules with variable density is characteristic; the smaller granules are denser. This is the less common type of PAS-positive mucoid cell found in the most anterior portion of the adenohypophysis (× 14,400). (Courtesy of Dr. D. W. McKeel.)

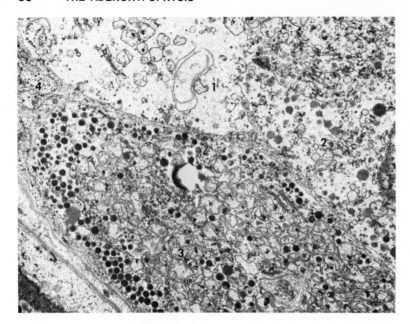

Figure 2–6. Electron micrograph of human adenohypophysis showing a chromophobe cell (1) and two types of cells (2 and 3) with intermediate-size granules. Cell 3 is packed with mitochondria. Cell 4 is a follicular or stellate cell with long processes enveloping cell 3 (× 14,400). (Courtesy of Dr. D. W. McKeel.)

stantly present in the pars tuberalis. The tinctorial characteristics of the corticotropic cells correspond to previously described β or R cells; the latter are subgroups of the basophilic cells of more primitive classification. In electron microscopic sections, corticotropic cells contain granules of varying size and density (Fig. 2–4).

The hyaline deposits which develop in corticotropic cells (Crooke's cells) in the presence of elevated plasma corticosteroid levels of any cause represent microtubular deposits and are not immunologically cross-reactive with ACTH antibodies.

Antisera raised against melanocyte stimulating hormone (MSH) appear to react with the corticotropic cells of the adeno- and neurohypophysis. While MSH and ACTH are probably secreted by the same cell, this assumption cannot be considered established. Secretion by a single cell would explain why the secretions of these two hormones change in parallel fashion in a number of disorders of the adrenal.

Nonsecretory Cells.   About one quarter of the pituitary cells contain no characteristic secretory granules (Fig. 2–6). These cells, which are classified as chromophobe cells in the older classification, may participate in pituitary function. Some chromophobe cells represent undifferentiated precursors of the secretory cells, and others are cells which have been temporarily depleted of stored secretion or reserve cells which are in a temporary resting state. Cytologists have recognized small granules with variable staining characteristics in most chromophobe cells and have designated these amphophil cells. The secretory potential of this group of cells has been established in certain corticotropin and prolactin secreting tumors of man.

Another cell of the human adenohypophysis is the follicular or stellate cell (Figs. 2–4 and 2–6). These cells have long cell processes adjacent to perivascular spaces and other processes in contact with those from other stellate cells to form primitive pituitary follicles. In certain areas microvilli and cilia may be present. There are few, if any, secretory granules seen by electron microscopy, and the function of stellate cells is still uncertain.

The frequency of the various pituitary cell types in the adenohypophyses of healthy human beings is unknown because there has been no recent systematic study in glands from individuals who have met sudden accidental death. Sommers examined the pituitaries of 273 adults and 28 children who died of varied causes. The results of differential cell counts are listed in Table 2–2.

TABLE 2–2.   PERCENTAGE OF DIFFERENT PITUITARY CELL TYPES IN MAN

Cell Type	Infants and Children (28)*	Adults (372)*	
		Men	Women
Acidophils	25.0 ± 6.7	34.8 ± 8.2	36.8 ± 6.3
Basophils	15.2 ± 7.1	21.7 ± 6.8	20.4 ± 7.3
Amphophils	22.6 ± 5.4	19.7 ± 6.5	17.8 ± 7.1
Chromophobes	35.9 ± 4.9	22.8 ± 3.9	23.6 ± 4.9
Hypertrophic amphophils	1.2 ± 0.6	1.4 ± 0.8	1.4 ± 1.0
Hyaline basophils	0.01 ± 0.003	0.06 ± 0.3	0.11 ± 0.3

*After Sommers. Per cent ± Standard Deviation.

THE PITUITARY HORMONES

The human adenohypophysis contains six hormones of established functional significance. These peptide and protein hormones as well as related hormones of the placenta can be assigned to three distinct families on the basis of molecular structure and biochemical evolution. Table 2–3 lists the members of the corticotropin, glycotropin, and somatotropin families and summarizes their basic chemical structures.

CHEMISTRY OF CORTICOTROPIN-RELATED PEPTIDE HORMONES

In all species thus far examined, corticotropin is a single peptide chain of 39 amino acids (Fig. 2–7). Species variations in sequence have been limited to the region of the chain from the twenty-fifth to the thirty-second residue.

The pituitaries of nearly all species contain two melanocyte stimulating peptides. The simplest is α MSH which contains 13 amino acids. The sequence of amino acids in α MSH when isolated from pig, cow, horse, and monkey pituitaries is identical. There is immunologic evidence of a similar peptide in the human pituitary. A second peptide, β MSH, exhibits species variations in size and amino acid sequence. In man this peptide contains 22 amino acids whose sequence is shown in Figure 2–7. The figure emphasizes the structural relationships between ACTH and the two MSH peptides. Noteworthy is the fact that the first 13 amino acids of ACTH are contained in the sequence of α MSH. Other studies have made it clear that the minimal unit responsible for MSH activity resides in amino acids 4 to 10 of ACTH and α MSH. This heptapeptide is also present in positions 11 to 17 of β MSH. Synthetic heptapeptide has definite, although weak, melanocyte stimulating activity.

Studies have also been carried out with fragments of the ACTH molecule which permit meaningful correlations between structure and function. The minimum requirement for biologic action resides in the first 13 amino acids beginning with the N-terminal amino acid. The addition of amino acid residues 14 through 20 progressively increases biologic activity up to that of the native hormone. Synthetic ACTH peptide containing the first 24 amino acids is available for clinical use. The ACTH peptide 1-26 is fully active in stimulating corticosteroid secretion but does not react with most antibodies developed in rabbits against porcine ACTH. The most potent immunologic determinants reside in the carboxyl tail of the peptide chain representing amino acids 22 to 39.

Pituitary extracts from many species have fat mobilizing actions, and two lipotropic peptides have been isolated from sheep adenohypophyses. Beta lipotropin is a polypeptide of 90 amino acids

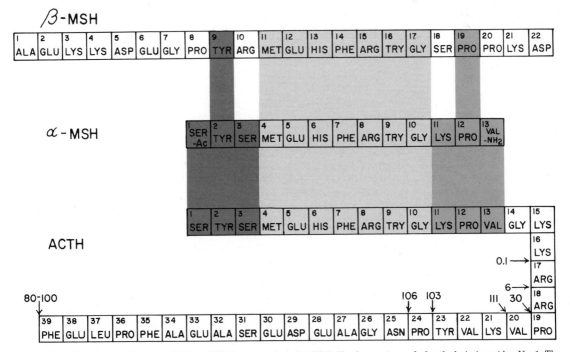

Figure 2–7. Structures of human β MSH, α MSH (presumed), and ACTH. The free amino end of each chain is residue No. 1. The figures are shaded to emphasize similar sequences of amino acids. The figures with arrows on the ACTH molecule indicate the biologic activity, according to Hofman, of the peptide beginning at the N terminal amino acid to the point indicated. The biologic activities are for porcine corticotropin and may be presumed identical to human corticotropin.

TABLE 2–3. COMPARISON OF COMPOSITION OF ADENOHYPOPHYSIAL HORMONES

Group	Hormones*	Amino Acids		Carbohydrate	Molecular Weight
I. *Corticotropin-Related Peptide Hormones*	1. α MSH (H)	13		0	1,823
	2. β MSH (H)	22		0	2,734
	3. Corticotropin (H)	39		0	4,507
Single peptide chain of 13 to 90 amino acids	4. α Lipotropin (O)	58		0	5,810
	5. β Lipotropin (O)	90		0	9,500
II. *Glycoprotein Hormones*	1. FSH (O)	236		18.2% 3.4% sialic acid	32,000
Two amino acid chains; sequence in α chain is similar or identical; more variability in β chain. All have carbohydrate substituents.	2. LH (O)	α 96	β 119	15.7% 0 sialic acid	30,000
	3. Chorionic gonadotropin (H)	α 92	β 139	31% 9% sialic acid	46,000
	4. Thyrotropin (B)	α 96	β 113	16.2% 0 sialic acid	26,600
	5. (Chorionic thyrotropin)	?		?	?
III. *Somatomammotropins*	1. Prolactin (O)	198		0	22,500
	2. Somatotropin (H)	191		0	21,700
One single peptide chain; two or three intramolecular S-S bonds.	3. (Chorionic somatomammotropin) (H)	19		0	21,600

*The letter in parentheses after the name of the hormone indicates source: H = human; O = ovine; B = bovine.

with a molecular weight of 9,500. Gamma lipotropin contains only 58 amino acids and has a molecular weight of 5,810. The first 58 amino acids from the amino end of the two molecules are identical. It is also significant that the sequence of amino acids 41 to 58 of the lipotropins is identical to that of β MSH. In addition to lipotropic activity, these peptides possess melanotropic and weak corticotropic actions. While the structural properties and biologic actions of these peptides are of great interest, their status as true endocrine secretions remains to be established. It is hoped that radioimmunoassays will soon answer the question of whether these peptides are present in plasma.

Corticotropin

Adrenal Actions. Corticotropin binds with specific receptors on the surface of the adrenal cortical cell. The affinity of binding of these receptors for ACTH is high (association constant about 10^{12}), which permits concentration of ACTH from plasma. When ACTH is bound to receptors in the presence of calcium, adenyl cyclase is activated which, in turn, increases the concentration of cyclic AMP in the adrenal cell. The net result of increased intracellular cyclic AMP is the phosphorylation of key enzymes and histones which lead to the biologic actions of the hormone. Increased steroidogenesis results from stimulation of the conversion of cholesterol to pregnenolone. The remaining enzymatic steps involved in formation of the 3-keto Δ 4-5 configuration in ring A and hydroxylations at 11 β, 21-OH, and 17 α-OH positions are not rate-limiting in the synthesis of cortisol. Cyclic AMP also stimulates RNA synthesis and synthesis of new adrenal proteins. This increases the synthetic machinery of the adrenal cell and increases adrenal weight.

The marked depletion of adrenal ascorbic acid following ACTH administration remains largely unexplained despite the fact that it provided the first practical end point for bioassay for corticotropin. Ascorbic acid is not required for steroidogenesis, and the vitamin may actually inhibit steroidogenesis. Loss of ascorbic acid from the adrenal may facilitate hormonal synthesis.

Extra-Adrenal Actions. Corticotropin has a number of actions on extra-adrenal tissues. It promotes lipolysis in fat cells and stimulates amino acid and glucose uptake in muscle. Large doses of corticotropin in adrenalectomized animals inhibit reduction of the Δ 4-5 double bond of cortisol in the liver and thereby prolong the plasma half-life of the hormone. In addition, corticotropin stimulates the pancreatic beta cell to secrete insulin and the somatotropic cells of the pituitary to secrete growth hormone.

While these varied extra-adrenal actions of corticotropin attest to the versatility of the corticotropin molecule, they are not evident at the plasma levels achieved during endogenous corticotropin release. Some of the effects can only be observed with isolated tissues *in vitro*. It is possible that the extreme hypersecretion of corticotropin which occurs in certain pituitary tumors (see Nelson's syndrome) could be having extra-adrenal effects in addition to contributing to hyperpigmentation.

Pituitary Storage. The amount of corticotropin stored in the adenohypophysis is small; the entire human gland contains only about 50 units, or 0.25 mg., of the active peptide. Probably the daily secretion only amounts to 1 to 5 units, but much larger amounts are secreted in conditions of stress.

Measurement. In the past, plasma corticotropin levels in man were measured by technically demanding bioassays in hypophysectomized rats. A particularly sensitive method was developed by Lipscomb and Nelson in which the ACTH-containing material was injected intravenously into hypophysectomized rats, and the corticosterone released into the left adrenal vein was measured.

Obviously the number of assays which can be performed in this way is limited.

The development of radioimmunoassays for corticotropin proved more difficult than the development of assays for other pituitary hormones because of the limited antigenicity of the hormone and the low concentrations of the hormone normally in plasma. Satisfactory assays have been reported by Berson and Yalow (7) and several other groups. An assay for ACTH has been described based on the competitive binding of labeled and unlabeled ACTH for the binding protein receptor action in cell membranes isolated from normal or tumorous adrenal cells. This assay has a high degree of correlation with the biologically active species of ACTH; it also has great sensitivity. Unfortunately, the difficulty involved in preparing stable membranes capable of specific binding of ACTH is so great that this assay approach has had only limited application.

Plasma Concentration.   As shown in Figure 2–8, the plasma corticotropin concentration of healthy adult subjects is usually less than 50 pg. per ml. Many hospitalized patients with the stress of nonendocrine illness have plasma ACTH levels up to 600 pg. per ml. Normally there is a diurnal pattern of plasma ACTH with the lowest levels reached between 6 P.M. and 11 P.M. Plasma levels begin to rise in the early morning hours and reach a peak between 6 A.M. and 8 A.M. The rise in plasma ACTH is closely followed by a rise in plasma cortisol.

In primary hypoadrenocorticism, plasma ACTH is often elevated to concentrations greater than 1,000 pg. per ml. Similar concentrations are encountered in plasma from patients with extrapituitary cancers producing ACTH and in patients with Cushing's disease after adrenalectomy.

Metabolism and Secretory Rate.   Corticotropin leaves the plama rapidly; the biologic half-life is approximately 25 minutes. The adrenal cortex has an unusual affinity for corticotropin, but it is unlikely that the adrenal is responsible for removing more than a relatively small fraction of corticotropin from the plasma. Based on a distribution equivalent to extracellular space, on the plasma concentration, and on a half-life of 25 minutes, the daily secretory rate is about 1 to 5 units per day (about 5 to 25 μg. of human ACTH).

Regulation.   The secretion of ACTH by the exterior pituitary is under dual control. The first type of control is "long loop" feedback inhibition of ACTH secretion by circulating cortisol. After adrenalectomy, cortisol levels fall, and ACTH secretion rises; the converse holds true after the administration of cortisol. The site of feedback control has received much study, but the results are inconclusive. Present evidence indicates that cortisol acts primarily on the pituitary corticotropic cells, but an additional site of feedback in the hypothalamus may well exist. The feedback control of the ACTH secretion process is similar to that of TSH secretion.

The second major level of ACTH regulation is ex-

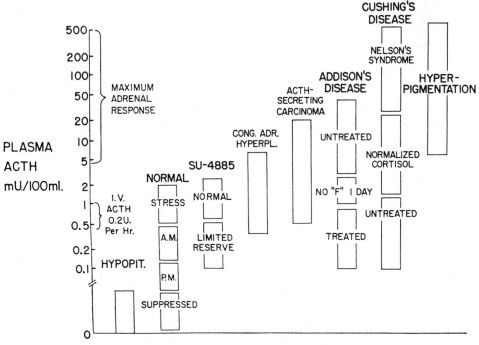

Figure 2–8.   A diagram illustrating the concentration of plasma ACTH in normal human beings and in a number of endocrine conditions. Nelson's syndrome refers to patients with pituitary tumors after adrenalectomy. Results on postoperative patients without hyperpigmentation or tumor who were receiving replacement cortisol are labeled "normalized cortisol." (Reproduced from Liddle, G. W., Island, D., et al.: *Recent Progr. Hormone Res. 18*:125, 1962, by permission of Academic Press Inc.)

erted by the hypothalamus through the secretion of corticotropin releasing hormone (CRF). This mechanism is involved in a number of neurogenic stimuli for ACTH release (e.g., circadian rhythm, response to pain, anxiety, pyrogen, hypoglycemia, vasopressin).

The possibility of a "short loop" feedback of ACTH inhibition on its own secretion in certain restricted experimental conditions has been entertained, but there is no evidence that this effect is significant in man.

Melanocyte Stimulating Hormones

Action.   The melanocyte stimulating hormones (MSH) disperse pigment granules of melanocytes in certain fish and amphibians. This action permits animals to blend inconspicuously with their environments. In these species, MSH is localized predominantly in the pars intermedia, and the release of MSH is under neurohumoral control. In human beings, MSH has no rapid effects on melanin pigment granule dispersal but increases pigmentation by promoting melanin synthesis. The existence of nonpigmentary effects of MSH in man remains to be established.

The human melanocyte stimulating hormone is released by the corticotropic cells found both in the adenohypophysis and, to some extent, within the neurohypophysis.

Pituitary Storage.   Human pituitaries contain about 300 to 400 μg. of MSH activity per gram of wet pituitary. Nearly all the material in the pituitary is β MSH with less than 3 per cent α MSH.

Measurement.   There exist sensitive bioassays for MSH based on the ability of pituitary plasma and urine extracts to cause dispersal of melanin granules in isolated frog skin. Radioimmunoassays exist for the separate measurement of α and β MSH.

Plasma Concentration.   Alpha MSH has not been detected in normal plasma. Beta MSH is present in extracts of normal plasma in a concentration of about 0.1 ng. per ml. Only a few samples have been assayed, and there is no information on the effects of age, sex, and race on MSH activity.

Greatly increased amounts of MSH are present in plasma under pathologic conditions. Patients with untreated Addison's disease have from 0.5 to 1.1 ng. per ml. of β MSH. In Cushing's syndrome, the MSH concentration can rise as high as 6 ng. per ml.

Equally high levels of MSH have been detected by the radioimmunoassay of β MSH in plasma of patients with ectopic tumors producing ACTH. This MSH secreted by tumors has a smaller molecular size than pituitary β MSH.

Metabolism and Secretion.   There is little information concerning the metabolism of β MSH in man. One can presume that the half-life would be 10 minutes. Estimates of total daily secretion in man are not available.

Regulation.   The regulation of MSH secretion has been extensively studied in lower animals. The predominant hypothalamic control is exerted by a MSH inhibiting factor. The existence of a MSH releasing factor is postulated by some. In man, MSH shares the same feedback inhibition by cortisol as does ACTH, so the secretion of the two hormones is usually closely interlocked.

CHEMISTRY OF THE GLYCOPROTEIN HORMONES (FSH, LH, TSH, HCG)

The glycoprotein hormones of the pituitary and placenta comprise a closely related family of hormones derived by biochemical evolution from a common primitive molecule. Included in this group of hormones are the thyrotropic hormone of the pituitary, the follicle stimulating and luteinizing gonadotropins of the pituitary, and the chorionic gonadotropic hormone (HCG) of the placenta. All these hormone molecules are made up of two peptide chains with carbohydrate substituent groups attached to each peptide chain which account for 15 to 31 per cent of the molecular weight. The sugars include fucose, mannose, galactose, glucosamine, and galactosamine. Sialic acid is inconstantly present. Even with homology of amino acid sequence, major differences in carbohydrate composition exist. Also, there is microheterogeneity of the carbohydrate components of a single hormone, which suggests that the addition of these components to the peptide chain is not under rigorous metabolic control.

Each of these hormones contains two peptide chains designated α and β. The amino acid sequences of the α chain appear to be identical or very similar for all these hormones (Fig. 2–9). The isolated α chains lack biologic activity. Hormonal specificity in the complete molecule is conferred by the β chains, which have greater differences in amino acid sequences between the various hormones. Even the chains of bovine TSH and LH have as many as 50 per cent of the amino acids identical or the result of simple base changes in DNA.

Proof that the hormonal specificity resides within the β chain has come from recombination experiments of the separate α and β chains. The separate β chain may have slight intrinsic biologic activity, but total activity is regained after the chains are recombined. Hybrids formed from the α chain of TSH and the β chain of LH possess luteinizing hormone activity. The converse recombination hybrid of α LH and β TSH results in a molecule with thyrotropic activity.

This new knowledge of the structure of the glycoprotein hormones explains the immunologic crossreactivity of these hormones. The role of the α chain, which is not involved in hormone specificity, is still unexplained. The fact that its peptide structure is retained in such diverse hormones as bovine TSH, ovine LH, and human chorionic gonadotropin indicates that few amino acid substitutions can be tolerated.

ALIGNMENT OF THE CHAINS OF THE TSH AND LH TO SHOW MAXIMUM HOMOLOGY

α (TSH and LH) NH₂-Phe-Pro-Asp-Gly-Glu-Phe-Thr-Met-⁸

TSH-β NH₂-Phe-Cys-Ile-Pro-Thr-Glu-Tyr-Met-Met-His-Val-Glu-Arg-¹³
LH-β Acyl-Ser-Arg-Gly-Pro-Leu-Arg-Pro-Leu-Cys-Gln-Pro-Ile-Asn-Ala-Thr-Leu-Ala-Ala-Glu-Lys-²⁰ (CHO)

α Gln-Gly-Cys-Pro-Glx-Cys-Lys-Leu-Lys-Glu-Asn-Lys-Tyr-Phe-Ser-Lys-Pro-Asx-Ala-Pro-²⁸

TSH-β Lys-Glu-Cys-Ala-Tyr-Cys- Leu-Thr-Ile-Asn-²³ (CHO)
LH-β Glu-Ala-Cys-Pro-Val-Cys- Ile-Thr-Phe-Thr-³⁰

α Ile-Tyr-Gln-Cys-Met-Gly-Cys-Cys-Phe-Ser-Arg-Ala-Tyr-Pro-Thr-Pro-Ala-Arg-Ser-Lys-⁴⁸

TSH-β Thr-Thr-Val-Cys-Ala-Gly-Tyr-Cys-Met-Thr-Arg-Asx-Val-Asx-Gly-Lys-Leu-Phe-Leu-Pro-⁴³
LH-β Thr-Ser-Ile-Cys-Ala-Gly-Tyr-Cys-Pro-Ser-Met-Lys-Arg-Val-Leu-Pro-Val-Ile-Leu-Pro-⁵⁰

α Lys-Thr-Met-Leu- Val-Pro-Lys-Asn-Ile-Thr-Ser-Glx-Ala-Thr-Cys-Cys-Val-Ala-Lys-⁶⁷ (CHOsα)

TSH-β Lys-Tyr-Ala-Leu-Ser-Gln-Asp-Val-Cys-Thr-Tyr-Arg-Asp-Phe-Met-Tyr-Lys-Thr-Ala-Glu-⁶³
LH-β Pro- Met-Pro- Gln-Arg-Val-Cys-Thr-Tyr-His-Glu-Leu-Arg-Phe-Ala-Ser-Val-Arg-⁶⁸

α Ala-The-Thr- Lys-Ala-Thr-Val-Met-Gly-Asn-Val-Arg-Val-Glx-Asn-His-Thr-Glx-Cys-⁸⁶ (CHOsβ)

TSH-β Ile-Pro-Gly-Cys-Pro-Arg-His-Val-Thr-Pro-Tyr-Phe-Ser-Tyr-Pro-Val-Ala-Ile-Ser-Cys-⁸³
LH-β Leu-Pro-Gly-Cys-Pro-Pro-Gly-Val-Asp-Pro-Met-Val-Ser-Phe-Pro-Val-Ala-Leu-Ser-Cys-⁸⁸

α His-Cys-Ser-Thr-Cys-Tyr-Tyr-His-Lys-Ser-COOH⁹⁶

TSH-β Lys-Cys-Gly-Lys-Cys-Asx-Thr-Asx-Tyr-Ser-Asx-Cys-Ile-His-Glu-Ala-Ile-Lys-Thr-Asn-¹⁰³
LH-β His-Cys-Gly-Pro-Cys-Arg-Leu-Ser-Ser-Thr-Asp-Cys-Gly-Pro-Gly-Arg-Thr-Glx-Pro-Leu-¹⁰⁸

TSH-β Tyr-Cys-Thr-Lys-Pro-Gln-Lys-Ser-Tyr-Met-COOH¹¹³
LH-β Ala-Cys-Asx-His-Pro-Pro-Leu-Pro-Asp-Ile-Leu-COOH¹¹⁹

Figure 2–9. The amino acid sequences of the α chain common to both bovine TSH and LH, and the separate β chains of TSH and LH. Chains are aligned to show homologies of structure. Amino acids which are identical are underlined with a solid line; closely related substitutions are underlined with a broken line. The positions of the carbohydrate side chains are indicated. (From data supplied by Dr. John G. Pierce and Dr. Darrell N. Ward.)

Gonadotropic Hormones (FSH and LH)

Actions. The pituitary gland contains two hormones whose primary action is on the gonads. The follicle stimulating hormone (FSH) stimulates follicular development in the ovary and gametogenesis in the testes. The luteinizing hormone (LH), sometimes called the *interstitial cell stimulating hormone* (ICSH), acts primarily in promoting luteinization of the ovary and Leydig cell function of the testes.

The urine of menopausal women contains substantial amounts of gonadotropic substances of pituitary origin. A relatively purified preparation has been isolated from urine and partially characterized; this urinary gonadotropin qualitatively resembles FSH but has less than 1/25 the biologic potency of the pituitary hormone. Moreover, the dose response curve in bioassays has a different slope. These findings indicate that a change in the structure of the molecule occurs in FSH either during its stay in the circulation or during its passage through the kidney.

The effects of gonadotropins are clearly recognized following administration to hypopituitary women. Follicle stimulating hormone, either isolated from human pituitaries or extracted from the urine of postmenopausal women, stimulates the development of one or more primordial follicles. After a period of 10 to 14 days of treatment with FSH, ovulation can be achieved by the addition of luteinizing hormone or chorionic gonadotropin. Under physiologic conditions, LH contributes to follicular development by synergizing with FSH. During the period of follicular development and growth, thecal cells are active in the secretion of estrogens. A surging secretion of LH and FSH at mid-cycle leads to ovulation. The function of the corpus luteum is maintained by LH. If pregnancy occurs, chorionic gonadotropin produced by trophoblastic cells maintains the corpus luteum of pregnancy. (This subject is discussed in detail in Chapter 7.)

The gonadotropic hormones can restore spermatogenesis and testosterone secretion in hypopituitary men. FSH is primarily concerned with the restoration of spermatogenesis and must be administered for 70 to 80 days, a time span much longer than that required for the development of the mature ovarian follicle in hypogonadotropic women.

Cellular Actions. The effects of LH and FSH on isolated ovaries, corpora lutea, and cultures of granulosa cells have been extensively studied.

In corpora lutea, LH (and HCG) promote steroidogenesis by stimulating the conversion of cholesterol to pregnenolone. Initially LH reacts with specific receptors on the cell surfaces of responsive cells. By mechanisms which remain to be defined, adenyl cyclase, also present in the plasma membrane, is activated, resulting in the accumulation of intracellular cyclic AMP. In turn, cyclic AMP directly or indirectly affects many intracellular processes, including activation of phosphorylase, ornithine decarboxylase, and the synthesis in other key proteins. The effects of LH on ovarian tissue can be reproduced by the addition of cyclic AMP or dibutyryl cyclic AMP.

The initial actions of LH on the Leydig cells of the testes are entirely comparable to those on the corpus luteum, but because of the enzymatic complement of the testes, the major product is testosterone rather than progesterone.

The actions of FSH are less well defined. It does stimulate testicular cyclic AMP but is without effect on corpus luteum cyclic AMP.

Pituitary Storage. The content of gonadotropins is low in the pituitaries of prepubertal children. In menstruating women, pituitary LH averages about 700 I.U. and the FSH about 200 I.U. Following menopause, the pituitary content of LH rises to about 1700 I.U., with a comparable rise in FSH. The pituitary gonadotropin content of men is not greatly different from that of menstruating women.

Measurement. Until recently, the bioassay of urinary gonadotropins was a standard procedure in clinical endocrinology. Gonadotropins are adsorbed from urine by kaolin or precipitated by alcohol. After minimal purification, the extracts are injected into immature rats and mice, and the ovaries or uteri are weighed. In most cases, the assay does not distinguish between FSH and LH. Improved specificity for FSH is achieved by addition of an excess of chorionic gonadotropin.

The most sensitive method for measuring LH by bioassay is the ovarian ascorbic acid depletion procedure of Parlow. In this assay, immature intact pseudopregnant rats receive the test material intravenously, and the depletion of ovarian ascorbate is determined. In another bioassay procedure, hypophysectomized rats are injected with the test material, and the gain in weight of the ventral prostate is determined.

At the present time, biologic assays of gonadotropins for clinical diagnosis are being abandoned because they are tedious, expensive, and inaccurate. The precision and simplicity of radioimmunoassays provide substantial advantages, despite the fact that biologic activity and immunologic activity do not always correlate. The radioimmunoassay of LH is highly satisfactory. Antibodies which react well with LH can be raised against the readily available chorionic gonadotropin. Highly purified human LH must be used for radiolabeling, but a cruder pituitary extract can be used for standardization.

The radioimmunoassay of FSH is more difficult than that of LH. Many antisera raised in rabbits against partially purified human FSH cross-react extensively with LH and are unsuitable for use. However, when a sufficient number of rabbits are immunized, a few show the desired specificity for FSH. One such antibody is available in the United States from the National Pituitary Agency. A purified human FSH preparation is required for radiolabeling, but less highly purified pituitary extracts of known biologic potency suffice for standards.

A major problem exists when attempts are made to correlate biologic and radioimmunologic assays for pituitary and urinary gonadotropins. It is evident that biologic activity can be lost to a variable extent without loss of immunologic activity. This has produced a highly confusing situation in regard to radioimmunoassays.

Different standards for radioimmunoassay have been used and the results expressed in several ways. The material currently being distributed by the National Pituitary Agency for standardization is a crude pituitary extract (LER 907), which has a biologic potency of 20 I.U. FSH and 48 I.U. LH per milligram when expressed in terms of the Second International Reference Powder (IRP) (a preparation of urinary gonadotropins). When the radioimmunologic potency is compared directly with the Second IRP, LER 907 contains about 219 I.U. per mg. of LH or five times its apparent biologic activity and 38 I.U. per mg. of FSH. Other workers are using highly purified FSH and LH preparations for standardization and expressing results on a weight basis. For the above reasons, comparison of results between laboratories is difficult, often impossible. For the time being, standards used for radioimmunoassay should have their potency expressed in terms of the radioimmunologic potency as compared to the Second IRP.

Plasma and Urine Gonadotropins. Gonadotropins are present in the plasma at all ages (Fig. 2–10). A twofold rise in gonadotropins occurs at the time of puberty. In ovulating women, there is a slight initial rise in FSH followed by a slow decline during the follicular phase of the cycle (Fig. 2–11). During the corresponding period, there is a sharp peak of excretion of both gonadotropins, with the greater rise of LH and a lesser rise in FSH. Except for the ovulatory spike, the concentrations of LH and FSH in men are not greatly different from those in women. There is little change in plasma gonadotropins in men as a function of age; only a slight increase in plasma LH occurs in the seventh and eighth decades. In women, however, a marked increase in both FSH and LH occurs after the menopause, usually in the fifth decade.

Following gonadectomy of men and women, there is a marked rise in plasma FSH and LH. In children with gonadal agenesis, the FSH begins to rise before the normal age of puberty, but the rise in LH is usually delayed beyond the age of 11 or 12 years.

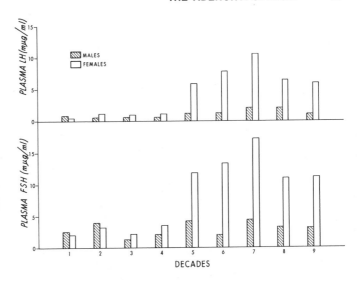

Figure 2–10. Plasma LH and FSH levels in normal males and females in relation to age. Each bar represents the mean value for five to ten individuals. All women in the fifth decade were postmenopausal, and this group had significantly higher mean LH and FSH levels than premenopausal women. The mean LH (but not FSH) level in men during the seventh and eighth decades was also found to be significantly higher (p < 0.02) than the mean level during the third and fourth decades. (Reproduced from *The Neuroendocrinology of Human Reproduction.* Mack, H. C., and Sherman, A. I. (eds.), Springfield, Ill., Charles C Thomas, 1971, with permission.)

In general, the urinary excretion of LH and FSH parallels plasma concentrations with the important exception that little gonadotropic hormone is found prepubertally (Fig. 2–12). After puberty, a tenfold rise in urinary LH occurs. It is still unexplained why urinary measurements should provide a better determinant of gonadotropic changes of puberty than plasma measurements.

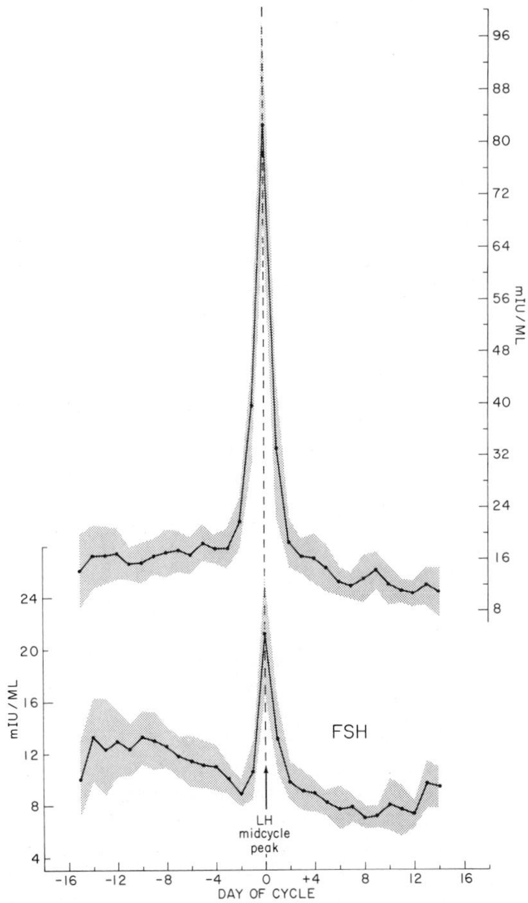

Metabolism and Secretory Rate. FSH and LH disappear from the plasma in a complex manner with a half-life of between 30 and 60 minutes. The urinary excretion of immunoassayable FSH may be as high as 36 per cent, but that of LH is considerably smaller, less than 5 per cent. Detailed studies of clearance of LH from the plasma have been conducted in women with the constant infusion techniques (20). The metabolic clearance rate is about 25 ml. per minute, and it is not affected by the gonadal function of the individual. Daily production rates of LH in normal women during most of the menstrual cycle are about 500 to 1,100 I.U. per day, with much higher levels occurring during the preovulatory period. In postmenopausal women, LH production is between 3,000 and 4,000 I.U. per day. When these production rates are compared to the scanty information concerning pituitary content of LH, it is evident that complete turnover of stored gonadotropin occurs every 12 to 24 hours, indicating that gonadotropin synthesis is an active process in the pituitary.

In contrast to the pituitary gonadotropins, the half-life of chorionic gonadotropin (HCG) in the plasma is much longer, about 8 hours by bioassay and considerably longer by radioimmunoassay. On the other hand, renal clearance of HCG is about 1 ml. per min., which is about seven times that of LH. The total daily production of HCG may reach as high as 30 mg. during the first trimester of pregnancy.

The marked differences in plasma and renal clearances of HCG and LH occur despite the fact that the amino acid sequences of the two peptides are closely similar. Differences in the carbohydrate substituents of the molecule are important determinants of metabolism. Chorionic gonadotropin differs from LH in its high sialic acid content (9 per cent). Enzymatic removal of the sialic acid greatly shortens plasma half-time and increases hepatic

Figure 2–11. Changes in serum LH and FSH during the menstrual cycle. This represents the average value for 16 normal menstrual cycles. (Reproduced from Ross, G. T., Cargille, C. M., et al.: *Recent Progr. Hormone Res.* 26:1, 1970, with permission.)

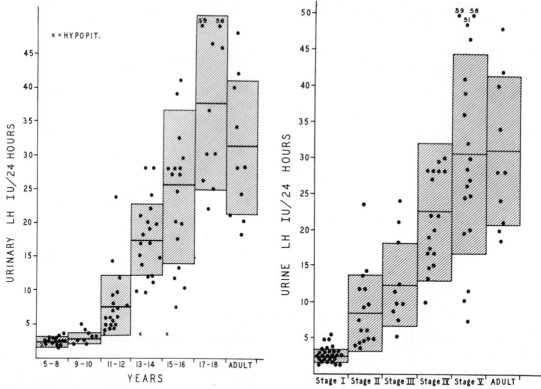

Figure 2–12. Urinary secretion of LH in normal boys and men. Changes in girls during puberty are similar but occur about one year earlier. Changes in urinary FSH show a less dramatic rise during puberty. (Reproduced from Baghdassarian, A., Guyda, H., et al.: *J. Clin. Endocr. 31*:428, 1970, with permission.)

extraction without affecting intrinsic biologic activity at the tissue level. The long half-life of HCG facilitates the rapid rise in plasma concentration early in pregnancy and may have teleologic significance.

Regulation. The secretion of FSH and LH is regulated by the hypophysiotropic hormone (or hormones) and by feedback inhibition by sex steroids. The chemical evidence indicates that a single hypothalamic hormone, the LH releasing hormone (LRH), also stimulates the release of FSH. The possibility of an additional hypophysiotropic hormone acting solely on FSH release has not been completely eliminated.

After gonadectomy, plasma FSH and LH concentrations rise markedly because of the absence of "feedback" inhibition of sex steroids. Estrogens are potent inhibitors of LH and FSH release, but testosterone is less effective. The role of other testicular steroids in pituitary FSH suppression remains conjectural. It is likely that sex steroids act on both the pituitary and the hypothalamus to modify gonadotropin secretion. If there proves to be only one gonadotropin releasing hormone, the differential secretion of FSH and LH which occurs in certain clinical states would require selective inhibition or facilitation of LH and FSH secretion by specific sex steroids acting directly on the pituitary. This hypothesis remains to be established.

Thyrotropin

Actions. Thyrotropin exerts profound effects on many aspects of thyroid function. Increases in thyroid size and vascularity are easily recognized after the administration of the hormone in experimental animals. Microscopically, the height of the follicular epithelium is increased, and the amount of colloid is reduced. Thyrotropin increases iodide uptake, thyroglobulin synthesis, iodotyrosine and iodothyronine formation, thyroglobulin proteolysis, and thyroxine and triiodothyronine release from the thyroid gland. After the binding of thyrotropin on the thyroid epithelium cell by specific receptors, adenyl cyclase located in the cell membrane is activated. As a consequence, there is an increase in intracellular cyclic AMP. This secondary messenger regulates the many intracellular reactors through phosphorylation of key proteins. Other alterations in thyroid cell biochemistry not directly related to hormone production and release follow TSH administration. There is an increase in oxygen uptake, phospholipid synthesis, RNA synthesis, and glucose utilization.

In experimental animals, thyrotropin preparations have a number of extrathyroidal effects. Thyrotropin promotes lipolysis in isolated adipose tissue. Administration of thyrotropin preparations to a number of animal species induces exoph-

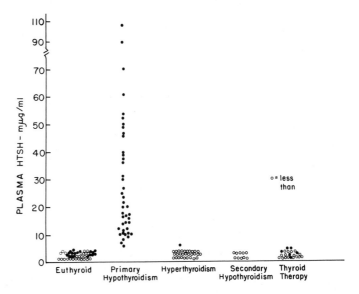

Figure 2–13. Plasma TSH measured by radioimmunoassay in hypothyroidism of several types and normal subjects. (Reproduced from Utiger, R. D., In *Current Topics in Thyroid Research.* New York, Academic Press Inc. 1965, p. 513, with permission.)

thalmos due to the deposition of mucopolysaccharide-rich edema fluid in the retro-orbital tissue. Thyrotropin itself may not be responsible for these effects on connective tissue because thyrotropin produced by mouse pituitary tumors does not induce exophthalmos. Separation of thyrotropic and exophthalmos-producing activity has been accomplished by chromatography of bovine pituitary extracts. Despite these experimental findings, their relevance to human exophthalmos is doubtful.

In man, exophthalmos occurs frequently during the course of hyperthyroidism and at times is associated with connective tissue abnormalities elsewhere (pretibial myxedema and acropathy). The plasma of such patients frequently contains a thyroid stimulating substance called LATS, which is a gamma globulin distinct from pituitary TSH. In addition, an exophthalmos producing substance (EPS) is demonstrable by bioassay in minnows. The relationship between LATS and EPS remains an enigma. It is likely that EPS of Graves' disease, like LATS, is not of pituitary origin.

Storage. There is little information concerning the concentrations of TSH in human pituitaries as a function of age and sex. Bioassay of a limited number of human pituitaries showed a content of about 4 I.U. This very low concentration has made the isolation or characterization of human TSH difficult.

Measurement. The detection of the small amount of thyrotropin in plasma by bioassay is a difficult task which has been achieved only in roughly quantitative terms. Bioassays have now been replaced by radioimmunoassays for studies of thyrotropin secretion in man.

Plasma Concentration. By radioimmunoassay normal human plasma contains less than 10 μU per ml. In about 10 per cent of normal individuals, thyrotropin is undetectable with current radioimmunoassays (Fig. 2–13). In patients with primary hypothyroidism, plasma thyrotropin concentrations are elevated as much as 50 times normal

(Fig. 2–14). With replacement treatment, TSH levels fall to normal; the rate of fall is dependent on the type and dosage of thyroid hormone administered. In most cases of hyperthyroidism, plasma TSH levels are low because of suppression by the elevated levels of circulating thyroid hormone.

Metabolism and Secretion. When I^{131}-thyrotropin is injected into normal adults, it is promptly distributed into a volume only slightly larger than the plasma volume. Over the next two hours, the disappearance is exponential with a mean half-life of about 50 minutes. On the basis of a mean plasma concentration of 2.7 μU per ml., Odell et al. (21) calculated pituitary secretion to be 165 mI.U. per day.

In hypothyroidism, disappearance of TSH from plasma is slow, but because of the high concentra-

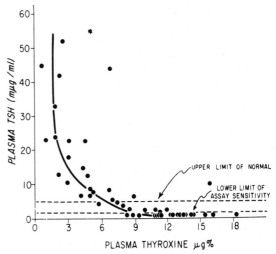

Figure 2–14. Relationship between plasma thyroxine and plasma TSH. (Reproduced from Reichlin, S., and Utiger, R. D.: *J. Clin. Endocr.* 27:251, 1967, with permission.)

tion of TSH in plasma, total secretory rate ranges from 390 to 23,025 mI.U. per day.

Regulation. The secretion of TSH by the adenohypophysis is determined partially by the level of circulating thyroid hormone and partially by thyrotropin releasing hormone (TRH). Following section of the pituitary stalk, thyroid activity is maintained at a higher level than after hypophysectomy, suggesting that at least minimal thyrotropin secretion persists under such conditions. The negative feedback control of thyrotropin secretion exercised by circulating thyroid hormone is exerted primarily at the pituitary level (see Chapter 12).

CHEMISTRY OF THE SOMATOMAMMOTROPIN FAMILY OF HORMONES

Characterization. Growth hormone (GH) and prolactin (Pr) of the pituitary and chorionic somatomammotropin (HCS) of the placenta have similar chemical structures and overlapping biologic actions. The amino acid structures of human growth hormone and chorionic somatomammotropin have been completely established. Both hormones contain 191 amino acids with two intramolecular S-S bonds in exactly the same location (between half-cystines at positions 53 and 165, and between 182 and 189) (Fig. 2–15).

Examination of the amino acid sequences reveals that 161 of the 191 amino acids are identical in the two hormones (Fig. 2–16). Of the remaining, 19 are highly compatible substitutions requiring only a simple base change in the DNA template, 4 are relatively compatible, and only 7 of the amino acid differences cannot be easily explained.

Human prolactin has chemical and immunologic resemblance to animal prolactins. Preliminary information indicates the structure has great simi-

larity to that of ovine prolactin, which has been completely characterized. Ovine prolactin is a simple protein slightly larger than GH. It contains 198 amino acids in a single peptide chain. Two intramolecular S-S bridges occupy the same relative positions as those in GH and HCS, and, in addition, there is a third disulfide bridge at the amino end of the molecule (Fig. 2–15). There are six regions of the ovine prolactin molecule comprising about 146 amino acids which appear to correspond closely to portions of the GH and HCS molecules (Fig. 2–16). Forty-nine of the amino acids in these sequences are identical, and an additional 68 are acceptable substitutions.

The structural homologies of these three hormones provide a strong indication that they evolved from a single progenitor hormone. Growth hormone and chorionic somatomammotropin are so closely related in structure that one may assume the evolutionary divergence of these two peptides is comparatively recent. Niall and associates (59) have identified an amino acid pattern which appears to repeat itself four times in each molecule (Fig. 2–15). From this they surmise that tandem duplication of the genetic information has occurred in the course of evolution of the primitive somatomammotropin.

Prolactin

Actions. Prolactin resembles growth hormone in that it acts directly on tissues and does not regulate the function of a secondary endocrine gland. The only established function of prolactin in man is in the initiation and maintenance of lactation. By itself, prolactin has little effect on the mammary gland; full lactation requires preparation by estrogens, progestins, corticosteroids, and insulin. When the gland has been primed, prolactin brings about milk secretion. In many species, milk cannot be removed by suckling unless oxytocin stimulates contraction in the myoepithelial cells of the mammary alveoli and ductules to force the milk into the larger collecting ducts and cisterns. In women, however, oxytocin is not required for successful nursing.

Prolactin acts directly on the mammary gland. This has been established by stimulating milk production through the introduction of prolactin into the major mammary duct of female rabbits primed with estrogens and progesterone. Prolactin can also induce milk formation when added to explants of mammary glands from pregnant mice *in vitro*.

The action of prolactin on the crop sac of pigeons and doves is a fascinating facet of comparative endocrinology. Following the hatching of the young, a nutritious material is formed by proliferation and desquamation of the crop epithelium. This crop "milk" is used for feeding the young. The action of prolactin on the crop sac is direct because local proliferation will surround an area of the crop sac into which prolactin is injected.

Prolactin has a luteotropic action on the ovary in

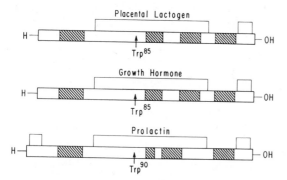

Figure 2–15. Diagram of basic structural properties of human chorionic somatomammotropin (HPL), human growth hormone, and ovine prolactin. The bars represent the peptide chains with the amino terminal to the left and the carboxyl terminal to the right. The shaded portions of each bar represent the recognizable areas, suggesting replicating sequences. The lines above the bars diagrammatically represent the position of disulfide bridges. (Reproduced from Niall, H. D., Hogan, M. L., et al.: *Proc. Nat. Acad. Sci.* USA **68**:866, 1971, with permission.)

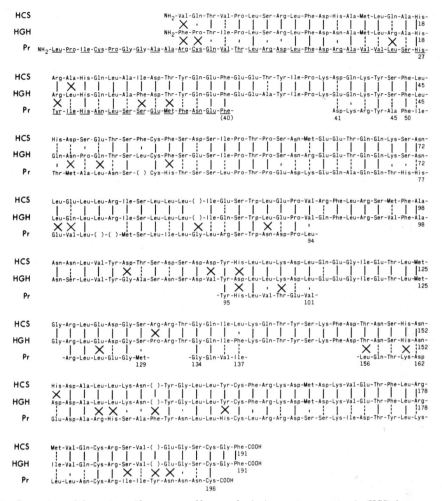

Figure 2–16. Comparison of the amino acid sequences of human chorionic somatomammotropin (HCS), human growth hormone (HGH), and prolactin (Pr). The first forty amino acids of the prolactin sequence are those of human prolactin. Homologous sections of the remaining amino acids are derived from the sequence of ovine prolactin. Homology is indicated as follows: identical pairs by a vertical bar, highly acceptable pairs by three dots, and acceptable pairs by a single dot. Nonhomologous pairs are indicated by a cross. [From data provided by Niall, H. D., Hogan M. L., et al.: *Recent Progr. Hormone Res.* 28 (in press, 1973).]

rats. Follicle stimulating and luteinizing hormones bring about follicular development, ovulation, and the initial development of the corpus luteum, but they are unable to sustain the secretory activity of the corpus luteum in the rat. Prolactin maintains luteal secretion but has no effect on ovarian follicles. By prolonging the secretory life of the corpus luteum, prolactin plays an important role in early pregnancy and during lactation. In other mammals, including ungulates, rabbits, guinea pigs, and probably man, prolactin does not have an important role in maintaining the secretory life of the corpus luteum.

Prolactin induces changes in maternal behavior which are important for the protection of the young. It promotes nesting behavior in some species of birds. Effects of prolactin on behavior have also been demonstrated in cold-blooded animals. For instance, small doses of prolactin stimulate the hypophysectomized eft stage of a terrestrial salamander to migrate to water.

Prolactin has general metabolic actions in the hypophysectomized animal which are unrelated to reproduction and which are similar to those of somatotropin. Under suitable experimental conditions, prolactin has been shown to be calorigenic and diabetogenic, to promote protein synthesis, and to increase the rate of chondroitin sulfate formation in cartilage. An increase in the weight of the liver and several other organs has been observed in prolactin-treated pigeons.

Similar growth hormone–like effects have been observed in man. The administration of large amounts of ovine prolactin to human beings with pituitary dwarfism has induced many of the metabolic changes previously observed with growth hormone. These include nitrogen retention, impairment of carbohydrate tolerance, hypercalciuria, and even skeletal growth; however, fat mobilization was not observed. The possible significance of these various actions of prolactin under physiologic conditions remains to be determined. As yet there is no known role of the hormone in the male sex.

Pituitary Storage. In most mammalian pituitaries, prolactin is an important protein constituent present in slightly lower concentration than growth hormone. Together the two hormones constitute one-third to one-half of pituitary protein and are easily recognized on electrophoretic separations of crude pituitary homogenates. Prolactin concentration is increased in pituitaries from adult female rats as compared to male rats. The human pituitary contains much less prolactin than that of other mammalian species. Only in pregnancy can a band associated with prolactin be recognized in electropherograms. Radioimmunoassays suggest that a single human pituitary only contains about 100 μg. of prolactin.

Measurement. Knowledge of the regulation of prolactin secretion in man has been greatly hampered until recently by the absence of suitable assays. To be sure, some information had been acquired by extraction of human plasma and assay of the extract for prolactin using the pigeon crop sac method. Within the last few years, adequate bioassays and radioimmunoassays have been developed. The new bioassays have used small explants of mammary gland generally obtained from mice in midpregnancy. A number of end points of prolactin action have been employed, including the histologic appearance of milk, the induction of the enzyme system concerned with lactose synthesis, and the synthesis of casein as demonstrated by P^{32} incorporation. Troublesome interference caused by the intrinsic prolactin activity of growth hormone is eliminated by immunologic neutralization. These assays have surprising sensitivity and can detect as little as 4 to 10 ng. of prolactin per milliliter of plasma. The assays, however, remain laborious and highly demanding in terms of technical skill.

The recent development of radioimmunoassays for prolactin has greatly expanded the potential for clinical studies of prolactin secretion. Friesen and coworkers (53) isolated small quantities of prolactin from cultures of primate pituitaries. This prolactin was used to raise antibodies and for radiolabeling. A very satisfactory mixed heterologous radioimmunoassay has been developed in the author's laboratory which only requires readily available animal prolactins. Porcine prolactin is labeled with I^{125}, and antiovine prolactin is produced in guinea pigs. Human prolactin competes well with porcine prolactin for binding by this antibody. Because chemically pure human prolactin is not yet readily available for standardization, it has been necessary to employ human plasma with very high prolactin content for standardization. Bioassay of the standard plasma allows presentation of results either as milliunits per ml. or as ng. per ml., based on the assumption that human prolactin has the same specific activity as animal prolactins.

Plasma Concentration. The mean plasma prolactin level of normal men is 6.2 $\pm$ 0.6 ng. per ml., while that for women is 9.0 $\pm$ 0.6 ng. per ml. (55) (Fig. 2–17). While the difference between the means is significant, there is a major overlap of the two groups. In women there is no significant alteration of prolactin levels during the menstrual cycle. The lack of a clear sex difference in prolactin levels raises the question of the essentiality of prolactin for human breast development.

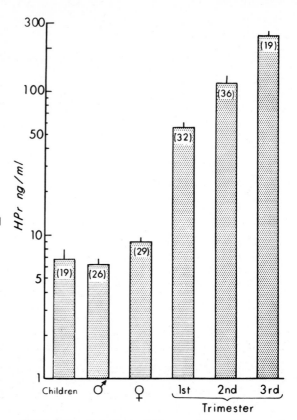

Figure 2–17. Prolactin levels in prepubertal children and adult men and women and in the three trimesters of pregnancy. (Reproduced from Jacobs, L. S., Mariz, I. K., et al.: *J. Clin. Endocr.* 34:484, 1972, with permission.)

In pregnancy, plasma prolactin begins to rise in the first trimester and increases progressively (Fig. 2–17). The rise in plasma prolactin almost exactly parallels the increase in placental somatomammotropin. The behavior of prolactin in human pregnancy is unusual because comparable rises in prolactin have not been found in pregnancy in other species, including the rhesus monkey. The rise in prolactin in human pregnancy may be the result of the very high level of estrogens which is present in the human species. During pregnancy, the combined effects of both pituitary and placental mammotropic hormones, estrogens, and progesterone develop the secretory apparatus of the breast for subsequent lactation but do not allow lactation. It is likely that the steroid hormones act both to stimulate mammary development and to inhibit the actual formation of milk. Following delivery, estrogens and progesterone levels fall rapidly, and the lactogenic action of prolactin is unopposed. During lactation, basal levels of prolactin in plasma are not greatly elevated after the immediate postpartum period. Soon after the start of nursing, there is a marked surge of prolactin secretion

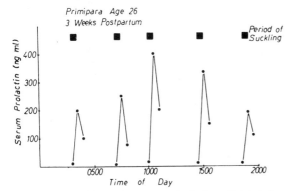

Figure 2–18. Changes in serum prolactin immediately before and after nursing in a 26-year-old woman three weeks after delivery. (Reproduced from Hwang, P., Guyda, H., et al.: *Proc. Nat. Acad. Sci.* USA 68:1902, 1971, with permission.)

(Fig. 2–18). This interval of prolactin secretion must act to prime the breast for the next period of nursing 4 to 6 hours hence. It is possible for lactation to continue more or less indefinitely as long as the repeated stimulus of nursing occurs. There are cases on record of the development of lactation in nonpuerperal women who allow infants to suckle repeatedly.

Metabolism and Secretion. The rate of disappearance of human prolactin from the plasma, its distribution in body fluids, and its secretory rate have not been definitively studied. The rapid fall in plasma prolactin concentrations after L-dopa administration suggests a half-life in the plasma of 20 to 30 minutes, a half-time very similar to GH.

Regulation. Radioimmunoassay of prolactin has established that the mechanical stimulation of the female breast for as little as 5 minutes leads to a massive secretion of prolactin (Fig. 2–19). Similar stimulation of the male breast does not result in prolactin secretion. Tactile stimulation of a nonmammary region of the same dermatome fails to stimulate prolactin. It is known that the breast, particularly the nipple and areolae, is richly endowed with specialized nerve endings. These sensory receptors initiate the impulses which eventually reach the area in the hypothalamus which regulates prolactin secretion.

In man, a number of drugs which affect dopaminergic mechanisms influence prolactin secretion by altering hypothalamic secretion of a prolactin inhibitory factor. Alpha methyldopa, an agent which inhibits dopamine synthesis, induces nonpuerperal lactation and hyperprolactinemia. On the other hand, levodopa, which crosses the blood-brain barrier and increases dopamine concentrations in hypothalamic neurons, inhibits normal prolactin secretion in normal women and also in many pathologic states associated with hyperprolactinemia (Fig. 2–20). The presumption is that this agent increases PIF secretion, although an alternative action directly on the pituitary is hard to rule out.

A variety of tranquilizing drugs, including the phenothiazines and reserpine, which interfere with dopaminergic transmission may induce nonpuerperal lactation and hyperprolactinemia in women. As a test of prolactin secretory reserve, 50 mg. of chlorpromazine is given intramuscularly, and samples are obtained hourly for 3 hours. Examples of normal responses are shown in Figure 2–21. The frequency with which abnormal responses occur in pituitary and hypothalamic disorders is under active investigation at the present time.

Recent evidence suggests that hypothalamic serotonin increases prolactin secretion. While this action of serotonin has not been established in man, it may explain the rise in plasma prolactin which follows tryptophan administration. This amino acid crosses the blood-brain barrier and is a precursor for serotonin.

In addition to a prolactin inhibiting factor, the hypothalamus may also contain prolactin releasing factors. The thyrotropin releasing hormone (TRH) is one such releasing substance. As shown in Figure 2–22, TRH is a potent stimulus for prolactin secretion in man. It is not at all clear why TRH should act to release both TSH and prolactin. Whether this surprising observation has any clinical or physiologic significance remains to be seen.

A number of nonspecific stimuli result in prolactin secretion, including surgical stress, uremia, and exercise. The physiologic significance of this prolactin secretion is obscure.

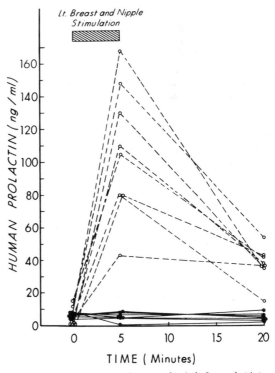

Figure 2–19. Changes in plasma prolactin before and at intervals after mechanical stimulation of breast and nipple in eight normal women (--○--) and eight normal men (-●-). [Reproduced from Kolodny, R. C., Jacobs, L. S., et al.: *Nature* (London) *238*: 284, 1972, with permission.]

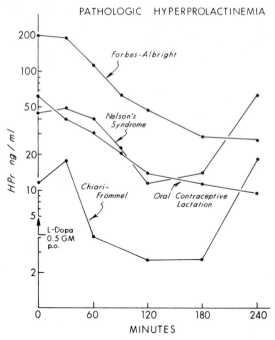

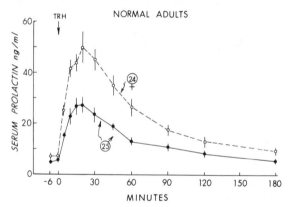

Figure 2–22. Serum prolactin changes after injection of TRH (100 to 400 μg.) into normal men (●) and women (○). [Reproduced from Jacobs, L. S., Snyder, R. D., et al.: *J. Clin. Endocr. 36:* 1973 (in press), with permission.]

Figure 2–20. Plasma prolactin concentrations before and after oral administration of L-dopa to four patients with different types of hyperprolactinemia. [Reproduced from Daughaday, W. H., and Jacobs, L. S.: *Proceedings, Fourth International Congress of Endocrinology*, 1972. (in press), with permission.]

Growth Hormone

Actions. Growth hormone influences many metabolic processes, but space does not permit more than a brief discussion of the major areas of action.

With the daily injection of growth hormone, actual growth of hypophysectomized rats is grossly detectable within a few days. Analysis of the carcass of such animals demonstrates that the predominant change in body composition is an increase in protein, often with a decrease in body fat. The anabolic effects of growth hormone are different from those produced experimentally by insulin.

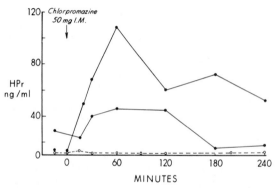

Figure 2–21. Changes in plasma prolactin following IM injection of 50 mg. of chlorpromazine. Results in two normal women (●) and in a patient with panhypopituitarism (○).

Many facets of protein metabolism have been examined after growth hormone administration, but the primary action of the hormone has not yet been localized. Soon after the administration of somatotropin to a deficient animal, the rate of conversion of amino acids to blood urea is decreased, and there is a marked decrease in plasma and urinary urea levels. Since somatotropin does not act primarily by inhibiting breakdown of amino acids, a role of growth hormone in stimulating protein synthesis has been sought. Entrance of amino acids into cells is accelerated by growth hormone, which results in a fall in the plasma level of amino acids.

The process of cellular penetration of amino acids can be distinguished from subsequent synthetic or catabolic fates by the use of the nonmetabolizable amino acid α isobutyric acid (AIB). This unnatural amino acid is transported into many cells of the body by the same mechanism utilized for the entry of glycine. Somatotropin given *in vitro* to hypophysectomized rats stimulates the accumulation of AIB in muscle, and growth hormone added *in vitro* has been reported to stimulate AIB uptake by the diaphragm. Despite these observations, it is unlikely that the augmented protein synthesis which follows growth hormone administration is the result of an increase in the intracellular pool of amino acids. Direct measurements of muscle intracellular amino acid pools after growth hormone administration to hypophysectomized rats have failed to demonstrate the predicted accumulation of intracellular amino acids. Other factors than the amino acid pool size must, therefore, regulate the rate of protein synthesis.

The effects of growth hormone on ribonucleic acid metabolism have received much attention. Hypophysectomy leads to a fall in total hepatic RNA synthesis, with a decrease in the number of ribosomes and the amount of messenger and transfer RNA. When growth hormone is given to hypophysectomized rats, there is stimulation of RNA synthesis and correction of two defects in protein synthesis. The immediate stimulation of protein synthesis appears to be the result of increased formation of messenger RNA. However, sustained protein synthesis requires all components of the protein synthetic apparatus. While these results have established definite effects of growth hormone on the subcellular protein synthesizing machinery, they fail to pinpoint a primary locus of growth hormone action.

Somatotropic control of synthetic reactions in connective tissues is clearly evident in the failure of skeletal growth in pituitary dwarfism and the overgrowth of skeletal and connective tissues in acromegaly. Proliferation of epiphysial cartilage virtually ceases after hypophysectomy, and the epiphysial growth plate becomes greatly narrowed. The ability of GH to correct the defects in cartilage growth is so consistent and sensitive that this response has been used extensively for the assay of growth hormone.

The stimulation of the synthetic processes of cartilage by growth hormone can be conveniently studied with S^{35}-sulfate. Sulfate incorporation into chondroitin sulfate is reduced about 70 per cent by hypophysectomy of rats but is restored within 24 hours by the administration of pituitary growth hormone. However, growth hormone is ineffective when added directly to isolated cartilage from hypophysectomized rats. Most significantly, normal plasma is capable of stimulating cartilage directly, whereas plasma from hypophysectomized rats is virtually inactive. These observations have led to extensive subsequent studies which strongly suggest that growth hormone exerts its effect on cartilage through a component of plasma, somatomedin (sulfation factor), which stimulates cartilage directly (Fig. 2–23).

While most studies of somatomedin have measured S^{35}-sulfate uptake by cartilage, it is now clear that the same material is responsible for the increased synthesis of collagen and other proteins in cartilage. Somatomedin also increases the synthesis of ribonucleic acids and promotes cell replication (DNA synthesis).

Progress has been made in characterizing somatomedin. In normal plasma it circulates with the large molecular-size plasma protein. It is likely that, in native plasma, somatomedin is bound to carrier protein. Somatomedin can be extracted from plasma in acid ethanol and purified by ion-exchange and gel filtration techniques. The biologically active purified material is a simple peptide with an estimated molecular weight of 4,000. Somatomedin has an insulin-like action on diaphragm and fat cells *in vitro* and is probably a major component of the insulin-like action of plasma which is not neutralized by anti-insulin plasma. The importance of somatomedin in mediating GH action on nonskeletal tissues is as yet unresolved.

The plasma of hypophysectomized patients contains little somatomedin. After the administration of GH, somatomedin is detectably increased in plasma within 4 hours and is usually present in normal concentrations by 24 hours. The site of somatomedin synthesis in man is not known, but

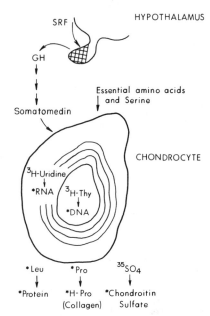

Figure 2–23. GH action on cartilage is mediated by somatomedin (sulfation factor). This peptide is produced by growth hormone action on liver and possibly kidney. It acts directly on chondrocytes to stimulate many aspects of cartilage metabolism necessary for cartilage replication and matrix formation.

animal experiments suggest that the liver is important. In acromegaly, increased concentrations of somatomedin can be demonstrated in about half the cases. Up to this time, the clinical application of somatomedin measurements have been limited because of the difficulty and imprecision of the method.

Hypophysectomy causes a decrease in the rate of synthesis and turnover of the acid mucopolysaccharides of skin. In the rat, growth hormone stimulates the synthesis of chondroitin sulfate more than hyaluronate.

Growth hormone induces a number of important alterations in fat metabolism. Mobilization of fat from the peripheral adipose depots occurs. This effect is associated with an increase in fat catabolism, which can be recognized by a lowering of the respiratory quotient and increased ketogenesis. The fat mobilized is transported in the plasma as nonesterified fatty acids. In human beings, the level of nonesterified fatty acids (NEFA) rises more than twofold between 1 and 2 hours after the injection of 1 mg. of human growth hormone. Under physiologic conditions in which GH is secreted without concomitant release of catecholamines, such as occurs during sleep, there is little change in plasma free fatty acids. Levels of FFA are not higher in the fasting state in acromegaly than in hyposomatotropic patients. These observations would suggest that endogenous GH is not of major significance in regulating lipolysis in man.

Abnormalities in carbohydrate metabolism are evident after hypophysectomy. The blood sugar level falls on fasting and may reach hypoglycemic levels. In addition, levels of glycogen in muscle as well as in liver fall. The hypoglycemic action of insulin is greatly increased by pituitary deficiency, and the ability to restore blood sugar levels after hypoglycemia is impaired. This defect is primarily the result of inadequate mobilization of the gluconeogenic precursors, alanine and glutamine, from muscle. Impaired gluconeogenic enzymatic machinery in the liver is of less importance.

Some of the disturbances in carbohydrate metabolism of hypopituitarism are the result of growth hormone deficiency, and some are the result of corticotropin deficiency. Treatment with adrenocortical steroids will restore normal levels of fasting blood sugar and liver glycogen, but abnormal sensitivity to insulin persists, indicating an important independent role of pituitary growth hormone.

Because of the diabetogenic effects of GH in whole animals, the divergent influences of growth hormone and insulin on isolated tissues have been much explored. Insulin facilitates the entrance of glucose into muscle and adipose tissue, while GH and adrenal steroids have little sustained action on this process. Administration of GH to hypophysectomized animals and man may result in a transient increase in glucose uptake, the so-called insulin-like action of GH. This effect is lost on repeated injections of GH. Both GH and corticosteroids appear to limit the rate of phosphorylation of glucose once it is within the muscle cell. Therefore, under conditions such as fasting, in which sugar penetration is the rate-limiting reaction, growth hormone does not greatly influence the rate of glucose utilization. When sugar penetration is greatly stimulated by insulin, the rate of phosphorylation becomes the rate-limiting factor, and the inhibitory effects of growth hormone become manifest. The exact nature of the inhibition of phosphorylating mechanisms induced by growth hormone remains elusive. These formulations, which are based on possible differences in the sites of action of growth hormone and insulin, provide an attractive explanation for many of the puzzling changes in glucose metabolism in hypopituitarism and the effects of growth hormone.

A relationship may exist between the lipolytic effects of growth hormone and the inhibition of glucose utilization. This has been called the "glucose–fatty acid cycle." Elevation of plasma free fatty acids in man and experimental animals inhibits glucose utilization. It has been difficult, however, to correlate the degree of inhibition of glucose utilization and the level of plasma free fatty acids. Intracellular free fatty acids or their acyl esters may be a more critical factor in glucose regulation than plasma free fatty acids. Intracellular fatty acids equilibrate slowly with plasma free fatty acids and would account for some of the discrepancies noted.

Actions in Man. Knobil and Greep, in 1957, demonstrated the potency of simian growth hormone in hypophysectomized monkeys, as compared to the ineffectiveness of nonprimate growth hormones. Soon thereafter, human growth hormone was prepared and tested in humans. With daily doses of 1 to 10 mg. per day, major metabolic changes are induced in hypopituitary patients and even in normal adult individuals. Nitrogen balance becomes strongly positive; plasma and urine urea values promptly fall. Although daily nitrogen retention decreases with continued growth hormone treatment, it is still adequate to maintain a greatly increased growth rate in pituitary dwarfs. Sodium, chloride, potassium, magnesium, and phosphorus are retained concomitant with the positive nitrogen balance (Fig. 2–24). Calcium may be retained by the body despite hypercalciuria. This unexpected finding is explained by increased gastrointestinal absorption of calcium. Plasma phos-

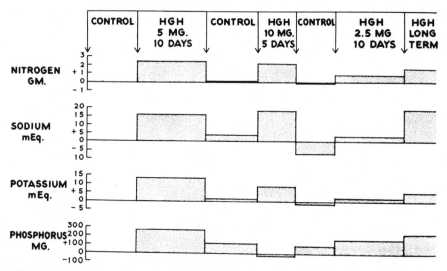

Figure 2–24. The effects of growth hormone treatment of an 11½-year-old girl with pituitary dwarfism on the balances of nitrogen, sodium, potassium, and phosphorus. Changes above the initial control baseline represent retention of the substance and below the line, loss. (Reproduced from Hutchings, J. J., et al.: *J. Clin. Endocr.* 19:759, 1959, with permission.)

phorus levels may rise after growth hormone administration, but this has been inconstant. Alkaline phosphatase levels are little changed.

In view of the well-documented diabetogenic effects of growth hormone in some experimental animals, carbohydrate metabolism has been carefully studied after growth hormone administration in man. When growth hormone is administered to fasting normal and hypophysectomized subjects, little change occurs in plasma glucose and insulin concentration. However, if glucose is administered 2 hours after growth hormone, glucose disappearance from plasma is inhibited. More prolonged administration of growth hormone does not produce diabetes unless very large doses are administered because of compensatory hyperinsulinism. The diabetogenic influence of growth hormone is most easily demonstrated when it is administered to hypophysectomized diabetic patients. In these patients, as little as 1 mg. of human growth hormone daily leads to exacerbation of diabetes and ketosis. These observations attest to the diabetogenic action of human growth hormone, which is masked in the presence of normal pancreatic reserve.

Pituitary Storage.   Fortunately, the human pituitary is particularly rich in growth hormone, and the somatotropic granule resists autolytic dissolution after death. While radioimmunoassays suggest a much higher content, the yield of somatotropin with present extraction methods is between 4 and 8 per cent of the dry weight of human pituitaries, equivalent to 3 to 5 mg. of hormone per gland. No significant changes in growth hormone content with age are evident. Octogenarians have nearly as much growth hormone as the rapidly growing child.

Measurement.   The biologic activity of growth hormone preparations is occasionally assayed by the ability of GH to stimulate body weight in hypophysectomized rats or in female rats whose growth has reached a plateau. A more sensitive method for assaying growth hormone depends upon administration of the hormone for 3 to 4 days and measurement of the width of the tibial epiphysial growth plate. The minimal dose required to achieve a signficant response with this assay is about 20 μg. of hormone per rat. This sensitivity is inadequate for the measurement of somatotropin in biologic fluids.

For clinical purposes, growth hormone is measured by one of several radioimmunologic methods. Results are expressed in terms of a highly purified growth hormone preparation. While immunologic activity of growth hormone does not correlate completely with biologic activity, this has not caused the problems which exist in LH radioimmunossay.

Plasma Concentration.   The level of circulating radioimmunoassayable GH in the well-rested adult prior to breakfast is less than 3 ng. per ml. However, with moderate exercise, such as is incurred by ambulatory patients coming to the hospital, higher values may be observed. The tendency for plasma GH levels to rise after exercise is greater in women than in men, so that a transient elevation to levels observed in acromegaly may be encountered. A rise in plasma growth hormone occurs in many individuals 2 to 4 hours after ingestion of a meal and during fasting prolonged beyond one night.

The effects of age on plasma growth hormone are of interest. In the first days of life, very high levels of GH occur, but there is great variability among infants. After 2 weeks of age, lower mean levels are found. In pubertal children, the basal plasma growth hormone concentration is not greatly different from that reported for adults, but more peaks of GH may occur during the day with physical activity. GH continues to be secreted after the period of skeletal growth has been completed. GH secretory responses to provocative stimuli are unimpaired even in elderly individuals.

The diurnal pattern of GH secretion has been characterized by obtaining blood samples every 20 or 30 minutes throughout the 24 hours under nonstressful conditions. During most of the day, plasma GH levels of normal adults are less than 3 ng. per ml., with one or two sharp spikes 3 to 4 hours after meals. The most consistent period of GH secretion for both children and adults occurs about 1 hour after the onset of deep sleep (Fig. 2–25). Subsequent smaller peaks of plasma GH may be observed later during the sleep period. The initial surge of GH secretion is correlated with the onset of stage III or IV sleep and not with any recognized general metabolic clues. Delay in the onset of deep sleep will correspondingly delay the onset of the GH peak. Plasma levels of glucose, fatty acids, and insulin are not changed by the sudden secretion of GH, but after the peak, the individual is more resistant to administered insulin, and glucose tolerance is slightly decreased. There is evidence that REM (rapid eye movement) sleep inhibits the GH peak and may be important in the termination of the sleep-related GH secretion. Despite the fact that a substantial fraction of total GH secretion occurs 1 to 2 hours after the onset of deep sleep, the significance of this pattern of GH secretion remains to be determined. It has been suggested that this GH secretion is important in anabolic and repair processes. There is great interest in determining whether abnormalities of GH secretion during sleep could influence skeletal growth.

Metabolism and Secretory Rate.   The turnover of growth hormone in the plasma is rapid. Administered hormone disappears from plasma with an initial half-life of about 20 to 25 minutes. A similar half-life in the disappearance of endogenous hormone has been reported following pituitary suppression with glucose or after hypophysectomy in acromegaly. The clearance rate for human growth hormone determined by the constant infusion method is between 100 and 150 ml. per square meter of body surface per minute. No consistent changes with age or sex exist. GH clearance is normal in acromegaly but is decreased in hypothyroidism and in many cases of diabetes mellitus. Markedly decreased clearance has been reported in a case of primordial dwarfism (Seckel dwarf).

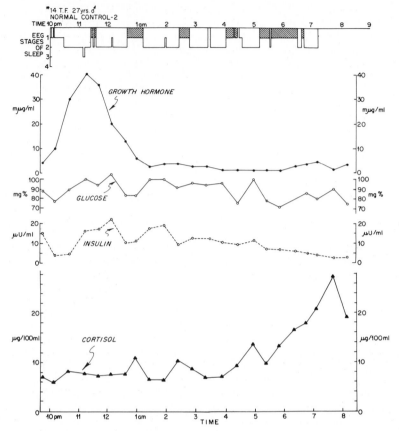

Figure 2–25. Changes in GH, glucose, insulin, and cortisol concentrations in plasma during the hours of sleep. The bars at the top of the graph indicate the stages of sleep. The shaded portions are periods of rapid eye movement sleep (REM). (Reproduced from Takahashi, Y., Kipnis, D. M., et al.: *J. Clin. Invest. 47*:2–79, 1968, with permission.)

Attempts have been made to estimate GH secretory rates on the basis of the basal GH levels and their metabolic clearance. This calculation disregards the marked fluctuation of plasma GH which may occur throughout the day and night. To obviate this difficulty, investigators have resorted to continuous or repetitive sampling to arrive at an integrated 24-hour GH concentration. This has been found to be 1.8 ± 1.0 (SD) mg. per ml. in men, somewhat higher in women, and 5.6 ± 3.6 mg. per ml. in preadolescent and adolescent boys. These results would suggest that normal GH secretion is between 0.75 and 3 mg. per day.

Attempts to estimate GH secretion by measuring the growth hormone activity in a 24-hour urine collection have not been successful. Investigators have detected material in the urine which reacts with antigrowth hormone plasma, but the immunologic identity of this material with purified hormone and the conditions of quantitative measurement have been a matter of dispute.

Regulation. The physiologic antagonism between growth hormone and insulin has been recognized since the days of Houssay. In human beings, the secretion of GH is an important defense mechanism against hypoglycemia (Fig. 2–26). To test the adequacy of the GH secretory response, 0.05 to 0.1 unit of insulin per kg. body weight is given intravenously with careful observation of the patient. The rise in plasma GH follows the nadir of blood sugar and reaches a maximum by 45 to 60 minutes. A rapid fall in blood sugar to less than 50 per cent of the initial level or below 50 mg. per 100 ml. represents an adequate stimulus for most subjects. A much smaller fall in blood sugar is adequate to stimulate GH release in many individuals. Administration of glucose with insulin prevents the rise in growth hormone levels in the plasma which is observed with insulin alone. The importance of glucose utilization by the growth hormone regulatory center is suggested by the observation that 2-deoxyglucose (which inhibits the utilization of glucose in the tissues) stimulates the secretion of growth hormone. It is of interest, but still unexplained, that obese patients do not respond to provocative stimuli with GH secretion as regularly as do individuals of normal weight.

Oral or intravenous administrations of amino acids stimulate GH secretion. Arginine is one of the most potent amino acids in causing growth hormone release (Fig. 2–27). This amino acid also stimulates the release of insulin, which precedes the release of growth hormone; the release of the two hormones is unrelated, however, since growth hormone secretion occurs in response to arginine in juvenile diabetics in whom the secretion of

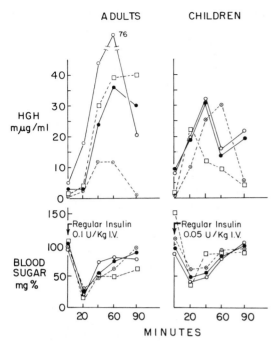

Figure 2-26. Plasma growth hormone concentrations in normal adults and children after the induction of hypoglycemia with insulin. (Courtesy of M. L. Parker.)

insulin is negligible. The reasonable suggestion has been made that the secretion of growth hormone induced by amino acids is a mechanism for stimulating protein synthesis when precursors are available.

As has already been mentioned, plasma growth hormone levels are elevated after exercise and after certain types of excitement. The effects of exercise have been correlated with increased levels of plasma free fatty acids, and the secretion of growth hormone may be important in initiating and sustaining lipolysis in adipose tissue. Provision of free fatty acids for the energy demands of exercise would spare the limited supplies of glucose.

The effects of other hormones on the secretion of growth hormone have received considerable attention. Plasma growth hormone levels are higher in many women after exercise, hypoglycemia, or arginine infusion than in men. This sex difference is due to estrogens. Relatively brief administration of potent estrogens will increase the growth hormone response induced in men by arginine administration. Corticosteroid excess occurring in spontaneous hyperadrenocorticism and after high-dose corticosteroid administration impairs the plasma growth hormone response to hypoglycemia and inhibits the sleep-related peak of growth hormone secretion.

Hypothyroidism in the rat greatly reduces the growth hormone content of the pituitary and the concentration of the hormone in plasma as detected by bioassay. In man, a similar but less profound change in growth hormone secretion occurs. Although the basal plasma levels of GH are not depressed in clinical hypothyroidism, the rise in plasma GH in response to hypoglycemia has been observed frequently to be subnormal in hypothyroid children.

Hypothalamic regulation of GH secretion can be altered by drugs which affect catecholamine neurotransmittors. Blockade of hypothalamic alpha adrenergic receptors with drugs such as phentolamine will decrease GH secretion in response to certain provocative stimuli. Beta adrenergic blockade, on the other hand, facilitates GH secretion. The administration of L-dopa by increasing hypothalamic release of dopamine and possibly norepinephrine leads to an acute discharge of GH. This response is useful in the diagnosis of hypopituitarism.

GH secretion after provocative stimuli is decreased by prior treatment with alpha adrenergic blocking drugs and potentiated by drugs which block beta adrenergic receptors in the hypothalamus.

HYPOPITUITARISM

Etiology. Primary hypopituitarism may result from surgical or radiation ablation, from nonsecretory pituitary tumors (discussed later), from metastatic tumors, from infarction, and from a number of infiltrative or granulomatous processes.

Pituitary infarction is most commonly associated with postpartum uterine hemorrhage, but it may occur from time to time in patients with extensive diabetic degenerative vascular disease and in patients with sickle cell anemia. Rare cases of hypopituitarism due to cavernous sinus thrombosis, temporal arteritis, carotid aneurysm, and trauma have been reported.

Sheehan's syndrome is a well-defined clinical entity accounting for the majority of cases of nonneoplastic spontaneous hypopituitarism in adult

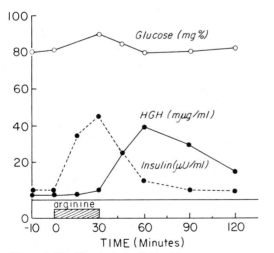

Figure 2-27. The typical effects of intravenous arginine (0.5 gm. per kg. body weight) on plasma glucose, human growth hormone (HGH), and insulin. (From Hammond, Parker, and Daughaday, unpublished.)

women. Normally hypertrophy of the pituitary takes place during pregnancy due to estrogen stimulation of lactotropic cell proliferation. After delivery, the succulent gland normally undergoes involution. Postpartum hemorrhage, with its attendant shock and frequent coagulation abnormalities, is the precipitating cause of ischemic necrosis. There is a correlation between the severity and duration of hypotension and the extent of the adenohypophysial lesion.

The exact pathogenesis of the pituitary vascular lesion is difficult to reconstruct. Sheehan (73) has postulated that severe arteriolar spasm develops in vessels supplying the critical hypothalamic areas from which hypothalamic-pituitary portal veins arise. This spasm leads to pituitary ischemia and thrombosis. When circulation is reestablished, pituitary hemorrhage develops. Disappearance of glandular elements after necrosis is so extensive that only small nests of recognizable pituitary cells may be found in condensed stroma lying in an otherwise empty sella turcica.

The neurohypophysis is generally spared because it is less dependent on the portal vessels for its nutrition; however, in unusual cases, damage to the neurohypophysis is extensive and diabetes insipidus results.

Rapid mammary involution and failure of lactation are the earliest recognizable evidences of hypopituitarism in patients surviving the period of postpartum shock. Normal strength and vigor are not regained in the puerperium. There follows a period of chronic debility and semi-invalidism with the features common to all hypopituitarism.

In early life, infiltration with cholesterol-laden histiocytes (Hand-Schüller-Christian disease) may lead to adenohypophysial and neurohypophysial damage. Pituitary infiltration by hemosiderin-laden macrophages (hemochromatosis) or by sarcoid granulomas can produce hypopituitarism in adults. Nontuberculous giant cell granuloma may involve the pituitary as well as the thyroid and adrenal glands. The resulting multiglandular syndrome presents difficult diagnostic problems. The pituitaries of certain patients examined at necropsy show only a diffuse fibrosis of uncertain origin.

Occasionally a patient with an enlarged sella turcica is found by pneumoencephalogram to have an empty sella. Adenohypophysial tissue is limited to a small rim about the periphery of the bony sella. Rarely, visual field defects occur. In most cases, signs of hypopituitarism are absent or minimal, and the enlarged sella turcica is discovered serendipitously because skull films are obtained for some unrelated complaint, but in other cases, clinical hypopituitarism is present. The cause of the empty sella syndrome remains obscure. Some have proposed that a defect in the diaphragma sellae leads to transmission of cerebrospinal fluid pressure to adenohypophysial tissue. It is hard to understand how CSF pressures sufficient to cause pituitary atrophy would occur in this way. Alternatively, some have suggested that pituitary cysts might be responsible for the enlargement of the sella. Rupture of the cyst would allow access to the cerebrospinal fluid and permit pneumoencephalographic recognition.

The diagnosis requires fractional pneumoencephalography with proper head positioning. Such studies are mandatory before radiation or surgical treatment is undertaken in patients with large sellae.

Tuberculosis and syphilis, once significant causes of hypopituitarism, are now very rarely seen. Isolated instances have been reported in which mycoses, brucellosis, and other infections have led to hypopituitarism.

In disease processes producing destruction in the pituitary, clinical manifestations of hypopituitarism are usually absent until about 75 per cent of the gland is destroyed. With more refined laboratory procedures, it is possible to detect lesser losses of functional reserve. As the extent of pituitary destruction increases, clinical evidences of hormonal deficiencies usually occur in the following order: (1) gonadotropins, (2) somatotropin (growth failure in children), (3) thyrotropin, (4) corticotropin, (5) prolactin. (Clinical evidence of prolactin deficiency is only recognized in postpartum necrosis of the pituitary. In other types of hypopituitarism, plasma prolactin is often normal or increased because of interruption of normal portal transport of prolactin inhibitory factor.) Exceptions to this sequence are frequent.

Pituitary hypofunction can result from disease processes attacking the hypothalamus which either destroy the ability to synthesize new hypophysiotropic hormones or impair the transport of these hormones to the pituitary. Disease processes which may produce secondary hypopituitarism include suprasellar tumors (craniopharyngiomas, optic gliomas, etc.), trauma, infection, hydrocephalus, congenital malformations, and granulomas (histiocytosis and sarcoid). While this mechanism of pituitary hypofunction has been suspected, it is only recently that evidence obtained by administration of TRH and LRH has definitely established the existence of secondary hypopituitarism. In most cases of secondary hypopituitarism involving more than one hormone, prolactin secretion is increased rather than decreased.

Clinical Features of Panhypopituitarism

Total deficiency of the adenohypophysis without replacement therapy is incompatible with survival in man. When hypopituitarism occurs as a result of tumor, infarction, or other disease, in contrast to total surgical hypophysectomy, hypopituitarism is usually incomplete and clinical manifestations are milder.

The clinical features of hypoadrenocorticism are most evident 4 to 14 days after withdrawal of maintenance therapy in a patient with total hypophysectomy. Nausea, vomiting, severe asthenia, and eventual collapse develop. Hyperthermia, often above 104°F, is common. Moderate hypotension during the early phases of corticosteroid withdrawal becomes severe and leads to death. The similarity of these clinical findings to those following adrenalectomy and the rapid clinical improvement after corticosteroid treatment are evidence that adrenal insufficiency is the most important element of the syndrome.

Despite corticosteroid deficiency, the hypophysectomized patient is able to conserve body sodium far better than the patient with Addison's disease. Hyponatremia, if it does occur, is more likely to be caused by excessive water retention than by sodium loss. Aldosterone excretion continues and actually increases if the patient is challenged with a low sodium diet. However, the excretion of aldosterone is lower than normal both on a normal salt diet and on a low sodium diet. There is evidence that the disturbance in mineralocorticoid excretion may become more severe as time passes.

Removal of the adenohypophysis does not prevent the appearance of diabetes insipidus in a patient with neurohypophysial damage but greatly decreases its severity. Urine volumes are seldom more than 4 to 5 liters a day, as compared to 6 to 10 liters in individuals with diabetes insipidus whose adenohypophysis is intact. The apparent improvement of diabetes insipidus in hypopituitarism can be attributed to the low rate of glomerular filtration resulting from growth hormone and adrenal steroid deficiencies and increased tubular reabsorption of water due to adrenal insufficiency. Conversely, treatment in patients with combined neural and adenohypophysial deficiency with cortisol or other cortical steroids will increase the severity of diabetes insipidus.

Hypo-osmolality without hypovolemia can occur within the first week after surgical hypophysectomy or cryohypophysectomy. Excessive administration of water to such patients can lead to dangerous water intoxication. In most cases, the hypo-osmolality is the result of inappropriate secretion of vasopressin. Adrenal insufficiency further impairs water diuresis. This limitation of free water clearance is a manifestation of cortisol and not mineralocorticoid deficiency. Whether this effect of cortisol is directly upon the renal tubule or whether cortisol lack promotes ADH secretion is still uncertain.

Four to eight weeks after the withdrawal of thyroid replacement from hypophysectomized patients, the clinical signs and symptoms of severe hypothyroidism appear. In spontaneous hypopituitarism, the appearance of clinical hypothyroidism may be delayed for 5 to 10 years. Torpor, cold intolerance, dryness of skin, and myxedema are indistinguishable in pituitary myxedema and in primary thyroidal hypofunction (Fig. 2–28). The serum protein–bound iodine reaches extremely low levels, 1 to 2 μg. per 100 ml., the basal metabolism is 25 to 35 per cent below normal, and the serum cholesterol level is usually elevated. Little radioiodine accumulates in the thyroid, and other deficiencies of iodine metabolism develop. The radioactive iodine uptake in the thyroid is restored to the normal range after 1 to 5 days of treatment with thyrotropin. Other laboratory tests of thyroid hypofunction are also corrected by thyrotropin.

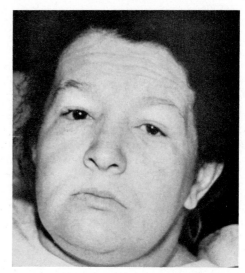

Figure 2–28. The facies of a patient with hypopituitarism. Note the myxedematous appearance and indolent expression.

Exceptional patients do not develop hypothyroidism after total hypophysectomy. Thyroid autonomy on the basis of a nodular goiter is the usual explanation. In a few cases, actual hyperthyroidism has been described. In several documented cases, this has been associated with plasma long-acting thyroid stimulator (LATS). This unusual situation provides evidence that LATS is not dependent on pituitary function.

The loss of pituitary gonadotropins after hypophysectomy leads to profound gonadal atrophy. In men, the testes are atrophic, soft, and less tender than normal to pressure. Libido and potency decrease; sperm disappear from the semen. In women, menstruation ceases; there is profound atrophy of the uterus and vagina, and libido decreases.

The overt changes in carbohydrate metabolism which occur after hypophysectomy are surprisingly few because of the compensatory decrease in insulin release. Fasting blood sugar values are lower than normal, but clinical hypoglycemia is rarely seen unless fever, diarrhea, or other stress is present. In patients who are receiving cortisone, it is difficult to demonstrate any real increase in insulin sensitivity using intravenous insulin tolerance tests.

Changes in carbohydrate metabolism are more easily recognized when hypophysectomy has been carried out on patients who previously had diabetes mellitus. The insulin requirement falls to less than one quarter the previous level. Severe, sometimes fatal, hypoglycemia is a major threat for diabetic patients who are hypophysectomized for degenerative complications. Amelioration of diabetes continues despite full maintenance doses of cortisone, indicating that GH deficiency is critical.

The appearance of the skin often provides the first clue to the presence of chronic hypopituitarism. A waxy character of the skin, often with myxedema, is most suggestive. In addition, the patient may appear to be prematurely aged because of fine wrinkles about the eyes and mouth. Melanin pigmentation usually decreases; even the areolae of the breast may become depigmented. The capacity to tan after exposure to sunlight is often lost or markedly decreased. The changes in skin pigmentation are of major diagnostic value and help to distinguish Sheehan's syndrome from Addison's disease.

Characteristic changes in body hair occur in hypopituitarism. Axillary and pubic hair becomes increasingly sparse, so that virtually none remains after several years of complete hypopituitarism (Fig. 2-29). In men, the rate of beard growth decreases; in both sexes, the total amount of general body hair is greatly lessened. The depilation of the eyebrows, so frequent in primary myxedema, also occurs in pituitary myxedema.

The notion that hypopituitarism frequently leads to cachexia persists despite much evidence to the contrary. Actually the extreme malnutrition which was described in some of the initial case reports of hypopituitarism is rarely encountered (Fig. 2-29). This emaciation was probably the result of lower standards of medical care and social welfare. Now patients with hypopituitarism are found to have a normal distribution of body weight.

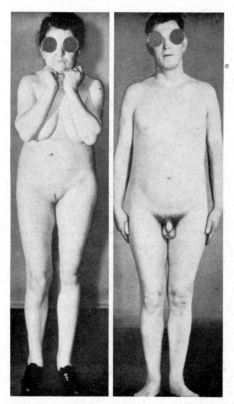

Figure 2-29. Left, hypopituitarism of 12 years' duration produced by postpartum necrosis of the adenohypophysis. Note good nutritional state, myxedematous facies, normal breasts, and absence of pubic hair. Right, hypopituitarism in a man produced by a chromophobe adenoma of the pituitary. Note the excellent nutritional state.

A moderate normocytic and normochromic anemia reflect bone marrow hypofunction in hypopituitarism. The adenohypophysis influences erythropoiesis indirectly. The humoral factor which stimulates red cell production, erythropoietin, is secreted predominantly by the kidneys, but the level or action of erythropoietin may be influenced by pituitary hormones.

Secondary hypothyroidism contributes to the anemia of hypopituitarism. In experimental animals and man, long-continued hypothyroidism may lead to decreased red cell production and a mild anemia. Thyroid replacement therapy in hypopituitarism usually is not sufficient to correct the anemia. In certain patients, the combination of thyroid and testosterone treatment will restore normal hemoglobin levels.

Other types of anemia can occur in hypopituitarism. Severe hemorrhage usually accompanies the onset of Sheehan's syndrome, and iron deficits may be imperfectly replaced. A number of patients with chronic hypopituitarism have pernicious anemia. Whether this association is fortuitous or not has not been determined.

Differential Diagnosis

Panhypopituitarism must be distinguished from a number of conditions commonly exhibiting similar clinical manifestations. Chronic malnutrition leads to decreased secretion of ACTH, TSH, and gonadotropins, but GH secretion may be increased. The term *anorexia nervosa* is applied to individuals whose malnutrition is attributable to a psychogenic disturbance in eating. The majority of cases of anorexia nervosa occur in unmarried women between the ages of 15 and 35 years. Anorexia nervosa is not a distinct psychiatric entity, but a clinical feature found in a number of psychic illnesses, including psychoneurosis and schizophrenia. For some patients, food and the process of eating have assumed an unacceptable sexual significance. Morbid fears of abdominal fullness as an indication of pregnancy may be expressed. In other patients, anorexia may be a more simple attention-seeking device. The disease can be distinguished from true hypopituitarism in most cases by (1) the infrequency of marked wasting in hypopituitarism, (2) preservation of axillary and pubic hair in anorexia nervosa, (3) higher levels of urinary steroid excretion in anorexia nervosa, and (4) normal or elevated concentration of plasma HGH.

Pituitary myxedema may be difficult to distinguish clinically from thyroidal myxedema because the general slowing of body processes, the cutaneous findings of myxedema, the loss of axillary and pubic hair, and the low excretion of urinary corticosteroids are common to both conditions. Plasma cortisol is usually normal in primary (thyroidal) myxedema and low in secondary (pituitary) myxedema.

The diagnosis of hypopituitarism is often suspected when testicular atrophy is combined with general debility in men with profound liver disease or myotonia atrophica. In most cases the underlying primary disease process can be recognized and simple hypopituitarism ruled out by laboratory procedures. Morphologic evidence of extensive pituitary destruction is rarely found at necropsy in these diseases.

Establishing the Diagnosis

An unequivocal diagnosis of panhypopituitarism must be established before a patient is committed to a lifetime of replacement therapy. Two lines of evidence help establish the diagnosis of hypopituitarism in a patient with compatible symptoms and physical findings: (a) evidence of a possible cause of pituitary damage, (b) laboratory evidence of hormonal deficiencies.

The great majority of cases of pituitary insufficiency of the adult are the result of pituitary tumor or postpartum necrosis of the pituitary. Careful roentgenograms of the sella turcica and determination of visual fields will usually demonstrate pituitary tumors of significance. When sellar enlargement is present, pneumoencephalograms are indicated to rule out the empty sella syndrome. Historical evidence of catastrophic postpartum collapse can be obtained in most patients with Sheehan's syndrome, but 20 or more years may intervene from the accident of pregnancy before the diagnosis of hypopituitarism is suspected.

Laboratory procedures for demonstrating hormonal deficiencies are now highly developed. It is unnecessary to document all the hormonal biochemical abnormalities existing in hypopituitarism, but procedures of proved differential value should be selected. Elaborate studies of carbohydrate and insulin tolerance are nonspecific and dangerous. Direct radioimmunoassay measurements of pituitary hormones in blood have made these indirect indices obsolete.

If urine and plasma corticosteroids are unequivocally low and a normal response to ACTH is present, it is safe to conclude that hypocorticotropism exists. When the corticosteroid levels are normal or borderline, documentation of impaired corticotropin secretory reserve requires the administration of metyrapone. By inhibiting 11-beta hydroxylase, this drug lowers cortisol secretion, thereby stimulating ACTH. The effects of increased endogenous ACTH are best documented by measuring the rise in plasma 11-deoxycortisol or by a rise in urinary 17–hydroxycorticosteroids (Porter-Silber chromogens) (Fig. 5–15). A failure of urinary 17-OH corticosteroids to double baseline values is evidence of decreased corticotropin reserve.

Metyrapone is given for 1 or 2 days in doses of 750 mg. by mouth every 4 hours to adults; children are given 15 mg. per kg. of body weight. Alternatively, metyrapone tartrate, 30 mg. per kg. of body weight, can be given intravenously for 4 hours, and urine 17-OH corticosteroids are measured on the day of administration.

The most direct method of distinguishing hypothyroidism which results from pituitary failure from that which is the result of primary thyroid disease is by measuring thyrotropin in the plasma (Fig. 2–13). In primary hypothyroidism, elevations of TSH invariably occur. When plasma TSH cannot be determined, thyroidal uptake of radioiodine can be measured before and after TSH administration (Fig. 2–30). The dose of TSH varies from clinic to clinic, but administration of 10 units of bovine

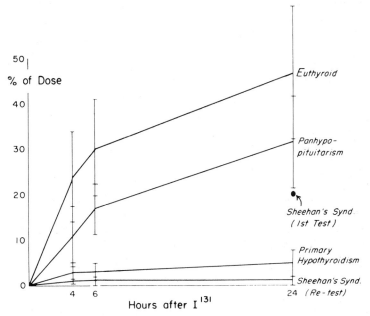

Figure 2–30.   Patients with hypothyroidism secondary to TSH deficiency respond with a major increase in radioiodine uptake after TSH injections (5 U. daily for 3 days), but those with myxedema caused by primary thyroid deficiency do not. Vertical bars indicate the standard deviation for each point. (From Taunton, O. D., McDaniel, H. G., et al.: *J. Clin. Endocr.* 25:266, 1965.)

TSH daily for 2 days should be sufficient to induce an increase in I^{131} thyroidal uptake to normal or supranormal levels. Unfortunately, the test is not entirely definitive. Some patients who have had hypopituitarism for many years have such complete thyroid involution that an increase in I^{131} thyroidal uptake may not be noted. If TSH levels are low in the presence of hypothyroidism, this could be the result of hypothalamic as well as pituitary disease. Differentiation of these two possibilities can be made by administering TRH. A rise in plasma TSH would indicate hypothalamic disease.

Growth hormone secretion can be evaluated best by measurement of plasma concentrations with immunoassay (see section on pituitary dwarfism).

Radioimmunoassays of LH and FSH in plasma urine are most helpful in the evaluation of hypopituitarism in women beyond the menopause. In this age group, gonadotropins are normally high. Gonadotropin measurements are less helpful in younger women and in men, in which cases clear distinctions between the levels observed in hypopituitary patients and in hospitalized nonendocrine patients are less evident. LH secretory capacity can be tested by measuring plasma LH before and after the administration of 100 mg. of clomiphene daily or after administration of luteinizing hormone releasing factor.

Measurements of plasma prolactin are of limited value in establishing the diagnosis of hypopituitarism. If all pituitary tissue has been destroyed, prolactin levels will be low, but many patients with partial hypopituitarism have normal or elevated plasma prolactin concentrations. This is most evident after stalk section, in which case plasma prolactin may be greatly elevated in the presence of clinical hypopituitarism. Elevated prolactin levels often are an indication of hypothalamic disease or interruption of the pituitary stalk.

Therapeutic Treatment. Replacement of pituitary hormones, although theoretically sound, has little practical use. The expense and discomfort of injections are objectionable. Human hormones are not generally available, but antibodies often develop to animal hormones which neutralize biologic activity. Fortunately, potent hormonal preparations are readily available to replace the secretions of the adrenals, thyroid, and gonads.

Experience dictates that a gradual restoration of thyroid hormone should be instituted. An initial dose of 30 mg. of desiccated thyroid (0.05 mg. of L-thyroxine) is prudent. Triiodothyronine would be preferable in the treatment of coma because of the faster onset of action, but it is not available in the United States for parenteral administration. Therefore, thyroxine must be given. The dose of desiccated thyroid is increased gradually over a period of 1 to 2 months to a full maintenance dose of 120 to 180 mg. (0.2 to 0.3 mg. L-thyroxine).

Replacement treatment with corticosteroids is mandatory if pituitary destruction is complete, and desirable if hypopituitarism is moderate. It may be reserved for periods of increased physiologic stress in mild hypopituitarism. Relatively small doses are required, 12.5 to 37.5 mg. of cortisone acetate or its equivalent of the newer synthetic analogues. During fever, gastrointestinal upsets, or surgical procedures, larger doses are indicated. There is no need to prescribe mineralocorticoids routinely to patients with hypopituitarism if they salt their foods normally.

The administration of androgens to men with hypopituitarism will usually improve general strength and vigor, as well as restore libido and potency. Methyltestosterone, in doses of 20 to 30 mg. daily by mouth, is sufficient. Some patients prefer to receive an intramuscular injection of a slowly absorbed preparation such as testosterone enanthate, 200 mg. every 2 to 3 weeks. Estrogen replacement is desirable in young women to correct vaginal mucosal atrophy and for its extragenital action on skin and bone.

Restoration of fertility is now possible with human pituitary gonadotropins. In women, preparatory treatment with FSH-containing preparations from human pituitaries or postmenopausal human urine for 10 to 14 days will stimulate ovarian follicular development. Ovulation is achieved by administration of human chorionic gonadotropin. Restoration of male fertility is more difficult and requires prolonged administration of FSH and chorionic gonadotropin preparations.

With replacement of all target gland hormonal deficiencies, the clinical response is gratifying to both patient and physician. The patient with severe hypopituitarism is transformed from a vegetating invalid to an active member of society. The signs of hypothyroidism disappear. Energy and strength increase nearly to normal. If provision is made for increased doses of corticosteroids during periods of metabolic stress, the prognosis for a long and useful life is excellent.

Isolated Hormonal Deficiencies

A deficiency in the release of a single pituitary hormone may occur. Hypogonadism may be the only clinically recognizable sign associated with incomplete pituitary destruction, but with more rigorous tests of pituitary reserve, other deficiencies are usually demonstrated. More interesting are the case reports of patients without gross destructive lesions of the pituitary who nonetheless exhibit clinical and laboratory signs of unihormonal insufficiency. It is likely that hypothalamic dysfunction accounts for some of these cases.

The evidence for selective deficiency in gonadotropic hormones is most clearly established. The condition known as hypogonadotropic eunuchoidism has been well characterized (Chapter 6). The analogous syndrome in women of amenorrhea secondary to decreased gonadotropin secretion is also well defined. Hypogonadotropic eunuchoidism associated with hyposmia (Kallman's syndrome) is a familial disorder in which other members of the family may be sexually normal but still have the hyposmia. Hypogonadotropic eunuchoidism is characterized by gonadal inactivity, little or no gonadotropins in urine and plasma, and responses of the gonad to exogenous gonadotropins.

Isolated deficiency of corticotropin secretion is a definite clinical entity. Symptoms such as weakness, hypoglycemia, weight loss, and decreased female sex hair suggest the diagnosis. The urinary steroid levels are low; they increase to normal after ACTH treatment but do not rise after administration of metyrapone. To make the diagnosis, clinical and laboratory evidence of other pituitary hormone deficiencies must be absent.

Isolated deficiency of TSH can lead to clinical hypothyroidism. For unknown reasons, isolated TSH deficiency has been reported in pseudohypoparathyroidism. The diagnosis can be accepted if the plasma TSH levels are low, if there is a definite increase in radioiodine uptake or plasma T_4 after administration of bovine TSH for one or more days, and if other pituitary functions are normal. Administration of thyrotropin releasing hormone (TRH) will cause TSH secretion in those patients in whom the defect in TSH secretion is the result of hypothalamic dysfunction.

The existence of isolated prolactin deficiency has recently been recognized by Turkington (63) in two patients who repeatedly failed to lactate after delivery. Basal prolactin levels are low, and no response to phenothiazine challenge occurs.

Isolated growth hormone deficiency has now been established in many cases of dwarfism. This will be described at length in the next section.

Pituitary Dwarfism

Deficiency of GH secretion by the fetal or maternal pituitary has little influence on fetal growth. Even anencephalic monsters lacking both brain and pituitary have relatively normal somatic size at birth. The growth hormone concentration of fetal plasma is high in the last months of gestation and may exert a slight effect on fetal growth because newborn infants with congenital growth hormone deficiency are statistically slightly shorter than the average normal infant. When carefully measured, growth velocity of hyposomatotropic dwarfs begins to lag within the early months of life. Physical growth continues at less than half the normal rate. The period of growth, however, is prolonged into the third and fourth decades, and height eventually reaches 4 to 5 feet.

The etiology of pituitary dwarfism is varied. Skull films will reveal evidence of craniopharyngioma or pituitary tumor in about a third of the cases. Most children with tumors will grow normally for a period of years with later failure of skeletal growth. In some patients, large areas of bone lysis in the skull, usually combined with diabetes insipidus, are diagnostic of histiocytosis. When the sella turcica is normal in size, the etiology of pituitary dwarfism usually cannot be determined.

In some patients, midline defects such as cleft palate, absence of the septum pellucidum, and nystagmus indicate involvement of the pituitary in a more general embryonic malformation. The basic defect in some may lie in the hypothalamic somatotropin-regulating centers.

A small fraction of the cases are familial. Analysis of a number of pedigrees of the familial form of hyposomatotropism indicates that it is transmitted by a recessive gene. The pituitary dysfunction is usually limited to the secretion of somatotropin. A delayed but otherwise normal puberty occurs. The affected women can become pregnant and deliver normal sized offspring. Lactation appears at the expected time because prolactin secretion is normal. The diagnosis of growth hormone deficiency in these patients has been unequivocally established by radioimmunoassay.

Most cases of pituitary dwarfism have no familial basis and are not the result of any recognizable disease process affecting the pituitary gland. In about a third of the cases, isolated GH deficiency is present. In the remaining cases, other pituitary deficiencies exist. Boys are affected twice as often as girls. Gestation and birth histories are generally normal, and the size and appearance of the infants at birth are unremarkable. Although growth failure may be recognized as early as 6 months, more frequently this is not recognized by pediatrician or parents until the child is 1 to 3 years of age. Body proportions and facial features remain immature. Many of the affected children are pudgy, with deposition of fat over the iliac crests and lower abdomen (Fig. 2–31). Primary teeth appear at the expected age, but the eruption of secondary teeth is delayed. In adult life, many pituitary dwarfs develop fine wrinkles about the mouth and eyes which give an appearance of immaturity combined with presenility.

General health often remains surprisingly good with normal responses to illness and trauma. Only about 10 per cent of the subjects suffer from symptomatic hypoglycemia. Low fasting blood sugars and impaired glucose tolerance are more common. The insulin response to glucose is usually subnormal.

Mental development usually keeps up with chronologic age, and, because of small stature, these children seem unusually bright. At first, adverse emotional reactions to small stature may not be recognized, but psychologic adjustment becomes increasingly difficult when their cohorts enter puberty.

Radiographic examination of the wrist is an important procedure in evaluating growth problems. In pituitary dwarfism, epiphysial maturation is retarded to the same extent as height.

While the clinical picture may suggest pituitary dwarfism, diagnosis can be accepted only when confirmed by radioimmunoassay. A single determination of plasma growth hormone in the basal state is of limited usefulness because the basal plasma levels of most normal children are so low that they cannot be differentiated with confidence from those of hypopituitary dwarfs. For this reason, growth hormone determinations should be carried out after provocative challenge. The greatest experience in this area has been derived from the induction of hypoglycemia with 0.05 to 0.1 unit

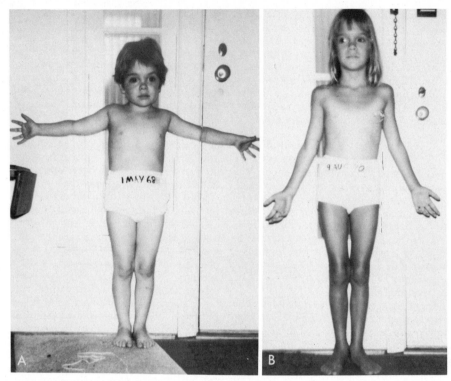

Figure 2–31. *A*, A 6-year-old girl with hyposomatotropic dwarfism secondary to a craniopharyngioma. Note infantile chubbiness and facial features. Height, 37 inches. *B*, Fifteen months later after she had been treated with 2.5 mg. of HGH twice weekly, her height had increased to 48¼ inches. In addition to her gain in height, note her obvious loss of infantile fat and more mature facial features.

regular insulin per kg. of body weight given intravenously (Fig. 2–20). A physician should be in attendance, and glucose should be available to abort serious symptoms. The administration of arginine has proved an equally effective stimulus for growth hormone secretion (Fig. 2–27). A dose of 0.5 gm. per kg. of neutralized arginine hydrochloride given intravenously over 30 minutes has proved just as helpful in the diagnosis of hypopituitarism and much better tolerated than insulin-induced hypoglycemia. The oral administration of L-dopa, 10 mg. per kg. of body weight in children and 0.5 gm. in adults, is an effective provocative challenge. Peak levels of GH are usually reached between 45 and 90 minutes. The patients should be lying down after L-dopa administration to prevent postural hypotension. Mild nausea may occur. Other provocative tests that have been advocated include Pyromen and glucagon administration. These agents have not been widely accepted. A rise of plasma GH to greater than 10 ng. per ml. is normal. Plasma levels between 5 and 10 ng. are equivocal, and levels less than 5 ng. per ml. are abnormal. In some normal patients, initial values may be elevated due to stress. A fall in subsequent plasma samples may occur. A substantial number of normal men and a few children will respond inadequately to pituitary stimulation. Pretreatment with 3 mg. of stilbestrol for 2 days may increase the growth hormone response.

Differential Diagnosis

Only a minority of children with short stature and normal body proportions who are brought to the physician have pituitary dwarfism.

A type of growth failure occurs in certain young children with bad home situations characterized by parental neglect and deprivation of love and affection. These children may exhibit distortions of appetite with perversions such as eating from garbage cans and stealing food. Abdominal bloating and a clinical picture resembling malabsorption may exist. With placement in a supportive environment, such as a metabolic ward or convalescent center, rapid acquisition of positive nitrogen balance and rapid resumption or "catch-up" growth may occur. There is incomplete evidence that this syndrome is the result of functional hyposomatotropism on the basis of psychic factors. The rapid reversibility of the "emotional deprivation" syndrome makes definitive study virtually impossible.

Functional GH deficiency may exist in certain patients with "constitutional" growth retardation. Some children are not as short as true pituitary dwarfs but show little or no rise in plasma GH after provocative tests unless primed with estrogens. Normal GH secretion follows puberty or androgen therapy, and relatively normal height is obtained. It is postulated that sex steroids sensitize the GH secretory mechanism.

A type of familial dwarfism exists which is indistinguishable clinically from pituitary dwarfism but characterized by high plasma GH concentrations (Laron dwarfism). Most reported cases have occurred in oriental Jews and other middle eastern peoples. The trait is transmitted as a mendelian recessive. Characteristically somatomedin (SF) concentrations are low and do not rise in response to GH (Fig. 2–32). Moreover, acute metabolic responses to GH are subnormal, and growth stimulation with prolonged therapy disappointing. This disorder can best be explained as a general disorder of GH receptors.

The growth disturbance in African pygmies is more complex. These people have normal plasma GH responses to provocative stimuli, and somatomedin concentrations are normal. They do show impaired nitrogen sparing and lipolytic actions of GH. Insulin secretion in response to glucose is subnormal and not improved by GH treatment. This disorder seems to be the result of a polygenic inheritance conferring resistance both to GH and somatomedin (SF) actions.

Hypothyroidism, starting either in infancy (cretinism) or in childhood (juvenile myxedema), is an important cause of growth retardation. The clinical features of hypothyroidism usually permit clinical diagnosis (Chapter 4). Bone maturation is greatly retarded in cretinism, and abnormal multicentric areas of epiphysial ossification may be present, most evident in the femoral head.

The short stature of patients with gonadal dysplasia is often confused with pituitary dwarfism. Growth retardation is only moderate, and bone maturation is little impaired. The diagnosis may be strongly suspected in short girls with primary amenorrhea and congenital anomalies, such as webbing of the neck, short metacarpal or metatarsal bones, increased carrying angle of the elbows, and coarctation of the aorta. Rarely the short stature may be associated with gonadal dysplasia without external congenital anomalies. Cytologic examination of the buccal smear should be included in the diagnostic evaluation of all stunted girls. The absence of the normal female chromatin body will permit unequivocal recognition of 80 per cent of individuals with gonadal dysplasia. In doubtful cases, complete characterization of the karyotype is desirable. Patients have been described with XO/XX or other X chromosomal mosaicism who present with short stature and few of the classical features of Turner's syndrome.

Growth failure can follow any serious systemic disease or nutritional deficiency in childhood. Prolonged corticosteroid therapy in children frequently causes growth impairment and delayed bone maturation. As corticosteroids can inhibit the release of growth hormone following hypoglycemia, it is possible that growth hormone insufficiency may contribute to the syndrome. However, the administration of growth hormone while corticosteroids are continued usually will not permit normal growth.

Retarded growth occurs in a number of congenital diseases, such as vitamin D–resistant rickets, Laurence-Moon-Biedl syndrome, mongolism, achondroplasia, neurofibromatosis, severe congenital heart disease, congenital hemolytic anemias, and progeria. Because the underlying disease is usually evident, distinguishing these disturbances in growth from pituitary dwarfism rarely presents problems.

Treatment. Administration of human growth hormone to pituitary dwarfs leads to a marked acceleration of growth with doses as small as 2.5 mg. twice a week (Fig. 2–33). Increases in height of 4 to 6 inches are frequently achieved within the first year. Thereafter, more moderate growth rates are encountered and higher doses of hormone may be required to maintain accelerated growth. An occasional child will respond initially but subsequently prove refractory. High levels of antibody against human growth hormone have been found in the plasma of a few such patients. In other cases, the refractoriness remains unexplained. Withholding the hormone for several months may restore the response to subsequent growth hormone administration.

Thus far supplies of human growth hormone in the United States have depended on a nationwide collection of cadaver pituitaries which has been conducted by the National Pituitary Agency. The growth hormone has been allocated for clinical investigation. Additional supplies of the hormone are urgently needed. The availability of synthetic growth hormone for therapeutic purposes is still years away.

Other therapeutic agents are of limited value in treatment of hyposomatotropism. Thyroid deficiency should be corrected, but overtreatment may cause excessive advancement of bone maturation. Cortisone treatment should be avoided, if possible, but may be required if hypoglycemia is a problem.

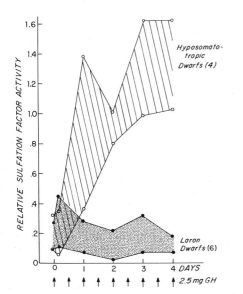

Figure 2–32. Comparison of somatomedin (sulfation factor) activity of hyposomatotropic and hypersomatotropic (Laron) dwarfs before and after twice-daily GH administration. (Reproduced from Daughaday, W. H., Laron, Z., et al.: *Trans. Ass. Amer. Physicians* 82:129, 1969, with permission.)

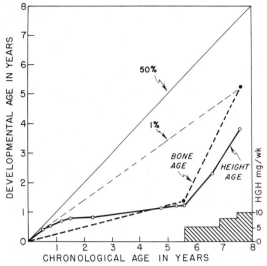

Figure 2–33. Extreme retardation of skeletal age and height age in a pituitary dwarf, plotted according to the convention of Lawson Wilkins. The rapid advancement of growth and bone maturation after treatment with human growth hormone is also shown. (Reproduced from Daughaday, W. H., and Parker, M. L.: *Disease-a-Month*, August, 1962, by permission of Year Book Medical Publishers, Inc.)

Androgenic steroids have a restricted use for patients who are refractory to human growth hormone or for children over 12 years for whom growth hormone is not available. If care is taken to prescribe a minimal dose of a metabolic androgen, stimulation of growth without undue virilization or prohibitive advance in bone maturation can be achieved. Eventual height may be increased slightly and growth obtained at a time appropriate for psychologic development. In the past, excessive doses have been used with the unfortunate result of premature closure of the epiphysis.

PITUITARY TUMORS

Pathology. Localized nests of cellular proliferation and small asymptomatic adenomas are found in one quarter of human pituitary glands examined at necropsy. Larger pituitary adenomas account for about 10 per cent of all intracranial tumors. Pituitary tumors have important complications of parasellar extension and dramatic syndromes of hormonal hypersecretion. Adenohypophysial tumors are still classified according to the staining characteristics of the secretory granules into chromophobe, acidophil, or basophil types, although more than one cell type may occur in an individual tumor. From a clinical point of view, it would be preferable to classify these tumors by their secretory products. It is convenient also to include craniopharyngiomas in a discussion of pituitary tumors; despite their origin from cells unrelated to the pituitary, the clinical problems presented by these tumors resemble those of chromophobe adenomas.

Chromophobe Adenomas. These account for 85 per cent of pituitary tumors. Men and women are affected with equal frequency. Chromophobe adenomas occur in individuals of all ages, but there is a definite predominance (78 per cent) in the third, fourth, and fifth decades; cases with onset before the age of 9 years are decidedly unusual. Chromophobe tumors rarely occur in siblings or parents of affected patients, but a tendency for individuals with parathyroid or islet cell adenomas to have pituitary adenomas (generally chromophobe) has been recognized. While chromophobe adenomas are usually considered nonsecretory, this is untrue in many cases in which radioimmunoassay evidence of secretion of one or more pituitary hormones can be found.

Chromophobe tumor cells often contain sparse fine granulation with the periodic acid-Schiff stain. Granules are more easily recognized and classified by electron microscopy (Fig. 2–34). Some chromophobe tumors become very large and extend into the posterior fossa or invade the hypothalamus and neighboring structures. Others may demonstrate their malignant nature by bursting the diaphragma sellae and widely infiltrating local tissues. Rarely, distant implantation of tumor in remote portions of the central nervous system takes place. Isolated examples of metastases in the liver and other organs outside the central nervous system have been reported.

Acidophilic adenomas account for 10 to 14 per cent of pituitary tumors, even though 37 to 49 per cent of the cells of the normal pituitary are acidophils. The sex and age distribution does not differ significantly from that reported for chromophobe adenomas. The acidophilic tumor cells contain the same secretory granules possessed by the normal lactotropic cell (Fig. 2–35) and somatotropic cell (Fig. 2–36), although greater variability in size and shape is evident by electron microscopy. On the whole, eosinophilic adenomas grow more slowly than chromophobe tumors, and distant metastases are practically never observed.

Basophilic adenomas of the pituitary are rarely of significant size and are infrequently recognized before necropsy. Their possible relation to Cushing's syndrome is discussed later in this chapter.

Craniopharyngiomas are the most important nonpituitary tumors arising in the vicinity of the sella turcica. They are believed to arise from remnants of Rathke's pouch. These tumors vary greatly in structure from simple cysts containing dark oily fluid to solid tumors composed of columnar cells on a basement membrane in a pattern which resembles adamantinomas. Occasionally squamous cells with masses of cornified tissue replace the columnar cells in areas of the tumor. They are more commonly suprasellar rather than intrasellar in location. The frequent occurrence of areas of calcification is a helpful diagnostic characteristic for the radiologist, suggesting craniopharyngioma rather than some other type of pituitary neoplasm.

Meningiomas, chordomas, teratoid tumors, and metastatic tumors of varied origin may involve the

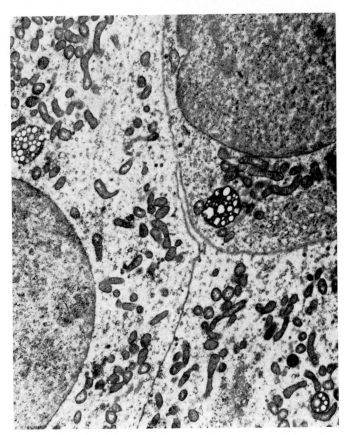

Figure 2–34. Chromophobe adenoma with parts of three cells evident. The nuclei are of regular outline. The mitochondria are numerous, and interspersed among them are round, dense foci of wear-and-tear pigment (lipofuscin). Part of the vesicles of the Golgi apparatus are present at the lower right. Scattered small granules are present in the cytoplasm, but very few in comparison to those of the normal pituitary basophil or acidophil (× 12,500). (Courtesy of Doctor Sarah Luse, Department of Pathology, Washington University School of Medicine.)

sella turcica and mimic chromophobe adenomas clinically.

Experimental Tumors. Pituitary tumors occur spontaneously or can be experimentally induced in a number of animal species, especially in rats and mice. In many cases, the tumor develops after the induction of a hypersecretory state. Thyroidectomy can lead to the development of TSH-secreting tumors in mice, and gonadectomy has led to pituitary tumors which secrete gonadotropins and corticotropin. Estrogen administration stimulates the pituitary lactotropic cells and has led to tumors which secrete prolactin and GH. The development of pituitary tumors with these endocrine manipu-

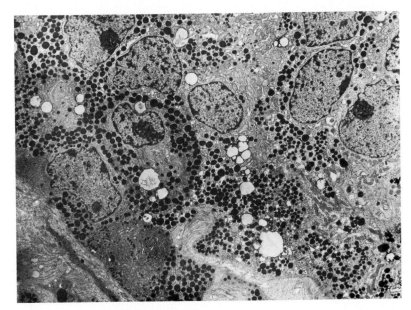

Figure 2–35. Electron micrograph of a lactotrope tumor cell from a patient with Forbes-Albright syndrome. Despite the similarity in appearance to the somatotrope cell, this tumor contained little or no growth hormone and easily detected prolactin. The granules are more varied in size and shape than somatotrope granules (× 4,680). (Courtesy of Dr. D. W. McKeel.)

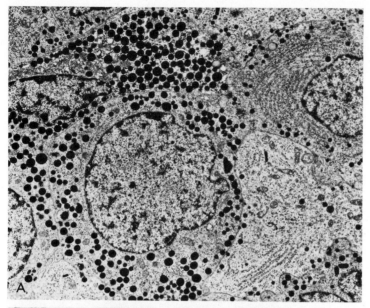

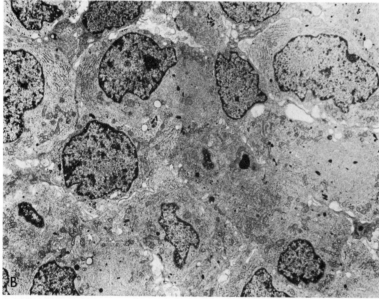

Figure 2–36. *A*, Electron micrograph of a somatotrope tumor cell from a patient with acromegaly. Note the uniform electron-dense granules, which are essentially normal in number and only slightly more variable in size than normal (× 10,080). *B*, Electron micrograph of a somatotrope tumor cell from a patient with acromegaly. Note the rare electron-dense secretory granules. Such tumors appear to consist of chromophobe cells by standard staining and light microscopy (× 4,680). (Courtesy of Dr. D. W. McKeel.)

lations is increased by radiation. At present, experimental pituitary tumors have been characterized which secrete MSH, ACTH, TSH, GH, and prolactin. Successful transplantation of some of these tumors requires a hormonally deficient recipient, indicating that tumor growth is not truly autonomous. Other tumors are not so fastidious and may be maintained in tissue culture. Secretory cell lines derived from single cells have been successfully propagated. The etiologic relation of hormonal hypersecretion to the experimental development of pituitary tumors may have relevance in man. Gonadectomy in man may be associated with increased incidence of pituitary tumors, and adrenalectomy in Cushing's syndrome probably predisposes to the development of ACTH-secreting tumors.

Local Manifestations. A pituitary tumor may bring the patient to the physician because of signs of an expanding intrasellar or parasellar mass or the effects of hormonal secretion. The local consequences of an enlarging pituitary mass are common to all tumor types and depend on the direction and extent of tumor growth. Initially, a pituitary tumor is confined to the sella turcica by the fibrous diaphragma sellae. Pressure of the expanding mass leads to erosion of the bony walls of the sella, which can be recognized by a ballooning of the sella on the roentgenogram of the skull. The floor of the sella is often depressed into the sphenoid sinus. The anterior and posterior clinoids rotate upward and away from the mass and become indistinct on x-ray films because of extensive osteoporosis.

The recognition of small degrees of sellar enlargement presents difficulties because of the normal variation in sellar size. Porosis of the clinoid processes takes place spontaneously with age and is accelerated by increased intracranial pressure. The upper limit of size of the sella is 12 mm. in depth and 15 mm. in length in the lateral x-ray projection. Measurement of the lateral area of the sella either with a planimeter or with semitransparent ruled paper provides a more accurate estimation of size. The area in normal adults is less than 130 square mm. Careful observations of the projected area of the sella turcica in children of different ages are reproduced in Figure 2–37. Moderate enlargement of the sella turcica can be demonstrated by such refined techniques in association with the pituitary hypertrophy which occurs in pregnancy or after prolonged hypothyroidism in children.

Loss of vision due to pressure on the optic nerves is one of the commonest complaints of patients with pituitary tumors. As the tumor presses upward from the bony confines of the sella turcica, the optic chiasm and optic nerves are at first displaced superiorly. Continued displacement is prevented by the anterior arterial arc of the circle of Willis (Fig. 2–1) which overlies the optic nerves and serves as a nonyielding constricting band against which the optic nerves are compressed. Most tumors protrude between the two arms of the optic nerves and exert pressure on the inferior medial aspects of the nerves. With this type of impingement, the earliest losses of visual field are recognized in the superior temporal quadrant. Later a quadratic loss of the visual field extends to hemianopsia. Further damage to the optic nerves leads to scotomas, loss of vision in the nasal fields, and finally total blindness.

Extensive damage to the optic nerve leads to pallor of the optic disk. Papilledema is rare. Anisocoria occurs if the loss in vision in one eye greatly exceeds that in the other. Because of the vagaries of tumor growth and the anatomic variations in the location of the optic chiasm, other patterns of visual loss may occur. Repeated examinations of the visual fields are an essential part of the management of pituitary tumors. Accurate measurements are particularly urgent during periods of radiation therapy, when swelling of the tumor can result in sudden worsening of vision.

Headaches are a troublesome complaint of more than three quarters of the patients with pituitary tumors. Traction on the diaphragma sellae or surrounding dural structures would appear to be the most common cause of headache. The lining of the sphenoid sinus and the walls of large blood vessels in the region of the sella are also capable of giving rise to painful sensations. The location of the headache is inconstant: in one large series of patients with chromophobe adenomas, 31 per cent were frontal, 19 per cent orbital, 16 per cent temporal, 10 per cent occipital, 7 per cent vertical, and 2 per cent generalized; in the remaining 15 per cent, the headaches were insufficiently characterized for tabulation. Most commonly, the headaches are of moderate severity and intermittent. Occasionally headaches are accompanied by nausea and vomiting.

Involvement of cranial nerves, other than the optic nerves, occurs infrequently (17 per cent of patients with chromophobe tumors) despite the proximity of the third, fourth, and sixth cranial nerves

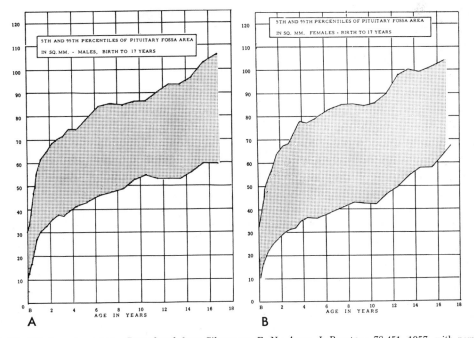

Figure 2–37. Pituitary fossa area. (Reproduced from Silverman, F. N.: *Amer. J. Roentgen. 78*:451, 1957, with permission.)

to any sellar mass expanding superiorly. Impairments of third nerve function are recognized more frequently than those of other cranial nerves. Occasionally the olfactory nerves or tracts are disrupted, with loss of the sense of smell.

Large pituitary tumors may compress or infiltrate the hypothalamus, producing a variety of manifestations, such as disturbances in appetite, sleep, and temperature regulation. Focal seizures, occasionally of the uncinate type, may take place. Deficiencies of adenohypophysial function occurring in suprasellar tumors may be the result of damage to the hypothalamic centers regulating adenohypophysial function.

Pituitary tumors may invade the large vessels that ring the sella turcica, with subsequent thrombosis or hemorrhage. The blood supply of pituitary tumors is easily impaired, and infarctions of tumors followed by cystic degeneration are common. Hemorrhage into a tumor, "pituitary apoplexy," leads to severe headache, abrupt loss of vision, mental obtundity, hypotension, and hyperthermia. Prompt evacuation of the clots and control of bleeding may save life and vision.

Hormonal Deficiencies.   Normal pituitary tissue may be compressed to a shell about a tumor mass, in which case the clinical evidences of hypopituitarism correlate roughly with the degree of destruction of normal tissue. Symptoms are usually not detected unless more than three quarters of the pituitary has been destroyed. Even with very large tumors, the signs of hormonal deficiency rarely equal in severity those which occur after hypophysectomy. Hypogonadism is usually the earliest sign of hypopituitarism, occurring in 69 per cent of men and 84 per cent of the women with chromophobe adenomas. Symptoms of hypothyroidism are present in 70 per cent of patients with chromophobe adenomas. Adrenal insufficiency rarely is symptomatic except under conditions of severe stress, but corticotropin reserve is commonly lost, as demonstrated by the failure of the urinary steroids to increase after the administration of metyrapone. The excretions of 17-ketosteroids and 17-hydroxycorticosteroids are generally low in patients with large tumors.

Disruption of the neurohypophysial regulation of water metabolism leading to diabetes insipidus only occurs in about 10 per cent of untreated cases of pituitary tumors. Patients with untreated acidophilic or basophilic tumors almost never have diabetes insipidus. Minor disturbances of water regulation are easily overlooked unless careful measurements of the osmolality of urine and plasma are made in the hydropenic state. Following surgical treatment of pituitary tumors, transitory or permanent diabetes insipidus frequently develops.

Endocrine Activity of Pituitary Tumors

Clinical syndromes of hypersecretion of four pituitary hormones have been recognized in association with pituitary neoplasms. These are the following: somatotropin (gigantism and acromegaly), prolactin (persistent lactation), corticotropin, and melanocyte stimulating hormone (pigmentation after treatment of Cushing's syndrome). Rarely, thyrotropin and gonadotropins may be secreted by tumors.

Hypersomatotropism

Clinical Characteristics.   The frequency of certain of the manifestations of acromegaly is given in Table 2–4. Excessive growth of the acral parts usually begins insidiously in the third to the fifth decade. Less commonly, the disease starts before puberty and leads to proportionate growth (gigantism). Rarely, more than one member of a family may suffer from the disease, but generally there is no recognizable hereditary influence.

The progressive facial and acral changes develop so gradually that neither family nor friends recognize the transformation until it is well advanced. A book of snapshot photographs taken over the years is more helpful than the patient's memory in charting the course of the disease (Fig. 2–38).

The variability of the course of acromegaly deserves emphasis. Overgrowth may be slight and the period of progression short. Harvey Cushing termed these cases "fugitive acromegaly." Even when the disease is more severe, there is a ten-

TABLE 2–4.   ACROMEGALY: FREQUENCY OF MANIFESTATIONS

	Per Cent
Parasellar Manifestations	
Enlarged sella	93 (80–93)
Headache	87 (75–87)
Visual impairment	62 (5–62)
Uncinate fits	7
Rhinorrhea	15
Pituitary apoplexy	(3)
Papilledema	3
Growth Hormone Excess	
Weight gain	39
Hypermetabolism	70
Hyperhidrosis	60
Impaired glucose tolerance	25 (37)
Clinical diabetes mellitus	12 (13)
Acral growth	100
Prognathism	Common
Arthritic complaints	(64)
Osteoporosis	Common
Soft tissue growth	100
Hypertrichosis	53
Pigmentation	40
Fibroma molluscum	27
Visceromegaly	Common
Goiter	25
Disturbances of Other Hormones	
Lactorrhea (?prolactin excess)	4
Hyperadrenocorticism	Rare
Hyperthyroidism	Rare
Increased libido	38
Decreased libido, male	23

Most of the data for the preparation of this chart were obtained from Davidoff. When other sources were used, the figures are placed in parentheses.

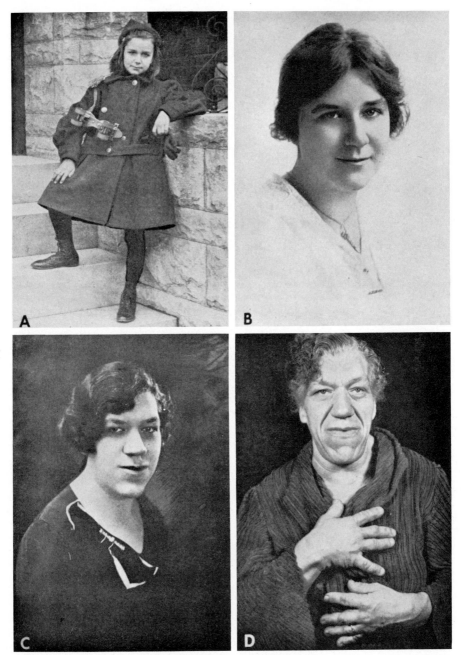

Figure 2–38. The progression of acromegaly is illustrated in these photographs. *A*, normal, age 9 years; *B*, age 16 years with possible early coarsening of features; *C*, age 33 years, well-established acromegaly; *D*, age 52 years, end stage acromegaly with gross disfigurement. (Reproduced from Clinical Pathological Conference. *Amer. J. Med. 20*:133, 1956, with permission.)

dency for obvious growth to cease after a period of years.

There are several explanations for this tendency of the disease to "burn out." In some cases, hormonal hypersecretion has ceased because of infarction of the tumor. In other cases, growth of acral parts is no longer observed despite continued presence of excessive growth hormone in the plasma. With constant hypersecretion of growth hormone, acral growth and soft tissue proliferation are not necessarily progressive. A similar plateauing of growth is observed with rats treated with growth hormone.

The pattern of growth induced by somatotropin hypersecretion is determined by age and genetic factors. Before epiphysial plates are fused, the long bones participate in proportionate growth and gigantism results. The extraordinary giants, such as the Alton giant, attained their great height because of the early onset and sustained hyper-

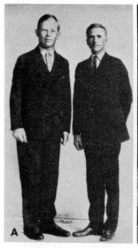
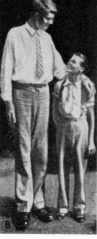
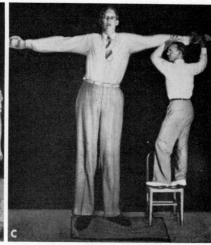

Figure 2-39. One of the most notable examples of growth hormone excess in the human was Robert Wadlow, later known as the "Alton Giant." Although weighing only 9 pounds at birth, he soon commenced to grow excessively and by 6 months of age weighed 30 pounds. At 1 year of age he had reached a weight of 62 pounds. Growth continued throughout his life. Shortly before his death, which occurred at the age of 22 years from cellulitis of the feet, he was found to be 8 feet 11 inches in height and 475 pounds in weight by the careful measurements of Doctor C. M. Charles (*A* and *B*, from Fadner, F.: Biography of Robert Wadlow, 1944. Courtesy of Bruce Humphries, Publishers. *C,* Courtesy of Doctors C. M. Charles and C. M. MacBryde.)

secretion of growth hormone (Figs. 2-39 and 2-40). The growing period of these giants is longer than in normal children because epiphysial closure may be delayed by hypogonadism. The giants who have survived into adult life have the long extremities of eunuchoidism combined with mildly acromegalic features. Almost all of the recorded giants of extreme height have died in early adult life of infection, progressing debility, or hypopituitarism.

When somatotropin hypersecretion occurs after puberty, there is little increase in height because the epiphysial plates have fused. Although bony and soft tissue overgrowth is observed clinically, the increase in total body mass is usually not great. Only about 40 per cent of acromegalic pa-

tients gain significant weight. Proliferation of bony and soft tissues is most evident clinically in the acral parts of the body (Fig. 2-41). The bones of the spadelike hands show cortical thickening with "tufting" of the tips of the distal phalanges on roentgenologic examination (Fig. 2-42). To a lesser extent, all of the skeleton shares in the process of increased periosteal bone formation. Osteophytic proliferations are common on the epiphyses of the long bones.

The bony deformities of the skull are most striking (Fig. 2-42). The mandible is noteworthy because its length as well as its thickness increases. The "lantern jaw" frequently results in overbite of the lower incisors beyond the upper incisors by as much as 1/2 inch. Women may note an inability to "bite a thread" early in their disease. Often the teeth are abnormally separated. Coarsening of the facial features due to overgrowth of the frontal, malar, and nasal bones completes the acromegalic facies. The calvarium is thickened; bony ridges and muscular attachments are often exaggerated. The frontal, mastoid, and ethmoid sinuses may be enlarged to a remarkable degree. Intriguing variations in the pattern of facial overgrowth are encountered. Some patients show an inordinate growth of a single facial feature, such as the jaw, orbital ridges, or nose, with little involvement of other bones of the face.

Articular symptoms, from mild arthralgias to severe crippling arthritis, are common in acromegaly. Bony overgrowth leads to distortion of the articular plate and abnormal joint mechanics. Vertebral overgrowth is most marked on the anterior surface of the bone. Articular cartilage proliferation initially widens the joint space (Fig. 2-43), but as the disease progresses, cartilage may become eroded, with resultant disabling arthritis

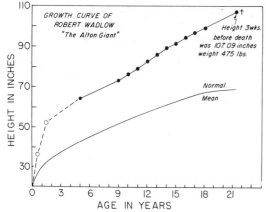

Figure 2-40. Growth curve of the Alton giant. The first two points (open circles) are estimates based on recorded weights and presumed normal body composition. (Reproduced from Daughaday, W. H., and Parker, M. L.: *Disease-a-Month,* August, 1962, by permission of Year Book Medical Publishers, Inc.)

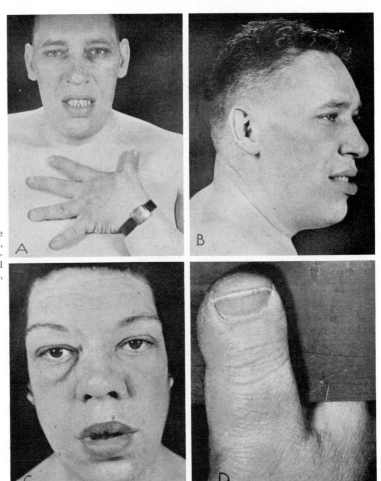

Figure 2–41. Acromegaly. *A* and *B*, Note the large and elongated head, large hand, nose, ears, and lips. There are also prognathism and slightly increased interdental spaces. *C*, Note the coarse features. *D*, Large, blunt-pointed thumb.

which is indistinguishable from osteoarthritis. Fibrous thickening of the joint capsule and related ligaments may contribute to the discomfort.

An important feature of the disease is the increase in the total mass of connective tissue in the body. As a result of this change, there is a disproportionate increase in the volume of interstitial fluid in acromegalic patients. Alterations in skin and subcutaneous tissue are easily observed in most acromegalic patients. The skin appears coarse and leathery, and there is exaggeration of all the normal skin pores and markings. Dermal proliferation of the scalp can lead to the formation of deep folds in the sagittal axis. Body hair is increased in amount and excessively coarse in texture. During the active phase of the disease, most patients complain of excessive sweating, and unusual oiliness of their skin may lead to an unpleasant odor. Moderate melanosis occurs in about half the patients. Another dermal manifestation of acromegaly is the occurrence of fibroma molluscum in about 27 per cent of the patients. The tongue is frequently enlarged and furrowed.

Involvement of peripheral nerves is common. Acroparesthesias are noted in about 20 per cent of the patients. In many cases, this complaint is due to entrapment of nerves by bony or soft tissue overgrowth. Compression of the median nerve in the carpal tunnel leads to weakness and sensory changes in the hands. Peripheral neuropathy can also be due to perineurial and endoneurial fibrous proliferation which may occur to such a degree that peripheral nerves are palpably enlarged.

Enlargement of the heart is found almost universally in acromegalic patients at necropsy, even in the absence of any functional impairment. Endocrine clinicians have been impressed that severe acromegalic patients often develop progressive congestive heart failure in the fifth and sixth decades. In some cases, the degree of hypertension or coronary arteriosclerosis is sufficient to explain the myocardial insufficiency. In other cases, a true chronic myocardiopathy is suspected. At necropsy the size of the myocardial fibers is increased, and the fibers are separated by interstitial fibrosis.

Hepatomegaly can often be detected on physical examination and is regularly observed at necropsy. The thyroid, parathyroid, spleen, and pancreas also are larger than normal.

A remarkable increase in the size of the kidneys can occur. The combined weight of the kidneys of one of our patients was 870 g., and there are

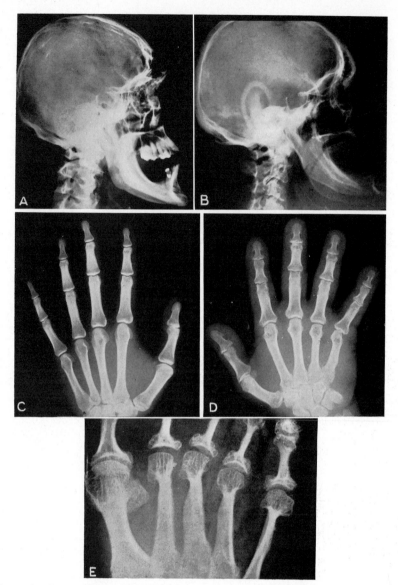

Figure 2–42. Note in *A* and *B* the enlarged sella turcica, large paranasal sinuses, and marked elongation of the mandible. *C* is the hand of a normal Norwegian-Swedish male who weighs 220 pounds and is 6 feet 4 inches in height. Though he is regarded as being "big-boned," or having a "big frame," there are many differences in the roentgenogram of his hand and that of the acromegalic hand, *D*, which shows marked thickening of the soft tissues, widened bones, periosteal reaction, small osteophytes, tufting and mushrooming of the terminal phalanges, and spur formation. In *E* note that the trabeculae in the bone ends are thickened and widely spaced, appearing porotic, while the shafts are narrow and dense; there is a sudden transition from a dense, narrow pipe-stem shaft to a squared and porotic bone end. (*E* is reproduced with modification from Kellgren, J. H., Ball, J., et al.: *Quart. J. Med. 21:*405, 1952, with permission.)

reports in the literature of even larger kidneys. The glomeruli may be twice normal in diameter, and comparable increases in the size of the renal tubules occur. Remarkable changes in renal function have been described. In a patient studied by Gershberg, the inulin clearance was 325 ml. per min. (normal value, 131 ml. per min.); the tubular reabsorption of glucose was 1068 mg. per min. (normal value 385 mg. per min.); the tubular secretion maximum for para-aminohippurate was 165 mg. per min. (normal value 76 mg. per min.).

Growth hormone increases tubular reabsorption of phosphate and leads to the mild hyperphosphatemia.

Impaired glucose tolerance is present in nearly half the cases of acromegaly, but clinical diabetes mellitus occurs in only about 10 per cent of patients. Even in those patients with normal glucose tolerance, plasma insulin response is increased, indicating insulin resistance. The insulin response to tolbutamide is also exaggerated.

It is widely suspected that diabetes only develops

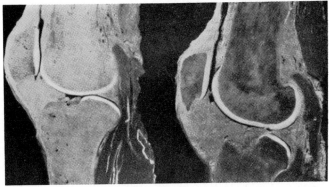

Figure 2–43. The knee on the left is normal, whereas the one on the right shows acromegalic arthropathy, with marked thickening of ligaments, meniscus, and fat pad. There is an enlarged femoral condyle with thickening of the articular cartilage. (Reproduced with modification from Kellgren, J. W., Ball, J., et al.: *Quart. J. Med. 21*:405, 1952, with permission.)

in those acromegalic patients who have a hereditary predisposition to diabetes; in the remaining patients, insulin secretory reserve is believed sufficient to overcome insulin antagonism. Rarely, severe insulin resistance may be encountered in acromegalic individuals with diabetes. Pathologically the islets of Langerhans may be enlarged and β cells packed with granules even in the presence of diabetes.

The frequency of degenerative diabetic complications occurring in acromegalic diabetes has aroused much interest. Diabetic retinopathy is not unusual, but only one patient at Barnes Hospital has developed pathologic changes of intercapillary glomerulosclerosis.

Growth Hormone Secretion. A number of patterns of GH hypersecretion occur in acromegaly. Plasma GH may be very slightly elevated (5 to 20 ng. per ml.) or may reach massive concentrations (> 1,000 ng. per ml.). Many patients exhibit little fluctuation of plasma GH throughout a 24-hour period. In other patients, GH levels are strikingly inconstant, with abrupt rises occurring at short intervals (Fig. 2–44). In almost all cases, the sleep-related peak of GH secretion is absent.

Peaks of GH secretion can be provoked in some acromegalic patients by mixed meals and arginine. The influence of changes of blood sugar on GH

secretion is of interest. Hypoglycemia can provoke increased GH secretion in some patients, and glucose administration may provoke a paradoxical rise in plasma GH. The GH responses to these metabolic stimuli require hypothalamic participation. Persistence of these responses suggests that a disorder of hypothalamic regulation exists in certain patients with hypersomatotropism. Recently growth hormone releasing activity has been described in plasma of patients with acromegaly. If hypothalamic regulation of GH secretion were normal in acromegaly, the high levels of GH present should inhibit growth hormone releasing factor and block the responses to metabolic stimuli. The existence of this type of short loop feedback for GH has been established in normal people receiving exogenous GH.

In addition to providing hints concerning the pathogenesis of acromegaly, GH measurements are of great practical value in diagnosis and the monitoring of therapeutic responses. Plasma GH measurement makes possible unequivocal diagnosis before significant acromegalic disfigurement. Blood should be obtained from hospitalized patients before breakfast in the basal state. Transient functional elevations of plasma GH occur in ambulatory patients, particularly in young women, and must be distinguished from pathologic hypersecretion. Functional GH secretion can be suppressed by obtaining samples of blood about 90 minutes after administration of 75 g. of glucose by mouth. Under these conditions, plasma GH normally is less than 5 ng. per ml. Levels between 5 and 10 ng. per ml. can be considered indeterminant, and higher values support the diagnosis of hypersomatotropism. Most acromegalic patients have substantially higher values. The highest levels that we have encountered are in excess of 1,000 ng. per ml.

The apparent lack of correlation of plasma GH levels and the stigmata of the disease has led to some misunderstandings. Often clinicians have not considered the important influence of duration of hypersomatotropism. Clinical manifestations of pathologic growth are cumulative, so that severe hypersomatotropism of short duration can be present with less marked acromegaly than mild hypersomatotropism of long duration. There are also age-dependent differences in tissue respon-

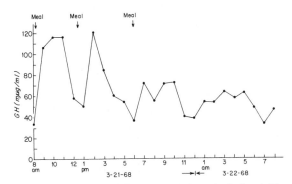

Figure 2–44. Serial GH measurements made during a 24-hour period in an acromegalic patient exhibiting marked instability of GH levels. Note rises of plasma GH occurring after meals and the absence of a defined sleep-related GH peak at night. (Reproduced from Cryer, P. E., and Daughaday, W. H.: *J. Clin. Endocr. 28*:386, 1969, with permission.)

siveness, younger patients being more responsive than older. In some patients, acromegalic changes represent the residual high tide mark of GH secretion in the past which has ebbed at the time of study. While not common, spontaneous improvement in hypersomatotropism can occur because of hemorrhagic infarction of tumors. Also, from what has been said, it should be remembered that one or two random GH measurements may not accurately reflect total GH secretion. Despite these limitations, GH measurements provide a much more reliable guide to therapy than minor fluctuations of symptoms and signs.

Secretion of Other Hormones. Certain clinical features suggest the existence of hyperthyroidism in acromegalic patients. Goiter is found in about a quarter of the patients, and excess sweating is a common finding in the active disease. Although the basal metabolic rate is commonly moderately elevated, more specific measurements of thyroid function (serum thyroxine, radioiodine uptake) have characteristically been normal. A decreased binding capacity of thyroid binding globulin and an increased capacity of thyroid binding prealbumin occur in some patients with acromegaly. Measurements of plasma TSH have thus far failed to show overproduction of this hormone. At operation or necropsy, the goiter has generally been found to be edematous without histologic evidence of hypersecretion. The hypermetabolism of acromegaly, therefore, seems to be a direct effect of growth hormone excess. Hypothyroidism may develop late in the course of acromegaly after normal pituitary tissue has been compressed by the adenoma or destroyed by treatment.

The occurrence of inapppropriate lactation in young women with acromegaly suggests excessive production of prolactin. Mild to moderate elevations of plasma prolactin are present in most acromegalic patients with nonpuerperal lactation. Most other acromegalic patients have plasma prolactin levels which are in the high normal range.

Corticotropin secretion is usually adequate to maintain basal cortisol secretion. Urinary 17-hydroxycorticosteroid excretion is usually normal, but a decrease in ACTH reserve may be uncovered with metyrapone administration. Failure of corticotropin secretion may complicate the later stages of the disease. Rarely, cases have been observed in which clinical and laboratory evidence of hyperadrenocorticism has been found in acromegaly.

It has been widely held, but never documented, that enhanced secretion of gonadotropins occurs early in the disease and leads to increased libido. This is proably incorrect, because it is doubtful if libido is greatly affected by greater than normal amounts of gonadal hormones. A mild increase in 17-ketosteroids may reflect altered metabolism of adrenal steroids.

Decreased gonadotropin secretion is the usual consequence of acidophilic tumors. Sexual immaturity is common in giants. About a third of men with acromegaly develop impotence, and nearly all women note menstrual irregularities or amenor-

rhea. Completion of normal pregnancy is unusual.

Associated Neoplasia. There is little solid evidence linking high levels of circulating growth hormone with an increased frequency of neoplasia. Experimentally, a variety of tumors have developed in rats receiving growth hormone injections for prolonged periods. Pituitary adenomas are associated with adenomas of the parathyroid, islets of Langerhans, and adrenal cortex in the polyendocrine adenomatosis syndrome. This possibility should be considered in evaluating patients with acromegaly.

Hypercorticotropism with Pituitary Tumors

In 1932 Harvey Cushing attributed secretory function to the small basophilic tumors of the pituitary in several patients with the clinical syndrome that was subsequently named after him. These tumors are a possible cause of increased corticotropin secretion in about one quarter of all patients with Cushing's syndrome.

Although the presence of pituitary tumors is occasionally recognized prior to treatment of Cushing's syndrome, the frequency of clinical detection is increased significantly after adrenalectomy. In one large series, pituitary tumors were present radiologically in 12 of 122 patients subjected to bilateral adrenalectomy. Several of these tumors showed unusual invasive properties; oculomotor nerve involvement developed in three patients and distant metastases in one. A tendency for hemorrhagic necrosis was also observed. In most reports, the cells of the tumors do not contain secretory granules.

The development of pituitary tumors in patients with Cushing's syndrome after adrenalectomy is heralded by intense pigmentation (Nelson's syndrome). The ACTH concentration of plasma is moderately elevated, even after corticosteroid administration. The pigmentation of this syndrome is due to increased plasma beta melanocyte stimulating hormone (β MSH). Although corticotropin has some MSH activity, most tumors secrete both peptides. The ratio of the two activities differs from patient to patient. Rarely patients have been described with pituitary tumors who had intense pigmentation but no evidence of adrenal dysfunction. Such tumors apparently secrete only MSH.

It is unknown whether there is any relation between corticotropin secreting chromophobe tumors of the pituitary and the small basophil tumors which have been recognized in the past. Adrenalectomy, by removing cortisol inhibition of corticotropin secretion, may induce tumor development or stimulate growth in an existing tumor. The rarity of pituitary tumors in Addison's disease, in which corticotropin secretion is also increased, is unexplained. It may be necessary to reevaluate the treatment of Cushing's syndrome, if the frequency of pituitary tumors continues to increase, and to aim treatment at controlling both the pituitary and adrenal components of the disease.

Prolactin-Secreting Pituitary Tumors

In 1954 Albright and his associates (52) defined the syndrome of nonpuerperal lactation with pituitary tumors unassociated with acromegaly (Forbes-Albright syndrome) and attributed the lactation to excessive prolactin secretion. This prediction has been amply confirmed with bioassay and radioimmunoassay of plasma prolactin. Clinically, most of these patients give a history of intermittent lactation and amenorrhea of long duration. Persistent lactation can follow puerperal lactation. One of our patients experienced premature thelarche in early childhood, and her pituitary tumor was not recognized until her early twenties. In most cases, lactation amounts to little more than a few milky drops on pressure. No increase in mammary tumors has been recognized, but this would be hard to establish from random reports. Growth hormone concentrations are normal or low, and the gonadotropin levels are usually low. Mild hirsutism and obesity are common and unexplained accompanying symptoms in this condition.

Histopathologically, most tumors do not contain secretory granules recognizable with histologic stains, but occasionally the tumors are frankly eosinophilic. Electron microscopic study of one of our tumors which contained prolactin with little or no growth hormone demonstrated large secretory granules similar to the prolactin-containing granules of other mammalian species (Fig. 2–35).

The newer prolactin assays have established that prolactin hypersecretion is common in pituitary tumors formerly considered nonsecretory; the actual incidence remains to be established. Increases in plasma prolactin concentrations are very impressive, often in excess of 500 ng. per ml. In only a fraction of women is lactation noted. Most men are asymptomatic, but a few have gynecomastia with or without lactation. The association of a pituitary tumor with high plasma prolactin concentrations does not establish secretion by a tumor. Craniopharyngiomas may be associated with elevations of plasma prolactin, and there is no evidence that the tumors have any secretory activity. Similarly, ACTH-secreting tumors may also be related to high plasma prolactin. In these cases, prolactin hypersecretion may arise from the normal remnant of pituitary tissue rather than the tumor. Hypothalamic damage or disruption of the pituitary portal circulation would lead to uninhibited oversecretion of the normal lactotropic cells. Pharmacologic tools now under investigation may allow us to distinguish primary oversecretion from that resulting from deficiency of prolactin inhibitory factor.

The differential diagnosis of nonpuerperal lactation includes many functional disturbances of the pituitary (Table 2–5). In most of the conditions listed, it is clear that lactation is due to increased prolactin secretion. The physiologic influence of estrogens, tranquilizing drugs, and alpha methyldopa has already been described, and the association of these substances with pathologic lactation is easily understood. Neurogenic impulses from the

TABLE 2–5. DIFFERENTIAL DIAGNOSIS OF GALACTORRHEA

I. *Primary Hypothalamic*
  1. Functional
    a. Postpartum
    b. Without pregnancy
  2. Destructive lesion of hypothalamic and pituitary stalk

II. *Drug-Induced*
  1. Tranquilizers
  2. Antidepressants
  3. Rauwolfia alkaloids
  4. α-Methyldopa

III. *Hormonal*
  1. Estrogens
  2. Hypothyroidism

IV. *Neurogenic*
  1. Mammary stimulation
  2. Chest wall lesions

V. *Secretory Tumors*
  1. Pituitary tumors
    a. Secretion of prolactin
    b. Secretion of prolactin and growth hormone
  2. Nonpituitary tumors with ectopic prolactin secretion

chest wall probably activate the same neural pathways involved in normal suckling. The association of lactation with certain cases of hypothyroidism suggests possible prolactin secretion in response to TRH secretion. This must remain a speculation, because an increased secretion of TRH in hypothyroidism remains to be established.

The time has come to drop the use of eponyms in naming the syndromes associated with inappropriate lactations, such as the Forbes-Albright syndrome, Chiari-Frommel syndrome (persistent lactation with amenorrhea following normal pregnancy), and del Castillo's syndrome (amenorrhea and lactation unassociated with preceding pregnancy). A functional classification such as is presented in Table 2–5 is recommended.

Secretion of Thyrotropin and Gonadotropin by Pituitary Tumors

Hypersecretion of thyrotropin and gonadotropins by pituitary tumors is seldom encountered in man. Two cases of pituitary tumors associated with mild hyperthyroidism and increases in plasma TSH have thus far been reported. The simple association of hyperthyroidism with pituitary tumor is not sufficient evidence to establish the presence of a secretory tumor. Most such patients probably have increased levels of LATS or autonomous thyroid nodules. The demonstration of increased levels of TSH in plasma and tumor by radioimmunoassay is essential.

Gonadotropin secretion by pituitary tumors has yet to be definitely established. There are case reports of patients with preexisting hypogonadism who have subsequently developed pituitary tumors which appeared to be functional because the urinary gonadotropins were elevated. These cases suggest that a chronic oversecretion of gonadotropins might lead to pituitary neoplasms. Such a sequence has been observed in mice following early gonadectomy.

Ablative Treatment of Pituitary Tumors

The goals of ablative treatment of pituitary tumors are to prevent parasellar extension and to correct hormonal hypersecretions without affecting secretion of other pituitary hormones. Unfortunately, these goals are difficult to achieve.

Radiation therapy has its greatest usefulness when pituitary enlargement is confined to the sella turcica. Gamma radiation administered by supravoltage sources has been used extensively. Control of tumor size and prevention of parasellar complications can usually be achieved, but many endocrinologists have been disappointed with the adequacy of control of hormonal hypersecretion. Reexamination of the results of treatment of acromegalic patients indicates that this poor reputation is probably undeserved. In one large series of patients, as many as 78 per cent of acromegalic patients had restoration of normal or near normal plasma concentrations of GH (less than 10 ng. per ml.). The response to therapy is slow, and two years may be required for any improvement. This experience may be unusually good, but the safety and general availability of gamma radiation recommend it for initial treatment for patients with mild to moderate hormonal hypersecretion and tumors without significant extrasellar extension. The details of therapy are not germane to this discussion, but there is little advantage in exceeding 5,500 R. The total dose of radiation should be given as a single course through multiple ports. With modern supravoltage equipment, early untoward reactions are rarely encountered, and late damage to cranial nerves and hypothalamic tissues is seldom recognized. Because the tumor is seldom eradicated, some of the benefit of irradiation may result from hypothalamic injury or pituitary portal vein thrombosis.

Treatment with accelerated proton beams permits a greater dose of radiation to be focused on the pituitary with less damage to intervening and neighboring tissue. Doses equivalent to 10,000 R. can be administered through multiple or rotational ports. The treatment carries a greater risk of cranial nerve and hypothalamic damage than was first claimed, but the overall responses to treatment appear quite satisfactory. A disadvantage of this form of treatment is the limited number of centers where it is available. It would appear to be a satisfactory form of treatment for patients with moderate or severe acromegaly and only moderate sellar enlargement. Because radiation damage is cumulative, proton beam radiation is not recommended after conventional gamma radiation.

Local implantation of radioactive isotopes of yttrium, gold, and strontium is seldom done in this country because of the frequency of rhinorrhea and meningitis.

Three modes of direct surgical treatment are available. The simplest of these is the stereotaxic placement of probes within the tumor and the destruction of the tumor by freezing from liquid nitrogen circulated through the probe or by heating by radiofrequency coils. In most cases, the contents of the sella turcica can be largely destroyed with little damage to surrounding tissues. In skilled hands, rhinorrhea and meningitis are infrequent. Cryosurgery is satisfactory for patients with acromegaly with small or moderately large tumors. Good hormonal control can be achieved in about 80 per cent of the cases. There is a higher incidence of diabetes insipidus and hypopituitarism in patients treated by cryohypophysectomy than in patients treated with gamma radiation.

The classical surgical approach to the pituitary is by the transfrontal route. This is recommended for tumors with considerable suprasellar extension with impingement on the optic nerves. Complete removal of the secretory tumor may not be possible. In acromegaly, excessive bleeding from the greatly thickened bone may occur.

There is renewal of interest in approaching the pituitary via the sphenoid sinus and removing the pituitary tumor by microsurgical techniques under direct microscopic visualization. Rhinorrhea and meningitis remain hazards, but with skillful surgeons they have not been prohibitive. Further technical improvements can be anticipated. This approach has the potential of removing small adenomas completely and leaving normal pituitary tissue behind. The improved visualization obtained has allowed Hardy (103) to recognize small fragments of secretory tissue overlooked by the suprasellar route.

Medical management of hormonal secretion by pituitary tumors is still experimental. The oral administration of medroxyprogesterone, 30 to 60 mg. per day, will lower plasma GH levels in about a quarter of the cases. A beneficial effect of chlorpromazine treatment has been reported in a single case. Levodopa in a daily dose of 1.5 to 3.0 g. per day will lower prolactin secretion by some tumors. Control of prolactin secretion has also been reported following the administration of newer ergot derivatives.

SECRETION OF PITUITARY HORMONES BY EXTRAPITUITARY TUMORS

Certain nonpituitary tumors acquire the capacity to manufacture and secrete peptide hormones. The anterior pituitary hormones which have been most commonly associated with extrapituitary tumors are corticotropin and MSH. Bronchogenic carcinomas, bronchial adenoma, thymomas, and pancreatic tumors have been responsible most frequently, but a great variety of other tumors have also been implicated. The hyperadrenocorticism of these cases is described more fully in Chapter 30. It is characterized by explosive onset, great severity, high frequency of electrolyte abnormalities, and pigmentation. Both corticotropin and

MSH have been found in the tumor and body fluids.

A thyrotropic substance appears to be released by certain choriocarcinomas and testicular tumors. Clinical signs of hyperthyroidism have been mild or difficult to detect, but the PBI and other indices of thyroid function have been abnormal. Thyrotropic activity has been demonstrated by bioassay, but the thyroid stimulating material does not react with radioimmunoassays for human thyrotropin. In certain cases, the thyrotropic substances can be measured with a bovine TSH assay.

Gonadotropin secretion regularly occurs with choriocarcinomas and certain teratomas, but as chorionic gonadotropin is the normal secretion of the tissue of origin, this cannot be considered in the same context as the secretion of hormones by tissues which normally have no hormonal activity. Of more interest are the reports of premature puberty in boys with hepatoblastomas and gynecomastia in men with bronchogenic carcinoma. Increased levels of gonadotropin have been detected in the urine, plasma, and tumor. The gonadotropin usually present in these cases has the immunologic properties of chorionic gonadotropin. It is possible that some tumors may secrete pituitary gonadotropins.

Bronchogenic and other carcinomas can produce GH. Plasma GH levels in such patients have only been moderately elevated (5 to 25 ng. per ml.) and are not suppressible with glucose. In some cases, GH has been demonstrated immunologically within the tumor. The GH secretion has not been associated with clinical manifestations.

Recently, several cases of hyperprolactinemia and inappropriate lactation have been described in patients with carcinoma (bronchogenic and renal). Release of prolactin by tumor fragments *in vitro* establishes the source of ectopic secretion.

REFERENCES

General Reviews

1. Harris, G. W., and Donovan, B. T.: *The Pituitary Gland.* Vols. 1–3. Berkeley, University of California Press, 1966.
2. Li, C. H.: Current concepts on the chemical biology of pituitary hormones. *Perspect. Biol. Med. 11*:498, 1968.
3. Rimoin, D. L., and Schimke, R. N.: *Genetic Disorders of the Endocrine Glands.* St. Louis, Mo., C. V. Mosby Co., 1971.

Anatomy

4. Bain, J., and Ezrin, C.: Immunofluorescent localization of the LH cell of the human adenohypophysis. *J. Clin. Endocr. 30*:181, 1970.
5. Bergland, R. M., Ray, B. S., et al.: Anatomical variations in the pituitary gland and adjacent structures in 225 human autopsy cases. *J. Neurosurg. 28*:93, 1968.
6. Phifer, R. F., Spicer, S. S., et al.: Specific demonstration of the human hypophyseal cells which produce adrenocorticotropic hormone. *J. Clin. Endocr. 31*:347, 1970.

ACTH and MSH

7. Berson, S. A., and Yalow, R. S.: Radioimmunoassay of ACTH in plasma. *J. Clin. Invest. 47*:2725, 1968.
8. Gill, G. N.: Mechanism of ACTH action. *Metabolism 21*:571, 1972.
9. Kaore, A., Nicholson, W. E., et al.: Radioimmunoassay of β-

MSH in human plasma and tissues. *J. Clin. Invest. 46*:1609, 1967.
10. Lefkowitz, R. J., Roth, J., et al.: ACTH receptors in the adrenal: Specific binding of ACTH-^{125}I and its relation to adenyl cyclase. *Proc. Nat. Acad. Sci. USA 65*:745, 1970.
11. Lerner, A. B., and McQuire, J. S.: Melanocyte stimulating hormone and adrenocorticotrophic hormone. *New Eng. J. Med. 270*:539, 1964.
12. Liddle, G. W., Island, D., et al.: Normal and abnormal regulation of corticotropin secretion in man. *Recent Progr. Hormone Res. 18*:125, 1962.
13. Metcalf, M. G., and Beaven, D. W.: The metopirone test of pituitary corticotrophin release. Evaluation of 101 tests. *Amer. J. Med. 45*:176, 1968.
14. Riniker, B., Sieber, P., et al.: Revised amino-acid sequences for porcine and human adrenocorticotrophic hormone. *Nature New Biol. 235*:114, 1972.
15. Shimizu, N., Ogata, E., et al.: Studies on the melanotropic activity of human plasma and tissues. *J. Clin. Endocr. 25*:984, 1965.

Gonadotropins

16. Amin, H. K., and Hunter, W. M.: Human pituitary follicle-stimulating hormone: distribution, plasma clearance and urinary excretion as determined by radioimmunoassay. *J. Endocr. 48*:307, 1970.
17. August, G. P., Grumbach, M. M., et al.: Hormonal changes in puberty: III. Correlation of plasma testosterone, LH, FSH, testicular size, and bone age with male pubertal development. *J. Clin. Endocr. 34*:319, 1972.
18. Baghdassarian, A., Guyda, H., et al.: Urinary excretion of radioimmunoassayable luteinizing hormone (LH) in normal male children and adults, according to age and stage of sexual development. *J. Clin. Endocr. 31*:428, 1970.
19. Johanson, A. J., Guyda, H., et al.: Serum luteinizing hormone by radioimmunoassay in normal children and adolescents. *J. Pediat. 74*:416, 1969.
20. Kohler, P. O., Ross, G. T., et al.: Metabolic clearance and production rates of human luteinizing hormone in pre- and postmenopausal women. *J. Clin. Invest. 47*:38, 1968.
21. Odell, W. D., Parlow, A. F., et al.: Radioimmunoassay for human follicle-stimulating hormone: Physiological studies. *J. Clin. Invest. 41*:2551, 1968.
22. Raiti, S., Johanson, A., et al.: Measurement of immunologically reactive follicle stimulating hormone in serum of normal male children and adults. *Metabolism 18*:234, 1969.
23. Ross, G. T., Cargille, C. M., et al.: Pituitary and gonadal hormones in women during spontaneous and induced ovulatory cycles. *Recent Progr. Hormone Res. 26*:1, 1970.
24. Saxena, B. B., Beling, C. G., and Gandy, H. W., (eds.), *Gonadotropins.* New York, Wiley-Interscience, 1972.
25. Vande Wiele, R. L., Bogumil, J., et al.: Mechanisms regulating the menstrual cycle in women. *Recent Progr. Hormone Res. 26*:63, 1970.
26. Wikramanayake, J. R., Keenan, J. R., et al.: Plasma and urinary luteinizing hormone levels in the diagnosis of endocrine disease. *Brit. Med. J. 1*:775, 1972.

TSH

27. Bowers, C. Y., Lee, K. L., et al.: A study on the interaction of the thyrotropin-releasing factor and L-triiodothyronine: Effects of puromycin and cycloheximide. *Endocrinology 82*:75, 1968.
28. Bowers, C. Y., Schally, A. V., et al.: Interactions of L-thyroxine or L-triiodothyronine and thyrotropin-releasing factor on the release and synthesis of thyrotropin from the anterior pituitary gland of mice. *Endocrinology 81*:741, 1967.
29. Cotton, G. E., Gorman, C. A., et al.: Suppression of thyrotropin (h-TSH) in serums of patients with myxedema of varying etiology treated with thyroid hormones. *New Eng. J. Med. 285*:529, 1971.
30. Fore, W., and Wynn, J.: The thyrotropin stimulation test. *Amer. J. Med. 40*:90, 1966.
31. Hall, R., Ormston, B. J., et al.: The thyrotrophin-releasing hormone test in diseases of the pituitary and hypothalamus. *Lancet I*:759, 1972.
32. Mayberry, W. E., Gharib, H., et al.: Radioimmunoassay for human thyrotropin: clinical value in patients with

normal and abnormal thyroid function. *Ann. Intern. Med.* 74:471, 1971.

33. Odell, W. D., Wilber, J. F., et al.: Studies of thyrotropin physiology by means of radioimmunoassay. *Recent Progr. Hormone Res.* 23:47, 1967.

34. Pastan, I., and Macchia, V.: Mechanism of thyroid-stimulating hormone action. Studies with dibutyryl 3',5'-adenosine monophosphate and lecithinase C. *J. Biol. Chem.* 242:5757, 1967.

35. Pierce, J. G.: Eli Lilly Lecture: The subunits of pituitary thyrotropin—their relationship to other glycoprotein hormones. *Endocrinology* 89:1331, 1971.

Growth Hormone

36. Abrams, R. L., Grumbach, M. M., et al.: The effect of administration of human growth hormone on the plasma growth hormone, cortisol, glucose, and free fatty acid response to insulin: Evidence for growth hormone autoregulation in man. *J. Clin. Invest.* 50:940, 1971.

37. Blackard, W. G., and Heidingsfelder, S. A.: Adrenergic receptor control mechanisms for growth hormone secretion. *J. Clin. Invest.* 47:1407, 1968.

38. Clemens, M. J., and Korner, A.: Amino acid requirement for the growth-hormone stimulation of incorporation of precursors into protein and nucleic acids of liver slices. *Biochem. J.* 119:629, 1970.

39. Cornblath, M., Parker, M. L., et al.: Secretion and metabolism of growth hormone in premature and full-term infants. *J. Clin. Endocr.* 25:209, 1965.

40. Daughaday, W. H., and Garland, J. T.: The sulfation factor hypothesis: recent observations, In *Growth and Growth Hormone.* Pecile, A., and Muller, E. E. (eds.), Amsterdam, Excerpta Medica, 1972.

41. Frantz, A. G., and Rabkin, M. T.: Effects of estrogen and sex difference on secretion of human growth hormone. *J. Clin. Endocr.* 25:1470, 1965.

42. Pecile, A., and Muller, E. E. (eds.), *Proceedings First International Symposium on Growth Hormone,* Milan, 1967, Excerpta Medica Foundation, Int. Congr. Series No. 158, 1968.

43. Pecile, A., and Muller, E. E. (eds.), *Proceedings Second International Symposium on Growth Hormone,* Milan, 1971, Excerpta Medica Foundation, Int. Congr. Series No. 236, 1972.

44. Raiti, S., and Blizzard, R. M.: Human growth hormone: current knowledge regarding its role in normal and abnormal metabolic states. *Advances Pediat.* 17:99, 1970.

45. Snipes, C. A.: Effects of growth hormone and insulin on amino acid and protein metabolism. *Quart. Rev. Biol.* 43:127, 1968.

46. Sonenberg, M., and Cohen, H.: Growth hormone. *Ann. N. Y. Acad. Sci.* 148:291, 1968.

47. Takahashi, Y., Kipnis, D. M., et al.: Growth hormone secretion during sleep. *J. Clin. Invest.* 47:2079, 1968.

Prolactin

48. Beck, J. C., Gonda, A., et al.: Some metabolic changes induced by primate growth hormone and purified ovine prolactin. *Metabolism* 13:1108, 1961.

49. Bern, H. A., and Nicoll, C. S.: The comparative endocrinology of prolactin. *Recent Progr. Hormone Res.* 24:681, 1968.

50. Daughaday, W. H., and Jacobs, L. S.: Human prolactin, In *Reviews of Physiology, Biochemistry and Experimental Pharmacology.* Berlin, Springer-Verlag, 1972.

51. Foley, T. P., Jr., Jacobs, L. S., et al.: Human prolactin and thyrotropin concentrations in the serum of normal and hypopituitary children before and after the administration of synthetic thyrotropin releasing hormone. *J. Clin. Invest.* 51:2143, 1972.

52. Forbes, A. P., Henneman, P. H., et al.: Syndrome characterized by galactorrhea, amenorrhea and low urinary FSH: Comparison with acromegaly and normal lactation. *J. Clin. Endocr.* 14:265, 1954.

53. Friesen, H., Guyda, H., et al.: Functional evaluation of prolactin secretion: a guide to therapy. *J. Clin. Invest.* 51:706, 1972.

54. Hwang, P., Guyda, H., et al.: A radioimmunoassay for human prolactin. *Proc. Nat. Acad. Sci., USA* 68:1902, 1971.

55. Jacobs, L. S., Mariz, I. K., et al.: A mixed heterologous radio-

56. Kleinberg, D. L., and Frantz, A. G.: Human prolactin: Measurement in plasma by *in vitro* bioassay. *J. Clin. Invest.* 50:1557, 1971.

57. Kolodny, R. C., Jacobs, L. S., et al.: Mammary stimulation causes prolactin secretion in non-lactating women. *Nature* (London) 238:284, 1972.

58. Lewis, U. J., Singh, R. N. P., et al.: Human prolactin: Isolation and some properties. *Biochem. Biophys. Res. Commun.* 44:1169, 1971.

59. Niall, H. D., Hogan, M. L., et al.: Sequences of pituitary and placental lactogenic and growth hormones: evolution from a primordial peptide by gene replication. *Proc. Nat. Acad. Sci. USA* 68:866, 1971.

60. Peake, G. T., McKeel, D. W., et al.: Ultrastructural, histologic and hormonal characterization of a prolactin-rich human pituitary tumor. *J. Clin. Endocr.* 29:1383, 1969.

61. Topper, Y. J.: Multiple hormone interactions in the development of mammary gland *in vitro. Recent Progr. Hormone Res.* 26:287, 1970.

62. Turkington, R. W., Underwood, L. E., et al.: Elevated serum prolactin levels after pituitary-stalk section in man. *New Eng. J. Med.* 285:707, 1971.

63. Turkington, R. W.: Phenothiazine stimulation test for prolactin reserve: The syndrome of isolated prolactin deficiency. *J. Clin. Endocr.* 34:247, 1972.

64. Turkington, R. W.: Inhibition of prolactin secretion and successful therapy of the Forbes-Albright syndrome with L-dopa. *J. Clin. Endocr.* 34:306, 1972.

65. Tyson, J. E., Hwang, P., et al.: Studies of prolactin secretion in human pregnancy. *Amer. J. Obstet. Gynec.* 113:14, 1972.

Hypopituitarism

66. Caplan, R. H., and Dobben, G. D.: Endocrine studies in patients with the "empty sella syndrome." *Arch. Intern. Med.* (Chicago) 123:611, 1969.

67. Cleveland, W. W., Green, O. C., et al.: A case of proved adrenocorticotropin deficiency. *J. Pediat.* 57:376, 1960.

68. Davis, B. B., Bloom, M. E., et al.: Hyponatremia in pituitary insufficiency. *Metabolism* 18:821, 1969.

69. Kovacs, K.: Necrosis of anterior pituitary in humans. *Neuroendocrinology* 4:201, 1969.

70. Merimee, T. J., Felig, P., et al.: Glucose and lipid homeostasis in the absence of human growth hormone. *J. Clin. Invest.* 50:574, 1971.

71. Odell, W. D.: Isolated deficiencies of anterior pituitary hormones: Symptoms and diagnosis. *J.A.M.A.* 197:1006, 1966.

72. Pearson, O. H. (ed.), *Hypophysectomy.* American Lecture Series No. 315. Springfield, Ill., Charles C Thomas, 1957.

73. Sheehan, H. L.: Simmond's disease due to postpartum necrosis of the anterior pituitary. *Quart. J. Med.* 8:277, 1939.

Hypopituitary Dwarfism

74. Daughaday, W. H., Laron, Z., et al.: Defective sulfation factor generation: A possible etiologic link in dwarfism. *Trans. Ass. Amer. Physicians* 82:129, 1969.

75. Goodman, H. G., Brumbach, M. M., et al.: Growth and growth hormone. II. Comparison of isolated growth-hormone deficiency and multiple pituitary hormone deficiencies in 35 patients with idiopathic hypopituitary dwarfism. *New Eng. J. Med.* 278:57, 1968.

76. Holmes, L. B., Frantz, A. G., et al.: Normal growth with subnormal growth hormone levels. *New Eng. J. Med.* 279:559, 1968.

77. Hoyt, W. F., Kaplan, S. L., et al.: Septo-optic dysplasia and pituitary dwarfism. *Lancet* I:893, 1970.

78. Laron, Z., Pertzelan, A., et al.: Administration of growth hormone to patients with familial dwarfism with high plasma immunoreactive growth hormone: Measurement of sulfation factor, metabolic and linear growth responses. *J. Clin. Endocr.* 33:332, 1971.

79. Parker, M. L., Mariz, I. K., et al.: Resistance to human growth hormone in pituitary dwarfism: Clinical and immunologic studies. *J. Clin. Endocr.* 24:997, 1964.

80. Raiti, S., Kowarski, A., et al.: Secretion of cortisol, cortico-

immunoassay for human prolactin. *J. Clin. Endocr.* 34:484, 1972.

sterone and aldosterone in children with hypopituitarism. *Johns Hopkins Med. J. 122*:229, 1968.

81. Rimoin, D. L., Merimee, T. J., et al.: Genetic aspects of clinical endocrinology. *Recent Progr. Hormone Res. 24*:365, 1968.

82. Soyka, L. F., Bode, H. H., et al.: Effectiveness of long-term human growth hormone therapy for short stature in children with growth hormone deficiency. *J. Clin. Endocr. 30*:1, 1970.

83. Tanner, J. M.: Human growth hormone. *Nature* (London) *237*:433, 1972.

Pituitary Tumors: General

84. Kernohan, J. W., and Sayre, G. P.: *Tumors of the Pituitary Gland and Infundibulum.* Washington, D.C., U. S. Armed Forces Institute of Pathology, 1956.

85. Robinson, J. L.: Sudden blindness in pituitary tumors. *J. Neurosurg. 36*:83, 1972.

86. Russfield, A. B.: Pituitary tumors, In *Pathology Annual.* Vol. 2. Sommers, S. C. (ed.), New York, Appleton-Century-Crofts, 1967.

Pituitary Tumors: Secretion

87. Hamilton, C. R., Adams, L. C., et al.: Hyperthyroidism due to thyrotropin-producing pituitary chromophobe adenoma. *New Eng. J. Med. 283*:1077, 1970.

88. Liddle, G. W., and Shute, A. M.: The evolution of Cushing's syndrome as a clinical entity. *Advances Int. Med. 15*:155, 1969.

89. Lindholm, J., Rasmussen, P., et al.: Chromophobe adenomas of the pituitary gland in Cushing's disease. *Acta Endocr.* (Kobenhavn) *62*:647, 1969.

90. Sawin, C. T., Abe, K., et al.: Hyperpigmentation due solely to increased plasma beta-melanotropin. *Arch. Intern. Med. 125*:708, 1970.

Pituitary Tumors: Acromegaly

91. Cryer, P. E., and Daughaday, W. H.: Regulation of growth hormone secretion in acromegaly. *J. Clin. Endocr. 29*:386, 1969.

92. Daughaday, W. H.: The Diagnosis of hypersomatotropism in man. *Med. Clin. N. Amer. 52*:371, 1968.

93. Fineberg, S. E., Merimee, T. J., et al.: Insulin secretion in acromegaly. *J. Clin. Endocr. 30*:288, 1970.

94. Hirsch, E. Z., Sloman, J. G., et al.: Cardiac function in acromegaly. *Amer. J. Med. Sci. 257*:1, 1969.

95. Ikkos, D.: Pathophysiological studies in acromegaly; pertaining to extracellular water, renal function and basal metabolism. *Acta Endocrinol.* (Kobenhavn) (Suppl. 25) *21*:1, 1956.

96. Kellgren, J. H., Ball, J., et al.: The articular and other limb changes in acromegaly. *Quart. J. Med. 21*:405, 1952.

97. Lawrence, A. M., Goldfine, I. D., et al.: Growth hormone dynamics in acromegaly. *J. Clin. Endocr. 31*:239, 1970.

98. Lawrence, A. M., and Kirsteins, L.: Progestins in the medical management of active acromegaly. *J. Clin. Endocr. 30*:646, 1970.

99. Luft, R., Cerasi, E., et al.: Studies on the pathogenesis of diabetes in acromegaly. *Acta Endocrinol.* (Kobenhavn) *56*:593, 1967.

100. Mastaglia, F. L., Barwick, D. D., et al.: Myopathy in acromegaly. *Lancet II*:907, 1970.

101. Nadarajah, A., Hartog, M., et al.: Calcium metabolism in acromegaly. *Brit. Med. J. 4*:797, 1968.

102. Wright, A. D., Hill, D. M., et al.: Mortality in acromegaly. *Quart. J. Med. 39*:1, 1970.

Pituitary Tumors: TREATMENT

103. Hardy, J.: Transphenoidal microsurgery of the normal and pathological pituitary. *Clin. Neurosurg. 16*:185, 1969.

104. Kramer, S., Southard, M., et al.: Radiotherapy in the management of craniopharyngiomas, further experiences and late results. *Amer. J. Roentgen. 103*:44, 1968.

105. Lawrence, A. M., Pinsky, S. M., et al.: Conventional radiation therapy in acromegaly. *Arch. Intern. Med. 128*:369, 1971.

106. Lawrence, J. H., Tobias, C. A., et al.: Successful treatment of acromegaly: Metabolic and clinical studies in 145 patients. *J. Clin. Endocr. 31*:180, 1970.

107. Matson, D. D., and Crigler, J. F., Jr.: Management of craniopharyngioma in childhood. *J. Neurosurg. 30*:377, 1969.

108. Roth, J., Gorden, P., et al.: Efficacy of conventional pituitary irradiation in acromegaly. *New Eng. J. Med. 282*:1385, 1970.

109. Zervas, N. T.: Stereotaxic radiofrequency surgery of the normal and the abnormal pituitary gland. *New Eng. J. Med. 280*:429, 1969.

Ectopic Hormones

110. Faiman, C., Colwell, J. A., et al.: Gonadotropin secretions from a bronchogenic carcinoma. *New Eng. J. Med. 277*:1395, 1967.

111. Liddle, G. W., Nicholson, W. E., et al.: Clinical and laboratory studies of ectopic humoral syndromes. *Recent Progr. Hormone Res. 25*:283, 1969.

112. Sparagana, M., Phillips, G., et al.: Ectopic growth hormone syndrome associated with lung cancer. *Metabolism 20*:730, 1971.

113. Turkington, R. W.: Ectopic production of prolactin. *New Eng. J. Med. 285*:1455, 1971.

CHAPTER 3

The Neurohypophysis

By Alexander Leaf and
    Cecil H. Coggins

The posterior lobe of the pituitary is not in itself a discrete endocrine organ. It is the distal component of a neurosecretory system that also includes the supraoptic and paraventricular nuclei of the hypothalamus and the neurohypophysial tract which carries axons from these nuclei to terminations in the median eminence, pituitary stalk, and posterior pituitary itself (Fig. 3–1). This chapter is concerned with the formation, release, and biologic actions of vasopressin (the human antidiuretic hormone) and oxytocin. It has become evident recently that portions of this functional unit are also involved in the formation and secretion of other hormones, chiefly those involved in regulating the secretions of the anterior pituitary. These will be discussed in Chapter 12.

ANATOMY

Although as early as 1901 Magnus and Schäfer (68) appreciated that extracts of posterior pituitary

gland had an effect on the rate of urine flow, it was their impression that the gland contained a substance with a diuretic action. It was not until 1913 when Farmi (34) and von den Velden (99) described the successful use of posterior pituitary extract in the treatment of diabetes insipidus that its antidiuretic properties were demonstrated. That the antidiuretic principle was associated with the posterior lobe alone was established by Geiling and associates (38). They found that in the whale, a species having anterior and posterior lobes widely separated anatomically, antidiuretic activity was limited to the posterior lobe. The classic studies of Ranson and his coworkers (35) in 1938 demonstrated the functional unity of the posterior pituitary gland and its hypothalamic connections and showed that, in the cat and monkey, diabetes insipidus is contingent upon the complete degeneration or removal of the neurohypophysis. The fascinating history of the identification of the hormonal constituents of the posterior pituitary and of their action was sketched by Sir Henry Dale (26).

It was thought formerly that the active hormones were produced within the pituicytes of the neurohypophysis and that the hypothalamic connections served only to regulate the release of these hormones. A considerable body of evidence, however, has led to the present interpretation that the hormones are synthesized in the ganglion cells of the hypothalamic nuclei and are transported down the axons of the neurohypophysial tract to terminations in the median eminence, pituitary stalk, and pars nervosa, where their release is influenced by the passage of impulses down the fibers of the neurohypophysial tract.

SYNTHESIS, TRANSPORT, AND STORAGE OF HORMONES IN THE HYPOTHALAMOHYPOPHYSIAL SYSTEM

Vasopressin and oxytocin have been extracted from the hypothalamic nuclei in concentrations

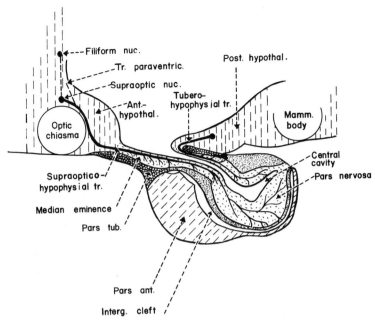

Figure 3-1. Diagrammatic representation of a sagittal section through the hypothalamus to illustrate the anatomic relations of the neurohypophysial tract.

clearly higher than those present elsewhere in the nervous system (7, 9, 10, 85). In addition, the ganglion cells of both the supraoptic and paraventricular nuclei contain distinctive dense granules. This neurosecretory material has been identified and characterized by a variety of staining and histochemical techniques (like the Gomori stain) and has also been found distributed down the neurohypophysial tract and in the posterior pituitary in concentrations which parallel the concentrations of extractable antidiuretic material from these same sites. The material is high in cystine, as are the hormones, and is thought to represent storage or transport forms of the hormones complexed to a matrix carrier of protein (11).

Rats with familial hypothalamic diabetes insipidus (Brattleboro strain) lack arginine vasopressin in their hypothalamic and posterior pituitary tissues as compared with normal rats and also have little or no neurosecretory material in their hypothalamus, neurohypophysial tract, and posterior pituitary (84). Sachs (79, 88) has shown that the guinea pig hypothalamus can incorporate labeled cystine or tyrosine into vasopressin *in vitro,* but the infundibular stem and posterior pituitary cannot. The rate of incorporation of labeled cystine into vasopressin increased when the guinea pigs had been dehydrated prior to the *in vitro* studies.

Since the hormone is synthesized in the hypothalamic nuclei but not in the posterior pituitary and is extractable from the latter, it must be transported from the former to the latter. In fact, this is the function of the neurohypophysial tract. After transection or compression of the pituitary stalk in a variety of vertebrates ranging from frog to man, the neurosecretory material has been observed to accumulate in the stalk on the hypothalamic side of the interrupted axons, suggesting that the granules migrate down the axons (7, 85). Distal movement of secretory granules down the axons of living supraoptic cells has also been observed in tissue culture (54).

Studies of the posterior pituitary from experimental animals that had been dehydrated (65, 74), given cinchoninic acid derivatives (17) or ether anesthesia (27), or been bled (27) have shown parallel decreases in neurosecretory material and assayable hormones and evidence of increased circulating antidiuretic activity. Similarly, the converse changes have been observed in hydrated animals (55). It has been more difficult to relate changes in the hypothalamic content of hormone to the functional state.

THE PHYSICAL STATE OF THE HORMONES

The long-standing controversy regarding the biologic form of the active principle seems now to be resolved. Early workers had found the active principles in urine or in pressed, fresh pituitary juices to be nondialyzable and from the latter source to be associated largely with a protein of some 30,000 molecular weight (67, 97). The isolation of vasopressin and oxytocin by du Vigneaud and associates (33) clearly established that the active principles were in fact small dialyzable peptides. Acher (2) has shown that the large molecule, which he has termed *neurophysin,* is a protein carrier molecule capable of binding oxytocin and vasopressin in a nondialyzable complex. The peptide hormones may bind electrostatically to the carrier protein (41, 42). Neurophysin is obtained from the posterior pituitary gland and may play a role in the storage of the hormones there. At the present time, evidence is conflicting as to the binding of the active peptides to proteins in the serum. Whether the neurophysin is secreted together with vasopressin and oxytocin, *with either*, or with neither is not known. The nondialyzable urinary component could be either neurophysin or some similar binding substance.

CHARACTERIZATION OF THE HORMONES

In 1954, 58 years after the first demonstration of the vasopressor potency of pituitary extracts, du Vigneaud and his associates (33) discovered the structure of vasopressin and oxytocin and synthesized oxytocin. This achievement was a milestone in endocrinology because for the first time a biologically active peptide hormone had been synthesized.

The structures of vasopressin and oxytocin are basically similar (Fig. 3–2). Both contain eight amino acid residues arranged with a five-member S-S bonded ring and a tail composed of three amino acids. The amino acid sequence of oxytocin differs from that of vasopressin in two locations, one in the peptide ring and one in the tripeptide tail. Arginine vasopressin has arginine in the tripeptide tail, whereas in lysine vasopressin, the lysine is substituted in this position for the arginine.

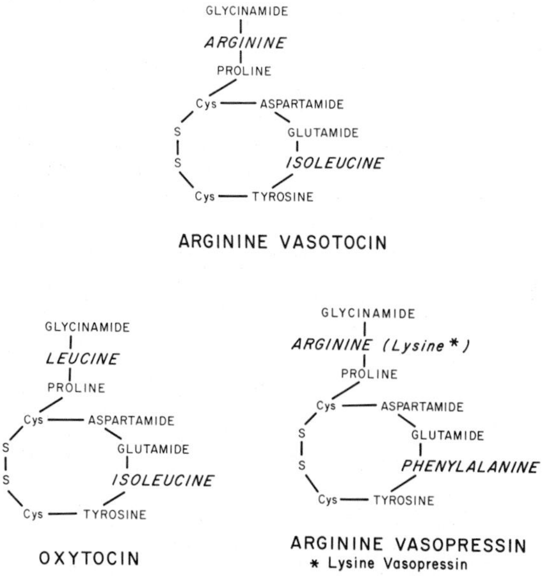

ARGININE VASOTOCIN

OXYTOCIN

ARGININE VASOPRESSIN
* Lysine Vasopressin

Figure 3–2. The structures of vasotocin, oxytocin, and vasopressin have an identical amino acid sequence except in two positions. Lysine vasopressin is unique in the pig family.

PHYLOGENETIC DISTRIBUTION AND FUNCTION OF THE HORMONES

Arginine vasopressin has been identified in a wide variety of mammals including such diverse types as whales, marsupials, and the spiny anteater, an egg-laying mammal (1, 83). The sole exception among the mammals thus far examined is the pig family in which lysine vasopressin is the active principle. The domestic pig and the hippopotamus possess only lysine vasopressin, whereas the wart hog and the peccary appear to possess both lysine and arginine vasopressin.

The identification and comparison of neurohormones in nonmammalian vertebrates similarly provides an interesting means of approach to evolutionary problems. This has been summarized recently by Sawyer (82) (see Figure 3–3). In nonmammalian vertebrates, arginine vasotocin replaces arginine vasopressin as a pressor substance. Oxytocin is present in bony fish, as well as in reptiles, birds, and Amphibia. Sawyer considers arginine vasotocin the prototype compound, as it appears to be present in all lower vertebrates thus far studied (83).

The function of neurohypophysial hormones in the phylogenetic sequence was investigated by Heller and Bentley (52). Below the Amphibia, no effect on water balance could be detected from homologous neurohypophysial extracts. In anurans, however, they found an increase in weight indicating water uptake through the skin. Arginine vasotocin, the naturally occurring hormone in this class, was the most potent physiologically.

The function of the neurohypophysial hormones in fish remains obscure. Sawyer has suggested that the fish neurohypophysis may serve solely to deliver neurosecretions which regulate the adenohypophysis.

MECHANISM OF RELEASE

Neurohypophysial hormones can be released rapidly into the circulation in response to a wide variety of stimuli, and stainable neurosecretory material can be depleted rapidly from the neurohypophysis. The exact mechanism by which this happens is not yet clear. Nerve impulses originating in the hypothalamus and conducted along the axons of the pituitary stalk or electrical stimulation of the axons result in depolarization of the neurosecretory terminals in the posterior pituitary and in the release of hormones through some calcium-dependent process (31, 32, 46, 91, 92, 93). Other conditions which should depolarize the neurosecretory terminals, e.g., high potassium concentrations, result in release of the hormones. Firm evidence is not yet available whether the hormone is released from the neurosecretory endings while still protein-bound or whether the process of release consists of breaking the bonds.

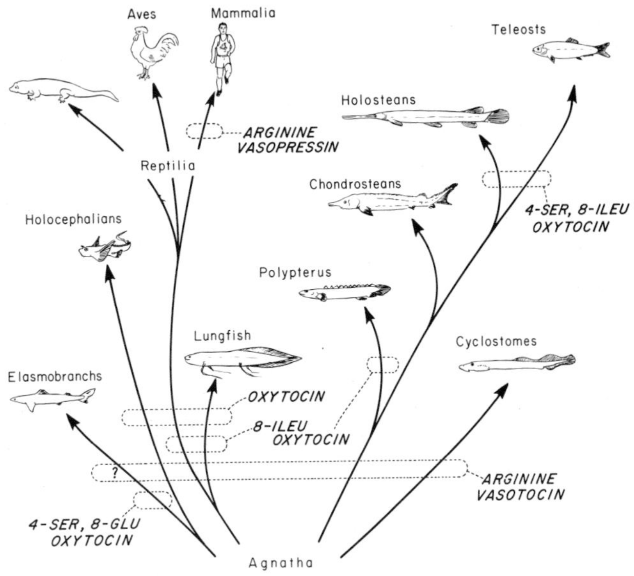

Figure 3–3. A representation of the probable evolutionary relationships between some major groups of vertebrates based on the chemical structure of their neurohypophysial hormones. (Reproduced with modification from Acher, R., Chauvet, J., et al.: *Bull. Soc. Chim. Biol.* 47:2279, 1965, and Sawyer, W. H.: *Endocrinology* 75:981, 1964, with permission.) The probable distributions of the hormones are indicated by the dotted circles. Acher has also identified 8-ileu oxytocin in amphibians.

VASOPRESSIN

Regulation of Secretion

Osmotic Stimuli

Although the term *vasopressin* denotes an action on blood pressure, it is clear that the major physiologic role of this hormone relates to its potent antidiuretic activity, hence its designation as the antidiuretic hormone. It had been known that dehydration provides the usual physiologic stimulus for release of the hormone. The classic studies of Verney in 1946 (98) established the role of the posterior pituitary in the conservation of body water. He demonstrated that an increase of only 1 to 2 per cent in the effective osmotic pressure of plasma in the distribution of the internal carotid artery resulted in the release of antidiuretic hormone and the formation of a concentrated urine. Thus isosmolar solutions of saline, sucrose, and dextrose were equally effective in eliciting an immediate antidiuresis, whereas urea was ineffective. Verney speculated that the osmoreceptors were not stimulated by solutes such as urea which penetrated cell membranes rapidly. In experiments of longer duration, dextrose also was less effective than isosmotic sodium chloride in producing antidiuresis.

It is generally accepted that the osmoreceptors are localized in the anterior hypothalamus. Verney described vesicular cells within the supraoptic nuclei which he thought might be the osmoreceptors. He speculated that an increase in tonicity or osmotic activity of the extracellular fluids might cause shrinkage of the cells and release of antidiuretic hormone. Bard (6) demonstrated that decorticated cats, with extensive lesions that isolated the anterior hypothalamus and pituitary from all neural connections, could still regulate their water balance appropriately. When deprived of water or infused with hypertonic saline, they diminished their urine volume and increased its specific gravity. Instillation of hypertonic saline through micropipets localized to the anterior hypothalamus also elicits antidiuresis.

Conversely, dilution of the plasma or body fluids suppresses release of antidiuretic hormone. In the absence of this circulating hormone, a profuse water diuresis occurs with excretion of a urine hypotonic to the body fluids. This allows excretion of a water load and serves to restore osmolarity of the body fluids to normal levels. Thus a negative feedback system exists, including the kidney and the central nervous system, which preserves within narrow limits the total solute concentration of the body fluids. Since we now know that the intracellular fluids share the same tonicity as the extracellular fluids, this same mechanism preserves a normal solute concentration or water activity throughout the body fluid compartments.

Relation to Thirst.   It is evident that renal conservation of water stimulated by the antidiuretic hormone could not alone prevent dehydration. The continuous obligatory loss of water via skin, lungs, and kidneys would result in progressive dehydration were not some mechanism available to alert the individual to the need for water. The thirst mechanism obviously serves this function. Today, largely as a result of the studies of Andersson (4), the close anatomic as well as physiologic relationship between the thirst and antidiuretic centers is appreciated. Andersson, and later Andersson and McCann, found that intrahypothalamic injections of small volumes of hypertonic saline (<0.01 ml. of 2 or 3 per cent sodium chloride solutions) into a medial part of the hypothalamus of goats often caused drinking of large volumes of water. A more reproducible method, which permitted more precise localization of the areas involved, proved to be electrical stimulation with carefully placed intra-hypothalamic electrodes. By this means, experimentally induced drinking could be repeated at will. Polydipsia commenced within a period of 5 seconds after the stimulation began and stopped as abruptly with cessation of the stimulus. The animals usually drank continuously while the stimulus was applied and, if the stimulus was prolonged, could be induced to drink volumes of water up to 40 per cent of total body weight in a short period of time. Such overhydration would result in hemolysis, hemoglobinuria, and other signs of severe water intoxication. The character of the response gave the observers the impression that the stimulus caused "a conscious urge to drink." The area involved was found to extend from the dorsal into the ventral hypothalamus.

An interesting association was found by Andersson and McCann between stimulation of thirst, antidiuresis, and ejection of milk. Stimulation in the anterior part of the "drinking area" was found to cause inhibition of water diuresis and ejection of milk simultaneously with polydipsia. Stimulation of the posterior part was not accompanied by evidence of release of neurohypophysial hormones. Stimulation within or in regions adjacent to the paraventricular and supraoptic nuclei or in the vicinity of the supraoptico-hypophysial tract caused, as expected, antidiuresis and milk ejection but failed to provoke polydipsia. Milk ejection in these experiments always occurred when antidiuresis was elicited. The proximity of the thirst and antidiuretic centers demonstrated in these studies, as well as their response to the same effective stimulus of increased solute concentration, indicates their close interrelationship. Whether there exist two separate centers which overlap or only a single center with nervous connections, stimulation of which may elicit separate responses, is not yet determined.

The role of the neurohypophysial-renal-thirst complex in regulation of concentration of the body fluids is summarized in Figure 3–4.

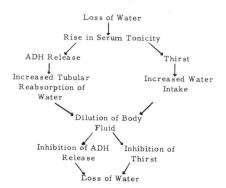

Figure 3–4. Illustrating the interrelationship between the vasopressin regulating system, the thirst center of the hypothalamus, oral intake, and renal excretion of water in maintaining a constant osmolarity of the body fluids.

Nonosmotic Stimuli

It is apparent that there are rich connections with other parts of the nervous system through which the release of vasopressin may be influenced. Pain and other emotional states have been associated with antidiuresis. Successful attempts to condition antidiuretic and diuretic responses have been claimed (23, 39, 57, 69). Stimulation of the ulnar nerve or vagus will elicit antidiuresis. In studies utilizing conscious monkeys, Hayward and Smith (51) have shown that antidiuresis similar to that induced by vasopressin can be elicited by electrical stimulation not only in the hypothalamus but in several areas remote to this, including the mesencephalic reticular formation. It has not been established in all instances, however, that the antidiuresis is truly due to release of antidiuretic hormone and is not merely the result of transient renal hemodynamic changes (see below).

In addition to neural stimuli arising outside the hypothalamus, release of vasopressin may be influenced by a number of pharmacologic agents. Alcohol may inhibit release of antidiuretic hormone, but the effect is a weak one and often obscured. Many other substances act to release antidiuretic hormone: cinchoninic acid (28), acetylcholine (75), nicotine (20), morphine (29), barbiturates (30), ferritin (5), bradykinin (78), and a variety of other substances which have been less well documented as causing antidiuresis through release of antidiuretic hormone.

It seems that the most important physiologic stimulus to secretion of vasopressin other than hypertonicity of extracellular fluids is a reduction in the effective plasma volume. Thus quiet standing, hemorrhage, tourniquets about extremities, reduced cardiac output, hypoalbuminemic states, and so forth, have been examined, and evidence has been elicited suggestive of antidiuretic hormone release (87). The antidiuretic response may occur even in the presence of hypotonicity of the body fluids, suggesting that volume control can override osmotic control. Though a vast literature exists in regard to the role of vasopressin in conserving body water in response to contraction of the effective plasma volume, the actual documentation of this relationship awaits a specific assay method for identification of circulating vasopressin.

Basis of Antidiuretic Action

An understanding of how vasopressin results in conservation of water requires knowledge of the renal countercurrent mechanism for concentrating and diluting the urine. Hargitay and Kuhn (48) suggested from theoretical considerations that a countercurrent mechanism was involved in the process of urinary concentration, and the first experimental evidence in support of this mechanism was obtained by Wirz (102). Further evidence was

DIURESIS ANTIDIURESIS

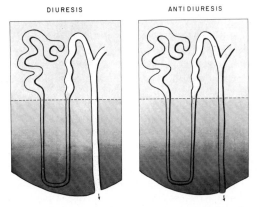

Figure 3–5. Schematic diagram of a nephron in diuresis and antidiuresis. From the glomerulus and proximal convoluted tubule in the renal cortex (above the broken line) the nephron proceeds to the loop of Henle which dips into the medulla. Returning from the medulla, the loop of Henle joins the distal convoluted tubule which empties into a collecting duct. The latter passes back through the hypertonic medulla to make its exit at the renal papilla. The density of stippling represents the osmolarity of the fluid in the interstitial tissues and tubules.

rapidly forthcoming from numerous laboratories, notably those of Gottschalk and Ullrich, so that at present a fairly complete description (Fig. 3–5) can be given of the renal concentrating and diluting mechanism, although a number of details remain to be settled [see Gottschalk (44) and Berliner (13)].

The ultrafiltrate which passes through the glomerular membrane is isosmotic with plasma and with the renal cortical interstitial fluid. The bulk of this filtrate, some 85 per cent, is reabsorbed as a passive process accompanying the active reabsorption of sodium as the filtrate passes through the proximal tubule. Since the epithelium of the proximal tubule has a high permeability to water, water moves out of the tubular lumen so that the luminal urine remains isosmotic with plasma. As the filtrate moves down the descending limb of the loop of Henle, it enters the hypertonic medullary zone and becomes progressively more concentrated as water moves out of the tubular lumen. This process of increasing concentration of the medullary interstitium and luminal contents proceeds to the tip of the loop. As the fluid begins to move up the ascending limb, its concentration falls gradually below that of the medullary interstitium as a result of an outward extrusion of sodium from lumen to interstitium without a proportionate movement of water. The extrusion of sodium from lumen to interstitium in the ascending limb of the loop of Henle provides the source for the hypertonicity of the medullary interstitial fluid and causes the urine entering the distal convoluted tubule to be hypotonic to the cortical interstitial fluid. To this point, the nephron handles the luminal contents similarly in both diuresis and antidiuresis. In the former condition, little water is reabsorbed during

further passage of luminal fluid through distal tubule and collecting duct, but sodium reabsorption continues. A very dilute urine results. During antidiuresis, the presence of antidiuretic hormone causes a marked increase in the permeability of the tubular lumen to water, so that equilibration of urine with interstitial fluid occurs. Since the collecting tubule passes down through the zone of marked interstitial fluid hypertonicity in the inner medulla and papillary tip, the urine enters the renal pelvis highly concentrated. Direct measurements of fluids from collecting tubules, tips of loop of Henle, and tips of vasa recta indicate that they are all of equal osmolarity at the same level. In man, concentrations of 1000 to 1200 mOsm. per kg. of water are maximal. In many mammals, very much higher concentrations can be achieved.

Largely from studies on isolated amphibian tissues—skin (96) and urinary bladder (63)—we know that vasopressin exerts its antidiuretic action by making the responsive epithelium more permeable to water and to urea. In the presence of vasopressin and an osmotic gradient, the renal tubular epithelium permits passage of large quantities of water with very little solute. The hormone alters the responsive plasma membrane at the luminal surface of the tubular cells to accommodate this bulk movement of water.

The nature of the membrane changes and the means by which they are induced by the hormone remain to be elucidated. Of special interest is the finding of Handler and Orloff (73) that 3′5′ cyclic adenosine monophosphate (3′5′ cyclic AMP), which has been implicated as an intracellular mediator of the action of several peptide hormones, mimics the action of vasopressin. Furthermore, increased tissue content of 3′5′ cyclic AMP has been noted following exposure of responsive tissues to vasopressin (47), and neurohypophysial hormones specifically will stimulate *in vitro* adenyl cyclase in membrane preparations from responsive tissues such as toad bladder. Although it appears to be an intermediate in the hormonal action, it still is not clear how this compound induces the changes in membrane permeability. It is remarkable that in *in vitro* systems the action of vasopressin occurs within seconds and can almost as promptly be terminated by removal of the hormone from the bathing medium. The action of the hormone also seems not to require energy but to effect changes in passive permeability in responsive epithelia. The hormonal effects are not blocked by inhibitors of protein or of DNA-dependent RNA synthesis.

No direct effect of vasopressin on sodium excretion has been observed in man. By its ability to cause water retention with expansion of body fluid volume, it may secondarily induce sodium excretion (64). Expansion of body fluid volume with water results in increased glomerular filtration rate and suppressed aldosterone secretion, a combination ideally suited to augment urinary sodium loss.

Other Physiologic and Pharmacologic Effects of Vasopressin

In spite of various claims in the past of an action of vasopressin on the formation or composition of sweat, more refined recent studies do not indicate any effect of the hormone on this function in man.

Although it has been shown that vasopressin can cause release of corticotropin from the anterior pituitary (72), adrenal steroidogenesis through a direct action on the adrenal cortex (56), release of radioactive iodine from the thyroid (37), and so forth, none of these effects appears to be significant physiologically.

When infused in quantities considerably larger than those required for maximal antidiuresis, vasopressin causes contraction of smooth muscle. Thus, effects on bowel and vasculature become evident. The vascular effects are widespread and result in a generalized increase in vascular resistance. In the anesthetized animal, this effect produces a rise in blood pressure, hence the name *vasopressin* and the standard pressor assay for this hormone. In the unanesthetized animal, compensatory reflexes prevent significant blood pressure elevation. The vasoconstriction is widespread, affecting both peripheral and visceral vessels (45). Cardiac output falls, and coronary vasoconstriction may constitute a hazard to elderly patients with coronary vascular disease if given large amounts of vasopressin. On the other hand, the vasoconstriction in the visceral blood vessels has led to the use of vasopressin and its analogues as an effective temporary means of controlling bleeding from the gastrointestinal tract, particularly from gastric or esophageal varices (71). The mechanism of action of vasopressin on smooth muscle is not known.

Fate of Vasopressin

The distribution and inactivation of vasopressin in the body have been the subjects of numerous studies with diverse and often conflicting results. Species differences, effects of physiologic versus pharmacologic concentrations on metabolism and removal of hormone from the blood, and above all the lack of reliable means of measuring the concentration of the hormone in biologic fluids have contributed to the state of confusion.

Estimates of the half-life of vasopressin in plasma have been indirectly derived (60, 81) and vary from about 1 minute in the rat to 10 to 20 minutes in man and some 7 minutes in the dog. However, in the rat the half-life of vasopressin has been estimated to vary from 0.6 minute at very high plasma levels of the hormone to 3.4 minutes at concentrations within the physiologic range. The rate of clearance of the hormone from plasma also depends on its concentration and its volume of distribution. Usually it is assumed that vasopressin is distributed in a volume equal to that of plasma, but this assumption lacks rigorous valida-

tion, as does the usual view that vasopressin in plasma is largely or entirely bound to protein.

The liver and kidneys were implicated by Ginsburg and Heller (40) as the major sites of inactivation of the hormone or of its removal from plasma. These workers found that in rats with high plasma levels of vasopressin the liver and kidneys cleared nearly all the vasopressin contained in plasma on a single circulation through the hepatic or renal vascular bed. The total clearance per minute by liver and kidneys equaled total plasma volume, and liver and kidneys contributed about equally to the disappearance of the hormone. Lauson (61, 62) has reexamined this matter more recently and concludes that at lower, more physiologic concentrations the hepatic portal extraction ratio for vasopressin averaged 12 per cent and that for the kidneys, some 25 per cent in hydrated, unanesthetized dogs.

Several estimations have been made of the fraction of vasopressin removed by the kidneys which appears in the urine. Sawyer (81) estimates that in the rat less than a quarter of the total vasopressin cleared appears in the urine; the remainder is probably inactivated. Thorn and Smith (93) found that 12 per cent of the synthetic arginine vasopressin injected intravenously is recoverable by bioassay from the urine. The total recoverable from urine appears by 100 minutes.

Whether other tissues inactivate the hormone is not known. In rats the absence of kidneys and liver reduced the rate of disappearance from plasma of high concentrations of vasopressin (Pitressin) by some eight- to tenfold. Whether the hormone is inactivated in serum has also been a controversial topic. High levels of oxytocinase and vasopressinase have been found in human plasma during pregnancy but not in plasma from nonpregnant women or from men (70, 95).

With the reliability of assay methods still uncertain (81), even the normal concentrations of antidiuretic hormone in the plasma are unsettled. In 1934 Theobald (89) estimated, from the antidiuresis resulting transiently after a single intravenous injection, that the physiologic level during antidiuresis in man must be about 2 microunits per ml. of arterial plasma. Many estimations since then by various assay methods fall within a factor of five of this estimate.

Diabetes Insipidus (Vasopressin Deficiency)

As would be surmised from its role in the regulation of water balance, deficiency of vasopressin for any reason will result in a diuresis of dilute urine. In the absence of sufficient intake of water, this will cause a rise in the total solute concentration or osmolality of the body fluids. Thus a failure of the kidney to concentrate urine in the presence of an increased effective solute concentration of the serum, together with the finding that the kidney can respond to exogenous vasopressin by producing a concentrated urine, constitutes the criterion for establishing the diagnosis of diabetes insipidus.

Destruction of the hypothalamic centers—supraoptic and paraventricular nuclei—or division of the supraoptico-hypophysial tract above the median eminence is associated with permanent diabetes insipidus. Transection of the tract below the median eminence or removal just of the posterior lobe produces only a transient polyuria; sufficient hormone can be released from fibers ending in the median eminence to prevent occurrence of frank diabetes insipidus.

Ranson and associates (35) utilized cats to demonstrate that animals with hypothalamic lesions sufficient to cause diabetes insipidus underwent a triphasic response to the surgical damage. Immediately following the lesion a polyuria and polydipsia commenced which lasted usually 4 to 5 days. After this a period of intense antidiuresis set in for some 6 days. This was followed by the permanent polyuria and polydipsia of established diabetes insipidus. The same pattern of response has been observed in humans following high pituitary stalk section (77). It is generally agreed that the initial diuretic phase results from acute damage to hypothalamic function so that stored hormone is not released. The antidiuretic stage results from degeneration of hormone-laden tissue with release of the contained hormone into the circulation. Administration of a water load during the antidiuretic phase will not induce the usual diuretic response. Removal of the posterior pituitary at the time of hypothalamic damage will prevent the antidiuretic phase (58). With lesser damage to the hypothalamus, the diabetes insipidus may never recur after the initial polyuria and polydipsia. This is seen after head trauma or neurosurgery. In early diabetes insipidus of traumatic origin, the attending physician is wise to avoid hasty prognostications regarding the permanence of the condition.

Clinical Causes

Diabetes insipidus may result from any condition that causes damage to the neurohypophysial system. Randall has suggested an etiologic classification of this condition with two major categories of primary and secondary diabetes insipidus (76). With primary diabetes insipidus he includes familial and idiopathic cases. Idiopathic cases constitute the major group in any such classification, comprising 45 per cent of Blotner's series (16). Idiopathic diabetes insipidus may become manifest at any age and affect either sex. It is unusual, however, for the idiopathic type to begin in infancy, although it may commence in early childhood. Familial diabetes insipidus, on the other hand, is very uncommon and must constitute less than 1 per cent of cases of diabetes insipidus. It may occur in infancy or childhood and may affect either males or females. The condition has been described in seven generations of one family (15). Familial diabetes insipidus is to be distinguished from nephrogenic diabetes insipidus (100); the latter is a renal tubular defect inherited largely by males wherein the affected tubules are unresponsive to antidiuretic hormone.

In the group with secondary diabetes insipidus, head trauma (accidental or neurosurgical) and neoplasms (primary or metastatic) constitute the major causes. In older series primary intracranial tumors constituted nearly one third of all cases. However the increasing incidence of automobile injuries and surgical pituitary stalk sections and other surgical procedures in the region of the neurohypophysial system has affected the frequency more recently. Of the metastatic tumors, breast cancer seems to have a special predilection for the hypothalamic area. Other etiologic factors contribute only small numbers to any series (90). However, sarcoid, birth injuries, eosinophilic granuloma, and a variety of local infections contribute recurring causes. Even with lesions in the hypothalamus, diabetes insipidus is a rare occurrence, presumably because only a small fraction of the system remaining will protect against manifest dysfunction.

Clinical Manifestations

The manifestations of diabetes insipidus are so dramatic that not infrequently intelligent adult patients can remember an exact day or even hour when the polyuria and polydipsia commenced. The fluid exchange may reach distressing proportions; urine volumes of 5 to 10 liters per 24 hours are usual, though rarely much greater volumes may be excreted. In normal man, urine flows of 12 ml. per minute may be attained readily during a brisk water diuresis. As such a diuresis is thought to result from a physiologic state of diabetes insipidus, it might be anticipated that the patient suffering from diabetes insipidus would persistently excrete urine at this rate, amounting to over 17 liters per day. Some increase in glomerular filtration rate accompanies the acute overhydration required to produce such rates of urine flow in the normal subject, whereas the filtration rate in the patient with diabetes insipidus is not increased and may be slightly below normal.

The specific gravity of the urine in diabetes is usually 1.001 to 1.005. The corresponding concentration will be about 50 to 200 mOsm. per kg. of water. With restriction of fluid intake, the specific gravity may reach 1.010 or even slightly higher with severe dehydration, and the concentration may increase to 300 mOsm. per kg. of water. Urine slightly hypertonic to the serum has been produced experimentally in the absence of antidiuretic hormone by great reduction in the glomerular filtration rate (12). The elaboration of hypertonic urine during severe dehydration by a patient with diabetes insipidus or with acute reduction of glomerular filtration rate due to any cause, such as syncope, need not therefore indicate some residual neurohypophysial function.

Aside from the annoyance of polyuria and polydipsia, there may be no other evidence of ill health or of other physiologic disturbance associated with this condition unless the patient suffers from the underlying disease which brought about destruction of the neurohypophysial system. The frequently encountered assumption that patients with diabetes insipidus suffer from severe dehydration is not supported by measurements of serum sodium or total solute concentrations. It is true that a slight elevation of sodium and total solute concentrations of serum has been demonstrated statistically. Barlow and de Wardener (8) found the plasma osmolality of patients suffering from diabetes insipidus to average 295 ± 15 mOsm. per kg. (SD), whereas that for normal subjects averaged 280 ± 6 mOsm. per kg. (SD). Since this statistically significant difference is associated with considerable overlap, this determination is of little help diagnostically in the individual case. As long as the patient's thirst center is undamaged, the total solute concentration of the body fluids will be preserved close to the normal limits but at the expense of polydipsia and the large fluid exchange which are characteristic of this condition.

The inability of the patient to demand or seek water during unconsciousness due to trauma or anesthesia may be fatal. This situation may occur at the onset of diabetes insipidus secondary to head trauma or intracranial surgery and is one of the causes of hypernatremia following head injury. A careful record of urine volumes and urine and serum concentrations in patients with acute head trauma and coma will prevent the occurrence of severe dehydration. Rarely, a patient with diabetes insipidus may also have destruction of the thirst center. Such a patient may suffer bouts of mental disturbance and high fever unless taught to take sufficient fluids and given replacement therapy. Markedly elevated serum sodium concentrations may be found in these rare cases.

Differential Diagnosis

A patient with persistent polyuria and urine of low concentration may have one or more of three basic disturbances: (1) inability of the kidney to elaborate a concentrated urine despite adequate vasopressin; (2) inadequate secretion of vasopressin; (3) persistent excessive water intake.

Any condition that disturbs the normal action of the renal concentrating mechanism so that it fails to respond to vasopressin may produce polyuria and a low urinary concentration. This renal unresponsiveness may arise from metabolic or structural changes in the kidney. Potassium depletion and hypercalcemia impair renal concentrating ability. Usually these conditions impair maximum concentrating ability but do not cause hypotonic urines. In a few patients, the polyuria and reduced urine concentration are sufficient to raise the possibility of diabetes insipidus. Structural and functional alterations in the medullary countercurrent systems interfere with concentrating ability so that many kinds of acute and chronic renal diseases are associated with failure to concentrate the urine. Urine volumes of 2 to 3 liters daily, together with nocturia, are common in renal disease but only rarely achieve levels to be confused with those of diabetes insipidus. Usually other stigmata of renal disease and impaired kidney function are evident by the time polyuria is noted. Polyuria may follow the oliguric stage in acute tubular necrosis, but this is transient and the clinical setting rarely leaves the cause of the polyuria in doubt. In the rare nephrogenic diabetes insipidus, which is hereditary and affects males, the disturbance occurs shortly after birth, and the defect is a failure of the renal tubules to respond to vasopressin (101). Patients with diabetes mellitus may have polydipsia and polyuria. The urine in this condition will have a high specific gravity, but its osmolality may not be much over 300 mOsm. per kg. This discrepancy between specific gravity and osmolality results from the large contribution glucose makes to specific gravity, even at relatively low concentrations.

Inadequate vasopressin secretion in the presence of an elevated serum osmolality has already been stated as the definition of diabetes insipidus.

For many years it was argued whether diabetes insipidus resulted from a primary polyuria or primary polydipsia. The increased understanding of the regulation of body fluid tonicity and of the physiologic action of purified antidiuretic hormone has left little doubt regarding the primacy of the polyuria in neurohypophysial insufficiency. However, clinicians are becoming increasingly aware of a group of patients, often referred to as compulsive water drinkers, whose primary disorder in water exchange is their polydipsia. Surprisingly, it may be quite difficult to distinguish by clinical or laboratory studies the cases of compulsive water drinking from the cases of diabetes insipidus. This is because of the effect on the renal concentrating mechanism of chronic ingestion of large volumes of water (see below).

A variety of special procedures have been devised to assist in a classification of patients with polyuria and polydipsia according to the three etiologic categories just mentioned. They are all designed basically to test whether the patient can respond to osmotic stimuli by elaboration of a concentrated urine and, if not, whether such failure is the consequence of lack of endogenous vasopressin or of a renal disturbance that blocks the normal response of the kidney tubule to the antidiuretic hormone.

The simplest test is to restrict water intake and observe changes in urine volume and concentration. This must be done under careful supervision with frequent weight checks made to avoid loss of more than 3 to 5 per cent of body weight, beyond which serious circulatory disturbances may occur. There should never be a need to prolong the period of water restriction beyond 24 hours to make a diagnosis, and it should of course be terminated earlier if weight loss of 3 to 5 per cent of body weight occurs. Small children or infants tolerate dehydration poorly and should be watched with special care. The volume and concentration of each passage of urine should be measured. A normal subject may be expected to reduce his urine flow to less than 0.5 ml. per minute and increase his urine concentration to greater than 800 mOsm. per kg. (this would correspond in the older clinical literature to specific gravities usually of 1.020 or above). In patients with true diabetes insipidus, it is expected that urine volumes well above this limit will persist, and urine concentration will remain below 200 mOsm. per kg. (specific gravities of 1.001 to 1.005) until advanced states of dehydration are present. Unfortunately the differences are often not so clear, and patients who have neurohypophysial insufficiency may concentrate their urines to 300 or 400 mOsm. per kg. (specific gravities of 1.008 to 1.014) with marked dehydration.

Another means of increasing plasma osmolality in order to examine the release of antidiuretic hormone is the infusion of hypertonic solutions, usually saline, intravenously. There are many variations of the original protocol of Hickey and Hare (53). The patient is hydrated initially with an infusion of dextrose and water at a rate sufficient (usually 8 to 10 ml. per minute) to induce a brisk diuresis (>5 ml. per minute). The intravenous solution is then switched to 2.5 per cent sodium chloride solution at a rate of 0.25 ml. per minute per kg. of body weight and continued for 45 minutes. Urine flow is measured by voidings at 15-minute intervals. If neurohypophysial function and renal function are normal, urine flow may be expected to fall sharply with the infusion of hypertonic saline. However, the large amounts of saline administered may cause an osmotic diuresis which obscures the expected antidiuresis. Furthermore, the volumes and rates of the saline infusions may precipitate congestive failure in some patients.

Pharmacologic means of eliciting secretion of antidiuretic hormone, as well as the physiologic stimulus of increased osmolarity of the plasma, have been used to test for availability of antidiuretic hormone.

It has been shown in both man and experimental animals that nicotine will cause antidiuresis by stimulating secretion of antidiuretic hormone from the neurohypophysis (19, 21, 66), and this has been used to assess neurohypophysial function in cases of suspected diabetes insipidus. Water diuresis is induced, and then nicotine is given intravenously in a dose of 0.5 to 1.0 mg. of nicotine base to nonsmokers and as much as 3.0 mg. to habitual smokers. With an adequate dose the patient will experience salivation, nausea, vomiting, flushing, dizziness, or syncope. It is necessary to measure urine concentration as well as to observe a sharp fall in the rate of urine flow; syncope may occur, causing a reduced urine flow secondary to the associated reduction in glomerular filtration rate. Little or no increase in urine concentration will occur in such an antidiuresis. Some patients will fail to respond to increased serum tonicity but will

still exhibit antidiuresis with nicotine. This has led to the possibility of dividing the group with diabetes insipidus into subclasses which have lesions affecting different steps in the water conserving system. Thus far this interesting possibility has not been exploited.

If the patient fails to elaborate a concentrated urine in response to osmotic stimuli, then it remains to show that his kidneys will respond to exogenous hormone, to establish a diagnosis of diabetes insipidus. For this purpose 5 milliunits per minute of aqueous Pitressin may be administered for at least 1 hour by a slow intravenous drip, or 5 units of the long-acting vasopressin tannate in oil may be administered intramuscularly. It should be pointed out that the response to even large single doses of aqueous Pitressin administered parenterally may be highly variable and often very transient. The same or lesser total amounts of hormone given by slow intravenous drip, or, better, as the slowly absorbed vasopressin tannate in oil, will afford much more reproducible and maximal antidiuresis. The vasopressin tannate in oil may be injected in the evening at 7 P.M. and the patient instructed to empty his bladder at bedtime. Urine specimens collected on the patient's arising the following morning and for 3 successive hours thereafter should exhibit maximal concentration. The subject should be deprived of fluid during this period for best evaluation of maximal concentrating ability.

These simple measures will readily distinguish diabetes insipidus from nephrogenic causes of diminished response to vasopressin. It is becoming increasingly evident that it is not as easy to distinguish true diabetes insipidus from compulsive water drinking. The difficulty is that continued polydipsia lowers the maximal urinary concentrations achievable following dehydration or infusions of hypertonic saline. Thus saturating amounts of vasopressin in a hydrated subject will not elicit as concentrated a urine as will dehydration in the normal subject. Also, in the subject with diabetes insipidus or compulsive water drinking, the time required by the kidney for recovery of maximal concentrating ability in the presence of excesses of exogenous hormone and dehydration is not well defined. When rats of the Brattleboro strain with hereditary, hypothalamic diabetes insipidus (49) were given a long-acting preparation designed to keep them continuously antidiuretic, it took some 3 weeks before urine concentrations rose to 2000 mOsm. per kg., which is not an inordinately high concentration for a rat. De Wardener has reviewed this problem of diagnosis (8) and has made several interesting observations and suggestions. He makes use of the observation that the normal subject excretes a more concentrated urine following dehydration than with vasopressin, whereas the patient with diabetes insipidus does the opposite. Thus he concludes that if after dehydration urine concentration is greater than that produced by vasopressin alone, then ability to secrete antidiuretic hormone is normal, however low urinary concentration may be. If, on the other hand, the urine concentration is substantially less with fluid deprivation than after vasopressin, the ability to secrete antidiuretic hormone is abnormal, irrespective of the high urine concentrations that are achieved. Using these criteria, de Wardener was able to distinguish in almost all cases between diabetes insipidus and compulsive water drinking. Not only do the laboratory studies indicate the presence of a physical disorder, but it should be remembered that compulsive water drinking severe enough to be confused with diabetes insipidus constitutes a severe psychogenic disorder. Clinical evaluation usually is rewarding in revealing many other neurotic symptoms that support the suspicion of a serious personality or behavioral disturbance.

Treatment

Since the patient with uncomplicated diabetes insipidus who has an intact thirst mechanism and an ample supply of water suffers no known harm but only inconvenience from lack of antidiuretic hormone, the indications for replacement therapy may not be pressing. The marked polydipsia and polyuria may be disturbing and distracting during the day and may prevent sleep at night. For reasons of convenience, replacement therapy is usually justified.

Fortunately there are several effective preparations available for the treatment of the distressing symptoms in the uncomplicated case of diabetes insipidus. The simplest preparation for the patient to self-administer is a nasal spray (aqueous Pitressin, 20 international units [pressor] per ml.). Applications every 2 to 6 hours will alleviate symptoms in most patients but may not permit an uninterrupted night's sleep. Moistening a pledget of cotton with this solution and inserting it into a nostril at bedtime may provide a longer period of antidiuresis. With coryza the hormone may be applied to the vaginal or buccal mucous membrane, as the small octapeptide apparently is absorbed readily through these surfaces. Posterior pituitary powder can be used by insufflation rather than the spray, but since patients frequently develop inflammation or irritation of mucous membranes, this form of therapy is being replaced by the spray.

Some patients find the nasal spray too troublesome or the relief provided of too short a duration. A longer-acting preparation, vasopressin tannate in oil, may be useful in such instances. This preparation is a suspension of 5 units of vasopressin tannate in 1.0 ml. of vegetable oil. One half to 1.0 ml. injected subcutaneously or intramuscularly will usually provide relief of symptoms for 24 to 72 hours. The dose should not be repeated until symptoms recur. This will prevent cumulative water retention and marked dilution of body fluids. Resistance to the antidiuretic effects of vasopressin do not occur. This long-acting preparation, however, is a suspension which must be warmed and shaken

vigorously before being injected. The authors have seen much documentation that confirms the absence of antidiuretic activity in the oil vehicle.

Aqueous Pitressin has almost no place in the therapy of uncomplicated diabetes insipidus. When administered parenterally by injection, it has a brief and variable period of antidiuretic activity because of its prompt absorption into the bloodstream and subsequent rapid inactivation. It is useful for diagnostic purposes, as described earlier, or for the management of the unconscious patient. Aqueous Pitressin added by an intravenous infusion may provide ideal therapy in diabetes insipidus following head trauma or surgery when the need for close control of diuresis may make a long-acting preparation undesirable.

In addition to specific hormonal replacement therapy, other measures are available which will ameliorate the symptoms. For any degree of limitation of the concentration of the urine, the urinary volume will depend upon the solute load that the patient excretes. Dietary restriction of protein and salt will therefore reduce the obligatory urinary volume in the patient with diabetes insipidus. Diuretics, particularly chlorothiazide, were first shown by Crawford and Kennedy (24) paradoxically to reduce the polyuria in diabetes insipidus. Patients using diuretics may decrease daily urine volume by one third to one half. It is evident that the effect of the diuretic correlates with the sodium deficit it induces (14, 50). The exact intrarenal mechanism by which the urine concentration increases is not clearly understood, but urine concentration need rise only from 100 to 200 mOsm. per kg. to reduce urine volumes by half. Dietary restrictions and the use of diuretics are the only measures that avail in nephrogenic diabetes insipidus.

Chlorpropamide, an oral hypoglycemic agent, has also been found to reduce the polyuria of diabetes insipidus of neurohypophysial origin. Single daily doses of 500 mg. produce an antidiuresis comparable to that of antidiuretics. Studies by Ozer and Sharp (74a) indicate that its antidiuretic effect is accomplished by three actions: it stimulates adenyl cyclase directly, enhances the response to vasopressin, and antagonizes prostaglandins which inhibit the activity of adenyl cyclase.

Relationship to Other Endocrine Glands

Ever since von Hann (100) suggested, as a result of her postmortem studies in man, that destruction of the posterior pituitary caused diabetes insipidus only if significant portions of the anterior pituitary gland remained intact, the interrelationship between antidiuretic hormone and other hormones has been investigated. Amelioration of clinical diabetes insipidus has been observed with development of anterior pituitary insufficiency. How this amelioration comes about, or to loss of what hormone of the anterior pituitary it is due, is not understood. Patients with anterior pituitary insufficiency generally are anorectic and present small solute loads for excretion. This will be reflected in a lowering of urine volume, even without a change in concentration of the urine. It is not known whether persistence of some anterior pituitary or adrenocortical activity is necessary to keep the urine dilute in the absence of vasopressin. The difficulty is that our methods for evaluating the presence of small residual amounts of either neurohypophysial activity or anterior pituitary and adrenocortical activity are insufficient to permit us to know what kidney function would be in the complete absence of hormones from both neuro- and adenohypophysis. Certainly patients with panhypopituitarism are seen who develop polyuria and polydipsia only when receiving adrenocortical replacement therapy with glucocorticoids. Part of the polyuria may result in the increased solute load associated with an improved appetite or from the increased renal blood flow and glomerular filtration rate that accompany steroid replacement in these patients. However, there appear to be additional, more subtle effects that may result from a reduction in sensitivity of the osmoreceptor in the subject who is treated with glucocorticoids and experiences no concomitant depression of thirst. The rise in serum tonicity fails to release antidiuretic hormone but stimulates thirst. The result is polydipsia with polyuria and an apparent antagonism of vasopressin by corticosteroids. Many studies, however, have demonstrated that adrenal steroids do not block the actions of vasopressin upon the kidney.

The thyroid hormones seem to have no direct effect upon water excretion by the kidney except as they may alter food ingestion and solute excretion or renal circulation and glomerular filtration rate. Similarly, the sex hormones have no direct effect on water excretion but may increase body water content secondary to enhancing sodium retention. Growth hormone may be required to preserve renal blood flow and glomerular filtration rate. Reductions in glomerular filtration rate will interfere with the ability to excrete water and produce a very dilute urine, as just discussed.

The Syndrome of Excessive Antidiuretic Hormone

The consequences of prolonged excessive exposure to vasopressin were investigated in normal human subjects following the administration of a long-acting preparation of vasopressin (64). On normal fluid intake, water retention occurred and with this, weight gain and dilution of the body fluids. By the third day of hormone administration, a very large diuresis of sodium occurred. The urinary sodium loss resulted from an increase in glomerular filtration rate and suppression of aldosterone secretion in consequence of the expansion of body fluid volume. Thus a state of hyponatremia with normal blood urea nitrogen and a competent circulatory system was produced. Furthermore, these subjects had considerable quantities of sodium in their urine and did not become edematous.

A similar constellation of findings was first described clinically by Schwartz and associates (86) in two patients with bronchogenic carcinomas. These patients, like the normal subjects given vasopressin, had hyponatremia, competent circulatory systems, and low concentrations of urea in the blood. In spite of the hyponatremia, the urine was not free of sodium as one would expect in patients with circulatory disturbances, such as, for example, congestive heart failure or cirrhosis, which may present with comparable levels of hyponatremia. Schwartz and associates postulated that an inappropriate and excessive secretion of antidiuretic hormone was responsible for the features described.

Since publication of this report, the syndrome has been described in a number of seemingly diverse conditions (43), most of which, however, have involved concomitant pulmonary or cerebral pathologic disturbances. Patients with tuberculous meningitis, brain tumors, head trauma, pneumonia, and intrathoracic tumors may all show this type of asymptomatic hyponatremia. Myxedema, acute intermittent porphyria, and cerebral dysrhythmia have also been associated with the syndrome.

What the nature of the antidiuretic substance is and whether it comes from neurohypophysial or other sources are not known in most instances. In two reported studies (3, 18), assays of tumor masses revealed them to possess antidiuretic activity of considerable potency and indicated that they, rather than the neurohypophysis, were the source of the antidiuretic activity.

As one might anticipate from the physiologic basis of this syndrome, the hyponatremia is very resistant to correction by administration of sodium chloride. The expanded state of extracellular fluid volume allows the patient to promptly excrete any administered sodium. On the other hand, strict limitation of fluid intake will correct all the physiologic disturbances despite persistence of the source of excessive antidiuretic activity.

OXYTOCIN

It has long been appreciated (25, 59) that, in addition to vasopressin, another principle was contained in the neurohypophysis which had its predominant effect in causing contraction of uterine musculature. This factor had been known as oxytocin, and with its isolation, together with that of vasopressin and subsequent synthesis by du Vigneaud (33), its separate chemical existence was established.

When synthetic oxytocin and vasopressin became available, it was found that each compound shared the physiologic actions of the other. Vasopressin is more potent in its antidiuretic and vasopressor effects but shares some oxytocic and milk ejection activity. The reverse is true for synthetic oxytocin, which has definite antidiuretic activity. Thus oxytocin is a hundredfold more potent than vasopressin in its milk ejection activity in the human (80), whereas vasopressin is more than a hundredfold more potent than oxytocin in eliciting antidiuresis in the dog (81). There is considerable species variation in such relative potencies, as well as differences dependent upon the test of function that is used.

Another feature of the physiologic action of these hormones that has been much discussed is the constancy or variability of their relative rates of secretion. Since species variability is great, a considerable literature may be summarized based on the studies of Gaitan and co-workers (22, 36) in the human. They studied a group of women during the last weeks of pregnancy or early puerperium, using their changes in uterine activity (and intramammary pressure) and in urine osmolality as criteria of oxytocin and vasopressin release, respectively. Suckling and mammary duct dilatation resulted in pronounced oxytocin and milk-ejecting activities but negligible antidiuresis. Conversely, nicotine and hypertonic saline resulted in marked antidiuresis but negligible oxytocin and milk-ejecting activities. These facts strongly suggest that oxytocin and vasopressin in man are released independently.

In spite of the many investigations of the physiologic actions of oxytocin, a definite function for this hormone has not been established in the human. Women with diabetes insipidus have accomplished normal delivery and have nursed their offspring. However, it has not been established that these patients were totally lacking in oxytocin. No known physiologic function for oxytocin exists in the male.

How oxytocin directly affects the uterine musculature and the myoepithelium surrounding the mammary ducts is not known. Estrogens enhance the responsiveness of uterine musculature to oxytocin, and the immature uterus is quite resistant to the hormonal effect. Paradoxically, the nonpregnant human uterus is consistently much more responsive to vasopressin than to oxytocin. The sensitivity of the human uterus to oxytocin increases in late pregnancy, and by term sensitivity is much greater to oxytocin than to vasopressin.

The pharmacologic uses of oxytocin are based mainly on the supposed physiologic actions on the uterus and mammary glands. Oxytocin may be administered to induce labor at term, to control postpartum hemorrhage, or to correct postpartum uterine atony. The action on the breast has been utilized in cases of difficult lactation in which it is felt that failure of the milk ejection reflex is at fault. It has also been used to relieve painful engorgement of the breasts during lactation. Either intranasal application or intramuscular injection has been successful in these circumstances. When oxytocin is given in large pharmacologic doses, it has a transient direct relaxing effect on vascular smooth muscle, producing a drop in peripheral vascular resistance and in blood pressure

with a compensatory tachycardia and increase in cardiac output. This effect is blocked by small doses of vasopressin.

REFERENCES

1. Acher, R., Chauvet, J., Chauvet, M. T., and Crepy, A. D.: Phylogénie des peptides hormonaux neurohypophysaires. *Bull. Soc. Chim. Biol.* 47:2279, 1965.
2. Acher, R., Manoussos, G., and Olivry, G.: Sur les relations entre l'ocytocine et la vasopressine d'une part et la protéine de van Dyke d'autre part. *Biochim. Biophys. Acta* 16:155, 1955.
3. Amatruda, T. T., Jr., Mulrow, P. J., Gallagher, J. C., and Sawyer, W. H.: Carcinoma of the lung with inappropriate antidiuresis. *New Eng. J. Med.* 269:544, 1963.
4. Andersson, B.: Polydipsia, antidiuresis and milk ejection caused by hypothalamic stimulation. In *The Neurohypophysis.* Heller, H. (ed.), London, Butterworth & Co., Ltd., 1957.
5. Baez, S., Mazur, A., and Shorr, E.: Role of the neurohypophysis in ferritin-induced antidiuresis. *Amer. J. Physiol.* 169:123, 1952.
6. Bard, P., Woods, J. W., and Bleier, R.: The locus and functional capacity of the osmoreceptors in the deafferented hypothalamus. *Trans. Ass. Amer. Physicians* 79:107, 1966.
7. Bargmann, W.: Relationship between neurohypophysial structure and function, In *The Neurohypophysis.* Heller, H. (ed.), London, Butterworth & Co., Ltd., 1957.
8. Barlow, E. D., and de Wardener, H. E.: Compulsive water drinking. *Quart. J. Med.* 28:235, 1959.
9. Barnafi, L., and Croxatto, H.: The concentration of vasopressin and oxytocin in the human hypothalamo-hypophysial system. *Experientia* 19:489, 1963.
10. Barnafi, L., and Croxatto, H.: Vasopressor and oxytocic activities in human hypothalamus, posterior and anterior lobes of the pituitary gland. *Acta Endocr.* 48:177, 1965.
11. Barnett, R. J., and Seligman, A. M.: Histochemical demonstration of sulfhydryl and disulfide groups of protein. *J. Nat. Cancer Inst.* 14:769, 1954.
12. Berliner, R. W., and Davidson, D. G.: Production of hypertonic urine in the absence of pituitary antidiuretic hormone. *J. Clin. Invest.* 36:1416, 1957.
13. Berliner, R. W., Levinsky, N. G., Davidson, D. G., and Eden, M.: Dilution and concentration of the urine and the action of antidiuretic hormone. *Amer. J. Med.* 24:730, 1958.
14. Blom, P. S., Rook, L., and Sonneveldt, H. A.: Sodium economy in the proximal and distal parts of the nephron studied in patients with diabetes insipidus. Their estimation under normal conditions and after salt restriction, chlorothiazide and a mercurial diuretic. *Acta Med. Scand.* 174:201, 1963.
15. Blotner, H.: The inheritance of diabetes insipidus. *Amer. J. Med. Sci.* 204:261, 1942.
16. Blotner, H.: Primary or idiopathic diabetes insipidus: a system disease. *Metabolism* 7:191, 1958.
17. Bodian, D.: Nerve endings, neurosecretory substance and lobular organization of the neurohypophysis. *Bull. Johns Hopkins Hosp.* 89:354, 1951.
18. Bower, B. F., Mason, D. M., and Forsham, P. H.: Bronchogenic carcinoma with inappropriate antidiuretic activity in plasma and tumor. *New Eng. J. Med.* 271:934, 1964.
19. Burn, G. P., and Grewal, R. S.: The antidiuretic response to and excretion of pituitary (posterior lobe) extract in man, with reference to the action of nicotine. *Brit. J. Pharmacol.* 6:471, 1951.
20. Burn, J. H., Truelove, L. H., and Burn, I.: The antidiuretic action of nicotine and of smoking. *Brit. Med. J.* 1:403, 1945.
21. Cates, J. E., and Garrod, O.: The effect of nicotine on urinary flow in diabetes insipidus. *Clin. Sci.* 10:145, 1951.
22. Cobo, E., Gaitan, E., Mizrachi, M., and Strada, G.: Neurohypophyseal hormone release in the human. I. Experimental study during pregnancy. *Amer. J. Obstet. Gynec.* 91:905, 1965.
23. Corson, R. A. D., Corson, E. O'L., Reese, W. G., Peters, J. E., and Seager, L. D.: Electrolyte excretion during positive

and negative conditioned responses in dogs. *Fed. Proc.* *18*:31, 1959.

24. Crawford, J. D., and Kennedy, G. C.: Chlorothiazide in diabetes insipidus. *Nature* (London) *183*:891, 1959.

25. Dale, H. H.: The action of extracts of the pituitary body. *Biochem. J.* *4*:427, 1909.

26. Dale, H. H.: Evidence concerning the endocrine function of the neurohypophysis and its nervous control, In *The Neurohypophysis,* Heller, H. (ed.), London, Butterworth & Co., Ltd., 1957.

27. Daniel, A. R., and Lederis, K.: Effects of ether anesthesia and haemorrhage on hormone storage and ultrastructure of the rat neurohypophysis. *J. Endocr.* *34*:91, 1966.

28. Dearborn, E. H., Lasagna, L., and Marshall, E. K., Jr.: On the mechanism of the antidiuretic action of cinchoninic acid derivatives. *J. Pharmacol Exp. Ther.* *106*:103, 1952.

29. de Bodo, R. C.: The antidiuretic action of morphine, and its mechanism. *J. Pharmacol. Exp. Ther.* *82*:74, 1944.

30. de Bodo, R. C., and Prescott, K. F.: The antidiuretic action of barbiturates (phenobarbital, Amytal, pentobarbital) and the mechanism involved in this action. *J. Pharmacol. Exp. Ther.* *85*:222, 1945.

31. Douglas, W. W., and Ishida, A.: The stimulant effect of cold on vasopressin release from the neurohypophysis *in vitro. J. Physiol.* (London) *179*:185, 1965.

32. Douglas, W. W., and Poisner, A. M.: Stimulus-secretion coupling in a neurosecretory organ: the role of calcium in the release of vasopressin from the neurohypophysis of the rat and its relation to the release of vasopressin. *J. Physiol.* (London) *172*:1–18, 19–30, 1964.

*33. du Vigneaud, V.: Hormones of the posterior pituitary gland: oxytocin and vasopressin, In *The Harvey Lectures 1954-1955.* New York, Academic Press Inc., 1956.

34. Farmi, F.: Über Diabetes insipidus und Hypophysistherapie. *Wien Klin. Wschr.* *26*:1867, 1913.

35. Fisher, C., Ingram, W. R., and Ranson, S. W.: *Diabetes Insipidus and the Neuro-hormonal Control of Water Balance.* Ann Arbor, Mich., Edwards Brothers Inc., 1938.

36. Gaitan, E., Cobo, E., and Mizrachi, M.: Evidence for the differential secretion of oxytocin and vasopressin in man. *J. Clin. Invest.* *43*:2310, 1964.

37. Garcia, J., Harris, G. W., and Schindler, W. J.: Vasopressin and thyroid function in the rabbit. *J. Physiol.* (London) *170*:487, 1964.

38. Geiling, E. M. K., and Oldham, F. K.: The site of formation of the posterior lobe hormones. *Trans. Ass. Amer. Physicians* *52*:132, 1937.

39. Gerbner, M., Altman, K., and Mészáres, I.: The mechanisms of the increase in diuresis induced by hypnotic suggestion. *J. Psychosom. Res.* *3*:282, 1959.

40. Ginsburg, M., and Heller, H.: The clearance of injected vasopressin from the circulation and its fate in the body. *J. Endocr.* *9*:283, 1953.

41. Ginsburg, M., and Ireland, M.: Binding of vasopressin and oxytocin to protein in extracts of bovine and rabbit neurohypophyses. *J. Endocr.* *30*:131, 1964.

42. Ginsburg, M., and Ireland, M.: The preparation of bovine neurophysin and the estimation of its maximum capacity to bind oxytocin and arginine vasopressin. *J. Endocr.* *32*:187, 1965.

*43. Goldberg, M.: Hyponatremia and the inappropriate secretion of antidiuretic hormone. *Amer. J. Med.* *35*:293, 1963.

*44. Gottschalk, C. W.: Osmotic concentration and dilution of the urine. *Amer. J. Med.* *36*:670, 1964.

45. Haddy, F. J., and Scott, J. B.: Cardiovascular pharmacology. *Ann. Rev. Pharmacol.* *6*:49, 1966.

46. Haller, E. W., Sachs, H., Sperelakis, N., and Share, L.: Release of vasopressin from isolated guinea pig posterior pituitaries. *Amer. J. Physiol.* *209*:79, 1965.

47. Handler, J. S., Butcher, R. W., Sutherland, E. W., and Orloff, J.: The effect of vasopressin and theophylline on the concentration of adenosine 3′,5′-phosphate in the urinary bladder of the toad. *J. Biol. Chem.* *240*:4524, 1965.

48. Hargitay, B., and Kuhn, W.: Das Multiplikationsprinzip als Grundlage der Harnkonzentrierung in der Niere. *Z. Elektro. Angew. Physik. Chem.* *55*:539, 1951.

49. Harrington, A. R., and Valtin, H.: Vasopressin effect on

urinary concentration in rats with hereditary hypothalamic diabetes insipidus (Brattleboro strain). *Proc. Soc. Exp. Biol. Med.* *118*:448, 1965.

50. Havard, C. W. H.: Thiazide-induced antidiuresis in diabetes insipidus. *Proc. Roy. Soc. Med.* *58*:1005, 1965.

51. Hayward, J. N., and Smith, W. K.: Antidiuretic response to electrical stimulation in brain stem of the monkey. *Amer. J. Physiol.* *206*:15, 1964.

*52. Heller, H., and Bentley, P. J.: Phylogenetic distribution of the effects of neurohypophysial hormones on water and sodium metabolism. *Gen. Comp. Endocr.* *5*:96, 1965.

53. Hickey, R. C., and Hare, K.: The renal excretion of chloride and water in diabetes insipidus. *J. Clin. Invest.* *23*:768, 1944.

54. Hild, W.: Das morphologische, kinetische und endocrinologische Verhalten von hypothalamischem und neurohypophysärem Gewebe *in vitro. Z. Zellforsch.* *40*:257, 1954.

55. Hild, W., and Zetler, G.: Vergleichende Untersuchungen über das Vorkommen das Hypophysenhinterlappenhormons im Zwischerhirn Säugetiere. *Deutsch Z. Nervenheilk.* *167*:105, 1952.

56. Hilton, J. G.: Adrenocorticotrophic action of antidiuretic hormone. *Circulation* *21*:1038, 1960.

57. Hofer, M. A., and Hinkle, L. A., Jr.: Production of conditioned diuresis in man. *J. Clin. Invest.* *42*:1421, 1963.

58. Hollinshead, W. H.: The interphase of diabetes insipidus. *Proc. Mayo Clin.* *39*:92, 1964.

59. Kamm, O., Aldrich, T. B., Grote, I. W., Rowe, L. W., and Bugbee, E. P.: The active principles of the posterior lobe of the pituitary gland. I. The demonstration of the presence of two active principles. II. The separation of the two principles and their concentration in the form of potent solid preparations. *J. Amer. Chem. Soc.* *50*:573, 1928.

*60. Lauson, H. D.: Vasopressin and oxytocin in the plasma of man and other mammals, In *Hormones in Human Plasma.* Antoniades, H. N. (ed.), Boston, Little, Brown & Co., 1960.

*61. Lauson, H. D.: Antidiuretic hormone. *Fed. Proc.* *24*:731, 1965.

62. Lauson, H. D., Bocanegra, M., and Beuzeville, C. F.: Hepatic and renal clearance of vasopressin from plasma of dogs. *Amer. J. Physiol.* *209*:199, 1965.

*63. Leaf, A.: Action of neurohypophyseal hormones on the toad bladder. *Gen. Comp. Endocr.* *2*:148, 1962.

64. Leaf, A., Bartter, F. C., Santos, R. F., and Wrong, O.: Evidence in man that urinary electrolyte loss induced by Pitressin is a function of water retention. *J. Clin. Invest.* *32*:868, 1953.

65. Leveque, T. F., and Scharrer, E.: Pituicytes and the origin of the antidiuretic hormone. *Endocrinology* *52*:436, 1953.

66. Lewis, A. A. G., and Chalmers, T. M.: A nicotine test for the investigation of diabetes insipidus. *Clin. Sci.* *10*:137, 1951.

67. MacArthur, C. G.: A new posterior pituitary preparation. *Science* *73*:448, 1931.

68. Magnus, R., and Schäfer, E. A.: The action of pituitary extracts upon the kidney. *J. Physiol.* (London) *27*:ix, 1901.

69. Marx, H.: Diuresis by conditioned reflex. *Amer. J. Physiol.* *96*:356, 1931.

70. Mendez-Bauer, C. J., et al.: Studies on plasma oxytocinase of pregnant women, In *Oxytocin.* Heller, H., and Caldeyro-Barcia, R. (eds.), London, Pergamon Press, 1961.

71. Merigan, T. C., Jr., Plotkin, G. R., and Davidson, C. S.: The effect of intravenous Pituitrin on hemorrhage from bleeding esophageal varices. *New Eng. J. Med.* *266*:134, 1962.

72. Nagareda, C. S., and Gaunt, R.: Functional relationship between the adrenal cortex and posterior pituitary. *Endocrinology* *48*:560, 1951.

73. Orloff, J., and Handler, J. S.: The cellular mode of action of antidiuretic hormone. *Amer. J. Med.* *36*:686, 1964.

74. Ortmann, R.: Über experimentelle Veränderungen der Morphologie des Hypophysenzwischenhirnsystems und die Beziehung der sog. "Gomori substanz" zum Adiuretin. *Z. Zellforsch.* *36*:92, 1951.

74a. Ozer, A., and Sharp, G. W. G.: Modulation of adenyl cyclase action in toad bladder by chlorpropamide:

Antagonism to prostaglandin E₁. *Europ. J. Pharmacol.*, 1973 (in press).

75. Pickford, M.: The inhibitory effect of acetylcholine on water diuresis in the dog, and its pituitary transmission. *J. Physiol.* (London) *95*:226, 1939.

76. Randall, R. V., Clark, E. C., and Bahn, R. C.: Classification of the causes of diabetes insipidus. *Proc. Mayo Clin. 34*:299, 1959.

77. Randall, R. V., Clark, E. C., Dodge, H. W., Jr., and Love, J. G.: Polyuria after operation for tumors in the region of the hypophysis and hypothalamus. *J. Clin. Endocr. 20*:1614, 1960.

78. Rocha e Silva, M., Jr., and Malnik, G.: Release of antidiuretic hormone by bradykinin. *J. Pharmacol. Exp. Ther. 146*:24, 1964.

79. Sachs, H., and Takabatake, Y.: Evidence for a precursor in vasopressin biosynthesis. *Endocrinology 75*:943, 1964.

80. Sala, N. L.: Milk-ejecting effect induced by various octapeptides in human beings. *Acta Physiol. Lat. Amer. 15*:191, 1965.

*81. Sawyer, W. H.: Neurohypophysial hormones. *Pharmacol. Rev. 13*:225, 1961.

82. Sawyer, W. H.: Vertebrate neurohypophysial principles. *Endocrinology 75*:981, 1964.

83. Sawyer, W. H.: Evolution of neurohypophysial principles. *Arch. Anat. Micr. Morph. Exp. 54*:295, 1965.

84. Sawyer, W. H., Valtin, H., and Sokol, H. W.: Neurohypophysial principles in rats with familial hypothalamic diabetes insipidus (Brattleboro strain). *Endocrinology 74*:153, 1964.

85. Scharrer, E., and Scharrer, B.: Hormones produced by neurosecretory cells. *Recent Progr. Hormone Res. 10*:183, 1954.

86. Schwartz, W. B., Bennett, W., Curelop, S., and Bartter, F. C.: A syndrome of renal sodium loss and hyponatremia, probably resulting from inappropriate secretion of antidiuretic hormone. *Amer. J. Med. 23*:529, 1957.

*87. Smith, H. W.: Salt and water volume receptors. *Amer. J. Med. 23*:623, 1957.

88. Takabatake, Y., and Sachs, H.: Vasopressin biosynthesis. III. *In vitro* studies. *Endocrinology 75*:934, 1964.

89. Theobald, G. W.: The alleged relation of hyperfunction of the posterior lobe of the hypophysis to eclampsia and the nephropathy of pregnancy. *Clin. Sci. 1*:225, 1934.

90. Thomas, W. C.: Diabetes insipidus (review). *J. Clin. Endocr. 17*:565, 1957.

91. Thorn, N. A.: Role of calcium in the release of vasopressin and oxytocin from posterior pituitary protein. *Acta Endocr. 50*:357, 1965.

*92. Thorn, N. A.: Antidiuretic hormone synthesis, release, and action under normal and pathological circumstances. *Advances Metab. Dis. 14*:39–75, 1970.

93. Thorn, N. A., and Smith, M. W.: Renal excretion of synthetic arginine-vasopressin injected into dogs. *Acta Endocr. 49*:388, 1965.

94. Thorn, N. A., Smith, M. W., and Skadhauge, E.: The antidiuretic effect of intravenous and intracarotid infusion of calcium chloride in hydrated rats. *J. Endocr. 32*:161, 1965.

95. Tuppy, H.: Biochemical studies of oxytocinase, In *Oxytocin.* Caldeyro-Barcia, R., and Heller, H. (eds.), London, Pergamon Press, 1961.

96. Ussing, H. H.: The alkali metal ions in isolated systems and tissues, In *Handbuch der Experimentellen Pharmakologie.* Berlin, Springer-Verlag, 1960.

97. van Dyke, H. B., Chow, B. F., Greep, R. O., and Rothen, A.: The isolation of a protein from the pars neuralis of the ox pituitary with constant oxytocic, pressor and diuresis-inhibiting activities. *J. Pharmacol. Exp. Ther. 74*:190, 1942.

*98. Verney, E. B.: The absorption and excretion of water: the antidiuretic hormone. *Lancet 2*:739–744, 781–783, 1946.

99. von den Velden, R.: Die Nierenwirkung von Hypophysenextrakten beim Menschen. *Klin. Wschr. 50*:2083, 1913.

100. von Hann, F.: Über die Bedeutung der Hypophysen-veränderungen bei Diabetes insipidus. *Frankfurt Z. Path. 21*:337, 1918.

101. Williams, R. H., and Henry, C.: Nephrogenic diabetes insipidus: transmitted by females and appearing during infancy in males. *Ann. Intern. Med. 27*:84, 1947.

102. Wirz, H., Hargitay, B., and Kuhn, W.: Lokalisation des Konzentrierungsprozesses in der Niere durch direkte Kryoskopie. *Helv. Physiol. Pharmacol. Acta 9*:196, 1951.

---

*These references are general reviews of various aspects dealt with in this chapter. They are recommended as source material to the reader who wishes to familiarize himself further with this subject. Also note that the American Journal of Medicine, Vol. 42, No. 5, May, 1967, is devoted to a symposium on the neurohypophysis.

CHAPTER 4

The Thyroid Gland

By Sidney H. Ingbar and
Kenneth A. Woeber

PHYLOGENY

In its phylogeny, its embryogenesis, and certain aspects of its function, the thyroid gland reveals its primitive relation to the gastrointestinal tract.

The ability of the thyroid to metabolize iodine

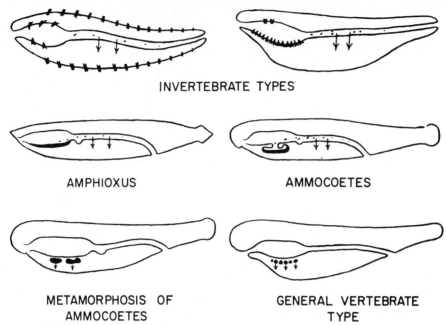

INVERTEBRATE TYPES

AMPHIOXUS

AMMOCOETES

METAMORPHOSIS OF
AMMOCOETES

GENERAL VERTEBRATE
TYPE

Figure 4–1. This figure summarizes the known distribution of iodoproteins (shown as solid black), iodotyrosine, and iodothyronine compounds in the animal kingdom, and suggests a pattern of evolution of thyroid function. Iodoproteins are quite generally found in most invertebrate phyla in fibrous, tough exoskeletal structures (top left) and in pharyngeal teeth (top right). It is supposed that when this readily available material first became of metabolic value to animals, its source was pharyngeal and it was hydrolyzed in the digestive tract to release its hormone. Once adaptive value developed, the pharyngeal source of iodoprotein was made large (second "invertebrate type"). Amphioxus and Ammocoetes both exhibit this type, except that the iodoprotein is no longer a sclero-protein but is associated with exocrine glandular activity. The advance of Ammocoetes over Amphioxus is in the separation of the iodoprotein-forming gland from the rest of the pharynx. At metamorphosis, the Ammocoetes' thyroid finally forms by closure of the duct and by dependence upon its own locally active protease for hydrolysis of the iodoprotein. It is at this point that an internally secreting thyroid, typical of all vertebrates, is differentiated. (From Gorbman, A.: *Comp. Endocr. 18*:266, 1958.)

and incorporate it into a variety of organic compounds is found widely throughout the animal and plant kingdoms. Monoiodotyrosine (MIT) and diiodotyrosine (DIT) have been found in a variety of invertebrate fauna, including mollusks, crustaceans, annelids, and insects, as well as in certain marine algae. In these lower forms, however, no recognizable thyroid tissue is present, and no effect of exposure to thyroid hormones has been demonstrated. Clearly recognizable thyroid tissue is, rather, confined to the vertebrates and is present in all species thereof. The evolutionary precursor of the vertebrate thyroid gland is probably characterized by specialized structures found in the protochordates, which are intermediate between invertebrate and vertebrate forms (Fig. 4–1). These marine forms, in addition to demonstrating iodoprotein in their cuticular exoskeleton, possess an endostyle, a tubular structure that secretes mucinous materials which pass by way of a duct into the pharynx and thence through the gastrointestinal tract. The endostyle of the protochordates is capable of concentrating iodine and carrying out organic iodinations that yield iodinated amino acids identical to those formed in the vertebrate thyroid, i.e., iodotyrosines, as well as L-thyroxine (T_4) or tetraiodothyronine and L-triiodothyronine (T_3) (Fig. 4–2). It is believed that these iodinated

materials are carried to the gastrointestinal tract together with other secretions and are then hydrolyzed and absorbed. What physiologic purpose they may subserve is unclear, however, since no effects of T_4 or of iodine itself have been noted in these animals. A closer link to the thyroid of higher vertebrates is evident in the ammocoete, the larval form of the lamprey. Here, the endostyle is also capable of carrying out iodinations, but prior to metamorphosis a protease appears in the endostyle that can hydrolyze the iodoprotein formed. Presumably, this permits the endostyle to lose its connection with the pharynx, as occurs during metamorphosis, and to assume its adult function as an endocrine organ which secretes iodothyronines.

Many fascinating peculiarities of iodine metabolism and idiosyncrasies in the response of the lower vertebrates to thyroid hormones have been observed. For example, in migrating amphibiotic species of teleosts, such as salmon and sea trout, there occurs in the blood a protein that is capable of binding inorganic iodide and providing a reservoir of this essential substrate for hormone formation as the fish moves from a marine environment to fresh water. In the marine lamprey, a similar function may be subserved by the notochord, which is capable of concentrating iodide from the plasma several hundredfold. Notochordal concentration of

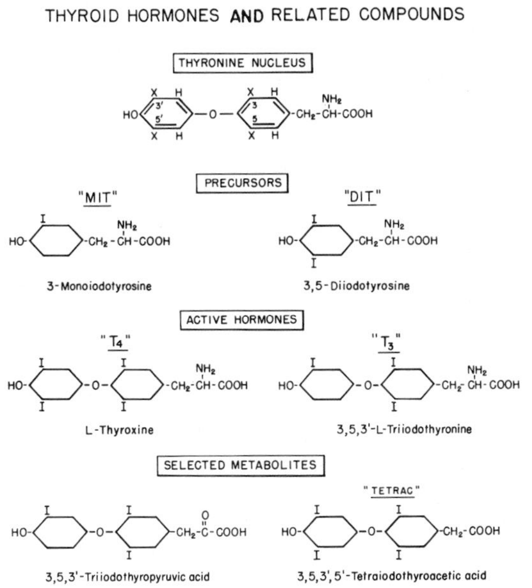

THYROID HORMONES **AND** RELATED COMPOUNDS

Figure 4–2. Structural formulas of thyroid hormones and related compounds. The structure of the thyronine nucleus of the hormonally active iodinated amino acids, T_4 and T_3, is shown above. Iodinated thyronines are formed through the oxidative coupling of the precursor iodotyrosines, MIT and DIT, in varying combination. $3,5,3'$-Triiodothyropyruvic acid is derived by oxidative deamination from T_3. "Tetrac" is derived from T_4 by oxidative deamination followed by decarboxylation.

iodide shows some features of thyroid iodide transport, since it is inhibited by thiocyanate. (For further details of these and other fascinating and provocative aspects of the comparative endocrinology of the thyroid, see review by Barrington, 1968.)

The phylogenetic association of the thyroid gland and the gastrointestinal (GI) tract is evident in several functional respects. Thus the salivary and gastric glands, like the thyroid, are capable of concentrating iodide in their secretions many times over, although iodide transport in these sites is not responsive to stimulation by thyrotropin (thyroid stimulating hormone, TSH). In the rare form of goitrous hypothyroidism due to lack of the thyroid iodide transport mechanism, salivary transport of iodide is also defective (Stanbury, 1972). The salivary gland also contains enzymic mechanisms similar to those in the thyroid that are capable of iodinating tyrosine when provided with hydrogen peroxide. Although it is unlikely that the salivary gland forms significant quantities of iodoproteins under normal circumstances, when completely thyroidectomized rats are given large doses of iodide, specific stigmata of hypothyroidism are reversed and synthesis of DIT and T_4 occurs, probably within a protein matrix (Taurog and Evans, 1967). Such iodoproteins may be formed in GI structures, pass into the lumen, and be digested, and the iodinated amino acids may well be absorbed. The functional similarity to that found in prevertebrates and in the ammocoete is thus apparent.

ANATOMICAL AND FUNCTIONAL EMBRYOLOGY

The human thyroid anlage is first recognizable at about one month after conception, when the embryo is approximately 3.5–4.0 mm. in length. An extensive discussion of its subsequent development is available (Boyd, 1964). Briefly, the primordium begins as a thickening of epithelium in the pharyngeal floor which later forms a diverticulum. With continuing development, the median diverticulum undergoes relative caudal displacement, and the primitive stalk connecting the primordium with the pharyngeal floor undergoes elongation (thyroglossal duct). During its caudal displacement, the primordium assumes a more bilobate shape, coming into contact and fusing with the ventral aspect of the fourth pharyngeal pouch. Normally, the thyroglossal duct undergoes dissolution and fragmentation by about the second month after conception, leaving at its point of origin a small dimple at the junction of the middle and posterior third of the tongue, the foramen cecum. Cells of the lower portion of the duct differentiate to thyroid tissue, forming the pyramidal lobe of the gland. Concomitantly, histologic alterations occur. Complex interconnecting cordlike arrangements of cells interspersed with vascular connective tissue replace the solid epithelial mass. These transform to tubulelike structures at about the third month of fetal life, and shortly thereafter, follicular arrangements devoid of colloid appear, followed by colloid-filled follicles.

Numerous studies have been conducted on the functional development of the thyroid in laboratory animals of various species. Although some discordance in the findings has been noted, several general features have emerged. Thyroprotein resembling thyroglobulin appears just prior to or at the time that follicular structure is first apparent. Evidently, this antecedes by a short period the capacity to collect iodine, although results of some studies suggest that early iodine accumulation is virtually concurrent with the appearance of MIT, DIT, T_4, and T_3. Other results suggest that iodide transport, organic binding (binding of iodine to tyrosine), and iodotyrosine-coupling functions appear in sequence. The continued anatomical and functional development of the thyroid after these functions have begun, and perhaps even before, is dependent upon TSH. Its origin is necessarily fetal since the placenta is impermeable to maternal TSH. (See Roques et al., 1972, for references.)

Because of obvious difficulties in studying this problem, the sequential development of the human fetal thyroid is less accurately defined. The capacity to synthesize thyroglobulin (the form in which the thyroid hormones are stored) has been demonstrated as early as the twenty-ninth day of gestation (Gitlin and Biasucci, 1969). Both T_4 and the T_4-binding globulin (TBG) have been identified in fetal serum as early as the eleventh week of gestation. The concentrations of both then rise progressively to term. The concentration of free T_4 also rises and may plateau at term levels by the end of the second trimester. In the single study in which it has been measured, T_3 was first detected in serum at about 24 weeks; it increased in concentration to term but nevertheless remained at a lower concentration than in maternal serum throughout. TSH has also been detected in fetal serum at about 11 weeks; its concentration rises rapidly so that by 16 weeks it has approached values found at term. These values are higher than those in normal children or in maternal serum, possibly as a result of what may be an abnormally low serum T_3 concentration (Greenberg et al., 1970; Fisher et al., 1973).

Abnormalities in the anatomical or biochemical development of the thyroid are reflected in certain disorders of postnatal life. Rarely, thyroid tissue may develop from remnants of the thyroglossal duct near the base of the tongue. Such lingual thyroid tissue may be the sole functioning thyroid present; its surgical removal will then lead to hypothyroidism. More commonly, elements of the thyroglossal duct may persist and later give rise to thyroglossal cysts, or thyroid tissue progenitors may migrate with adjacent cardiovascular structures to occupy a place within the mediastinum. Functionally, the patterns of iodine metabolism in certain defects of hormone synthesis apparent after birth may represent or mimic a particular stage in the functional development of the fetal thyroid. Examples are evident in genetically determined goiters or in tumors of the mature gland that are not capable of carrying out organic iodinations or of synthesizing active hormones from precursor iodotyrosines.

ANATOMY AND HISTOLOGY

The thyroid is normally one of the largest of the endocrine organs, weighing approximately 20 g. in North American adults. Moreover, the potential of the thyroid for growth is tremendous. Goiters weighing many hundred grams are not rare. The normal thyroid is made up of two lobes joined by a thin band of tissue, the isthmus. The latter is approximately 0.5 cm. thick, 2 cm. wide, and 2 cm. high. The individual lobes normally display a rather pointed superior pole and a poorly defined blunt inferior pole merging medially with the isthmus. Each lobe is approximately 2.0 or 2.5 cm. in both thickness and width at its largest diameter and is approximately 4.0 cm. in length. Occasionally, especially when the remainder of the gland is goitrous, a pyramidal lobe is discernible as a fingerlike projection directed upward from the isthmus, generally just lateral to the midline, usually on the left. The right lobe of the thyroid is normally more vascular than the left, is often the larger of the two, and tends to enlarge more in disorders associated with a diffuse increase in size.

The thyroid is closely affixed to the anterior and lateral aspects of the trachea by loose connective tissue. The upper margin of the isthmus generally lies just below the cricoid cartilage, which therefore provides a convenient landmark for locating the gland. The lobes themselves lie along the lower half of the lateral margins of the thyroid cartilage. Lying between the thyroid gland and the subcutaneous tissue are the thin infrahyoid muscles. Lateral to the gland are the carotid sheaths and sternocleidomastoid muscles, while the recurrent laryngeal nerves lie in the grooves between the lateral lobes and the trachea. Two pairs of parathyroid glands are normally situated on or beneath the posterior surface of the thyroid lobes.

Two main pairs of vessels constitute the major arterial blood supply. The superior thyroid arteries, arising from the external carotids, and the inferior thyroid arteries from the subclavians enter their respective poles. The thyroid gland is exceptionally well vascularized. Estimates of thyroid blood flow range from 4 to 6 ml./min./g., well in excess of the blood flow to the kidney (3 ml./min./g.). In severe hyperplasia as in diffuse toxic goiter, blood flow rates greater than 1 liter/min. may occur. Increased flow is evident clinically in the presence of a thrill or audible bruit over the gland or in its immediate vicinity. There is rich lymphatic drainage. Its function relative to the endocrine activity of the gland is uncertain, but reports suggest that the lymph contains a higher concentration of newly released radioiodine than does thyroid venous blood, probably in the form of iodoprotein.

The thyroid receives its nerve supply from both adrenergic and cholinergic nervous systems, the former arising from the cervical ganglia and the latter from the vagus nerve. Afferent fibers pass through the laryngeal nerves and regulate an active vasomotor system. An unusual feature is the presence of contractile endothelial cushions in the arteriolar endothelium. It has been thought that the sole function of neurogenic stimuli is the regulation of blood flow to the thyroid. Although acute changes in blood flow do not appear to alter the rate of hormonal release, the rate of perfusion influences the delivery of TSH, iodide, and metabolic substrates and may eventually influence glandular function and growth. Recent ultrastructural and autoradiographic studies have revealed, in addition, a network of adrenergic fibers terminating near the basement membrane of the follicular wall. These findings, together with new evidence that adrenergic and other amines influence thyroid iodine metabolism in isolated thyroid cells and *in vivo*, indicate that the adrenergic nervous system can influence thyroid function through a direct effect on the function of the follicle cell. This is discussed more fully in a later section on factors that affect thyroid function.

The thyroid is invested with a thin fibrous capsule that penetrates the gland, forming irregular pseudolobules. The gland itself is firm yet resilient. The cut surface of a normal gland has a spotted beefy red appearance. Minute vesicles (the follicles) from which the amber-colored, sticky colloid exudes are more or less evenly distributed throughout.

With light microscopy, the gland is seen to be composed of closely packed sacs, called acini or follicles, which are invested with a rich capillary network. The interior of the follicle is filled with the clear, proteinaceous colloid, which normally is the major constituent of the total thyroid mass. The diameter of the follicles varies considerably, even within a single gland, but averages about 200 μ. As might be expected, the iodine-accumulating function of the individual follicle varies with its surface area. The wall of the follicle is lined by a single layer of closely packed cuboidal cells, approximately 15 μ high. The cell height of the acinar epithelium varies with the degree of glandular stimulation, becoming columnar when active and flat when inactive. The epithelium rests upon a well-defined basement membrane that stains positively with reagents for mucopolysaccharides and separates the follicular cells from the surrounding capillaries. From 20 to 40 follicles are demarcated by connective tissue septa to form a lobule supplied by a single artery. The function of an individual lobule may vary from that of its neighbors. This and other evidence of functional heterogeneity of the thyroid has been reviewed by Wollman (1965).

With electron microscopy, the thyroid is seen to have many features in common with other secretory cells but some which are peculiar to the thyroid. From the apical aspect of the follicular cell, numerous microvilli extend into the colloid (Fig. 4–3). There is considerable evidence that it is at or near this surface of the cell that such crucial reactions as iodination and the initial phase of hormone secretion, namely colloid resorption, occur. The nucleus of the follicular cell has no distinctive features. The cytoplasm contains an extensive endoplasmic reticulum (ER) laden with microsomes. The ER is distinctive in being composed of a network of wide irregular tubules which probably contain the precursor of thyroglobulin. The carbohydrate component of thyroglobulin is probably added to this precursor in the Golgi apparatus which is located apically. Membrane-limited dense granules, believed to be lysosomes, and mitochondria are scattered throughout the cytoplasm. Upon stimulation by TSH, the follicular cell undergoes changes in its ultrastructure. These include enlargement of the Golgi apparatus, formation of pseudopodia at the apical surface, and appearance

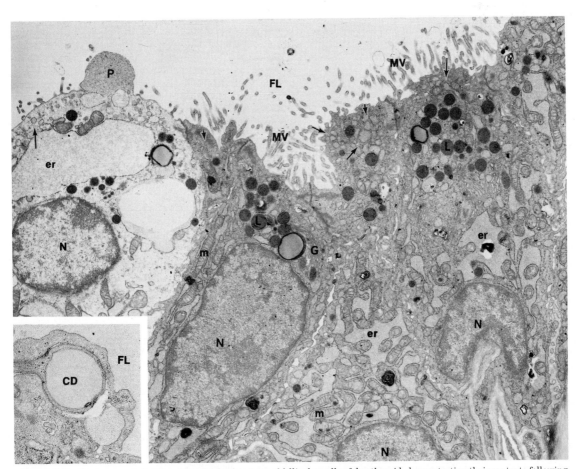

Figure 4–3. Low-powered electron micrograph of a group of follicular cells of dog thyroid, demonstrating their contents following stimulation with thyroid stimulating hormone (TSH). A number of microvilli (MV) projecting into the follicular lumen (FL) are demonstrated. In the cytoplasm, numerous single membrane-limited vacuoles, representing colloid droplets (arrows), are seen. Besides nuclei (N), Golgi apparatus (G), endoplasmic reticulum (er) and mitochondria (m), numerous lysosomes (L) are also seen. A pseudopod is shown (inset) with colloid droplet (CD) formation. Note that the material in the droplets is similar to that found in the follicular lumen (FL). (Electron micrograph and its interpretation kindly provided by Dr. Nicholas A. Panagiotis.)

in the apical portion of the cell of many droplets that contain colloid taken up from the follicular lumen.

In addition to the follicular cell, the thyroid contains a population of other cells, variously termed parafollicular, light, or C cells. Although the existence of these cells has been recognized for nearly 100 years, it is only recently that they have aroused interest when it was shown that they produce a calcium-lowering polypeptide, calcitonin. These cells are believed to arise during embryonic development from the last pair of pharyngeal pouches, and in mammals they are incorporated into the thyroid gland. They are located in the follicular epithelium as well as in the interstitium, but they never border on the follicular lumen. The C cell is ovoid and has an irregular nucleus and many cytoplasmic granules. Electron microscopy reveals a well-developed ER, numerous free ribosomes, and a prominent Golgi apparatus. Mitochondria are more numerous than in the adjacent follicular cells. The cytoplasmic granules are membrane-limited and dense and are believed to be secretory. The administration of calcium results in degranulation of the cytoplasm. In addition to its distinctive histologic appearance, the C cell differs from the follicular cell in its high activity of α-glycerophosphate dehydrogenase (αGPD). (For a more extensive discussion of the ultrastructure of the thyroid and extensive references to the literature, see Fawcett et al., 1969.)

IODINE METABOLISM: THE SYNTHESIS, SECRETION, AND METABOLISM OF THE THYROID HORMONES

In the most general sense, the function of the thyroid in higher forms, including man, is to secrete such quantities of hormone as are necessary to meet the demands of the peripheral tissue. This section will deal with the overall metabolism of one of the major components of the thyroid hormones, iodine; the reactions by which iodine is incorporated into them; the synthesis of the specific protein, thyroglobulin, which serves as a matrix in which the hormones are formed and stored; and the processes by which the hormones are released into the blood. Consideration will also be given to the peripheral transport of the hormones and the avenues along which they are excreted or degraded. A subsequent section will deal with the regulation of thyroid function.

Extrathyroidal Metabolism of Iodide

Formation of normal quantities of thyroid hormone ultimately depends upon the availability of adequate quantities of exogenous iodine. Although efficient mechanisms exist to conserve iodine in the presence of iodine deficiency, such mechanisms do not entirely succeed in preventing depletion of iodine stores, which ultimately may lead to insuffi-

cient production of hormone. In normal circumstances, iodine balance is maintained from dietary sources, i.e., food and water, but increasingly, especially in more highly developed cultures, iodine may enter the body via medications, diagnostic agents, and food supplements. Such increments in available iodine modify both the metabolism of iodine and the clinical tests by which it is assessed and hence will be discussed more fully in the section on laboratory tests.

It is difficult to assign normal limits to the daily dietary intake of iodine since this varies widely throughout the world, depending on the iodine content of soil and water and upon culturally established dietary preferences. Even in any single area, considerable variation in iodine intake can be expected among different individuals and in the same individual from day to day. In most areas of the United States, for example, dietary iodine intake now approximates 500 μg. daily, while in Japan, where large quantities of foods rich in iodine are characteristically consumed, intakes as high as several milligrams per day are commonplace. In other areas of the world, iodine intakes substantially less than those of the United States are apparently well tolerated without overt widespread thyroid dysfunction. As with pharmacologically induced alterations in iodine intake, such variations in the common dietary intake, when sustained, are reflected in differences in the kinetics of iodine metabolism and hence must be taken into account in assigning normal limits to tests designed to evaluate thyroid function. Figure 4-4 is a schema of the major pathways of overall iodine metabolism, summarizing the movement of iodine into, out of, and among the various compartments of body iodine. The numerical values presented are approximations to the normal means in the United

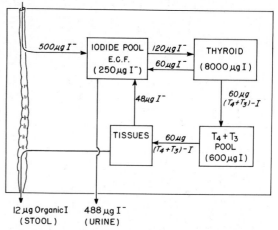

Figure 4-4. Diagram depicting normal pathways of iodine metabolism in a state of iodine balance. Note that most (approximately 90%) of body iodine store is present in the thyroid (chiefly in the organic form). Approximately 10% is present as iodide. Arrows indicate daily flux of iodine from one compartment to another. In this example, one-fifth of the iodide entering the iodide space (120/608) is accumulated by the thyroid. Peak thyroid uptake of I^{131} should be 20%, and the rate of turnover of thyronine-iodine peripherally 10%/day.

States, but even here rather wide variations are encountered. Iodine used in the synthesis of thyroid hormone is drawn from the inorganic iodide of the extracellular fluid (ECF). There are several sources from which this iodide is in turn replenished. Some iodide is apparently secreted back into the circulation by the thyroid itself, especially by the hyperactive thyroid. Iodide also enters the ECF from peripheral tissues which have carried out the deiodination of thyroid hormones. Ultimately, however, the diet is the most important source of iodine. Iodine is ingested in both the inorganic and the organically bound form. The rapidity of absorption of organically bound iodine and the form in which it is absorbed are uncertain, but eventually the iodine is made available as inorganic iodide. Iodide itself is rapidly and efficiently absorbed from the GI tract, and little is lost in the stool.

In the body, iodide is largely confined to the ECF; however, the iodide distribution space, which averages approximately 20 liters in the adult, has three extensions beyond the true ECF. Thus iodide is found in red blood cell water and is concentrated in the intraluminal fluids of the GI tract, notably the saliva and gastric juice, from which it is ultimately reabsorbed and reenters the ECF. In addition, until bound to organic compounds (chiefly tyrosine), iodide brought into the thyroid by active transport is in essence a portion of the extracellular iodide, since, like iodide in the other two extensions of the extracellular iodide space, it is in rapid equilibrium with iodide in the main compartment. The concentration of iodide in the ECF is normally quite low, approximately 1.0–1.5 μg./100 ml., indicating a peripheral pool of approximately 250 μg. Thus only a very small percentage of total body iodine is present in the iodide compartment, and this is turned over, i.e., removed and replenished, several times daily.

There are two main sites for the removal of iodide from the ECF. Small quantities of iodide are lost in expired air and through the skin, but the major clearance of iodide occurs via the thyroid and the kidneys. The processes by which thyroid clearance occurs and the subsequent fate of the iodide thereby removed will be considered in detail later. An appreciation of the renal mechanism for iodide clearance is important, since renal removal of iodide determines the availability of iodide to the thyroid (and vice versa). Although iodide is almost completely filterable at the glomerulus, the renal iodide clearance rate in adults normally approximates 30–40 ml./min. Thus filtered iodide is largely reabsorbed, but available evidence indicates that such reabsorption is passive rather than active. In man, unlike in other animals, the renal iodide clearance rate is unaffected by the excretion of chloride or other anions and is apparently independent of the plasma iodide concentration and hence the filtered load. Iodide clearance is minimally affected by the rate of urine flow per se and is uninfluenced by physiologic agents, such as TSH, or drugs, such as thiocyanate, that alter thyroidal iodide transport. As with other urinary components that are passively reabsorbed, the renal clearance of iodide varies with changes in glomerular filtration rate (GFR), the iodide clearance increasing or decreasing disproportionately when GFR is acutely increased or decreased, respectively. Thus, when intrinsic renal function is normal, the kidneys can be considered passive participants in iodide metabolism, not really sharing in the physiologic adjustments designed to maintain thyroidal homeostasis under abnormal circumstances.

Normally about 500 μg. of iodine is cleared into the urine daily, almost entirely in the inorganic form. This quantity is only slightly less than the average daily dietary intake, reflecting the scant loss of iodine through other avenues. Among these, the GI tract is the most important, about 12 μg. of iodine being lost in the stool daily, mainly in the organic form. Under abnormal circumstances, substantial losses of iodine may occur. In nephrosis or other proteinuric states, T_4 and T_3 are excreted in the urine in association with their transport proteins. Iodinated tyrosines are lost in the urine in the rare familial disorder in which the enzyme iodotyrosine dehalogenase is lacking from both the thyroid and peripheral tissues. Fecal loss of organic iodine may be excessive when GI absorption is impaired (Hiss and Dowling, 1962), as in chronic diarrheal states or under the influence of certain dietary constituents, such as soybean products (Pinchera et al., 1965). Finally, notable losses of iodine in both organic and inorganic form may occur through lactation.

The second major site of removal of iodide from the ECF is the thyroid. Iodide removed from the plasma by the thyroid is not irreversibly lost, however, since ultimately it will be secreted into the circulation as either iodinated thyronines, T_4 and T_3, or as inorganic iodide. The thyroid contains by far the largest pool of body iodine, under normal circumstances approximately 8000 μg., most of which is in the form of iodinated amino acids. Normally this pool of iodine turns over quite slowly (about 1 per cent/day).

Synthesis and Secretion of the Thyroid Hormones

The structural formulas of the thyroid hormones, their precursors, and several related compounds are shown in Figure 4–2, and the major steps in the synthesis and secretion of the hormones are shown in Figure 4–5. It is convenient to consider the metabolism of iodine leading to the biosynthesis of thyroid hormones as occurring in three sequential stages: (1) active transport of iodide into the thyroid, (2) oxidation of iodide and iodination by the oxidized form of tyrosyl residues within thyroglobulin to yield the hormonally inactive iodotyrosines, and (3) coupling of iodotyrosines to form the hormonally active iodothyronines, notably T_4 and T_3. The hormones thus formed are held in peptide linkage within the specific thyroprotein, thyroglobulin, which is the major component of the intra-

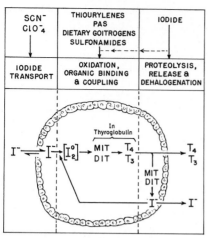

Figure 4–5. Diagram of the major steps in thyroid hormone biosynthesis. In this diagram, the follicular outline is intended merely to differentiate the intrathyroid from the interstitial compartment and should not be construed as indicating that the reactions shown necessarily occur in the follicular lumen. Note that the concentration of intrathyroid iodide maintained by the iodide transport mechanism is greater than that in the extracellular fluid. The processes of iodide oxidation, organic-binding, and coupling of iodotyrosines are grouped together since they appear to be closely related oxidative reactions. The precise proportions of the iodide liberated from iodotyrosines by dehalogenation that are reused or released into the extracellular fluid are unknown. Shown above are the major inhibitors of the several steps in hormone biosynthesis. Large quantities of iodide inhibit organic binding and coupling (dashed lines), but this effect is usually transient. Although not shown, the lithium ion, like iodide, is an inhibitor of proteolysis and release.

follicular colloid. Release of hormones, in addition, involves two additional groups of reactions: (1) hydrolysis of thyroglobulin by a thyroid protease and by peptidases, liberating free iodinated amino acids; and (2) passage of iodothyronines into the blood, while the iodotyrosines undergo intrathyroid deiodination.

Iodide Transport

Except when the plasma concentration of inorganic iodide is greatly increased, synthesis of adequate quantities of hormone requires that iodide enter the thyroid more rapidly than would be possible by simple diffusion from the ECF. The thyroid, however, contains a mechanism, variously known as the iodide-concentrating, -transport, or -trapping mechanism, that subserves this end and provides sufficient iodide substrate for subsequent steps in hormone formation (comprehensively reviewed by Wolff, 1964). Iodide transported into the gland either is oxidized and organified or is free to diffuse back into the ECF. Under normal circumstances, at least in many animals and probably in man, the rate of inward clearance of iodide exceeds the combined rates of organic binding* and back

diffusion, with the result that intrathyroid concentration gradients for iodide in excess of unity are maintained within the gland. Such gradients are often referred to as thyroid/plasma (T:P) or thyroid/serum (T:S) ratios. When, through the action of pharmacologic inhibitors or spontaneous disease, iodide transport is defective, goiter and hypothyroidism result. Both can be overcome by increasing the plasma iodide concentration, however, allowing adequate quantities of iodide to enter the gland by simple diffusion.

Since organic-binding reactions normally proceed rapidly, T:P ratios for inorganic iodide in unblocked glands are ordinarily low. Therefore, the activity of the thyroid iodide transport mechanism per se is best assessed when organic binding is inhibited by appropriate pharmacologic means. Under these circumstances, the ability of the thyroid to maintain concentration ratios for inorganic iodide is often remarkable. In the highly stimulated thyroid of the rat or mouse, for example, such as develops during prolonged iodide deficiency or during administration of antithyroid drugs, T:P concentration ratios of several hundredfold have been reported. Ratios are also increased in the diffuse toxic goiter of Graves' disease, often greatly so. The ability of the thyroid to transport inorganic iodide and to maintain concentration gradients for iodide is not unlimited, however. Rather, there exists a maximum rate of iodide transport, the magnitude of which will vary with the functional state of the thyroid. Thus progressive increases in the concentration of inorganic iodide in the plasma are associated with progressively declining values for T:P ratios, while the concentration of iodide actively transported into the thyroid increases progressively and ultimately reaches a maximum. Both these maxima and T:P concentration ratios at normal plasma iodide concentration serve as indices of the activity of the iodide transport mechanism, and almost always these indices vary together.

The precise locus of the iodide concentrating mechanism within the thyroid is uncertain. When I^{131}* is administered acutely to animals in which organic binding of thyroid iodide is blocked, radioautographs of thyroids removed within a few minutes reveal that most iodide is distributed rather uniformly throughout the follicular lumen; however, small amounts are also found at the apical portion of the acinar epithelial cell. The latter finding, together with the observation that isolated acinar cells grown in tissue culture are capable of maintaining concentration gradients for inorganic iodide, indicates that the locus of the iodide concentrating mechanism is within the

---

*For brevity, "organic binding," "organic iodine," "organified," and similar terms are often used. These expressions signify that iodide is bound to organic compounds, chiefly as iodotyrosine.

*Since the last edition of this book was published, the convention for notation of isotopes has been changed so that what had been designated I^{131} is now designated ^{131}I. However, since the habits of decades are not easily expunged, most readers think "I^{131}" while reading "^{131}I." Accordingly, we have chosen to employ the older notation in this chapter. Unfortunately, as a consequence, purists will be required to think "^{131}I" while reading "I^{131}."

thyroid epithelial cell itself. The interior of the acinar cell maintains a negative electrical potential in relation to both the interstitial tissue and the follicular lumen. Presumably, iodide is actively transported into the cell against this negative potential and then diffuses along the electrochemical gradient into the luminal area.

The exact biochemical mechanism of active iodide transport is unknown. However, like other active transport mechanisms, thyroid iodide transport is an energy-requiring process, highly dependent upon continued generation of phosphate bond energy. Iodide transport is inhibited by anoxia, by inhibitors of oxidative metabolism, and by agents that inhibit oxidative phosphorylation. In addition, active iodide transport is closely related to the function of the sodium (Na^+)-, potassium (K^+)-dependent ATPase system. Ouabain and other cardiac glycosides that inhibit this system also inhibit iodide transport, an effect that can be overcome by increasing the concentration of K^+ in the medium in which thyroid tissue is incubated. Although TSH increases the activity of both the iodide transport and ouabain-sensitive ATPase systems, the two do not respond in parallel in other circumstances. Hence the precise nature of their relationship remains uncertain. ATPase, acting on ATP at the cell membrane, may make phosphate bond energy available for iodide transport. Alternatively, reversible exchange of iodide for phosphate in a specific carrier may take place. The nature of the iodide carrier is unknown, but lecithins capable of reversibly binding iodide have been extracted from thyroid tissue (Schneider and Wolff, 1965).

The thyroid mechanism for concentrating iodide is apparently shared by other monovalent anions, including perchlorate and pertechnetate. These and other anions act as competitive inhibitors of iodide transport, a property that may relate to similarity of their partial specific molecular volumes. Thiocyanate, another monovalent anion that inhibits iodide transport, is not itself concentrated within the thyroid and may possibly act by uncoupling thyroid oxidative phosphorylation. The ability of perchlorate and thiocyanate to inhibit iodide transport is the basis for their use in the perchlorate- or thiocyanate-discharge tests for defects in the thyroid organic-binding mechanism, and concentration of the radioactive anion pertechnetate makes this a valuable agent for thyroid imaging (see later section on thyroid function tests).

The activity of the iodide transport mechanism is influenced by a variety of physiologic factors. Among these, TSH is generally held to be the most important. Under most circumstances, iodide transport is enhanced by TSH and diminished by hypophysectomy. However, other humoral factors, some of which remain undefined, also influence iodide transport. In hypophysectomized rats, T:P ratios decrease, but not as much as those in intact rats whose secretion of TSH is inhibited by exogenous thyroid hormone. Moreover, administration of exogenous hormone to hypophysectomized

rats does not decrease their T:P values to the lower values seen in the intact animal in which TSH secretion is suppressed. The activity of the iodide transport mechanism is also modified by an internal autoregulatory system, with the result that its intrinsic activity and its responsiveness to TSH stimulation vary inversely with the glandular content of organic iodine (reviewed by Ingbar, 1972).

The ability of the thyroid to concentrate iodide is shared by other tissues of endodermal origin, notably the salivary and gastric glands. The effect of metabolic inhibitors and inhibitory anions on iodide transport in these other tissues is similar to that on iodide transport in the thyroid. Rarely goitrous hypothyroidism in man may stem from the absence of an effective thyroid iodide transport mechanism, in which case salivary and gastric concentration of iodide is also lacking.

In addition to iodide brought into the thyroid by active transport from the ECF, iodide is generated in the thyroid by the deiodination of iodotyrosines liberated during the hydrolysis of thyroglobulin. A portion of this iodide is reorganified, while the remainder is lost from the gland as the so-called "iodide leak." Whether such iodide is functionally distinct from that which enters the gland through active transport and whether it persists in the thyroid long enough to constitute a second or "internal iodide pool" is a matter of current disagreement.

Oxidation of Iodide and Organic Iodinations

After its transport into or regeneration within the thyroid, iodide enters into a series of reactions which ultimately lead to the synthesis of the active thyroid hormones. (For a review of the organic-binding and coupling mechanisms, see DeGroot et al., 1970.) The first of these reactions involves oxidation of iodide and incorporation of the resulting intermediate into the hormonally inactive precursors, MIT and DIT. Iodide thus metabolized is removed from the iodide pool and can no longer be discharged by thiocyanate, perchlorate, or other inhibitors of iodide transport. In most species, oxidation of iodide is normally rapid but probably not instantaneous, since newly transported iodide can be found in the gland by direct analysis. After administration of I^{131}, the isotope is almost immediately found in organic combination, mainly in soluble thyroprotein, principally thyroglobulin, and to a limited extent in subcellular particulate proteins and lipids. Formation of iodinated nucleic acids has also been reported. These iodinated products are probably the result of random rather than specifically directed iodinations. The earliest products of thyroid iodinations are mono- and diiodotyrosyl groups in thyroglobulin and, to a much lesser extent, in particulate iodoprotein. Traces of iodohistidine are also found.

There is conclusive evidence that the iodinations that lead to formation of iodotyrosines occur within a preformed thyroprotein molecule rather than in free amino acids that are then incorporated into protein. Puromycin, in concentrations sufficient to block thyroprotein synthesis completely, fails to inhibit the formation of MIT and DIT. Furthermore, tRNA for MIT and DIT is lacking in the thyroid. Although evidence concerning the cellular locus of the iodinating reactions is somewhat contradictory, radioautographic evidence, as well as the demonstration that ghosts of isolated thyroid cells that are virtually devoid of intracellular contents are capable of carrying out organic iodinations, suggests that iodinations occur at the cell-colloid interface.

There is general agreement that oxidation of thyroid iodide is mediated by a peroxidase. Enzymes with peroxidatic activity have been demonstrated in the thyroid of many species, including man, especially in particulate subcellular fractions. A peroxidase in hog thyroid has been substantially purified and appears to be a heme protein; this accounts for the requirement of organic iodinations for molecular oxygen and their ready inhibition by cyanide and azide. In vitro, thyroid peroxidase, when afforded a source of hydrogen peroxide, readily iodinates thyroglobulin as well as other proteins. The reaction catalyzed by peroxidase in vitro has many properties of the iodination reaction in vivo, including inhibition by antithyroid agents and by high concentrations of iodide (Wolff-Chaikoff effect). The evanescent product of the peroxidation of iodide, i.e., the active iodinating form, is uncertain, but may be the iodinium ion (I^+), or a free radical of iodine. Current evidence suggests that the hydrogen peroxide that serves as the oxidant of iodide is generated through the auto-oxidation of flavin enzymes acting as NADH- and particularly NADPH-oxidases. In this way, generation of hydrogen peroxide is linked to electron transfers consequent to substrate oxidations within the thyroid. Oxidation of amines, notably tyramine, may also serve as a source of reduced flavoproteins that give rise to hydrogen peroxide.

It is uncertain whether a second enzyme, designated "tyrosine iodinase," is necessary to direct the actual iodination of tyrosyl groups by the activated form of iodine as some have suggested. None seems necessary in vitro, but this does not preclude the presence of such an enzyme in vivo. As judged from studies in vitro, soluble inhibitors of organic iodinations, principally ascorbic acid and reduced glutathione, exist in thyroid tissue. These may inhibit iodinations by reducing either the oxidized form of iodine or hydrogen peroxide itself. Thus mitochondrial systems may provide a source of hydrogen peroxide and microsomal structures the iodide-peroxidase, while the cytoplasmic fraction may contain regulatory inhibitors of organic iodinations.

Organic iodinations are conditioned by the extent of thyroid stimulation by TSH. They are retarded in the hypophysectomized rat and are promptly increased by administration of TSH. Iodinations are susceptible to inhibition by a great number of pharmacologic agents, including the usual antithyroid drugs, most of which have intrinsic reducing activity. Iodinations are also inhibited by freezing, cooling, or storage of the thyroid tissue. Defects in the organic-binding mechanism of variable severity occur in humans and lead to the development of goitrous hypothyroidism or, if less severe, to goiter without hypothyroidism. In certain instances of this type, the thyroid is found to be lacking in peroxidase. In others, peroxidase is present, and the defect may reside in inadequate production of hydrogen peroxide or abnormalities in thyroglobulin that render it less readily iodinated.

Formation of Iodothyronines

Oxidation and organic binding of thyroid iodide to yield iodotyrosines are followed by the synthesis of the hormonally active iodothyronines, T_4 and T_3. Since noniodinated thyronine cannot be demonstrated in thyroglobulin, it seems certain that T_4 and T_3 must arise from iodinated precursors. Synthesis of T_4 from DIT requires the fusion of two DIT molecules to yield a structure with two diiodinated rings linked by an ether bridge. Concomitantly, there occurs a net loss of the alanine side chain from the ring that ultimately contains the phenolic hydroxyl group (beta or outer ring). This reaction is commonly termed the coupling reaction. In aqueous media, this or analogous reactions take place when DIT or derivatives of DIT are allowed to stand under oxidative conditions. Nevertheless, the manner in which T_4 is synthesized in vivo remains uncertain. Two general hypotheses have received major consideration. The first is that T_4 and T_3 are formed by the interaction of a peptide-bound DIT with an oxidation product of DIT or MIT, respectively. In the case of DIT, the suggested product is 3,5-diiodo-4-hydroxy-phenylpyruvic acid (DIHPPA). In vitro, DIHPPA has been shown to be a product of oxidative systems that yield T_4 from DIT. Moreover, when DIHPPA is added to solutions of DIT, T_4 is formed, with pyruvic acid and ammonia as by-products. Additional studies in vitro have revealed formation of labeled T_4 when thyroglobulin is incubated with labeled DIHPPA. As small quantities of DIHPPA and its monoiodinated analogue, MIHPPA, the suggested precursor of T_3, have been found in thyroid tissue, this mechanism of synthesis of iodothyronines in vivo seems quite possible. It is attractive since it does not require the extensive structural alterations in the thyroglobulin molecule during iodothyronine synthesis required by the alternative hypothesis.

The most commonly held view concerning the synthesis of T_4 and T_3 differs from that described above in that it requires the coupling of two iodotyrosines, both of which are initially held in peptide bond within the thyroglobulin molecule. A free radical mechanism whereby two molecules of DIT yield T_4 via a quinol ether intermediate has been proposed, but it is apparent that, whatever the intermediates in the reaction, coupling of two peptide-bound iodotyrosines would require disruption of the peptide bonds holding the iodotyrosyl group that yields the beta ring of the thyronine nucleus. This would obviously require substantial changes in the structure of thyroglobulin as iodothyronines are formed. Such rearrangements are possible, however, since T_4 can be formed *in vitro* during iodination of thyroglobulin or even of proteins that are not normally iodinated, such as casein, insulin, or albumin. Moreover, both *in vivo* and *in vitro*, the enhanced synthesis of iodothyronines that accompanies increasing iodination of thyroglobulin is associated with an increase in both the sedimentation constant of the protein and its stability to conditions that induce dissociation. These changes are consistent with the occurrence of a major change in the structure of the protein consequent to the synthesis of T_4 and T_3.

Whatever its mechanism, synthesis of iodothyronines requires oxidative conditions. There is increasing thought that the reaction is mediated by a peroxidase, perhaps the same peroxidase that mediates the initial oxidation of iodide, since there are interesting similarities between the two reactions. Virtually all agents that inhibit organic binding also inhibit coupling. In addition, cell-free particulate fractions can yield T_4 from free DIT when provided with a source of hydrogen peroxide. Moreover, synthesis of labeled iodothyronines from prelabeled iodotyrosines is demonstrable when prelabeled thyroglobulin is incubated with thyroid peroxidase and a source of hydrogen peroxide in the absence of free iodide. Despite this evidence that peroxidase may mediate both the organic-binding and the coupling mechanisms, there are certain physiologic differences between the two. The coupling reaction is much more sensitive to a variety of factors. Inhibition of coupling with continued generation of MIT and DIT occurs in response to small doses of antithyroid agents or during the acute response to large amounts of iodide. Iodine deficiency and lack of TSH impair the synthesis of iodothyronines relatively more than the synthesis of iodotyrosines. Thermal injury to the thyroid does the same. A more complete dissociation of coupling and organic iodinations may be evident in the fetal chick thyroid, in which synthesis of iodotyrosines is said to antecede synthesis of iodothyronines by nearly a day. Finally, a failure of coupling may be the cause of certain cases of goitrous hypothyroidism in man. Here, inadequate secretion of iodothyronines occurs, and although the thyroid contains ample iodotyrosines, little T_4 and T_3 are found. It is thus uncertain whether the organic-binding and coupling reactions are indeed separate or whether they are mediated by a similar mechanism. Perhaps they are the same but are differentially affected by other factors, possibly the inherent oxidative potential of the gland.

Storage and Release of Hormones

The thyroid is unique among the endocrine glands by virtue of the large store of hormone that it contains and the slow overall rate at which the hormone normally turns over. This aspect of thyroid hormone economy has homeostatic value in that the large hormone reservoir provides prolonged protection against depletion of circulating hormone should synthesis cease. In normal man, administration of completely blocking doses of antithyroid agents for as long as two weeks results in little lowering of the serum T_4 concentration, and plasma concentrations of TSH are not increased. Thus an important aspect of hormone economy is the storage function of the thyroid. Analyses reveal that the normal thyroid contains about 8000 μg. of iodine, of which as much as 10 per cent may be inorganic. Direct analyses of human thyroids performed when iodine intake was generally lower indicated that the organic iodine is constituted as follows: MIT, 17–28 per cent; DIT, 24–42 per cent; T_4, 35 per cent; T_3, 5–8 per cent. More recent analyses show that the $T_4 : T_3$ ratio may be even higher than the foregoing figures indicate (Chopra et al., 1973). It is not certain whether this reflects more refined analytic techniques or the effect of a general increase in dietary iodine intake.

Thyroglobulin is the storage form of the thyroid hormone. Although it has been thought that thyroglobulin is excluded completely from the peripheral blood, immunochemical analyses suggest that the protein may be present in the plasma of about 60 per cent of normal individuals (0.01–0.15 μg./ml.) (Torrigiani et al., 1969). Direct cannulation reveals that the lymphatics are the avenue through which thyroglobulin normally enters the blood. It is very unlikely, however, that peripheral hydrolysis of thyroglobulin contributes significantly to the T_4 and T_3 found in the blood. Rather, T_4 and T_3 enter the blood directly after their liberation from thyroglobulin by proteolytic cleavage within the follicular cell.

The mechanisms whereby this cleavage occurs have been extensively clarified by submicroscopic, histochemical, and biochemical studies, and the sequence is best observed after stimulation of the resting thyroid by TSH (see review by Dumont, 1971). Within a few minutes after such stimulation, formation of pseudopodia is evident at the apical surface of the follicular cell, followed by endocytosis of colloid to yield multiple vesicles (colloid droplets). That these vesicles contain colloid is evident in that they are PAS-positive and contain C^{14}-amino acids or radioiodine previously allowed to accumulate in the luminal contents. The process of endocytosis apparently involves destabilization of the apical membrane, since membrane stabilizers, such as chlorpromazine, inhibit this process. The process is not confined to thyroglobulin, since isolated thyroid cells are capable of accumulating latex particles, and this process is stimulated by factors that enhance the endocytosis of colloid. Concomitantly with endocytosis, there occurs a migration of dense bodies, rich in esterases and acid phosphatase and apparently identical with lysosomes, from the basal toward the apical end of the cell. Fusion of lysosomes with colloid droplets occurs. The resulting "phagolysosomes" have histochemical characteristics of both component particles and are likely the site of the physiologically active protease. The latter is an acid hydrolase similar in properties to cathepsin D. Hydrolysis of thyroglobulin is thought to occur in the phagolysosomes, which gradually regain the ultrastructural properties and basal location of lysosomes as hydrolysis is completed. Microtubular and microfilamentous structures, similar to those found in other organs, are present in the thyroid cell. They are apparently involved in the secretory process, since inhibitors of both the former (vincristine, vinblastine, colchicine) and the latter (cytochalasin B) inhibit the secretory process.

Studies *in vitro* with subcellular fractions of thyroid tissue containing phagolysosomes have shed light on the biochemical processes by which thyroglobulin is hydrolyzed. It appears that hydrolysis is facilitated by reduction of disulfide bonds in thyroglobulin, this being effected by a transhydrogenase that uses reduced glutathione (GSH). The availability of GSH, in turn, depends upon the activity of a second enzyme, glutathione reductase, that uses NADPH to reduce oxidized glutathione. If true, the proposed mechanism would link the secretory process to intermediary metabolism and biologic oxidations within the gland.

Although it had been thought that iodothyronines liberated by this process were entirely free to enter the blood, there being no mechanism within the gland to effect their degradation, it now appears that the thyroid is capable of deiodinating T_4 and T_3 by a mechanism that may involve a peroxidase reaction. Generation of T_3 from T_4 by this mechanism has been demonstrated (Haibach, 1971), but it is unlikely that this pathway is normally operative within the thyroid to any great extent. In the rat, for example, the $T_3:T_4$ ratio in the thyroid venous effluent is similar to that in the gland as a whole, and, as will be seen below, little T_3 is apparently secreted by the normal human thyroid. Whether significant quantities of T_3 are generated from T_4 within the thyroid when secretion of T_3 relative to T_4 is disproportionately great is uncertain.

Iodotyrosines liberated from thyroglobulin are subject to the action of a microsomal iodotyrosine dehalogenase, an NADPH-dependent enzyme found in the peripheral tissues as well as in the thyroid. This enzyme liberates iodide from MIT and DIT and normally prevents their entry into the blood in appreciable quantities. It is inactive against peptide-bound iodotyrosines or free iodothyronines, and hence differs from the mechanism for T_4 deiodination described above. Activity of the thyroid iodotyrosine deiodinase system is enhanced by TSH administration, possibly because of increased NADPH generation, rather than an increase in enzyme concentration. Iodide liberated from MIT and DIT is partly used for hormone synthesis and partly lost from the gland as "iodide leak." It comprises or contributes to the iodide measured in the so-called internal or second iodide pool.

There is much evidence that the thyroid does not behave as a single homogeneous functioning unit.

Radioautographic studies reveal variations in function among different areas of the gland and in different follicles. In addition, it seems clear that the thyroid contains at least two pools of organic iodine which turn over at different rates. One pool, representing more newly iodinated materials, is smaller but turns over more rapidly than the other, larger pool of older hormone (last come—first served). This may result from the contiguity of the sites for iodination and colloid resorption. In truth, there may be many iodine pools in the thyroid turning over at different rates, just as there are many subtle differences in the thyroglobulin molecules within a single thyroid (reviewed by Rosenberg and Bastomsky, 1965).

The storage function of the thyroid may not be perfectly maintained under even normal circumstances. Thus, as noted above, some thyroglobulin can be detected in the blood of most normal individuals, and the frequency with which it is detected is increased in pregnancy. Increased concentrations are present in the serum of patients with nontoxic goiter or hyperthyroidism. In the latter disorder, concentrations of thyroglobulin display a moderately close correlation with the serum PBI, an observation consonant with the enhancement of thyroglobulin release by TSH stimulation in the animal. Uncertainty exists as to the extent to which iodotyrosines are normally released from the thyroid. From iodine analyses of chromatograms of extracts of serum, and from direct immunoassay, it appears that substantial concentrations of iodotyrosines are present in the blood of normal individuals. Doubt about the validity of this finding, however, arises from the fact that iodotyrosines are removed from the blood so rapidly that an improbably high secretion rate would be required to maintain the concentrations apparently measured. Moreover, in experimental animals, significant quantities of labeled iodotyrosines are not found in the venous effluent from prelabeled thyroids. For the present, therefore, this question remains unresolved.

Clear-cut disturbances of the storage mechanisms comprise an important category of thyroid dysfunction. Large quantities of thyroglobulin are released from the gland during surgical manipulation or radiation thyroiditis, and possibly in patients with subacute thyroiditis. In both forms of thyroiditis, T_4 and T_3 may be released transiently into the blood in sufficient quantities to produce thyrotoxicosis. Relatively high concentrations of thyroglobulin are also found in the blood of some patients with papillary carcinoma of the thyroid. An abnormal iodoprotein resembling albumin in many of its properties is found in the blood of some patients with hyperthyroidism, thyroid neoplasm, and varying types of dyshormonogenesis. It is also found in certain varieties of nontoxic goiter, occasionally in association with hypothyroidism. In the latter instances, hypothyroidism is thought to result from diversion of thyroid iodine metabolism from normal channels to the secretion of the hormonally inactive iodoprotein. Another variety of goitrous hypothyroidism is associated with deficiency of iodotyrosine dehalogenase within the thyroid. Owing to the absence of the enzyme from peripheral tissues as well, the iodotyrosines lost from the gland fail to undergo deiodination peripherally and are excreted into the urine either unchanged or as their keto-acid metabolites. The resulting losses of iodine produce a state of conditioned iodine deficiency, which is in large part responsible for development of the goiter and can be overcome by dietary iodine supplementation (Stanbury, 1972). A similar disorder can be produced in animals by administration of the inhibitors of iodotyrosine dehalogenase, mono- or dinitrotyrosine (Green, 1971). The extent to which mild forms of the disorder are responsible for sporadic nontoxic goiter in man is unknown.

The process of proteolysis and release of thyroid hormones is inhibited by a variety of agents. Most important among these is iodine. The ability of iodine to inhibit these processes is responsible for the rapid improvement in thyrotoxicosis that iodine produces in the hyperthyroid patient. The mechanism whereby this effect is mediated is uncertain, but recent findings in the authors' laboratory suggest that it may occur through an inhibition of glutathione reductase. A similar effect on hormone release is produced by the lithium ion, which is therefore also effective in the treatment of hyperthyroidism. The action of lithium on the thyroid is complex. It inhibits both the increase in adenylate cyclase induced by TSH and the stimulation of I^{131} release from prelabeled thyroids by dibutyryl cyclic AMP. (See Emerson et al., 1973, for references on the effects of lithium.)

Thyroid Iodoproteins

Thyroglobulin is the principal iodoprotein of the thyroid gland. It constitutes virtually all of the follicular colloid and is therefore the major component of the normal thyroid mass. It is furthermore the repository of virtually all the active hormones, T_4 and T_3, within the gland and of most of their immediate precursors, MIT and DIT. Retention within the gland of this large protein permits maintenance of the unique storage function of the thyroid. Because of its distinctive character and the relative ease with which it can be isolated in highly purified form, it has been a source of interest not only to thyroidologists but also to biochemists and immunochemists and, more recently, to molecular biologists. (For a detailed review of the chemistry and synthesis of thyroglobulin, see Edelhoch, 1965.) Thyroglobulin is a glycoprotein containing approximately 10 per cent by weight of carbohydrates, which include glucosamine, mannose, fucose, galactose, and sialic acid. Its molecular weight is approximately 660,000, and its sedimentation constant ($S^0_{20,w}$) approximately 19. Terminal amino acid analysis suggests that thyroglobulin is composed of four peptide chains. Individual chains may exist in the 6-7S (monomeric) or 12S (dimeric) form in saline extracts of the thyroid. However, iodoproteins with sedimentation constants of 27S and 32S are also found. The latter may represent more highly iodinated forms of the 19S molecule.

The thyroglobulin molecule contains approximately 120 tyrosyl residues, of which a varying but relatively small portion are naturally iodinated. During iodination *in vitro*, even when excess iodine is added, approximately 30 per cent of the tyrosyl residues remain uniodinated, but these can be iodinated when the molecule is unfolded in 8 M urea. Small amounts of T_4 are formed *in vitro* during the iodination of thyroglobulin but not if the molecule has been subjected to enzymatic digestion, suggesting that peptide chain length is an important factor in T_4 formation. Although suggested by earlier work, it does not seem likely that iodinated amino acids exist as end groups in the thyroglobulin molecule. Results of some studies suggest that in natural thyroglobulin T_4 is commonly surrounded by particular amino acids, indicating that T_4 formation is favored by a unique amino acid sequence at the site of coupling. The I/N ratio in thyroglobulin is highly variable among different species and among animals of the same species. In addition, even within a single animal, thyroglobulin can be shown by chromatographic techniques to be heterogeneous. Later portions of the chromatographic eluate contain relatively more iodine and possibly more T_4, and contain more of the heavy components. The more highly iodinated thyroglobulin is less susceptible to dissociation by dilution or exposure to alkaline pH.

The site and mode of synthesis of thyroglobulin have been studied both by radioautography and by biochemical analysis following administration of labeled amino acids and sugars. Pulse-chase experiments show that labeled amino acids are quickly incorporated into 3-8S and 12S proteins. Soon thereafter, 17-18S proteins are seen to be labeled, and a shift of activity from the 12S to the former zone progressively occurs. By contrast, the 3-8S fraction does not appear to be a source of labeled amino acid for the heavier fractions. The 17-18S "prethyroglobulin" is transformed to 19S "mature thyroglobulin" through iodination, and further iodination is thought to produce the 27S variety. Synthesis of the peptide skeleton of thyroglobulin occurs in the rough ER of the follicular cell, where a portion of the carbohydrate components may be added. The partly synthesized molecule then moves through the channels of the ER to the Golgi apparatus where glycosidation is completed. The protein then moves to the apex of the cell, where at least much of the iodination takes place at or near the cell-colloid interface.

In recent years, great attention has been focused on the nonthyroglobulin proteins of normal and diseased glands, particularly the soluble protein(s) with a sedimentation coefficient of approximately 4 (4S or S-1 iodoprotein). Small quantities of this protein are found in normal thyroids of both man and other species, and larger quantities have been detected in a wide variety of thyroid disorders, particularly those associated with glandular hyperfunction, irrespective of the rate of T_4 and T_3 synthesis. Thus the protein is abnormally abundant in frankly dyshormonogenetic goiters with or without hypothyroidism, in some cases of simple nontoxic goiter, in the diffuse toxic goiter of Graves' disease, in endemic goiter, and in Hashimoto's disease. A similar protein is also found in some thyroid neoplasms. Very often in these conditions an abnormal iodoprotein of similar properties appears in the serum, producing an unusually large discrepancy between the protein-bound iodine (PBI) and T_4-iodine concentrations. The iodoprotein in both serum and thyroid has the electrophoretic mobility of serum albumin; hence, that form found in the thyroid has been designated thyralbumin. This finding has stimulated much effort to ascertain whether the protein is in fact identical to serum albumin and whether it is synthesized *de novo* in the thyroid or merely iodinated therein. These questions have been approached using a variety of techniques, including amino acid analysis, assessment of immunologic cross-reactivity, determination of solubility characteristics, and studies of the incorporation of labeled precursors *in vitro*. The data generated have often been at variance with one another, rendering firm conclusions difficult. It appears, however, that the 4S iodoprotein may consist of two varieties, one of which is clearly synthesized within the thyroid and differs from serum albumin immunologically and in amino acid content. The other appears to be indistinguishable from serum albumin and may merely represent protein that has entered the thyroid from the blood and undergone iodination. From studies in patients with nontoxic goiter, it appears that the secretion of the 4S iodoprotein is under physiologic control, since its release from the thyroid is enhanced by TSH and decreased by suppressive doses of T_4. This is consistent with either of the foregoing suggestions concerning the origin of such proteins. In rare cases, the thyroid and, less frequently, the plasma contain an iodoprotein similar or identical in properties to the T_4-binding prealbumin. (For references in this area, see Furth et al., 1970; Jonckheer and Karcher, 1971; and Otten et al., 1971.)

Transport, Turnover, and Metabolism of the Thyroid Hormones

Hormone Transport

Extracellular Binding Proteins. Upon entering the blood, the major secretory products of the normal thyroid gland, T_4 and T_3, are bound to particular proteins in a firm but reversible bond (see review by Woeber and Ingbar, 1973, for more extensive discussion and references). Much of what is known about the specific binding of the thyroid hormones, including its initial demonstration, has been derived from study of serum enriched with labeled hormone by the technique of zonal electrophoresis, particularly in filter paper, but also in starch, agar, or polyacrylamide gels. Although

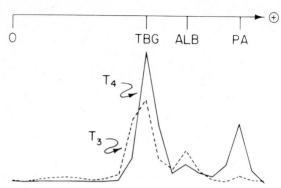

Figure 4–6. Diagram depicting the electrophoretic migration of radioiodine-labeled T_4 and T_3 in normal human serum. TBG, thyronine-binding globulin; ALB, albumin; PA, prealbumin, also known as T_4-binding prealbumin (TBPA). T_4 is bound predominantly by TBG, to a lesser extent by TBPA, and to a slight extent by albumin. T_3 is bound by TBG and by albumin, but little, if at all, by TBPA.

these electrophoretic techniques result in some distortions of the hormone-protein interactions, they are quantitative rather than qualitative. Electrophoretic studies have disclosed two plasma proteins with which T_4 is mainly associated, a T_4-binding inter-α globulin (TBG) and a T_4-binding prealbumin (TBPA). To a limited extent, T_4 is also bound to albumin. T_3, on the other hand, is bound mainly by TBG and, to a small extent, by albumin (Fig. 4–6). Despite some data suggesting that T_3 might be bound to a slight extent by TBPA, the bulk of evidence suggests that, for practical purposes, T_3 is not bound by TBPA at all. In view of the fact that TBG binds both T_4 and T_3, a more appropriate designation than the commonly employed T_4-binding globulin would be "thyronine-binding globulin," a term that would not necessitate altering the universally accepted abbreviation, TBG.

TBG has been isolated from human plasma by several groups of workers. From their studies, it appears that its molecular weight is approximately 60,000 and its concentration in normal plasma approximately 2 mg./100 ml. This quantity is capable of binding approximately 20 μg. of T_4. TBG is a glycoprotein which contains about 9 moles of neuraminic acid per mole. Treatment of the protein with bacterial neuraminidase alters its electrophoretic mobility but does not influence its ability to bind T_4. In normal man, its half-time in plasma is about five days (Cavalieri, unpublished observations).

TBPA has also been isolated from human plasma, in which it exists in part as a complex with retinol (Vitamin A)-binding protein. Its molecular weight is approximately 50,000 and its concentration in plasma approximately 25 mg./100 ml. This quantity of TBPA can bind about 200 μg. of T_4. TBPA is poor in carbohydrate but rich in tryptophan. In normal man, its half-time in plasma is about two days.

Although both TBG and TBPA are capable of binding T_4 avidly, their binding sites exhibit substantially different properties. The TBG molecule appears to have one thyronine binding site. Its affinity for T_3 is, however, less than that for T_4, the equilibrium constant for the latter reaction being about 10^{10} liters/mole. TBG binds the dextro-isomer of T_4 apparently as well as it binds the naturally occurring levo-isomeric form. Deamination of the iodothyronine molecule greatly reduces the binding to TBG; the acetic and propionic acid analogues of T_4 and T_3 are bound by TBG little if at all. Binding of T_4 by TBG is inhibited by a variety of organic compounds, including diphenylhydantoin, tetrachlorthyronine, salicylate, anilinonaphthalenesulfonic acid, and o,p'-DDD (dichloro-diphenyldichloroethane).

Like TBG, the TBPA molecule has but one major binding site, the equilibrium constant for the interaction with T_4 being about 10^8 liters/mole. D-Thyroxine is not bound appreciably by TBPA, and deamination of the alanine side chain yields products that interact much more strongly than do the parent compounds. Thus tetraiodothyroacetic acid (tetrac) and tetraiodothyropropionic acid are bound to TBPA more strongly than is T_4. Moreover, the triiodinated analogues, unlike T_3 itself, are bound by TBPA quite strongly. A variety of organic compounds are potent inhibitors of the T_4-TBPA interaction; these include barbital, salicylate and some of its congeners, 2,4-dinitrophenol, and penicillin.

Owing to the quantitatively variable results provided by different electrophoretic techniques, there has been considerable confusion as to the relative importance of TBG and TBPA in determining the overall intensity of T_4 binding in plasma. However, by means of refined electrophoretic techniques and of immunochemical removal of TBPA from serum by a specific antibody, it has been possible to demonstrate that TBG is normally responsible for the transport of most of the T_4 (about 75 per cent) and, with the serum T_4 concentration, is by far the major determinant of the free T_4. TBPA plays a far lesser role, except when TBG is lacking, and even then, rather marked variations in TBPA influence the concentration and turnover of T_4 only slightly. Much effort has been directed toward the elucidation of the function of the T_4-binding proteins. Certain conclusions seem indisputable. Thus, as a result of their interaction with the transport proteins, the iodinated amino acids acquire macromolecular properties which profoundly alter their metabolism. The neglible normal urinary excretion of T_4 and T_3 is almost certainly due to their limited filterability at the glomerulus. Furthermore, as will be seen, values for the volume of distribution and rate of turnover of the hormones are also affected by their protein associations, so that they resemble more closely those of the plasma proteins than those of unbound amino acids.

In vitro, the interaction between the thyroid hormones and their binding proteins has been found to conform to a reversible binding equilibrium which can be expressed by conventional equilibrium equations. For those formulations which follow, T_4 is used as the hormone prototype, with the understanding that similar interactions apply in the case of T_3. In addition, TBG is used as the prototype binding protein, in view of the predominant role that it plays in hormone transport. The interaction between T_4 and TBG can be expressed as follows:

$$T_4 + TBG \overset{k}{\rightleftharpoons} T_4 \cdot TBG$$

Here, TBG represents the unoccupied binding sites of the protein; k, the equilibrium constant for the interaction; and $T_4 \cdot TBG$, the binding sites on TBG occupied by T_4. This interaction can also be expressed by the mass-action relationship, wherein

$$\frac{(T_4 \cdot TBG)}{(T_4)\,(TBG)} = k$$

rearranging,

$$\frac{(T_4)}{(T_4 \cdot TBG)} = \frac{1}{(TBG)k}$$

These expressions predict that T_4 will exist in the plasma in both the bound and free forms. That this is the case has been demonstrated by direct analysis. Although the concentration of free T_4 in normal human serum cannot be measured directly, the proportion of hormone that is free can be measured by radioisotopic techniques, and the concentration can then be calculated as the product of the total hormone concentration and the fraction that is free. In normal serum, the free T_4 is approximately 0.03 per cent of the total, and its absolute concentration is about 2 ng./100 ml.

It is also evident from the preceding formula that the proportion of free hormone is inversely related to the concentration of unoccupied binding sites and their binding affinity for the hormone in question. For example, the lesser affinity of TBG for T_3 results in a proportion of free T_3 (0.30 per cent) that is about ten times that of T_4.

Studies *in vitro* in which T_4 has been allowed to interact with both plasma and tissues have led to an expansion of the formulation as follows:

$$T_4 \quad \begin{matrix} + TBG \overset{k_1}{\rightleftharpoons} T_4 \cdot TBG \\[6pt] + CBP \overset{k_2}{\rightleftharpoons} T_4 \cdot CBP \overset{k_3}{\rightarrow} \end{matrix}$$

Here, CBP represents the unoccupied binding sites on cellular binding proteins; k_2, their affinity for T_4; $T_4 \cdot CBP$, occupied binding sites on CBP; and k_3, the rate of irreversible metabolism or degradation of T_4 affixed to the cell.

This formulation indicates that it is the free hormone that is available to the tissues and that can, therefore, both induce metabolic effects and undergo degradation. The bound form of the hormone then acts merely as a metabolically inert reservoir. It also follows that it should be the concentration of the free hormone that acts as an important determinant of the metabolic state and that homeostatic mechanisms would seek to defend. On the other hand, the proportion of free hormone, in determining the fraction of the total hormone that is available to the tissues, greatly influences the kinetics of hormone metabolism.

This formulation, which has come to be known as the "free thyroxine hypothesis," is better termed the "free thyroid hormone hypothesis" in view of the important metabolic role that is undoubtedly played by T_3. In addition, although the formulation attributes an important role to free T_4 and T_3 as determinants of hormone metabolism, it by no means precludes an important role for cellular factors. Indeed, the participation of cellular factors is explicitly included.

Cellular Binding Proteins. The free thyroid hormone hypothesis implies the existence within the cell or on its surface of sites with which T_4 and T_3 engage in a reversible binding interaction. The identification, isolation, and characterization of such binding proteins has received increasing attention within the recent past. Electrophoretic studies in supporting media which themselves do not interact with the hormones have revealed in the cytosol from rat and human liver the presence of two groups of binding proteins, one of which binds T_4 but not T_3, while the other binds T_3 but not T_4 (Hamada and Ingbar, unpublished observations). Apparently specific binding proteins for T_4 and T_3 have also been found in the cytosol from rat kidney, myocardium, skeletal muscle, and brain. The binding affinities and capacities of these proteins have not yet been determined. Of additional interest is the recent demonstration of the presence of apparently saturable binding sites for T_3 in the nuclei of rat liver and kidney cells. Although nuclear binding of T_4 was observed, binding sites for this hormone appeared less avid and less readily saturable (Oppenheimer et al., 1972).

Hormone Turnover

The availability of high specific activity preparations of labeled thyroid hormones has made possible studies of the metabolism of the hormones in man and experimental animals *in vivo*. (For a review of this subject with extensive references, see Oppenheimer et al., 1969, and Nicoloff et al., 1972.) Although such studies *in vivo* have several limitations, they have provided useful information concerning the overall metabolism of the hormones both in normal and in disease states. In man, with few exceptions, studies of hormone metabolism have been conducted by observing the fate of a single injection of hormone containing radioiodine only in the 3' position (Fig. 4–7). Such studies provide evidence of the overall distribution and turnover of the intact hormone molecule and of the fate of the labeled iodine atoms, but give no information concerning the metabolism of the remainder of the hormone molecule. Nevertheless, in a state of physiologic equilibrium, the quantity of hormone degraded or excreted per unit time must equal the rate of hormone secretion, which can be

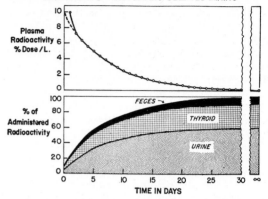

SCHEMA OF THE DISTRIBUTION & FATE OF A SINGLE DOSE OF THYROXINE-I^{131} DISPLAYING DELAYED MIXING

Figure 4–7. Fate of the radioiodine in a single intravenous injection of labeled T_4 in a normal subject. After an initial period of mixing within its distribution space, the labeled T_4 disappears from plasma at an exponential rate. Ultimately, approximately 15% of administered radioactivity appears in the feces, almost entirely in the organic form. The remainder of the hormone is deiodinated, and the labeled iodine released is apportioned between the thyroid and urine. (From Ingbar, S. H., and Freinkel, N.: *J. Clin. Invest. 34*:808, 1955.)

measured indirectly in this manner. Furthermore, in a homeostatically regulated system, the rate of hormone disposal may well determine the requisite rate of hormone manufacture. Hence considerable interest is focused upon such measurements. As judged from such studies, T_4 in the normal adult has a volume of distribution of approximately 10 liters; that is, the extrathyroidal amount of T_4 is equivalent to the quantity that would be contained in 10 liters of plasma. Since the normal concentration of T_4 in plasma approximates 8 $\mu g./100$ ml., the extrathyroidal pool of T_4 is approximately 800 μg. In the young or middle-aged adult, the fractional rate of turnover of T_4 in the periphery is normally about 10 per cent/day (half-time, 6.7 days). Thus about 1 liter of the peripheral T_4 distribution space is cleared of hormone daily, a volume that contains approximately 80 μg. of T_4. The fractional rate of turnover and rate of clearance of T_4 are much smaller than those of other hormones. The slower turnover of T_4 is doubtless a reflection of the predominant extent to which T_4 is bound, leaving only a small fraction free for metabolic turnover. If only the free T_4, which is about 1/3000 of the total, is available for metabolic turnover, then the rate of clearance of free T_4 would be at least 3000 liters/day or more than 120 liters/hr.

The foregoing values are based upon single compartmental analysis of the kinetics of labeled T_4 metabolism. This type of analysis appears to be justified in the case of a hormone whose turnover is slow, as is the case with T_4.

Of the labeled iodine present in the administered T_4, about 80 per cent is ultimately removed from the thyronine nucleus, forming iodide that is either accumulated by the thyroid or excreted in the urine. Recent evidence discussed more fully below indicates that approximately half of the T_4 metabolized in this way (about 40 per cent of the total) gives rise to T_3, which is then further metabolized. The remaining 20 per cent of T_4-radioiodine is lost in the stool in organic form. This portion arises mainly from excretion of T_4 into the bile, where it appears both in the free form and as a conjugate of glucuronic acid with the phenolic hydroxyl group. Since it has been estimated that in man as much as one-third of the removal of T_4 from the plasma occurs via biliary excretion, a portion (one-third to one-half) of the biliary content of T_4 and its metabolites must undergo reabsorption. In the rat, biliary excretion of T_4 is more active than in man, and a more extensive enterohepatic circulation apparently exists, especially when the concentration of T_4 in the plasma is increased. In man, by contrast, the relative contributions to T_4 disposal of deiodination and fecal excretion are not appreciably altered by the increases in circulating T_4 that occur in the thyrotoxic state.

The kinetics of T_3 metabolism differ markedly from those of T_4, owing in part to differences in intensity of their binding to TBG. A single dose of labeled T_3 is rapidly cleared from the plasma as a result of both widespread distribution and rapid cellular degradation. As judged from single compartmental analysis, the volume of distribution of T_3 in the normal adult is about 40 liters and its fractional rate of turnover about 60 per cent/day. Hence the total daily clearance rate is about 24 liters. As with T_4, about 80 per cent of the administered T_3 is ultimately deiodinated, the remaining 20 per cent appearing in the bile as conjugates with glucuronate and sulfate. In the hands of some but not all investigators, noncompartmental analysis yields similar results with respect to the clearance rate in normal adults (see Nicoloff et al., 1972, and Surks et al., 1973). Some uncertainty exists concerning the magnitude of the extrathyroidal T_3 pool and the absolute rate of disposal therefrom, owing to uncertainty concerning the precise range of the normal serum T_3 concentration. However, if as seems likely the mean normal serum T_3 concentration is approximately 120 ng./100 ml., then the normal pool would contain approximately 48 μg. of T_3, and the daily disposal rate would be about 30 μg. daily.

From the foregoing values, it is seen that T_4 is to a large extent an extracellular rather than intracellular hormone, while the converse is true for T_3. This difference cannot reside solely in the difference in their extracellular binding, since there are also differences in their relative tissue distributions. Thus, in the case of T_4, the exchangeable hepatic distribution volume can comprise as much as 30 per cent of the total, while in the case of T_3, the hepatic component is relatively smaller and the renal component relatively greater.

Pathways of Hormone Metabolism

Except for a search for specific metabolites of T_4 and T_3, studies in man do not lend themselves to an elucidation of the mechanisms and pathways for thyroid hormone metabolism. Such studies are best conducted either in whole animals or in excised tissues therefrom. Nevertheless, findings of exceptional importance to an understanding of normal and disordered thyroid hormone economy have emerged from studies conducted in man. Principal among these is the recent demonstration that the major source of T_3 in the peripheral tissues of man is not direct secretion from the thyroid but generation through the peripheral deiodination of T_4. Long-standing speculation as to whether T_4 gives rise to T_3 during its peripheral metabolism was laid to rest by the demonstration that athyreotic patients given a mixture of highly purified stable and radioiodine-labeled T_4 as replacement therapy displayed in their serum substantial quantities of stable and labeled T_3 (Braverman et al., 1970). Subsequent studies by more complex techniques which permit calculation of the fractional rate of conversion of T_4 to T_3 and the absolute quantity of T_3 derived therefrom have fully confirmed this finding and have indicated that a minimum of about 40 per cent of T_4 is metabolized via monodeiodination to T_3 (Surks et al., 1973). The tissues in which T_4 to T_3 conversion takes place *in vivo* are unknown; however, generation of T_3 from T_4 in vitro has been demonstrated in human fibroblasts, in liver and kidney cells in culture, and in freshly isolated human leukocytes.

Several important concepts have emerged from these findings. First, when allowance is made for the daily disposal of T_4, its fractional conversion to T_3, and the smaller molecular weight of T_3 relative to T_4, it can be calculated that approximately 27 μg. of T_3 are produced daily from T_4. This value is only slightly less than the total daily production and disposal rate for T_3 described above. This indicates that only a small proportion at most of T_3 is normally secreted by the thyroid. The implication that a high T_4:T_3 ratio is the normal pattern of thyroid secretion is in accord with recently refined analyses of normal thyroid tissue which reveal an unexpectedly high T_4:T_3 ratio (Chopra et al., 1973).

Second, the large proportion of T_4 metabolized to T_3, together with a 2–3 times greater biologic potency of T_3, has led to the suggestion that virtually all of the metabolic action of T_4 is derived from the T_3 generated therefrom. Viewed in this light, T_4 need have no intrinsic biologic activity but would merely serve as a stable prohormone for the evanescent, physiologically active metabolite, T_3. Consonant with this concept are observations that agents, such as the thiouracils, which partly inhibit the deiodination of T_4 and its conversion to T_3, also diminish the metabolic potency of T_4. Such observations do not provide a crucial test of this hypothesis, however. They reveal only that T_4 gains potency through its conversion to T_3 and do not indicate whether T_4 has intrinsic, though lesser, biologic activity. This question remains open, and its answer is being actively pursued.

A third outgrowth of the observation that virtually all T_3 normally arises in the periphery from T_4 is the conclusion that adequate maintenance therapy of the hypothyroid patient does not require either administration of both hormones or provision of T_4 in quantities substantially greater than those normally secreted. This is discussed further in the section concerning the treatment of hypothyroidism.

The experiments that have demonstrated the peripheral conversion of T_4 to T_3 have also revealed that tetrac is a normal metabolite of T_4 in man. Similar findings have been made in animals.

Studies in man using T_4 labeled either with radioiodine in the inner ring or with C^{14} have revealed rates of disappearance from plasma that are similar to those of T_4 containing radioiodine in the outer or phenolic ring. Such findings suggest, first, that neither ring is preferentially deiodinated and, second, that significant quantities of long-lived products are not generated. After complete deiodination of T_4, the resulting excretory products retain the ether link of the original thyronine nucleus intact (Surks and Oppenheimer, 1971).

Studies of the products of the deiodination of T_3 in man are much more difficult to perform in view of its much faster rate of metabolism relative to T_4. The major product that has been identified is an iodoprotein that is manufactured peripherally, that appears in the plasma, and that, by electrophoretic analysis, resembles serum albumin. The turnover rate of the iodoprotein is much slower than that of T_3, with the result that after a single injection of labeled T_3 the iodoprotein becomes an increasingly prominent component of the plasma radioactivity with the passage of time. Nevertheless, the proportion of the administered radioiodine that appears in the plasma as iodoprotein is exceedingly small. As would be expected, the iodoprotein is insoluble in organic solvents, and hence the iodine contained therein is referred to as nonextractable iodine or NEI.

The foregoing discussion has been concerned with the fate of the approximately 80 per cent of T_4 and T_3 that is metabolized via deiodinative pathways. The remaining 20 per cent of both hormones ultimately appears in the stool as either free hormone or conjugates with glucuronate or sulfate. Sulfoconjugation is a particularly prominent mechanism in the case of T_3.

Studies of thyroid hormone metabolism in animals or *in vitro* have complemented findings obtained in man. In the rat as in man, T_3 is generated peripherally from T_4, and an iodoprotein appears in plasma as a product of deiodination. In addition, studies in the living rat suggest that removal of iodine atoms from T_4 occurs in random order. On the other hand, in rat and dog liver, iodines in the outer ring of T_4 are apparently removed more readily than those in the inner ring. Organ-related differences may occur, however, since, in the intact dog, iodines in the inner ring are apparently removed more rapidly than those in the outer ring. These observations suggest that deiodination may not be the result of a truly random process. The question is one of extreme importance with regard to the mechanism of T_3 generation from T_4. If deiodination is truly random, then the proportion of all T_4 undergoing deiodination that is metabo-

lized via T_3 must be fixed at 50 per cent, regardless of the operation of factors that change the overall rate of deiodination. If, however, deiodination is not random, then the possibility emerges that the generation of T_3 from T_4 is a specific process that undergoes a specific change in rate during various physiologic states.

Studies of the metabolism of T_4 and T_3 in the rat have revealed the formation of tissue iodoproteins whose rate of formation is proportional to the rate of hormone deiodination. In liver, they are found predominantly in the microsomal fraction, which is the site of greatest deiodinative activity. Hydrolysis of iodoproteins yields iodide, iodotyrosine, and, most interestingly, the original iodothyronine studied. Generally similar iodoproteins are formed *in vitro* during deiodination of T_4 by all tissues studied. The physiologic significance of tissue iodoproteins arising during the metabolism of T_4 and T_3 is unknown.

The capacity to deiodinate T_4 and probably T_3 is a property of all tissues studied *in vitro* to date. In most, the greatest deiodinative activity is found in the microsomal fraction. However, no specific deiodinase for T_4 or T_3 has been isolated. Indeed, tissue preparations *in vitro* in which deiodination of thyroid hormones has been studied have exhibited peculiar properties, including activation by short periods of boiling. This may indicate that deiodination in such systems is a mixture of enzymic deiodination and direct chemical deiodination, the latter perhaps representing a technical artifact. There is considerable evidence that deiodination is an oxidative process, possibly mediated by tissue peroxidases and inhibited by catalase. Teleologically, this is an attractive hypothesis, since the degradation of thyroid hormones would thereby be linked to oxidative processes in the cell. The possibility is intriguing that enzymes similar to those which mediate iodinations in the thyroid also catalyze hormonal deiodination in the periphery.

Alterations in the Transport, Turnover, and Metabolism of the Thyroid Hormones

The free thyroid hormone hypothesis assigns to the concentration of free hormone a role as a major determinant of the quantity of hormone available to the cells and, hence, the absolute rate of hormone turnover and the metabolic state of the patient. It assigns to the proportion of free hormone a role as a major determinant of the proportionate distribution and metabolism of hormone. In addition, the hypothesis encompasses the operation of cellular factors that may influence the distribution, effectiveness, and metabolism of the hormone, independently of alterations in extracellular binding. Studies in man have disclosed the existence and consequences of abnormalities in both these major aspects of hormone metabolism.

Extracellular Abnormalities. Abnormalities in the interaction between the thyroid hormones and their binding proteins, predominantly TBG, are of two types: those that result primarily from a change in the number or affinity of available bind-

SCHEMA OF THE CONSEQUENCES OF A PRIMARY
INCREASE IN THE BINDING ACTIVITY OF TBG

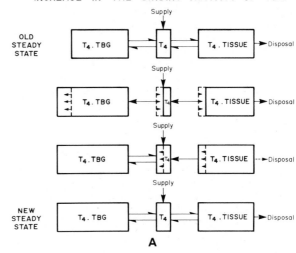

SCHEMA OF THE CONSEQUENCES OF A PRIMARY
DECREASE IN THE BINDING ACTIVITY OF TBG

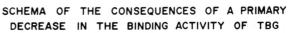

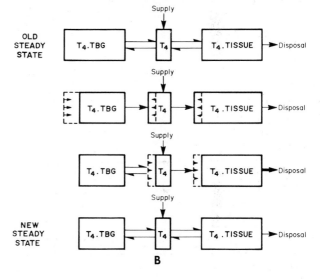

Figure 4–8. $T_4 \cdot TBG$ and T_4 indicate concentrations in plasma of bound and free T_4, respectively. $T_4 \cdot$ tissue indicates the concentration of exchangeable T_4 within the cellular compartment. Increases (*A*) or decreases (*B*) in TBG are associated with the following consequences when a new steady state is attained: normal concentration of free T_4 in plasma; normal concentration of T_4 in the cellular compartment; normal rate of disposal, equal to supply; and, respectively, increased or decreased concentration of bound hormone in plasma.

ing sites, and those that result primarily from a change in the concentration of the hormone. The static, kinetic, and physiologic consequences of these two types of change differ greatly from one another.

These differences can best be appreciated by considering the sequential perturbations that follow abnormalities of each type (Fig. 4–8). If, for example, some factor were to increase the concentration in plasma of TBG, the number of unoccupied binding sites would increase, resulting initially in a shift of hormone from the free to the bound state and a decrease in the quantity of hormone removed from the plasma. With a normal or perhaps increased influx of T_4 into the plasma, the total concentration of hormone would increase progressively until such time as the concentration of free hormone and, as a result, the absolute rate of hormone turnover are restored to their initial values. At this time, the total and bound concentrations of

hormone, which are numerically almost equal, would be increased; hence, the proportion of free hormone would be decreased, and this would be reflected *in vivo* in a decreased volume of distribution and fractional turnover rate of the hormone in plasma. This sequence is almost precisely that which has been observed for both T_4 and T_3 in a variety of states associated with an increased TBG in plasma. The converse consequences would be predicted and have been observed in states associated with decreased TBG (see Table 4–3 and section on laboratory tests for a description of the circumstances in which TBG is altered).

Thus it can be seen that, although primary alterations in TBG alter the total concentration of hormone in plasma and its kinetics of metabolism, they do not ultimately influence the absolute quantity of hormone that enters the cell, acts, and is degraded in unit time. Therefore, they do not influence the total turnover of hormone or the metabolic state of the patient. These remain a function of the rate of hormone production or supply, and when homeostatic mechanisms are normal, hormone production and the metabolic state of the patient will be normal too.

Far different consequences follow a primary alteration in the rate of hormone supply. For example, in hyperthyroid states, hypersecretion of hormone leads to an increase in total hormone concentration. As a result, the concentration of unoccupied binding sites on TBG decreases, and the concentrations of both free and bound hormone rise. As a consequence of the fixed quantity of TBG available, the mass action expression dictates that the concentration of free hormone would increase to a disproportionately great extent and that the proportion of free hormone would therefore rise. *In vivo,* these changes would be reflected in increased fractional and absolute rates of hormone turnover, and in a hypermetabolic state. Converse con-

sequences occur when the supply of hormone is decreased as in hypothyroidism. Here, as in the case of primary alterations in hormone binding, the flux of hormone to the tissues and the metabolic state of the patient are again determined by the rate of hormone production. In the final analysis, therefore, barring metabolically wasteful loss of hormone, the metabolic state of the patient is determined by the rate of hormone production. The effect of alterations in binding is merely to change the concentration, partition, and clearance rate of the hormone for a given rate of hormone production.

Cellular Abnormalities. As predicted by the free thyroid hormone hypothesis, factors intrinsic to the cell may, in certain circumstances, play a primary role in mediating alterations in the distribution and metabolism of the thyroid hormones and their concentrations in the blood (Fig. 4–9). This was first demonstrated in the case of pheno-

SCHEMA OF THE CONSEQUENCES OF A PRIMARY INCREASE IN TISSUE BINDING

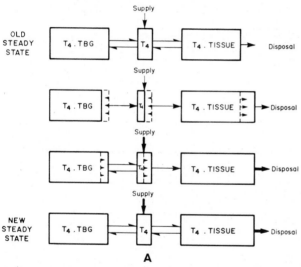

A

SCHEMA OF THE CONSEQUENCES OF A PRIMARY DECREASE IN TISSUE BINDING

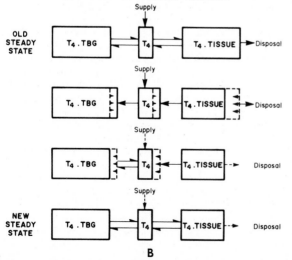

B

Figure 4–9. $T_4 \cdot$TBG and T_4 indicate concentrations in plasma of bound and free T_4, respectively. $T_4 \cdot$ tissue indicates the concentration of exchangeable T_4 within the cellular compartment. Increases (*A*) or decreases (*B*) in tissue binding are associated with the following consequences when a new steady state is attained: normal bound and free T_4 concentrations in plasma; and increased or decreased exchangeable cellular T_4 and T_4 disposal rate, with hormone supply adjusted to equal disposal. The conditions depicted in *A* resemble those induced by phenobarbital.

barbital, an agent known to induce hypertrophy of the smooth endoplasmic reticulum (Oppenheimer et al., 1971). In rats, phenobarbital produces an increase in the liver:plasma concentration ratio for T_4 but not for T_3. The peripheral clearance of the two hormones is increased, that for T_4 resulting from an increase in both fecal and deiodinative removal, and that for T_3 from an increase in the fecal component alone. Despite these losses of T_4, its concentration in plasma is maintained as a result of compensatory hyperfunction of the thyroid. These changes occur without a net change in extracellular hormone binding, indicating that they are cellular in origin. The foregoing response to phenobarbital typifies the effect of an increase in the cellular disposal of T_4 in which disposal is not associated with metabolic action and in which the pituitary and hypothalamus do not appear to be primarily affected.

Diphenylhydantoin, like phenobarbital, accelerates the peripheral metabolism of T_4, an effect that is demonstrable both in the rat and in man. Here, too, the effect cannot be ascribed to an alteration in the extracellular binding of hormone. Indeed, the concentration of total and free T_4 are subnormal, while the total disposal of hormone (and TSH secretion as well as thyroid function) remains unchanged. Kinetic studies indicate that diphenylhydantoin accelerates the peripheral generation of T_3 from T_4 and increases the concentration of free T_3, and that this may be responsible for the maintenance of normal pituitary and thyroid function despite the low serum T_4 concentration (Cullen et al., 1972). The findings in the case of diphenylhydantoin exemplify a situation in which cellular factors lower the serum concentration of T_4 without eliciting a pituitary response because of diversion of T_4 disposal into metabolically more efficient pathways.

A number of other circumstances in man are associated with alterations in peripheral hormone metabolism that are apparently primary within the cell. In patients with Graves' disease, accelerated fractional turnover rates of T_4 and T_3 have been demonstrated long after a eumetabolic state has been restored by treatment. With advancing age, both fractional turnover and absolute disposal rates for T_4 progressively decline (Oddie et al., 1966). Similarly, the decreasing concentration of T_3 in serum in the presence of unchanged serum T_4 concentration suggests a decreasing fractional conversion of T_4 to T_3 with advancing age (Brunelle and Bohuon, 1972). In none of the foregoing circumstances are alterations in the extracellular binding of hormone demonstrable.

REGULATION OF THYROID FUNCTION

In common with other endocrine organs, the function of the thyroid gland is closely regulated in order that constancy of the internal metabolic milieu be maintained. Regulation of the thyroid, however, seems more complex and more extensive

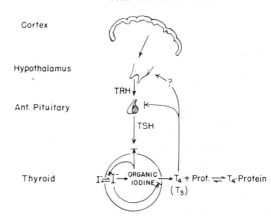

Figure 4–10. Diagram of the factors that regulate thyroid function. Thyroid hormones (T_4 and T_3) in the pituitary, as reflected by their unbound concentrations in blood, inhibit secretion of thyroid stimulating hormone (TSH). The TSH releasing hormone (TRH) sets the threshold in the pituitary at which this negative feedback occurs. Factors regulating the secretion of TRH are uncertain but may include influences from higher centers and a stimulatory effect of the thyroid hormones. Autoregulatory control of thyroid function is also shown. High concentrations of intrathyroid iodide decrease the rate of release of thyroid iodine. In addition, the magnitude of the organic iodine pool inversely influences the iodide transport mechanism and the response to TSH.

than that of other endocrine organs. Figure 4–10 is a schema of regulatory mechanisms affecting the thyroid as currently conceived. Like the gonads and adrenal cortices, the thyroid participates with the hypothalamus and pituitary in a classic type of feedback control. In addition, intrinsic regulatory mechanisms exist within the thyroid that create an inverse relationship between glandular organic iodine and the activity of hormonogenetic mechanisms. Such autoregulatory mechanisms are apparently found in no other endocrine gland. Teleologically, they subserve an important purpose, for in the case of no other endocrine gland is the rate of hormone synthesis potentially so susceptible to acute fluctuations in the availability of a requisite substrate such as iodine. Furthermore, relative to other hormones with effects on metabolic processes (e.g., insulin, glucocorticoids, parathyroid hormone), the effects of thyroid hormones, although less dramatic, are much longer lasting. Hence, it is homeostatically important that fluctuation in hormone secretion be prevented, if possible, rather than merely compensated for after it has occurred. This is achieved in part by the storage function of the gland. A large intraglandular store of hormone that buffers the effect of acute increases or decreases in hormone synthesis can thus be maintained. Autoregulatory mechanisms within the gland, in turn, tend to maintain the constancy of the thyroid hormone pool. Finally, the classic feedback mechanism senses variations in the availability of thyroid hormones and their metabolic impact at the periphery; it is generally concerned, therefore, with correcting abnormalities in the effective concentration of thyroid hormones in the blood, however small, once they have occurred.

The Hypothalamic-Pituitary-Thyroid Complex

A large body of anatomical and physiologic evidence has over the years indicated the existence of a close functional relationship between the thyroid and the pituitary. More recently, the classical concept of an independent pituitary-thyroid axis has been modified to accommodate evidence of a similar nature with respect to the hypothalamus, leading to the concept of a hypothalamic-pituitary-thyroid complex. (See Ch. 12 and review by Reichlin et al., 1972.) Inferential evidence for the secretion by the pituitary of a thyroid stimulator and for the secretion by the hypothalamus of a pituitary stimulator has culminated in the isolation in pure form of the postulated stimulators, i.e., thyroid stimulating hormone (TSH) and TSH releasing hormone (TRH), respectively. Moreover, an understanding of the evident feedback influence of the thyroid hormones on the pituitary and hypothalamus at both the physiologic and molecular levels is being approached.

It has long been known that the pituitary exerts a stimulatory influence on the thyroid. Removal of the pituitary leads to thyroid atrophy, diminished thyroid blood flow, and decreased function. Concentrations of thyroid hormone in the blood decline. Conversely, extracts of pituitary produce thyroid growth, hypervascularity, and increased function. Moreover, the administration of antithyroid agents leads to the development of thyroid enlargement (goiter) in the intact animal, but not when the pituitary has been removed. Similarly, a variety of observations has indicated a reciprocal effect of the thyroid hormones upon the pituitary. Removal of the thyroid or functional failure is accompanied by an increase in pituitary size and weight and by the appearance in the anterior pituitary of large numbers of finely granulated, PAS-positive "thyroidectomy" cells. These changes are reversed by the administration of thyroid hormone. In long-standing hypothyroidism in man, pituitary growth may be sufficient to cause enlargement of the pituitary fossa with compression of adjacent structures similar to that which occurs with tumors of the pituitary. Thyroidectomy or the imposition of factors that restrict thyroid function results in increased concentrations of bioassayable and, more recently, radioimmunoassayable TSH in plasma.

Evidence for a role of the hypothalamus derives from experiments involving stimulation or ablation of specific areas within the hypothalamus. Electrical stimulation of the anterior hypothalamus activates the pituitary thyrotropic cells, increases the plasma TSH concentration, and leads to functional and histologic evidence of thyroid activation. Conversely, destructive lesions in the anterior hypothalamus or section of the pituitary stalk result in decreased thyroid activity. Subsequent to these observations, hypothalamic extracts of increasing potency were prepared that in remarkably small quantities had the capability of causing the release of TSH from the pituitary both *in vitro* and *in vivo*.

Although these findings indicate that the hypothalamus exerts a stimulatory influence on TSH secretion, there is substantial evidence that the feedback influence of the thyroid hormones on TSH secretion is exerted mainly within the pituitary itself rather than via the hypothalamus. For example, direct instillation of systemically ineffective quantities of T_4 into the pituitary inhibits thyroid function, and implantation of thyroid tissue into the pituitary results in atrophy of the pituitary thyrotropic cells. Furthermore, TSH secretion can be either inhibited by excess of thyroid hormone or enhanced by deficiency of thyroid hormone, even when the pituitary is separated from its hypothalamic connections or when the hypothalamic areas that appear to influence TSH secretion are destroyed. Finally, the thyroid hypofunction that results from the destruction of such hypothalamic areas is less severe than that which results from hypophysectomy, and the degree of residual function in the former circumstance can be varied by raising or lowering the concentration of thyroid hormone in the blood. These observations indicate that the hypothalamus exerts a modulating influence on TSH secretion, even though it is not the ultimate arbiter of feedback control.

A deeper understanding of these complex interactions is emerging as a result of the availability of chemically synthesized TRH and of sensitive and specific assays for the measurement of TSH in plasma. The monumental contributions of Guillemin, Burgus, Schally, Bowers, and their respective co-workers led to the identification of the hypothalamic TSH-releasing principle as a tripeptide amide, pyroglutamyl-histidyl-prolinamide. TRH is capable of stimulating the synthesis of TSH and its release from the pituitary. It is effective both *in vivo* and, when incubated with pituitary tissue, *in vitro*. Even when administered systemically by intravenous injection, it is remarkably effective; as little as 1 ng. in the mouse and 6 μg. in man is capable of eliciting an increase in plasma TSH concentration. The action of TRH on the pituitary may be mediated by an adenylate cyclase–cyclic AMP system, since TRH increases the pituitary content of cyclic AMP, and the latter compound is capable of reproducing the TSH-releasing effect of TRH. The response to TRH requires Ca^{2+} and oxidative metabolism within the pituitary but not new protein synthesis. TRH is rapidly removed from the plasma, owing in part to renal excretion and in part to rapid degradation within the plasma itself.

The most remarkable feature of the action of TRH is its susceptibility to inhibition by T_4 or T_3, either administered *in vivo* or added *in vitro* to pituitary explants, but this inhibition can be overcome by increasing the dose of TRH. Consonant with the action of thyroid hormones to enhance protein synthesis in other tissues is the finding that the inhibitory effect of T_4 and T_3 on the response to TRH is abolished by inhibitors of protein synthesis. The counterpart of these effects is evident in man and forms the basis for TRH testing, in which excess of thyroid hormone diminishes and deficiency enhances the pituitary response to TRH (see section on laboratory tests). The poise of the pituitary between normal responsiveness and diminished responsiveness is exquisitely balanced, since very small doses of thyroid hormone, sufficient only to produce barely detectable changes in plasma concentration, greatly diminish the response to exogenous TRH.

The foregoing observations provide a firm basis for the earlier hypothesis that feedback control of thyroid function is exerted at the level of the pituitary and that the hypothalamus, presumably through secretion of TRH, determines the set-point of the feedback threshold. A further complexity in the hypothalamic regulation of the pituitary-thyroid axis arises from the fact that a hypothalamic enzyme system that is capable of synthesizing TRH from precursor amino acids (TRH synthetase) is more active than normal in tissue from T_4-treated animals and less active in tissue from their hypothyroid counterparts. These findings suggest a positive feedback of thyroid hormone on TRH synthesis to accompany the negative feedback on the pituitary TRH response.

The highly specific effect of the thyroid hormones on the pituitary response to TRH makes this a desirable system in which to study the more general question of the nature of the active thyroid hormone. Although demonstrated in other tissues, monodeiodination of T_4 to yield T_3 is most readily demonstrable in the pituitary. The question arises, therefore, whether T_4 must undergo deiodination to T_3 within the pituitary in order to effect its inhibition of the TRH response. Some data bearing upon this question have been obtained. Propylthiouracil has been shown to inhibit both the peripheral deiodination of T_4 and the general metabolic response to this hormone, though not to T_3. It is of interest, therefore, that minute doses of propylthiouracil in the rat induce an acute increase in plasma TSH and the release of radioiodine from the thyroid. In addition, small doses of propylthiouracil diminish the inhibitory effect of T_4 on the pituitary response to TRH. These observations are consonant with the conclusion that T_3 is the major form in which the thyroid hormones are effective within the pituitary. They do not, however, exclude the possibility that T_4 itself has an independent action.

A final fascinating aspect of the action of TRH is the fact that, in addition to causing the release of TSH from the pituitary, it also stimulates the secretion of prolactin. Moreover, this effect is modulated by the state of thyroid function in a manner analogous to the effect of TRH on the release of TSH. The functional significance of this response, as well as its biochemical basis, is unknown. In some patients with acromegaly, TRH stimulates the release of growth hormone, an effect that is not apparent in the normal pituitary gland.

Thyroid Autoregulation

The pronounced changes in thyroid iodine and intermediary metabolism, size, and histology that accompany variations in the secretion of TSH suggest that TSH is the major regulator of thyroid structure and function. There is ample evidence, however, that the thyroid is the seat of a group of intrinsic responses that modify several aspects of its own function, most importantly its responsiveness to TSH. In contrast to the classical feedback control effected via TSH, which seeks to defend the plasma or tissue concentrations of the thyroid hormones, these so-called autoregulatory mechanisms seek to maintain constancy of thyroid hormone stores. They are, therefore, most clearly evident in situations in which thyroid iodine content is varied by changes in iodine ingestion or by abnormalities in thyroid iodine utilization. Moreover, the induction of severe intrathyroidal iodine deficiency by low-iodine regimens combined with propylthiouracil greatly sensitizes the thyroid of the hypophysectomized rat to the growth-stimulating effect of a wide range of TSH doses. The intermediary metabolism of the thyroid is also subject to autoregulatory influences, since variations in the organic iodine content of the thyroid in hypophysectomized rats are associated with inverse changes in the rate of glucose dissimilation and incorporation of glucose into CO_2, lactate, lipid, and nucleic acid.

The actual extent to which these autoregulatory responses are operative in diverse states of thyroid function is uncertain. Nevertheless, it appears likely that their participation as a first line of defense of thyroid homeostasis is extensive. In man, increases in iodine ingestion are not accompanied by either increased serum hormone or decreased TSH concentrations. Hence, the decreased efficiency of thyroid iodide extraction manifested in the lowered I^{131} uptake that follows excessive iodine ingestion is doubtless mediated by autoregulatory inhibition of iodide transport. Conversely, acute iodide depletion is associated with an enhanced autoregulatory response. In the iodine-deficient rat, goiter development antecedes any demonstrable increase in serum TSH concentration. Similarly, in both sporadic nontoxic goiter and the goiter associated with moderate iodine deficiency, serum TSH concentration is usually normal. Such findings support the logical hypothesis that, by enhancing the morphologic and functional response to TSH, autoregulatory mechanisms are a major factor in the ability of the thyroid to overcome the influence of factors that impair hormone synthesis.

Operationally, autoregulatory responses are those that are demonstrable when the level of TSH is constant, i.e., when TSH either is totally lacking or is provided in standard quantities. Although a variety of intrathyroidal processes are influenced by iodine (see section on the pharmacology of iodine), the classic type of autoregulatory response is that which affects the activity of the thyroid iodide transport mechanism, as judged from both thyroid/serum iodide concentration ratios and iodide transport maxima. In the hypophysectomized rat, regardless of whether standard doses of TSH are administered, variations in the dietary iodine intake are associated with inverse changes in iodide transport activity. However, the inhibition of iodide transport induced by supplemental iodine, whether given chronically or acutely, is abolished if administred iodide is prevented from binding to tyrosine by concomitant administration of propylthiouracil. This and other evidence indicates that it is organic rather than inorganic iodine that exerts an autoregulatory influence on iodide transport. Although an iodinated inhibitor of iodide transport has been postulated as the responsible agent, no such inhibitor has been specifically demonstrated.

The organic iodine content of the thyroid also influences glandular morphology. Thyroids of hypophysectomized rats subjected to prolonged iodine deficiency are larger than those of iodine-sufficient hypophysectomized controls. Moreover, in hypophysectomized rats, depletion of thyroid iodine greatly increases the growth response of the thyroid to standard doses of TSH (Bray, 1968). (For a more extensive discussion of autoregulation, see Ingbar, 1972.)

FACTORS THAT INFLUENCE THYROID HORMONE ECONOMY

The widespread metabolic role of the thyroid hormones, the diverse processes involved in the synthesis and secretion of the hormones, and the complex mode of regulation of thyroid function suggest that a great many factors could influence one or more aspects of thyroid hormone economy. This is indeed the case. In general, the factors can be considered in the following categories: endogenous variables, pharmacologic agents, environmental alterations, and dysfunction or diseases of other organ systems.

Thyrotropin (Thyroid Stimulating Hormone, TSH)

In many respects, TSH can be considered the major regulator of the anatomical and functional state of the thyroid. Removal of TSH stimulation is followed by decreased synthesis and secretion of hormone, hypovascularity, and atrophy, whereas converse effects are produced by stimulatory doses of TSH. As indicated earlier, it is not certain that all adjustments in thyroid function in response to a variety of stimuli are mediated by changes in the rate of TSH secretion. Intrinsic autoregulatory mechanisms may be the first sensors of changes in the rate of hormone synthesis and may respond appropriately to alter thyroid sensitivity to constant degrees of TSH stimulation. If this response is inadequate to maintain continued secretion of requisite quantities of hormone, modification of the rate of TSH secretion follows.

TSH is a glycopeptide secreted by the adenohypophysis and is probably present in all vertebrates. Highly purified preparations have been obtained from a number of mammalian species, including man. TSH has a molecular weight of approximately 28,000 and is a polypeptide containing approximately 15% carbohydrate. The most highly purified preparations available have been found to be heterogeneous with regard to electrophoretic and chromatographic behavior, but the chemical composition and specific hormonal activity of the several fractions are similar. The potency of highly purified preparations of TSH can be as high as 70 I.U./mg. Although the human thyroid is capable of response to bovine and ovine TSH, essentially no immunologic reaction occurs between these preparations and antisera against human TSH. Hence, the antigenic and physiologic determinants of the TSH molecule are distinct from each other.

Recent studies of the structure and composition of TSH and other glycopeptide hormones, carried out principally in Pierce's laboratory (1971a, 1971b), have provided further information concerning their structure. TSH, as well as luteinizing hormone (LH) and human chorionic gonadotropin (hCG), can be dissociated by propionic acid into two subunits, the α and β subunits. Studies with bovine hormone indicate that the α subunits of TSH and LH are identical in amino acid sequence, or nearly so, and the same can be said of the α subunits of human TSH, LH, and hCG. Greater differences are evident in the composition of the specific β subunits of these hormones, though strong similarities nevertheless exist. The physiologic activity of the isolated subunits is negligible, but activity can be restored by recombination of corresponding specific subunits. Of even greater interest is the observation, based largely on experiments with bovine TSH and LH and hCG, that recombination of α subunits of any of the hormones with a specific β subunit yields physiologic activity corresponding to that of the parent hormone of the β subunit. Immunologic specificity, like physiologic activity, appears to reside in the β subunits. Similar relationships appear to apply in the case of ovine follicle stimulating hormone (FSH). These studies afford a fascinating insight into structure-function relationships among the glycopeptide hormones. Further, they raise the possibility that certain disturbances of function may result from abnormalities in the synthesis or secretion of particular subunits. They afford, moreover, the opportunity to explore such abnormalities by specific radioimmunoassay of the isolated subunit components.

The technique of radioimmunoassay has provided a tool for studies of the concentration and rate of secretion of TSH in normal man and of the effects of various factors that influence these functions. The major effects of TRH and the modifying influence of thyroid hormones on the response of TSH to TRH are discussed in the preceding section. The mean normal concentration of TSH in human serum is approximately 2.3 μU./ml. (Human Research Standard A). Studies with radioiodine-labeled hormone in man indicate that the half-time of TSH in plasma is normally about one hour and its volume of distribution approximately 6% of body weight. From these values, it can be calculated that the daily secretory rate of TSH is approximately 170 mU. (Odell et al., 1967). Values for plasma half-time are prolonged in hypothyroidism, but because of the usual great increase in serum concentration, secretory rates are greatly increased. In hyperthyroidism, the plasma half-time is shortened, but secretory rates are negligible since TSH cannot be detected in serum.

Although TSH is capable of inducing lipolysis *in vitro,* its major effects *in vivo* are on the structure and function of the thyroid gland. The effect of TSH on intrathyroid iodine metabolism is to enhance essentially all processes leading to the synthesis and secretion of hormone (see review by Rosenberg and Bastomsky, 1965). Abolition of TSH secretion by hypophysectomy or suppression is followed by decreased activity of the thyroid iodide transport mechanism. In addition, organic binding is inhibited, as indicated both by kinetic analysis and by an increase in the proportion of newly accumulated intrathyroid iodine present in the inorganic form. A decreased fraction of organified iodine is present as iodothyronines, indicating a decrease in the rate of coupling of iodotyrosines. In the intact animal, the fractional release of glandular I^{131} is retarded, indicating a decrease in proteolysis of thyroglobulin. Following administration of TSH, iodide transport activity is increased—under most circumstances, after a brief intitial period of inhibition. Organic-binding reactions are also enhanced, and a very prompt stimulation of the coupling reaction occurs. Proteolysis of thyroglobulin and release of glandular iodine are accelerated. Finally, the rate of iodotyrosine dehalogenation is increased, possibly because of increased availability of NADPH, rather than an increase in concentration of the enzyme. Clinically, the effects of TSH on iodine metabolism are evident in increased thyroid I^{131} uptake and thyroid iodide clearance rate, an increase in the rate of release of glandular I^{131}, and an increase in serum T_4 and T_3 concentrations. When the thyroid is responsive, BMR is increased within a few hours after administration of TSH, an effect that may reflect the increased secretion of T_3.

In view of suggestive evidence that the several stages in thyroid hormone synthesis may be closely linked to or dependent upon thyroid energy metabolism, considerable interest has centered upon the effects of TSH on glandular intermediary metabolism. In brief, TSH stimulates thyroid oxygen consumption, glucose assimilation, and glucose oxidation via the hexose monophosphate shunt and glycolytic and tricarboxylic acid cycles. As a consequence, production of carbon dioxide and lactate from exogenous glucose is increased. Oxygen consumption and carbon dioxide production are increased by TSH in the absence of exogenous glucose, indicating increased oxidation of endogenous substrate. TSH acutely increases the total thyroid content of NADP and also increases the $NADP^+/NADPH$ ratio. TSH also has a pronounced and rapid effect on phospholipid metabolism. Accelerated turnover of thyroid phospholipids is evident, particularly among the phosphomonoinosi-

tides, changes in phosphatidic acid and phosphatidyl serine being less prominent. Incorporation of glucose and glycerol carbon into thyroid phospholipids is also accelerated. The glandular concentration of inorganic phosphate is increased by TSH, reflecting hydrolysis of organic phosphates. This may serve as a stimulus to oxidative metabolism. TSH stimulates the synthesis of purine and pyrimidine precursors and their incorporation into nucleic acids. Uptake of α-aminoisobutyrate by thyroid cells is enhanced by TSH, and leucine incorporation is accelerated in the thyroid of rats given TSH. Thus TSH stimulates both catabolic and anabolic processes in the thyroid, the former presumably supplying energy requisite for the latter.

The mechanism(s) whereby TSH produces the foregoing effects on thyroid iodine and intermediary metabolism has long been sought. It appears, however, that the effects of TSH on the thyroid can be explained in large measure at least by mediation through the ubiquitous second messenger, cyclic AMP. Activation of the thyroid by TSH requires binding of the hormone to the plasma membrane of the thyroid cell, the presumed locus of adenylate cyclase. Both *in vivo* and *in vitro,* TSH promptly stimulates thyroid adenylate cyclase activity and increases the concentration of cyclic AMP. The presumed effectors of the cyclic AMP response, i.e., protein kinases, are present in thyroid tissue. Finally, under appropriate conditions of study, virtually all effects of TSH on thyroid iodine and intermediary metabolism that have been examined can be reproduced by cyclic AMP or its dibutyryl derivative. All of the foregoing provide compelling evidence that cyclic AMP is the mediator of TSH action. Recent studies indicate that prostaglandins are in some way involved in the action of TSH, but their role is as yet uncertain. The vast literature that has rapidly accumulated in this field has been comprehensively reviewed by Dumont (1971).

Iodine

In addition to its role as a requisite substrate for thyroid hormone biosynthesis, iodine participates in a number of clinically important interactions with the thyroid. Elucidation of the nature and mechanism of these interactions has for some years constituted a fascinating avenue of clinical and physiologic exploration. (See Ingbar, 1972, for a more extensive consideration of the various effects of iodine on the thyroid.)

Effects on Thyroid Hormone Synthesis

The effect of iodine on the rate of thyroid hormone synthesis depends on the amount and duration of iodine administration. When administered acutely, small to moderate amounts of stable iodine do not influence the percentage of thyroid uptake of concomitantly administered I^{131}. In addition, direct analysis reveals little change in the fraction of accumulated iodine that has undergone organification or in the proportions of the several iodinated amino acids formed. Hence these small acute doses result in an increased rate of thyroid hormone synthesis, at least for a time.

With progressively larger acute doses of iodide, more complex consequences result. The quantity of iodine that undergoes organification displays a biphasic response to increasing doses of iodide, at first increasing, then declining as a result of at least a relative blockade of organic binding. This decreasing yield of organic iodine from increasing doses of iodide is termed the acute Wolff-Chaikoff effect. The mechanism of the acute effect is uncertain, but it has been shown that this effect depends upon the establishment within the thyroid of a sufficiently high concentration of inorganic iodide. Under these conditions, the reactive form of iodine generated by oxidative mechanisms may complex with iodide, perhaps to form iodine itself (I_2), which is relatively inefficient in iodinating tyrosine. In common with other situations in which the proportionate rate of organic binding is decreased, as when propylthiouracil is administered, qualitative changes in hormone synthesis also occur. Of that iodine that is bound to organic compounds, little if any is incorporated into T_4 and T_3, a subnormal proportion appears as DIT, and MIT becomes the major product formed. It is unlikely that organic-iodinations are completely inhibited during the acute Wolff-Chaikoff effect, but from chromatographic evidence it appears that synthesis of the hormonally active iodothyronines is abolished. Thus the thyroid rejects both quantitatively and qualitatively the large quantity of iodide acutely administered, and the massive increase in thyroid hormone formation that would otherwise occur is prevented.

In man, induction of at least a partial blockade of organic binding by an acute dose of iodide is what is responsible for the iodide discharged from the thyroid during the iodide-perchlorate discharge test. In normal man, somewhat more than 2 mg. of iodide must be given acutely in order to induce a Wolff-Chaikoff effect and hence to inhibit the uptake and organic binding of a concomitantly administered dose of I^{131}. That is why substantially smaller doses of iodide are employed in the iodide-perchlorate discharge test. Abnormal sensitivity to the Wolff-Chaikoff effect in terms of the dose of iodide required for its elicitation is conditioned by one or both of two factors. Susceptibility is increased when the iodide transport mechanism is activated. Here the increase in intrathyroid iodide concentration produced by a given dose of iodide is enhanced. This may explain the enhanced susceptibility of some patients with Graves' disease or of normal individuals given TSH. Susceptibility is also increased when there is an underlying defect in the organic-binding mechanism. This likely accounts for the increased susceptibility seen in patients who have previously developed goiter during chronic iodide administration or for that seen in many patients with Hashimoto's disease or with Graves' disease previously treated with surgery, I^{131}, or antithyroid drugs. Such patients are likely to develop goiter if given iodides chronically, and in them the defective organic-binding mechanism may be a forerunner of eventual thyroid failure.

When moderate or large doses of iodide are administered repeatedly, the relative inhibition of organic binding and inhibition of iodothyronine formation are at least partly relieved. This so-called "escape or adaptation" phenomenon occurs because, with continued iodine administration, iodide transport activity decreases, and the thyroid iodide concentration becomes insufficient to maintain a full Wolff-Chaikoff effect. This response is demonstrable in the hypophysectomized animal and hence is a manifestation of the thyroid autoregulatory inhibition of iodide transport discussed earlier. It allows synthesis of iodothyronines to resume, despite continued iodine administration, and thereby forestalls the development of goitrous hypothyroidism. The reduction in iodide transport which permits adaptation reduces the thyroid iodide clearance rate and hence the thyroid I^{131} uptake. Nevertheless, the quantity of iodine accumulated and organified is well in excess of normal, though the rate of secretion of T_4 is not enhanced. Hence it is evident that during chronic iodine administration the thyroid forms and releases noncalorigenic forms of iodine. Probably much of the iodine lost from the gland in this manner is iodide. In normal individuals the magnitude of this so-called "iodide leak" varies directly with the dietary iodine intake (Wartofsky and Ingbar, 1971). In rare instances, adaptation does not occur, and synthesis of hormone is chronically inhibited, leading to the development of goiter and hypothyroidism (iodide myxedema). This disorder, to which patients with Hashimoto's disease and certain patients with Graves' disease are prone, is discussed more fully in the section dealing with disorders that lead to hypothyroidism.

Effect on Thyroid Hormone Release

In the clinical setting, probably the most important effect of pharmacologic doses of iodine on the thyroid is their ability to induce a prompt inhibition of hormone release. When the thyroid iodine is labeled with I^{131} and large doses of antithyroid agents are administered to prevent recycling of I^{131} released from the gland, administration of iodine is followed soon thereafter by a decrease in the rate of disappearance of I^{131} from the gland (Fig. 4-11). This effect is most clearly evident in hyperfunctioning thyroids but can also be demonstrated in the normal thyroid, though with some difficulty because of the relatively slow initial rate of radioiodine turnover. Alternative methods of analysis, involving measurement of the serum T_4 concentration and rate of disappearance from serum of exogenous radioiodine-labeled T_4, have shown that iodine not only decreases the fractional turnover of thyroid radioiodine but also decreases the actual T_4 secretion rate (Wartofsky et al., 1970).

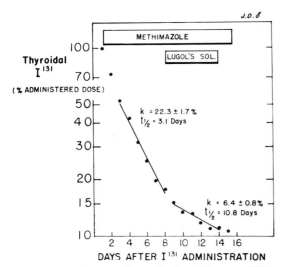

Figure 4–11. Effect of iodine on the thyroid turnover of I^{131} in a patient with Graves' disease. The initial turnover rate of 22.3%/day is much faster than that observed in normal patients and is abruptly slowed by the administration of Lugol's iodine.

This effect of iodine is doubtless the mechanism whereby iodine rapidly lowers the serum T_4 concentration and acutely alleviates thyrotoxicity in the patient with diffuse toxic goiter. The response to iodine in this disorder cannot be ascribed to the persistence of an acute Wolff-Chaikoff effect with inhibition of T_4 synthesis, since the ameliorative effect is much more rapid than that produced by even large doses of antithyroid agent. Neither can the response to iodine be ascribed to an effect on the peripheral metabolism or metabolic effectiveness of T_4, since none can be demonstrated. In most patients with otherwise untreated diffuse toxic goiter, the decrease in serum T_4 concentration during iodine administration does not continue into the hypothyroid range, but rather stabilizes at a normal or high normal value. The reason for this is uncertain, but in normal individuals the decline in serum T_4 and T_3 concentrations induced by iodine appears to elicit an increase in TSH secretion that counteracts the effect of iodine (Vagenakis et al., 1973). Whether normalization of the serum T_4 concentration by iodine in the thyrotoxic patient also elicits secretion of TSH has not been studied.

The mechanism by which iodine inhibits secretion of T_4 is unknown. Clearly the effect is mediated at the thyroid level rather than through an action on TSH in view of its occurrence in Graves' disease. Moreover, the effect is demonstrable in the autonomously hyperfunctioning thyroid nodule, in which disorder the secretion of TSH is also lacking. The effect of iodine on the secretory mechanism is not confined to an effect on the release of T_4 itself but is likely an effect on the mechanism of proteolysis, since iodine acutely inhibits "iodide leak" (Wartofsky and Ingbar, 1971). It is not known at what biochemical stage iodine acts, but it appears to act at some stage distal to the initial effect of cAMP. Recent evidence suggests that iodine

may inhibit the enzyme glutathione reductase (Hati and Ingbar, unpublished observations). This enzyme conditions the intrathyroid concentration of reduced glutathione, and this, in turn, is thought to facilitate reduction of disulfide bonds in thyroglobulin, making it more susceptible to the action of the thyroid protease (Balasubramaniam et al., 1965).

Involution of Thyroid Hyperplasia

One of the most important and enigmatic effects of iodine on the thyroid is its ability to diminish the hypervascularity and hyperplasia that characterize the diffuse toxic goiter of Graves' disease. This effect, which greatly facilitates surgical therapy of this disorder, is not an obligatory action of iodide on the thyroid, since intense hyperplasia characterizes the thyroid gland of patients with iodide myxedema. In the latter disorder, pharmacologic quantities of iodide inhibit hormone synthesis, while in Graves' disease some binding of iodine to organic compounds doubtless occurs, even during treatment with antithyroid agents. The involuting effect of iodine may reflect an autoregulation of thyroid intermediary metabolism, since the rat thyroid which is rich in iodine uses glucose less efficiently and forms therefrom less carbon dioxide, lactate, and lipid than does the thyroid which is poor in iodine (unpublished observations of Nagataki). Decreased energy metabolism in the thyroid may retard anabolic processes necessary for maintenance of hyperplasia, while decreased production of acid metabolites may be responsible for the reduction in vascularity that iodine produces.

Adrenergic Nervous System and Bioactive Amines

The effects of the adrenergic nervous system and of catecholamines on various aspects of thyroid function have long been a subject of interest. Studies of varying design in varying species have yielded variable results. As a consequence, there has been considerable doubt as to whether the adrenergic nervous system has any significant influence on thyroid function. Considerable clarification, however, has come in recent years, principally from the studies of Melander and co-workers. These investigators have shown that the extent of adrenergic innervation of the thyroid varies from species to species and with the age of the animal, possibly explaining the variable results obtained by other investigators. In the mouse, abundant adrenergic fibers terminate in the thyroid, both in conjunction with arterioles and close to the basement membrane of the follicular cell. Stimulation of the cervical sympathetic trunks in mice whose thyroid glands have been prelabeled with I^{131} and then suppressed by exogenous T_4 induces formation of colloid droplets and an increase in blood I^{131} concentration. Unilateral stimulation induces colloid droplet formation only within the distribution of the stimulated nerve. Conversely, as judged from the rate of decrease of blood I^{131} in mice whose thyroids have been prelabeled but not suppressed by T_4, either surgical or chemical sympathectomy decreases transiently the rate of thyroid I^{131} release. A direct stimulatory effect of catecholamines on thyroid hormone secretion is indicated by the demonstration that epinephrine, norepinephrine, and tyramine induce release of I^{131} from the prelabeled and T_4-suppressed thyroid of the mouse. The effect of these agents is inhibited by α-receptor antagonists. Direct stimulatory effects of the same monoamines on thyroid adenylate cyclase activity as well as on iodine and intermediary metabolism have been demonstrated by other workers in isolated thyroid cells. Evidence of a role for indolamines in influencing thyroid function has also been obtained. The thyroid of the rat is rich in mast cells, which contain 5-hydroxytryptamine (serotonin, 5-HT) as well as histamine, though evidence exists that the latter compound is inactive. Administration of agents that degranulate mast cells induces in T_4-pretreated rats the formation of colloid droplets and increase the blood I^{131} concentration. No such change is seen in T_4-pretreated mice, however, whose thyroids contain fewer mast cells. The mast cell within the rat thyroid, but not in extrathyroidal tissues, is depleted of 5-HT within a few minutes after injection of TSH. Finally, both 5-HT and related indolamines stimulate both the formation of colloid droplets and the release of I^{131} from the thyroid of T_4-pretreated mice. They also enhance adenylate cyclase activity as well as iodine and intermediary metabolism of isolated bovine thyroid cells. These effects, like those of the catecholamines, are inhibited by α-receptor antagonists. An interaction between TSH and catecholamines is indicated by two observations. First, the stimulatory effect of TSH on I^{131} release from the thyroid of T_4-pretreated mice is partly inhibited by α-receptor antagonists. Second, pretreatment of similar mice with α-receptor antagonists inhibits the response to subsequently administered TSH.

All of the foregoing findings indicate the likelihood that the norepinephrine released from adrenergic nerve terminals within the thyroid and the indolamines contained within thyroid mast cells may significantly influence thyroid function by a direct effect on the thyroid follicular cell, by an interaction with TSH, and, possibly, by an effect on the thyroid vasculature and blood flow (see review by Melander, 1971).

Effects of catecholamines on thyroid hormone economy in man, as might be expected, have been less well defined. Acute administration of epinephrine, depending on the timing and magnitude of the dose, may either increase or decrease the thyroid I^{131} uptake, and thyroid function is normal in most patients with pheochromocytoma. No significant alterations in thyroid function or serum T_4 concentration are seen in patients given the usual pharmacologic doses of adrenergic antagonists. Epinephrine has been reported to decrease the fractional turnover rate of T_4, but it has no consistent effect on the PBI. It does, however, increase the BMR in euthyroid, and especially thyrotoxic, subjects but has little effect in patients with hypothyroidism until they are treated. In patients with hypothyroidism, administration of L-dopa rapidly depresses the elevated serum TSH concentration, but no abnormalities of thyroid function are evident in normal individuals given L-dopa chronically (Rapoport et al., 1973).

Antithyroid Agents

A wide variety of chemical agents have the ability to inhibit one or more reactions required in the synthesis of thyroid hormones. When the effect of such agents is sufficient to reduce the secretion of thyroid hormones to subnormal levels, secretion of TSH is increased, and goiter ensues. Hence such agents are commonly termed goitrogens. In clinical practice, goitrogenic agents are encountered as drugs used in the treatment of hyperthyroidism, as pharmacologic agents used for other purposes but which happen to have antithyroid properties, and as goitrogens occurring naturally in foodstuffs. The present section will provide a classification of several varieties of antithyroid agents and their mode of action. Since the use of antithyroid drugs in the treatment of hyperthyroidism is discussed in a later section, special attention will be given to those agents that are not used in the control of hyperthyroidism but are nevertheless encountered clinically.

From the standpoint of the aspects of iodine metabolism which they inhibit, antithyroid agents can be grouped into two classes: agents that inhibit thyroid iodide transport and those that inhibit the complex of reactions involved in organic binding and coupling processes. Without clear exception, inhibitors of iodide transport belong to the class of monovalent anions; of these, thiocyanate and perchlorate have been used clinically. Other anions that inhibit thyroid iodide transport have been discussed in the section on hormone biosynthesis. Because of their toxicity, neither thiocyanate nor perchlorate is any longer widely used in the treatment of hyperthyroidism, although they are usually effective agents in this respect. Perchlorate has enjoyed some vogue as a therapeutic agent but should probably not be used, since it sometimes produces irreversible aplastic anemia (Krevans et al., 1962). Inhibitors of iodide transport decrease hormone synthesis by limiting T:P concentration ratios for iodide, thereby reducing the intrathyroid iodide concentration. This is effective when the plasma iodide concentration is normal or low; however, should the patient be exposed to excessive amounts of iodine, hormone overproduction will resume. Thus control may be unpredictable and, furthermore, these agents cannot be used with iodine in preparing patients for subtotal thyroidectomy.

The second class of antithyroid agents consists of compounds that inhibit the thyroid organic bind-

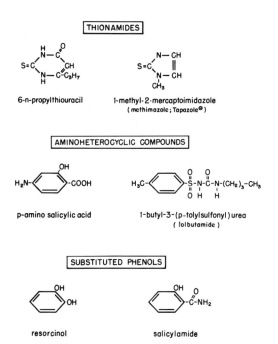

Figure 4–12. Structural formulas of some representative antithyroid compounds.

ing and coupling reactions. Although a great many compounds exert this effect, with few exceptions they can be classified into three main groups, according to their basic chemical structure: thionamides, aminoheterocyclic compounds, and substituted phenols (Fig. 4–12). In the case of the thionamides, it was initially thought that these agents exert their antithyroid action solely by inhibiting the initial oxidation and binding of iodide in the thyroid. Later it was learned that the inhibitory action of these agents is directed, in order of decreasing sensitivity, at the coupling of iodotyrosines, the iodination of MIT to form DIT, and lastly, the formation of MIT. Subsequent studies have shown a similar order of sensitivity in the action of all agents that ultimately (at their highest doses) inhibit organic binding per se.

As a class, the thionamide compounds, which include the classic antithyroid agents, are the most potent inhibitors of thyroid hormone formation known, and are characterized by the following substituent grouping,

$$S = C \Big\langle \begin{matrix} N- \\ \\ R- \end{matrix}$$

in which R may be a sulfur, oxygen, or nitrogen atom. In contrast to the action of agents that inhibit thyroid iodide transport, the action of the thionamides is not prevented by large doses of iodide, although it is decreased somewhat.

The aminoheterocyclic compounds are in general far less potent than the thionamides and are not used in the treatment of hyperthyroidism. Their effects on the thyroid are sometimes manifest, however, during their use in the treatment of other disease. Para-aminosalicylic acid, used as an antituberculosis agent, is goitrogenic in rats, lowers thyroid I^{131} uptake in man, and occasionally produces goiter with or without hypothyroidism. The hypoglycemic sulfonylureas, tolbutamide and especially carbutamide, decrease I^{131} uptake in man, although they are not sufficiently potent to be goitrogenic in man. The goitrogenic effect of para-aminosalicylic acid and the sulfonylureas, like that of the thionamides, is slightly decreased by large amounts of iodine. An additional group of agents in this class is the sulfonamides. Although they have not been shown to be goitrogenic in man, interest in them arises from the fact that their goitrogenic potency is usually increased by supplemental iodide. This and other evidence indicates that the mechanism of action of the sulfonamides differs from that of the thionamides and of other aminoheterocyclic compounds.

The final major category of antithyroid agents that inhibit organic binding is that of the substituted phenols. Agents of interest in this group include resorcinol, a cutaneous antiseptic that has produced goitrous hypothyroidism in man. Closely related to resorcinol are the congeners of salicylic acid. The latter is devoid of antithyroid action, although it does inhibit the binding of T_4 by TBPA. Several derivatives of salicylic acid, particularly those with an additional hydroxyl substitution, have moderate antithyroid potency and are also able to inhibit T_4 binding by TBPA. Agents of this class, such as salicylamide, are used clinically because of their antirheumatic, antipyretic, and especially their analgesic effect (see Woeber and Ingbar, 1965, for references). Whether they exert a significant antithyroid action in ordinary clinical use is uncertain.

A number of other agents of diverse chemical nature also have antithyroid activity. Phenylbutazone decreases the thyroid uptake of I^{131} and has been reported to produce goitrous hypothyroidism in man. Strangely, the latter effect is said to be transient. Iodopyrine, an antiasthmatic preparation containing iodine and antipyrine (phenazone), has been reported to produce goiter in about 30 per cent of patients (Begg and Hall, 1963). This high incidence of goiter is due to a synergistic action of iodide upon the antithyroid effect of antipyrine, which is itself a goitrogen (Pasternak et al., 1969). Cobalt, which is incorporated in some hematinic preparations, occasionally produces goitrous hypothyroidism, often in children. The mechanism of action of cobalt is uncertain, but it may act by blocking organic-binding reactions. High levels of dietary calcium have been said to be goitrogenic, but the mechanism of goitrogenesis is unclear. An antithyroid action in animals has been ascribed to certain antibiotics of the tetracycline group; published results have been conflicting.

The final category of antithyroid agents comprises those that occur naturally in foods. These are widely distributed in the family Cruciferae or Brassicaceae, particularly in the genus Brassica. Included are cabbages, turnips, kale, kohlrabi, rutabaga, mustard, and a number of plants not eaten by humans but which serve as animal fodder. It is likely that some thiocyanate is present in such plants (particularly cabbage), especially in the leaves. In addition to some thiocyanate, the seeds, roots, and perhaps leaves also contain another variety of potential goitrogens or "progoitrins" in the form of various thioglycosides. The progoitrins are themselves not goitrogenic but become so when acted upon either by a heat-labile thioglycosidase, myrosinase, also present in the plant, or by the glycosidases liberated by intestinal bacteria. In the case of turnips, the active goitrogen has been shown to be L-5-vinyl-2-thiooxazolidone. Actively goitrogenic isothiocyanates have been isolated from other plants of the same family. Except for thiocyanate, dietary goitrogens influence thyroid iodine metabolism in the same manner as do the thionamides, which they resemble chemically. The role of dietary goitrogens in the induction of disease in humans is uncertain; their effect may depend upon the concomitant iodine intake. Although humans rarely if ever eat goitrogenic foods in quantities sufficient to lead to goiter, the possibility of endemia due to transmission of sufficient quantities of the goitrogen in milk has been raised. (For extensive discussion of this subject, the reader is referred to reviews by Clements, 1960, and Greer et al., 1964.)

Sex and Sex Hormones

A relationship between the thyroid and the gonads is suggested by the far more frequent occurrence of thyroid disorders in women than in men and by the common appearance of goiter during puberty, pregnancy, and the menopause. This apparent relationship has engendered many studies to assess the effect of the administration of sex hormones on thyroid function.

In man, the administration of small doses of estrogens leads to an acute decrease in the serum TSH concentration, from which an escape occurs by the second or third day of continued administration. This effect of estrogens, which resembles that induced by glucocorticoids, appears to be exerted through an inhibition of endogenous TRH release. Testosterone and progesterone in essentially physiologic doses do not appear to influence TSH secretion (Gross et al., 1971).

The administration of estrogens or androgens has no consistent effect on the thyroid I^{131} uptake but causes alterations in the binding of thyroid hormones in plasma. Estrogens increase the concentration of TBG and elevate the serum T_4 and T_3 concentrations, whereas androgens induce converse effects, although they appear to increase the

concentration of TBPA. The kinetic consequences of these alterations in hormone transport have been discussed in an earlier section.

Thyroid function and the peripheral metabolism of the thyroid hormones appear to be essentially independent of the sex of the individual. There is no appreciable variation in thyroid I^{131} uptake during different phases of the menstrual cycle. The normal ranges for the serum T_4 and T_3 concentrations are the same in nonpregnant women and men. The BMR tends to be somewhat higher in men than in women, probably because of the relatively greater muscle mass in men.

Pregnancy and the Newborn State

Pregnancy affects virtually all aspects of thyroid hormone economy. The thyroid gland is enlarged, and a bruit, reflecting the increased blood flow, may be present. The thyroid I^{131} uptake and the thyroid iodide clearance rate are increased. These alterations are largely due to the iodine deficiency state that occurs during pregnancy as a result of an increase in renal iodide clearance (Aboul-Khair et al., 1964). The concentration in serum of pituitary TSH is normal in pregnancy. The normal placenta elaborates a thyroid-stimulating peptide, termed human chorionic thyrotropin (hCT), that cross-reacts immunologically with bovine but not human pituitary TSH (Hershman and Starnes, 1969). The physiologic role of hCT in pregnancy is uncertain. The thyroid I^{131} uptake and the thyroid and renal iodide clearance rates return to nonpregnant levels within six weeks after delivery.

The serum T_4 concentration increases during the first month of pregnancy to values between 7 and 12 μg./100 ml. and remains at this level until after delivery. The serum T_3 concentration also increases during pregnancy but to a lesser extent than does the serum T_4, with the result that the $T_4:T_3$ ratio in serum is greater than that in the nonpregnant state (Larsen, 1972). The increase in serum T_4 and T_3 concentrations is due to the increased concentration of TBG in plasma, resulting in all likelihood from the increased secretion of estrogens. The proportion of free T_4, whether assessed directly or indirectly by an uptake test *in vitro*, is decreased. However, the absolute concentration of free T_4 or the free T_4 index, representing the product of the serum T_4 concentration and either the proportion of free hormone or the value for the uptake test, remains essentially normal. Although the proportion of free T_3 is also decreased, it is not yet certain whether the absolute concentration of free T_3 is normal or decreased in pregnancy. As a result of the decrease in the proportion of free T_4, the volume of distribution and fractional rate of turnover of T_4 are decreased, but the total daily disposal of hormone remains essentially unchanged (Dowling et al., 1967). The serum T_4 and T_3 concentrations, as well as the concentration of TBG, return to nonpregnant levels within six weeks after delivery.

The basal metabolic rate (BMR) increases during the second trimester, and values of $+20-30$ per cent are common at term. The increase in BMR is due to the increase in the total mass of body tissue.

All the changes in thyroid function that accompany normal pregnancy are exaggerated in molar pregnancy: the serum T_4 concentration is usually well in excess of 12 μg./100 ml., and the thyroid I^{131} uptake is increased to distinctly hyperthyroid levels. Despite the increased serum T_4 concentration, the increase in TBG in molar pregnancy is less than that in normal pregnancy, with the result that the absolute concentration of free T_4 exceeds nonpregnant values. This syndrome of thyroid hyperfunction results from secretion by the molar tissue of a thyroid-stimulating peptide, termed molar thyrotropin, that does not cross-react immunologically with either human or bovine TSH. Despite the laboratory evidence of hyperthyroidism, patients with molar pregnancy usually display little clinical evidence of thyrotoxicosis (Galton et al., 1971).

Little information is available on the kinetics of transplacental passage of thyroid hormones in man. If, as seems likely, thyroid hormone–plasma protein interactions largely determine such passage, one would expect net transfer of hormone from fetus to mother, since throughout pregnancy the concentration of TBG in maternal plasma exceeds that in the fetus. This is important because it indicates that the maternal supply of hormone may not necessarily be adequate to support the development of a fetus whose thyroid is not functioning.

At delivery, the concentration of T_4 in cord serum is only slightly less than that in maternal serum, but the proportion of free T_4 is greater because of a smaller increase in TBG relative to maternal serum. As a result, the absolute concentration of free T_4 exceeds that in maternal serum. By contrast, the concentrations of total and free T_3 in cord serum are much lower than those in maternal serum, being in the distinctly hypothyroid range (Abuid et al., 1973). This provides strong evidence that the passage of T_3 from mother to the fetus is at most very limited. As a result, the $T_4:T_3$ ratio in cord serum is greatly increased. The concentration of TSH in cord serum exceeds that in maternal serum.

After delivery, the serum TSH concentration in the neonate increases rapidly to a peak at 30 minutes of extrauterine life and then declines, returning to its initial value within 48 hours (Fisher and Odell, 1969). The rapid increase in serum TSH is believed to be due in part to the cooling that follows emergence into the extrauterine environment. In response to the increase in TSH secretion, the serum T_3 and T_4 concentrations increase rapidly, reaching a plateau by 24 hours of life. At the plateau, both are in the distinctly hyperthyroid range, the T_3 concentration being at least four times greater than its initial value in cord serum and the T_4 concentration two times greater (Abuid et al., 1973).

Age

The increased values for the serum T_4 and T_3 concentrations in the neonate (see preceding section) gradually decline, reaching the normal adult range toward the end of the first year. The thyroid I^{131} uptake is also increased in the neonate, reflecting the transient increase in TSH secretion.

From childhood through senescence, the serum T_4 concentration is essentially independent of age, whereas the mean value for the serum T_3 concentration declines to approximately two-thirds that in normal adults by the ninth decade (Brunelle and Bohuon, 1972). The thyroid I^{131} uptake, clearance rate, and turnover rate decrease slightly with age, resulting in part from the decrease in the total daily disposal of T_4 that occurs with age and in part from an age-dependent decrease in renal iodide clearance. From infancy through senescence, both the total daily disposal of T_4 and the BMR decrease progressively with age, probably reflecting alterations in the cellular metabolism of thyroid hormones (Oddie et al., 1966). In men, but apparently not in women, the peak increment in the response of the serum TSH concentration to TRH declines progressively with advancing age (Snyder and Utiger, 1972b).

In adolescent girls, a small goiter is often found without evidence of altered metabolism. This goiter may reflect the response to an increased peripheral demand for hormone, since in some of these girls, the thyroid I^{131} uptake and total daily disposal of T_4 are increased (unpublished data from the authors' laboratory). In old age, the thyroid often tends to be firm and slightly irregular, and histologic examination may reveal an increase in fibrous tissue.

Glucocorticoids

Both ACTH, through its action on the adrenal cortex, and glucocorticoids influence thyroid function. Early work demonstrated that pharmacologic doses of these agents decrease the thyroid I^{131} uptake, clearance rate, and turnover rate in man. In addition, it was demonstrated that these alterations could be reversed by the administration of exogenous TSH, suggesting that these agents suppress pituitary TSH secretion. This was confirmed by recent studies in which it was shown that the administration of pharmacologic doses of glucocorticoid reduces serum TSH concentrations in both normal and hypothyroid patients, an effect that is believed to be mediated through an inhibition of endogenous TRH release (Wilber and Utiger, 1969). When glucocorticoids are withdrawn, the serum TSH concentration rebounds to values in excess of pretreatment values. With continued administration of glucocorticoids, there occurs an escape from the suppression of serum TSH concentration in some but not all patients. The decrease in thyroid secretory rate resulting from the suppression of pituitary TSH secretion is in all likelihood responsible for the slight decrease in serum T_4 concentration that glucocorticoids induce in normal subjects, since no change in serum T_4 concentration is seen in hypothyroid patients maintained on a constant daily dose of exogenous hormone.

Pharmacologic doses of glucocorticoids decrease the concentration in serum of TBG and increase that of TBPA but do not affect the proportion or absolute concentration of free T_4. Consistent with the latter finding is the observation that glucocorticoids do not induce significant alterations in the metabolic disappearance of T_4. However, they do retard the distributive disappearance of T_4, probably by decreasing the hepatic binding of hormone (Kumar et al., 1968).

Stress

Studies of the effects of various stressful situations on thyroid hormone economy in man are scanty, and the results thereof are often contradictory. Nervous stress has been reported to result in an increased PBI in some studies but not in others. Exercise stress produces no significant changes in serum T_4 or TSH concentration but leads to an increase in the total daily disposal of T_4. Values for the latter function are higher in athletes than in nonathletes (Terjung and Tipton, 1971).

Studies of the effects of surgical stress are complicated by the fact that the effects of anesthesia and of surgery per se have to be identified. For example, ether anesthesia appears to cause an influx of T_4 into the circulation from tissue sites other than the thyroid (Fore et al., 1966). Surgery does not appear to be accompanied by an acceleration of T_4 turnover.

In man as well as in the rhesus monkey, acute bacterial sepsis is accompanied by an acceleration of T_4 and T_3 turnover. In the monkey, these alterations result from a primary increase in the cellular uptake of hormones, perhaps by circulating and fixed phagocytic cells (DeRubertis and Woeber, 1973).

Environmental Temperature

Exposure of human subjects to cold for several days results in an increase in serum T_4 concentration which is evident by 24 hours and which reaches a maximum by three days. The thyroid I^{131} uptake and clearance rate also increase. These alterations may represent a compensatory response to a depletion of the peripheral hormone pool, resulting from an increased rate of T_4 metabolism by the peripheral tissues. By contrast, short-term exposure to cold is not accompanied by an increased serum TSH concentration in adult subjects. In the newborn, on the other hand, brief cooling provokes an increase in serum TSH concentration, suggesting that the hypothalamus is initially responsive to the cold stimulus but becomes refractory with age. (See Fisher and Odell, 1971, for a discussion of this subject.)

In man, no consistent alterations in thyroid hormone economy have been observed in cold climates because clothing and heating prevent significant cold stress. Similarly, no consistent alterations have been observed in hot climates.

Liver Disease

The hepatobiliary system is an important site for the distribution and metabolism of the thyroid hormones (Oppenheimer et al., 1969). In man, as much as one-third of the total extrathyroidal pool of T_4 is located within the liver, and as much as one-third of the clearance of T_4 from the plasma occurs via biliary excretion, the T_4 appearing both in the free form and as a conjugate with glucuronic acid. Net reabsorption occurs from the gut, as is evidenced by the increase in fecal T_4 excretion that follows the administration of complexing agents, such as cholestyramine. The liver is also the site of synthesis of TBG and TBPA. Consequently, liver disease may cause profound alterations in serum hormone concentrations and in the kinetics of peripheral hormone metabolism. For example, in cirrhosis, diminished synthesis of TBG results in a decreased serum T_4 concentration and in an increased proportion of free hormone. Whether or not this decrease in plasma binding of hormone leads to an increase in the fractional turnover rate of T_4 will depend upon the severity of the impairment in the hepatic uptake and metabolism of T_4 that has been demonstrated in this disorder. On the other hand, in infectious hepatitis, the concentration of TBG in plasma may be increased, leading to an increase in serum T_4 concentration and to a decrease in the fractional turnover rate of T_4. In cholestatic states, regurgitation of metabolically inactive thyroid hormone conjugates as well as free hormone may be accompanied by an increase in PBI and perhaps in serum T_4 concentration (Vannotti and Beraud, 1959). Finally, in patients with cirrhosis, the thyroid I^{131} uptake is often increased, reflecting the iodine-deficient state that may result from a salt-restricted or inadequate diet.

Cardiac and Renal Disease

Because of impairment of glomerular filtration, renal iodide clearance is reduced in severe cardiac or renal disease. The resulting increase in plasma iodide leads to a decrease in the rate of clearance by the thyroid of administered I^{131}. Owing to delayed renal excretion of the I^{131}, thyroid I^{131} accumulation continues beyond the usual 24 hours, approaching a plateau at 48 or 72 hours. On the other hand, if salt restriction is accompanied by a deficient iodine intake, retardation of thyroid I^{131} accumulation may not be observed, and the uptake at 24 hours may be normal or increased. In cardiac failure, the increased work of breathing results in an increased BMR.

In anephric patients undergoing regular dialysis, iodine metabolism is essentially normal, dialysis substituting for the impaired renal iodide clearance. Studies of the kinetics of peripheral T_4 metabolism have revealed normal values for the distribution volume and fractional turnover rate of T_4, but the total daily disposal of T_4 is increased as a result of increased fecal excretion of hormone. The concentrations of TBG, T_4, and TSH in serum are normal (Oddie et al., 1970b).

In the nephrotic syndrome, there occur some stigmata of hypothyroidism as well as complex changes in peripheral T_4 metabolism. Values for the BMR and serum T_4 concentration are usually subnormal, and the serum cholesterol concentration is increased. To what extent these alterations reflect an actual deficiency in the quantity of hormone available to the tissues is uncertain, since measurements of neither the absolute concentration of free T_4 nor the serum T_3 concentration have been reported. Urinary loss of TBG and TBPA leads to decreased concentrations of these proteins in plasma. The decreased serum T_4 concentration characteristic of this disorder may result from urinary loss of hormone in association with the binding proteins as well as from the decrease in hormone binding. As a result of these alterations, the fractional turnover rate of T_4 is increased. The total daily disposal of T_4 is normal or decreased, but since a fraction thereof may represent unchanged T_4 in the urine, it is possible that the quantity of hormone delivered to the tissues is subnormal. However, the compensatory thyroid hyperfunction that would be expected if the latter were the case is usually not seen, since values for the thyroid I^{131} uptake are not usually increased.

Malnutrition

Severe malnutrition, whether due to starvation, anorexia nervosa, or malabsorption, results in a variable degree of hypothalamic or pituitary dysfunction which may be accompanied by a decreased thyroid I^{131} uptake and serum T_4 concentration. The BMR is usually low, but this may be due in part to the loss of muscle mass.

Miscellaneous Disorders

A wide variety of systemic illnesses are accompanied by a modest decrease in the serum T_4 concentration, though the values usually remain within the normal range. The decrease in serum T_4 concentration is associated with an increase in the proportion of free hormone, so that the concentration of free hormone may be normal or increased. These alterations appear to be due at least in part to a decreased concentration of TBG in plasma (Bellabarba et al., 1968).

An increase in BMR occurs in fever, anemia, myelo- and lymphoproliferative disorders, acromegaly, pheochromocytoma, and cardiac or pulmonary insufficiency. The hypermetabolism in these disorders appears to be entirely extrathyroidal in origin.

LABORATORY TESTS OF THYROID HORMONE ECONOMY

There are more methods available for assessing the state of thyroid function and hormone economy than for any other endocrine gland (see classification of commonly employed tests in Table 4–1). In the next section, these methods are described in detail in terms of their physiologic basis and aberrations in disease states. The reasons for emphasis on testing procedures are as follows. First, laboratory procedures of increasing specificity and sensitivity have made possible diagnosis of thyroid dysfunction in patients in whom clinical findings are marginal or are obscured by coincidental nonthyroidal disorders. Second, even when the clinical picture seems clear and the diagnosis straightforward, the physician often seeks both the reassurance of confirmatory laboratory findings and the advantage of obtaining pretreatment baseline values. Furthermore, the very profusion of testing procedures indicates that each procedure has inherent limitations. Thus no single procedure is uniformly reliable in the diagnosis of all disorders of thyroid function, and virtually all procedures are subject to alteration by endogenous or exogenous factors that complicate their interpretation. Such factors may cause the several indices to diverge from the normal in a conflicting way. Nevertheless, through an appreciation of the specific physiologic datum which each test provides and the factors that may influence the results obtained, it is usually possible, through careful selection and

TABLE 4–1. COMMONLY EMPLOYED LABORATORY TESTS OF THYROID HORMONE ECONOMY

1. *Direct Tests of Thyroid Function*
   Thyroid uptake of I^{131}, RAIU

2. *Tests Related to the Concentration and Binding of the Thyroid Hormones in Blood*
   Measurements of Hormone Concentration
     Serum T_4 concentration by competitive protein binding (displacement) analysis, T_4(D)
     Serum T_3 concentration by radioimmunoassay, T_3(RIA)
     Serum protein–bound iodine, PBI
   Measurements of Hormone Binding
     Per cent free T_4, %FT_4
     Resin T_3 uptake *in vitro*, RT_3U
     Free T_4 concentration, FT_4
     Free T_4 index, T_4-RT_3 index

3. *Tests that Assess the Metabolic Impact of the Thyroid Hormones*
   Basal metabolic rate, BMR
   Serum cholesterol concentration
   Achilles reflex time

4. *Tests that Assess the Mechanisms for Regulating Thyroid Function*
   Thyroid suppression test
   TSH-stimulation test
   Serum TSH concentration
   TRH-stimulation test

5. *Miscellaneous Tests*
   External scintiscanning
   Tests for thyroid autoantibodies

interpretation, to achieve at least a reasonably thorough understanding of the physiopathologic aberration present in specific diseases states or individual patients. It is to emphasize this dependence of clinical interpretation on physiologic understanding that laboratory procedures are not discussed immediately after the description of the disease states but rather here, immediately after reviewing the physiology and biochemistry of the thyroid and its hormones.

Laboratory procedures can be divided into four major categories: (1) direct tests of thyroid function that provide quantitative or qualitative information or both about hormone synthesis and secretion; (2) tests related to the concentration and binding of the thyroid hormones and other iodinated materials in the blood; (3) tests that assess the impact of the thyroid hormones upon the tissues (metabolic indices); and (4) tests that assess the mechanisms for regulating thyroid function. There are in addition a variety of miscellaneous tests that do not fit into the other categories. A system of abbreviations has been adopted by the American Thyroid Association to identify some of the commonly used tests (Solomon et al., 1972). Although not used in this chapter, these abbreviations are frequently used in the literature and therefore are given in Table 4–1.

Direct Tests of Thyroid Function

Although many tests are available from which the state of thyroid function can be inferred, it is only with the aid of radioactive isotopes of the stable form of iodine, I^{127}, that the function of the gland can be evaluated directly. This fact has led to a profusion of testing procedures that assess some aspect of the thyroid metabolism of radioiodine, most common among them being measurement of the fractional uptake of a single dose of radioiodine. In the past, these tests were most commonly used in the diagnosis of hyper- or hypothyroidism. Two factors have led to a diminishing use in this regard, however. The first is the improvement in indirect methods for assessing thyroid status, either through specific measurement of the thyroid hormones in blood or through assessment of the state of mechanisms for regulating thyroid function. The second is the progressive decline in normal values for thyroid radioiodine uptake consequent to the widespread increase in daily dietary iodine intake that has followed the enrichment of foods, particularly bread, with iodine (Oddie et al., 1970a; Caplan and Kujak, 1971; Ghahremani et al., 1971). The latter has greatly reduced the usefulness of measurements of thyroid radioiodine uptake in the diagnosis of hypothyroid states. Nevertheless, measurements of thyroid radioiodine metabolism are of substantial or critical importance in a number of circumstances, including confirmation of thyroid hyperfunction, evaluation of thyroid supressibility, affirmation or exclusion of a diagnosis of thyrotoxicosis factitia, assessment of the thyroid's responsiveness to exogenous TSH, exploration of biosynthetic defects within the thyroid, and diagnosis of subacute thyroiditis. Because of this broad scope and because of the unique physiologic information that is conveyed, this category of tests will be discussed in some detail.

Three radioisotopes of iodine have found particular use in clinical practice and laboratory investigation, I^{131}, I^{132}, and I^{125}. Of these, I^{131} (physical half-life, 8 days) is by far the most widely used, but special characteristics of I^{132} and I^{125} make them particularly suitable in special circumstances. The short physical half-life of I^{132} (2.3 hours) makes this isotope particularly useful when repeated doses of radioiodine are required, while I^{125} (physical half-life, 60 days) has been particularly recommended for localization of functioning thyroid tissue by scintiscanning procedures. All are synthetic isotopes available as inorganic iodide of high specific activity, i.e., high ratio of radioactivity to chemical iodine content. Physiologically, all are indistinguishable from the naturally occurring stable isotope, I^{127}. All are emitters of gamma radiation, which makes possible their external measurement in sites of concentration *in vivo*, such as the thyroid gland or aberrant thyroid tissue.

Measurements of Thyroid Radioiodine Accumulation

Physiologic Basis. When tracer quantities of inorganic radioiodine are administered either orally or intravenously, the isotope quickly becomes uniformly mixed with the endogenous stable iodide within the iodide distribution space.* Immediately upon its entrance into the plasma, I^{131} begins to be removed by its two major sites of clearance, the thyroid and the kidneys. As this process continues, the plasma concentration of I^{131} declines exponentially. Normally, very low values are reached by 24 hours, and inorganic I^{131} is virtually undetectable in the plasma by 72 hours after its administration. Since the quantity of I^{131} that enters the thyroid (or urine) during any time period is proportional to the concentration of I^{131} in the plasma, the thyroid content of I^{131} increases rapidly during the early hours, then at a decreasing rate until a virtual plateau is reached. The proportion of administered I^{131} ultimately accumulated by the thyroid is a function of the relative rates of clearance of iodide by the thyroid and kidneys. The relation is simply expressed as follows:

$$\% \text{ uptake at plateau} = \frac{C_T}{C_T + C_K} \times 100$$

where C_T represents the thyroid iodide clearance rate and C_K the renal iodide clearance

---

*In the ensuing discussion, for purposes of brevity reference will be made to the most commonly used radioisotope of iodine, I^{131}; however, all considerations apply equally to other radioisotopes of iodine.

rate. Since the normal thyroid iodide clearance rate is approximately 0.4 liter/hr. and the renal iodide clearance 2.0 liters/hr., the ultimate uptake of I^{131} normally approximates 17 per cent of the administered dose (range, approximately 5–30 per cent).

The plateau value of the percentage thyroid uptake of I^{131} indicates the statistical likelihood that any molecule of iodide leaving the extracellular fluid will be accumulated by the thyroid and hence indicates the percentage of all the iodide removed from the ECF during any time period that is taken up by the thyroid. Measurements of the percentage thyroid uptake of I^{131} are generally made at 24 hours not only as a matter of convenience but also because the value at 24 hours is usually near its plateau except in unusual circumstances noted below.

The configuration of the curve describing the cumulative urinary excretion of I^{131} with time is similar to that which describes the thyroid collection of the isotope. In most circumstances, values for the two functions maintain a constant ratio that is the same as the ratio of their rates of iodide clearance.

Usually, measurements of thyroid I^{131} uptake are taken to be an index of thyroid hormone synthesis and, by inference, release into the blood. Clearly, however, the thyroid I^{131} uptake reveals only the efficiency of the gland relative to that of the kidney in removing iodide from the blood. A direct assessment of the efficiency of the thyroid with respect to iodine accumulation independent of that of the kidney is the measurement of thyroid iodide clearance rate, which relates the quantity of I^{131} accumulated during a standard time period to the concentration of I^{131} in the blood during the same period. However, neither the percentage uptake of I^{131} nor the thyroid iodide clearance rate provides information about the absolute quantity of iodine accumulated. Inferences concerning the latter can be drawn only if it is assumed that the flux of stable iodide into and out of ECF or the concentration of stable iodide in the blood is normal. Further assumptions inherent in equating any of the foregoing functions with the rate of hormone synthesis and release are that (1) at the time the measurement is made, significant quantities of I^{131} have not been released from the gland; (2) the I^{131} retained is being used for the formation and release of hormonally active products; and (3) the iodine accumulated is not being used merely to replenish depleted thyroid hormone stores. Instances in which these several assumptions are not valid and means by which they can be tested will be discussed later.

Thyroid Uptake of I^{131} (RAIU). This is the most commonly used isotopic procedure for the assessment of thyroid function per se. The 24-hour interval is generally selected not only because of its convenience to the patient but also because the value is then at or near its plateau except in severe abnormal states. Except in the latter circumstances, when measurements are best made at a far different time interval, it is not necessary that the uptake be determined at precisely 24 hours. Little difference will be noted if the uptake is measured any time during the day following the day on which the isotope was administered.

With the counting equipment currently available, the uptake can conveniently be determined with sufficient statistical accuracy following doses of 5–15 μCi. of I^{131}. The dose is usually given orally. There is no requirement that the patient be fasting before receiving the isotope or that special dietary precautions be observed thereafter. No restrictions on the activity of the patient need be imposed. No adverse reactions occur. An occasional patient will complain of symptoms allegedly induced by the I^{131}, but these are doubtless psychogenic and reflect apprehension about exposure to radiation. Still other patients will feel greatly improved by the testing procedure. At the designated time interval, the thyroid content of I^{131} is determined with a suitable detector, and this is compared with the I^{131} content of the administered dose (counting standard), positioned so as to simulate the geometric relationship of the patient's thyroid to the detector.

Because of the varying sensitivity of different counting devices to scattered or secondary radiation, variations in the geometry of the counting apparatus, and variations in iodine intake, the range of normal values for the uptake at any time interval varies among laboratories and should be determined individually. In general, the range of normal values is approximately 5–30 per cent. Higher values indicate thyroid hyperfunction; this usually but not always reflects hormone overproduction and a thyrotoxic state. (See Table 4–2 for a classification of factors affecting the 24-hour uptake.)

Sometimes under certain conditions it is best to measure the uptake before 24 hours after administration of the isotope. In states of severe thyroid hyperfunction, the uptake may be exceedingly rapid, plateau values being reached within a few hours or less. Thereafter, release of accumulated I^{131}, either as true hormone in severe thyrotoxicosis or as some hormonally inactive product, may be so rapid that the value for the uptake at 24 hours is well below its maximum and occasionally within the normal range. In thyrotoxicosis this is rare, and the clinical manifestations in such cases are so clear as to make the diagnosis obvious. Nevertheless, some laboratories choose to measure the uptake at an earlier time when hyperthyroidism is suspected. Recent data suggest that the upper limit of normal at 4 hours is approximately 12 per cent (Ghahremani et al., 1971). As with the 24-hour uptake (or with all other diagnostic procedures, for that matter), clinically difficult cases with borderline thyrotoxicosis often display values at or just above the upper limit of the normal range.

Thyroid Iodide Clearance Rate. In accumulating iodide and incorporating it into organic compounds that remain in the gland for some time, the thyroid can be considered to clear iodide from the plasma much as does the kidney. If the quantity of I^{131} accumulated by the thyroid during any time interval and the mean plasma concentration of I^{131}

TABLE 4–2. FACTORS THAT INFLUENCE THE 24-HOUR THYROID I^{131} UPTAKE

1. *Factors that Increase Uptake*
   Reflecting increased hormone synthesis
     Hyperthyroidism
     Response to glandular hormone depletion
       Recovery from thyroid suppression
       Recovery from subacute thyroiditis
       Antithyroid agents
     Excessive hormone losses
       Nephrosis
       Chronic diarrheal states
       Soybean ingestion
   Not reflecting increased hormone synthesis
     Iodine deficiency
       Dietary supply
       Excessive loss (dehalogenase defect, pregnancy)
     Hormone biosynthetic defects

2. *Factors that Decrease Uptake*
   Reflecting decreased hormone synthesis
     Primary hypofunction
       Thyroprivic hypothyroidism
       Antithyroid agents
       Some hormone biosynthetic defects
       Hashimoto's disease
       Subacute thyroiditis
     Secondary hypofunction
       Trophoprivic hypothyroidism
       Exogenous thyroid hormones
   Not reflecting decreased hormone synthesis
     Increased availability of iodine
       Dietary or pharmacologic supply
       Cardiac or renal insufficiency
     Increased hormone release
       Very severe hyperthyroidism (rare)

iodide during that interval are measured, the thyroid iodide clearance rate can be calculated from the conventional clearance formula:

$$\text{Thyroid iodide clearance rate } (C_T) = \frac{\text{Thyroid } I^{131} \text{ accumulation rate}}{\text{Plasma iodide}^{131} \text{ concentration}}$$

Since the calculation relates the rate of thyroid I^{131} uptake to the plasma iodide^{131} concentration, the measurement is uninfluenced by the rate of removal of iodide from the plasma by the kidneys. For this reason, the thyroid iodide clearance rate is considered by many to be the most direct index of thyroid activity with regard to iodine accumulation. Normal values for this function have not been established since the increase in dietary iodine intake has occurred but are probably of the order of 6 ml./min. Clearance rates are increased in states of thyroid hyperfunction, often to extremely high values, as in patients with severe thyrotoxicosis.

Clearance measurements require intravenous administration of I^{131}, serial counting of radioactivity in the thyroid, and analysis of plasma samples for iodide^{131}. They have not, therefore, gained wide clinical use despite efforts to simplify the procedure. Nevertheless, they remain important investigative tools.

Absolute Iodine Uptake. As already mentioned, isotopic measurements of thyroid iodine accumulation only provide information about rates of movement (e.g., clearance rates) or proportionate distribution (e.g., percentage uptake) of iodine. Al-though isotopic procedures are widely used alone because of their relative simplicity, the information that both the clinician and the physiologist truly desire, i.e., the absolute rate of iodine accumulation, requires conjoint measurement of radioactive and stable iodine. Such measurements are not generally employed clinically but have nevertheless provided important information of both a clinical and physiologic nature. Furthermore, the principles upon which measurements of absolute iodine uptake are based are diagnostically applicable in the difficult clinical case.

Several methods are available for measuring the absolute rate of thyroid iodine uptake or AIU. All are based on the inability of organs that metabolize iodide to distinguish between radioactive iodine and the stable form, I^{127}. The simplest method for measuring the absolute iodine uptake derives from the following consideration. During any time period after administration of I^{131},

$$\frac{\text{Thyroid } I^{131} \text{ accumulation}}{\text{Thyroid } I^{127} \text{ accumulation (AIU)}} = \frac{\text{Urinary } I^{131} \text{ content}}{\text{Urinary } I^{127} \text{ content}}$$

Rearranging,

$$\text{AIU} = \frac{\text{Urinary } I^{127} \text{ content} \times \text{thyroid } I^{131} \text{ accumulation}}{\text{Urinary } I^{131} \text{ content}}$$

Although measurements of thyroid and urinary I^{131} and of urinary I^{127} can be made at any time after administration of the isotope, they are usually performed at either 24 hours or within a few hours after the isotope is given. Normal values for the absolute iodine uptake obtained by this method now average about 120 μg. iodine/24 hr. This method is quite simple, requires no venipuncture, and can be used to ascertain whether abnormal values for thyroid I^{131} uptake are the result of reciprocal alterations in the extracellular iodide content.

Urinary Excretion of Radioiodine. Since the thyroid and kidneys are the main avenues for the removal of iodide from the plasma, the maximum urinary excretion and maximum thyroid accumulation of radioiodine together should approach 100 per cent of the administered dose. Accordingly, it should be possible to estimate the thyroid uptake of I^{131} from measurements of urinary I^{131} excretion. Normally the sum of thyroid and urinary I^{131} at 24 hours is at least 90 per cent of the dose. Thus values for urinary excretion of less than 60 per cent indicate an increased thyroid uptake and values greater than 85 per cent, a decreased thyroid uptake of I^{131}.

Although this method has the advantage of not requiring that the patient be brought to the radioisotope laboratory for epithyroid counting, several important disadvantages limit its clinical usefulness. First, incomplete urinary collections will lead to overestimation of thyroid activity. This will also be true in any condition in which renal excretion of I^{131} at 24 hours is considerably less than its ultimate maximum value.

On the other hand, in severe hyperthyroidism,

rapid release of labeled hormone from the gland may lead to underestimation of thyroid I^{131} uptake if epithyroid counting is employed; here, urinary excretion of I^{131} may reflect total thyroid accumulation of I^{131} more accurately. In this circumstance, the sum of thyroid and urinary I^{131} will be inordinately low; however, the concentration of protein-bound I^{131} (PBI^{131}) in the plasma will be greatly increased. A subnormal value for the sum of thyroid and urinary I^{131} (<70 per cent) will also occur when I^{131} is accumulated by ectopic thyroid tissue, such as struma ovarii or functioning metastatic tumors. Such lesions should be sought by external counting over multiple sites or by scinti-scanning procedures after large doses of radio-iodine.

States Associated with Increased Radioiodine Accumulation

Although an increased thyroid I^{131} uptake may reflect the overproduction and ultimate release of excessive quantities of thyroid hormone, it is important to recognize that many other factors will produce a similar abnormality of uptake tests. An increased uptake will occur whenever the thyroid iodide clearance rate is increased relative to that of the kidney. Such may reflect not hyperthyroidism but a compensatory response to factors tending to produce hypothyroidism. The following are the more important clinical states associated with an increased uptake of I^{131}.

Hyperthyroidism. Except in the case of T_3 toxicosis (see below), hyperthyroidism is almost invariably associated with an increased uptake, unless body iodide stores are increased. Such increases in uptake are evident at all times of measurement except in patients with severe thyrotoxicosis, in whom release of hormone is so rapid that the thyroid content of I^{131} has declined to the normal range by the time the measurement is made; this is rare and is usually associated with flagrant thyrotoxicosis. Unfortunately, in cases that are clinically marginal, uptake values are often within or just above the upper limit of the normal range, as would be expected.

Alterations in Hormone Synthesis. Uptake of I^{131} is increased in the absence of hyperthyroidism in a number of disorders in which accumulated iodine is inefficiently or ineffectively used to synthesize and secrete active hormone. Here, the impairment in iodine use leads to enhanced sensitivity to TSH, hypersecretion of TSH, or both; this in turn produces both goiter and stimulation of all steps in hormone synthesis capable of response. As a result, synthesis of normal quantities of hormone may resume; the patient will be metabolically normal but goitrous. Alternatively, secretion of hormone may remain inadequate, and the patient will display goitrous hypothyroidism. This sequence occurs as a consequence of defects in the organic-binding or coupling mechanisms or in the structure of the thyroglobulin molecule. It is also a consequence of disorders in which hormonally inactive products are released from the gland in the form of iodotyrosines (dehalogenase defect) or iodoproteins, including thyroglobulin. The magnitude of the increase in uptake and the time at which the plateau is achieved vary with the nature and severity of the disorder. In general, the increase in uptake is greater and the plateau occurs earlier in disorders characterized by intrathyroid enzymic abnormalities than in those associated with iodoprotein release. (See Stanbury, 1972, for references and illustrated functional patterns.) Differentiation of the foregoing states from hyperthyroidism is generally not difficult since, in the former, clinical evidence of hyperthyroidism will be lacking and indeed hypothyroidism may be present. Furthermore, the serum T_4 concentration will be normal and the serum TSH concentration sometimes increased. The increased uptake in patients with biosynthetic aberrations will, in almost all instances, be decreased by suppressive doses of exogenous hormone; this will not occur in patients with thyrotoxicosis. Finally, in the patient with thyrotoxicosis, the serum TSH concentration will not increase after administration of TRH, while the response in a patient with a biosynthetic defect will be normal or exaggerated.

Iodine Deficiency. Increases in thyroid iodide clearance rate and I^{131} uptake occur in response to acute or chronic iodine deficiency. Such deficiency can be demonstrated by measurement of urinary iodine excretion, values lower than 100 μg./day indicating a deficiency state. Chronic iodine deficiency is most often the result of an inadequate content of iodine in the food and water on which the patients subsist (endemic iodine deficiency). In the United States, this situation was formerly common in the Great Lakes area, but here and in the other areas of the world its frequency has been greatly reduced by the use of iodized salt. Deficiency of iodine may also result from other than environmental factors. Patients with cardiac, renal, or hepatic disease may develop iodine deficiency if given diets severely restricted in salt. Iodine deficiency not uncommonly occurs in patients with thyrotoxicosis treated with antithyroid drugs; this may forestall recurrence of thyrotoxicity when treatment is withdrawn (Harden et al., 1966). Thyroid hyperfunction in the normal pregnant woman is the result of increased renal iodide clearance. Iodine deficiency evidently plays a role in the goitrous hypothyroidism associated with deficiency of thyroid and peripheral iodotyrosine dehalogenase in which large quantities of iodine are lost in the urine as iodotyrosines.

In severe iodine deficiency, in addition to the quantitative adjustments in thyroid avidity for iodide which the increased I^{131} uptake reflects, a qualitative adaption occurs in which T_3 is preferentially synthesized and secreted. As a result, the ratio of T_3 to T_4 in the plasma is increased (DeLange et al., 1972a). This mechanism has important adaptive value, since for each atom of iodine secreted the calorigenic impact is approximately four times as great when the iodine is affixed to T_3 than when it is part of T_4.

Response to Thyroid Hormone Depletion. Withdrawal of factors that lead to thyroid hormone depletion is associated with a rebound increase in thyroid hormone synthesis without an associated increase in hormone release. If hormone depletion has been produced by factors that lead to decreased hormone supply to the tissues, such as antithyroid drugs, the rebound response may reflect in part enhanced TSH stimulation and in part an autoregulatory response to depletion of thyroid hormone stores. In other instances, only the latter mechanism appears responsible. Rebound increases in uptake of I^{131} are seen after withdrawal of antithyroid therapy, after relief of subacute thyroiditis, and after prolonged suppression of thyroid function by exogenous hormone. A striking increase in uptake is evident in patients with iodide-induced myxedema following cessation of iodide administration. The duration of the rebound is variable and probably depends on the time required to replenish thyroid hormone stores. Generally its duration is no longer than several weeks, but after withdrawal of prolonged thyroid suppression, an abnormally high uptake may persist for many weeks. Differentiation from thyrotoxicosis is evident from the history and from differences in the values of other conventional indices of thyroid function.

Excessive Hormone Losses. Instances in which excessive losses of thyroid hormone occur may be associated with a compensatory increase in hormone synthesis that is, in turn, evident in an increased uptake of I^{131}. The outstanding example of this sequence occurs in nephrosis, in which excessive losses of hormone in the urine in association with urinary loss of binding protein take place. In addition, diminished binding of T_4 in the plasma in nephrosis may lead to excessive loss of hormone via the feces. Some patients with nephrosis display an increased uptake, presumably as a result of the loss of hormonal iodine. A similar sequence may occur when losses of hormone via the GI tract are abnormal, such as in chronic diarrheal states or during ingestion of soybean, which binds hormone in the gut.

States Associated with Decreased Radioiodine Accumulation

Hypothyroidism. Insufficient production of thyroid hormone leading to hypothyroidism is usually reflected in a decreased thyroid I^{131} uptake. When hypothyroidism results from insufficient functioning tissue (thyroprivic hypothyroidism), values for thyroid I^{131} uptake tend to be lower than when hypothyroidism results from insufficient stimulation by TSH (trophoprivic hypothyroidism). This difference has been obscured, however, by the recent increase in dietary iodine intake. By contrast, hypothyroidism that results from qualitative abnormalities in hormone synthesis is usually associated with growth of thyroid tissue (goitrous hypothyroidism); here, the avidity for iodine is often high. An exception to the latter rule

is the rare form of goitrous hypothyroidism due to absence of the iodide transport mechanism.

The syndrome of decreased thyroid reserve is a special instance of thyroprivic hypothyroidism in which destruction of functioning thyroid tissue is incomplete. Uptake values within the normal range are often seen, but these fail to increase after administration of exogenous TSH. Moreover, the concentration of endogenous TSH in serum is usually increased.

Relatively transient decreases in uptake associated with decreased hormone formation characteristically occur in patients with subacute thyroiditis. Here, the serum T_4 concentration is normal or increased and, together with the classic clinical findings, serves to differentiate this disorder from a true hypothyroid state.

Exogenous Thyroid Hormone. Except in those disorders in which homeostatic control is disrupted (Grave's disease, autonomously functioning thyroid nodules), administration of physiologic replacement doses of thyroid hormone will suppress secretion of TSH and lead to lowering of the thyroid I^{131} uptake, usually to values below 5 per cent if complete replacement doses are administered. Suppression of uptake can be effected by adequate quantities of any thyroactive material and, depending on the dose administered, a eumetabolic or hypermetabolic state will be present. When suppression is effected by T_4 or thyroid extract, the serum T_4 concentration will be normal or increased, but when suppression is effected by T_3, the serum T_4 concentration will be subnormal. The patient whose thyroid is suppressed by exogenous hormone is physiologically similar to the patient with trophoprivic hypothyroidism. Reversal of the decreased uptake by exogenous TSH or a subnormal value for serum TSH concentration will readily distinguish these two states from thyroprivic hypothyroidism but not from each other.

Exposure to Excessive Iodine. Exposure to excessive iodine and expansion of body iodide stores is probably the most common cause for a subnormal thyroid I^{131} uptake. Such decreases are "spurious" in the clinical sense, since they do not indicate decreased absolute iodine uptake and decreased hormone production. They are not spurious in the physiologic sense, however, since they reflect a desirable homeostatic response to overavailability of the iodide substrate.

The decreased fractional uptake of iodide resides in an autoregulatory inhibition of the iodide transport mechanism as a result of the increase in the glandular stores of organic iodine. In addition, when plasma iodide concentrations are sufficiently high, dilution of the administered isotope by stable iodide would lead to a decreased percentage accumulation of the isotope. As indicated in an earlier section, the compensatory response to excessive iodine stores is not perfect, and total iodine accumulation during continued overabundance of iodide will exceed normal values. Nevertheless, the excess iodine is not incorporated into active hormone but is organified and then lost from the gland largely as iodide itself (Wartofsky and Ingbar, 1971).

A decreased thyroid I[131] intake can be produced by the introduction of excessive quantities of iodine into the body in any form — inorganic, organic, or elemental. Special offenders in this regard are organic iodinated dyes used as x-ray contrast media. The duration of suppression of the uptake varies from individual to individual and with the compound administered, depending on its rapidity of excretion or deiodination. In general, dyes used for pyelography are cleared relatively rapidly, while those used in cholecystography persist longer and may influence the uptake for several months. Inorganic iodide may be ingested directly, usually as an expectorant, and following a single large dose, a decreased uptake may persist for several days. Following chronic ingestion of iodide, depression of the uptake may persist for many weeks. It should be noted in this regard that Lugol's solution or saturated solution of potassium iodide (SSKI) in the dosage usually given will deliver up to about 500 mg. of iodine daily. In addition to iodide per se and iodinated dyes, excessive quantities of iodine may be encountered in a variety of other forms, including vitamins and mineral preparations, vaginal or rectal suppositories, and iodinated antiseptics. Some preparations of barium sulfate used in x-ray diagnosis may contain substantial quantities of iodine, as may certain preparations of bromsulfophthalein. In the northeastern United States and Canada, some patients may snack on a dried seaweed preparation rich in iodine known as "dults." Inhibition of uptake resulting from excess stable iodine is of shorter duration in hyperthyroid than in normal individuals.

The measurement of urinary iodine excretion provides a useful means for establishing the existence of excessive body iodide stores. Values in excess of 1000 μg. daily suggest that a subnormal thyroid I[131] uptake need not indicate hypothyroidism.

Decreased Renal Iodide Clearance. Reduction in renal iodide clearance rate, whether it be due to renal or cardiac insufficiency, will result in an increased plasma inorganic iodide concentration if dietary iodine intake remains unchanged. Thus, unless thyroid function is correspondingly decreased, absolute iodine uptake will be abnormally large. In most instances, a compensatory decrease in thyroid iodide clearance rate is effected, but this may be insufficient to keep absolute iodine uptake within normal limits. Although the maximum uptake would be expected to be normal in patients whose renal function is decreased, the proportionate reduction in thyroid and renal iodide clearance rates will result in a slow clearance of I[131] from the plasma, and maximum values for the uptake will not be achieved by 24 hours. Rather, the uptake at 24 hours tends to be subnormal and will increase to a normal value by 48–72 hours. Although this is the usual sequence in patients with impaired renal function, the maximum uptake is occasionally increased. The factors underlying this unexpected occurrence are unknown.

Measurements of Thyroid Radioiodine Turnover and Release

Physiologic Basis. Following accumulation and organification of radioiodine, release from the thyroid of labeled products occurs. With the aid of radioiodine, the fractional rate of release or turnover of thyroid iodine can be inferred either from direct observation of the rate of I[131] disappearance from the gland or from the rate of appearance of iodinated products in the blood. There are, however, several problems involved in drawing conclusions about the absolute rate of release of thyroid hormone from observations of the types just described. First, any inference concerning the quantity of hormone released requires knowledge of the iodine content of the pool or pools whose turnover is being measured; this is rarely available. Furthermore, the earlier, tacitly accepted concept that the entire thyroid behaves as a homogeneous entity is no longer tenable. Both anatomical and functional heterogeneity exists in the thyroid. Hence the iodine released is likely drawn from at least several pools of varying iodine content and turnover rate. Finally, other products (including iodide, iodotyrosines, and thyroglobulin or other iodoproteins) may be released. Their release would, of course, be reflected in the loss of I[131] from the gland or the appearance of radioiodinated materials in the blood.

Thyroid Release of I[131]. In this technique, a moderately large dose of I[131] (50 μCi. or more) is administered and allowed to accumulate in the thyroid. Serial epithyroid counts will then reveal the rate of release of accumulated I[131]. In order that the curve describing release of the initially accumulated I[131] not be obscured by reaccumulation of I[131] already secreted by the gland, completely blocking doses of an antithyroid agent are generally administered. When this is done, the curve of epithyroid counts closely conforms to a single exponential function of time, indicating the release of a constant fraction of thyroid I[131]/unit time. When corrected for physical decay of the isotope, such observations indicate a rate of turnover of accumulated I[131] in normal humans of about 1 per cent daily. The rate of glandular I[131] turnover is accelerated, often greatly so, in states associated with thyroid hyperfunction. In view of the considerable period of time and multiple observations required by this technique, it is rarely used for clinical diagnosis, particularly since indirect methods involving measurement of hormonal radioiodine in blood are available. The technique has, however, been very effectively employed in physiologic studies. TSH can be shown to enhance acutely, and iodide to retard acutely, the rate of I[131] release (Fig. 4–11).

Serum Protein-bound I[131]. An alternative to the direct measurement of thyroid I[131] release is the measurement of the radioiodinated products of glandular secretion in the serum. Radioiodinated T_4 and T_3 secreted from the gland are bound to plasma proteins and hence are measurable as protein-bound I^{131} (PBI^{131}). This can be separated from radioiodide by trichloroacetic acid precipitation of serum or by exposure of the serum to an ion-exchange resin. The concentration of PBI^{131} in serum is related to the administered dose of I^{131} in samples of serum obtained at 24, 48, or 72 hours after radioiodine administration. High values are indicative of thyroid hyperfunction but not necessarily of hyperthyroidism, since the PBI^{131} will be increased whenever the turnover of the thyroid organic iodine pool is rapid. A typical example is the case of the functioning thyroid remnant, in which high values for the PBI^{131} may be associated with frank hypothyroidism. The PBI^{131} does not discriminate well between normal patients and patients with thyroid hypofunction.

Tests Related to the Concentration and Binding of Thyroid Hormones in Blood

Measurements of the serum concentrations of the two thyroid hormones and of the extent of their association with plasma proteins have become the most commonly employed tests for differentiating among the hypothyroid, euthyroid, and hyperthyroid states. This has resulted from the development of highly sensitive and specific methods for measuring T_4 and T_3 in blood and from a better understanding of the factors other than alterations in the rate of hormone production that influence their concentrations. Because of their wide use and clinical importance, their physiologic interest, and the large number of factors that influence their interpretation, these tests will be considered in detail.

Physiologic Basis

Until quite recently, the thyroid hormones in the blood could be measured only by virtue of their iodine content. This basically nonspecific procedure was rendered somewhat more valuable by the fact that the hormones are bound to plasma proteins, a fact which made possible separation of hormonal iodine from inorganic iodide through measurement of the protein-bound iodine or PBI. The latter, however, did not serve to differentiate between hormonal iodine and a variety of exogenous or endogenous products that contained iodine and that were either bound to protein or were proteins themselves. The development of methods for measuring T_4 specifically constituted a giant step forward in the accuracy of clinical diagnosis and in physiologic understanding (Fig. 4–13). Concomitantly, the PBI was relegated to infrequent use except in special circumstances discussed below.

The ability to measure T_3, which followed by several years the ability to measure T_4, further refined diagnostic accuracy but also increased complexity, since the concentrations of the two hormones do not always deviate from normal to the same extent or in the same direction. Instances in which this is the case are discussed below. Finally, the interaction between both T_4 and T_3 and plasma proteins renders interpretation of alterations in the concentration of these hormones in blood more complex, since changes in concentration may reflect a primary alteration in hormone binding rather than in hormone supply.

It is important to understand how these two causes of an altered hormone concentration differ from one another in terms of the concentration of free hormone, the kinetics of hormone metabolism, and the metabolic state of the patient. In the following discussion, T_4 will be employed as the prototype, since both the interaction between T_4 and its

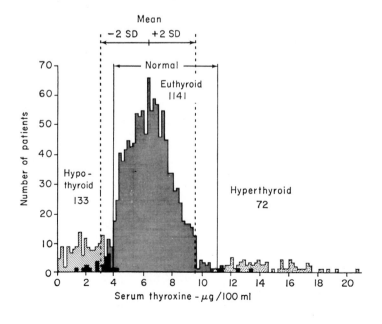

Figure 4–13. Distribution of values for serum T_4 concentration in euthyroid, hypothyroid, and hyperthyroid patients. Because the euthyroid values are not normally distributed, the normal range is arbitrarily selected and appears preferable to the mean ±2 (SD). (From Murphy, B. E. P.: *Recent Progr. Hormone Res.* 25:563, 1969.)

major binding protein in plasma, TBG, and the kinetic consequences thereof appear to be the same for both hormones. In all states of thyroid dysfunction leading to secretion of abnormal quantities of T_4, the normal homeostatic mechanism that regulates thyroid function is disrupted, with the result that either excessive or insufficient secretion of hormone continues. In hyperthyroidism, for example, excessive quantities of hormone are released into the circulation. Since the removal of hormone from the blood is a first-order reaction (a constant proportion being removed per unit time), entry of hormone into the blood will initially exceed removal, and hence the concentration of hormone will rise. This increase will continue until removal and entry are once again in equilibrium, at which time the concentration of hormone in the blood will be increased. The consequences of such an increase on the protein-binding interaction are best seen by examining the binding equilibrium:

$$T_4 + TBG \rightleftharpoons T_4 \cdot TBG$$

and

$$\frac{(T_4 \cdot TBG)}{(T_4)(TBG)} = k$$

In this formulation, $(T_4 \cdot TBG)$ represents the concentration of bound T_4; (T_4), the concentration of free T_4; and (TBG), the concentration of unoccupied protein-binding sites. The constant, k, represents the equilibrium constant for the interaction between T_4 and TBG. In hyperthyroid states, the concentration of binding proteins does not increase proportionately to the increase in hormone concentration; indeed, the concentration of binding sites decreases as a result of decreased TBG and perhaps TBPA. The foregoing formulation indicates, therefore, that the concentrations of both total and free T_4 increase, but that the relative increase in free T_4 exceeds the increase in total hormone, so that the proportion of free T_4 increases. The increased proportion of free T_4 results in an increased proportion of extracellular hormone degraded daily. In addition, the absolute concentration of free T_4 having increased, more hormone is available to the cells, more hormone is degraded daily, and the metabolic state of the patient increases. The consequences of decreased secretion of hormone are the converse of those found in hyperthyroidism.

Far different consequences follow primary changes in the concentration of TBG (Fig. 4–8). When this is increased, for example, T_4 initially shifts from the free to the bound form, because of the increase in binding sites. This decrease in free hormone concentration results in decreased hormone disposal, while secretion of hormone is undiminished. Hence the concentration of hormone in the ECF increases until the binding equilibrium again provides a normal concentration of free hormone and a normal rate of hormone disposal. Here too, as in hyperthyroidism, the total concentration of hormone at physiologic equilibrium is increased, but, in contrast, the absolute concentration of free

hormone and the metabolic state of the patient are normal. Since the total concentration of hormone is increased and the concentration of free hormone normal, the proportion of free hormone is decreased, and hence the fractional turnover rate of hormone diminished. Provided that entry of hormone via secretion or ingestion is held constant, increased hormone binding will result in increased circulating hormone and restoration of physiologic equilibrium. For example, in patients with hypothyroidism receiving constant doses of exogenous hormone, increases in TBG are associated with an increased serum T_4 concentration. It is not clear to what extent homeostatic mechanisms act to speed restoration of physiologic equilibrium in normal individuals by increasing hormone secretion. Converse effects are associated with primary decreases in hormone binding.

Considerable attention has been paid to the differentiation between the proportion of free hormone and the absolute concentration of free hormone. The proportion of free hormone per se has no direct relation to the metabolic state of the patient but influences the kinetics of hormone metabolism. Its clinical importance stems from the fact that several tests have been designed to detect alterations in the proportion of free hormone. When such tests are used for the diagnosis of hyper- or hypothyroidism, abnormalities are presumed to result from primary changes in the concentration of hormone in the blood. From the foregoing discussion, however, it is evident that alterations similar to those produced by primary thyroid disorders also occur when the concentration of TBG is abnormal. Differentiation between these alternatives can be achieved by calculating the absolute concentration of free hormone as the product of the total concentration and the proportion that is free. This will be normal in circumstances associated solely with a change in TBG and abnormal in situations resulting primarily from a change in hormone supply. In both categories, the metabolic state of the patient will usually correlate well with the absolute concentration of free hormone, suggesting that the latter is a physiologically important variable.

Despite the foregoing, it is clear that measurements of the absolute concentrations of free T_4 and free T_3 do not in all circumstances provide clarification of the metabolic state of the patient. If, as some have suggested, T_4 is lacking in intrinsic biologic activity and is active only by virtue of its conversion to T_3, then the correlation noted between the absolute concentration of free T_4 and the metabolic state of the patient probably stems from a correlation between the concentration of free T_4 and the rate of generation of T_3. In this case, the proximate correlation would be between the metabolic state of the patient and the absolute concentration of free T_3. On the other hand, if, as seems likely, T_4 has some intrinsic metabolic activity, problems are posed in circumstances, such as incipient thyroid failure and endemic goiter, in which changes in the absolute concentrations of free T_4 and free T_3 are in discordant directions. For example, there is currently no indication as to the increase in the concentration of free T_3 that is required to offset a decrease in the concentration of free T_4.

It has also become clear that the absolute concentration of free hormone is not the sole determinant of the rate of hormone disposal, since alterations in the activity of factors within the cell itself also influence hormone turnover. Such influences are operative in some patients with Graves' disease and are also seen in patients receiving drugs, such as diphenylhydantoin or phenobarbital, that accelerate cellular disposal of hormone, possibly through the induction of a variety of microsomal enzymes (Cullen et al., 1972; Oppenheimer et al., 1971). Despite the foregoing complexities, it should be emphasized that in the great majority of clinical circumstances measurements of the concentration of total and free T_4 and, when necessary, T_3 will provide important and accurate information concerning the thyroid status of the patient.

Measurements of Hormone Concentration

Serum T_4 Concentration. Several methods are available for the specific measurement of T_4 in serum. Of these, the most common are variants of the competitive protein-binding technique first introduced by Murphy and Pattee. In this technique, the T_4 is extracted from the serum either with organic solvents or by exposure of the serum to adsorptive material. With radioiodine-labeled T_4 as a tracer, the extracted T_4 is allowed to interact with a standard quantity of TBG, and the apportionment of the hormone between the bound and free forms is determined. This apportionment is indicative of the quantity of T_4 in the serum extract when related to a standard curve prepared by interacting known quantities of T_4 with the standard solution of TBG.

The extreme specificity of the interaction between T_4 and TBG renders this method highly specific in the clinical setting. Although T_3 also interacts with TBG, its affinity for the protein is so much less than that of T_4 that concentrations of T_3, even when greatly increased, do not influence the analysis for T_4. The great variety of iodinated compounds that create such difficulty in the interpretation of the PBI have no influence on the measurement of T_4 by this technique. Normal values for the serum T_4 concentration by this technique vary between 4 and 11 μg./100 ml. Values are sometimes reported in terms of T_4-iodine; these are derived by multiplying the measured T_4 concentration by 0.65, which is the mole fraction of T_4 that is iodine.

The serum T_4 concentration can also be measured conveniently by radioimmunoassay. Values obtained by this technique accord well with those obtained by the competitive protein-binding analysis discussed above. Other methods employ column or thin-layer chromatography to separate T_4 from other iodinated materials, the iodine content being determined in the T_4 eluate. As these chromato-graphic methods ("T_4 by column") do not afford a clear separation of T_4 from high concentrations of iodinated contaminants, such as radiographic contrast media, they are now used with decreasing frequency.

Serum T_3 Concentration. The first methods available for measuring T_3 in serum on a routine basis were introduced by Naumann, Werner, Sterling, and their respective co-workers and used the competitive protein-binding principle, similar to that employed for the measurement of serum T_4. Although these methods were important in stimulating interest in this subject, experience has shown them to be more difficult to perform and less likely to be accurate than measurements of T_3 by radioimmunoassay. This follows from the fact that, if TBG is to be used as the standard binding protein, the serum extract containing T_3 must be entirely freed of T_4 under conditions in which no T_3 is generated artifactually from the far higher concentrations of T_4 present in serum. Consequently, radioimmunoassay of T_3 is now invariably employed. Antibody for the assay is prepared by immunizing rabbits with a complex of T_3 covalently bonded to a protein, such as bovine serum albumin. T_3 is then measured either in an extract of serum or in whole serum itself. In the latter case, an inhibitor of T_3 binding to TBG must be added to make T_3 entirely available to the antibody. Although normal values for the serum T_3 concentration by radioimmunoassay initially varied widely, there is a growing consensus that the mean normal value is approximately 120 ng./100 ml. (see Surks et al., 1972, for references). The mean normal value for serum T_3 concentration declines with advancing age to approximately two-thirds of that for young adults by the ninth decade (Brunelle and Bohuon, 1972).

Serum PBI. Although the mainstay of thyroid diagnosis for many years, measurements of PBI are now infrequently performed. The serum PBI measures iodine in T_4, the exceedingly small quantity of iodine in T_3, a great variety of iodinated materials of exogenous origin that are bound to protein, and a class of compounds, usually of endogenous origin, termed iodoproteins, in which iodine is covalently bound within the peptide sequence of the protein molecule. Hence, when exogenous contaminants are absent, the difference between the PBI and the T_4-iodine is an index of the iodine contained in iodoproteins. Such iodoproteins are commonly found in the sera of patients with Hashimoto's disease and subacute thyroiditis and may also be present in the sera of patients with nontoxic goiter and thyroid neoplasms. Here, measurement of the PBI–T_4-iodine difference may be of diagnostic value. Thus the PBI is no longer used as a measure of hormonal iodine but rather as a measure of nonhormonal iodine in the blood.

Measurements of Hormone Binding

As indicated earlier, the importance of tests that reflect hormone binding in serum stems from the fact that they afford the most convenient means of determining whether a change in the total concentration of hormone is due to a change in its binding or a change in its production rate. The tests assume critical importance, therefore, in differentiating hyper- and hypothyroidism from the euthyroid state.

Proportion and Concentration of Free T_4 and T_3.   The concentrations of free T_4 and T_3 in serum are too low to be measured directly by any available technique. The proportion of free T_4 or T_3 can be measured, however, with the aid of the appropriate synthetic radioiodine-labeled hormone. The serum is enriched with a tracer quantity of the labeled hormone, and this is quickly distributed between the free and bound forms in a manner analogous to the behavior of the endogenous hormone. Since the free hormone is capable of passing through a dialysis membrane while the bound is not, the former can be assessed by means of ultrafiltration or dialysis techniques.

Since the methods of analysis vary somewhat, principally in whether whole or dilute serum is used, normal values for the proportion of free T_4 have varied among laboratories but generally range between 0.02 and 0.04 per cent of the total. Because of its lesser affinity for TBG, the proportion of free T_3 is normally about ten times that of T_4, i.e., 0.30 per cent of the total. The absolute concentrations of free T_4 and free T_3 can readily be calculated as the product of their respective total concentrations and the proportion of each that is free. Normal values approximate 2 ng./100 ml. for free T_4 and 0.4 ng./100 ml. for free T_3.

In Vitro Uptake Tests.   Since direct measurements of the proportion of free T_4 and T_3 are time-consuming and cumbersome, a variety of simpler methods have been devised. In common with measurements of the proportion of free T_4 and T_3, these provide evidence of the overall intensity of hormone binding in serum. They serve as an index, therefore, of the proportion of free T_4 and T_3. Such tests are performed by enriching the patient's serum with a tracer quantity of radioiodine-labeled hormone and incubating the serum with an insoluble particulate material that is capable of binding the hormone and competing with the binding proteins in the serum phase. After a standard interval, the proportion of labeled hormone bound by the particulate phase is determined. This varies inversely with the concentration and binding affinity of unoccupied binding sites on the individual binding proteins, principally TBG. Labeled T_3 is usually used in preference to labeled T_4 because of its less intense binding; this yields a higher uptake onto the particulate material, thereby reducing counting error. Variations in the techniques used stem principally from differences in the particulate material used. Among these are anion exchange resins, either in granular form or impregnated in a sponge, coated charcoal, or Sephadex. The normal values must be determined for each laboratory in which the test is performed.

The product of the *in vitro* uptake value and the serum total T_4 concentration provides a so-called

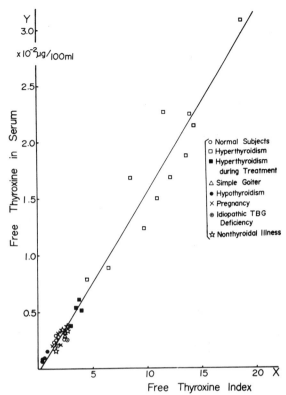

Figure 4–14. In the study from which this figure was derived, serum T_4 concentration was estimated from measurements of the PBI. The correlation between free T_4 concentration measured by dialysis and the free T_4 index is clearly demonstrated. Linearity of the relationship was achieved by calculating the free T_4 index as follows: PBI × RT_3U/1-0.6 RT_3U. Note that values for both functions in circumstances in which TBG is altered are in the normal range. (From Hamada, S., Nakagawa, T., et al.: *J. Clin. Endocr. 31*:166, 1970.)

"free T_4 index" which is analogous to and varies with the absolute concentration of free T_4 (Fig. 4–14). Such calculations can be performed regardless of whether T_3 or T_4 was used as the labeled hormone, but normal values for the indices obtained with labeled T_3 will be much higher than those obtained with T_4. Abnormalities in the free T_4 index have the same significance as changes in the absolute concentration of free T_4. Although measurements of a "free T_3 index" have not been reported, it is to be expected that this would vary in a manner analogous to the absolute concentration of free T_3. Kits have been developed which measure directly a free T_4 index in that the total T_4 concentration is "corrected" for variations in the concentration of TBG. It is not recommended, however, that measurements of a free T_4 index be made to the exclusion of measurements of serum total T_4 concentration.

T_4-Binding Capacities of TBG and TBPA.   It is occasionally desirable to verify the results of indirect methods of assessing hormone binding by measuring directly the T_4-binding capacities of TBG and TBPA. The test sample of serum is enriched with both labeled T_4 and varying concentrations of stable T_4, and aliquots are then subjected to filter-paper electrophoresis. From the percentage distribution of the labeled hormone among the binding proteins and the known total concentration of hormone in each specimen, the absolute quantity of T_4 bound by each protein per unit volume of serum can be determined. At sufficiently high concentrations of added T_4, maximum binding capacities are determined. Under most analytic conditions, the T_4-binding capacity of TBG averages approximately 20 μg. T_4 per 100 ml. of serum. The binding capacity of TBPA is far more subject to variations based upon methodologic differences, mean normal values ranging from 150–300 μg./100 ml. Measurements of T_4-binding capacity are time-consuming and are generally carried out only in specialized laboratories. They are, however, of value in providing direct confirmation of abnormalities in hormone binding suggested by more indirect techniques.

The recent purification of TBG and production of antibodies thereto has made possible measurement of the concentration of this protein in serum by radioimmunoassay. Such assays have demonstrated a good concordance between the T_4-binding capacity of TBG in abnormal states and the actual concentration of the protein in serum (Levy et al., 1971).

Disorders Associated with Increased Serum T_4 and T_3 Concentrations

In the majority of thyroid disorders, the serum concentrations of T_4 and T_3 either are both normal or diverge from normal in the same direction (see review by Larsen, 1972, for references concerning the serum T_3 concentration in various states). This is true of the disorders discussed both in this section and in the immediately ensuing section that describes disorders associated with decreased concentrations of the hormones in serum. Disorders in which serum T_4 and T_3 are divergent are discussed in a separate section.

As indicated earlier, increases in serum T_4 and T_3 concentrations may result primarily from alterations in their supply or from alterations in hormone binding.

Increased Hormone Supply. An increase in serum T_4 concentration is the mark of hyperthyroidism, regardless of whether this reflects the presence of Graves' disease, toxic multinodular goiter, toxic adenoma, or those rare varieties of hyperthyroidism that occur in diseases associated with ectopic or inappropriate thyroid stimulators (molar pregnancy, choriocarcinoma within the uterus or testis, and TSH-producing pituitary tumors). Patients with mild clinical manifestations are likely to have marginal elevations of serum T_4, and values above 20 μg./100 ml. are rarely seen except in the most severe cases.

To date, there are no known examples of hyperthyroidism associated with an increase in serum T_4 concentration without an accompanying increase in serum T_3 concentration. Indeed, in the

case of the common causes of hyperthyroidism, both the serum T_3 concentration and the T_3 production rate are disproportionately increased relative to the increases seen in T_4. Although it is possible that the enhanced production of T_3 results from increased peripheral generation from T_4, it is likely that direct hypersecretion of T_3 plays a more prominent role.

Owing to the increase in hormone concentration and, frequently, to a decrease in the concentration of TBG, the proportions of free T_4 and free T_3, as well as their *in vitro* uptake values, are increased. Calculated values of absolute concentrations of free T_4 and free T_3 and their corresponding indices would be increased more markedly.

Modest increases in serum T_4 concentration are frequently seen in hypothyroid patients receiving what has been considered to be the requisite maintenance dose of L-thyroxine (300 μg. daily). In such patients, the serum T_3 is derived entirely through generation from T_4 in the peripheral tissues, and its concentration is in the slightly low to low-normal range. In view of recent evidence, it is likely that doses of L-thyroxine that elevate the serum T_4 concentration are slightly in excess of physiologic requirements (Braverman et al., 1973). Serum T_4 and, in all likelihood, serum T_3 concentrations are increased both in patients with thyrotoxicosis factitia resulting from the ingestion of thyroid extract or L-thyroxine and in patients with thyrotoxicosis resulting from hyperfunction of ectopic thyroid tissue. Indices of hormone binding will be similar to those seen in thyrotoxicosis of thyroidal origin. In the absence of coincidental thyroid disease, these disorders can be distinguished from hyperthyroidism by the presence of a suppressed thyroid I^{131} uptake and atrophy of the thyroid gland.

Increased Hormone Binding. A variety of clinical states is associated with an increase in the concentration of TBG in plasma (Table 4–3). In these situations, a number of secondary consequences occur (Fig. 4–8). Most important clinically are the secondary increase in serum T_4 concentration and the decrease in the proportion of free T_4 and in values for *in vitro* uptake tests. The absolute concentration of free T_4 is normal and the

TABLE 4–3. CIRCUMSTANCES ASSOCIATED WITH ALTERATIONS IN THE CONCENTRATION OF TBG

1. *Increased Concentration of TBG*
   Pregnancy
   Neonatal state
   Estrogens and hyperestrogenemic states
   Oral contraceptives
   Acute intermittent porphyria
   Infectious hepatitis
   Genetic determination

2. *Decreased Concentration of TBG*
   Androgenic or anabolic steroids
   Large doses of glucocorticoids
   Active acromegaly
   Nephrotic syndrome
   Major illnesses
   Genetic determination

metabolic state of the patient unchanged. Kinetically, the fractional rate of turnover and rate of clearance of T_4 peripherally are decreased, but because of the increased content of the peripheral T_4 pool, total disposal of hormone is normal.

The most common natural cause of increased TBG is normal pregnancy. The increase is often demonstrable as early as the first week after the first missed menstrual period. The T_4-binding capacity of TBG then rises rapidly from its normal value of approximately 20 μg./ml., reaching a maximum of approximately 50 or 60 μg./100 ml. during the second or third month and remaining constant thereafter. Values for the serum T_4 concentration increase *pari passu* and during normal pregnancy range between 7 and 12 μg./100 ml. Somewhat lesser elevations of serum T_4 concentration are seen in the cord blood of the neonate. Post partum, the binding capacity of TBG and the serum T_4 concentration decline progressively, returning to normal values in 4–6 weeks. Changes in other transport proteins are evident in pregnancy; thus concentrations of corticosteroid binding globulin and ceruloplasmin are also increased.

The early increase in TBG and serum T_4 concentration often fails to occur in women destined to undergo spontaneous abortion by the tenth or twelfth week of pregnancy. However, when pregnancy persists beyond this period, the usual increase in TBG is seen, even though abortion may occur subsequently. It seems fairly certain that early fetal loss is not the result of an inadequate TBG response to normal stimuli but that such stimuli are themselves inadequate because of intrinsic abnormality of the conceptus.

The increased TBG of the pregnant woman and the neonate is almost surely due to increased secretion of estrogen, since large doses of natural or synthetic estrogens within a few weeks increase TBG and the serum T_4 concentration to values found during normal pregnancy. This response is seen in both men and women. Comparable values are achieved with smaller doses of estrogen but more slowly. A very frequent cause of an increased TBG and serum T_4 concentration is the oral contraceptive agents; these vary in their potency in this regard, depending upon their constituent hormones (Winikoff and Taylor, 1966).

In the authors' experience, estimation of TBG has proved to be of value in differentiating true precocious puberty from pseudoprecocious puberty caused by estrogen-secreting tumors. In the latter disorders, but not in the former, abnormally high values for TBG, consistent with those observed during pregnancy, have been found.

An increase in TBG and serum T_4 concentration has been found in some patients with acute intermittent porphyria, especially women. The reason for this exceptionally interesting finding is unclear (Hollander et al., 1967).

Patients with infectious hepatitis not infrequently display an increase in TBG. The serum PBI and presumably the serum T_4 concentration are elevated. Some of the elevation of PBI may be due to biliary reflux of conjugated T_4.

An increase in TBG may accompany the prolonged administration of perphenazine (Trilafon).

Rarely, increased TBG is the result of a familial disorder that appears to be transmitted as an X chromosome-linked trait. It is usually discovered by finding an elevated TBG and serum T_4 concentration, evidence of unsaturation of the binding proteins, normal thyroid function, and a euthyroid state. There is no evidence of excessive estrogen secretion, and the concentration of other estrogen-sensitive transport proteins is not abnormal.

Although not studied in all circumstances associated with an increase in TBG, serum T_3 concentration is increased during pregnancy and estrogen treatment and in patients with an idiopathic increase in TBG. It appears, however, that the increase in serum T_3 concentration is less marked than that of T_4. Absolute rates of T_3 disposal are normal in patients with increased TBG, suggesting that the kinetic consequences of the altered binding of T_3 are similar to those for T_4 (Nicoloff et al., 1972). A notable exception to the concordant behavior of serum T_4 and T_3 concentrations in association with increased TBG occurs in the neonate. Here, although serum T_4 concentrations are higher than they are later in life, the serum T_3 concentrations are distinctly lower (Abuid et al., 1973).

Disorders Associated with Decreased Serum T_4 and T_3 Concentrations

Decreased Hormone Supply. Decreases in serum T_4 concentration characterize hypothyroid states. Similarly, serum T_3 concentrations are decreased in frank hypothyroidism, although often not to as great an extent as the serum T_4 concentration. Moreover, in mild or incipient thyroid failure, in the presence of a clinical state that appears to be normal, the serum T_4 concentration may be low while the serum T_3 concentration is normal or slightly elevated. Thus a decreased serum T_4 concentration in the absence of a decrease in TBG is not necessarily indicative of a subnormal metabolic state.

When the serum T_4 concentration is low as a result of thyroid failure, both the proportions and absolute concentrations of free T_4 and free T_3, as well as their related indices, would be expected to be subnormal. Although this is often the case, a surprisingly high proportion of patients with primary hypothyroidism display values for both the proportion of free T_4 and *in vitro* uptake tests that are within the normal range. The reason for this diagnostic overlap is uncertain. Even here, however, values for the absolute concentration of free T_4 and the free T_4 index are subnormal because of the decrease in serum total T_4 concentration.

When the normal thyroid is suppressed by physiologic replacement doses of sodium T_3 (liothyronine), secretion of T_4 is inhibited and the serum T_4 concentration declines. The latter can be used instead of the thyroid I^{131} uptake as an index of thyroid suppression. Treatment of hypothyroidism with liothyronine leads to an analogous situation in which the patient may be metabolically normal or even thyrotoxic despite a subnormal serum T_4 concentration. In addition, as would be expected, a decreased serum T_4 concentration is also found in intrinsically euthyroid individuals with thyrotoxicosis factitia due to liothyronine ingestion. Values for the serum T_3 concentration in patients taking liothyronine vary greatly with the interval between ingestion of the hormone and sampling of the blood, owing to the rapid absorption of liothyronine and its subsequent rapid clearance from the blood. After a single oral dose of 100 μg., values for the serum T_3 concentration reach a peak in approximately 2–4 hr. and then decline rapidly, returning to control values by the next day (Lieblich and Utiger, 1972). An even more rapid clearance would be expected if the patient were thyrotoxic.

Decreased Hormone Binding. The consequences of a decrease in the concentration of TBG are the direct antithesis of those associated with increased TBG (Fig. 4–8; Table 4–3). Patients are metabolically normal, although the serum T_4 concentration is in the hypothyroid range. In the majority of reported cases, thyroid function is normal. The proportion of free T_4 is increased, as are values for *in vitro* uptake tests. The absolute concentration of free T_4 is normal. Kinetically, the fractional rate of T_4 turnover and the T_4 clearance rate are increased, but daily T_4 disposal is normal.

Pharmacologic doses of testosterone and several of its derivatives with predominant androgenic or anabolic activity decrease TBG greatly, usually to values one-half or one-third of normal. Values of the serum T_4 concentration decrease *pari passu,* but rarely decline into the frankly hypothyroid range. It is of interest that these agents also increase the binding capacity of TBPA. This may account for the failure of the serum T_4 concentration to decrease more markedly, since TBPA has been shown to increase the amount of its T_4-binding when TBG is decreased.

Very high doses of ACTH or glucocorticoids decrease TBG and increase TBPA. Values of the serum T_4 concentration often decline but do not reflect sustained thyroid hypofunction. Similar changes in TBG, TBPA, and serum T_4 concentration are seen in some patients with Cushing's syndrome (Oppenheimer and Werner, 1966).

Decreases in TBG and serum T_4 concentration are seen in some patients with active acromegaly. As in the case of glucocorticoid excess, the mechanism of this change is unknown.

Urinary loss of TBG (and TBPA) in nephrotic states leads to decreased concentrations of these proteins in the plasma. The decrease in serum T_4 concentration characteristic of this disorder may result from urinary loss of hormone, as well as from the change in hormone binding. Neither measurements of the absolute concentration of free T_4 nor measurements of serum T_3 concentration have been reported; hence it is not certain whether the quantity of hormone available to the tissues is normal or decreased. The compensatory hyperfunction of the thyroid that would be expected if the latter were the case is usually not seen, since thyroid I^{131} uptakes are not usually increased.

In severe illnesses, the serum T_4 concentration may be slightly or moderately decreased, usually in association with a decrease in the concentration of TBG (Bellabarba et al., 1968). The proportion of free T_4 is increased, often to a greater extent than the lowering of the serum T_4 concentration. As a result, the absolute concentration of free T_4 is frequently increased, sometimes into the hyperthyroid range. Whether this represents a readjustment of the homeostatic set point or an abnormality in the production or metabolism of T_3 is uncertain.

In rare instances, a decreased concentration of TBG in serum occurs as an X chromosome–linked heritable trait. The extent of the abnormality is more striking in males than in females in accord with the Lyon hypothesis. Affected individuals display a decrease in serum T_4 concentration, together with an increase in the proportion of free T_4. The result of these changes is a free T_4 concentration in the low-normal range. Total T_4 production and disposal are normal, as is the patient's metabolic state. Concentrations of other estrogen-sensitive transport proteins in serum, such as corticosteroid-binding globulin and ceruloplasmin, are normal.

In conditions associated with decreased TBG in which appropriate analyses have been made, serum T_3 concentrations like those of serum T_4 have been found to be subnormal. Alterations in the kinetics of T_3 metabolism associated with decreased TBG resemble those seen in the case of T_4 (Nicoloff et al., 1972).

Disorders Associated with Divergent Serum T_4 and T_3 Concentrations

Although increasing the number of laboratory tests that the physician may feel obliged to request and in some respects complicating the interpretation of measurements of serum T_4 concentration, measurements of serum T_3 concentration have made possible clarification of several previously perplexing situations. In the main, these are situations in which the serum T_3 concentration is unusually high in relation to the serum T_4 concentration. (Additional discussion will be found in the appropriate parts of the clinical section; also see Larsen, 1972, for a well-referenced review.)

T_3-Toxicosis. Thyrotoxicosis associated with increased concentrations of T_3 in serum together with only slightly elevated, normal, or occasionally low serum concentrations of T_4 is a recently recognized entity, termed T_3-toxicosis. As discussed above, the serum T_3 concentration usually is inordinately increased in the common variety of thyrotoxicosis in which the serum T_4 concentration is high, but in T_3-toxicosis, the magnitude of this discrepancy is greatly exaggerated. This great discrepancy suggests that the elevated serum T_3 does not arise from the peripheral conversion of T_4 to T_3 but rather results from predominant hypersecretion of T_3 relative to T_4. In support of this view is the finding that hyperfunctioning thyroid nodules, a relatively common cause of T_3-toxicosis, frequently contain an abnormally high $T_3 : T_4$ ratio in their thyroglobulin. The frequency of T_3-toxicosis in relation to the common variety is not known, but it has been described in association not only with toxic nodular goiter but also with the diffuse toxic goiter of Graves' disease. Values for the proportion of free T_4 and *in vitro* uptake tests are usually normal.

Some patients with T_3-toxicosis, if left untreated, will subsequently develop the common variety of hyperthyroidism in which both the serum T_3 and T_4 concentrations are increased. This observation has raised the possibility that very mild or entirely asymptomatic hyperthyroidism associated only with an increase in serum T_3 concentration may be a forerunner of frank hyperthyroidism of the usual variety in many and perhaps all patients.

In patients with Graves' disease who have been in remission following a course of antithyroid therapy, increases in serum T_3 concentration may similarly herald the reemergence of frank thyrotoxicosis.

T_3-Euthyroidism. As mentioned above, the serum T_3 concentration not infrequently is decreased to a lesser extent than is the serum T_4 concentration in patients who are clinically hypothyroid. There are, in addition, some patients who appear clinically euthyroid and in whom the serum T_4 concentration is low, but in whom the serum T_3 concentration is normal or near normal. The presumption is that in such instances the normal clinical state is being largely maintained by relative hypersecretion of T_3. These situations may therefore be collectively termed T_3-euthyroidism. This syndrome is seen most frequently in patients with Graves' disease who have undergone ablative treatment, particularly with radioiodine, and it also occurs in patients with Hashimoto's disease. Many of these patients display slight elevations of serum TSH concentration and hence may be slightly hypothyroid, though not sufficiently so to evoke frank clinical manifestations. On the other hand, it could be reasoned that the hypersecretion of TSH is a compensatory mechanism sufficient to maintain a euthyroid state through stimulation of relatively predominant T_3 secretion.

Endemic Goiter. A special case of T_3-euthyroidism is the patient with severe iodine deficiency. Many patients in regions of iodine deficiency display very low serum T_4 concentrations but nevertheless appear eumetabolic. This is probably explained by the elevated serum T_3 concentration, which in such regions varies inversely with the serum T_4 concentration (DeLange et al., 1972a). In such patients, serum TSH concentrations are also increased. The relative hypersecretion of T_3 that occurs in areas of iodine deficiency represents an efficient mechanism for the defense of metabolic status since the calorigenic yield of an iodine atom in T_3 is approximately four times that of an iodine atom in T_4.

Tests that Assess the Metabolic Impact of the Thyroid Hormones

Abnormalities in the quantity of thyroid hormones available to the tissues are associated with alterations in a vast number of metabolic processes. Certain of these altered reactions or the biochemical or physiologic changes that they produce are susceptible to measurement in a clinical setting. Therefore they provide a a potential means of determining whether the supply of hormone is inadequate or excessive in relation to tissue needs and responsiveness. Measurement of these "metabolic indices" provides a means of assessing one aspect of thyroid economy not directly measurable by tests of any other type. Such tests should and often do correlate most closely with the symptomatic state of the patient.

Although procedures of this genre were for a long period the only available laboratory aids in the diagnosis of hyperthyroidism or hypothyroidism, their use is decreasing. Such disfavor is partly justified, largely because the metabolic indices are often influenced by other physiologic factors or diseases and hence may be considered nonspecific. Other more "specific" indices, such as the serum T_4 concentration or thyroid uptake of I^{131}, may be equally nonspecific under certain circumstances but are probably less often so. To a certain extent, psychological factors have also influenced the choice of testing procedures. Conventional metabolic indices such as the BMR or serum cholesterol concentration are neglected, while more recently described metabolic or physiologic indices, which may be equally nonspecific, enjoy a vogue of popularity. Tests such as the BMR and serum cholesterol measurement are often criticized because of the wide range of normal values; such criticism is unjustified. In the BMR, for example, the normal range may lie between -20 per cent and $+5$ per cent. If the serum T_4 concentration and 24-hour thyroid I^{131} uptake were calculated as a percentage variation from a mean normal value, as is the case with the BMR, the normal range would be found to vary between $+50$ and -50 per cent.

In the past we have held the view that metabolic indices, notably the BMR, retain considerable clinical usefulness, particularly in the case of mild or questionable hypo- or hyperthyroidism. It could be argued that this is no longer the case. Thus, mild hypothyroidism may best be diagnosed by an elevated serum TSH concentration; however, it could equally well be argued that the hypersecretion of TSH merely indicates a compensatory response to a failing thyroid and that some metabolic index is required to ascertain whether the compensation is complete. In the case of hyperthyroidism, it would appear that diminished pituitary responsiveness to TRH is a very sensitive index of hormone excess. What is uncertain, however, is whether the threshold of excess is the same for the pituitary as for other tissues. Moreover, until there is clarification of the suggestion that in Graves' disease an abnormal response to TRH may occur in an entirely euthyroid patient, the specificity of this test for hyperthyroidism per se must remain in question.

For the foregoing reasons, great value would devolve on any test which could clearly differentiate between the normal state and instances of mild disease difficult to recognize on clinical grounds. It is most unlikely that one will discover an all-or-none metabolic response to slight excess or deficiency of a normal bodily constituent, i.e., thyroid hormone. By the same token, it is probably a forlorn hope to seek clear-cut abnormalities of any metabolic index in a patient whose metabolic disturbance is only mild.

Basal Metabolic Rate (BMR)

The classic metabolic action of the thyroid hormones is their calorigenic effect, increasing energy expenditure and heat production; this is manifest in the weight loss, increased caloric requirement, and heat intolerance of the thyrotoxic patient. The classic test that reflects this effect is the measurement of the basal metabolic rate or BMR. Since it is impractical to measure heat expenditure directly, the test actually measures oxygen consumption under specified conditions. The caloric equivalent of the oxygen consumed depends upon the nature of the substrates being metabolized and whether anabolic or catabolic reactions predominate. Under the prescribed basal conditions, however, this varies within narrow limits. The assumption is made that the energy equivalent of 1 liter of oxygen (at standard temperature and pressure) is 4.83 Cal., corresponding to a respiratory quotient of 0.82.

Under basal conditions, approximately 25 per cent of oxygen consumption represents energy expenditure in visceral organs, including liver, kidney, and heart; 10 per cent in brain; 10 per cent in respiratory activity; and the remainder in skeletal musculature. Since oxygen consumption is related to functioning tissue mass, efforts have been made to develop a reliable index thereof. The one universally used is the estimated body surface area, based on measurements of height and weight. Basal oxygen consumption is relatively much higher in males than in females, and it declines rapidly from infancy to the third decade and more slowly with age thereafter. Therefore, after standardization for surface area, values in the individual patient are compared with established normal means for persons of the same sex and age. Finally, values are expressed as a percentage difference from the appropriate normal mean. The normal range of BMR is generally considered to be −10 per cent to +10 per cent. Under optimal conditions, somewhat lower values are obtained only if the patient is in a truly basal state. He must be at rest, warm and comfortable, and emotionally at ease, and he must not have eaten for at least 12 hours. The oxygen consumption is then measured by means of a closed, oxygen-filled spirometer with coupled kymograph, carbon dioxide and moisture in the expired breath being removed by soda lime.

The greatest source of error in the determination of the BMR is failure of the patient to achieve a truly basal state. Apprehension concerning either the apparatus or the implications of a possible abnormal result elevate the BMR. These are accentuated by inexperienced or injudicious technicians. Whenever feasible, the test should be repeated on a second day, since more reliable results are generally obtained when the patient is accustomed to the procedure. As a result, the test has maximum reliability when used repeatedly to follow the course of therapy. The effect of psychological factors can be reduced by administration of small doses of a sedative before the test, but hypnotic doses should not be used. Induction of barbiturate narcosis for measurement of the "somnolent metabolic rate" does not seem worth the risk involved.

Small outward leaks, such as occur when the patient has a perforated eardrum or when the mouth or nose pieces fit poorly, are common causes of spurious increases in BMR. This problem is especially prominent in edentulous patients. Spurious decreases in BMR are produced by incomplete absorption of carbon dioxide and moisture caused by defective soda lime. Here, the kymographic tracing will reveal progressive tachypnea as the test proceeds. A variety of systemic disorders is associated with abnormalities in BMR; these are listed in Table 4–4.

Since most errors in BMR determinations increase the measured value, the test is most useful in excluding the diagnosis of significant thyrotoxicosis. No more than approximately 5 per cent of patients with this disorder will have results within the normal range. A normal value provides reasonable evidence against this diagnosis, although it is always possible that the patient's normal value is even lower. In severe hypothyroidism,

TABLE 4–4. EXTRATHYROIDAL FACTORS AFFECTING THE BASAL METABOLIC RATE

Extrathyroidal factors increasing *the basal metabolic rate*
   Errors in preparation of patient: anxiety, inadequate rest, recent food ingestion, drugs (caffeine, epinephrine, ephedrine, dextroamphetamine, thyroid hormones, aminophylline), smoking
   Errors during test: surrounding noise, extremes in room temperature, uncomfortable table or bed, insufficient elevation of patient (cardiac or obese subjects), tight nose piece, girdle or collar, leakage of oxygen around mouth piece or around perforated eardrum, beginning test with chest overexpanded, irregular breathing habits
Disorders of:
   Nervous system: anxiety neuroses, mania, disorders of heat center, disorders causing involuntary motions, such as tics, tremors, choreiform activities.
   Cardiovascular system: congestive heart failure, hypertension, aortic stenosis, arteriovenous aneurysm, coarctation of aorta, Paget's disease (increased circulation)
   Respiratory system: various obstructions of tracheobronchial tree, emphysema, lung diseases
   Blood and/or lymph nodes: leukemia, polycythemia, severe anemia, lymphoma
   Endocrine system: acromegaly, pheochromocytoma, pregnancy, diabetes insipidus, adrenal hyperfunction
   Skin: many skin diseases are associated with excessive heat loss
   Fever
Extrathyroidal factors decreasing *the basal metabolic rate*
   Technical errors: excessively used soda lime, beginning test with underexpansion of chest
   Disorders of the patient: starvation, malnutrition, anorexia nervosa, postinfectious asthenia, Addison's disease, nephrosis, shock

values as low as −40 per cent or −45 per cent are seen, but a substantial proportion of patients (up to 20 per cent) may have values in the normal range. (Excellent discussions of the principles underlying the measurement of BMR and the techniques employed therein are to be found in Peters and Van Slyke, 1946, and Becker, 1971.)

Serum Cholesterol Concentration

The concentration of cholesterol in serum varies rather widely among normal individuals and is influenced by age, sex, and dietary intake of both fat and total calories. As a consequence, this traditional metabolic index is rarely employed at present as a primary diagnostic aid in thyroid disease. Nevertheless, in primary hypothyroidism, the serum cholesterol concentration is usually increased, and this may be used as a secondary diagnostic test. The presence of a normal serum cholesterol in a clearly hypothyroid patient should suggest the possibility of pituitary failure, since values are not usually increased in trophoprivic hypothyroidism. Serial measurements of serum cholesterol are also of aid in following the response to a therapeutic trial of thyroid medication. In patients who truly have primary hypothyroidism, a striking decrease will occur within a few weeks, a response that will not occur in normal individuals. In thyrotoxic states, a demonstrable decrease in serum cholesterol concentration does not occur with sufficient frequency to make the test of diagnostic value.

Achilles Reflex Time

In approximately 90 per cent of patients with hypothyroidism, there occurs a visible delay in the relaxation phase of the deep tendon reflexes. A complex apparatus for timing objectively the several phases of the deep tendon reflex has been employed in some clinics for many years. Recently, however, several simpler devices have been introduced that could make measurement of reflex time a feasible office diagnostic procedure. The kinemometer is an apparatus for measuring the current induced in a coil by a magnet strapped to the sole. The photomotograph records variations in the current output of a photoelectric cell as the foot moves through the path of a beam of light. With either apparatus, an ECG can be used to record the current produced and make a permanent record in which the duration of the reflex components can be measured.

The duration of the Achilles tendon reflex is prolonged in hypothyroidism and shortened in hyperthyroidism. These differences are not due to differences in the neural component of the arc but to differences in the speed of both muscular contraction and relaxation, particularly the latter. The phase of the tendon reflex recommended to be measured varies among different laboratories and with different instruments.

A considerable dispute exists in the literature concerning the efficacy of measurements of the Achilles reflex time as a diagnostic measure. There is general agreement that the test has little value in the diagnosis of hyperthyroidism, since as many as 78 per cent of the values may fall within the normal range. As regards hypothyroidism, opinions vary, as little as 2.5 per cent overlap with the normal range being reported by some workers and as much as 38 per cent by others. Delayed relaxation of the deep tendon reflexes has also been reported in pregnant women, in patients with pernicious anemia, myotonia congenita, and other myotonic disorders, and in some psychotic patients. Delay is also said to follow the administration of glucose, potassium, reserpine, and propranolol. Of particular importance is the observation that hypothermic states other than hypothyroidism may cause a prolongation of the deep tendon reflexes (for discussion and references, see Waal-Manning, 1969). We have had relatively little experience with measurement of the Achilles reflex time as a diagnostic tool, although an instrument has been available in the laboratory for several years.

Enzyme Concentrations in Blood

In view of the abnormalities of muscular function in both hyperthyroidism and hypothyroidism, recently investigators have been concerned with the activity in serum of several enzymes of muscular origin. Values of the creatine phosphokinase in serum are significantly increased in patients with hypothyroidism and may be slightly lowered in patients with hyperthyroidism. Increased values for SGOT and LDH have been reported to occur in patients with severe hypothyroidism. In the presence of heart disease associated with hypothyroidism, LDH isoenzymes one and two may be increased (Aber et al., 1966). In thyrotoxicosis, the red cell content of carbonic anhydrase B may be decreased (Funakoshi and Deutsch, 1971).

Tests that Assess the Mechanisms for Regulating Thyroid Function

The synthesis and secretion of normal quantities of thyroid hormone depend upon the normality of function at each of the successive links in the homeostatic regulatory chain. Hypothalamic and pituitary mechanisms for regulating the secretion of TSH must be normally responsive to variations in the availability of thyroid hormone, the pituitary must be capable of secreting TSH in response to appropriate stimuli, and the thyroid must retain both its dependence upon and responsiveness to TSH. Finally, there must not be, as there may be in Graves' disease, the interposition of an extraneous thyroid stimulator, formation of which is not regulated by the usual mechanisms of feedback control. When any of these prerequisites for the maintenance of homeostasis is lacking, either excess or insufficient production of hormone occurs. Such is in fact the case in several of the major diseases of the thyroid. Consequently, tests designed to challenge regulatory control have assumed great importance in both clinical diagnosis and physiopathologic investigation. Currently, there are available means for assessing the responsiveness of the pituitary to TRH; the basal concentration of serum TSH, an index of the rate of TSH secretion; the responsiveness of the thyroid to TSH; and the ability of exogenous thyroid hormone to bring the thyroid to a state of diminished activity. Although these procedures permit the evaluation of much of the regulatory system, at least one major link remains to be closed, i.e., the ability to measure the concentration of TRH in plasma or its rate of secretion.

Thyroid Suppression Test

When normal individuals are given TH (thyroid hormone) in quantities adequate to meet peripheral requirements, suppression of endogenous thyroid function occurs. Such suppression, which is the result of decreased secretion of TSH, is associated with both a decrease in the rate of hormone secretion, as indicated by a decrease in the thyroid release of I^{131}, and a decrease in hormone synthesis, as indicated by a lowering of the thyroid I^{131} uptake. This principle forms the basis for the thyroid suppression test, which has proved to be of exceptional value in diagnosing the patient with suspected thyrotoxicosis and in establishing the presence of Graves' disease.

Implicit in the presence of thyrotoxicosis resulting from thyroid hyperfunction (as opposed to excessive quantities of exogenous hormone) is the existence of disrupted homeostatic control. Without such disruption, overproduction of hormone could not persist. Since excessive quantities of endogenous hormone fail to suppress thyroid function, it would follow that exogenous hormone would be similarly ineffective. This line of reasoning has been so universally accepted and so uniformly borne out by clinical experience that virtually all are now agreed that a normal suppressive response to TH eliminates the possibility that the patient has active thyrotoxicosis. The thyroid suppression test is therefore of special value in patients with marginal clinical findings and laboratory tests suggestive of mild thyrotoxicosis. A normal suppressive response excludes the diagnosis of thyrotoxicosis. As will be seen in this discussion, an abnormal response is consistent with, but not pathognomonic of, thyrotoxicosis.

An abnormal suppression test will occur in thyrotoxicosis of endogenous origin, regardless of the underlying disease. Thus it occurs in patients with the diffuse toxic goiter of Graves' disease and in patients with toxic multinodular goiter. Lack of suppression is also seen in patients with autonomously hyperfunctioning adenomas. None of these lesions is TSH-dependent, and consequently exogenous hormone does not decrease their function.

Thus it is to be emphasized that an abnormal suppression test in the presence of thyrotoxicosis does not indicate that the patient necessarily has Graves' disease. Other features, such as a diffusely active goiter or coexistent ophthalmopathy or both, would be necessary to make this diagnosis.

Although an abnormal suppression test in the presence of thyrotoxicosis is not pathognomonic of Graves' disease, an abnormal suppression test in the absence of thyrotoxicosis is almost always indicative of Graves' disease. It has been noted that abnormal suppression tests in Graves' disease may persist for varying periods, occasionally for many years, after thyrotoxicosis has been relieved either spontaneously or as a result of treatment (Fig. 4-15). Furthermore, abnormal suppression tests occur in about one-half of patients with active ophthalmopathy of Graves' disease, even when thyroid function is normal. Demonstration of an abnormal suppressive response in such patients greatly weighs in favor of the ophthalmopathy being due to Graves' disease, rather than to an intracranial or intraorbital lesion. The fact that an abnormal thyroid suppression test may occur in Graves' disease in the absence of frank thyrotoxicosis indicates that this abnormal response is a reflection of a more basic pathogenetic element in this disorder. Indeed, it is the demonstration that the result of a suppression test can be normal when LATS is demonstrable in the serum that has led to the current doubt concerning the pathogenetic importance of LATS (see section on the pathogenesis of Graves' disease).

It has been reported that in a small proportion of patients with nontoxic goiter, Hashimoto's disease, and iodide goiter and myxedema, thyroid function is not suppressible by exogenous hormone. At present, there is no way to be certain whether or not such patients may also have underlying Graves' disease. Since the presence of LATS in

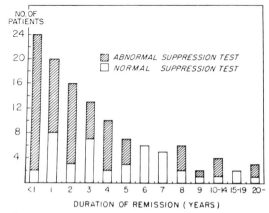

Figure 4-15. Persistence of abnormal T_3 suppression test following relief of thyrotoxicosis in patients with Graves' disease. Patients in this series had relief of thyrotoxicosis following surgical, radioiodine, or antithyroid therapy, or following spontaneous remission. Note the prolonged persistence of an abnormal suppression test in some patients despite maintenance of a normal metabolic state. (Figure constructed from data presented by Werner, S. C.: *J. Clin. Invest.* 35:57, 1956.)

serum is virtually pathognomonic of Graves' disease, though not necessarily pathogenetic, assays for LATS in the sera of such patients would be of considerable interest.

In patients with known Graves' disease, a normal result generally indicates that the disease is in an inactive phase, and hence the suppression can be used prognostically. In patients receiving antithyroid therapy, a normal result increases the likelihood that a prolonged remission will follow cessation of treatment. In using the suppression test in this manner, the antithyroid drug need not be discontinued while the test is being conducted, since with doses of antithyroid drug sufficient to render the patient euthyroid, active uptake of I^{131} by the thyroid persists, and suppression of uptake can therefore be tested.

The technique of carrying out the suppression test varies somewhat among different laboratories. Sodium T_3 (liothyronine) is universally used as the suppressive agent, and the lowering of the thyroid radioiodine uptake is most commonly employed as an index of suppression. The recommended dosage of liothyronine varies between 75 and 100 μg. daily and the duration of administration between 8 days and 2 weeks. The authors prefer the larger dose of liothyronine in view of evidence suggesting that 75 μg. daily may not constitute a full physiologic replacement dose (Cotton et al., 1971). Others have suggested that suppressibility be tested by the administration of a single large dose of L-thyroxine, thereby forestalling a spurious nonsuppression owing to failure of the patient to take the hormone (Wallack et al., 1970).

It is generally considered that a reduction of the 24 hr. I^{131} uptake to less than half of its initial value before liothyronine administration constitutes a normal response. The same criterion is applied in the case of 20-min. I^{131} uptake. In view of the decline in normal values for radioiodine uptake, interpretation of the suppression based on this function has become more difficult. However, since the suppressive response to liothyronine is associated with a decrease in the secretion of T_4, a reduction in serum T_4 concentration can also be used as an index of suppression.

Since the test is usually conducted in patients with mild hyperthyroidism, not being required in the presence of flagrant disease, little if any risk is incurred by the larger dose of liothyronine. However, in elderly patients or those with heart disease, the thyroid suppression test should not be performed. In these circumstances, the TRH stimulation test, which is described later in this section, should be undertaken if thyrotoxicosis is strongly suspected.

TSH Stimulation Test

Until recently, the TSH stimulation test has played a prominent role in the diagnosis of several varieties of thyroid hypofunction. The test depends upon the fact that the normal or potentially normal thyroid responds to an increase in stimulation by TSH with an increase in both iodine accumulation and hormone release. On the other hand, a thyroid that is failing or has failed because of intrinsic disease should be maximally stimulated by endogenous TSH, provided that the patient's hypothalamic and pituitary function is intrinsically normal. Thus the TSH test has been employed to differentiate between thyroprivic and trophoprivic varieties of hypothyroidism. The test has also been of value in demonstrating the presence of so-called decreased thyroid reserve, in which the maximum functional capacity of the thyroid has already been evoked by endogenous TSH in order to yield a normal or near-normal rate of hormone production (see section on hypothyroidism). Finally, the test can be used to disclose whether the thyroid of a patient receiving exogenous TH is capable or incapable of response to TSH. In the former circumstance, the patient either is normal or has trophoprivic hypothyroidism; in the latter circumstance, thyroprivic hypothyroidism, but not decreased thyroid reserve, is likely to be present.

With the development of methods for measuring the concentration of TSH in serum and for assessing the pituitary responsiveness to TRH, the usefulness of the TSH stimulation test has become restricted. Thus, in the presence of frank hypothyroidism, the basal concentration of TSH in serum will serve to differentiate the thyroprivic from the trophoprivic varieties. Moreover, mild thyroprivic hypothyroidism will be evident in an elevated basal TSH concentration and an exaggerated response to TRH. Currently, therefore, the TSH stimulation test can be used when measurements of serum TSH concentration are unavailable or when the degree of impairment in thyroid function is sufficiently slight that basal TSH concentrations are increased only marginally, if at all. The latter situation is in essence a variety of decreased thyroid reserve.

Several variants of the TSH stimulation test have been used clinically. These may be categorized as 1-day tests, 3-day tests, or a combination of the two. For the diagnosis of decreased thyroid reserve, the 1-day test seems adequate, since normal individuals respond well to a single injection of TSH, whereas those with decreased thyroid reserve have, in the authors' experience, failed to respond even to repeated TSH stimulation. Hence, the 1-day test is adequate to establish this diagnosis. The usual 1-day test is conducted as follows. The thyroid I^{131} uptake is measured 3 hours after an oral dose of the isotope and blood is drawn for measurement of the serum T_4 concentration. Either 5 U. or 10 U. of bovine TSH, to which the human thyroid is normally responsive, is given intramuscularly immediately thereafter. Approximately 24 hours after the first dose of I^{131}, a second specimen of blood is drawn for measurement of serum T_4 concentration, and the epithyroid radioactivity is determined. This provides a measurement of basal 24 hr. uptake and also a "residual count" to be subtracted from subsequent measurements of thyroid radioactivity. A second dose of I^{131} is then administered, and its accumulation in the thyroid measured at 3 hours and, if desired, at 24 hours. In normal individuals, there is an approximate twofold increase in the uptake after TSH and at least a 2.0 μg./100 ml. increase in the serum T_4 concentration.

Significant untoward reactions to TSH are quite uncommon. Virtually all patients experience some discomfort at the site of injection. Less common reactions include nausea and vomiting, pain and tenderness in the region of the thyroid or salivary glands, fever, urticaria, symptoms of thyrotoxicosis, dysrhythmias, and angina. Death has occurred in rare instances. Generally, however, the test is well tolerated, even in patients with hypopituitarism. The possibility that adrenal crisis may be produced by thyroid activation or by an allergic reaction in patients with concomitant deficiency of ACTH has been frequently discussed. Although this response must be quite rare, it is desirable that the patient who is to undergo a TSH test be given glucocorticoids if hypopituitarism is strongly suspected. (For further discussion of variants of the TSH stimulation test and their clinical applicability, see Burke, 1968.)

Serum TSH Concentration

The development of a sensitive and highly specific radioimmunoassay for measuring the concentration of pituitary TSH in serum has provided a powerful tool for the diagnosis and management of several thyroid disorders (Mayberry et al., 1971; Hershman and Pittman, 1971; Utiger, 1971) (Fig. 4–16). In addition, classic concepts concerning the regulatory control of thyroid function have been largely confirmed, and the assay has also provided the index of response for the TRH stimulation test described below.

As with all radioimmunoassays, values obtained in different laboratories vary somewhat. Nevertheless, with the antisera currently available, direct assays of normal serum yield values near the lower limit of detectability, and while the mean normal value is about 3 μU./ml. (Human Research Standard A), values in approximately 10 per cent of normal individuals are below the limit of detection. As a consequence, the test does not discriminate between normal and subnormal values. This relative lack of sensitivity has made it difficult to ascertain whether TSH secretion undergoes significant diurnal variation, and conflicting reports concerning this question have appeared (Webster et al., 1972). Nevertheless, it is clear that measurable variations in serum TSH concentration do not occur under ambient circumstances, and that stimuli, such as hypoglycemia, arginine, and chlorpromazine, that elicit the secretion of some pituitary hormones, do not evoke the release of TSH.

Except in rare instances of hyperthyroidism associated with pituitary tumors, values in virtually all cases of hyperthyroidism reported to date have been in this indeterminate normal or low range. Since this is true regardless of the underlying eti-

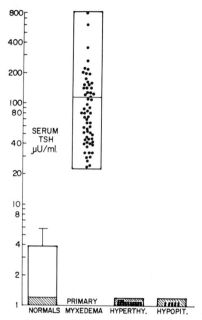

Figure 4–16. Serum TSH concentrations in various circumstances. Cross-hatched areas indicate values not distinguishable from zero. In primary hypothyroidism of mild degree, less marked elevations of serum TSH concentration are observed. (From Hershman, J. M., and Pittman, J. A.: *Ann. Intern. Med.* 74:481, 1971.)

ology, hypersecretion of pituitary TSH, at least in an immunoreactive form, can be dismissed as a pathogenetic factor.

By contrast, the serum TSH concentration is invariably increased in patients with hypothyroidism of primary thyroidal origin, the extent of the increase closely correlating with the severity of the disease. Hence, values may range from those that are minimally elevated in very mild hypothyroidism to those that are in excess of 1000 μU./ml. in patients with severe disease. In patients with Hashimoto's disease and in patients who have been treated with radioiodine or surgery for hyperthyroidism, i.e., patients with limited functioning thyroid mass, values for serum TSH concentration may be increased although the patients are clinically euthyroid and values for the serum T_4 and T_3 concentrations are in the normal range. Such findings are indicative of early thyroid failure for which increased stimulation by TSH is able to compensate. This is not necessarily indicative of decreased thyroid reserve, since, in some instances, such patients are capable of responding to further TSH stimulation.

The association of a normal or undetectable serum TSH concentration with clear-cut hypothyroidism is diagnostic of trophoprivic hypothyroidism, but within this category, testing of the TSH response to exogenous TRH is necessary to differentiate the pituitary and hypothalamic varieties.

Although enhanced secretion of TSH is commonly implicated in its pathogenesis, simple or nontoxic goiter is not usually associated with an increased serum TSH concentration. However, when the pathogenetic factors that lead to simple goiter are sufficiently severe to produce hypothyroidism (goitrous hypothyroidism), then increased serum TSH concentrations emerge. In endemic goiter associated with severe iodine deficiency, serum TSH concentrations are often high and may be in part responsible for the hypersecretion of T_3 that occurs in these circumstances. In areas of less severe iodine deficiency, endemic goiter is associated with normal serum TSH concentrations, much as it is in sporadic nontoxic goiter discussed above. In the human neonate, the serum TSH concentration increases greatly during the first few hours following parturition, returning to normal values during the first day post partum. This response is thought to be due to the entry of the neonate into the relatively cool extrauterine environment. Cold exposure in the adult, however, has no apparent effect.

Except when massive doses of hormone are administered acutely, treatment of patients with hypothyroidism progressively lowers the elevated serum TSH concentration, but normal levels are not attained for several weeks. After withdrawal of replacement liothyronine, in patients with hypothyroidism, a progressive increase in serum TSH concentration begins within a few days. By contrast, when patients have been treated for long periods with L-thyroxine, return of the serum TSH concentration to elevated values may require a few weeks, even though the serum T_4 and T_3 concentrations have fallen to subnormal values in the interim.

Although pituitary extracts containing TSH and peptic digests of purified TSH are capable of inducing exophthalmos in test animals, no increase in TSH concentration has been detected in the serum of patients with the active ophthalmopathy of Graves' disease. Nor has the β subunit of TSH been detected in excess, despite the fact that it is a component of the presumed exophthalmogenic peptic fragment (for a further discussion of subunits, see earlier section on TSH).

Values for TSH concentration are normal in the serum of pregnant women despite the fact that the normal placenta produces a thyroid-stimulating peptide termed human chorionic thyrotropin (hCT). The physiologic role of hCT in pregnancy is uncertain, but this material is of interest immunochemically since it cross-reacts with bovine but not human pituitary TSH. In this respect, it is similar to the thyrotropin found in the sera of some patients with thyroid neoplasms. Despite the occurrence of thyroid hyperfunction and occasional frank thyrotoxicosis in some patients with trophoblastic tumors, assays for pituitary TSH in serum reveal no increase. Rather, this syndrome results from secretion by the tumors of a thyroid-stimulating peptide termed molar thyrotropin that does not cross-react immunologically with either human or bovine TSH (Hershman and Higgins, 1971).

TRH Stimulation Test

To a large extent, the synthesis and secretion of pituitary TSH are dependent upon the tonic stimulation by a hypothalamic neurohumor designated TSH releasing hormone (TRH) (see earlier section on regulation of thyroid function). The response of the pituitary to TRH is modulated by an action of the thyroid hormones within the pituitary, an excess of hormone inhibiting and insufficiency enhancing the secretory response. For these reasons, the availability of synthetic TRH suitable for use in humans makes it possible to assess either the functional integrity of the thyrotropic cell or the operation of factors that influence the stimulatory response (Anderson et al., 1971; Snyder and Utiger, 1972a, b).

In man, when given in sufficient dosage, TRH is effective whether administered orally, intramuscularly, or intravenously. However, the greatest experience has been accumulated with intravenous use. Doses of TRH varying between approximately 6 and 400 μg. produce a graded response in increasing the serum TSH concentration, but larger doses are apparently without additional effect (Fig. 4–17). Consequently, the dose of 400 μg. is recommended for the intravenous TRH stimulation test. In normal individuals, a dose of this magnitude produces a prompt rise in serum TSH concentration that is maximum between 20 and 40 minutes and then declines rapidly. The peak increment of the normal response averages about 15 μU./ml., no significant sex difference being observed in young adults. In men, but apparently not in women, the peak increment declines progressively with age, a factor which should be borne in mind when interpreting the results of the test in the elderly male. Increments in serum T_4 and particularly T_3 concentrations frequently occur after TRH administration, but the increments are small and inconstant and hence are not of diagnostic value.

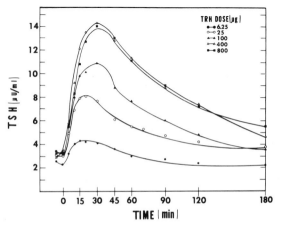

Figure 4–17. Response of serum TSH concentration to intravenous TRH in the dosage shown in normal subjects. (From Snyder, P. J., and Utiger, R. D.: *J. Clin. Endocr. 34*:380, 1972.)

As would be expected, in hypothyroidism of primary thyroidal origin, the response of serum TSH to TRH is accentuated, peak increments being increased, often greatly so, and the duration of the response prolonged. Since the concurrence of a high basal serum TSH concentration in association with hypothyroidism will already establish the diagnosis of hypothyroidism of primary thyroidal origin, the principal diagnostic value of the TRH stimulation test will be present in those patients in whom the disorder is mild and the increase in basal serum TSH marginal. When hypothyroidism is present without an increase in basal serum concentration, a diagnosis of trophoprivic hypothyroidism is indicated, and here a lack of response of the serum TSH to TRH will establish the diagnosis of intrinsic pituitary disease rather than hypothalamic dysfunction. In patients with pituitary disease, a subnormal response to TRH indicates impairment of thyrotropic function, even though clinical and laboratory evidence of hypothyroidism is lacking.

Perhaps even more important than its diagnostic capability in hypothyroidism is the value of the TRH stimulation test in the diagnosis of states of TH excess. All available information indicates that the response of the serum TSH concentration to TRH is greatly depressed or totally abolished in patients with thyrotoxicosis regardless of its underlying cause. That the test is highly sensitive to very slight increments in the availability of TH is indicated by the observation that in the normal individual the response to TRH is promptly and markedly diminished by very small doses of exogenous hormone, insufficient to raise the serum T_4 and T_3 concentrations appreciably, and certainly insufficient to raise them above the normal range. Indeed, in a sense, the test may be too sensitive, since the response characteristic of thyrotoxicosis may be seen in patients lacking both clinical and laboratory evidence of thyrotoxicosis, for example, in some patients with autonomously functioning thyroid adenomas. A similar sensitivity to small excess of TH may explain the lack of TRH responsiveness that has been reported to occur in some patients with apparently euthyroid Graves' disease. On the other hand, the sensitivity of the test makes possible a favorable diagnostic use when it is applied to the symptomatic patient with borderline routine laboratory values. As a corollary, the TRH stimulation test should be used instead of the T_3-suppression test in the elderly patient or the patient with coexisting cardiac disease who is suspected of having thyrotoxicosis.

Currently, the usefulness of the TRH stimulation test is somewhat limited by the relative unavailability of TSH radioimmunoassays. Although this situation is likely to improve, a recent modification of the conventional test affords promise of eliminating the necessity of serum TSH analyses in many instances. When a large dose (2 mg.) of TRH is administered intramuscularly to normal individuals, a distinct and readily detectable increase in serum T_4 concentration, averaging approximately 2 μg./100 ml., is evident in samples obtained at 4–5 hr. (Azizi et al., 1973). This readily apparent secondary stimulation of the thyroid is doubtless the result of a greater and more prolonged stimulation of TSH secretion than is induced by the intravenous administration of TRH. Where hypo- or hyperthyroidism is suspected, failure of the serum T_4 concentration to increase will indicate the diagnosis without the necessity of measuring the serum TSH concentration. The latter measurement is only necessary to distinguish among the several varieties of hypothyroidism.

TRH is virtually free of adverse effects. Some patients describe a sensation of flushing or a desire to urinate following its administration, but more severe untoward reactions have not been reported.

Miscellaneous Tests

External Scintiscanning

Localization of the site of radioiodine accumulation in the thyroid or elsewhere is sometimes of great value in the diagnosis or management of the patient with thyroid disease and is facilitated by the technique of scintiscanning. Here, a mechanical device moves a highly collimated (focused) scintillation detector back and forth across the area of study in a series of parallel tracks moving progressively downward from above. A printing device that moves in concert with the detector is activated to record a mark whenever a predetermined number of counts has been received. In this way, a visual representation of the localization of radioactivity in the area being scanned is obtained, areas of greatest radioactivity corresponding to areas of greater density in the scan. Modifications of the foregoing apparatus make it possible to print a mark whose color varies with the counting rate, producing the so-called "color scan." Still other modifications make use of a light source that moves synchronously with the detector and whose intensity is proportional to the counting rate. The light exposes a sheet of x-ray film, and the degree of darkening of the final image corresponds roughly to the counting rate at the appropriate site in the thyroid ("photo scan").

Scintillation cameras are devices that view the entire field of interest and translate the counting rates from specific areas of the field into photographic images or into images on a fluoroscopic screen that can be viewed directly or photographed. Sophisticated instruments permit the quantitation of radioactivity in specific areas and can record the information obtained on magnetic tape for later study.

Although I[131] has been the isotope most commonly used for scintiscanning, I[125] and particularly Tc[99m]-pertechnetate are increasingly used because of their physical and biochemical properties. The physical half-life of I[125] (60 days) is longer than that of I[131] (8 days), but its lower radiation energy delivers less radiation to the thyroid. In addition, its softer emission permits better delineation of superficial lesions. Tc^{99m}-pertechnetate is a monovalent anion that, in common with iodide, is actively concentrated by the thyroid gland but is organically bound only to a negligible extent. Its short physical half-life (6 hours), together with its transient stay within the thyroid, makes the radiation delivered to the thyroid by a standard dose about one ten-thousandth that of I^{131}. Conversely, very large doses (1 mCi.) can be administered, permitting high counting rates and often an adequate image of the thyroid when the fractional uptake is too low to permit scintiscanning with radioiodine (Strauss et al., 1970). Pertechnetate is usually given as a single intravenous bolus, and scanning can be carried out within the first 30 minutes. By means of the scintillation camera, serial images can therefore be obtained, providing information about the dynamics of isotope accumulation. By contrast, in the case of radioiodine, the dose administered ($50-100\mu Ci.$) is so small that an adequate image is usually not obtained for many hours after the radioiodine is administered. Moreover, both organic binding and retention of the resulting radioiodinated product are required for a satisfactory scintiscan image.

The scintiscanning technique can be used to provide some evidence, though not accurate, of overall thyroid size. More importantly, it is used to define areas of increased or decreased function ("hot" or "cold" areas, respectively) relative to the function of the remainder of the gland, provided that these are about 1 cm. or more in diameter (Fig. 4–18). Although small cold nodules may be obscured by overlying functioning tissue, demonstration that a palpable nodule is nonfunctioning increases the likelihood that it may be malignant. Conversely, functioning nodules, particularly if they are either more active than surrounding tissue or the sole functioning tissue, are unlikely to be malignant. Superior discrimination of lesions can be achieved if the gland is scanned in the lateral as well as the anteroposterior dimension. Accurate interpretation also requires careful correlation between the findings on palpation and on the scintiscan.

Scintiscanning may also reveal substernal goiters or the location of ectopic thyroid tissue in the tongue, chest, or ovary and can detect functioning metastases of thyroid carcinoma. Occasionally, a nodule that appears "cold" by radioiodine scintiscanning demonstrates uptake of pertechnetate, apparently as a result of retention of the transport function while the organic binding function that is required for visualization with radioiodine is lost. (For a comprehensive and well-illustrated discussion of scintiscanning, see Johnson, 1971.)

Assessment of Organic Binding of Iodide

In normally functioning or generally hyperfunctioning thyroids, oxidation of iodide and organic binding are sufficiently rapid that relatively little free iodide is present in the thyroid at any time. Consequently, little loss of iodide from the normal thyroid can be demonstrated following the administration of agents, such as perchlorate, that inhibit iodide transport and thereby discharge accumulated iodide. When organic binding is incomplete, however, substantial accumulation of iodide occurs, and significant discharge follows inhibition of iodide transport. Two tests of the integrity of the organic-binding mechanism have been devised, the standard perchlorate discharge test and the iodide-perchlorate discharge test. In the former, a dose of radioiodine is allowed to accumulate in the thyroid, and after measurement of the thyroid I^{131} content, a blocking dose of perchlorate is administered. A significant decrease in epithyroid radioactivity within one hour constitutes a positive response and indicates a defect in organic binding when the plasma stable iodide, and hence the intrathyroid iodide concentration, is normal or near normal. The iodide-perchlorate discharge test affords a more severe challenge to the organic-binding mechanism, since an acute load of stable iodide is administered with the radioiodine. As a result, the concentration of intrathyroid iodide is greatly increased, and even a mild impairment of organic binding will leave a significant portion of thyroid radioiodine unbound and susceptible to discharge. Hence, subtle defects can be demonstrated by means of this test. However, the interpretation of the iodide-perchlorate discharge test is more complex than is that of the standard test. When entirely normal individuals are given sufficient quantities of stable iodide, an acute inhibition of organic binding (acute Wolff-Chaikoff effect) ensues, and a variable proportion of thyroid iodide becomes dischargeable. Although the dose of stable iodide used in the iodide-perchlorate discharge test is less than that required to induce an inhibition of organic binding in the normal gland, it may be sufficient to do so in the stimulated gland in which iodide transport activity is increased. This may explain the positive tests that are seen in some patients with hyperthyroidism and in some normal individuals who have been given TSH. (For details of the testing procedures and further discussion of findings, see Suzuki and Mashimo, 1972.)

A positive response to the standard test is seen in patients with a genetically determined defect in organic binding, in some patients with Hashimoto's disease, and in patients with diffuse toxic goiter shortly after treatment with radioiodine. A positive response to the iodide-perchlorate discharge test is seen more commonly or more strikingly in all of the foregoing disorders, as well as in some patients with untreated hyperthyroidism and those previously treated surgically or with radioiodine or antithyroid drugs. A positive response to the iodide-perchlorate discharge test is thought to be a possible forerunner of thyroid failure and an indication that the patient will be prone to develop hypothyroidism if iodides are given chronically (Braverman et al., 1971).

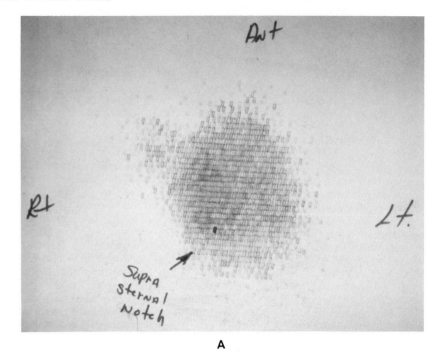

Figure 4–18. Scans of hyperfunctioning and nonfunctioning thyroid nodules. *A*, Scan of hyperfunctioning follicular adenoma arising at the junction of the isthmus and left lateral lobe. Function of the extranodular tissue is almost completely suppressed. *B*, Scan of nonfunctioning thyroid nodule in the corpus of the left lateral lobe. At operation, the lesion was a papillary carcinoma.

Tests for Thyroid Antibodies

Autoimmunity is thought to play a role in the pathogenesis of Hashimoto's disease, primary thyroprivic hypothyroidism, and Graves' disease. In part, this relationship has been suspected because of the frequent demonstration of thyroid au-toantibodies in the sera of patients with these diseases.

Four types of thyroid autoantibody have been demonstrated:

1. An antithyroglobulin antibody detectable by the agar gel diffusion precipitin technique, by the agglutination technique using tanned red cells or

particles of latex, by the fluorescent antibody technique using fixed sections of thyroid tissue, or by radioimmunoassay.

2. An antibody directed against a microsomal component of thyroid cells demonstrable by complement-fixation, by the fluorescent antibody technique using unfixed tissue, or by radioimmunoassay. This antibody may be the same as that which produces a cytotoxic effect in thyroid cells in tissue culture.

3. An antibody directed against a colloid antigen distinct from thyroglobulin, demonstrable by the fluorescent antibody technique using fixed tissue.

4. An antibody reacting with a nuclear component of thyroid cells detectable by the fluorescent antibody technique using unfixed sections of thyroid tissue.

These autoantibodies are immunoglobulins, and, except for the antinuclear antibody, are organ-specific. Only the antithyroglobulin and antimicrosomal antibodies have been used as diagnostic tools to any extent, owing to the fact that the tests for their detection in serum are more readily available.

A sensitive technique for detecting antithyroglobulin antibody is the tanned red cell agglutination test. Either sheep red cells or group O human cells are treated with tannic acid and then coated with thyroglobulin. Agglutination of these sensitized cells occurs when they are exposed to serum containing antithyroglobulin antibody. Antimicrosomal antibody is most readily detected by the ability of the patient's serum to fix complement, as indicated by a hemolytic system, in the presence of a microsomal fraction of thyroid cells.

Low titers of antithyroglobulin antibody may be detected by the tanned red cell agglutination test in the serum of normal individuals, particularly women. The frequency increases with age, approaching 20 per cent by the eighth decade (Howel Evans et al., 1967). The presence of antibody appears to correlate with the presence of focal thyroiditis histologically. Complement-fixing antibody is found in a very low percentage of men and in less than 10 per cent of women without clinically evident thyroid disease. Such individuals often display evidence of other disorders in which autoimmune phenomena occur, such as progressive hepatitis, rheumatoid arthritis, or systemic lupus erythematosus. The frequency of complement-fix-

ing antibody also increases with age, particularly in women (Howel Evans et al., 1967).

Recently, highly sensitive and specific radioimmunoassays have been developed for measuring antithyroglobulin and antimicrosomal antibodies in serum (Mori and Kriss, 1971). With these more sensitive methods, antibodies are detectable in the serum of as many as 24 per cent of normal individuals without clinically evident thyroid disease.

The approximate frequency of thyroid autoantibodies in the sera of patients with Hashimoto's disease, Graves' disease, and primary thyroprivic hypothyroidism as reported in the literature is given in Table 4–5. The reported frequencies are conditioned by the sensitivities of the tests employed. The highest titers occur in adult patients with Hashimoto's disease, but high titers are also seen in some patients with Graves' disease or primary thyroprivic hypothyroidism. In young patients with Hashimoto's disease, however, antibody titers may be low. The frequency of thyroid autoantibodies in patients with nontoxic goiter or thyroid cancer appears to be no greater than that in normal individuals without clinically overt thyroid disease.

The measurement of thyroid autoantibodies has its greatest application in the diagnosis of Hashimoto's disease. Nevertheless, in view of their high incidence in other diseases, the presence of thyroid autoantibodies must be interpreted in conjunction with the clinical picture. Measurement of thyroid autoantibodies is also helpful in the euthyroid patient with unilateral exophthalmos, since the presence of autoantibodies suggests Graves' disease rather than an intraorbital or intracranial lesion as the cause of the exophthalmos.

Thyroid Biopsy

Biopsy of the thyroid is not infrequently an exceedingly valuable diagnostic aid. It may serve to differentiate between benign and malignant neoplasms, chronic thyroiditis, and nontoxic multinodular goiter. It is also sometimes useful in establishing the diagnosis of subacute thyroiditis in atypical cases. Two types of biopsy are performed, closed and open. Closed biopsy is performed with a Vim-Silverman needle under local anesthesia after a small skin incision has been made. Although needle biopsy is used fre-

TABLE 4–5. THE INCIDENCE OF THYROID AUTOANTIBODIES IN VARIOUS THYROID DISORDERS

	Antithyroglobulin Antibody Tests		Antimicrosomal Antibody Tests	
	TRC	RIA*	CFT	RIA*
	% positive		% positive	
Hashimoto's disease	71†	86	92†	95
Graves' disease	50‡	89	35‡	98
Primary thyroprivic hypothyroidism	43†	67	80†	75

*From Mori, T., and Kriss, J. P.: *J. Clin. Endocr. 33*:688, 1971.
†From Evered, D. C., Ormston, B. J., et al.: *Brit. Med. J. 1*:657, 1973.
‡From Howel Evans, A. W., Woodrow, J. C., et al.: *Lancet 1*:636, 1967.
TRC: tanned red cell; RIA: radioimmunoassay; CFT: complement-fixation test.

quently in some clinics, the authors have not employed this technique extensively. There is general agreement that lesions suspected of being malignant should not be subjected to biopsy in this manner, since seeding of carcinoma along the needle track commonly occurs. In addition, bleeding is a hazard in the case of highly vascular glands. The main use of the needle biopsy is in establishing the diagnosis of Hashimoto's disease. Although positive tests for thyroid antibodies in conjunction with the appropriate clinical picture are highly suggestive of the presence of Hashimoto's disease, the occurrence of thyroid antibodies in other disorders, particularly in Graves' disease, makes thyroid biopsy the truly definitive diagnostic measure.

Open biopsy can be performed under either local or general anesthesia. The former should not be used if carcinoma, or another lesion requiring further surgical therapy, is anticipated. When, however, the biopsy is mainly for diagnostic purposes, local anesthesia suffices and yields more adequate specimens than does needle biopsy. This can be done on an outpatient basis. Biopsy under general anesthesia should be performed when carcinoma is suspected. Here a wider incision should be made, and the suspected lesion should be excised *in toto* and subjected to examination by frozen section.

EFFECTS OF THYROID HORMONES ON METABOLIC PROCESSES

In the sections that follow this one, the multiplicity of physiologic and biochemical derangements that are clinically evident in states of hyperthyroidism or hypothyroidism will be discussed, together with the specific disease states that produce them. This section will summarize the major metabolic effects of the thyroid hormones and the main theories concerning the cellular or molecular basis of thyroid hormone action. (For the reader interested in a more extensive discussion of these subjects, see reviews by Hoch, 1962, and Wolff and Wolff, 1964.)

Effects on Calorigenesis

One classic action of the thyroid hormones (TH) is their stimulatory effect on calorigenesis. This is reflected in increased oxygen consumption in the whole animal or in isolated tissues *in vitro*. This response occurs after a latent period of several hours or days and is evident in most tissues, the spleen, brain, and testis being notable exceptions (Fig. 4–19). T_3 causes a more prompt but somewhat shorter-lived effect than does T_4. The lag preceding these calorigenic responses has led to the suggestion that metabolic transformation of the thyroid hormones necessarily precedes induction of metabolic action. Other responses *in vivo*, however, such as increased heart rate, decreased cardiac glycogen content, and increased sensitivity to the lipolytic effect of epinephrine, precede any increase in oxygen consumption. Furthermore, several actions of the thyroid hormones *in vitro* that seem to bear a relationship to effects *in vivo* are demonstrable following a negligible lag.

The precise mechanism of the calorigenic effect of the thyroid hormones is uncertain. The calorigenic response can be inhibited or promptly reversed, however, by inhibitors of protein or nucleic acid synthesis, suggesting that it represents, at least partly, the energy requirement of protein synthe-

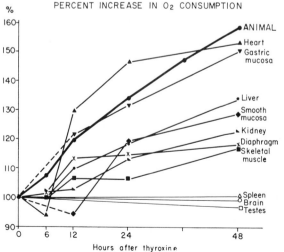

Figure 4–19. The metabolic response to thyroxine. After the injection of a single large dose of thyroxine, tissues were removed at various intervals. Their oxygen consumption rate was measured and is expressed as a percentage of the initial level. Myocardial tissue is very sensitive; the metabolic increase in this tissue actually exceeds the increase in the overall body metabolic rate. Certain tissues are shown to be unresponsive to thyroxine. The lag period can also be seen (see text). (From Barker, S. B., and Klitgaard, H. M.: *Amer. J. Physiol. 170*:81, 1952.)

sis. Many factors condition the magnitude of the calorigenic response to thyroid hormones. Advancing age and adrenergic blockade are associated with decreased reactivity. The hypothyroid patient shows a greater than normal response to a standard dose, while the converse is true in the hyperthyroid patient. These differing responses are perhaps explained on the basis of the differing proportionate increment in available hormone evoked by a standard dose.

Effects on Protein Metabolism

The pronounced effects that the thyroid hormones exert on protein metabolism may be fundamental to many of the metabolic actions of the hormones. Stimulation of protein synthesis by thyroid hormones may be directly responsible for a portion of their calorigenic effect, as previously indicated, while enhanced synthesis of specific enzymes may result in other metabolic sequelae. The relation of enhanced protein synthesis to the intrinsic mechanism of thyroid hormone action is discussed in this section.

The effect of thyroid hormones on protein metabolism depends upon the metabolic state of the recipient organism and the size of the administered dose. In thyroidectomized rats, moderate doses of T_4 increase protein synthesis and decrease nitrogen excretion. Larger doses inhibit protein synthesis and increase the concentration of free amino acids in plasma, liver, and muscle. A similar biphasic response of protein synthesis has been noted in rabbit bone marrow slices incubated in varying concentrations of T_4 *in vitro*. In rats, optimal doses of TH are necessary for the elicitation of the full growth response to growth hormone (GH); the nature of the interaction of these hormones is uncertain.

Variations in overall growth rate are probably the most general reflection of the effects of thyroid hormones on protein synthesis, and here too the effects are biphasic. In immature animals and young patients, growth is retarded by hypothyroidism, is restored by replacement doses, and is inhibited by excessive doses of hormone. In the thyrotoxic state, nitrogen excretion is increased, but it is not clear whether the catabolic response to thyroid hormones is an obligatory effect or is due to negative caloric balance. In adult patients with hypothyroidism, studies with N^{15}-glycine indicate a decreased rate of protein synthesis, and observations with I^{131}-labeled serum albumin indicate that the synthesis and degradation of this protein are retarded. These functions in the hypothyroid patient are restored to normal by replacement doses of TH.

Effects on Carbohydrate Metabolism

Thyroid hormones affect virtually all aspects of carbohydrate metabolism. Many of their influences are dependent upon or modified by other hormones, in particular the catecholamines and insulin. Thyroid hormones appear to regulate

the magnitude of the glycogenolytic and hyperglycemic actions of epinephrine, possibly by enhancing responsiveness of the adenylate cyclase–cyclic AMP system, and to potentiate the effects of insulin on glycogen synthesis and glucose utilization. Some of the effects of thyroid hormones depend upon the dose, and as a result, biphasic actions have been observed. For example, in rats, small doses of T_4 increase glycogen synthesis in the presence of insulin, whereas large doses increase hepatic glycogenolysis, causing glycogen depletion. This biphasic action of T_4 modifies the subsequent glycogenolytic response to epinephrine, small doses of T_4 enhancing and large doses depressing the response. Large doses of T_4 enhance gluconeogenesis by increasing the availability of precursors, such as lactate and glycerol. Thyroid hormones enhance the rate of intestinal absorption of glucose and galactose. They also increase the rate of uptake of glucose by adipose tissue and muscle and potentiate the effect of insulin in this respect. Insulin degradation appears to be increased by thyroid hormones, and this may account for the diminished sensitivity to exogenous insulin that is sometimes seen in thyrotoxicosis. The converse changes occur in hypothyroidism.

Effects on Lipid Metabolism

Thyroid hormones appear to stimulate virtually all aspects of lipid metabolism, including synthesis, mobilization, and degradation. In general, degradation is affected more than synthesis, the net effect in states of hormone excess being a decrease in the stores of most lipids and usually their concentrations in plasma. This is true for triglycerides, phospholipids, and cholesterol. Converse changes are seen in states of TH deficiency.

Most closely related to the changes in energy metabolism that accompany states of TH excess or deficiency are changes in the metabolism of fatty acids at their sites of storage and degradation. Thyroid hormones increase lipolysis in adipose tissue both by a direct effect through the adenylate cyclase–cyclic AMP system and by sensitizing the tissue to other lipolytic agents, such as catecholamines, GH, glucocorticoids, and glucagon. Oxidation of FFA is also increased, and this enhancement may account for some of the calorigenic action of thyroid hormones.

Hepatic synthesis of triglycerides is increased, probably as a result of the increased availability of FFA and glycerol mobilized from adipose tissue. Concomitantly, removal of triglycerides from plasma is accelerated, possibly because of an increase in lipoprotein lipase.

A classic effect of thyroid hormones is to lower the concentration of cholesterol in plasma. This is probably the result of a variety of actions. Synthesis of cholesterol is enhanced at the stage of conversion of β-hydroxy-β-methylglutaryl-coenzyme A to mevalonate, probably by increasing the activity of the enzyme concerned. Thyroid hormone action on the elimination of cholesterol is effected by an increase in both the fecal excretion of cholesterol and its conversion to bile acids. A further effect of the thyroid hormones is to enhance the turnover of low density apolipoprotein to which are bound cholesterol and phospholipids. (For references, see Challoner and Allen, 1970, and Nikkilä and Kekki, 1972.)

Effects on Vitamin Metabolism

Because of their stimulatory effect on metabolic processes, thyroid hormones increase the demand for coenzymes and the vitamins from which they are derived. In hyperthyroidism, the requirements for water-soluble vitamins, such as thiamine, riboflavin, vitamin B_{12}, and vitamin C, are increased, and their tissue concentrations are reduced. The conversion of some water-soluble vitamins to the coenzyme form may be impaired in hyperthyroidism, possibly as a result of defective energy transfers. For example, phosphorylation of pyridoxine to pyridoxal-5-phosphate (codecarboxylase) and synthesis of pyridine nucleotides (NAD and NADP) from nicotinamide appear to be defective in tissues of hyperthyroid animals. On the other hand, the synthesis of some coenzymes from vitamin requires thyroid hormones. For example, the synthesis of flavin mononucleotide and flavin adenine dinucleotide from riboflavin requires the stimulatory effect of thyroid hormones on the enzyme flavokinase (Rivlin and Langdon, 1969).

The metabolism of fat-soluble vitamins is also influenced by thyroid hormones. They are required for the synthesis of vitamin A from carotene and for the conversion of vitamin A to retinene, the pigment required for dark adaptation. In hypothyroidism, the serum carotene concentration is increased and may give the skin a yellow tint, and clinical manifestations of vitamin A deficiency may occur. In hyperthyroidism, the requirement for vitamin A is increased and the tissue concentration is reduced. Vitamins D and E appear to be deficient in hyperthyroid animals.

THEORIES CONCERNING THE MECHANISM OF ACTION OF THYROID HORMONES

There is an appealing parsimony in the concept that the manifold physiologic and biochemical effects of the thyroid hormones reflect a single action, or perhaps a few basic actions, at the cellular or molecular level. That this may be the case is suggested by the very diversity of hormonal effects, since it is very unlikely that a distinct mechanism is responsible for each. More likely, many of the effects observed are merely secondary consequences of a more fundamental action. Furthermore, most actions of the thyroid hormones are demonstrable only after a considerable latent period, suggesting that they are anteceded by some more proximate event. This perhaps explains the inability of thyroactive materials to reproduce in

vitro the great majority of hormonal effects elicited *in vivo*. Nevertheless, despite the literally hundreds, and perhaps thousands, of studies designed to clarify the mode of action of the thyroid hormones, the data as yet do no more than indicate potentially fruitful avenues for future study.

The activity of a great many enzymes involved in substrate dissimilation or electron transport has been shown to be responsive to variations in the supply of TH to the intact organism or to tissue preparations *in vitro*. To date, however, it has not been possible to construct and support a hypothesis by which the many metabolic effects of the thyroid hormones could be explained by a primary action on specific enzymes or enzyme complexes. It is the general feeling at present that while these changes in enzyme activity may indeed influence or sustain the pattern of metabolic response to thyroid hormones, they are unlikely to be the primary initiators of thyroid hormone action. The possibility that the thyroid hormones may themselves function as oxidation-reduction catalysts has also received consideration, but the importance of this mechanism is difficult to evaluate.

In view of the fact that increased oxygen consumption is one of the cardinal effects of the thyroid hormones, great attention has been directed toward the effects of thyroid hormones on mitochondria, since they are the locus of terminal oxidation of metabolites and transfer of electrons to oxygen along the respiratory chain. It is here, too, that oxidations are most efficiently linked or coupled to the generation of the high-energy phosphate bonds of ATP, a form that can be utilized for the performance of physical or chemical work. An additional relevant feature of mitochondrial respiration is that the rate of generation of high-energy phosphate in some way regulates inversely the rate of substrate oxidation and oxygen utilization. Normally, the rate of oxidation is highly dependent upon the availability of ADP or other phosphate acceptors. When this is the case, respiration is said to be "tightly controlled."

An early theory concerning the mechanism of stimulation of oxygen consumption and energy expenditure by thyroid hormones suggested that thyroid hormones uncouple oxidative phosphorylations, i,e., decrease the rate of high-energy phosphate-bond generation in relation to the rate of prevailing oxidations (P:O ratio). Under these conditions, oxygen consumption is increased, but the yield of usable energy is relatively decreased. However, interest in this possibility has waned in view of the finding that mitochondria from skeletal muscle of thyrotoxic patients do not display uncoupling, nor do mitochondria from animals brought from a hypothyroid to a euthyroid state. Moreover, other agents, such as 2, 4-dinitrophenol (DNP), that uncouple oxidative phosphorylations fail to mimic fully the metabolic and physiologic effects of the thyroid hormones and, unlike T_4, fail to support growth or amphibian metamorphosis.

A variety of other mitochondrial effects of the thyroid hormones have been observed. *In vivo*, T_4 induces an increase in the number and size of mitochondria and in the number of mitochondrial cristae. It induces swelling of mitochondria *in vitro* with loss of mitochondrial constituents, an effect seen in T_4-responsive tissues but not in tissues whose oxygen consumption fails to increase in response to T_4, such as brain, testis, and spleen. In hypothyroid animals, T_4 promptly stimulates mitochondrial respiration in the absence of added ADP (state 4 respiration) (Hoch, 1967), and later it stimulates ADP-dependent respiration (state 3) as well. Some evidence suggests that the stimulation of state 4 respiration may reflect the action of a specific mitochondrial protein whose synthesis is induced by thyroid hormones (Kaplay and Sanadi, 1971). T_4 and T_3, both *in vitro* and *in vivo*, promptly stimulate mitochondrial protein synthesis, and both, after several days, increase the carrier-mediated uptake of ADP by rat liver mitochondria, an effect thought to mediate enhanced ATP generation. It is not known whether or how the foregoing effects are interrelated, but their net result would presumably be an enhanced rate of oxygen consumption, an increased number of respiratory units, and an increased availability of high-energy phosphate (energy charge) within the cell.

Not directly related to effects on the mitochondria, but perhaps coordinated with mitochondrial function, is the recently described effect of thyroid hormones to increase the activity of plasma membrane-bound, Na^+, K^+-dependent, ouabain-sensitive ATPase (Ismail-Beigi and Edelman, 1971). Inhibition of this system by ouabain results in abolition of much, though not all, of the TH-mediated increase in oxygen consumption to an extent which varies among different tissues. The increase in ATPase activity may be secondary to the enhanced transport of ADP into the mitochondrion, with a resulting increase in energy charge (Babior et al., 1973), but whether this is true or not, the resultant of both effects would be an increased turnover of high-energy phosphate and increased substrate oxidations.

In view of the profound effects of the thyroid hormones on growth and other aspects of protein metabolism, a second major thrust of research concerning the mechanism of thyroid hormone action has been in the area of the mechanisms of protein synthesis. *In vivo*, thyroid hormones enhance the incorporation of amino acids into tissues that are otherwise T_4-responsive. It may be presumed that the enhanced protein synthesis that this represents, if appropriately directed, could explain the increased synthesis of specific enzymes that thyroid hormones induce. The demonstration that inhibitors of protein synthesis inhibit the calorigenic action of thyroid hormones is consonant with the concept that the stimulation of protein synthesis and the stimulation of respiration induced by T_4 are causally related. In addition to the stimulation of mitochondrial protein synthesis noted above, there are two other sites where an effect on the protein synthetic mechanism has been detected. In studies of hypothyroid animals given exogenous hormone, a stimulation of the mechanism for protein synthesis at the transcriptional level preceded the increase in oxygen consumption. The effects observed were an increase in the activity of nuclear RNA-polymerase followed by an increase in the synthesis of RNA, particularly ribosomal RNA (Tata and Widnell, 1966). Subsequently, it was demonstrated that the thyroid hormones have an even earlier effect on protein synthesis at the level of translation. Within a few minutes after administration of hormone or its addition *in vitro*, enhanced transfer to ribosomal protein of amino acid bound to tRNA can be demonstrated (Sokoloff et al., 1968). It appeared that this effect could be demonstrated only in the presence of mitochondria, but whether this reflects the release of a stimulatory mitochondrial factor, as has been suggested, or merely the provision of ATP is uncertain (Carter et al., 1971).

Among the other effects of thyroid hormones which have to date been less thoroughly explored are several that appear to occur at the plasma membrane of the cell. These include stimulation of adenylate cyclase and enhancement of amino acid transport in certain tissues, as well as the effects on the Na^+, K^+-dependent ATPase already described.

For the present, it is uncertain whether the thyroid hormones exert a single action from which all others follow, or, as seems more likely to the authors, several actions, each of which has a multiplicity of consequences. It is obvious, however, that in the intact organism thyroid hormones act upon the whole cell and that there occurs a considerable degree of interdependence and cooperativity between the various effects observed.

AN APPROACH TO THE CLINICAL DIAGNOSIS OF THYROID DISEASE

Diseases of the thyroid gland almost always manifest themselves through symptoms resulting from excessive or insufficient production of thyroid hormone, through local symptoms in the neck, principally goiter (but occasionally pain or compression of adjacent structures), or, in the case of Graves' disease, through exophthalmos. Although the physician's attention is directed initially at the major clinical evidence, he seeks ultimately to establish both a functional and an anatomical diagnosis; i.e., he seeks to define the patient's metabolic state and to ascertain the nature of the lesion in the thyroid gland. These two aspects of the complete diagnosis are not arrived at independently, because the functional state will delimit the possible anatomical diagnoses and vice versa.

A functional diagnosis of thyroid disease is based upon a carefully taken history, a thorough search for the physical signs of hypothyroidism or thyrotoxicosis, and an intelligent appraisal of the results of laboratory tests. Characteristic alterations in these aspects will be found in the discussions of the various disease states. Although conditioned by the functional diagnosis, the anatomical diag-

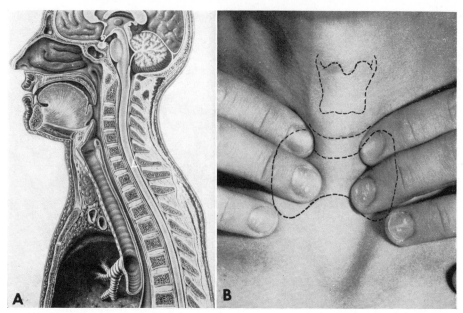

Figure 4–20. *A*, This sagittal section demonstrates the relations of the isthmus of the normal thyroid gland. The superior border is inferior to the cricoid cartilage. The inferior thyroid border is essentially at the level of the superior surface of the manubrium. The inferior portions of the lateral lobes (not shown) extend more inferiorly than the isthmus. (Reproduced by permission of Merck & Co., Inc.).

B, The cricoid cartilage is regarded as a very important landmark. Especially when the thyroid gland is suspected as being essentially normal or subnormal in size the cricoid should be located. This is easily accomplished. The index fingers are then inserted so that their superior portion rests against the inferior portion of the cricoid, while the inferior portion of these fingers is over the superior portion of the thyroid. The second and third fingers are rotated over other portions of the gland, evaluating its size, contour, consistency, possible adherence to surrounding structures, and other features. Since there is marked variation among different subjects in the length and thickness of the neck and in the length of the trachea superior to the level of the manubrium, there is variation in the relative position of the thyroid. In some cases, essentially all of the thyroid rests posterior to the sternum. In most instances, however, by having the patient extend his neck maximally (short of markedly tightening the neck muscles) and by having him swallow repeatedly, it is possible to palpate most or all of the gland. One point deserving emphasis is the fact that in spite of marked variations in neck-chest relations, thyroid tissue, when present, is found within 1 cm. of the cricoid. By concentrating the palpation meticulously in the area where the thyroid is normally found, with very rare exceptions it is possible to outline small as well as enlarged glands.

nosis will depend largely upon the examination of the thyroid gland itself (Fig. 4–20).

Local examination of the neck is best accomplished with the patient seated in a good light with the neck moderately extended. The patient should be provided with a glass of water to facilitate swallowing. The physician should first inspect the neck from the front and sides. The presence of old surgical scars, distended veins, and redness or fixation of the overlying skin should be noted. If a mass is present, attention should be directed to its location and to whether or not it moves on swallowing. Movement on swallowing is a characteristic feature of the thyroid gland and is due to the fact that the gland is ensheathed by the pretracheal fascia; this feature distinguishes a goiter from most other masses arising in the neck. However, if a goiter is so large that it occupies all the available space in the neck, or if the thyroid gland is the seat of an invasive carcinoma or Riedel's thyroiditis that has led to fixation to adjacent structures, movement on swallowing may be lost. The physician should also inspect the dorsum of the tongue, which is the origin of the thyroglossal duct and occasionally the seat of a goiter (lingual goiter).

Palpation of the neck is best accomplished by standing behind the seated patient and palpating with the fingertips of both hands. The position of the cricoid cartilage is first determined; this is an important landmark, since the superior border of the isthmus lies just below it. The isthmus is a band of tissue crossing the front of the trachea and joining the two lateral lobes on either side of the trachea. The examiner then attempts to outline the thyroid gland and to determine the limits of the lower borders of the lateral lobes, while the patient swallows sips of water at appropriate intervals. A normal thyroid gland can usually be felt on palpation. The examiner should note the shape of the gland, its size in relation to normal and its consistency. The normal gland is rubbery. Whereas the diffuse colloid goiter and the hyperplastic gland of Graves' disease tend to be softer than normal, the gland of Hashimoto's disease tends to be firmer than normal, and the gland that is the seat of carcinoma or Riedel's thyroiditis may be "stony" hard. Irregularities of the surface, variations in consistency, and tender areas should be noted. If nodules are palpated, their shape, size, position, and consistency in relation to the surrounding tissue should be determined. A search should be made for the pyramidal lobe; this is a band of tissue extending upward from the isthmus to the right or left of the midline. The pyramidal lobe may be mistaken for the pretracheal or "delphian" lymph node that sometimes accompanies thyroid carcinoma or thyroiditis. Another midline mass that may lead to confusion is a thyroglossal cyst, but since this often remains attached to the base of the tongue by the obliterated thyroglossal duct, it moves upward when the tongue is protruded. During palpation a vascular thrill may be felt and, in the absence of cardiac disease, is very suggestive of hyperthyroidism. Finally, palpation should always include examination of the regional lymph nodes.

Ausculation of the neck should be performed since it gives some indication of the vascularity of the gland. A systolic or continuous bruit is commonly heard over a hyperplastic gland. However, care should be taken to distinguish a thyroid bruit from a murmur transmitted from the base of the heart or from a venous hum that can be obliterated by compression of the external jugular vein or by turning the head.

Two useful clinical maneuvers that are often neglected are transillumination and the arm-raising test. Transillumination is readily performed with a penlight and serves to distinguish between cystic and solid masses in the thyroid. Since the normal tissues of the neck transilluminate to some extent, the transillumination in the lesion should be compared with that in an indifferent area. The arm-raising test is useful in the patient in whom a retrosternal goiter is suspected. The basis for this maneuver is that if the size of the thoracic inlet is already reduced by a retrosternal goiter, raising both arms until they touch the sides of the head will further narrow the thoracic inlet and cause congestion of the face and respiratory distress (Pemberton's sign).

In addition to examination of the thyroid gland and regional lymph nodes, evidence of compression or displacement of adjacent structures should also be sought. Hoarseness may indicate compression of the recurrent laryngeal nerve, usually by a malignant thyroid neoplasm, and this should be confirmed by laryngoscopy. Displacement of the trachea may be evident, and inspiratory stridor may indicate compression of the trachea. Radiologic examination is a useful adjunct, since it may reveal retrosternal extension of a goiter, displacement or narrowing of the trachea, and, during a barium swallow, displacement of the esophagus. Calcification in the thyroid gland may also be seen and, by its nature, aid in distinguishing between benign and malignant lesions.

THYROTOXICOSIS

The term thyrotoxicosis refers to the biochemical and physiologic complex that results when the tissues are presented with excessive quantities of the thyroid hormones. The authors prefer the general term thyrotoxicosis rather than hyperthyroidism to describe this syndrome, since it need not originate in the thyroid gland. The term hyperthyroid-

What is a ⊕ Plummer's Sign

ism is best reserved for the usual instances in which thyrotoxicosis results from overproduction of hormone by the thyroid itself. There are several causes of thyrotoxicosis, the most important and intriguing being Graves' disease. Overproduction of hormone may also arise in patients with preexisting nontoxic multinodular goiter or with one or more autonomously functioning adenomas within the gland. Less commonly, thyrotoxicosis may result from hyperfunction of ectopic thyroid tissue or from ingestion of large quantities of exogenous hormone (thyrotoxicosis factitia). The nature of the manifestations of thyrotoxicosis depends upon the severity of the syndrome, the age of the patient, and the presence or absence of disease in other organ systems. Additional clinical features are conditioned by the specific disorder producing the thyrotoxicosis.

Hashimoto may be harder
auscultate the gland   ? hoarse

Peripheral Manifestations of Thyrotoxicosis

vide Pemberton's Sign.

Skin and Appendages

Thyrotoxicosis leads to a variety of changes in the skin and its appendages. Most characteristic is the warm moist feel of the skin that results from cutaneous vasodilation and excessive sweating as part of the hyperdynamic circulatory state. The hands are usually warm and moist, but the texture of the skin in this area is often altered by occupational or environmental factors; hence, texture is best assessed on the inner aspect of the arm or thigh or over the thorax. Classically, the elbows are smooth and pink. The complexion is rosy and the patient blushes readily. Palmar erythema, indistinguishable from "liver palms," is common, and there may be some telangiectasia. Increased diffuse pigmentation is found occasionally and may resemble that found in Addison's disease, but the authors have not noted buccal pigmentation in uncomplicated thyrotoxicosis. Patchy vitiligo may also occur. Increased pigmentation may result from hypersecretion of ACTH secondary to accelerated metabolism of cortisol.

The hair is fine and friable and does not retain a wave; some may fall out. The nails are often soft and friable. A characteristic finding is Plummer's nails, a term applied to separation of the distal margin of the nail from the nail bed with irregular recession of the junction (onycholysis). Dirt often accumulates under the nail. Usually these changes are best seen in the fourth finger and are frequently accompanied by a thin shiny appearance of the skin surrounding the nail.

Eyes

Retraction of the upper eyelid, evident as the presence of a rim of sclera between the lid and the limbus, is a very frequent manifestation of all forms of thyrotoxicosis, irrespective of the underlying cause. It is responsible for the bright-eyed "stare" of the patient with thyrotoxicosis. Accompanying lid retraction are the phenomena of lid lag, in which the upper lid lags behind the globe when the patient is asked to gaze slowly downward, and globe lag, in which the globe lags behind the upper lid when the patient gazes slowly upward. The movements of the lids are jerky and spasmodic, and a fine tremor of the lightly closed lids can often be observed. These ocular manifestations appear to be the result of increased adrenergic activity, since they are ameliorated by adrenergic antagonists. It is important to differentiate these ocular manifestations, which occur in all forms of thyrotoxicosis, from those of infiltrative ophthalmopathy, which are characteristic of Graves' disease.

Cardiovascular System

Alterations in cardiovascular function are among the most prominent manifestations of thyrotoxicosis. Increased circulatory demands result from both the hypermetabolism and the need to dissipate the excess heat produced. At rest, peripheral vascular resistance is decreased, and cardiac output is increased as a result of an increase in both stroke volume and heart rate (Graettinger et al., 1959). At first, the thyroid hormones were considered to exert their inotropic and chronotropic effects largely through the adrenergic nervous system by sensitizing a catecholamine-responsive adenylate cyclase–cyclic AMP system in the myocardium. It has recently been shown, however, that they exert direct inotropic and chronotropic effects independent of the adrenergic nervous system (Buccino et al., 1967; Grossman et al., 1971a), which appear to be mediated by activation of a thyroid hormone–specific adenylate cyclase–cyclic AMP system. Nevertheless, an increase in adrenergic activity does also appear to be involved in the maintenance of the hyperdynamic circulatory state of thyrotoxicosis, since some amelioration of the hemodynamic manifestations accompanies treatment with adrenergic antagonists. The mechanism ultimately responsible for the increased adrenergic activity is uncertain, however. (See Levey, 1971, for an extensive review of the literature.)

Clinically, tachycardia is almost always present, even at rest. Tachycardia during sleep (pulse rate greater than 90 beats/min.) serves to distinguish tachycardia of thyrotoxic origin from that of psychogenic origin. The pulse pressure is widened as a result of both an increase in systolic and a decrease in diastolic pressure. The increased force of cardiac contraction is often felt by the patient as palpitation and is evident on inspection or palpation of the precordium. Owing to the diffuse and forceful nature of the apex beat, the heart often seems enlarged, but x-ray study generally does not confirm this impression. Heart sounds are loud and ringing, and a systolic or even a late diastolic or presystolic murmur may be present at the apex. A scratchy systolic sound along the left sternal border, resembling a pericardial friction rub, may also be heard. These physical signs abate when a normal metabolic state is restored.

Cardiac arrhythmias are common with thyrotoxicosis and are almost invariably supraventricular. Approximately 10 per cent of patients with thyrotoxicosis manifest atrial fibrillation and a similar percentage of patients with otherwise unexplained atrial fibrillation prove to be thyrotoxic. Paroxysmal supraventricular tachycardia may be manifested or may be suggested by the history.

The adequacy of the circulation is a question of great importance in the patient with thyrotoxicosis. The arteriovenous oxygen difference is generally normal, but the significance of this is obscured since, for purposes of heat loss, a considerable proportion of the cardiac output may be directed to the skin, in which relatively little oxygen consumption occurs. Although the cardiovascular cost of a standard work load or metabolic challenge is increased, this is adequately met if the patient is not or has not previously been in heart failure. Thus, in most patients without underlying heart disease, cardiac competence is maintained. Mild edema not uncommonly occurs in the absence of heart failure. Nevertheless, thyrotoxicosis may indeed lead to congestive heart failure, but even so, the circulation time may remain shortened. Heart failure usually occurs in patients with preexisting heart disease, but the presence of heart disease often cannot be determined until after thyrotoxicosis is relieved. There is little doubt that pure thyrocardiac disease does occur, but only uncommonly, and usually in association with atrial fibrillation. Since the latter decreases the efficiency of the cardiac response to any increased circulatory demand, it may play a prominent role in bringing about cardiac failure. Attempts to convert atrial fibrillation to sinus rhythm are usually of no avail while thyrotoxicosis is present. Regardless of the type of rhythm the response to digitalis is decreased, possibly because of accelerated metabolism of the drug (Doherty and Perkins, 1966), and large quantities are required to produce a clinical effect. Resistance to digitalis, as well as failure of cardiac decompensation to respond to a usually adequate regimen, should suggest the possibility of thyrotoxicosis.

The frequency of coronary artery disease in patients with thyrotoxicosis is uncertain. Frank myocardial infarction is uncommon; however, when angina pectoris is present, it is aggravated by thyrotoxicosis and relieved by treatment.

Respiratory System

Dyspnea is a common symptom of thyrotoxicosis and need not be due to heart failure. Studies of pulmonary function have revealed several factors that may contribute to this symptom. Vital capacity is commonly reduced; this appears to result mainly from weakness of the respiratory muscles, but decreased pulmonary compliance may also play a role. During exercise, ventilation is increased out of proportion to the increase in oxygen uptake; diffusing capacity of the lung is normal, however. The alterations in pulmonary function return to normal when a normal metabolic state is restored (Stein et al., 1961).

Alimentary System

Increase in appetite, both at mealtimes and between meals, is a common symptom of thyrotoxicosis, but the mechanism whereby this occurs is unknown. Except in unusual cases, increased intake of food is inadequate to meet the increased caloric requirements, and weight is lost at a variable rate. In the occasional, usually younger, patient with mild disease, weight gain may occur instead. Anorexia, rather than hyperphagia, sometimes accompanies severe forms of thyrotoxicosis. It also occurs in some older patients and contributes to the picture of "masked" thyrotoxicosis.

The commonest symptoms referable to the GI tract are those related to bowel function. Frank diarrhea is rare; more often, stools are merely less well formed and the frequency of bowel movements is increased. When constipation has anteceded the development of thyrotoxicosis, bowel function may return to normal. Anorexia, nausea, and vomiting are uncommon, but when they occur, it is usually in patients with severe disease. These symptoms, as well as abdominal pain, may be forerunners of thyroid storm. The frequency with which they are manifestations of associated hypercalcemia is unknown.

The function of the GI tract in thyrotoxicosis has not been thoroughly studied. No explanation is available for the increase in GI motility, since increased adrenergic activity should have the opposite effect. Peptic ulcer is said to be uncommon in patients with thyrotoxicosis, perhaps because a high proportion of patients display gastric achlorhydria. In the majority, acid secretion returns after relief of the thyrotoxicosis, but in some it does not. Circulating autoantibodies against gastric parietal cells are found in approximately one-third of patients with Graves' disease, and approximately 3 per cent have been reported to have frank pernicious anemia (Ardeman et al., 1966). It is commonly thought that intestinal absorption is accelerated in thyrotoxicosis, but evidence for this is sparse. In experimental animals, intestinal absorption of xylose is unaffected by induction of thyrotoxicosis, and no evidence for an increased rate of absorption of xylose has been found in thyrotoxic humans. It is commonly stated that the oral glucose tolerance curve displays a high early peak in patients with thyrotoxicosis, but, in fact, the glycemic peak is frequently delayed (Woeber et al., 1966).

Hepatic dysfunction occurs in thyrotoxicosis, particularly when the disease is severe; hypoproteinemia, increases in serum transaminase and alkaline phosphatase, and mild BSP retention may occur. In milder cases, no dysfunction may be evident. In the most severe cases, hepatomegaly and jaundice may be found. Gynecomastia is present in about 5 per cent of men with thyrotoxicosis. In thyrotoxicosis, splanchnic oxygen consumption is increased, while blood flow is essentially unchanged. As a result, the arteriovenous oxygen difference across the splanchnic bed is increased; hence, hypoxia may contribute to hepatic dysfunction. Hypoxia, together with the state of relative caloric deprivation, may partly account for the depletion of hepatic glycogen which is evident both in the response to glycogenolytic agents and on direct analysis. In the absence of severe thyrotoxicosis or congestive heart failure, the liver may appear normal on light microscopic examination. In severe cases, however, centrilobular fatty infiltration may occur, together with patchy portal fibrosis, lymphocytic infiltration, and proliferation of bile ducts. Ultramicroscopic examination of the liver reveals enlarged mitochondria and hypertrophic smooth endoplasmic reticulum (Klion et al., 1971).

Nervous System

Alterations in the function of the nervous system are an almost invariable accompaniment of thyrotoxicosis and are most commonly manifested by nervousness, emotional lability, and hyperkinesia. The nervousness of the thyrotoxic patient is not that of the patient who is chronically anxious but rather is characterized by restlessness, shortness of attention span, and a need to be moving around and doing, despite a feeling of fatigue. Unlike the patient with neurocirculatory asthenia, the thyrotoxic patient wishes to be active but is hampered by fatigability; he is tired from the neck down, rather than from the top of the head down. Fatigue may be a manifestation of muscle weakness and the insomnia of which patients with thyrotoxicosis commonly complain. In some patients, asthenia and fatigue are so severe that overall activity is decreased.

Emotional lability is also a prominent symptom. Patients lose their tempers easily and have episodes of crying without apparent reason. Crying may be evoked by merely questioning the patient about this symptom. In rare cases, severe psychic disturbance may occur; manic-depressive, schizoid, or paranoid reactions may emerge during thyrotoxicosis. These sometimes fail to regress when a normal metabolic state is restored.

The hyperkinesia of the thyrotoxic patient is characteristic to those who are familiar with the disease. During the interview, the patient cannot sit still; he drums on the table, taps his foot, or shifts positions frequently. Movements are quick, jerky, exaggerated, and often purposeless. In children, in whom such manifestations tend to be more severe, Sydenham's chorea may be suggested. Examination also reveals a fine, rhythmic tremor of the hands, tongue, or lightly closed eyelids. With the aid of a magnifying glass, a tremor of the eyeballs may be seen. The tremor of thyrotoxicosis may sometimes mimic that of parkinsonism, while preexisting parkinsonian tremor is accentuated during thyrotoxicosis. In patients with convulsive disorders, the frequency of seizures is increased. The electroencephalogram reveals an increase in fast wave activity, and in experimental animals, the convulsive threshold is decreased.

The physiologic basis of the findings referable to the nervous system is not well understood. In part, they may reflect increased adrenergic activity since some improvement occurs during treatment with adrenergic antagonists (Grossman et al., 1971b). Although the cerebral blood flow of thyrotoxic patients is increased, arteriovenous oxygen difference is diminished, and oxygen extraction is unchanged. This correlates well with failure of T_4 to increase the oxygen consumption of brain tissue in animals. Nevertheless, failure of oxygen consumption to increase does not exclude the likelihood that other alterations in cerebral metabolism are induced by thyroid hormone.

Muscle

Weakness and fatigability are frequent complaints of the patient with thyrotoxicosis. In most instances, these are not accompanied by any objective evidence of local disease of muscle save for the generalized wasting that is associated with loss of weight. Often the weakness is most prominent in the proximal muscles of the limbs, with the result that the patient experiences difficulty in climbing stairs or in maintaining the leg in an extended position. The latter maneuver can be employed to assess the degree of muscle weakness. In occasional cases, involvement of muscle is associated with wasting that again tends to be proximal and is out of proportion to the overall loss of weight (thyrotoxic myopathy). Here, in the extreme form, the patient may be unable to rise from a sitting or lying position and may be virtually unable to walk. This disorder may resemble progressive muscular atrophy or polymyositis, but fasciculation is absent and, on biopsy, little if any inflammatory change is evident. Instead, atrophy of muscle and infiltration by fat cells and lymphocytes are present. Electron microscopy reveals abnormal mitochondria and focal dilations of the transverse tubular system (Engel, 1972). Electromyograms reveal a decreased duration of mean action potentials and an increased percentage of polyphasic potentials (Ramsay, 1966). The biochemical basis of the muscular weakness is uncertain but may be related to the impaired ability of thyrotoxic muscle to phosphorylate creatine. Creatinuria is present and creatine tolerance is diminished.

Myopathy affects men with thyrotoxicosis more commonly than women and may overshadow the other manifestations of the syndrome. In the most severe forms, the myopathy may involve the more distal muscles of the extremities, as well as muscles of the trunk and face. Although involvement of ocular muscles is unusual, the disorder may mimic myasthenia gravis; Graves' disease and myasthenia do occur together with inordinate frequency. In uncomplicated thyrotoxic myopathy, some improvement of muscular strength may follow administration of edrophonium, but, unlike that in myasthenia, the response is incomplete. Muscular strength returns to normal when a normal metabolic state has been restored, but muscle mass takes longer to recover.

Graves' disease occurs in about 3–5 per cent of patients with myasthenia gravis, and about 1 per cent of patients with Graves' disease develop myasthenia gravis. These associations are of interest in view of the frequent association of thymic enlargement with Graves' disease. Unlike thyrotoxic myopathy, the association of myasthenia gravis with Graves' disease has a distinct female sex preponderance similar to that of uncomplicated Graves' disease. The effect of both thyrotoxicosis and its alleviation on the course of myasthenia gravis is variable, but in the majority of instances, myasthenia is accentuated during the thyrotoxic state and improves when a normal metabolic state is restored (Namba and Grob, 1971).

Periodic paralysis of the hypokalemic type may occur together with thyrotoxicosis, and its severity is greatly accentuated by the latter disorder. The coincidence of the two disorders is particularly common in Japanese and Chinese patients, in whom the incidence of periodic paralysis has been reported to be as high as 13 per cent in men and 0.4 per cent in women with thyrotoxicosis (McFadzean and Yeung, 1967).

Skeletal System: Calcium and Phosphorus Metabolism

The interrelationships between the thyroid gland, bone, and mineral metabolism are complex, varied, and poorly understood. Changes in the structure of bone or the metabolism of calcium and phosphorus in thyrotoxicosis have in the past been ascribed to direct effects of thyroid hormone either on bone or on the excretion or absorption of mineral, perhaps with secondary alterations in parathyroid activity. The demonstration, however, that the thyroid gland secretes a humoral product (calcitonin) that has effects generally antagonistic to those of parathyroid hormone has complicated already clouded physiopathologic interrelationships, since nothing is known of the effect of those disorders that lead to thyrotoxicosis on the ability of the thyroid gland to produce calcitonin. Hence a consideration of the changes in mineral metabolism that accompany thyrotoxicosis must be largely descriptive.

Thyrotoxicosis is generally associated with increased excretion of calcium and phosphorus in urine and stool. Excessive loss of mineral is sometimes associated with radiologically demonstrable demineralization of bone and occasionally with pathologic fractures, especially in elderly women. In such instances, the histologic appearance of bone is variable, suggesting osteitis fibrosa, osteomalacia, or osteoporosis. Osteoporosis has been traditionally ascribed to loss of protein matrix, but severely negative calcium balance has been found in some patients who are in virtual nitrogen equilibrium, making this explanation unlikely. Urinary excretion of hydroxyproline is invariably increased in thyrotoxicosis, indicating increased turnover of collagen. Kinetic studies indicate an increase in the exchangeable calcium pool and acceleration of both bone resorption and accretion, the former especially so.

Hypercalcemia sometimes occurs, but the precise incidence of this complication is uncertain. However, it may occur in as many as 20 per cent of patients. In rare cases, hypercalcemia may be sufficient to induce anorexia, nausea, vomiting, polyuria, or even renal failure. The serum alkaline phosphatase concentration is usually normal, but occasionally it may be increased. Hence the findings in serum may closely simulate those in primary hyperparathyroidism, but indices of tubular reabsorption of phosphate or the response to calcium infusion are inconsistent with parathyroid hyperfunction and autonomy. Very rarely, thyrotoxicosis and true primary hyperparathyroidism coexist (reviewed extensively by Michie et al., 1971).

The average height is above normal in thyrotoxic children. Maturation of bone may be stimulated so that bone age is advanced, but usually this is not of marked degree.

Renal Function: Water and Electrolyte Metabolism

In the absence of associated hypercalcemia or diabetes mellitus, thyrotoxicosis produces no symptoms referable to the urinary tract save for mild polyuria. Nevertheless, rates of renal blood flow and glomerular filtration as well as tubular reabsorptive and secretory maxima are increased. Total body water and exchangeable potassium (K^+) are decreased, possibly because of a decrease in lean body mass, but exchangeable sodium (Na^+) tends to be increased (Wayne, 1960). Serum Na^+, K^+, and chloride (Cl^-) concentrations are normal, however. In thyrotoxicosis, exchangeable magnesium (Mg^{2+}) is normal, but serum Mg^{2+} concentration is often decreased and urinary Mg^{2+} excretion increased (Jones et al., 1966).

Hematopoietic System

In most patients with thyrotoxicosis, the red cells are normal as judged by the usual indices. In response to the increased oxygen requirements of the thyrotoxic state, the red cell mass is increased. This is associated with erythroid hyperplasia and may account for a moderate increase in the fecal excretion of urobilin. In thyrotoxicosis, oxygen release from hemoglobin is increased. This has been ascribed to the increased content of 2,3-diphosphoglyceric acid in the red cell in this dis-

order, since 2,3-disphosphoglyceric acid enhances the dissociation of oxygen from hemoglobin by virtue of its ability to bind to hemoglobin and stabilize its reduced form (Miller et al., 1970). Thyroid hormones increase the content of 2,3-diphosphoglyceric acid in normal red cells *in vitro*, perhaps by stimulating directly diphosphoglycerate mutase activity (Snyder and Reddy, 1970). Other red cell abnormalities in thyrotoxicosis include a reduced content of the B isoenzyme of carbonic anhydrase (Funakoshi and Deutsch, 1971) and an increased content of Na^+, suggesting impaired activity of the Na^+, K^+ pump (Goolden et al., 1971).

Approximately 3 per cent of patients with Graves' disease have pernicious anemia, and a further 3 per cent are reported to have intrinsic factor autoantibodies with normal absorption of vitamin B_{12}. Circulating autoantibodies against gastric parietal cells have been reported to occur in about one-third of patients with Graves' disease (Ardeman et al., 1966). In thyrotoxicosis, requirements for vitamin B_{12} and folic acid appear to be increased. Rarely, thyrotoxicosis is associated with a mild, hypochromic anemia that is characterized by adequate stores of iron in the marrow and a response to large doses of pyridoxine.

In about 10 per cent of patients with thyrotoxicosis, the total white cell count is low because of a decrease in neutrophils. The absolute lymphocyte count is normal or increased, leading to a relative lymphocytosis. Monocytes may also be increased, and, in the authors' clinic, the absolute eosinophil count was often increased. Splenic enlargement occurs in about 10 per cent of the patients, and thymic and lymph node enlargement is said to be common. It is not known whether these abnormalities are a reflection of the autoimmune aspects of Graves' disease, but this is unlikely, since comparable alterations do not occur in Hashimoto's disease. Alternatively, these alterations may result from mild adrenocortical insufficiency or from a direct effect of thyroid hormone on lymphoid tissue.

Blood platelets and the intrinsic clotting mechanism are normal. However, the concentration of factor VIII is often increased, and this returns to normal when the thyrotoxicosis is treated (Simone et al., 1965). The increase in factor VIII may reflect increased adrenergic activity, since infusion of epinephrine into normal subjects produces a similar effect.

Pituitary and Adrenocortical Function

In some respects, the thyrotoxic state imposes a challenge on pituitary and particularly adrenocortical function. In thyrotoxicosis, the metabolic transformations leading to the inactivation of cortisol are accelerated. These include reduction of the A ring, which is rapidly followed by conjugation, and oxidation of the 11-hydroxy group to a keto group as a result of an increase in 11β-hydroxysteroid dehydrogenase activity; the 11-keto compounds are less active than their 11-hydroxy precursors (Hellman et al., 1970). As a result of these changes the disposal of cortisol is accelerated, but its rate of secretion is also increased so that plasma cortisol concentration remains normal. The urinary excretion of 17-hydroxycorticosteroids (17-OHCS) is normal or slightly increased, whereas the urinary excretion of 17-ketosteroids (17-KS) may be moderately reduced.

The foregoing alterations require that some degree of adrenocortical hyperfunction be sustained in thyrotoxic patients and may account for the finding of increased concentrations of ACTH-like activity in plasma. Pituitary-adrenal function is adequate for basal demands, as indicated by normal plasma cortisol concentrations, and the response to an acute challenge, such as is imposed by metyrapone or hypoglycemia, is generally adequate (Giustina et al., 1971). However, the response to the 2-day ACTH test is often subnormal on the second day, indicating some limitation of adrenocortical reserve.

The rate of turnover of aldosterone is increased, but its plasma concentration is normal (Luetscher et al., 1963). Plasma renin activity is increased, and sensitivity to angiotensin II is reduced (Hauger-Klevene et al., 1972).

The response of plasma growth hormone (GH) concentration to insulin-induced hypoglycemia is subnormal in patients with thyrotoxicosis, particularly those with severe disease (Giustina et al., 1971). This observation need not indicate deficient GH production but rather may reflect depletion of pituitary stores from prolonged caloric inadequacy or accelerated removal of GH from plasma. Suppression of plasma GH concentration by induced hyperglycemia has been reported to be incomplete in thyrotoxicosis; this may also reflect prolonged caloric deprivation (Vinik et al., 1967).

Catecholamines

An important but poorly understood association between the adrenergic nervous system and the thyroid hormones is evident in the thyrotoxic state. Many of the effects induced by excessive quantities of the thyroid hormones are reminiscent of those induced by epinephrine, including tachycardia, increased cardiac output, and enhanced glycogenolysis, lipolysis, and calorigenesis. Moreover, some of the clinical manifestations of thyrotoxicosis, among them eyelid retraction, tremor, excessive sweating, and tachycardia, are at least partly alleviated by adrenergic antagonists that either deplete tissue stores or block the action of catecholamines. These observations have been interpreted as indicating that a state of increased adrenergic activity exists in the thyrotoxic organism.

The mechanism ultimately responsible for the increased adrenergic activity has not been elucidated. Plasma catecholamine concentrations and urinary catecholamines and their major metabolites are normal in thyrotoxicosis. Moreover, in thyrotoxic patients, urinary catecholamines are not reduced by treatment with propranolol, a beta-receptor adrenergic antagonist (Bayliss and Edwards, 1971). Since the catecholamines exert their action through the mediation of an adenylate cyclase–cyclic AMP system, it is conceivable that the thyroid hormones, by virtue of their ability to stimulate protein synthesis, may increase the quantity of adenylate cyclase in the tissue and in this way induce an increase in adrenergic activity.

Reproductive Function

Thyrotoxicosis beginning in early life may be associated with delayed sexual maturation, although general physical development is normal and skeletal growth is often accelerated. Thyrotoxicosis occurring after puberty also influences reproductive function, especially in women. An increase in libido sometimes occurs in both sexes, and in women menstrual function is usually disturbed. The intermenstrual interval may be either prolonged or shortened, while menstrual flow at first is diminished and ultimately ceases altogether. Fertility may be reduced, and if conception takes place, abortion may result.

In some patients, cycles are predominantly anovulatory, but in most ovulation occurs, as indicated by a secretory endometrium. In the former, failure of production of or response to luteinizing hormone (LH) may be responsible, but the cause of the menstrual abnormalities in the latter group is unclear. In some patients with amenorrhea, urinary excretion of follicle stimulating hormone (FSH) is increased.

In thyrotoxicosis, there occur both quantitative and qualitative alterations in the metabolism of gonadal steroids that may be of fundamental importance. With respect to the quantitative alterations, thyrotoxicosis, whether spontaneous or induced by T_3, is accompanied by a great increase in the binding activity of testosterone-estradiol binding globulin in plasma. As a result, the plasma concentrations of both testosterone and estradiol are increased, but their unbound fractions are decreased. The increased binding in plasma is responsible for the decreased metabolic clearance rate of testosterone and the resulting increase in plasma LH concentration in thyrotoxicosis. In the case of estradiol, however, the metabolic clearance rate is normal, suggesting that tissue metabolism of the hormone is increased (Olivo et al., 1970; Ruder et al., 1971).

With respect to the qualitative alterations, thyrotoxicosis favors metabolism of estradiol and estrone via 2-oxygenation over that via 16 α-hydroxylation, with the result that formation of 2-hydroxyestrone and its derivative, 2-methoxyestrone, is increased, while formation of estriol is decreased. In the case of androgens, thyrotoxicosis favors metabolism of testosterone to androsterone over that to etiocholanolone. These alterations occur in both spontaneous thyrotoxicosis and that induced by T_3, whereas the converse alterations occur in hypothyroidism (Hellman et al., 1970).

The physiologic significance of these alterations is uncertain, but it is of interest that androsterone has a hypocholesterolemic action, suggesting that some metabolic effects of the thyroid hormones may be mediated by alterations in the metabolism of other hormones.

Energy Metabolism: Protein, Carbohydrate, and Lipid Metabolism

The intrinsic effects of the thyroid hormones on intermediary metabolism are discussed in an earlier section. This section will deal largely with the manner in which these effects are clinically evident in the patient with thyrotoxicosis.

The stimulation of energy metabolism and heat production is reflected in the increased BMR, increased appetite, and heat intolerance and in the slightly elevated basal body temperature of the patient with thyrotoxicosis. Despite the increased food intake, however, a state of chronic caloric and nutritional inadequacy almost always ensues.

Both the synthesis and degradation of protein are increased, the latter to a relatively greater extent than the former, with the result that there is net degradation of tissue protein. This is evident in the negative nitrogen balance, loss of weight, muscle wasting and weakness, and mild hypoalbuminemia.

The oral glucose tolerance curve is often abnormal in patients with thyrotoxicosis and varies from one in which the peak glycemia is increased and somewhat delayed to one that is frankly diabetic in form. Plasma insulin concentrations, however, are increased, suggesting the existence of insulin antagonism. The pathogenesis of these alterations remains to be defined. Preexisting diabetes mellitus is aggravated by thyrotoxicosis, perhaps as a result of increased degradation of insulin. (See Doar et al., 1969, for a review of carbohydrate metabolism in thyrotoxicosis.)

Both the synthesis and degradation of triglycerides and of cholesterol are increased in thyrotoxicosis, but the net effect is principally one of lipid degradation. This is reflected in an increase in plasma free fatty acids (FFA) and glycerol and a decrease in serum cholesterol; serum triglycerides, however, may be variable but are usually slightly decreased. Post-heparin lipolytic activity has been reported as being both decreased and increased. The mobilization of FFA in response to fasting, catecholamines, and GH is accentuated, and the oxidation of FFA is enhanced. These alterations, which appear to be due to activation of adenylate cyclase, result in a tendency to ketosis and to fatty infiltration of the liver, depending upon the degree of caloric inadequacy. (See Nikkilä and Kekki, 1972, for a review of lipid metabolism in thyrotoxicosis.)

Composite Clinical Picture and Laboratory Tests in Thyrotoxic States

The immediately foregoing section described the effects of an excess of thyroid hormones on the major organ systems. While these effects are in general common to thyrotoxic states regardless of their underlying etiology, their frequency and intensity as well as the other findings with which they are associated are greatly influenced by the nature of the disorder underlying the thyrotoxicosis. To a large extent, the same may be said of the results of the laboratory tests. Consequently, it is propitious to consider the clinical picture, characteristic laboratory findings, and differential diagnosis of thyrotoxic states as they relate to each of the specific etiologies. This approach is undertaken not merely as a matter of literary convenience but to emphasize the differences among the various forms of thyrotoxicosis that have an important bearing upon the clinical course, diagnosis, and treatment.

Graves' Disease

The disease known as Graves' disease in the English-speaking world and as Basedow's disease on the continent of Europe has been known for over a hundred years, but in areas of iodine abundance it has remained the most enigmatic, and, from the clinical standpoint, the most important of all thyroid diseases.

Graves' disease is a multisystem disease characterized by diffuse goiter, thyrotoxicosis, infiltrative ophthalmopathy, and occasionally by infiltrative dermopathy. As knowledge has increased, however, it has become apparent that in the individual patient these features may occur singly or in varying combination and that the full syndrome may never develop. Since other diseases may also produce goiter, thyrotoxicosis, or ophthalmopathy, a need existed for some means by which Graves' disease could clearly be identified. Tests designed to assess the integrity of homeostatic control of thyroid function, such as the thyroid suppression test, have afforded some help in this regard. An abnormal suppression test is common to all varieties of hyperthyroidism. Except in the case of autonomously functioning foci, it is only in Graves' disease that homeostatic disruption can thus be demonstrated in the absence of thyrotoxicosis.

More recently, another specific criterion has been recognized. This is the presence in serum of an immunoglobulin G, termed the long-acting thyroid stimulator (LATS), a material that to date has been found in significant concentration only in Graves' disease, in some euthyroid relatives of patients with Graves' disease, and in the occasional patient with Hashimoto's disease. LATS may be found in the serum in various forms of Graves' disease.

Graves' disease may occur at any age but appears most commonly in the third and fourth decades. It is several times more common in women than in men and often occurs in several members of the same family. In the patient with Graves' disease, there often occur generalized lymphoid hyperplasia, lymphocytic infiltration of the thyroid and retro-orbital tissues, and circulating autoantibodies directed against thyroid tissue components. In addition, both in patients with Graves' disease and in some of their relatives, there is often clinical and serological evidence of certain disorders of a presumed autoimmune nature, such as Hashimoto's disease, pernicious anemia, rheumatoid arthritis, myasthenia gravis, systemic lupus erythematosus, and idiopathic adrenal insufficiency. This means that Graves' disease must be considered among the group of disorders displaying an autoimmune component, probably conditioned by genetic factors.

Pathogenesis

Early observations in animals indicating that crude extracts of anterior pituitary could produce thyroid hyperplasia and hyperfunction led to the inference that hypersecretion of a thyroid-stimulating material from the pituitary was the proximate cause of Graves' disease. For many years, numerous methods were employed and great effort was expended in attempts to demonstrate increased quantities of thyroid-stimulating material, such as TSH, in the body fluids of patients with Graves' disease. The inconclusiveness of these initial efforts led to the alternative postulate that the disorder might arise from some primary abnormality within the thyroid itself.

A crucial turning point in this controversy took place in 1956 when Adams and Purves, using a new technique for the assay of TSH, discovered in the serum of patients with Graves' disease a thyroid stimulator (LATS) that differed from TSH principally in the longer duration of its action in the test animal. The assay depended upon the ability of the test material to induce an increase in the blood radioiodine of guinea pigs whose thyroid glands had previously been labeled with I^{131} and were then suppressed by exogenous thyroid hormone (Fig. 4–21). The assay has since been modified by McKenzie for performance in mice, and variations of the McKenzie technique have become the standard. In this system, TSH either added to serum or present therein as a result of primary hypothyroidism produces an increase in blood radioiodine that is greatest at about two hours and declines thereafter; the increase in blood radioiodine produced by LATS is maximum between 8 and 16 hours. The relative magnitudes of the values at the early and late time periods are considered to indicate whether a stimulator more closely resembles TSH or LATS. The discovery of LATS became even more significant with the observation that TSH was invariably undetectable by sensitive radioimmunoassay in the serum of actively thyrotoxic patients, indicating that TSH was not pathogenetically involved. Since these initial observations, additional information concerning the action of LATS has been obtained. Its longer duration of action than that of TSH has been shown to result from a slower removal from the blood of the recipient animal. *In vivo*, sera containing LATS are capable of inducing thyroid hyperplasia and increased

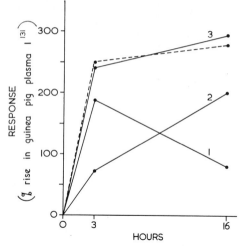

Figure 4–21. The 3-hour and 16-hour responses to standard TSH (1), to serum from a case of thyrotoxicosis with exophthalmos (2), and to a mixture of the two (3). The broken line represents the arithmetical sum of curves (1) and (2). (From Adams, D. D.: *J. Clin. Endocr. 18*:699, 1958.)

iodine accumulation, and their action is independent of the pituitary, since it occurs even when the recipient animal is hypophysectomized. In addition, LATS, like TSH, induces resorption of colloid and proteolysis of thyroglobulin and stimulates thyroid glucose oxidation and phospholipid synthesis. There is evidence to suggest that these effects, like those of TSH, may be mediated through activation by LATS of an adenylate cyclase–cyclic AMP system in thyroid tissue.

Great interest derived from the observation that essentially all LATS activity in serum resided in the 7S IgG fraction and that its biological activity could be prevented by treatment with antibody directed against this class of proteins. Moreover, lymphocytes from patients with Graves' disease were found capable of synthesizing LATS in tissue culture when stimulated with phytohemagglutinin. These observations led to almost universal acceptance of the concept that LATS is an autoantibody directed against some component of the thyroid. A search was therefore undertaken to ascertain the nature of the presumed "LATS antigen." Early observations indicated that either the soluble or microsomal fraction of thyroid homogenates might contain the LATS antigen, since incubation of sera containing LATS with these fractions led to an inhibition or abolition of the LATS effect. In the case of the microsomes, LATS seemed to be adsorbed from the serum, since LATS activity could subsequently be eluted from the particles by chaotropic agents capable of disrupting antigen-antibody complexes. More recent evidence suggests that these effects may have been due to contamination of the foregoing fractions by fragments of plasma membrane (Schleusener et al., 1971); this accords with the likelihood that the effects of LATS are mediated by adenylate cyclase, which is membrane-bound. Also of great interest was the observation that human retro-orbital adipose and muscle tissue failed to neutralize LATS (Shillinglaw and Utiger, 1968).

Studies *in vivo*, though difficult to perform, suggest that LATS has a stimulatory effect in the human thyroid. However, the most convincing evidence relating LATS to the hyperthyroidism of Graves' disease was provided by the rare disorder of neonatal thyrotoxicosis. In this syndrome, infants born to mothers with Graves' disease whose sera contained LATS in high titer display in the postnatal period goiter, ophthalmopathy, and manifestations of thyrotoxicosis. LATS is initially demonstrable in the sera of such infants, presumably as a result of transplacental passage. The disorder undergoes spontaneous resolution in association with the disappearance of LATS from the serum, and the latter takes place with a half-time similar to that of IgG.

On the basis of this evidence, there was nearly general acceptance of the hypothesis that LATS must play an important pathogenetic role in the hyperthyroidism of Graves' disease. However, a variety of early data, as well as more recent findings, have raised doubt concerning the validity of this conclusion. First, it was recognized that LATS could be demonstrated in the sera of only about two-thirds of actively thyrotoxic patients with Graves' disease, even when tenfold IgG concentrates of serum were tested. Second, in the sera of thyrotoxic patients, the titer of LATS did not correlate well with the degree of thyrotoxicosis or with thyroid size. Rather, it appeared to relate to the number of manifestations of Graves' disease present. Finally, it has been assumed that the pathogenetic factor in diffuse toxic goiter would manifest itself in nonsuppressibility of thyroid function. However, recent studies have demonstrated the presence of LATS in the sera of some patients with Graves' disease whose thyroid function is normally suppressible. Hence, if LATS does play a pathogenetic role, other factors must also be operative.

The most recent line of interest with respect to the pathogenetic influence of humoral antibodies in Graves' disease follows from the relatively early observations that the sera of some patients with this disorder contain an IgG that prevents the neutralization of LATS by human, but not mouse, thyroid tissue (LATS protector; Adams and Kennedy, 1971). More recent studies have provided evidence to suggest that LATS protector may have stimulatory activity which, like its protector activity, is specific for human thyroid tissue (Shishiba et al., 1973). Concurrent with these developments, interest has evolved in the possibility that cell-mediated rather than humoral autoimmunity may be causally related to the hyperthyroidism of Graves' disease. Evidence to suggest this possibility has come from studies that demonstrate the capability of thyroid fractions to elicit migration inhibitory factor (MIF) from the lymphocytes of patients with Graves' disease (Lamki et al., 1973). All these observations are currently in the early phase of their exploitation, and conclusions concerning the pathogenesis of the diffuse toxic goiter of Graves' disease must again be delayed.

Uncertainty also prevails with respect to the pathogenesis of the ophthalmopathy of Graves' disease. Older observations indicated that extracts of pituitary containing TSH-like activity were capable of producing exophthalmos in test animals. Similar exophthalmogenic activity has been demonstrated in the sera of some patients with the ophthalmopathy of Graves' disease. It appears from recent observations that the activity of pituitary extracts resides in a portion of the TSH molecule. An active fragment of TSH lacking thyroid-stimulating activity but possessing exophthalmogenic activity can be isolated from peptic digests of TSH (Kohn and Winand, 1971). This fragment is a glycopeptide consisting in part of the β subunit of TSH. Although this finding affords an intriguing avenue for further study, it is difficult to reconcile with the apparent inhibition of TSH secretion in thyrotoxic ophthalmopathic patients with Graves' disease, with the absence of measurable quantities of β subunit by radioimmunoassay of the sera of patients with ophthalmopathy (Kourides et al., 1973), and with the well-documented instances in which ophthalmopathy has emerged in patients with spontaneous or postoperative panhypopituitarism.

Also difficult to place in context but of considerable interest are observations that the IgG fraction of the serum of some patients with ophthalmopathy contains a factor that is different from LATS and that stimulates the uptake of radiosulfate by the intraorbitally situated Harderian gland of mice (Singh and McKenzie, 1971). This response is thought to reflect the action of an exophthalmogenic principle. It is apparent that resolution of the pathogenesis of the ophthalmopathy of Graves' disease is not yet in sight. There has, in addition, been no tangible progress toward elucidation of the pathogenesis of the dermopathy in Graves' disease. (For comprehensive reviews of the pathogenesis of Graves' disease, see McKenzie, 1972, and Solomon and Chopra, 1972.)

Constitutional Factors

Whatever its ultimate pathogenesis, both the emergence of clinically evident Graves' disease and its subsequent course are modified by such factors as heredity, sex, and perhaps emotion. The tendency of Graves' disease to occur in several members of the same family and sometimes in several generations is well recognized. Several extensive studies have given statistical support to this concept (Martin and Fisher, 1945). In addition, a higher concordance rate of Graves' disease has been noted in monozygotic than in dizygotic twins. The foregoing statistics were based upon the appearance of overt thyroid disease in relatives. Studies conducted in the authors' clinic have revealed a high incidence of abnormalities in iodine metabolism in euthyroid relatives, some of whom were goitrous. Thyroid I^{131} uptakes were increased in approximately 20 per cent of the relatives studied, especially in sisters and daughters of the propositi. An increase in the fractional rate of peripheral turnover of T_4 was also noted, similar to that observed in clinically overt Graves' disease. Considered together, these findings leave little doubt of an inherited susceptibility to Graves' disease, but the precise mode of its transmission is uncertain.

The hereditary factor in Graves' disease also appears to involve autoimmune aspects. This is suggested by the increased incidence in patients with Graves' disease or in members of their families of other autoimmune disorders or manifestations, such as Hashimoto's disease or pernicious anemia, and of autoantibodies against thyroid tissue components, gastric parietal cells, and intrinsic factor (Howel Evans et al., 1967). Recently LATS has been found in a significant proportion of euthyroid relatives of patients with Graves' disease (Wall et al., 1969).

A strong relationship also exists between sex and both the frequency and the clinical manifestations of Graves' disease. Overall, the disorder is many times more common in women than in men (approximately 7:1). Furthermore, it tends to become manifest during such times as puberty, pregnancy, and the menopause. Although men are less often affected, in them the disease tends to occur at a later age, to be more severe, and relatively more often to be accompanied by significant ophthalmopathy. It is not known whether the influence of sex in Graves' is a direct result of genetic determinants or of physiologic factors related to reproductive function. The female sex preponderance is consonant with the autoimmune aspects, since most disorders considered to be of an autoimmune nature occur most commonly in women. The foregoing evidence for the operation of autoimmune and genetic factors has led to a concept that Graves' disease is the result of a genetically determined defect of immunologic surveillance. This unifying concept, which implicates an immunologic defect as the inherited factor, ignores the absence of evidence of immunologic disorder in nontoxic goiter and thyroid carcinoma. Yet a marked preponderance of females is seen in both the latter disorders, and a familial relationship exists between nontoxic goiter and Graves' disease (see review by Skillern, 1972).

From the earliest descriptions of Graves' disease, the possible role of emotional factors in its emergence has been suggested. Those who see the disease frequently are repeatedly impressed by instances in which Graves' disease becomes evident either after a severe emotional stress, such as the actual or threatened separation from an individual upon whom the patient is emotionally dependent, or after an acute fright, such as an automobile accident. It has also been suggested that patients with Graves' disease may be drawn from a population with a characteristic pattern of personality, but some data do not support this hypothesis (Hermann and Quarton, 1965). The difficulties of conducting controlled studies in this field are obvious, but such are what is needed if conclusions concerning the role of emotional factors in the pathogenesis of overt Graves' disease are to be drawn. Beyond this, there would be required an elucida-

tion of the physiopathologic mechanism whereby evocative emotional factors express their effect.

Natural History and Course

The course of the thyrotoxic component of untreated Graves' disease is variable and often erratic. In some patients the thyrotoxic component is persistent, though it may vary in severity; in others it may be cyclic, exhibiting exacerbations of varying frequency, intensity, and duration. This cyclic feature has an important bearing on the treatment of the disorder and must also be encompassed by any comprehensive theory of its pathogenesis. With the passage of time, which may vary from a few months to many years, the thyrotoxic component tends to "burn itself out." Thyroid function is not under normal homeostatic control in most phases of Graves' disease, and this can be detected clinically in an abnormal thyroid suppression test. Hence it has become possible to correlate the major clinical manifestations of the disease with this aspect of its underlying pathogenesis. Such correlations reveal that the suppression test is invariably abnormal in the untreated patient who is thyrotoxic. It may be either normal or abnormal following relief of thyrotoxicosis, either spontaneously or as a result of any form of treatment. The authors have found it helpful, therefore, to classify the activity of the thyroid component of Graves' disease according to the following categories: (1) an active phase during which the untreated patient is thyrotoxic and in which the suppression test is abnormal; (2) a latent phase during which the untreated patient is not thyrotoxic but in which the suppression test is abnormal; (3) an inactive phase during which the untreated patient is not thyrotoxic and in which the suppression test is normal.

Although the ophthalmopathy of Graves' disease often commences together with the thyrotoxic component, this association is frequently lacking. Thus thyrotoxic patients may be initially free of ophthalmopathy but may develop this manifestation months or years later or not at all. Conversely, the disease may begin with ophthalmopathy and only later, if at all, be associated with thyrotoxicosis. Moreover, although the suppression test is often abnormal in patients with active ophthalmopathy, this is true in only about half the cases. Conversely, the suppression test may be abnormal in patients in whom activity of the ophthalmopathy has subsided. These facts suggest that if the thyroid and ophthalmopathic components of Graves' disease are indeed manifestations of a single disease process rather than manifestations of closely related but separate diseases, they nevertheless tend to run separate courses.

Histopathology

A convenient designation for the thyroid gland of Graves' disease during the period of active thyrotoxicosis is the term *diffuse toxic goiter*, which denotes that the gland is both enlarged and uniformly affected. Diffuse toxic goiters vary in consistency from softer than normal to firm and rubbery. The outer surface is usually smooth but may be somewhat lobular; rarely, if ever, is it grossly nodular in the early stages of the disease prior to treatment. The cut surface is red and glistening. Microscopically, the follicles are small, are lined by hyperplastic columnar epithelium, and contain scant colloid that displays much marginal scalloping and vacuolization (Fig. 4–22). The nuclei are vesicular, are basally situated, and exhibit mitoses. Papillary projections of the hyperplastic epithelium into the lumina of the follicles are common. Vascularity is increased, and there is an infiltration to a varying degree of lymphocytes and plasma cells. These collect in aggregates forming lymphoid follicles. When the patient is treated with iodine, the thyroid undergoes a process termed *involution*, in which the hyperplasia and increased vascularity abate, the papillary projections recede, and the follicles enlarge and become

filled with colloid. An extensive treatise on the fine structure of the thyroid in Graves' disease has been published (Heimann, 1966). No characteristic alterations have been described in the pituitary in Graves' disease.

In patients with *infiltrative ophthalmopathy*, the volume of the orbital contents is increased, owing to an increase in the retrobulbar connective tissue as well as to an increase in the mass of the extraocular muscles. Some of the increase in connective tissue is due to edema resulting from the increased content in the ground substance of hyaluronic acid, which is hydrophilic. The extraocular muscles are swollen, and the fibers display loss of striation, fragmentation, and lymphocytic infiltration. The lacrimal glands may also be involved. Ultimately, fibrosis of the tissues occurs.

In infiltrative dermopathy, the content of hyaluronic acid in the dermis is increased with resulting edema; the collagen fibers are separated and fragmented, and there is lymphocytic infiltration.

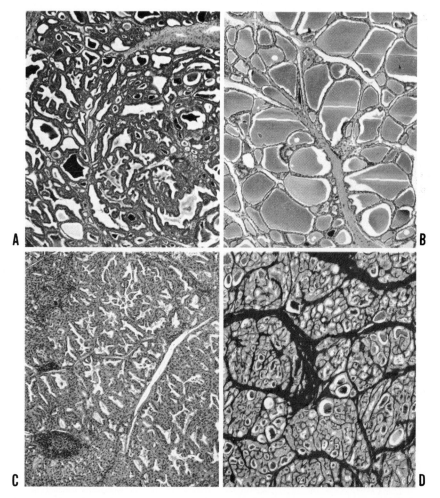

Figure 4–22. Sections of thyroid gland of four patients with Graves' disease. *A*, Untreated. *B*, After therapy with potassium iodide for 3 weeks. *C*, After treatment with thiouracil for 5 weeks. *D*, Three months after last of three treatments with radioiodine. Note the marked hypertrophy and hyperplasia of the acinar cells and scant amount of colloid in sections *A*, *C*, and *D*. A lymph follicle is present in *C*. Note the broad bands of scar tissue in *D*. Section *B* is almost normal in appearance. Each patient, except the first one, was euthyroid at the time of thyroidectomy.

Physiopathology

Virtually every aspect of thyroid hormone economy is abnormal in patients with the diffuse toxic goiter of Graves' disease. Physiopathologic abnormalities can be divided into three categories: those related to the overproduction of hormone, those related to the peripheral metabolism of hormone, and those reflecting disruption of the normal homeostatic control of thyroid function.

In the first category, the disturbance is one that ultimately leads to hypersecretion of the thyroid hormones. The thyroid iodide clearance rate is increased from its normal range of approximately 6–7 ml./min. to values that vary with the severity of the disorder but that may approach 2 liters/min. in the most severe cases. As a result of the increased thyroid iodide clearance rate, the absolute uptake of iodine is enhanced. The great increase in iodide clearance rate must reflect enhanced thyroid blood flow, even if extraction of iodine is assumed to be complete. Hypervascularity of the thyroid in turn may be due to humoral or neurogenic mechanisms but is almost certainly due at least in part to the increased rate of energy metabolism in the gland itself. The enhanced thyroid iodide clearance rate is usually the result of an increase in both the overall glandular mass and its unit functional activity. Iodide transport and probably organic binding are accelerated. The increase in iodide transport is responsible at least in part for the enhanced susceptibility of the thyroid gland of Graves' disease to the inhibitory effects of iodide on organic-binding reactions; this is evident in a positive iodide-perchlorate discharge test (Suzuki and Mashimo, 1972). As judged from the normal ratio of iodotyrosines to iodothyronines, the rate of the coupling reaction must also be increased. The content of the glandular iodine pool is generally normal. Both direct measurements and estimates based upon the appearance of PBI^{131} in the blood after administration of inorganic I^{131} indicate that the rate of turnover and release of the glandular iodine pool is increased, often greatly so. As judged from kinetic studies, the major product of glandular secretion is T_4, but the ratio of T_3 to T_4 in the thyroid secretion is increased. In some instances, T_3 appears to be the major secretory product, with the result that the serum T_3 concentration alone is increased, the serum T_4 concentration being normal (T_3-toxicosis) (see Sterling et al., 1970; Hollander et al., 1972). An iodinated protein similar in properties to serum albumin is also secreted, but the relative proportion of iodine released in this form is uncertain.

Thyroid hormone–protein interactions in the plasma are disturbed, the proportion of total T_4 and T_3 in the free or unbound state being increased. This change results from a decrease in the binding capacity of TBG, as well as from the increase in the concentrations of the two hormones. The fractional rates of turnover of T_4 and T_3 are increased, often greatly so, and this, together with the increased amounts of hormone in the peripheral pool, leads to an increase in total daily disposal of T_4 and T_3. In the most severe cases, values for this function may increase from the normal of approximately 80 μg. of T_4 and 30 μg. of T_3 daily to values in excess of 500 μg. for both hormones. The total daily disposal of T_3 is disproportionately increased relative to that of T_4, indicating that the production rate of T_3 is disproportionately increased. Whether this results solely from a preferential increase in thyroid secretion of T_3 or whether there is in addition a disproportionate increase in the peripheral conversion of T_4 to T_3 is uncertain. In any event, since the metabolic potency of T_3 is about three times greater than that of T_4, T_3 is responsible for the bulk of thyroid hormone action in thyrotoxicosis. As judged from studies with the labeled hormones, the proportionate disposal of T_4 and T_3 by deiodination relative to fecal excretion is not altered.

The foregoing abnormalities in the kinetics of hormone turnover in the patient with active thyrotoxicosis irrespective of its underlying cause are probably the result of several factors, including both the disturbance in hormone binding and the hypermetabolism. In addition, in Graves' disease, several lines of evidence suggest that an intrinsic abnormality in the peripheral metabolism of T_4 exists. For example, an acceleration of the fractional rate of turnover of T_4 has been found in some patients long after the thyrotoxicosis had been relieved and also has been noted in some euthyroid relatives of patients with Graves' disease. Recently persistent acceleration of the fractional rate of turnover of T_3 has also been shown to be present in patients with Graves' disease after a normal metabolic state had been restored with treatment (Woeber et al., 1970). The relationship of this abnormality to the other physiopathologic alterations in Graves' disease is unclear.

The disturbance of homeostatic control that makes possible the development of thyrotoxicosis has not been elucidated. This aspect of the physiopathology has been considered in the section dealing with the pathogenesis of Graves' disease. However, it is important to note that the normal pituitary-thyroid feedback control is functioning appropriately. With very rare exceptions, radioimmunoassay reveals no detectable TSH in the blood of thyrotoxic patients, but elevated concentrations are present if they are rendered hypothyroid. Clinically this is manifested by further thyroid enlargement and the appearance or accentuation of a bruit which signal developing hypothyroidism in a patient receiving antithyroid drugs. (See Ingbar, 1961, Alexander et al., 1962, and Nicoloff et al., 1972, for an extensive discussion of the physiopathology of Graves' disease.)

Clinical Picture

Graves' disease is most commonly manifest in patients in the third and fourth decades of life. The disease is rare before the age of 10 years, and although unusual, it is being diagnosed with increasing frequency in the elderly. Like other diseases of the thyroid, it displays a striking female sex preponderance of approximately 7:1. The whole syndrome comprises diffuse goiter, thyrotoxicosis, infiltrative ophthalmopathy, and occasionally infiltrative dermopathy. Since the infiltrative ophthalmopathy and dermopathy may occur independently of the former two manifestations, they will be discussed separately.

Diffuse Toxic Goiter. (Since hyperthyroidism occurs in diseases other than Graves' disease, and since Graves' disease may be present in the absence of thyrotoxicosis, the term diffuse toxic goiter is a convenient nosological entity in that it connotes the presence of thyrotoxicosis resulting specifically from Graves' disease.) Most commonly, the symptoms of diffuse toxic goiter begin gradually, the patient noting nervousness, irritability, palpitation, fatigue, heat intolerance, weight loss, or change in menstrual pattern. Any one of these symptoms may predominate (Table 4–6). Enlargement of the thyroid may be noted as a fullness in the neck or rarely may produce obstructive symptoms. In about one-third of the cases, ocular manifestations begin coincidentally with the onset of thyrotoxicosis. Some of these are manifestations of thyrotoxicosis itself, whereas others are due to the ophthalmopathy and will be discussed later. Symptoms may remain mild or may progress to a florid state characterized by aggravation of the foregoing complaints together with weakness, insomnia, voracious appetite, and excessive sweating.

Several features of the foregoing symptoms merit further consideration. Nervousness, which is probably the most common symptom, may manifest itself in various ways, notably as a feeling of apprehension and inability to concentrate. Emotional lability and irritability may lead to difficulty in interpersonal relationships and to inappropriate spells of crying or euphoria. Fatigability frustrates the desire of the patient to be continuously active. Weakness is noted particularly on climbing stairs, and this activity, as well as others, is prone to produce breathlessness. Heat intolerance, associated with increased sweating, is also a prominent symptom and may be a cause of familial discord. The patient prefers a cooler environment than do others around him and may lower the thermostat, open the windows, sleep with fewer blankets, or kick off the covers while asleep. The patient usually prefers winter to summer and often finds hot weather intolerable. The change in menstrual pattern usually takes the form of oligomenorrhea with a variable intermenstrual period, occasionally progressing to amenorrhea. Frank diarrhea is uncommon, but increase in the frequency of bowel movements and softening of the stools is often noted. Palpitation may be continuous or episodic, suggesting paroxysmal dysrhythmia. Although weight loss despite increase in appetite is common, the occasional patient notes a gain in weight, while in more severe cases the appetite may be decreased. Women may complain of excessive fineness of the hair and of its inability to hold a wave. The skin may become more pigmented. The ocular manifestations of thyrotoxicosis per se are due to spasm and retraction of the eyelids and are noted as a bright-eyed, staring appearance.

Although this symptom complex may develop over a period of months or even years before the patient is first seen, the disease is sometimes fulminant in its emergence, the florid clinical picture developing within a few weeks or less. In such patients, emotional stress may be a forerunner. In some patients with preexisting heart disease, mild or moderate thyrotoxicosis may precipitate heart failure, which then overshadows the manifestations of thyrotoxicosis. In others, severe weakness and wasting of muscles may dominate the clinical picture. The last two forms are often designated "masked" hyperthyroidism. This term is often taken to indicate that the characteristic clinical manifestations of thyrotoxicosis are lacking, but this is usually not the case, as a careful history and examination will disclose.

TABLE 4–6. INCIDENCE OF SYMPTOMS AND SIGNS OBSERVED IN 247 PATIENTS WITH THYROTOXICOSIS

Symptom	Per Cent	Symptom	Per Cent
Nervousness	99	Increased appetite	65
Increased sweating	91	Eye complaints	54
Hypersensitivity to heat	89	Swelling of legs	35
Palpitation	89	Hyperdefecation (without diarrhea)	33
Fatigue	88	Diarrhea	23
Weight loss	85	Anorexia	9
Tachycardia	82	Constipation	4
Dyspnea	75	Weight gain	2
Weakness	70		

Sign	Per Cent	Sign	Per Cent
Tachycardia*	100	Eye signs	71
Goiter†	100	Atrial fibrillation	10
Skin changes	97	Splenomegaly	10
Tremor	97	Gynecomastia	10
Bruit over thyroid	77	Liver palms	8

*In other studies thyrotoxic patients with normal pulse rate have been observed.

†The data shown in this table are taken from Williams, R. H.: *J. Clin. Endocr.* 6:1, 1946. In the experience of the present authors, enlargement of the thyroid is lacking in approximately 3 per cent of patients with thyrotoxicosis.

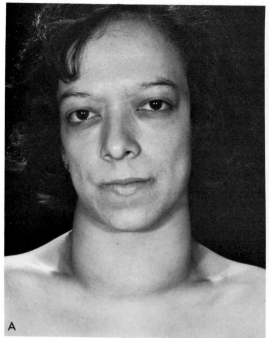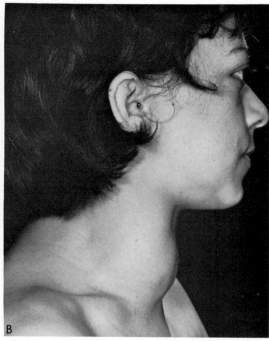

Figure 4–23. Massive thyroid enlargement due to diffuse toxic goiter. Note the sulcus between the thyroid and the lateral aspect of the neck in *B*, as well as the dilated veins overlying the thyroid gland. The patient was severely thyrotoxic and maintained a PBI of 40 μg./100 ml. while receiving 1200 mg. of propylthiouracil daily. The only ocular abnormality was slight widening of the right palpebral fissure, without true exophthalmos.

The characteristic physical signs in the patient with diffuse toxic goiter are manifold. Apart from the goiter and exophthalmos, which in themselves may suffice to establish a clinical diagnosis, other aspects of the patient's appearance and behavior may be virtually pathognomonic of thyrotoxicosis. The patient usually displays an exaggerated alertness, fidgets, responds quickly to questions or commands, is bright-eyed, may appear flushed, and often looks younger than would be expected from the chronological age.

The thyroid is enlarged in most patients but not invariably, since thyrotoxicosis in Graves' disease may occur in association with a gland of normal size in approximately 3 per cent of cases; in the authors' experience, this has most often been the case in older patients, usually men. The thyroid gland is most commonly 2–3 times normal size, but it may be massively enlarged (Fig. 4–23). Its consistency varies from one that is somewhat softer than normal to one that is firm and rubbery. The enlargement is usually symmetrical, but sometimes the right lateral lobe is larger than the left. The surface of the gland is usually smooth but may feel lobular. Especially in more severe cases, a thrill may be felt, usually over the upper poles, and a bruit may be audible. This is usually continuous but may sometimes be heard only in systole and is most readily detected at the upper or lower poles. It should not be confused with a venous hum or murmur arising from the base of the heart. A thrill or bruit is highly suggestive but not pathognomonic of hyperthyroidism.

Spasm and retraction of the eyelids lead to wid-

ening of the palpebral fissure, with the result that sclera is exposed above the superior margin of the limbus. The retraction may be asymmetrical. When the patient looks downward, the upper lid lags behind the globe, exposing more of the sclera, and when he gazes upward, the globe often lags behind the lid (lid lag and globe lag). The movements of the lids are jerky and spasmodic, and a tremor of the lightly closed lids can often be elicited.

The remaining peripheral manifestations of thyrotoxicosis were discussed in detail according to the individual organ systems in a previous section. Among these are the warm, smooth, moist texture of the skin, Plummer's nails, physical signs of a hyperdynamic circulation, tremor of the hands and tongue, muscular wasting, and hyper-reflexia.

In general, men tend to develop the disease at a somewhat older age than women, and although the degree of thyroid hyperfunction is often more severe in men, the severity of the symptoms is often less. Men also seem especially prone to develop myopathy as well as the more severe forms of ophthalmopathy. In older patients the circulatory manifestations may predominate, while the nervous manifestations, which are especially prominent in children and young adults, are lacking. Ophthalmopathy is less common in the elderly patient, who is also more prone to display muscular weakness, prostration, and anorexia (apathetic hyperthyroidism).

Infiltrative Ophthalmopathy and Dermopathy. Ophthalmic changes are a major manifestation of Graves' disease. As has been suggested, it is impor-

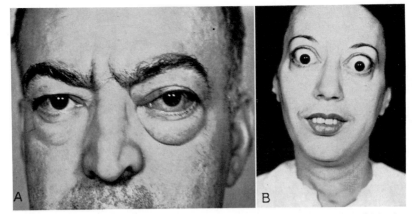

Figure 4–24. Patient A was euthyroid and had marked orbital swelling, exophthalmos, conjunctival injection, and chemosis. The proptosis, limitation of extraocular movements, edema, and other manifestations of infiltrative ophthalmopathy are much more marked in *A* than in *B*, who had mild hyperthyroidism, with slight diffuse enlargement of the thyroid, marked widening of the palpebral fissures, with marked stare and proptosis.

tant to differentiate between the ocular changes that result from thyrotoxicosis per se and those that not only are more proximately related to the disease process but also may pose serious problems in treatment and prognosis. It is the latter form which has been designated *infiltrative ophthalmopathy*. The thyrotoxic ocular manifestations have already been described. If present alone, these usually abate when the thyrotoxicosis is relieved. Infiltrative ophthalmopathy on the other hand follows a course that is not uncommonly independent of the thyrotoxic aspect and is to a large extent uninfluenced by its treatment (Fig. 4–24). It occurs in about 50 per cent of cases.

The symptoms associated with infiltrative ophthalmopathy are diverse and may appear in varying combinations. Early symptoms often include a sense of irritation in the eyes, resembling that caused by a foreign body, and excessive tearing that is often made worse by exposure to cold air or wind, especially if exophthalmos is present. Injection of the conjunctivae may be noted. Exophthalmos, which is frequently slightly asymmetrical but sometimes greatly so, may also be noted and may be accompanied by a feeling of pressure behind the globes. When exophthalmos is pronounced, the patient may be forced to sleep with his eyes partly open. Exophthalmos may be masked by periorbital edema, which is a common accompaniment and source of complaint. Patients frequently report that their vision is blurred and that their eyes tire easily. Double vision may be noted either in combination with the foregoing symptoms or alone. In severe cases, visual acuity may be decreased or lost, or the patient may display symptoms resulting from corneal ulceration or infection.

The ocular findings are quite variable (Fig. 4–25). Exophthalmos is probably the most common manifestation. This is usually bilateral but often is slightly asymmetrical. True unilateral exophthalmos is rare and usually occurs in the absence of thyrotoxicosis; most often the other eye is eventu-

ally affected. Exophthalmos is very frequently accompanied by periorbital edema which tends to obscure its degree. For this reason and because of their importance in following the course of the disease, objective measurements of the degree of exophthalmos must be made. These can be accomplished with the aid of either the Hertel or the Luedde exophthalmometer. These instruments conveniently and accurately permit measurement of the distance between the lateral angle of the bony orbit and an imaginary perpendicular tangent to the most anterior part of the cornea. Generally this distance does not exceed 16 mm., but 20 mm. is considered the upper limit of normal. In severe exophthalmos, readings may be as high as 30 mm. A rough estimation of the degree of exophthalmos may be obtained by standing behind the seated patient and looking downward from above to ascertain the extent to which the eyes protrude beyond the plane of the forehead.

In addition to being edematous, the lids are often reddened, and enlarged lacrimal glands may cause a bulging of their surface. The extent to which the upper and lower lids can be completely apposed should be determined, since failure of apposition will promote drying and ulceration of the cornea. Injection of the bulbar conjunctiva is commonly seen and in more severe cases is accompanied by edema or frank chemosis, in which the edematous conjunctiva is seen to bulge from under the lids and around the corneal limbus.

Weakness of the extraocular muscles is an important finding that is most commonly evident in an inability to achieve or maintain convergence. Limitation of upward gaze and especially of superolateral gaze may be present. Occasionally there is complete paralysis of upward gaze; in such cases, a characteristic position of the head is assumed in which the neck is extended to make possible a field of vision above the horizontal. Rarely is downward or inward gaze severely affected. Ophthalmoplegic manifestations usually occur in association with other signs of infiltrative ophthal-

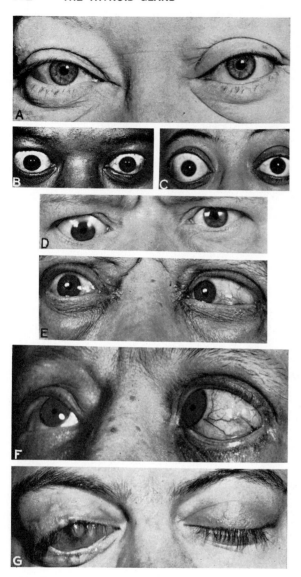

Figure 4–25. Infiltrative ophthalmopathy. *A*, Palpebral edema. This patient's eyeballs protruded anteriorly 1 cm. more than normal, but there is no "pop-eye" appearance, owing to edema of the surrounding structures. *B*, Marked widening of palpebral fissures; slight palpebral swelling. *C*, Unequal degrees of ophthalmopathy. *D*, Unilateral lid retraction. *E*, Palpebral swelling, due presumably to fat pads and edema; paralysis of right external rectus muscle. *F*, Marked conjunctival injection and chemosis, together with ophthalmoplegia. *G*, Failure to close lids on right due to marked exophthalmos, corneal scarring, and panophthalmitis; eye had to be enucleated.

mopathy but may occur alone. In some cases, only a single muscle is affected (Fig. 4–26).

Some indication of the severity of the infiltrative process in the orbit is provided by an assessment of intraorbital tension. Although an instrument for this purpose has been devised (orbitonometer), clinical assessment will usually suffice. This can be accomplished by having the patient close the eyes lightly and by determining the ease with which the globe can be displaced posteriorly by pressure from the thumb.

The manifestations of the most extreme form of ophthalmopathy or its complications are often catastrophic. These include subluxation of the globe and ulceration or infection of the cornea secondary to incomplete apposition of the lids. This may lead to panophthalmitis and destruction of one or both eyes. Ophthalmoscopic examination may reveal venous congestion and papilledema;

these findings may be accompanied by visual field defects.

An uncommon manifestation of Graves' disease is *infiltrative dermopathy*. It occurs in about 5–10 per cent of cases and is almost always accompanied by infiltrative ophthalmopathy, usually of severe degree. This lesion appears as a violaceous induration of the skin over the pretibial area (pretibial myxedema) and over the dorsa of the feet usually in the form of individual plaques but occasionally becoming confluent. Rarely it is seen on the face or dorsa of the hands. Clubbing of the digits and osteoarthropathy are occasionally associated manifestations (thyroid acropachy).

Laboratory Tests

In the classic case of moderate or severe diffuse toxic goiter, results of laboratory tests are clearly

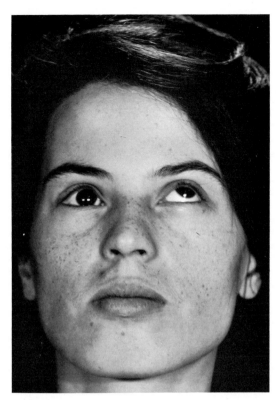

Figure 4–26. Ophthalmoplegia due to Graves' disease. The patient was severely hyperthyroid. Other than slight conjunctival injection, the only ocular abnormality was paralysis of upward gaze on the right.

abnormal and are consonant with the physiopathology of this disorder. The increase in thyroid iodide clearance rate is reflected in the increased thyroid I^{131} uptake, and the enhanced turnover of glandular iodine is evident in high values for PBI^{131} in the blood. Hypersecretion of hormone leads to an increase in the concentrations in serum of T_4 and T_3, but the latter is disproportionately increased relative to the former. Occasionally, this discrepancy is exaggerated, the serum T_4 concentration being normal and the serum T_3 concentration alone being elevated (T_3-toxicosis) (Sterling et al., 1970; Hollander et al., 1972); in this circumstance, the thyroid I^{131} uptake may also be within the normal range. In conjunction with the increased concentrations of T_4 and T_3 in the blood, a decreased binding capacity of TBG produces an increase in both the proportions and absolute concentrations of free T_4 and T_3 and abnormally high values for the *in vitro* uptake test and free T_4 index. Metabolic indices, such as the BMR and serum cholesterol concentration, reflect the action of excessive amounts of thyroid hormone on the peripheral tissues. It is unusual for the BMR to exceed +60 per cent; higher values suggest either absence of a basal state or an artifact. The thyroid suppression test is invariably abnormal in the actively thyrotoxic patient, including the patient with T_3-toxicosis. LATS is present in the serum of about two-thirds of actively thyrotoxic patients, and moderately high titers of other thyroid autoantibodies

are found in the serum in approximately 40 per cent of cases.

An extensive discussion of the physiologic basis of these tests and the manner in which they are affected by factors other than thyroid disease have been presented in an earlier section. Nevertheless it is important to consider some practical aspects of the use of these tests in the diagnosis of diffuse toxic goiter. It is neither desirable nor usually feasible that all the major laboratory tests be used to assist in the diagnosis. It is often asked, therefore, what may be the single best test for this purpose. Measurement of the serum T_4 concentration alone will probably establish or exclude the diagnosis in the greatest number of cases. In order to exclude the possibility that the increase in serum T_4 concentration is the result of an increase in hormone binding in the blood, concomitant measurement either of the *in vitro* uptake of T_3 or T_4 or of the proportion of free T_4 should be performed and the free T_4 index or concentration calculated. If the latter functions are increased, a diagnosis of thyrotoxicosis is virtually assured. In the unusual instance in which values for the serum total or free T_4 concentrations are not increased, measurement of serum T_3 concentration should be performed.

Measurement of thyroid I^{131} uptake is also of value, and its diagnostic accuracy may approach that of the serum T_4 concentration alone. In view of the several other thyroid disorders that may increase the thyroid I^{131} uptake, however, it seems unlikely that its accuracy would approach that of the use of an *in vitro* uptake test together with measurement of serum T_4 concentration. The accuracy of the *in vitro* uptake tests per se does not warrant their use as the sole diagnostic procedure. The diagnostic accuracy of the BMR when carefully performed may approach that of the thyroid I^{131} uptake or serum T_4 concentration. However, it is unlikely that this demanding procedure will be resurrected from its place at the periphery of the diagnostic scrap heap. Unfortunately, in the mild form of this or other thyroid disorders in which the diagnostic tests are most greatly needed, their values are likely to be only slightly abnormal, if at all. When such is the case in the patient with possible thyrotoxicosis, the value of the thyroid suppression test is at its greatest. Although an abnormal response is not pathognomonic of thyrotoxicosis, especially if the patient is known to have Graves' disease, a normal response would clearly exclude the diagnosis. On the other hand, absent responsiveness to TRH would strongly suggest at least mild thyrotoxicosis. In view of the poor correlation between the presence or absence of thyrotoxicosis and the presence or absence of demonstrable LATS, assay for LATS should not be performed as a means of diagnosing hyperthyroidism.

Differential Diagnosis

The patient who displays all the major manifestations of Graves' disease, namely thyrotoxicosis, goiter, and infiltrative ophthalmopathy, does not pose a diagnostic problem. In some patients, however, one of the major manifestations either dominates the clinical picture or is present alone, and the disorder may mimic some disease other than Graves' disease. Since the major manifestations are so different, the conditions from which they require differentiation will be considered separately.

A variety of disorders have features that resemble those of thyrotoxicosis in a general way. The most frequent disorder that simulates thyrotoxicosis is *neurasthenia*. As in Graves' disease, the commonest cause of thyrotoxicosis, the patient with neurasthenia is usually a young woman who complains of fatigue, palpitation, nervous irritability, and insomnia. Fatigue is pronounced and differs from that in thyrotoxicosis in that it is not accompanied by a desire to be active. The patient is both listless and fatigued and often feels tired on awakening. In the patient with neurasthenia, tachycardia is common during examination, but, in contrast to what is found in thyrotoxicosis, the sleeping pulse rate is normal. The palms are characteristically cool and clammy, rather than warm and moist. Hyper-reflexia is present in both disorders. In neurasthenia, goiter is absent and laboratory indices of thyroid function are normal. Chronic pulmonary disease may require differentiation from thyrotoxicosis. Here, retention of carbon dioxide may lead to a warm flushed skin, tremulousness, and a bounding pulse. Mild exophthalmos may also be present. Very often these patients receive iodides as an expectorant, and this not only invalidates the thyroid I^{131} uptake, but also may lead to goiter (iodide goiter). The BMR is increased by respiratory insufficiency. Nevertheless, the serum T_4 concentration will accurately reflect the metabolic state of the patient.

Pheochromocytoma may closely resemble thyrotoxicosis in that adrenergic overactivity and hypermetabolism are common to both. Similarities include nervous irritability, eyelid retraction, tremulousness, excessive sweating, and tachycardia. Like the patient with thyrotoxicosis, the patient with pheochromocytoma may have weight loss despite a good appetite, and hyperglycemia with glucosuria. However, in the patient with pheochromocytoma, diastolic hypertension is present, and urinary excretion of vanillylmandelic acid is increased, features that are lacking in thyrotoxicosis. In the patient with pheochromocytoma, goiter is absent, and, with very rare exceptions, the laboratory indices of thyroid function are normal.

In *diabetes mellitus*, weight loss despite a good appetite, polyuria, muscle wasting, and occasionally diarrhea may suggest thyrotoxicosis. Moreover, the incidence of goiter in patients with diabetes mellitus is higher than in the general population. However, other features of thyrotoxicosis are usually lacking, and laboratory indices of thyroid function are normal.

Myeloproliferative disorders are accompanied by hypermetabolism, which may be manifested by increased sweating and weight loss and by tachy-cardia, especially if anemia is present. This disorder, therefore, may bear a superficial resemblance to thyrotoxicosis, but goiter is absent and laboratory indices of thyroid function are normal.

Cirrhosis of the liver may require differentiation from thyrotoxicosis, since patients with cirrhosis often display weight loss, excessive sweating, a bounding pulse, and occasionally mild exophthalmos. Furthermore, the thyroid I^{131} uptake may be increased in cirrhosis as a result of iodine deficiency secondary to an inadequate diet. However, the serum T_4 concentration is normal, goiter is generally absent, and the I^{131} uptake returns to normal when a nutritious diet is given.

One disorder that simulates thyrotoxicosis clinically is unlikely to be encountered because of its rarity, but is nevertheless of great theoretical interest. A single case has been reported of a woman who displayed severe hypermetabolism (in the range of +200 per cent), weight loss despite good appetite, profuse sweating, and progressive asthenia associated with myopathy. These symptoms had been present since childhood. Goiter was absent, and the thyroid I^{131} uptake was normal. The disorder was ascribed to structural abnormalities in the mitochondria leading to loosening of respiratory control (Luft et al., 1962).

Thyrotoxic myopathy may require differentiation from progressive muscular atrophy or polymyositis. In *progressive muscular atrophy*, fasciculation is present and the deep tendon jerks are diminished or absent. *Polymyositis* may resemble thyrotoxic myopathy, but muscle biopsy discloses inflammatory and degenerative changes. In both progressive muscular atrophy and polymyositis, other features of thyrotoxicosis are lacking and laboratory indices of thyroid function are normal.

The diffuse goiter of Graves' disease will rarely be confused with that of other thyroid diseases if thyrotoxicosis is present. Possible exceptions include the rare case of Hashimoto's disease, in which features of thyrotoxicosis are present (which may in fact represent the concurrence of the two disorders), and the early stage of subacute thyroiditis. In the latter disorder, clinical manifestations of thyrotoxicosis, enlargement of the thyroid, and elevation of the serum T_4 concentration may be present, but the frequent asymmetry and exquisite tenderness of the thyroid together with the subnormal thyroid I^{131} uptake serve to distinguish this from diffuse toxic goiter. When Graves' disease is in a latent or inactive phase and thyrotoxicosis is absent, the diffuse goiter usually persists and may require exclusion of Hashimoto's disease or simple nontoxic goiter as possible diagnoses. The goiter of Hashimoto's disease tends to be somewhat lobulated and firmer than that of Graves' disease. Thyroid autoantibodies are more commonly found in the serum in Hashimoto's disease, and the titers are generally much higher. In the absence of thyrotoxicosis, the diffuse goiter of Graves' disease cannot be distinguished on clinical grounds from the diffuse stage of nontoxic goiter. If the disease is in a latent phase, an abnormal thyroid suppression test will indicate underlying Graves' disease, but if the disease is inactive, the two disorders will be indistinguishable. Indeed, in some patients, active Graves' disease may first emerge from a background of what appeared to be simple nontoxic goiter.

The exophthalmos of Graves' disease, if bilateral and associated with thyrotoxicosis past or present, does not require differentiation from exophthalmos of other origin. Although purely unilateral exophthalmos does occur in Graves' disease, it is uncommon; hence, careful clinical evaluation and x-ray examination of the orbit are indicated to exclude a local cause. When exophthalmos occurs in the patient who has not been thyrotoxic, consideration must be given to other diseases that may produce either unilateral or bilateral exophthalmos. These include orbital neoplasms, caroticocavernous fistulae, thrombosis of the cavernous sinus or ophthalmic vein, retrobulbar hemorrhage, leukemic infiltration of the orbit, and pseudotumor cerebri. Mild bilateral exophthalmos, generally without infiltrative signs, is occasionally present on a familial basis and also sometimes occurs in patients with Cushing's syndrome, cirrhosis, uremia, or chronic pulmonary disease. In the absence of thyrotoxicosis, demonstration of an abnormal thyroid suppression test or the presence of thyroid autoantibodies in the serum strongly suggests that the ophthalmic disorder is a manifestation of Graves' disease. The absence of thyroid autoantibodies or a normal suppression test does not exclude Graves' disease as the cause of the exophthalmos, but should intensify the search for another origin.

Treatment of Thyrotoxicosis

Although considerable progress has been made in recent years toward an understanding of the etiology of Graves' disease, this progress has not yet led to the development of therapeutic measures aimed at the basic pathogenetic factors in the disease. In a very real sense, existing therapies for both the thyrotoxic and the ophthalmopathic manifestations are merely palliative in that they may relieve but do not cure the disease. The lack of general agreement as to which of the several therapies is the best reflects the fact that, although they all may be satisfactory, none is ideal. Since the therapeutic problems posed by the thyrotoxicosis and the ophthalmopathy differ so widely and since they run independent courses, their treatment will be discussed separately.

As indicated earlier, the thyrotoxicosis of Graves' disease is due to an abnormal rate of hormone synthesis and release. All major forms of treatment exert their effects by imposing restraints on the rate of hormone secretion. This is accomplished either by means of antithyroid agents that inhibit one or more stages in hormone synthesis or release or by so reducing the quantity of thyroid tissue that overproduction of hormone is no longer possible.

Antithyroid Agents. The first stage in hormone biosynthesis that is susceptible to chemotherapeutic inhibition is the iodide transport mechanism. Both thiocyanate and perchlorate, agents that inhibit thyroid iodide transport, have been employed successfully. However, theoretical and practical disadvantages attend their use. The ameliorative effect of these agents in thyrotoxicosis depends upon their ability to decrease the net flux of iodide into the thyroid, thereby limiting the quantity of substrate available for subsequent steps in hormone biosynthesis. Such treatment, however, leaves the patient at the mercy of his iodine intake, since if plasma inorganic iodide concentration is increased, sufficient iodide can enter the thyroid by simple diffusion to permit reestablishment of an excessive rate of hormone formation. Furthermore, this consideration makes it impossible to use iodine together with these agents in the preparation of the patient for subtotal thyroidectomy. In addition, a variety of serious adverse reactions may be produced by these drugs. The untoward effects of thiocyanate led to its abandonment years ago, and although perchlorate has enjoyed a period of popularity, its use now appears to be precluded by reports of the development of irreversible aplastic anemia (Krevans et al., 1962).

The major agents employed in the chemotherapy of thyrotoxicosis are drugs of the thionamide class having the chemical structure shown in Figure 4–12. The agents most commonly employed are propylthiouracil and methimazole (Tapazole) and the related drug, carbimazole (Neomercazole). The mode of action of these agents on hormone biosynthesis is complex. Although initially considered to exert their antithyroid action solely by inhibiting the oxidation and organic binding of thyroid iodide, they are now known to inhibit the coupling of iodotyrosines primarily and the formation of DIT and MIT secondarily. Thus they are capable of producing an inhibition of hormone synthesis of far greater degree than the inhibition of total iodine accumulation. This fact is of importance in interpreting values for the thyroid I^{131} uptake during treatment with these drugs, since uptakes may remain elevated despite the fact that the patient has been restored to a normal metabolic state.

Few data concerning the distribution and metabolism of these compounds are available. In man, the plasma concentration of methimazole peaks at about 60 minutes after a single oral dose and then declines with a half-life of about 6 hours; at 24 hours little can be detected in the plasma (Pittman et al., 1971). The half-time in plasma of propylthiouracil is even shorter. Accordingly, these compounds should be administered at relatively frequent intervals. Of great importance is the fact that they are capable of crossing the placenta and inhibiting fetal thyroid function. They are also excreted in breast milk and can thereby be transmitted to nursing infants. They are accumulated by the thyroid and metabolized by transsulfuration, a feature that may be closely related to their mode of action. In the hyperactive thyroid gland, the thyroid metabolism of thiourea, a related compound, is enhanced. (See Marchant et al., 1972, for a discussion and references concerning the distribution and metabolism of these compounds.)

The initial dose of propylthiouracil most commonly employed by the authors is 100–150 mg. given orally at intervals of 6 hours. Although this dosage is effective in most patients, in some no therapeutic response is seen. It is unlikely, however, that a true state of complete resistance to these agents ever occurs, although in some patients remarkably large doses of up to 1200 mg. daily may be required. This relative lack of effect usually occurs in patients with severe thyroid hyperfunction and large thyroid glands, possibly because of a more rapid degradation of the drug either within the gland or extrathyroidally. When large doses are required, it is often advantageous to increase the frequency of administration to intervals of 4 hours instead of or in addition to the size. The response to effective antithyroid therapy invariably occurs only after a latent period. This follows from the fact that these agents inhibit the synthesis but not the release of hormone, and hence a reduction in the supply of hormone to the tissues must await depletion of glandular hormone stores.

Several factors influence the duration of the latent period. Among these are the quantity of hormone initially present in the thyroid, its inherent rate of release, and the degree of blockade of new hormone synthesis that is achieved. In the thyroid rich in iodine, such as occurs when the patient has received medications containing iodine, the clinical response to antithyroid agents may be delayed for long periods, even months. As would be expected, the latent period is shortened by the administration of large doses (more than 600 mg. daily of propylthiouracil), and such should be used when a more rapid therapeutic response is required. Generally some improvement will occur within the first two weeks; the patient may note a decrease in nervousness and palpitations, an increase in strength, and a gain in weight during this period. Usually, a normal metabolic state can be restored within about six weeks. At this time, the dosage can often be reduced by approximately one-third and a normal metabolic state thereafter maintained.

During treatment, the size of the thyroid decreases in approximately half of the patients. In others it may remain unchanged, while in the remainder it enlarges. The latter change signals either an intensification of the disease process, which often requires that the dosage of drug be increased, or the production of hypothyroidism due to excessive dosage, which will be discussed shortly. Obviously, it is important to differentiate between these extremes. Clinical criteria should be the main guidelines by which the adequacy of treatment is judged, but confirmation may be sought in the serum T_4 concentration. Mild thyrotoxicosis may persist despite a serum T_4 concentration in the normal range, since the peripheral turnover of T_4 may remain accelerated for some time, and since the serum T_3 concentration may still be increased. The latter phenomenon may also account for the maintenance of a normal metabolic state in the face of a subnormal serum T_4 concentration (Sterling et al., 1971). By contrast, an elevation of the thyroid I^{131} uptake may persist despite adequate treatment, illustrating the primary action of the antithyroid agent on the later steps in hormone biosynthesis. Careful measurements of the BMR, if available, are an effective means of following the course of treatment.

The antithyroid agents have the potential of inducing hypothyroidism if given in excessive quantities over prolonged periods. When this occurs, the patient often complains of excessive gain in weight, sluggishness, and fatigue. Signs of mild hypothyroidism may be present, especially a delay in the relaxation phase of the deep tendon jerks. Important signs of incipient hypothyroidism are enlargement of the thyroid gland and the appearance or accentuation of a bruit. These result from hypersecretion of TSH and, together with hypothyroidism, can be reversed either by reducing the dosage of the antithyroid drug or by administering supplemental thyroid hormone. To forestall this development, which may have adverse effects on preexisting ophthalmopathy, some physicians employ supplemental thyroid hormone routinely. Although the authors do not regularly prescribe this regimen, they see no contraindication to its use.

A central question in the long-term use of antithyroid drugs is the period over which treatment should be continued. No arbitrary answer can be given, but the problem is best understood in the light of the physiopathology of the disorder. In the authors' opinion, there is no reason to believe that antithyroid therapy alters the course of the underlying disease process. If this is true, then persistence of remission following withdrawal of treatment will occur only if the disorder through its natural evolution has entered a latent or inactive phase. This may be difficult to discern while the patient is receiving treatment; however, decrease in the size of the thyroid suggests that this has occurred.

The thyroid-suppression test is of some assistance in this regard, since a normal response indicates that the disease is inactive. In some clinics, suppression tests are performed at intervals of about six months, and treatment is withdrawn when the test reverts to normal. It is not necessary that antithyroid medication be discontinued while suppression is being attempted, or even while the thyroid I^{131} uptakes in the test are being measured. In a general way, the suppression test may also be used as an indicator of the likelihood of recurrence of thyrotoxicosis following withdrawal of antithyroid therapy. Long-term remission is more likely to occur in patients who demonstrate a substantial degree of thyroid suppression than in those who do not; however, this correlation is imperfect. Moreover, some patients in whom the suppression test is abnormal remain in clinical remission for long periods after therapy is withdrawn (Alexander et al., 1970). Generally, then, treatment is continued for 12 months or longer and then withdrawn over several weeks rather than abruptly. This often permits an immediate exacerbation to be detected while some antithyroid effect is still maintained.

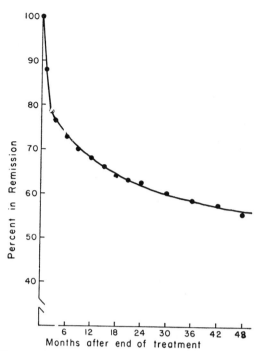

Figure 4-27. The percentage of patients in remission as a function of the interval after the cessation of a single course of antithyroid therapy of at least 6 months' duration. Note the biphasic nature of the curve. The initial rapid decline is produced by prompt recrudescence of hyperthyroidism following withdrawal of therapy. These patients were apparently in an active phase of their disease when treatment was discontinued. The second phase of the curve depicts progressive recurrence of hyperthyroidism in patients who were presumably in a latent or inactive phase of their disease when treatment was discontinued. (From Solomon, D. H., Beck, J. C., et al.: *J.A.M.A., 152:*201, 1953.)

There is considerable agreement in the literature concerning the late results of long-term antithyroid therapy. In studies with a follow-up period of four years or more, the incidence of prolonged remission after withdrawal of antithyroid therapy ranges between 45 and 72 per cent. The results of an early study are depicted in Figure 4-27, which demonstrates the percentage of patients remaining in remission from thyrotoxicosis following withdrawal of treatment (Solomon et al., 1953). The curve displays two components, the first representing an early exacerbation of thyrotoxicosis in one group, and the second a more gradual incidence of recurrence in the other. It may be presumed that in the first group the disease was in an active phase when therapy was withdrawn. In the second group, the disease was probably either latent or inactive but returned to an active phase at some later period. These studies also revealed that a progressively smaller proportion of patients displayed sustained remission of thyrotoxicosis following second and third courses of treatment. This finding may be interpreted as indicating that patients who require successive doses of therapy represent a population in which the disease more closely approaches a continuously active phase. In a later study from the same laboratory (Hershman, 1966), 54 per cent of 176 patients with either diffuse or multinodular toxic goiter experienced re-

missions. In three quarters of these patients, remissions lasted 10–20 years, and in the remainder they lasted 6–9 years. No significant difference was noted between the results obtained in patients with diffuse goiter and those with multinodular goiter. The age of the patient also did not appear to influence the results, but a decrease in glandular size during treatment correlated significantly with subsequent long-term remission. In the opinion of the authors and others, the likelihood of a sustained remission following long-term antithyroid therapy is less in those patients who initially manifest severe disease and an unusually large goiter.

Although prolonged remission following withdrawal of antithyroid therapy is the result of passage of the disease into a latent or inactive phase, other factors may be operative during the first several months after treatment is discontinued. Recent studies indicate that a state of iodine deficiency develops during treatment with antithyroid drugs. Following their withdrawal, this is manifested by a tendency for the plasma inorganic iodine concentration to be subnormal. The degree of iodine deficiency may condition both the frequency and the rapidity of relapse, since a greater incidence of relapse has been noted in patients in whom, after antithyroid therapy was discontinued, plasma inorganic iodide did not become subnormal or in those given small supplements of iodine (Harden et al., 1966). Some physicians have advocated the use of small doses of supplemental iodine during long-term antithyroid therapy; the foregoing findings appear to contraindicate this regimen. In addition, if the foregoing relationship holds, one might well question whether the recent general increase in dietary iodine intake will not adversely affect the frequency and duration of long-term remission following antithyroid therapy.

Methimazole (Tapazole) is the alternative antithyroid agent most commonly used in the United States. Its potency is generally considered to be about 10 times that of propylthiouracil, and hence the doses given are one-tenth those described earlier. It is the authors' impression, however, that this ratio underestimates the potency of methimazole. Except for the dosage, the use of methimazole is similar in all respects to that of propylthiouracil.

Adverse reactions occur in a small percentage of patients taking antithyroid drugs of the thionamide class (Table 4-7). The most significant of these are skin rash, drug fever, and agranulocytosis. Of these, the last reaction is the most serious and occurs in a fraction of 1 per cent of the pa-

TABLE 4-7.   PER CENT INCIDENCE OF TOXIC REACTIONS

	All Reactions	Agranulocytosis
Methimazole	7.1	0.1
Carbimazole	1.9	0.8
Propylthiouracil	3.3	0.4
Methylthiouracil	13.8	0.5

tients. Agranulocytosis, like the other adverse reactions, generally occurs within the first few weeks or months of treatment. It is accompanied by fever and sore throat, and hence, when therapy is begun, the patient should be instructed to discontinue the drug and notify the physician immediately should these symptoms develop. This precaution is more important than the frequent measurement of leukocyte counts, since agranulocytosis may develop within a day or two. Should agranulocytosis occur, the drug should be discontinued immediately and the patient should be isolated and given glucocorticoids and antibiotics. Almost invariably recovery will occur. Thereafter the patient should never be given the offending drug again, but the alternative drug may be given a cautious trial.

Granulocytopenia may also occur during antithyroid therapy and is sometimes a forerunner of agranulocytosis. On the other hand, mild granulocytopenia may be merely a manifestation of thyrotoxicosis. For this reason, granulocytopenia detected during the first few weeks of therapy may present the physician with a difficult decision—whether or not treatment should be continued. In this circumstance, serial measurements of the white cell count should be made, and if these display a downward trend, the antithyroid drug should be discontinued. Usually, however, serial measurements will reveal a return of the white cell count to normal, and treatment need not be interrupted. Skin rash, which may take many forms, is the most common type of reaction, and in the authors' experience occurs more frequently with methimazole than with propylthiouracil.

In addition to these reactions, others may occur, but fortunately even less frequently. These include arthralgia, myalgia, neuritis, hepatitis with evidence of cholestasis, thrombocytopenia, loss of or abnormal pigmentation of the hair, loss of taste sensation, enlargment of lymph nodes or salivary glands, edema, and toxic psychoses. The nature of the pathologic disturbances underlying these reactions is not known, although some, including the skin rash, may disappear despite continuance of treatment. Nevertheless, since it is known that drugs of the thionamide class can produce periarteritic lesions, it is the authors' view that most of the foregoing reactions are an indication for withdrawal of the drug and its replacement by an alternative agent. If the latter should produce similar reactions as is sometimes the case, thyrotoxicosis is treated by surgery or radioiodine.

Iodine. Iodine, which until 1943 was the major chemotherapeutic agent for thyrotoxicosis, is now rarely used as sole therapy. The mechanism of action of iodine in relieving thyrotoxicosis differs greatly from that of the thionamides. Although quantities of iodine in excess of several milligrams are capable of inducing an acute inhibition of organic binding (acute Wolff-Chaikoff effect), this is a transient phenomenon which, in all likelihood, does not contribute to the therapeutic action of iodine. Rather, the major action of iodine is to inhibit hormonal release, as several lines of evidence indicate.

First, administration of iodine is associated with an increase in glandular organic iodine stores. Second, the beneficial effect of iodine is evident much more quickly than is the effect of even large doses of agents that inhibit hormonal synthesis. Finally, in patients with diffuse toxic goiter, kinetic analysis demonstrates that iodine acutely retards the rate of secretion of T_4; this effect is rapidly lost when iodine is withdrawn (Wartofsky et al., 1970). These features of its action provide both the disadvantages and advantages of iodine therapy. The enrichment of glandular organic iodine stores that occurs when this agent is given alone may greatly retard the clinical response to subsequently administered antithyroid therapy, and furthermore, the decrease in thyroid I^{131} uptake that iodine produces will prevent the use of radioiodine as treatment for a period of weeks or more. In addition, if iodine is withdrawn, resumption of a rapid rate of release from an enriched glandular hormonal pool may produce a severe exacerbation of thyrotoxicosis. Still another reason for not using iodine alone is that in some patients the therapeutic response is either incomplete or lacking and that, even if initially effective, iodine may lose its effect with time. (This phenomenon, which has been termed "iodine escape," should not be confused with the escape from the acute Wolff-Chaikoff effect; see section on thyroid autoregulation.) On the other hand, the rapid slowing of hormonal release that iodine induces makes it a more effective agent than the thionamide drugs when rapid relief of thyrotoxicosis is mandatory. Therefore, aside from its use in the preparation of the patient for subtotal thyroidectomy, iodine is mainly useful for patients with actual or impending thyrotoxic crisis, severe thyrocardiac disease, or acute surgical emergencies—all conditions in which thyrotoxicosis is life-threatening.

If iodine is to be used in these circumstances, it is highly desirable that it be administered with large doses of an antithyroid drug, as the severity of the thyrotoxicosis would itself indicate. The dose of iodine as iodide required for control of thyrotoxicosis is not entirely certain but has been estimated to be approximately 6 mg. daily, a quantity far less than that usually given. Six milligrams of iodide would be contained in approximately one-eighth of a drop of saturated solution of potassium iodide (SSKI) or eight-tenths of a drop of Lugol's solution; many physicians, however, prescribe 5-10 drops of one of these agents three times daily. Although it is advisable to administer amounts larger than the suggested minimum effective dose, the huge quantities of iodine commonly administered are distinctly disadvantageous in that they are more likely to produce adverse reactions, including iodide myxedema. The authors recommend the use of two drops of saturated solution of potassium iodide (SSKI) three times daily. In patients who are so ill that medications cannot be taken by mouth, antithyroid agents can be triturated and administered by stomach tube; iodine can be given by the same route. When use of a stomach tube is contraindicated, thionamide drugs cannot be administered, since preparations for parenteral use are not available. Here, the disadvantages attendant upon the administration of iodine may be accepted if the clinical situation is sufficiently serious, and a preparation of sodium iodide is available for intravenous use. Adverse reactions to iodine are unusual and, although varied, are generally not serious. These include skin rash, which may be acneiform, drug fever, sialadenitis, conjunctivitis and rhinitis, lesions resembling those of periarteritis or thrombotic thrombocytopenic purpura, and a leukemoid eosinophilic granulocytosis. Sialadenitis may respond to reduction of the dosage; in the case of the other reactions, iodine should be withdrawn. As will be discussed later, iodine appears to be particularly effective when given after the administration of a therapeutic dose of I^{131}. This combination may be very useful when rapid alleviation of thyrotoxicosis is required.

Like iodine, lithium carbonate also inhibits thyroid hormone secretion and has been used effectively in several patients to alleviate thyrotoxicosis. Unlike iodine, however, it has the advantage that it does not interfere with the accumulation of a subsequently administered dose of radioiodine (Temple et al., 1972).

Surgery. As mentioned earlier, there is no reason to believe that antithyroid agents used in treating thyrotoxicosis have any direct effect on the thyroid that persists after the treatment is discontinued. By contrast, the other major types of therapy, i.e., surgery and radioiodine, exert their effects through the permanent removal or destruction of thyroid tissue, rendering the gland incapable of producing excessive quantities of hormone. This effect is likely to be long-lasting, and hence these forms of ablative therapy are referred to as "definitive treatment." Thus, as regards their duration of effect, antithyroid therapy and ablative therapy are diametrically different, and their opposite properties may be considered advantageous or disadvantageous, depending upon one's point of view.

The impermanence of antithyroid therapy leads to a relatively frequent recurrence of thyrotoxicosis, while with ablative therapy recurrence is uncommon. On the other hand, antithyroid therapy never produces permanent hypothyroidism, while with ablative therapy the incidence of permanent hypothyroidism may be distressingly or unacceptably high. The effectiveness of surgery in relieving hyperthyroidism is unquestioned. In most series, the incidence of recurrent hyperthyroidism following subtotal thyroidectomy in adults is less than 10 per cent. On the other hand, the combined incidence of postoperative hypothyroidism and other surgical complications is relatively high, rendering surgery less than ideal as a form of treatment.

Table 4–8 is taken from a report in which the results of surgery for hyperthyroidism in eight series are summarized (Hershman, 1966). The major postoperative complication is permanent hypothyroidism, which in the series cited ranged between 4 per cent and approximately 30 per cent.

TABLE 4–8. RANGE OF RESULTS OF SURGERY FOR HYPERTHYROIDISM, AS REPORTED FROM EIGHT CLINICS

	Per Cent
Mortality	0.0– 3.1
Recurrent hyperthyroidism	0.6–17.9
Vocal cord paralysis	0.0– 4.4
Permanent hypoparathyroidism	0.0– 3.6
Permanent hypothyroidism	4.0–29.7

From Hershman, J. M.: *Ann. Intern. Med. 64*:1306, 1966.

It is worthy of note that the highest incidence of permanent postoperative hypothyroidism was reported from those clinics in which internists did the follow-ups on the patients. In a more recent study conducted by internists, a mean incidence of 28 per cent was found in patients followed for 1–16 years, and the incidence in patients followed for 10 years was 43 per cent (Nofal et al., 1966).

Although it has been assumed that hypothyroidism will usually develop within one year after operation if it is to occur at all, recently reported series indicate a progressive increase in the cumulative incidence with time similar to that produced by radioiodine but of lesser magnitude. It may be presumed that the overall incidence of some impairment of thyroid function is even higher than that of frank hypothyroidism since subtotal thyroidectomy is one important cause of decreased thyroid reserve. The increasing incidence of hypothyroidism with time may result from progressive restriction of blood supply or from autoimmune destruction of the thyroid remnant. If, as suggested earlier, eventual thyroid failure is a frequent consequence of the Graves' disease process itself, the large increase in cumulative incidence of hypothyroidism with time that follows both surgery and radioiodine therapy is both expected and unavoidable. Treatment that destroys thyroid tissue would obviously accelerate the emergence of hypothyroidism resulting from the disease process itself.

It is generally agreed that an inverse relationship obtains between the incidence of recurrence and that of hypothyroidism, and that the relative incidence of the two partly depends upon the quantity of thyroid tissue left in place. What is more remarkable than the fact that some patients develop a recurrence and others hypothyroidism is that among patients whose thyroid glands vary greatly in size and degree of hyperfunction and who are operated upon by surgeons whose techniques must vary to a considerable extent a normal metabolic state is restored, at least for long periods, in most patients. It has been held that this favorable outcome of surgery may result because the amount of tissue remaining after operation is alone insufficient to sustain a normal metabolic state and hence becomes stimulated by the necessary quantity of endogenous TSH. In this way, the patient's homeostatic mechanism provides the adjustment in thyroid function that the surgeon, quite naturally, could not. This hypothesis is supported by the demonstration of TSH in the sera of patients restored to a normal metabolic state by surgery. Furthermore, it explains the more frequent return of the thyroid suppression test to normal after operation (or radioiodine) than after antithyroid treatment, since that component of function, being sustained by TSH, would obviously be suppressible.

Bleeding into the operative site is the most serious postoperative complication, since it can rapidly produce death by asphyxia. This complication requires immediate evacuation of the hematoma and ligation of the bleeding vessel. Damage to the recurrent laryngeal nerve is one of the major complications of thyroid surgery and, if unilateral, it results in dysphonia that usually improves in a few weeks but which may leave the patient slightly hoarse. If damage is bilateral, obstruction of the airway will usually occur within a few hours, producing severe stridor; tracheostomy is then required, and at this time the nature of the damage to the nerves should be sought.

Hypoparathyroidism is another major complication; it may be either transient or permanent. Transient hypoparathyroidism results from two factors: inadvertent removal of some parathyroids and impairment of blood supply to those that remain. Depending upon the severity of these insults, symptoms and signs of hypocalcemia will appear, usually within 1–7 days after operation. The earliest indication of hypoparathyroidism may be anxiety and mental depression, followed by paresthesia and evidence of heightened neuromuscular excitability, such as Chvostek's and Trousseau's signs and carpopedal spasm. The serum calcium is subnormal and the inorganic phosphate increased, and the urine Sulkowitch test is negative. When hypoparathyroidism is first evident, if severe it should be treated with intravenous calcium gluconate or calcium chloride. Milder cases can be treated with oral calcium chloride in a dose of 1 g. three times daily. Initially it is impossible to ascertain whether the hypoparathyroidism will be permanent or whether it will regress within a few weeks, as usually occurs.

Recently it has been suggested that the hypocalcemia that occurs in the thyrotoxic patient in the immediate postoperative period is not due to transient hypoparathyroidism, since it occurs more frequently here than after surgery for other thyroid disorders. Rather it has been ascribed to retention of calcium by bone in the thyrotoxic patient, but what initiates this phenomenon has not been determined (Michie et al., 1971). The incidence of permanent hypoparathyroidism varies in a general way with the proportion of the thyroid removed and hence with the incidence of postoperative hypothyroidism. The incidence of mild hypoparathyroidism (or diminished parathyroid reserve) detectable years after operation is probably greater than is generally supposed, and it may be as high as 24 per cent (Davis et al., 1961). The treatment of permanent hypoparathyroidism is discussed in Chapter 11.

It is clear that the hazards of subtotal thyroidectomy are inversely related to the experience and skill of the surgical team. Consequently, as surgery is less frequently performed, the hazards attendant upon it increase. For these reasons, it is impossible to generalize about the frequency of complications, and statistics drawn from the former era in which surgery was commonly applied are probably no longer applicable.

Preoperative use of the antithyroid agents has greatly decreased the morbidity and mortality of surgery for diffuse toxic goiter. This results from the ability of these drugs to deplete glandular hormone stores and secondarily to restore the patient to an entirely normal metabolic state before operation. On the other hand, these agents do not have the favorable influence on the hyperplasia and hypervascularity of the gland that is exerted by iodine. Iodine induces a process termed involution that is characterized by a decrease in height of the follicular cells, enlargement of follicles with retention of colloid, and last, but most important, reduction of hypervascularity. Hence, the aim of preoperative management is to restore a normal metabolic state with antithyroid agents and then to bring about involution of the gland with iodine. Achievement of these objectives makes the patient a better operative and postoperative risk in all respects. In the authors' clinic, patients who are to undergo subtotal thyroidectomy are first given antithyroid therapy in the manner described earlier. Often, relatively large doses are given, either to hasten the clinical response or because the patients for whom surgery is recommended are frequently those with severe disease or very large goiters. After a normal metabolic state has been restored, saturated solution of KI is given as two drops three times daily for a further 7–10 days. During this period, a preexisting bruit or thrill may decrease in intensity or disappear entirely; the gland usually becomes firmer and may appear to have enlarged.

Within this general approach, there are several specific guidelines that should be followed. First, no definite date for surgery should be set until the patient has been restored to a normal metabolic state. Much too often, the operation is planned well in advance, and the patient is given a standardized regimen that is largely independent of his clinical progress. Second, therapy with iodine should not be started until metabolic control has been produced by the antithyroid drug; iodine should not be relied upon to complete an as yet incomplete response to antithyroid therapy. This is true because if the antithyroid drug is not entirely effective the additional iodine will enrich glandular hormone stores. Finally, for closely related reasons, antithyroid agents should not be withdrawn when therapy with iodine is begun.

Radioiodine. Until quite recently, radioiodine was considered by many the ideal form of treatment for diffuse toxic goiter, because it is economical, simple to administer, essentially free of immediate complications, and effective over long periods of time. Since radioiodine provides a form of ablative therapy, it was not surprising that a certain proportion of patients developed therapeutic hypothyroidism, but this proportion was thought to be acceptably small. Some concern was also felt for the possibility that this form of therapy might lead to thyroid carcinoma, leukemia, or transmissible genetic damage. Therefore, in many clinics the use of radioiodine was restricted initially to patients more than 40 years of age. However, during the 25 years or so that radioiodine has been in use, only a few cases of thyroid carcinoma have been reported in patients treated with radioiodine (McDougall et al., 1971b), and the incidence of leukemia is not increased (Saenger et al., 1968). Furthermore, the incidence of genetic damage in the offspring of patients treated with radioiodine does not appear to be increased (Hayek et al., 1970). Consequently, the age limit for the use of radioiodine has been lowered progressively, so that in some clinics it is employed regularly in young adults and even children. This has not been the practice in the authors' clinic, in view of the feeling that both the amount and duration of experience in this regard are insufficient to permit definite conclusions.

During the early years of radioiodine therapy, attempts were made to standardize the radiation delivered to the thyroid gland by varying the dose of radioiodine according to the size of the gland, the uptake of I^{131}, and its subsequent rate of release. It has become apparent, however, that such calculations do not provide uniform results, probably owing largely to variations in individual sensitivity. Hence most clinics have settled upon an arbitrary dose of approximately 140–160 μCi./g. of estimated glandular weight.

Until the early 1960's most reports indicated that the incidence of postradioiodine hypothyroidism following doses of this magnitude was approximately 7–12 per cent, most of this occurring during the first year or two after treatment. Although an occasional patient developed hypothyroidism later, this was considered an uncommon occurrence. In 1961, however, there appeared the first of several reports that by now have completely altered this view. Not only is the incidence of hypothyroidism higher during the first year or two after treatment than originally thought, but it continues to increase at a rate of approximately 3 per cent/yr. thereafter (Beling and Einhorn, 1961). Thus the incidence of postradioiodine hypothyroidism at five years is approximately 30 per cent and at 10 years approximately 40 per cent, although values as high as 70 per cent have been reported (Dunn and Chapman, 1964; Nofal et al., 1966) (Fig. 4–28).

There is little doubt that the early beneficial effect of radioiodine and the early induction of hypothyroidism both depend upon radiation-induced destruction of thyroid parenchyma. Within the first few weeks after treatment, there occur epithelial swelling and necrosis, disruption of follicular architecture, edema, and infiltration with leukocytes (radiation thyroiditis). Resolution of the acute inflammation is followed by fibrosis, vascular narrowing, and lymphocytic infiltration. These structural changes account for the early response

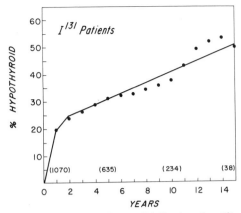

Figure 4-28. Incidence of postradioiodine hypothyroidism in relation to the duration of follow-up. Total number of patients followed for each of the indicated time periods is shown in parentheses. (From Dunn, J. T., and Chapman, E. M.: *New Eng. J. Med.* 271:1037, 1964.)

to radioiodine, be it favorable or excessive. In themselves, however, they do not appear sufficient to account for the increasing incidence of hypothyroidism with time, and more subtle factors appear to be operative.

A subtle functional abnormality is the defective organic binding of thyroid iodide that follows apparently successful therapy; this is evident in the frequently abnormal iodide-perchlorate discharge test and the enhanced susceptibility to iodide-induced hypothyroidism (Braverman et al., 1971). This phenomenon may be but one of several abnormalities that eventually produce thyroid failure. Among these may be damage to the nucleus of the follicular cell, leading to failure of normal replication, progressive autoimmune destruction, or progressive restriction of blood supply. Such factors would summate with factors related to the disease process itself which lead to eventual thyroid failure.

In view of the foregoing, it is unlikely that the early ablative effects can be obtained free of subsequent late effects. If this be true, then doses of radioiodine sufficient to exert an early therapeutic action would inevitably be associated with a high incidence of delayed hypothyroidism.

This statement summarizes the therapeutic dilemma with respect to radioiodine therapy. From various clinics, several approaches to this dilemma have emerged. Some authorities continue to administer the conventional dose because of its relatively rapid and high effectiveness and because hypothyroidism, when it eventually occurs, is readily treated. A disadvantage of such an approach is that the onset and progression of hypothyroidism may be very insidious, that careful and prolonged follow-up of patients may not be possible, and that the patient may not associate symptoms arising as a complication of therapy long removed with that therapy. A rebuttal in favor of using this approach would be that the dangers of persistent or recurrent thyrotoxicosis in the patient lacking follow-up exceed those of hypothyroidism, especially if the patient is elderly.

A second approach seeks to forestall the eventual development of clinical hypothyroidism through the routine administration of replacement doses of thyroid hormone following radioiodine therapy. If this approach is to be used, it should only be done after a eumetabolic state has been achieved. It can be argued, however, that in anticipation of employing replacement therapy the physician may administer inordinately large doses of radioiodine hoping to obtain sure control of the thyrotoxicosis. Moreover, patients frequently tire of taking medication and discontinue it, despite urging to the contrary. The consequence of these factors would be a high frequency of hypothyroidism.

Other approaches seek to minimize the incidence of hypothyroidism in patients treated with radioiodine. One such approach involves the use of I^{125}, whose β emission has a lower energy and shorter path length than that of I^{131}. These characteristics of I^{125} might permit irradiation of the apical portion of the follicular cell adjacent to the I^{125} in the colloid, with resulting impairment of hormone biosynthesis, while at the same time sparing the basally situated nucleus and its replicative machinery. A recent report has provided evidence that I^{125} effectively controls thyrotoxicosis, but the incidence of hypothyroidism appears to be as great as that following I^{131} (McDougall et al., 1971a).

A final approach employs smaller than usual doses of radioiodine. The rationale of such an approach is that the small dose may be sufficient to prevent both the high incidence of delayed hypothyroidism, which constitutes the chief disadvantage of conventional doses, and the late recurrence of thyrotoxicosis, which constitutes the chief disadvantage of antithyroid drug therapy. Although it is recognized that such small doses are likely insufficient to control thyrotoxicosis acutely, such control can be achieved by the administration of antithyroid drugs or stable iodine after radioiodine has been given (Smith and Wilson, 1967; Hagen et al., 1967).

The efficacy of this approach is not yet certain. Retrospective analysis indicates that the frequency of hypothyroidism varies directly with the magnitude of the dose used (Hershman, 1966). Moreover, in a controlled prospective study, the effects of a single conventional dose of approximately 140 μCi./g. of estimated glandular weight were compared with the effects of half the dose (Smith and Wilson, 1967). Although the therapeutic effect of radioiodine appeared more slowly in the patients receiving the half-dose and a greater proportion required antithyroid drug therapy until this became apparent, the incidence of remission after two years was essentially the same as that in the patients receiving the conventional dose, and recurrence of thyrotoxicosis was no more common. Of great importance was the finding that with the full dose group, the incidence of hypothyroidism was 8 per cent at one year and 29 per cent at five years, whereas in the half-dose group, the corresponding values were 4 per cent and 7 per cent. These results are in general agreement with those of another study (Hagen et al., 1967). However, recent data suggest that, although the use of low doses of I^{131} reduces the incidence of hypothyroidism during the first five years, after five years the cumulative incidence with time is similar to that observed with conventional doses (Glennon et al., 1972). It is apparent, therefore, that further observations of this type are required. The authors' viewpoints with regard to these approaches are discussed in the section concerning choice of therapy.

Several additional hazards may attend the use of radioiodine, particularly large doses. The parathyroids are exposed to radiation in patients treated with radioiodine, but the appearance of clinically overt hypoparathyroidism is rare. However, there is evidence to suggest that parathyroid reserve is diminished in some patients (Orme and Conolly, 1971). The effect of radioiodine on other tissues that concentrate iodide, such as the salivary and gastric glands, has received little attention. Another potential hazard of radioiodine therapy, namely radiation thyroiditis, may influence the therapeutic regimen. This complication may lead to an exacerbation of thyrotoxicosis about 10–14 days after the radioiodine is administered. Serious consequences occasionally have resulted in patients with severe thyrotoxicosis or thyrocardiac disease; these include precipitation of thyrotoxic crisis and aggravation of cardiac insufficiency. In cases of this type, therefore, it is advisable to administer antithyroid drugs for several weeks before radioiodine is given in order to deplete glandular hormone stores. This prevents an outpouring of hormone should radiation thyroiditis occur. The antithyroid agent is withdrawn 2–3 days before administration of the radioiodine and, if the clinical condition warrants, it can be given again several days later.

Adrenergic Antagonists. Agents that either deplete tissues of their catecholamine content (reserpine or guanethidine) or block the response to catecholamines at the receptor site (propranolol) are capable of antagonizing to a variable extent some of the manifestations of thyrotoxicosis. Hence they are useful adjuncts in the management of patients with this disorder. Tremulousness, palpitation, excessive sweating, eyelid retraction, and heart rate decrease, and the BMR is sometimes lowered. When administered in sufficient dosage, these agents have effects that are rapidly manifest and appear to be mediated solely through the adrenergic nervous system, since the serum T_4 concentration does not change.

Adrenergic antagonists have their greatest use in patients with severe thyrotoxicosis, such as those with impending or actual thyrotoxic crisis (see section dealing with special aspects of thyrotoxicosis). They are also of value, however, in patients with less severe disease in whom tremor, tachycardia, palpitation, or nervousness are particularly troublesome. Adrenergic antagonists have also been used in patients with thyrocardiac disease in whom tachycardia of either sinus or ectopic origin is contributing to cardiac insufficiency. These agents should be used with caution, however, since by depressing myocardial contractility they may aggravate cardiac insufficiency. Moreover, since it has been shown that thyroid hormone also has a direct effect on the myocardium independent of the adrenergic nervous system, the authors prefer to use iodine in conjunction with large doses of an antithyroid drug for rapid control of thyrotoxicosis in the patient with severe thyrocardiac disease. Adrenergic antagonists should be considered as adjunctive rather than primary tools in the treatment of thyrotoxicosis. They are most frequently useful in the interval during which the response to antithyroid or radioiodine therapy is being awaited.

Of the agents available, the authors generally prefer propranolol, as it is relatively free of adverse effects. It can be given either orally in a dose of 10–40 mg. every six or eight hours or, if indicated, intravenously in a dose of 2 mg. with electrocardiographic monitoring. Because of its central depressant action, reserpine may be useful in the patient in whom nervousness is a prominent symptom. It can be given either orally in a dose of 0.25 mg. every eight hours or, if indicated by the severity of the disease, intramuscularly in a dose of 2.5 mg. every six or eight hours. Reserpine is contraindicated in patients with preexisting mental depression or peptic ulcer. Guanethidine has the disadvantage that doses required to produce a beneficial effect (50–150 mg. daily) often cause troublesome postural hypotension. (See Riddle and Schwartz, 1970, for references.)

General Measures. Several general measures often contribute substantially to the well-being of the thyrotoxic patient. Removal of the patient from what may be a troubled domestic or occupational environment to the restful atmosphere of a hospital may in itself be accompanied by a moderate decrease in the BMR and subsidence of thyrotoxic manifestations. In addition, a dietary regimen rich in protein, calories, and vitamins serves to repair the general and specific nutritional deficiencies that thyrotoxic patients frequently develop. Psychotherapy has been recommended, but whether its contribution to the patient's well-being is greater than it would be in other diseases is uncertain.

Choice of Therapy. The choice of therapy for thyrotoxicosis is often difficult in actuality, but it becomes even more difficult when considered in a hypothetical setting, since a variety of factors other than those immediately related to the disease itself interplay with the disease to modify the therapeutic decision. Among these are emotional attitudes, economic considerations, and factors within the family and home. Their impact will be discussed as they become pertinent to each of the therapeutic possibilities.

The authors' choice of therapy in diffuse toxic goiter is one which accommodates factors related to the natural history of the disease, the advantages and disadvantages of the several therapeutic modalities discussed above, and the factors pertinent to the population group in which the patient falls. It has been thought that the operative and immediate postoperative risks of surgery, as well as the discomfort and expense that surgery entails, are justified by the frequency with which a long-lasting remission of thyrotoxicosis can be achieved without a high incidence of hypothyroidism. However, the recently detected incidence of hypothyroidism of up to 30 per cent has modified this view. Admittedly it is likely that the incidence of postoperative hypothyroidism could be reduced if less thyroid tissue were removed at operation, but all available data suggest that the incidence of postoperative recurrence would increase as a result to an extent that is currently unpredictable. Hence the authors recommend surgery only in patients for whom shortcomings of other modes of therapy have special importance. As will be seen, this conclusion gives surgery a significant role in the treatment of diffuse toxic goiter.

In the authors' opinion, therefore, radioiodine and antithyroid therapy become the mainstays of treatment, and the major choice rests between these two. The data currently available do not suggest that radioiodine carries an appreciable risk of thyroid carcinoma or leukemia. Furthermore, in patients who either by choice or by age will no longer become parents, the possibility of transmissible genetic damage induced by radioiodine does not exist. Consequently, the only tangible disadvantage to radioiodine therapy in such patients is the possibility that hypothyroidism will develop. Because of their relatively limited life expectancy and because of their susceptibility to serious complications of thyrotoxicosis, e.g., thyrocardiac disease, patients over 55 years of age should be given full or conventional doses of radioiodine. Supplemental thyroid hormone therapy is not routinely given for the reasons described earlier. Patients between 35 or 40 and 55 years of age are usually given the small-dose radioiodine regimen with supplemental antithyroid drug or iodine. Alternatively a conventional course of antithyroid therapy alone may be used, especially if the disease is mild and the thyroid is small.

Considerations peculiar to the treatment of thyrotoxicosis in children and adolescents are discussed in a later section dealing with special aspects of thyrotoxicosis. Hence the remainder of this section will be confined to the choice of therapy in young adults. Although the genetic and carcinogenic risks of radioiodine do not appear significant, it should be remembered that it has taken approximately 20 years to recognize that radioiodine frequently produces hypothyroidism within 5–10 years after its administration. By analogy, it may require 40 years to detect more subtle complications that occur 20 years after treatment. These considerations impel the authors toward a general choice of antithyroid therapy in the younger age group.

This overall recommendation is modified by several factors, however. Many patients urgently wish to be freed of the manifestations of their disease as quickly as possible. Here surgery is advised if the patient persists in this desire after the relative risks of surgery have been explained. Surgery is also recommended in the young adult who, because of inherent unreliability or other personal factors, is unwilling or unable to take medication or to be examined regularly. Such patients should be hospitalized until surgery has been performed, since they may avoid treatment altogether if left to their own devices. Surgery is also the treatment of choice for the young adult who has reacted adversely to both propylthiouracil and methimazole. Subtotal thyroidectomy is usually performed in young adults with severe disease or very large goiters (often accompanied by loud bruits), since in the experience of the authors and others these patients are less likely to experience a prolonged remission following withdrawal of antithyroid therapy. Surgery is also strongly considered for thyrotoxicosis that recurs after a single course of antithyroid therapy, and in this age group it will be recommended if two or more recurrences have taken place. The foregoing indications for surgical therapy in young adults are overruled, however, if a previous subtotal thyroidectomy has been performed, since the incidence of complications following secondary thyroid surgery is greatly increased. Finally, in the occasional young adult, it becomes necessary to remove a diffuse toxic goiter because of obstructive symptoms or cosmetic disfigurement.

Treatment of Infiltrative Ophthalmopathy and Infiltrative Dermopathy

Infiltrative ophthalmopathy varies in severity from a mild form, which is common, to a severe form that may threaten the vision and even the life of the patient. Fortunately the latter form is rare, since it presents difficult problems in the selection among and timing of many suggested modes of treatment. The variety of treatments that have been proposed and the continuing, often heated, discussion of their relative efficacy bespeak the general inadequacy of all, the most effective being merely palliative. The natural course of the disorder, which is highly variable and characterized by unaccountable exacerbations and remissions, makes conclusions about the efficacy of most treatments difficult or even dubious. This is all the more the case since the number of patients afflicted with the severe form is relatively small and since the severity of this form makes controlled studies difficult to perform. A further source of confusion is the variable terminology for describing the manifestations of ophthalmopathy and the lack of rigid criteria for defining their severity. General use of a recent classification that defines these variables is therefore strongly recommended (Werner, 1969).

The first question that arises is the effect that various forms of treatment for thyrotoxicosis may have on the course of the ophthalmopathy. Although opinions vary widely, it does not appear that subtotal thyroidectomy, radioiodine therapy, or antithyroid therapy in themselves significantly influence the course of the ophthalmopathy except as they may lead to the development of hypothy-

roidism. Almost all would agree that hypothyroidism has an adverse effect upon the disorder and should be avoided. When hypothyroidism occurs it should be treated fully, but there is no evidence that exogenous thyroid hormone in the absence of hypothyroidism favorably influences the ophthalmopathy. Similarly, no evidence exists for a favorable action of iodine once widely used. Indeed, in patients with Graves' disease, especially those treated with radioiodine, this agent may actually induce a hypothyroid state (iodide myxedema).

The measures used in treatment can be divided into those that are largely symptomatic (useful mainly in the mild form) and those that attempt to arrest or reverse the progression of the disorder, either by an attack on its presumed pathogenesis or by mechanical means. In milder forms of the disorder, little treatment is required. The patient who experiences photophobia and sensitivity to wind or cold air is benefited by wearing dark glasses, which also afford protection from foreign bodies. Elevation of the head of the bed at night and instillation of lubricants, such as 1 per cent methylcellulose, may benefit the patient whose lids do not appose completely during sleep. Mild or moderate infiltrative changes may also be benefited by restriction of salt intake and administration of diuretics. Since the ophthalmic manifestations tend to be self-limited and the progression to a more severe form uncommon, such measures usually suffice to tide the patient over until the disorder regresses spontaneously.

The appearance of increasing proptosis, with increasing inability to appose the lids, or of such severe infiltrative manifestations as chemosis, indicates progression of the disorder and warrants the use of more vigorous therapeutic measures. In this stage of the disorder, when the condition is serious but not desperate, several methods of treatment have been proposed. It is in relation to the efficacy of these that the greatest doubt exists. Changes of this type, even when severe, may respond favorably and rapidly to the administration of prednisone in massive doses (120–140 mg. daily) (Werner, 1966). If improvement occurs, the daily dose is decreased to the lowest level at which improvement is maintained. The latter is still likely to be large, but it is hoped that a halt to the progression or actual regression of the disease will occur before untoward effects make withdrawal of the drug necessary. In an attempt to circumvent the inevitable side effects of large doses of glucocorticoids given systemically, periodic injection of depot preparations of glucocorticoids given subconjunctivally or into the retro-orbital space have been advocated. Such treatment may have a dramatic effect on irritative symptoms as well as on diplopia, but its efficacy varies, and mild systemic effects of the glucocorticoids are sometimes seen. Moreover, this treatment entails the risk of puncture of the globe or a retro-orbital hematoma.

As an alternative to glucocorticoid therapy, external radiation to the orbits or to the pituitary has been employed. The value of such treatment is not definitely established, since reported results have been variable. Very recently, highly collimated supervoltage radiation of the retro-orbital space has been applied, with seemingly rapid and beneficial effects upon infiltrative and inflammatory manifestations (Donaldson et al., 1972). Relatively few patients have been treated, however, and this mode of therapy requires further evaluation.

On the basis of available evidence, there appears to be no merit to the suggestion that infiltrative ophthalmopathy is benefited or its progression retarded by total ablation of the thyroid, whether performed surgically or by radioiodine or by a combination of the two.

In view of the foregoing considerations, the authors recommend a trial of oral glucocorticoid therapy for patients with severe or progressive ophthalmopathy. If effective doses cannot be tolerated, a course of external radiation may be attempted. Local measures should be employed, along with these major forms of treatment. Ulceration and infection of the cornea should be treated with antibiotics, lubricants, and protective shields. An attempt to appose the lids by means of sutures (tarsorrhaphy) is often ineffective, as the sutures may tear out and result in scarring.

If glucocorticoid therapy and external radiation fail to halt progression of the disease, and if loss of vision is threatened either by ulceration or infection of the cornea or by changes in the retina or optic nerve, orbital decompression is performed. Classically this has involved removal of either the lateral wall or the roof of the orbit. More recently, good results have been reported with the transantral approach, in which the lateral wall of the ethmoid sinus and the roof of the maxillary sinus are removed (Ogura et al., 1971).

The management of the patient with severe ophthalmopathy should never be undertaken by the internist or endocrinologist or by the ophthalmologist acting alone. Close and coordinated observation with respect to the effects of medical therapy and the progress of the disease is necessary to determine whether and when the surgical approach to treatment, which almost invariably halts the progress of the disease and preserves vision if performed in time, should be employed.

Treatment of infiltrative dermopathy is seldom necessary. However, if this manifestation is severe, a topical glucocorticoid preparation along with an occlusive dressing will produce regression of the lesion.

Toxic Multinodular Goiter

Toxic multinodular goiter is a disorder in which hyperthyroidism arises in a multinodular goiter, usually of long standing. It is uncertain whether it represents one disease, perhaps Graves' disease, or whether it is the clinical expression of one of several pathogenetic factors. The authors feel it important to avoid the term "toxic nodular goiter," since this term encompasses both toxic multinodular goiter, as here described, and toxic adenoma of the thyroid gland, which will be discussed in a succeeding section.

Pathogenesis and Histopathology

The pathogenesis of toxic multinodular goiter cannot be considered apart from the clinical history of patients with this disorder or from the patterns of thyroid function with which it is associated. Here a nontoxic multinodular goiter, usually of long standing, invariably antedates development of hyperthyroidism. It is presumed that the pathogenesis and histopathology of the preexisting nontoxic goiter are those described in the later section dealing with this disorder. What causes the preexisting nontoxic goiter to lose its normal homeostatic regulation, thereby making possible the development of hyperthyroidism, is unknown. The patterns of function displayed by toxic multinodular goiters, however, suggest that either of two mechanisms is responsible. In radioautographs and in scintiscans, two basic patterns are discernible. The first is a diffuse but somewhat uneven localization of I^{131} that is not appreciably altered by the administration of either TSH or exogenous thyroid hormone. Histopathologic examination reveals multiple aggregates of small follicles with hyperplastic epithelium, interspersed with variably sized nodules composed of large follicles that appear inactive and accumulate little radioiodine. The latter may represent the nodular areas of the preexisting nontoxic goiter. The functional characteristics suggest that, in this type of toxic multinodular goiter, all areas capable of functioning are functioning, and none is dependent upon TSH. Whether this autonomous function originates in the thyroid gland itself or is due to an external stimulator, such as LATS, is not known. Assays for LATS in a large group of patients with lesions of this type are required, as positive assays would strongly indicate that this type represents Graves' disease. If this were to be the case, the rarity of ophthalmopathy in this disorder would require explanation.

What appears to be the second type of toxic multinodular goiter is also distinguished by its functional pattern. Here radioiodine becomes localized in one or more discrete nodules, while iodine accumulation in the remainder of the gland is suppressed. No further suppression is produced by exogenous thyroid hormone, but TSH stimulates accumulation of iodine in the areas previously inactive. Histopathologically, the functioning areas resemble adenomas in being reasonably well demarcated from surrounding tissue. They generally consist of large follicles, sometimes with hyperplastic epithelium, but the correlation of architecture with functional state is not good. The remaining tissue appears inactive, and zones of degeneration are present in both functioning and nonfunctioning areas. These findings suggest that areas that are functioning can do so without TSH and may therefore be termed areas of "adenomatous hyperfunction." The remaining areas, in contrast, retain their dependency upon TSH, their function being suppressed as a consequence of hyperfunction in the autonomous zones. It is most unlikely that function in this type of gland is sustained by an external stimulator of normal or abnormal origin. Hence, from the physiopathologic standpoint, this disorder resembles most closely the normal thyroid that harbors a solitary hyperfunctioning adenoma. Whether the hyperfunctioning areas represent true adenomas in a biologic sense is unknown.

Physiopathology

Little careful work has been done to correlate other aspects of the physiopathology of toxic multinodular goiter with the patterns of function that have been described. The major finding of certainty is the disruption of homeostatic regulation, regardless of its origin, that is evident in the failure of thyroid function to be suppressed by exogenous thyroid hormone. Several lines of evidence indicate that the extent of overproduction of thyroid hormone in toxic multinodular goiter is usually mild relative to that which occurs in classic Graves' disease. First, the clinical manifestations of thyrotoxicosis are rarely flagrant. Second, the serum T_4 concentration is often only marginally increased. Finally, the thyroid I^{131} uptake is not greatly increased and may even be within the normal range. The relative mildness of the hyperthyroidism is not inconsistent with either of its presumed pathogenetic origins. The effectiveness of any stimulus to hyperfunction may well be blunted in a thyroid that is the seat of a preexisting nontoxic goiter, since the latter disorder results from some inherent impairment in the efficiency of the gland with respect to hormone synthesis; this explanation is of course speculative.

A disproportionate increase in the synthesis and secretion of T_3 could explain the occurrence of thyrotoxicosis, albeit mild, with essentially normal values for thyroid I^{131} uptake and serum T_4 concentration (T_3-toxicosis) (Sterling et al., 1970; Hollander et al., 1972). An additional factor relates to the age of the patient in whom this disorder usually occurs. Requirements for thyroid hormone normally decrease with advancing age (Oddie et al., 1966), and, in elderly individuals, values for serum T_3 concentration are normally about two-thirds those in young adults (Brunelle and Bohuon, 1972). Hence, even small increases in the concentration of hormone in serum may lead to thyrotoxicosis.

Clinical Picture

Toxic multinodular goiter is a common complication of its nontoxic precursor, but its precise incidence in the latter disorder is unknown. It usually occurs after the age of 50 in patients who have had multinodular goiter for many years. Like its forerunner, it is many times more common in women than in men. Toxic multinodular goiter is almost never accompanied by infiltrative ophthalmopathy, but when it is, it doubtless represents the emergence of frank Graves' disease.

The clinical manifestations of thyrotoxicosis in toxic multinodular goiter tend to differ in predominance from those in the diffuse toxic goiter of Graves' disease. Cardiovascular manifestations tend to predominate, possibly because of the age of the patient. These may include atrial fibrillation or tachycardia, with or without heart failure. Frequently, a decreased response to digitalis first alerts the physician to the presence of thyrotoxicosis. Weakness and wasting of muscles are common. The nervous manifestations are less prominent than in the younger patient with thyrotoxicosis, but emotional lability may be pronounced. Because of the physical characteristics of the thyroid gland as well as its not infrequent retrosternal extension, obstructive symptoms are more common than in diffuse toxic goiter. On palpation, the characteristics of the goiter are the same as those of the more common nontoxic multinodular goiter discussed later.

Laboratory Tests and Differential Diagnosis

The main clinical problem is to determine whether the patient with a multinodular goiter is thyrotoxic. Laboratory tests may or may not be of assistance in this regard. The thyroid I^{131} uptake may be of little value unless distinctly elevated, because thyrotoxicosis may exist in association with values that are normal or only slightly increased. Difficulty also arises from the fact that slight increases in thyroid I^{131} uptake are seen in some patients with nontoxic multinodular goiter. Similar difficulties arise in connection with the serum T_4 concentration; often thyrotoxicosis is present in association with values that are only slightly increased or at the upper limit of normal. A value for the serum T_3 concentration that is normal for young adults represents an increase in the elderly patient (Brunelle and Bohuon, 1972). Measurements of the BMR should be helpful but often are not because of coexisting cardiac or respiratory disease, anxiety, or edentia. The thyroid suppression test may be of value, but should not be performed in the elderly patient or the patient with overt heart disease. It is in these situations that the TRH-stimulation test has its greatest usefulness. This test is virtually free of untoward effects, and lack of responsiveness to TRH is seen with only slight increases in the concentration of hormone in serum (see section on laboratory tests).

Treatment

Radioiodine appears to be the treatment of choice for the majority of patients with toxic multinodular goiter, despite the fact that there is considerable disagreement among the various clinics concerning the magnitude and number of doses required to achieve a therapeutic response. In general, the experience along the eastern seaboard of the United States indicates that the responsiveness to radioiodine of toxic multinodular goiter differs little from that of diffuse toxic goiter. On the other hand, in areas where goiter tends to be endemic, such as the Great Lakes area of the United States, toxic multinodular goiter is said to be very resistant to radioiodine. Although no correlative studies necessary to support this hypothesis have been reported, it might be suggested that the type that readily responds to radioiodine is that which resembles diffuse toxic goiter in displaying a relatively diffuse accumulation of iodine. The more resistant variety, on the other hand, may be that associated with adenomatous hyperfunction, in which focal accumulation of radioiodine occurs; here, tissue previously suppressed may regain function and ultimately achieve autonomy after the hyperactive tissue has been destroyed.

Because of the age of the patient and variations in sensitivity to radioiodine, the small-dose regimen that has been recommended by some clinics for the treatment of diffuse toxic goiter is not recommended for the treatment of toxic multinodular goiter. Instead, conventional doses should be administered. In any event, these are likely to be larger than those used in diffuse toxic goiter, because the percentage uptake of I^{131} tends to be lower and the size of the gland greater. Many patients with this disorder have underlying heart disease. Therefore, it is recommended that the administration of radioiodine be preceded by a course of antithyroid therapy until a eumetabolic state is achieved. Medication is then discontinued for 2–3 days before administering radioiodine. Several days thereafter, the antithyroid drug is reinstituted so that control of thyrotoxicosis is maintained until radioiodine exerts its effect. After 6–8 weeks, the antithyroid drug is withdrawn, and if thyrotoxicosis recurs, a second course of therapy should be given. Surgical therapy is recommended after adequate preoperative preparation in patients in whom obstructive manifestations are present or in whom it is feared that such manifestations may result from the temporary enlargement of the thyroid that radioiodine sometimes produces.

Toxic Adenoma

A third and far less common form of hyperthyroidism is that sometimes produced by one or more autonomous adenomas of the thyroid gland. As herein employed, the term refers to adenomas present in a thyroid that is otherwise intrinsically normal, differentiating this lesion from areas of adenomatous hyperfunction within a toxic multinodular goiter. The disorder is usually caused by a single adenoma that is palpable as a solitary nodule and hence is sometimes referred to as "hyperfunctioning solitary nodule" or "toxic nodule." Occasionally, two or three adenomas of similar character are present.

Pathogenesis, Histopathology, and Physiopathology

Toxic adenomas are true follicular adenomas of the thyroid gland (for histopathologic characteristics see section dealing with thyroid neoplasms); hence, their basic pathogenesis is unknown.

By definition, the adenoma is capable of functioning without stimulation by TSH, and assays reveal no LATS in the blood (McKenzie, 1966). The natural course of the lesion is one of slow, progressive growth and increasing function evolving over many years. At first, it may be present as a small nodule or may be impalpable, but in either case, it may be detectable in the scintiscan as a localized area of increased radioiodine accumulation. Upon the administration of exogenous TH (thyroid hormone) the function of the remainder of the gland is suppressed, but function in the adenoma persists. Later, with further growth, a progressively increasing share of glandular function is assumed by the adenoma, with the result that the remaining tissue is increasingly suppressed. Ultimately, atrophy and complete suppression of the remainder of the gland occur, and the scintiscan reveals function only in the adenoma ("hot" nodule) (Fig. 4–18). Although it is likely that continued growth of the adenoma is associated with secretion of excessive quantities of hormone, some time may pass before overt thyrotoxicosis is manifest. The extranodular tissue generally retains its capacity to function if TSH is provided, either by exogenous administration or as a result of ablation of the nodule. Some adenomas of this type secrete T_3 predominantly, and some, in addition to the normal thyroid hormones, secrete an iodinated protein that is measurable as protein-bound iodine (PBI), leading to a disproportionate elevation of the latter relative to T_4-iodine.

Clinical Picture

Toxic adenoma occurs in a younger age group than does toxic multinodular goiter, often being seen in patients in their thirties or forties. Frequently, a history of a long-standing, slowly growing lump in the neck is obtained. Rarely does the lesion develop sufficient function to produce thyrotoxicosis until it has achieved a diameter of 2.5–3 cm. Not infrequently, the lesion may undergo central necrosis and hemorrhage; as a result, the thyrotoxicosis may be relieved, the remainder of the thyroid may resume its function, and the adenoma may appear on the scintiscan as a cold area, suggesting a thyroid carcinoma. Calcification in the area of hemorrhage may take place and be evident on x-ray examination.

The peripheral manifestations of toxic adenoma are generally milder than those of diffuse toxic goiter and are notable for the absence of infiltrative ophthalmopathy and myopathy; cardiovascular manifestations, however, may be prominent. On examination, the nodule is usually felt as a smooth, well-defined, round or ovoid mass that is firm and moves freely on swallowing. Often, the remainder of the gland is not palpable. A bruit is never present.

Laboratory Tests

The results of laboratory tests depend upon the stage of the disorder. At first, laboratory indices are normal, except that the thyroid I^{131} uptake cannot be completely suppressed with exogenous TH; the function that remains during suppression is localized in the adenoma, as shown by the scintiscan (Fig. 4–18). Later, suppressibility is lost as function is confined to the adenoma, but clear evidence of hyperfunction is lacking. At this stage, an increase in thyroid I^{131} uptake may be found, but the serum T_4 and T_3 concentrations, as well as metabolic indices, will usually be normal. At this point, in view of the suppression of extranodular function, an absent response to TRH administration would be expected. When thyrotoxicosis supervenes, the thyroid I^{131} uptake is more greatly increased, the serum T_4 and T_3 concentrations are increased, and the metabolic indices are consistent with thyrotoxicosis. The degree of thyroid hyperfunction may not be accurately reflected by measurement of the 24-hr. thyroid I^{131} uptake. Measurement of the uptake at an earlier period, e.g., at 4 hours, frequently reveals a relatively greater increase in the uptake at this time, and the PBI^{131} is often inordinately high, indicating a rapid release of iodinated products from the adenoma. Occasionally, values for serum T_4 concentration are normal, and the serum T_3 concentration alone is increased (T_3-toxicosis) (Sterling et al., 1970; Hollander et al., 1972). In this event, the thyroid I^{131} uptake may be normal. Relative to its overall rate of occurrence, toxic adenoma is the most frequent cause of T_3-toxicosis.

Treatment

The hyperfunctioning adenoma that has suppressed the remainder of the thyroid gland should be treated with ablative therapy, regardless of whether or not the patient is overtly thyrotoxic, since the likelihood of eventual thyrotoxicosis is high. Although the lesion may seem especially amenable to treatment with radioiodine because of the highly localized accumulation of iodine, the authors prefer excision of the adenoma unless surgery is contraindicated. Radioiodine frequently fails to eliminate the nodule entirely, whereas surgery in essence cures the disease. Furthermore, rare cases of hyperfunctioning thyroid carcinomas have been reported (Sung and Cavalieri, 1973). Before surgery, exogenous TSH should be administered (for three days if necessary) in order that the scintiscan may verify the functional capability of the extranodular tissue; almost invariably, potential function is present. The rare instance in which

the extranodular tissue is unresponsive to TSH may be analogous to the unresponsiveness sometimes found in long-standing hypopituitarism. In patients with this finding, replacement therapy with TH will probably be required postoperatively, but in the great majority of patients, normal function will be reestablished in the residual tissue after the adenoma has been removed.

The thyroid that is the seat of a toxic adenoma is not diffusely hypervascular, and hence preoperative preparation with iodine is not required, but in the patient with overt thyrotoxicosis, restoration to a normal metabolic state with an antithyroid drug before surgery is desirable.

Thyrotoxicosis Factitia

This term designates thyrotoxicosis that arises from the ingestion, usually chronic, of excessive quantities of thyroid hormone rather than from overactivity of the thyroid gland and is therefore an example of thyrotoxicosis without hyperthyroidism. The disorder usually occurs in women, often those with a background of underlying psychiatric disease, and especially in paramedical personnel who have access to TH or in patients for whom TH medication has been prescribed in the past. Generally, the patient is aware that she is taking TH but may adamantly deny this to be the case. In other instances, large doses of TH or other thyroactive material, such as iodocasein, may be given to the patient without her knowing their nature, usually as part of a regimen for weight reduction.

Symptoms are those typical of thyrotoxicosis and may be severe. In the absence of preexisting disease of the thyroid, diagnosis is made from the combination of typical thyrotoxic manifestations, together with thyroid atrophy and hypofunction. Infiltrative ophthalmopathy never occurs, but lid lag, stare, and other "thyrotoxic" eye signs may be present. Hypofunction of the thyroid gland is evidenced by subnormal values for the thyroid I^{131} uptake which can be increased by the administration of TSH. Values for the serum T_4 concentration are increased unless the patient is taking T_3, in which case they will be subnormal. Metabolic indices are in accord with the thyrotoxic state.

The disorder may be confused with the rare cases of thyrotoxicosis caused by ectopic thyroid tissue, but strong evidence for the latter can be obtained by the demonstration of low values for the sum of thyroid and urinary I^{131} after a tracer dose, high values for the serum PBI^{131}, and, in particular, localization of the ectopic focus by external scintiscanning.

Treatment consists of withdrawing the offending medication. Psychotherapy may be desirable in certain instances.

Miscellaneous Thyrotoxic States

Rarely, hyperthyroidism is associated with an increased serum TSH concentration. In three reported cases, there was an associated pituitary tumor (Hamilton et al., 1970), while in a fourth no such lesion was demonstrable, and the disorder was believed to result from excessive secretion of TRH (Emerson and Utiger, 1972). Hyperthyroidism may also result from the production of a thyroid stimulator at some site other than the pituitary. The latter has been reported in association with metastatic embryonal carcinoma of the testis and with hydatidiform mole and choriocarcinoma. In the hydatidiform mole, the TSH-like material is immunologically distinct from pituitary TSH and from the normal chorionic thyrotropin and differs from LATS in not being an immunoglobulin G and having a shorter duration of action (Hershman and Higgins, 1971). Laboratory indices are consistent with the hyperthyroid, thyrotoxic state, but clinical manifestations of thyrotoxicosis may not be prominent, and the thyroid gland may not be enlarged (Galton et al., 1971).

Thyroid tissue is not infrequently present in teratomas, especially in the ovary (struma ovarii), and, rarely, such foci may produce thyrotoxicosis (Perlmutter and Mufson, 1951). The distinguishing features of such lesions are discussed under Thyrotoxicosis Factitia.

Special Aspects of Thyrotoxicosis

Thyrotoxicosis in Childhood and Adolescence

Thyrotoxicosis in childhood and adolescence is almost always the result of Graves' disease. Although thyrotoxicosis in this age group comprises only a small proportion of all cases, it is worthy of special consideration because treatment is less satisfactory than it is in adults. Hence there is more uncertainty and greater disagreement concerning its optimal management. (For a discussion of the management of neonatal and childhood thyrotoxicosis, see Hayles, 1972.) Several factors weigh against the use of radioiodine in children. First, the enhanced carcinogenic potential of radiation in the thyroid gland of the infant or child seems clearly established by the very high correlation between childhood thyroid carcinoma and a history of x-ray therapy to the neck or chest (Winship and Rosvoll, 1961). Second, among all patients with thyrotoxicosis, fear of transmissible genetic damage is most cogent among those treated in childhood or adolescence, although recent data suggest that this may not be significant (Hayek et al., 1970). Finally, the authors consider postradioiodine hypothyroidism to be a particularly undesirable complication in children, since inadequate or interrupted therapy can have profound effects on growth and development and on scholastic performance. For these reasons, it is felt that radioiodine should not be used in the treatment of childhood thyrotoxicosis.

The choice between surgical and antithyroid therapy is a difficult one. The data indicate a lower incidence of long-term remission following antithyroid therapy than is the case in adults, although some believe that thyrotoxicosis often undergoes remission after adolescence. On the other hand, most surgical series reveal a relatively high incidence of postoperative hypothyroidism, which is no more desirable after surgery than after radioiodine administration. Recurrences are also more frequent, presumably as a result of attempts to avoid hypothyroidism. Furthermore, the occasional operative death seems more tragic in a child than in an adult, and such complications as hypoparathyroidism and recurrent laryngeal nerve damage need to be borne over a longer life span. On the basis of these considerations, the authors favor the use of antithyroid therapy and recommend a course of 1–2 years' duration. Supplemental TH therapy is desirable, since it forestalls the possibility of therapeutic hypothyroidism and has no adverse side effects. In contrast to the recommendation in young adults, a second course of antithyroid therapy is regularly employed if recrudescence or relapse occurs after the first course. If sustained remission does not follow a second course of therapy and, particularly, if the patient has passed through adolescence during this period, surgery would be indicated.

Thyrotoxicosis in Pregnancy

Thyrotoxicosis occurring during pregnancy is almost always due to Graves' disease. Difficulty in conception and fetal wastage are increased in women with thyrotoxicosis. Nevertheless, an occasional patient will become pregnant despite antecedent untreated hyperthyroidism. More commonly, a woman being treated for thyrotoxicosis will become pregnant, or hyperthyroidism will appear after pregnancy is under way. Whatever the sequence, the concurrence of thyrotoxicosis and pregnancy presents features of special concern from both the diagnostic and therapeutic standpoints.

Pregnancy and hyperthyroidism have many features in common. Both are accompanied by thyroid enlargement, manifestations of a hyperdynamic circulation, and hypermetabolism. Amenorrhea may occur in thyrotoxicosis not associated with pregnancy. In the two conditions, the serum T_4 and T_3 concentrations, the thyroid I^{131} uptake, and the BMR may be comparably increased. Laboratory tests useful in this differentiation are measurements of the proportion of free T_4 in serum or *in vitro* uptake tests. These reflect the increased hormone binding in plasma in pregnancy and the decreased binding in thyrotoxicosis. A positive pregnancy test will complete the diagnostic differentiation. A more difficult diagnostic problem is whether or not a pregnant woman is mildly thyrotoxic. Increases in serum T_4 concentration above 12 μg./100 ml. and failure of *in vitro* uptake tests to display their usual subnormal values, resulting in calculated values for the free T_4 index that are above the normal range, and values for the BMR in excess of +30 per cent are in accord with a diagnosis of thyrotoxicosis. In the normal pregnant woman, homeostatic regulation of thyroid function is apparently intact. Since I^{131} is not wittingly administered to pregnant women, changes in the thyroid I^{131} uptake cannot be used as an index of thyroid suppression. In the authors' experience, however, substantial decreases in serum T_4 concentration can be induced by the administration of T_3, though values as low as those in nonpregnant women receiving T_3 may not be found. Hence the thyroid suppression test may be of value in the marginal case. In this situation, the TRH-stimulation test would also be useful, since only slight increases in the quantity of hormone available to the tissues result in a diminished response to TRH.

An even greater problem is posed by the management of thyrotoxicosis during pregnancy. Surgery during the last trimester and probably during the first trimester as well appears to be contraindicated because of the likelihood of inducing premature labor. Although surgery may be successful during the middle trimester, it is best to avoid any major surgical procedure during pregnancy if possible. Since antithyroid treatment poses no greater risk to the mother or fetus than does surgery, and possibly poses less risk, medical therapy is the method of choice.

The problem is the selection of the optimal form of medical therapy. There are two major schools of thought, one advocating antithyroid drugs in quantities just sufficient to control the thyrotoxicosis, the other advocating supplementation of antithyroid drugs with replacement doses of TH (thyroid hormone). The divergence of these views stems from inadequate knowledge of crucial aspects of TH economy in human pregnancy. Mainly, it is uncertain to what extent TH traverses the placenta, either from mother to fetus or vice versa. Since it is known that the antithyroid agents can readily cross the placenta and produce goitrous hypothyroidism in the fetus, the extent to which maternal hormone of either endogenous or exogenous origin protects against this becomes a critical consideration. Although passage of labeled hormone from mother to fetus at term has been demonstrated, this indicates merely hormone exchange and not net transfer. Since it is generally assumed that TH–plasma protein interactions largely condition such transplacental passage of TH as may occur, one would expect net transfer of hormone from fetus to mother rather than the reverse, since during pregnancy the binding activity of maternal plasma exceeds that of the fetus.

In any case, the results of both regimens are quite similar. Data suggesting that the combined approach may produce somewhat more favorable results may merely reflect the fact that studies of the efficacy of antithyroid drugs alone have been largely retrospective. No prospective study comparing the effects of the two regimens is presently available. All agree, however, that when maternal hypothyroidism is induced, the incidence of goitrous hypothyroidism in the fetus is increased, sometimes with catastrophic consequences. The authors believe that the regimen employing antithyroid agents alone is the more desirable of the two, provided that care is exercised. In this regimen, the dose of antithyroid agent should be adjusted so that the patient is in a state consistent with normal pregnancy. The clinical manifestations of the mild hypermetabolism and the increased circulatory burden of normal pregnancy should not be construed as indicating inadequate treatment. The serum T_4 concentration should be maintained between 9 and 13 μg./100 ml., the free T_4 index in the upper normal range, and the BMR during the latter half of pregnancy at +20–30 per cent. Attention to these criteria will require frequent observation of the patient, but this may be a major advantage of the regimen rather than a disadvantage. Once the correct dosage of the antithyroid drug has been determined, supplementation with TH will do no harm and conceivably could be of benefit. However, a regimen that depends primarily on the use of supplemental TH may have two disadvantages. First, it may discourage frequent observations, since it may be felt that the hormone needs of mother and fetus are being met. Second, it may encourage the use of larger doses of antithyroid agent than are otherwise needed; this would be detrimental if transfer of TH from mother to fetus is indeed limited.

Iodine should not be used as adjunctive or sole therapy in the pregnant woman because of the likelihood of inducing iodide goiter in the fetus. Mothers receiving antithyroid agents during the postpartum period should not breast-feed their infants, since these are excreted in the milk in quantities sufficient to produce goitrous hypothyroidism in the newborn.

Assay for LATS in the serum of pregnant women with known Graves' disease may be of value, since neonatal thyrotoxicosis is prone to occur in the newborn of mothers in whom titers of LATS in serum are high.

Thyrotoxic Crisis

Thyrotoxic crisis or storm is an extreme accentuation of thyrotoxicosis. It is an uncommon but exceedingly serious complication, usually occurring in association with Graves' disease but sometimes with toxic multinodular goiter. Before the availability of adequate means for achieving full preoperative control, crisis frequently followed subtotal thyroidectomy ("surgical crisis"); currently "medical crisis" is the more common. Thyrotoxic crisis is almost always of abrupt onset and occurs in patients of any age and either sex in whom preexisting thyrotoxicosis has been treated either incompletely or not at all. Crisis is almost always evoked by a precipitating factor, such as infection, trauma, or surgical emergencies or operations. Less common precipitating factors include radiation thyroiditis, diabetic ketoacidosis, toxemia of pregnancy, and parturition. The clinical picture is dominated by manifestations of severe hypermetabolism. Fever is almost invariably present and may be extreme; profuse sweating occurs. Marked tachycardia of sinus or ectopic origin may be accompanied by pulmonary edema or congestive heart failure. Early, tremulousness and restlessness are invariably present; delirium or frank psychosis occasionally occurs. Nausea, vomiting, and abdominal pain are common early manifestations. As the disorder progresses, apathy, stupor, and coma may supervene, and the blood pressure, which is initially well maintained, may fall to hypotensive levels. If the condition goes unrecognized, it is invariably fatal. This clinical picture in a patient either with a history of preexisting thyrotoxicosis or with goiter or exophthalmos or both is sufficient to establish the diagnosis, and treatment, which is urgently required, should not await laboratory confirmation.

There are no foolproof criteria by which severe thyrotoxicosis complicated by some other serious disease can be distinguished from thyrotoxic crisis induced by that disease. In any event, the differentiation between these alternatives is of no great significance, since treatment of the two is the same. Treatment of thyrotoxic crisis aims to correct both the severe thyrotoxicosis and the precipitating illness and to provide general supportive therapy. The therapy of crisis per se consists of efforts to inhibit both hormone synthesis and release and to antagonize the adrenergically mediated aspects of peripheral TH action. Large doses of an antithyroid agent (200 mg. of propylthiouracil every four hours) are given by mouth or stomach tube. This serves to initiate therapy for the postcrisis period and to prevent enrichment of glandular hormone stores by the iodine, whose administration is of more immediate importance. The latter agent, administered either as saturated solution of potassium iodide (SSKI, 5 drops every 4 hours by mouth) or as sodium iodide (1–2 g. by slow intravenous infusion), is intended to retard acutely the release of hormone from the thyroid. Propranolol (2 mg. intravenously with electrocardiographic monitoring, followed by 10–40 mg. every six or eight hours by mouth) should be administered to antagonize the adrenergic component of the disorder (Das and Krieger, 1969). Supportive measures that may be of great importance include the administration of hydrocortisone (100–300 mg. daily) and correction of the inevitable dehydration and possible hyponatremia. Glucose should be administered together with large amounts of vitamins of the B complex. A vigorous attack on the hyperpyrexia should be made. In milder cases, aspirin may suffice, but more often wet packs, fans, or ice packs may be required. If heart failure or pulmonary congestion is present, digitalis and diuretics are indicated.

Regimens similar to the foregoing have reduced the mortality rate in this disorder to approximately 20 per cent, a figure that is still disturbingly high. When treatment is successful, improvement is usually manifest within 1–2 days, and recovery occurs within a week. Thereafter, therapy directed at the long-term management of the thyrotoxicosis is required.

THYROID HORMONE DEFICIENCY

A large number of structural or functional abnormalities may lead to insufficient synthesis of thyroid hormones. Efforts to classify the causes of hypothyroidism into mutually exclusive categories invariably fail. One convenient classification divides types of hypothyroidism into those that are associated with loss or atrophy of thyroid tissue (thyroprivic hypothyroidism) and those that are associated with compensatory goitrogenesis (goitrous hypothyroidism). In the latter disorders, the abnormality is biochemical in nature, and the thyroid, at least initially, is anatomically intact. However, this classification makes no allowance for hypothalamic or pituitary hypothyroidism or for the hypothyroidism associated with Hashimoto's disease; in the latter disorder, there is a destruction of thyroid tissue together with goiter as well as distinct abnormalities in hormone biosynthesis. In the following section, causes of hypothyroidism will be discussed in the following sequence: (a) hypothyroidism associated with loss or absence of functioning thyroid tissue (thyroprivic hypothyroidism); (b) hypothyroidism due to insufficient stimulation of an intrinsically normal gland as a result of hypothalamic or pituitary disease (trophoprivic hypothyroidism); and (c) disorders of a primarily biochemical nature that may lead to hypothyroidism (goitrous hypothyroidism). Hashimoto's disease will be discussed in a separate section dealing with thyroiditis.

Peripheral Manifestations of Thyroid Hormone Deficiency

The clinical state that results from all these disorders whenever production of thyroid hormones (TH) is insufficient is termed hypothyroidism and is manifest in all organ systems. These manifestations are to a large extent independent of the underlying disorder in the thyroid gland, but are more closely related to the degree of hormone deficiency.

Skin and Appendages

In the dermis as well as in other tissues an accumulation of hyaluronic acid alters the composition of the ground substance. This material binds water, producing the mucinous edema that is responsible for the thickened features and puffy appearance of the patient with full-blown hypothyroidism and gives this severe degree of hypothyroidism its classic designation, *myxedema.* The myxedema is characteristically boggy and nonpitting and is most apparent around the eyes, on the dorsa of the hands and feet, and in the supraclavicular fossae. It causes enlargement of the tongue and thickening of the pharyngeal and laryngeal mucous membranes. A histologically similar type of deposit may occur in patients with Graves' disease usually over the pretibial area (infiltrative dermopathy or pretibial myxedema). In addition to having a puffy appearance, the skin in hypothyroidism is pale and cool as a result of cutaneous vasoconstriction. Anemia commonly accompanies hypothyroidism and contributes to the pallor; not uncommonly, hypercarotenemia gives the skin a yellow tint. The secretions of the sweat glands and sebaceous glands are reduced, leading to dryness and coarseness of the skin which, in extreme cases, may resemble that seen in ichthyosis.

Because of the skin's slow rate of growth, wounds of the skin tend to heal slowly. A bruising tendency is common in hypothyroidism and results from an increase in capillary fragility.

Characteristic changes are also seen in the skin appendages in hypothyroidism. Head and body hair is dry and brittle, lacks luster, and tends to fall out. Loss of hair from the temporal aspects of the eyebrows is a common feature. Growth of hair is greatly retarded so that haircuts and shaves are required less often. The nails are brittle and grow abnormally slowly.

In pituitary hypothyroidism, the changes in the skin and its appendages are less striking than in thyroprivic hypothyroidism. Although the skin is pale and cool, it tends to be thinner and finely wrinkled, and myxedematous infiltration of the tissues is less prominent than in thyroprivic hypothyroidism. Depigmentation of areas that are normally pigmented, such as the areolae, frequently occurs in pituitary but not thyroprivic hypothyroidism.

Histopathologic examination of the skin in hypothyroidism reveals hyperkeratosis with plugging of hair follicles and sweat glands. The dermis is edematous, and the connective tissue fibers are separated by an increase in the normal amount of metachromatically staining, PAS-positive mucinous material. This mucinous material consists of protein complexed with two mucopolysaccharides, hyaluronic acid and chondroitin sulfate B, especially the former. It is mobilized early during treatment with thyroid hormone, leading to an increase in the urinary excretion of nitrogen and hexosamines.

Cardiovascular System

In hypothyroidism, the cardiac output at rest is decreased because of a reduction in both stroke volume and heart rate, reflecting the loss of the inotropic and chronotropic effects of thyroid hormones. Peripheral vascular resistance at rest is increased, and blood volume is reduced. These hemodynamic alterations result in a narrowing of pulse pressure, a prolongation of circulation time, and a decrease in blood flow to the tissues. The decrease in cutaneous circulation is responsible for the coolness and pallor of the skin and the sensitivity to cold. In most tissues, the decrease in blood flow is proportional to the decrease in oxygen consumption, so that the mixed arteriovenous oxygen difference remains essentially normal. Despite the hemodynamic alterations at rest, which resemble those of congestive heart failure, cardiac output increases normally and peripheral vascular resistance decreases normally in response to exercise (Graettinger et al., 1958).

In thyroprivic hypothyroidism, the heart is enlarged (Fig. 4–29) and the heart sounds are diminished in intensity. These findings appear to be due largely to effusion into the percardial sac of fluid rich in protein and mucopolysaccharides, but dilation of a "flabby" myocardium may also be a factor. Although pericardial effusion is common, it is very rarely of a degree sufficient to cause tamponade. In

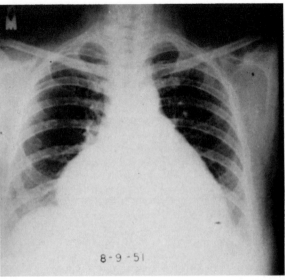 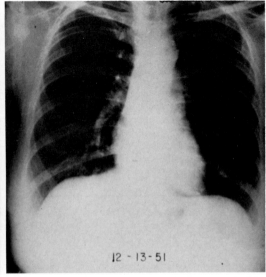

Figure 4–29. Chest roentgenograms in a patient with myxedema heart disease. The patient had signs of severe congestive heart failure and was treated with thyroid hormone alone. Within four months, the heart had returned to normal size and there was no evidence of underlying heart disease.

pituitary hypothyroidism, the heart is frequently small.

Angina pectoris is uncommon in hypothyroidism. Because of this, thyroid ablation has been used in the treatment of intractable angina. Rarely is typical angina present in the hypothyroid state, and occasionally it disappears when the eumetabolic state is restored. More commonly, angina either appears or is worsened during treatment of the hypothyroid state with TH. There has been much discussion as to whether the hypercholesterolemia that accompanies primary hypothyroidism accelerates the development of coronary atherosclerosis. Recent necropsy data suggest that the hypercholesterolemia of hypothyroidism predisposes to coronary atherosclerosis only in the presence of hypertension; in normotensive hypothyroid patients, the degree of coronary atherosclerosis appears to be no greater than that in age- and sex-matched normotensive control subjects (Steinberg, 1968).

Electrocardiographic (ECG) changes are common and include sinus bradycardia, prolongation of the PR interval, low amplitude of the P wave and QRS complex, alterations of the ST segment, and flattened or inverted T waves. Pericardial effusion is probably responsible in part for the ECG changes.

The concentrations in serum of such enzymes as creatine phosphokinase, glutamic oxalacetic transaminase, and lactic dehydrogenase may be increased in hypothyroidism. Furthermore, the isoenzyme pattern of lactic dehydrogenase may be reminiscent of that seen in acute myocardial infarction, suggesting that a specific form of myocardiopathy exists in hypothyroidism (Aber et al., 1966).

In hypothyroidism, the large heart, together with the hemodynamic and ECG alterations and the serum enzyme changes, has been termed *myxedema heart*. There has been considerable discussion as to whether myxedema heart ever is the sole cause of heart failure. If it is, this must be quite rare, since in hypothyroidism the usual hemodynamic response to exercise differs from that observed in heart failure. Furthermore, the response of pulse pressure to the acute reduction in filling pressure induced by the Valsalva maneuver differs in the two situations. In the patient with hypothyroidism, as in the normal, the Valsalva maneuver leads to a decrease in pulse pressure, whereas in the patient with heart failure, the pulse pressure does not decrease, but displays a so-called "square-wave" response. In the absence of coexisting organic heart disease, treatment with TH corrects the hemodynamic, ECG, and serum enzyme alterations of myxedema heart and restores heart size to normal (Fig. 4–29).

On pathologic examination, the pericardial sac contains an increased amount of fluid that is rich in protein and mucopolysaccharides. The heart is dilated and the myocardium is pale and flabby. Coronary atherosclerosis is commonly present. Histopathologic examination of the myocardium reveals interstitial edema and swelling of the muscle fibers with loss of striations.

Respiratory System

Pleural effusions are common in hypothyroidism. Usually, these are evident only on radiologic examination but rarely may be of a degree sufficient to cause dyspnea. Lung volumes are usually normal in hypothyroidism, but maximum breathing capacity and diffusing capacity are reduced (Wilson and Bedell, 1960). In severe hypothyroidism, myxedematous involvement of respiratory muscles as well as depression of the respiratory center may lead to alveolar hypoventilation and carbon dioxide retention, which in turn may contribute to the development of myxedema coma.

Alimentary System

Although most patients show a modest gain in weight, the appetite is characteristically reduced. Contrary to popular conception, gross obesity is never a feature of hypothyroidism per se. Such weight gain as occurs is due largely to retention of fluid by the hydrophilic mucopolysaccharide deposits in the tissues. Peristaltic activity is decreased and, together with the decreased food intake, is responsible for the frequent complaint of constipation. The latter may be extreme, leading to fecal impaction. Gaseous distention of the abdomen may occur (myxedema ileus) and, if accompanied by colicky pain and vomiting, may mimic mechanical ileus. Clinically discernible ascites in the absence of other cause is unusual in hypothyroidism, but it may occur, usually in association with pleural and pericardial effusions. Like effusions into the other serous cavities, the ascitic fluid is rich in protein and mucopolysaccharides.

Achlorhydria after maximum histamine stimulation reportedly occurs in about one-half of patients with primary hypothyroidism. Even in the absence of overt anemia, many of these patients absorb vitamin B_{12} poorly and have low concentrations of vitamin B_{12} in serum. The impaired absorption of vitamin B_{12} is corrected by ingesting intrinsic factor (Tudhope and Wilson, 1962). Circulating antibodies against gastric parietal cells have been found in about one-third of patients with primary hypothyroidism and probably reflect the presence of an atrophic gastric mucosa (Ardeman et al., 1966). Overt pernicious anemia is reported in about 12 per cent of patients with primary hypothyroidism (Tudhope and Wilson, 1962). The coexistence of pernicious anemia as well as other presumed autoimmune diseases with primary hypothyroidism supports the view that autoimmunity plays a primary role in the pathogenesis of primary hypothyroidism.

The effects of hypothyroidism on intestinal absorption are complex. Although the rates of absorption of many substances are decreased, the total amount that is eventually absorbed may be normal or even increased, because the decreased motility of the bowel may allow more time for absorption to occur. Overt malabsorption occasionally occurs.

Liver function tests are normal in hypothyroidism. Cholecystography often reveals a distended gallbladder that contracts sluggishly, but whether these changes predispose to the development of gallstones is unknown. Radiologic examination of the abdomen may reveal a greatly distended colon (myxedema megacolon).

Histopathologic examination of the GI tract frequently reveals atrophy of the gastric and intestinal mucosa and myxedematous infiltration of the bowel wall. The colon may be greatly distended. The volume of fluid in the peritoneal cavity is usually increased. The liver and pancreas are normal.

Nervous System

TH is essential for the development of the CNS. Deficiency of TH beginning in fetal life or at birth results in retention of the infantile characteristics of the brain, hypoplasia of cortical neurons with poor development of cellular processes, retarded myelination, and reduced vascularity (Eayrs, 1960, 1966). If the deficiency is not corrected in early postnatal life, irreversible damage results. Deficiency of TH beginning in adult life causes manifestations of lesser severity that usually respond adequately to treatment with TH. The cerebral circulation shares in the hemodynamic alterations of hypothyroidism in that cerebral blood flow is reduced. Cerebral oxygen consumption, however, may be normal; this is in accord with the observation that the oxygen consumption *in vitro* of isolated brain tissue, unlike that of most other tissues, is not stimulated by administration of thyroid hormones. Consequently, the decrease in cerebral blood flow may lead to cerebral hypoxia.

One of the characteristic features of hypothyroidism is a general slowing of all intellectual functions, including speech. There is loss of initiative. Slow-wittedness and memory defects are common. Lethargy and somnolence are prominent. Dementia may occur and in the elderly patient may be mistaken for senile dementia. Psychiatric reactions are not uncommon and are usually of the paranoid or depressive type, but agitated states have also been described (myxedema madness). Headache occurs quite frequently. Cerebral hypoxia resulting from the circulatory alterations may predispose to confusional attacks and syncope. Syncope may be prolonged, leading to stupor or coma. Other factors predisposing to coma in hypothyroidism include exposure to severe cold, infection, trauma, hypoventilation with carbon dioxide retention, and depressant drugs. Epileptic fits have been reported and are especially liable to occur in myxedema coma (Jellinek, 1962). Night blindness is common and is due to deficient synthesis of retinene, the pigment required for dark adaptation. Hearing loss of the perceptive type is frequently present. Perceptive deafness may also occur in association with a defect in the organic binding of thyroidal iodide (Pendred's syndrome) or with endemic cretinism, but in these instances, it is not due to hypothyroidism per se. Thick slurred speech and hoarseness are common and are due to myxedematous infiltration of the tongue and larynx, respectively. All movements are slow and clumsy, and pronounced ataxia of cerebellar type may occur. Numbness and tingling of the extremities are frequent complaints; in the fingers, these symptoms are often due to compression by mucinous deposits in and around the median nerve in the carpal tunnel (carpal tunnel syndrome). The tendon jerks are slow, especially during the relaxation phase, producing the characteristic "hung-up reflexes"; this phenomenon appears to result from a decrease in the rate of muscle contraction and relaxation, rather than from a delay in nerve conduction. The presence of extensor plantar responses or diminished vibration sense should alert the physician to the possibility of coexisting pernicious anemia.

Electroencephalographic changes are common and include slow α-wave activity and general loss of amplitude. The concentration of protein in spinal fluid is often increased, but the pressure is normal.

On histopathologic examination, the nervous system is edematous, with mucinous deposits in and around nerve fibers. There may be foci of degeneration and an increase in glial tissue. The cerebral vessels commonly show atherosclerosis. (See review by Sanders, 1962, for an extensive discussion of the neurologic manifestations of myxedema.)

Muscle

Stiffness and aching of muscles are common complaints of the hypothyroid patient. Slowness of muscle contraction and relaxation is characteristic and is responsible for the slowness of movement and the delayed tendon jerks. These changes are aggravated by cold. Muscle strength is usually normal. Muscle mass may be slightly increased, and the muscles tend to be firmer than normal. Rarely, a great increase in muscle mass accompanied by slowness of muscular activity may be the predominant manifestation of hypothyroidism (the Kocher-Debre-Semelaigne or Hoffman syndrome).

Urinary excretion of creatine is reduced and creatine tolerance is increased, but these changes are generally not of a magnitude sufficient to afford a clear separation from normal values. The concentrations in serum of some enzymes of muscular origin, such as creatine phosphokinase and glutamic oxalacetic transaminase, are increased.

On histopathologic examination, the muscles appear pale and swollen. The muscle fibers may show swelling, loss of normal striations, and separation by mucinous deposits, but often no definite abnormalities are present.

Skeletal System: Calcium and Phosphorus Metabolism

TH is essential for the normal growth and maturation of the skeleton. The effect on growth appears to be due to a stimulation of protein synthesis as well as to a potentiation of both the secretion and action of GH. Before puberty, TH is the major prerequisite for normal maturation of bone. Deficiency of TH beginning in early life leads to both a delay in the development of and an abnormal, stippled appearance of the epiphysial centers of ossification (epiphysial dysgenesis). Linear growth is severely impaired, leading to dwarfism in which the limbs are disproportionately short in relation to the trunk. Bone age is always retarded in relation to chronological age.

Data concerning the effects of hypothyroidism on calcium and phosphorus metabolism in man are scanty. In general, urinary excretion of calcium is decreased, whereas fecal excretion of calcium and urinary and fecal excretion of phosphorus are variable. Calcium balance is also variable, and the changes reported are slight. The exchangeable pool of calcium and its rate of turnover are consistently reduced. These changes reflect decreases in the rates of bone formation and resorption. Aching and stiffness of the joints are not uncommon complaints, and joint effusions are occasionally seen.

Concentrations of calcium and phosphorus in serum are usually normal, but alkaline phosphatase is characteristically low in infantile and juvenile hypothyroidism. Bone density may be increased on radiologic examination. The radiologic appearances of the skeletal abnormalities of cretinism and juvenile hypothyroidism are discussed in the section dealing with these disorders.

Renal Function: Water and Electrolyte Metabolism

As part of the hemodynamic alterations that accompany hypothyroidism, renal blood flow and GFR are decreased, and tubular reabsorptive and secretory maxima are reduced. Blood urea nitrogen and serum creatinine, however, are normal. Urine flow is reduced, and the excretion of a water load may be delayed, resulting in a reversal of the normal diurnal pattern of urine excretion. The delay in water excretion appears to be due to decreased volume delivery to the distal diluting segment of the nephron as a result of the diminished renal perfusion rather than to an inappropriate secretion of antidiuretic hormone (De Rubertis et al., 1971). It is reversed by treatment with TH. The ability to concentrate urine may be slightly impaired. Proteinuria of mild degree may occur. (See DiScala and Kinney, 1971, and De Rubertis et al., 1971, for extensive discussions of renal function in hypothyroidism.)

The impaired renal excretion of water along with retention of water by the hydrophilic deposits in the tissues results in an increase in total body water, even though plasma volume is reduced. This increase accounts for the hyponatremia that is commonly noted, since exchangeable Na^+ is increased in hypothyroidism. Exchangeable K^+ is usually normal in relation to lean body mass. The serum Mg^{++} concentration may be increased, but exchangeable Mg^{++} and urinary Mg^{++} excretion are decreased (Jones et al., 1966).

Hematopoietic System

In hypothyroidism, several hematologic abnormalities may occur. In response to the diminished oxygen requirements, the red cell mass is decreased; this is evident in the mild normocytic, normochromic anemia that often occurs. Less commonly, the anemia is macrocytic, and usually, though not invariably, this results from deficiency of vitamin B_{12}. Reference has already been made to the high incidence of pernicious anemia (and of achlorhydria and vitamin B_{12} deficiency without overt anemia) in patients with primary hypothyroidism (see Alimentary System). The defective absorption of vitamin B_{12} in primary hypothyroidism cannot be ascribed to lack of TH per se, since it is not found to the same extent in the hypothyroid state that follows radioiodine treatment of thyrotoxicosis and is not corrected by treatment with TH. In fact, defective absorption of vitamin B_{12} may develop or progress during treatment of hypothyroidism. Since this abnormality appears to be corrected by intrinsic factor, the macrocytic anemia that is sometimes seen in patients with primary hypothyroidism is more likely to be the result of deficiency of vitamin B_{12} than of TH per se (Tudhope and Wilson, 1962). Nevertheless, TH may be required for an optimum hematologic response to vitamin B_{12}. Folate deficiency resulting from malabsorption or dietary inadequacy may also be responsible for a macrocytic anemia. Both the frequent menorrhagia and the defective absorption of iron resulting from achlorhydria may lead to a microcytic, hypochromic anemia.

The total and differential white cell count is usually normal, and platelets are adequate in hypothyroidism. An aspirate of bone marrow often has a gelatinous consistency, and the bone marrow may be hypocellular. If pernicious anemia or significant folate deficiency is present, the characteristic changes in the peripheral blood and bone marrow will be found. The intrinsic clotting mechanism may be defective because of decreased concentrations in plasma of factors VIII and IX (Simone et al., 1965), and this, together with an increase in capillary fragility, may account for the bleeding tendency that sometimes occurs.

Pituitary and Adrenal Function

In hypothyroidism, the rate of turnover of cortisol is decreased. This alteration is due to a decrease in the rate of oxidation of cortisol to its inactive 11-keto metabolites as a result of a decrease in 11-β-hydroxysteroid dehydrogenase activity (Hellman et al., 1970). As a result of the decreased rate of turnover of cortisol, the 24-hour urinary excretion of 17-OHCS and 17-KS is decreased, but the plasma cortisol concentration is usually normal. The responses of the urinary 17-OHCS to exogenous ACTH and metyrapone are usually normal in thyroprivic hypothyroidism, but occasionally sluggish responses are observed (Kaplan, 1965). The response of plasma cortisol to insulin-induced hypoglycemia may be impaired in some patients with thyroprivic hypothyroidism, and the response of plasma GH is usually subnormal (Vince et al., 1970). In severe, long-standing, thyroprivic hypothyroidism, secondary depression of pituitary and adrenal function may occur, and adrenal insufficiency may be precipitated by stress or by rapid replacement therapy with TH.

The rate of turnover of aldosterone is decreased, but the plasma concentration is normal (Luetscher et al., 1963). Plasma renin activity is decreased and sensitivity to angiotensin II is increased (Hauger-Klevene et al., 1972).

The 24-hour urinary excretion of catecholamines and their metabolites is essentially normal in hypothyroidism. The metabolic and hemodynamic responses to exogenous catecholamines are depressed and are restored by treatment with TH.

On histopathologic examination, the pituitary in thyroprivic hypothyroidism shows an increase in the number of sparsely granulated cells which are probably actively secreting TSH. In thyroprivic hypothyroidism dating from infancy or childhood, the pituitary may be distinctly enlarged. The adrenals are usually normal but occasionally show cortical atrophy.

Reproductive Function

In both sexes, TH influences sexual development and reproductive function. Thyroprivic hypothyroidism from infancy, if untreated, leads to sexual immaturity, while hypothyroidism beginning before puberty causes a delay in the onset of puberty followed by anovulatory cycles. Thyroprivic hypothyroidism has been reported in association with precocious sexual development and galactorrhea. To what extent this rare consequence is the result of the enhanced responsiveness of prolactin to TRH in hypothyroidism is unclear.

In adult women, hypothyroidism is commonly associated with diminished libido and failure of ovulation. Secretion of progesterone fails and endometrial proliferation persists, resulting in excessive and irregular menstrual bleeding. These changes may be due to a failure of secretion of luteinizing hormone (LH). In severe, long-standing, thyroprivic hypothyroidism, secondary depression of pituitary function may occur, leading to ovarian atrophy and amenorrhea. Amenorrhea accompanied by galactorrhea and a high plasma prolactin concentration has been reported (Edwards et al., 1971). Fertility is reduced in hypothyroidism, but if conception does take place, abortion often results. In men, hypothyroidism may be accompanied by diminished libido, impotence, and oligospermia.

The metabolism of both androgens and estrogens is altered in hypothyroidism. Secretion of androgens is decreased, and the metabolic transformation of testosterone is shifted toward etiocholanolone rather than androsterone (Hellman et al., 1970). In man, androsterone decreases serum cholesterol, but whether deficiency of androsterone in hypothyroidism is at all responsible for the increase in serum cholesterol remains to be determined. With respect to estradiol and estrone, hypothyroidism favors metabolism of these steroids via 16α-hydroxylation over that via 2-oxygenation, with the result that formation of estriol is increased at the expense of 2-hydroxyestrone and its derivative, 2-methoxyestrone (Hellman et al., 1970). The binding activity of testosterone-estradiol binding globulin in plasma is decreased, with the result that the plasma concentrations of both testosterone and estradiol are decreased, but their unbound fractions are increased (Olivo et al., 1970). The alterations in steroid metabolism disappear when the euthyroid state is restored.

Values for urinary or plasma gonadotropins are usually in the normal range in thyroprivic hypothyroidism. In postmenopausal women with this disorder, these values are somewhat lower than those in euthyroid women of the same age, but they are nevertheless distinctly increased. This provides a valuable means of differentiating thyroprivic from pituitary hypothyroidism.

Histopathologic examination of the ovaries and testes may reveal degenerative changes, especially if hypothyroidism began before puberty. In long-standing postpubertal hypothyroidism the ovaries may be atrophied.

Energy Metabolism: Protein, Carbohydrate, and Lipid Metabolism

The intrinsic effects of TH on intermediary metabolism are discussed under Effects of Thyroid Hormones on Metabolic Processes. This section will deal with the manner in which these effects are clinically evident in the patient with hypothyroidism.

The decrease in energy metabolism and heat production of the hypothyroid patient is reflected in the low BMR, decreased appetite, cold intolerance, and slightly low basal body temperature.

In hypothyroidism, both the synthesis and degradation of protein are decreased, the latter especially so, with the result that nitrogen balance is usually slightly positive. The decrease in protein synthesis is reflected in retardation of both skeletal and soft tissue growth. In addition, TH deficiency is accompanied by both a decrease in the secretion and a lessened effectiveness of GH.

Permeability of capillaries to protein is increased, accounting for the high concentration of protein in effusions into serous cavities and perhaps in spinal fluid. In addition, the total exchangeable albumin pool is increased, as a result of the relatively greater decrease in albumin degradation than in albumin synthesis. A greater than normal proportion and quantity of exchangeable albumin is localized in the extravascular space. The total concentration of serum proteins may be increased.

The oral glucose tolerance curve is characteristically flat and the insulin response delayed. These alterations may be due to a decreased rate of absorption of glucose from the gut. The disappearance from plasma of an intravenous load of glucose is delayed, reflecting the slow rate of uptake of glucose by the tissues. Degradation of insulin is slower than normal, with the result that there may be an increased sensitivity to exogenous insulin. This, as well as the decrease in appetite, presumably accounts for the diminished insulin requirement that occurs when hypothyroidism supervenes in a patient with preexisting diabetes mellitus.

Both the synthesis and degradation of lipid are depressed, the latter especially so, with the result that the net effect is one of lipid synthesis. The decrease in lipid degradation may reflect a decrease in post-heparin lipolytic activity, as well as a decreased delivery of lipid to degradative sites. Although an increase in serum cholesterol is the most commonly recognized abnormality of lipid metabolism in thyroprivic (but not pituitary) hypothyroidism, serum phospholipid phosphorus and serum triglycerides are also increased, and the concentration in serum of low-density lipoproteins (LDL) is increased. Plasma FFA are decreased and the mobilization of FFA in response to fasting, catecholamines, and GH is impaired. (See Nikkilä and Kekki, 1972, for a review of lipid metabolism.)

Composite Clinical Picture of Hypothyroidism

Adult Hypothyroidism

The onset of hypothyroidism is usually so insidious that the classic clinical manifestations may take months or years to appear and frequently go unnoticed by persons well acquainted with the patient. The gradual development of the hypothyroid state is due to a slow progression both of thyroidal hypofunction and of the clinical manifestations after thyroidal failure is complete. This course is in contrast to the more rapid development of the hypothyroid state that occurs either when replacement therapy is discontinued in a patient with treated thyroprivic hypothyroidism or when the

thyroid gland of a normal subject is surgically removed. In these circumstances, the BMR decreases to about -20 per cent, and symptoms of mild hypothyroidism appear within three weeks. After six weeks, the BMR has decreased to -30 per cent, and manifestations of frank hypothyroidism are present; by three months, full-blown myxedema is usually evident.

The early symptoms of hypothyroidism are variable and nonspecific. Tiredness and lethargy are very common and lead to difficulty in performing a full day's work. Constipation may either develop or, if already present, become worse. Sensitivity to cold may be an early manifestation; its presence is often suggested by the use of more blankets on the bed or a preference for warm weather. Women may complain of menstrual disturbance, especially menorrhagia, or difficulty in conceiving because of anovulatory cycles. Loss of libido occasionally occurs in both men and women (Table 4-9). At this stage of the disease, the BMR is moderately decreased. With progression of the disease, the BMR falls to its minimum value, usually between -35 and -45 per cent, but the clinical picture continues to evolve slowly. Drowsiness and slowing of intellectual and motor activity appear. The patient becomes apathetic and listless and loses interest in his work and environment. Women frequently complain of hair loss, brittle nails, and dry skin. Despite a reduction in appetite, modest weight gain often occurs. The voice becomes husky, which may be attributed to laryngitis. Periorbital puffiness may be noticed by the patient or his family (Figs. 4-30 and 4-31). Mucus collects in the eyes, and the lids are often stuck together when the patient awakens in the morning. Stiffness and aching of muscles are sometimes prominent symptoms and may be attributed to "rheumatism." Numbness and tingling of the fingers may occur. Progressive deafness may lead the patient to seek medical advice. Eventually, the picture of full-blown myxedema results, with thickened features, enlarged tongue, hoarseness, nonpitting edema, and extreme mental and physical lethargy. Mild

TABLE 4-9. SYMPTOMATOLOGY OF MYXEDEMA
(77 Cases: 64 Women, 13 Men)

Symptom	Per Cent of Cases	Symptom	Per Cent of Cases
Weakness	99	Constipation	61
Dry skin	97	Gain in weight	59
Coarse skin	97	Loss of hair	57
Lethargy	91	Pallor of lips	57
Slow speech	91	Dyspnea	55
Edema of eyelids	90	Peripheral edema	55
Sensation of cold	89	Hoarseness or aphonia	52
Decreased sweating	89	Anorexia	45
Cold skin	83	Nervousness	35
Thick tongue	82	Menorrhagia	32
Edema of face	79	Palpitation	31
Coarseness of hair	76	Deafness	30
Pallor of skin	67	Precordial pain	25
Memory impairment	66		

After Means.

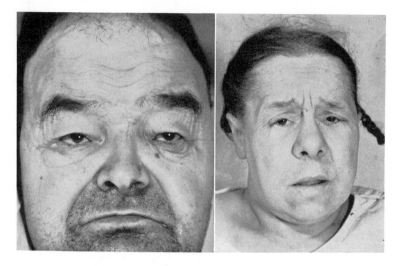

Figure 4–30. Typical facial appearance of myxedematous patients.

hypothermia may call the physician's attention to the diagnosis. Many of the structural and functional manifestations presented in the preceding section become evident, but occasionally those arising in a particular organ predominate. The patient, if untreated, may remain in this state for many years, finally passing into a state of myxedema coma or succumbing to an intercurrent infection or a vascular occlusion.

Infantile Hypothyroidism and Cretinism

Hypothyroidism is seldom apparent at birth. The age at which symptoms of hypothyroidism appear will depend upon the degree of impairment of thyroid function in the infant. Severe hypothyroidism beginning in infancy is termed cretinism. As the age of onset increases, the clinical picture of cretinism merges imperceptibly with that of juvenile hypothyroidism. Retardation of mental development and growth is the hallmark of cretinism. Since these changes only become manifest in later

infancy and are by then largely irreversible, early recognition of the hypothyroid state is crucial if eventual intellectual attainment and growth are to be normal. An early clue may be the abnormally long persistence of physiologic jaundice in the newborn. During the first few months of life, symptoms suggestive of hypothyroidism include feeding problems, failure to thrive, constipation, a hoarse cry, and somnolence. In succeeding months, especially in severe cases, protuberance of the abdomen, dry skin, poor growth of hair and nails, and delayed eruption of the deciduous teeth become evident. Retardation of mental and physical development is manifested by delay in reaching the normal milestones of development, such as holding up the head, sitting, walking, and talking.

Linear growth is severely impaired, resulting in dwarfism, with the limbs disproportionately short in relation to the trunk. Closure of the fontanelles is delayed, leading to a head that is large in relation to the body. The naso-orbital configuration of the infant is retained. Maldevelopment of the femoral epiphyses results in a waddling gait. The

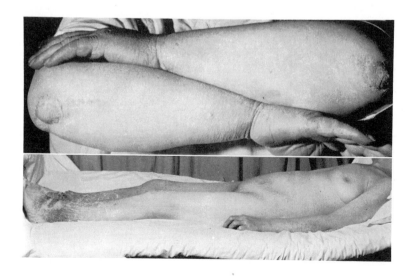

Figure 4–31. Dry, scaly skin with marked hyperkeratosis over the elbows and legs.

teeth are malformed and readily become carious. The appearance of the fully developed cretin is characteristic, with broad flat nose, widely set eyes, periorbital puffiness, large protruding tongue, sparse hair, rough skin, short neck, and protuberant abdomen with an umbilical hernia. Mental deficiency is always present and is usually severe.

Radiologic examination of the skeleton is diagnostic of cretinism. The skull shows a poorly developed base, delayed closure of the fontanelles, widely set orbits, and a short flat nasal bone. The pituitary fossa may be enlarged. Shedding of deciduous teeth and eruption of permanent teeth are delayed. A radiologic feature that is virtually pathognomonic of hypothyroidism in infancy and childhood is epiphysial dysgenesis (Wilkins, 1941). This abnormality may affect any center of endochondral ossification, depending on the age of onset of the hypothyroid state but is usually best seen in larger centers, such as the femoral and humeral heads and the navicular bone of the foot. The center of ossification appears late, with the result that bone age is retarded in relation to chronological age. When the center eventually appears, instead of a single center, multiple small centers are scattered through a misshapen epiphysis. These small centers of ossification eventually coalesce, forming a single center that has an irregular outline and a stippled appearance ("stippled epiphysis"). Epiphysial dysgenesis is evident only in centers that would normally undergo ossification at a time after the onset of the hypothyroidism. After a normal metabolic state has been restored by treatment, development of the centers destined to ossify at a later age proceeds normally.

Hypothyroidism beginning in childhood is termed juvenile hypothyroidism. The clinical manifestations of this state are intermediate between those of infantile and adult hypothyroidism, in that the developmental retardation is not as severe as that of cretinism and the manifestations of full-blown adult myxedema are rarely seen. Growth and sexual development are predominantly affected. Linear growth is severely retarded, resulting in dwarfism in which the limbs are disproportionately short in relation to the trunk. The rate of linear growth is characteristically less than that of weight gain. Maturation of the facial bones is impaired, so that the naso-orbital configuration of the infant or young child is retained. Eruption of permanent teeth is delayed. Sexual maturation is retarded, and the onset of puberty is delayed. The result is a child who appears much younger than his chronological age (Fig. 4–32). Rarely, precocious puberty and galactorrhea occur. Intellectual performance is distinctly poor, but the severe mental deficiency that characterizes cretinism is not found. The clinical manifestations of adult hypothyroidism are present to a varying, but usually milder, degree. On radiologic examination, epiphysial dysgenesis may be present, and epiphysial union is always delayed, resulting in a bone age that is retarded in relation to chronological age.

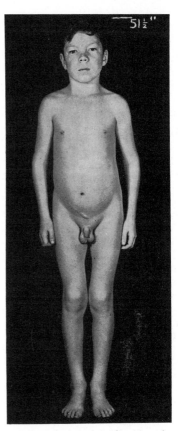

Figure 4–32. Juvenile hypothyroidism in a boy, aged 17. Dwarfism and delayed sexual development are apparent. Trunk is longer than legs. Appearance is youthful.

Laboratory Tests

A decrease in the concentration of circulating thyroid hormones is common to all forms of hypothyroidism and is evidenced by subnormal values for the serum T_4 and T_3 concentrations and usually the PBI. If abnormal iodinated materials are present in the serum, however, the PBI will be normal or increased. Alterations in the TH–plasma protein interaction reflect the decrease in hormone concentration as well as a slight increase in the binding capacity of TBG and frequently, but not invariably, result in a low value for the *in vitro* uptake test or the proportion of free T_4. The BMR is decreased in all forms of hypothyroidism. The serum TSH concentration, as measured by radioimmunoassay, is invariably increased in hypothyroidism of primary thyroidal origin and is hyper-responsive to TRH administration. By contrast, in pituitary hypothyroidism, serum TSH is not increased and does not respond to TRH administration. The serum cholesterol concentration is increased to values usually in excess of 300 mg./100 ml., but in pituitary hypothyroidism the values may be normal or even low. In cretinism, hypercholesterolemia may not appear until late infancy; as a result, a normal value for serum cholesterol during the first several months of life does not exclude the diagnosis. Other manifestations of the hypothyroid state include both increased serum concentrations of such enzymes as creatine phosphokinase, SGOT, and LDH, and an abnormally long Achilles reflex time, as assessed by kinemometry or photomotography. In infantile and juvenile hypothyroidism, the serum alkaline phosphatase concentration does not display the usual increase seen during the period of active growth.

The foregoing laboratory indices are common to all forms of hypothyroidism and reflect the inadequate secretion of thyroid hormones. Tests that employ I^{131} and assess the function of the thyroid gland per se display a variable pattern, depending upon the underlying thyroid disorder. When the amount of thyroid tissue is reduced (thyroprivic hypothyroidism), the thyroid I^{131} uptake is subnormal. However, the diagnostic value of this finding is minimized by the recent decline in the range of normal values that has resulted from the increase in dietary iodine intake. On the other hand, in disorders in which hypothyroidism results primarily from biochemical rather than anatomical failure and in which compensatory goitrogenesis usually occurs, the thyroid I^{131} uptake may be normal or increased. Specific functional patterns are discussed later in relation to the several causes of hypothyroidism. Laboratory tests that aid in differentiating between primary and pituitary hypothyroidism are discussed in the section dealing with the latter disorder.

Differential Diagnosis

The clinical picture of fully developed myxedema is usually characteristic enough to leave the diagnosis in little doubt. In its milder forms, hypothyroidism may require differentiation from several other states in which the appearance of the patient may be similar. The fact that these disorders, like hypothyroidism, tend to occur in elderly patients is partly responsible for any diagnostic uncertainty. In some elderly patients, slowing of mental and physical activity, dry skin, and loss of hair, especially from the lateral third of the eyebrows, may mimic similar findings in hypothyroidism. Furthermore, elderly patients often become hypothermic on exposure to cold. In elderly patients, the results of the conventional laboratory tests, such as the thyroid I^{131} uptake and serum T_4 concentration, are not significantly different from those in younger individuals, but the overall turnover of thyroid hormone is substantially decreased. The clinical features just described, therefore, may reflect a diminished flux of hormone to the tissues. In the patient with chronic renal insufficiency, anorexia, torpor, edema, periorbital puffiness, sallow complexion, and anemia may suggest hypothyroidism. In addition, decreased thyroid clearance of iodide secondary to renal retention may lead to a subnormal uptake of I^{131} when measured at 24 hours. However, retinopathy, azotemia, an abnormal urinalysis, and hypertension provide a clear differentiation between the two diseases. The dif-

ferentiation of nephrotic states from hypothyroidism is more difficult. Here, waxy pallor, edema, hypercholesterolemia, and hypometabolism may suggest hypothyroidism. In addition, a decrease in serum T_4 concentration results from both excretion of T_4-binding proteins in the urine and excessive losses of T_4 into the urine and possibly the feces. However, massive proteinuria and severe hypoproteinemia do not occur in hypothyroidism. Furthermore, in nephrotic states the thyroid I^{131} uptake is normal or increased, and indices of the TH–plasma protein interaction, such as the *in vitro* uptake test and the proportion of free T_4, indicate a decrease in overall hormone binding. In pernicious anemia, psychiatric abnormalities, a lemon-yellow tint of the skin, and numbness and tingling of the extremities may mimic similar findings in hypothyroidism. On the other hand, histamine-fast achlorhydria and mild macrocytosis in hypothyroidism may suggest pernicious anemia. Although there is a clinical and immunologic overlap between primary hypothyroidism and pernicious anemia, this association is not invariable, and when pernicious anemia occurs alone, it is not accompanied by specific clinical stigmata and laboratory evidence of thyroid hypofunction.

Mongolism (Down's syndrome) resembles cretinism in that it is accompanied by retardation of mental development and shortness of stature. The differentiation of these two diseases is not difficult and can usually be made on clinical grounds alone. The infant with mongolism is more active, lacks the dry skin of the cretin, and displays specific stigmata, such as obliquely set eyes, epicanthal folds, white flecks in the iris (Brushfield's spots), inward-curving fifth fingers, and abnormal palmar and plantar creases. In addition, analysis of the chromosomes usually reveals either trisomy-21 or 15/21 translocation. Epiphysial dysgenesis and laboratory evidence of thyroidal hypofunction are lacking in mongolism. Dwarfism resulting from cretinism or juvenile hypothyroidism differs from dwarfism of other causes, such as hypopituitarism, rickets, and achondroplasia, in that it is accompanied by mental retardation and other manifestations of hypothyroidism, retarded bone age, and epiphysial dysgenesis. Replacement therapy with thyroid hormone restores growth in hypothyroid dwarfism but is ineffective in dwarfism due to other causes. The dysgenesis of the femoral epiphysis seen in hypothyroidism resembles that of Legg-Perthes' disease, but evidence of thyroidal hypofunction is lacking in the latter disorder.

Thyroprivic Hypothyroidism

This section will deal with a variety of disorders characterized by loss or atrophy of thyroid tissue that results in decreased production of TH despite presumably maximum stimulation of the thyroid remnant by TSH. The disorders that fall into this category include primary hypothyroidism, the hypothyroid state that follows therapeutic ablation of the thyroid gland by surgery or radioiodine (postablative hypothyroidism), and sporadic athyreotic cretinism.

Primary Hypothyroidism

Although primary hypothyroidism is an uncommon disorder, it is by far the most common cause of hypothyroidism in the adult patient. It is several times more common in women than in men and occurs most often between the ages of 40 and 60. The cause is unknown.

The presence of circulating thyroid autoantibodies in up to 80 per cent of the patients as well as the clinical and immunologic overlap with presumed autoimmune diseases suggests, however, that it might represent the end-stage of an autoimmune thyroiditis in which goiter either was absent or had gone unnoticed. The functional state of "decreased thyroid reserve" represents, in all likelihood, a phase in the evolution of this disorder.

On histopathologic examination, the small thyroid remnant consists largely of fibrous tissue, with an occasional thyroid follicle and focus of lymphocytic infiltration.

The clinical manifestations and composite clinical picture of primary hypothyroidism were presented in an earlier section. In patients with this disorder, in contrast to the normal, the thyroid is usually impalpable, but occasionally a fibrous band may be felt in the region of the isthmus.

Typical laboratory indices discussed earlier include a low serum T_4 concentration and a high serum TSH concentration that is hyper-responsive to TRH administration. Values for the *in vitro* uptake test and the proportion of free T_4 are often subnormal but may be in the normal range. Thyroid autoantibodies are detectable in the serum in up to 80 per cent of the patients but may be absent in long-standing disease. The serum cholesterol concentration is usually increased.

Postablative Hypothyroidism

One type of postablative hypothyroidism is that which follows total or subtotal thyroidectomy. Although functioning remnants may be present, as indicated by foci of radioiodine accumulation, hypothyroidism invariably develops after total thyroidectomy. This procedure, which is associated with a high incidence of recurrent laryngeal nerve palsy and postoperative hypoparathyroidism, was formerly employed in the management of intractable angina pectoris, but it has been supplanted by radioiodine. It is sometimes performed in patients with thyroid carcinoma. A high incidence of hypothyroidism follows subtotal resection of the goiter in Hashimoto's disease. Except for relief of obstruction or suspicion of carcinoma, surgery is not indicated in this disease.

By far the most common type of postoperative hypothyroidism is that which follows subtotal resection of the diffuse goiter in Graves' disease. Its incidence is determined by the amount of tissue removed and varies inversely with the incidence of recurrent hyperthyroidism. In addition, autoimmune destruction of the thyroid remnant may sometimes be a factor, since a correlation has been shown to exist between the presence of circulating thyroid autoantibodies in thyrotoxicosis and the development of hypothyroidism after surgery (Green and Wilson, 1964). Hypothyroidism often becomes manifest during the first year after surgery, but, as in the case of postradioiodine hypothyroidism, there also occurs a progressively rising incidence with time. A survey of the surgical literature indicates a modal incidence of about 10 per cent. However, since most patients who develop hypothyroidism seek medical rather than surgical advice, these figures may be an underestimation. In reports from clinics in which internists do the follow-up studies, the incidence may approach 30 per cent or more (Hershman, 1966; Nofal et al., 1966). In some patients, mild hypothyroidism appears during the early postoperative period and then goes into remission. In adults, therefore, it may be justified to withhold replacement therapy for one or two months, provided that close observation is maintained. In children, treatment should be instituted whenever hypothyroidism supervenes.

Hypothyroidism may follow destruction of thyroid tissue with radioiodine. Its incidence is determined in large part by the dose of radiation delivered to the thyroid, but it is also influenced by variations in individual susceptibility that are conditioned by other factors, including autoimmune phenomena (Green and Wilson, 1964). Recent reports indicate that the incidence of postradioiodine hypothyroidism increases progressively with time. Thus the data currently available indicate an incidence at 10 years of approximately 40 per cent, although values as high as 70 per cent have been reported. (See Dunn and Chapman, 1964, and Nofal et al., 1966, for data and references. See also the section on Graves' disease.)

The clinical manifestations and laboratory indices of postablative hypothyroidism are similar to those of primary hypothyroidism of comparable severity and duration. In addition to frank hypothyroidism, both surgical and radioiodine therapy may lead to the development of decreased thyroid reserve. Some patients with postablative reduction of the serum T_4 concentration to less than normal values are clinically eumetabolic, probably as a result of a compensatory increase in T_3 secretion and serum T_3 concentration.

Sporadic Nongoitrous (Athyreotic) Cretinism

If thyroid tissue is completely absent, severe hypothyroidism will appear soon after birth and, if untreated, will lead to cretinism. This is the most common variety of cretinism occurring in regions of iodine abundance. A developmental defect is generally held responsible for the congenital absence of thyroid tissue. Transplacental passage of maternal thyroid autoantibodies does not appear to lead to autoimmune destruction of the fetal thyroid gland (Parker and Beierwaltes, 1961).

Hypothyroidism, usually beginning later in infancy or childhood, may be associated with failure of the thyroid gland to descend properly during embryologic development. Thyroid tissue may then be found anywhere along its route of descent from the foramen cecum at the junction of the anterior two-thirds and posterior third of the tongue (lingual thyroid) to the normal site or below. As part of the developmental defects, the ectopic thyroid tissue may fail to attain a size sufficient to meet the hormonal demands of the growing child.

The laboratory indices are similar to those of other forms of thyroprivic hypothyroidism. External scintiscanning after the administration of radioiodine or Tc^{99m}-pertechnetate may be used to reveal or confirm the location of ectopic thyroid tissue and to demonstrate the absence of functioning thyroid tissue from its normal location.

Trophoprivic Hypothyroidism

A thorough discussion of the evolution and clinical picture of pituitary insufficiency is presented in Chapter 2. This section will deal mainly with the features that may serve to differentiate hypothyroidism of primary thyroidal origin from that arising from disease in higher centers. When the intrinsically normal thyroid gland is deprived of TSH stimulation as a result of hypothalamic or pituitary disease, partial atrophy of the thyroid and decreased production of TH occur. In most cases, the hyposecretion of TSH is accompanied by decreased secretion of other pituitary hormones, with the result that evidence of gonadal and adrenocortical insufficiency is also present. Instances in which hyposecretion of TSH is the sole demonstrable abnormality (unitropic deficiency) are quite rare. Hypothyroidism resulting from pituitary insufficiency varies widely in severity, from instances in which it is mild and overshadowed by features of gonadal and adrenocortical failure to instances in which the features of the hypothyroid state are the predominant manifestations.

The differentiation of pituitary from thyroprivic hypothyroidism is important because, in the former, treatment with TH alone fails to correct the associated endocrine abnormalities and, indeed, by precipitating acute adrenocortical insufficiency, may be dangerous. Three major aspects serve to differentiate pituitary from thyroprivic hypothyroidism: (1) features arising from the cause of the pituitary insufficiency itself; (2) differences in the clinical manifestations; and (3) differences in the laboratory indices.

In most cases, pituitary hypothyroidism results either from postpartal pituitary necrosis (Sheehan's syndrome) or from tumors of the pituitary or adjacent structures. The tumors most commonly responsible are chromophobe adenomas of the pituitary or craniopharyngiomas (suprasellar cysts).

Postpartal pituitary necrosis is strongly suggested by a history of bleeding or shock after delivery necessitating blood transfusion, followed by deficient lactation, persistent amenorrhea, and loss of libido and of pubic and axillary hair. Symptoms of hypothyroidism may appear rapidly, in contrast to their usual slow evolution in thyroprivic hypothyroidism. Although these are the usual manifestations of Sheehan's syndrome, many years may elapse before symptoms of pituitary insufficiency appear. The presence of a tumor in the region of the pituitary is suggested by headache, especially if retro-orbital in location, by visual field defects, and by enlargement of the pituitary fossa. Intracranial pressure may be increased, and diverse neurologic manifestations may occur if the tumor extends widely beyond the pituitary fossa. Radiologic examination of the skull usually reveals enlargement of the pituitary fossa and erosion of the clinoid processes. A craniopharyngioma is strongly suggested by suprasellar calcification. Cerebral angiograms may aid in the demonstration of a tumor or of an aneurysm of the internal carotid artery, which in rare instances may cause pituitary insufficiency.

The clinical manifestations of pituitary hypothyroidism tend to differ in certain respects from those of thyroprivic hypothyroidism. Although the skin is pale and cool, it tends to be thinner and finely wrinkled, and myxedematous infiltration of the tissues is less prominent than in thyroprivic hypothyroidism. Depigmentation of areas that are normally pigmented, such as the areolae, frequently occurs. The texture of the hair is finer than that in thyroprivic hypothyroidism. Enlargement of the tongue, which is a striking feature of thyroprivic hypothyroidism, is less prominent in pituitary hypothyroidism. Other differentiating features of pituitary insufficiency may result from inadequate secretion of other pituitary hormones, notably gonadotropins and corticotropin. In women of premenopausal age, amenorrhea rather than menorrhagia occurs, and the breasts are atrophic. As regards manifestations of adrenocortical hypofunction, some similarities may exist. Loss of axillary and pubic hair is common in women with either disease. In pituitary hypothyroidism, however, the heart is usually small, and the blood pressure is low. Furthermore, manifestations of hypoglycemia are not uncommon in pituitary hypothyroidism but are rare in thyroprivic hypothyroidism.

Very often, when the foregoing features are inconclusive, differentiation of pituitary from thyroprivic hypothyroidism will depend upon the results of laboratory tests. Indices of thyroid function tend to differ in the extent to which they are abnormal. In pituitary insufficiency, the serum T_4 concentration is usually not as low as in thyroprivic hypothyroidism, values at or near the lower limit of the normal range commonly being found. The same is true of the thyroid I^{131} uptake, but for reasons discussed earlier the test has little diagnostic value except as part of the TSH-stimulation test. The serum cholesterol concentration, which is usually increased in thyroprivic hypothyroidism, is low in pituitary hypothyroidism. Although the BMR is usually not as low in pituitary hypothyroidism as it is in thyroprivic hypothyroidism, it is often lower than the clinical state would suggest, owing to the associated deficiency of cortisol. In difficult cases, the demonstration of circulating thyroid autoantibodies may provide a rapid means of differentiating these disorders, since even low titers are rarely found in hypothyroidism of pituitary origin.

Measurement of serum TSH concentration by radioimmunoassay provides the most direct means of differentiating between pituitary and thyroprivic hypothyroidism. In pituitary hypothyroidism, serum TSH is usually undetectable but always within the normal range, whereas in thyroprivic hypothyroidism, the serum TSH concentration is invariably increased, often greatly so (Mayberry et al., 1971; Hershman and Pittman, 1971; Utiger, 1971) (Fig. 4–16). In addition, measurements of serum TSH concentration in conjunction with the administration of TRH now permit the differentiation of hypothyroidism of pituitary origin from that of hypothalamic origin (Fig. 4–17). In the latter but not the former variety, serum TSH should increase in response to TRH, and several such cases of hypothalamic hypothyroidism have recently been reported (Kaplan et al., 1972). In the event that radioimmunoassay of TSH is not available, the TSH-stimulation test provides the next direct means of differentiating pituitary and thyroprivic hypothyroidism. Since a thyroid long deprived of TSH stimulation may not respond to a single dose of exogenous TSH, the three-day test should be employed. The procedure for the performance of this test and the occasional adverse reactions that accompany it are outlined in the section dealing with laboratory tests. In pituitary (but not thyroprivic) hypothyroidism, the administration of TSH usually increases the thyroid I^{131} uptake and sometimes the serum T_4 concentration. Occasionally, in long-standing pituitary hypothyroidism, loss of responsiveness to exogenous TSH may occur and may lead to an erroneous diagnosis of thyroprivic hypothyroidism (Taunton et al., 1965).

Measurement of the urinary excretion or plasma concentration of gonadotropins can provide a means of differentiating pituitary from thyroprivic hypothyroidism. In postmenopausal women with thyroprivic hypothyroidism, the values may be somewhat lower than those found normally at the same age, but they remain, nevertheless, distinctly elevated. In women of premenopausal age, the values are less discriminatory, since they are normally much lower. In pituitary hypothyroidism, gonadotropins are usually absent from the plasma or urine.

Tests of the pituitary-adrenal axis are generally less useful. Although values for the basal 24-hour urinary excretion of 17-OHCS and 17-KS are characteristically reduced in hypopituitarism, subnormal values are also usually encountered in thyroprivic hypothyroidism. The latter results, at least in large part, from decreased metabolic disposal of cortisol, with the result that the plasma cortisol concentration is usually normal despite a decreased rate of cortisol secretion. In pituitary hypothyroidism, the plasma cortisol concentration is usually low. Further evidence may be obtained by assessing the response of the urinary 17-OHCS to metyrapone. In thyroprivic hypothyroidism, the response is usually normal, the maximum increase in 17-OHCS occurring on the day after the administration of metyrapone. In some cases of thyroprivic hypothyroidism, however, the response is either subnormal or delayed, the maximum increase in 17-OHCS occurring two or three days after the administration of metyrapone (Kaplan, 1965). By contrast, in pituitary hypothyroidism, the response to metyrapone is usually subnormal, reflecting the diminished reserve of corticotropin.

In pituitary insufficiency, the increase in plasma GH concentration that normally occurs in response to insulin-induced hypoglycemia either is blunted or fails to occur. Subnormal responses are also usually seen in thyroprivic hypothyroidism, and hence this test does not provide a useful means of differentiating between these two varieties of hypothyroidism.

Goitrous Hypothyroidism

This section will deal with a variety of disorders characterized by a relatively or absolutely impaired ability to synthesize thyroid hormone, either because of some extrinsic factor or because of an intrinsic, usually heritable, defect in hormone biosynthesis. Inadequate synthesis of hormone leads to hypersecretion of TSH, which in turn produces both goiter and stimulation of all steps in hormone biosynthesis capable of response. This compensatory response may be inadequate, and goiter with hypothyroidism or cretinism results. In many instances, however, the compensatory response overcomes the impairment in hormone biosynthesis, and the patient is eumetabolic but goitrous. The latter condition, termed simple or nontoxic goiter, will be discussed in a later section.

Endemic Goiter

The term endemic goiter denotes any goiter occurring in a region where goiter is prevalent. Classically, endemic goiter occurs in areas of environmental iodine deficiency and has been ascribed to this pathogenic factor; however, as will be indicated, other factors may also be operative. Endemic goiter is most prevalent in mountainous areas, such as the Alps, Himalayas, and Andes, but may also occur in nonmountainous regions. In the United States, goiter was formerly common in the region around the Great Lakes, but here as in other areas of endemic disease, its incidence has been greatly reduced by the use of iodized salt. The belief that iodine deficiency plays a major role in the genesis of endemic goiter is supported by an inverse correlation between the iodine content of soil and water and the incidence of goiter, the kinetics of iodine metabolism in patients with this disorder, and a decrease in incidence with iodine prophylaxis. On the other hand, both the isolated geographic locale and the cultural patterns of some populations in areas of severe endemic incidence favor inbreeding, with the result that genetically determined abnormalities in hormonal biosynthesis may also play a role. The frequent occurrence of deaf-mutism, mental retardation, and motor defects in the populations of such areas also support this view. Furthermore, severe iodine deficiency and its associated abnormalities in the kinetics of iodine metabolism may occur in the absence of goiter. Endemic goiter may display a spotty incidence, even within an area of known iodine deficiency; the role of dietary minerals or naturally occurring goitrogens and of pollution of water supplies has been questioned in instances of this type. Indeed, in the Cauca valley of Colombia, water-borne goitrogens have been implicated (Wahner et al., 1971), and in Idjwi Island, Republic of the Congo, a dietary goitrogen may be involved (DeLange et al., 1972b).

A variety of abnormalities in iodine metabolism occur in patients with endemic goiter. The majority are consistent with the expected effects of iodine deficiency. Others, such as those indicating the existence of heterogeneous pools of thyroidal iodine and the secretion of butanol-insoluble iodinated products, are probably mere exaggerations of processes occurring in the normal gland but made more prominent by prolonged hyperfunction. To date, no abnormality clearly due to a primary defect in iodine metabolism has been described in endemic goiter. Thyroid iodide clearance rates and I^{131} uptakes are increased inversely with the decrease in urinary stable iodine excretion. The absolute iodine uptake is normal or low. The thyroid hyperfunction can be suppressed by exogenous hormone, indicating that it represents a homeostatic compensatory response. In areas of only moderate iodine deficiency, the serum T_4 concentration is usually in the lower range of normal; in areas of severe endemia, however, the values may be distinctly decreased. Nevertheless, most patients in these areas do not appear to be clinically hypothyroid, a discrepancy that is due to an increase in the synthesis of the calorigenically more efficient hormone, T_3, at the expense of T_4 (DeLange et al., 1972a).

The severity of goiter is not uniform among all inhabitants of an area of endemic incidence. As a group, goitrous inhabitants display lower serum T_4 concentrations and higher serum TSH concentrations than do nongoitrous inhabitants, indicating a less efficient adaptation to the iodine deficiency, but what underlies this difference in adaptive response is unclear. (For a discussion of the functional abnormalities in endemic goiter and references to earlier work, see DeLange et al., 1971 and 1972a, b).

The gross and histopathologic appearance of endemic goiter depends upon the duration of the goiter and the severity of the pathogenetic insult.

In the initial stages, the stimulus of iodine deficiency leads to hypertrophy and hyperplasia of the epithelial cells lining the follicles. The cells increase in height and number and may protrude into the follicular lumen, forming papillary projections. The amount of colloid in the follicles decreases. The hyperplasia is accompanied by an increase in vascularity. This is the diffuse hyperplastic goiter that is usually seen in children in endemic areas. If the iodine intake is increased, the hypertrophy and hyperplasia of the epithelial cells disappear, and colloid reaccumulates in the follicles. This process of involution leads to a return of the gland to normal size if the hyperplasia is of relatively short duration but probably results in a diffuse colloid goiter if the hyperplastic phase has been present for years. In long-standing goiter, repeated cycles of hyperplasia and involution eventually lead to the formation of nodules of involuted tissue surrounded by more hyperplastic tissue, and a multinodular goiter results. Localized hyperplasia with the formation of encapsulated adenomas (adenomatous hyperplasia) is a less common cause of nodularity in endemic goiter; it may be difficult to distinguish this lesion from true neoplasia. Nodules often undergo hemorrhagic or cystic degeneration and may become calcified or ossified.

The incidence and severity of endemic goiter, as well as the metabolic state of the goitrous patient, depend mainly on the degree of iodine deficiency. In the absence of hypothyroidism, the effects of the goiter are mainly disfiguring. When the goiter has become nodular, however, hemorrhage into a nodule may cause acute pain and swelling, mimicking subacute thyroiditis or neoplasia. Occasionally, a goiter may cause symptoms by compressing adjacent structures, such as the trachea, esophagus, and recurrent laryngeal nerves.

The development of hyperthyroidism is unusual in patients with endemic goiter. This is in contrast to the tendency of multinodular goiter in nonendemic regions to produce hyperthyroidism in later life. It seems likely that iodine deficiency protects some patients with endemic goiter from developing hyperthyroidism. The incidence of thyrotoxicosis in an endemic goiter region has been reported to increase following the introduction of measures to increase iodine intake (Connolly et al., 1970). The induction by iodine of hyperthyroidism in a patient with endemic goiter is known as the jod-Basedow phenomenon. The incidence of thyroid carcinoma in endemic goiter is probably not increased; the suggestion that it may be increased seems largely due to the difficulty in distinguishing adenomatous hyperplasia from true neoplasia.

The incidence of endemic goiter has been greatly reduced in many areas by the introduction of iodized salt. In the United States, table salt is enriched with KI to a concentration of 0.01 per cent, which, if the intake of salt is normal, would provide an iodine intake of approximately 500 μg. daily, which is considered to represent the desired amount in an adult (Oddie et al., 1970a). In areas where the salt is crude and moist, iodine added as potassium iodide may be lost by sublimation; in this instance, potassium iodate is preferable since it is more stable. In primitive communities, an annual injection of iodized oil is an effective means of administering iodine.

The administration of iodine has little if any effect on a colloid or multinodular goiter, but it will cause the early hyperplastic goiter to regress. Similarly, TH usually has no effect on goiters of long standing or on established mental or skeletal changes, but it should be given in full replacement doses if there is evidence of hypothyroidism; this is of paramount importance in pregnant women. Surgical treatment is indicated if the adjacent structures are compressed or if the goiter is either very large or enlarging rapidly.

Endemic Cretinism

Endemic cretinism is a specific developmental disorder that occurs in regions of severe endemic goiter. Both parents of an endemic cretin are usually goitrous. In addition to the classic features of cretinism described earlier, endemic cretins often display deaf-mutism and impairment of motor function. These may be hereditary, but it is thought by some that they result from a severely deficient supply of maternal TH in early fetal life before fetal thyroid function begins. The retardation of skeletal development is due largely to postnatal hypothyroidism. Consequently, defective mental and neurologic development may occur without dwarfism if severe deficiency of TH is largely restricted to early fetal life (Choufoer et al., 1965).

Goiter is commonly absent in endemic cretinism, and at necropsy the thyroid is frequently atrophic. This has been ascribed either to exhaustion atrophy, resulting from continuous overstimulation, or to pituitary failure. Neither explanation seems wholly satisfactory.

The role of iodine deficiency and hypothyroidism in the pathogenesis of endemic cretinism has been questioned on the grounds that some endemic cretins do not display evidence of hypothyroidism. However, absence of hypothyroidism at the time of testing does not exclude severe deficiency of TH in fetal or early postnatal life when the availability of iodine may have been much reduced.

Goiter Due to Antithyroid Agents

The ingestion of compounds with antithyroid potency is an occasional cause of goiter with or without hypothyroidism. Apart from the agents commonly used in the treatment of thyrotoxicosis, antithyroid agents may be encountered either as drugs used in the treatment of disorders unrelated to the thyroid gland or as agents occurring naturally in foodstuffs. Drugs that have occasionally been reported to produce goitrous hypothyroidism include para-aminosalicylic acid, phenylbutazone, cobalt, and topically applied resorcinol. Like the commonly used antithyroid agents, these drugs exert their effect by interfering with both the organic binding of iodine and the later steps in hormone biosynthesis. Antithyroid agents readily cross the placenta and are excreted in breast milk. Consequently, administration of an antithyroid agent to a pregnant or lactating woman for the treatment of thyrotoxicosis may lead to goitrous hypothyroidism in the infant. The goiter and hypothyroidism in the infant are usually self-limited, disappearing soon after birth or after the child is weaned. Occasionally, however, a large neonatal goiter may cause respiratory distress and death from asphyxia.

Antithyroid agents, whose chemical nature has been discussed in an earlier section, occur naturally in certain plants, particularly those of the family Cruciferae. Some of these are eaten by man; among them, rutabaga and white turnip appear to be richest in goitrogen. It is uncertain, however, whether goitrogenic quantities of such foods are ever directly ingested. Rather, such foods may accentuate the effects of dietary iodine deficiency. In addition, it has been suggested that when cows are allowed to graze in pastures contaminated with cruciferous weeds, the transmission of the goitrogen in milk may cause goiter in children. (For more extensive discussions, see reviews by Clements, 1960, and Greer et al., 1964.)

Although soybean is not an antithyroid agent, soybean products in feeding formulas formerly led to goiter in children by enhancing fecal loss of hormone which, together with the low iodine content of soybean products, produced a state of iodine deficiency (Pinchera et al., 1965). Feeding formulas containing soybean products are now enriched with iodine.

Only limited data concerning the effects of pharmacologic and dietary goitrogens on thyroid iodine metabolism in man are available. Subnormal values for the 24-hour thyroid I^{131} uptake may occur in patients being treated with para-aminosalicylic acid or resorcinol. Soybean goiter may be associated with an increased thyroid I^{131} uptake.

Both the goiter and the hypothyroidism usually subside after the antithyroid agent is withdrawn, but if continued administration of pharmacologic goitrogens is required, replacement therapy with TH will cause the disorder to regress.

Iodide Goiter and Hypothyroidism

In rare instances, goiter and hypothyroidism, either alone or in combination, are induced by the chronic administration of iodine in either organic or inorganic form. This is seen most commonly in patients with chronic respiratory disease, since these patients are often given potassium iodide as an expectorant. Iodide goiter develops in only a small proportion of patients given iodine. By contrast, it has been reported that the incidence of goiter may be as high as 30 per cent in asthmatic patients given iodopyrine, a compound of iodine and phenazone (Begg and Hall, 1963). This inordinately high incidence is due to a synergistic action of iodine upon the antithyroid effect of phenazone, which is itself a goitrogen (Pasternak et al., 1969). The development of iodide goiter has also been reported to follow the single administration of radiographic contrast media from which iodide is released slowly over a long period. Iodide goiter without hypothyroidism occurs endemically in Hokkaido, where seaweed is consumed in large quantity.

From the majority of reported cases, it appears that, except in instances associated with iodopyrine ingestion, iodide goiter occurs only when an underlying intrathyroidal defect is already present. The disorder affects women more commonly than men. Patients with Hashimoto's disease appear to be especially susceptible, as do patients with Graves' disease, particularly after treatment with radioiodine (Braverman et al., 1971). A defect in organic binding is demonstrable by the iodide-perchlorate discharge test after iodine has been withdrawn and the patient restored to a normal metabolic state. In some instances, the thyroid suppression test is abnormal. Of particular importance is the fact that goiter and often hypothyroidism commonly occur in newborn infants of women given iodine during pregnancy, and death from neonatal asphyxia has been reported (Fig. 4–33). In such cases, the mother is usually free of goiter. Owing to the effects on the fetus, pregnant women should

not be given large doses of iodine. It is not known whether iodide goiter in the newborn results from an inherent hypersensitivity of the fetal thyroid or from the fact that the placenta appears to concentrate iodide severalfold.

As was discussed in the section dealing with factors that influence TH economy, large doses of iodine induce an acute inhibition of organic binding that in the normal individual abates, despite continued iodine administration (acute Wolff-Chaikoff effect and escape). Iodide goiter appears to result from a more pronounced inhibition of organic binding and a failure of escape to occur. As a consequence of decreased hormone synthesis, iodide transport is enhanced, and since inhibition of organic binding is a function of the intrathyroidal concentration of iodide, a vicious circle is set in motion.

The disorder usually appears as a goiter with or without hypothyroidism; rarely, iodine may produce hypothyroidism unaccompanied by goiter. The disorder usually develops slowly. The thyroid is firm and diffusely enlarged, often greatly so. Histopathologic examination reveals hyperplasia that is often intense.

The laboratory indices in patients with iodide goiter are superficially confusing but in fact are entirely consistent with the physiopathology of this disorder. While iodine is being administered, the thyroid I^{131} uptake within the first few hours after its administration is often high, reflecting both the large size of the thyroid and the hyperactive iodide transport mechanism. Since organic binding is inhibited, however, inorganic I^{131} is not retained and the thyroid uptake at 24 hours is subnormal. The serum TSH concentration is increased, while the serum T_4 concentration is normal or subnormal, in accord with the metabolic state of the patient. The 24-hour urinary iodine excretion and the serum inorganic iodide concentration are greatly increased.

The disorder regresses after iodine is withdrawn. TH may be given in addition to hasten regression. (For more extensive discussions of iodide goiter and iodide myxedema, see Wolff, 1969, and Braverman et al., 1971).

Defects in Hormone Biosynthesis

Genetically determined defects in hormone biosynthesis are rare but fascinating causes of goitrous hypothyroidism. Since an extensive review of this topic is available, these defects will be considered only briefly here (Stanbury, 1972). Several members of a family are usually affected. In most instances, the defect appears to be transmitted as an autosomal recessive characteristic. Individuals who display goitrous hypothyroidism are presumably homozygous for the abnormal gene, whereas euthyroid relatives with slightly enlarged thyroids are presumably heterozygous. In the latter, appropriate functional testing may disclose a milder abnormality of the same biosynthetic step that is grossly defective in the homozygous individual. In

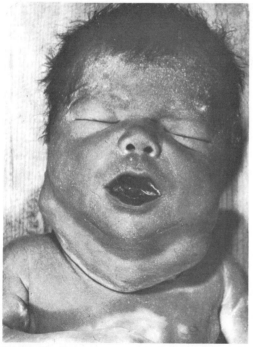

Figure 4–33. Large goiter in newborn which caused death by asphyxiation. The mother had received an iodine-containing medication for asthma during pregnancy. (From Galina, M. P., Avnet, N. L., et al.: *New Eng. J. Med.* 267:1124, 1962.)

contrast to nontoxic goiter, which is many times more common in females than in males, these defects as a group affect females only slightly more commonly than males.

It is important to realize that although goiter may be present at birth, it more commonly does not appear until several years later. Therefore, the absence of goiter in a child with functioning thyroid tissue does not necessarily exclude the presence of hypothyroidism. Initially, the goiter is diffusely hyperplastic, often intensely so, suggesting papillary carcinoma; eventually, it becomes nodular. In general, the more severe the biosynthetic defect, the earlier the goiter appears, the larger it is likely to be, and the greater is the likelihood of the early emergence of manifestations of hypothyroidism. In severe cases, cretinism commonly results (sporadic goitrous cretinism).

Five specific defects in hormone synthesis have been identified.

Iodide Transport Defect. This defect, which is exceptionally rare, is characterized by nonfunction of the iodide transport mechanism which is specifically reflected in a very low thyroid I^{131} uptake. Impaired iodide transport is also demonstrable in other tissues, such as salivary gland and gastric mucosa, that share a similar embryologic origin with the thyroid and normally also transport iodide actively. The administration of iodine, by raising the plasma concentration of inorganic iodide, will increase the intrathyroidal concentration of iodide sufficiently to permit the production of normal quantities of hormone and will thereby cause regression of both goiter and hypothyroidism.

Organic-Binding Defect. This defect is characterized by a relative or absolute inability of the thyroid to carry out organic iodinations. The resulting goiter and enhancement of iodide transport lead to a rapid thyroid accumulation of I^{131}, but this can be discharged almost completely by perchlorate. A milder form of this defect also occurs; when associated with nerve deafness, it is known as Pendred's syndrome. The deafness, which may either be present at birth or develop during early childhood, is not due to hypothyroidism per se, since most patients with this syndrome, though goitrous, are euthyroid.

Iodotyrosine Coupling Defect. In this defect, there appears to be an inability to couple iodotyrosines to form iodothyronines. The rate of thyroid accumulation of I^{131} is very rapid, approaching 100 per cent of the administered dose within the first two hours. Kinetic analysis reveals a very rapid turnover and recycling of thyroid iodine. Analysis of thyroid tissue in this disorder reveals little or no T_4 and T_3, most of the organic iodine being in the form of MIT and DIT. Of the several defects in hormone biosynthesis, this is the least well characterized, and indeed, some question has been raised whether the postulated abnormality truly exists.

Iodotyrosine Dehalogenase Defect. The pathogenesis of goiter and hypothyroidism in this defect is more complex than that in the other defects described. The major abnormality is an impairment of both intrathyroidal and peripheral deiodination of iodotyrosines, presumably because the enzyme is absent in these tissues. As a consequence of both intense thyroid stimulation and lack of intrathyroidal recycling of iodide derived from dehalogenation, I^{131} is rapidly accumulated by the thyroid gland and rapidly released; labeled MIT and DIT are found in the blood and, together with their deaminated derivatives, in the urine. Hypothyroidism is presumed to result from an intense stimulation of the thyroid release mechanism, leading to the release of large quantities of MIT and DIT, together with iodine deficiency secondary to the loss of these iodotyrosines in the urine. The goiter and hypothyroidism are relieved by the administration of large doses of iodine. The most specific test for the presence of this defect is the appearance in the urine of a large proportion of unchanged MIT or DIT after their systemic administration. A milder defect of similar type is seen in some patients with notoxic goiter and even in nongoitrous relatives of patients with the severe defect.

Abnormal Secretion of Iodoproteins. Release of abnormal iodinated proteins or polypeptides occurs in a variety of thyroid diseases, including Hashimoto's disease, benign adenomas, diffuse toxic goiter, thyroid carcinoma, and endemic goiter. In addition, release of similar compounds appears to be the sole or major physiopathologic abnormality leading to goiter with or without hypothyroidism. Goiter presumably develops because these calorigenically inactive compounds comprise a major proportion of the products of hormone biosynthesis. Reflecting the diversion of iodine into hormonally inactive iodoproteins, the thyroid I^{131} uptake is increased. Recent evidence suggests that a small quantity of similar iodoproteins is present in the serum of normal individuals. Hence the abnormality in the goitrous group appears to be quantitative rather than qualitative. In their physical properties, these compounds usually resemble serum albumin, but an iodoprotein resembling prealbumin has been described in some cases. A more extensive discussion of the nature of these iodoproteins and their relation to intrathyroidal proteins other than thyroglobulin appears in the section dealing with thyroid iodoproteins. Formation and release of these compounds are under the control of TSH, since exogenous TSH increases and exogenous TH decreases their concentration in serum. The severity of the defect ranges from that sufficient to cause frank cretinism to that only sufficient to cause nontoxic goiter in the adult. At least in some instances the disorder is familial, but the frequency with which this is the case has not been established.

In all the biosynthetic defects, the serum T_4 concentration is decreased. Tests that assess the TH–plasma protein interaction and the metabolic indices will reflect the decreased concentration of hormone in the blood. In the disorder characterized by abnormal secretion of iodoproteins, the serum PBI overestimates the true concentration of hormone, resulting in an abnormally large PBI-T_4-iodine difference. The serum TSH concentration is increased.

In addition to the foregoing biosynthetic defects, congenital hypothyroidism has been reported to result from an apparent failure of the thyroid to respond to TSH (Stanbury, 1972) and from an apparent resistance of the peripheral tissues to thyroid hormones (Refetoff, 1970). In the former disorder, goiter is absent, and there is no response to exogenous TSH. In the latter disorder, serum T_4 and T_3 concentrations are increased, and there is no response to large doses of exogenous thyroid hormones.

Treatment of Hypothyroidism

Treatment in the Adult

Hypothyroidism in the adult is generally one of the most gratifying diseases to treat because of the ease and completeness with which it responds to the administration of TH. Treatment is carried out with one of two general types of preparation, either synthetic hormone or thyroprotein derived from animal thyroid glands. In the former category, sodium L-thyroxine (levothyroxine), sodium L-triiodothyronine (liothyronine), or a combination of the two (liotrix) have been employed. In the second category, thyroid extract, USP, is most commonly used. This preparation is a powder derived from dried, defatted thyroid glands that needs to be standardized only with respect to its organic iodine content (0.2 per cent). A preparation of purified porcine thyroglobulin is also available, and its biologic activity is standardized according to its ability to inhibit propylthiouracil-induced goiter in the rat. The British Pharmacopoeia prescribes that thyroid extract be standardized according to "thyroxine" iodine content, i.e., the content of iodinated materials precipitated from a hydrolysate of the extract at pH 3.5. Recent studies indicate that preparations of natural origin may vary considerably in regard to the proportion of total organic iodine present as T_4 and T_3, as well as the ratio between these hormones themselves. Consequently, wide variations in biologic potency may occur among different preparations or different batches of the same preparation, despite their conforming to prescribed standards (Mangieri and Lund, 1970).

Over the years, there has been a distinct trend away from the use of the natural preparations and towards the newer synthetic preparations, in view of their uniform potency and, as a result, their more predictable effects. More recently acquired information has had a major impact upon the choice among synthetic agents. It was formerly believed that therapy with levothyroxine required the administration of doses sufficient to yield serum T_4 concentrations above the normal range, since the metabolic contribution normally provided by T_3 was felt to be lacking. This was considered a disadvantage of levothyroxine therapy in that the metabolic state of the patient and the

serum T_4 concentration were thought to be partly dissociated. Indeed, liotrix was formulated with the intention of circumventing this difficulty. The recent demonstration that most of the T_3 in serum is derived from the metabolism of T_4 and, as a corollary, that serum T_3 concentrations are nearly normal in patients receiving replacement doses of T_4 has to a large extent eliminated the rationale both for the use of liotrix and for the maintenance of elevated serum T_4 concentrations when levothyroxine is employed. A recent study has demonstrated that disposal rates for T_4 and T_3 are considerably greater than normal when patients are given the maintenance dose of levothyroxine formerly prescribed, i.e., 300 μg. daily (Braverman et al., 1973). Other studies have shown in addition that serum TSH concentrations are brought into the normal range by doses as low as 200 μg. (Cotton et al., 1971). Such doses maintain serum T_4 concentrations that are above the mean but still within the normal range. Thus a major presumed disadvantage of levothyroxine therapy has been shown not to apply.

Several positive advantages attend the use of levothyroxine. First, in contrast to the patient treated with liothyronine, the patient treated with levothyroxine develops a substantial peripheral pool of T_4 that turns over more slowly than does T_3 and that, therefore, provides a buffer against lapses in the ingestion of medication. Second, this pool of T_4 acts as a continuous source, thereby maintaining a constant serum T_3 concentration. This is in contrast to the recurrent peaks in serum T_3 concentration that attend the administration of thyroid extract, liotrix, or liothyronine (Surks et al., 1972). Such peaks make assessment of the proper dosage through measurement of hormone concentration extremely difficult and, moreover, may have adverse effects, especially in the older patient or in the patient with cardiac disease. This consideration accords with the experience of Smith et al. (1970), who noted a higher incidence of adverse effects with a combined T_4-T_3 preparation. In view of the foregoing, the authors believe that levothyroxine is the agent of choice in the maintenance therapy of hypothyroidism. For those who, despite the foregoing, wish to use a preparation other than levothyroxine, the approximate therapeutic equivalence of these agents when administered orally should be noted: levothyroxine, 100 μg.; liothyronine, 25 μg.; liotrix, 1 unit; and thyroid extract, 1 grain.

When first diagnosed, hypothyroidism is usually of long standing and seldom requires prompt reversal. Consequently, although a few authorities may disagree, the consensus is that the restoration of a normal metabolic state should be undertaken gradually. The untreated patient with hypothyroidism is inordinately sensitive to small doses of TH. The initial daily dose, therefore, should not exceed 50 μg. of levothyroxine. Caution is of paramount importance in the hypothyroid patient with heart disease and in the patient with severe long-standing hypothyroidism, because overenthusiastic treatment may precipitate heart failure or myocardial infarction in the former, or may provoke relative adrenocortical insufficiency in the latter. In these instances, an initial daily dose of 12.5 or 25 μg. of levothyroxine is recommended. Thereafter, the daily dose is increased by increments of 25 or 50 μg. at two- to three-week intervals until a normal metabolic state is attained. The final maintenance dose required is that which maintains the serum T_4 concentration around 9 μg./100 ml. (approximately 200 μg. daily).

The interval between the initiation of treatment and the appearance of the first evidences of improvement depends upon the size of the dose given. An early clinical evidence of response is the occurrence of diuresis, and this is accompanied by loss of weight and some regression of puffiness. Even earlier, the serum Na^+ increases if hyponatremia was present initially. Thereafter, pulse rate and pulse pressure increase, appetite improves, and constipation may disappear. Psychomotor activity increases, and the delay in the deep tendon jerks disappears. Hoarseness abates slowly, and the changes in the skin and hair generally require several months to disappear.

It is not always easy to define the optimal maintenance dose of TH for the individual patient. The clinical state of the patient is generally the best means of determining when a satisfactory dose has been achieved. Nevertheless, even when the patient appears metabolically normal, a small increase in the dose may produce still further improvement without producing thyrotoxicity. Metabolic indices, such as the BMR and serum cholesterol, afford confirmation of the metabolic state of the patient. There is a tendency among physicians to rely too heavily upon the serum T_4 concentration as an indicator of the adequacy of treatment. It should be recalled that the normal range of the serum T_4 concentration is rather wide and in the individual patient will encompass rather wide variations in metabolic state. Within the limitations imposed by the type of thyroid preparation administered, the serum T_4 concentration should be employed as a confirmatory rather than as a primary indicator of the metabolic state.

Several other interesting features attend the treatment of hypothyroidism. In contrast to what might be expected, there is no evidence that the requisite maintenance dose of TH undergoes seasonal variation. In addition, patients with hypothyroidism display a great propensity to discontinue their medication when they are feeling better or when their supply of hormone is exhausted; this occurs even when the patient has been informed that treatment is required indefinitely. In this way, a single patient with myxedema may serve to familiarize successive groups of medical students with the features of this disease. A final feature of great interest is the fact that, in the usual patient with myxedema, manifestations of thyrotoxicosis are readily induced by doses of TH only slightly in excess of those that provide optimum maintenance. This is in contrast to the relatively large doses of hormone that are required to induce thyrotoxicosis in the usual normal individu-al. The factors underlying this difference are unknown.

Restoration of a normal metabolic state, although the specific objective in treating hypothyroidism, is sometimes accompanied by adverse effects. These include production or aggravation of angina pectoris, heart failure or, rarely, severe psychiatric disturbance. In such instances, the more general objective of therapy enunciated by Means should be sought, i.e., the maximum metabolic restoration consistent with the well-being of the patient.

Besides myxedema coma, which is discussed later, there are a few instances in which it seems mandatory to alleviate hypothyroidism rapidly. Inordinate sensitivity to CNS depressants and lack of sensitivity to pressor amines make the patient with hypothyroidism a very poor operative risk. In addition, such patients withstand acute infections poorly and may descend rapidly into myxedema coma as a result. Consequently, in these circumstances, rapid repletion of the peripheral hormone pool is necessary. This can be accomplished by a single intravenous dose of 500 μg. of levothyroxine (Holvey et al., 1964). Alternatively, by virtue of its rapid onset of action, liothyronine can be used if the patient is able to take medication by mouth, as an intravenous preparation is not available. This is administered orally in a dose of 25 μg. every 6 hours. With both agents, the initial effect is achieved within several hours and is evident as an increase in BMR and in the ECG as a restoration of the normal configuration of the ST segment and T wave. Oral therapy with levothyroxine is instituted as soon as possible, as outlined earlier. Because of the possibility that acute increases in metabolic rate will overtax existing pituitary-adrenocortical reserve, supplemental glucocorticoid should be administered. Finally, in view of the tendency of hypothyroid patients to retain water, vigorous hydration with hypotonic or isotonic fluids should be avoided.

When hypothyroidism results from the administration of iodine or drugs with antithyroid activity, withdrawal of the offending agent will usually suffice to relieve both the hypothyroidism and the accompanying goiter.

Treatment in the Infant and Child

In the cretin, the critical factor determining eventual intellectual attainment is the age at which adequate treatment with thyroid hormone was begun. In general, if severe hypothyroidism did not begin *in utero*, the chances of normal intellectual development are good if vigorous treatment is begun before the age of four months. By contrast, normal physical development may occur even when treatment is begun later in infancy with doses of TH that are inadequate for normal intellectual development. Thus, in assessing the response to treatment in infancy, it is essential that attention be paid to the ages at which the various milestones of development are attained. Because of its uniform potency, levothyroxine is the TH preparation of choice. On a unit weight basis, infants and children require larger doses than do adults. Kinetically, this is reflected in a more rapid fractional rate of turnover of T_4. Treatment is begun with a daily dose of 25 μg. of levothyroxine, and this is increased by increments of 25 μg. at one-week intervals, so that the infant will be receiving a daily dose of 100 μg. after 3–4 weeks. Thereafter, the daily dose of levothyroxine is increased slowly so as to maintain the serum T_4 concentration between 9 and 12 μg./100 ml.; however, if the clinical response is unsatisfactory, even larger doses are administered. In the infant, intellectual development is the crucial guide to the adequacy of the treatment; it is better to give too much than too little hormone. In the older child, the rate of skeletal growth and maturation and the time of dental eruption and sexual maturation are important guidelines in treatment. The maintenance dose of TH in the older child approximates that in the adult.

Special Aspects of Hypothyroidism

Mild Hypothyroidism, Metabolic Insufficiency, and Decreased Thyroid Reserve

The problem of mild hypothyroidism is one that has long vexed both the physician and the clinical physiologist. Until recently, it was uncertain that such a clinical state did in fact occur; this is now accepted. It is highly probable that the greatest proportion of TH therapy administered in the United States is used in treating what is thought to be mild rather than severe thyroid insufficiency. As will become evident, it is the authors' view that, in most instances, the disorders being treated are not truly thyroidal in origin or at least have not been conclusively shown to be so. From the evolution of hypothyroidism in patients with Hashimoto's disease or progressive thyroprivic hypothyroidism, the clinical picture resulting from clearly demonstrable but incomplete thyroid hormone deficiency can be derived. Symptoms include mild lassitude, fatigue, slight anemia, constipation, apathy, slight cold intolerance, menstrual irregularities, inability to conceive, dry skin, some loss of hair, and slight to moderate weight gain. These symptoms, however, are not pathognomonic of hypothyroidism since they also occur either singly or in varying combinations in other disorders of organic or psychogenic origin. With regard to the latter, they constitute the typical picture of the commonly ecounntered "tired housewife syndrome." Needless to say, similar symptoms are also encountered in single women or even in men.

Many patients with such complaints have been treated with thyroid hormones. Frequently, adequate laboratory documentation of TH deficiency is lacking, or at most, a moderately low BMR is de-

monstrable. The response to TH therapy is sometimes gratifying, at least initially, but often symptomatic improvement disappears after a time, unless the dose is increased. In this way, the total dosage progressively increases until the amounts given exceed those required for complete hormone replacement in frank myxedema. Eventually, even such large doses may fail to alleviate the symptoms. This alone suggests that the symptoms do not arise from deficiency of TH. Some patients report that omission of a single dose of TH results in a rapid emergence (often within hours) of the previous symptoms and that these are equally rapidly relieved by a single dose. These responses are inconsistent with the time of onset and duration of action of thyroid hormones.

As indicated earlier, patterns of thyroid dysfunction have not, by and large, been defined in the majority of patients with the foregoing clinical course. Efforts to do so have led to the suggestion that there may be a type of disturbance in TH economy in which the majority of laboratory function tests are normal. This suggested syndrome, about which much has been written, has been termed metabolic insufficiency or nonmyxedematous hypometabolism. Here, the foregoing symptoms are present to variable degrees. The BMR is by definition decreased (usually slightly to moderately), but evidence of thyroid hypofunction, as judged from the serum T_4 concentration or thyroid I^{131} uptake, is lacking. It was suggested that the underlying abnormality in such patients is an inability of the tissues to respond to T_4, either endogenous or exogenous, while responsiveness to T_3 is retained; hence treatment with T_3 was advocated. From the outset, it seemed unlikely that the majority of patients ascribed to this category could be suffering from such a defect, since one would have expected compensatory goitrogenesis and thyroid hyperfunction if supplies of hormone to the tissues were inadequate. Neither of these findings was present, however. Moreover, it has been shown in doubleblind studies that, in patients satisfying the criteria for the diagnosis of metabolic insufficiency, the symptomatic response to placebo is at least as good as that to T_3 (Levin, 1960; Sikkema, 1960). Hence there appears to be no reason at present to retain the concept of such a syndrome or to treat its supposed symptom complex with T_3. Studies of the rate of peripheral conversion of T_4 to T_3 in patients with the typical clinical picture will be required to ascertain whether such a syndrome exists.

Despite the foregoing, it is clear that true mild hypothyroidism does exist. In view of the relatively nonspecific way in which it is clinically manifest, it is mandatory that the diagnosis be adequately documented. This not only will avoid administration of intrinsically ineffective therapy but also will tend to prevent overlooking the true cause of the patient's symptoms. Hypothyroidism resulting from peripheral refractoriness to adequate amounts of hormone, if it exists at all, must be exceedingly rare. Hence mild hypothyroidism results from incomplete failure of TH production. This may lead to laboratory values that are at the lower limit of or still within the normal range. Often, only the BMR is slightly lowered, but the serum cholesterol concentration is occasionally increased. To the extent that production of TH is insufficient, the endogenous TSH mechanism must be activated and the serum TSH concentration increased, as is the serum T_3 concentration not infrequently. As a result, the degree of endogenous stimulation of the thyroid must be increased, and little, if any, further stimulation would follow the administration of exogenous TSH. Accordingly, an increased serum TSH concentration or a subnormal response to exogenous TSH will permit the diagnosis of mild hypothyroidism due to "decreased thyroid reserve" to be made on the basis of objective criteria. In practice, such patients usually have Hashimoto's disease or have had partial thyroid ablation by surgery or radioiodine. In the remaining instances, the patients may be presumed to be in an early stage of primary thyroprivic hypothyroidism. In such cases, the response to TH is as would be expected, in that the patients respond well to small doses and the response is maintained. Nevertheless, full replacement doses are usually given, because the underlying disorder is generally progressive.

Not infrequently, the physician is confronted with a patient in whom the diagnosis of hypothyroidism, often mild, has already been made, and the patient has been given replacement therapy. In this circumstance, it is impossible to determine from the clinical or laboratory findings whether TH replacement is truly required, since a normal thyroid would have been suppressed. Often, a strong indication that the patient is not truly hypothyroid can be obtained from the nature of his initial complaints or from peculiarities in the response to treatment, as already described. Documentation of true thyroid insufficiency can generally be achieved by two means. First, TH can be withdrawn and the functional state of the thyroid assessed some time later. When the thyroid is intrinsically normal, the I^{131} uptake returns within a few weeks to normal or elevated values; the serum T_4 concentration may be low for a time but will return to normal. The serum cholesterol remains essentially unchanged in contrast to the increase that occurs in true hypothyroidism. Although patients become psychologically dependent upon the medication and expect a return of symptoms when it is withdrawn, this can often be forestalled by firm reassurance to the contrary. Alternatively, TH therapy may be continued and the intrinsic functional capacity of the thyroid assessed with exogenous TSH, as has been described earlier. A brisk response suggests that no underlying thyroid disorder exists.

Myxedema Coma

Myxedema coma is the ultimate stage of severe long-standing hypothyroidism in which mental obtundation and physiologic retardation are profound. This state, which invariably affects the elderly patient, occurs most commonly during the winter months and is associated with a very high mortality rate. It is usually, but not always, accompanied by a subnormal temperature, values as low as 23.3° C. having been recorded. Since the ordinary clinical thermometer is graduated only to 32.4 or 34.5° C., and since a nurse may fail to shake down the mercury below 37° C., the true depth of the hypothermia may not be appreciated. The external manifestations of severe myxedema, as well as bradycardia and severe hypotension, are invariably present. The characteristic delay in the deep tendon jerks may be lacking since the patient is often areflexic. Epileptic fits may accompany the comatose state (Jellinek, 1962).

Although the pathogenesis of myxedema coma is not known, several factors predispose to its development. Prominent among these are exposure to cold, infection, trauma, and CNS depressants. Alveolar hypoventilation, leading to carbon dioxide retention and narcosis, and dilutional hyponatremia resembling that seen during inappropriate secretion of antidiuretic hormone are common accompaniments of myxedema coma and may contribute importantly to the clinical state.

From the foregoing, it appears that the diagnosis of myxedema coma should be obvious. Nevertheless, this is not the case. Elderly patients may resemble patients with myxedema, and after a brainstem infarction, they may be both comatose and hypothermic. In addition, hypothermia of any cause, most commonly exposure of the elderly to cold, may induce physiologic alterations suggestive of myxedema. The importance of this difficulty in diagnosing myxedema coma is that a delay in therapy greatly worsens the prognosis. Consequently, the diagnosis should be made on clinical grounds and therapy initiated without awaiting the results of confirmatory tests, such as the serum T_4 concentration.

The treatment of myxedema coma consists of the administration of TH and of attempts to correct the associated physiologic disturbances. Because of the exceedingly sluggish circulation and severe hypometabolism, absorption of therapeutic agents from the gut or from subcutaneous or intramuscular sites is unpredictable; hence, all medications should be administered intravenously if possible. TH is best given as a single intravenous dose of 500 μg. of levothyroxine (Holvey et al., 1964). This serves to rapidly replete the peripheral hormone pool and is often followed by some improvement within several hours. Hydrocortisone (100 mg. daily) should also be administered because of the likelihood of associated adrenocortical insufficiency, especially as the metabolic rate increases. Intravenous fluids should be administered cautiously because of the danger of water intoxication. Hypertonic saline and glucose may be required to alleviate severe dilutional hyponatremia and the occasional hypoglycemia. A critical element in therapy is support of respiratory function by means of assisted ventilation and controlled oxygen administration. External warming should be avoided since it may lead to vascular collapse, but further heat loss should be prevented. An increase in temperature is seen within 24 hours in response to levothyroxine. General measures applicable to the comatose patient, such as frequent turning, prevention of aspiration, and attention to fecal impaction and urinary retention, should be undertaken. Finally, the physician should be alert to the presence of coexisting disease, such as infection and cardiac or cerebrovascular disease. Ideally, the management of the patient with myxedema coma should be undertaken in an intensive care unit. As soon as the patient is able to take medication by mouth, treatment with oral levothyroxine should be instituted.

Although myxedema coma has carried a uniformly poor prognosis, survivals have been achieved with the therapeutic regimen outlined above. (See Royce, 1971, for an excellent review of myxedema coma.)

SIMPLE OR NONTOXIC GOITER: DIFFUSE AND MULTINODULAR

Simple or nontoxic goiter may be defined as any thyroid enlargement that is not associated with thyrotoxicosis or hypothyroidism and does not result from an inflammatory or neoplastic process. The term is usually restricted to that form which occurs sporadically, i.e., in nonendemic regions.

Pathogenesis and Physiopathology

It is generally agreed that nontoxic goiter represents a compensatory response to any of a variety of factors that impair the efficiency of the thyroid in manufacturing adequate quantities of hormone. It had been thought that when such factors are operative, hypersecretion of TSH results, leading to a stimulation of thyroid growth and an increase in the activity of processes concerned with hormone biosynthesis that are capable of response. As a consequence of the resulting increases in thyroid mass and unit functional activity, a normal rate of hormone secretion is restored, and the patient is eumetabolic but goitrous. Thus, this disorder differs only in degree from goitrous hypothyroidism and can be presumed to result from the same specific etiologic factors. These have been discussed in the previous section.

This concept of the pathogenesis of nontoxic goiter has been rendered tenuous, however, by the recent demonstration that neither the serum concentration nor the production rate of TSH is increased in patients with the established disorder (Beckers and Cornette, 1971). Nonetheless, some participatory role of TSH in the maintenance of goiter is indicated by the regression of goiter that sometimes follows the administration of suppressive doses of TH (thyroid hormone). Two possible mechanisms may serve to accommodate these seemingly divergent findings. Of these, the one having the greatest experimental support derives from the observation that in hypophysectomized

rats the response of thyroid weight to standard doses of TSH is augmented by prior thyroid iodine depletion (Bray, 1968). Hence, any factor that impairs normal iodine usage may lead to gradual development of goiter in response to normal concentrations of TSH. A second possibility is that the primary goitrogenic stimulus is no longer present at the time of study, and that the residual normal TSH concentration is responsible for the maintenance of, but not the initiation of, the goiter.

Owing to the fact that the functional disturbance is milder than in goitrous hypothyroidism, the role of some contributory factors is more clearly evident. Prominent among these is the striking female sex preponderance (7–9:1). By contrast, as might be expected, the role of heredity is less readily apparent, although it is evident in some families and in large statistical studies. Owing to its more subtle nature, the functional defect is more difficult to define, and vigorous efforts directed at its elucidation are not justified. Although mild degrees of iodine deficiency can be readily detected, this is rarely a cause of sporadic nontoxic goiter in most areas of the world. In some areas of the world, dietary goitrogens have been implicated (Clements, 1960; Greer et al., 1964); in the remainder, the precise etiology is obscure but presumably resides in biosynthetic defects within the thyroid. In this group, possibly the most common abnormality is the secretion of an abnormal iodoprotein (Greenspan et al., 1963). In addition, defective organic binding has been described in goitrous euthyroid patients, as in patients with Pendred's syndrome or their relatives. The frequency of abnormal coupling or deiodinative mechanisms as a cause of nontoxic goiter is unknown.

Histopathology

The histopathologic evolution of nontoxic goiter from its initial diffuse form to its late multinodular stage is similar to that described for endemic goiter in the preceding section (Fig. 4–34).

Clinical Picture

The clinical features of nontoxic goiter are those that result from thyroid enlargement. Most commonly, the effect either is merely disfiguring or is felt as a tightening of garments worn about the neck. With larger goiters, displacement or compression of the esophagus or trachea may occur, leading to dysphagia, a choking sensation, and inspiratory stridor. Narrowing of the thoracic inlet may compromise the venous return from the head, neck, and upper limbs sufficiently to produce venous engorgement. This obstruction is accentuated when the patient's arms are raised (Pemberton's sign); dizziness and even syncope may result. Compression of the recurrent laryngeal nerve leading to hoarseness suggests carcinoma rather than nontoxic goiter. Hemorrhage into a nodule or cyst produces acute, painful enlargement locally and, if

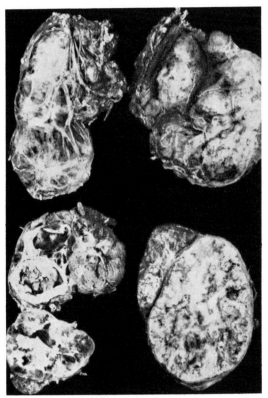

Figure 4–34. Outer and cut surface of a nontoxic nodular goiter observed by patient for 15 years. Note variations in size and structure of the nodules; there are thick areas of fibrous tissue, flecks of calcium, scattered areas of thyroid tissue, cysts, and small hemorrhages.

crucially situated, can enhance or induce obstructive symptoms.

Nontoxic goiter seems to occur more commonly during adolescence, pregnancy, and at the time of the menses. The pathogenetic relationship of these events to the development of goiter is unknown. In some patients, the goiter that appears at these times later regresses; in others, the goiter persists. Patients often have the impression that their thyroid enlarges during times of emotional stress or during the menses, but this is not well documented. During prolonged follow-up by the authors of a group of patients with nontoxic adolescent goiter, diffuse toxic goiter has supervened with an inordinately high frequency, in some cases even when suppressive doses of TH were being administered. This suggests that some varieties of nontoxic diffuse goiter may be precursors of Graves' disease. Thyrotoxicosis may also develop spontaneously as a complication of the late multinodular stage of the disease (toxic multinodular goiter: see section dealing with disorders that lead to thyrotoxicosis). In addition, thyrotoxicosis has been reported to develop in a high proportion of patients with apparent nontoxic goiter given large doses of stable iodine, even in an area of iodine sufficiency (Vagenakis et al., 1972). Although the pathogenesis of either the spontaneous or iodine-

induced thyrotoxicosis is unclear, it seems apparent that an underlying autonomy of function must be present in both.

Laboratory Tests

The most consistent group of tests in nontoxic goiter are the metabolic indices, which reflect a normal rate of hormone secretion. Other laboratory tests may diverge from those found in nongoitrous euthyroid patients in a manner that depends upon the presumed etiology of the goiter. In some patients, the thyroid I^{131} uptake is increased, presumably reflecting either mild iodine deficiency or the diversion of iodine into calorigenically inactive materials. Usually, however, the thyroid I^{131} uptake is normal. Most commonly, values for the serum T_4 and PBI concentrations are also normal, but the PBI may be increased if iodoproteins are released into the blood. Little is known as yet of the serum T_3 concentration in this disorder. Tests that assess the TH plasma protein interaction are almost invariably normal.

Differential Diagnosis

The differential diagnosis of nontoxic goiter can be considered from both functional and anatomical aspects. As indicated earlier, the disorder differs from goitrous hypothyroidism only in degree, and hence a functional spectrum ranging between frank hypothyroidism and euthyroidism would be expected. Some patients therefore may be marginally hypothyroid. On the other hand, the physiopathology of the goiter may be such as to lead some function tests, especially the thyroid I^{131} uptake and PBI, to display values similar to those found in hyperthyroidism. In nontoxic goiter, however, values for the serum T_4 concentration will be normal. Furthermore, in nontoxic goiter the I^{131} uptake will almost always be suppressible by exogenous TH.

From the anatomical standpoint, the diffuse stage of nontoxic goiter resembles most closely the thyroid of either Graves' disease or Hashimoto's disease. If the Graves' disease is not in an actively thyrotoxic phase and if the ocular manifestations are lacking, there is no way to differentiate the two disorders save for the possible presence of an abnormal thyroid suppression test in the patient with Graves' disease. Diffuse nontoxic goiter is sometimes difficult to differentiate from Hashimoto's disease. Functional patterns in the two may be quite similar. The thyroid of Hashimoto's disease is usually more firm, and its margins and surface are more irregular, but this is not invariably the case. Demonstration of high titers of thyroid autoantibodies or hypergammaglobulinemia is often of assistance, but biopsy of the thyroid may be required.

In its multinodular stage, nontoxic goiter may suggest the possibility of thyroid carcinoma. The approach to this differential diagnosis is discussed in the section dealing with thyroid neoplasms.

Treatment

Treatment of simple goiter is directed at removing the stimulus to thyroid hyperplasia. This can be accomplished either by alleviating an external restraint to hormone formation or by supplying sufficient quantities of exogenous hormone to inhibit secretion of TSH, thereby putting the thyroid at rest. In the occasional instance, withdrawal of a pharmacologic goitrogen will suffice. Since iodine deficiency is not a common causative factor, at least in the United States, administration of iodine is generally ineffective, and its use is to be deplored in view of its demonstrated ability to induce thyrotoxicosis. As the etiology of the goiter is usually obscure, suppressive therapy with thyroid hormone is the treatment of choice, since its action is independent of the origin of the goiter. Successful therapy requires that doses of hormone sufficient to produce a maximum state of thyroid inactivity be given. Levothyroxine is administered in a dose of 200–300 μg. daily. Adequacy of dosage is assessed by measurement of the thyroid I^{131} uptake. Lowering of the uptake indicates at least partial suppression, and values below 5 per cent complete suppression of endogenous thyroid function. The latter is the therapeutic objective and can usually be achieved without inducing thyrotoxicosis, especially if the suppressive dose is approached in gradual increments. In younger patients, the authors usually initiate treatment with 200 μg. of levothyroxine daily, checking the uptake at four-week intervals and increasing the daily dose by 50 μg. as needed. Doses greater than 300 μg. daily have not been required if function is destined to be suppressed at all. In older patients or in those suspected to have heart disease, the initial dose is smaller and is increased more gradually. If function cannot be completely suppressed, a scintiscan is indicated. This may reveal areas that have been suppressed intermingled with foci of presumed autonomous function. Having lost their dependency upon homeostatic restraints, these autonomous foci have the potential of eventually inducing thyrotoxicosis.

Considerable variation is present in the reported results of suppressive therapy. In some clinics very favorable results are obtained, complete regression having been reported in 33 per cent of diffuse and 24 per cent of multinodular nontoxic goiters. Partial regression was noted in 34 per cent of diffuse and over 50 per cent of multinodular goiters (Astwood et al., 1960). Unfortunately, the experience of the present authors and others has not been as favorable. The diffuse form generally responds well, particularly when cases with Hashimoto's disease are excluded. In the multinodular stage, there is most commonly some decrease in overall thyroid size and occasionally in the size of individual nodules. Generally, however, regression of thyroid enlargement leaves most nodules unchanged or more prominent than they were before. Hence in the authors' view, the rationale for thyroid therapy in multinodular nontoxic goiter is to prevent further extension rather than to cause reversion of the pathologic process. By decreasing vascularity, suppressive therapy may also reduce the risk of hemorrhage. Furthermore, when symptoms of pressure are present, even a small decrease in thyroid size may afford relief. It is not known whether suppressive therapy forestalls the subsequent development of hyperfunction leading to thyrotoxicity in the multinodular nontoxic gland.

It is impossible to predict whether, as is sometimes the case, regression of goiter will persist if suppression is withdrawn; few if any data concerning this point are available. If, however, recurrence takes place, suppressive therapy should be reinstituted and continued indefinitely.

Surgery of simple nontoxic goiter is physiologically unsound, since it further restricts the ability of the thyroid to meet hormone requirements. Nevertheless, surgery may become necessary because of persistence of obstructive symptoms despite a trial of exogenous TH. As discussed in the section dealing with thyroid neoplasms, surgery is sometimes indicated because a carcinoma is thought to be present in a multinodular goiter. It should never be performed for prophylaxis of carcinoma, however. In view of the physiopathology, surgery should always be followed by full replacement therapy with TH in order to inhibit regrowth of the goiter.

THYROID NEOPLASMS

The subject of thyroid neoplasms is one which has received attention far beyond its importance as a cause of morbidity in the general population. An important reason for this concern is the prevalence of thyroid nodules in the general population. This has been estimated to be as high as 4 per cent on the basis of palpatory findings (Sokal, 1959). The incidence of thyroid nodules is even higher at necropsy. In itself, this would not represent a problem, however, were it not for the fact that the nodule is a highly nonspecific mode of manifesting a variety of different diseases with differing implications concerning the patients' ultimate well-being. Most important in contributing to the voluminous literature bearing upon the problem of thyroid neoplasms is the inadequacy of current knowledge in this area. These inadequacies stem from the relative inability to distinguish the various diseases on clinical and sometimes histopathologic grounds, to ascertain with certainty their relative frequencies, and to achieve a general agreement on their ultimate prognosis and optimum treatment. It is perhaps ironic that the vast literature on thyroid nodules reflects not our great knowledge but our considerable ignorance of this area. The authors' approach to the diagnosis and management of the nodular thyroid gland will be presented at the end of this section. First, it is necessary to consider the characteristics of that variety of thyroid nodule which is of greatest concern, the thyroid neoplasm.

Benign Neoplasms

Benign neoplasms of the thyroid gland are termed adenomas. The problem of their intrinsic causation and the biologic properties that cause their behavior to differ from that of normal tissue, on the one hand, or that of malignant neoplasms, on the other, are unknown but represent basic questions in oncology. Nevertheless, adenomas have the properties of being well encapsulated, of not invading adjacent tissues or metastasizing to noncontiguous areas, of displaying few mitoses, and, in the case of endocrine adenomas, of being at least relatively free of the usual homeostatic restraints on growth and function. The most clearcut lesions of the thyroid that display these properties are those that arise in glands that are otherwise entirely normal. Much of the confusion concerning thyroid nodules arises from the fact that lesions that are anatomically similar or identical (differing architecturally from surrounding tissue and separated therefrom by fibrous tissue) are found in the late stage of nontoxic multinodular goiter. Because of this similarity, they are often termed adenomas, and the disorder itself is termed *adenomatous goiter.* In most instances, it is not known whether these are true adenomas in the basic biologic sense and whether they arise *de novo* or as a consequence of the hyperplastic stimulus that is thought to underly the pathogenesis of nontoxic goiter. Lacking such basic biologic criteria, the authors feel that the term adenoma, be it in a normal or an otherwise diseased gland, should be applied to lesions that display the anatomical properties just described, together with evidence of some degree of autonomy of growth and function. A further source of confusion, on the other hand, is the fact that, in the case of thyroid neoplasms, the architecture of benign and malignant lesions may be so similar that even careful histopathologic examination fails to reveal local evidence of malignancy, although the tumor displays evidence of malignancy by its clinical course. Finally, as is the case with neoplasms in other organs, it is uncertain whether benign neoplasms of the thyroid gland ever undergo malignant transformation.

The clearly defined benign neoplasms of the thyroid can be classified according to their histopathologic characteristics.

Histopathology (Fig. 4–35)

Embryonal Adenoma. Here, the histopathologic appearance resembles that of the embryonic thyroid prior to the development of follicles in that the cells are closely packed, forming a cordlike or trabecular pattern. For this reason, the lesion is sometimes termed a *trabecular adenoma.*

Fetal Adenoma. This lesion is characterized by an architecture that resembles the fetal thyroid in its stage of early follicle formation. The cells are arranged in a tubular pattern, but colloid is scant or absent.

Microfollicular Adenoma. This lesion is composed of small, closely packed follicles lined by a cuboidal epithelium and containing little colloid.

Macrofollicular Adenoma. Here well-formed follicles are present. These are usually large, well filled with colloid, and lined by a flat epithelium. Small follicles and areas of epithelial hyperplasia are often present. Another term applied to this lesion is *colloid adenoma.*

Papillary Cystadenoma. This lesion, although classified as an adenoma, is typically unencapsulated, merges into the adjacent tissue, and often cannot be distinguished on histopathologic grounds from low-grade papillary carcinoma. It is composed of columnar epithelium that is thrown into folds, forming papillary projections with connective tissue stalks and cystlike cavities. Follicular elements may be present to a varying degree.

Hürthle Cell Adenoma. This rare lesion is composed of large, pale, acidophilic cells that are usually arranged in a trabecular pattern.

The foregoing classification suggests that adenomas are uniform in structure, but in fact their architecture is often variegated; macrofillicular, microfollicular, and fetal elements are often found in the same lesion. In addition, multiple adenomas of differing histopathologic types are not infrequently present in the same gland, often in opposite lobes.

Clinical Picture and Laboratory Tests

The chief importance of thyroid adenomas lies in the need to differentiate them from carcinoma and in their ability in some instances to produce sufficient hormone to suppress the remaining thyroid tissue and induce a thyrotoxic state. The former problem is discussed later in this section in that part dealing with the management of the nodular thyroid gland, and the latter problem has been presented in the earlier section dealing with disorders that lead to thyrotoxicosis. However, some other features of thyroid adenomas merit consideration. The majority are predominantly follicular in type and are able to accumulate and retain radioactive iodine, a feature that aids in distinguishing them from most carcinomas. Functioning adenomas may retain their ability to respond to TSH but, as indicated earlier, are not dependent upon TSH for maintenance of their function. Such lesions tend to secrete abnormal iodoproteins that increase the serum PBI, causing the difference between the PBI and T_4-iodine concentration to widen. They are also prone to secrete T_3 in abnormally high proportion to T_4 and may be the source of T_3-toxicosis.

In general, adenomas grow slowly and produce no symptoms. When less than 1 cm. in diameter, they are generally not palpable, but as they become larger they are likely to be noted as a lump in the neck. Not infrequently, however, they are the site of local hemorrhage that leads to acute painful enlargement, mimicking subacute thyroiditis. Resolution of the hemorrhage is often followed by loss of function and by development of either a cyst

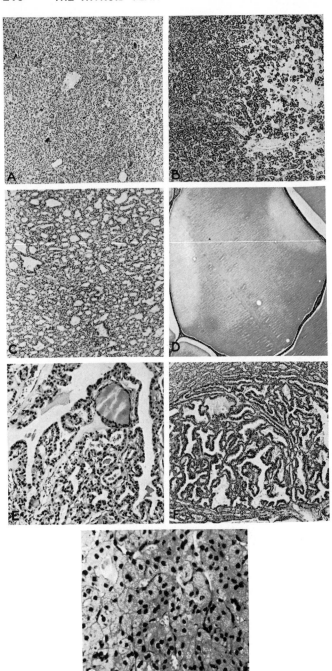

Figure 4–35. Thyroid adenomas. *A*, Embryonal (×80). *B*, Fetal (×80). *C*, Micro-follicular (×80). *D*, Macrofollicular (×60). *E* and *F*, Papillary cystadenomas (×40). *G*, Hürthle cell (×450).

or a nodule of very firm consistency that may be mistaken for carcinoma.

Malignant Neoplasms

Virtually all malignant neoplasms of the thyroid are epithelial in origin and hence are carcinomas. Of these, two general types occur, those arising from follicular epithelium and, less often, those arising from parafollicular (C-cell) elements.

Rarely, the thyroid is the seat of a metastatic deposit or of a fibrosarcoma or lymphosarcoma, both of which are highly malignant.

Carcinoma of Follicular Epithelium: Histopathology and Clinical Features

A variety of classifications have been proposed, but the one most commonly used is that of Woolner and associates (1961). This classification demar-

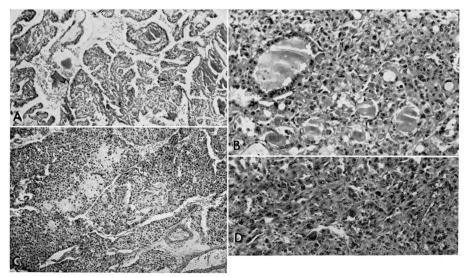

Figure 4-36. Thyroid carcinomas. *A*, Papillary carcinoma. *B*, Follicular carcinoma. *C*, Solid carcinoma with amyloid stroma. (From Hazard, J. B., Hawk, W. A., et al.: *J. Clin. Endocr. 19*:152, 1959.) *D*, Anaplastic carcinoma.

cates three categories of carcinoma of follicular origin: papillary, follicular, and anaplastic (Fig. 4-36). A fourth category, that of medullary carcinoma or solid carcinoma with amyloid stroma, is discussed separately because of its parafollicular origin and distinctive manifestations.

Papillary Carcinoma. In most series, thyroid carcinoma that is either purely or predominantly papillary in structure is by far the most common, accounting for about one-half of all thyroid carcinomas. Papillary carcinoma may occur at any age, but it is seen more frequently in children and young adults than are the other types of thyroid malignancy; almost one-half of the cases occur before the age of 40 (Fig. 4-37). Women are affected 2-3 times more commonly than men. Young patients with this disease sometimes give a history of having received x-ray therapy during childhood for cervical lymphadenitis or thymic enlargement, suggesting that radiation in the vicinity of the thyroid gland may play a pathogenetic role. In general, papillary carcinoma is the most slow-growing of all thyroid carcinomas, often remaining localized to the thyroid gland for many years. It tends to spread via the intraglandular lymphatics from its primary site to other parts of the thyroid and to the pericapsular and regional lymph nodes, where it may remain localized for years. Sometimes, the metastases in the cervical lymph nodes so overshadow the primary lesion that their true nature is overlooked. In the past, such lesions were thought to arise from the fourth pharyngeal pouch; these were called "lateral aberrant thyroids." Hematogenous spread to distant sites such as lung is uncommon. The growth of papillary carcinoma is thought by some to depend partly upon TSH stimulation; this view stems from the observation that the administration of suppressive doses of TH (thyroid hormone) sometimes leads to regression of metastases from a primary lesion that was predominantly papillary in type. It should be

noted, however, that most papillary carcinomas contain follicular elements, and the metastases may be composed predominantly of the latter. Papillary carcinoma has a tendency to become more malignant with advancing age; indeed, it has been suggested that the highly malignant anaplastic carcinomas do not arise *de novo* but develop from preexisting low-grade papillary or follicular

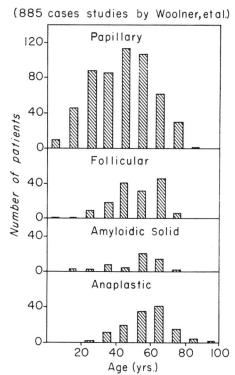

Figure 4-37. Age incidence of thyroid carcinoma of various types. (Taken from the data of Woolner, L. B., Beahrs, O. H., et al.: *Amer. J. Surg. 102*:354, 1961.)

carcinomas (Russell et al., 1963). The age of the patient appears to be more important than any other factor in determining the prognosis in papillary carcinoma (McKenzie, 1971).

Grossly, the carcinoma varies greatly in size and is usually unencapsulated. On histopathologic examination, it is composed of columnar epithelium that is thrown into folds, forming papillary projections with connective tissue stalks. There is frequently a mixed papillary and follicular pattern, the former predominating. Occasionally, there are foci of large cells with well-defined nuclei and pale, acidophilic cytoplasm (Hürthle cells). Concentrically layered deposits of calcium (psammoma bodies) are commonly found. There may be gross or microscopic foci of carcinoma in other parts of the gland, resulting from spread via the intraglandular lymphatics.

Clinically, papillary carcinoma usually appears either as an asymptomatic nodule in an otherwise normal thyroid or as an enlargement of the regional lymph nodes, sometimes without a palpable thyroid nodule. Invasion of adjacent structures and distant metastases are late manifestations.

Since papillary carcinoma accumulates iodine less efficiently than does the surrounding normal thyroid tissue, it will appear as a "cold" area in the thyroid scintiscan, provided that it is large enough to allow resolution by the scanner and is not surrounded by a large amount of functioning tissue (Fig. 4–18). Radiologic examination of the neck may disclose concentrically layered calcium in the psammoma bodies.

Follicular Carcinoma. In most series, thyroid carcinoma that is either purely or predominantly follicular in structure comprises about one-quarter of all thyroid carcinomas. It occurs in an older age group than papillary carcinoma, the majority of cases occurring after the age of 40 (Fig. 4–37). Women are affected 2–3 times more commonly than men. As in papillary carcinoma, there may be a history of radiotherapy to the neck area during infancy or childhood. Its degree of malignancy varies but generally exceeds that of papillary carcinoma. Follicular carcinoma seldom spreads to the regional lymph nodes, but invasion of blood vessels with hematogenous spread to distant sites, particularly bone, lung, and liver, often occurs relatively early. As is the case in primary papillary carcinoma, the metastases sometimes regress under the influence of suppressive doses of TH. Follicular carcinoma occasionally becomes more malignant with advancing age.

Grossly, follicular carcinoma varies in size and is typically encapsulated. The histopathologic appearance of the lesion varies from area to area. In some areas, it resembles normal thyroid tissue except that the follicles are smaller and contain subnormal amounts of colloid, while in other areas it is composed of solid sheets of cells. The cells exhibit mitoses to a varying degree. There may be foci of Hürthle cells; rarely, these are the predominant type of cell. In many follicular carcinomas, papillary elements are present to a varying degree. Invasion of blood vessels and adjacent thyroid parenchyma is often observed. The degree of invasiveness, which is greatest in the older age group of patients (McKenzie, 1971), largely determines the prognosis in follicular carcinoma. In minimally invasive lesions, a 10-year survival rate of 86 per cent has been reported, whereas the comparable figure for the more invasive variety is only 44 per cent (Woolner et al., 1961). The metastases may display either a follicular or a mixed follicular and papillary pattern. In some cases, the histologic appearance of a metastatic lesion so closely resembles that of normal thyroid tissue that the term benign metastasizing struma has been applied to this lesion.

The clinical features of follicular carcinoma differ in several respects from those of the usual case of papillary carcinoma. In some patients, a goiter has been present for many years. The carcinoma usually consists of a single nodule or mass that is stony hard in consistency; sometimes it involves one whole lobe. Pain and invasion of adjacent structures are late manifestations. The regional lymph nodes are seldom enlarged. Occasionally, either a pathologic fracture due to a metastatic deposit in bone or a pulmonary metastatic nodule is the major manifestation.

Follicular carcinoma differs from the other types of thyroid malignancy in that it may accumulate iodine almost as efficiently as does the surrounding normal tissue. The metastatic deposits also may accumulate iodine if they are composed predominantly of follicular elements. Rarely, function in the metastases may be sufficient to produce thyrotoxicosis, including T_3-toxicosis (Sung and Cavalieri, 1973).

Anaplastic Carcinoma. Anaplastic carcinoma comprises about 10 per cent of all thyroid carcinomas. It usually occurs after the age of 50 and is slightly more common in women. It is a highly malignant lesion, rapidly invading adjacent structures and metastasizing extensively throughout the body.

Grossly, anaplastic carcinoma is unencapsulated and extends widely, distorting the shape of the thyroid. Its consistency varies, being stony hard in some areas and soft or friable in others. Evidence of invasion of adjacent structures, such as skin, muscle, nerve, blood vessels, larynx, and esophagus, is common. On histopathologic examination, the lesion is composed of atypical cells that exhibit numerous mitoses and form a variety of patterns. Spindle-shaped cells and multinucleate giant cells are usually the predominant types of cell. In some cases, small cells predominate; as a result, there may be difficulty in distinguishing the lesion from lymphosarcoma. Rarely, the lesion is composed of clear cells, resembling hypernephroma, or large epithelial cells (epidermoid carcinoma). Areas of necrosis and polymorphonuclear infiltration are frequently present. Sometimes elements of papillary or follicular carcinoma can be detected, suggesting that they may be the precursors of anaplastic carcinoma (Russell et al., 1963).

The usual clinical complaint is of a rapid, often painful enlargement of a mass that has been present in the thyroid gland for many years. The mass rapidly invades adjacent structures, causing hoarseness, inspiratory stridor, and difficulty in swallowing. On examination, the skin overlying the mass is often warm and discolored. The mass is large and tender and is often fixed to adjacent structures, with the result that it moves poorly on swallowing. It is stony hard in consistency, but some areas may be soft or fluctuant. The regional lymph nodes are enlarged, and there may be evidence of distant metastases. The patient usually succumbs within several months after the diagnosis has been made. In general, anaplastic carcinomas do not accumulate iodine.

Carcinoma of Parafollicular Origin (Medullary Carcinoma, Solid Carcinoma with Amyloid Stroma)

This is the most distinctive type of thyroid carcinoma, although it comprises only about 5–10 per cent of the cases. It usually occurs after the age of 50 and is slightly more common in women. It is more malignant than follicular carcinoma. Solid carcinoma readily invades the intraglandular lymphatics, spreading to other parts of the gland and to the pericapsular and regional lymph nodes. In this respect it resembles papillary carcinoma, but unlike the latter it also spreads via the bloodstream to distant sites, particularly lung, bone, and liver.

Grossly, solid carcinoma is firm and usually unencapsulated. On histopathologic examination, it is composed of cells that vary widely in morphologic features and arrangement. Round, polyhedral, and spindle-shaped cells form a variety of patterns, but formation of papillary folds or follicles is not seen. The cells may appear undifferentiated and exhibit mitoses, but, unlike the findings in anaplastic carcinoma, necrosis and polymorphonuclear infiltration are absent. There is an abundant hyaline connective tissue stroma that gives the staining reactions for amyloid; apart from plasmacytoma, this feature is unique to solid thyroid carcinoma. Gross or microscopic foci of carcinoma are often evident in other parts of the gland. Invasion of blood vessels may be seen. The histopathologic appearance of the metastases closely resembles that of the primary lesion.

Clinically, solid carcinoma first appears either as a hard nodule or mass in the thyroid gland or as an enlargement of the regional lymph nodes. Occasionally, a metastatic lesion in a distant site is found first. As in the preceding types of thyroid malignancy, invasion of adjacent structures is a late manifestation of the disease. As in the case of papillary carcinoma, it accumulates iodine poorly and, provided that it is large enough, appears as a "cold" area in the thyroid scintiscan (Fig. 4–18).

Medullary carcinoma has recently aroused much interest because of several remarkable properties. Perhaps the most interesting feature, which derives from its parafollicular origin, is the propensity to secrete calcitonin. Elevated concentrations of radioimmunoassayable calcitonin are frequently measurable in the blood or can be elicited by the infusion of calcium. Cushing's syndrome and carcinoid syndrome have been reported in association with medullary carcinoma, apparently because of secretion by the tumor of ACTH and serotonin respectively. The secretion of histaminase and prostaglandins has also been reported. These tumors may also be associated with pheochromocytoma (usually bilateral), hyperparathyroidism, multiple neuromas, and a Marfanoid appearance. Finally, although the disease may occur sporadically, it is frequently familial and is apparently inherited as an autosomal dominant characteristic. In relatives of patients with this disorder, who therefore are at high risk, measurement of calcitonin should be carried out periodically, since an increased serum calcitonin concentration is a forerunner of clinically overt disease. When increased levels of calcitonin are found, prophylactic total thyroidectomy is indicated. (For a thorough discussion of this disorder, see the review by Melvin et al., 1972).

Laboratory Tests

In general, patients with thyroid carcinoma are eumetabolic, and the indices of overall thyroid function are normal. Thyroid carcinomas that accumulate radioiodine may also secrete an iodoprotein with many of the properties of serum albumin. Of particular interest is the finding that the serum of approximately one-third of patients with carcinoma of follicular origin contains a material that cross-reacts immunologically with bovine but not human TSH. The concentration in serum of this material is not decreased by suppressive doses of thyroid hormone. A material with similar properties has been found in both the blood and tumor tissue of some patients with nonthyroid carcinoma. (See Greenspan et al., 1972, for references.)

Diagnosis and Management of the Nodular Thyroid Gland

In essence, the problem of the nodular thyroid gland is the problem of thyroid carcinoma in all its ramifications. These can be resolved into three component questions: (1) Is the nodular thyroid in question likely to harbor a carcinoma? (2) If carcinoma is present, what is likely to be its course, either without treatment or after various forms of treatment? (3) What are the hazards of treatment relative to the likely benefits?

There is little general agreement concerning the answers to these questions, and as already indicated, such disagreement stems from the inadequacy of the data available. Unless metastasis or local extension is or becomes evident, no purely clinical means exists for establishing or excluding the presence of carcinoma in a thyroid nodule. Hence the diagnosis ultimately depends upon histopathologic examination of the excised lesion. Since this diagnostic technique is also a principal mode of therapy, the natural history of proven carcinomas must inevitably be altered. On the other hand, if the nature of the lesion is not proven, conclusions concerning either the natural course of the supposed carcinoma or the efficacy of nonsurgical therapy must be presumptive, since the diagnosis is not known with certainty. Furthermore, since the diagnostic and therapeutic surgical measures are themselves not without risk, they are almost invariably employed in a highly selected group of patients, and hence the true incidence of carcinoma in the nodular thyroid gland is obscured.

The question of the incidence of carcinoma in the nodular thyroid has been a focus of overriding attention during the past 25 years. During the early 1940's and since, a large number of reports, mainly emanating from surgical clinics, indicated a high incidence of carcinoma in nodular goiter. In surgically excised nontoxic multinodular goiter, an incidence as high as 15 per cent was reported. In seemingly uninodular glands, an even higher incidence approaching 25 per cent was reported. Shortly thereafter, however, an examination of necropsy statistics revealed that carcinoma of the thyroid gland is only rarely a cause of death, despite the fact that nodular goiter is quite common in the general population (Sokal, 1959). In the intervening years, great effort has been devoted to the resolution of this discrepancy. Several possible explanations have emerged. First, it is abundantly evident that a major factor is the ability of the physician to select from among all patients with nodular goiter a group in which the likelihood of carcinoma is far greater than in the remaining patients. The tendency for surgery to be performed in this high-risk group unquestionably accounts in large part for the high incidence of carcinoma in surgical series. A second factor may be the difficulty in differentiating benign from malignant neoplasms on histopathologic grounds. Finally, since surgery provides both diagnosis and some measure of treatment, it is possible that the discrepancy between thyroid carcinoma as a cause of death and as a cause of operation reflects a favorable result of excision. Whether these factors taken together would completely resolve the foregoing discrepancy is uncertain.

On the basis mainly of biopsy, the incidence of carcinoma in nodular goiter has been estimated in a USPHS survey to be 25 new cases per million population per year. Since the incidence of nodular goiter is thought to be 40,000 per million population at any time, the likelihood of finding carcinoma in nodular goiter appears to be very low (approximately 0.06 per cent). However, this figure does not truly reflect the incidence, because thyroid cancer is more likely to be diagnosed in a recently diagnosed nodular goiter. Hence some estimate of the annual incidence rate of nodular goiter is required. If it can be assumed that the average patient with nodular goiter survives with his goiter for 40 years, then the incidence of newly diagnosed nodular goiter would be approximately 1000 per million population per year, and an approximate incidence of carcinoma in relation to newly discovered nodular goiter of 2.5 per cent would be derived. This figure can be taken as a rough approximation of the relative rates of appearance of the two disorders. Beyond this, factors of selection become apparent. There are no data concerning the proportion of patients with nodular goiter who go to their local physicians for treatment of this lesion. Similarly, there are no data concerning the frequency with which the general physician refers such patients to special clinics for diagnosis and care. As already indicated, in such clinics a further process of selection occurs. However, in a study in which a histopathologic diagnosis of nodular goiter was obtained in the majority of 235 patients referred by physicians to a special clinic, the overall incidence of carcinoma proved to be approximately 7 per cent (Shimaoka et al., 1962). This figure is remarkably similar to that found in a consecutive series of approximately 100 patients referred to the authors' clinic some years ago. In the former series of 235 patients, approximately 15 per cent were designated as suspected of or probably having a malignancy, and of these, 40 per cent proved to have thyroid carcinoma. Only 2 per cent of those classified as probably benign proved to be malignant. This high degree of diagnostic accuracy was also evident in the smaller series studied by the present authors.

What then is the basis upon which a reasonable judgment concerning the likelihood of carcinoma in a nodular goiter can be made? Such judgment is derived from a constellation of findings, among which some weigh for and some against a clinical diagnosis of carcinoma. The age of the patient is an important determinant. In papillary carcinoma, which is by far the most common type of thyroid malignancy, almost half the cases are discovered before the age of 40, yet most nonmalignant nodules in the thyroid occur after the age of 40. Hence the younger the patient, the greater is the likelihood that a nodular thyroid harbors a malignancy. The sex of the patient is also an important consideration. The overall incidence of nodular goiter is far greater in women than in men (approximately 7-9:1), but the sex ratio in carcinoma is far lower. Hence the ratio of malignant to benign nodules is far higher in men than in women. There is substantial evidence and quite general agreement that the incidence of carcinoma is distinctly greater in nodules that are clinically solitary than in the nodules of a multinodular gland. This is true despite the fact, first, that a considerable proportion of glands considered to be uninodular on palpation prove at surgery to contain more than one nodule, and second, that thyroid carcinoma is not infrequently found in more than one site within the gland, owing to intraglandular lymphatic spread. An additional criterion of importance is the functional activity of the nodule as judged by scintiscan. The limitations that the size and location of a "cold" nodule impose on its detection by scintiscan have been discussed and should be borne in mind. Furthermore, it is clear that nonfunctioning nodules may represent areas of hemorrhagic or cystic degeneration either in benign adenomas or in nodular areas within a nontoxic multinodular goiter. Nevertheless, the great majority of carcinomas appear as inactive areas in the scintiscan, and hence this finding, although by no means pathognomonic, is highly suspicious. Finally, several clinical criteria are of importance. Although unusual, a history of radiation to the head, neck, or chest during childhood suggests the likelihood of carcinoma, as does a history of recent painless growth or a nodule of a very firm or stony hard consistency. Radiologic examination of the neck may provide ancillary evidence of papillary carcinoma if the calcification of psammoma bodies is detected. The foregoing criteria considered either alone or in combination do not provide a definite diagnosis of thyroid carcinoma; for this, histopathologic examination is required. They do, however, serve to distinguish a high-risk group in whom the likelihood of carcinoma outweighs the hazards of excisional biopsy. Needle biopsy of the thyroid gland should not be performed in suspected malignancy because of the likelihood of seeding carcinoma along the needle track.

Criteria such as fixation, vocal-cord paralysis, or extension to regional lymph nodes are indeed characteristic of thyroid carcinoma but are late manifestations. To the extent that there is any merit to early diagnosis, and this is disputed by some, the physician must not await the appearance of these signs.

From the foregoing considerations, the following general guidelines have been adopted in the authors' clinic. In a man, most solitary nodules should be removed unless the patient is very old or a specific contraindication to operation exists. Removal becomes especially urgent if the patient is under 40, if the lesion is found to be nonfunctioning, or if doubt exists concerning its function. In a woman under 40, a solitary nodule should be removed if there is doubt whether it is functioning. In a woman over 40, a solitary nodule should be removed if it is clearly nonfunctioning. In either sex, if the nodule is clearly functioning, a trial of suppressive therapy with TH may be undertaken, provided that the other clinical criteria suggestive of malignancy are not present. If suppressive therapy induces regression of the nodule, it should be continued indefinitely. If the nodule fails to regress after several months, surgery may be undertaken, but if the nodule enlarges during suppressive therapy, surgery is definitely indicated. If a solitary nodule in either sex is functioning to an extent sufficient to suppress the adjacent tissue, the nodule is very unlikely to be malignant, but surgery may be indicated if the patient is thyrotoxic. A similar approach should be followed if only two or three nodules are felt in an otherwise normal thyroid gland. A thyroid that is generally enlarged and is the seat of multiple well-defined nodules very likely represents the late stage of simple or nontoxic goiter (nontoxic multinodular goiter). This is a very common disorder in women but is unusual in

men. In the authors' view, the high incidence of malignancy in multinodular goiter removed at surgery merely reflects a much higher degree of selection than is applied in patients with solitary nodules. Furthermore, areas of nonfunction not uncommonly are present. Hence unless a particular area has undergone recent growth or there is evidence suggestive of local spread or invasion, suppressive therapy with TH is used (see section dealing with simple or nontoxic goiter).

Treatment of Thyroid Carcinoma

The foregoing section has provided guidelines for the selection of patients in whom surgery is indicated for diagnosed nodular goiter suspected of being the seat of carcinoma. When surgery is performed, it should be carried out under general anesthesia through a wide incision and the suspicious lesion removed *in toto* together with a generous margin of surrounding tissue. Under no circumstances should the lesion be transsected *in situ*. Examination by frozen section is mandatory unless local invasion or metastases are clearly evident. If this examination indicates carcinoma, the authors feel that total thyroidectomy and removal of the pericapsular lymph nodes should be performed in view of the high incidence of intraglandular lymphatic spread (Russell et al., 1963). Admittedly, the incidence of complications, such as injury to the recurrent laryngeal nerve and hypoparathyroidism, is higher following total than subtotal thyroidectomy. These risks are not great, and owing to the gravity of the disease, the more extensive procedure seems justified. Not all, however, would agree with this view. In the case of most thyroid carcinomas, the regional lymph nodes should be removed if enlarged, but radical dissection should not be performed. In the case of medullary carcinoma, however, a more aggressive approach to cervical metastases is probably justified. If anaplastic carcinoma is found, local removal to prevent or alleviate obstruction to vital function should be performed, but efforts to remove the tumor *in toto* should not be made. If the examination by frozen section is equivocal, total thyroidectomy is deferred pending the result of the permanent sections.

Several general principles underlie the subsequent management of thyroid carcinoma. First, both the predominant histopathologic type of metastatic deposits and their functional capability with respect to iodine accumulation may differ from those of the primary lesion. Second, accumulation within the tumor of sufficient radioiodine may eradicate the disease locally. Third, stimulation by TSH may serve to initiate or enhance radioiodine accumulation. Fourth, some tumors may be TSH-dependent with respect to growth as well as iodine accumulation.

These principles are expressed in several ways. First, attempts to treat with radioiodine alone have proved disappointing. Even in metastatic lesions that do accumulate radioiodine, the uptake is often so low as to preclude a therapeutic effect from doses that do not produce untoward effects elsewhere. Hence total thyroidectomy should be performed not only for the reasons cited earlier with respect to intraglandular spread but also to induce hypothyroidism, thereby permitting hypersecretion of endogenous TSH to elicit the full functional potential of residual lesions. Therefore, subsequent to total thyroidectomy, approximately six weeks are allowed to elapse, at which time a large tracer dose (1–2 mCi.) is administered and activity either in the thyroid bed or in metastatic foci sought by scintiscanning techniques. If such activity is present, a large dose (variously 50–250 mCi. among different clinics) of radioiodine is administered. It has been recommended by some that vigorous diuresis to produce a state of acute iodine deficiency be performed before administration of radioiodine in order to increase uptake by the lesion without increasing the total body radiation dose (Hamburger, 1969). Several days after the final dose of radioiodine, therapy with fully suppressive doses of levothyroxine (300 μg. or more daily) is instituted. Thereafter, the patient is seen at 2- to 3-month intervals, and careful examination is made to ascertain whether local recurrence or regional lymph node involvement has become manifest. If not, the patient is kept on suppressive therapy until 4 weeks before the next scintiscan examination, at which time the levothyroxine is replaced with an equivalent dosage of liothyronine. The latter is withdrawn about 10 days before the administration of the scan dose of radioiodine. This regimen substitutes T_3 for T_4 in the peripheral hormone pool, allowing a more rapid return of TSH hypersecretion than would be the case if levothyroxine had been employed. The objective is to maximize the effect of TSH on iodine accumulation while minimizing any possible effects on tumor growth. This routine is carried out after a 6-month interval if the last scan was positive and after an interval of one year if it was not.

If interim clinical examination reveals local recurrence or regional spread, surgical excision rather than radioiodine therapy is often desirable. Scintiscanning should be carried out postoperatively to ascertain whether removal of functioning tissue was complete.

The mainstays of postoperative therapy, as described above, are radioiodine and suppressive therapy. The doses of radioiodine usually required for treatment are inordinately high. Consequently, radiation sickness, neutropenia, or thrombocytopenia may occur acutely, while pulmonary fibrosis, mutagenic effects, and leukemia have been reported to occur later. Nevertheless, radioiodine therapy in conjunction with surgery has been reported to result in a significantly higher survival rate than that following surgery alone (Varma et al., 1970).

Although a rational basis exists for the use of suppressive thyroid therapy in the treatment of thyroid carcinoma, it is as yet too early to evaluate its impact upon the course of this disease. Several instances of remarkable regression of lesions have been reported (Molnar et al., 1963). However, in the case of the most common type, papillary carcinoma, the prognosis for prolonged survival is usually excellent irrespective of the form of treatment. The data of Woolner and associates (1961) indicate an overall 10-year survival rate of 82 per cent following surgery alone. This figure is very similar to the results ascribed to surgery followed by suppressive therapy (Crile, 1964). Experience with suppressive therapy in follicular carcinoma is even more limited, and the ultimate role of suppressive thyroid therapy in the treatment of thyroid carcinoma awaits more extensive evaluation.

THYROIDITIS

Hashimoto's Disease (Lymphocytic Thyroiditis, Struma Lymphomatosa)

The original description of this chronic disorder of the thyroid with its distinctive histologic appearance was given by Hashimoto in 1912. Until the demonstration of circulating thyroid autoantibodies, Hashimoto's disease could be diagnosed with certainty only by biopsy of the thyroid. The demonstration of high titers of circulating autoantibodies in most patients with Hashimoto's disease has led to the use of the term *autoimmune thyroiditis* to describe this disorder.

Hashimoto's disease is a common disorder affecting women many times more often than men. It occurs most frequently between the ages of 30 and 50 but may occur during any period of life. It is, in all likelihood, the most common cause of sporadic goiter in children. There is often a family history of Hashimoto's disease, goiter, primary hypothyroidism, or Graves' disease, and even in relatives without overt thyroid disease circulating autoantibodies may be detected. There is evidence to suggest that cell-mediated immunity plays an important role in the pathogenesis of Hashimoto's disease. (See Lamki et al., 1973, for references.)

Histopathology

The glandular tissue is pale and firm. The histopathologic changes vary in type and extent but in general consist of a combination of diffuse lymphocytic infiltration, obliteration of thyroid follicles, and fibrosis (Fig. 4–38). In most cases, there is destruction of epithelial cells and degeneration and fragmentation of the follicular basement membrane. The remaining epithelial cells may be larger and show oxyphilic changes in the cytoplasm; these so-called Askanazy cells are virtually pathognomonic of this disease. In some cases epithelial hyperplasia may be a prominent feature. Colloid is sparse. The interstitial tissue is infiltrated with lymphocytes which may form typical lymphoid follicles with germinal centers. Plasma cells may be prominent. Fibrosis is generally

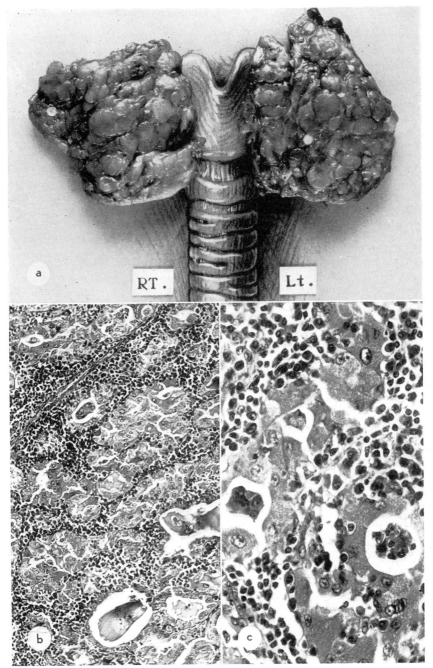

Figure 4-38. Hashimoto's disease. *A*, Note exaggeration of normal lobular pattern. *B*, Interfollicular infiltration by lymphocytes and plasma cells. *C*, Granular, oxyphilic changes in the cytoplasm of the follicular epithelium (Askanazy cells). (From Woolner, L. B., McConahey, W. M., and Beahrs, O. H.: *J. Clin. Endocr. 19*:53, 1959.)

present, especially in the older lesions, but not to the extent seen in Riedel's thyroiditis.

Lymphocytic infiltration of a focal or diffuse nature may be found in the thyroid gland of Graves' disease, in thyroid neoplasms, and in simple or nontoxic goiter. In the past, a diagnosis of coexisting Hashimoto's disease was not made unless Askanazy cells or lymphoid follicles were present. Since the lymphocytic infiltration in these other diseases has been shown usually to be associated with circulating thyroid autoantibodies, the pathogenetic mechanisms leading to lymphocytic infiltration in all these disorders may be similar. In the case of Graves' disease, lymphocytic infiltration and associated autoantibodies may favor the development of hypothyroidism after partial thyroidectomy or radioiodine therapy (Green and Wilson, 1964).

Physiopathology

A variety of abnormalities in hormone biosynthesis may be seen in patients with Hashimoto's disease. (See Buchanan et al., 1965, for references.) These include a defect in organic binding of thyroid iodide, as evidenced by a positive percholorate discharge test, and an accelerated turnover of a depleted organic iodine pool, as evidenced by a high PBI[131]. In addition, abnormal release of iodoproteins occurs; in their physical properties, these may resemble either thyroglobulin or the albumin-like iodoprotein found in the sera of patients with other thyroid disorders. The foregoing abnormalities in hormone biosynthesis may occur in clinically normal individuals who either are relatives of patients with Hashimoto's disease or have circulating thyroid autoantibodies.

Because of the faulty synthesis of hormone, hypersecretion of TSH results, producing functional evidence of thyroid hyperactivity without thyrotoxicosis. Maximal stimulation by endogenous TSH may take place, with the result that no further stimulation is brought about by exogenous TSH (decreased thyroid reserve).

A high proportion of patients with Hashimoto's disease develop iodide myxedema when iodide is taken chronically. Results of the iodide-perchlorate discharge test in such patients are abnormal, indicating an underlying defect in the organic-binding mechanism in the presence of an iodide load. This defect presumably accounts for the susceptibility to iodide myxedema (Braverman et al., 1971).

Clinical Picture

Goiter is the outstanding clinical feature of Hashimoto's disease. It usually appears gradually and is often found during examination for some other complaint. In occasional instances, however, the thyroid enlarges rapidly, and when accompanied by pain and tenderness, the disorder may mimic de Quervain's or subacute thyroiditis. Sometimes symptoms of mild thyrotoxicosis appear during the early phase of the disease. About 20 per cent of the patients are hypothyroid when first seen. The goiter is generally moderate in size and firm in consistency and moves freely when the patient swallows. Its surface is either smooth or scalloped, but well-defined nodules are unusual. Both lobes are enlarged, but one is often larger than the other. Enlargement of the pyramidal lobe is common. Compression of adjacent structures, such as trachea, esophagus, and recurrent laryngeal nerves, occurs rarely. Enlargement of regional lymph nodes may be present but is unusual.

Although primary (thyroprivic) hypothyroidism is thought to be the end-result of autoimmune destruction of the thyroid, the clinical entity of Hashimoto's disease has not been observed to progress to classic thyroprivic hypothyroidism in the individual patient. Indeed, the histopathologic picture tends to remain rather static, except for some increase in fibrous tissue (Vickery and Hamlin, 1961). Clinically, the goiter tends either to remain unchanged or to enlarge gradually over many years if left untreated. The clinical features of hypothyroidism commonly develop over several years in those patients who are euthyroid when first seen.

Several studies have suggested that there is an increased incidence of thyroid neoplasia in the thyroid of Hashimoto's disease. In most instances, the neoplasm is papillary in type and of low-grade malignancy (Woolner et al., 1959). Prolonged observation of patients with Hashimoto's disease, however, has failed to show the emergence of clinically overt thyroid malignancy (Crile and Hazard, 1962).

Hashimoto's disease may coexist with pernicious anemia, and even in the absence of overt anemia, circulating autoantibodies against gastric parietal cells may be found. Other diseases presumed to have an autoimmune basis, such as idiopathic adrenal atrophy, Sjögren's syndrome, rheumatoid arthritis, progressive hepatitis, and systemic lupus erythematosus, appear to occur in patients with Hashimoto's disease and in their relatives more often than can be accounted for by chance.

Laboratory Tests

The results of the common tests of thyroid function are variable, depending upon the stage of the disease. At first, the tests indicate the presence of thyroid hyperfunction without overproduction of metabolically active hormone. The thyroid I^{131} uptake is often increased and the PBI slightly elevated, but the serum T_4 concentration is normal, and hence the PBI-T_4-iodine difference is abnormally large. These changes reflect the secretion of abnormal iodoproteins. At this stage, the patient is eumetabolic, as indicated by a normal BMR, and the glandular hyperfunction reflects hypersecretion of TSH since it is suppressed by exogenous hormone. With the passage of time, evidence of hyperfunction diminishes, and the thyroid I^{131} uptake, PBI, and serum T_4 concentration progressively approach subnormal values, but the serum T_3 concentration may be increased. During this period, serum TSH may be increased, and the response to exogenous TSH may be subnormal, indicating diminished thyroid reserve. Ultimately, laboratory indices and the clinical state of the patient will reflect inadequate secretion of hormone.

The diagnosis of Hashimoto's disease is confirmed by the finding of high titers of thyroid autoantibodies in the serum. When both the tanned red cell agglutination and complement fixation tests are carried out, virtually all patients with this disease have circulating autoantibodies, and in most patients these are present in high titer (more than 1:25,000 in the tanned red cell test). In young patients, however, typical Hashimoto's disease may be present with lower titers of autoantibodies; hence in this group, low titers do not exclude the diagnosis. Abnormal sero-flocculation tests, reflecting an increase in immunoglobulin concentration, are associated with titers of autoantibody and have been advocated as a screening test. A serologic test for syphilis may be falsely positive.

Since the diagnosis of Hashimoto's disease in most patients can readily be confirmed by thyroid antibody tests and since such tests seem at least as reliable as needle biopsy, the latter is probably no longer an important adjunct in diagnosis. When a neoplastic lesion is suspected, open biopsy under general anesthesia is preferable because needle biopsy is often misleading and may result in seeding of a carcinoma along the needle track.

Differential Diagnosis

The differentiation of Hashimoto's disease from other uncomplicated disorders of the thyroid has been greatly facilitated by the demonstration that high titers of thyroid autoantibodies occur commonly in Hashimoto's disease but less frequently in other thyroid disorders. The frequent coexistence of hypothyroidism with Hashimoto's disease also serves to distinguish this disease from others, such as nontoxic goiter and thyroid neoplasm, from which it must be differentiated. Differentiation of Hashimoto's disease from diffuse nontoxic goiter is often difficult on clinical grounds, although the goiter in the latter disorder tends to be softer than that of Hashimoto's disease. In addition, the results of tests of thyroid function may not be helpful, since, in common with Hashimoto's disease, the thyroid I^{131} uptake may be increased and the PBI-T_4-iodine difference disproportionately large in nontoxic goiter. In adolescent patients, the differentiation from a diffuse nontoxic goiter is even more difficult because in this age group Hashimoto's disease may not be accompanied by the high titers of autoantibodies found in adult patients. Biopsy of the thyroid gland will then be necessary to establish the diagnosis. The presence of well-defined nodules will generally serve to distinguish nontoxic multinodular goiter from Hashimoto's disease.

The differentiation between Hashimoto's disease and thyroid carcinoma can often be made on clinical grounds alone. A goiter that is the seat of a thyroid carcinoma is usually nodular and firm or hard and may become fixed to adjacent structures. Compression of the recurrent laryngeal nerve with consequent hoarseness is virtually pathognomonic of thyroid carcinoma. A history of a recent enlargement of the goiter is more frequent in thyroid carcinoma than in Hashimoto's disease. Enlargement of regional lymph nodes is common in thyroid carcinoma but unusual in Hashimoto's disease. Finally, in the case of thyroid carcinoma, external scintiscanning of the thyroid may reveal areas of nonfunction, whereas in Hashimoto's disease activity is usually present throughout the gland.

Treatment

In many patients, no treatment is required because the goiter is small and the disease asymptomatic; however, it could be argued that suppressive doses of thyroid hormone might interrupt the cycle of autoimmune insult to the gland. In other patients, treatment with TH (thyroid hormone) is directed at alleviating goiter or hypothyroidism or both. Treatment is indicated in patients in whom the goiter is pressing on adjacent structures or is unsightly. This is most likely to be effective in the patient with goiter of recent onset. In long-standing goiter, treatment with TH is often ineffective, possibly because of more fibrosis in the gland. In patients in whom the onset of the disease is acute and accompanied by pain and tenderness, glucocorticoids together with TH have been reported to be beneficial. Glucocorticoids cause regression of the goiter and decrease autoantibody titers, but in view of both their untoward side effects and the fact that the activity of the disease returns after treatment is withdrawn, these agents are not recommended in the management of the usual case. Full replacement doses of TH should be given when frank hypothyroidism supervenes or when diminished thyroid reserve has been demonstrated. Although surgery is a popular form of treatment in some centers, the authors feel that it is justified only if pressure symptoms or unsightly enlargement persists after a trial of TH. TH should be continued after surgery, because hypothyroidism inevitably results.

Subacute Thyroiditis

Subacute thyroiditis has been termed granulomatous, giant-cell, or de Quervain's thyroiditis. It does not appear to belong to the autoimmune group of diseases; available evidence suggests that it might be a viral infection of the thyroid gland. It often follows an upper respiratory illness, and a tendency to a seasonal and geographic aggregation of cases has been noted. The mumps virus has been implicated in some cases, and there is some evidence suggesting that Coxsackie, influenza, and ECHO viruses and adenoviruses may also be etiologic agents (Volpé et al., 1967).

This disease is uncommon, but it is likely that mild cases are mistakenly diagnosed as pharyngitis. Women are far more frequently affected than men, and the maximum incidence is in the fourth and fifth decades.

Histopathology (Fig. 4–39)

The histopathologic changes are distinctive and quite different from those seen in Hashimoto's disease (Meachim and Young, 1963). The lesions are patchy in distribution and characteristically vary in their stage of development from area to area. In affected areas, follicles are infiltrated with cells predominantly of the mononuclear type.

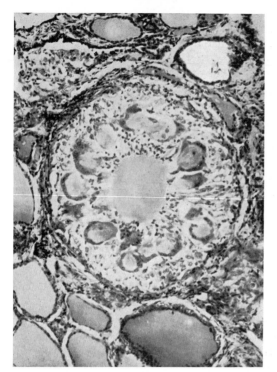

Figure 4–39. Subacute thyroiditis. Intrafollicular giant-cells surrounding a central core of colloid. (From Meachim, G., and Young, M. H.: *J. Clin. Path. 16*:189, 1963.)

These infiltrated follicles show disruption of epithelium, partial or complete loss of colloid, and fragmentation and duplication of the basement membrane. To this extent, the histopathologic appearance may resemble that seen in Hashimoto's disease. A more characteristic feature of the disease is seen in the well-developed follicular lesions and consists of a central core of colloid surrounded by the multinucleate giant cells, from which stems the designation "giant-cell" thyroiditis. Colloid may be found in the interstitium or within the giant cells (colloidophagy). The follicular changes progress to form granulomas. Interfollicular fibrosis and an interstitial inflammatory reaction are present to varying degrees. When the disease has subsided, an essentially normal histologic appearance is restored.

Physiopathology

In subacute thyroiditis, the destruction of follicular epithelium results in a diminution of hormone biosynthesis. This is reflected in the very low thyroid I^{131} uptake of virtually all patients during the active phase of the disease. Moreover, the loss of follicular integrity may allow the passage into the circulation of variable quantities of abnormal iodinated materials as well as stored hormone. These abnormal iodinated materials lead to a disproportionate increase in the PBI relative to the T_4-iodine concentration, causing an abnormal dis-

crepancy between the results of these tests. Later in the disease when the glandular store of hormone is depleted, the PBI and serum T_4 concentrations may approach subnormal values. The release of thyroglobulin may give rise to circulating autoantibodies during the active phase of the disease.

Clinical Picture

The characteristic feature of this disease is the gradual or sudden appearance of pain in the region of the thyroid gland accompanied in severe cases by fever. The pain, which is aggravated by turning the head or swallowing, characteristically radiates to the ear, the jaw, or the occiput and may mimic disorders arising in these areas. Hoarseness and dysphagia may be present. Patients frequently complain of palpitation, nervousness, and particularly lassitude; lassitude is often extreme and unexpectedly great, considering the local nature of the disease. Although severe cases may appear with acute manifestations, in milder cases, which are often wrongly diagnosed, symptoms may have been present for months. On palpation, at least a part of the thyroid is slightly to moderately enlarged, firm, often nodular, and usually exquisitely tender, one lobe being generally more severely affected than the other. The overlying skin may be warm and red. Occasionally, the locus of maximal involvement migrates over the course of a few weeks to other parts of the gland. The disease usually subsides within a few months, leaving no residual deficiency of thyroid function. In rare cases, the disease may smolder with repeated exacerbations over many months, with hypothyroidism as the end-result.

Laboratory Tests

The association of a very low thyroid I^{131} uptake with a normal or high serum T_4 concentration is characteristic of the early phase of this disease. Subnormal values for thyroid I^{131} uptake are usually found, even when only one part of the gland is affected clinically, but occasionally, especially in milder cases, uptake in unaffected parts of the gland may persist, as can be demonstrated in the scintiscan. The PBI is often disproportionately higher than the T_4-iodine concentration, indicating the presence in serum of abnormal iodinated materials. Later in the disease, values for the PBI and serum T_4 concentration may be subnormal. Exogenous TSH may increase the uptake, but the response is subnormal. The BMR may be normal or high. Recovery of thyroid function is revealed by return of the I^{131} uptake toward normal. Circulating thyroid autoantibodies are present in low titer in a minority of cases and disappear when the disease subsides. During the acute phase, the sedimentation rate is increased, often inordinately so, and is a useful index of the progress of the disease. The leukocyte count is usually normal.

Differential Diagnosis

Subacute thyroiditis must be differentiated mainly from acute hemorrhagic degeneration in a preexisting thyroid nodule, from Hashimoto's disease of acute onset, and from acute pyogenic thyroiditis. Differentiation from hemorrhage into a nodule will present no difficulty when this occurs in a multinodular goiter, because other nontender nodules will be felt. Decision is more difficult when there is hemorrhage into a solitary nodule. In both varieties of hemorrhage, however, function in the remainder of the gland persists, and marked elevation of the sedimentation rate is rarely present. Hashimoto's disease of acute onset may be accompanied by pain and tenderness in the thyroid gland, but the gland is usually diffusely affected, and the thyroid I^{131} uptake is not decreased. Acute pyogenic thyroiditis is distinguished by the presence of a septic focus elsewhere, by a greater inflammatory reaction in the tissues adjacent to the thyroid, and by much greater leukocytic and febrile responses. In the authors' experience, a normal thyroid I^{131} uptake is preserved in acute pyogenic thyroiditis.

Treatment

Many forms of treatment have been recommended for subacute thyroiditis, including thionamide drugs, TSH, and suppressive doses of TH. The evidence that these agents influence the course of the disease is unconvincing. In mild cases, aspirin is generally adequate to control the symptoms. In more severe cases, glucocorticoids (e.g., prednisone up to 40 mg. daily) rapidly alleviate the clinical manifestations but do not influence the underlying disease process. Hence the symptoms may be exacerbated if treatment is withdrawn too early, but they will again respond if treatment is reinstituted. It has been suggested that a relapse can be avoided if glucocorticoid therapy is continued at a dose that maintains the patient in an asymptomatic state until the thyroid I^{131} uptake has returned to normal (Vagenakis et al., 1970). The application to the thyroid area of small doses of x-ray often produces clinical improvement and was formerly a popular mode of therapy. However, because of a significant failure rate and the greater effectiveness of glucocorticoids, it is no longer frequently used. Thyroidectomy is contraindicated in this disease. (See Greene, 1971, for a review of subacute thyroiditis with extensive references.)

Riedel's Thyroiditis

Riedel's thyroiditis is very rare and is observed chiefly in middle-aged women. The etiology is unknown. In the past, Riedel's thyroiditis was considered to be an advanced state of Hashimoto's disease, but it is now generally considered to be a separate disease entity. It is characterized by extensive fibrosis of the thyroid gland and adjacent structures and may be associated with fibrosis elsewhere, especially in the retroperitoneal area (Turner-Warwick et al., 1966).

Symptoms develop insidiously and are related chiefly to compression of adjacent structures, in particular the trachea, esophagus, and recurrent laryngeal nerves. Constitutional symptoms of inflammation are uncommon. The thyroid gland is moderately enlarged and stony hard. The enlargement is usually asymmetrical. The stony hard consistency of the gland and the invasion of adjacent structures suggest carcinoma, but there is no enlargement of regional lymph nodes. The temperature, pulse, and leukocyte count are normal. Hypothyroidism occurs occasionally.

The thyroid I^{131} uptake may be normal or low. Some patients have circulating thyroid autoantibodies but much less frequently and in lower titer than is usually seen in Hashimoto's disease.

Treatment with TH relieves the hypothyroidism but has no effect on the goiter. If pressure symptoms are prominent, partial thyroidectomy is indicated.

Acute Pyogenic Thyroiditis

Acute pyogenic thyroiditis is a rare disorder that is due to infection of the thyroid by pyogenic organisms. It is characterized by severe pain and tenderness in the region of the thyroid, accompanied by dysphagia, fever, and malaise. There are signs of acute inflammation in the gland and usually in the surrounding tissues. The disease responds to treatment with the appropriate antibiotic. Surgical drainage is indicated only when fluctuation is present.

REFERENCES

Aber, C. P., Noble, R. L., et al.: Serum lactic dehydrogenase isoenzymes in "myxoedema heart disease." *Brit. Heart J. 28*:663, 1966.

Aboul-Khair, S. A., Crooks, J., et al.: The physiological changes in thyroid function during pregnancy. *Clin. Sci. 27*:195, 1964.

Abuid, J., Stinson, D. A., et al.: Serum triiodothyronine and thyroxine in the neonate and the acute increases in these hormones following delivery. *J. Clin. Invest. 52*:1195, 1973.

Adams, D. D., and Kennedy, T. H.: Evidence to suggest that LATS protector stimulates the human thyroid gland. *J. Clin. Endocr. 33*:47, 1971.

Alexander, W. D., Harden, R. M., et al.: Thyroid suppression by triiodothyronine as a guide to duration of treatment of thyrotoxicosis with antithyroid drugs. *Lancet 2*:1041, 1966.

Alexander, W. D., Koutras, D. A., et al.: Quantitative studies of iodine metabolism in thyroid disease. *Quart. J. Med. 31*:281, 1962.

Alexander, W. D., McLarty, D. G., et al.: Prediction of the long-term results of antithyroid drug therapy for thyrotoxicosis. *J. Clin. Endocr. 30*:540, 1970.

Anderson, M. S., Bowers, C. Y., et al.: Synthetic thyrotropin-releasing hormone. A potent stimulator of thyrotropin secretion in man. *New Eng. J. Med. 285*:1279, 1971.

Ardeman, S., Chanarin, I., et al.: Addisonian pernicious anemia and intrinsic factor antibodies in thyroid disorders. *Quart. J. Med. 35*:421, 1966.

Astwood, E. B., Cassidy, C. E., et al.: Treatment of goiter and thyroid nodules with thyroid. *J.A.M.A.* 174:459, 1960.

Azizi, F., Portnay, G., et al.: Pituitary-thyroid response to intramuscular TRH (abstract). *Clin. Res.* 21:484, 1973.

Babior, B. M., Creagan, S., et al.: Stimulation of mitochondrial adenosine diphosphate uptake by thyroid hormones. *Proc. Nat. Acad. Sci. U.S.A.* 70:98, 1973.

Balasubramaniam, K., Deiss, W. P., Jr., et al.: Effect of thyrotropin on iodoprotein of thyroid cell fractions. *Endocrinology* 77:54, 1965.

Barrington, E. J. W.: Phylogenetic perspectives in vertebrate endocrinology, In *Perspectives in Endocrinology.* Barrington, E. J. W., and Jorgensen, C. A. (eds.), New York, Academic Press, 1968.

Bayliss, R. I. S., and Edwards, O. M.: Urinary excretion of free catecholamines in Graves' disease. *J. Endocr.* 49:167, 1971.

Becker, D. V.: Metabolic indices, In *The Thyroid.* Werner, S. C., and Ingbar, S. H. (eds.), New York, Harper and Row, 1971.

Beckers, C., and Cornette, C.: TSH production rate in nontoxic goiter. *J. Clin. Endocr.* 32:852, 1971.

Begg, T. B., and Hall, R.: Iodide goiter and hypothyroidism. *Quart. J. Med.* 32:351, 1963.

Beling, U., and Einhorn, J.: Incidence of hypothyroidism and recurrences following I¹³¹ treatment of hyperthyroidism. *Acta Radiol.* 56:275, 1961.

Bellabarba, D., Inada, M., et al.: Thyroxine transport and turnover in major nonthyroidal illness. *J. Clin. Endocr.* 28:1023, 1968.

Boyd, J. D.: Development of the human thyroid gland, In *The Thyroid Gland.* Pitt-Rivers, R., and Trotter, W. R. (eds.), Washington, Butterworths, 1964.

Braverman, L. E., Ingbar, S. H., et al.: Conversion of thyroxine (T₄) to triiodothyronine (T₃) in athyreotic human subjects. *J. Clin. Invest.* 49:855, 1970.

Braverman, L. E., Vagenakis, A. G., et al.: Effects of replacement doses of sodium L-thyroxine on the peripheral metabolism of thyroxine and triiodothyronine in man. *J. Clin. Invest.* 52:1010, 1973.

Braverman, L. E., Vagenakis, A. G., et al.: Studies on the pathogenesis of iodide myxedema. *Trans. Ass. Amer. Physicians* 84:130, 1971.

Bray, G. A.: Increased sensitivity of the thyroid in iodine-depleted rats to the goitrogenic effects of thyrotropin. *J. Clin. Invest.* 47:1640, 1968.

Brunelle, P., and Bohuon, C.: Baisse de la triiodothyronine serique avec l'âge. *Clin. Chim. Acta* 42:201, 1972.

Buccino, R. A., Spann, J. F., Jr., et al.: Influence of thyroid state on the intrinsic contractile properties and energy stores of the myocardium. *J. Clin. Invest.* 46:1669, 1967.

Buchanan, W. W., Harden, R. M., et al.: Abnormalities of iodine metabolism in euthyroid, non-goitrous women with complement-fixing antimicrosomal thyroid autoantibodies. *J. Clin. Endocr.* 25:301, 1965.

Burke, G.: The thyrotrophin stimulation test. *Ann. Intern. Med.* 69:1127, 1968.

Caplan, R. H., and Kujak, R.: Thyroid uptake of radioactive iodine. A reevaluation. *J.A.M.A.* 215:916, 1971.

Carter, W. J., Faas, F. H., et al.: Thyroxine stimulation of protein synthesis in vitro in the absence of mitochondria. *J. Biol. Chem.* 246:4973, 1971.

Challoner, D. R., and Allen, D. O.: An in vitro effect of triiodothyronine on lipolysis, cyclic AMP-¹⁴C accumulation and oxygen consumption in isolated fat cells. *Metabolism* 19:480, 1970.

Chopra, I. J., Fisher, D. A., et al.: Thyroxine and triiodothyronine in the human thyroid. *J. Clin. Endocr.* 36:311, 1973.

Choufoer, J. C., Van Rhijn, M., et al.: Endemic goiter in Western New Guinea. II. Clinical picture, incidence and pathogenesis of endemic cretinism. *J. Clin. Endocr.* 25:385, 1965.

Clements, F. W.: Naturally occurring goitrogens. *Brit. Med. Bull.* 16:133, 1960.

Connolly, R. J., Vidor, G. I., et al.: Increase in thyrotoxicosis in endemic goiter area after iodination of bread. *Lancet* 1:500, 1970.

Cotton, G. E., Gorman, C. A., et al.: Suppression of thyrotropin (h-TSH) in serums of patients with myxedema of varying etiology treated with thyroid hormones. *New Eng. J. Med.* 285:529, 1971.

Crile, G., Jr.: Late results of treatment for papillary cancer of the thyroid. *Ann. Surg.* 160:178, 1964.

Crile, G., Jr., and Hazard, J. B.: Incidence of cancer in struma lymphomatosa. *Surg. Gynec. Obstet.* 115:101, 1962.

Cullen, M. J., Burger, A. G., et al: Effects of diphenylhydantoin on peripheral thyroid hormone economy and the conversion of T₄ to T₃ (Abstract). *Israel J. Med. Sci.* 8:11, 1972.

Das, G., and Krieger, M.: Treatment of thyrotoxic storm with intravenous administration of propranolol. *Ann. Intern. Med.* 70:985, 1969.

Davis, R. H., Fourman, P., et al.: Prevalence of parathyroid insufficiency after thyroidectomy. *Lancet* 2:1432, 1961.

DeGroot, L. J., Nagasaka, A., et al.: Biosynthesis of thyroid hormone. *Excerpta Medica Int. Congr. Ser.* 238:53, 1970.

DeLange, F., Camus, M., et al.: Circulating thyroid hormones in endemic goiter. *J. Clin. Endocr.* 34:891, 1972a.

DeLange, F., Ermans, A. M., et al.: Endemic cretinism in Idjwi Island (Kivu Lake, Republic of the Congo). *J. Clin. Endocr.* 34:1059, 1972b.

DeLange, F., Hershman, J.M., et al.: Relationship between the serum thyrotropin level, the prevalence of goiter and the pattern of iodine metabolism in Idjwi Island. *J. Clin. Endocr.* 33:261, 1971.

DeRubertis, F. R., and Woeber, K. A.: Accelerated cellular uptake and metabolism of L-thyroxine during acute *Salmonella typhimurium* sepsis. *J. Clin. Invest.* 52:78, 1973.

DeRubertis, F. R., Michelis, M. F., et al.: Impaired water excretion in myxedema. *Amer. J. Med.* 51:41, 1971.

DiScala, V. A., and Kinney, M. J.: Effects of myxedema on the renal diluting and concentrating mechanism. *Amer. J. Med.* 50:325, 1971.

Doar, J. W. H., Stamp, T. C. B., et al.: Effects of oral and intravenous glucose loading in thyrotoxicosis. Studies of plasma glucose, free fatty acid, plasma insulin and blood pyruvate levels. *Diabetes* 18:663, 1969.

Doherty, J. E., and Perkins, W. H.: Digoxin metabolism in hypo- and hyperthyroidism. *Ann. Intern. Med.* 64:489, 1966.

Donaldson, S. S., Bagshaw, M. S., et al.: Supervoltage orbital radiotherapy for Graves' ophthalmopathy. Forty-Eighth Meeting, American Thyroid Association, 1972, p. 55.

Dowling, J. T., Appleton, W. G., et al.: Thyroxine turnover during human pregnancy. *J. Clin. Endocr.* 27:1749, 1967.

Dumont, J. E.: The action of thyrotropin on thyroid metabolism. *Vitam. Horm.* 29:287, 1971.

Dunn, J. T., and Chapman, E. M.: Rising incidence of hypothyroidism after radioactive-iodine therapy in thyrotoxicosis. *New Eng. J. Med.* 271:1037, 1964.

Eayrs, J. T.: Influence of the thyroid on the central nervous system. *Brit. Med. Bull.* 16:122, 1960.

Eayrs, J. T.: Thyroid and central nervous development. *The Scientific Basis of Medicine Annual Reviews.* The Athlone Press, Univ. of London, 1966, p. 317.

Edelhoch, H.: The structure of thyroglobulin and its role in iodination. *Recent Progr. Hormone Res.* 21:1, 1965.

Edwards, C. R. W., Forsyth, I. A., et al: Amenorrhoea, galactorrhoea, and primary hypothyroidism with high circulating levels of prolactin. *Brit. Med. J.* 3:462, 1971.

Emerson, C. H., and Utiger, R. D.: Hyperthyroidism and excessive thyrotropin secretion. *New Eng. J. Med.* 287:328, 1972.

Emerson, C. H., Dyson, W. L., et al.: Serum thyrotropin and thyroxine concentrations in patients receiving lithium carbonate. *J. Clin. Endocr.* 36:338, 1972.

Engel, A. G.: Neuromuscular manifestations of Graves' disease. *Mayo Clinic Proc.* 47:919, 1972.

Fawcett, D. W., Long, J. A., et al: The ultrastructure of endocrine glands. *Recent Progr. Hormone Res.* 25:315, 1969.

Fisher, D. A., and Odell, W. D.: Acute release of thyrotropin in the newborn. *J. Clin. Invest.* 48:1670, 1969.

Fisher, D. A., and Odell, W. D.: Effect of cold on TSH secretion in man. *J. Clin. Endocr.* 33:859, 1971.

Fisher, D. A., Dussault, J. H., et al.: Serum and thyroid gland triiodothyronine in the human fetus. *J. Clin. Endocr.* 36:397, 1973.

Fore, W., Kohler, P., et al.: Rapid redistribution of serum thyroxine during ether anesthesia. *J. Clin. Endocr.* 26:821, 1966.

Funakoshi, S., and Deutsch, H. F.: Human carbonic anhydrases. V. Levels in erythrocytes in various states. *J. Lab. Clin. Med.* 77:39, 1971.

Furth, E. D., Agrawal, R. B., et al.: Secretion of iodoalbumin and iodoprealbumin by a congenital goiter containing thyroglobulin and the iodoalbumins. *J. Clin. Endocr.* 31:60, 1970.

Galton, V. A., Ingbar, S. H., et al.: Alterations in thyroid hormone economy in patients with hydatidiform mole. *J. Clin. Invest.* 50:1345, 1971.

Ghahremani, G. G., Hoffer, P. B., et al.: New normal values for thyroid uptake of radioactive iodine. *J.A.M.A. 217:*337, 1971.

Gitlin, D., and Biasucci, A.: Ontogenesis of immunoreactive thyroglobulin in the human conceptus. *J. Clin. Endocr.* 29:849, 1969.

Giustina, G., Reschini, E., et al.: Growth hormone and cortisol responses to insulin-induced hypoglycemia in thyrotoxicosis. *J. Clin. Endocr.* 32:571, 1971.

Glennon, J. A., Gordon, E. S., et al.: Hypothyroidism after low-dose I[131] treatment of hyperthyroidism. *Ann. Intern. Med.* 76:721, 1972.

Goolden, A. W. G., Bateman, D., et al.: Red cell sodium in hyperthyroidism. *Brit. Med. J. 1:*552, 1971.

Graettinger, J. S., Muenster, J. J., et al.: A correlation of clinical and hemodynamic studies in patients with hypothyroidism. *J. Clin. Invest.* 37:502, 1958.

Graettinger, J. S., Muenster, J. J., et al.: A correlation of clinical and hemodynamic studies in patients with hyperthyroidism with and without congestive heart failure. *J. Clin. Invest.* 38:1316, 1959.

Green, M., and Wilson, G. M.: Thyrotoxicosis treated by surgery or iodine-131. With special reference to development of hypothyroidism. *Brit. Med. J. 1:*1005, 1964.

Green, W. L.: Effects of 3-nitro-L-tyrosine on thyroid function in the rat: an experimental model for the dehalogenase defect. *J. Clin. Invest.* 50:2474, 1971.

Greenberg, A. H., Czernichow, P., et al.: Observations on the maturation of thyroid function in early fetal life. *J. Clin. Invest.* 49:1790, 1970.

Greene, J. N.: Subacute thyroiditis. *Amer. J. Med.* 51:97, 1971.

Greenspan, F. S., Lowenstein, J. M., et al.: Abnormal iodoprotein in non-toxic goiter. *New Eng. J. Med.* 269:830, 1963.

Greenspan, F. S., Lowenstein, J. M., et al.: Immunoreactive material to bovine TSH in plasma from patients with thyroid cancer. *J. Clin. Endocr.* 35:795, 1972.

Greer, M. A., Kendall, J. W., et al.: Antithyroid compounds, In *The Thyroid Gland.* Pitt-Rivers, R., and Trotter, W. R. (eds.), Washington, Butterworths, 1964.

Gross, H. A., Appleman, M. D., et al.: Effect of biologically active steroids on thyroid function in man. *J. Clin. Endocr.* 33:242, 1971.

Grossman, W., Robin, N. I., et al.: The enhanced myocardial contractility of thyrotoxicosis. Role of the beta adrenergic receptor. *Ann. Intern Med.* 74:869, 1971a.

Grossman, W., Robin, N. I., et al.: Effects of beta blockade on the peripheral manifestations of thyrotoxicosis. *Ann. Intern. Med.* 74:875, 1971b.

Hagen, G. A., Ouellette, R. P., et al.: Comparison of high and low dosage levels of I[131] in the treatment of thyrotoxicosis. *New Eng. J. Med.* 277:559, 1967.

Haibach, H.: Evidence for a thyroxine deiodinating mechanism in the rat thyroid different from iodotyrosine deiodinase. *Endocrinology* 88:918, 1971.

Hamburger, J. I.: Diuretic augmentation of I[131] uptake in inoperable thyroid cancer. *New Eng. J. Med.* 280:1091, 1969.

Hamilton, C. R., Adams, L. C., et al.: Hyperthyroidism due to thyrotropin-producing pituitary chromophobe adenoma. *New Eng. J. Med.* 283:1077, 1970.

Harden, R. M., Alexander, W. D., et al.: Quantitative studies of iodine metabolism after longterm treatment of thyrotoxicosis with antithyroid drugs. *J. Clin. Endocr.* 26:397, 1966.

Hauger-Klevene, J. H., Brown, H., et al.:Plasma renin activity in hyper- and hypothyroidism: Effect of adrenergic blocking agents. *J. Clin. Endocr.* 34:625, 1972.

Hayek, A., Chapman, E. M., et al.: Long-term results of treatment of thyrotoxicosis in children and adolescents with radioactive iodine. *New Eng. J. Med.* 283:949, 1970.

Hayles, A. B.: Problems of childhood Graves' disease. *Mayo Clinic Proc.* 47:850, 1972.

Heimann, P.: Ultrastructure of human thyroid. A study of normal thyroid, untreated and treated diffuse toxic goiter. *Acta Endocr.* (Kbh) 53 (Suppl. 110):1, 1966.

Hellman, L., Bradlow, H. L., et al.: Recent advances in human steroid metabolism. *Advances Clin. Chem.* 13:1, 1970.

Hermann, H. T., and Quarton, G. C.: Psychological changes and psychogenesis in thyroid hormone disorders. *J. Clin. Endocr.* 25:327, 1965.

Hershman, J. M.: The treatment of hyperthyroidism. *Ann. Intern. Med.* 64:1306, 1966.

Hershman, J. M., and Higgins, H. P.: Hydatidiform mole—a cause of clinical hyperthyroidism. *New Eng. J. Med.* 284: 573, 1971.

Hershman, J. M., and Pittman, J. A.: Utility of the radioimmunoassay of serum thyrotrophin in man. *Ann. Intern. Med.* 74:481, 1971.

Hershman, J. M., and Starnes, W. P.: Extraction and characterization of a thyrotropic material from the human placenta. *J. Clin. Invest.* 48:923, 1969.

Hiss, J. M., and Dowling, J. T.: Thyroxine metabolism in untreated and treated pancreatic steatorrhea. *J. Clin. Invest.* 41:988, 1962.

Hoch, F. L.: Biochemical actions of thyroid hormones. *Physiol. Rev.* 42:605, 1962.

Hoch, F. L.: Early action of injected L-thyroxine on mitochondrial oxidative phosphorylation. *Proc. Nat. Acad. Sci. USA* 58:506, 1967.

Hollander, C. S., Mitsuma, T., et al.: Clinical and laboratory observations in cases of triiodothyronine toxicosis confirmed by radioimmunoassay. *Lancet* 1:609, 1972.

Hollander, C. S., Scott, R. L., et al.: Increased protein-bound iodine and thyroxine-binding globulin in acute intermittent porphyria. *New Eng. J. Med.* 277:995, 1967.

Holvey, D. N., Goodner, C. J., et al.: Treatment of myxedema coma with intravenous thyroxine. *Arch. Intern. Med.* 113:89, 1964.

Howel Evans, A. W., Woodrow, J. C., et al.: Antibodies in the families of thyrotoxic patients. *Lancet* 1:636, 1967.

Ingbar, S. H.: Autoregulation of the thyroid. Response to iodide excess and depletion. *Mayo Clinic Proc.* 47:814, 1972.

Ingbar, S. H.: Physiological considerations in the treatment of diffuse toxic goiter. *Arch. Intern. Med.* 107:932, 1961.

Ismail-Beigi, F., and Edelman, I. S.: The mechanism of the calorigenic action of thyroid hormone. *J. Gen. Physiol.* 57:710, 1971.

Jellinek, E. H.: Fits, faints, coma, and dementia in myxoedema. *Lancet* 2:1010, 1962.

Johnson, P. M.: Thyroid and whole body scanning, In *The Thyroid.* Werner, S. C., and Ingbar, S. H. (eds.), New York, Harper and Row, 1971.

Jonckheer, M. H., and Karcher, D. M.: Thyroid albumin. I. Isolation and characterization. *J. Clin. Endocr.* 32:7, 1971.

Jones, J. E., Desper, P. C., et al.: Magnesium metabolism in hyperthyroidism and hypothyroidism. *J. Clin. Invest.* 45:891, 1966.

Kaplan, N. H.: Methopyrapone test in primary hypothyroidism. *J. Clin. Endocr.* 25:146, 1965.

Kaplan, S. L., Grumbach, M. M., et al.: Thyrotropin-releasing factor (TRF) effect on secretion of human pituitary prolactin and thyrotropin in children and in idiopathic hypopituitary dwarfism: further evidence for hypophysiotropic hormone deficiencies. *J. Clin. Endocr.* 35:825, 1972.

Kaplay, S. S., and Sanadi, D. R.: Thyroxine-induced mitochondrial protein and its effect on respiration. *Arch. Biochem. Biophys.* 144:440, 1971.

Klion, F. M., Segal, R., et al.: The effect of altered thyroid function on the ultrastructure of the human liver. *Amer. J. Med.* 50:317, 1971.

Kohn, L. D., and Winand, R. J.: Relationship of thyrotropin to exophthalmos-producing substance. *J. Biol. Chem.* 246:6570, 1971.

Kourides, I. A., Weintraub, B. D., et al.: Purification of the beta subunit of human thyrotropin (HTSH-β) and development of a specific radioimmunoassay (RIA) (abstract). *Clin. Res.* 21:496, 1973.

Krevans, J. R., Asper, S. P., Jr., et al.: Total aplastic anemia following use of potassium perchlorate in thyrotoxicosis. *J.A.M.A.* 181:162, 1962.

Kumar, R. S., Musa, B. U., et al.: Effect of prednisone on thyroxine distribution. *J. Clin. Endocr.* 28:1335, 1968.

Lamki, L., Row, V. V., et al.: Cell-mediated immunity in Graves' disease and in Hashimoto's thyroiditis as shown by the demonstration of migration inhibition factor (MIF). *J. Clin. Endocr.* 36:358, 1973.

Larsen, P. R.: Triiodothyronine: review of recent studies of its physiology and pathophysiology in man. *Metabolism* 21: 1073, 1972.

Levey, G. S.: Catecholamine sensitivity, thyroid hormone and the heart. *Amer. J. Med.* 50:413, 1971.

Levin, M. E.: "Metabolic insufficiency": a doubleblind study using triiodothyronine, thyroxine and a placebo: psychometric evaluation of the hypometabolic patient. *J. Clin. Endocr. 20*:106, 1960.

Levy, R. P., Marshall, J. S., et al.: Radioimmunoassay of human thyroxine-binding globulin (TBG). *J. Clin. Endocr. 32*:372, 1971.

Lieblich, J., and Utiger, R. D.: Triiodothyronine radioimmunoassay. *J. Clin. Invest. 51*:157, 1972.

Luetscher, J. A., Cohn, A. P., et al.: Aldosterone secretion and metabolism in hyperthyroidism and myxedema. *J. Clin. Endocr. 23*:873, 1963.

Luft, R., Ikkos, D., et al.: A case of severe hypermetabolism of nonthyroid origin with a defect in the maintenance of mitochondrial control: a correlated clinical, biochemical, and morphological study. *J. Clin. Invest. 41*:1776, 1962.

McDougall, I. R., Greig, W. R., et al.: Radioactive iodine (^{125}I) therapy for thyrotoxicosis. Background and evaluation in 148 patients. *New Eng. J. Med. 285*:1099, 1971a.

McDougall, I. R., Kennedy, J. S., et al.: Thyroid carcinoma following iodine-131 therapy. Report of a case and review of the literature. *J. Clin. Endocr. 33*:287, 1971b.

McFadzean, A. J. S., and Yeung, R.: Periodic paralysis complicating thyrotoxicosis in Chinese. *Brit. Med. J. 1*:451, 1967.

McKenzie, A. D. : The natural history of thyroid cancer. *Arch. Surg. 102*:274, 1971.

McKenzie, J. M.: Does LATS cause hyperthyroidism in Graves' disease? (a review biased toward the affirmative). *Metabolism 21*:883, 1972.

McKenzie, J. M.: Hyperthyroidism caused by thyroid adenomata. *J. Clin. Endocr. 26*:779, 1966.

Mangieri, C. N., and Lund, M. H.: Potency of United States Pharmacopeia desiccated thyroid tablets as determined by the antigoitrogenic assay in rats. *J. Clin. Endocr. 30*:102, 1970.

Marchant, B., Alexander, W. D., et al.: The accumulation of ^{35}S-antithyroid drugs by the thyroid gland. *J. Clin. Endocr. 34*:847, 1972.

Martin, L., and Fisher, R. A.: The hereditary and familial aspects of exophthalmic goiter and nodular goiter. *Quart. J. Med. 14*:207, 1945.

Mayberry, W. E., Gharib, H., et al.: Radioimmunoassay for human thyrotrophin. Clinical value in patients with normal and abnormal thyroid function. *Ann. Intern. Med. 74*:471, 1971.

Meachim, G., and Young, M. H.: De Quervain's subacute granulomatous thyroiditis: histological identification and incidence. *J. Clin. Path. 16*:189, 1963.

Melander, A.: Thyroid hormone secretion. Its regulation by intrathyroidal amines. *Acta Physiol. Scand., 83*(Suppl. 370):1, 1971.

Melvin, K. E. W., Tashjian, A. H., Jr., et al.: Studies in familial (medullary) thyroid carcinoma. *Recent Progr. Hormone Res. 28*:399, 1972.

Michie, W., Stowers, J. M., et al.: Mechanism of hypocalcemia after thyroidectomy for thyrotoxicosis. *Lancet 1*:508, 1971.

Miller, L. D., Sugarman, H. J., et al.: Increased peripheral oxygen delivery in thyrotoxicosis: role of red cell 2,3-diphosphoglycerate. *Ann. Surg. 172*:1051, 1970.

Molnar, G. D., Colby, M. Y., et al.: Demonstration of thyroid-stimulating-hormone dependence in a case of metastatic carcinoma of thyroid origin. *Mayo Clinic Proc. 38*:280, 1963.

Mori, T., and Kriss, J. P.: Measurements by competitive binding radioassay of serum anti-microsomal and anti-thyroglobulin antibodies in Graves' disease and other thyroid disorders. *J. Clin. Endocr. 33*:688, 1971.

Namba, T., and Grob, D.: Myasthenia gravis and hyperthyroidism occurring in two sisters. *Neurology 21*:377, 1971.

Nicoloff, J. T., Low, J. C., et al.: Simultaneous measurement of thyroxine and triiodothyronine peripheral turnover kinetics in man. *J. Clin. Invest. 51*:473, 1972.

Nikkilä, E. A., and Kekki, M.: Plasma triglyceride metabolism in thyroid disease. *J. Clin. Invest. 51*:2103, 1972.

Nofal, M. M., Beierwaltes, W. H.: Treatment of hyperthyroidism with sodium iodide I^{131}. *J.A.M.A. 197*:605, 1966.

Oddie, T. H., Fisher, D. A., et al.: Iodine intake in the United States: A reassessment. *J. Clin. Endocr. 30*:659, 1970a.

Oddie, T. H., Flanigan, W. J., et al.: Iodine and thyroxine metabolism in anephric patients receiving chronic peritoneal dialysis. *J. Clin. Endocr. 31*:277, 1970b.

Oddie, T. H., Meade, J. H., Jr., et al.: An analysis of published data on thyroxine turnover in human subjects. *J. Clin. Endocr. 26*:425, 1966.

Odell, W. D., Utiger, R. D., et al.: Estimation of the secretion rate

of thyrotropin in man. *J. Clin. Invest. 46*:953, 1967.

Ogura, J., Wessler, S., et al.: Surgical approach to the ophthalmopathy of Graves' disease. *J.A.M.A. 216*:1627, 1971.

Olivo, J., Southren, A. L., et al.: Studies of the protein binding of testosterone in plasma in disorders of thyroid function: Effect of therapy. *J. Clin. Endocr. 31*:539, 1970.

Oppenheimer, J. H., and Werner, S. C.: Effect of prednisone on thyroxine-binding proteins. *J. Clin. Endocr. 26*:715, 1966.

Oppenheimer, J. H., Koerner, D., et al.: Specific nuclear triiodothyronine binding sites in rat liver and kidney. *J. Clin. Endocr. 35*:330, 1972.

Oppenheimer, J. H., Shapiro, H. C., et al.:Dissociation between thyroxine metabolism and hormonal action in phenobarbital-treated rats. *Endocrinology 88*:115, 1971.

Oppenheimer, J. H., Surks, M. I., et al.: The metabolic significance of exchangeable cellular thyroxine. *Recent Progr. Hormone Res. 25*:381, 1969.

Orme, M. C. L'E., and Conolly, M. E.: Hypoparathyroidism after iodine-131 treatment of thyrotoxicosis. *Ann. Intern. Med. 75*: 136, 1971.

Otten, J., Jonckheer, M., et al.: Thyroid albumin. II. In vitro synthesis of a thyroid albumin by normal human thyroid tissue. *J. Clin. Endocr. 32*:18-26, 1971.

Parker, R. H., and Beierwaltes, W. H.: Thyroid antibodies during pregnancy and in newborn. *J. Clin. Endocr. 21*:792, 1961.

Pasternak, D. P., Socolow, E. L., et al.: Synergistic interaction of phenazone and iodide on thyroid hormone biosynthesis in the rat. *Endocrinology 84*:769, 1969.

Perlmutter, M., and Mufson, M.: Inhibition of a cervical thyroid gland by a functioning struma ovarii. *J. Clin. Endocr. 11*:621, 1951.

Peters, J. P., and Van Slyke, D. D.: *Quantitative Clinical Chemistry.* Baltimore, Williams and Wilkins, 1946.

Pierce, J. G.: Eli Lilly Lecture: The subunits of pituitary thyrotropin—their relationship to other glycoprotein hormones. *Endocrinology 89*:1331, 1971a.

Pierce, J. G., Liao, T., et al.: Studies on the structure of thyrotropin: its relationship to luteinizing hormone. *Recent Progr. Hormone Res. 27*:165, 1971b.

Pinchera, A., MacGillivray, M. H., et al.: Thyroid refractoriness in an athyriotic cretin fed soybean formula. *New Eng. J. Med. 273*:83, 1965.

Pittman, J. A., Beschi, R. J., et al.: Methimazole: Its absorption and excretion in man and tissue distribution in rats. *J. Clin. Endocr. 33*:182, 1971.

Ramsay, I. D.: Muscle dysfunction in hyperthyroidism. *Lancet 2*:931, 1966.

Rapoport, B., Refetoff, S., et al.: Suppression of serum thyrotropin (TSH) by L-dopa in chronic hypothyroidism: interrelationships in the regulation of TSH and prolactin secretion. *J. Clin. Endocr. 36*:256, 1973.

Refetoff, S.: Resistance to the intracellular action of thyroid hormones. Program, Fifty-second meeting, The Endocrine Soc., Abstract 111, 1970, p. 92.

Reichlin, S., Martin, J. B., et al.: The hypothalamus in pituitary-thyroid regulation. *Recent Progr. Hormone Res. 28*:229, 1972.

Riddle, M. C., and Schwartz, T. B.: New tactics for hyperthyroidism: sympathetic blockade. *Ann. Intern Med. 72*:749, 1970.

Rivlin, R. S., and Langdon, R. G.: Effects of thyroxine upon biosynthesis of flavin mononucleotide and flavin adenine dinucleotide. *Endocrinology 84*:584, 1969.

Roques, M., Torresani, J., et al.: Relationship between thyroglobulin synthesis, iodine metabolism, and histogenesis in the developing rabbit fetal thyroid gland. *Gen. Comp. Endocr. 19*:457, 1972.

Rosenberg, I. N., and Bastomsky, C H.: Thyroid. *Ann. Rev. Physiol. 27*:71, 1965.

Royce, P. C.: Severely impaired consciousness in myxedema—a review. *Amer. J. Med. Sci. 261*:46, 1971.

Ruder, H., Corvol, P., et al.: Effects of induced hyperthyroidism on steroid metabolism in man. *J. Clin. Endocr. 33*:382, 1971.

Russell, W. O., Ibanez, M. L., et al.: Thyroid carcinoma. Classification, intraglandular dissemination, and clinicopathological study based upon whole organ sections of 80 glands. *Cancer 16*:1425, 1963.

Saenger, E. L., Thoma, G. E., et al.: Incidence of leukemia following treatment of hyperthyroidism. *J.A.M.A. 205*:855, 1968.

Sanders, V.: Neurologic manifestations of myxedema. *New Eng. J. Med. 266*:547 and 599, 1962.

Schleusener, H., Murthy, P. V. N., et al.: Studies on the thyroid gland component inhibiting LATS. *Metabolism 20*:299, 1971.

Schneider, P. B., and Wolff, J.: Thyroidal iodide transport. VI. A possible role for iodide-binding phospholipids. *Biochim. Biophys. Acta* 94:114, 1965.

Shillinglaw, J., and Utiger, R. D.: Failure of retro-orbital tissue to neutralize the biological activity of the long-acting thyroid stimulator. *J. Clin. Endocr.* 28:1069, 1968.

Shimaoka, K., Badillo, J., et al.: Clinical differentiation between thyroid cancer and benign goiter. *J.A.M.A.* 181:179, 1962.

Shishiba, Y., Shimizu, T., et al.: Direct evidence for human thyroidal stimulation by LATS-protector. *J. Clin. Endocr.* 36:517, 1973.

Sikkema, S. H.: Triiodothyronine in the diagnosis and treatment of hypothyroidism: failure to demonstrate the metabolic insufficiency syndrome (controlled study). *J. Clin. Endocr.* 20:545, 1960.

Simone, J. V., Abildgaard, C. F., et al.: Blood coagulation in thyroid dysfunction. *New Eng. J. Med.* 273:1057, 1965.

Singh, S. P., and McKenzie, J. M.: ^{35}S-sulfate uptake by mouse Harderian gland: effect of serum from patients with Graves' disease. *Metabolism* 20:422, 1971.

Skillern, P. G.: Genetics of Graves' disease. *Mayo Clinic Proc.* 47:848, 1972.

Smith, R. N., and Wilson, G. M.: Clinical trial of different doses of I^{131} in treatment of thyrotoxicosis. *Brit. Med. J.* 1:129, 1967.

Smith, R. N., Taylor, S. A., et al.: Controlled clinical trial of combined triiodothyronine and thyroxine in the treatment of hypothyroidism. *Brit. Med. J.* 4:145, 1970.

Snyder, L. M., and Reddy, W. J.: Mechanism of action of thyroid hormones on erythrocyte 2, 3-diphosphoglyceric acid synthesis. *J. Clin. Invest.* 49:1993, 1970.

Snyder, P. J., and Utiger, R. D.: Response to thyrotropin releasing hormone (TRH) in normal man. *J. Clin. Endocr.* 34:380, 1972a.

Snyder, P. J., and Utiger, R. D.: Thyrotropin response to thyrotropin releasing hormone in normal females over forty. *J. Clin. Endocr.* 34:1096, 1972b.

Sokal, J. E.: The problem of malignancy in nodular goiter—recapitulation and a challenge. *J.A.M.A.* 170:405, 1959.

Sokoloff, L., Roberts, P. A., et al.: Mechanisms of stimulation of protein synthesis by thyroid hormones in vivo. *Proc. Nat. Acad. Sci. USA* 60:652, 1968.

Solomon, D. H., and Chopra, I. J.: Graves' disease—1972. *Mayo Clinic Proc.* 47:803, 1972.

Solomon, D. H., Beck, J. C., et al.: Prognosis of hyperthyroidism treated by antithyroid drugs. *J.A.M.A.* 152:201, 1953.

Solomon, D. H., Benotti, J., et al.: A nomenclature for tests of thyroid hormones in serum: report of a committee of the American Thyroid Association. *J. Clin. Endocr.* 34:884, 1972.

Stanbury, J. B.: Familial goiter, In *The Metabolic Basis of Inherited Disease.* Stanbury, J. B., Wyngaarden, J. B., et al. (eds.), New York, McGraw-Hill, 1972.

Stein, M., Kimbel, P., et al.: Pulmonary function in hyperthyroidism. *J. Clin. Invest.* 40:348, 1961.

Steinberg, A. D.: Myxedema and coronary artery disease—a comparative autopsy study. *Ann. Intern. Med.* 68:338, 1968.

Sterling, K., Brenner, M. A., et al.: The significance of triiodothyronine (T$_3$) in maintenance of euthyroid status after treatment of hyperthyroidism. *J. Clin. Endocr.* 33:729, 1971.

Sterling, K., Refetoff, S., et al.: T$_3$ thyrotoxicosis. Thyrotoxicosis due to elevated serum triiodothyronine levels. *J.A.M.A.* 213:571, 1970.

Strauss, H. W., Hurley, P. J., et al.: Advantages of ^{99m}Tc pertechnetate for thyroid scanning in patients with decreased radioiodine uptake. *Radiology* 97:307, 1970.

Sung, L. C., and Cavalieri, R. R.: T$_3$ thyrotoxicosis due to metastatic thyroid carcinoma. *J. Clin. Endocr.* 36:215, 1973.

Surks, M. I., and Oppenheimer, J. H.: Metabolism of phenolic- and tyrosyl-ring labeled L-thyroxine in human beings and rats. *J. Clin. Endocr.* 33:612, 1971.

Surks, M. I., Schadlow, A. R., et al.: A new radioimmunoassay for plasma L-triiodothyronine: Measurements in thyroid disease and in patients maintained on hormonal replacement. *J. Clin. Invest.* 51:3104, 1972.

Surks, M. I., Schadlow, A. R., et al.: Determination of iodothyronine absorption and conversion of L-thyroxine (T$_4$) to L-triiodothyronine (T$_3$) using turnover rate techniques. *J. Clin. Invest.* 52:805, 1973.

Suzuki, H., and Mashimo, K.: Significance of the iodide-perchlorate discharge test in patients with ^{131}I-treated and untreated hyperthyroidism. *J. Clin. Endocr.* 34:332, 1972.

Tata, J. R., and Widnell, C. C.: Ribonucleic acid synthesis during the early action of thyroid hormones. *Biochem. J.* 98:604, 1966.

Taunton, O. D., McDaniel, H. G., et al.: Standardization of TSH testing. *J. Clin. Endocr.* 25:266, 1965.

Taurog, A., and Evans, E. S.: Extrathyroidal thyroxine formation in completely thyroidectomized rats. *Endocrinology* 80:915, 1967.

Temple, R., Berman, M., et al.: The use of lithium in Graves' disease. *Mayo Clinic Proc.* 47:872, 1972.

Terjung, R. L., and Tipton, C. M.: Plasma thyroxine and thyroid-stimulating hormone levels during submaximal exercise in humans. *Amer. J. Physiol.* 220:1840, 1971.

Torrigiani, G., Doniach, D., et al.: Serum thyroglobulin levels in healthy subjects and in patients with thyroid disease. *J. Clin. Endocr.* 29:305, 1969.

Tudhope, G. R., and Wilson, G. M.: Deficiency of vitamin B$_{12}$ in hypothyroidism. *Lancet* 1:703, 1962.

Turner-Warwick, R., Nabarro, J. D. N., et al.: Riedel's thyroiditis and retroperitoneal fibrosis. *Proc. Roy. Soc. Med.* 59:596, 1966.

Utiger, R. D.: Thyrotrophin radioimmunoassay: another test of thyroid function. *Ann. Intern. Med.* 74:627, 1971.

Vagenakis, A. G., Abreau, C. M., et al.: Prevention of recurrence in acute thyroiditis following corticosteroid withdrawal. *J. Clin. Endocr.* 31: 705, 1970.

Vagenakis, A. G., Downs, P., et al.: Control of thyroid hormone secretion in normal subjects receiving iodides. *J. Clin. Invest.* 52:528, 1973.

Vagenakis, A. G., Wang, C., et al.: Iodide-induced thyrotoxicosis in Boston. *New Eng. J. Med.* 287:523, 1972.

Vannotti, A., and Béraud, T.: Functional relationships between the liver, the thyroxine-binding protein of serum, and the thyroid. *J. Clin. Endocr.* 19:466, 1959.

Varma, V. M., Beierwaltes, W. H., et al.: Treatment of thyroid cancer. Death rates after surgery and after surgery followed by sodium iodide I^{131}. *J.A.M.A.* 214:1437, 1970.

Vickery, A. L., and Hamlin, E., Jr.: Struma lymphomatosa (Hashimoto's thyroiditis): observations on repeated biopsies in 16 patients. *New Eng. J. Med.* 264:266, 1961.

Vince, F. P., Boucher, B. J., et al.: The response of plasma sugar, free fatty acids, 11-hydroxycorticosteroids and growth hormone to insulin-induced hypoglycaemia and vasopressin in primary myxoedema. *J. Endocr.* 48:389, 1970.

Vinik, A., Pimstone, B., et al.: Impairment of hyperglycemic-induced growth hormone suppression in hyperthyroidism. *J. Clin. Endocr.* 28:1534, 1968.

Volpé, R., Row, V. V., et al.: Circulating viral and thyroid antibodies in subacute thyroiditis. *J. Clin. Endocr.* 27:1275, 1967.

Waal-Manning, H. J.: Effect of propranolol on the duration of the Achilles tendon reflex. *Clin. Pharmacol. Ther.* 10:199, 1969.

Wahner, H. W., Mayberry, W. E., et al.: Endemic goiter in the Cauca Valley. III. Role of serum TSH in goitrogenesis. *J. Clin. Endocr.* 32:491, 1971.

Wall, J. R., Good, B. F., et al.: Long-acting thyroid stimulator in euthyroid relatives of thyrotoxic patients. *Lancet* 2:1024, 1969.

Wallack, M. S., Adelberg, H. M., et al.: A thyroid suppression test using a single dose of L-thyroxine. *New Eng. J. Med.* 283:402, 1970.

Wartofsky, L., and Ingbar, S. H.: Estimation of the rate of release of non-thyroxine iodine from the thyroid glands of normal subjects and patients with thyrotoxicosis. *J. Clin. Endocr.* 33:488, 1971.

Wartofsky, L., Ransil, B. J., et al.: Inhibition by iodine of the release of thyroxine from the thyroid glands of patients with thyrotoxicosis. *J. Clin. Invest.* 49:78, 1970.

Wayne, E. J.: Clinical and metabolic studies in thyroid disease. *Brit. Med. J.* 1:78, 1960.

Webster, B. R., Guansing, A. R., et al.: Absence of diurnal variation of serum TSH. *J. Clin. Endocr.* 34:899, 1972.

Werner, S. C.: Classification of the eye changes of Graves' disease. *J. Clin. Endocr.* 29:982, 1969.

Werner, S. C.: Prednisone in emergency treatment of malignant exophthalmos. *Lancet* 1:1004, 1966.

Wilber, J. F., and Utiger, R. D.: The effect of glucocorticoids on thyrotropin secretion. *J. Clin. Invest.* 48:2096, 1969.

Wilkins, L.: Epiphysial dysgenesis associated with hypothyroidism. *Amer. J. Dis. Child.* 61:13, 1941.

Wilson, W. R., and Bedell, G. N.: The pulmonary abnormalities in myxedema. *J. Clin. Invest.* 39:42, 1960.

Winikoff, D., and Taylor, K.: Oral contraceptives and thyroid function tests. *Med. J. Aust. 2:*108, 1966.

Winship, T., and Rosvoll, R. V.: Childhood thyroid carcinoma. *Cancer 14:*734, 1961.

Woeber, K. A., and Ingbar, S. H.: Antithyroid effect of noncalorigenic congeners of salicylate, with observations on the influence of serum proteins on the potency of antithyroid agents. *Endocrinology 76:*584, 1965.

Woeber, K. A., and Ingbar, S. H.: The interactions of the thyroid hormones with binding proteins, In *Thyroid. Handbook of Physiology.* Greer, M. A., and Solomon, D. H. (eds.), Washington, American Physiological Society, 1973.

Woeber, K. A., Arky, R., et al.: Reversal by guanethidine of abnormal oral glucose tolerance in thyrotoxicosis. *Lancet 1:*895, 1966.

Woeber, K. A., Sobel, R. J., et al.: The peripheral metabolism of triiodothyronine in normal subjects and in patients with hyperthyroidism. *J. Clin. Invest. 49:*643, 1970.

Wolff, E. C., and Wolff, J.: The mechanism of action of the thyroid hormones, In *The Thyroid Gland.* Pitt-Rivers, R., and Trotter, W. R. (eds.), Washington, Butterworths, 1964.

Wolff, J.: Iodide goiter and the pharmacologic effects of excess iodide. *Amer. J. Med. 47:*101, 1969.

Wolff, J.: Transport of iodide and other anions in thyroid gland. *Physiol. Rev. 44:*45, 1964.

Wollman, S. H.: Heterogeneity of the thyroid gland, In *Current Topics in Thyroid Research.* Cassano, C., and Andreoli, M. (eds.), New York, Academic Press, 1965.

Woolner, L. B., Beahrs, O. H., et al.: Classification and prognosis of thyroid carcinoma. A study of 885 cases observed in a thirty-year period. *Amer. J. Surg. 102:*354, 1961.

Woolner, L. B., McConahey, W. M., et al.: Struma lymphomatosa (Hashimoto's thyroiditis) and related thyroidal disorders. *J. Clin. Endocr. 19:*53, 1959.

CHAPTER 5

The Adrenals

By Grant W. Liddle
and Kenneth L. Melmon

Part I:
The Adrenal Cortex

By Grant W. Liddle

THE NORMAL ADRENAL CORTEX

Embryology

During the fourth to sixth week of fetal life, cells from the coelomic mesoderm of the posterior abdominal wall near the mesonephros form a cluster between the root of the mesentery and the genital ridge to establish the fetal adrenal cortex. Some five weeks later, small basophilic cells appear

233

around the fetal cortex; these are the forerunners of the permanent adrenal cortex.

During the seventh week of embryonic development, the fetal adrenal cortex is invaded by cells migrating from the neural crest; these "sympathogonia" are forerunners of the adrenal medulla. They undergo further differentiation to form either ganglion cells or chromaffin cells; the latter secrete catecholamines.

The adrenal glands are relatively large structures during fetal life and undergo rapid involution during the first few months of extrauterine life (1). Much of the bulk of the fetal adrenal cortex is attributable to an inner zone of large acidophilic cells arranged in anastomosing cords, separated by large, thin-walled sinusoidal capillaries. The fetal cortex is ACTH-dependent and is relatively small in the absence of a functioning pituitary.

Anatomy

The adrenal glands are paired, convoluted, somewhat pyramidal structures which, as their name implies, are situated atop the kidneys. The outer portion, or cortex (approximately 80 per cent by weight in the normal adult), is firm and golden yellow; the inner portion, or medulla, is soft and reddish-brown in color. Normally, each gland weighs about 5 g.; they are smaller in conditions associated with a deficiency of ACTH and may become as much as four times larger in response to a chronic excess of ACTH.

The adrenals are supplied by numerous small arteries arising from the phrenic arteries, the aorta, and the renal arteries and occasionally by branches from the ovarian, spermatic, or intercostal arteries as well. These vessels penetrate the gland along connective tissue trabeculae and break up into a network of sinusoidal capillaries that extend radially into large venous lacunae in the medulla. Venules collect into a large central vein, which runs as an axis through the gland and empties, on the left, into the renal vein and, on the right, into the inferior vena cava. Anatomic variations are relatively common.

Histologically, the human adrenal has three zones: an outer *zona glomerulosa*, a middle *zona fasciculata*, and an inner *zona reticularis*, so named because of the arrangement of the cells in each zone (Fig. 5–1). The narrow subcapsular zona glomerulosa consists of relatively small, compact cells grouped in ill-defined clusters. Electron microscopy reveals elongated mitochondria with transverse shelflike infoldings of the inner mitochondrial membrane ("cristae"). The wider zona fasciculata consists of larger lipid-laden cells radially arranged in parallel cords. Here the mitochondria are more nearly spherical, and the cristae appear as short tubular invaginations of the inner membrane. The zona reticularis consists of anastomosing networks of cells which resemble those of the zona fasciculata except for the fact that they contain less lipid. Here the mitochondria are elongated and contain a mixture of tubular and flattened cristae. Differences in mitochondrial morphology are thought to be of aid in determining the origins of cells in adrenal neoplasms.

Biochemical Basis of Steroidogenesis

The adrenal cortex is able both to synthesize cholesterol and to take it up from the circulation. The cholesterol thus accumulated is then available for conversion into steroid hormones. The total process entails dozens of enzymatically governed chemical transformations. There is much that remains unknown about the natural processes of steroidogenesis because they are functions of subcellular organization, which is all too readily disrupted by experimental manipulation.

In certain cells, and presumably in the adrenal cortex, cholesterol is synthesized from acetate through a long series of reactions involving acetyl coenzyme A, mevalonic acid, squalene, lanosterol, zymosterol, and desmosterol as some of the intermediates. Whether cholesterol synthesis by the adrenal is as important quantitatively as cholesterol uptake from plasma has never been established with certainty, but both processes are known to occur, and under special circumstances it has been possible to demonstrate that the accumulation of cholesterol by the adrenal is stimulated by ACTH (2).

Normally, the rate-limiting step in biosynthesis of steroids is the conversion of cholesterol to pregnenolone.* Under all circumstances, an abundance of cholesterol is found in the adrenal cortex, most of it within cytoplasmic lipid droplets. Unless the adrenal cell is stimulated by one or another extraadrenal regulator, there is little utilization of the available cholesterol, and the formation of adrenal cortical steroids is minimal. In the presence of an adrenal stimulator, however, cholesterol is utilized to form 20α-hydroxycholesterol, which is then converted to 20α,22-dihydroxycholesterol, which then undergoes scission between carbon atoms 20 and 22 to yield *pregnenolone* and isocaproic aldehyde. The best known pathway of steroid biosynthesis involves the conversion of cholesterol to pregnenolone, which is readily transformed by a series of stable enzymes into the major biologically active corticosteroids (3). The major steps involved in the derivation of these hormonal steroids are depicted in Figure 5–2. In a side reaction, some cholesterol is converted to 17α-hydroxycholesterol, then to 17α,20-dihydroxycholesterol, then to 17α-hydroxypregnenolone, a possible precursor of the abundant but weak adrenal androgen, *dehydroepiandrosterone* (DHEA), as well as of the important glucocorticoid, *cortisol*.

The conversion of pregnenolone to cortisol by the zona fasciculata first entails the dehydrogenation of the 3β-hydroxyl group of pregnenolone to form

---

*For the sake of convenience, commonly used trivial names are employed in this chapter. Their equivalents in standard chemical nomenclature are listed in Table 5–1.

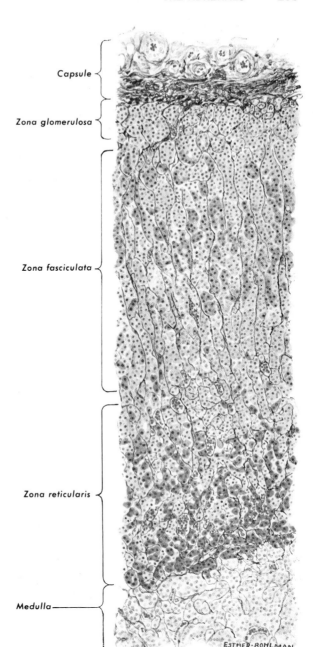

Figure 5-1. Adrenal histology shown in cross section. Mallory-azan stain. (Modified from Maximow and Bloom.)

Capsule

Zona glomerulosa

Zona fasciculata

Zona reticularis

Medulla

ESTHER·BOHLMAN

pregn-5-ene-3,20-dione. This then undergoes isomerization, with a shift of the double bond from the 5-6 position to the 4-5 position, forming *progesterone*. Two closely related enzymes are necessary for the conversion of pregnenolone to progesterone. The first is 3β-hydroxysteroid dehydrogenase, which oxidizes the 3β-ol to a 3-oxo group. The second is a Δ^5-3-oxosteroid isomerase, which catalyzes the migration of the double bond from the 5–6 to the 4–5 position. Progesterone is converted to 17α-hydroxyprogesterone by the action of a 17α-hydroxylase system. The 17α-hydroxyprogesterone is converted to 17α,21-dihydroxyprogesterone (11-deoxycortisol or "substance S" of Reichstein) by the 21-hydroxylase system. Finally, substance S is

converted to cortisol (Compound F) by the action of 11β-hydroxylase.

The zona fasciculata also forms a small amount of corticosterone as a by-product of cortisol synthesis. The pathway is identical except that progesterone escapes 17α-hydroxylation and proceeds directly to the 21-hydroxylase reaction and finally undergoes 11β-hydroxylation. It thus differs from cortisol only in that it lacks a 17α-hydroxyl group, but this structural difference accounts for a very great difference in the biologic potency of the two hormones.

The conversion of pregnenolone to aldosterone by the zona glomerulosa entails a series of enzymatically regulated steps similar to those involved

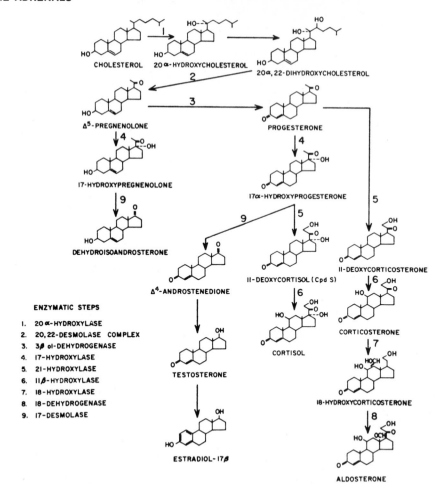

ENZYMATIC STEPS

1. 20 α-HYDROXYLASE
2. 20,22-DESMOLASE COMPLEX
3. 3β ol-DEHYDROGENASE
4. 17-HYDROXYLASE
5. 21-HYDROXYLASE
6. 11β-HYDROXYLASE
7. 18-HYDROXYLASE
8. 18-DEHYDROGENASE
9. 17-DESMOLASE

Figure 5–2. Major biosynthetic pathways for adrenal steroids. (From Temple, T. E., and Liddle, G. W.: *Ann. Rev. Pharmacol.* *10*:199, 1970.)

in cortisol synthesis but with three crucial differences. The zona glomerulosa lacks 17α-hydroxylase and, therefore, lacks the capacity to form 17α-hydroxyprogesterone; it is for this reason alone that the zona glomerulosa cannot synthesize cortisol. Instead it forms corticosterone, and some of this steroid is acted on by 18-hydroxylase to form 18-hydroxycorticosterone, and then by 18-hydroxysteroid dehydrogenase to form aldosterone. 18-Hydroxysteroid dehydrogenase is found only in the zona glomerulosa, and this is the reason that only the zona glomerulosa has the capacity to synthesize aldosterone.

Although among the products of the human adrenal cortex only cortisol and aldosterone appear to be essential for good health, the adrenal also produces a number of by-products, including androgens and estrogens. Quantitatively, the most important of these is dehydroepiandrosterone (DHEA), which is derived from 17α-hydroxypregnenolone by the action of 17-desmolase, an enzyme which cleaves two adjacent hydroxylated carbon atoms, in this case carbons 17 and 20. Much of the dehydroepiandrosterone formed by the adrenal is secreted without further modification, but a very

small amount is converted to the classical androgens, androst-4-ene-3,17-dione and testosterone. Any of these can undergo 11β-hydroxylation, and any can appear as a sulfate esterified at the 3-position. Although there is no doubt that the human adrenal can synthesize minute amounts of estrogen, the structural identity has been difficult to establish. It is reasonable to think that mechanisms known to be operative in gonadal tissue also work in the adrenal with enzymatic conversion of androst-4-ene-3, 17-dione to its 19-hydroxy derivative, then cleavage of the angular hydroxymethyl group, leaving an 18-carbon steroid with a phenolic ring A, the basic structure of the natural estrogens.

Under normal circumstances, the enzymatic transformation of pregnenolone to cortisol, corticosterone, aldosterone, and dehydroepiandrosterone occurs so rapidly that only these products accumulate in quantities sufficient to result in physiologically important secretion. As we shall see later, impairment of any of these enzymatic transformations can result in accumulation and secretion of biosynthetic intermediates in quantities sufficient to be of pathophysiologic importance.

TABLE 5–1. TRIVIAL NAMES OF ADRENAL HORMONES AND RELATED SUBSTANCES

Cyclic AMP: Adenosine-3',5'-monophosphate
ACTH: Adenocorticotropic hormone, corticotropin
MSH: Melanocyte-stimulating hormone, melanotropin
CRF: Corticotropin-releasing factor
Aldosterone: Pregn-4-ene-11β, 21-diol-3,20-dione-18-al
Androsterone: (5α)androstan-3-ol-17-one
Cortisol: Hydrocortisone; pregn-4-ene-11β, 17α,21-triol-3,20-dione
Cortisone: Pregn-4-ene-17α,21-diol-3,11,20-trione
Corticosterone: Pregn-4-ene-11β,21-diol-3,20-dione
Cortol: 5β-Pregnane-3α, 11β, 17, 20α, 21-pentol
Cortolone: Pregnane-3α, 17α, 20α, 21-tetrol-11-one
DHEA: Dehydroepiandrosterone, DHIA, dehydroisoandrosterone; androst-5-en-3β-ol-17-one
DOC: Deoxycorticosterone, 11-deoxycorticosterone; pregn-4-ene-21-ol-3,20-dione
Etiocholanolone: (5β)androstan-3-ol-17-one
17-Hydroxypregnenolone: Pregn-5-ene-3β, 17α-diol, 20-one
17-Hydroxyprogesterone: Pregn-4-en-17α-ol-3,20-dione
Pregnanetriol: Pregnane-3α,17α,20-triol
Pregnenolone: Pregn-5-en-3β-ol-20-one
Progesterone: Pregn-4-ene-3,20-dione
Substance S: 11-deoxycortisol, pregn-4-ene-17α,21-diol-3,20-dione
Tetrahydroaldosterone: Pregnane-3α,11β,21-triol-20-one-18-al
THE: Tetrahydrocortisone; pregnane-3α,17α,21-triol-11,20-dione
THF: Tetrahydrocortisol; pregnane-3α,11β,17α, 21-tetrol-20-one
THS: Tetrahydro S; pregnane-3α,17α,21-triol-20-one

Regulators of Adrenal Cortical Function

Adrenocorticotropic Hormone (ACTH)

The major regulator of adrenocortical growth and secretory activity is the anterior pituitary hormone, ACTH. This is one of many hormones now known to act through the mediation of cyclic AMP (see Ch. 16). ACTH attaches to receptors on the surface of the adrenal cortical cell and activates the enzyme, adenylate cyclase, which converts adenosine triphosphate (ATP) to adenosine 3',5'-monophosphate (cyclic AMP). This interesting compound serves as a cofactor in activating key enzymes of the adrenal cortex, called protein kinases. The most thoroughly studied protein kinases are composed of two subunits that are metabolically inactive when combined with each other. One subunit serves as a receptor for cyclic AMP, and the other is potentially catalytic. The attachment of cyclic AMP to the receptor results in dissociation of the receptor subunit from the catalytic subunit, which then acts to catalyze the transfer of phosphate groups from ATP to certain proteins. (By definition, "protein kinase" is an enzyme which catalyzes the transfer of phosphate radicals from ATP to a protein.) When phosphorylated, these proteins take on biologic activities that would otherwise be inapparent. Presumably, these phosphorylated proteins, directly or indirectly, stimulate the rate-limiting step in steroidogenesis and, in addition, induce adrenocortical growth.

ACTH has also been demonstrated to have a

TABLE 5–2. SOME EFFECTS OF ACTH

Adrenal
1. Maintenance of gland size
2. Depletion of ascorbic acid
3. Activation of adenylate cyclase
4. Accumulation of cholesterol
5. Conversion of cholesterol to pregnenolone
6. Maintenance of enzymes active in converting pregnenolone to hormonal steroids.

Extra-adrenal
1. Melanocyte stimulation
2. Activation of tissue lipase

number of effects on extra-adrenal tissues (Table 5–2), but their physiologic importance may be questioned inasmuch as they require high concentrations of ACTH. These extra-adrenal actions have also been shown to be mediated by cyclic AMP.

Structure-Function Relationships of ACTH and Its Analogues

Peptide chemists of the past three decades have defined the structure of ACTH and have provided numerous modifications of the natural hormone, which have been utilized in studies of structure-function relationships (4, 5). Several mammalian species have been found to produce corticotropic hormones that are single-chain polypeptides containing 39 amino acids (Fig. 5–3).

In all species that have been studied, the N-terminal 24 amino acids are the same, but minor species differences occur in amino acid composition in the 25–39 portion of the molecule.

The biologically active "core" of ACTH is its N-terminal 26 amino acids; this fragment of the hormone is almost equal to the complete molecule in biologic potency. In other words, as one shortens the 39-amino acid ACTH molecule by removing amino acids from the C-terminus, little or no change in potency occurs with removal of the C-terminal 13 amino acids. Thereafter, biologic potency is progressively reduced, so that the N-terminal 17 amino acid sequence has only about 5 per cent of that of the intact molecule. Removal of the seventeenth amino acid results in a fiftyfold loss of potency. Further shortening of the sequence results in further loss of adrenal-stimulating activity. The shortest fragment that has been found to have adrenocorticotropic activity is the N-terminal 10 amino acid sequence, which has only about 0.002 per cent of the biologic potency of the whole ACTH molecule (5).

Comparatively minor modifications of the N-terminal portion of the ACTH molecule may severely reduce biologic potency. Oxidation of the N-terminal serine to a glyoxylyl residue virtually destroys the adrenal-stimulating activity of ACTH, but substitution of a glycyl residue for the N-terminal serine has little or no effect on biologic potency. From such observations, it has been inferred that an intact α-NH$_2$ group, though not necessarily

AMINO ACID SEQUENCES OF HUMAN ADRENOCORTICOTROPIC AND MELANOCYTE
STIMULATING HORMONES

a-MSH
Acetyl-Ser.Tyr.Ser.Met.Glu.His.Phe.Arg.Trp.Gly.Lys.Pro.Val-NH$_2$
        1   2   3   4   5   6   7   8   9   10   11   12   13

β-MSH
Ala.Glu.Lys.Lys.Asp.Glu.Gly.Pro.Tyr.Arg.Met.Glu.His.Phe.Arg.Trp.Gly.Ser.Pro.Pro.Lys.Asp
  1   2   3   4   5   6   7   8   9   10   11   12   13   14   15   16   17   18   19   20   21   22

Figure 5-3.

ACTH
Ser.Tyr.Ser.Met.Glu.His.Phe.Arg.Trp.Gly.Lys.Pro.Val.Gly.Lys.Lys.Arg.Arg.
  1   2   3   4   5   6   7   8   9   10   11   12   13   14   15   16   17   18   Pro 19
                                                                                         Val 20
                                                                                         Lys 21

Phe.Glu.Leu.Pro.Phe.Ala.Glu.Ala.Ser.Glu.Asp.Glu.Ala.Gly.Asn.Pro.Tyr.Val
 39   38   37   36   35   34   33   32   31   30   29   28   27   26   25   24   23   22

a serine group, is requisite for biologic ACTH activity. Certain structural features of the ACTH molecule which were once thought to be essential for biologic activity are now known not to be absolutely essential. For example, the methionine residue in the fourth position from the N-terminus was formerly considered to be essential for full biologic activity, since its conversion to a sulfoxide by treatment with hydrogen peroxide was accompanied by loss of adrenal-stimulating activity. It is now known, however, that, in synthetic preparations of ACTH, an isoleucine can be substituted for the methionine without loss of biologic potency.

Several synthetic analogues of ACTH have had C-terminal amide groups rather than terminal carboxyl structures. In general, the amidated peptides have shown greater potency than their carboxylated congeners.

There is suggestive evidence that one fate of circulating ACTH is enzymatic cleavage of the 16–17 Lys-Arg bond by the plasmin-plasminogen system, leaving two fragments with practically no biologic activity but retaining immunoreactivity to antibodies directed toward the N-terminal and C-terminal portions of the ACTH molecule, respectively (6). The precise fate of ACTH as a chemical entity is unknown, but after it is injected, it is removed from the circulation by many tissues, the circulating half-time in man being of the order of 10 minutes. If ACTH is added to whole blood in the absence of tissues, its disappearance half-time is of the order of 48 minutes; if added to an acid or buffered aqueous solution containing no proteolytic enzymes, it is stable for days.

Dynamics of Adrenal Response to ACTH

In animals, the adrenal response to ACTH can be evaluated in terms of (1) an increase in cyclic AMP content, which occurs almost instantly and reaches a maximum within three minutes; (2) an increase in steroid secretion, which appears within about three minutes after a "pulse" of ACTH, peaks at about ten minutes, and wanes over a period of ten minutes or more, depending upon the dose of ACTH; (3) a decrease in adrenal ascorbic acid content, which is most marked an hour or two after the injection; or (4) an increase in adrenal size, which is apparent over a period of a day or more. In man, the only practical way to appraise the adrenal response to ACTH is to measure steroids, particularly plasma cortisol or the urinary metabolites of cortisol, the so-called 17-hydroxycorticosteroids. Although other indices of the secretory response to ACTH have been employed in the past, they are little used at the present time.

If a subject with normal adrenals receives, on separate occasions, several intravenous infusions of ACTH, both the total magnitude and the duration of the adrenal secretory responses are directly proportional to the dose of ACTH. The family of curves describing this relationship are represented in Figure 5–4.

A finite quantity of ACTH stimulates more cortisol secretion if it is administered slowly than if administered quickly. This is one of the main reasons underlying the development of depot preparations of ACTH for intramuscular injection. This relationship is represented in Figure 5–5, showing that 32 U. of ACTH infused intravenously over a 3-hour period stimulates only a small increase in 17-hydroxycorticosteroids on the day of injection. The same dose infused over a 12-, 24-, or 48- hour period stimulates proportionately larger increases in urinary 17-hydroxycorticosteroids.

Repetitive treatment with ACTH enhances the responsiveness of the adrenal to standard ACTH stimulation. For example, if one administers 50 U. of ACTH as an 8-hour intravenous infusion on five successive days, urinary 17-hydroxycorticosteroids are likely to be about twice as high on the fifth day as on the first. The increase in responsiveness is retained only for a short time. It can still be demonstrated if one gives another infusion after a lapse of one or two days but will have disappeared if one waits more than a week before giving the next infusion of ACTH. Conversely, if one suppresses endogenous ACTH for a time by administering dexamethasone, there is a decrease in adrenal responsiveness. If one measures 17-hydroxycorticosteroids in response to a standard 8-hour infu-

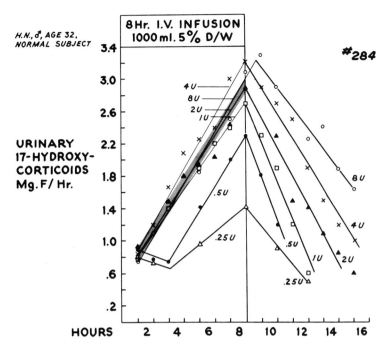

H.N., ♂, AGE 32, NORMAL SUBJECT

Figure 5-4. Hourly steroidogenic response to various doses of α-corticotropin (hog, administered by an 8-hour intravenous infusion. (From DiRaimondo, V. C., et al.: *Metabolism* 4:110, 1955.)

sion of ACTH on day 1, then gives dexamethasone on days 2 and 3 and tests the 17-hydroxycorticosteroid response to ACTH on day 4, the response will be only half as great as on day 1.

For practical considerations, there is a threshold dose of ACTH below which the adrenal response is almost imperceptible, and there is a larger dose that induces a "maximal" adrenal secretory response. This simply refers to the fact that, beyond a certain point in the dose-response curve, further increments in ACTH dosage do not induce further increments in cortisol secretion. Between these limits there is a rectilinear relationship between the log-dose of ACTH and the magnitude of the steroid secretory response. Perceptible stimulation of steroidogenesis occurs with plasma ACTH concentrations in the neighborhood of 0.1 mU. per 100 ml. (10 pg. per ml.). Such concentrations can be achieved by the infusion (or secretion) of a mere 0.5

mU. per minute or 0.2 U. over an 8-hour period. Almost maximal adrenal stimulation occurs with about thirty times this amount of ACTH, a plasma concentration of about 3 mU. per 100 ml. resulting from an infusion of about 6 U. per 8-hour period. These facts have had many practical implications for our understanding of pituitary-adrenal relationships in many clinical disorders. A preliminary view of the plasma ACTH concentrations encountered under various normal and abnormal clinical conditions is presented in Figure 5–6.

Regulation of ACTH Secretion

Since the normal adrenal secretes significant quantities of cortisol only in response to ACTH, it is possible to transform the question, "What regulates cortisol," into the question, "What regulates ACTH secretion?" If one interrupts the portal vessels which pass from the hypothalamus to the anterior pituitary, pituitary-adrenal function usually diminishes to minimal levels. This plus the fact that hypothalamic extracts contain a "corticotropin releasing factor" or "CRF" has led to the concept that the secretion of ACTH is governed largely by the hypothalamus (7). CRF is thought to act by stimulating cyclic AMP formation within ACTH-secreting cells. This is not the whole story, however, for there is experimental and clinical evidence that corticosteroids act, at least in part, at the level of the anterior pituitary to suppress ACTH secretion. Recent experiments have suggested that the hypothalamic secretion of CRF is stimulated by cholinergic neurons and inhibited by adrenergic neurons.

For practical purposes, the secretion of ACTH by

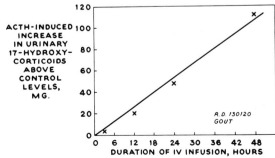

STEROIDOGENIC EFFECTIVENESS OF ACTH AS A FUNCTION OF DURATION OF INFUSION (EACH INFUSION 32 USP UNITS, X-5229)

Figure 5-5.

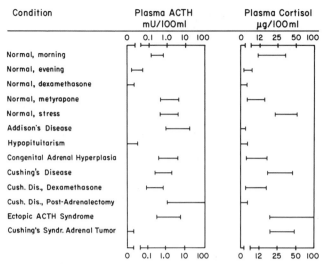

Figure 5–6. Typical values for plasma ACTH in various clinical states.

the normal pituitary may be considered to be governed by three factors: cortisol-like steroids, a "biologic clock," and stress. Each factor will be described separately, and some observations regarding their interaction will be summarized.

Negative Feedback Action of Corticosteroids. If other things are equal, the higher the level of cortisol-like steroids, the less ACTH is secreted. Of the products of the human adrenal cortex, only cortisol itself has much ACTH-suppressing activity. There are, however, a multitude of synthetic corticosteroids which share this along with the other biologic properties of cortisol. If cortisol levels are supraphysiologic, ACTH secretion is suppressed, and the adrenal ceases its secretory activity until cortisol levels return to normal. Conversely, if cortisol levels are subnormal, the anterior pituitary is released from this suppressive influence, ACTH levels rise, and the adrenal secretes cortisol until normal blood levels are restored. This is a classic example of a negative feedback or "servomechanism," which is important in maintaining homeostasis.

Pituitary-Adrenal Rhythms. The normal individual has higher blood ACTH levels in the morning than in the evening. This accounts for the well-known diurnal rhythms in cortisol secretion, plasma cortisol concentration, and 17-hydroxycorticosteroid excretion. The regularity of this rhythm is a function of one's sleep-wake habits. Normal subjects who sleep regularly at the same hours each day develop ACTH-cortisol secretory patterns characterized by a sharp increase during the third to fifth hours of sleep, reaching a maximum shortly after the hour of awakening, and falling irregularly throughout the waking day to reach minimal values during the few hours before and after resumption of sleep (Fig. 5–7). The timing and duration of the pituitary-adrenal secretory cycle can be altered by consistent revision of the timing and duration of the sleep-wake schedule (8). The presence of a rhythm in ACTH secretion has been demonstrated not only in subjects with normal adrenal

function but also in patients with primary adrenal insufficiency (9). Thus patients with Addison's disease who teleologically "need" more cortisol at all hours of the day, as evidenced by their round-the-clock elevations of ACTH, nevertheless have distinctly higher plasma ACTH levels in the morning than in the evening.

Pituitary-Adrenal Responses to Stress. Superimposed upon all other regulators of ACTH secretion is the stimulatory influence of *stress*. Regardless of the time of day and regardless of the level of plasma cortisol, the normal individual responds to a major stress (such as a laparotomy) with a brisk increase in ACTH secretion and a consequent increase in cortisol secretion. Among the stresses that have been shown to induce increased pituitary-adrenal activity are severe trauma, pyrogens, acute hypoglycemia, injections of histamine, electroconvulsive treatments, and acute anxiety. It has been observed that plasma cortisol concentrations are generally elevated in dying patients.

It appears that the "biologic clock" and "stress" work through the central nervous system to stimu-

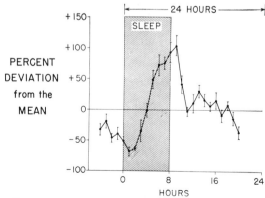

Figure 5–7. Temporal pattern of plasma cortisol concentrations in normal subjects who sleep at regular hours. (From Orth, D. N., Island, D. P., et al.: *J. Clin. Endocr.* 27:549, 1967.)

late ACTH secretion and that cortisol works at the level of the pituitary (and possibly at CNS levels as well) to suppress ACTH secretion. Although much remains to be learned about the precise mechanisms through which each factor regulates ACTH secretion, it can be said that the three act as physiologic vectors. Other things being equal, the lower the plasma cortisol, the greater will be the secretion of ACTH. Other things being equal, the greater the stress, the greater will be the secretion of ACTH. And other things being equal, ACTH is secreted most abundantly during the late hours of sleep and the early hours of the waking day.

Secretion of ACTH by Neoplasms. As will be discussed in detail under the heading "Cushing's Syndrome," ACTH is sometimes secreted in unregulated fashion by tumors arising in various extrapituitary sites. These tumors appear to be unresponsive to stress. They fail to conform to the influence of biologic clocks. With very rare exceptions they appear to be uninfluenced by circulating corticosteroid levels.

Pituitary tumors often secrete ACTH in semiautonomous fashion. Their responses to stress are ambiguous: they seem to secrete ACTH in response to severe surgical stress but not in response to hypoglycemia or pyrogens. They do not conform to the influence of the normal biologic clock. They are somewhat suppressible, but not to a normal degree, by elevated concentrations of corticosteroids.

Measurement of ACTH

Extracts of pituitary tissue have long been assayable for their content of ACTH by a variety of methods which, though reliable and specific, lack the sensitivity needed to detect ACTH in plasma. Most of these methods have depended directly on an adrenal response to ACTH. In order to be certain that the assay animal was responding to the ACTH in the test material and not to endogenous ACTH secreted in response to stress, most assay methods have employed hypophysectomized animals incapable of secreting endogenous ACTH. The adrenal responses that have provided quantitative indices of the amount of ACTH in the test dose have included the following:

1. *Adrenal weight.* ACTH prevents the loss of adrenal weight that would otherwise occur in the hypophysectomized animal.

2. *Adrenal ascorbic acid depletion.* ACTH stimulates the discharge of ascorbic acid from the adrenal gland of the hypophysectomized rat.

3. *Corticosteroid secretion.* ACTH stimulates increases in plasma cortisol, plasma corticosterone, urinary 17-hydroxycorticosteroids, and urinary 17-ketosteroids in various species.

4. *Thymic weight, liver glycogen, circulating eosinophils.* The corticosterone that is secreted in response to ACTH causes involution of the thymus gland, deposition of glycogen in the liver, and decreases in circulating eosinophils of the hypophysectomized rat.

In order to assay the ACTH content of plasma, it has generally been necessary to concentrate the hormone by some extraction procedure prior to assay (10). This has been achieved by the use of agents such as oxycellulose, the cation exchange resin Amberlite IRC-50, or Quoso. The ACTH content of 5 to 50 ml. of plasma can then be assayed in one of the following systems:

1. Measurement of the acute increase in plasma corticosterone of the hypophysectomized rat.

2. Measurement of corticosterone production by freshly prepared suspensions of adrenal cells.

3. Radioimmunoassay: measurement of the degree of displacement of radioactive ACTH from specific ACTH antibodies by the nonradioactive ACTH in the test material (11).

Recent improvements in the last two methods have made it possible to assay ACTH in unextracted plasma, but the procedures are not easy and, reliably performed, are of extremely limited availability.

The Renin-Angiotensin System

A major regulator of aldosterone production by the zona glomerulosa is the renin-angiotensin system (12). Renin is an enzyme that is released into the circulation by the juxtaglomerular apparatus of the nephron. The action of renin is to cleave a plasma globulin, "renin substrate," to release the decapeptide, *angiotensin I*. This substance is further hydrolyzed to an octapeptide, *"angiotensin II,"* by a "converting enzyme" which is found in abundance in the lung. Angiotensin II has been known for many years to be an extremely potent vasoconstrictor; in recent years it has been found to stimulate the formation of aldosterone.

Mode of Action and Temporal Aspects

The precise mechanism through which angiotensin stimulates aldosterone biosynthesis has not been elucidated. Whatever the mechanism of its action, angiotensin appears to stimulate the conversion of cholesterol to pregnenolone, which then serves as a precursor of the progesterone → desoxycorticosterone → corticosterone → 18-hydroxycorticosterone → aldosterone pathway (13). The onset of action is rapid and is demonstrable within minutes of the time the adrenal is exposed to angiotensin; it ceases within minutes after angiotensin has been removed. If other factors are held constant, the aldosterone secretory response of the adrenal is proportional to the dose of angiotensin.

Angiotensin itself is a very labile peptide which, in plasma and tissues, is quickly destroyed by angiotensinases. The circulating half-time of angiotensin is only of the order of one minute, in contrast to that of renin, which has a circulating half-time in man of more than ten minutes. Renin substrate appears to be abundantly available under all circumstances *in vivo*; plasma concentrations are particularly high during pregnancy and during treatment with supraphysiologic doses of estrogen (e.g., oral contraceptives). Plasma renin activity (PRA) as it is ordinarily measured in clinical laboratories is elevated under these circumstances, as is the aldosterone secretion rate (14).

Regulation of Renin Secretion

A whole host of circumstances leads to increased renin secretion, but many of them can be viewed as working through a smaller number of final common pathways.

Renal cell suspensions have been shown to increase their production of renin in the presence of cyclic AMP, epinephrine, or norepinephrine (15). It has been speculated that these effects of the catecholamines in renin-producing cells (like those in other tissues) might be mediated by cyclic AMP. *In vivo*, exogenous epinephrine and norepinephrine stimulate renin release, and there is indirect evidence that endogenous catecholamines and the sympathetic nervous system may mediate the stimulation of renin secretion by painful stimuli, upright posture, and hypovolemia (16).

One of the earliest facts established concerning the regulation of renin was that it is increased by compromising the blood flow to the kidney. This obviously occurs when a renal artery is constricted or becomes stenotic as a consequence of some disease, such as atherosclerosis or fibromuscular dysplasia. It occurs in a more subtle way whenever intravascular volume is reduced by exsanguination, dehydration, sodium depletion, or hypoalbuminemia. It can also occur when blood is sequestered on the venous side of the circulation by processes such as constriction of the vena cava, hepatic cirrhosis, or congestive heart failure. It has been shown experimentally that it is the decrease in perfusion pressure of the kidney rather than the decrease in the volume of blood flow that serves as the stimulus to renin release (17), and it is considered likely that baroreceptors associated with the juxtaglomerular apparatus mediate this response.

The regulation of renin secretion is more intricate than this, however, for it has also been shown that the magnitude of sodium flux in the region of the macula densa of the ascending limb of Henle's loop is also a determinant of renin secretion. In many circumstances, a change in perfusion and a change in macula densa sodium flux work together to regulate renin secretion, and it has been necessary to devise experiments of great elegance to demonstrate that the two mechanisms can operate independently of each other (18).

A diurnal rhythm has been demonstrated in plasma renin activity. If other factors such as diet and posture are held constant, plasma renin activity is lower in the afternoon than in the forenoon in normal subjects who habitually sleep at night and are awake during the day. It seems probable that this rhythm is controlled by the nervous system, that it is related to a similar rhythm in renal function (glomerular filtration and solute excretion

tend to be greater during the afternoon than during the forenoon), and that it in turn leads to a diurnal rhythm in aldosterone secretion, which is generally greater in the forenoon than in the afternoon.

A variety of other agents have also been shown to influence renin secretion. Angiotensin II itself has a direct inhibitory effect on renin secretion, thus completing the circuit in a "short loop" negative feedback system. Potassium depletion has a tendency to increase renin secretion and potassium loading to suppress it, but these effects may be obscured by changes in sodium metabolism, since potassium loading leads to increased sodium excretion and potassium depletion leads to sodium retention. Adrenergic blocking agents tend to decrease renin secretion. Agents that induce acute vasodilation, such as nitroprusside, increase renin secretion. Diazoxide, an arteriolar relaxant, increases renin secretion not only when administered systemically but also when injected directly into one renal artery. Potent diuretics such as furosemide induce acute increases in renin secretion. In general, if one wishes to appraise a patient's renin production in a meaningful way, it is best for him to receive no medications or to have the medications administered according to a well-standardized protocol.

From the standpoint of practical adrenal physiology, the most interesting determinant of renin secretion is aldosterone, which acts indirectly to suppress renin secretion and thus acts even more indirectly to suppress the further secretion of aldosterone, thus completing the circuit in a "long loop" negative feedback system. The relationships between renin and aldosterone are illustrated in Figure 5–8. The administration of aldosterone or the autonomous secretion of aldosterone by an adrenal adenoma results in sodium retention which, in the presence of a normal osmoregulatory mechanism, necessarily results in water retention. The resultant expansion of the extracellular fluid compartment is associated with some expansion in blood volume, which is interpreted by the arterial side of the circulation as an increase in "effective" blood volume. This brings about an increase in perfusion pressure of the kidney, resulting in suppression of renin secretion. Thus in "primary aldos-

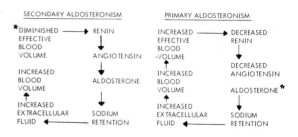

Figure 5–8. Typical relationships between renin and aldosterone secretion in secondary aldosteronism as contrasted with primary aldosteronism. In each part of the diagram, the asterisk represents the primary physiologic abnormality: diminished effective blood volume in secondary aldosteronism, and autonomous secretion of aldosterone in primary aldosteronism.

teronism," one finds a combination of high aldosterone secretion rate and low plasma renin activity (19). In contrast, there are several physiologic disorders in which there are decreases in effective blood volume. These are associated with increased secretion of renin and increased generation of angiotensin, which stimulates increased secretion of aldosterone. Again, the aldosterone promotes retention of sodium and water and expansion of the extracellular fluid compartment, culminating in a compensatory increase in blood volume and effective blood volume. This sequence is commonly referred to as "secondary aldosteronism." These relationships between renin and aldosterone can be generalized. An increase in renin-angiotensin activity, regardless of the cause, tends to increase aldosterone secretion; and a primary excess of any mineralocorticoid tends to suppress renin production. (See also Ch. 20.)

Measurement of Renin and Angiotensin

Angiotensin can be assayed in terms of its pressor activity in anesthetized, nephrectomized, pentolinium-blocked rats (20). Properly performed, this is a very sensitive and reliable assay method. It does not distinguish between angiotensin I and angiotensin II, since the former is quickly converted to the latter by a "converting enzyme" which is found in the lungs in very significant quantities. For most practical purposes, this distinction is unimportant.

The development of specific antibodies to angiotensin I and angiotensin II has made it possible to measure one or the other of these peptides by radioimmunoassay (21). Because the angiotensins are so labile in plasma and because they are generated in untreated plasma, great care must be taken in collection and storage of specimens for angiotensin assay, including special attention to the inactivation of renin, the inactivation of angiotensinases, and sequestration of angiotensin on special resins.

Renin can be assayed by incubating the specimen under standard conditions in the presence of the plasma α_2-globulin, renin substrate, and then measuring the amount of angiotensin I that is generated. The angiotensin may be measured either by bioassay or radioimmunoassay. There is generally enough renin substrate in normal plasma so that renin can be assayed by incubating plasma without the special addition of substrate. When the assay is performed in this way, one ordinarily refers to the result as "plasma renin activity" (PRA). More specific assays of renin require kinetic analysis of the rate of generation of angiotensin I from precisely controlled quantities of renin substrate under standard conditions. Following the same principles, renin substrate can also be assayed by quantifying the rate of generation of angiotensin I that is catalyzed by a known quantity of renin (14).

Other Regulators of Adrenal Function

Electrolytes are of some practical importance in regulating the secretion of aldosterone, over and above their effects on extracellular fluid volume and renin production. Increases in potassium concentration stimulate and hypokalemia tends to minimize aldosterone biosynthesis (22). Sodium concentration has also been shown to modify aldosterone secretion, at least in experimental situations: hyponatremia stimulates aldosterone secretion. These regulators tend to function as negative feedback regulators of aldosterone secretion, since potassium excretion is promoted by aldosterone, and aldosterone secretion is in turn suppressed by potassium depletion; sodium excretion is decreased by aldosterone, and aldosterone secretion is in turn stimulated by hyponatremia. (It should be noted, however, that hyponatremia is often a consequence of persistent antidiuretic hormone action and is accompanied by bodily fluid expansion which tends to suppress rather than stimulate aldosterone secretion. Thus the relationships noted above have often had to be demonstrated by carefully designed experiments in which one factor was held constant while the other was varied.)

Melanocyte-stimulating hormone (MSH) and its structural analogues have slight corticosterone-stimulating activity in the rat, and Rudman has even shown that, in the rabbit, β-MSH has the same order of adrenal stimulating potency as ACTH (23). It remains to be shown that MSH has significant adrenal-stimulating activity in human physiology. Certain prostaglandins have been shown by Kaplan's group to have steroidogenic activity *in vitro* (24). Whether they have importance in normal physiology or in pathologic situations remains uncertain. In extremely large doses, vasopressin has direct adrenal-stimulating activity; it also stimulates the release of ACTH. Calcium ions are necessary for the steroidogenic action of ACTH, but as yet no clinical perturbation of calcium metabolism has been shown to be extreme enough to affect the rate of steroidogenesis.

Although it has no obvious effect on steroidogenesis, growth hormone has been demonstrated to promote an increase in adrenal size and, perhaps related to this, to stimulate ornithine decarboxylase activity in the adrenal. In both of these actions, growth hormone acts synergistically with ACTH. There is perhaps another pituitary factor which promotes the conversion of corticosterone to aldosterone *in vitro*.

Other factors have been shown to modify adrenal function under experimental conditions, but their possible physiologic significance remains to be established.

Metabolic Fates of Adrenal Steroids

Transcortin: Steroid Binding Globulin (25)

Once secreted, cortisol becomes associated with "transcortin," a plasma glycoprotein with high affinity for cortisol, progesterone, deoxycorticosterone, corticosterone, and some but not all synthetic corticosteroid analogues. Under most physiologic circumstances, about 75 per cent of the plasma cortisol is tightly but reversibly bound to transcortin, one molecule of cortisol to one molecule of transcortin. About 15 per cent of the plasma cortisol is loosely bound to albumin; about 10 per cent of the plasma cortisol is unbound. It is this unbound fraction that is free to move into cells either to exert metabolic effects or to be transformed into an inactive metabolite. The reversibility of the binding of cortisol to transcortin is such that the transcortin-bound fraction and total plasma cortisol can fall from high normal values (e.g., 25 μg. per 100 ml.) to low values (e.g., 5 μg. per 100 ml.) within a period of less than three hours as the unbound fraction is cleared by the liver, provided there is no newly secreted cortisol to add to the pool size.

In normal pregnancy, and during treatment with supraphysiologic doses of estrogen, although cortisol secretion rates are not increased, plasma cortisol concentrations are increased two- to threefold, owing to increased plasma concentrations of transcortin.

Diseases characterized by hypoalbuminemia (e.g., the nephrotic syndrome) are usually characterized by subnormal plasma transcortin levels and correspondingly low plasma cortisol concentrations. Certain families have a genetically-determined absence of transcortin and extremely low levels of plasma cortisol. These deviations from normal do not appear to have any serious consequences with regard to the efficacy of cortisol, the adrenal production of cortisol, or the ultimate metabolism of cortisol. The teleologic importance of transcortin is, therefore, open to doubt; nevertheless, its presence makes life easier for the adrenal physiologist, since it results in the development of higher (and therefore more readily measurable) plasma concentrations of cortisol than would occur otherwise.

In Cushing's syndrome (clinical hypercortisolism), the hypersecretion of cortisol tends to overload the binding capacity of transcortin, so that an abnormally high proportion of the plasma cortisol is unbound. Unbound cortisol is more readily excreted in the urine than is protein-bound cortisol; therefore, patients with Cushing's syndrome often have distinctly supernormal levels of urinary cortisol, a fact that has been turned to diagnostic use by some.

Transcortin concentrations, unlike cortisol concentrations, are quite constant throughout the day and from day to day. They are not affected by hyper- or hypocortisolism. When subjects are treated with estrogen, transcortin concentrations rise to a plateau within three to five days. After estrogen is withdrawn, transcortin decreases with a half-time of four to five days, and levels are normal within two weeks.

Although certain other steroids do have affinity for transcortin, they are ordinarily secreted in such small quantities that they do not seriously compete with cortisol for binding sites on the protein molecule. Aldosterone, for example, has some affinity for transcortin but less than that of cortisol; moreover, in comparison with cortisol, plasma concentrations are extremely low. Dehydroisoandrosterone, androstenedione, and the various steroid conjugates have little affinity for transcortin. Testosterone and estradiol have little affinity for transcortin but happen to have high affinity for yet another plasma protein (Chs. 6 and 7).

Extra-Adrenal Metabolism of Corticosteroids

The metabolic inactivation of hormonal steroids is, in the main, unrelated to the mechanism through which steroids exert their physiologic effects. The latter subject will be considered later. There is no evidence that the human body can destroy the basic steroid nucleus. Furthermore, intact, biologically active corticosteroids are excreted in various bodily fluids only in trace quantities. The general fate of corticosteroids is to undergo inactivation by enzymes which introduce oxygen or hydrogen atoms at one or more positions. They are then conjugated to form water-soluble derivatives which are excreted in the urine.

The major organ for inactivating steroids is the liver, and the major process through which corticosteroids are inactivated involves the enzymatic reduction of the 4–5 double bond in "ring A" to form the dihydrosteroid derivative, which is generally devoid of biologic activity. The dihydro derivative is quickly converted to a tetrahydro derivative by the enzymatic reduction of the 3-oxo group to a 3-hydroxyl group. This derivative is then readily conjugated with glucuronic acid, forming a water-soluble product which is rapidly excreted by the kidneys.

Thus a major derivative of cortisol is tetrahydrocortisol glucuronide (Fig. 5–9). A major derivative of aldosterone is tetrahydroaldosterone glucuronide. A major derivative of corticosterone is tetrahydrocorticosterone glucuronide. DOC is excreted as tetrahydro-DOC glucuronide, and 11-deoxycortisol (substance S) is excreted as tetrahydro-S glucuronide.

Cortisol can be converted to cortisone by the action of 11β-hydroxysteroid dehydrogenase, and cortisone is then metabolized and excreted as tetrahydrocortisone glucuronide. In similar fashion, corticosterone can be converted to its 11-oxo analogue, "compound A," which is then metabolized and excreted as tetrahydro-A glucuronide.

Cortisol and other steroids with 20-oxo groups can be acted on by enzymes which convert the 20-oxo to 20-hydroxyl groups. These steroids, too, are subject to ring-A reduction, conjugation, and excretion as glucuronides. Thus cortisol can be converted to cortol glucuronide, progesterone to pregnanediol glucuronide, and 17-hydroxyprogesterone to pregnanetriol glucuronide.

A number of other pathways of metabolic inactivation are known. One involves a desmolase re-

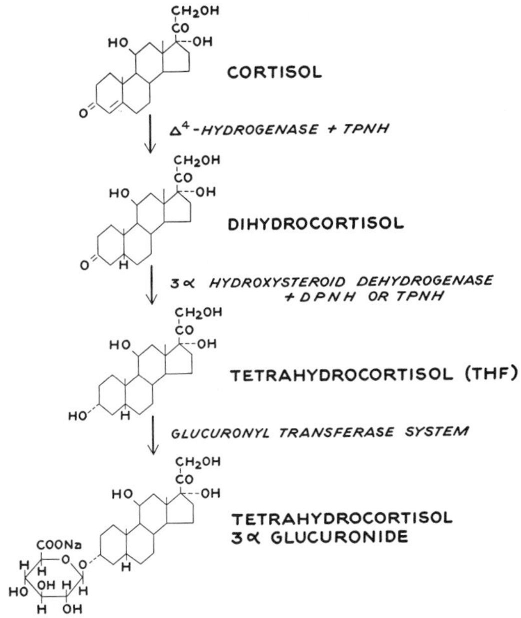

CORTISOL

Δ^4-HYDROGENASE + TPNH

DIHYDROCORTISOL

3α HYDROXYSTEROID DEHYDROGENASE + DPNH OR TPNH

TETRAHYDROCORTISOL (THF)

GLUCURONYL TRANSFERASE SYSTEM

TETRAHYDROCORTISOL 3α GLUCURONIDE

Figure 5–9. Steps in the metabolism of cortisol by the liver and its excretion by the kidney.

action which cleaves the 17–20 carbon linkage, yielding 17-ketosteroids. This reaction is limited to steroids which have 17α-hydroxyl groups and 20-oxo groups. Cortisol is one such steroid, and approximately 5 per cent of cortisol appears in the urine as a 17-ketosteroid.

A small proportion of cortisol is metabolized by hydroxylation at 6α-position. This pathway is greatly enhanced by drugs which induce hepatic 6α-hydroxylase, such as phenobarbital and o,p'-DDD (3,3 bis [p-aminophenyl] butanone-2). This pathway is also increased during pregnancy.

Aldosterone, in addition to being susceptible to ring-A reduction, which results in the formation of tetrahydroaldosterone, is also susceptible to conjugation with glucuronic acid at the 18-oxo position. This is formed both in the liver and in the kidney. It is very water-soluble and is readily excreted into the urine. It can be cleaved by acid, yielding free aldosterone, and this fact is often used to advantage in the clinical measurement of urinary aldosterone.

Dehydroepiandrosterone (DHEA), the major C-19 product of the human adrenal is, in the main, conjugated with sulfuric acid. DHEA sulfate is bound to plasma protein, and in this form it is not readily excreted but circulates in higher concentrations than any other steroid. DHEA is the principal precursor of the urinary 17-ketosteroids. Its metabolism is complex, but a major portion of the DHEA is oxidized at the 3-position to form androst-5-ene-3,17-dione. This is then acted on by an isomerase to form androst-4-ene-3,17-dione, which then undergoes the now familiar reduction of ring A to the tetrahydro derivatives, androsterone and etiocholanolone. A portion of these metabolites are conjugated with glucuronic acid but a larger portion with sulfate. The urinary sulfates can be

hydrolyzed enzymatically or with acid in order to liberate the water-insoluble steroids preparatory to their measurement as 17-ketosteroids. It will be noted that DHEA is metabolized to the same excretory end-products as testosterone. DHEA itself has little if any androgenic activity, but a small proportion of it is metabolized to testosterone and thus assumes biologic importance as an androgen. It has become traditional to minimize the value of urinary 17-ketosteroids as an index of androgen production; indeed, testosterone is such a potent androgen that it can induce full virilization without giving rise to enough urinary 17-ketosteroids to be clearly detectable. Nevertheless, when clear-cut virilization is due to an excess of *adrenal* steroids, DHEA is usually produced in sufficient quantities to elevate the urinary 17-ketosteroids. The measurement of urinary 17-ketosteroids, therefore, is of practical clinical value in evaluating patients with virilizing disorders.

Although the liver is the major extra-adrenal site of corticosteroid metabolism, it is not the only one. Other tissues, including muscle, skin, fibroblasts, intestine, and lymphocytes, can carry on oxidation-reduction reactions at the 3-, 11-, 17-, and 20-positions of the corticosteroid molecule, all positions where oxygen functions can exist either as oxo or hydroxyl groups.

The numerous minor pathways of corticosteroid metabolism lie beyond the scope of the present chapter. The interested reader will find a wealth of information on the entire subject of extra-adrenal metabolism of corticosteroids in a recent article by Peterson (26).

Functions of Adrenal Steroids

Molecular Biology of Steroid Action

It is currently thought that steroids of all groups exert their biologic effects in the following way (27). As lipid-soluble substances, steroid hormones can diffuse freely through cell membranes, reaching the cytoplasm. A target tissue of a particular steroid has cytoplasmic receptor proteins which exhibit high affinity for the steroid in question. The steroid-receptor complex migrates into the nucleus, where it becomes attached to specific areas of the chromatin and serves to de-repress or activate certain genes, allowing their expression in the formation of new RNA. The new RNA controls the formation of new proteins, some of which are important in cell structure and some in cell replication. Some are enzymes regulating metabolic functions of the cells, and some are transported out of the target cells as secretory products. Certain steroids compete with others in their affinity for the cytoplasmic receptors and, in doing so, act as biologic antagonists. In many instances, steroids which have similar biologic effects probably share the same receptor proteins and work through the same intracellular mechanisms. The mechanism outlined above requires a finite period of time to operate; therefore, there is a measurable latent period before the metabolic effects of a steroid can be observed, usually of hours' duration.

It is known that some target tissues can metabolize tropic steroids, rendering them either more or less active biologically. It has been suggested that testosterone is activated through its conversion to dihydrotestosterone by androgen-sensitive cells (28). It is also probable that some steroid transformation products are devoid of biologic activity. This would represent one possible mechanism of limiting or terminating the effect of a steroid hormone within the target tissue. In any event, the duration of the stimulating effect of a steroid hormone is limited to a finite period of several hours (or perhaps a very few days in some cases). Unless there is a continuing supply of the steroid hormone, the formation of new RNA ceases, followed by disappearance of the associated proteins and cessation of the characteristic metabolic response of the target tissue.

The fact that certain tissues are "targets" for steroid hormone action and others are not apparently depends upon the fact that target tissues have cytoplasmic receptors for the particular steroid and others do not. The *type* of metabolic response is determined by the part of the genome that is functionally modified by the steroid-receptor complex and the type of RNA that is transcribed as a consequence.

Biologic Effects of Glucocorticoids (29)

The term "glucocorticoid" has been applied to steroids that have distinct effects on carbohydrate metabolism, including promotion of gluconeogenesis, promotion of liver glycogen deposition, and elevation of blood glucose concentrations. Of the naturally occurring steroids, only cortisol, cortisone, corticosterone, and 11-dehydrocorticosterone ("compound A") have appreciable glucocorticoid activity. Of these, cortisol is the most potent. In certain species, such as the rat, which lack the capacity to synthesize cortisol, however, corticosterone is the most important glucocorticoid. Cortisone and compound A lack inherent glucocorticoid activity but are potentially active because they are convertible in the body to cortisol and corticosterone, respectively.

A large number of synthetic analogues of cortisol have been shown to have glucocorticoid activity; several are more potent than cortisol itself. Their relative potencies are listed in Table 5-3, and the structural features which determine glucocorticoid potency are reviewed in Figure 5-10.

More or less in proportion to their potency in affecting carbohydrate metabolism, all of the glucocorticoids also possess the following biologic properties, some of which are of considerable clinical importance.

1. *Protein-wasting activity.* Glucocorticoids accelerate the breakdown of proteins such as albumin. They inhibit amino acid uptake and protein synthesis by many extrahepatic tissues. Glucocor-

TABLE 5-3. RELATIVE POTENCIES OF STEROIDS

	Gluco-corticoid Activity	Mineralo-corticoid Activity
Cortisol	1	1
Cortisone	0.7	0.7
Corticosterone	0.2	2
11-Deoxycorticosterone	nil	20
Aldosterone	0.1	400
Fludrocortisone	10	400
Prednisone	4	0.7
Prednisolone	4	0.7
Dexamethasone	30	2
Triamcinolone	3	nil
6α-Methylprednisolone	5	0.5

ticoids accelerate the uptake of amino acids by the liver, which utilizes some of them to synthesize albumin. But the liver also deaminates amino acids to form urea and substrates for energy metabolism, and this process is accelerated by glucocorticoids (gluconeogenesis). If present chronically in supraphysiologic quantities, glucocorticoids suppress growth hormone secretion and inhibit somatic growth; the latter effect cannot be completely overcome by the administration of growth hormone.

2. *ACTH-suppressing activity.* All glucocorticoids suppress the synthesis and secretion of ACTH. There is experimental evidence indicating that this action of the steroids is exerted, at least partially, at the level of the pituitary itself, but it is possible that glucocorticoids also act to suppress CRF.

3. *Anti-inflammatory activity.* When present in supraphysiologic amounts, glucocorticoids inhibit inflammatory and allergic reactions. There are, of course, many components to the inflammatory response to tissue injury, and glucocorticoids act to suppress the response at multiple points. Glucocorticoids have been shown to stabilize lysosomes; these are intracellular packages of proteolytic en-

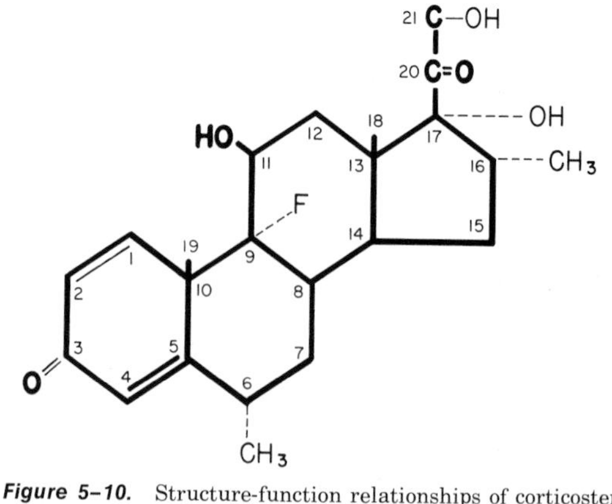

Figure 5-10. Structure-function relationships of corticosteroids. The bold lines and letters indicate the structure of pregn-4-ene, 11β-ol-3,20-dione, which is common to all steroids that have been shown to have glucocorticoid activity in man. Substituents which individually are nonessential but which, if present, enhance glucocorticoid activity are represented by light lines and letters.

zymes which, when released as a consequence of cellular injury, cause damage to neighboring cells. Glucocorticoids inhibit the diapedesis of leukocytes across capillary walls and their migration through tissues. They inhibit granuloma formation. As a consequence of these actions, glucocorticoids may interfere with host responses to bacterial infection and suppress delayed sensitivity reactions.

Closely related to their anti-inflammatory actions are the immunosuppressive actions of the glucocorticoids. These steroids are lympholytic. They cause decreases in circulating lymphocytes and diminish the size of lymph nodes, thymus, and spleen. Antibody production is decreased.

4. *Miscellaneous Activities.* Glucocorticoids also have a multitude of other activities, including the induction of several enzymes, stimulation of hematopoiesis, promotion of fat deposition in faciocervicotruncal areas, promotion of uric acid excretion, facilitation of free-water excretion, promotion of appetite, reduction of circulating eosinophils, and maintenance of muscular work capacity.

Biologic Effects of Mineralocorticoids

The term "mineralocorticoid" has been applied to steroids that have distinct effects on ion transport by epithelial cells, resulting in sodium conservation and loss of potassium. Many naturally occurring steroids have this property, but the most potent and, teleologically, the most useful is aldosterone. The second most potent is 11-deoxycorticosterone (DOC), followed in order of potency by 18-hydroxy-DOC, corticosterone, and cortisol.

A large number of synthetic corticosteroid analogues have been shown to have mineralocorticoid activity; some are even more potent than aldosterone. Their relative potencies are listed in Table 5-3. In addition, estrogens and androgens may promote sodium retention under certain circumstances, but the mechanism may be different from that of the mineralocorticoids.

Epithelial cells of the renal tubules, sweat glands, and glands of the alimentary system have enzymatically controlled mechanisms for transporting electrolytes across cell membranes. The electrolyte "pumps" respond to mineralocorticoids by conserving sodium and chloride and by wasting bodily potassium. A good example of such a system is found in the distal convoluted tubule of the mammalian nephron. Here, even in the absence of a mineralocorticoid, a cation exchange mechanism brings about reabsorption of sodium ions from fluid in the lumen of the tubule and secretion of potassium and hydrogen ions into the lumen. These processes are accelerated by mineralocorticoids. Absence of mineralocorticoid activity may result in lethal wastage of sodium and retention of potassium. Sufficient mineralocorticoid helps the body to achieve electrolyte homeostasis, but an overabundance of mineralocorticoid can cause potassium depletion and excessive sodium retention, leading to edema, hypertension, and suppression of renal production of renin.

Biology of Adrenal Androgens and Estrogens

Under normal circumstances, adrenocortical production of androgen and estrogen is trivial in comparison with the production of these hormones by the gonads. A pathologic excess of adrenal androgen, however, can induce virilization (the development of masculine secondary sex characteristics). In the adult male, the effects of adrenal androgen escape notice since he is already fully virilized, but in the female or immature male they can be very conspicuous. Adrenal virilism in the female fetus can induce the formation of a urogenital sinus (rather than separate external orifices of the urinary and genital systems), labial fusion, and clitoral hypertrophy. Such ambiguity of the external genitalia is referred to as "pseudohermaphroditism." In children of either sex, an excess of adrenal androgen can cause phallic hypertrophy, increased muscularity, rapid somatic growth, and precocious development of pubic, axillary, and facial hair. In addition, the affected individual can develop acne, coarsening of the voice, and recession of scalp hair. The various manifestations of childhood virilism appear chronologically in the order listed above. Women with adrenal virilism may experience clitoral hypertrophy, hirsutism, balding, coarsening of the voice, and suppression of estrogen effects, resulting in amenorrhea, infertility, and breast atrophy.

Feminization due to adrenal estrogen is extremely rare. It might be unnoticed in mature women, but in men and children it would lead to enlargement of the breasts and (in young girls) maturation of the uterus and vagina.

Although normal amounts of adrenal androgen and estrogen have trivial effects with respect to the development of secondary sex characteristics, they may have some importance in supporting the growth of certain tumors, specifically, mammary and prostatic carcinomas. Some such tumors regress initially following gonadectomy and then again following adrenalectomy. Mammary tumors that respond to adrenalectomy can be identified in advance by demonstrating the presence of cytoplasmic estrogen-receptor proteins in biopsy specimens (30).

Measurement of Adrenal Steroids

Steroids can be extracted from plasma, urine, or adrenal tissue with an organic solvent such as dichloromethane and then quantified by any of several procedures. Most of the quantification procedures are not entirely specific for one steroid; therefore, partial purification using differential solvent extraction or chromatography might be necessary preliminary to quantification.

Cortisol

Cortisol, as well as certain related steroids, can be measured colorimetrically because its dihy-

droxy-acetone side chain reacts with phenylhydra-
zine in sulfuric acid to give a yellow color, the intensity of which is proportional to the amount of
cortisol in the specimen. This method was developed by Porter and Silber (31); therefore, the
steroids measured by this procedure are often referred to as "Porter-Silber chromogens." These
steroids are also referred to as "17,21-dihydroxy-
20-ketosteroids," "17-hydroxycorticosteroids," or
"17-OHCS." Since cortisol, cortisone, 11-deoxycor-
tisol ("substance S") and their tetrahydro derivatives all have 17,21-dihydroxy-20-keto side chains,
they are all measurable as Porter-Silber chromogens (Figs. 5–11, 5–12, and 5–13). Of all these
steroids, however, the only one that occurs in normal human plasma to any significant degree is cortisol. Cortisone will not be encountered unless it is
administered as such. 11-deoxycortisol is normally
barely detectable, but it is abundantly secreted in
some cases of adrenal carcinoma, in subjects
treated with an 11β-hydroxylase inhibitor
(metyrapone), and in patients with congenital
adrenal hyperplasia due to 11β-hydroxylase
deficiency. The tetrahydro derivatives of cortisol,
cortisone, and 11-deoxycortisol are so quickly
converted to water-soluble glucuronides that
they do not interfere with the measurement of
cortisol. Therefore, for most practical purposes,
measurements of plasma Porter-Silber chromogens
are equivalent to measurements of plasma cortisol.

A rapid, relatively specific method for measuring
cortisol is the fluorometric method of Mattingly
(32), based on the fact that cortisol fluoresces when
incubated in ethanolic sulfuric acid. This property
is shared by corticosterone, but the latter is
present in human plasma in only about one-tenth

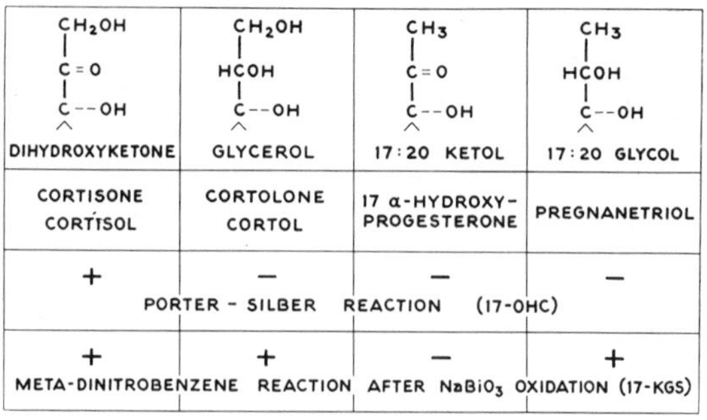

Figure 5–12. Characteristic side-chain groups and the practical tests specific for them.

the concentration of cortisol. For most practical
purposes, therefore, measuring fluorogenic steroids in human plasma is equivalent to measuring
plasma cortisol.

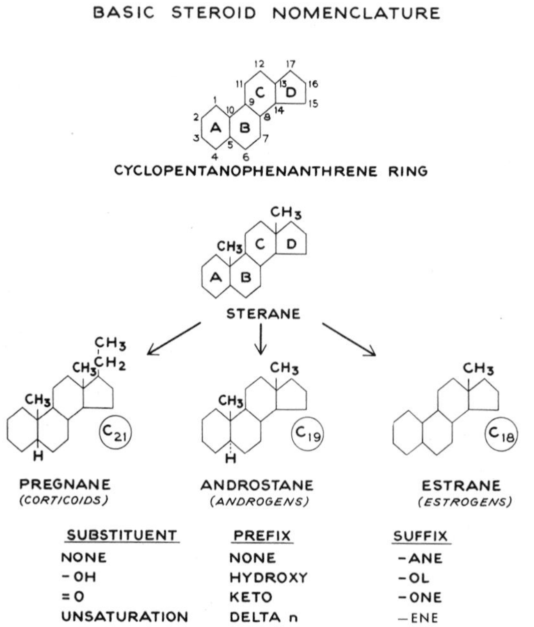

A technically difficult but very sensitive method
for measuring cortisol is the double-isotope derivative method originally devised by Peterson.
Recently, several groups have developed radioimmunoassays for cortisol which, although
technically exacting, are so sensitive that they permit the measurement of cortisol in smaller specimens than possible heretofore.

As stated previously, unaltered cortisol appears
in the urine in only very limited quantities. Even
so, this has been turned to diagnostic use since
there is a proportionately great increase in urinary
cortisol in clinical hypercortisolism, when the
amount of free plasma cortisol (as opposed to protein-bound cortisol) is excessive. Under these circumstances, urinary cortisol increases from its
usual value of less than 150 μg. per day to several
hundred or even several thousand μg. per day.
After suitable extraction and purification, urinary
cortisol can be measured by any of the procedures
described above.

Urinary 17-Hydroxycorticosteroids
(17-OHCS)

Although cortisol appears in the urine in only
very limited quantities, its major metabolites, tetrahydrocortisol glucuronide and tetrahydrocortisone glucuronide, appear in quantities equivalent
to about 30 per cent of the cortisol secretory rate.
These glucuronides are so water-soluble that they
escape extraction with the organic solvents. Hydrolytic cleavage of the glucuronides with glucuronidase releases the free steroids, which can
then be extracted with organic solvents and quantified as 17-OHCS by the Porter-Silber method.
Urinary 17-OHCS as determined in this way provide an extremely useful index of cortisol secretion. The method is not entirely specific for cortisol
metabolites, however, since the tetrahydro derivative of 11-deoxycortisol, "tetrahydro S," is also
excreted in the urine as a glucuronide, is liberated
by glucuronidase, is extracted with organic solvents, and is measurable as a Porter-Silber chro-

BASIC STEROID NOMENCLATURE

Figure 5–11. Basic concepts in steroid biochemistry and
nomenclature.

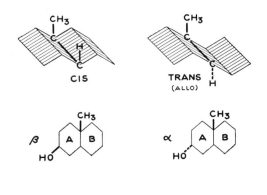

Figure 5–13. Diagrammatic representation of stereoisomerism of the steroid molecule.

mogen. It is simple to distinguish "tetrahydro S" from cortisol metabolites, however, because the tetrahydro S is so nonpolar that it is extractable from urine with carbon tetrachloride, while cortisol metabolites are not. By extracting the urinary glucuronidase-hydrolysate first with carbon tetrachloride and then with dichloromethane, one can readily fractionate the "total 17-OHCS" into 11-deoxycortisol metabolites and cortisol metabolites. In practice, there are occasions when it is important to know how much of the total 17-OHCS are derivatives of these two hormonal steroids, but there are other occasions (e.g., during metyrapone tests) when it is sufficient to know the total.

Aldosterone and Its Derivatives

Compared with cortisol, the measurement of aldosterone presents a technical challenge because of its much lower concentration in biologic fluids. Normal plasma concentrations are of the order of 10 ng. per 100 ml. (compared with cortisol, which is normally present in concentrations of about 10 μg. per 100 ml.). Urinary free aldosterone values are generally less than 1 μg. per day. Aldosterone is unique in that a considerable portion (approximately 10 per cent) of the hormonal steroid is excreted as a water-soluble 18-oxo-conjugate (glucuronide) (33). When hydrolyzed by incubation with acid, aldosterone is released and can be extracted and measured by a variety of methods. The advantage of working with this metabolite rather than free aldosterone is that it appears in the urine in quantities of the order of 10 μg. per day.

The double isotope derivative method (34) for measuring aldosterone involves the following steps. First, to the "unknown" specimen is added a trace amount of H[3]-labeled aldosterone to permit monitoring of recoveries at the conclusion of extensive purification. Second, the aldosterone-containing extract is subjected to various chromatographic procedures known to separate this from other steroids. Third, the "aldosterone fraction" is allowed to react with C[14]-labeled acetic anhydride

under conditions that convert aldosterone (both H[3]-labeled aldosterone and that of biologic origin) to aldosterone-C[14]-acetate. Fourth, the products of acetylation are then subjected to further chromatography employing systems known to separate aldosterone acetates from other steroid acetates. Fifth, when repeated chromatography in various systems reveals that the ratio of C[14] to H[3] is constant, the purification is considered to be complete, and the quantity of aldosterone in the original specimen is computed from the amount of H[3]-labeled aldosterone added as tracer, the degree of "dilution" of H[3]-aldosterone-C[14]-acetate with aldosterone-C[14]-acetate, and the various dilutions and aliquots that were employed.

Recently, radioimmunoassays for aldosterone (35) have been developed with sensitivity comparable to that of the double-isotope derivative method. Since antisera are rarely specific for any particular steroid, cross reactions with other structurally related steroids are common, and care must be taken to separate aldosterone from other potentially interfering steroids before quantification by radioimmunoassay is attempted. The principles and techniques of radioimmunoassay have been described in detail elsewhere.

Another aldosterone metabolite, tetrahydro-aldosterone glucuronide, can also be measured following cleavage of the steroid from glucuronic acid using glucuronidase, extraction with dichloromethane, extensive purification, and measurement of "blue tetrazolium-reducing" activity.

17-Ketosteroids

The oldest practical chemical method for measuring adrenal steroids was that devised by Callow in 1940, employing the Zimmermann reaction for 17-ketosteroids. The most abundant urinary 17-ketosteroids are androsterone and etiocholanolone, which appear in the urine principally as water-soluble conjugates (largely sulfates). The main precursor of the urinary 17-ketosteroids is dehydroepiandrosterone, but testosterone, androstenedione, and cortisol are included among a large number of minor precursors of this group of hormone metabolites. The steroid sulfates are hydrolyzed by exposure to acid. The steroids are then extracted with an organic solvent such as ether and estimated colorimetrically by the metadinitrobenzene ("Zimmermann") reaction. Although androsterone and etiocholanolone are derivatives of hormones originating either in adrenal or gonadal tissue, their 11-oxygenated analogues are derived exclusively from adrenal steroids. This distinction, if desired, can be made by chromatographic separation of the various 17-ketosteroids.

17-Ketogenic Steroids (17-KGS)

Not to be confused with 17-ketosteroids are the 17-*ketogenic* steroids—those that can be converted into 17-ketosteroids by treatment with the oxidizing reagent, sodium bismuthate (36). These steroids include those with dihydroxyacetone side chains, glycerol side chains, or 17:20 glycol side chains attached to carbon 17. The first group includes cortisol, cortisone, 11-deoxycortisol and their respective tetrahydo derivatives. The second group includes derivatives of these steroids which have undergone reduction of the 20-keto group (e.g., cortol and cortolone). The third group includes pregnanetriol. Interestingly, the precursor of pregnanetriol, 17α-hydroxyprogesterone, is *not* a 17-ketogenic steroid. Despite its obvious lack of specificity, the 17-ketogenic steroid method has enjoyed widespread use in certain regions in the evaluation of adrenal steroid production.

Steroid Secretory Rates

An important new dimension in steroid methodology was developed during the late nineteen-fifties and early nineteen-sixties in the laboratories of Peterson, Lieberman, Tait, and Cope with the demonstration that production rates of many steroids can be measured if one has an isotopically labeled form of the steroid and if one can isolate and quantify some unique metabolite of the steroid in question. A known amount of the labeled steroid is administered. Urine is then collected over a sufficient period to allow the labeled steroid to mix with the body pool of secreted steroid and to be metabolized and excreted. The unique urinary metabolite is then quantified and its specific activity then provides a measure of the amount of steroid secreted during the period of the study, utilizing the principle that the secreted steroid, being unlabeled, would dilute the labeled steroid, thus decreasing its specific activity. The general formula is as follows:

Secretory rate (mg.) =

$$\frac{\text{Total counts of tracer injected (cpm.)}}{\text{Specific activity of metabolite (cpm./mg.)}}$$

This method must observe several rigorous conditions to give valid data, but it has proven extremely useful in providing information concerning production rates of cortisol, aldosterone, corticosterone, 11-deoxycorticosterone, 11-deoxycortisol, and 18-hydroxycorticosterone.

It is also possible to measure the secretion rate of a steroid by the straightforward method of administering a tracer dose of the steroid and then determining the rate at which the labeled steroid is diluted with unlabeled steroid within the circulation. If one assumes that the metabolic clearance rate is the same for labeled and unlabeled steroid alike, then the decrease in specific activity of the steroid is a function of secretion of new, unlabeled steroid into the miscible pool (37).

After a labeled steroid has been distributed throughout the miscible pool, it is characteristically cleared from the plasma at a relatively constant rate. This is referred to as the "metabolic clearance rate," and for most corticosteroids, it is

normally of the order of 1,000 liters per day. The ratio of the secretion rate for a given steroid (μg. per day) divided by the metabolic clearance rate (liters per day) equals the mean plasma concentration of the steroid throughout the day (μg. per liter) (38).

Measurement of Other Steroids

Not only the steroids listed above but also several others as well have been measured by a variety of techniques. Thus 11-deoxycorticosterone, 11-deoxycortisol, and progesterone in plasma have been measured by methods in which the steroids are first extracted from plasma, partially purified, and measured by a "competitive binding method" in which the endogenous steroid displaces labeled steroid from (or competes with it for) binding sites on transcortin. The principle is similar to that underlying radioimmunoassay except that a natural "binding protein" rather than an antibody is employed. Similar assays have been employed for certain estrogens and androgens using testosterone-binding globulin rather than transcortin. In addition, trace quantities of several steroids have been quantified by gas-liquid chromatography. Recently, radioimmunoassays have been developed for pregnenolone and 17-hydroxypregnenolone. The adaptability of these various methods for the measurement of various steroids seems to be unlimited.

Normal Values in Adults

Normal values for the concentrations of several steroids in human plasma and normal values for secretion rates and excretion rates are listed in Table 5–4. It should be remembered that the actual values are functions of the physiologic state of the subject, the test conditions, the adequacy of collection and preservation of the specimens, and the care with which the laboratory procedure is performed. It is known that disparities between plasma and urinary steroid levels are common in pregnancy, estrogen therapy, hypothyroidism, hy-

TABLE 5–4. SECRETION AND EXCRETION RATES OF CERTAIN STEROIDS BY NORMAL ADULTS

Steroid	Secretion Rate mg./day
Cortisol	12–30
Corticosterone	1–4
Aldosterone	0.05–0.15
DOC	0.05–0.2
DHEA	15–50

Steroid	Excretion Rate mg./day
17-OHCS	4–12
17-KS	7–20
Pregnanetriol	0.5–2.5

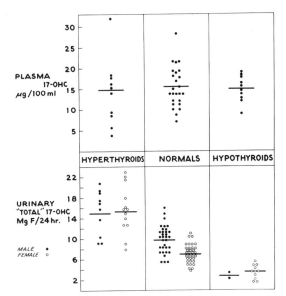

Figure 5–14. The effect of different thyroid states on adrenocortical function. While plasma cortisol levels are essentially identical in all states, the urinary excretion is in the range of Cushing's syndrome in the group with hyperthyroidism and low in hypothyroidism. (After DiRaimondo and Sagan.)

perthyroidism, and hepatic insufficiency (Fig. 5–14). It is strongly recommended that the physician have full knowledge of the physiologic condition of the subject and that he have a close working relationship with the laboratory so as to minimize the likelihood of misleading results.

Tests of Adrenal Reserve, Pituitary (ACTH) Reserve, and Pituitary-Adrenal Suppressibility

The normal pituitary-adrenal system has reserve capacity to secrete its hormones with more than ordinary intensity if properly stimulated. On the other hand, under appropriate conditions, it can be suppressed to such a degree that it virtually ceases to function. There are a number of clinical situations in which it is useful to know whether an individual has normal adrenal reserve, normal ACTH-secreting reserve, or normal pituitary-adrenal suppressibility. Therefore, standard tests of each of these functions have been developed.

Adrenal Reserve

The responsiveness of the adrenal to ACTH can be assessed by measuring plasma or urinary steroids before and again during the administration of ACTH. The most secure method of testing adrenal reserve is to infuse ACTH (corticotropin) intravenously at the rate of about 5 units per hour for 8 hours (39). Plasma should be collected prior to the beginning of the infusion and again after at least one hour of the infusion but before the termination of the infusion. Urine should be collected for

24 hours prior to the ACTH infusion and again for 24 hours commencing with the start of the infusion. The time of day is not of critical importance in standardizing this test; however, the interpretation of control values should take into consideration the fact that plasma cortisol concentrations are normally in the range of 10 to 25 μg. per 100 ml. in the morning and less than 10 μg. per 100 ml. late in the evening. Regardless of the control value, however, the individual with normal adrenal reserve exhibits an increase of 10 to 25 μg. per 100 ml. during the first hour and 15 to 40 μg. per 100 ml. by the eighth hour of an ACTH infusion. Urinary 17-OHCS values are normally proportional to body size, and it is useful to relate them to urinary creatinine for individuals of all ages and sizes. Under control conditions, normal individuals should excrete 3 to 7 mg. of 17-OHCS per g. of creatinine. In response to a standard 8-hour infusion of ACTH, urinary 17-OHCS should increase to 12 to 25 mg. per g. of creatinine. In response to ACTH infusion, urinary 17-ketosteroids should increase by a factor of 1.5 to 2.5 relative to control values, which are normally 4 to 10 mg. per g. of creatinine under control conditions.

There are a number of modifications of the test for adrenal reserve, including the use of intramuscular injections rather than intravenous infusions of ACTH. The critical feature of the test, however it might be performed, is that a substantial increase in adrenal steroids must occur in response to ACTH if one is to prove the existence of adrenal reserve. There have been cases in which adrenal insufficiency was mistakenly diagnosed when the real difficulty was that the ACTH was of poor quality and was ineffective when administered intramuscularly.

Pituitary (ACTH) Reserve

If a particular individual's adrenals are responsive to exogenous ACTH (as described above), then it is possible to utilize his adrenals to appraise changes in endogenous ACTH. In other words, by applying a stimulus to ACTH secretion and measuring changes in adrenal steroids, one can evaluate the integrity of the subject's ACTH secretory mechanism. If the individual responds normally to such a stimulus, it may be assumed that he possesses both pituitary reserve and adrenal reserve. If he responds normally to exogenous ACTH but not to the stimulus to ACTH secretion, it may be assumed that he lacks normal pituitary reserve. In the absence of intact adrenals, however, it is impossible to evaluate pituitary reserve using this group of tests.

Metyrapone is widely used in testing pituitary-adrenal reserve (40). This drug inhibits 11β-hydroxylase, the enzyme that catalyzes the final step in cortisol biosynthesis. A metyrapone–induced decrease in cortisol secretion results in a compensatory increase in ACTH secretion which stimulates further steroid biogenesis. Since inhibition of 11β-hydroxylation is usually incomplete,

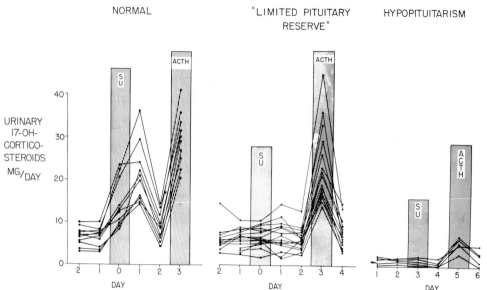

Figure 5–15. Typical responses of urinary 17-OHCS during treatment with standard doses of SU (metyrapone) or ACTH in normal subjects, in patients with limited pituitary reserve, and in patients with frank hypopituitarism. (From Liddle, G. W., Island, D., et al.: *Recent Progr. Hormone Res. 18*:125, 1962.)

the increased formation of cortisol precursors eventuates in partial restoration of cortisol secretion to normal, but this is accomplished only at the cost of increased pituitary secretion of ACTH and increased adrenal secretion of 11-deoxycortisol. An increase in 11-deoxycortisol alone does not mean that there has been an increase in pituitary-adrenal activity in response to metyrapone; it only means that cortisol secretion has been inhibited and that the cortisol precursor rather than cortisol itself is being released by the adrenal. An increase in total 17-hydroxycorticosteroids, comprising cortisol, 11-deoxycortisol, and their respective metabolites, however, indicates that there has been an increase in ACTH secretion and a consequent increase in adrenal secretory activity (Fig. 5–15).

A standard test of pituitary-adrenal reserve is performed by administering metyrapone in oral doses of 10 mg. per kg. of ideal body weight every 4 hours for 6 doses. The normal response consists of a twofold (or greater) increase in total urinary 17-OHCS on either the day of treatment or on the subsequent day.

Various modifications of this test have been developed. In some, the metyrapone is given intravenously. In some, the test period is shortened. In some, the response is assessed in terms of increases in plasma ACTH, urinary 17-ketogenic steroids, urinary 17-ketosteroids, plasma 11-deoxycortisol ("S"), or urinary "tetrahydro S." When critically performed, they all give essentially the same information. The most common mistakes have arisen from shortening the test so much that a full response is not elicited or from measuring "S" or its metabolites alone without taking into consideration the total adrenal output of 17-hydroxycorticosteroids (see above).

Certain precautions should be taken in performing a metyrapone test. First, the patient should not simultaneously receive drugs that suppress ACTH secretion (exogenous glucocorticoids) or drugs that accelerate the metabolism of metyrapone (e.g., diphenylhydantoin) (41). Patients with manifestations of adrenal insufficiency should be observed closely during performance of a metyrapone test so that supportive treatment may be provided if the patient develops hypotension or vomiting. If absorbed too rapidly, metyrapone causes transient vertigo. This can be prevented by administering the tablets with a meal or 200 ml. of milk.

A variety of mildly stressful stimuli have also been utilized in testing pituitary-adrenal reserve. These have included insulin-induced hypoglycemia, intravenous injection of pyrogens, and intravenous injection of vasopressin. The first causes sweating, tremulousness, and mental confusion. The second causes a chill and fever. The third causes abdominal cramping. All of them cause increases in ACTH secretion, with consequent increases in plasma cortisol concentrations within approximately one hour. The ACTH stimulation is so transient that urinary steroids are not appreciably affected. Despite the discomfort they cause, these stimuli have practical utility in that they permit relatively quick testing of pituitary-adrenal reserve.

Dexamethasone Suppression Tests

Glucocorticoids suppress the secretion of ACTH and thereby curtail the secretion of cortisol and its by-products. Thus, under normal circumstances, cortisol is self-regulating. In Cushing's syndrome, however, the pituitary-adrenal system loses its normal sensitivity to the suppressive action of glucocorticoids and, as a result, cortisol is excessively secreted. Standard pituitary-adrenal sup-

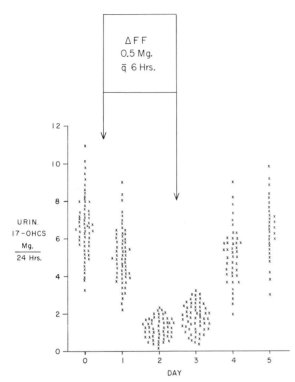

Figure 5–16. Normal responses of urinary 17-OHCS during treatment with standard doses of ΔFF (dexamethasone). From Liddle, G. W., Island, D., et al.: *Recent Progr. Hormone Res. 18*: 125, 1962.)

pression tests have been developed to aid in the elucidation of this condition (42). Dexamethasone is used as the suppressive agent because it is so potent biologically that only very small amounts of it are required to suppress ACTH. Such small amounts of the exogenous steroid do not interfere with the chemical measurement of endogenous steroids.

Normal nonstressed subjects respond to dexamethasone in doses of 0.5 mg. every 6 hours with virtually complete cessation of ACTH and cortisol secretion (Fig. 5–16). Urinary 17-OHCS fall to less than 2.5 mg. per day by the second day of treatment, and plasma cortisol falls to less than 5 μg. per 100 ml. If in response to these small doses of dexamethasone, 17-OHCS are not profoundly suppressed, one must suspect the presence of Cushing's syndrome. The cause of the Cushing's syndrome can often be determined by the use of a "high-dose" suppression test in which dexamethasone is given in doses of 2.0 mg. every 6 hours for 8 doses (see below).

Pharmacologic Inhibition of Adrenal Steroid Biosynthesis

Several drugs have been shown to inhibit one or another of the enzymatically controlled steps through which cholesterol is converted to hormonal steroids (43). Figure 5–17 depicts structural formulas of the most important of these agents; some have yet to be assigned official pharmaceutical names. Enzyme inhibition results in decreased formation of steroids appearing in the pathway beyond the inhibited step and increased secretion of steroids occurring just prior to the inhibited step. If cortisol biosynthesis is inhibited, there ensues a compensatory increase in ACTH secretion, which results in accelerated formation of all steroids formed by the zona fasciculata. With increased formation of precursors, cortisol secretion may return toward normal, but this is achieved only at the cost of increased secretion of ACTH and increased biosynthesis of steroid precursors. Similarly, if mineralocorticoid secretion is impaired by an adrenal inhibitor, there will be a compensatory increase in renin-angiotensin production and increased formation of steroids appearing in the aldosterone biosynthetic pathway prior to the inhibited step. Thus pharmacologic inhibition of an adrenal enzyme may result in a distorted pattern of steroid secretion, and the biologic consequences of adrenal inhibition can be understood in terms of the biologic activities of steroids that are deficiently secreted and the biologic activities of steroids that are excessively secreted.

Amino-glutethimide has been shown to inhibit the conversion of cholesterol to pregnenolone, presumably by inhibiting the enzyme 20α-hydroxylase. It thus curtails the biosynthesis of all hormonal steroids and leads to accumulation of cholesterol within the adrenal cortex. Clinically, it has found limited use as an inhibitor of mineralocorticoid secretion in patients with steroid hypertension and as an inhibitor of cortisol secretion in patients with Cushing's syndrome.

Cyanoketone has been shown to inhibit the conversion of Δ^5-3β-ol steroids to Δ^4-3-oxo steroids, presumably by inhibiting the enzyme, 3β-hydroxysteroid dehydrogenase. Consequently, pregnenolone cannot be converted efficiently to progesterone or its potent corticosteroid derivatives, all of which have Δ^4-3-oxo configurations.

SU-9055 and SU-8000 (Fig. 5–17) have been shown to inhibit 17α-hydroxylase and, thereby, to curtail the production of cortisol. They also inhibit aldosterone production by interfering with oxidation at the carbon-18. As a consequence of the latter action, they induce sodium excretion in patients with primary or secondary aldosteronism.

Metyrapone and SKF 12185 (Fig. 5–17) have been shown to inhibit 11β-hydroxylase and thus to curtail the conversion of 11-deoxycortisol to cortisol and DOC to corticosterone. The former property has been exploited in establishing metyrapone as an agent for testing pituitary-adrenal reserve (see above). These agents have also seen limited use in the treatment of hypercortisolism.

Heparin and heparinoids have been shown to alter the histochemical appearance of the zona glomerulosa and to inhibit aldosterone secretion. The precise mechanism is unknown. These agents have seen limited use in the treatment of primary and secondary aldosteronism.

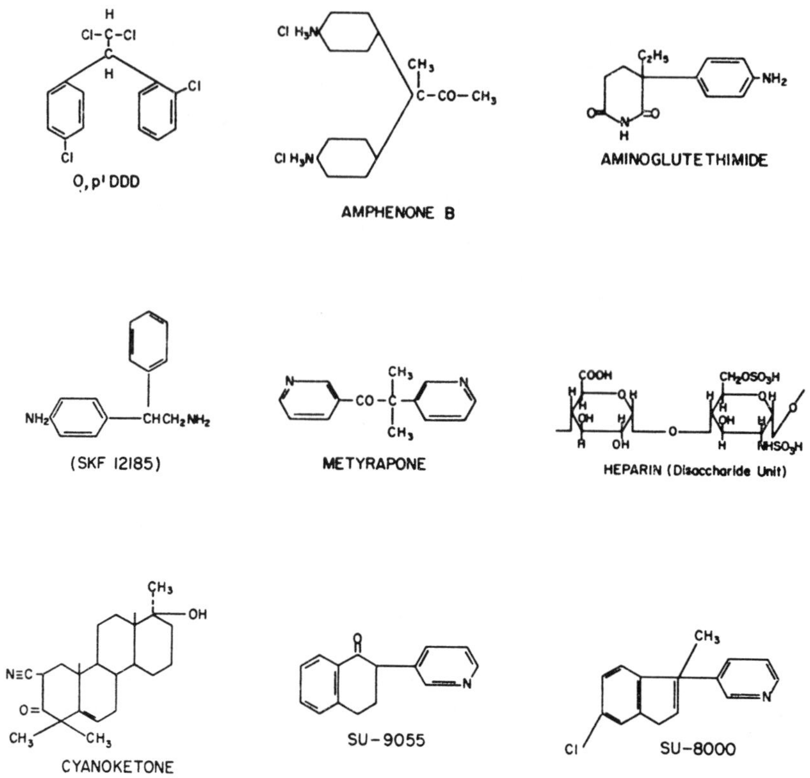

Figure 5-17. Structures of several inhibitors of adrenal steroid biosynthesis. (From Temple, T. E., and Liddle, G. W.: *Ann. Rev. Pharmacol. 10*:199, 1970.)

The cells of the zona fasciculata and zona reticularis of dog and man are selectively destroyed by o,p'-DDD, thus compromising the capacity of the adrenal to secrete cortisol. Although certain enzyme systems (e.g., 11β-hydroxylase) precede others in their loss of efficiency, it has not been shown that o,p'-DDD is a selective inhibitor of any particular enzyme in the same sense that metyrapone and cyanoketone are. This drug is of established value in the treatment of adrenocortical carcinoma and of Cushing's syndrome.

Amphenone B, one of the earliest known adrenal inhibitors, interferes with a number of steps in the steroid biosynthetic scheme. It has been used clinically to reduce aldosterone, cortisol, and adrenal estrogen production, but its clinical use has been abandoned because of its numerous side effects.

Aldosterone Antagonism

Certain steroids, even though lacking intrinsic corticosteroid activity, have the capacity of blocking the actions of corticosteroids. The best-known example of such a phenomenon is the action of spironolactone as an aldosterone antagonist. This is merely a particular instance of a more general phenomenon of mineralocorticoid antagonism by progesterone and a group of synthetic steroidal lactones (44). These agents have little or no effect of

their own on electrolyte excretion but, when administered in the presence of mineralocorticoids, they antagonize the sodium-retaining, potassium-losing actions of these steroids (Fig. 5–18). The steroidal lactones have been shown to promote sodium excretion and diminish potassium excretion in both primary and secondary aldosteronism and to correct edema, hypertension, and hypokalemia when these abnormalities are dependent upon mineralocorticoids. It has been suggested that the steroidal lactones compete with mineralocorticoids for attachment to their receptor proteins in target tissues.

ADRENAL CORTICAL DISEASES

In the main, adrenal cortical diseases assume importance only when they lead to increased or decreased production of steroid hormones. Accordingly, this section will be organized in such a way as to give emphasis to the fact that the major endocrinopathies represent either overproduction or underproduction of particular hormones. By far the most important hormones of the human adrenal cortex are cortisol and aldosterone, and these hormones will be given most attention, while others will be considered as by-products which only occasionally assume importance in clinical medicine.

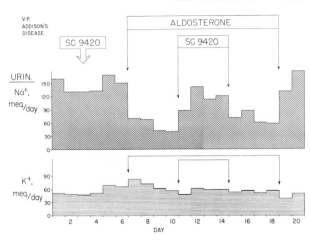

Figure 5–18. SC-9420 (spironolactone) is without discernible natriuretic effect in the absence of mineralocorticoids, as, for example, when it is administered to an addisonian patient who is maintained solely on a liberal sodium intake and a glucocorticoid. When the same patient is maintained on aldosterone, however, treatment with spironolactone exerts an obvious natriuretic effect.

Adrenal Cortical Hyperfunction

The hyperfunctioning adrenal cortex can produce syndromes of hypercortisolism, mineralocorticoid excess, virilism, or feminization. Mixed syndromes may occur.

Hypercortisolism (Cushing's Syndrome)

Although the medical literature had previously been sprinkled with reports of similar cases, it was not until Cushing's report (45) of cases of "pituitary basophilism" in 1932 that this clinical entity attracted major attention. In Cushing's view, the syndrome of central obesity, cutaneous striae, osteoporosis, weakness, hypertension, diabetes, plethora, and hirsutism was of pituitary origin; but others emphasized the role of the adrenal cortex in the pathogenesis of the syndrome. In 1942, Fuller Albright (46) pointed out that the distinctive features of Cushing's syndrome could best be attributed to the "sugar hormone" of the adrenal cortex, the hormone that favored gluconeogenesis, protein wasting, and diabetes; he contrasted this syndrome of glucocorticoid excess with that of adrenal androgen excess in which there are conspicuous signs of protein anabolism. With Daughaday's development of a method for measuring formaldehydogenic steroids, it became possible to demonstrate that C-21-oxygenated steroids were elevated in the urine of patients with Cushing's syndrome. Subsequent evolution of more specific methods for measuring corticosteroids finally made it possible to demonstrate that the chemical common denominator of all cases of spontaneous Cushing's syndrome was an excess of cortisol. Cortisone and other synthetic glucocorticoids have given rise to iatrogenic Cushing's syndrome, but the only glucocorticoid produced in significant quantities by the human adrenal cortex is cortisol itself. Brief elevations of cortisol do not cause clinically recognizable Cushing's syndrome; rather, Cushing's syndrome is a result of a chronic excess of this steroid.

General Features of Hypercortisolism

Cushing's syndrome occurs sporadically in all races, all ages, and both sexes, but it has been reported with greatest frequency in women between the ages of 20 and 60. Typically it is characterized by weight gain, and, in contrast to certain other endocrinopathies such as acromegaly and virilism, the gain in weight is due principally to accumulation of adipose tissue, particularly in the facial, nuchal, truncal, and girdle areas. This is sometimes referred to as centripetal or "buffalo" obesity (Fig. 5–19).

Equally characteristic of hypercortisolism is evidence of protein wasting. In mild cases or those of only a few months duration, this may amount to nothing more than a tendency to bruise easily. In more severe, chronic cases, the skin may be so thin and fragile that it is denuded by removal of a strip of adhesive tape or some other trivial injury. Insignificant trauma may result in formation of purpura, especially common on the dorsal aspects of the hands or forearms. Where the weakened integument is stretched by underlying accumulation of adipose tissue, it may become so thin that streaks of capillaries become visible—the pink or purple striae of classic Cushing's syndrome.

Occasionally, muscle wasting progresses to the point where it is objectively apparent; frequently it results in such severe weakness that the patient cannot rise from a deep-knee bend without assistance.

Attrition of bone matrix results in generalized osteoporosis. A particularly vulnerable part of the skeleton is the vertebral column, where weakening of the vertebral bodies may permit bulging of the intervertebral discs, giving a "codfish vertebrae" appearance in lateral radiographic views. Compression fractures may occur with anterior wedging of the vertebral bodies, resulting in kyphosis, loss of height, and backache. The osteoporotic process is generalized, and radiographic evidence of it is frequently encountered in the skull and extremities; pathologic fractures of the extremities have occurred in several cases.

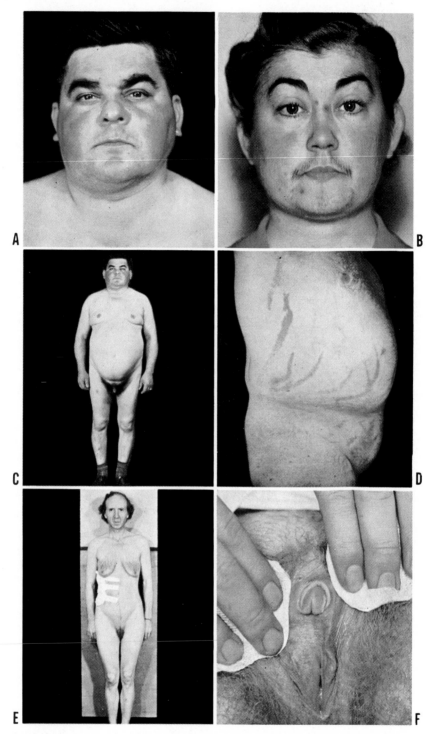

Figure 5–19. *Cushing's Syndrome. A,* Round, fiery-red face; short, thick neck. Typical moon face. *B,* Red moon face with hirsutism. *C,* Truncal obesity with prominent abdomen and relatively thin extremities. *D,* Purplish-red striae and protuberant abdomen.

Adrenogenital syndrome. E, Masculine figure with prominent muscles, partial baldness, and excessive hair on the breasts. *F,* Enlarged clitoris in the same case.

Perhaps as a consequence of osteoporosis, modest hypercalciuria is common, with urinary calcium values of 150 to 300 mg. per day. Renal stones occur in approximately 20 per cent of long-standing cases of Cushing's syndrome.

Surgeons frequently find the tissues of patients with chronic or severe Cushing's syndrome to have poor tensile strength so that they tear easily, retain sutures poorly, and heal slowly. Superficial wounds may also heal slowly and become sites of indolent infection and ulceration; this is especially common in pretibial areas.

Growth is arrested, and this is an important aspect of Cushing's syndrome in children and adolescents, for if the epiphyses of the long bones close before the Cushing's syndrome is corrected, shortened stature will be inevitable. As a rule, one can be fairly confident that an obese child who is growing rapidly does not have Cushing's syndrome, but the syndrome must be suspected in obese children who grow slowly.

In addition to centripetal obesity and protein wasting, the patient with Cushing's syndrome usually has impaired glucose tolerance. The usual pattern is not that of frank diabetes mellitus with glycosuria and elevated fasting blood glucose (these occur in about 20 per cent) but rather a failure of the blood glucose to return to fasting levels during the second and third hours of a standard glucose tolerance test. Approximately 90 per cent of patients with Cushing's syndrome will have at least mild impairment of glucose tolerance.

Whether it is due entirely to hypercortisolism or is due partly to excessive secretion of associated steroids, the majority of patients with Cushing's syndrome have high blood pressure. In association with this, they may have left ventricular hypertrophy and increased susceptibility to occlusion of major arteries. Edema and hypokalemia (unprovoked by diuretics) occur in only a minority of patients with Cushing's syndrome, but these abnormalities are common in those patients whose steroid levels are especially high.

Other common manifestations of hypercortisolism include heightened color of face and neck, downy hirsutism, oligomenorrhea, mild erythrocytosis, lymphopenia, and eosinopenia. About 30 per cent of patients have superficial fungal infections such as tinea versicolor. Serum gamma globulin concentrations and serum protein-bound iodine concentrations are often slightly subnormal. Many patients with Cushing's syndrome are emotionally labile and easily irritated. A few are psychotic, and the psychotic patterns have most frequently resembled schizophrenia, hypomania, or depression. Patients with Cushing's syndrome often have difficulty in limiting the spread of infections.

In the past, death commonly resulted among patients with Cushing's syndrome from infections with pyogenic organisms, hypertensive-arteriosclerotic cardiovascular disease, and suicide.

Many patients with hypercortisolism have some associated excess of adrenal androgen. Unless the androgen excess is extreme, the clinical manifestations amount to nothing more than some hirsutism in androgen-sensitive areas, acne, and oligomenorrhea. Extreme excesses of adrenal androgen might result in temporal hair recession, coarsening of the voice, and clitoral hypertrophy.

Although a minority of patients with Cushing's syndrome present most of the clinical features described above, many of them present a less complete clinical picture. Rather than persisting in uncertainty and rather than devoting an inordinate amount of effort to nonspecific tests, it is often wise to proceed directly to the most efficient methods available for proving or disproving the diagnosis of hypercortisolism. For this purpose it is desirable to measure the cortisol in specimens of plasma obtained late in the evening and to measure 17-OHCS in 24-hour collections of urine. If the bedtime plasma cortisol concentration is greater than 7 μg. per 100 ml., and if the urinary 17-OHCS are greater than 7 mg. per g. of creatinine, one should proceed with a "small-dose" dexamethasone suppression test (see above). If in response to dexamethasone, 0.5 mg. every 6 hours for two days, plasma cortisol does not fall to less than 5 μg. per 100 ml. and urinary 17-OHCS to less than 2.5 mg. per g. of creatinine, one is entitled to diagnose hypercortisolism.

An erroneous diagnosis of "non–Cushing's syndrome" might be made through laboratory errors or if the patient were almost normally sensitive to dexamethasone (perhaps 2 per cent of cases). An erroneous diagnosis of Cushing's syndrome might be made (1) through laboratory error, (2) if the patient were severely stressed, (3) if the dexamethasone were not administered, or (4) if the patient were inadvertently given exogenous cortisol, ACTH, cortisone, or spironolactone (which interferes with chromogenic and fluorogenic measurements of cortisol).

Patients with Cushing's syndrome lack the normal diurnal rhythm in cortisol secretion. In contrast to normal individuals who have relatively high plasma cortisol values early in their waking day and low values as the hour of sleep approaches, patients with Cushing's syndrome have relatively high values at all hours (47). It is decidedly unusual for patients with Cushing's syndrome to have any plasma cortisol values below 7 μg. per 100 ml. Plasma cortisol concentrations in Cushing's syndrome usually range from about 15 to 35 μg. per 100 ml. regardless of the time of day. Obviously, this permits considerable overlap with normal morning values, which usually range from about 12 to 25 μg. per 100 ml. In contrast, there is usually clear separation of Cushing's syndrome values from the normal range of 1 to 8 μg. per 100 ml. late in the evening. Therefore, in screening for Cushing's syndrome, there is little value in measuring plasma cortisol in the morning but great value in measuring it late in the evening.

Because certain factors modify the binding of plasma cortisol or alter the extra-adrenal metabolism of cortisol, it is advisable to employ more than one chemical dimension in establishing a diagnosis of Cushing's syndrome. One should demonstrate that plasma cortisol is relatively high and that it remains so late in the day, but one should also employ some index of cortisol production rate (such as urinary 17-OHCS excretion), and one should confirm the basic fact that there is abnormal resistance to suppression by performing a "small-dose" dexamethasone test (see above).

The following modification of the "small dose" dexamethasone test deserves special mention because of its simplicity and economy in ruling out Cushing's syndrome when this diagnosis is considered improbable from the outset. By giving 1 mg. of dexamethasone at midnight and sampling blood for cortisol measurement eight hours later, one can, in about 90 per cent of non–Cushing's syndrome patients, exclude the diagnosis of hypercortisolism by demonstrating a plasma cortisol value of less than 5 μg. per 100 ml. Patients whose plasma cortisol values are not so suppressible may then be tested further with the more discriminating 2-day test using dexamethasone, 0.5 mg. every 6 hours for 8 doses.

Differential Diagnosis of Cushing's Syndrome

There are three major varieties of Cushing's syndrome. They are all characterized by the clinical features described in the preceding section as well as by increased production of cortisol, hypercortisolemia with loss of the normal diurnal rhythm, increased renal excretion of free cortisol, increased renal excretion of 17-OHCS, and abnormal resistance to the suppressive influence of small doses of dexamethasone. These features are present regardless of whether the primary cause of the hypercortisolism is autonomous function by an adrenal neoplasm, excessive stimulation of the adrenals by pituitary ACTH, or excessive stimulation of the adrenals by ectopic ACTH. The optimal treatment of each of these disorders is different; therefore, specific diagnosis is important. The differential diagnosis rests on the steroid secretory response to a "large-dose" dexamethasone test, the measurement of plasma ACTH, and a clinical appraisal for evidence of a neoplasm.

Adrenal Neoplasms that Secrete Cortisol Autonomously. Occasionally, clones of adrenal cortical cells lose their dependence upon ACTH and acquire the capacity to grow and secrete cortisol autonomously. Morphologically, these cells may behave like carcinomas which grow exuberantly, invade, and metastasize; or they may behave like benign adenomas. They are usually unilateral but rarely bilateral; or they may have the appearance of microadenomas in both adrenal glands. When the secretion of cortisol by such clones of cells exceeds that of normal adrenal glands, clinical and chemical hypercortisolism occurs, secretion of ACTH by the otherwise normal pituitary gland ceases, and the ACTH-dependent portions of the adrenals become atrophic.

In this disorder, the administration of large doses of dexamethasone is without effect on plasma cortisol or urinary 17-OHCS or 17-KS (Fig. 5–20). The explanation is simple: the only way in which dexamethasone has been shown to modify steroid secretion is by suppressing ACTH secretion. In patients with Cushing's syndrome due to autonomous cortisol secretion, ACTH is already suppressed, and dexamethasone has no way of affecting adrenocortical activity. Occasionally, one encounters an adrenal tumor that exhibits spontaneous day-to-day fluctuations in cortisol secretion, and inadequate study might lead one to the erroneous conclusion that dexamethasone had caused a fall in the steroid output by the tumor. There has never been a case of Cushing's syndrome due to an adrenal neoplasm in which steroid production has been shown to be reproducibly suppressed on repeated testing with dexamethasone.

Although valid measurements of plasma ACTH are not generally available, when these determinations have been performed, they have revealed that patients with Cushing's syndrome due to adrenal tumors have subnormal values. Indeed, any other finding would require special explanation.

A corollary to the rule that these patients have suppression of their ACTH-secretory mechanisms is the extensively verified fact that they fail to respond to standard metyrapone tests of pituitary reserve; unlike normal individuals, they do not exhibit increases in their *total* urinary 17-OHCS when given metyrapone to block the final step in cortisol biosynthesis (40). The importance of focusing attention on changes in *total* 17-OHCS rather than "tetrahydro S" alone in interpreting the metyrapone test becomes obvious here. An adrenal tumor that autonomously secretes cortisol will,

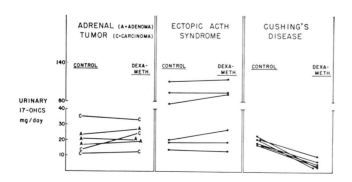

Figure 5–20. Results of dexamethasone suppression test, using 2 mg. of dexamethasone every 6 hours for 2 days, in patients with hypercortisolism due to adrenal tumor, secretion of ectopic ACTH, or inappropriate secretion of pituitary ACTH. (From Liddle, G. W.: "Cushing's Syndrome," In *The Adrenal Cortex.* Eisenstein, A. B. (ed.), Boston, Little, Brown and Co., 1967.)

under the inhibitory influence of metyrapone, autonomously secrete 11-deoxycorticol ("S") in its stead. An increase in urinary "tetrahydro S," therefore, does not necessarily indicate an increase in pituitary-adrenal activity. In any event, a *failure* to respond to metyrapone with an increase in total 17-OHCS is a reliable diagnostic feature of Cushing's syndrome due to adrenal (tumor) autonomy.

To say that a group of adrenal cells can function autonomously in the absence of ACTH is not equivalent to saying that they would be unresponsive to ACTH if ACTH were present. About 50 per cent of patients with Cushing's syndrome due to benign adrenal neoplasms show vigorous responses to standard ACTH tests. Proof that these responses come from the tumors themselves, rather than from the nontumorous portions of the adrenal, is based on the observation that surgical removal of the tumors results in adrenal insufficiency with subnormal responsiveness to ACTH. The remaining 50 per cent of benign adrenal tumors and over 90 per cent of adrenal carcinomas are unresponsive to standard infusions of ACTH (48).

Patients with hypercortisolism secondary to excess ACTH usually have elevated urinary 17-ketosteroids more or less in proportion to the elevation of their 17-OHCS. Patients with Cushing's syndrome due to autonomous adrenal tumors may have subnormal, normal, or supernormal 17-KS. A grossly disproportionate increase in "S" production or a grossly disproportionate degree of virilism relative to the severity of the hypercortisolism should make one alert to the probability of an adrenal carcinoma.

Until proven otherwise, a patient with elevated, arrhythmic plasma cortisol, elevated urinary 17-OHCS, absolute resistance to the suppressive influence of dexamethasone, unresponsiveness to metyrapone, and subnormal plasma ACTH must be considered to have an adrenal tumor. Usually cortisol-secreting adrenal tumors can be located preoperatively by physical examination or radiographic studies. Most adrenal carcinomas are so inefficient in synthesizing cortisol that, by the time they have attracted medical attention through causing Cushing's syndrome, they are more than 6 cm. in diameter. Some are massive enough to be palpable through the abdominal wall. Many are large enough to cause displacement of the kidney, as seen by intravenous urography. Most can be made visible by careful adrenal arteriography. Most benign adenomas that cause Cushing's syndrome are 2 to 6 cm. in diameter and can usually be seen during adrenal arteriography. Other methods of revealing the tumors have also been used but are probably less reliable. Microadenomas of the adrenals cannot be seen by any available methods.

Unless the tumor is obviously nonresectable or the patient's general condition is too precarious to permit major surgery, every patient with a diagnosis of an adrenal tumor should be offered an adrenal exploration. A useful method is to have two surgeons operate simultaneously through bilateral flank incisions so that both adrenals can be examined before a decision is made regarding definitive therapy. If a tumor is found on only one side, as will be the case more than 90 per cent of the time, that adrenal should be removed and the contralateral adrenal left intact. If bilateral adenomas are found, both adrenals should be removed. If no discrete adenomas are found, both adrenals should be removed in the expectation that they will show microadenomatosis. At this point it is obvious why the preoperative diagnosis of adrenal autonomy must be as firm as possible, since treatments other than adrenalectomy are usually preferable for the other varieties of Cushing's syndrome (49).

It is imperative that a patient undergoing resection of adrenal tumors receive cortisol substitution therapy during and after the operation, until his remaining atrophic adrenal tissue has been demonstrated to be functioning adequately. Water-soluble esters of glucocorticoids should be given intravenously or intramuscularly until the patient can dependably take medications by mouth. If dexamethasone is used (in order to permit early evaluation of the completeness of removal of autonomous adrenal tissue), the dose should be 1/25 that suggested for hydrocortisone. On the day of the operation, the dose of steroid should be equivalent to 400 mg. of hydrocortisone (100 mg. every 6 hours, beginning with the operation). On each succeeding day, the dose may be decreased by a twofold factor until the total daily dose is 50 mg. This dose might well be given for two weeks, in two or three divided doses. Then one might give 30 mg. daily for two months, 20 mg. in the morning and 10 mg. late in the day. Thereafter, one might give 20 mg. once each morning for six months, by the end of which time pituitary-adrenal recovery should be demonstrable both clinically and chemically. To prove the latter, endogenous plasma cortisol concentrations should be at least 12 μg. per 100 ml. 24 hours after the last morning dose of exogenous hydrocortisone. By giving the exogenous hydrocortisone in the amount of 20 mg. per day, one can prevent symptoms of adrenal insufficiency; by giving it as a single dose only once each morning, one can avoid perpetuating the suppression of pituitary-adrenal function.

In the event that total adrenalectomy is necessary, lifelong treatment with glucocorticoids, sodium chloride, and usually mineralocorticoids must be employed as outlined in the section on the treatment of Addison's disease.

Patients with adrenal carcinomas should be observed periodically for evidence of recurrence of the tumor. Recurrence after 12 years of clinical and chemical "cure" has been reported. A patient with definite evidence of a nonresectable adrenal carcinoma may be treated with the adrenocorticolytic drug, o,p'-DDD (50). To date, this drug has never cured an adrenal carcinoma; nevertheless, it is the only agent that has been shown to have a selective effect in destroying adrenal tissue. In doses of 6 to 10 g. per day, o,p'-DDD has been shown to induce objective regression of tumor size in about one-third of patients with an adrenal carcinoma and to curtail steroid production not only in these but also in an additional one-third as well. Objective remissions are usually of three months' to three years' duration. The side effects—anorexia, nausea, vomiting, diarrhea, lethargy, and ataxia—are often troublesome and may require reduction of dosage or even total withdrawal of the drug. If one has the good fortune of inducing a remission, it is possible that, with prolonged therapy, the zona fasciculata of the nontumorous adrenal may also be destroyed. Therefore, it is wise to add to the regimen a daily dose of dexamethasone, 0.5 mg., in order to forestall possible adrenal insufficiency. Symptoms of the latter might be difficult to evaluate in patients receiving a drug that causes anorexia and nausea.

When the major symptoms of nonresectable adrenal carcinomas are due to the excessive production of corticosteroids, treatment with metyrapone can be employed to curtail the production of 11 β-hydroxysteroids such as cortisol. In doses of 1 to 3 g. per day, metyrapone will usually bring plasma cortisol into an acceptable range of 10 to 20 μg. per 100 ml. In countries where it is marketed, aminoglutethimide can be employed to curtail the production of steroids of all classes. The usual dose of aminoglutethimide is 0.75 to 1.0 g. per day; larger doses often cause ataxia.

Unless resected, an adrenal carcinoma sooner or later progresses relentlessly, invading the neighboring abdominal organs, occluding the inferior vena cava, metastasizing to the liver where it may cause massive hepatomegaly, and metastasizing to the lungs where it leads to progressive respiratory embarrassment. One rarely sees major involvement of bones, skin, brain, or other organs. The downhill course of the patient with an adrenal carcinoma is characterized by abdominal distention, ascites, edema of the lower extremities, anorexia, nausea, vomiting, dyspnea, wasting, weakness, and progressive debility. Occasionally, early or late, the patient's course may be punctuated by spontaneous rupture of the tumor, abdominal pain, and hemorrhagic shock.

In contrast to the salubrious prognosis of the patient with a benign adrenal tumor, in whom surgical cure of the tumor and gradual recovery of normal pituitary-adrenal function is the rule, the prognosis of the patient with an adrenal carcinoma must remain guarded. Approximately one-half of these tumors are incompletely resectable by the time the diagnosis is made. Another fourth appear to be resectable initially but subsequently prove otherwise. The remaining fourth can be cured by surgical removal of the primary adrenal tumor.

"Cushing's Disease": Hypercortisolism Secondary to Inappropriate Secretion of ACTH By the Pituitary. From a basic physiologic point of view, "Cushing's disease" stands in sharp contrast to hypercortisolism due to adrenal autonomy, although the clinical features of hypercortisolism are much the same in either disorder. "Cushing's syndrome" is the generic term applied to the constellation of clinical and chemical abnormalities resulting from a chronic excess of glucocorticoids. The more specific term, "Cushing's disease," is applied to those cases of Cushing's syndrome in which hypercortisolism is secondary to inappropriate secretion of ACTH by the pituitary. Patients with this disorder have *relatively* high plasma ACTH concentrations. Their adrenal secretory activity is at least partially suppressible with large doses of dexamethasone, and they have vigorous pituitary-adrenal responses to metyrapone. Furthermore, normalization of their plasma cortisol concentrations (by adrenalectomy followed by chronic cortisol substitution therapy) is followed by supernormal elevations of plasma ACTH. In all these respects (51), patients with Cushing's disease differ from those with truly *primary* adrenal hyperfunction, i.e., those with adrenal neoplasms that autonomously secrete cortisol.

A diagnosis of Cushing's disease can be made with a high degree of confidence if all the following criteria are satisfied: (1) there are definite clinical features of hypercortisolism, (2) plasma cortisol fails to fall to less than 8 μg. per 100 ml. late in the day, (3) urinary 17-OHCS are elevated under basal conditions and fail to fall to less than 2 mg. per g. of creatinine on the second day of treatment with dexamethasone, 0.5 mg. every 6 hours, (4) urinary 17-OHCS fall reproducibly in response to large doses of dexamethasone (2 mg. every 6 hours for two days).

The dexamethasone suppression test can be of extremely great value (42) when used under controlled conditions and in combination with a specific method for measuring urinary 17-OHCS. In checking the validity of the methods one can, from time to time, carry out dexamethasone suppression tests in nonstressed subjects who do not have Cushing's syndrome. On either the small or the large dose of dexamethasone, urinary 17-OHCS should invariably fall to less than 2 mg. per g. of creatinine on the second day of treatment. Failure to do so should alert one to the fact that a methodological problem exists; the possibilities include failure of the subject to take the dexamethasone, lack of specificity of the laboratory method for measuring 17-OHCS, or the presence of interfering medications. In the last category one might include corticotropin, cortisone, hydrocortisone, spironolactone, a variety of psychoactive drugs, and a few fungicides. Obviously, such sources of error should be scrupulously avoided in testing a patient suspected of having Cushing's syndrome.

The principal use of the small-dose dexamethasone test is to separate patients with true hypercortisolism from those without. Any nonstressed individual who does not show profound suppression of 17-OHCS in response to small doses of dexamethasone should be suspected of having Cushing's syndrome. It has sometimes been said that a "normal" response is a 50 per cent (or greater) decrease below control 17-OHCS, but this is erroneous, for patients with Cushing's disease not infrequently qualify as "normal" under the "50 per cent rule." For example, a decrease in urinary 17-OHCS from control values of 14 mg. per g. of creatinine down to 7 mg. per g. of creatinine during treatment with small doses of dexamethasone would be fairly typical of Cushing's disease.

The only purpose of the large-dose dexamethasone test is to separate patients with Cushing's disease from those with other varieties of Cushing's syndrome. Reproducible reduction of urinary 17-OHCS, on repeated testing with large doses of dexamethasone, should be interpreted to mean that adrenal function is pituitary-dependent. The degree of suppression is not crucial, as long as it is beyond the day-to-day fluctuations observed during control periods. In response to large doses of dexamethasone, some patients with Cushing's disease exhibit decreases in urinary 17-OHCS to less than 2 mg. per g. of creatinine, and most exhibit decreases to less than 50 per cent of their control values. A few, however, have been known merely to exhibit decreases to 70 to 80 per cent of their control values.

If in response to *small* doses of dexamethasone, one observes *distinct* but incomplete suppression of 17-OHCS, it is not necessary to employ large doses. That is to say, in many patients with Cushing's disease, one can demonstrate an abnormal degree of resistance to suppression, yet the obvious presence of suppressibility, with small doses of dexamethasone alone.

The following ancillary tests may be performed in characterizing the pituitary-adrenal function of the patient with Cushing's disease (Fig. 5–21): (1) *metyrapone test:* patients with Cushing's disease exhibit increases in *total* 17-OHCS, in contrast to patients with Cushing's syndrome due to adrenal neoplasms; (2) *ACTH infusion test:* patients with Cushing's disease exhibit distinct increases in 17-OHCS, in contrast to some patients with adrenal neoplasms; (3) *plasma ACTH assay:* patients with Cushing's disease have concentrations within the normal range or higher, in contrast to patients with adrenal neoplasms. These ancillary tests do not provide definitive information for separating patients with Cushing's disease from those with the ectopic ACTH syndrome (see below). This distinction must be based on the results of the dexamethasone test and morphologic evidence of a tumor.

Once a diagnosis of Cushing's disease has been established, it may be worthwhile to obtain radiographic views of the sella turcica in search of a pituitary tumor. At least 10 per cent of patients with Cushing's disease have pituitary adenomas (usually chromophobic) that are large enough to cause sellar erosion. If they are not apparent initially, they may become so with continued observation. It is uncertain how many of those with normal-appearing sellae have small chromophobe or basophil adenomas of the type described by Cushing, since most of the patients who have been diagnosed as having Cushing's disease by modern methods are still living and have not undergone hypophysectomy; therefore, their pituitaries have not been carefully examined. From the standpoint of their responses to various endocrinologic manipulations, patients with Cushing's disease with obvious pituitary tumors are indistinguishable from those without.

Treatment of Cushing's Disease. Since the advent of synthetic corticosteroids for use in substitution therapy, it has been feasible to treat Cushing's disease by bilateral adrenalectomy or hypophysectomy. To create a situation in which the patient has lifelong dependency on substitution therapy, however, is not an ideal solution to the problem. For some patients, a better outcome has been achieved with pituitary irradiation (49). In about one-third of patients, it has been possible to correct hypercortisolism without producing endocrinologic deficiencies by irradiating the pituitary with up to 5,000 r. Recently, cyclotrons have been employed to deliver twice as many rads to the pituitary, and the success rate has been twice as high. The great advantage of a mode of therapy which leaves the patient independent of lifelong cortisol substitu-

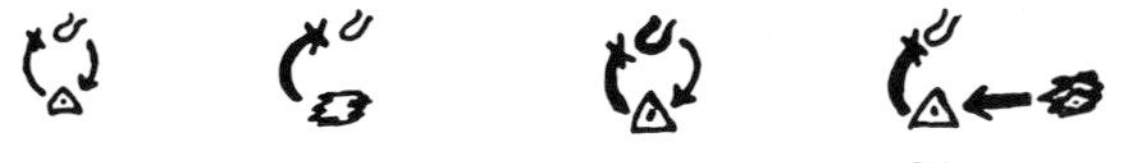

	NORMAL	ADRENAL TUMOR	"CUSHING'S DISEASE"	ECTOPIC ACTH SYNDROME
PLASMA CORTISOL	10-25 μg% RHYTHMIC	HIGH NO RHYTHM	HIGH, NO RHYTHM	HIGH, NO RHYTHM
PLASMA ACTH	0.1 - 0.4 mU%	LOW	HIGH	HIGH
17-OHCS RESPONSE TO ACTH	3-5 FOLD RISE	+,0	+	+,0
RESPONSE TO METYRAPONE	2-4 FOLD RISE	0	+	+,0
RESPONSE TO DEXAMETHASONE	0-3 mg/d	NO FALL	PARTIAL FALL	NO FALL
PLASMA ACTH AFTER ADRENALECTOMY, ON NORMAL CORTISOL	NORMAL	LOW	HIGH	HIGH

Figure 5–21. Typical ACTH, cortisol, and urinary 17-OHCS values in normal subjects and in subjects with various types of Cushing's syndrome under basal conditions and in response to various treatments. (From Liddle, G. W.: *Amer. J. Med. 53:*638, 1972.)

tion therapy is obvious, and pituitary irradiation is now recommended as the primary treatment of choice for most patients with Cushing's disease. Conventional irradiation (up to 5,000 r.) does not result in hypopituitarism, but as dosage advances to 10,000 r., the risk of hypopituitarism becomes appreciable.

A number of medical centers have developed methods for achieving partial hypophysectomy with the hope that the cells responsible for secreting ACTH inappropriately might be destroyed without totally destroying the functional capacity of the anterior pituitary. Perhaps the most elegant of these employs a trans-sphenoidal approach under a dissecting microscope. Other methods that have been used with some success include either cryohypophysectomy or implantation of radioactive gold or yttrium seeds via a trans-sphenoidal approach. Trans-sphenoidal surgery involves some risk of cerebrospinal fluid rhinorrhea and meningitis as well as some uncertainty as to the success of curing hypercortisolism without causing hypopituitarism. Hypophysectomy via craniotomy has had only limited use in the treatment of Cushing's disease. Although this method may cure the Cushing's disease, it does so at the price of causing hypopituitarism. In one reported case (52) of Cushing's disease, pituitary *stalk section* failed to correct the abnormalities of pituitary-adrenal function, even though it did induce hypopituitarism with respect to TSH and gonadotropin production. In general, procedures that carry a high risk of producing hypopituitarism are not ideal for growing children or for adults who wish to preserve reproductive potential.

Bilateral adrenalectomy has been in vogue as a major treatment for Cushing's disease ever since synthetic cortisone became generally available in 1950. It has the advantages of speed and certainty; the source of endogenous cortisol can be removed with only a very slight chance of late recurrence due to growth of accessory adrenal tissue. The main disadvantages are that (1) the operation itself is a major procedure, and this is of particular concern if the patient's condition is already precarious; (2) the patient is left dependent on steroid substitution therapy for the remainder of his life; (3) there is risk of subsequent growth of a pituitary adenoma.

Unilateral adrenalectomy as the sole procedure is not adequate therapy for Cushing's disease; the pituitary merely secretes additional ACTH, and the remaining adrenal secretes approximately as much cortisol as the two adrenals had secreted prior to the operation. Subtotal adrenal resection, leaving a remnant of one adrenal, has occasionally been successful, but it is not recommended since the outcome is unpredictable. Some patients develop adrenal insufficiency, and others sooner or later experience recurrence of Cushing's syndrome. Re-exploration in an attempt to remove all adrenal tissue is then technically difficult and usually unsuccessful.

On an investigational basis, "medical adrenalectomy" has been performed in selected cases of Cushing's disease by administering the adrenocorticolytic agent, o,p'-DDD in doses of 2 to 5 g. per day for several months (53). In these doses, the side effects are usually tolerable. Plasma cortisol can be brought to within the desired range of 5 to 10 μg. per 100 ml. without concomitant aldosterone deficiency. The degree of response is not totally predictable, and when plasma cortisol reaches normal, it is advisable to discontinue administration of o,p'-DDD and institute supportive treatment with dexamethasone 0.5 mg. daily. The administration of o,p'-DDD alters the extra-adrenal metabolism of cortisol, and for several weeks following a course of o,p'-DDD administration, urinary 17-OHCS are deceptively low (54). Plasma cortisol levels must be followed as the index of adrenal function.

During and following any attempt at hypophysectomy or adrenalectomy, the patient should receive glucocorticoid substitution therapy until it has been established that his postoperative endogenous cortisol production is adequate.

Although mild cases of Cushing's disease do not require urgent treatment, severe cases should be treated without undue delay. While bringing the hypercortisolism under control, it is often desirable to minimize protein wasting by providing a high protein intake (at least 100 g. per day). The desirability of a high potassium, high calcium, low sodium intake should be considered. If frank diabetes exists, it should be brought under control with diet and insulin. Infections should be treated, when possible, with specific antibiotics. Hypomania may be treated with reserpine, 1 mg. per day orally for up to a week. More serious psychiatric disturbances should receive the attention of a psychiatric consultant.

The Ectopic ACTH Syndrome.   The third major variety of spontaneous hypercortisolism stems from the production of ACTH by a nonpituitary neoplasm and is usually referred to as "the ectopic ACTH syndrome." In some cases, the clinical manifestations of this variety of hypercortisolism are indistinguishable from those of an adrenal neoplasm and Cushing's disease. Occasionally, the typical clinical features of Cushing's syndrome are remarkably severe in patients with the ectopic ACTH syndrome. In the majority of cases, however, the "typical" features of obesity, striae, plethora, osteoporosis, and renal stones are absent, and the clinical picture is dominated by wasting, weakness, and other manifestations of rapidly advancing malignancy. Often the condition is initially suspected on the basis of persistent hypokalemia in a patient with a tumor, and the suspicion is confirmed by finding extremely high plasma cortisol and urinary 17-OHCS. The clinical spectrum of the ectopic ACTH syndrome is so broad that, in order not to overlook a case, one must follow the dictum, "If one sees hypercortisolism, he should look for a tumor; if one sees a tumor, he should look for hypercortisolism."

Final proof that a patient has the ectopic ACTH syndrome depends upon the demonstration that he has excessive cortisol production and that he has a nonpituitary tumor that contains a higher concentration of ACTH than is found in the plasma. A presumptive diagnosis of the ectopic ACTH syndrome may be based on the following findings: (1) high plasma cortisol and urinary 17-OHCS, (2) failure of dexamethasone in large doses to suppress the output of 17-OHCS reproducibly, and (3) "normal" or elevated plasma ACTH concentrations (Fig. 5–22).

If the patient appears to have the ectopic ACTH syndrome, a search for a tumor should be conducted. A majority will be found in the thorax, with "oat-cell" (small-cell) carcinoma of the lung being the single most common variety. The search should not end there, however, for tumors arising in a wide variety of locations have been found to produce ectopic ACTH (Table 5–5). Even the adrenal should not be overlooked, for at least four ACTH-secreting tumors of the adrenal have been reported—two pheochromocytomas, one paraganglioma, and one adrenocortical carcinoma. Approximately 10 per cent of the reported cases of the ectopic ACTH syndrome have apparently been cured by surgical removal of the tumor. In the others, the tumors proved to be incompletely resectable. This bleak statistic is weighted heavily by the fact that oat-cell carcinoma of the lung, which is almost never curable, accounts for such a high percentage of the total number of cases. If surgical cure cannot be effected, palliative treatment with adrenal inhibitors may be used to curtail the excessive secretion of cortisol and improve the metabolic status of the patient. If the course of the neoplastic disease is favorable enough to permit one to prognosticate survival for a year or more, bilateral adrenalectomy or its "medical equivalent" with o,p'-DDD might be considered as methods for controlling the hypercortisolism.

Virilism and Mineralocorticoid Excess Associated with Cushing's Syndrome. Even though the patient's clinical picture may be dominated by signs of virilism or by signs of mineralocorticoid excess rather than by typical features of Cushing's syndrome, it is important that every patient with such disorders be evaluated for possible hypercortisolism, for the choice of therapy will be critically

TABLE 5–5. SOURCES OF ECTOPIC ACTH IN 100 CASES

Tumor	Number
Carcinoma of lung	52
Carcinoma of pancreas (including carcinoid)	11
Thymoma	11
Benign bronchial adenoma (including carcinoid)	5
Pheochromocytoma	3
Carcinoma of thyroid	2
Carcinoma of liver	2
Carcinoma of prostate	2
Carcinoma of ovary	2
Undifferentiated carcinoma of mediastinum	2
Carcinoma of breast	1
Carcinoma of parotid gland	1
Carcinoma of esophagus	1
Paraganglioma	1
Ganglioma	1
Primary site uncertain	3

affected by this information. When androgens or mineralocorticoids are produced in association with excess cortisol, the patient should be considered to have some variety of Cushing's syndrome and be managed according to the principles outlined above. But if there is excessive production of androgens or mineralocorticoids (particularly DOC) without hypercortisolism, the patient may have congenital adrenal hyperplasia, a condition that is best treated by administering cortisol; or he may have a neoplasm that can be treated by unilateral adrenalectomy or gonadectomy without danger of postoperative adrenal insufficiency. It is important to remember that all three varieties of Cushing's syndrome are often associated with some evidence of androgen or mineralocorticoid excess, and occasionally these features dominate the clinical picture in each variety of hypercortisolism.

Special Problems Related to Cushing's Syndrome

The Structure of Ectopic ACTH. Ever since the discovery that certain nonpituitary tumors synthesize "ectopic ACTH," attempts have been made to determine whether or not the tumor product has the same structure as pituitary ACTH. Unfortunately, the quantities of ectopic ACTH that have been available for study have been so small that it has been impossible to purify and sequence the material. As outlined in Table 5–6, however, a great many tests have been performed that indicate similarity between ectopic ACTH and pituitary ACTH (55). The two hormones can be extracted and partially purified by the same methods. They are both inactivated by the same chemical agents. Ectopic ACTH has all the biologic properties of pituitary ACTH. Various antisera that bind or neutralize pituitary ACTH also bind or neutralize ectopic ACTH. Recent work by Orth has shown that the production of ectopic ACTH is accompanied by the production of smaller polypeptides, which may be the N-terminal and C-terminal halves of the whole ACTH molecule (56). The C-terminal "fragment" is devoid of biologic activity and is detectable only

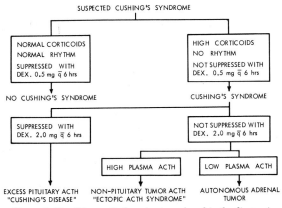

Figure 5–22. Diagnostic flow sheet employed in the diagnosis of Cushing's syndrome.

TABLE 5–6. PROPERTIES COMMON TO PITUITARY ACTH AND TUMOR ACTH

1. Stimulation of adrenocortical enlargement
2. Stimulation of corticosterone secretion in hypophysectomized rat
3. Stimulation of adrenal ascorbic acid depletion in hypophysectomized rat
4. Stimulation of cortisol, corticosterone, and 17-ketosteroid production in man
5. Melanocyte-stimulating activity *in vitro* in frog skin preparation and in hypophysectomized frog
6. Release of free fatty acids in adipose tissue incubates
7. Extractable from tissue with glacial acetic acid
8. Precipitable from acetic acid with acetone-plus-ether
9. Adsorbable onto IRC-50 from dilute acetic acid
10. Can be eluted from IRC-50 with 50% acetic acid
11. Adsorbable onto oxycellulose from dilute acetic acid
12. Can be eluted from oxycellulose with 0.1 N HCl
13. Behavior during counter-current distribution
14. Separable from MSH by chromatography on SE-Sephadex
15. Dialyzable only in acid medium
16. Inactivation by trypsin and chymotrypsin
17. Lability in unheated human plasma
18. Relative stability in acid and lability in alkali
19. Inactivated by hydrogen peroxide; reactivated by cysteine
20. Irreversibly inactivated by periodate
21. Neutralization by ACTH antisera
22. Stimulation of adrenal cyclic AMP
23. Affinity for N-terminal ACTH antibody
24. Affinity for C-terminal ACTH antibody
25. Affinity for central ACTH antibody
26. Behavior on Sephadex G-50 Fine

because it reacts with "C-terminal" ACTH antibodies. The N-terminal "fragment" is practically devoid of adrenal-stimulating activity but appears to have some melanocyte-stimulating activity. Such "fragments" of ACTH have not been found in pituitary tissues. In addition to ACTH and ACTH "fragments," the tumors have also been found to produce immunoreactive α MSH (57) and immunoreactive β MSH (58); these two hormones are also found in human pituitaries. In summary, all available evidence is consistent with the view that ectopic ACTH is identical to pituitary ACTH but that its production by nonpituitary tumors is accompanied by the production of abnormal ACTH analogues.

Recovery From Pituitary-Adrenal Suppression. It has long been known that exogenous corticosteroids induce adrenal atrophy and that cortisol secreted by an adrenal tumor induces atrophy of the nontumorous portions of the adrenal cortex. The adrenal atrophy has been attributed to suppression of ACTH. It has been observed repeatedly that recovery from severe prolonged pituitary-adrenal suppression does not occur readily; in fact, it may be many months before the patient who has been cured of an adrenal adenoma recovers normal pituitary-adrenal function. The question of whether the limiting factor in recovery is at the level of the pituitary or the adrenal was investigated by Graber (59), who made serial measurements of plasma cortisol and ACTH in several patients before and after removal of adrenal tumors (Fig. 5–23). Prior to removal of the adrenal tumor, cortisol levels were supernormal, and ACTH levels were suppressed. During the first month after

removal of the tumor, cortisol levels were subnormal; despite this fact, ACTH levels also remained subnormal, indicating that the chronically suppressed pituitary did not readily return to normal after correction of hypercortisolism. During the ensuing four months, ACTH levels rose to normal and then to supernormal values, but cortisol values remained subnormal, indicating that adrenal responsiveness lags behind pituitary recovery. Finally, cortisol levels rose to normal and then ACTH levels fell back to normal. At this point, normal responses to metyrapone and ACTH were demonstrable. The entire recovery process required at least nine months in patients who had suffered profound pituitary-adrenal suppression for periods in excess of a year.

Pituitary Tumors Following Bilateral Adrenalectomy. Prior to adrenalectomy, plasma ACTH and MSH levels are only modestly elevated in patients with Cushing's disease (10). Apparently pituitary production of ACTH is partially restrained, even in these patients, by the supraphysiologic levels of cortisol, for normalization of plasma cortisol (by bilateral adrenalectomy and subsequent administration of physiologic doses of cortisol) results in distinct elevation of ACTH and MSH levels to about 2 to 20 times the normal range (60). In time, a minority of these patients will go on to develop astronomical elevations of plasma ACTH and MSH (100 to 1,000 times normal). Such patients become deeply pigmented, and many of them can be demonstrated to have chromophobe adenomas that erode the sella turcica and occasionally impinge on the optic chiasm, expand into the third ventricle, or invade the cavernous sinus or sphenoid sinus, sometimes causing death by occluding vessels of the circle of Willis. This complication of Cushing's disease has rarely been seen in patients who have received pituitary irradiation as their primary mode of therapy. In view of the invasive tendencies of these adenomas, it is probably wise to treat them aggressively by proton beam irradiation or surgical excision whenever they become evident as mac-

PATIENTS RECOVERING FROM
PROLONGED PITUITARY-ADRENAL SUPPRESSION

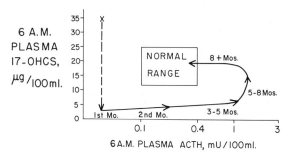

Figure 5–23. Relationship between plasma ACTH and plasma 17-OHCS (cortisol) concentrations during recovery from severe, prolonged pituitary-adrenal suppression with exogenous corticosteroids or autonomously secreted cortisol.

roscopic tumors, without waiting for them to invade adjacent structures. In summary, any patient with Cushing's disease who, following bilateral adrenalectomy, develops intense hyperpigmentation should have plasma ACTH or MSH assayed. If these values are astronomical, despite adequate cortisol substitution therapy, the patient should have radiographic studies for a possible chromophobe adenoma. If an adenoma is found, it should be removed, if feasible.

Hormonal Basis of Hyperpigmentation in Cushing's Disease, the Ectopic ACTH Syndrome, and Addison's Disease. As long as the adrenal glands are intact, ACTH and MSH do not rise to extremely high levels; they could not do so without causing fulminant hyperadrenocorticism. Modest elevations in ACTH and MSH usually cause little or no hyperpigmentation. Once the adrenal glands have been largely or totally resected or destroyed, however, ACTH and MSH levels may rise to very high levels, leading to melanin deposition and striking hyperpigmentation. The hormonal basis of such hyperpigmentation has been investigated by Abe (58), who has inferred that beta-MSH is probably the major agent leading to hyperpigmentation in Addison's disease or in adrenalectomized patients with Cushing's disease or the ectopic ACTH syndrome. This inference rests on the facts that β-MSH is an extremely potent pigmentary hormone and that these patients have elevations in plasma β MSH which are in a general way correlated with the severity of the hyperpigmentation. ACTH too has some melanocyte-stimulating activity, and, on a molar basis, plasma ACTH concentrations are approximately as high as β MSH concentrations. In melanocyte-stimulation assays, however, ACTH is far less potent than β MSH (5). Another pigmentary hormone, α MSH, is approximately as potent as β MSH, but it has not been found in measurable concentrations in the plasma of hyperpigmented patients. Although β MSH might be the agent that is largely responsible for hyperpigmentation in patients with compromised adrenocortical function, it has not been shown to have a role in other conditions associated with hyperpigmentation (58).

Paradoxical Responses to Dexamethasone. A few cases have been described in which patients with Cushing's syndrome have been observed to show paradoxical *increases* in adrenal function during treatment with dexamethasone. Since there is no known mechanism through which dexamethasone could directly stimulate steroid biosynthesis, these "paradoxical" increases have, until recently, remained unexplained. In a recent study of a patient with hypercortisolism and a "paradoxical response" to dexamethasone, Brown (61) discovered that the patient had enigmatic increases in adrenal function not only when treated with dexamethasone but also when observed during extended control periods as well. Detailed study revealed that this patient had striking periodic increases in cortisol secretion, with plasma and urinary steroids rising to extremely high peaks, then returning to modestly elevated levels, in cycles lasting about 11 days. ACTH concentrations were elevated. The patient proved to have a chromophobe adenoma that had extended into the third ventricle; removal of the adenoma and the pituitary cured the hypercorticism. Although there is no available explanation for the periodicity of pituitary-adrenal function, the very fact that such a phenomenon can occur might lead one to question whether apparently "paradoxical responses" to dexamethasone are really *responses* or merely *coincidences*. Perhaps the best way to solve this problem is to carry out protracted studies of patients with apparently paradoxical responses to dexamethasone in order to determine whether they might have spontaneous increases in adrenal function, even when they are not receiving dexamethasone, and to determine whether dexamethasone when given at irregular intervals invariably brings about increased adrenocortical function. Intermittent (if not periodic) hormonogenesis has been observed rarely in patients with hypercortisolism due to an adrenal neoplasm, to pituitary neoplasm, and to the ectopic ACTH syndrome. Such irregularities only serve to emphasize the fact that one must insist on reproducibility of a suppression or stimulation test before reaching a firm conclusion about the suppressibility or responsiveness of the pituitary-adrenal system in any particular case.

Hyperaldosteronism

Although aldosterone is physiologically useful in maintaining fluid and electrolyte homeostasis (62), an excess can lead to potassium depletion and undesirable expansion of the extracellular fluid compartment; the latter may result in edema or hypertension. When hypersecretion of aldosterone occurs as a consequence of the adrenal-stimulating action of angiotensin, it is referred to as "secondary aldosteronism." When it occurs as a consequence of a primary adrenal abnormality (best illustrated by the autonomous function of an adrenal adenoma), it is referred to as "primary aldosteronism."

Atypical forms of hyperaldosteronism which do not fit neatly into either of these categories have been described. Laidlaw and co-workers (63) have described a familial disorder in which hypersecretion of aldosterone appeared to be ACTH-dependent. This is rare, however, and ordinarily ACTH has only a minor effect on aldosterone secretion, not one leading to clinical disease. It is also known that some patients with all the clinical and chemical features of primary aldosteronism have non-adenomatous adrenal glands, and this has raised the question of whether some factor other than angiotensin, ACTH, or potassium might be stimulating their aldosterone-secreting cells. At the moment, this entity remains idiopathic (64).

Secondary Aldosteronism

As listed in Table 5-7, there are numerous clinical and experimental situations in which increased activity of the renin-angiotensin system

TABLE 5–7. STIMULI TO RENIN SECRETION

1. Dehydration
2. Sodium depletion
3. Serum albumin depletion
4. Exsanguination
5. Upright posture
6. Renal artery stenosis
7. Cardiac failure
8. Constriction of inferior vena cava
9. Hepatic cirrhosis
10. Surgical operations
11. Catecholamines
12. Renal nerve stimulation
13. Potassium depletion
14. Diazoxide and other direct vasodilators

results in secondary increases in aldosterone secretion. Anything that compromises the blood supply to the kidney is likely to bring about an increase in renin secretion. This is readily perceived as the mechanism through which experimental or pathologic constriction of the renal artery results in hyper-reninism. It may also be the mechanism through which a reduction in "effective" blood volume results in increased renin secretion. In general, those conditions which are associated with (1) depletion of extracellular fluid volume (severe water deprivation or sodium depletion), (2) reduction of plasma volume (hypoalbuminemia), or (3) sequestration of blood on the venous side of the circulation (caval constriction or hepatic cirrhosis) all result in increased renin and aldosterone production. Even the assumption of upright posture after a period of recumbency results in pooling of blood in the dependent portions of the body, decreased cardiac output, decreased renal blood flow, increased renin production, and increased secretion of aldosterone. In all the conditions listed above, the increase in aldosterone secretion may be viewed, teleologically, as a compensatory mechanism designed to maintain effective blood flow to various organs, including the kidney. An increase in aldosterone promotes sodium retention, which is accompanied by water retention and expansion of the extracellular fluid compartment. The intravascular compartment participates in this volume expansion, and there is some increase in arterial pressure and blood flow to various organs. There may be so much expansion of extracellular volume that edema becomes apparent. The distribution of the edema will be determined by the nature of the primary circulatory disorder.

A special case of secondary aldosteronism is that of Bartter's syndrome, characterized by renal juxtaglomerular cell hyperplasia, hyper-reninemia, hyperaldosteronism, hypokalemia, and failure to thrive (65). Blood pressure tends to be low and relatively unresponsive to exogenous angiotensin. There is uncertainty as to whether the primary abnormality is a sodium-wasting nephropathy or a refractoriness of blood vessels to the pressor action of angiotensin.

Another rare cause of secondary aldosteronism is that occurring in association with a renin-secreting tumor of the kidney (66).

Increases in plasma renin activity and aldosterone secretion occur normally in pregnancy and during treatment with supraphysiologic doses of estrogen (e.g., with oral contraceptives). The increase in plasma renin activity is thought to be related to estrogen-induced increases in the hepatic production of renin substrate (14). It has not been established that the hyper-reninism or hyperaldosteronism of pregnancy are deleterious. In fact, patients with pre-eclampsia tend to have lower plasma renin activity than do women with uncomplicated pregnancies (67).

From the foregoing, it should be obvious that secondary aldosteronism is extremely common, occurring as it does in normal pregnancy, in healthy individuals in response to sodium loss, and in a wide variety of diseases. It should also be obvious that the diagnostic value of an aldosterone measurement is nil unless one knows a great deal about the physiologic status of the patient at the time the crucial specimen is collected.

Secondary aldosteronism is not a specific entity but rather a component of the pathophysiology of a multitude of clinical disorders. An appreciation of the role of aldosterone in various states is fundamental to a clear understanding of disturbed physiology, but secondary aldosteronism does not itself call for specific diagnosis and treatment. Although aldosterone plays a role in the pathogenesis of edema-forming disorders, it should be remembered that these are primarily circulatory disorders, that the hypersecretion of aldosterone is simply a response to the circulatory disorder, and that the distribution of edema fluid will be determined by the nature of the circulatory disorder. Therapeutic attention should generally be focused on the circulatory abnormality. Restriction of sodium intake and treatment with diuretics, while relieving certain congestive symptoms, may further compromise effective blood volume, calling forth even greater secretion of renin and aldosterone. Secondary aldosteronism rarely leads to potassium depletion unless the patient is treated with diuretics. With continued diuretic treatment of the edematous patient, increases in endogenous aldosterone may reduce the natriuretic effectiveness of diuretic agents while accentuating their effectiveness as kaliuretic agents. The mineralocorticoid antagonist, spironolactone, can be used to potentiate the natriuretic action of other diuretics while diminishing their kaliuretic effects (68).

Although it is not necessary to prove that a patient has secondary aldosteronism in order to manage him properly, it has been of great academic interest to investigate aldosterone production and metabolism in various disorders. Normal well-hydrated adults secrete from 40 to 200 μg. of aldosterone per day in response to plasma renin activity ranging from 100 to 800 ng. per 100 ml. of plasma (the amount of angiotensin I generated during a three-hour incubation). Higher aldosterone secretion rates may be said to represent hyperaldosteronism, and, if they are accompanied by higher levels of plasma renin activity, it may be assumed that they represent secondary aldosteronism. The

METABOLISM OF ALDOSTERONE

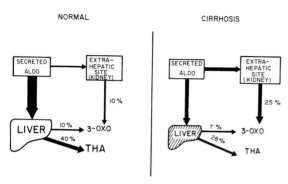

NORMAL   CIRRHOSIS

Figure 5–24. A diagrammatic representation of the concept that aldosterone is metabolized by the liver to two products, tetrahydroaldosterone (THA) and aldosterone-18-glucuronide (3-oxo); in addition, a small proportion of circulating aldosterone is converted by the kidney to 3-oxo. Cirrhosis decreases the capacity of the liver to metabolize aldosterone; therefore, more 3-oxo is formed by the kidney. The percentages should not be interpreted literally.

combination of supernormal renin and subnormal aldosterone is seen in primary adrenal insufficiency. Conversely, an elevation of aldosterone accompanied by subnormal plasma renin activity is seen in primary aldosteronism. It is, therefore, the *combination* of high plasma renin activity and high aldosterone secretion rate that enables one to diagnose secondary aldosteronism with confidence. Plasma concentrations of aldosterone are ordinarily in excess of 20 ng. per 100 ml., and urinary excretion of the acid-hydrolyzable conjugate of aldosterone is ordinarily in excess of 20 μg. per day in secondary aldosteronism. The quantitative relationships between secretion rates, plasma concentrations, and excretion rates are altered in certain diseases. Luetscher (69) has shown that patients with impaired hepatic blood flow or impaired hepatic function have diminished metabolic clearance rates of aldosterone; therefore, plasma concentrations of aldosterone in such patients can be high relative to the aldosterone secretion rate. Bledsoe (70) has shown that the liver and kidney compete with each other as sites for the metabolism of aldosterone. The liver forms both tetrahydroaldosterone and the acid-labile conjugate of aldosterone, but the kidney forms only the latter. Hepatic insufficiency gives an advantage to the kidney, and, for this reason, patients with hepatic insufficiency excrete an abnormally high proportion of aldosterone as the acid-hydrolyzable conjugate. Therefore, urinary "aldosterone," as it is usually measured, is excessively high relative to aldosterone secretion rates or plasma aldosterone concentrations in patients with liver disease (Fig. 5–24).

Primary Aldosteronism

Autonomous secretion of aldosterone gives rise to the clinical syndrome of primary aldosteronism.

The term "primary" implies that the fundamental physiologic disorder is within the adrenal cortex itself, in contradistinction to "secondary" aldosteronism, in which the basically normal adrenal cortex secretes a superabundance of aldosterone in response to a stimulus originating outside of the adrenal. Usually the source of aldosterone is a solitary adrenal adenoma. Occasionally, there are multiple adenomas, or the adrenal cortex appears hyperplastic or normal. In extremely rare instances, the source of aldosterone is an adrenocortical carcinoma.

The pathophysiology of primary aldosteronism (71) can be understood in terms of the known effects of this hormone on electrolyte metabolism. Aldosterone acts on epithelial cells of the nephron, sweat glands, salivary glands, and the gastrointestinal tract to promote the conservation of sodium chloride and the excretion of potassium. As a consequence of sodium retention, there is a modest expansion of extracellular fluid volume. Arterial blood pressure increases and may in time result in all the familiar features of hypertensive cardiovascular disease. Renin production is characteristically suppressed. As a consequence of potassium wastage, there may be hypokalemic alkalosis, alterations in myocardial electrophysiology, skeletal muscular weakness, and kaliopenic nephropathy. The hypokalemic alkalosis may give rise to tetany with muscle cramps and paresthesias. Cardiac abnormalities include depression of S-T segments and T waves and the appearance of U waves in the electrocardiogram. Premature ventricular contractions are frequently noted. The author has seen three patients who experienced near-fatal runs of ventricular fibrillation with repeated episodes of syncope before they were recognized as having the hypokalemia of primary aldosteronism. Skeletal muscular weakness may be so severe that the patient experiences episodic paralysis of the extremities associated with hyporeflexia. Kaliopenic nephropathy is characterized by loss of renal concentrating capacity; even after the injection of vasopressin, urine specific gravity might not exceed 1.020. Subjectively, the patient may note nocturia. It should be remembered that a majority of patients with primary aldosteronism do not have clear-cut *symptoms* of potassium depletion. The symptoms listed above are rare unless the hypokalemia is relatively severe (less than 3.0 mEq. per liter).

For practical purposes, the diagnosis of primary aldosteronism begins with the recognition that a patient has high blood pressure. Any hypertensive patient who has unprovoked hypokalemia should be evaluated carefully for primary aldosteronism. The diagnosis is established by demonstrating that, under standard conditions, aldosterone secretion (or excretion) is elevated and plasma renin activity is subnormal. Each of these points requires some elaboration.

Hypokalemia as a diagnostic criterion for primary aldosteronism is a convenience rather than a necessity. Primary aldosteronism can cause hypertension, can be diagnosed by measuring aldosterone and plasma renin activity, and can be cured by removing an adrenal adenoma in patients who have never been known to be hypokalemic (72). Several studies have shown, however, that so-called "normokalemic" primary aldosteronism is a rare occurrence, while essential hypertension (from which it must be distinguished) is extremely common. It is generally not practical to carry out standard aldosterone studies in normokalemic hypertensives in search of the rare individual with normokalemic primary aldosteronism. It has been stated that only about 1 per cent of patients with normokalemic hypertension have primary aldosteronism. In contrast, among the relatively small subset of patients with unprovoked hypokalemia and hypertension, one may expect that approximately 50 per cent will prove to have primary aldosteronism.

Only "unprovoked" hypokalemia is of value in diagnosing primary aldosteronism. When a patient has lost potassium through vomiting, diarrhea, or the use of diuretics, potassium repletion should be accomplished and the patient observed further for the possible development of unprovoked hypokalemia.

Plasma renin activity (PRA) is characteristically subnormal in patients with primary aldosteronism. In order for it to be of diagnostic value, it is essential that the specimen be obtained under carefully controlled conditions. In anyone, sodium loading and recumbency will decrease renin production, and sodium depletion and upright posture will elevate renin production. In order to bring out the differences between patients with primary aldosteronism and those without, it is best to stimulate renin production in a standard fashion. One method is to restrict sodium intake to 10 mEq. per day for three days and on the third day have the patient upright (standing, sitting, or walking) for three hours prior to drawing blood for assay. Another method is to administer 40 mg. of furosemide (a potent diuretic) at 6 A.M. and have the patient upright from 8 to 11 A.M., at which time blood is drawn for assay. In either case, patients with primary aldosteronism still have low plasma renin activity levels after such maneuvers, while the majority of patients with other varieties of hypertensive disease will have clearly higher values. Each laboratory must standardize its own method and determine empirically what represents "normal" and what represents "suppressed" plasma renin activity. Under the conditions described above, the author's laboratory has found PRA values of less than 300 ng. per 100 ml. (ng. of generated angiotensin per 3-hr. incubation) in most patients with primary aldosteronism. Normal subjects and most hypertensive subjects studied under the same conditions have PRA values greater than 600. The finding of suppressed PRA has come to be a sine qua non in the diagnosis of primary aldosteronism (73).

It has been proposed that measurement of PRA under standard conditions might be a useful screening procedure in searching for patients with primary aldosteronism. This proposal is not without merit, but it has been found that at least 20 per cent of patients with essential hypertension have PRA levels comparable to those of patients with primary aldosteronism. Since this group of patients makes up 20 per cent of the hypertensive population and primary aldosteronism only 1 per cent, it is apparent that the PRA assay by itself is not a very efficient way of separating patients with primary aldosteronism from those without. It should be mentioned that PRA is suppressed not only in primary aldosteronism but also in other clinical disorders characterized by hypertension and potassium depletion, including pseudoaldosteronism (74), licorice intoxication, and disorders characterized by DOC hypersecretion. In summary, although suppressed PRA is a sine qua non in the diagnosis of primary aldosteronism, the vast majority of patients with suppressed PRA do not have primary aldosteronism.

Aldosterone secretion or *excretion rates* must be elevated under standard test conditions if one is to satisfy contemporary criteria for diagnosing primary aldosteronism. The standard test conditions for diagnosing primary aldosteronism include the administration of a diet containing at least 100 mEq. of sodium per day for several days, while withholding diuretics or other medications that might elevate aldosterone production. If, under these conditions, the aldosterone secretion rate exceeds 200 μg. per day or aldosterone excretion exceeds 20 μg. per day, primary aldosteronism must be seriously suspected. Although elevated aldosterone secretion or excretion must be considered a sine qua non in diagnosing primary aldosteronism, it is not by itself sufficient, because, as stressed in foregoing paragraphs, secondary aldosteronism is far more common than primary aldosteronism. The combination of elevated aldosterone production and low PRA is pathognomonic of primary aldosteronism. Ordinarily, the steps in diagnosis are the observation of hypertension, then hypokalemia, then suppressed PRA, then elevated aldosterone output.

The standard treatment for primary aldosteronism is surgical removal of the adenoma (Fig. 5–25) or adenomas, if present, and removal of 1½ adrenal glands (in search of small adenomas) if none can be seen or palpated. If hyperaldosteronism persists following this operation, it can be controlled by chronic treatment with spironolactone.

For patients with primary aldosteronism who are not satisfactory surgical candidates, spironolactone may be given in initial doses of 400 mg. daily for 6 weeks and 100 or 200 mg. daily thereafter in order to control their hypertension and hypokalemia. Side effects of lassitude, impotency, gynecomastia, and oligomenorrhea are not infrequent.

Role of the Adrenal Cortex in Essential Hypertension

"Essential hypertension" is, by definition, idiopathic. Yet there is increasing evidence that it is not a single disorder but rather a manifestation of a number of different disorders. Some patients

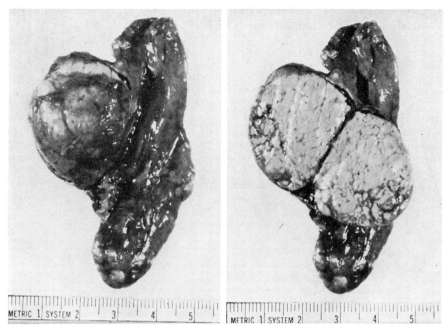

Figure 5–25. Typical aldosteronoma, canary yellow, weighing 5 g. and measuring approximately 2 cm. in diameter. Removal in patient led to regression of all the symptomatology within 4 weeks.

with "essential hypertension" behave in many ways as though they have an excess of some mineralocorticoid. First, they have low PRA. Second, Woods and co-workers (75) demonstrated that these patients, but not those with hypertension and normal renin, experience amelioration of their hypertension when treated with aminoglutethamide, an inhibitor of steroid biosynthesis. Third, it has been shown by several groups that these patients experience amelioration of their hypertension when treated with spironolactone, an antagonist of mineralocorticoid actions (Fig. 5–26).

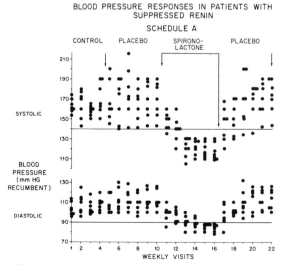

Figure 5–26. Effects of spironolactone, 400 mg. per day, on the systolic and diastolic blood pressures of seven patients with the syndrome of essential hypertension and suppressed PRA.

Fourth, it has been shown by Gunnells and co-workers (76) that these patients experience amelioration of their hypertension following bilateral adrenalectomy. Finally, it has been shown by Adlin and co-workers (77) that these patients have lower salivary sodium/potassium ratios than do patients with essential hypertension and normal renin. It remains to be shown what mineralocorticoid (if any) is responsible for the syndrome of essential hypertension with suppressed renin. Nevertheless, patients who have been properly categorized in this way have approximately a 90 per cent chance of responding to spironolactone, 400 mg. daily for six weeks, with significant reduction of their blood pressures (78). Once a full response has been achieved, the dose of spironolactone can be reduced to 100 or 200 mg. daily with satisfactory control of the blood pressure.

There is another disorder which has all the clinical hallmarks of primary mineralocorticoid excess, with hypertension, urinary wastage of potassium, and suppression of plasma renin activity, but which is clearly not due to an excess of mineralocorticoids. This is a familial disorder in which the renal tubules reabsorb sodium and excrete potassium excessively. The tendency to retain sodium results in hypertension, suppression of renin production, and suppression of aldosterone secretion to negligible values. The tendency to excrete potassium results in hypokalemic alkalosis. Because mineralocorticoid production is negligible, neither adrenal inhibitors nor mineralocorticoid antagonists are useful in favorably altering electrolyte excretion. Triamterene, a pteridine derivative which is not a mineralocorticoid antagonist but which does block sodium-potassium exchange by the distal tubule, is used in the treatment of this disorder, which has been referred to as "pseudoaldosteronism" (74).

Virilizing Tumors, Feminizing Tumors, and "Nonfunctioning" Tumors of the Adrenal Cortex

Normal virilization and feminization are attributable to gonadal function, but when these phenomena occur inappropriately (virilization in women or children or feminization in men or children), they might alert the physician to the possibility of an adrenal neoplasm. As emphasized in foregoing paragraphs, any patient with signs of androgen excess should be studied for possible hypercortisolism, since proper understanding of the mechanisms involved and proper treatment will follow the lines outlined for Cushing's syndrome if hypercortisolism does in fact exist, regardless of the severity of the accompanying androgen excess. If cortisol levels are normal but urinary 17-ketosteroids are distinctly elevated and not suppressible to less than 5 mg. daily after several successive days of treatment with dexamethasone, 0.5 mg. every 6 hours, the probability of an adrenal or gonadal tumor is high enough to justify anatomical studies, such as culdoscopy in search of an ovarian tumor, or adrenal arteriography in search of an adrenal tumor.

Feminizing adrenal tumors are extremely rare. Depending on the age and sex of the patient, they might enter into the differential diagnosis of Klinefelter's syndrome, precocious puberty, or ectopic gonadotropin production (see Chs. 6 & 7). Establishment of the diagnosis might be accomplished in the following steps: observation of abnormal feminization, then the demonstration of subnormal gonadotropin levels and supra-normal estrogen levels, and, finally, radiographic demonstration of an adrenal mass.

Adrenal cortical tumors that are "nonfunctioning" in the sense that they produce no biologically active or chemically identifiable steroids are very rare. Most so-called nonfunctioning adrenal tumors that have been mentioned in the literature have not actually been carefully studied prior to their removal or the death of the patient. Some androgen-secreting adrenal tumors have been mistakenly considered to be nonfunctioning because they caused no symptoms; however, since the patients were already fully virilized men, there was no way in which an excess of adrenal androgen could express itself in terms of symptoms. The fact that the tumors were not truly nonfunctioning became clear when chemical measurements of steroids (e.g., urinary 17-ketosteroids) were performed. The more thoroughly one surveys patients with adrenal tumors, the more likely it is that the tumors will be found to secrete steroids, even though the steroids might cause no symptoms. It is conceivable that some adrenal tumors are truly "nonfunctioning" with respect to steroid secretion; a tumor that lacked the enzymatic machinery for converting cholesterol to pregnenolone might, for example, be considered to be truly nonfunctioning.

Adrenal Cortical Hypofunction

Adrenal insufficiency can occur as a result of a primary adrenal abnormality which impairs the capacity of this gland to secrete cortisol or aldosterone or both in response to adrenal stimulators, or it can occur as a result of the lack of adrenal stimulators. In certain disorders there are deficiencies of both cortisol and aldosterone; in other disorders production of only one hormone is impaired. A primary deficiency of cortisol results in a compensatory increase in ACTH production. In analogous fashion, a primary deficiency of aldosterone usually results in a compensatory increase in renin production.

Primary Adrenal Insufficiency (Addison's Disease)

Clinical and Chemical Features of Primary Adrenal Insufficiency

Destruction of the adrenal cortex, regardless of the nature of the underlying process, leads to Addison's disease. The major clinical manifestations are attributable to deficiencies of aldosterone (Table 5–8) and cortisol (Table 5–9). In addition, loss of adrenal androgen in women with Addison's disease may result in diminished growth of axillary hair.

Lack of aldosterone results in impaired ability to conserve sodium and excrete potassium. As long as the patient has a very high sodium intake (an occasional patient actually experiences salt craving), his lack of aldosterone may be of little consequence; however, on a moderate or restricted sodium intake, he soon becomes seriously depleted of sodium. This predicament can be quickly worsened if the patient experiences anorexia, vomiting, diarrhea, or excessive sweating. Without aldosterone or aldosterone substitution therapy, it is virtually impossible for the addisonian patient to diminish his urinary sodium to less than 50 mEq. per day. Excretion of sodium in excess of intake results in a

TABLE 5–8. MANIFESTATIONS OF ALDOSTERONE DEFICIENCY

A. Inability to conserve sodium
  Decreased extracellular fluid volume
  Weight loss
  Hypovolemia
  Hypotension
  Decreased cardiac size
  Decreased cardiac output
  Decreased renal blood flow
  Prerenal azotemia
  Increased renin production
  Decreased pressor response to catecholamines
  Weakness
  Postural syncope
  Shock
B. Impaired renal secretion of potassium and hydrogen ions
  Hyperkalemia
    Cardiac asystole
  Mild acidosis

TABLE 5–9. MANIFESTATIONS OF
CORTISOL DEFICIENCY

1. *Gastrointestinal:* anorexia, nausea, vomiting, hypochlorhydria, abdominal pain, weight loss
2. *Mental:* diminished vigor, lethargy, apathy, confusion, psychosis
3. *Energy metabolism:* impaired gluconeogenesis, impaired fat mobilization and utilization, liver glycogen depletion, fasting hypoglycemia
4. *Cardiovascular-renal:* impaired ability to excrete "free water," impaired pressor responses to catecholamines, hypotension
5. *Pituitary:* unrestrained secretion of ACTH and MSH, resulting in mucocutaneous hyperpigmentation
6. *Impaired tolerance to stress:* any of the above manifestations might become more pronounced during trauma, infection, or fasting

decrease in extracellular fluid, weight loss, a decrease in plasma volume, a decrease in blood pressure, a decrease in cardiac output, a decrease in heart size, an increase in renin production, a decrease in renal blood flow, azotemia, generalized weakness, and postural syncope. Lack of aldos-

terone also favors the development of hyperkalemia and mild acidosis, in part due to diminished glomerular filtration rate and in part due to diminished cation exchange by the distal convoluted tubule.

Lack of cortisol results in anorexia, abdominal pain, wasting of fat depots, apathy, weakness, fasting hypoglycemia, diminished ability to excrete free water, hyponatremia, increased production of ACTH and MSH, hyperpigmentation, (Fig. 5–27), and diminished ability to withstand a variety of physiologic stresses.

A combined deficiency of aldosterone and cortisol, therefore, culminates in the clinical picture so graphically described by Addison (79):

"The patient, in most of the cases I have seen, has been observed gradually to fall off in general health; he becomes languid and weak, indisposed to either bodily or mental exertion; the appetite is impaired or entirely lost; . . . the pulse small and feeble . . . excessively soft and compressible; the body wastes . . . slight pain or uneasiness is from time to time referred to the region of

Figure 5–27. *A,* Addison's disease secondary to tuberculosis of the adrenals. Note diffuse brown pigmentation of variable intensity. The scars above and lateral to each breast are pigmented. *B,* Contrasting skin changes in two patients with adrenocortical insufficiency of differing etiology. Note the absence of pigmentation in the male suffering from a chromophobe adenoma of the pituitary contrasted with the presence of hyperpigmentation and vitiligo in the female with adrenocortical atrophy of unknown cause.

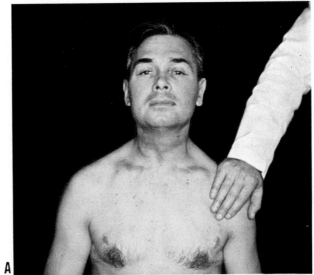

A

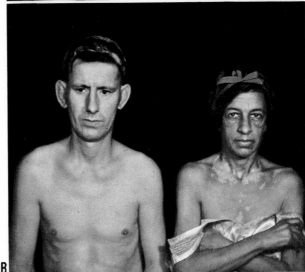

B

the stomach, and there is occasionally actual vomiting . . . it is by no means uncommon for the patient to manifest indications of disturbed cerebral circulation. . . . We discover a most remarkable, and, so far as I know, characteristic discoloration taking place in the skin — sufficiently marked indeed as generally to have attracted the attention of the patient himself, or of the patient's friends. . . . It may be said to present a dingy or smoky appearance, or various tints or shades of deep· amber or chestnut brown. . . . The body wastes . . . the pulse becomes smaller and weaker, and . . . the patient at length gradually sinks and expires."

Formerly, the principal cause of Addison's disease was tuberculous destruction of the adrenal glands. In parts of the world where the incidence of tuberculosis has diminished in recent decades, idiopathic atrophy of the adrenals has become the most common cause of Addison's disease. There is evidence suggesting that "idiopathic atrophy" might represent autoimmune destruction of the adrenal cortex (80).

Patients with idiopathic adrenal atrophy are at increased risk with respect to "autoimmune" destruction of other tissues as well, and the physician should be alert to the possibility that they might in time develop hypothyroidism, diabetes mellitus, hypoparathyroidism, primary ovarian failure, or pernicious anemia. Conversely, patients with these disorders are at increased risk with respect to the development of Addison's disease.

In some regions where systemic fungal infections (such as histoplasmosis) are common, these may be as important as tuberculosis or autoimmune disease in the etiology of Addison's disease. Rare causes of Addison's disease include amyloidosis, adrenal apoplexy, (Waterhouse-Friderichsen syndrome, Fig. 5-28), and metastatic carcinoma involving the adrenals. Nowadays, of course, bilateral adrenalectomy is performed in the treatment of several diseases, and this must be reckoned as a relatively common cause of the addisonian state. For the sake of completeness, one might mention that prolonged treatment with o,p'-DDD can result in adrenal atrophy and cortisol deficiency (81) and that treatment with heparinoids can result in structural changes in the zona glomerulosa and reversible aldosterone deficiency (82). There is a familial disorder characterized by the combined abnormalities of diffuse demyelinization of the central nervous system (leukodystrophy) and Addison's disease, a disorder that appears to be limited to boys and young men. There have also been reports of children with congenital aplasia of the zona fasciculata and zona reticularis. Their miniature adrenal cortices are composed of zona glomerulosa cells which secrete aldosterone but not cortisol.

In most cases Addison's disease is insidious in its evolution, adrenal destruction is a gradual process, and compensatory increases in ACTH and renin enable the adrenal for a time to secrete enough cortisol and aldosterone to satisfy physiologic requirements in the absence of some intercurrent stress, such as vomiting, infection, trauma, or a surgical operation. When more than 90 per cent of the adrenal cortex has been destroyed, however, homeostatic compensation can no longer be achieved, and

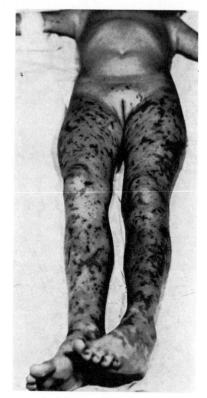

Figure 5-28. Waterhouse-Friderichsen syndrome of 2 days' duration. Note hemorrhagic lesions in the skin.

the patient develops the clinical disease as it was seen by Addison. "Addisonian crisis" is the term applied to the patient whose hypotension progresses to shock and, if untreated, to death. Addisonian crisis is characterized by anorexia, vomiting, abdominal pain, apathy, confusion, and extreme weakness.

Diagnosis

The diagnosis of Addison's disease should be considered whenever one sees a patient with any of the features mentioned in the foregoing paragraphs. It should be strongly considered whenever one sees a patient with the tetralogy of hypotension, weight loss, anorexia, and weakness. Each of these manifestations is so characteristic of untreated Addison's disease that one can be fairly secure that a patient is not (at that moment) suffering from this disorder if one can be certain that the patient is hypertensive, that he is gaining weight, that he has a hearty appetite, or that he has normal vigor. Hyperpigmentation is not emphasized as much by contemporary endocrinologists as it was in Addison's original descriptions of this disease; its presence may be a useful clue, but its absence does not exclude the diagnosis of Addison's disease.

Modern methods make it possible to prove or disprove the diagnosis of Addison's disease without employing a large number of laboratory tests. It is only necessary to measure "adrenal reserve" by the technique outlined on p. 250. If the clinical suspicion of Addison's disease is correct, it may be highly desirable to institute treatment without delay. Fortunately, if one employs the following protocol it is possible to diagnose and treat Addison's disease simultaneously.

1. Draw 10 ml. of blood for plasma cortisol assay.

2. Start a rapid intravenous infusion of physiologic saline; add (as soon as available) dexamethasone phosphate, 4 mg. (1 ml. of the pharmaceutical solution), and 25 I.U. corticotropin. This first liter of saline with dexamethasone and corticotropin should be infused within the first hour.

3. At the end of the infusion, draw a second 10-ml. specimen of blood for plasma cortisol assay.

4. Administer additional 5 per cent dextrose in saline as rapidly and as long as indicated for treatment of dehydration and shock.

5. Start a 24-hour urine collection for 17-OHCS assay.

6. Inject intramuscularly 80 I.U. of corticotropin (suspended in gelatin or complexed with zinc). As an alternative, one might add corticotropin to each liter of intravenous saline so that at least 3 I.U. are infused every hour for at least eight hours.

7. Obtain a third blood specimen for plasma cortisol assay between the sixth and eighth hours of treatment with corticotropin.

If the patient does have Addison's disease, one should see distinct clinical improvement in response to treatment with saline and dexamethasone. In addition, all plasma cortisol values should be less than 15 μg. per 100 ml., including those obtained after the administration of corticotropin. Furthermore, the urinary 17-OHCS value should be less than 10 mg. per 24 hours, despite the administration of corticotropin. Steroid responses indicative of intact adrenocortical reserve exclude the diagnosis of Addison's disease. If one is to follow the combined diagnostic-therapeutic protocol outlined above, it is imperative that no hydrocortisone or cortisone be administered. These steroids will be detected in the assays for plasma cortisol and urinary 17-OHCS; dexamethasone will not. If dexamethasone is not available, the clinician must make a decision as to whether it is more important at the moment to follow the diagnostic protocol alone (giving ACTH with saline and measuring the steroid response) or to follow a modified therapeutic protocol by giving saline and hydrocortisone (or cortisone) and deferring the crucial diagnostic maneuvers until a later date.

In patients whose symptoms are so mild and stable that they do not seem to require saline and dexamethasone, the diagnosis of Addison's disease can be established or excluded merely by testing adrenocortical reserve as outlined above.

Treatment of Primary Adrenal Insufficiency

Management of Addisonian Crisis. Typical addisonian crisis is the outcome of combined cortisol deficiency, aldosterone deficiency, extracellular volume depletion, and (often) some precipitating stress. This is a life-threatening medical emergency which calls for rapid intravenous infusion of physiologic saline, parenteral administration of glucocorticoids, and specific treatment for any recognizable precipitating stress. It can usually be assumed that the patient in addisonian crisis is depleted of 20 per cent of his extracellular fluid volume. Unless there is some obvious contraindication, this deficit should be corrected as rapidly as possible by intravenously infusing physiologic saline. An adult might require as much as 3 liters of saline over a period of a few hours; a child might require proportionately less in terms of volume, but vigorous therapy is just as urgent as in the adult. One obviously cannot repair a sodium deficit without giving enough sodium. One does not depend upon sodium-*retaining* steroids to replenish sodium stores once they have become depleted. As long as one gives enough saline in treating addisonian crisis, it is relatively unimportant whether one establishes mineralocorticoid substitution therapy immediately or waits until the patient's condition has stabilized. Such flexibility is not justified with respect to glucocorticoid replacement therapy. There is little to fear from giving intravenously a single 100-mg. dose of hydrocortisone phosphate or a single 4-mg. dose of dexamethasone phosphate, and such treatment immediately provides circulating glucocorticoid concentrations comparable to those of severely stressed patients with intact adrenal function. Such injections, therefore, are recommended routinely as part of the treatment for addisonian crisis. Once the addisonian patient has received enough saline to replete his extracellular volume and enough glucocorticoid to mimic the normal adrenal response to severe stress, he should be considered for the moment to be "endocrinologically normal," and the remainder of his medical problems should be managed as they would be in patients without Addison's disease.

Management of Addisonian Patients During Surgical or Other Stresses. Patients undergoing adrenalectomy or addisonian patients who are subjected to surgical operations or other major stresses should be treated with adequate doses of cortisol; by "adequate" is meant at least as much as an endocrinologically normal individual would secrete in response to similar stresses. In response to major stresses, people with intact adrenals might secrete more than 100 mg. per day but probably never more than 300 mg. per day. Therefore, it is often recommended that severely stressed addisonian patients be given hydrocortisone phosphate in divided doses totaling not less than 300 on the day of stress. Since most surgical stresses are of brief duration, it is advisable to decrease the dose of hydrocortisone by 50 per cent each day until the maintenance level has been reached (about 30 mg. daily). Minor stresses or those of short duration might well be managed by administering a single 100-mg. dose of hydrocortisone or an equivalent amount of some other glucocorticoid (Table 5–3).

In treating acute stresses it is permissible to err on the side of overtreatment, inasmuch as brief excesses of glucocorticoids are relatively innocuous and provide much security against any possibility of adrenal insufficiency. If stresses are protracted, however, one must consider the dangers of over-treatment as well as those of undertreatment. In treating the chronically stressed addisonian patient, one might give between 20 and 100 mg. of hydrocortisone daily, depending upon the severity of the stress. If the stress is an infection, one might assume that glucocorticoid therapy is adequate if the temperature is less than 38° C but inadequate if it exceeds 39° C. In this situation, one would not wish to give too much glucocorticoid for fear of interfering with host defense mechanisms and of creating a false sense of security by masking signs of infection. On the other hand, one would not wish to give too little steroid and leave the patient vulnerable to the stress imposed by the infection.

Stressed patients usually cannot be relied upon to take full diets; therefore, in the absence of normal adrenal function, they may quickly become dangerously depleted of sodium. This can be avoided by giving any addisonian patient at least 1 liter of physiologic saline intravenously every day until he is taking a full diet. Here it is wise to err on the side of oversolicitude, since ill patients may not consume full diets even though these are prescribed. Until the patient has fully demonstrated that he is eating heartily, he should continue to receive his daily liter of saline.

Management of Intercritical Addison's Disease. It is essential that the addisonian patient be thoroughly indoctrinated in how to care for himself during intervals between crises. With minor modifications, he should take cortisol (or its glucocorticoid equivalent) in doses of 20 mg. each morning and 10 mg. each evening, and Florinef (fludrocortisone) in doses of 0.1 mg. per day. He should carry a sterile syringe containing 4 mg. of dexamethasone phosphate (in 1 ml. of water) for emergency injection. He should have an identification card giving his name, physician's name, and the following statement: "I have Addison's disease. In an emergency involving loss of consciousness, injury, or vomiting, I should immediately be given an intramuscular injection of dexamethasone phosphate (with my personal belongings). Call a physician without delay." His diet should include a liberal amount of sodium (at least 150 mEq. per day); moreover, in the event of diarrhea or profuse sweating, he should take supplemental sodium chloride. The dose of fludrocortisone should be cautiously decreased if the patient exhibits edema, hypertension, or hypokalemia and increased if he exhibits hypotension or hyperkalemia. Some patients who have had hypertension prior to the development of Addison's disease require no mineralocorticoid substitution therapy and may respond to ordinary doses of fludrocortisone by becoming hypertensive. Although some addisonian patients may not require mineralocorticoid therapy, they all require liberal intakes of sodium chloride.

It should be remembered that Addison's disease is often a complication of some other disease. If appropriate investigations reveal evidence of tuber-culosis or disseminated histoplasmosis, these infections should be specifically treated. If the Addison's disease is thought to be due to autoimmune atrophy of the adrenals, the patient should be observed from time to time for evidence of hypothyroidism, hypoparathyroidism, or diabetes mellitus so that these conditions might be treated before they become incapacitating or life-threatening.

In growing children, it is of utmost importance that the dose of steroid employed in glucocorticoid substitution therapy be carefully regulated so as to avoid adrenal insufficiency, on the one hand, and retardation of linear growth, on the other. Growth retardation is a very sensitive index of glucocorticoid excess and can occur in the virtual absence of obesity, impairment of glucose tolerance, ecchymoses, or other common signs of Cushing's syndrome. An initial maintenance dose of hydrocortisone might be 20 mg. per square meter of body surface per day (in two or three doses given principally in the morning), but one must be prepared to adjust the dosage from time to time according to the empirical requirements of the individual patient.

Secondary Adrenal Insufficiency

Cortisol deficiency can occur as a consequence of ACTH deficiency. The clinical manifestations of ACTH deficiency are listed in Table 5–9, with the exception that cutaneous hyperpigmentation is not present, since in this variety of adrenal insufficiency, the pigmentary hormones ACTH and beta-MSH are low rather than high.

Plasma cortisol concentrations and urinary 17-OHCS and 17-ketosteroids are characteristically subnormal and rise only sluggishly in response to standard test doses of ACTH. The fact that they rise at all, however, sets this condition apart from primary adrenal insufficiency, in which adrenocortical reserve is negligible. With prolonged treatment with ACTH, patients with secondary adrenal insufficiency can generate normal or supernormal adrenal steroid levels, but these cannot be maintained after exogenous ACTH has been withdrawn (Fig. 5–29).

The distinction between primary and secondary adrenal insufficiency is important for two practical reasons. First, in primary adrenal insufficiency, cortisol deficiency is usually accompanied by aldosterone deficiency, but in secondary adrenal insufficiency, the aldosterone-secretory mechanism is usually intact, and mineralocorticoid substitution therapy is not required. Second, while primary adrenal insufficiency should alert the physician to the possible coexistence of tuberculosis, histoplasmosis, amyloidosis, or autoimmune disorders, secondary adrenal insufficiency should alert the physician to the possibility that the patient might have deficiencies of multiple pituitary hormones as well as to the possibility that the disease leading to pituitary destruction might endanger neighboring neural structures. The recognition of a pituitary tumor or cyst might lead to early treatment (either

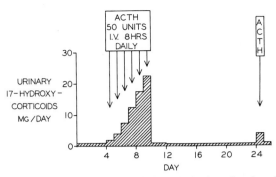

RESPONSE TO ACTH IN HYPOPITUITARISM

Figure 5–29. In patients with hypopituitarism, the adrenal steroidogenic response to a standard test dose of ACTH is subnormal. Repetitive treatment with ACTH enhances adrenal responsiveness, but if exogenous ACTH is withdrawn, adrenal reserve becomes subnormal again.

culty in making this diagnosis since there will be a history of Cushing's syndrome followed by steroid withdrawal. Basal levels of plasma cortisol and urinary 17-OHCS are subnormal, and the adrenal cortical responses to standard test doses of ACTH are subnormal. In time, complete recovery of pituitary-adrenal function can be anticipated, but this may require as long as a year. During this period, the patient should receive protective doses of glucocorticoids during major stresses. Even in the absence of severe stress, some patients require daily steroid therapy in order to avoid symptoms of weakness, myalgia, anorexia, and despondency. Such steroid therapy should be given as single morning doses of hydrocortisone in order to minimize the possibility of continued suppression of ACTH secretion. As time passes, the daily dose of hydrocortisone can be diminished gradually and finally withdrawn altogether.

surgical or radiologic) in time to prevent encroachment on such structures as the optic chiasm or the circle of Willis. A detailed discussion of hypopituitarism is to be found in Chapter 2. In treating secondary adrenal insufficiency, one aims to provide exogenous glucocorticoids in quantities similar to those secreted by patients with intact adrenal function; the doses and indications are the same as those outlined above for the treatment of primary adrenal insufficiency. As in the case of primary adrenal insufficiency, it is essential that the patient be well-educated as to his need for glucocorticoid therapy; he should carry an identification card and an emergency supply of injectable dexamethasone phosphate or hydrocortisone phosphate.

A special case of secondary hypocortisolism is that resulting from chronic suppression of ACTH by cortisol from an adrenal neoplasm or by exogenous glucocorticoids. There should be no diffi-

Limited ACTH Reserve

Any disease that can cause frank hypopituitarism can also cause a milder degree of pituitary dysfunction, a condition referred to as "limited pituitary reserve." Such patients secrete enough ACTH to maintain adrenal responsiveness to standard test doses of ACTH, but they are incapable of increasing their ACTH secretion normally in response to stress or in response to some stimulus designed to test ACTH reserve. In the latter category are insulin, pyrogens, and metyrapone (Fig. 5–15). Based on the results of standard metyrapone tests, patients with a variety of endocrinologic disorders have been found to have limited pituitary reserve (Table 5–10).

Routine treatment of "limited pituitary reserve" is not necessary, but the physician should be prepared to administer glucocorticoids if the patient with "limited pituitary reserve" is subjected to a major stress.

TABLE 5–10. RESULTS OF PITUITARY-ADRENAL EVALUATION IN 266 PATIENTS WITH VARIOUS ENDOCRINE-METABOLIC DISORDERS

| | | Pituitary-Adrenal Status | |
	Normal	*Limited Pituitary Reserve*	*Frank Insufficiency*
Pituitary dwarfism	0	2	5
Sheehan's syndrome	0	2	7
Craniopharyngioma	1	0	6
Chromophobe adenoma	12	26	6
Acromegaly	14	5	0
After pituitary irradiation	33	23	0
Low-FSH eunuchoidism	5	2	0
Metastases to pituitary	0	1	1
Cachexia	6	6	0
Post-traumatic diabetes insipidus	3	2	0
Cushing's syndrome, adrenal tumor	0	11	0
Cushing's syndrome, pituitary	29	1	0
Congenital adrenal hyperplasia (non–salt losers)	7	0	0
Primary aldosteronism	5	0	0
Primary hypothyroidism	34	2	0
Graves' disease	8	1	0

Mixed Hypo- and Hyperadrenocorticism: Congenital Adrenal Hyperplasia

The secretion of the important adrenocortical hormones, cortisol and aldosterone, requires the integrity of biosynthetic pathways involving a long series of enzymatically regulated steps. If, through a genetic error, any one of these enzymes is defective, the corresponding biosynthetic step will be impeded, derivatives of that step will be diminished, and precursors immediately preceding the impeded step will accumulate in increased quantities. If the cortisol pathway is impeded, there will be a compensatory increase in ACTH secretion (83). If mineralocorticoid production is impeded, there will be a compensatory increase in renin-angiotensin production. Increased stimulation of the adrenal by its tropic hormones results in increased formation of steroid precursors up to the impeded step. If the impediment is incomplete, then the increase in precursors may lead to normal or nearly normal production of cortisol or aldosterone, but this compensation will be accomplished at the price of a continuing increase in the production of tropic hormones and a continuing excess of pre-impediment precursors and byproducts. Some of these precursors and byproducts have biologic activities which assume clinical importance when they are secreted in excessive amounts even though they are of little or no clinical importance when secreted in normal quantities. The clinical manifestations of a genetic error in adrenal metabolism depend upon the severity of the cortisol or aldosterone deficiency, on the one hand, and, on the other hand, upon the properties of the steroid precursors and byproducts that are excessively secreted.

Because the inefficient adrenal glands are chronically stimulated by relatively high concentrations of adrenotropic hormones, they become hyperplastic. For this reason, these disorders have come to be grouped under the heading "congenital adrenal hyperplasia." The disorders appear to be inherited through autosomal recessive genes. In any one family, the affected siblings have similar adrenal steroid patterns and similar degrees of severity of the disorder.

There are now six known varieties of congenital adrenal hyperplasia, each attributable to inefficiency of a specific enzymatically regulated step in cortisol or aldosterone biosynthesis. Certain enzymes are unique to the cortisol pathway, others are unique to the aldosterone pathway, and still others are found in both. Therefore, in various types of congenital adrenal hyperplasia, one can find deficiencies of either cortisol or aldosterone or both, depending upon the specific biosynthetic error. Certain enzymes of the adrenal cortex are also found in the gonads. Inborn errors affecting these enzymes result not only in derangements of adrenal function but also in gonadal function as well.

Treatment of congenital adrenal hyperplasia is directed toward supplying physiologic quantities of the deficient steroids. Such treatment should re-strain the overproduction of tropic hormones, thus correcting the adrenal hyperplasia and the hypersecretion of steroid precursors and byproducts (83). In patients with severe deficiencies of cortisol and aldosterone, treatment with glucocorticoids, mineralocorticoids, and sodium chloride should be similar to that employed in Addison's disease, including special supplements during major stresses.

Deficiency of 20-Hydroxylase (Cholesterol Desmolase)

The earliest step in the conversion of cholesterol to hormonal steroids is hydroxylation at carbon 20, with subsequent cleavage of the 20–22 side chain (a desmolase reaction) to form pregnenolone. This process is thought to be essential for the formation of all adrenal and gonadal steroids. An inborn error in the enzyme system governing this reaction is thought to be the cause of a rare form of congenital adrenal hyperplasia, first described by Prader (84), in which the adrenal glands are massively enlarged and laden with cholesterol. Infants with this disorder have female external genitalia even though they may have XY genotypes, and this has been taken as evidence that their gonads were incapable of synthesizing normal quantities of androgen. The poor survival of these infants has permitted little accumulation of biochemical data, but one would expect all steroids in blood and urine to be subnormal (Fig. 5–30) and ACTH secretion to be abnormally high. Appropriate treatment should be directed at correcting the deficiencies of cortisol and aldosterone and should include, at the appropriate age, the use of estrogens and progestins.

Deficiency of 3 β-Hydroxysteroid Dehydrogenase

An important step in the formation of all potent adrenal and gonadal steroids is dehydrogenation of

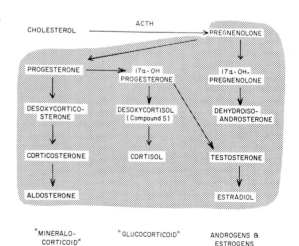

Figure 5–30. Consequences of impaired conversion of cholesterol to pregnenolone: a deficiency of all steroids within the shaded area.

the 3 β-hydroxyl group of the Δ⁵ steroids. This facilitates the isomerase reaction through which the Δ⁵ double bond is shifted to the Δ⁴ position. Bongiovanni (85) was the first to describe a form of congenital adrenal hyperplasia caused by a defect in this process. Affected patients produce little in the way of Δ⁴ steroids, such as cortisol, but increased quantities of Δ⁵ steroids, such as DHEA (Fig. 5–31).

Clinically, patients with this disorder manifest cortisol and aldosterone deficiency; in addition, however, neonates of either sex have ambiguous external genitalia. Failure of the genetic males to develop normal external genitalia has been attributed to inability of their gonads to produce fetal androgen (presumably a Δ⁴ steroid, probably testosterone). Partial masculinization of the external genitalia of the genetic females has been attributed to their hypersecretion of weak adrenal androgens, possibly DHEA.

Treatment of this disorder is directed toward physiologic replacement of the deficient glucocorticoids and mineralocorticoids. Initially, glucocorticoid therapy might consist of cortisone acetate, 25 mg. intramuscularly every 48 hours, and deoxycorticosterone pivalate, 25 mg. intramuscularly once a month. Sodium chloride may be added to the formula or withheld, depending upon the state of hydration, blood pressure, and serum electrolyte concentrations.

The developmental aspects of sexual ambiguity, the differential diagnosis, and therapeutic management are discussed in Chapter 8.

Deficiency of 17α-Hydroxylase

An essential step in the formation of cortisol, estrogens, androgens, and 17-ketosteroid precursors is 17α-hydroxylation of either progesterone or pregnenolone. This step is not involved in the biosynthesis of important mineralocorticoids. Be-

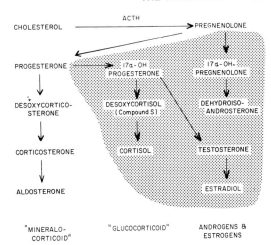

Figure 5–32. Consequences of 17α-hydroxylase deficiency: impaired formation of all steroids within the shaded area.

cause patients with genetic deficiencies of 17-hydroxylase are incapable of secreting cortisol with normal efficiency, they have compensatory increases in ACTH secretion. Under the influence of high levels of ACTH, their adrenals synthesize large quantities of the 17-deoxycorticosteroids, DOC and corticosterone (86). In affected males, failure of the fetal testis to secrete androgen results in failure to develop masculine external genitalia. In females, failure of the ovary to secrete estrogen results in failure to develop secondary sex characteristics at the normal age of puberty.

Chemically (Fig. 5–32), this disorder is characterized by (1) subnormal levels of plasma cortisol, urinary 17-OHCS, and 17-ketosteroids; (2) supernormal levels of plasma ACTH, DOC, and corticosterone; (3) subnormal levels of plasma renin activity and aldosterone; (4) subnormal levels of estrogen and testosterone; and (5) supernormal levels of pituitary gonadotropins (after the normal age of puberty).

Clinically, this disorder is characterized by hypertension and sexual infantilism in phenotypic females.

Therapy is directed toward adequate replacement of glucocorticoids and estrogens. With adequate treatment, hypersecretion of DOC is suppressed and hypertension is corrected.

Deficiency of 21-Hydroxylase (Fig. 5–33)

This is the most common variety of congenital adrenal hyperplasia. An essential step in the biosynthesis of all glucocorticoids and mineralocorticoids is enzymatic hydroxylation at carbon 21. Because patients with 21-hydroxylase deficiency are incapable of synthesizing cortisol with normal efficiency, there is a compensatory increase in ACTH, leading to adrenal hyperplasia and excessive secretion of 17α-hydroxyprogesterone, the precursor of urinary pregnanetriol. The adrenal androgen, DHEA, is excessively secreted, leading

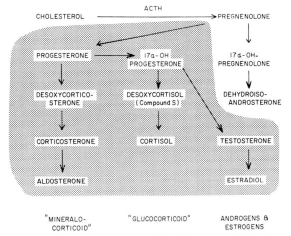

Figure 5–31. Consequences of 3β-hydroxysteroid dehydrogenase deficiency: impaired formation of all steroids within the shaded area.

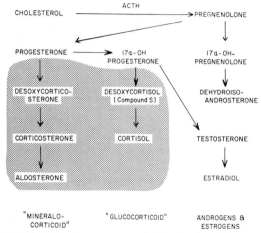

Figure 5-33. Consequences of 21-hydroxylase deficiency: impaired formation of all steroids within the shaded area.

plastic, and they develop facial hirsutism and temporal balding. Once glucocorticoid substitution therapy is instituted, the processes of virilization are arrested and normal feminization proceeds. If the female child has matured under the influence of adrenal androgen to such a degree that her bone age exceeds 13 years by the time glucocorticoid therapy is instituted, she is likely then to develop feminine secondary sex characteristics even though her chronological age may be only 8 or 9 years. It thus appears that sex hormones exert a "positive feedback" effect on maturation of the gonadotropin-regulating mechanism. Infertility was the rule in congenital adrenal hyperplasia until glucocorticoid therapy was instituted to suppress excessive adrenal androgen production. With glucocorticoid therapy, patients with this disorder are now often able to have children.

to virilization and increased excretion of 17-ketosteroids. If the enzymatic defect is severe enough, it results in a frank deficiency of aldosterone, which in turn leads to hyperkalemia and to sodium depletion, dehydration, hypotension, and compensatory hyper-reninemia.

This disorder occurs in mild form in certain families and with life-threatening severity in others. The severe form is characterized by early virilization, leading, in female fetuses, to marked masculinization of the external genitalia with formation of a urogenital sinus, partial fusion of labioscrotal folds, and marked clitoral hypertrophy. The condition is aptly described as "female pseudohermaphrotidism," and the affected female infant may be mistaken for a male with bilateral cryptorchidism and hypospadia. The correct diagnosis can be made quickly by noting that an older sibling had virilizing congenital adrenal hyperplasia, that the karyotype is that of a normal female, that urinary pregnanetriol and 17-ketosteroid levels are elevated, and that, unless treated with sodium and mineralocorticoids, the child readily displays salt wasting and peripheral vascular collapse. In males, the diagnosis is not so obvious since the external genitalia are normal; unless there is a family history of the disorder, the diagnosis is often not suspected until the tendency toward salt wasting becomes clinically evident. Salt-wasting congenital adrenal hyperplasia is often fatal unless diagnosed promptly and treated adequately with glucocorticoids, mineralocorticoids, and sodium chloride in much the same way as for Addison's disease.

Milder forms of virilizing congenital adrenal hyperplasia may be unnoticed (except, in some cases, for clitoral hypertrophy) until some time between the ages of 2 and 10 years when affected males or females attract attention because of rapid somatic growth, muscularity, early appearance of pubic and axillary hair, acne, coarsening of the voice, and cessation of linear growth due to closure of epiphyses of the long bones. Affected females do not develop normal secondary sex characteristics; they fail to menstruate, their breasts remain hypo-

Deficiency of 11β-Hydroxylase

The final step in the biosynthesis of cortisol and corticosterone is the introduction of an hydroxyl function in 11β-position. 11β-Hydroxylase is found only in the adrenal cortex. A deficiency of 11β-hydroxylase activity results in diminished secretion of cortisol, a compensatory increase in ACTH secretion, and a consequent increase in biosynthesis and secretion of 11-deoxysteroids (88).

The chemical hallmarks (Fig. 5-34) of 11β-hydroxylase deficiency, then, are as follows:

1. *Subnormal plasma cortisol, urinary tetrahydrocortisol, and urinary tetrahydrocortisone.* Depending upon the severity of the enzymatic defect, these steroids may be negligible, subnormal, or normal in quantity (the last situation representing a mild defect and fully effective homeostatic compensation).

2. *Supernormal plasma 11-deoxycortisol and 11-deoxycorticosterone (DOC) and supernormal urinary excretion of the tetrahydro derivatives of these steroids.*

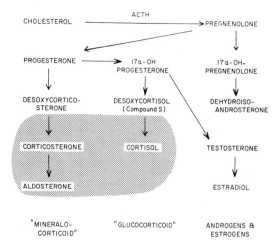

Figure 5-34. Consequences of 11β-hydroxylase deficiency: impaired formation of all steroids within the shaded area and increased formation of those not shaded.

3. *Supernormal excretion of 11-deoxy-17-ketosteroids.* These are derived largely from DHEA and appear in the urine as androsterone and etiocholanolone. Total urinary 17-ketosteroids are increased even though 11-oxygenated 17-ketosteroids are diminished.

4. *Supernormal plasma ACTH and β-MSH.*

5. *Subnormal plasma renin activity and aldosterone secretion rates.*

The clinical manifestations of 11β-hydroxylase deficiency are as follows:

1. *Virilization.* This results from overproduction of adrenal androgen and may take the form of pseudohermaphroditism (in females), rapid somatic growth but early closure of epiphyses, phallic hypertrophy, early appearance of pubic and axillary hair, and (in females) mammary hypoplasia and amenorrhea.

2. *Hypertension.* This results from overproduction of DOC and can lead to the usual complications of hypertensive cardiovascular disease.

It is possible to mistake this disorder (with its virilism, hypertension, and elevated 17-hydroxycorticosteroids) for Cushing's syndrome, but the latter is characterized by glucose intolerance, central obesity, and protein wasting, none of which is characteristic of 11β-hydroxylase deficiency. In 11-β-hydroxylase deficiency, 17-OHCS and 17-ketosteroids are profoundly suppressible with small doses of dexamethasone, in contrast to the resistance to suppression seen in patients with Cushing's syndrome or those with virilizing adrenal or ovarian tumors.

Treatment of 11β-hydroxylase deficiency consists of the administration of glucocorticoids in doses sufficient to suppress ACTH and thus suppress the secretion of DOC and adrenal androgens. Successful treatment leads, within several days, to correction of the hypertension and arrest of the virilization. As in other varieties of congenital adrenal hyperplasia, overtreatment with glucocorticoids might lead to inhibition of linear growth. Even though aldosterone production is subnormal, it is more than compensated for by DOC production, and mineralocorticoid substitution therapy is not a consideration in this variety of congenital adrenal hyperplasia.

Deficiency of 18-Hydroxysteroid Dehydrogenase

The final step in aldosterone biosynthesis is the removal of two hydrogen atoms from 18-hydroxycorticosterone, converting it to 18-aldo-corticosterone (aldosterone). The enzyme system that performs this function, 18-hydroxysteroid dehydrogenase, is limited to the zona glomerulosa and has no known function apart from the biosynthesis of aldosterone.

Deficiency of 18-hydroxysteroid dehydrogenase would be expected to result in aldosterone deficiency, sodium depletion, potassium retention, dehydration, hypotension, and increased plasma renin activity. As a consequence of the sodium

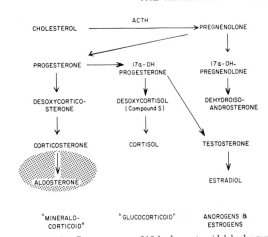

Figure 5–35. Consequences of 18-hydroxysteroid dehydrogenase deficiency: impaired formation of 18-hydroxycorticosterone with resultant impairment of aldosterone synthesis.

depletion, hyperkalemia, and hyper-reninemia, one would expect accelerated biosynthesis of aldosterone precursors, culminating in supernormal secretion of 18-hydroxycorticosterone. Precisely this chemical-clinical syndrome has been described by Ulick (89) and has been attributed to 18-hydroxysteroid dehydrogenase deficiency (Fig. 5–35). Appropriate therapy consists of supplemental sodium chloride and mineralocorticoid substitution therapy, following the same principles advocated in the treatment of Addison's disease. Glucocorticoid substitution therapy is unnecessary.

PHARMACOLOGIC USE OF ACTH AND STEROIDS AS ANTI-INFLAMMATORY AND IMMUNOSUPPRESSIVE AGENTS

Although glucocorticoids are essential for survival and must be administered in the treatment of adrenal insufficiency, this represents only a very small portion of the total usage of such agents in contemporary medical practice. In "supraphysiologic" doses, glucocorticoids have anti-inflammatory and immunosuppressive actions which have made them useful as therapeutic agents in a wide variety of diseases (Table 5–11). In addition to their uses as anti-inflammatory and immunosuppressive agents, glucocorticoids are efficacious in elevating the blood glucose in patients with hypoglycemia. Regardless of the therapeutic indication for which glucocorticoids are used, whenever they are given in supraphysiologic doses for prolonged periods of time they suppress inflammation and ACTH secretion; promote protein wasting; tend to antagonize the action of insulin; stimulate the deposition of fat in facial, cervical, and truncal depots; cause involution of lymphoid tissues; and inhibit antibody production. All available glucocorticoids share all these properties and differ from each other only with respect to potency (Table 5–3).

When injected into extravascular sites, various esters of the glucocorticoids have different rates of absorption and, therefore, different durations of ac-

TABLE 5–11. NONENDOCRINE DISORDERS IN WHICH GLUCOCORTICOIDS ARE THERAPEUTICALLY EFFECTIVE

1. Rheumatoid arthritis
2. Psoriatic arthritis
3. Gouty arthritis
4. Bursitis and tenosynovitis
5. Systemic lupus erythematosus
6. Acute rheumatic carditis
7. Pemphigus
8. Erythema multiforme
9. Exfoliative dermatitis
10. Mycosis fungoides
11. Allergic rhinitis
12. Bronchial asthma
13. Atopic dermatitis
14. Serum sickness
15. Allergic conjunctivitis
16. Uveitis
17. Retrobulbar neuritis
18. Sarcoidosis
19. Löffler's syndrome
20. Berylliosis
21. Idiopathic thrombocytopenic purpura
22. Autoimmune hemolytic anemia
23. Lymphomas
24. Immune nephritis
25. Tuberculous meningitis
26. Urticaria
27. Chronic active hepatitis
28. Ulcerative colitis
29. Regional enteritis
30. Nontropical sprue
31. Dental postoperative inflammation
32. Cerebral edema
33. Subacute nonsuppurative thyroiditis
34. Malignant exophthalmos
35. Hypercalcemia
36. Trichinosis
37. Myasthenia gravis

tion (Table 5–12). Those that are slowly absorbed are ideal when one desires a sustained effect but a low blood concentration. Those that are most rapidly absorbed can be used as alternatives to orally or intravenously administered steroids, providing peak blood concentrations quickly, followed by rapid dissipation of the steroids and their effects.

The untoward metabolic effects of corticosteroids are those of prolonged usage. There is no contraindication to a single dose of corticosteroid. In general, the briefer the course of corticosteroid therapy, the less likely one is to encounter any undesirable effects. In deciding whether or not to employ anti-inflammatory steroids for more than a few days, the physician must consider whether the disease he is attempting to suppress is more dangerous than the Cushing's syndrome that he might in-

TABLE 5–12. STEROID ESTERS FOR EXTRAVASCULAR INJECTION

Acid Group	Period of Absorption
Succinate	Minutes to hours
Phosphate	Minutes to hours
Acetate	Days to weeks
Diacetate	Days to weeks
Hexacetonide	Weeks
Pivalate	Weeks

duce. Corticosteroid therapy should supplement rather than supplant other standard therapeutic measures. When needed to save a life or prevent serious incapacitation, corticosteroids should be used without hesitation in whatever dosage is necessary.

Illnesses that are of short duration, such as urticaria, serum sickness, trichinosis, or other relatively acute allergic reactions will often respond dramatically to large doses of corticosteroids; moreover, if the illnesses are self-limited, treatment can be limited to a period of hours or days.

Certain other disorders can be controlled satisfactorily by giving corticosteroids intermittently, for example, a single large dose on alternate days or moderate doses for three consecutive days, followed by four days without steroids. In general, intermittent therapy is less likely than is continuous therapy to cause pituitary-adrenal suppression or the severe protein wasting of Cushing's syndrome. Intermittent therapy is not always effective in controlling inflammatory or immunologic disorders, however, and in each case it must be ascertained empirically whether the therapeutic objectives can be attained by using such a treatment schedule.

Whenever a disease process can be treated adequately by local administration of corticosteroids, this is ordinarily preferable to systemic treatment. Even if the administered steroid is ultimately totally absorbed into the systemic circulation, it will, nevertheless, be present in maximal concentrations at the point of application, thereby conferring a maximum of local benefit without necessarily producing commensurate systemic side effects. This principle has been used with some success in the treatment of certain ophthalmologic disorders, allergic dermatoses, allergic rhinitis, bronchial asthma, and arthritis.

Triamcinolone acetonide and fluorometholone are said to exhibit much higher ratios of potency (relative to hydrocortisone) when administered percutaneously than when administered systemically.

Certain groups of patients are especially vulnerable to the unwanted side effects of corticosteroids. Patients who are elderly, debilitated, or poorly nourished are especially vulnerable to the protein-wasting effects of corticosteroids. Supraphysiologic doses of corticosteroids cause growth retardation in children, a problem that has no counterpart in adults. Gonadectomized or postmenopausal women are especially likely to develop osteoporosis during treatment with glucocorticoids. Latent diabetes can be converted into frank diabetes by glucocorticoid therapy. Peptic ulcers may perforate or hemorrhage during treatment with glucocorticoids. Because of the special hazards accompanying corticosteroid therapy in these groups of patients, it is imperative that the therapeutic indications be clear cut and that the steroid dosage be kept as low as is consistent with achieving one's therapeutic objectives if one is to use steroids at all.

Because anti-inflammatory agents draw no distinction between the "useful" inflammation that walls off infection and "useless" inflammation, one should be reluctant to initiate steroid therapy for more than emergency purposes in patients who have infections for which specific antibiotics are not available. Even when specific antibiotic therapy is available, one should not use glucocorticoids in the presence of infection unless the therapeutic indications are compelling. A special dilemma arises whenever a patient who is already on steroid therapy acquires an infection. Here it is usually wise to continue steroids lest the stress of infection be poorly tolerated. Nevertheless, the dose of glucocorticoid should be held to the minimum that will forestall adrenal insufficiency and general clinical deterioration, and specific antibiotics should be employed without delay.

While one can often safely treat diseases of brief duration with corticosteroids, there is a risk of incurring a long-term commitment when one treats a chronic disease such as rheumatoid arthritis or intractable bronchial asthma. What started as "short-term" therapy has often led to long-term therapy in such patients. When patients learn that steroids confer dramatic relief of their symptoms, they may be strongly tempted to abandon nonsteroidal therapeutic measures. If steroids must be used they should, if possible, be employed topically, briefly, intermittently, and in the lowest dosage consistent with achieving the desired objectives of preventing incapacitation due to inflammatory or immunologic disease.

Particularly after prolonged usage, abrupt withdrawal of corticosteroids may result in manifestations of adrenal insufficiency and exacerbation of inflammatory processes. Gradual withdrawal of steroids is, therefore, often advisable. Each week the daily dose may be decreased by an amount of steroid equivalent to 5 mg. of hydrocortisone. Once physiologic levels are reached, the patient may be given a single daily dose of hydrocortisone, 20 mg. each morning, for several months. This will not perpetuate the manifestations of Cushing's syndrome but will prevent adrenal insufficiency while permitting gradual recovery of normal pituitary-adrenal reserve.

Corticotropin (ACTH) may be used as an alternative to exogenous glucocorticoids in most of the conditions under consideration. Its anti-inflammatory, immunosuppressive action is mediated by the cortisol that is secreted in response to ACTH. The cortisol secretory response to ACTH is a function of the type of ACTH preparation, the route of administration, and the duration of treatment. ACTH can be absorbed after intranasal application, but the conventional routes of administration are intravenous or intramuscular. A pulse of ACTH given intravenously results in a brief increase in plasma cortisol lasting approximately an hour (more or less, depending upon the dose). A sustained intravenous infusion of ACTH results in a sustained cortisol secretory response lasting for the duration of the ACTH infusion plus an hour or two. The most convenient method of administering ACTH is by intramuscular injection.

In this method, depot preparations of ACTH are most commonly employed. These are either gelatin suspensions or zinc hydroxide precipitates of ACTH. Depending upon the dose, they are absorbed from an intramuscular injection site over a period of about 8 to 16 hours.

In previously untreated patients with normal adrenals, 100 U. of depot ACTH will result in the secretion of approximately 100 mg. of cortisol during the ensuing 16 hours. Patients with adrenal atrophy secondary to prolonged steroid therapy will have much smaller responses, perhaps only 30 mg. of cortisol during the ensuing 16 hours. Patients with adrenal hyperplasia secondary to prolonged ACTH therapy will have much larger responses, perhaps as much as 300 mg. of cortisol during the ensuing 16 hours. One of the disadvantages of ACTH therapy compared with exogenous steroid therapy is the unpredictability of the cortisol secretory response. It should be apparent from the above that there might be as much as a tenfold range of cortisol secretory responses to the same dose of ACTH depending upon the responsiveness of the adrenals. Another disadvantage of ACTH as compared with exogenous steroids is the fact that ACTH must be given parenterally, while steroids may conveniently be administered orally. An advantage of ACTH is that it maintains adrenal responsiveness rather than inducing adrenal atrophy, so that prolonged substitution therapy is not necessary after one elects to withdraw supraphysiologic doses of the hormone. As with cortisol itself, one often encounters an undesirable degree of sodium retention and potassium depletion when ACTH is used in high doses over prolonged periods. If there is a clinical indication for extremely large doses of glucocorticoids, such as in the treatment of the crises of disseminated lupus erythematosus, one should employ corticosteroids rather than ACTH since the adrenal glands are capable of secreting only 10 to 20 mg. of cortisol per hour even with continuous maximum ACTH stimulation, and this may not be sufficient to control the inflammatory, immunologic disorder.

Although all available glucocorticoids are similar in suppressing inflammation, suppressing ACTH secretion, promoting protein wasting, elevating blood glucose, and promoting obesity, they differ significantly in their electrolyte-regulating properties. Cortisone and hydrocortisone ordinarily cause significant sodium retention and potassium depletion when administered in excess of 75 mg. daily. Equivalent glucocorticoid doses of prednisone, prednisolone, and dexamethasone have only about 20 per cent as much electrolyte-regulating activity as hydrocortisone, and triamcinolone has virtually no sodium-retaining activity.

REFERENCES

1. Villee, D. B.: The development of steroidogenesis. *Amer. J. Med.* 53:533, 1972.

2. Dexter, R. N., Fishman, L. M., et al.: Stimulation of adrenal cholesterol uptake from plasma by adrenocorticotrophin. *Endocrinology* 87:836, 1970.

3. Samuels, L. T., and Uchikawa, T.: Biosynthesis of adrenal steroids, In *The Adrenal Cortex.* Eisenstein, A. B. (ed.), Boston, Little, Brown, and Co., 1967, p. 61.

4. Kappeler, H.: Aspects of synthetic ACTH, MSH, and derivatives thereof. *Proceedings Second International Congress of Endocrinology.* Part II. Amsterdam, Excerpta Medica Foundation, 1964, p. 1173.

5. Ney, R. L., Ogata, E., et al.: Structure-function relationships of ACTH and MSH analogues. *Proceedings Second International Congress of Endocrinology.* Part II. Amsterdam, Excerpta Medica Foundation, 1964, p. 1184.

6. Besser, G. M., Orth, D. N., et al.: Dissociation of the disappearance of bioactive and radioimmunoreactive ACTH from plasma in man. *J. Clin. Endocr.* 32:595, 1971.

7. Ganong, W. F.: The central nervous system and the synthesis and release of ACTH, In *Advances in Neuroendocrinology.* Nalbandov, A. V. (ed.), Urbana, University of Illinois Press, 1963, p. 92.

8. Orth, D. N., Island, D. P., et al.: Experimental alteration of the circadian rhythm in plasma cortisol (17-OHCS) concentration in man. *J. Clin. Endocr.* 27:549, 1967.

9. Graber, A. L., Givens, J. R., et al.: Persistence of diurnal rhythmicity in plasma ACTH concentrations in cortisol-deficient patients. *J. Clin. Endocr.* 25:804, 1965.

10. Ney, R. L., Shimizu, N., et al.: Correlation of plasma ACTH concentration with adrenocortical response in normal human subjects, surgical patients, and patients with Cushing's disease. *J. Clin. Invest.* 42:1669, 1963.

11. Berson, S. A., and Yalow, R. S.: Methods in investigative and diagnostic endocrinology: Vol. 2A, In *Peptide Hormones.* Berson, S. A., and Yalow, R. S. (eds.), New York: American Elsevier Publishing Co., 1973.

12. Davis, J. O., Higgins, J. T., et al.: Relation of renin and angiotensin II to aldosterone secretion and sodium excretion, In *Aldosterone.* Baulieu, E. E., and Robel, P. (eds.), Oxford: Blackwell, Scientific Publications, 1964, p. 175.

13. Kaplan, N. M., and Bartter, F. C.: The effect of ACTH, renin, angiotensin II and various precursors on biosynthesis of aldosterone by adrenal slices. *J. Clin. Invest.* 41:715, 1962.

14. Skinner, S. L.: Improved assay methods for renin "concentration" and "activity" in human plasma. *Circ. Res.* 20:391, 1967.

15. Michelakis, A. M., Caudle, J., et al.: *In vitro* stimulation of renin production by epinephrine, norepinephrine and cyclic AMP. *Proc. Soc. Exp. Biol. Med.* 130:748, 1969.

16. Gordon, R. D., Kuchel, O., et al.: Role of the sympathetic nervous system in regulating renin and aldosterone production in man. *J. Clin. Invest.* 46:599, 1967.

17. Vander, A. J.: Effect of catecholamines and the renal nerves on renin secretion in anesthetized dogs. *Amer. J. Physiol.* 209:689, 1965.

18. Davis, J. O.: Mechanisms of renin release. *Proceedings Fourth International Congress of Endocrinology.* Amsterdam: Excerpta Medica Foundation, 1973.

19. Lever, A.: Discussion, In *Aldosterone.* Baulieu, E. E., and Robel, P. (eds.), Oxford: Blackwell Scientific Publications, 1964, p. 455.

20. Boucher, R., et al.: New procedures for measurement of human plasma angiotensin and renin activity levels. *Canad. Med. Ass. J.* 90:194, 1964.

21. Haber, E., et al.: Application of a radioimmunoassay for angiotensin I to the physiologic measurements of plasma renin activity in normal human subjects. *J. Clin. Endocr.* 29:1349, 1969.

22. Laragh, J. H., and Stoerk, H. C.: A study of the mechanism of secretion of the sodium-retaining hormone (aldosterone). *J. Clin. Invest.* 36:383, 1957.

23. Rudman, D., Del Rio, A. E., et al.: Effect of porcine beta melanocyte-stimulating hormone on blood lymphocyte count and serum corticosterone concentration of the rabbit. *Endocrinology* 86:1410, 1970.

24. Saruta, T., and Kaplan, N. M.: Adrenocortical steroidogenesis: the effects of prostaglandins. *J. Clin. Invest.* 51:2246, 1972.

25. Sandberg, A. A., and Slaunwhite, W. R., Jr.: Physical state of adrenal cortical hormones in plasma, In *The Human Adrenal Cortex.* Christy, N. P. (ed.), New York: Harper and Row, 1971, p. 69.

26. Peterson, R. E.: Metabolism of adrenal cortical steroids, In *The Human Adrenal Cortex.* Christy, N. P. (ed.), New York: Harper and Row, 1971, p. 87.

27. Feldman, D., Funder, J. W., et al.: Subcellular mechanisms in the action of adrenal steroids. *Amer. J. Med.* 53:545, 1972.

28. Bruchovsky, N., and Wilson, J. D.: The conversion of testosterone to 5-alpha-androstan-17-beta-ol-3-one by rat prostate in vivo and in vitro. *J. Biol. Chem.* 243:2012, 1968.

29. Baxter, J. D., and Forsham, P. H.: Tissue effects of glucocorticoids. *Amer. J. Med.* 53:573, 1972.

30. Jensen, E. V., and DeSombre, E. R.: Estrogen receptors in breast cancer. *Proceedings Fourth International Congress of Endocrinology.* Amsterdam: Excerpta Medica Foundation, 1973.

31. Porter, C. C., and Silber, R. H.: A quantitative color reaction for cortisone and related 17,21-dihydroxy-20-ketosteroids. *J. Biol. Chem.* 185:201, 1950.

32. Mattingly, D.: A simple fluorimetric method for the estimation of free 11-hydroxycorticoids in human plasma. *J. Clin. Path.* 15:374, 1962.

33. Underwood, R. H., and Tait, J. F.: Purification, partial characterization and metabolism of an acid-labile conjugate of aldosterone. *J. Clin. Endocr.* 24:1110, 1964.

34. Kliman, B., and Peterson, R. E.: Double isotope derivative assay of aldosterone in biological extracts. *J. Biol. Chem.* 235:1639, 1960.

35. Ito, T., et al.: A radioimmunoassay for aldosterone in human peripheral plasma including a comparison of alternate techniques. *J. Clin. Endocr.* 34:106, 1972.

36. Norymberski, J. K.: Determination of urinary corticosteroids. *Nature* (London) 170:1074, 1952.

37. Peterson, R. E.: The miscible pool and turnover rate of adrenocortical steroids in man. *Recent Progr. Hormone Res.* 15:231, 1959.

38. Tait, J. F.: Review. The use of isotopic steroids for the measurement of production rates in vivo. *J. Clin. Endocr.* 23:1285, 1963.

39. Renold, A. E., Jenkins, D., et al.: The use of intravenous ACTH: a study in quantitative adrenocortical stimulation. *J. Clin. Endocr.* 12:763, 1952.

40. Liddle, G. W., Estep, H. L., et al.: Clinical application of a new test of pituitary reserve. *J. Clin. Endocr.* 19:875, 1959.

41. Jubiz, W., Levinson, R. A., et al.: Absorption and conjugation of metyrapone during diphenylhydantoin therapy. Mechanism of the abnormal response to oral metyrapone. *Endocrinology* 86:328, 1970.

42. Liddle, G. W.: Tests of pituitary-adrenal suppressibility in the diagnosis of Cushing's syndrome. *J. Clin. Endocr.* 12:1539, 1960.

43. Temple, T. E., and Liddle, G. W.: Inhibitors of adrenal steroid biosynthesis. *Ann. Rev. Pharmacol.* 10:199, 1970.

44. Liddle, G. W.: Specific and non-specific inhibition of mineralocorticoid activity. *Metabolism* 10:1021, 1961.

45. Cushing, H.: The basophil adenomas of the pituitary body and their clinical manifestations (pituitary basophilism), *Bull. Johns Hopkins Hosp.* 50:137, 1932.

46. Albright, F.: Cushing's syndrome. *Harvey Lect.* 38:123, 1942–43.

47. Lindsay, A. E., et al.: The diagnostic value of plasma and urinary 17-hydroxycorticosteroid determinations in Cushing's syndrome. *Amer. J. Med.* 20:15, 1956.

48. Scott, H. W., Jr., Foster, J. H., et al.: Cushing's syndrome due to adrenocortical tumor. *Ann. Surg.* 162:505, 1965.

49. Orth, D. N., and Liddle, G. W.: Results of treatment in 108 patients with Cushing's syndrome. *New Eng. J. Med.* 285:243, 1971.

50. Hutter, A. M., Jr., and Kayhoe, D. E.: Adrenal cortical carcinoma. *Amer. J. Med.* 41:581, 1966.

51. Liddle, G. W., Island, D., et al.: Normal and abnormal regulation of corticotropin secretion in man. *Recent Progr. Hormone Res.* 18:125, 1962.

52. Liddle, G. W.: Pathogenesis of glucocorticoid disorders. *Amer. J. Med.* 53:638, 1972.

53. Temple, T. E., Jones, D. J., et al.: Use of o,p'DDD to correct hypercortisolism without inducing aldosterone deficiency in the treatment of Cushing's disease. *New Eng. J. Med.* 281:801, 1969.

54. Bledsoe, T., Island, D. P., et al.: An effect of o,p'-DDD on the extra-adrenal metabolism of cortisol in man. *J. Clin. Endocr.* 24:1303, 1964.

55. Liddle, G. W., Nicholson, W. E., et al.: Clinical and laboratory studies of ectopic humoral syndromes. *Recent Progr. Hormone Res.* 25:238, 1969.

56. Orth, D. N., Nicholson, W. E., et al.: Biologic and immunologic characterization and physical separation of ACTH and ACTH fragments in the ectopic ACTH syndrome. *J. Clin. Invest.* 52:1756, 1973.

57. Abe, K., Island, D. P., et al.: Radioimmunologic evidence for α-MSH (melanocyte stimulating hormone) in human pituitary and tumor tissues. *J. Clin. Endocr.* 27:46, 1967.

58. Abe, K., Nicholson, W. E., et al.: Radioimmunoassay of β-MSH in human plasma and tissues. *J. Clin. Invest.* 46:1609, 1967.

59. Graber, A. L., Ney, R. L., et al.: Natural history of pituitary-adrenal recovery following long-term suppression with corticosteroids. *J. Clin. Endocr.* 25:11, 1965.

60. Williams, W. C., Jr., Island, D., et al.: Blood corticotropin (ACTH) levels in Cushing's disease. *J. Clin. Endocr.* 21:426, 1961.

61. Brown, R. D., Van Loon, G. R., et al.: Cushing's syndrome with periodic hormonogenesis: one explanation for paradoxical response to dexamethasone. *J. Clin. Endocr.* 36:445, 1973.

62. Luetscher, J. A.: Studies of aldosterone in relation to water and electrolyte balance in man. *Recent Progr. Hormone Res.* 12:175, 1956.

63. Sutherland, D. J. A., et al.: Hypertension, increased aldosterone secretion and low plasma renin activity relieved by dexamethasone. *Canad. Med. Ass. J.* 95:1109, 1966.

64. Laragh, J. H., Ledingham, J. G. G., et al.: Secondary aldosteronism and reduced plasma renin in hypertensive disease. *Trans. Ass. Amer. Physicians.* 80:168, 1967.

65. Bartter, F. C., et al.: Hyperplasia of the juxtaglomerular complex with hyperaldosteronism and hypokalemic alkalosis. Angiotensin II. *Amer. J. Med.* 33:811, 1962.

66. Schambelan, M., and Biglieri, E. G.: Renin secreting tumor as a cause of hypertension. *Proceedings Fourth International Congress of Endocrinology.* Amsterdam: Excerpta Medica Foundation, 1973.

67. Brown, J. J., et al.: Plasma renin concentration in hypertensive disease of pregnancy. *Lancet* 2:1219, 1965.

68. Liddle, G. W.: Aldosterone antagonists. *Arch. Intern. Med.* (Chicago) 102:998, 1958.

69. Luetscher, J. A., Dowdy, A. J., et al.: Studies of secretion and metabolism of aldosterone and cortisol. *Trans. Ass. Amer. Physicians* 75:293, 1962.

70. Bledsoe, T., Liddle, G. W., et al.: Comparative fates of intravenously and orally administered aldosterone: evidence for extrahepatic formation of acid-labile conjugate in man. *J. Clin. Invest.* 45:264, 1966.

71. Conn, J. W.: Primary aldosteronism, a new clinical syndrome. *J. Lab. Clin. Med.* 45:3, 1955.

72. Conn, J. W., Rovner, D. R., et al.: Normokalemic primary aldosteronism. *J.A.M.A.* 195:21, 1966.

73. Conn, J. W.: Plasma renin activity in primary aldosteronism. Importance in differential diagnosis and in research of essential hypertension. *J.A.M.A.* 190:222, 1964.

74. Liddle, G. W., Bledsoe, T., et al.: A familial renal disorder simulating primary aldosteronism but with negligible aldosterone secretion. *Trans. Ass. Amer. Physicians* 76:199, 1963.

75. Woods, J. W., Liddle, G. W., et al.: Effect of an adrenal inhibitor in hypertensive patients with suppressed renin. *Arch. Intern. Med.* (Chicago) 123:366, 1969.

76. Gunnells, C. J., et al.: Hypertension, adrenal abnormalities and alterations in plasma renin activity. *Ann. Intern. Med.* 73:901, 1970.

77. Adlin, E. V., Channick, B. J., et al.: Salivary sodium-potassium ratio and plasma renin activity in hypertension. *Circulation* 39:685, 1969.

78. Carey, R. M., Douglas, J. G., et al.: The syndrome of essential hypertension and suppressed plasma renin activity. *Arch. Intern. Med.* (Chicago) 130:849, 1972.

79. Addison, T.: On the constitutional and local effects of disease of the suprarenal capsules, London: Highley, 1855.

80. Blizzard, R. M., and Kyle, M.: Studies of the adrenal antigens and antibodies in Addison's disease. *J. Clin. Invest.* 42:1653, 1963.

81. Southren, A. L., Tochimoto, S., et al.: Remission in Cushing's syndrome with o,p'-DDD. *J. Clin. Endocr.* 26:268, 1966.

82. Laidlaw, J. C., Abbott, E. C., et al.: The influence of a heparin-like compound on hypertension, electrolytes and aldosterone in man. *Trans. Amer. Clin. Climat. Ass.* 77:111, 1965.

83. Bartter, F. C., and Albright, F.: The effects of adrenocorticotropic hormone and cortisone in adrenogenital syndrome associated with congenital adrenal hyperplasia: An attempt to explain and correct its disordered hormonal pattern. *J. Clin. Invest.* 30:237, 1951.

84. Prader, V. A., and Gurtner, H. P.: Das syndrom des Pseudohermaphroditismus masculinus bei kongenitaler Nebennierenrinden-Hyperplasie ohne Androgenuberproduktion (adrenaler Pseudohermaphroditismus masculinus). *Helv. Paediat. Acta* 10:397, 1955.

85. Bongiovanni, A. M., Eberlein, W. R., et al.: Disorders of adrenal steroid biogenesis. *Recent Progr. Hormone Res.* 23:375, 1967.

86. Biglieri, E. G., Herron, M. A., et al.: 17-Hydroxylation deficiency in man. *J. Clin. Invest.* 45:1946, 1966.

87. Bongiovanni, A. M., Eberlein, W. R., et al.: Disorders of adrenal steroid biogenesis. *Recent Progr. Hormone Res.* 23:375, 1967.

88. Eberlein, W. R., and Bongiovanni, A. M.: Plasma and urinary corticosteroids in the hypertensive form of congenital adrenal hyperplasia. *J. Biol. Chem.* 223:85, 1956.

89. Ulick, S., Gautier, E., et al.: An aldosterone biosynthetic defect in a salt-losing disorder. *J. Clin. Endocr.* 24:669, 1964.

Part II:
Catecholamines and the Adrenal Medulla*

By Kenneth L. Melmon

*Original work discussed in this report was supported by USPHS Grants HL-09964, GM-01791, and GM-16496 and a special fellowship 1-FO-HL-50,244-01.

INTRODUCTION

Catecholamines are dihydroxylated phenolic amines. The most prominent members of this fam-

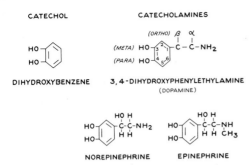

Figure 5–36. Biochemical structure of a catechol (left) and of the endogenous catecholamines (right). Carbon chain and phenolic ring positions are indicated on the dopamine structure.

ily are dopamine, norepinephrine, and epinephrine (Fig. 5–36). Each of the three has different and characteristic physiologic functions, pharmacologic actions, sites of production, and pathways of metabolism. As a group they are synthesized in the brain, in sympathetic nerve ends, and in cells of neural crest origin throughout the body. When released from storage sites in nerve endings and adrenal medulla, they have profound effects on smooth muscle, adipose tissue, myocardium, the liver, the brain, formed elements of the blood, a number of hormone-producing organs, and the myometrium. All effects are exaggerated when catecholamines are administered or released in unusually large quantities. During certain diseases small quantities may produce an exaggerated effect, as for instance, in patients with sympathetic denervation of any cause, myocardiopathies, or some dietary deficiency syndromes. Conversely, the effects of catecholamines are diminished in patients with endocrinopathies such as myxedema and Addison's disease.

In the last twenty years scientists have elucidated the biochemical nature, the modes of synthesis and degradation, and the physiologic significance of catecholamines, as well as the pathologic changes they induce. All the enzymes involved in the synthesis of catecholamines have been isolated. Characterization of the enzymes has permitted identification of rate-limiting steps and observations on responses to drugs that interfere with catecholamine synthesis, breakdown, or peripheral effects. The information integrated from these sources has enabled us to distinguish between drugs that interfere with the catecholamine effects or synthesis and drugs that must be incorporated into the pathways of synthesis and transformed to false neurotransmitters before producing pharmacologic effects. We can now undertake a rational and methodical search for agents that can predictably alter catechol synthesis, release, or tissue response. In addition, we can begin to understand the symptoms, biochemical alterations, and complications produced by tumors that elaborate excessive amounts of catecholamines.

It is hard to think of any field in biology that has moved more rapidly or had more applied relevance to man. We now can define the molecular nature of catecholamine effects and change at will the synthesis, storage, release, reuptake, metabolism, and elimination of the amines. We can even begin to change specific functions of specific amines in individual tissues. We also have become aware of many of the interrelationships of catecholamines with other endocrine systems and attuned to the possibility of highly selective and therapeutically effective alteration of endocrine systems via perturbation of the catecholamine system. Now an endocrinologist must become familiar with all aspects of catecholamine physiology, chemistry, and pathology to understand the function of many endocrine organs.

This chapter primarily summarizes the well-founded data on the synthesis, degradation, and pharmacologic and physiologic significance of catecholamine substances, the diseases characterized by extreme sensitivity or insensitivity to catecholamines, the unusual interrelationships between catecholamines and other biologically active substances, the diseases produced by tumors derived from cells of neural crest origin, and the rationale for the use or avoidance of certain agents during the treatment of pheochromocytoma. In addition, the extraordinarily exciting (even if in some cases less firmly established) developments related to each of these areas are discussed. For instance, new discoveries suggest possibilities for understanding both the chemical basis of central nervous system function and the implications of interrelationships of catecholamines with leukocytes. A feasible search for drugs that will alter autonomic nervous system function in given areas of specific organs can be initiated.

CATECHOLAMINES

Synthesis

Catecholamine synthesis occurs exclusively in the brain (483), sympathetic nerve endings (341), and sites of chromaffin tissue (482), including the adrenal medulla, organ of Zuckerkandl, and ectopic rests of neural crest tissue. The main mammalian pathway starts with tyrosine, which is abundant in human tissue and is derived either from the diet (the probable main source) or via para-hydroxylation of phenylalanine by phenylalanine hydroxylase, mainly in the liver (Fig. 5–37). Only recently has the interplay between phenylalanine hydroxylase and norepinephrine been appreciated. As norepinephrine accumulates in tissues, it inhibits formation of tyrosine. The inhibition is competitive with respect to one co-factor (pteridine) and noncompetitive with respect to the substrate, phenylalanine (64). In diseases such as phenylketonuria, accumulation of phenylalanine may interfere with the action of tyrosine hydroxylase, the rate-limiting enzymatic step in the synthesis of catecholamines.

Subsequent steps in the mammalian synthesis of catecholamines include the meta-hydroxylation of tyrosine to dopa (by tyrosine hydroxylase), decar-

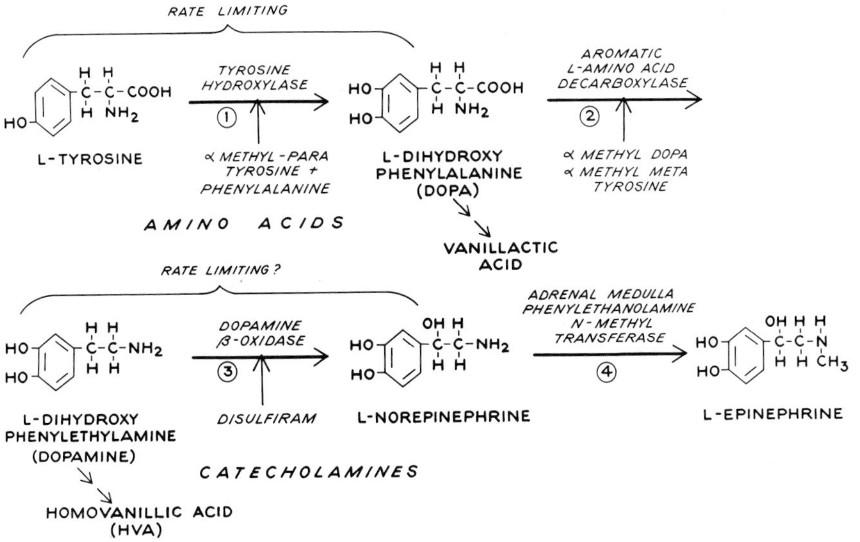

Figure 5-37. Biosynthesis of catecholamines in the brain, adrenal medulla, and sympathetic nerve endings. Rate-limiting steps are those in which only minimal inhibition of enzymes will result in significantly diminished synthesis (1 and ?3). Heavy horizontal arrows represent major steps documented in man. Vertical arrows represent inhibition of specific steps.

boxylation of dopa to dopamine (by L-amino acid decarboxylase), and beta-hydroxylation of dopamine to norepinephrine (by dopamine beta-oxidase). The latter step may also be rate-limiting in some circumstances but does not seem as critical as the conversion of tyrosine to dopa. Norepinephrine can be converted to epinephrine by the N-methylating enzyme, phenylethanolamine-N-methyl transferase found only in the adrenal medulla or organ of Zuckerkandl (and in very small amounts in the brain). The synthesis and metabolism of catecholamines have been recently reviewed (13, 353, 404).

Figure 5-38 illustrates some alternate pathways in the synthesis of catecholamines. Most of the proposed steps have been demonstrated in subprimates. One pathway demonstrated in rabbits involves direct synthesis of catecholamines from tyramine, which is then hydroxylated in two positions—first by dopamine beta-hydroxylase and later in the meta position of the phenolic ring to form norepinephrine. Some alternate pathways have been postulated but not proved operative in man (404).

Figure 5-39 illustrates the distribution within the neuron of the enzymes for synthesis. Note that

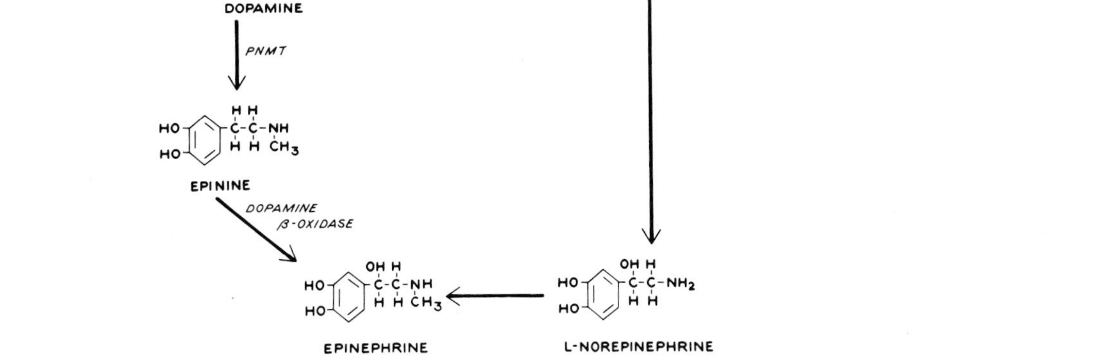

Figure 5-38. Possible alternate routes of catecholamine synthesis.

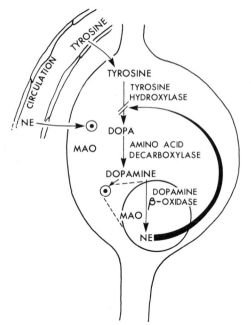

Figure 5–39. The biosynthesis of norepinephrine in the sympathetic nerve. Abbreviations: NE, norepinephrine; MAO, monoamine oxidase. [Reproduced from Axelrod, J., and Kopin, I. J. The uptake, storage, release, and metabolism of noradenaline sympathetic nerves, In *Mechanisms of Synaptic Transmission, Progress in Brain Research,* Vol. 31. Akert, K., and Wasser, P. G. (eds.), Amsterdam, Elsevier, 1969, Fig. 2, p. 24.]

the rate-limiting enzyme (tyrosine hydroxylase) is located in the mitochondria within the cytoplasm and is separated from the end product of synthesis (norepinephrine) by the granules containing dopamine beta-hydroxylase. The distribution of the enzymes implies that: (1) sufficient quantities of tyrosine must be transported to the site of the tyrosine hydroxylase enzyme before dopa (4,5-dihydroxyphenylalanine) can be formed; (2) dopamine must be actively transported into the granule before norepinephrine can be synthesized; and (3) either norepinephrine must be released from the granule or extraneuronal norepinephrine taken up into the cytoplasm if there is to be either feedback inhibition of the rate-limiting step in synthesis or the production of epinephrine. The only important intraneuronal degradative enzyme for catecholamines is cytoplasmic monoamine oxidase.

The major pathway described above is normally operative in all tissues which synthesize catecholamines. However, local conditions in each organ apparently regulate the rate of synthesis, release, uptake, and metabolism of the catecholamines. In most tissues, the control of synthesis depends on the rate of turnover (e.g., increased during sympathetic nerve stimulation) of catecholamines in that tissue. In brain and adrenal medulla, a number of physiologic factors in addition to nerve stimulation may profoundly influence rates of synthesis. For practical purposes, it is reasonable to think of the synthesis, release, effects, and metabolism of catecholamines in the central nervous system as being independent of their analogous counterparts in the peripheral sympathetic nervous system.

Tyrosine Hydroxylase

Tyrosine hydroxylase has been demonstrated in the adrenal medulla, brain, and sympathetically innervated tissues by Nagatsu, Levitt, and Udenfriend (343). The enzyme, purified from several tissues and even crystallized from bacteria, has similar characteristics in various animal tissues. It requires oxygen to incorporate into tyrosine to form dopa (112), a reduced pteridine co-factor [oxygen also affects the affinity of pteridine for the enzyme (225)], and perhaps iron (Fe^{++}) (467). Experiments *in vitro* using perfusions of guinea pig hearts demonstrated that the rates of tyrosine conversion to norepinephrine were dependent on tyrosine concentration and were maximal at substrate concentrations of 5×10^{-4}M tyrosine (281). The apparent K_m for the overall reaction (tyrosine→ norepinephrine) was comparable to that observed for conversion of tyrosine to dopa by purified tyrosine hydroxylase. When isolated guinea pig heart was perfused in turn with varying concentrations of radiolabeled tyrosine, dopa, and dopamine, the conversion to norepinephrine reached ordinary maximum rates only with the first of these substrates. Furthermore, some studies found that the actual and calculated degrees of tyrosine hydroxylase inhibition *in vivo* were almost identical, a circumstance which can only be explained if the enzyme is rate limiting. The absence of appreciable amounts of dopa or dopamine in most sympathetically innervated tissues provides further evidence for the rate-limiting activities of tyrosine hydroxylase.

Synthesis may be slowed by manipulations other than limitation of substrate availability. The level of the pteridine co-factor may be critically controlled by shifting concentrations of dihydropteridine reductase (340); catecholamines at low concentrations (2×10^{-5}M) also can markedly inhibit tyrosine hydroxylase. However, increased tissue concentrations of dihydropteridine reductase can overcome enzyme inhibition by catecholamines. Thus at least three endogenous factors seem to influence the usual rate of catecholamine production: (1) tyrosine concentration in the intraneuronal site (depends on an active transport system that may be altered by disease, unnatural extracellular accumulation of large quantities of alternate amino acids that may compete for the same transport system, or toxic levels of some drugs that interfere with transport); (2) concentration of the pteridine co-factor; and (3) concentration of norepinephrine in the milieu of the enzyme.

Physiologic and pharmacologic manipulations which release catecholamines from their storage sites may also influence the rate of synthesis (8, 166, 335, 398, 471, 475). Stimulation of the sympathetic nerves to a variety of organs releases catecholamines and may be associated with a considerable increase in norepinephrine synthesis. Neither the actual depolarization of the nerve nor any blood-borne factor (398) seems to trigger the acceleration of norepinephrine synthesis. The increased synthesis does not depend on tyrosine

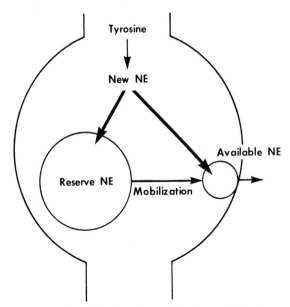

Figure 5–40. Selective release of newly synthesized norepinephrine (NE). NE which is released by nerve stimulation comes from a small, immediately "available" store. Both newly synthesized NE and NE mobilized from the reserve stores are used to replenish the NE in the available store. While new NE can also enter the reserve store, it is a greater fraction of the smaller available store. [Reproduced from Axelrod, J., and Kopin, I. J. The uptake, storage, release, and metabolism of noradrenaline in sympathetic nerves, In *Mechanisms of Synaptic Transmission, Progress in Brain Research.* Vol. 31. Akert, K., and Wasser, P. G. (eds.), Amsterdam, Elsevier, 1969, Fig. 4, p. 28.]

transport or effector organ activity (398). Rather, the synthesis rate appears to rise as the newly formed norepinephrine, comprising the majority of readily released catecholamines, is released from the cells (Fig. 5–40) (166, 474). The increase in rate of synthesis is not necessarily accompanied by an overall depletion of intracellular norepinephrine or by an increase in the total amount of tyrosine hydroxylase in the stimulated nerve (8). The rapid synthesis is probably due to removal of the feedback inhibition of existing tyrosine hydroxylase as cytoplasmic (not total) concentrations of catecholamine fall (471).

When nerve stimulation is intense or protracted (hours), when reflux nervous stimulation is provoked by drugs that block sympathetic action, or when partial chemical or surgical sympathectomy is performed, the increased rate of catecholamine synthesis in the affected nerves or residual nervous system is accompanied by an increase in the activity of tyrosine hydroxylase (335, 471). This additional compensatory mechanism for catecholamine synthesis can be blocked by agents inhibiting protein synthesis and, therefore, is presumably due to an increase in the rate of synthesis of tyrosine hydroxylase (339). In summary, a prime stimulatory factor in the synthesis of catecholamines probably is reduction of the concentration of cytoplasmic norepinephrine. A second factor involves increased synthesis of the rate-limiting enzyme. The molecular stimulus for increased enzyme synthesis is not known. However, several intriguing

facts have led Axelrod and his co-workers to suggest that in the adrenal medulla there may be a cholinergic receptor or an unidentified neurotransmitter that mediates the increase in tyrosine hydroxylase (338). It is not known whether such cholinergic receptors influence synthesis of tyrosine hydroxylase in other parts of the sympathetic nervous system.

At one time it was thought that catecholamines were primarily synthesized in the nerve bodies of the sympathetic neuron and gradually migrated down the axon. Although this may be true, another explanation seems plausible. The induction of tyrosine hydroxylase by reserpine in various segments of sciatic nerves indicates a proximal to distal transport of the enzyme. The apparent rate of enzyme transport is not sufficient to account for the total increase in enzyme in the nerve terminals. Thus local synthesis *de novo* of both enzyme and catecholamines may account for the catecholamines in the nerve terminals (473).

Once tyrosine hydroxylase was established as the rate-limiting factor in the physiologic pathway for catecholamine synthesis, progress was rapid: (1) specificity of the enzyme was found to be quite high; (2) derivatives of tyrosine were correctly predicted as inhibitors; and (3) alpha-methyltyrosine was discovered as a potent competitive inhibitor of catecholamine synthesis *in vitro* and *in vivo* (Fig. 5–37) (442). In addition, halogenated derivatives of tyrosine, one a precursor of thyroid hormone (3-iodotyrosine), were found to inhibit tyrosine hydroxylase, a fact that potentially linked synthesis of thyroxine with synthesis of catecholamines (229, 308, 441). Also it was found that 5-halogenated tryptophan could inhibit tyrosine hydroxylase, thus linking the catecholamine pathway with serotonin. Finally, catechol derivatives themselves have significant inhibitory effects on tyrosine hydroxylase [e.g., 3,4-dihydroxyphenylpropylacetamide (H22/54)].

Aromatic L-Amino Acid Decarboxylase

Aromatic L-amino acid decarboxylase is found in large quantities in the cytoplasm of many tissues and has high affinity for a number of primary phenolic L-amino acids also found in tissues (294). The enzyme requires pyridoxal 5-phosphate as a co-factor. Unlike the production of dopa, which may be severely impaired by minor decreases in concentration of the substrate for tyrosine hydroxylase, decarboxylation of dopa proceeds at a high rate even when dopa concentrations are low. Under ordinary circumstances, the rate of dopa formation by tyrosine hydroxylase cannot approach the capacity of the decarboxylase to rapidly convert the amino acid into the first catecholamine, dopamine. Because of the enzyme's high affinity for its substrate and a high V_{max} (maximum velocity), even very potent inhibitors do not decrease the rate of catecholamine synthesis *in vivo*. Therefore, the enzyme plays a negligible role in regulating the synthesis of norepinephrine.

As with inhibitors of tyrosine hydroxylase, among the earliest known decarboxylase inhibitors were derivatives of the substrate dopa, alpha-methyldopa and alpha-methyldopa hydrazine. Because the decarboxylase lacked the substrate specificity of tyrosine hydroxylase, other derivatives of native L-amino acids were tried. Thus alpha-methylmetatyrosine, tryptophan derivatives, and a host of hydrazine compounds were found capable of decreasing decarboxylase activity *in vitro* and *in vivo*. Those which have proved most useful clinically are alpha-methyldopa and alpha-methyldopa hydrazine (MK-485). Both drugs substantially inhibit decarboxylase activity *in vivo*, but neither used alone decreases catecholamine synthesis. An additional recent finding is that some decarboxylase inhibitors predominantly affect the enzyme in peripheral tissues but are insufficiently distributed to central nervous tissues to inhibit the enzyme there. When, for instance, MK-485 is administered to man, it will block decarboxylase activity outside the brain. If the amino acid dopa were then administered, far more than the ordinary amount would reach the brain; less than normal amounts of dopamine and its metabolites would be made in the periphery, but excessive dopa, dopamine, and metabolites would accumulate in the brain (187, 360, 441).

Dopamine Beta-hydroxylase

Once dopamine has been formed, it is actively transported by an ATP-dependent mechanism into "cytoplasmic particles" (44, 493) present in sympathetic nerve endings and the adrenal medulla. The transport can be inhibited by norepinephrine itself (452). The particles or granules harbor dopamine beta-hydroxylase (277), a copper-containing mixed-function oxidase enzyme (161) which requires ascorbic acid and oxygen to hydroxylate dopamine to norepinephrine. In recent years, the enzyme has been purified, crystallized, and characterized, and antibodies have been produced to it (167, 256, 404). The dopamine beta-hydroxylase apparently is contained on the inner surface of the sac-like granule or vesicle which, surrounded by a semipermeable membrane (31), behaves as an osmotic system. At least 40 per cent of the enzyme is in association with the granule wall protein. This portion has much higher activity than does a water-insoluble portion that is not associated with the granule membrane but is within the granule. In the granule, the enzyme is associated with a macromolecule (M.W. 2.9×10^5) termed chromogranin A (203, 204). This water-insoluble substance may be composed of subunits of dopamine beta-hydroxylase, and when it comes in contact with ATP, the enzyme and chromogranin become solubilized, and the enzyme becomes activated. ATP also has a functional relationship with storage of catecholamines in the granules.

A number of assays for dopamine beta-hydroxylase have been devised. The enzyme has been found in human and rat plasma; its concentration seems dependent on the integrity and activity of the sympathetic nervous system (327). When the sympathetic nervous system is destroyed or its function is inhibited by preventing release of catecholamines from storage sites, the amount of circulating enzyme is low (508, 509). Increased sympathetic nervous activity has the opposite effect. The characteristics of the circulating enzyme are similar to those of enzyme obtained from the adrenal medulla and sympathetic nerves (508). If evidence suggesting that catecholamines are released by a process of exocytosis (417) involving extrusion of the whole vesicle including the membrane is true (see the following), then the assay of circulating dopamine beta-hydroxylase may complement direct measurements of catecholamines in the blood. If exocytosis is operative both in the nerve endings and adrenal medulla, such measurements may reflect the functional state of the sympathetic nervous system in physiologic and disease states. In many diseases in which abnormalities of the autonomic nervous system are suspected (idiopathic orthostatic hypotension, familial dysautonomia, hypertension, and infantile hypoglycemia), measurements of circulating catecholamines or their metabolites are not sufficiently accurate to indicate with certainty that a lesion exists. In addition, some diseases of the autonomic nervous system may indicate primary alterations of enzymatic contents of the storage vesicle which would not be reflected in routine measurements of the end products.

The control of synthesis of dopamine beta-hydroxylase seems related to the same factors favoring synthesis of tyrosine hydroxylase. Unlike tyrosine hydroxylase, the dopamine-converting enzyme is lost from the neuron when catecholamines are released. It is not surprising, therefore, that factors which increase release of catecholamines from the neuron also stimulate the synthesis of the enzyme (261). As is the case with any of the enzymes in the synthetic or metabolic pathway for catecholamines, the actual chemical signal for initiating or stopping synthesis of dopamine beta-hydroxylase is not known.

There is little substrate specificity of dopamine beta-hydroxylase; it will hydroxylate many phenylethylamines including epinine (Fig. 5–38), forming epinephrine and octopamine. Tyramine is probably a better substrate for the enzyme than dopamine. Substrate activity occurs only in the presence of an aromatic ring, with a side chain of two or three carbon atoms terminating with an amino group. Phenylalkylamines with two carbon side chains are better substrates than are those with three carbon atoms, and primary amines are better than secondary.

There is considerable pragmatic importance to the nonspecificity of many of the steps in the transport of substrates and the synthesis of intermediates of catecholamines. Amino acid transport into the neuron is active but nonspecific with regard to eventual substrates for L-amino acid decarboxylase; once in the cytoplasm, a number of amino acids will be decarboxylated to their corresponding amines. Many of these can be actively transported into the vesicle containing dopamine beta-hydroxylase, where some will be converted into beta-hydroxylated products; these intragranular amines may not be catecholamines, but many have pharmacologic properties (404). Some displace norepinephrine (the natural neurotransmitter) from storage sites. Others, if bound within the granule, may be released by nerve stimulation and produce their own characteristic effects. These latter unnatural substances have become classified as "false" neurotransmitters, but they have considerable pharmacologic importance themselves.

There are several natural endogenous inhibitors of dopamine beta-hydroxylase. These are of low molecular weight (M.W. 750 to 1,200) and contain carbohydrate, phosphate, and trace amounts of nitrogen. They have a distinctive ultraviolet spectrum and apparently work by chelation of enzyme-bound Cu^{++}. They are found in many tissues (344) and probably in blood. We know little about the controls for their synthesis (89) or their physiologic importance. It is likely that they have physiologic or pathologic importance, since, in many circumstances, dopamine beta-hydroxylase appears to be rate-limiting in the synthesis of catecholamines.

The rate-limiting characteristics of dopamine beta-hydroxylase have been revealed by use of competitive inhibitors (derivatives of phenylethylamines) which are themselves substrates for the enzyme (404). In certain experimental settings, these inhibitors result in decreased content of tissue (primarily brain) norepinephrine with a reciprocal but nonstoichiometric increase in dopamine. The incomplete replacement of norepinephrine by dopamine has been taken to indicate that binding of dopamine in the neuronal vesicle is not as avid as binding of norepinephrine (470). Another interpretation may be that other unidentified substances are accumulated in the nerve ending as a result of inhibition of the enzyme. With stimulation of the affected neurons, release of dopamine and norepinephrine is in perfect proportion to their ratios in the involved neurons. This further indicates that release of amines is in quanta by extrusion of intact vesicles from the nerve (470). The ability to selectively deplete norepinephrine from the central nervous system helped to elucidate its individual role in the central nervous system (228, 461, 467).

A caveat related to inhibitors of dopamine beta-hydroxylase seems warranted. Disulfiram (Antabuse) is an inhibitor of dopamine beta-hydroxylase (182). *In vivo,* the drug is reduced to a chelating agent and has been reported to decrease norepinephrine levels in the heart and brain. One interpretation of these results would be that dopamine beta-hydroxylase is a rate-limiting step. However, the chelating properties affect Fe^{++} and thereby also inhibit tyrosine hydroxylase, a known rate-limiting step (467). These results should serve as a reminder that many drugs have multiple actions which must be investigated. An additional example concerns another "dopamine beta-hydroxylase inhibitor," 5-butylpicolinic acid (Fusaric acid)

(211). When given to animals, it decreases their brain norepinephrine levels, increases serotonin (which should be unaffected by the inhibitor) by 25 per cent, but does not change dopamine concentrations. The combination of decreased norepinephrine, normal dopamine, and raised serotonin cannot be fully explained on the basis of inhibition of dopamine beta-hydroxylase. Further investigations may reveal additional useful actions of the inhibitor that are not obvious today.

Phenylethanolamine-N-methyl Transferase

In selected tissues, synthesis of catecholamines can continue beyond norepinephrine to epinephrine. In man, only the chromaffin cells nearest the adrenal cortex (and some in the brain) appear to have the cytoplasmic enzyme capable of N-methylating norepinephrine. This enzyme, since it has relatively nonspecific requirements for substrate, was named phenylethanolamine-N-methyl transferase (PNMT) by Axelrod (10) who first characterized it. It predominantly methylates phenylethanolamines, which include endogenous beta-hydroxycatecholamines (e.g., norepinephrine and octopamine), their methoxyamine metabolites (e.g., normetanephrine), drugs structurally related to phenylethanolamine (e.g., norephedrine and amphetamine), and even some secondary beta-hydroxylated amines (e.g., epinephrine and neosynephrine). The substrate with the lowest K_m is norepinephrine, the apparently preferred substrate.

The sulfhydryl-containing enzyme has an absolute requirement for a methyl-group donor (S-adenosylmethionine), oxygen, and probably Mg^{++}. Norepinephrine and most of its substrates competitively inhibit the enzyme's function, but its product, epinephrine, is its most potent and noncompetitive inhibitor. Ordinary concentrations of unbound epinephrine in the cell cytoplasm are probably sufficient to regulate the minute-to-minute function of the enzyme. The details of the enzyme's affinity for various substrates, of its chemical and physical properties, of its synthesis and action, and of its distribution in mammals still are under investigation.

Why Is the Adrenal Cortex Contiguous With the Medulla?
An examination of the development of the mammalian adrenal gland must suggest that these two parts are together for a biologic reason. Mammals are unique among vertebrates in possessing an adrenal gland organized into layers. The layers are derived from two separate embryologic regions, and venous drainage from the cortex literally bathes the medullary cells with blood containing the highest concentration of steroid of any fluid (Fig. 5–41). Even so, it has never been apparent that the adrenal medulla has an important function different from that of other sympathetic ganglia. Removing the medulla does not seem to critically threaten the life of man, yet there are physiologic conditions (e.g., during sud-

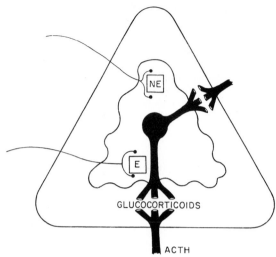

Figure 5–41. Schematic diagram illustrating the anatomical relationship between the adrenal cortex and medulla, and the intramural adrenal portal vascular system. An "epinephrine cell" is shown lying near an adrenal sinusoid, and a "norepinephrine cell" is shown at some distance from the sinusoid. Both receive a preganglionic cholinergic innervation. (Reproduced from Pohorecky, L. A., and Wurtman, R. J.: *Pharmacol. Rev.* *23*:1, 1971. Copyright © The Williams & Wilkins Co., Baltimore.)

den hypoglycemia or acute stress) which benefit from release of epinephrine from the medulla.

Investigators have found a number of facts that physiologically link the adrenal cortex and medulla:

1. Hypophysectomized rats make little epinephrine.

2. Administration of adrenal corticotropic hormone (ACTH) restores normal epinephrine content to the adrenal glands of hypophysectomized animals.

3. Administration of other pituitary tropic hormones does not produce the same changes as in 2.

4. In the rabbit and other species, the mature adrenal gland contains almost solely epinephrine, but extra-adrenal chromaffin cells do not.

5. Fetal adrenal medullary cells do not contain epinephrine until the cortical cells are mature.

6. Dogfish chromaffin cells were removed from direct contact with adrenocortical cells and contained only norepinephrine. The anatomical pattern of the adrenal cortex and these biologic observations spurred Wurtman and Axelrod (524) to find that PNMT was present only in the adrenal medulla and probably was responsible for the formation of epinephrine from norepinephrine. The two workers subsequently confirmed that each manipulation which increased or decreased epinephrine appropriately altered PNMT within the gland. They and others indicated that, if the synthesis of PNMT were blocked by inhibitors of protein synthesis, so would epinephrine synthesis be inhibited.

Many of the factors controlling PNMT synthesis seemed to originate in the adrenal cortex. If an animal was hypophysectomized, his adrenal epinephrine and PNMT decreased as glucocorticoid content of the body dropped. If either ACTH (but

not other tropic hormones) or corticosteroids (dexamethasone and to some extent aldosterone, but not androgenic or estrogenic steroids) were given to the animals, the PNMT and epinephrine levels returned toward normal. Other enzymes involved in the synthesis or metabolism of catecholamines were unaffected by these manipulations.

A few problems arose as the relationship between the cortex and medulla was further probed. Other nonsteroidal hormones (insulin and glucagon) have been found to stimulate PNMT. Also aminoglutethimide, a drug that suppresses glucocorticoid secretion from the adrenal cortex, can increase PNMT. Finally, nerve stimulation to the adrenal medulla appears to be an independent and important system of control. During such direct or indirect stimulation, PNMT levels, like those of tyrosine hydroxylase and dopamine beta-hydroxylase, rise (472).

There can be no question that adrenal cortical steroids, under certain circumstances, can profoundly influence medullary chromaffin cells. How critical this function is to man or animals is unknown. In dogs, large doses (300 mg. intravenously with 100 mg. every hour) of hydrocortisone have no observed effect on catecholamine secretion rates. The only noticeable effects of the steroids were seen when they augmented epinephrine release during hypovolemia (200). However, in human beings with Cushing's disease, there is poor correlation between ACTH or glucocorticoid concentrations and PNMT concentrations (240).

As yet there are no other known reasons for the intimate association of the adrenal cortex with the medulla. No further functions of the medulla have been influenced by the cortical hormones, though most have been tested. Conversely, however, few if any of the effects of catecholamines, their precursors or metabolites, on cortical function have been explored. One could argue that the pattern of blood flow from cortex to medulla would not suggest that medullary activities influence the cortex. However, teleologically the two portions of the gland are likely to be together for some reason. [The interested reader is directed to the following literature for extended knowledge of this area (369, 370, 522, 524)].

At least one clinical corollary arises from our interest in PNMT. The distribution of PNMT is unique in man. It is found in the organ of Zuckerkandl during the first year of life only and from then on primarily in the adrenal medulla (53). Therefore, whenever clinical disease, such as a pheochromocytoma, is associated with excess epinephrine, either of those locations is a likely source. So far there has been only one exception to this rule (133), when the pheochromocytoma was found in the thorax.

False Neurotransmitters

General Concepts

Some biologists question whether norepinephrine and epinephrine are the only physiologic

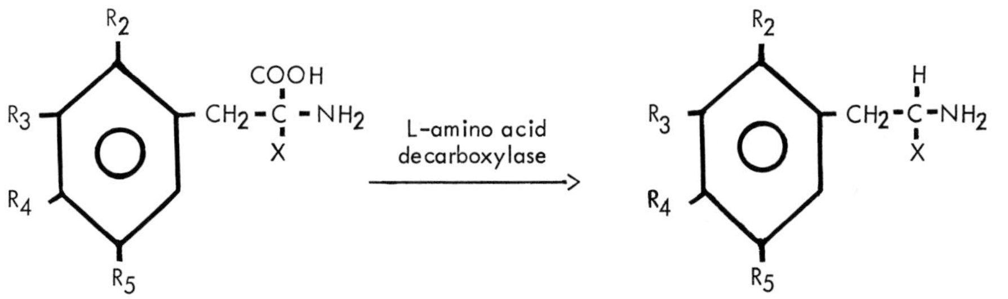

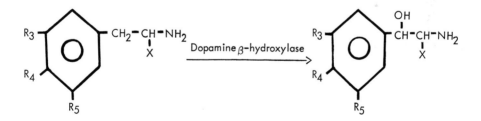

R2	R3	R4	R5	X	Product
-	-	OH	-	-	Tyramine
-	OH	-	-	-	m-Tyramine
-	OH	OH	-	-	Dopamine
OH	-	OH	OH	-	6-Hydroxydopamine
-	OH	OH	OH	-	5-Hydroxydopamine
-	OH	OCH₃	OH	-	3,5-Dihydroxy-4-methoxyphenylethylamine
-	OH	-	-	CH₃	α-Methyl-m-Tyramine
-	OH	OH	-	CH₃	α-Methyl Dopamine
OH	-	-	-	-	0-Tyramine

Figure 5–42. Substrates for aromatic L-amino acid decarboxylase and the product that would be produced in the cell. (Reproduced with modification from Kopin, I. J.: *Fed. Proc. 30*:904, 1971, with permission.)

transmitters released from sympathetic nerve endings during physiologic stimuli. Few doubt that the amines are transmitters released from the nerves or that they can produce the majority of changes associated with activation of the sympathetic system (131, 223).

However, as was mentioned above, the process of synthesis of catecholamines is nonspecific at a number of steps; unnatural amino acids (250) can be transported into the neuron, where they can be nonspecifically decarboxylated (Fig. 5–42); the resulting amines often can serve as unnatural substrates for dopamine beta-hydroxylase (Fig. 5–43). As will be discussed, the process of storage and

R3	R4	R5	X	Product
-	-	-	-	Phenylethanolamine
-	OH	-	-	Octopamine
OH	-	-	-	m-Octopamine
OH	OH	-	-	Norepinephrine
OH	OH	OH	-	5-Hydroxynorepinephrine
-	OH	-	CH₃	α-Methyloctopamine
OH	-	-	CH₃	Metaraminol
OH	OH	-	CH₃	α-Methylnorepinephrine
-	-	-	CH₃	Norephedrine
OH	OH	OCH₃	-	5-Methoxynorepinephrine
OH	OCH₃	OH	-	4-Methoxy-3,5-dihydroxyphenylethanolamine

Figure 5–43. Phenylethanolamine-type substrates that can gain access to the intraneuronal vesicle containing dopamine beta-hydroxylase. The products will only be found in the sympathetic nerve or adrenal chromaffin cell where the enzyme is exclusively harbored. Only the beta-hydroxylated amines are released as transmitters during nerve stimulation (155). (Reproduced with modification from Kopin, I. J.: *Fed. Proc. 30*:904, 1971, with permission.)

release of the catecholamines also is nonspecific. Therefore, the unnatural amines conceivably can be used as substitute or false neurotransmitters.

The criteria for a false neurotransmitter have been reviewed frequently in the last few years (91, 106, 246, 247, 248, 250). Generally, although they are not normally present in the sympathetic neurons in significant quantity, they can be made to accumulate in the nerve endings at the same site as the natural transmitter. The accumulation may follow administration of the substance itself, a precursor, or a drug that allows an endogenous compound to form the false neurotransmitter. The false neurotransmitter must be held in the same storage sites, released by the same nerve stimulation, and depleted by drugs that deplete norepinephrine. The released substance does not, however, have to have the same pharmacologic properties as the native transmitter. In addition, the pharmacologic effects of a false neurotransmitter may not be due to its activity as a stimulator of an effector cell but rather to its effects on synthesis, storage, or release of the native transmitter (477). I will discuss only those drugs and transmitters that have been found clinically useful. As might be expected, they affect the cardiovascular system and clinically have so far been used in the management of hypertension. The heuristic qualities (both positive and negative) of the false neurotransmitter concept will be weighed in this section. By following the history of researching the actions of some antihypertensive drugs, the reader should understand the practical importance of the concept.

Alpha-methyldopa (Methyldopa) and Alpha-methylnorepinephrine

Methyldopa was first studied as an antihypertensive drug because it was known to inhibit aromatic L-amino acid decarboxylase *in vitro*. The effects in animals were discouraging, but Oates and co-workers (278, 352) found that the L-or S-enantiomer inhibited decarboxylase, decreased tissue stores of norepinephrine, and lowered arterial pressure in patients with essential hypertension. The latter two actions were considered to be caused by diminished catecholamine synthesis at step 2 in Fig. 5–37 (the conversion of dopa to dopamine). Then it was discovered that (1) norepinephrine depletion produced by methyldopa exceeds the duration of decarboxylase inhibition; (2) metabolism of catecholamines as reflected by vanillylmandelic acid excretion in urine was not significantly changed after administration of methyldopa; and (3) agents producing more profound decarboxylase inhibition did not alter the rate of synthesis, size of stores, or turnover of catecholamines, nor did they affect arterial blood pressure (278, 433). Since decarboxylation is not a rate-limiting step in the biosynthesis of catecholamines, its inhibition cannot be expected to affect the net synthesis of the end product.

After effective doses of methyldopa were administered to animals, alpha-methylnorepinephrine

was found in brain tissue. The amino acid drug presumably is taken into the sympathetic neurons where it undergoes decarboxylation and subsequent beta-hydroxylation to alpha-methylnorepinephrine by the same enzymes that convert dopa to norepinephrine (Figs. 5–37 and 5–44) (433). The newly formed alpha-methylnorepinephrine then can displace norepinephrine, can be stored in the storage granules, and be released in place of norepinephrine by nerve stimulation (78).

Although the false neurotransmitter concept is scientifically valuable and has practical implications, it has failed to explain satisfactorily the mechanism of action of methyldopa (15). Alpha-methylnorepinephrine is almost as potent a vasoconstrictor and cardioaccelerating agent as norepinephrine when tested in many animals, but in man it may be somewhat less potent than norepinephrine. The peripheral sympathetic blockade produced by methyldopa may be related to inhibition of tyrosine hydroxylase in the nerve ending by alpha-methylnorepinephrine. As we have seen, inhibition of this rate-limiting step in the synthesis of catecholamines results in a decrease in the amount of transmitter available for release (246). Another possibility is that alpha-methylnorepinephrine, although less available for release by nerve stimulation, is nevertheless capable of displacing the native neurotransmitters from binding sites within the cell. None of these explanations is proved, and the actual mechanism is unknown. Indeed, it is likely that methyldopa has important effects on arterial blood pressure through direct dilation of peripheral vessels (324), through inhibiting the secretion of renin (165), and through action on the central nervous system.

Alpha-methylmetatyrosine and Metaraminol

Following the discovery that alpha-methylnorepinephrine qualified as a false neurotransmitter, the breadth of the concept was tested in a prospective manner. Additional analogs of tyrosine, dopa, dopamine, and norepinephrine were investigated (54). Alpha-methylmetatyrosine was found to be transported into the nerve endings and brain and transformed into meta-hydroxynorephedrine (metaraminol) by the same enzymes that form norepinephrine from tyrosine (Figs. 5–37 and 5–44). The endogenously formed metaraminol is a false neurotransmitter: it stoichiometrically displaces norepinephrine from the storage sites and is released by stimulation of nerves (91). Such findings emphasize the assets of a hypothesis in helping to design studies on the mechanism of action of a drug.

Infused metaraminol is taken up by the adrenergic neuron and directly displaces norepinephrine from the granules. When clinically useful doses are rapidly infused, metaraminol is initially an effective pressor agent. However, tachyphylaxis to the pressor effects of metaraminol occurs later, an effect that can be explained by the false neurotrans-

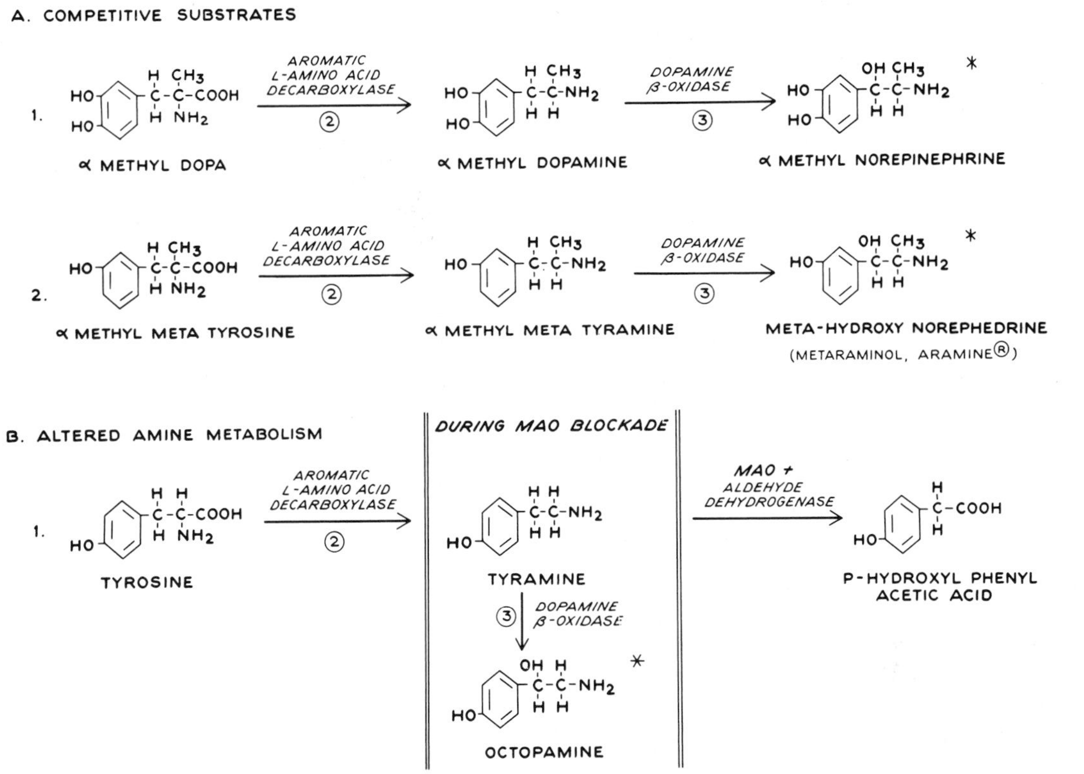

A. COMPETITIVE SUBSTRATES

1. α METHYL DOPA → (AROMATIC L-AMINO ACID DECARBOXYLASE ②) → α METHYL DOPAMINE → (DOPAMINE β-OXIDASE ③) → α METHYL NOREPINEPHRINE *

2. α METHYL META TYROSINE → (AROMATIC L-AMINO ACID DECARBOXYLASE ②) → α METHYL META TYRAMINE → (DOPAMINE β-OXIDASE ③) → META-HYDROXY NOREPHEDRINE (METARAMINOL, ARAMINE®) *

B. ALTERED AMINE METABOLISM

1. TYROSINE → (AROMATIC L-AMINO ACID DECARBOXYLASE ②) → **DURING MAO BLOCKADE** → TYRAMINE → (MAO + ALDEHYDE DEHYDROGENASE) → P-HYDROXYL PHENYL ACETIC ACID

TYRAMINE → (DOPAMINE β-OXIDASE ③) → OCTOPAMINE *

Figure 5–44. Formation of false neurotransmitters (indicated by asterisk). Some are formed by incorporation of a pharmacologic compound into the metabolic pathway for catecholamine synthesis (A.1 and A.2); others are formed independently of catecholamine production (B.1).

mitter hypothesis. Metaraminol has less than 5 per cent of the potency of norepinephrine; when most of the norepinephrine in the nerve ending has been replaced, stimulation of the nerve results in minimal release of native transmitters, and a partial blockade of the sympathetic nervous system is established. Further doses of metaraminol fail to release adequate amounts of the potent neurotransmitter, resulting not only in refractory responses to metaraminol but also in the appearance of a new drug effect, hypotension. Patients treated with metaraminol have large concentrations of the drug in their sympathetic tissues (106). An infusion of norepinephrine reestablishes the stores of norepinephrine and restores the hypertensive response to metaraminol.

Metaraminol given in repeated small doses does not produce hypertension because the quantity of catecholamines released after a single dose is small, but eventually the cumulative effects seriously deplete stores of catecholamines and reduce the blood pressure of patients with essential hypertension. Although use of metaraminol as an antihypertensive drug is not seriously suggested, knowledge of its mechanism of action can help explain an otherwise paradoxical response. Both metaraminol and alpha-methylmetatyrosine, therefore, can be antihypertensive agents in man (91, 106, 216). Again, a valid hypothesis not only may explain an observed effect but also may be used to predict future observations (regardless of

how unexpected they may seem). If the hypothesis fails to predict a response, either the hypothesis or the observation is incorrect. Usually the hypothesis is more vulnerable.

Observing the effects of metaraminol allows us to further define the usefulness of the false neurotransmitter hypothesis:

1. Metaraminol does not cross the blood-brain barrier; therefore, attention can be focused entirely upon peripheral mechanisms of sympathetic blockade, which do not differ from the effects of agents that also act on the central nervous system.

2. Metaraminol has only one hydroxyl group on the aromatic ring, proving that the catechol (dihydroxyphenyl) structure is not an absolute requirement for a false neurotransmitter.

Monoamine Oxidase Inhibitors

Originally used as antidepressants, monoamine oxidase (MAO) inhibitors were found to produce postural hypotension that correlated with the degree of inhibition of MAO *in vivo* (355). Although monoamine oxidase does not primarily inactivate circulating catecholamines, it does metabolize the amines accessible to it in the cell's cytoplasm (249). When MAO is blocked, the amount of norepinephrine as well as other amines [e.g., octopamine (325)] in the storage granules increases. When these amines enter the granule, they become potential false neurotransmitters which might either compete with norepinephrine for release or act in the nerve ending to disrupt normal catecholamine synthesis, storage, or release. Octopamine may be the key false neurotransmitter during MAO inhibition. It is formed by beta-hydroxylation of tyramine, the product of decarboxylation of tyrosine, and is less than 1 per cent as potent as norepinephrine (Fig. 5–44). Normally tyramine and octopamine are rapidly destroyed by MAO, but, when protected from oxidation during MAO inhibition, both can accumulate. Thus after any standard nerve stimulation, a finite amount of transmitter leaves the nerve ending, but the amount of potent transmitter may be diluted by the impotent false neurotransmitter, octopamine. The resulting sympathetic blockade appears to account for the antihypertensive action of MAO inhibition (252).

Infused tyramine in normal persons releases norepinephrine from nerve endings and results in a brief rise of arterial pressure. Because tyramine is rapidly destroyed by MAO, its effects are transient. When catecholamine stores are increased, as in patients with pheochromocytomas, an infusion of tyramine produces a brief but exaggerated rise of arterial blood pressure. When catecholamine stores are increased and tyramine is protected from destruction, relatively small amounts of infused or ingested tyramine can provoke severe prolonged hypertension. Hypertensive reactions have been reported after ingestion of tyramine-containing foods, including aged cheese, wine, beer, marmite, pickled herring, broad beans, or chicken liver. In addition to tyramine-containing foods, commonly used catecholamine-releasing drugs (amphetamine, ephedrine, phenylpropanolamine, mephentermine, metaraminol, methylphenidate, and phenmetrazine) can produce hypertensive reactions during MAO inhibition.

Guanethidine

Guanethidine has many properties common to the false neurotransmitters. Guanethidine is actively transported into the nerve ending by the transport system for norepinephrine. Like norepinephrine its uptake is blocked by cocaine, imipramine and its derivatives, and amphetamine (322). The drug is bound to the norepinephrine storage sites (84); it releases norepinephrine from the nerve ending (81), and because it does not inhibit monoamine oxidase in the nerve, the net effect is depletion of catecholamines (257). Guanethidine can be released by reserpine or by nerve stimulation and its effects prevented or reversed by imipramines, cocaine, ephedrine, amphetamine, tyramine, or metaraminol, the same list of drugs that either release or block uptake of norepinephrine (323).

In spite of its similarity to classic false neurotransmitters, guanethidine produces sympathetic inhibition prior to major decreases in catecholamine stores, and the sympathetic inhibition disappears before the amine content is noticeably depleted. Guanethidine probably not only depletes but also interferes with release of norepinephrine during physiologic stimulus of the nerve. Perhaps it causes a persistent and direct depolarization of the sympathetic nerve ending, which in turn initially discharges catecholamines and results in adrenergic inhibition (84). This hypothesis is consistent with the observation that large parenteral doses of guanethidine release enough norepinephrine to induce hypertension while simultaneously blocking the response to postganglionic nerve stimulation. Hypertensive response to agents that deplete adrenergic neuronal stores of norepinephrine (279) should be expected, particularly in patients with expanded stores of catecholamines (e.g., caused by a pheochromocytoma, neuroblastoma, or monoamine oxidase inhibitor), and should be treated when necessary with the most specific therapy known: alpha-adrenergic blocking agents. Comprehensive reviews of antihypertensive agents and false neurotransmitters along with discussions of the possible role of the sympathetic nervous system in essential hypertension have recently appeared (49, 155, 159, 198, 313, 348).

6-Hydroxydopamine

Drugs that affect the sympathetic nervous system as false neurotransmitters are useful to more than the clinician. Selective and specific methods of manipulating the autonomic nervous system (151) yield specific lessons. For instance, surgical ablation of a spinal cord gives considerably less information than does a surgical sympathectomy about the specific function of the autonomic nervous system. On the other hand, information about the sympathetic nervous system was gained from the finding that antisera to a sympathetic nerve growth factor could ablate the entire sympathetic system in newborn animals (222). Certain drugs (e.g., reserpine, methyldopa, alpha-methylmetatyrosine) can alter stores of catecholamines and give an idea of the function of sympathetic nerve endings (158); a major advance was the realization that 6-hydroxydopamine was one of the unnatural substances that could be transported into the nerve ending and could interfere with uptake, synthesis, storage, and release of the native transmitter.

When the amine is given to animals, it specifically enters adrenergic neurons. When given intraperitoneally, it produces a selective peripheral sympathectomy, sparing the adrenal gland and the central nervous system (58, 268). Within hours of administration, it begins to destroy the nerve ending in a characteristic fashion (125, 163); a rapid depletion of endogenous norepinephrine is associated with a preferential release of microsomal contents of the neuron (containing the catecholamine storage vesicles) and loss of tyrosine hydroxylase (232, 471). Following the loss of the neurotransmitter, the actual nerve ending degenerates. This stage of diminished uptake of exogenous catecholamines correlates with hypersensitivity of the effector organs to the amine (63, 193, 220, 342). Later some neurons regenerate, and their ability to take up (and therefore biologically inactivate) catecholamines returns before synthesis of the catechols is reestablished at normal rates.

When given intracisternally, the drug is also taken up into specific sites in the brain but produces no peripheral effects. Although some doses exhaust both norepinephrine and dopamine, careful regulation depletes norepinephrine more than dopaminergic sites (57, 147, 484, 485). Serotoninergic sites are not affected. The study of behavioral changes correlated with isolated changes in norepinephrine or dopamine content of brain has helped to identify both the presence and function of specific sets of adrenergic neurons (67). Although these findings may not directly interest the non-biologic investigator, they suggest the best use of, and therapeutic effects of, catecholamine precursors in patients with Parkinson's disease.

The mechanism of action of 6-hydroxydopamine has been partially elucidated. When given to animals, the precursor 6-hydroxydopa enters primarily the peripheral sympathetic nerves and must be decarboxylated to be effective (33). Although the amine enters the catecholamine storage vesicle, this is not essential for its action (163). Perhaps its biochemical effects are related to its ability to generate hydrogen peroxide (202). The peroxide damages biogenic amine uptake systems in synaptosomes (pinched-off nerve endings), and both peroxide generation and the effects of 6-hydroxydopamine are partially prevented by catalase.

Physiologic Factors That Affect Catecholamine Synthesis

As methods for studying the synthesis and disposition of catecholamines have developed (137, 297, 422), physiologic controls of synthesis have come to light. Nerve stimulation has been mentioned as a vital factor in catecholamine synthesis (326, 422). Mild stimulation increases tyrosine hydroxylase activity by releasing the most recently synthesized pool of catecholamines, reducing feedback inhibition of the activity of the enzyme. Intense or protracted stimulation increases synthesis of both tyrosine hydroxylase and dopamine beta-hydroxylase and is in part responsible for intensified production of catecholamines (326).

The physiologic factors of moment-to-moment control of the synthesis in the brain seem more complex. There is a diurnal variation (control mechanism unknown) in concentration of catecholamines in the brain (532) and perhaps in peripheral tissues (523). The pool of catecholamines in the brain is greatest at night, and the amines seem to have a function (not fully defined) in such cyclical processes as sleep, arousal, temperature regulation, and even eating and drinking. There is some evidence that the functions of one subcategory of nerve ending (e.g., a serotoninergic or

dopaminergic ending) can control the functions of another subcategory (e.g., one containing norepinephrine) (364). What other factors enter into the control of brain amine synthesis and whether similar factors control synthesis in both the brain and periphery remains to be seen.

The basal synthesis rate of catecholamines seems to be variably affected by the function of "unassociated" endocrine systems. Normal maintenance of adrenal tyrosine hydroxylase requires ACTH (336); follicle stimulating hormone (FSH) but not luteinizing hormone (LH) controls the turnover of norepinephrine in selected parts of the brain (3), and dopamine and serotoninergic nerves apparently regulate LH release in rats (418). Angiotensin may have a stimulative effect [perhaps by releasing some of the newly synthesized norepinephrine or by inhibiting its uptake into nerve endings (46, 116, 358, 362)] on norepinephrine production in the peripheral sympathetic nerves.

When man (184, 533) or animals are subjected to extraordinary stresses (e.g., childbirth, burns, cold, hypoxia, immobilization, isolation, or physical exercise), the rate of synthesis of catecholamines increases greatly (258, 259, 260, 262, 263, 264, 335, 361, 450, 460, 511). The increase is associated with an increase in production of synthesizing enzymes and sometimes may be limited by the availability of substrate for the enzymes. The synthesis rate is integrated with, but not entirely dependent upon, production of ACTH, corticosteroids, and perhaps other tropic hormones produced by the pituitary (260, 361). At least two additional mechanisms may be influencing the overall synthesis and effect of the catecholamines: (1) as the stress continues, the sensitivity of effector organs to catecholamines may gradually increase, requiring less and less released catecholamine to elicit any given effect (258); (2) metabolic compensatory responses related to such factors as heat production may alter (increase or decrease) the need for release of catecholamines (259, 262, 460). Any loss of the nerves from the sympathetic nervous system—by accident, surgery, chemical ablation, or perhaps some diseases affecting the integrity of the nerves—will increase production of the catecholamines in the remaining intact areas (264, 335).

Many commonly used drugs, common diseases, or complex physiologic activities such as fighting (511) alter the synthesis of catecholamines. However, their actions are often complex, affecting not only synthesis but also storage, release, metabolism, and excretion of the amines. They will therefore be discussed after an explanation of these other factors.

Storage and Release of Catecholamines

The presence of "cytoplasmic particles" in the adrenal medulla and sympathetic nerve endings was reported first by Blaschko and Welch in 1953 (44) and confirmed shortly afterward by von Euler and Hillarp (493). In addition to their importance in synthesis, these granules play a major role in the storage and biologic inactivation of catecholamines (373). Storage of catecholamines is probably related to hydrogen bonding of the catecholamines to the phosphorus moiety of adenosine-triphosphatase (ATP) and to a specific intragranular protein (497). The granules then are a storehouse of potentially active catecholamines, which, if left free in the cytoplasm, would be metabolized by MAO (Fig. 5–38) (249).

The biochemical composition of the granules (their complement of amino acids, electron carriers, lipids, and electrolytes), as well as their morphologic characteristics and appearance on electron microscopy, is remarkably constant regardless of the organ or species of origin (43, 156, 438, 455, 469, 494, 531). Even neoplastic tissue (pheochromocytoma) has "normal" granules (43, 438, 455, 531). The development of the granules in the early embryologic life of rats correlates with the ability to take up and then synthesize catecholamines (99). The granules are almost certainly responsible for the major part (more than 80 per cent) of binding of catecholamines in any tissue (428), although some tissues (e.g., skeletal muscle) may be able to bind the amines at extragranular sites. The granules are found only in chromaffin-derived cells and are physically distinct from the mitochondria and lysosomes. Although the granules have similar physical properties, some evidence indicates that their function varies, depending on their location in specific organs (34, 75). For example, granules obtained from different segments of the same blood vessel will have different amine content.

The granules are relatively nonspecific as to the amines they will transport and bind (468) (see false neurotransmitters). The concentrating process in all granules studied is active and energy-consuming, shows preference for the L-isomers of the respective amines, is dependent on Na^+, ATP, and Mg^{++}, and is inhibited by ouabain (an inhibitor of the Na-K ATPase pump), K^+, and Ca^{++} (36, 47, 217, 287, 289, 496). Despite the pump's ability to transport an amine against a concentration gradient, low levels of amine in a fluid perfusing a tissue will result in disproportionately low final concentrations in the granule. In a perfusate containing low concentrations, the transported amines are rapidly metabolized, and accumulation will be apparent only when large quantities are transported. Interestingly, the pump is stimulated by O-methylated metabolites of catecholamines, a fact which might encourage conservation of the amines after a sudden-burst or sustained release (221). As more is known about transport processes, it appears that specific drugs may be designed to selectively inhibit transport into either dopamine or norepinephrine-containing neurons (215). Finally, in some diseases such as pheochromocytoma the ratio of norepinephrine plus epinephrine to ATP is increased (420, 454), which tends to promote a leak of catechols and a more rapid than normal turnover of formed catecholamines (105).

Two pools of catecholamines have been postu-lated (12): one that is kept from active metabolism by cytoplasmic enzymes and has a half-life approaching 24 hours, and a second smaller pool that is readily available for release from the nerve ending and has a half-life of only 2 hours. The second pool has been termed the "easily releasable" pool because it is readily diminished by physiologic stimulation and pharmacologic agents such as tyramine (70). It is composed primarily of the most recently synthesized amines (37, 251) and is probably concentrated in peripheral portions of nerve endings; it equilibrates only slowly with the first or "tightly bound" pool. There is no convincing evidence that the two pools are anatomically separate (520).

Ordinarily nerve stimulation (a propagated impulse) is necessary to release catecholamines from both anatomical storage sites into the plasma (209). The actual chemical mediation of the release appears to be linked to the presence of acetylcholine or the influx of calcium ions into the granule or both (68, 128, 236, 400). The process is energy-dependent, requiring glycolysis or oxidative metabolism (399). Not all catecholamine release is via stimulation of sympathetic nerves; at least a small reserve can be released by stimulation of the vagus nerve (488).

One mechanism of release from both sympathetic nerves and the adrenal medulla appears similar to the secretory process of a number of exocrine glands (417). The hormone can be released in quanta along with the chemical constituents of the vesicle (40). The migration of the vesicle to the cell surface, where it is extruded by exocytosis, seems dependent on contraction of the microfibrils of the cells (371); the microfibrils may perform a similar function in the release of histamine from mast cells, insulin from the pancreas, and granules from leukocytes during phagocytosis. Release of catecholamines is inhibited by colchicine, vinblastine, and vincristine (all of which interfere with the microtubules) and is potentiated by deuterium oxide, which also potentiates histamine and insulin release. The release of catecholamines from the adrenal gland can be selective: in man, release of epinephrine is not necessarily associated with concomitant release of norepinephrine (405). How the adrenal receives signals to call for release of one amine instead of the other is not known.

Apparently not all release involves exocytosis (40, 416); not only is there a constant leak of catecholamines into the circulation, but some unusual chemicals such as acetaldehyde, which accumulates during metabolism of alcohol or in diabetics, can promote release of catecholamines without exocytosis (416). These situations are not associated with protein release from the granules, though they appear to depend on the direct action of chemicals on the granules. Whether or not acidemia or hypoxemia provokes release of catecholamines entirely by reflex stimulation of nerves is unknown but is not likely (346).

Sympathomimetic amines such as tyramine and amphetamine release bound norepinephrine from the storage vesicles, indirectly causing a rise in blood pressure (69). Tyramine and reserpine both reduce catecholamine (or false neurotransmitter) content in tissues but by different mechanisms. The tyramine rapidly releases relatively large quantities of catecholamines that leave the nerve unmetabolized and produce a pressor effect. The tyramine is metabolized later (249). On the other hand, reserpine both abolishes the ability of the nerve vesicle to bind norepinephrine (214) and releases catecholamines more slowly than tyramine. The released catecholamines are likely to be oxidized in the nerve ending by intraneuronal MAO, and the metabolites that are physiologically inactive produce no pharmacologic effects when released from the axon.

Once the catecholamines are released, they act on effector sites (457, 458) and are then either rapidly destroyed by plasma enzymes, rebound by granules, or excreted in the urine. What is known of the physiochemical mechanism of action of catecholamines has been described in a comprehensive review (30) and related papers (435, 436, 437).

Inactivation of Catecholamines

Reuptake of Catecholamines

Four mechanisms exist to biologically inactivate catecholamines. Probably the most important is the "reuptake" of the catecholamines by postganglionic neuron storage granules (209), a fact supported by two observations:

1. Agents (e.g., guanethidine, cocaine, imipramine) which block reuptake of catecholamines into sympathetic nerve endings potentiate the response of tissues to sympathetic nerve stimulation or catecholamine infusion (Fig. 5–45) (208, 227, 274, 453, 478, 495).

2. When tissues have been deprived of sympathetic innervation and, therefore, of postganglionic neuron storage granules, the response of the effectors to administered catecholamines is enhanced (207). The granules bind catecholamines without destroying the molecule, thus allowing later release of the same catecholamines.

The process of uptake by transport across the neuronal membrane and into the nerve vesicle is distinct from the process of storage in the vesicle. Drugs which interfere with one may have little or no effect upon the other. Reserpine, which interferes with storage of norepinephrine, affects uptake minimally, and cocaine and tricyclic antidepressants (imipramine) which block uptake have no obvious effect on storage. A third separate process is synthesis. Drugs that influence synthesis need not also influence uptake or storage of catecholamines. Only inhibition of uptake is associated with striking supersensitivity to norepinephrine.

Metabolism of Norepinephrine and Epinephrine by Peripheral Tissues

Two of the mechanisms of inactivation are enzymatic. For some time the physiologic importance of these two metabolic pathways has been controversial. Apparently, however, catechol-O-methyl

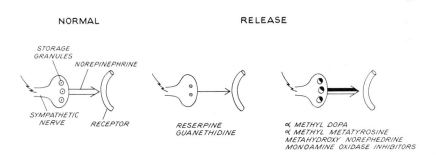

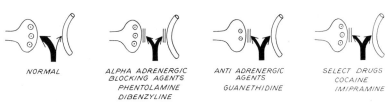

Figure 5–45. Schematic diagram of the mechanisms by which pharmacologic agents alter the effect of endogenous or exogenous catecholamines. Some agents (*top*) act by diminishing the stores of catecholamines in nerve endings (guanethidine), by promoting formation of false neurotransmitters (methyldopa), or by being accumulated themselves as false neurotransmitters (metahydroxy norephedrine). Other agents (*bottom*) act by inhibiting uptake of catecholamines into storage sites or into both storage and effector sites (phentolamine, Dibenzyline). When uptake into storage sites is blocked (imipramine), uptake into effector sites is greatly increased.

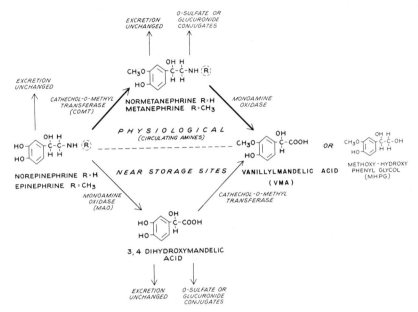

Figure 5–46. Biochemical pathways for the metabolism of catecholamines. Heavy diagonal arrows indicate the major sequence of metabolism of catecholamines released into the circulation. Light diagonal arrows indicate the sequence of metabolism of catecholamines released intracellularly. Vertical arrows indicate minor mechanism of excretion or metabolism of specific intermediary products.

transferase (COMT), found in plasma, liver, and kidneys, is responsible for the initial enzymatic inactivation of physiologic amounts of circulating catecholamines (11, 16, 18, 77, 176, 412, 479) (Fig. 5–46). When COMT is inhibited by an agent such as pyrogallol, O-methylation of the catecholamines is blocked, and the effect of sympathetic nerve stimulation or of administered catecholamines is somewhat prolonged (11, 16, 18, 77, 176, 412, 479).

Such is not the case when monoamine oxidase is inhibited. Blockage of MAO, although it alters the response to sympathetic stimulation, does not change the degree or duration of tissue reaction to administered catecholamines (191). Despite its presence in plasma (9, 164, 174, 293, 385, 481) and the fact that it may be induced by the presence of substrate (334, 381), apparently MAO plays a minor role in the metabolism of circulating catecholamines. Monoamine oxidase is thought responsible for the rapid inactivation of catechols in the cytoplasm of the nerve endings (249). Inhibition of MAO by pargyline or equivalent agents results in an increase in stored catecholamines and other biologically important amines (see discussion on false neurotransmitters).

Regardless of which of the two enzymes, COMT or MAO, accounts for the initial inactivation of catecholamines, vanillylmandelic acid (VMA) is the end product. Conjugated forms of normetanephrine or metanephrine make up a relatively small portion of the metabolized catecholamines.

The fourth, and minor, mechanism for the biologic inactivation of physiologic amounts of catecholamines is their metabolism or excretion unaltered by the kidney (237, 411, 458).

Synthesis and Metabolism of Catecholamines in the Central Nervous System

General Considerations

When this chapter was last written, no more than the beginning of our understanding of brain amines was available. We were sure of basic similarities between the synthesis, storage, release, and metabolism of catecholamines in the CNS and the peripheral tissues. However, we were also sure that transport of the amines or their metabolites from brain to blood or blood to brain was limited (176). The two areas were therefore potentially autonomous regarding the dynamics of catecholamines. Histochemical studies and tagging of endogenous norepinephrine with radioactive precursors of catecholamines or catecholamines themselves proved to be valid procedures for studying normal and drug-induced changes in the uptake, storage, and release of norepinephrine and dopamine in the CNS (412). Histofluorescent techniques have shown that the brain contains tracts with high concentrations of either norepinephrine, dopamine, or serotonin in nerve endings (77). These endings are highly branched and have a beaded appearance as have peripheral nerves, and any one nerve coapts with a host of other cells (9). Norepinephrine nerve terminals are distributed in many regions of the brain and spinal cord but are concentrated in the hypothalamus, while dopaminergic nerves are mainly in the caudate nucleus and striatum (164). During intraventricular administration of radioactive H^3-norepinephrine, some amine is taken up and bound in the nerve terminals (probably in the varicosities of the nerve endings). Unequal localization of the H^3-norepinephrine in various brain areas correlates closely with the usual distribution of norepinephrine in the periventricular and ventromedial nucleus of the hypothalamus, the median forebrain bundle, certain tracts in the spinal cord and the optical dendritic layer of the hippocampus (174, 381). When labeled dopamine is injected intraventricularly in animals, it too distributes unequally as H^3-dopamine into the area of dopaminergic endings—the corpus striatum (where it is present in ten times the concentration of norepinephrine) and substantia nigra. The H^3-dopamine reaching other sites is converted into H^3-norepinephrine. When animals are pretreated with drugs that block uptake of norepinephrine (e.g., imipramine), the H^3-norepinephrine level, but not the H^3-dopamine level, decreases. These observations may indicate that the norepinephrine formed from dopamine is spontaneously released from the neuron and recaptured by uptake. In the presence of imipramine, the released norepinephrine is not recaptured and is lost to metabolism (9).

All the enzymes necessary for synthesis of dopamine and norepinephrine are found in the brain (9), although PNMT is present only in traces. After injection of precursors of dopamine and norepinephrine, the amines appear in proportion to their ordinary distribution and with few exceptions are metabolized in a fashion analogous to the metabolism in peripheral tissues (55, 381, 382, 410, 411).

A variety of techniques (inhibition of synthesis, or tracing the appearance or disappearance of labeled amine) reveal important differences in the turnover rate of catecholamines in various brain areas (9). Norepinephrine use in the brain varies; for example, it is increased during electroconvulsive shock (237), paradoxical sleep (376), and different stages of the estrus cycle (4). Furthermore, lesions demonstrate a likely function by the amines; most striking is the finding that dopamine plays a role in the pathogenesis of Parkinson's disease (see the following).

Drugs that Affect Catecholamines in the Brain

Centrally and peripherally acting agents commonly used in medicine can alter the uptake, synthesis, storage, release, and metabolism of catecholamines (90, 380, 413, 466). As in peripheral sympathetic nerves, accumulation of catecholamines in the brain is a complex process that can be altered at any step. Some drugs have simple actions, others complex. Imipramine and related antidepressant drugs block uptake of norepinephrine across the neural membrane (Fig. 5–47), thus making more released neurotransmitter available for adrenergic receptors (173). Bretylium blocks re-

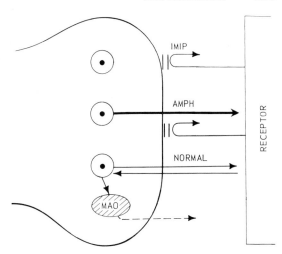

Figure 5–47. The effect of antidepressant drugs, amphetamine (AMPH) and imipramine (IMIP) on the uptake and release of norepinephrine in central adrenergic neurons. (Reproduced from Axelrod, J.: *Physiologist 11*:63, 1968, with permission.)

lease of norepinephrine during propagated nerve impulses in the peripheral nervous system (254, 255), and the ions lithium and bromide do the same in the central nervous system; structurally related ions do not block release (188, 235) (see also Chapter 29). In the peripheral nervous system, alpha-adrenergic blocking agents prevent uptake of amines and so reflexly increase synthesis rates within the neuron by compensatory increases in axonal tyrosine hydroxylase (111). Reserpine slowly releases catecholamines from the nerve endings of the central nervous system and periphery. Since the release is associated with falling intraneuronal (cytoplasmic) norepinephrine, it too reflexly stimulates norepinephrine synthesis by increasing axonal tyrosine hydroxylase activity (175, 337).

Undoubtedly amphetamine produces the most complex effects on catecholamine synthesis. Like imipramine, it blocks uptake of catecholamines. Predominantly in the central nervous system, it increases norepinephrine release as it inhibits intraneuronal monoamine oxidase (Fig. 5–47). Via MAO inhibition, relatively more than usual amine accumulates in the cytoplasm (e.g., more than after reserpine treatment) (275). [Tyramine and metaraminol behave similarly but in peripheral nerves only (253, 275).] Amphetamine also directly inhibits both tyrosine hydroxylase and dopamine beta-hydroxylase. Secondarily it decreases catecholamine synthesis as the intracytoplasmic amine content rises and suppresses tyrosine hydroxylase (56, 253). Octopamine, metaraminol, and alpha-methyldopa also produce this type of effect (230, 253). After prolonged administration of amphetamine, reflex sympathetic activity in the brain overcomes the drug's short-term effects, and synthesis of tyrosine hydroxylase and more rapid synthesis of catecholamines commence (299).

Chlorpromazine uniquely decreases the synthesis of norepinephrine by blocking dopamine uptake into storage granules, where it would come into contact with dopamine beta-hydroxylase. The result is that dopamine accumulates rapidly because it does not enter into feedback inhibition of tyrosine hydroxylase (227, 349, 350, 351).

Pharmacologic and Physiologic Actions of Catecholamines

General Considerations

Norepinephrine and epinephrine circulate in quantities sufficient for biologic activity. Concentrations in arterial blood are usually less than those in venous blood.

The two major sources of circulating norepinephrine are the sympathetic nerve endings and, to a much lesser degree, the adrenal medulla (49). The sympathetic nerve endings constantly "leak" norepinephrine into the venous blood, but the most profound increases in venous concentration occur during intense sympathetic nerve stimulation. Norepinephrine is also released from nerve endings and the adrenal medulla by endogenous hormones, such as bradykinin and histamine, and by many drugs, including tyramine, many clinically useful pressor agents, such as metaraminol (Aramine), mephentermine (Wyamine), and ephedrine, and some of the hypotensive agents, such as reserpine, alpha-methyldopa, and guanethidine.

Epinephrine is intermittently released almost exclusively by the adrenal medulla. The central nervous system, although it contains large amounts of catecholamines, neither contributes substantially to the circulating catecholamines (176) nor receives them readily across the blood-brain barrier (506).

Once released into the circulation, catecholamines have a short half-life, rarely exceeding two or three circulation times (14). In recent studies in man, infused H^3-norepinephrine has been shown to have a half-life (in tissues) of about 8 hours, and its metabolite VMA a half-life of about 11 to 16 hours (124). These studies provided reasonably valid assay systems for determining the kinetics of catecholamines in man; they indicated that assays of total urinary norepinephrine plus normetanephrine excretion per day should be a reasonable measure of peripheral sympathetic nerve activity (298). The techniques are now being used to study possible alterations of uptake, binding, release, or metabolism in disease states such as hypertension, familial dysautonomia, and Zetterstrom's syndrome (59, 170, 185). There are at least two advantages to such an approach over the techniques of simply measuring concentrations of amine in blood or excretion of amine or metabolites in urine: (1) the studies of kinetics are more likely to be sensitive to small but physiologically important lesions; and (2) careful analysis of data might pinpoint the etiology of a lesion (i.e., uptake, binding, release, synthesis, metabolism, or excretion) (124, 298).

TABLE 5–13. CLASSIFICATION OF MAJOR ALPHA AND BETA ADRENERGIC RESPONSES ELICITED BY CATECHOLAMINES

Effects	Alpha	Beta
Vascular		
Constriction, veins and arteries	+	0
Dilatation, arteries	0	+
Cardiac		
Increase in heart rate	0	+
Increase in atrial contractility and conduction rate	0	+
Increase in conduction velocity of A-V node	0	+
Increase in ventricular contractility, automaticity, and conduction velocity	0	+
Pulmonary		
Dilatation of bronchial musculature	0	+
Metabolic		
Increase in blood glucose and free fatty acid levels; inhibition of insulin release	0	+

Catecholamines in circulation either bind to receptor sites in various organs, where they produce their physiologic effect, or are inactivated. Their fate depends on enzyme composition and innervation of the organ to which they are distributed, acid-base balance in the body, presence or absence of a disease capable of modifying their effect, and the pharmacologic state of the body at the time of their release. Although the duration and magnitude of effect vary with different doses, catecholamines elicit a predictable response. Pharmacologists have separated these responses into alpha and beta receptor-mediated effects (Table 5–13) (243).

Receptors for Catecholamines

The idea that a released neurotransmitter resulted in a physiologic change, via its interaction with a specific portion of the effector cells, came from Cannon and Rosenbleuth (76). They postulated that a single transmitter (or, in modern terms, first messenger) contacted effector cells and produced one of two substances, sympathin E if the response was "excitatory" or sympathin I if the response was "inhibitory." The concept of a single transmitter was questioned when two transmitters (epinephrine and norepinephrine) were found to be released from various sympathetic nerve tissues. The concept was abandoned when it was decided that the tissue membranes were probably the most important discriminatory factors in any given response.

Ahlquist noted that different tissues produced their characteristic responses when exposed to any of a number of sympathomimetic agents (1). The responses were reproducible in any given tissue; the potency ranking of the agents was also reproducible. This led him to a tentative conclusion, that at least two types of receptors existed for catecholamines. He defined the alpha receptor as one which was found in a tissue that responded most to epinephrine or norepinephrine and least to equimolar doses of isoproterenol (epinephrine > norepinephrine >> isoproterenol) and the beta receptor as one which was found in a tissue that responded most to isoproterenol and less to equimolar concentrations of epinephrine or norepinephrine, with phenylephrine being the least potent sympathomimetic amine in this series (isoproterenol >> epinephrine or norepinephrine > phenylephrine).

The theory gained additional attention from the fact that ergot and its derivatives specifically blocked the effects of the sympathomimetic drugs in tissues with alpha receptors, but could not inhibit responses to the same drugs in tissues with beta receptors. Later it was discovered that derivatives of isoproterenol—first those whose phenyl hydroxyl groups were replaced by chloride (DCI) and then the derivatives, propranolol and pronethalol, which did not stimulate tissues themselves—could block beta receptor reactions to stimulation but not alpha receptor activity (390).

Despite Ahlquist's warnings, many medical scientists concluded that the receptors were concrete identifiable structures, that only alpha receptors were stimulated by norepinephrine or phenylephrine, and that only beta receptors were stimulated by isoproterenol; this oversimplification has led to considerable confusion in medical literature.

All drugs tested produced some effects on each tissue tested. That is, isoproterenol, norepinephrine, and epinephrine, if used in sufficient concentration, could stimulate both alpha and beta receptors. Therefore, the response to a single agent (particularly *in vivo*) could not characterize the receptors that are stimulated to produce the effect. Also, although the classical alpha blockers (such as phentolamine, dihydroergotamine, and Dibenzyline) and beta blockers (such as propranolol and pronethalol) specifically blocked their respective receptors, their actions *in vivo* or at high concentrations *in vitro* might be nonspecific and depend on some other pharmacologic property. Thus, although propranolol may have a salutary effect on some clinical condition (e.g., tachycardia), the response per se does not mean that the drug is working by its receptor-blocking qualities nor that the pathogenesis of the clinical condition lies in an abnormality of the sympathetic nervous system or the receptors (50, 162).

Using two procedures, pharmacologists have begun to rigorously classify responses of various tissues. They first determine the concentration-response curves of a given effector system (cell, tissue, organ, or organ system) for a series of sympathomimetic drugs. Then they establish the quantitative capacity of a series of antagonists to reduce the sensitivity of the responding tissues to an agonist (162, 330). By the latter procedure, they establish a series of dissociation constants (K_B) for the receptor-antagonist complexes (162). Major advantages attend this careful approach.

1. The chemical characteristics of receptors can begin to be understood. The alpha receptors, regardless of tissue or species of origin, appear to have strikingly similar potency orders of agonists and K_B for antagonists (162). In contrast, the beta receptors seem to represent a broad spectrum of chemical or physical types; the potency orders of agonists and K_B vary in different tissues, or even in the same tissue, when different responses are studied (162, 282). On this basis, some have begun to subcategorize beta receptors into β_1 (beta receptors in the heart) and β_2 (those in the vascular and tracheal smooth muscle). The consensus is that this classification is premature. However, the benefit of such critical scrutiny is obvious: the structure-activity relationships of given agonists or antagonists are being worked out (265), and agents to produce or inhibit specific responses in specific tissues are becoming available (282). The clinician can hope to obtain drugs which will selectively effect only certain functions of the effectors. For instance, it might be highly desirable to stimulate cardiac rate without producing vasodilation (e.g., in patients with myocardial failure) or to inhibit catecholamine-induced cardioacceleration while producing bronchodilation (e.g., in asthmatics). Drugs that can be used to produce these selective effects are becoming available (282).

2. By insolubilizing some drugs with a high affinity for receptors, we can isolate the chemical components of cells that make up the receptor (150, 273). Furthermore, we have already begun to separate those cells with receptors to specific agonists from suspension of cells with similar morphologic characteristics (310, 315, 510). Thus the function of those agonists in cells previously not known to respond to catecholamines will be more readily defined.

3. Finally we are beginning to understand and apply data that define the molecular interactions of catecholamines with other hormones (e.g., corticosteroids) or drugs (e.g., tolbutamide) (148, 434). This would be impossible if a chemically defined receptor were not in the offing.

The following are the present working definitions of the alpha and beta receptors (162):

Adrenergic receptors classified as "*alpha*" mediate responses which are characterized by a relative potency series in which epinephrine and norepinephrine are highest, phenylephrine somewhat lower, and isoproterenol very low, and by a susceptibility to blockade by a number of the so-called "classical" adrenergic blocking agents (e. g., phentolamine, dihydroergotamine, and phenoxybenzamine).

... All responses mediated by receptors in the *beta* class are characterized by: *1*) a potency ratio for the four amines studied in which isoproterenol is always highest and phenylephrine lowest (although epinephrine may be higher or lower than norepinephrine); *2*) a susceptibility to blockade by pronethalol and propranolol at relatively low concentrations; and *3*) a lack of susceptibility to blockade by potent *alpha* receptor agonists (e.g., phentolamine and phenoxybenzamine) at considerably higher concentrations.

A few representative cardiorespiratory responses produced by catecholamines are listed in Table 5–13. An exhaustive list of the pharmacologic actions of catecholamines and a classification of their alpha and beta mediation is beyond the scope of this chapter but is the subject of frequent and good reviews (131, 219, 223) and a number of other chapters in this book (Chapters 4, Part I of 5, 9, 10, 12 to 15, 18 to 20, 22, 24, and 29).

Cyclic 3',5'-Adenosine Monophosphate and Catecholamines

Knowing what the catecholamines can do and that the various responses are mediated through alpha or beta receptors does not mean that the actual mechanism of their effect is known. There are several determinants of a cell's response: the catecholamine must be released and make its way to the cell; the cell must possess a proper receptor to accept the messenger; the cell's initial response to the messenger appears to be dependent on some intracellular second messenger; and the ultimate response depends on the transfer of the second messenger to the cellular machinery that carries on the response.

In some cells, a response may go unnoticed because we do not know what to measure (e.g., the effects of catecholamines on avian or amphibian red blood cells); however, in most instances the *effect* is known, but the mechanism of its initiation is not. Recently it has become apparent that the second messenger for at least some responses to catecholamines is cyclic 3',5'-adenosine monophosphate (286, 387, 388, 456, 457, 458). As discussed in other chapters, cyclic AMP appears to be a key second messenger for a variety of hormones.

Cyclic AMP was discovered during studies of the effects of epinephrine on hepatic glycogenolysis (387). Cyclic AMP is now established as a likely second messenger following receptor stimulation by catecholamines. Elegant studies convincingly linked the production of glucose by the liver with stimulation of the beta receptor and accumulation of cyclic AMP. The present minimal criteria for determining whether cyclic AMP mediates the effect of any catecholamine include the following: the agonist drug or hormone must produce a specific effect, which is specifically blocked by an antagonist, and the stimulation should correlate with (1) a rise in intracellular cyclic AMP; (2) a drop in cyclic AMP when the response is blocked; (3) a mimicking of the effect of the agonist by cyclic AMP or a derivative, dibutyryl cyclic AMP, more capable of entering cells; and (4) the ability of drugs (e.g., xanthine derivatives such as theophylline) that prevent intracellular enzymatic breakdown of cyclic AMP to potentiate the effects of the agonist at doses that only potentiate accumulation of intracellular cyclic AMP. In recent years one more test has occasionally been added: nonspecific stimulants of adenyl cyclase that result in accumulation of intracellular cyclic AMP (e.g., cholera toxin, which stimulates adenyl cyclase in all tissues in which it has been tested) should produce the same cellular effect as the agonist (285). Of course, the ultimate aim of investigators is to isolate the cell machinery and show that cyclic AMP initiates the effect in a cell-free system. In the case of the hepatocyte, such has been done.

The majority of the above criteria have been applied to a few select actions of catecholamines on beta receptors, including (1) hepatic glycogenolysis, (2) lipolysis in the adipocyte, (3) the positive inotropic response in the heart, (4) relaxation of uterine muscle, (5) release of insulin from the pancreas, and (6) inhibition of leukocytic release of histamine provoked by IgE (48), of cytolysis of mast cells by sensitized lymphocytes (205), and of antibody release from some lymphocytes (426). The latter may indicate that we are beginning to understand some new anti-inflammatory actions of catechol and indole amines (5, 6, 189).

It is likely that more effects of catecholamines mediated by stimulation of beta receptors will be linked to cyclic AMP [e.g., calorigenic effects of catecholamines, vascular and bronchial dilation, lactic acid production by skeletal muscle (51), effects on some hormone-producing glands such as the pineal, and many of the actions of catecholamines on brain (389, 423).] The nucleotide has a host of pharmacologic effects which, if listed, might supply an outline for a text of endocrinology (197). In fact, some investigators have speculated that the beta receptor is actually adenyl cyclase (386). Although there are several theoretical reasons why the receptor per se may not be adenyl cyclase alone, it already seems apparent that, at least in myocardial tissue, the beta receptor is intimately, physically associated with some components of the cyclic AMP-generating system (273). Table 5–14 lists some tissues in which adenyl cyclase is stimulated by catecholamines.

Sympathomimetic amines do not stimulate alpha receptors via a mediating step involving activation of cellular adenyl cyclase. In fact, the opposite perhaps occurs. Stimulation of alpha receptors in the pancreas limits insulin release (150), in the adipocyte inhibits lipolysis, in the dorsal frog skin antagonizes skin darkening effect, in the platelet inhibits platelet aggregation (see prostaglandins for further discussion), and in toad bladder reduces permeability to water. In each preparation, stimulation and the effect are associated with reduction of cyclic AMP concentrations. The mechanism of this reduction is not known. It was probably fortunate that responses to beta stimulation were studied before those to alpha stimulation. In a number of experimental settings in the study of the alpha receptor, pharmacologic manipulations first had to be performed to raise concentrations of cyclic AMP. Only then could stimulation of the alpha receptor be correlated with noticeable decreases in cyclic AMP. Such observations make it less easy to accept cyclic AMP as the second messenger for alpha receptor stimulation than it is to accept it as the second messenger for beta stimulation. Perhaps a decrease in the nucleotide concen-

TABLE 5–14. SOME CELLS AND TISSUES IN WHICH ADENYL CYCLASE IS STIMULATED BY CATECHOLAMINES (387)

Liver	Adipose tissue
Spleen	Pancreatic islets
Cardiac muscle	Avian and amphibian but not
Skeletal muscle	human erythrocytes
Smooth muscle	Leukocytes
Brain	Parotid gland
Pineal	Lung

tration could be a signal for activity in the cells; perhaps another mediator is the true messenger. One candidate now being considered is cyclic guanosine monophosphate (cyclic GMP) (17).

Finally, it is important to realize that the response of tissues to catecholamines can be modulated by other chemically unrelated endocrines. For instance, estrogenic steroids and progesterones modify the response of the uterus to catecholamines during the normal menstrual cycle (386, 387). Glucocorticoids modify the response of adipocytes and vascular tissue to catecholamines by entirely different mechanisms (233, 419). The effects of some steroids on the oviduct and the prostate can be reversed by beta blocking drugs at reasonable doses ($>10^{-4}$ to 10^{-5}M.) (39). Serotonin and dopamine may modify the effects of sympathomimetic agents on insulin release (377). Many of these interactions are discussed in other chapters but are mentioned here to draw attention once again to the complexity of interrelationships that must always be considered when interpreting the action of catecholamines *in vitro*.

Pharmacologic Effects of Dopamine

No longer can dopamine be considered only as a chemical precursor of norepinephrine. In the last few years, the pharmacologic effects of the amine have been studied, and they are distinct from those of norepinephrine and epinephrine. The differences between the pharmacologic properties of dopamine and those of the two endogenous catecholamines may have clinical importance.

Peripheral Effects. Dopamine selectively dilates the renal arteries, increases inotropic and chronotropic actions on the heart, and produces mild, clinically undetectable arterial constriction (19, 42, 61, 80, 168, 319). When in a steady state of concentration in blood, the drug produces dose-related increases in cardiac output, minor changes in blood pressure, and major increases in renal blood flow, glomerular filtration rate, and sodium diuresis. Most of these effects are inhibited by haloperidol, a drug that does not inhibit the vascular or metabolic effects of isoproterenol or the vasodilatory effects of bradykinin (530). The latter studies indicate that a specific receptor for dopamine probably is available in some peripheral tissues, but they do not imply that all of the amine's effects are exclusively mediated by stimulation of those receptors. Although dopamine does not produce the majority of metabolic effects associated with its beta-hydroxylated relatives (305), what metabolic effects it does have (e.g., on inhibition of insulin release) are mediated either by its ability to release catecholamines or to mimic the effects of norepinephrine. Its ability to inhibit insulin release is in turn blocked by alpha-adrenergic blocking drugs (377). When given intravenously (e.g., as in the treatment of shock in man), dopamine may produce a transitory increase in blood pressure by the same mechanism that affects insulin release. This arterial constriction can be prevented by giv-

ing the drug slowly, administering an alpha blocking agent or, as has been recently noted, administering the drug as the amino acid, L-dopa (153).

L-dopa generally produces the same cardiovascular and metabolic effects as dopamine. The amino acid is readily decarboxylated, particularly in noncentral nervous system tissues. If decarboxylation is inhibited, the majority of L-dopa's direct pharmacologic effects are also inhibited (356). The drug, unlike dopamine, can enter the brain. There its amine (produced both by enzymatic and nonenzymatic decarboxylation) (403) produces minor negative inotropic and chronotropic effects on the heart (356). However, the effects of L-dopa on the function of certain areas of the brain are profound, and its proper use has resulted in one of the most exciting therapeutic stories (74, 95, 98, 144, 178, 241, 421, 440, 521).

Dopamine and the Central Nervous System. The articles and reviews listed above provide detailed and interesting reading. They explain the diversified work leading to the present use of L-dopa in the treatment of Parkinson's disease. The critical steps in that work will be reviewed. Only those points not covered or referenced in the reviews are referenced below.

Initially, study of the function of the basal ganglia was carried out by physiologists who were more or less limited to creating surgical lesions and studying the functional results. Few if any useful models of parkinsonism were developed. By chance, pharmacologists discovered that a number of drugs could create a condition like Parkinson's syndrome. These drugs (haloperidol, reserpine, and phenothiazines) were dissimilar in chemical structure but all had effects on the central nervous system that only recently have been mechanistically defined. Simultaneously, with developing investigation of these three drugs, evidence began to indicate a role for acetylcholine in the central nervous system.

Belladona was tried 75 to 100 years ago in some patients with Parkinson's disease and was sometimes beneficial. Neither the reason it worked in some but not others nor its mechanism of action was known. Investigation at first was limited to drug screening. A number of additional anticholinergic drugs were tried with variable but more or less useful results. Later, cholinomimetic drugs (e.g., tremorine) were injected into the central nervous system where they reproduced a tremor like that in Parkinson's disease. Until 1967, no one was sure that the beneficial effects of the anti-parkinsonism drugs (anticholinergic drugs) were based on their effects on the central nervous system. Then it was clearly shown that physostigmine given centrally reproduced the syndrome, and only those anticholinergic drugs that were transported into the central nervous system (e.g., benztropine and scopolamine but not quarternary anticholinesterases) would ameliorate symptoms.

Working with these drugs, Duvoisin made a major breakthrough when he pinpointed the corpus striatum as the locale where the drugs had their beneficial effects. Later, this area was found to contain the highest concentrations of choline acetylase, acetylcholine, and acetylcholinesterase of any region in the brain. Duvoisin was among the first to conclude that cholinergic activity was important in ordinary function of the extrapyramidal areas and to suggest that the influence of the cholinergic system was probably balanced by another brain chemical, dopamine.

Investigation of the function of the adrenergic neurons in the central nervous system paralleled study of the function of acetylcholine. Some expected that the functions of dopamine, which had been measured in the central nervous system, would be different from those of the other adrenergic neurotransmitter, norepinephrine. In the cardiovascular system, dopamine's effects were different from those of norepinephrine and epinephrine, and in the brain dopamine comprised about 50 per cent of the total catecholamines. It did not seem logical that so much should be there simply as a substrate for catecholamine synthesis when the rate-limiting step in synthesis was tyrosine hydroxylase, not dopamine beta-oxidase. The turnover of dopamine was faster in areas where it was concentrated than in areas where norepinephrine was predominant (127). The opposite would have been expected if the dopamine were serving only as a precursor to norepinephrine. Then Carlsson's group and others found that most of the dopamine in the brain was concentrated in very few areas, primarily in the corpus striatum where the ratio of dopamine to norepinephrine was 100/1. In the caudate nucleus of some animal species, dopamine concentration was 10 μg. per g., and norepinephrine was 0.1 μg. per g. Conversely, in the hypothalamus of the same animals, the ratio was reversed, 1/10.

Using fluorescent staining techniques, catecholamines (norepinephrine and dopamine) were found in the neuron bodies of the substantia nigra of nonprimates, but not in the corpus striatum. At the same time, it was shown that lesions in the substantia nigra produced degeneration of nerves in that area, loss of dopamine from axons of the corpus striatum, and a tremor that resembled parkinsonism; analogous experiments in subhuman primates produced the same results. Furthermore, stimulation of the nerves of the substantia nigra resulted in release of dopamine from the area of the corpus striatum, while chlorpromazine could block uptake of dopamine on the receptor areas of the nerves. Pharmacologic inhibition (by haloperidol) of the effects of dopamine produced a tremor. Reserpine-depleted dopamine and norepinephrine, and dopamine-like drugs (apomorphine) had beneficial effects in patients with Parkinson's syndrome (97).

A unifying hypothesis linking dopamine to the function of the extrapyramidal system was on the way. Some experiments using reserpine and other drugs in the mouse selectively replenished dopamine in the brain, while also reawakening the animal and restoring normal extrapyramidal function (102). It remained only to find that humans with Parkinsonism had consistent lesions in the substantia nigra. The same area showed abnormally low concentrations of dopamine and its metabolite, homovanillic acid (HVA), without profound depletion of norepinephrine and serotonin. The pathogenesis seemed certain.

It was later found that the decarboxylase enzyme and amine metabolizing enzymes remained in the area of the lesions and that administration of dopa (which crossed the blood-brain barrier) could reverse the central effects of reserpine and chlorpromazine (an adverse drug reaction had proved beneficial) (213). The way was paved for a proper therapeutic trial with dopa in man (309). When prolonged high doses of dopa were administered to patients with Parkinson's disease, most were noticeably improved and some "cured." They became indistinguishable from normal individuals until the drug was withdrawn (94, 307, 451, 526, 527), at which time the symptoms returned (379).

The present hypothesis proposes that acetylcholine and dopamine interact to control the function of the extrapyramidal system. The system can be rebalanced either by returning the malfunctioning component to normal (ideal) or inhibiting the function of the normal component to bring it into harmony with the other (e.g., use of anticholinergic drugs in parkinsonism). Combinations of both approaches are rational and efficacious. To say that such advances could have been made or understood without knowing the details of catecholamine synthesis, storage, release, effect, and metabolism would be foolish.

L-dopa is well absorbed (363). It must be given in large doses to ensure that adequate amounts will penetrate the brain (525); it must be spontaneously or enzymatically decarboxylated before it works; and its effects are consistent with its inhibitory function (283, 284). The deficiency of tyrosine hydroxylase that produces the lesion in parkinsonism need not be inherited. Any abnormality that results in degenerative lesions of the adrenergic nerves will decrease the tissue content of tyrosine hydroxylase (see synthesis of catecholamines) (183, 303). In a great number of patients with Parkinson's disease or syndrome, L-dopa is effective; it even works in those patients with magnesium poisoning that results in physical and chemical lesions similar to those in parkinsonism (94).

There are unwanted side effects from use of the drug (66, 82, 149, 194, 224, 302, 401, 402), apparently including some peripheral effects of dopamine and its common and uncommon (476) metabolites. If the peripheral effects of dopamine were detrimental, decarboxylase inhibitors might be expected to preferentially inhibit metabolism of dopa in non-brain tissues (23, 24, 71, 186, 187, 505). Such tests of decarboxylase inhibition will have to be carefully watched because there is evidence that some beneficial effects of dopa are mediated by the peripheral effects of some of its metabolites (72, 439). In addition, it has been learned that diets should probably be controlled (507) and that monoamine oxidase inhibitors can cause hypertension in people taking dopa (218). When dopamine is formed rapidly, it accumulates and probably displaces norepinephrine from its storage sites in the same way as would tyramine (see section on false neurotransmitters).

Hypotension may also be a problem during chronic administration of the drug (73, 130, 145, 290, 306, 424). The mechanism of action is not certain but could include arterial dilation of the renal vascular system, the naturetic effects of the dopa, and its central negative inotropic and chronotropic actions. Also actions of unusual metabolites of the drug or amine may cause the hypotension. We are a long way from fully understanding all we need to know about the drug's action (2, 21, 61, 192, 226, 526). If the hypotension is related to the peripheral actions of dopamine or its metabolites, perhaps peripheral decarboxylase inhibitors will be useful to counter it. Otherwise, decreasing the dose of dopa and adding adjunctive drugs seems inevitable (52). One adjunctive drug may be a dopamine derivative that crosses the blood-brain barrier and has no peripheral effects (22, 366). Others might be drugs like amantadine which, though not a catecholamine, seems to enhance accumulation of dopamine in the brain (501). Still others might be the anticholinergic drugs with a mechanism of action very different from that of dopa.

Although the advances in therapy and their basis on a solid scientific hypothesis are appealing and rewarding, we must not be prematurely convinced. There are some inconsistencies in the data which demand careful study (74, 241, 403).

There are at least two additional clinical applications of our knowledge of the chemistry and pharmacology of dopa and dopamine.

1. The decreased renal arterial vascular resistance and lack of major peripheral vascular pressor effects from dopamine may explain the relative infrequency of hypertension in patients with neuroblastomas, tumors frequently associated with increased urinary excretion of dopamine and its metabolite, homovanillic acid.

2. In cases of suspected neural crest tumors, increased excretion of dopamine or homovanillic acid or both may herald the malignant spread of a pheochromocytoma or of tumors of more primitive types (discussed later) (101).

Alterations During Disease and Drug Therapy

In several pathologic states, the responses to endogenous or exogenous catecholamines may be altered (Table 5–15). For example, in patients with various types of cardiomegaly, the increased mass of myocardium may "dilute" nerve endings capable of biologically inactivating catecholamines, whereas effector sites remain stable (154). This explanation, although plausible, is unproven, and chemical alterations in binding sites as well as defects in synthesis of catecholamines have been detected in some cardiac diseases (e.g., congestive heart failure) (87, 88, 115, 372). The increased sensitivity to catecholamines after surgical sympathetic denervation or in disease states such as

TABLE 5–15. SOME CONDITIONS CHARACTERIZED BY ALTERED SENSITIVITY TO CATECHOLAMINES

Conditions Associated with Increased Sensitivity
Cardiomegaly
  Congestive heart failure
  Hypertrophy—secondary to physical obstruction or increase in peripheral vascular resistance
  Myocardiopathy of various etiologies
Thyrotoxicosis (?)*
Sympathetic denervation
  Diabetes mellitus
  Surgical or anesthetic procedures
  Orthostatic hypotension
Nutritional abnormalities
  Scurvy
Unclassified diseases
  Hyperkinetic cardiovascular disorders
  Familial dysautonomia
Drugs
  Imipramine
  Some antiadrenergic drugs (e.g., guanethidine and reserpine)

Conditions Associated with Decreased Sensitivity
Acidosis—metabolic or respiratory
Myxedema
Adrenal insufficiency

Conditions Associated with Paradoxical Effects
Diseases
  Carcinoid syndrome
Drug administration
  Phenothiazines

---

*There is considerable debate about the sensitivity of patients with thyrotoxicosis to catecholamines. The rate of turnover and the binding properties by the neurons may be altered, and excessive adrenergic activity may result. However, recently acquired data makes it unlikely that there is true hypersensitivity in response to exogenous catecholamines (276).

diabetes mellitus also may be related to a decrease in the uptake of catecholamines into storage sites (207). The same phenomenon occurs in patients taking drugs that block catecholamine uptake into storage sites but do not affect receptor areas (208, 447, 514), and this may be an operative factor in thyrotoxicosis or during administration of thyroid hormone (276). Not all drugs that alter the effects of catecholamines are similar in chemical structure to catecholamines, nor are they all used for their effects on the sympathetic nervous system (Fig. 5–45).

Major alterations in the receptor tissue could cause decreased responsiveness to catecholamines, as in such diseases as metabolic or respiratory acidosis, myxedema, and adrenocortical insufficiency. In rare clinical conditions and during administration of certain drugs, catecholamines may elicit a hypotensive rather than hypertensive response. The occurrence of such paradoxical effects is seen most strikingly in the carcinoid syndrome (described in Chapter 29).

For many years, there has been a suspicion that some abnormality of the sympathetic nervous system or change in the sensitivity of effector organs for the actions of catecholamines might participate in the pathogenesis of essential hypertension in humans (103, 318). Although there is recent evidence that abnormalities in the storage of catecholamines in the central nervous system of a strain of rats may result in familial hypertension (292, 357,

529), there is no evidence that such abnormalities are shared by hypertensive man. Catecholamines may influence the production of angiotensin (517) or other vasoactive peptides that may affect blood pressure (301). However, though various abnormalities in storage, synthesis, or release of catecholamines have been described in experimental and human hypertension (117, 118, 121, 123, 124, 139, 291, 318, 347), neither these abnormalities nor consistent abnormalities of the sympathetic nervous system have been etiologically related to essential hypertension in man (210, 348).

Diseases Associated with Abnormalities of the Adrenal Medulla

No known diseases are caused by adrenal medullary insufficiency. After bilateral adrenalectomy, urinary excretion of epinephrine falls rapidly, but excretion of norepinephrine and its metabolic products remains relatively unchanged (492). The physiologic function of the adrenal medulla is difficult to determine since it is a minor source of catecholamines (489). Tumors at that site often produce distinctive and clinically important syndromes. The most prominent tumor, the pheochromocytoma, has served as a model for application of the previously discussed facts to life-threatening clinical disease (430).

Pheochromocytoma

Pheochromocytomas [or functioning paragangliomas (280, 445)], although found in less than 1 per cent of the hypertensive population (119, 206), have several clinically important aspects:

1. Associated hypertension is usually curable.

2. The presence of these tumors may herald other occult, potentially fatal, but curable diseases.

3. Their manifestations may suggest other diseases of altered metabolism such as diabetes mellitus, thyrotoxicosis, anxiety states, Cushing's syndrome, and the carcinoid syndrome.

4. A rational, specific approach to diagnosis and therapy is available.

5. Family studies disclose a high incidence of pheochromocytoma in kindreds, inheritance as an autosomal dominant trait, and need for genetic counseling (79, 475). Questions regarding gene expressivity and the etiology of certain types of neoplasia may be answered by further investigation of such families (408, 512).

Pathogenesis of the Symptoms of Pheochromocytomas. The common manifestations of a pheochromocytoma (Table 5–16) may result directly from the physical presence of the tumor but more often are related to production of increased amounts of catecholamines. The reasons for increased production of catecholamines from tumor tissue are numerous and have recently been studied. Some have noted abnormally rapid turnover rates, particularly in tumors in children and in small tumors in adults (393, 407, 408, 427). The

TABLE 5–16. COMMON MANIFESTATIONS OF PHEOCHROMOCYTOMAS AND UNUSUAL COMBINATIONS OF SYMPTOMS LEADING TO ERRONEOUS DIAGNOSIS*

Signs and Symptoms Attributable to Catecholamine Secretion

Hypertension	
Sweating	
Paroxysmal attacks of blanching or flushing	
Palpitations and tachycardia	Commonly found in pheochromocytomas
Headache	
Anorexia, weight loss, psychic changes	
Evidence of hypermetabolism, increased fasting blood glucose level	
Decreased gastrointestinal motility	
Postural hypotension	
Increased blood pressure, palpitations, headache, sweating, evidence of hypermetabolism and psychic changes	Suggesting toxemia of pregnancy
Increased fasting blood glucose level and abnormal results in glucose tolerance tests	Suggesting diabetes mellitus
Psychosis, tremulousness, increased respiratory rate	Suggesting functional hyperventilation
Decreased gastrointestinal motility and resultant constipation	Suggesting Hirschsprung's disease
Increased basal metabolic rate, increased oxygen consumption, weight loss, psychosis, tremulousness, increased respiratory rate	Suggesting thyrotoxicosis

*Data obtained from review of 67 consecutive patients with pheochromocytomas seen recently at the University of California Medical Center.

biochemical properties of the tumor's chromaffin cells and granules are remarkably similar to normal cell properties. The storage mechanisms as far as they have been studied are also normal. Therefore, the unusual secretion rates must be linked to lack of ordinary control mechanisms regulating synthesis or release of norepinephrine or its precursors. A malignant tissue may be autonomous in its growth characteristics, but other explanations for excessive production of amines have also been advanced:

1. Ordinary concentrations of noreprinephrine in the cell do not seem to inhibit the tumor's tyrosine hydroxylase (345, 397). This could mean that the enzyme is unusual (has a different K_m for its substrate) or that once the amines are formed they are held in compartments that do not allow feedback inhibition of normal enzyme (518). The relative contribution of each factor to the abnormalities of synthesis has not yet been determined.

2. In addition, the tumor metabolizes a substantial proportion of the amines it produces. These metabolites have been shown to prevent ordinary feedback inhibition of tyrosine hydroxylase by norepinephrine (221).

Most symptoms can be readily explained on the basis of the pharmacologic effects of catecholamines. The increase in peripheral vascular resistance is a well-recognized aspect of the disease. The hypertension may be sustained or paroxysmal, probably depending on whether the tumor's secretion of catecholamines, particularly norepinephrine, into the blood is sustained or comes in "spurts" (329). One of the most common symptoms is sweating (160, 375), which may be episodic and associated with profound flushing or blanching, or continuous and subtle, provoking comments on the need for frequent showers and shampoos. Palpitations and tachycardia are also prominent symptoms. Weight loss, tremulousness, and other evidence of hypermetabolism may be the direct effects of catecholamines. Less easy to explain, but an important symptom, is the existence of postural hypotension in the hypertensive patient. The most plausible explanation for its presence is a catecholamine-induced decrease in plasma and total blood volumes. Such reductions in plasma volume, however, are less frequent than the orthostatic hypotension (432). In contrast, postural hypotension is a frequent finding in aldosteronism, a disease characterized by increases in plasma volume (38). The analogy with the aldosterone-producing tumor can be extended, since patients with such tumors also have impaired sympathetic reflexes as a result of decreased total body potassium (38). Severe potassium deficiency, however, has not been documented frequently in patients with a pheochromocytoma (see p. 308). Another mechanism that may contribute to the orthostatic hypotension is the ganglionic blocking activity of excessive amounts of catecholamines.

The basis for the central nervous system manifestations of a pheochromocytoma is not clear. Catecholamines can affect the central nervous system, producing changes in sleep patterns (353), psychosis, tremulousness, and hyperventilation. Although little is known about the total brain content of catecholamines in patients with a pheochromocytoma, an increase could be expected despite the fact that circulating catecholamines have difficulty passing the blood-brain barrier. Over long periods, the increased concentrations of catecholamines in blood could force upward the usual equilibrium of catecholamines in the central nervous system.

Catecholamines produce myocarditis and myocardial necrosis in patients with pheochromocytomas; the mechanism of production is unknown. However, at least one effect of high catecholamine (isoproterenol) concentrations on the heart is to create a defective storage of endogenous amines in the heart (333). In addition, high concentrations of free fatty acids caused by the metabolic activity of catecholamines may contribute to myocardial lesions (212). This complication, which may be manifested by arrhythmia or congestive failure and nonspecific electrocardiographic changes, may be a direct toxic effect of catecholamines or may be mediated by the increased work demanded of the myocardium (143, 242, 462, 487). Arrhythmia may also be caused by the direct chronotropic effects of the catecholamines, reflex baroreceptor-mediated bradycardia secondary to sudden increases in blood pressure (120), or, rarely, by sudden decreases in blood pressure following spontaneous necrosis of the tumor (157).

Differential Diagnosis. A pheochromocytoma may be manifested by relatively few symptoms or by an unusual combination of symptoms (378, 384), leading at times to an erroneous diagnosis (Table 5–16). For example, the occurrence of polyuria (on the basis of the antidiuretic hormone secreting activity of norepinephrine) or polydipsia in association with an increase in the fasting blood glucose level (443) in a patient without hypertension or other symptoms characteristic of a pheochromocytoma may lead to a diagnosis of nonketotic diabetes. Likewise, a diagnosis of functional hyperventilation syndrome has been made in patients with a pheochromocytoma because their initial symptoms were psychosis, nervousness, or hyperventilation in the absence of sustained hypertension. Severe constipation resulting from the inhibitory effects of catecholamines on intestinal motility, although unusual, also may be a manifestation of a pheochromocytoma. This finding has been interpreted to indicate Hirschsprung's disease and has led to unnecessary and hazardous operative procedures. When combinations of symptoms are incorrectly interpreted, diabetes mellitus, thyrotoxicosis, or even toxemia of pregnancy (269) may be considered the most "obvious" diagnosis. Because their manifestations can be mimicked in part by the pharmacologic effect of catecholamines, such diseases must be considered in the differential diagnosis of a pheochromocytoma.

Associated Diseases. Certain diseases are frequently associated with a pheochromocytoma but may be occult at the time the tumor is detected. For example, the incidence of neuroectodermal syndromes is increased in this selected hypertensive population. Neurofibromatosis, the most common of these conditions, is found in about 5 per cent of patients with pheochromocytomas (32, 85, 177). Patients with Lindau's disease, which is characterized by retinal hemangioblastomas, cerebellar, medullary, and spinal cord hemangioblastomas, and cysts in the lung, liver, pancreas, kidneys, and epididymis, as well as by hypernephromas, also have a high incidence of pheochromocytomas (314). Sturge-Weber disease, hereditary cerebellar ataxia with telangiectasia of the conjunctiva, and tuberous sclerosis are other neuroectodermal syndromes whose manifestations may coexist with those of neurofibromatosis and Lindau's disease. Most of these diseases are familial, inherited in the same genetic pattern as pheochromocytomas (autosomal dominant trait). An increased incidence of pheochromocytomas might be expected in such patients. Therefore, when any one of these syndromes is diagnosed, the patient and his family should be carefully screened both for other manifestations of the primary disease and for a pheochromocytoma.

Also associated with pheochromocytomas is a rare form of medullary carcinoma of the thyroid (25, 238, 271, 414, 429, 449). The two tumors may be associated by their apparent derivation from neuroblastic or neural crest cells (415, 463). The C cells of the medullary carcinoma release calcitonin into the blood (35, 238, 317, 480, 519). The resultant hypocalcemia (45, 465) may be protracted and may account for subsequent parathyroid hyperplasias and adenomas (238, 300, 316, 359). Cushing's syndrome has also been described in association with the double tumors. The ACTH apparently is released from either the thyroid or an adrenal medullary tumor (126, 179, 238). The thyroid medullary tumor also has the endocrinologic potential to secrete prostaglandin, which might contribute to the diarrhea and flushing reported in some patients (515, 516). Patients with pheochromocytomas may have other manifestations of thyroid disease and chromosomal abnormalities, but so far these rarely appear (28, 320).

The pheochromocytoma may elaborate an erythrocyte-stimulating factor, causing an absolute increase in red blood cell mass (396). In rare cases, pheochromocytoma is associated with an astrocytoma in the brain (which may account for headache in some patients) or with xanthine oxidase deficiency, as reported by Engelman et al. (143).

Physical Examination. The findings by physical examination are relatively nonspecific. Pheochromocytomas may occur at any age, although the majority of patients are in the fourth to sixth decade. There is no sex predilection. Most patients seek medical advice because of symptoms associated with hypertension or other pharmacologic effects of catecholamines. In the 5 per cent who also have neuroectodermal disorders, the most striking physical findings may be associated with these diseases. These findings include neurofibromas, café-au-lait or "port wine" spots, telangiectasia over the conjunctiva, and central nervous system disturbances referable to the cerebellum, medulla, or spinal cord. The latter may include compression by the tumor or syringomyelia. The common physical findings directly attributable to the pheochromocytoma are sticky, moist hair, profuse sweating, retinal changes consistent with hypertension, nodules in the thyroid, rapid heart rate with a left ventricular thrust, and enlargement of the heart if catechol myocardiopathy or congestive heart failure is present. Abdominal organs are usually not palpable unless coexistent Lindau's disease has produced significant cystic disease of the liver or pancreas.

The tumor is present in the abdominal cavity in 95 per cent of affected patients but is palpable in only about 15 per cent. In about 50 per cent, however, pressure on the abdomen will produce a rise in blood pressure or an increase in sweating. If the primary tumor is in the neck, it usually can be palpated; if it is in the chest, it can be detected in most instances by roentgenography. If the primary tumor is in the bladder or pelvic region, it may be manifested by micturition syncope or paroxysms of hypertension associated with micturition. In some cases, palpation over the bladder may provoke these symptoms. When the tumor has metastasized into bone, it can often be palpated in the rib area, or pain may be evoked when pressure is applied over the affected skeletal parts.

Neurologic findings are relatively nonspecific and include the psychotic manifestations of the disease, evidence of metastatic or associated primary lesions in the brain, and electrolyte abnormalities secondary to associated hyperparathyroidism. Neurologic abnormalities related to Parkinson's disease are not seen with a pheochromocytoma or a neuroblastoma, however, and dopamine levels in various brain areas have not been measured.

In summary, the diagnosis of a pheochromocytoma is dependent on the physician's awareness of the subtleties of its manifestations. Thus any patient of any age should be suspected of having a pheochromocytoma if he has moderate to severe sustained or intermittent hypertension in combination with excessive sweating, orthostatic hypotension, headache, hypermetabolism, weight loss, psychic changes, or an elevated fasting blood glucose level. A full spectrum of symptoms may not be apparent when the patient is first seen, and in many cases the initial diagnosis is essential hypertension, hyperthyroidism, diabetes mellitus, psychoneurosis, idiopathic orthostatic hypotension, or functional bowel problems. That more attention must be paid to "insignificant" symptoms is emphasized by the high mortality during operative procedures on patients with unsuspected pheochromocytoma.

Diagnostic Procedures. The diagnosis may be suspected on the basis of the history and initial physical findings but cannot be definitive until laboratory tests have been performed.

Routine Laboratory Tests. Routine laboratory data may give initial confirmation to the physician's suspicion. The hematocrit may be increased because of (1) a decrease in plasma volume and relative increase in red cell mass due to the direct effects of catecholamines; or (2) the elaboration by the tumor of large amounts of erythrocyte-stimulating factor. The latter, although relatively infrequent, has been well demonstrated by Rosse and Waldmann (396). The presence of a coexistent tumor may also result in an increase in red cell mass. For example, in a patient with a pheochromocytoma and Lindau's disease, excessive amounts of erythrocyte-stimulating factor may be produced by a cerebellar hemangioblastoma with associated cysts or by an associated hypernephroma, which is more common in patients with Lindau's disease than in the general population (314). There are no consistent abnormalities in leukocyte or platelet counts, although leukocytosis is not rare and can be caused by catecholamines (448). For unknown reasons, but probably because the hypertension is of short duration, urinalysis does not usually reveal evidence of renal failure. The urine may contain glucose if the fasting blood glucose level is sufficiently increased.

The demonstration of increases in fasting blood glucose and free fatty acid levels (136) will also help to confirm the diagnosis. Serum concentrations of electrolytes and alkaline phosphatase will be altered if hyperparathyroidism is present. Slight decreases in serum potassium levels in some patients have been noted (311). In one of five patients studied, the serum potassium concentration was consistently below 3 mEq. per liter. The mechanism of the decrease is not obvious; it may be related to aldosterone abnormalities, but this hypothesis has not been fully investigated. The serum potassium concentration is clinically important since low potassium levels in association with hypertension are found in patients with aldosterone-producing tumors, but it is normal or only slightly low in most patients with a pheochromocytoma.

Roentgenography. Roentgenographic studies often help to locate the tumor (96, 122, 383, 504). Routine x-ray films of the chest, together with oblique views, may reveal a paravertebral tumor mass. Scout films of the abdomen will locate the tumor in about 20 per cent of patients. Intravenous pyelograms with or without tomography of the perirenal area will place the tumor in about 50 per cent of cases. Retroperitoneal infusion of carbon dioxide is occasionally useful. Because it is laborious to perform and is associated with a low but definite incidence of complications (e.g., hypertensive crisis), gas insufflation should be reserved for selected patients whose tumors have escaped surgical detection or are by chemical tests judged to be small. The danger of catecholamine effects during this procedure may be avoided by pretreatment with alpha blocking agents. Selective arteriography and venography have been used recently to demonstrate primary and metastatic lesions (312) but, like retroperitoneal gas studies, should be limited to difficult cases. These procedures may be successful because pheochromocytomas are often highly vascular and the tumor will appear as a "blush" in arteriograms and venograms.

Definitive Chemical Tests. Although the routine procedures are useful in locating a primary tumor or areas of metastases, they are not specific for pheochromocytomas. Certain chemical tests devised in recent years, however, provide unequivocal data for a definitive diagnosis of pheochromocytomas (132, 137, 138, 171, 406, 409). Blood catecholamine concentrations are still difficult to measure and are usually done only in research laboratories. Nevertheless, the clinician can gain much information from standard quantitative tests for measuring the urinary excretion of catecholamines and their metabolites metanephrine, normetanephrine, and vanilmandelic acid (VMA). Experience at the University of California Medical Center has shown that the most reliable methods are those of Crout and Pisano and their collaborators (104, 108, 367, 368). The normal range of catecholamine concentrations in urine, blood, and adrenal medulla and of urinary VMA and normetanephrine are listed in Table 5–17.

For determinations on urine, 24-hour specimens are collected in 15 ml. of 6 N hydrochloric acid. Because a variety of tests exist and because the methods used in different laboratories differ in specificity, certain drugs and foods should be withdrawn before urine specimens are collected. Administration of exogenous catecholamines such as vasopressors, even for nasal stuffiness, highly

TABLE 5–17. NORMAL RANGE OF CATECHOLAMINE AND METABOLITE CONCENTRATIONS*

Urine
  Catecholamines††
    Norepinephrine: 10 to 70 μg. per 24 hr.
    Epinephrine: 0 to 20 μg. per 24 hr.
  Normetanephrine and metanephrine:
    <1.3 mg. per 24 hr.
  Vanillylmandelic acid: 1.8 to 9.0 mg. per 24 hr.
  Dopamine: <200 μg. per 24 hr.
Blood (Plasma)
  Catecholamines: <1 μg. per liter
  Norepinephrine: 0.2 ± 0.08 μg. per liter plasma**
  Epinephrine: 0.05 ± 0.03 μg. per liter plasma**
  Dopamine beta-hydroxylase: 116 ± 1.8 N moles per ml. per 20 min.†
Adrenal Medulla
  Norepinephrine: 0.04 to 0.16 mg. per g.
  Epinephrine: 0.22 to 0.84 mg. per g.

*Since the values obtained in different laboratories vary considerably, only a general range can be given.
**Engelman, K., and Portnoy, B.: *Circ. Res.* 26:53, 1970.
†Weinshilboum, R., and Axelrod, J.: *Circ. Res.* 28:307, 1971.
††In most patients with pheochromocytomas, total catecholamine excretion is >300 μg. per day.

fluorescent compounds (e.g., tetracyclines), and certain antihypertensive drugs like alpha-methyldopa, which are catechols themselves or form catecholamines, may influence the results of catecholamine determinations. Such drugs, however, have no appreciable effect on VMA and metanephrine determinations and, if clinically advisable, need not be withdrawn before such tests. Long-term administration of reserpine or guanethidine usually has no significant effect on the results of such assays. Monoamine oxidase inhibitors, however, may result in a misleading increase in urinary metanephrine and decrease in VMA excretion. Because several of the screening tests for VMA detect other phenolic acids, the patient should omit coffee, vanilla, certain vegetables and citrus fruits, and chocolates from his diet before urinary VMA determinations. Other drugs used in the therapy of hypertension and its complications, including hydrochlorothiazide, hydralazine, and digitalis, do not affect the assay. Alpha-methyldopa in patients with no pheochromocytoma may lower VMA excretion. Phentolamine, phenoxybenzamine, and propranolol will not interfere with the chemical tests and may be used during diagnostic procedures.

What are the most reliable chemical tests for the detection of a pheochromocytoma? Sjoerdsma et al. (432), in evaluating the data on 24-hour urinary excretion of catecholamines and methoxylated metabolites in 62 patients with pheochromocytomas, found normal or near-normal values for VMA in three cases, for metanephrine in two cases, and for catecholamines in two cases. In the three cases of normal VMA excretion, metanephrine and catecholamine levels were abnormally high. One of the two patients with normal catecholamine levels excreted abnormally high amounts of catecholamines for short periods after histamine stimulation and after spontaneous attacks of hypertension; total 24-hour catecholamine levels for this patient, however, appeared normal, the normal or subnormal periods of excretion compensating for the periods of abnormally high "spurts." In another series of 67 patients with pheochromocytomas studied recently at the University of California Medical Center, the only six who excreted normal amounts of VMA showed increased urinary catecholamine excreted over 24 hours.

In some patients, it is preferable to collect timed samples during a period of hypertension and express the excretion rates of the catecholamines and their metabolites in μg. per hr. Normal rates (μg. per hr.) are as follows: total free catecholamines, 2.5 $\pm$ 0.8 with 22 per cent being epinephrine; total free and conjugated metanephrines and normetanephrines, 16$\pm$5 with 35 per cent being metanephrine; VMA 240$\pm$120 (means $\pm$ one standard deviation). Catecholamine excretion in excess of 10 μg. per hr., metanephrine in excess of 60 μg. per hr., or VMA in excess of 500 μg. per hr. should be taken to indicate a pheochromocytoma until proven otherwise. In some patients under severe stress or with other diseases characterized by excessive sympathetic nervous system activity (e.g., congestive heart failure, acute myocardial infarction, or recent surgical procedures), the "normal" values will be exceeded.

Dividing the 24-hour urine collection into day and night samples may be useful in determining pheochromocytomas, since normally the patient's upright position during the day is more likely to increase catecholamine excretion than is the supine position at night (199); in patients with pheochromocytomas, there should be little difference between the two periods of collection.

In summary, the initial screening test for pheochromocytomas should estimate the 24-hour excretion of vanillylmandelic acid or normetanephrine-metanephrine. In 80 or 90 per cent of patients, either test will confirm the diagnosis of a pheochromocytoma. These tests are cheaper, more reliable, and technically less difficult than urinary catecholamine determinations. Negative results would suggest repeating the tests, and, if necessary, determining urinary catecholamine excretion. If all three tests give negative results but the diagnosis is still suspect, urine collected over a 2- or 3-hour period after a spontaneous attack of hypertension or after administration of histamine with or without simultaneous use of an alpha blocking agent should be assayed for catecholamine content. In such cases a control sample should be tested for comparison.

After a definitive diagnosis of a pheochromocytoma has been made, the ratio of norepinephrine to epinephrine in the urine may aid in locating the tumor. For example, the N-methylating enzyme for the conversion of norepinephrine to epinephrine is found predominantly in the adrenal medulla and the organ of Zuckerkandl (10). Therefore, when epinephrine constitutes more than 20 per cent of the total catecholamines in the urine, the tumor is almost invariably located in one of these two sites (296). When norepinephrine alone is increased, the tumor probably will be found in

the adrenal, possibly in other intra-abdominal sites, and occasionally in extra-abdominal sites.

The pattern of urinary catecholamine and metabolite excretion varies considerably from patient to patient, although it depends in part on the size of the pheochromocytoma. Thus the ratio of urinary norepinephrine plus epinephrine to metabolites, particularly VMA, may predict the size of the mass (109). A low ratio of urinary VMA to norepinephrine plus epinephrine will indicate a tumor with a low content of norepinephrine and epinephrine (less than 100 mg.), usually weighing less than 5 g. Such tumors have a rapid rate of catecholamine synthesis and, for some reason, readily release the amines as biologically active norepinephrine or other catecholamines into the circulation. Patients with such tumors will manifest symptoms before the mass becomes large. Tumors with a high content of catecholamines (100 mg. to 10 g.) bind amines well (probably by virtue of near-normal ATP concentrations), have a slow rate of catecholamine turnover, metabolize catecholamines within the tumor substance, and release metabolites as well as catecholamines into the circulation. Symptoms in such patients will not appear until sufficient amounts of active catecholamines have been released into the blood. By the time symptoms occur, the tumor is large (weighing 50 g. or more), and the ratio of VMA to norepinephrine plus epinephrine in the urine is usually high.

Two additional substances have diagnostic application in families with medullary-thyroid carcinomas and bilateral pheochromocytomas. High plasma concentration of calcitonin provides evidence of the medullary thyroid carcinoma (464); increased plasma concentrations of histaminase or diamine oxidase may indicate metastasis (29). The latter patients often have abnormal responses to intradermally injected histamine (26).

Pharmacologic Testing. In recent years, pharmacologic tests have become safer but less necessary and less popular for screening purposes. If the patient is hypertensive, phentolamine (Regitine), an alpha blocking agent, may be used in both a diagnostic and a therapeutic capacity to lower the blood pressure. If a pheochromocytoma is present, however, even small doses of phentolamine, 1 mg. or less, may produce profound and prolonged hypotension (Fig. 5–48), creating a risk of cerebral or myocardial infarction. Therefore, instead of the recommended dose of 5 mg., the initial dose of phentolamine in patients with suspected pheochromocytomas should be less than 1 mg. A fall in blood pressure of 35/25 mm. Hg, lasting at least 4 minutes but persisting up to 2 or 3 hours, is indicative of a pheochromocytoma. The test is only 75 per cent accurate; false positive results are frequent, especially in patients with azotemia or in those under sedation or being treated for hypertension. Some of the false positive tests may be eliminated by also measuring changes in circulating insulin and blood glucose. When the phentolamine is given, patients with pheochromocytomas will show

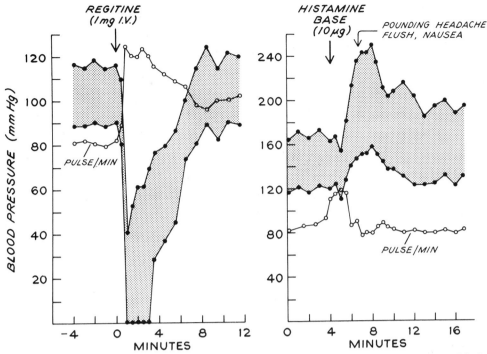

Figure 5–48. Responses to administration of phentolamine (Regitine) (1 mg.) and histamine (10 μg.) in patients with pheochromocytoma, showing that even small amounts of these agents (20 per cent of the doses usually recommended for pharmacologic testing) can cause profound changes in blood pressure.

a rise in insulin and a fall in glucose that accompany a fall in blood pressure (444).

In a normotensive patient, either of two pharmacologic agents may be used to provoke an attack of hypertension or, in the presence of alpha adrenergic blockade, increase urinary catecholamine excretion. Both histamine (by producing reflex sympathetic discharge) and tyramine (by direct action) release the catecholamine stores of normal sympathetic nerve endings. In a patient with a pheochromocytoma, these stores are increased because the nerve endings constantly are exposed to abnormally high concentrations of catecholamines in plasma. The uptake process expands their releasable store. Since pheochromocytoma tissue probably is not innervated, histamine would not be expected to affect the tumor itself. Although the effect of tyramine on tumor tissue has not been defined, its direct action on release of catecholamines from tissues would likely effect release from the tumor.

The clinical usefulness of the histamine test currently is limited to patients with negative urinary catecholamine tests or those on whom other diagnostic tests could not be performed during spontaneous hypertension. Although histamine can be used to provoke an attack, the initial dose should be smaller (less than 25 μg.) than the usual amount recommended for pharmacologic testing. An alpha blocking agent should be used immediately for any large unexpected rise in blood pressure (Fig. 5–48). Urine collected for a 2-hour period before and after the histamine test should be assayed for catecholamine content (not for metabolites). The histamine test rarely gives false negative results.

The tyramine test described by Engelman, Sjoerdsma, and their co-workers (134, 141, 432) depends on direct release of catecholamines from nerve endings. Rapid intravenous administration of tyramine in graded doses of up to 2 mg. will produce an increase in blood pressure within 45 to 60 seconds, which reaches a peak at 1 to 1½ minutes. The response lasts less than 3 minutes. A rise of 20 to 80 mm. Hg in systolic pressure and about 40 mm. Hg in diastolic pressure is considered a positive response (Fig. 5–49). If the increase is prolonged or unusually or dangerously high, phentolamine will reverse it rapidly. False negative results are seen in about 25 per cent of patients with pheochromocytomas, most frequently in those with the familial variety of the tumor associated with a medullary carcinoma of the thyroid, precisely the setting for which a simple screening test would be most desirable. False negative results are also possible in the patient taking hydrochlorothiazide or phenoxybenzamine. Nevertheless, the tyramine test may be preferable to the histamine test that often produces untoward effects.

A third test in the normotensive patient is glucagon administration. The peptide is normally released from pancreatic islet cells during hypoglycemia. Its release or administration is associated with considerable increases in catecholamines in the peripheral and adrenal venous blood (272). The drug has so far produced no false positive results;

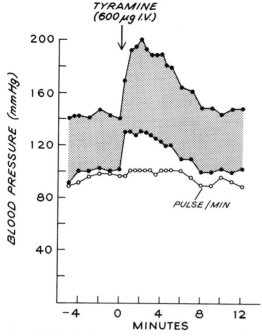

Figure 5–49. Results of a tyramine test in a patient with pheochromocytoma, showing a positive response (rise of about 80 mm. Hg in systolic pressure and 40 mm. Hg in diastolic pressure within 45 to 60 seconds after intravenous administration of the drug).

however, it seldom has been tried in patients with pheochromocytomas (270, 272). If its effects are limited to the adrenal, it would likely affect tumors only in that site and would not influence the same pools of catecholamines affected by histamine and tyramine. Only additional work will determine where glucagon fits in the diagnostic armamentarium.

Pharmacologic tests are also important to exclude pheochromocytomas in patients with hypertension before they are treated with antiadrenergic drugs. As shown in Fig. 5–45, many agents frequently used in treating hypertension, such as reserpine, alpha-methyldopa and guanethidine, have in common the property of releasing stored catecholamines. In normotensive human subjects, administration of guanethidine in large amounts has resulted in paradoxical hypertension instead of hypotension. Even less potent catecholamine releasers like reserpine and alpha-methyldopa have produced pressor responses in normal individuals (92, 279). Since abnormally large stores of catecholamines are characteristic of a pheochromocytoma, affected patients can be expected to react adversely to these drugs. Therefore, when patients with moderate to severe hypertension are seen for the first time, they must be tested for a pheochromocytoma before treatment is instituted. If a patient is hospitalized because of malignant acceleration of hypertension but has not been seen previously, he should be tested with phentolamine before treatment is attempted. If the test is positive, phentolamine can be continued on a maintenance basis until further studies can be completed (see section on therapy).

If the test results are equivocal, potent, rapid-acting ganglionic blocking agents (e.g., trimethaphan) should be administered rather than antiadrenergic agents that can release catecholamines. [The trimethaphan would not be expected to affect circulating catecholamines. However, it would be beneficial in a patient, even one with a pheochromocytoma, in whom the majority of catecholamines were released from normal nerve endings; if the majority of amines were coming from the adrenal tumor (a postganglionic structure), the ganglionic blocker would probably not be of help.] When phentolamine tests are negative, antiadrenergic agents can be administered with relative safety.

To summarize, about 90 per cent of pheochromocytoma cases can be diagnosed by a single test for urinary norepinephrine and epinephrine, normetanephrine plus metanephrine, or VMA levels. The size of the tumor can be estimated from the ratio of urinary VMA to norepinephrine plus epinephrine, and the location of the tumor can be predicted if large amounts of epinephrine are being secreted. Pharmacologic tests are adjuvants to diagnosis for the other 10 per cent of pheochromocytoma cases. Tyramine and histamine tests should be performed with caution; ordinarily they are not used in patients with blood pressure above 170/100 mm. Hg. Adrenergic blocking agents, which act by inhibiting the effects of circulating catechols at the receptor site, should be used only when the blood pressure is high.

Special Procedures. Blood volume determinations may allow judgment of the need for fluid replacement before and during removal of the tumor. Previously, reductions in both total blood volume and plasma volume were assumed to be the major cause of the orthostatic or postoperative hypotension frequently seen in patients with pheochromocytomas. Sjoerdsma et al. (432) altered this assumption; only 4 of their 15 patients with pheochromocytomas showed a decrease in plasma volume greater than 2 standard deviations below the mean value in normal subjects. In addition, using chromium[51]-labeled red cells, only 3 of the 15 showed a reduction in total blood volume greater than 2 standard deviations below normal. Nevertheless, replacement or even overreplacement of blood estimated by preoperative testing or lost at operation can be of major importance in preventing postoperative hypotension and surgical mortality (62, 180). Biskind, Meyer, and Beadner (39) reported that profound hypotension develops in more than 50 per cent of patients after resection of a pheochromocytoma and will be a frequent cause of death if pressor agents alone are used for its control.

Determining blood catecholamine concentrations at different levels during catheterization of the inferior or superior vena cava is a useful procedure in the rare cases in which the tumor cannot be located by other means (353). It is a difficult technical procedure, and the data must be interpreted with skill. The findings may be misleading because of intermittent secretion of catecholamines by the tumor or falsely elevated or lowered catecholamine concentrations caused by laminar flow in different vessels. The test can falsely suggest only a single tumor if most of the catecholamine increase is localized in a narrow portion of the vessel, when actually the single vein is being fed by multiple tumors. Remember that 80 per cent of all pheochromocytomas originate in the adrenal glands, and 95 per cent are located in the abdominal or pelvic regions. Remember also that in 10 per cent of adult patients, and more frequently in children, the tumors arise bilaterally or from multiple foci. In addition, bilateral medullary hyperplasia may be responsible for excessive catecholamine excretion (129, 328). These observations indicate that most if not all surgical procedures must be designed to explore the entire abdominal cavity. The catheterization procedure for determining blood catecholamine concentrations should be restricted to those cases in which a tumor is not found by careful exploration of the abdomen or is suspected to be elsewhere than in the abdominal cavity.

Therapy. *General.* Therapy for the patient with a pheochromocytoma has two distinctive phases: (1) the preparation of the patient for surgical removal of the tumor, and (2) the chronic management of the patient with a malignant pheochromocytoma or the patient unable to undergo a definitive surgical procedure. Effective control of blood pressure, blood volumes, and myocardial damage enables the patient to sustain the surgical and postsurgical course. Untreated patients frequently die from cardiovascular complications directly related to the pheochromocytoma.

Two major classes of drugs are used in treatment. The most widely employed are the alpha adrenergic blocking agents (172, 201), which inhibit the effects of catecholamines but do not alter their synthesis or degradation. Both phentolamine, a short-acting agent, and phenoxybenzamine hydrochloride (Dibenzyline), a haloalkylamine which must be metabolized before it becomes an effective alpha blocker, are used. The choice of agents for presurgical therapy appears relatively unimportant. If the patient is generally well and requires only moderate control of blood pressure for a short time, phentolamine is the drug of choice. When given intravenously, phentolamine acts quickly and for short periods, allowing minute-to-minute control of catecholamine effect. When given orally, however, it has several disadvantages for prolonged use. It is well absorbed but may produce severe nausea or gastric irritation; it must be given every 4 to 6 hours, which requires waking the patient during the night; and its effect may be uneven, resulting in variations in blood pressure from normotensive to severely hypertensive. Therefore, in most medical centers, Dibenzyline is given instead in single oral doses (40 to 100 mg.) every 12 hours. Despite initial fears, experience has indicated that this drug can be given until the time of operation without causing severe hypotension which might be unresponsive to administration of adrenergic pressor agents after removal of the tumor.

With both drugs, effectiveness of therapy can be judged by the return of blood pressure to normal, freedom from hypertensive attacks, a decrease in sweating, and in many instances a return to normal of fasting blood glucose and plasma free fatty acid levels (486). Most patients are treated for periods of 10 days to 2 weeks before surgery, although patients with severe catecholamine-induced cardiomyopathy may require longer. Two of the patients described by Engelman and Sjoerdsma (140, 143) required up to 6 months of presurgical treatment. The drugs may block some but not all of the effects of catecholamines. In several clinical cases, these agents have blocked the cardiovascular effects of catecholamines but not the gastrointestinal effects (432). In other patients, free fatty acid and fasting blood glucose levels and oxygen consumption did not return to baseline, although palpitations disappeared and peripheral vascular resistance returned to normal (486). Thus the disadvantage of alpha blocking agents lies in their apparent inability to reverse all the beta receptor–mediated effects of catecholamines.

The beta adrenergic blocking agents may be very helpful in selected patients with cardiac arrhythmia who are not responsive to alpha adrenergic blocking agents and efforts to reduce blood pressure. Neither our own clinical experience nor the publications dealing with beta blocking drugs have convincingly documented a routine need for propranolol or pronethalol in the preoperative management of patients with pheochromocytoma (65, 100, 172, 353, 395). Patients with pheochromocytomas can be extraordinarily sensitive to either alpha or beta adrenergic blocking agents. A patient should be started on 20 mg. of phenoxybenzamine daily and the dose increased by 10 to 20 mg. per day until the cardiovascular manifestations are controlled. If arrhythmia persists after a maximally tolerable dosage schedule of the alpha blocking agent, propranolol in low doses of 10 to 40 mg. should control the arrhythmia. Propranolol should not be considered until an effective regimen with phenoxybenzamine has been established. If propranolol were used alone, severe hypertension could result as the alphamimetic activity of the circulating catecholamines would continue unopposed by the blocking agent and unbalanced by beta receptor-mediated vasodilation.

A second major class of drugs, now available for the treatment of pheochromocytomas, acts at the rate-limiting step in the biosynthesis of catecholamines. The effect of these drugs is to decrease total catecholamine synthesis and, at least theoretically, prevent symptoms caused by excessive production of catechols. One such agent, alpha-methyltyrosine, inhibits tyrosine hydroxylase (442). Engelman, Sjoerdsma, and their collaborators used the drug on 19 patients with pheochromocytomas, including 4 with malignant pheochromocytomas (142, 431). They found decreases in the synthesis of catecholamines by the tumor and reductions of up to 70 to 80 per cent in urinary excretion of catecholamines and their metabolites. We obtained similar results with alpha-methyltyrosine in the treatment of three patients with malignant pheochromocytomas (312). The decreased catecholamine excretion was accompanied by general improvement in the clinical status of the patient and decreases in blood pressure, pulse rate, sweating, and oxygen consumption. In the past few years, the drug has been further tested (135, 172, 231). The initial impressions of its effectiveness in patients with pheochromocytoma hold true. Some have used it to inhibit catecholamine synthesis only when conventional adrenergic blocking agents were inadequate to control the effects of catecholamines. Not surprisingly, alpha-methyltyrosine has little effect on patients with essential hypertension whose synthesis of catecholamines appears normal. As the drug inhibits catecholamine synthesis, undesirable effects seem inevitable. Sedation is common and is followed by insomnia when the drug is withdrawn. Anxiety, diarrhea, and galactorrhea are common. Tremors similar to those in Parkinson's disease have been seen during chronic administration of the drug. For the present, the conservative and sparing use of the drug appears warranted.

One other compound, disulfiram (Antabuse), an inhibitor of dopamine beta-oxidase, is commercially available but has not yet been used in the therapy of pheochromocytomas. Preparations of other agents that act by inhibiting tyrosine hydroxylase or dopamine beta-oxidase undoubtedly will be introduced. Whether such agents will be of value in the treatment of patients with malignant pheochromocytomas remains to be seen.

To repeat, beta blocking agents and catecholamine synthesis inhibitors are useful for the short-term preoperative care of patients with pheochromocytomas and for patients with malignant lesions or those who cannot tolerate operative procedures. If metastasis has occurred, symptomatic treatment is the only alternative. No data have been reported that strongly support the use of antitumor agents in this disease. Because of the neural crest origin of the tumor cells, pheochromocytomas would be expected to be highly resistant to radiation and most antitumor drugs, and thus far they have proved so in practice.

After the patient has been asymptomatic for one week and ancillary diagnostic procedures have defined the presence, probable location, and biochemical characteristics of the tumor, surgical resection is the next step. Because patients with pheochromocytomas often have gallstones, gallbladder function should be evaluated before the operation. Simultaneous cholecystectomy and removal of a pheochromocytoma has been reported (432), but it would seem prudent to perform the procedures separately.

Colonic enemas should be avoided before removing an abdominal pheochromocytoma since they may induce a hypertensive crisis. However, since the colon must be manipulated during the abdominal exploratory procedure, it may be reasonable to have the patient take a clear fluid diet for one to two days before surgery. Antibiotics also have been used to prepare the bowel.

Anesthetic Considerations. A narcotic analgesic used in conjunction with scopolamine has been favored for preanesthetic medication (395). Atropine is occasionally followed by tachycardia (395) and phenothiazine by shock (60), and both should therefore be avoided.

Before intubation or induction of anesthesia, an intra-arterial needle should be inserted into either the radial or brachial artery as determined by results of the Allen test to allow constant monitoring of blood pressure. Electrocardiographic leads and a catheter for determining the central venous pressure (354) should also be positioned for use. Careful monitoring of pressures is particularly important during early induction of anesthesia and tracheal intubation, when the blood pressure may rise. During periods of increased blood pressure, repeated doses of 1 to 5 mg. of phentolamine should be given intravenously (Fig. 5–50). Beta blocking agents such as propranolol have been found helpful in controlling arrhythmia (295, 432). The central venous pressure serves as an index of cardiac competency and adequate maintenance of blood volume.

The choice of anesthetic probably is inconsequential. Halothane has been used at the National Institutes of Health because it elicits little or no sympathoadrenal activity as measured by changes in plasma norepinephrine levels (41, 93, 331, 374, 432). It has the drawback, however, of being able to potentiate catecholamine-induced arrhythmia (196) and probably should not be used unless an effective beta blocking agent is available for its control (101). If such agents are not available, lidocaine (446) may be given intravenously if arrhythmia occurs. Anesthetics known to cause increased sympathetic activity and possible hypertension (e.g., ether and cyclopropane) probably

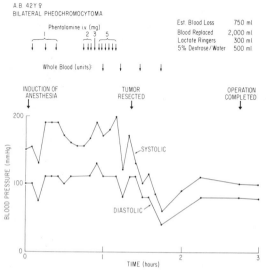

Figure 5–50. Effect of repeated doses of phentolamine on blood pressure levels of a patient with bilateral pheochromocytoma during surgical removal of the tumors. (Reproduced from Sjoerdsma, A., Engelman, K., et al.: *Ann. Intern. Med.* 65:1302, 1966, by permission of authors and publisher.)

should be avoided. In most hospitals, thiopental sodium and nitrous oxide are reasonable choices, since neither one is known to release catecholamines or potentiate the arrhythmic effects of catecholamines. Curare can be used for muscle relaxation. Theoretical reasoning aside, the practical choice of anesthetics varies widely, and no particular agent is uniquely safe or hazardous (107, 239). Paying attention to the fundamentals of oxygenation and proper intravascular fluid volume leads to relatively favorable responses regardless of the anesthetic used. Blood replacement should be started soon after anesthesia and surgical intervention and continued at a rate that will not dangerously increase central venous pressure.

Surgical Considerations. Most surgeons choose an abdominal incision for a patient with a possible pheochromocytoma (107, 365). When the pheochromocytoma is found in the adrenal, a "radical" adrenalectomy, with removal not only of the gland but also of adjacent areolar tissue (often the site of neural crest rests or other primary tumors), is the preferred procedure. Episodes of hypertension may occur during intubation, induction of anesthesia, peritoneal incision, manipulation and isolation of the tumor, and palpation of other organs that may contain tumor masses. Such episodes can be readily managed by repeated injection of phentolamine, as described previously, or constant infusions of phentolamine. The surgeon should palpate the gallbladder for the presence of stones or evidence of chronic cholecystitis.

If blood volume has been adequately maintained and the patient well managed during surgery, there is little risk of postoperative hypotensive episodes which cannot be controlled by further blood replacement or the use of small amounts of pressor agents. Of the 32 patients with pheochromocytomas operated on most recently at the University of California Medical Center, use of pressor agents has been required in only a few. Corticosteroid replacement must be planned if a bilateral adrenalectomy is carried out.

Several days after the operation, 24-hour urinary excretion of catecholamines and metabolites should be measured to determine whether the surgical procedure has been successful. If VMA levels are still abnormally high after the first postoperative week, further evaluation is indicated, and additional surgical procedures should be con-

sidered. Once the urinary catecholamine and metabolite levels return to normal, the patient can be discharged. The patient should be reevaluated at regular intervals, since additional primary pheochromocytomas may occur. This is particularly true in young patients and in families where more than one member has had a pheochromocytoma.

Other Tumors Arising from Sympathetic and Adrenal Medullary Tissue

Since it is derived from neural crest tissue, the adrenal medulla is occasionally the site of tumors other than pheochromocytomas. Although found most commonly in the adrenal medulla, they may occur in other retroperitoneal and retropleural sites (513). Such tumors also occur in other sites of neural crest origin, such as the brain, sympathetic ganglia, and celiac plexus. The neoplasms are of two main types: neuroblastomas and ganglioneuromas (Fig. 5–51). The neuroblastomas are usually large. They occur in the neonate and child and rarely in the adult (29, 86, 146, 195, 288, 502). The young also are predisposed to the ganglioneuroma, but it occurs more frequently in the adult. There may be a familial predisposition to neuroblastomas (86). The tumor cells of both neoplasms are small and round, have hyperchromatic nuclei, and are dispersed in rosettes among more highly differentiated cellular elements. They derive chiefly from sympathogonia and sympathoblasts. Since pheochromoblasts and sympathoblasts are difficult to differentiate, neuroblastomas probably arise from both cell types. Such tumors metastasize early, either by direct spread into contiguous tissues or by embolization to lymph nodes, liver, other abdominal organs, and bone. The most common symptom of neuroblastomas (and occasionally ganglioneuromas) is diarrhea (392). Hypertension, although it does occur, is infrequent. For the neuroblastoma, early radical surgical resection, radiation therapy, and administration of antitumor agents may result in a cure (267, 459, 490). Treatment is most successful when metastasis is confined to the abdomen, but occasional instances of very wide-spread disease may have a favorable prognosis following vigorous therapy (113).

The ganglioneuroma is derived from sympa-

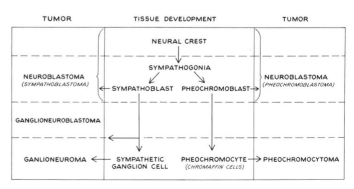

Figure 5–51. Embryologic derivation of endocrinologically functioning tumors of neural crest origin. The ganglioneuroblastoma is derived from cell types intermediate between those of the neuroblastoma and pheochromocytoma.

thetic ganglion cells and is composed of organized, mature cells. This tumor usually develops during youth but also occurs frequently in adulthood. If detected early enough, it can be treated successfully by surgical extirpation, but it may become anaplastic and degenerate into a malignant neuroblastoma. Pathologists have classified a tumor with cellular elements intermediate between those of neuroblastoma and ganglioneuroma as a ganglioneuroblastoma (321). This differentiation is largely on a histologic basis. The ganglioneuroblastoma may behave like either a ganglioneuroma or a neuroblastoma. There have been instances of actual maturation of a neuroblastoma to a ganglioneuroma (7).

The pheochromocytoma, neuroblastoma, ganglioneuroblastoma, and ganglioneuroma have a common embryologic origin. Therefore, the finding by Mason et al. (304) of increased excretion of pressor amines in the urine of an infant with a neuroblastoma is not surprising. Later studies have shown that patients with neuroblastomas and subsequently cultured neuroblastoma cells (181) frequently excrete a variety of chemical precursors of catecholamines, as well as their metabolic products (20, 169, 190, 266, 498, 499). In one reported series of 73 patients with neuroblastoma (234), increased urinary excretion of VMA was found in 69 patients; dopamine excretion was increased in 32 of 36 patients tested, and the oxidation product of dopamine, homovanillic acid, was increased in 24 of 36. Subsequent experience has confirmed the usefulness of measuring urinary catecholamines both to detect and follow the effects of therapy in patients with neuroblastoma (152, 332). The radiologic techniques used to discover pheochromocytomas are applicable to neuroblastomas and ganglioneuromas. New procedures that depend on the cell's ability to take up methionine are promising (114).

Experience with neural crest tumors other than pheochromocytomas has led to two important observations. First, it appears that the more primitive the tumor cell, the more likely it is that the tumor will elaborate the precursors of catecholamines and their metabolic products. Thus the neuroblastoma is associated almost invariably with a high urinary output of VMA and frequently with elaboration of dopamine and homovanillic acid (234). In contrast, dopamine and homovanillic acid usually are not excreted by patients with pheochromocytomas unless the tumors have become malignant (234, 499). Second, as the cell type approaches a more mature form of differentiation, the frequency with which biologically active substances are excreted diminishes. In the primitive cell tumor, the tumor substance actually may be able to produce catecholamines, but the binding properties of the tumor are impaired. A good rule of thumb is that increased excretion of dopa, dopamine, or homovanillic acid is suggestive of the malignant rather than benign form of neural crest tumors and that, in the case of the neuroblastoma and the ganglioneuroma, the more primitive form is more likely to be associated with increased excretion of vanillylmandelic acid. An exception to the rule is the finding that urinary excretion of dopa and its metabolites may be elevated in patients with melanomas (503).

Another point of interest is that apparently little or no correlation exists between the clinical symptoms, such as chronic diarrhea, hypertension, or abnormalities in serum glucose levels (425), and the excretion of known catecholamines or their metabolites in patients with either neuroblastomas or ganglioneuromas. One possible explanation for the lack of correlation may be the metabolism of most of the biologically active amines within the tumor cell. However, a more likely explanation is that we have not identified all the biologically active substances that the tumor cells can produce. Some authorities believe that the pheochromocytoma may be an incomplete expression of pluriglandular adenomatosis because it is associated with other endocrinopathies (110). The pheochromocytoma has been shown to be capable of producing more than one class of endocrine hormone, i.e., erythrocyte-stimulating factor, a protein or peptide quite different from the simple amines it characteristically produces. It seems equally possible that neuroblastomas and ganglioneuromas may produce their symptoms by elaboration of a biologically active substance as yet unidentified. The tumors apparently are responsible for the symptoms, since removal of the primary or metastatic masses is followed by lessening of the diarrhea and hypertension, and often the patient becomes asymptomatic (244, 245). Thus such tumors may be analogous to the carcinoid tumor, which can elaborate a spectrum of biologically active substances. The neural crest tumors may be able to produce hormones by some mechanism completely unrelated to their usual cell function. That such a phenomenon can occur is shown by the description in Chapter 29 of tumors histologically unrelated to the carcinoid tumor which produce symptoms indistinguishable from those of the carcinoid syndrome. Whether the symptoms result from the release of endogenous vasoactive substances by the tumor or whether the tumor actually produces biologically active compounds remains to be determined.

REFERENCES

1. Ahlquist, R. P.: *Amer. J. Physiol. 153*:586, 1948.
2. Alton, H., and Goodall, M.: *Biochem. Pharmacol. 18*:1373, 1969.
3. Anton-Tay, F., Pelham, R. W., et al.: *Endocrinology 84*:1489, 1969.
4. Anton-Tay, F., and Wurtman, R. J.: *Science 159*:1245, 1968.
5. Assem, E. S. K., Pickup, P. M., et al.: *Brit. J. Pharmacol. 39*:212P, 1970.
6. Assem, E. S. K., and Schild, H. O.: *Brit. J. Pharmacol. 42*:620, 1971.
7. Aterman, K., and Schueller, E. F.: *Amer. J. Dis. Child. 120*:217, 1970.
8. Austin, L., Livett, B. G., et al.: *Life Sciences 6*:97, 1967.
9. Axelrod, J.: Proc. of Third Intl. Cong. of Endocrinology, Mexico, 1968, p. 286.
10. Axelrod, J.: *J. Biol. Chem. 237*:1657, 1962.

11. Axelrod, J.: *The Physiologist 11*:63, 1968.
12. Axelrod, J., In *Symposium on the Clinical Chemistry of Monamines*, Manchester, England, 1962. Varley, H., and Gowenlock, A. H. (eds.), Amsterdam, Elsevier Publishing Company, 1963, p. 5.
13. Axelrod, J., and Kopin, I. J., In *Progress in Brain Research.* Vol. 31. Akert, K., and Waser, P. G. (eds.), Amsterdam, Elsevier Publishing Company, 1969, p. 21.
14. Axelrod, J., Weil-Malherbe, H., et al.: *J. Pharmacol. Exp. Ther. 127*:251, 1959.
15. Ayitey-Smith, E., and Varma, D. R.: *Brit. J. Pharmacol. 40*:186, 1970.
16. Bacq, A. M., Gosselin, L., et al.: *Science 130*:453, 1959.
17. Ball, J. H., Kaminsky, N. I., et al.: *J. Clin. Invest. 51*:2124, 1972.
18. Ball, P., Knuppen, R., et al.: *Europ. J. Biochem. 21*:517, 1971.
19. Barnardo, D. E., Baldus, W. P., et al.: *Gastroenterology 58*:524, 1970.
20. Barontini de Gutiérrez Moyano, M., Bergadá, C., et al.: *J. Pediat. 77*:239, 1970.
21. Bartholini, G., Da Prada, M., et al.: *J. Pharm. Pharmacol. 20*:228, 1968.
22. Bartholini, G., Kuruma, I., et al.: *Nature* (London) *230*:533, 1971.
23. Bartholini, G., and Pletscher, A.: *J. Pharmacol. Exp. Ther. 161*:14, 1968.
24. Bartholini, G., and Pletscher, A.: *J. Pharm. Pharmacol. 21*:323, 1969.
25. Bartlett, R. C., Myall, R. W. T., et al.: *Oral Surg. 31*:206, 1971.
26. Baum, J. L.: *New Eng. J. Med. 284*:963, 1971.
27. Baylin, S. B., Beaven, M. A., et al.: *New Eng. J. Med. 283*:1239, 1970.
28. Becker, C. E., Rosen, S. W., et al.: *Ann. Intern. Med. 70*:325, 1969.
29. Becker, J. M., Schneider, K. M., et al.: *Progr. Clin. Cancer 4*:382, 1970.
30. Belleau, B.: *Pharmacol. Rev. 18*:131, 1966.
31. Belpaire, F., and Laduron, P.: *Biochem Pharmacol. 17*:411, 1968.
32. Benedict, P. H., Szabó, G., et al.: *J.A.M.A. 205*:618, 1968.
33. Berkowitz, B. A., Spector, S., et al.: *Experientia* (Basel) *26*:982, 1970.
34. Berkowitz, B. A., Tarver, J. H., et al.: *J. Pharmacol. Exp. Ther. 177*:119, 1971.
35. Bernier, J. J., Rambaud, J. C., et al.: *Gut 10*:980, 1969.
36. Berti, F., and Shore, P. A.: *Biochem. Pharmacol. 16*:2271, 1967.
37. Besson, M. J., Cheramy, A., et al.: *Proc. Nat. Acad. Sci.* USA *62*:741, 1969.
38. Biglieri, E. G., and McIlroy, M. B.: *Circulation 33*:78, 1966.
39. Biskind, G. R., Meyer, M. A., et al.: *J. Clin. Endocr. 1*:113, 1941.
40. Bittner, G. D., and Kennedy, D.: *J. Cell Biol. 47*:585, 1970.
41. Black, G. W., and McArdle, L.: *Brit. J. Anaesth. 34*:2, 1962.
42. Black, W. L., and Rolett, E. L.: *Amer. Heart J. 75*:233, 1968.
43. Blaschko, H., Jerrome, D. W., et al.: *Clin. Sci. 34*:453, 1968.
44. Blaschko, H., and Welch, A. D.: *Arch. Exp. Path. Pharmakol. 219*:17, 1953.
45. Block, M. A.: *G.P. 39*:105, 1969.
46. Boadle, M. C., Hughes, J., et al.: *Nature* (London) *222*:987, 1969.
47. Bogdanski, D. F., and Brodie, B. B.: *Life Sci. 5*:1563, 1966.
48. Bourne, H. R., Lichtenstein, L. M., et al.: *J. Immun. 108*:695, 1972.
49. Bourne, H. R., and Melmon, K. L.: *Rational Drug Ther. 5*:#4, 1971.
50. Bourne, H. R., Thomson, P., et al.: *Arch. Intern. Med.* (Chicago) *125*:1063, 1970.
51. Bowman, W. C., and Nott, M. W.: *Pharmacol. Rev. 21*:27, 1969.
52. Braham, J.: *Brit. Med. J. 2*:540, 1970.
53. Brantigan, C. O., and Katase, R. Y.: *Surgery 65*:898, 1969.
54. Breese, G. R., Chase, T. N., et al.: *J. Pharmacol. Exp. Ther. 165*:9, 1969.
55. Breese, G. R., Chase, T. N., et al.: *Biochem. Pharmacol. 18*:863, 1969.
56. Breese, G. R., Kopin, I. J., et al.: *Brit. J. Pharmacol. 38*:537, 1970.
57. Breese, G. R., and Traylor, T. D.: *J. Pharmacol. Exp. Ther. 174*:413, 1970.
58. Brimijoin, S., and Molinoff, P. B.: *J. Pharmacol. Exp. Ther. 178*:417, 1971.
59. Broberger, O., and Zetterstrom, R.: *J. Pediat. 59*:215, 1961.
60. Brody, I. A.: *J.A.M.A. 169*:1749, 1959.
61. Brooks, H. L., Stein, P. D., et al.: *Circ. Res. 24*:699, 1969.
62. Brunjes, S., Johns, V. J., Jr., et al.: *New Eng. J. Med. 262*:393, 1960.
63. Brus, R., Hess, M. E., et al.: *Europ. J. Pharmacol. 10*:323, 1970.
64. Bublitz, C.: *Biochem. Pharmacol. 20*:2543, 1971.
65. Buist, N. R., Mijer, F., et al.: *Arch. Dis. Child. 41*:435, 1966.
66. Bunney, W. E., Jr.: *Amer. J. Psychiat. 127*:361, 1970.
67. Burkard, W. P., Jalfre, M., et al.: *Experientia* (Basel) *25*:1295, 1969.
68. Burn, J. H.: *Nature* (London) *231*:237, 1971.
69. Burn, J. H., and Rand, M. J.: *Brit. J. Pharmacol. 15*:56, 1960.
70. Burn, J. H., and Rand, M. J.: *J. Physiol.* (London) *144*:314, 1958.
71. Butcher, L. L., and Engel, J.: *Brain Res. 15*:233, 1969.
72. Butcher, L. L., and Engel, J.: *J. Pharm. Pharmacol. 21*:614, 1969.
73. Calne, D. B., Brennan, J., et al.: *Brit. Med. J. 1*:474, 1970.
74. Calne, D. B., and Sandler, M.: *Nature* (London) *226*:21, 1970.
75. Campos, H. R., and Crout, J. R.: *Fed. Proc. 29*:545, 1970.
76. Cannon, W. B., and Rosenbleuth, A.: *Autonomic Neuroeffector Systems.* New York, MacMillan Company, 1948.
77. Carlsson, A., Falck, B., et al.: *Acta Physiol. Scand.* (Suppl. 196) *56*:1, 1962.
78. Carlsson, A., Lundborg, P., et al.: *J. Pharmacol. Exp. Ther. 158*:175, 1967.
79. Carman, C. T., and Brashear, R. E.: *New Eng. J. Med. 263*:419, 1960.
80. Carvalho, M., Vyden, J. K., et al.: *Amer. J. Cardiol. 23*:217, 1969.
81. Cass, R., Kuntzman, R., et al.: *Proc. Soc. Exp. Biol. Med. 103*:871, 1960.
82. Celesia, G. G., and Barr, A. N.: *Arch. Neurol.* (Chicago) *23*:193, 1970.
83. Chalmers, J. P., Baldessarini, R. J., et al.: *Proc. Nat. Acad. Sci.* U.S.A. *68*:662, 1971.
84. Chang, C. C., Costa, E., et al.: *J. Pharmacol. Exp. Ther. 147*:303, 1965.
85. Chapman, R. C., Kamp, V. E., et al.: *Amer. J. Med. 26*:883, 1959.
86. Chatten, J., and Voorhess, M. L.: *New Eng. J. Med. 277*:1230, 1967.
87. Chidsey, C. A., and Braunwald, E.: *Pharmacol. Rev. 18*:685, 1966.
88. Chidsey, C. A., Kaiser, G. A., et al.: *J. Clin. Invest. 43*:2386, 1964.
89. Chubb, L. W., Preston, B. N., et al.: *Biochem. J. 111*:243, 1969.
90. Clouet, D. H., and Ratner, M.: *Science 168*:854, 1970.
91. Cohen, R. A., Kopin, I. J., et al.: *Ann. Intern. Med. 65*:347, 1966.
92. Cohn, J. N.: *New Eng. J. Med. 275*:643, 1966.
93. Cooperman, L. H., Engelman, K., et al.: *Anesthesiology 28*:575, 1967.
94. Cotzias, G. C.: *Hosp. Pract.,* p. 35, Sept. 1969.
95. Cotzias, G. C.: *J.A.M.A. 210*:1255, 1969.
96. Cotzias, G. C., and Papavasiliou, P. S.: *J.A.M.A. 207*:1353, 1969.
97. Cotzias, G. C., Papavasiliou, P. S., et al.: *New Eng. J. Med. 282*:31, 1970.
98. Cotzias, G. C., Papavasiliou, P. S., et al.: *New Eng. J. Med. 280*:337, 1969.
99. Coyle, J. T., and Axelrod, J.: *J. Neurochem. 18*:2061, 1971.
100. Crago, R. M., Eckholdt, J. W., et al.: *J.A.M.A. 202*:870, 1967.
101. Crandell, D. L., and Myers, R. T.: *J.A.M.A. 187*:12, 1964.
102. Creveling, C. R., Daly, J., et al.: *Biochem. Pharmacol. 17*:65, 1968.
103. Crout, J. R., In *Hormones and Hypertension.* Manger, W. M. (ed.), Springfield, Illinois, Charles C Thomas, Publisher, 1966, p. 3.
104. Crout, J. R., In *Standard Methods of the American Association of Clinical Chemists.* Vol. III. Seligson, D. (ed.), New York, Academic Press, Inc., 1960, p. 62.
105. Crout, J. R.: *Pharmacol. Rev. 18*:651, 1966.
106. Crout, J. R.: *Circ. Res.* (Suppl. 1) *18* & *19*:120, 1966.
107. Crout, J. R., and Brown, B. R., Jr.: *Anesthesiology 30*:29, 1969.

108. Crout, J. R., Pisano, J. J., et al.: *Amer. Heart J. 61*:375, 1961.
109. Crout, J. R., and Sjoerdsma, A.: *J. Clin. Invest. 43*:94, 1964.
110. Cushman, P., Jr.: *Amer. J. Med. 32*:352, 1962.
111. Dairman, W., Gordon, R., et al.: *Molec. Pharmacol. 4*:457, 1968.
112. Daly, J., Levitt, M., et al.: *Arch. Biochem. Biophys. 126*:593, 1968.
113. D'Angio, G. J., Evans, A. E., et al.: *Lancet 1*:1046, 1971.
114. D'Angio, G. J., Loken, M., et al.: *Radiology 93*:615, 1969.
115. Danowski, T. S., Heineman, A. C., Jr., et al.: *Metabolism 13*:747, 1964.
116. Davila, D., and Khairallah, Ph.A.: *Arch. Int. Pharmacodyn. 193*:307, 1971.
117. de Champlain, J., Krakoff, L. R., et al.: *Life Sci. 5*:2283, 1966.
118. de Champlain, J., Mueller, R. A., et al.: *Circ. Res. 25*:285, 1969.
119. De Graeff, J., and Horak, B. J. V.: *Acta Med. Scand. 176*:583, 1964.
120. Delaney, J. P., and Paritzky, A. Z.: *New Eng. J. Med. 280*:1394, 1969.
121. DeQuattro, V.: *Circ. Res. 28*:84, 1971.
122. DeQuattro, V., Margolin, A. H., et al.: *J. Clin. Endocr. 30*:138, 1970.
123. DeQuattro, V., Nagatsu, T., et al.: *Circ. Res. 24*:545, 1969.
124. DeQuattro, V., and Sjoerdsma, A.: *J. Clin. Invest. 47*:2359, 1968.
125. Devine, C. E.: *Proc. Univ. Otago Med. Sch. 47*:4, 1969.
126. Donahower, G. F., Schumacher, O. P., et al.: *J. Clin. Endocr. 28*:1199, 1968.
127. Dorris, R. L., and Shore, P. A.: *J. Pharmacol. Exp. Ther. 179*:15, 1971.
128. Douglas, W. W., and Rubin, R. P.: *J. Physiol.* (London) *159*:40, 1961.
129. Drukker, W., Fomijne, P., et al.: *Brit. Med. J. 1*:186, 1957.
130. Duvoisin, R. C.: *Brit. Med. J. 3*:47, 1970.
131. Edis, A. J., and Shepherd, J. T.: *Arch. Intern. Med.* (Chicago) *125*:716, 1970.
132. Engelman, K.: *Bull. N. Y. Acad. Sci. 45*:851, 1969.
133. Engelman, K., and Hammond, W. G.: *Lancet 1*:609, 1968.
134. Engelman, K., Horwitz, D., et al.: *New Eng. J. Med. 278*:705, 1968.
135. Engelman, K., Horwitz, D., et al.: *J. Clin. Invest. 47*:577, 1968.
136. Engelman, K., Mueller, P. S., et al.: *New Eng. J. Med. 270*:865, 1964.
137. Engelman, K., and Portnoy, B.: *Circ. Res. 26*:53, 1970.
138. Engelman, K., Portnoy, B., et al.: *Amer. J. Med. Sci. 255*:259, 1968.
139. Engelman, K., Portnoy, B., et al.: *Circ. Res.* (Suppl. 1) *26 & 27*:141, 1970.
140. Engelman, K., and Sjoerdsma, A.: *Ann. Intern. Med. 61*:229, 1964.
141. Engelman, K., and Sjoerdsma, A.: *J.A.M.A. 189*:81, 1964.
142. Engelman, K., and Sjoerdsma, A.: *Circ. Res.* (Suppl. 1) *18*:104, 1966.
143. Engelman, K., Watts, R. W. E., et al.: *Amer. J. Med. 37*:839, 1964.
144. Ernst, A. M.: *Acta Physiol. Pharmacol. Neerl. 15*:141, 1969.
145. *J.A.M.A. 215*:1969, 1971 (by an author group).
146. Evans, A. E., D'Angio, G. J., et al.: *Cancer 27*:374, 1971.
147. Evetts, K. D., Uretsky, N. J., et al.: *Nature* (London) *225*:961, 1970.
148. Fain, J. N.: *Fed. Proc. 29*:1402, 1970.
149. Federal Drug Administration Current Drug Information: *Ann. Intern. Med. 73*:445, 1970.
150. Feldman, J. M., and Lebovitz, H. E.: *J. Pharmacol. Exp. Ther. 179*:56, 1971.
151. Finch, L., and Leach, G. D. H.: *J. Pharm. Pharmacol. 22*:354, 1970.
152. Finklestein, J. Z., and Gilchrist, G. S.: *Calif. Med. 116*:27–36, 1972.
153. Finlay, G. D., Whitsett, T. L., et al.: *New Eng. J. Med. 284*:865, 1971.
154. Fischer, J. E., Horst, D. W., et al.: *Nature* (London) *207*:951, 1965.
155. Fischer, J. E., Weise, V. K., et al.: *Amer. J. Med. Sci. 255*:158, 1968.
156. Flatmark, T., Lagercrantz, H., et al.: *Biochim. Biophys. Acta 245*:249, 1971.
157. Forde, T. P., Yormak, S. S., et al.: *Amer. Heart J. 76*:388, 1968.
158. Forsyth, R. P.: *Fed. Proc. 31*:1240, 1972.
159. Forsyth, R. P., Hoffbrand, B. I., et al.: *Circulation 44*:119, 1971.
160. Foster, K. G., Ginsburg, J., et al.: *Clin. Sci. 39*:823, 1970.
161. Friedman, S., and Kaufman, S.: *J. Biol. Chem. 240*:552, 1965.
162. Furchgott, R. F.: *Fed. Proc. 29*:1352, 1970.
163. Furness, J. B., Campbell, G. R., et al.: *J. Pharmacol. Exp. Ther. 174*:111, 1970.
164. Fuxe, K.: *Acta Physiol. Scand.* (Suppl. 247) *64*:39, 1965.
165. Gaffney, T. E., Sigell, L. T., et al.: *Progr. Cardiovasc. Dis. 12*:52, 1969.
166. Gewirtz, G. P., and Kopin, I. J.: *J. Pharmacol. Exp. Ther. 175*:514, 1970.
167. Gibb, J. W., Spector, S., et al.: *Molec. Pharmacol. 3*:473, 1967.
168. Gifford, R. M., MacCannell, K. L., et al.: *Canad. J. Physiol. Pharmacol. 46*:847, 1968.
169. Gitlow, S. E., Bertani, L. M., et al.: *Cancer 25*:1377, 1970.
170. Gitlow, S. E., Bertani, L. M., et al.: *Pediatrics 46*:513, 1970.
171. Gitlow, S. E., Mendlowitz, M., et al.: *Amer. J. Cardiol. 26*:270, 1970.
172. Gitlow, S. E., Pertsemlidis, D., et al.: *Amer. Heart J. 82*:557, 1971.
173. Glowinski, J., and Axelrod, J.: *Nature* (London) *204*:1318, 1964.
174. Glowinski, J., and Iversen, L. L.: *J. Neurochem. 13*:655, 1966.
175. Glowinski, J., Iversen, L. L., et al.: *J. Pharmacol. Exp. Ther. 151*:385, 1966.
176. Glowinski, J., Kopin, I. J., et al.: *J. Neurochem. 12*:25, 1965.
177. Glushien, A. S., Mansuy, M. M., et al.: *Amer. J. Med. 14*:318, 1953.
178. Godwin-Austen, R. B., Tomlinson, E. B., et al.: *Lancet 2*:165, 1969.
179. Goldberg, W. M., and McNeil, M. J.: *Canad. Med. Ass. J. 96*:1577, 1967.
180. Goldfien, A.: *Anesthesiology 24*:462, 1963.
181. Goldstein, M., Anagnoste, B., et al.: *Science 160*:767, 1968.
182. Goldstein, M., Anagnoste, B., et al.: *Life Sci. 3*:763, 1964.
183. Goodall, McC., and Alton, H.: *J. Clin. Invest. 48*:2300, 1969.
184. Goodall, McC., and Alton, H.: *J. Clin. Invest. 48*:1761, 1969.
185. Goodall, McC., Gitlow, S. E., et al.: *J. Clin. Invest. 50*:2734, 1971.
186. Goodwin, F. K., and Brodie, H. K.: *Lancet 1*:1339, 1970.
187. Goodwin, F. K., Brodie, H. K., et al.: *Lancet 2*:908, 1970.
188. Goodwin, J. S., Katz, R. I., et al.: *Nature* (London) *221*:556, 1969.
189. Gözsy, B., and Kátó, L.: *Int. Arch. Allerg. 30*:553, 1966.
190. Greenberg, R. E., and Gardner, L. I.: *J. Clin. Invest. 39*:1729, 1960.
191. Griesemer, E. C., Barsky, J., et al.: *Proc. Soc. Exp. Biol. Med. 84*:699, 1953.
192. Guldberg, H. C., and Yates, C. M.: *Brit. J. Pharmacol. Chemother. 33*:457, 1968.
193. Haeusler, G., Haefely, W., et al.: *J. Pharmacol. Exp. Ther. 170*:50, 1969.
194. Hakanson, R., Lundquist, I., et al.: *Europ. J. Pharmacol. 1*:114, 1967.
195. Hale, J. E.: *Brit. J. Surg. 57*:551, 1970.
196. Hall, K. D., and Norris, F. H., Jr.: *Anesthesiology 19*:631, 1958.
197. Hardman, J. G., Robison, G. A., et al.: *Ann. Rev. Physiol. 33*:311, 1971.
198. Harris, R. E., Forsyth, R. P., In *High Blood Pressure.* Mayer, J. H., Onesti, G., and Kim, K. E. (eds.), New York, Grune & Stratton, 1973 (in press).
199. Harrison, T. S., Bartlett, J. D., Jr., et al.: *New Eng. J. Med. 277*:725, 1967.
200. Harrison, T. S., Chawla, R. C., et al.: *New Eng. J. Med. 279*:136, 1968.
201. Harrison, T. S., Dagher, F. J., et al.: *Med. Clin. N. Amer. 53*:1349, 1969.
202. Heikkila, R., and Cohen, G.: *Science 172*:1257, 1971.
203. Helle, K. B.: *Biochim. Biophys. Acta 245*:80, 1971.
204. Helle, K. B., and Brodtkorb, E.: *Biochim. Biophys. Acta 245*:94, 1971.
205. Henney, C. S., Bourne, H. R., et al.: *J. Immun. 108*:1526, 1972.

206. Hermann, H., and Mornex, R.: *Human Tumours Secreting Catecholamines.* Oxford, Pergamon Press, 1964.
207. Hertting, G., Axelrod, J., et al.: *Nature* (London) *189*:66, 1961.
208. Hertting, G., Axelrod, J., et al.: *J. Pharmacol. Exp. Ther. 134*:146, 1961.
209. Hertting, G., Potter, L. T., et al.: *J. Pharmacol. Exp. Ther. 136*:289, 1962.
210. Hickler, R. B., and Vandam, L. D.: *Anesthesiology 33*:214, 1970.
211. Hidaka, H.: *Nature* (London) *231*:54, 1971.
212. Hoak, J. C., Warner, E. D., et al.: *Arch. Path. 87*:332, 1969.
213. Hollister, L. E., In *Clinical Pharmacology — Basic Principles in Therapeutics.* Melmon, K. L., and Morrelli, H. F. (eds.), New York, The MacMillan Company, 1972.
214. Holzbauer, M., and Vogt, M.: *J. Neurochem. 1*:8, 1956.
215. Horn, A. S., Coyle, J. T., et al.: *Molec. Pharmacol. 7*:66, 1971.
216. Horowitz, D., and Sjoerdsma, A.: *Life Sci. 3*:41, 1964.
217. Horst, W. D., Kopin, I. J., et al.: *Amer. J. Physiol. 215*:817, 1968.
218. Hunter, K. R., Boakes, A. J., et al.: *Brit. Med. J. 3*:388, 1970.
219. Innes, I. R., and Nickerson, M., In *The Pharmacological Basis of Therapeutics.* 4th ed. Goodman, L. S., and Gilman, A., (eds.), New York, The MacMillan Company, 1970, p. 478.
220. Iversen, L. L.: *Europ. J. Pharmacol. 10*:408, 1970.
221. Iversen, L. L., Fischer, J. E., et al.: *J. Pharmacol. Exp. Ther. 154*:56, 1966.
222. Iversen, L. L., Glowinski, J., et al.: *Nature* (London) *206*:1222, 1965.
223. James, T. N., Bear, E. S., et al.: *Arch. Intern. Med.* (Chicago) *125*:512, 1970.
224. Jenkins, R. B., and Groh, R. H.: *Lancet 2*:177, 1970.
225. Joh, T. H., Kapit, R., et al.: *Biochim. Biophys. Acta 171*:378, 1969.
226. Johansson, B., and Roos, B. E.: *Europ. J. Clin. Pharmacol. 3*:232, 1971.
227. Johnson, D. G., Thoa, N. B., et al.: *J. Pharmacol. Exp. Ther. 177*:146, 1971.
228. Johnson, G. A., Boukma, S. J., et al.: *J. Pharmacol. Exp. Ther. 171*:80, 1970.
229. Johnson, G. A., Kim, E. G., et al.: *Biochem. Pharmacol. 16*:401, 1967.
230. Johnson, G. E., and Pugsley, T. A.: *Brit. J. Pharmacol. 39*:167, 1970.
231. Jones, N. F., Walker, G., et al.: *Lancet 2*:1105, 1968.
232. Jonsson, G., and Sachs, C.: *Europ. J. Pharmacol. 9*:141, 1970.
233. Kalsner, S.: *Circ. Res. 24*:383, 1969.
234. Kaser, H.: *Pharmacol. Rev. 18*:659, 1966.
235. Katz, R. I., Chase, T. N., et al.: *Science 162*:466, 1968.
236. Katz, R. I., and Kopin, I. J.: *J. Pharmacol. Exp. Ther. 169*:229, 1969.
237. Kety, S. S., Javoy, F., et al.: *Proc. Nat. Acad. Sci. USA 58*:1249, 1967.
238. Keynes, W. M., and Till, A. S.: *Quart. J. Med. 40*:443, 1971.
239. Kirkendall, W. M., Liechty, R. D., et al.: *Arch. Intern. Med.* (Chicago) *115*:529, 1965.
240. Kitabchi, A. E., and Williams, R. H.: *J. Clin. Endocr. 28*:1082, 1968.
241. Klawans, H. L., Jr.: *Dis. Nerv. Syst. 29*:805, 1968.
242. Kline, I. K.: *Amer. J. Path. 38*:539, 1961.
243. Koelle, G. B., In *The Pharmacological Basis of Therapeutics.* Goodman, L. S., and Gilman, A. (eds.), New York, The MacMillan Company, 1965, p. 399.
244. Kogut, M. D., and Kaplan, S. A.: *J. Pediat. 60*:694, 1962.
245. Kontras, S. B.: *Cancer Chemother. Rep. 16*:443, 1962.
246. Kopin, I. J.: *Ann. Rev. Pharmacol. 8*:377, 1968.
247. Kopin, I. J., In *Psychopharmacology: A Review of Progress, 1957-1967.* Efron, D., (ed.), Dept. of HEW, US Govt. Pub. No. 1836, 1968, p. 57.
248. Kopin, I. J.: *Proc. 3rd Intl. Pharmacol. Mtg. 10*:83, 1966.
249. Kopin, I. J.: *Pharmacol. Rev. 16*:179, 1964.
250. Kopin, I. J.: *Fed. Proc. 30*:904, 1971.
251. Kopin, I. J., Breese, G. R., et al.: *J. Pharmacol. Exp. Ther. 161*:271, 1968.
252. Kopin, I. J., Fischer, J. E., et al.: *J. Pharmacol. Exp. Ther. 147*:186, 1965.
253. Kopin, I. J., Weise, V. K., et al.: *J. Pharmacol. Exp. Ther. 170*:246, 1969.
254. Krauss, K. R., Carpenter, D. O., et al.: *J. Pharmacol. Exp. Ther. 173*:416, 1970.
255. Krauss, K. R., Kopin, I. J., et al.: *J. Pharmacol. Exp. Ther. 172*:282, 1970.
256. Kumagai, H., Matsui, H., et al.: *Biochem. Biophys. Res. Commun. 34*:266, 1969.
257. Kuntzman, R., and Jacobson, M. M.: *J. Pharmacol. Exp. Ther. 141*:166, 1963.
258. Kvetnansky, R., Gewirtz, G. P., et al.: *Amer. J. Physiol. 220*:928, 1971.
259. Kvetnansky, R., Gewirtz, G. P., et al.: *Endocrinology 89*:50, 1971.
260. Kvetnansky, R., Gewirtz, G. P., et al.: *Endocrinology 87*:1323, 1970.
261. Kvetnansky, R., Gewirtz, G. P., et al.: *Molec. Pharmacol. 7*:81, 1971.
262. Kvetnansky, R., Silbergeld, S., et al.: *Psychopharmacologia* (Berlin) *20*:22, 1971.
263. Kvetnansky, R., Weise, V. K., et al.: *Endocrinology 89*:46, 1971.
264. Kvetnansky, R., Weise, V. K., et al.: *Endocrinology 87*:744, 1970.
265. Labows, J., Swern, D., et al.: *Chem. Biol. Interact. 3*:449, 1971.
266. LaBrosse, E. H.: *J. Clin. Endocr. 30*:580, 1970.
267. Langman, M. J. S.: *Arch. Dis. Child. 45*:385, 1970.
268. Laverty, R., and Phelan, E. L.: *Proc. Univ. Otago Med. Sch. 47*:18, 1969.
269. Lawee, D.: *Canad. Med. Ass. J. 103*:1185, 1970.
270. Lawrence, A. M.: *Ann. Intern. Med. 66*:1091, 1967.
271. Leading Article: *Brit. Med. J. 2*:549, 1965.
272. Lefebvre, P. J., Cession-Fossion, A., et al.: *Lancet 2*:1366, 1966.
273. Lefkowitz, R. L., and Haber, E.: *Proc. Nat. Acad. Sci. USA 68*:1773, 1971.
274. Leitz, F. H., and Stefano, F. J. E.: *Europ. J. Pharmacol. 11*:278, 1970.
275. Leitz, F. H., and Stefano, F. J. E.: *J. Pharmacol. Exp. Ther. 178*:464, 1971.
276. Levey, G. S.: *Amer. J. Med. 50*:413, 1971.
277. Levin, E. Y., Levenberg, B., et al.: *J. Biol. Chem. 235*:2080, 1960.
278. Levine, R. J., and Sjoerdsma, A.: *J. Pharmacol. 146*:42, 1964.
279. Levine, R. J., and Strauch, B. S.: *New Eng. J. Med. 275*:946, 1966.
280. Levit, S. A., Sheps, S. G., et al.: *New Eng. J. Med. 281*:805, 1969.
281. Levitt, M., Spector, S., et al.: *J. Pharmacol. Exp. Ther. 148*:1, 1965.
282. Levy, B., and Wilkenfeld, B. E.: *Fed. Proc. 29*:1362, 1970.
283. Libet, B.: *Fed. Proc. 29*:1945, 1970.
284. Libet, B., and Tosaka, T.: *Proc. Nat. Acad. Sci. USA 67*:667, 1970.
285. Lichtenstein, L. M., Bourne, H. R., et al.: *J. Clin. Invest., 52*:698, 1973.
286. Liddle, G. W., and Hardman, J. G.: *New Eng. J. Med. 285*:560, 1971.
287. Lightman, S. L., and Iversen, L. L.: *Brit. J. Pharmacol. 37*:638, 1969.
288. Lingley, J. F., Sagerman, R. H., et al.: *New Eng. J. Med. 277*:1227, 1967.
289. Lishajko, F.: *Acta Physiol. Scand. 76*:159, 1969.
290. Liu, P. L., Krenis, L. J., et al.: *Anesthesiology 34*:4, 1971.
291. Louis, W. J., Krauss, K. R., et al.: *Circ. Res. 27*:589, 1970.
292. Louis, W. J., Spector, S., et al.: *Circ. Res. 24*:85, 1969.
293. Lovenberg, W., and Beaven, M. A.: *Biochim. Biophys. Acta 251*:452, 1971.
294. Lovenberg, W., Weissbach, H., et al.: *J. Biol. Chem. 237*:89, 1962.
295. Lucchesi, B. R.: *J. Pharmacol. Exp. Ther. 148*:94, 1965.
296. Lulu, D. J.: *Arch. Surg. 99*:641, 1969.
297. Maas, J. W.: *J. Pharmacol. Exp. Ther. 174*:369, 1970.
298. Maas, J. W., and Landis, D. H.: *J. Pharmacol. Exp. Ther. 177*:600, 1971.
299. Mandell, A. J., and Morgan, M.: *Nature* (London) *227*:75, 1970.
300. Manning, P. C., Molnar, G. D., et al.: *New Eng. J. Med. 268*:68, 1963.
301. Margolius, H. S., Geller, R., et al.: *Lancet 2*:1063, 1971.
302. Martin, W. E.: *Clin.-Alert,* No. 151, July 16, 1971.
303. Martin, W. E.: *Lancet 1*:1050, 1971.

304. Mason, G. A., Hart-Mercer, I., et al.: *Lancet 2*:322, 1957.
305. McDonald, R. H., Jr., Goldberg, L. I., et al.: *J. Clin. Invest. 43*:1116, 1964.
306. McDowell, F. H., and Lee, J. E.: *Ann. Intern. Med. 72*:751, 1970.
307. McDowell, F., Lee, J. E., et al.: *Ann. Intern. Med. 72*:29, 1970.
308. McGeer, E. G., McGeer, P. L., et al.: *Life Sci. 6*:2221, 1967.
309. Melmon, K. L.: *Calif. Med. 117*:77, 1972.
310. Melmon, K. L., Bourne, H. R., et al.: *Science 177*:707, 1972.
311. Melmon, K. L., Goldfien, A., et al.: Unpublished data.
312. Melmon, K. L., Holland, P., et al.: Unpublished data.
313. Melmon, K. L., Nies, A. S., et al.: In *Principles of Cardiology*. Austin, G., Cohen, L., et al. (eds.), Grune & Stratton, 1973 (in press).
314. Melmon, K. L., and Rosen, S. W.: *Amer. J. Med. 36*:595, 1964.
315. Melmon, K. L., Weinstein, J., et al.: *J. Clin. Invest.* 1973 (in press).
316. Melvin, K. E. W., and Tashjian, A. H., Jr.: *Proc. Nat. Acad. Sci. USA 59*:1216, 1968.
317. Melvin, K. E. W., Voelkel, E. F., et al., In *Calcitonin, 1969, Proc. of Second International Symposium, London*. Taylor, S., and Foster, G. (eds.), New York, Springer-Verlag, 1970, p. 487.
318. Mendlowitz, M., Wolf, R. L., et al.: *Amer. Heart J. 79*:401, 1970.
319. Meyer, M. B., McNay, J. L., et al.: *J. Pharmacol. Exp. Ther. 156*:186, 1967.
320. Miller, G. L., and Wynn, J.: *Arch. Intern. Med.* (Chicago) *127*:299, 1971.
321. Mindell, H. J., and Kupic, E. A.: *Amer. J. Roentgen. 106*:208, 1969.
322. Mitchell, J. R., Arias, L., et al.: *J.A.M.A. 202*:149, 1967.
323. Mitchell, J. R., Cavanaugh, J. H., et al.: *J. Clin. Invest. 49*:1596, 1970.
324. Mohammed, S., Gaffney, T. E., et al.: *J. Pharmacol. Exp. Ther. 160*:300, 1968.
325. Molinoff, P., and Axelrod, J.: *Science 164*:428, 1969.
326. Molinoff, P. B., Brimijoin, S., et al.: *Proc. Nat. Acad. Sci. USA 66*:453, 1970.
327. Molinoff, P. B., Weinshilboum, R., et al.: *J. Pharmacol. Exp. Ther. 178*:425, 1971.
328. Montalbano, F. P., Baronofsky, I. D., et al.: *J.A.M.A. 182*:264, 1962.
329. Moorhead, E. L., Caldwell, J. R., et al.: *J.A.M.A. 196*:1107, 1966.
330. Moran, N. C.: *Ann. N. Y. Acad. Sci. 139*:545, 1967.
331. Morrow, D. H., and Morrow, A. G.: *Anesthesiology 22*:537, 1961.
332. Moyano, M. B., Bergada, C., et al.: *J. Pediat. 77*:239, 1970.
333. Mueller, R. A., and Axelrod, J.: *Circ. Res. 23*:771, 1968.
334. Mueller, R. A., de Champlain, J., et al.: *Biochem. Pharmacol. 17*:2455, 1968.
335. Mueller, R. A., Thoenen, H., et al.: *Science 158*:468, 1969.
336. Mueller, R. A., Thoenen, H., et al.: *Endocrinology 86*:751, 1970.
337. Mueller, R. A., Thoenen, H., et al.: *J. Pharmacol. Exp. Ther. 169*:74, 1969.
338. Mueller, R. A., Thoenen, H., et al.: *Europ. J. Pharmacol. 10*:51, 1970.
339. Mueller, R. A., Thoenen, H., et al.: *Molec. Pharmacol. 5*:463, 1969.
340. Musacchio, J. M., D'Angelo, G. L., et al.: *Proc. Nat. Acad. Sci. USA 68*:2087, 1971.
341. Musacchio, J. M., and Goldstein, M.: *Biochem. Pharmacol. 12*:1061, 1963.
342. Nadeau, R. A., de Champlain, J., et al.: *Canad. J. Physiol. Pharmacol. 49*:36, 1971.
343. Nagatsu, T., Levitt, M., et al.: *J. Biol. Chem. 239*:2910, 1964.
344. Nagatsu, T., Rust, L. A., et al.: *Biochem. Pharmacol. 18*:1441, 1969.
345. Nagatsu, T., Yamamoto, T., et al.: *Biochim. Biophys. Acta 198*:210, 1970.
346. Nahas, G. G., Zagury, D., et al.: *Amer. J. Physiol. 213*:1186, 1967.
347. Nakamura, K., Gerald, M., et al.: *Naunyn Schmiedebergs Arch. Pharm. 268*:125, 1971.
348. Nies, A. S., In *Clinical Pharmacology: Basic Principles in Therapeutics*. Melmon, K. L., and Morrelli, H. F. (eds.), New York, The MacMillan Company, 1972, p. 142.
349. Nyback, H., and Sedvall, G.: *J. Pharmacol. Exp. Ther. 162*:294, 1968.
350. Nyback, H., and Sedvall, G.: *Europ. J. Pharmacol. 10*:193, 1970.
351. Nyback, H., Sedvall, G., et al.: *Life Sci. 6*:2307, 1967.
352. Oates, J. A., Gillespie, L., et al.: *Science 131*:1890, 1960.
353. Odell, W. D.: *Calif. Med. 117*:32, 1972.
354. Orkin, L. R.: *Clinical Management of the Patient in Shock*. Philadelphia, F. A. Davis Company, 1965, p. 193.
355. Orvis, H. H., Tamanga, I. G., et al.: *Ann. N. Y. Acad. Sci. 107*:958, 1963.
356. Osborne, M. W., Wenger, J. J., et al.: *J. Pharmacol. Exp. Ther. 178*:517, 1971.
357. Ozaki, M., Suzuki, Y., et al.: *Jap. Circ. J. 32*:1367, 1968.
358. Palaic, D., and Khairallah, P. A.: *Biochem. Pharmacol. 16*:2291, 1967.
359. Paloyan, E., Scanu, A., et al.: *J.A.M.A. 214*:1443, 1970.
360. Parks, L. C., Watanabe, A. M., et al.: *Lancet 2*:1014, 1970.
361. Paul, M. I., Kvetnansky, R., et al.: *Endocrinology 88*:338, 1971.
362. Peach, M. J., Bumpus, F. M., et al.: *J. Pharmacol. Exp. Ther. 167*:291, 1969.
363. Peaston, M. J. T., and Bianchine, J. R.: *Brit. Med. J. 1*:400, 1970.
364. Persson, T., and Waldeck, B.: *Europ. J. Pharmacol. 11*:315, 1970.
365. Pertsemlidis, D., Gitlow, S. E., et al.: *Ann. Surg. 169*:376, 1969.
366. Pinder, R. M.: *Nature* (London) *228*:358, 1970.
367. Pisano, J. J.: *Clin. Chim. Acta 5*:406, 1960.
368. Pisano, J. J., Crout, J. R., et al.: *Clin. Chim. Acta 7*:285, 1962.
369. Pohorecky, L. A., and Wurtman, R. J.: *Pharmacol. Rev. 23*:1, 1971.
370. Pohorecky, L. A., and Wurtman, R. J.: *Nature* (London) *219*:392, 1968.
371. Poisner, A. M., and Bernstein, J.: *J. Pharmacol. Exp. Ther. 177*:102, 1971.
372. Pool, P. E., Covell, J. W., et al.: *Circ. Res. 20*:349, 1967.
373. Potter, L. T., and Axelrod, J.: *J. Pharmacol. Exp. Ther. 142*:299, 1963.
374. Price, H. L., Linde, H. W., et al.: *Anesthesiology 20*:563, 1959.
375. Prout, B. J., and Wardell, W. M.: *Clin. Sci. 36*:109, 1969.
376. Pujol, J. F., Mouret, J., et al.: *Science 159*:112, 1968.
377. Quickel, K. E., Jr., Feldman, J. M., et al.: *Endocrinology 89*:1295, 1971.
378. Ramsay, I. D., and Langlands, J. H.: *Lancet 2*:126, 1961.
379. Rao, N. S.: *Lancet 2*:470, 1970.
380. Reis, D. J., and Fuxe, K.: *Proc. Nat. Acad. Sci. USA 64*:108, 1969.
381. Reivich, M., and Glowinski, J.: *Brain 90*:633, 1967.
382. Rennick, B., and Quebbemann, A.: *Amer. J. Physiol. 218*:1307, 1970.
383. Reuter, S. R.: *New Eng. J. Med. 278*:1423, 1968.
384. Richards, P., Adamson, A. R., et al.: *Lancet 2*:820, 1969.
385. Robinson, D. S., Lovenberg, W., et al.: *Biochem. Pharmacol. 17*:109, 1968.
386. Robison, G. A., Butcher, R. W., et al.: *Ann. N. Y. Acad. Sci. 139*:703, 1967.
387. Robison, G. A., Butcher, R. W., et al.: *Cyclic AMP*. New York, Academic Press Inc., 1971.
388. Robison, G. A., Butcher, R. W., et al., In *Fundamental Concepts in Drug-Receptor Interactions*. Morgan, J. A., and Triggle, D. J. (eds.), New York, Academic Press Inc., 1970, p. 59.
389. Robison, G. A., Schmidt, M. J., et al., In *Role of Cyclic AMP in Cell Function. Advances in Biochemical Psychopharmacology*. Vol. 3. Greengard, P., and Costa, E. (eds.), New York, Raven Press, 1970, p. 11.
390. Robison, G. A., and Sutherland, E. W.: *Circ. Res.* (Suppl. 1) *26 & 27*:147, 1970.
391. Rosenfeld, M. G., and O'Malley, B. W.: *Science 168*:253, 1970.
392. Rosenstein, B. J., and Engelman, K.: *J. Pediat. 63*:217, 1963.
393. Rosenthal, I. M., Greenberg, R., et al.: *Amer. J. Dis. Child. 112*:389, 1966.
394. Ross, E. J., Edwards, D., et al.: *Proc. Roy. Soc. Med. 55*:427, 1962.
395. Ross, E. J., Prichard, B. N. C., et al.: *Brit. Med. J. 1*:191, 1967.

396. Rosse, W. F., and Waldmann, T. A.: *Blood 24*:739, 1964.
397. Roth, R. H., Stjarne, L., et al.: *J. Lab. Clin. Med. 72*:397, 1968.
398. Roth, R. H., Stjarne, L., et al.: *J. Pharmacol. Exp. Ther. 158*:373, 1967.
399. Rubin, R. P.: *J. Physiol. 202*:197, 1969.
400. Rubin, R. P.: *Pharmacol. Rev. 22*:389, 1970.
401. Sacks, O. W., and Kohl, M.: *Lancet 2*:215, 1970.
402. Sacks, O. W., Messeloff, C., et al.: *Lancet 2*:1231, 1970.
403. Sandler, M.: *Lancet 1*:784, 1971.
404. Sandler, M., and Ruthven, G. R. J., In *Progress in Medicinal Chemistry*. Vol. 6. Ellis, G. P., and West, G. B. (eds.), London, Butterworth and Co., 1969, p. 200.
405. Sapira, J. D., and Bron, K.: *J. Clin. Endocr. 33*:436, 1971.
406. Sato, T., and DeQuattro, V.: *J. Lab. Clin. Med. 74*:672, 1969.
407. Sato, T., Ono, I., et al.: *Jap. Heart J. 12*:214, 1971.
408. Sato, T., Yoshinaga, K., et al.: *Jap. Heart J. 11*:423, 1970.
409. Sato, T., Yoshinaga, K., et al.: *Jap. Heart J. 7*:419, 1966.
410. Schanberg, S. M., Breese, G. R., et al.: *Biochem. Pharmacol. 17*:2006, 1968.
411. Schanberg, S. M., Schildkraut, J. J., et al.: *Biochem. Pharmacol. 17*:247, 1968.
412. Schanberg, S. M., Schildkraut, J. J., et al.: *J. Pharmacol. Exp. Ther. 157*:311, 1967.
413. Schildkraut, J. J., Winokur, A., et al.: *Science 168*:867, 1970.
414. Schimke, R. N., and Hartmann, W. H.: *Ann. Intern. Med. 63*:1027, 1965.
415. Schimke, R. N., Hartmann, W. H., et al.: *New Eng. J. Med. 279*:1, 1968.
416. Schneider, F. H.: *J. Pharmacol. Exp. Ther. 177*:109, 1971.
417. Schneider, F. H., Smith, A. D., et al.: *Brit. J. Pharmacol. 31*:94, 1967.
418. Schneider, H. P. G., and McCann, S. M.: *Endocrinology 86*:1127, 1970.
419. Schonhofer, P. S., Skidmore, I. F., et al.: *Naunyn Schmiedebergs Arch. Pharm. 273*:267, 1972.
420. Schumann, H. J.: *Klin. Wschr. 38*:11, 1960.
421. Schwarz, G. A., and Fahn, S.: *Med. Clin. N. Amer. 54*:773, 1970.
422. Sedvall, G. C., Weise, V. K., et al.: *J. Pharmacol. Exp. Ther. 159*:274, 1968.
423. Seeds, N. W.: *Science 174*:292, 1971.
424. Shanks, R. G.: *Brit. Med. J. 3*:403, 1970.
425. Shapiro, M., Simcha, A., et al.: *Israel J. Med. Sci. 2*:705, 1966.
426. Shearer, G., Melmon, K. L., et al.: *J. Exp. Med. 136*:1302, 1972.
427. Sheps, S. G., Tyce, G. M., et al.: *Circulation 34*:473, 1966.
428. Silberstein, S. D., Johnson, D. G., et al.: *Proc. Nat. Acad. Sci. USA 68*:1121, 1971.
429. Sipple, J. H.: *Amer. J. Med. 31*:163, 1961.
430. Sjoerdsma, A., In *Proc. 3rd Intl. Pharmacological Mtg., July 24-30, 1966.* Vol. 3. Oxford, Pergamon Press, 1968, p. 65.
431. Sjoerdsma, A., Engelman, K., et al.: *Lancet 2*:1092, 1965.
432. Sjoerdsma, A., Engelman, K., et al.: *Ann. Intern. Med. 65*:1302, 1966.
433. Sjoerdsma, A., Vendsalu, A., et al.: *Circulation 28*:492, 1963.
434. Skidmore, I. F., Schonhofer, P. S., et al.: *Pharmacology 6*:330, 1971.
435. Smissman, E. E., and Borchardt, R. T.: *J. Med. Chem. 14*:377, 1971.
436. Smissman, E. E., and Borchardt, R. T.: *J. Med. Chem. 14*:383, 1971.
437. Smissman, E. E., and Borchardt, R. T.: *J. Med. Chem. 14*:702, 1971.
438. Smith, A. D., In *The Interaction of Drugs and Subcellular Components on Animal Cells.* Campbell, P. N. (ed.), London, Churchill, 1968, p. 239.
439. Sourkes, T. L.: *Biochem. Med. 3*:321, 1970.
440. Sourkes, T. L., and Poirier, L. J.: *Advances Pharmacol. 6*:335, 1968.
441. Spector, S.: *Pharmacol. Rev. 18*:599, 1966.
442. Spector, S., Sjoerdsma, A., et al.: *J. Pharmacol. Exp. Ther. 147*:86, 1965.
443. Spergel, G., Bleicher, S. J., et al.: *New Eng. J. Med. 278*:803, 1968.
444. Spergel, G., Levy, L. J., et al.: *J.A.M.A. 211*:266, 1970.
445. Spitzer, R., Borrison, R., et al.: *Radiology 98*:577, 1971.
446. Sprouse, J. H., Galindo, A. H., et al.: *Anesthesiology 24*:141, 1963.
447. Stafford, A.: *Brit. J. Pharmacol. 21*:361, 1963.
448. Steel, C. M., French, E. B., et al.: *Brit. J. Haemat. 21*:413, 1971.
449. Steiner, A. L., Goodman, A. D., et al.: *Medicine 47*:371, 1968.
450. Steinsland, O. S., Passo, S. S., et al.: *Amer. J. Physiol. 218*:995, 1970.
451. Stellar, S., Mandell, S., et al.: *J. Neurosurg. 32*:275, 1970.
452. Stjarne, L.: *Acta Physiol. Scand. 67*:441, 1966.
453. Stjarne, L., Roth, R. H., et al.: *Biochem. Pharmacol. 17*:1464, 1968.
454. Stjarne, L., Von Euler, U. S., et al.: *Biochem. Pharmacol. 13*:809, 1964.
455. Strieder, N., Ziegler, E., et al.: *Biochem. Pharmacol. 17*:1553, 1968.
456. Sutherland, E. W.: *J.A.M.A. 214*:1281, 1970.
457. Sutherland, E. W., and Rall, T. W.: *Pharmacol. Rev. 12*:265, 1960.
458. Sutherland, E. W., and Robison, G. A.: *Pharmacol. Rev. 18*:145, 1966.
459. Sutow, W. W., Gehan, E. A., et al.: *Pediatrics 45*:800, 1970.
460. Svensson, T. H.: *Naunyn Schmiedebergs Arch. Pharm. 271*:111, 1971.
461. Svensson, T. H., and Waldeck, B.: *Europ. J. Pharmacol. 7*:278, 1969.
462. Szakacs, J. E., and Cannon, A.: *Amer. J. Clin. Path. 30*:425, 1958.
463. Talmadge, R. V., and Munson, P. L. (eds.): *Fourth Parathyroid Conference.* Chapel Hill, North Carolina, Excerpta Medica Foundation, 1971.
464. Tashjian, A., Howland, B., et al.: *New Eng. J. Med. 283*:890, 1970.
465. Tashjian, A. H., and Melvin, K. E. W.: *New Eng. J. Med. 279*:279, 1968.
466. Taylor, K. M., and Snyder, S. H.: *Science 168*:1487, 1970.
467. Taylor, R. J., Stubbs, C. S., et al.: *Biochem. Pharmacol. 18*:587, 1969.
468. Thoa, N. B., Eccleston, D., et al.: *J. Pharmacol. Exp. Ther. 169*:68, 1969.
469. Thoa, N. B., Johnson, D. G., et al.: *Europ. J. Pharmacol. 15*:29, 1971.
470. Thoenen, H., Haefely, W., et al.: *J. Pharmacol. Exp. Ther. 156*:246, 1967.
471. Thoenen, H., Mueller, R. A., et al.: *Nature* (London) *221*:1264, 1969.
472. Thoenen, H., Mueller, R. A., et al.: *Biochem. Pharmacol. 19*:669, 1970.
473. Thoenen, H., Mueller, R. A., et al.: *Proc. Nat. Acad. Sci. USA 65*:58, 1970.
474. Thoenen, H., Mueller, R. A., et al.: *J. Pharmacol. Exp. Ther. 169*:249, 1969.
475. Tisherman, S. E., Gregg, F. J., et al.: *J.A.M.A. 182*:152, 1962.
476. Tissot, R., Bartholini, G., et al.: *Arch. Neurol.* (Chicago) *20*:187, 1969.
477. Torchiana, M. L., Porter, C. C., et al.: *Arch. Int. Pharmacodyn. 174*:118, 1968.
478. Trendelenburg, U.: *J. Pharmacol. Exp. Ther. 125*:55, 1959.
479. Trendelenburg, U., Hohn, D., et al.: *Naunyn Schmiedebergs Arch. Pharm. 271*:59, 1971.
480. Tubiana, M., Milhaud, G., et al.: *Brit. Med. J. 4*:87, 1968.
481. Tufvesson, G.: *Scand. J. Clin. Lab. Invest. 23*:71, 1969.
482. Udenfriend, S., and Wyngaarden, J. B.: *Biochim. Biophys. Acta 20*:48, 1956.
483. Udenfriend, S., and Zaltzman-Nirenberg, P.: *Science 142*:394, 1963.
484. Ungerstedt, U.: *Europ. J. Pharmacol. 5*:107, 1968.
485. Uretsky, N. J., and Iversen, L. L.: *Nature* (London) *221*:557, 1969.
486. Vance, J. E., Buchanan, K. D., et al.: *J. Clin. Endocr. 29*:911, 1969.
487. Van Vliet, P. D., Burchell, H. B., et al.: *New Eng. J. Med. 274*:1102, 1966.
488. Vassalle, M., Mandel, W. J., et al.: *Amer. J. Physiol. 218*:115, 1970.
489. Vassalle, M., Stuckey, J. H., et al.: *Amer. J. Physiol. 217*:930, 1969.
490. *Amer. J. Dis. Child. 119*:308, 1970 (by an author group).
491. von Euler, U. S.: *Science 173*:202, 1971.
492. von Euler, U. S., Franksson, C., et al.: *Acta Physiol. Scand. 31*:1, 1954.
493. von Euler, U. S., and Hillarp, N. A.: *Nature* (London) *177*:44, 1956.

494. von Euler, U. S., and Lishajko, F.: *Acta Physiol. Scand.* 77:298, 1969.
495. von Euler, U. S., and Lishajko, F.: *Acta Physiol. Scand.* 74:501, 1968.
496. von Euler, U. S., and Lishajko, F.: *Acta Physiol. Scand.* 71:151, 1967.
497. von Euler, U. S., Lishajko, F., et al.: *Acta Physiol. Scand.* 59:495, 1963.
498. Von Studnitz, W.: *Scand. J. Clin. Lab. Invest.* (Suppl. 48) 12:58, 1960.
499. Von Studnitz, W.: *Klin. Wschr. 40*:163, 1962.
500. Von Studnitz, W.: *Pharmacol. Rev. 18*:645, 1966.
501. von Voigtlander, P. F., and Moore, K. E.: *Science 174*:408, 1971.
502. Voorhess, M. L.: *Pediat. Clin. N. Amer. 13*:3, 1966.
503. Voorhess, M. L.: *Cancer 26*:146, 1970.
504. Wallace, S., Hill, C. S., et al.: *Radiol. Clin. N. Amer. 8*:463, 1970.
505. Watanabe, A. M., Parks, L. C., et al.: *J. Clin. Invest. 50*:1322, 1971.
506. Weil-Malherbe, H., Axelrod, J., et al.: *Science 129*:1226, 1959.
507. Weil-Malherbe, H., and van Buren, J. M.: *J. Lab. Clin. Med.* 74:305, 1969.
508. Weinshilboum, R., and Axelrod, J.: *Circ. Res. 28*:307, 1971.
509. Weinshilboum, R., and Axelrod, J.: *Science 173*:931, 1971.
510. Weinstein, J., Melmon, K. L., et al.: *J. Clin. Invest.*, 1973 (in press).
511. Welch, B. L., and Welch, A. S., In *Communications in Behavioral Biology,* Part A. Vol. 3. New York, Academic Press Inc., 1969, p. 125.
512. Wermer, P.: *Amer. J. Med. 35*:205, 1963.
513. Weston, J. A., and Butler, S. L.: *Develop. Biol. 14*:246, 1966.
514. Whitby, L. G., Hertting, G., et al.: *Nature* (London) *187*:604, 1960.
515. Williams, E. D.: *Proc. Roy. Soc. Med. 59*:602, 1966a.
516. Williams, E. D., Karin, S. M. M., et al.: *Lancet 1*:22, 1968.
517. Winer, N., Chokshi, D. S., et al.: *Circ. Res. 29*:239, 1971.
518. Winkler, H., and Smith, A. D.: *Lancet 1*:793, 1968.
519. Woodhouse, N. J. Y., Gudmundsson, T. V., et al.: *J. Endocr.* (Suppl.) *45*:xvi, 1969.
520. Wurtman, R. J.: *New Eng. J. Med. 273*:637, 693, 746, 1965.
521. Wurtman, R. J.: *New Eng. J. Med. 282*:45, 1970.
522. Wurtman, R. J., and Axelrod, J.: *Science 150*:1464, 1965.
523. Wurtman, R. J., and Axelrod, J.: *Life Sci. 5*:665, 1966.
524. Wurtman, R. J., and Axelrod, J.: *J. Biol. Chem. 241*:2301, 1966.
525. Wurtman, R. J., Chou, C., et al.: *J. Pharmacol. Exp. Ther.* 174:351, 1970.
526. Wurtman, R. J., and Rose, C. M.: *Science 169*:395, 1970.
527. Wycis, H. T., Cunningham, W., et al.: *J. Neurosurg. 32*:281, 1970.
528. Yahr, M. D., Duvoisin, R. C., et al.: *Arch. Neurol. 21*:343, 1969.
529. Yamori, Y., Lovenberg, W., et al.: *Science 170*:544, 1970.
530. Yeh, B. K., McNay, J. L., et al.: *J. Pharmacol. Exp. Ther.* 168:303, 1969.
531. Yokoyama, M., and Takayasu, H.: *Urol. Int. 24*:79, 1969.
532. Zigmond, M. J., and Wurtman, R. J.: *J. Pharmacol. Exp. Ther. 172*:416, 1970.
533. Zuspan, F. P.: *J. Clin. Endocr. 30*:357, 1970.

CHAPTER 6

The Testes

By C. Alvin Paulsen

INTRODUCTION

The development of specific, sensitive radioimmunoassay and competitive protein-binding methods for measuring the gonadotropin and sex-steroid levels present in serum have vastly improved our understanding of testicular control mechanisms. This information, in combination with structure-function correlative data derived from testicular biopsy specimens, including chromosomal analyses, is progressively removing the uncertainties that surround the pathogenesis of male hypogonadism.*

This section will deal with testicular physiology and the diagnosis and treatment of disorders in which fetal *somatic* development has been essentially normal. The reader is referred to Chapter 8 for the important embryologic and clinical discussion of sex differentiation and gonadal development. Reference should also be made to the reviews of Smith (1) and of Rimoin and Schimke (2) to gain appreciation of the numerous syndromes involving somatic and gonadal disorders present in the prepuberal and adolescent male.

Finally, because of its social importance, approaches to male contraception will be discussed.

PHYSIOLOGIC ASPECTS OF TESTICULAR FUNCTION

Histology: Stages, Cycles, and Duration of Spermatogenesis; Role of Sertoli Cells; Developmental Considerations; Pituitary-Gonadal Control Mechanisms

The testes serve two roles, one *hormonal* and the other *reproductive*. The first involves the synthesis and secretion of testosterone by the interstitial cells of Leydig, which are found interspersed in groups between the seminiferous tubules (Fig. 6–1, *A*). The second function involves spermatogenesis, which is the development and maturation of the germ cells in the epithelium of the seminiferous tubules. From the spermatogonia, which line the basement membrane of the tubules, through the spermatocyte and spermatid series to the mature spermatozoa, which are seen nearest the lumen, spermatogenesis is an active and orderly process in the normal adult male.

Clermont's studies have paved the way for a much clearer understanding of human spermatogenesis (3). He has demonstrated that the germinal epithelium is arranged into six stages (Fig. 6–2). Each stage is composed of a specific cellular constellation representing a particular degree of maturation. Altogether stages I-VI*, in sequence, constitute the total functional unit. This unit has been designated as one cycle. If newly formed, pale, type A spermatogonia are followed, maturation progresses in order through each stage several times before the spermatogonia finally emerge as mature spermatozoa.

In contrast to that of other mammals, the human germinal epithelium in individual seminiferous

---

*Hypogonadism is defined as a decrease in testicular function. This may involve testosterone secretion or spermatogenesis or both. Hypogonadism may be due to an intratesticular disease, or it may be secondary to pituitary or hypothalamic failure.

*The original numbers for each stage were retained by Clermont, even though later kinetic studies indicated that spermatogenesis should be defined as beginning in stage V.

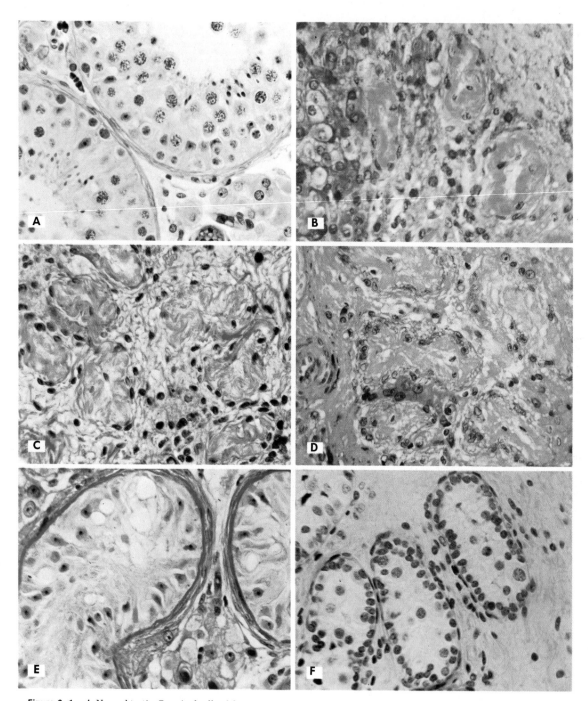

Figure 6–1. *A,* Normal testis. Germinal cells of the seminiferous tubules are undergoing active spermatogenesis. Sertoli cells; type A, B spermatogonia; zygotene, pachytene primary spermatocytes, and various types of spermatids can be readily identified. (Refer to Figure 6–2 for characteristics of each cell type.) The basement membrane and tunica propria surround the tubules. Groups of Leydig cells may be seen in the interstitial spaces and are characterized by a prominent nucleolus and abundant cytoplasm (× 600).

B, Klinefelter testis. In this example, the tubules (blue) are devoid of germinal or Sertoli cells. The tubular membranes have undergone complete hyalinization. Leydig cells are in adenomatous "clumps." A portion of one such aggregate may be seen in the left-hand portion of the photomicrograph (× 600).

C, Klinefelter testis. In this case, the tubules are characteristically hyalinized but the Leydig cells are diffusely spread throughout the biopsy specimen (× 600).

D, Postmumps orchitis testis. Complete hyalinization of the seminiferous tubules has occurred. Although not depicted, Leydig cells are grouped in adenomatous "clumps" similar to those observed in the usual case of Klinefelter's syndrome. However, in contrast to the picture noted in Klinefelter's syndrome (*B* and *C*), elastic and reticular fibers are present around the thickened tunica propria (× 600).

tubules lacks a uniform wave of spermatogenesis; thus when a single tubule is examined in cross section, two or more stages may be present side by side in pie-shaped fashion.

The duration of human spermatogenesis has been determined by Heller and Clermont, who used tritiated thymidine and autoradiographic techniques (4). They found that each cycle lasts about 16 days and that the individual stages occupy different periods in any given cycle. It appears that the beginning of spermatogenesis is at a point midway through stage V. This is when the pale, type A spermatogonia first appear. The end of spermatogenesis is some four cycles later, midway through stage II. The interval is 74 ± 4-5 days. The time periods for spermatogenesis vary from species to species. This should be kept in mind when interpreting basic studies on spermatogenesis. In subhuman primates, the duration is 36-39 days (5). In the mouse and the ram, the intervals are 33.5 and 49 days, respectively.

The Sertoli cells also line the basement membrane of the seminiferous tubule. They contain considerable glycogen in their cytoplasm and are considered to serve a supportive and nutritive function for the germinal epithelium. A hormone-secreting role has also been attributed to them. Although direct evidence for this is lacking, electron microscopic studies have revealed that the organelles that could be involved in such a function are present (6). Further ultrastructure studies have emphasized the close role between the germ cells in varying degrees of maturation and the Sertoli cell (7, 8) by demonstrating that the Sertoli cell encloses the primary spermatocytes, spermatids, and probably the more mature spermatogonia.

Another important observation is that an extensive lymphatic sinusoidal system lies within the interstitial spaces (9). The Leydig cells are more closely related to these lymphatics than to the venules; from this it can be assumed that the lymphatic system plays an important role in the transport of testosterone to the seminiferous tubules, epididymis, and other portions of the immediate reproductive tract. The spermatic veins undoubtedly play the major role in delivering testosterone to more distant target sites. Estimates of human intratesticular testosterone levels (normal adult males) approximate 55,300 ng./100 g. (assume 1 g. = 1 ml. plasma) (10), lymphatic fluid (rams) 33,000 ng./100 ml. (11), spermatic vein 49,700 ng./100 ml. (12), and peripheral venous blood 670 ng./100 ml.

(13). Both spermatogenesis and testosterone secretion are under control of the gonadotropic hormones secreted by the anterior pituitary. Follicle stimulating hormone (FSH) acts on the germinal epithelium to promote full spermatogenesis and interstitial cell stimulating hormone (ICSH)*—or, as it is better known today, luteinizing hormone (LH) induces the Leydig cells to secrete androgens and estrogens. In the male, the action of prolactin (HPr) on the testis is unknown (Fig. 6–3).

The gonadotropins are glycoproteins composed of α and β subunits. Intact LH cross-reacts with human chorionic gonadotropin (hCG) in immunoassay systems, because the α subunits of each gonadotropin share similar antigenic properties. When antisera to purified β subunits of hCG are used, assay specificity is improved. The β subunits are antigenically specific for their respective hormones, e.g., anti-β subunit hCG does not cross-react with LH. In the diagnosis and management of trophoblastic disease or testicular germinal cell carcinomas, an understanding of this concept is very important (Ch. 2 and 7).

Leydig cells can be identified in the fetal testicular interstitium. Sometime in the first neonatal month they revert to mesenchymal cells. This initial development is most likely due to the influence of maternal chorionic gonadotropin, which is known to act like LH in inducing Leydig cell stimulation. This hypothesis is supported by van Wagenen and Simpson, who observed that the number and differentiation of fetal Leydig cells reach maximum between the third and fourth months of gestation (14) and thereafter regress. This sequence corresponds to the titer of chorionic gonadotropin during pregnancy, which reaches its highest value during the third month.

New information based on the sensitive assay systems for serum FSH and LH determinations clearly shows that these gonadotropins are secreted in small amounts during the prepuberal years. Moreover, the hypothalamic-pituitary-testicular axis is operational to a limited degree during this period. For example, agonadal prepuberal boys exhibit higher titers of FSH and LH than do intact prepuberal boys of the same age (15–19).

---

*Traditionally ICSH refers to the gonadotropic hormone in the male which stimulates the Leydig cells, and LH refers to the gonadotropin which acts on the ovary. Since these "two" hormones are undoubtedly the same chemically, the term LH will be used throughout the text to avoid confusion.

Figure 6–1. **Continued**
  E, Sertoli-cell-only testis. The seminiferous tubules are somewhat reduced in size but the tubular membranes are not sclerosed. Sertoli cells, with their characteristic nucleoli and brush borders, are the only cells within the tubules. The Leydig cells appear normal (× 600).
  F, Hypogonadotropic eunuchoid testis. Typical immature seminiferous tubules containing undifferentiated germinal epithelium can be seen. Mesenchymal precursors of Leydig cells are interspersed between the tubules (× 600).
  Photomicrograph of specimen depicted in *A* was stained with iron hematoxylin and eosin; the remainder were stained with Masson modified trichrome.
  The author acknowledges the assistance of Dr. John Jewell of Ayerst Laboratories in the preparation of this plate.

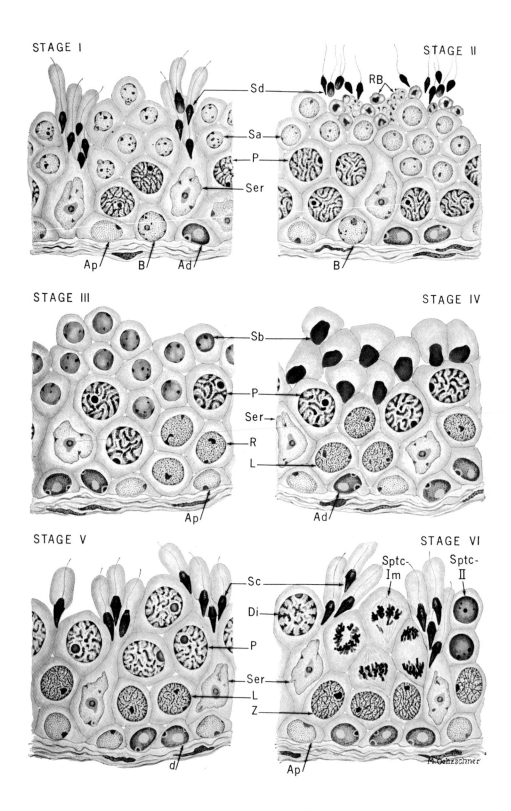

Figure 6–2.   The six stages of spermatogenesis. Together these stages represent one cycle of the germinal epithelium. Ser, Sertoli cell; Ad and Ap, *dark* and *pale* type A spermatogonia; B, type B spermatogonia; R, resting or preleptotene spermatocytes; L, leptotene spermatocytes; Z, zygotene spermatocytes; P, pachytene spermatocytes; Im, primary spermatocytes in division; II, secondary spermatocytes; Sa, Sb, Sc, Sd, spermatids in various steps of spermiogenesis; and RB, residual bodies. Unlike in other mammals, the stages of spermatogenesis in the human are intermixed within the same tubule. (From Clermont, Y.: *Amer. J. Anat. 112*:35, 1963.)

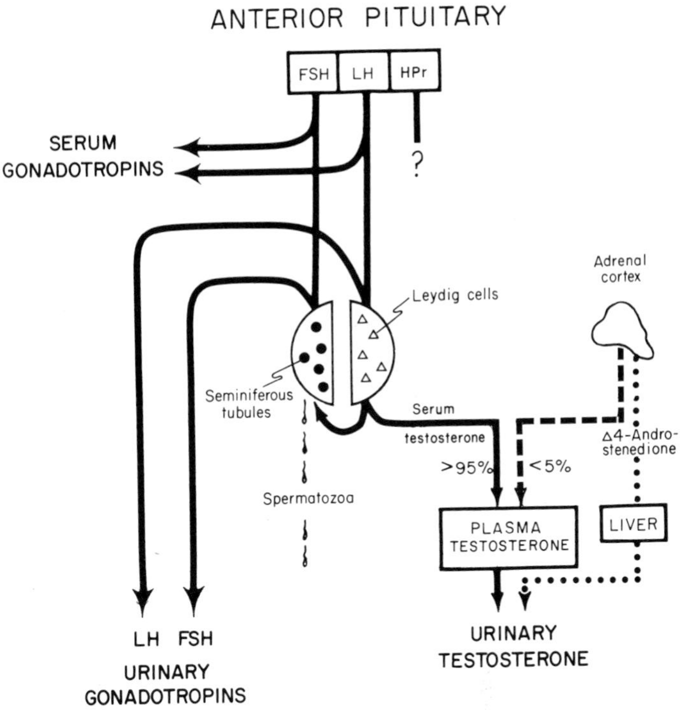

Figure 6-3. The pituitary-gonadal axis of the normal male. In contrast to that in the female, the function of human prolactin (HPr) in the male is not known. LH stimulates the Leydig cells to mature and secrete testosterone. FSH acts on the germinal epithelium to promote full spermatogenesis. Also shown is the relationship between the testes and the adrenal cortex with respect to the formation of plasma and urinary testosterone "pools." Normally the adrenal cortex secretes little testosterone into the plasma. Similarly, the Δ^4-androstenedione derived from the adrenal cortex forms only a small portion of the total urinary testosterone moiety. Before appearing in the urine, adrenal cortical Δ^4-androstenedione is transformed by the liver into testosterone glucuronide.

Castration performed in animals before puberty also raises the serum gonadotropin levels (20).

The histologic pattern of the prepuberal testis is relatively stable until approximately age 6 (21–23). From then until the onset of puberty, minimal growth changes occur. The seminiferous tubules acquire a lumen, and the gonocytes start to proliferate, the nuclei organizing into two layers. During this period, the interstitial cells change only slightly.

At the time of puberty, which normally varies from age 9–16, pituitary gonadotropin secretion increases, stimulating testicular maturation. LH acts directly on the interstitial mesenchymal elements, causing them to secrete testosterone and estrogen as they are developing into mature Leydig cells. FSH acts on the seminiferous tubules to induce and maintain normal spermatogenesis.

When introduced into male animals (24), radioactive labeled LH localizes in the Leydig cells and to a lesser extent in the cells of the peritubular membranes. With respect to FSH, specific testicular binding has been demonstrated, but the site or sites of action have not been precisely defined (25). It may be that Sertoli cells are the exclusive targets. On the other hand, additional portions of the seminiferous tubular complex may also be involved (26, 27). At no time does the maturing germ cell appear to concentrate FSH. There is evidence that FSH increases testicular adenyl cyclase (28, 29), and protein synthesis is stimulated within the seminiferous tubules by FSH administration (30, 31). These important basic studies still leave unresolved the question as to which steps of human spermatogenesis are *FSH-dependent* and which are *FSH-independent.*

It is interesting to note that certain data indicate that FSH is synergistic to the action of LH on Leydig cell steroidogenesis (32, 33, 34). Perhaps the same holds true for spermatogenesis, with reversed roles for FSH and LH in terms of importance.

According to present concepts, the mechanism for LH action on the seminiferous tubules would be via stimulation of endogenous testosterone secretion. Indeed, the importance of testosterone as a regulator of human spermatogenesis is probably greater than has been appreciated—witness the high intratesticular testosterone concentration (p. 325) and the extensive animal data which bear on this point (35).

In addition to the development of the secondary sex characteristics, such as growth of facial and body hair, enlargement of the external genitalia, lowering of the voice, recession of scalp hair, and development of muscle (Table 6–1), testosterone also stimulates growth of the seminiferous tubule. Estrogens are also secreted by the testis (36, 37, 38); presumably this takes place within the Leydig cells (39). The role of estrogens in the function of the male reproductive tract is not clear.

If gonadotropin secretion ceases after puberty, as in severe adult panhypopituitarism, secondary testicular atrophy follows. The germinal elements slough, the germinal epithelium atrophies, and finally the seminiferous tubules become totally hyalinized. Likewise, Leydig cell function ceases, and these cells revert to fibroblastic elements (Fig. 6–4).

When the seminiferous tubular and Leydig cell functions of the testes are primarily damaged to a severe degree or absent, increased FSH and LH

TABLE 6–1. PUBERAL CHANGES DUE TO TESTOSTERONE SECRETION

External genitalia
  The penis and scrotum increase in size and become pigmented. Rugal folds appear in the scrotal skin.

Hair growth
  Mustache and beard develop and scalp line undergoes recession. Pubic hair grows upward into the typical diamond-shape pattern of the male escutcheon. Axillary, body, extremity, and anal hair appears.

Linear growth
  Until puberty, linear growth is fairly stable at about 2 inches per year. At puberty there is a growth spurt which increases the rate to about 3 inches per year.

Accessory sex organs
  The prostate becomes palpable and the other organs, such as the seminal vesicles, enlarge over the next 4 to 5 years. Secretory activity develops.

Voice
  The voice pitch is lowered because of enlargement of the larynx and thickening of the vocal cords.

Psyche
  More aggressive attitudes are manifest; libido and sexual potentia develop.

titers are found in the serum and urine. Examples of this condition include patients with Klinefelter's syndrome and ones with functional prepuberal castration. Selective loss of testicular function, as in severe damage to the seminiferous tubules with retention of normal Leydig cell function, results in elevated FSH levels and normal LH levels, e.g., Sertoli-cell-only syndrome (Fig. 6–5).

As a general rule, the endocrine system is regulated by negative feedback; control of testicular function appears to fall into this category. According to the negative feedback concept, the target gland regulates the secretion of its pituitary tropic hormone by means of the hormone or hormones it produces. If the target gland increases the production of its hormone, then the pituitary is inhibited. On the other hand, when the production of hormone by the target gland decreases or is absent, the secretion of its tropic hormone is increased.

In the testis, the interrelationship between LH and testosterone appears to be reasonably straightforward (Fig. 6–5). When Leydig cells are damaged so that testosterone levels *decrease*, LH levels *increase*. On the other hand, when testosterone levels *increase*, LH levels *decrease*. The problem lies in understanding the regulatory mechanism for FSH secretion. Theoretically, the seminiferous tubules should produce a separate hormone that acts on the pituitary to control FSH levels. Unfortunately, the existence of such a substance has not been established. In light of this uncertainty, an inspection of the various theories put forth to account for FSH secretion seems worthwhile.

Basically two hypotheses have been proposed: (1) negative feedback, and (2) utilization.

With respect to negative feedback, Mottram and Cramer (40), followed by McCullagh (41), suggested that the germinal epithelium secreted a nonandrogenic, nonestrogenic, water-soluble substance designated "inhibin" which affected gonadotropin secretion. Later del Castillo et al. (42) proposed that the Sertoli cells secreted an estrogen that controlled "FSH" secretion. Howard et al. (43) modified this concept by suggesting that Δ^5-pregnenolone was the inhibitory substance. Lacy (44) and Johnsen (45, 46) each have outlined a more elaborate scheme. Lacy hypothesized that the Sertoli cells phagocytize the residual bodies shed by the mature spermatids and are involved in FSH control. He suggested that the residual bodies contained a precursor substance which enabled the Sertoli cells to secrete the final inhibitory product. The nature of this compound Lacy has not identified.

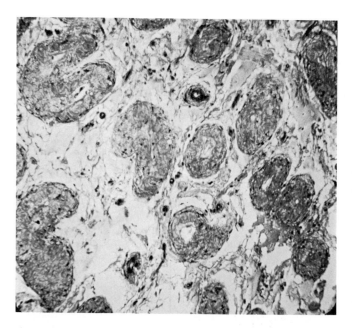

Figure 6–4. Postpuberal pituitary failure testis. In this patient effective gonadotropin and ACTH secretion was not present. Complete hyalinization of the seminiferous tubules is evident. Leydig cells are absent and only a few fibroblasts can be seen in the interstitium ($\times$ 250).

PITUITARY-GONADAL AXIS IN NORMAL AND SELECTED EXAMPLES OF HYPOGONADAL MALES

Figure 6–5. The influence of pituitary and testicular function on gonadotropin secretion and excretion. When hypothalamic-pituitary function is defective, as in the congenital disorder hypogonadotropic eunuchoidism, the gonadotropic hormones are not secreted. Testicular function is not stimulated, the testis remains immature, and serum and urinary gonadotropins are below normal levels. When the testes are primarily damaged so that the germinal epithelium *and* Leydig cells are involved, as in the functional prepuberal castrate, FSH and LH levels in blood and urine are increased. If the testes are damaged selectively, such as in the majority of patients with Sertoli-cell-only syndrome, only FSH levels are increased.

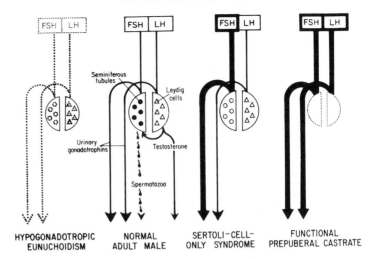

HYPOGONADOTROPIC EUNUCHOIDISM   NORMAL ADULT MALE   SERTOLI-CELL-ONLY SYNDROME   FUNCTIONAL PREPUBERAL CASTRATE

Johnsen also focused on the later phases of spermatogenesis. He proposed that either the phagocytized residual bodies or the mature spermatozoa alter the secretory function of the Sertoli cells by direct contact. This results in the release of estrogens into the circulation, which in turn inhibits FSH. To comply with these two conjectures, an inverse relationship between spermatogenesis (especially the later stages) and FSH secretion should exist. Leonard et al. (47) (Fig. 6–6) and de Kretser et al. (48) have documented that such a relationship does not exist. Although their conclusions reject the feedback theory as interpreted by Lacy, Johnsen, and Franchimont et al. (49), they do not exclude the Sertoli cell as a so-called "independent station" to control FSH (Fig. 6–7).

With regard to utilization, Heller and Nelson (50) and Heller et al. (51) proposed that the germinal epithelium used up FSH in some way, thereby controlling FSH levels encountered in the pituitary, serum, and urine. Accordingly, if the testes were primarily damaged, less "utilization" would occur. This would result in increased serum and urine FSH titers.

The utilization theory contains major flaws. First, it is not likely that the testes metabolize the necessary quantity of gonadotropin required to fit the concept. For example, in the case of the ovary, the LH gradient across that gland is small (52, 53). Second, it is difficult to conceive that "utilization" alone could inform the pituitary gland as to the functional status of the testis.

This discussion does not imply that testosterone and estrogens cannot suppress pituitary FSH secretion, for they do have this ability at pharmacologic levels, and at levels still within the physiologic range, modulation of FSH and LH occurs (54). However, LH secretion is more readily depressed by testosterone administration than is FSH secretion (55, 56). This seems to hold true for each of the known androgens and estrogens. On the other hand, the inhibiting substance from the seminiferous tubules should readily inhibit FSH secretion and exert minimal changes in LH secretion at physiologic or near physiologic dose levels.

Our understanding of the control mechanisms for LH and FSH secretion has been further complicated by the isolation and purification of LH releasing hormone (LHRH) from the hypothalamus (porcine) (57). Matsuo et al. (58, 59) synthesized this decapeptide after identifying its structure. Kastin et al. (60) and numerous workers have demonstrated that synthetic LHRH releases both LH and FSH into the circulation of men and women. To date, a separate FSH releasing hormone has not been isolated. Earlier animal studies with less pure hypothalamic extracts suggested that such a hormone exists. It is clear that our perception of the highly integrated hypothalamic-pituitary-gonadal axis will require further investigation,

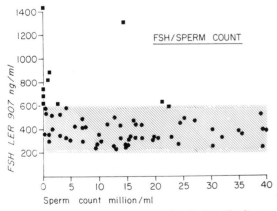

Figure 6–6. Mean sperm counts of patients with oligo- or azoöspermia compared with their serum FSH titers. (FSH levels are expressed with reference to standards of the National Pituitary Agency. LER 907 refers to the fact that the preparation was prepared in the laboratories of L. E. Reichert.) Cross-hatched area indicates the normal adult male range for serum FSH. Note that the second highest FSH titer was present in a male with 15 million/ml. mean sperm density. (From Leonard, J. M., et al.: *J. Clin. Endocr. 34*:209, 1972.)

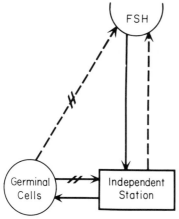

Figure 6–7. Schematic depiction of "independent" station concept. FSH interacts with the independent station (IS), which in turn imparts energy to germ cell maturation. Specific germ cells or germ cells *in toto* do not directly influence IS or FSH secretion control mechanisms. The integrity of IS controls FSH secretion. Sertoli cells are best candidates for role of IS. (From Leonard, J. M., et al.: *J. Clin. Endocr. 34*:209, 1972.)

and considerable conceptual modification will be necessary before all the pieces fall into place (Ch. 2, 7, and 12).

Testicular Steroidogenesis, Intracellular Metabolism and Action of Testosterone and Dihydrotestosterone, General Aspects of Androgen Metabolism, Clinical Effects of Testosterone

Testosterone, the principal androgen produced by the Leydig cells, is a 17β-hydroxylated, C-19 steroid (61, 62). Studies on steroidogenesis indicate that similar precursors are involved in the synthesis of testicular androgens, ovarian steroids, and adrenal corticosteroids (63–69). In the testis, two pathways exist from Δ^5-pregnenolone to testosterone (Fig. 6–8) (66, 69, 70). LH apparently acts on a specific Leydig cell adenyl cyclase to initiate androgen production. Cholesterol synthesis takes place on or near the smooth endoplasmic reticulum; cholesterol is then transported to the mitochondria, where pregnenolone is generated (71). This process apparently stimulates microsomal activity, and testosterone emerges as the final product. Testosterone is transported in the plasma by a β-globulin designated testosterone binding globulin (TBG). It is estimated that about 97–99% of the circulating testosterone is bound, the remainder present as a free component. This latter fraction is assumed to be the metabolically active portion of the total testosterone level (72, 73, 74).

When testosterone reaches the cells of the target glands, such as the prostate, an enzyme, 5α-reductase, transforms testosterone into dihydrotestosterone (DHT). This reaction takes place in the cytoplasm and nuclear membrane. DHT is rapidly attached to a specific binding protein that possesses a high affinity for DHT. This is in contrast to the low affinity that exists between testosterone

and its binding protein (TBG) (75). With respect to the next metabolic event, O'Malley has concluded that steroids participate in the transcription of new DNA (76). During these intracellular processes, a metabolite, androstanediol, is formed. Although the role of that steroid has not been assigned, testosterone and DHT appear to be the important androgens.

Testosterone does not behave exclusively as a prehormone for DHT, since not all androgen target tissues contain the enzyme, 5α-reductase. For example, testosterone exerts a "direct" effect on muscle and bone. These tissues also respond to DHT; DHT has some limitation in its androgenic properties, however, since male mating behavior cannot be restored when DHT is administered to the castrated male rat. On the other hand, testosterone administration does restore male behavior.

Tissues other than Leydig cells have the ability to transform steroid precursors, such as acetate and cholesterol, to testosterone as well as to change testosterone into various metabolites (9, 77, 78, 79). These sites include the seminiferous tubules and epididymis. The significance of these extra Leydig cell sources of testosterone production remains to be determined. The most likely reason for this phenomenon is to ensure a high local concentration of testosterone rather than to be important to the systemic androgenic pool. This contention is based on data which show that the combined contribution of these sites to the plasma testosterone pool is less than 5% of that secreted by the

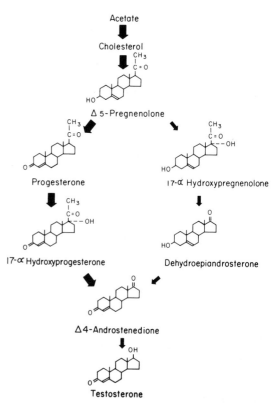

Figure 6–8. Steroid pathways for testosterone production by the testis. The heavy arrows indicate the preferred pathway.

testes, except when adrenal cortical hyperplasia or an adrenal cortical tumor is present (80).

When androgen target tissues do not respond to endogenous or exogenous testosterone, a state of end-organ resistance or insensitivity exists. This may be expressed selectively; for example, the relative lack of facial hair present in the American Indian. Alternatively, the entire body may be involved, e.g., patients with testicular feminization syndrome (Ch. 8). Bullock and Bardin have performed studies in rats and mice (both in normal strains and in strains exhibiting the equivalent of human testicular feminization) that provide an explanation for target tissue resistance to testosterone and other androgens. It appears that in this genetic disorder there is an absence of cytosol receptor proteins for testosterone and DHT (81). Therefore, these androgens cannot initiate their metabolic functions within the cell. Previously, investigators had considered that an absence of the enzyme, 5α-reductase, was responsible for the testosterone resistance, but later experiments have failed to substantiate that proposal (Ch. 8).

DHT is synthesized by the testis in addition to being produced within androgen target tissues. The testicular contribution is probably less than 10% of the total DHT produced daily. The testis also secretes at least two additional androgens, namely Δ^4-androstenedione and dehydroepiandrosterone. These steroids are less potent than are testosterone or DHT.

Hudson's studies demonstrated that spermatic vein blood from normal adult males contained testosterone, Δ^4-androstenedione, and dehydroepiandrosterone in concentrations of 47.9, 2.9, and 4.5 μg./100 ml., respectively (12). In contrast, the adrenal cortex secretes dehydroepiandrosterone and Δ^4-androstenedione as its major androgens (Ch. 5). The mean testicular testosterone production rate for normal males is approximately 7.0 mg./day.

It has been suggested that alterations in testicular steroidogenesis analogous to those encountered in congenital adrenal hyperplasia might explain the decreased testosterone production present in such genetic conditions as Klinefelter's syndrome. To date, proof of this is lacking. On the other hand, Biglieri's studies in a hypogonadal female show that enzyme deficiency can be responsible for gonadal disease (82). His patient exhibited hypertension, and sexual development was absent. Since her adrenals secreted corticosterone and desoxycorticosterone but no cortisol, and her ovaries failed to produce estrogens in the face of high endogenous gonadotropins, a 17β-hydroxylase deficiency existed in both organs. Additional examples of this syndrome have been reported, including partial enzymatic deficiencies in males. These patients all have ambiguous genitalia, as one would expect in a disorder with androgen deficiency present in early fetal life. Another example of an enzymatic disorder leading to pseudohermaphrodism is the abnormality observed in 17β-hydroxysteroid dehydrogenase deficiency (83, 84) (Ch. 8).

Testosterone is secreted episodically throughout the day, so that multiple peaks can be observed if frequent blood sampling is performed (85). Still uncertain is the question whether testosterone secretion follows a diurnal pattern which is physiologically important. In part, this uncertainty is based on the fact that most studies did not require sufficiently frequent blood sampling (12, 86, 87). Moreover, Lipsett has suggested that the high metabolic clearance rate for testosterone, coupled with the fact that there are significant changes in hepatic blood flow even during mild exercise, may mask diurnal changes in testosterone secretion (88). Finally, data do not exist with respect to the pattern of "free" testosterone levels throughout a time period such as 24 hours.

Total serum testosterone levels remain in the normal adult male range with advancing age (12). However, if the "apparent free testosterone concentration" (AFTC) is measured by equilibrium dialysis methods, decreased titers are noted in aged men (89). This agrees with data demonstrating a decreased testosterone clearance rate (90) and consequently a calculated lower production rate for older men (91) (p. 346, Male Climacteric).

Other instances associated with depressed testosterone levels include mental stresses (92) and states of peer dominance (93). The latter study was performed in monkeys. It has also been reported that surgical stress may lower testosterone levels (94).

The last stages of androgen metabolism require discussion, since the details are relevant to the diagnostic approach to evaluating Leydig cell function. Testosterone and DHT are broken down into various metabolites, mainly 17-KS (95–99). Following this, the 17-KS are conjugated with glucuronic and sulfuric acid and then excreted in the urine. In contrast to estrogens, the testosterone metabolites are found in the bile or feces in only small amounts (100, 101).

Of the total urinary 17-KS production, the testes account for approximately 30%. The adrenal cortex contributes the remaining 70%. Androsterone, etiocholanolone, and epiandrosterone are mainly derived from testosterone metabolism, whereas *dehydro*epiandrosterone primarily emanates from the adrenal cortex. Because of the metabolic interconversion between testicular and adrenal androgens and nonandrogenic 17-KS, the origin of any given urinary 17-KS is lost (102, 103).

It should be remembered that not all 17-KS are androgens, and not all androgens are 17-KS. For example, etiocholanolone has no androgenic activity, and testosterone is not a 17-KS. As mentioned previously, the androgenic effect of the total adrenal steroid output is considerably less than that of the testes. Therefore, the adrenal cortex is not capable of substituting for normal Leydig cell function if the latter is impaired.

Testosterone is also converted to estrogenic substances, mainly estradiol and estrone (98, 104, 105). This represents a relatively minor aspect of its overall metabolism, and whether this conversion has physiologic significance is not known.

With the onset of puberty, testosterone stimulates the development of the male secondary sex characteristics (106). Thus pubic hair begins to grow at the base of the penis as one of the first signs of beginning puberty. Other changes that occur at this time are listed in Table 6–1.

The potent protein anabolic action exerted by testosterone accounts mainly for the growth changes noted at puberty and maintains the muscle mass and bone tissue of the adult male. Retention of nitrogen, potassium, phosphorus, and calcium is a manifestation of this action. Studies in dogs indicate that both *increased* protein synthesis and *decreased* amino acid catabolism are responsible for the nitrogen-retaining effect of testosterone (107).

Decreased creatinuria is observed during testosterone therapy, which probably indicates that more creatine is available to ATP to form creatine phosphate. This substance is important in carbohydrate metabolism of muscle.

When elaboration of the male hormone ceases after puberty has been completed, regression of the secondary sex characteristics occurs very slowly. This is due to the fact that abrupt, complete, Leydig cell failure is uncommon, except in surgical or traumatic castration, and to the fact that very little androgen is required to maintain the secondary sex characteristics once they have fully developed. Thus it may be 10–20 years after the onset of the testicular androgen failure before the deficiency is obvious upon clinical examination. Other evidences of androgen withdrawal include increased irritability, mental depression, hot flashes, more passive behavior, and decreased libido and sexual potential. After orchiectomy most, if not all, of the features of androgen deficiency are invariably present. It is of interest that an occasional orchiectomized patient, in the absence of replacement therapy, will retain minimal libido and sexual potential, especially if heterosexual patterns have been well established.

METHODS FOR THE DIAGNOSIS OF HYPOGONADISM

Clinical Examination

If testicular failure occurs before puberty and if testosterone production is not normal, the puberal changes enumerated in Table 6–1 will not develop. Thus the patient will display obvious features of eunuchoidism (Table 6–2). In addition to sexual infantilism, the delay in epiphysial closure allows continued long-bone growth, which results in the typical eunuchoidal habitus.

The picture described usually presents no problem in clinical recognition. However, the detection of Leydig cell failure occurring after puberty may be difficult unless the testicular damage is severe, or unless sufficient time has elapsed to allow regression of the male secondary sex characteristics, or both. The symptoms of impotence and decreased libido that develop after Leydig cell failure are also encountered frequently in emotional disorders. This tends to limit their value as diagnostic points

TABLE 6–2. CLINICAL FEATURES OF EUNUCHOIDISM

Eunuchoidal skeleton
  Span more than 2 inches greater than height. Soles to symphysis more than 2 inches greater than symphysis to head. Delay in closure of epiphyses.

Lack of adult male hair distribution
  Sparse or absent facial and body hair. Scant pubic and axillary hair. Failure of scalp hair to recede.

High-pitched voice

Infantile genitalia
  Small penis, testes, and scrotum.

Poor muscular development
  Decreased muscle mass. Diminished endurance and strength.

(see Adult Leydig Cell Failure). When isolated damage to the seminiferous tubules occurs postpuberally, the testes become small and soft, and infertility is usually the chief complaint. Normally the testis measures 4.6 cm. in length (range 3.6–5.5) and 2.6 cm. in width (range 2.1–3.2). Age per se does not influence testicular size; therefore, the significance of small testes in men over 50 years is the same as in younger adults (108).

Examination of the Seminal Fluid

Functional evaluation of the seminiferous tubules is easily accomplished by seminal fluid analysis. This is specific, provided that the ductal system has developed normally and has not been altered by infection.

The only satisfactory way to obtain seminal fluid is to have the patient masturbate into a clean glass container and then submit the fresh specimen for examination within an hour. Condom sheaths cannot be used, since sperm motility decreases markedly upon contact with the sheath. Interrupted coitus as a means of collecting the seminal fluid is also unsatisfactory since the initial portion of the ejaculate, which contains the highest density of sperm, may be lost.

Immediately after ejaculation, coagulation of the seminal fluid occurs, followed in 15–30 minutes by liquefaction. In some specimens, liquefaction is incomplete or fails to occur. To these specimens several drops of a solution of 5% alpha-amylase in Locke's solution may be added to break up the coagulum (109). This can be done without harming motility.

Estimation of motility is made by examining a drop of undiluted seminal fluid, using the 40× objective and recording the percentage of motile forms. The quality of motility can be graded from 1 to 3. Spermatozoa with grade 3 motility tend to move rapidly across the field, whereas spermatozoa with grade 1 motility remain in one spot, exhibiting motion of the tail only. For research purposes, more elaborate techniques have been devised for evaluating motility (110). Seminal fluid volume may be determined by use of a suitable graduated cylinder.

Sperm counts are made in the following manner: draw thoroughly mixed seminal fluid up to the 0.5 mark of a white cell pipet, then dilute to the 11 mark with 1% Chloramine-T solution. Methylene blue, in a small amount, may be added to effect better contrast. Shake for 2 minutes, spread the diluted specimen over a 0.1-mm. deep Neubauer counting chamber, and count the total number of sperm in 32 large squares. Add 5 zeros to the total to obtain the number of spermatozoa per ml. Make note of the percentage of abnormal forms (111, 112). The normal volume of the ejaculate ranges from 2.5 to slightly over 6.0 ml. Motile forms should represent 60% or more of the total, with the majority of these being of grade 3 quality. The normal range for sperm counts is usually considered to be from 50 million to over 100 million/ml.

MacLeod, however, suggests that fertility is not impaired until the density drops to below 20 million/cm.[3] (113, 114). More than half the sperm should have a normal morphology.

For greater accuracy and efficiency, an electronic particle counter may be used to estimate sperm concentration (115, 116). Although the apparatus is relatively expensive, many clinical laboratories use this method for counting blood cells. In order to process seminal fluid, the 50 μ aperture tube is used instead of the 100 μ tube.

The importance of assessing the sperm morphology should not be overlooked — for example, the relationship between an increase in tapered forms and a varicocele that exists in some infertile men (p. 36, Male Infertility). Briefly, the seminal fluid smear is prepared similar to the way a blood smear is made. After the slide is air-dried, the smear is stained with PAS. For normal males, the per cent distribution of the various sperm shapes is as follows: oval = 73, large = 2.7, small = 8.6, taper = 6.1, amorphous = 8.6, duplicate = 1.0, and immature = <0.5. These values are based on the classification of MacLeod (117). In addition, it is necessary to differentiate the immature germ cells from any white blood cells that may be present in the seminal fluid. If the latter are present, an unsuspected infection of the genital tract may exist and require treatment.

Urinary Hormone Assays

Gonadotropins. The physiologic information derived from the various procedures for measuring urinary gonadotropin titers requires comment because of some confusion. There are two basic bioassay methods: those that measure total gonadotropin potency — FSH *plus* LH — and those that specifically measure FSH or LH levels. The total or general gonadotropin assays (GGA) make use of changes in ovarian weight of the immature female rat or in uterine weight of the immature female mouse as their end-point. Unfortunately, the mouse uterine weight method was initially described as an "FSH" assay. This erroneous concept still remains in the minds of many clinicians and laboratories and, of course, is present in the literature. Since there are assay techniques to measure the specific gonadotropins, the GGA method should be discarded.

When measuring gonadotropins, attention should be paid to the possibility that spuriously low values may be obtained. This is particularly important when intratesticular disease coexists. The reasons for this artifact include (1) exogenous sex hormone administration; (2) hormone-secreting tumors, such as an estrogen-producing adrenal carcinoma; (3) primary myxedema; (4) protein catabolic states, and (5) congenital or acquired brain lesions, which may or may not be associated with mental retardation.

Urinary FSH. Biologically active FSH levels can be measured using the Steelman-Pohley method (118) after kaolin-acetone precipitation (119). Titers are expressed as I.U./24 hr.; the second international reference preparation (IRP) should be used as the reference standard. The normal adult male range is from 3.8–25.0 I.U./24 hr.*

If only a 12-hour aliquot is used, FSH may not be detected at all times in normal men.

Urinary LH. LH titers may be estimated in urine by using the immature hypophysectomized male rat as the assay model. Increments in the ventral prostate weight serve as the end-point. This assay procedure is costly and relatively insensitive to changes in LH titers; thus it has been replaced by the more sensitive radioimmunoassay techniques.

Urinary 17-KS. Although the determination of urinary 17-KS excretion is quite popular in evaluating gonadal status, it has no value in this instance.

This is primarily because about 70% of the urinary 17-KS originate from precursors secreted by the adrenal cortex. Separating the individual 17-KS prior to measurement accomplishes little, since interconversion between steroids secreted by the testes and adrenal cortex occurs before excretion. Thus in individual patients the determination of 17-KS excretion does *not* indicate whether testosterone production is normal or deficient. 17-KS assays should be reserved for potential adrenal cortical disorders (Ch. 5).

Urinary Testosterone. Methods are available for measuring testosterone glucuronide excretion titers. Since urinary testosterone is not derived exclusively from the testes, the parameter also lacks precision in terms of being a reliable index of Leydig cell function. Lipsett et al. (86, 88) have shown that androstenedione secreted by the adrenal cortex is converted by the liver into testosterone glucuronide, which is then excreted into the urine (Fig. 6–3). Therefore, the measurement of urinary testosterone may seriously overestimate testosterone secretion. Apparently this problem is not as important in normal men as it is in women. However, Hudson has encountered this discrepancy in some hypogonadal males (12). Clearly, more specific methods such as one of the techniques for measuring serum testosterone are preferred.

Serum Gonadotropins. Through the efforts of the National Pituitary Agency (NPA) and the many investigators that prepared materials and gave counsel, reagents are readily available for estimating serum gonadotropins. For extensive details of these procedures, the reader is referred to the First Karolinska Symposium (120).

Serum LH. Serum LH may be measured by the double antibody radioimmunoassay method of Morgan et al. (121) as adapted by Midgley for LH (122). Either the second IRP or LER 907 can serve as standards. When the second IRP is used directly in the assay system, the normal adult male range is from 4–24 mI.U./ml.

Conversion factors to express results in ng./ml. LER 907 vary from laboratory to laboratory.*

Serum FSH. Serum FSH can be measured by the radioimmunoassay method of Midgley (123).

---

*All normal adult male hormone titers listed in this chapter are based on the experience of the author's laboratory unless otherwise cited.

*In our laboratory, 1 mg. LER 907 equals 219 I.U. of second IRP-hMG in terms of LH, and 38 I.U. of second IRP-hMG in terms of FSH.

Normal adult male values depend on the immuno-chemical preparation used for iodination and the specifications of each "batch" of antisera. Normal adult male values are 190–600 ng./ml. LER 907; 869-2 used for iodination and batch No. 1 anti-sera (NPA) used for first antibody. Normal adult male values are 50–450 ng./ml.; 1366 used for iodination and batch No. 3 antisera (NPA).

Clomiphene Test. Occasionally, patients with hypogonadotropic eunuchoidism or lesions involving anterior pituitary function exhibit serum FSH or LH values that overlap with the lower titers of the normal adult male range. To overcome this problem, clomiphene citrate is administered in a dose of 50 mg. twice daily for 7 days. The minimum normal response during clomiphene administration has been defined as an increase over control levels of 30% for LH and 22% for FSH (124).

Serum Testosterone. The total serum testosterone concentration can be measured by several reliable techniques. These include the following methods: double isotope derivative (12, 125), competitive protein-binding (126), and radioimmunoassay (127). If these are performed with appropriate extraction and purification procedures, the results obtained with each method are for practical purposes equivalent. Normal adult male values range from 0.26–1.44 μg./100 ml. It is not practical to estimate the AFTC (apparent free testosterone concentration) (p. 331) for routine purposes.

Testicular Biopsy

When oligospermia or azoöspermia is present, a testicular biopsy specimen must be obtained and examined to allow full appreciation of the nature and extent of the defect. For example, when azoöspermia is due to ductal obstruction, the biopsy specimen is normal. The appearance of the biopsy specimen also permits the physician to determine whether therapeutic measures are worthwhile in male infertility. Finally, it may be necessary to obtain testicular material for sex chromosomal analysis (p. 335, Klinefelter's syndrome). In addition to these reasons, the testicular biopsy procedure is primarily for research purposes. The aim is to establish the histologic criteria of hypogonadism with more precision and to define the effects of contraceptive, therapeutic, and other agents on testicular function. Quantitation of the germinal epithelium is an important feature of the biopsy examination. Several techniques have been used.

It should be pointed out that testicular biopsy is not without some hazard. Studies in normal volunteers demonstrated that sperm counts decreased in about 45% of men following testicular biopsy (128). This complication is usually temporary and the alteration in sperm production relatively minor. In our experience, patients or normal volunteers for research studies have not received permanent harm from a biopsy unless the epididymis was inadvertently entered. Therefore, careful attention to procedural details and proper selection of patients is important.

A testicular biopsy can be readily performed under local anesthesia on an outpatient basis (129, 130). The skin and subcutaneous tissue are infiltrated with a 2% procaine solution after premedication with Demerol, atropine, and secobarbital. With one assistant holding the testis in proper orientation, so as to avoid the epididymis, the operator makes a small incision in the scrotum. Next, the subcutaneous tissue and tunica vaginalis are incised and spread for exposure. With the sharp point of a scalpel blade, a 5-mm. incision is made in the tunica albuginea. A small amount of seminiferous tubular tissue extrudes through the incision. This tissue is then excised with a razor blade. The razor blade is used to avoid crushing of the tubules. The specimen is immediately placed into freshly prepared Cleland's or Bouin's solution for fixation. Unless bleeding persists from the small vessels lying along the undersurface of the tunica albuginea, closure of this layer is not required. The tunica vaginalis and scrotum are closed and a Lister-type of scrotal suspensory is used to support the testis and hold the dressing. The patient must be advised to avoid strenuous activities for the next week in order to prevent hematoma formation. Ordinarily the patient can return to light activity in 2 days.

Examination of epithelial cells obtained by *buccal smear* is a practical screening method that provides evidence for the number of X chromosomes present (absent X chromosomes = "negative" chromatin pattern; one or more X chromosomes = "positive" chromatin pattern). If special stains and the fluorescent microscope are used, detection of the Y chromosome is possible. In the presence of a difficult diagnostic problem or chromosomal mosaicism, it is necessary to submit peripheral blood or gonadal tissue to *short-term tissue culture.* This technique enables the physician to have the entire *autosomal* and *sex chromosomal configuration* demonstrated (Chs. 7 and 8).

CLASSIFICATION OF MALE HYPOGONADISM

Any classification of male hopogonadism suffers from the uncharted complexities of control mechanisms and the uncertainties of pathogenesis that still exist. For the present, a modification of the classification proposed by Heller and Nelson (131) serves a useful purpose in that it directs the clinician toward the site of pathologic change in most instances (Table 6–3). Thus in severe primary testicular failure—the *hypergonadotropic* syndromes—serum FSH and LH titers are elevated. Sometimes selective elevation of either FSH or LH levels will be seen (Fig. 6–5). The term *eugonadotropic* syndromes applies to men who exhibit intrinsic disruption of spermatogenesis, but the damage does not include the independent station; therefore FSH levels remain normal. In the *hypogonadotropic* syndromes, there is decreased pituitary function with impaired secretion of the gonadotropic hormones. Occasionally, selective involvement of LH secretion will occur. Moreover, the pituitary failure may be monotropic in nature, i.e., limited to the gonadotropins, or it may be more complicated and involve any combination of the other tropic hormones up to the entire group. The last condition is designated panhypopituitarism. Finally, it should be pointed out that the three major categories contain examples of both hereditary and acquired disorders.

TABLE 6–3. MALE HYPOGONADISM

Eugonadotropic "syndromes"
  Adult seminiferous tubule failure

Hypergonadotropic syndromes
  Klinefelter's syndrome
    Classic form
    Variant forms
  "XYY" syndrome
  Sertoli-cell-only syndrome
  Reifenstein's syndrome
  Functional prepuberal castrate syndrome
  "Male" Turner's syndrome
  Adult seminiferous tubule failure
  Orchitis
    Epidemic Parotitis
    Gonorrhea
    Leprosy
  Irradiation
  Myotonia dystrophica
  Adult Leydig cell failure

Hypogonadotropic syndromes
  Hypogonadotropic eunuchoidism
    Classic form
    Variant forms
  Delayed puberty

Prepuberal panhypopituitarism
  (Pituitary dwarfism)

Postpuberal pituitary failure
  Selective pituitary failure
  Panhypopituitarism

PITUITARY-GONADAL AXIS IN
ADULT SEMINIFEROUS TUBULE FAILURE

(With retention of Leydig cell function)

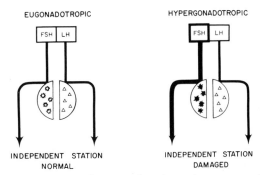

Figure 6–9. In the eugonadotropic syndrome, spermatogenesis is abnormal, but the damage is not severe enough to affect the integrity of the independent station (IS). Serum FSH titers are normal. When damage is more severe and IS is also damaged, serum FSH levels are elevated.

Eugonadotropic Syndromes

This category has been added to focus attention on the fact that the majority of infertile men with oligospermia, or rarely azoöspermia, demonstrate normal serum FSH, LH, and testosterone levels (Fig. 6–6). Furthermore, these patients are characteristically free of endocrinopathy. This patient group represents a mild form of seminiferous tubule failure in which the normal interaction between central FSH secretory mechanisms and the testicular independent "station" is retained (Figs. 6–7, 6–9). It is likely that the condition of many of these patients will deteriorate with time, and eventually their FSH levels will rise. No data exist to confirm this contention. It seems reasonably clear from several recent studies of infertile males that, although FSH levels are not directly related to sperm counts, normal FSH levels are associated with lesser degrees of oligospermia (132, 133). The exception to this is "obstructive" azoöspermia. Also, it has been observed that normal FSH levels are present in patients with minimal tubular-membrane hyalinization and fibrosis and some evidence of active spermatogenesis, particularly in the early phases (i.e., spermatogonial cells are *not* grossly depleted in numbers).

Aside from "obstructive" azoöspermia, two other entities belong in this category, namely D/D 13–15 translocation and varicocele. These conditions will be discussed further under male infertility along with the present status of its treatment (p. 361).

Hypergonadotropic Syndromes

Klinefelter's Syndrome (Seminiferous Tubule Dysgenesis, Puberal Seminiferous Tubule Failure, Sclerosing Tubular Degeneration, Primary Microorchidism;* Figs. 6–1, B and C, 6–10, 6–11, and Table 6–4)

This syndrome represents the most common example of male hypogonadism (134, 136). It is characterized by varying degrees of seminiferous tubule failure and decreased Leydig cell function. In 1942 Klinefelter, Reifenstein, and Albright described the characteristics exhibited by certain hypogonadal males (137). As the pathogenesis has become better understood, the original description has been expanded to include additional features (138, 139). The presence of supernumerary X chromosomes is considered to be the fundamental underlying etiologic factor. Patients with Klinefelter's syndrome may be divided into two major categories: the classic form and the variant forms (Table 6–4). In the classic form, the salient features include small *firm* testes, varying degrees of eunuchoidism, azoöspermia, gynecomastia, mental abnormalities, chromatin-positive buccal smear pattern, and elevated serum FSH and LH titers. With the advent of chromosome analysis, an XXY sex chromosomal complement has been demonstrated in the tissues of most of these patients.

Males considered to have a variant form of Kline-

---

*Various other designations have been suggested for patients with Klinefelter's syndrome. These are included for the reader's information. The author prefers the term Klinefelter's syndrome since the other terms are too limited in their scope or could apply equally well to other forms of primary testicular disease. For example, seminiferous tubule dysgenesis could refer to Klinefelter's syndrome or Sertoli-cell-only syndrome, or both.

TABLE 6–4. KLINEFELTER'S SYNDROME

| | Classic Form | Variant Forms | | | | |
| | | Mutant or Phenocopy | YY Group | Poly X + Y Chromosome Group | | |
				Mosaicism	Mosaicism	Poly X + Y Disorder
Karyotype Findings	XXY	XY	XXYY	XXY/XX XXY/XY XXY/XYY XXY/XXYY XxY/XY/Xx	XXXY/XY XXXY/XXY XXXY/XXY/XY XXXXY/XXXY XXXXY/XXXXY/XXXY	XXXY XXXYY XXXXY XXXxY
Clinical and Laboratory Findings	1. Prepuberal: No definite decrease in germinal cells. Hyalinization or fibrosis of tubular membranes not present. 2. Cryptorchidism: Incidence not increased. 3. Subnormal intelligence (varying degrees—usually mild). 4. Bone abnormalities: Not consistent. 5. Buccal smear: One sex chromatin body.	This type is rare. Strict diagnostic criteria should be maintained. By definition, then, all patients with the typical clinical and laboratory features of Klinefelter's syndrome except for buccal smear and chromosome analysis. The latter should demonstrate an XY sex chromosomal pattern in blood, skin, and testes.	Not common. Clinical and laboratory features similar to those seen in classic form except for the following: 1. More severe degree of mental retardation. 2. Tendency to be tall, e.g., over 6 ft. 3. Increased incidence of (a) antisocial behavior (?) (b) varicose veins	Clinical and pathologic features vary. In patients with sex chromosomal mosaicism, spermatogenesis may be active and sperm present in the ejaculate. Thus the testes may be virtually normal in size. This is particularly true when the normal stem cell line (XY) is present in the testis. Patients with other forms of mosaicism usually demonstrate testicular damage that extends to that observed in the classic form.		1. Prepuberal: Definite decrease in immature germinal cells, with hypoplastic tubules and increased connective tissue stroma. 2. Cryptorchidism: Increased incidence. 3. Subnormal intelligence (severe). 4. Bone abnormalities: Radioulnar synostosis and other abnormalities of the elbow. 5. Buccal smear: Two sex chromatin bodies in XXXY and XXXXY; three sex chromatin bodies in XXXXY.

Similar Postpuberal Features

1. Eunuchoidism (varying degrees).
2. Gynecomastia.
3. Azoöspermia.
4. Elevated serum gonadotropins.
5. Small, firm testes (variable size in mosaicism).
   a. Hyalinization and fibrosis of seminiferous tubules (almost all tubules severely involved).
   b. Leydig-cell hyperplasia and decreased function.
   c. Absence of elastic fibers around tunica propria of hyalinized tubules.

felter's syndrome usually manifest different clinical features from those with the classic form. These differences include both number and severity of abnormal findings. In this variation, the pathologic features are influenced by the presence of sex chromosomal patterns other than "pure" XXY and the specific tissue or tissues that contain the abnormal stem cell line(s). For example, in sex chromosomal mosaicism in which there is more than one stem cell line, if one of the stem cell lines is normal (XY), gonadal function may be virtually normal (136, 140). On the other hand, if more than two X chromosomes plus the Y chromosome are present as a single stem cell line, the pathologic changes are more severe and widespread (141).

Available data indicate that the presence of abnormal numbers of X chromosomes in testicular tissue is the focal point for the seminiferous tubule and Leydig cell changes observed in Klinefelter's syndrome. Chromosomal analysis of skin or peripheral blood or both from some patients may reveal a normal male sex chromosomal pattern, but if the testes contain a supernumerary X chromosomal complement, testicular dysgenesis typical for Klinefelter's syndrome develops.

Some investigators have also classified patients with Klinefelter's syndrome as chromatin-positive or chromatin-negative (based on their buccal smear chromatin pattern) (142, 143). The presence or absence of sex chromatin in this instance indicates the number of X chromosomes in the buccal mucosa only and not in other tissues of the body, including the testes. Therefore, such a classification lacks the proper line of division.

Information about the incidence of Klinefelter's syndrome has been gathered essentially only from patients who demonstrate a chromatin-positive buccal smear pattern. Large scale surveys of phenotypic males have supplied the data indicating the frequency of this syndrome in the general population. In newborn infants, the incidence of chromatin-positive buccal smear patterns is 0.21% (134). A similar incidence has been found in the adult male population (0.15–0.24%) (135, 136). That the frequency in the adult population is not decreased confirms the absence of associated lethal anomalies in these patients.

The incidence of Klinefelter's syndrome is significantly higher in mentally retarded individuals (144, 145). The frequency varies from 0.45–2.38% in this segment of the population. These data emphasize the relationship of mental deficiency to this syndrome.

One can appreciate from the foregoing figures that Klinefelter's syndrome represents a relatively common disorder. Furthermore, if one considers the variant forms that exhibit a chromatin-negative buccal smear pattern and sex chromosomal mosaicism, the actual incidence of this syndrome becomes even higher.

Clinical Manifestations, Classic Form.   The finding of small firm testes, gynecomastia, and decreased androgenicity suggests the presence of Klinefelter's syndrome (Figs. 6–10 and 6–11). Al-

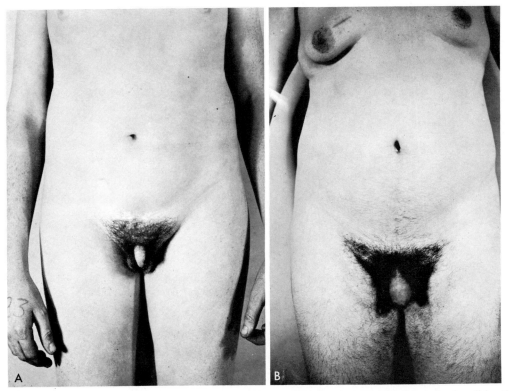

Figure 6–10.   Two untreated patients having Klinefelter's syndrome, who demonstrate the variations in Leydig cell function observed in this entity.

A, The small penis, decreased pubic hair, and sparse body hair indicate minimal androgen secretion. *B,* Normal penile development and adequate pubic and body hair growth indicate essentially normal androgen production by the testis. Gynecomastia is also present.

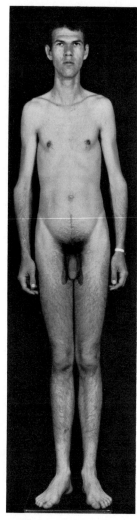

Figure 6–11. Example of variant form; this 21-year-old patient demonstrated XXY/XY mosaicism in all tissues examined. Note the eunuchoidal skeletal features, particularly with regard to the lower extremities. Plasma testosterone levels were 0.42 μg./100 ml., which accounts for the greater androgenicity. His testes were somewhat larger than those encountered in patients with the classic form of the syndrome. Seminal fluid examination revealed a sperm count of 300,000/ml.

though the disorder is congenital, these relatively specific features are not evident prior to puberty. It has been suggested that the prepuberal Klinefelter testis contains fewer cellular elements in the undifferentiated germinal epithelium. However, even if this is true, the testis is not abnormally small at this time. Certain signs, such as subnormal intelligence or a tendency toward eunuchoidal skeletal proportions, may be present before puberty, but these are not specific enough to cause one to suspect the diagnosis.

At puberty, when pituitary gonadotropin secretion is initiated, the basically abnormal testis undergoes typical pathologic changes. It fails to increase in size and becomes firmer in consistency. This is due to progressive fibrosis and hyalinization of the seminiferous tubules, which ordinarily comprise 85% of the volume of the normal testis.

Thus testicular size in these patients rarely exceeds 2.0 × 1.5 × 1.5 cm. In contrast, the longest dimension of the normal adult testis is at least 3.5 cm. (108, 146). Leydig-cell function is impaired to varying degrees in these patients. This results in incomplete development of secondary sex characteristics. Some patients exhibit little evidence of androgen production. In others, the androgen deficiency is so subtle that superficial evaluation may result in the erroneous conclusion that testosterone production is normal. Indeed, a dichotomy between serum testosterone levels and secondary sex characteristics exists in many patients. It may be that the "AFTC" (p. 331) is decreased in such patients, and the observation that "total" serum testosterone levels are normal is misleading. There may be another reason for this phenomenon. Since Leydig cell reserve is impaired in these patients, i.e., response to hCG administration is less than normal (13), the testosterone secretory spikes observed in normal males may not be present in patients with Klinefelter's syndrome. Extensive metabolic studies will be required to clarify this issue.

Whereas androgen deficiency is the usual finding, the development of eunuchoidal skeletal measurements in Klinefelter's syndrome appears to be on another basis. Usually, skeletal changes of this type are considered to arise from a delay in long bone epiphysial closure secondary to testosterone deficiency. Normal thyroid, adrenocortical, and growth hormone production is also required. However, in most patients with Klinefelter's syndrome, the excessive long bone growth is initiated prior to puberty (147, 148), and the bone age is usually appropriate for the patient's chronologic age. Furthermore, the linear growth of the long bones in the lower extremities is greater than it is in the upper extremities. This results in a span:height ratio of 1 or less. In patients whose eunuchoidal skeletal measurements are exclusively secondary to androgen deficiency, the situation is different. The long bones of the upper and lower extremities grow in a comparable fashion. This results in a span at least 2 inches greater than the height, and the ratio therefore is greater than 1. The basis for the skeletal changes in patients with Klinefelter's syndrome may be related to an abnormal sex chromosome constitution in the osseous tissue. Data are lacking on this point.

Bilateral gynecomastia is present in most patients. Usually, this is evident grossly either by inspection or by palpation. Microscopic examination of breast biopsy specimens sometimes is required for detection. When the gynecomastia is minimal, it may be overlooked by improper palpation. The cause for the gynecomastia remains obscure. Microscopically, it is characterized by hyperplasia of the interductal tissue. In contrast, gynecomastia associated with systemic estrogen administration or increased endogenous estrogen production exhibits ductal hyperplasia. (See discussion of gynecomastia on page 358 for further details.)

Subnormal intelligence, defined as an I.Q. of less

than 80, may be evident in many patients with Klinefelter's syndrome (149). When the general population is considered and not that residing in mental institutions, the precise incidence is not known, since detailed intelligence tests are not usually carried out. In some series, though, the incidence approaches 15–25%. Even though the remaining patients may demonstrate normal intelligence, in our experience most of them exhibit character or personality disorders. When the affected individual reaches the age of puberty, he realizes he is different from his contemporaries. Physical exposure in communal locker rooms makes him vulnerable to ridicule because of his enlarged breasts or abnormal sexual development. The continued lack of androgens with consequent poor muscular development limits his physical capabilities. This tends to confirm in his mind that he is an inadequate individual. If his parents fail to understand the problem and do not seek proper medical advice, further difficulties in interpersonal relationships arise. Thus it is no wonder that many of these patients have behavioral disorders, neuroses, or frank psychoses. Of course, a basic defect in the metabolic processes of the CNS could also exist. Again this could be due to the presence of supernumerary X chromosomes in that tissue.

Occasionally a patient with a classic form of the syndrome may progress through puberty in reasonably normal fashion. Then at some later time he undergoes the typical pathologic changes in his testes. Such an individual may have virtually complete maturation of his secondary sexual characteristics. He relates that his testes became smaller for no apparent reason, or he may state that the diminution in testicular size resulted from trauma. This type of history naturally is misleading to the examiner unless further studies, such as a buccal smear or a testicular biopsy, are performed. Although it has not been documented for patients with the classic form, this type of patient may produce progeny prior to development of his testicular damage. Therefore, the history of having had children should not dissuade the physician from considering the possibility of Klinefelter's syndrome.

A greater incidence of other systemic disorders in patients with Klinefelter's syndrome has also been suggested (139, 150–152). These include diabetes mellitus, emphysema, chronic bronchitis, neoplasia, and various autoimmune or allergic disorders. Whether or not Klinefelter's syndrome is associated with a predisposition for these diseases awaits extensive epidemiologic study.

Variant Forms of Klinefelter's Syndrome — Poly X + Y. The majority of male patients with more than two X chromosomes have been discovered prepuberally by buccal smear surveys done in mental institutions; therefore, the overwhelming preponderance of mental retardation in these subjects may simply be a reflection of this situation.

XXXXY Disorder. The more constant features consist of severe mental retardation (highest I.Q., 53), prepuberal testicular damage, scrotal hypoplasia, cryptorchidism, and various osseous abnormalities, such as proximal radioulnar synostosis and overgrowth of the radial or ulnar heads or both. Somewhat more variable features include retarded linear growth, bone age, motor development, and coordination. These patients tend to be thin and frequently come to clinical attention with epicanthal folds, hypertelorism, cubitus valgus, and incurving of the fifth digit (141).

XXXY Disorder. Patients afflicted with this chromosomal pattern present a clinical picture somewhere between the classic form of Klinefelter's syndrome and the XXXXY disorder (153). The incidence and degree of mental retardation resemble those encountered in patients with the XXXXY disorder. Similarly, radioulnar synostosis and cryptorchidism are frequently present in these patients. However, the pre- and postpuberal testes resemble those encountered in patients with the classic form of Klinefelter's syndrome (XXY).

Mosaicism. The clinical picture is quite variable in patients with more than one stem cell line. In some the damage is severe and resembles that seen in the classic form of the syndrome. The majority of patients with mosaicism exhibit less severe changes (Fig. 6–11), particularly if the normal stem cell line (XY) is present. Indeed, normal gonadal function during young adult life with successful fertility has been documented in this type of patient. Sometimes mental retardation may be the only clinical feature.

Clearly, then, the patient in the variant category of Klinefelter's syndrome with sex chromosomal mosaicism presents the greatest challenge insofar as detection and proper diagnosis are concerned. It is important to remind the reader that in this category all the tissues available for study (i.e., skin, blood, and testes) need *not* demonstrate the multiple stem cell pattern or even an abnormal stem cell line.

The concept of mosaicism (154) along with the broad spectrum of abnormalities observed in Klinefelter's syndrome is fundamental to the understanding of genetic diseases related to chromosomal defects. For a more extensive discussion, the reader is referred to several review articles (13, 155, 156).

Mutant or Phenocopy. Rarely, a patient demonstrates all the classic features of Klinefelter's syndrome without any abnormality in the number of X chromosomes. Tissue culture studies of skin, blood, and testicular material reveal a normal XY chromosomal pattern. To prevent confusion in dealing with these patients, strict diagnostic criteria should be followed. Otherwise, various ill-defined examples of postpuberal testicular disorders could be placed into this category.

YY Group. Although not a common variant of the syndrome, patients in this category may have some characteristic clinical features (157, 158). For example, they tend to be tall, i.e., over 6 feet, and saphenous vein varicosities appear more frequently than expected. The testicular damage is similar to that observed in the classic form. A rather uniform behavioral pattern of mental instability associated with aggressiveness and antisocial tendencies has been documented. Since most of these patients have been detected in surveys performed in mental or penal institutions, it will be necessary to investigate the general population before this influence of supernumerary YY chromosomes can be established as a fact.

XX (?). Whether a separate category should exist for patients who demonstrate a "pure" XX sex chromosomal pattern is not settled. Some investigators have suggested that the short arms of the Y chromosome may be translocated onto autosomes. Proof for this is lacking. Also to be resolved is the question as to how testes develop, even imperfectly, in the absence of a Y chromosome. Apparently the incidence of finding an XX chromosomal pattern is 1:9000 phenotypic males. These males are somewhat shorter in height than is the typical patient with Klinefelter's syndrome. Otherwise the pathologic characteristics resemble those of patients with XXY/XY mosaicism (159).

Laboratory Findings. Testicular biopsy specimens reveal two main features: hyalinization of the seminiferous tubular membranes and adenomatous "clumping" of the Leydig cells. In the usual case, virtually all the tubules are severely hyalinized and acellular (Fig. 6–1, *B* and *C*). Occasionally certain areas of the testes have tubules with complete spermatozoa. This finding is more common when sex chromosomal mosaicism of the XXY/XY variety is present. Apparently, the dilution of the abnormal stem cell line by the normal (XY) stem cell line exerts a favorable influence. Consequently, the testicular damage with respect to spermatogenesis is less. There are not sufficient data to conclude that the same condition holds true for Leydig cell function (13, 155). In all forms of the syndrome, the disturbance in androgen steroidogenesis is reflected by the adenomatous clumping of Leydig cells which tend to be less granular than normal and to contain less lipid material. Fibroblastic and intermediate forms of these cells are increased also. Before this syndrome was well recognized, these adenomatous clumps when quite extensive were mistaken for interstitial cell tumors. Rarely, the interstitial cells may be sparse and difficult to identify (160, 161). Here the transition to the fibroblastic forms may have been more rapid and complete (162, 163).

Special stains demonstrate the absence of elastic fibers in and around the thickened tunica propria. This finding supports the congenital nature of this entity, as elastic fibers normally appear during puberal maturation (164). Furthermore, it aids in differentiating Klinefelter's syndrome from mumps orchitis, myotonia dystrophica, etc., which may present a similar histologic pattern (Fig. 6–1, *F*).

Azoöspermia is the characteristic finding in the classic form of Klinefelter's syndrome. Occasionally, as mentioned previously, spermatogenesis will be less damaged. This results in the finding of viable sperm in the ejaculate. Sperm counts in patients with XXY/XY mosaicism may be normal at some point in their lives, since fertility has been documented (165, 166). However, in our experi-

ence, severe oligospermia is invariably present at the time of physician contact. The reason for this is obvious; examination of gonadal function is usually deferred until complaints referable to reproductive function are presented to the physician. No unique diagnostic changes occur in the seminal fluid volume or in the various constituents of the seminal fluid plasma. In general, when androgen deficiency is severe, the volume of the ejaculate is small and the fructose and phosphatase content decreased.

In 1950, Plunkett and Barr demonstrated a positive chromatin pattern in patients having this syndrome (167). Using a buccal smear to detect the condensed X chromosome is an invaluable aid to diagnostic screening for this syndrome. As mentioned previously, this laboratory test has limitations when sex chromosomal mosaicism is present.

Chromosome analysis by means of short-term tissue culture affords the most complete information regarding the presence of Klinefelter's syndrome. However, this procedure is laborious and costly and should be reserved for the difficult diagnostic problems. (See Chapter 8 for details of technique.)

Serum and urinary gonadotropin titers are usually elevated in these patients. In one series of 26 patients, the mean serum LH titer ranged from 19.5 to >128 mI.U./ml. (13). Only three patients exhibited values below 24 mI.U./ml. (p. 333). Serum FSH levels are generally above 1200 ng. LER 907/ml. in our experience. Urinary FSH titers have been found to range from 56 to 205 I.U./24 hr. (13). Naturally, patients whose pathologic features are delayed until later in life will probably pass through a phase of normal gonadotropin levels. In prepuberal or young adolescents with Klinefelter's syndrome, gonadotropin levels have not been studied.

Leydig cell function may be difficult to assess clinically, particularly if secondary sex characteristics have developed significantly during puberty. The determination of serum testosterone levels permits a more specific assessment. As mentioned previously (p. 333), urinary testosterone levels may provide only limited interpretation in dealing with hypogonadal males.

In normal men, plasma testosterone levels vary from approximately 0.23 to 1.44 μg./100 ml. Testosterone levels in patients with Klinefelter's syndrome generally lie in the lower part of the normal range or lower (12). In one study of 25 patients with either the classic or variant forms of the syndrome, plasma testosterone levels varied from 0.05 to 0.86 μg./100 ml. (13). Testosterone titers in the so-called chromatin-positive and chromatin-negative patients were not different.

In normal males, urinary testosterone varies from 30 to 86 μg. per 24 hours. Although patients with Klinefelter's syndrome have not been studied extensively by this new procedure, it would be expected that urinary testosterone levels, like plasma levels, would vary from low to normal.

Administration of human chorionic gonadotropin (hCG) as a Leydig cell stimulation test does not appear to be useful in diagnosing Klinefelter's syndrome. Originally it was suggested that a single injection of 2000 to 5000 I.U. hCG increased plasma testosterone levels significantly in normal men (86) but not in patients with Klinefelter's syndrome (88, 168). We have found that some normal men do not respond to the single dose of hCG and that four daily injections are required for a satisfactory "test." Patients with Klinefelter's syndrome may respond satisfactorily the first day but later plateau in terms of their plasma testosterone levels. This signifies limited Leydig cell reserve (13). Although important for studying physiologic principles, these findings add little to the diagnostic evaluation at the present time.

Interestingly, some patients demonstrate a disturbance in thyroid function (169). Lower than normal 24-hour radioactive iodine uptake values have been reported in a few patients. Clinically they were euthyroid, and the protein-bound iodine level was within normal limits. When TSH was administered, normal or less than normal increments in the radioactive iodine uptake occurred. Additional investigation is needed before these observations can be fully understood.

Treatment of patients with Klinefelter's syndrome is directed toward correcting the androgen deficiency that is usually present. In this regard, androgen replacement therapy produces adequate sexual maturation. (See p. 355 for additional comments on testosterone therapy in general.)

The infertility is irreversible, and the gynecomastia is not amenable to medical therapy. When the latter is sufficient to cause social embarrassment, plastic surgery should be performed.

Summary. Early detection is an important goal in this syndrome. This will avoid many of the social adjustment problems that otherwise develop for these patients. Furthermore, if the mental behavior is too disorganized, expert psychiatric attention should be made available as early as possible. To achieve this goal of early detection, the clinician needs to suspect Klinefelter's syndrome if one or more of the following conditions are present: (1) boys with scholastic problems, (2) inadequate and somewhat delayed sexual maturation, (3) long-leggedness, (4) behavioral problems at home or school or both. Some investigators have added to the above listing smaller than normal genitalia for the individual's age (170). This may be quite difficult to ascertain prepuberally.

XYY Syndrome

The occurrence of XYY in the general population is between 0.01–0.02% (171, 172). Testicular function (spermatogenesis) may be normal, minimally impaired, or severely damaged (173, 174). Retention of normal spermatogenesis in most patients is considered to be related to the observation that the extra Y chromosome is usually deleted during spermatogonial mitosis (175). Thus, the genetic material with the germ cells regains "balance." Initially, investigators proposed that the YY con-figuration resulted in increased testosterone levels. However, later studies have demonstrated normal testosterone levels in these men (173, 176). Serum FSH and LH levels are usually normal but may be elevated when testicular damage is present. In one series, 1 of 7 patients studied demonstrated elevated FSH and LH titers. Testicular function was severely damaged in that patient (132).

Histologically, there is no distinct pattern seen in the testicular biopsy specimen (174). Spermatogenic arrest at the primary spermatocyte level may be detected. More severe damage may be seen with greater depletion of germ cells, or tubules containing only Sertoli cells may be present (see below).

Two additional features are considered to be part of this syndrome; namely, increased height and pustular acne (177). With respect to the increased linear growth, this finding is apparently independent of the gonadal status.

Finally, controversy surrounds the mental behavior in men with XYY. Surveys in penal institutions and mental institutions have uncovered evidence that these patients may be more aggressive, hostile, and antisocial than would be expected if the general population of XY men were examined (145, 178–181). As stated previously, documentation of the mental behavior of XYY men in the general population will be required before appropriate conclusions can be drawn on this point.

No known treatment is available to improve fertility in those patients with impaired spermatogenesis.

Sertoli-Cell-Only Syndrome (Germinal Cell Aplasia)

Testes of normal consistency but slightly smaller in size than normal, azoöspermia, and elevated FSH titers constitute the classic features of this relatively uncommon disorder. Since androgen production usually remains intact, LH titers are normal (Fig. 6–5), and the only presenting complaint is infertility. Occasionally, testosterone levels will be lower than normal. Gynecomastia is not a part of the clinical picture but may occur in the same frequency as observed in normal males (p. 358). Abnormalities in sex chromosomal configuration are uncommon (see page 342).

Inspection of the testicular biopsy specimen shows the seminiferous tubules to be moderately reduced in size and devoid of germ cells (Fig. 6–1, D). There may be some thickening of the tunica propria, but significant peritubular sclerosis and hyalinization are not present. Leydig cells are morphologically normal. Although cells may appear to be increased in number, adenomatous clumping does not occur.

Some workers have considered that congenital absence of germ cells is the basis for this syndrome, but no direct evidence for this exists. Even though the biopsy specimen may uniformly demonstrate the absence of the germinal epithelium, an occasional patient will have a few sperm in his ejaculate (43, 163). In other patients, an isolated tubule may be found containing some germinal elements. These variant features are usually observed in the youngest individuals having this syndrome.

Thus the germinal epithelium may be essentially normal until puberty, when spermatogenesis is initiated. Then, because of inherent defects, the gametocytes slough away from the tubular walls into the lumen. This process includes the spermatogonia, so that the germinal epithelium cannot be replenished. Finally the tubules are populated only by Sertoli cells.

The pathogenesis of this entity remains unknown, except in several instances. An XYY sex chromosomal pattern was detected in 1 of 10 patients in one report (132). Extensive chromosomal studies have not been conducted in most clinics, but XYY as a causal factor is probably not common. Also, Kjessler lists the few reports where some chromosomal aberration was detected (185).

Serum gonadotropin assays and buccal smear examinations, including the use of fluorescent stains, are diagnostic aids in evaluating the patient with almost normal-sized testes and azoöspermia. The information obtained should enable the clinician to discriminate between patients with ductal obstruction and those patients with Sertoli-cell-only syndrome or a variant of Klinefelter's syndrome. It may be necessary to obtain a testicular biopsy so that definitive separation between the patient with ductal obstruction and the patient with complete germinal cell arrest can be achieved. The reason for this is that some patients in the latter category will have normal gonadotropins.

It should be emphasized at this time that patients with other gonadal disorders may also have seminiferous tubules that contain only Sertoli cells (51). But, in addition, the testes are usually smaller, the microscopic pattern is not as uniform, and, in contrast to the Sertoli-cell-only syndrome, severe sclerosis and hyalinization are predominant features. For example, in Klinefelter's syndrome, 90% of the tubules may be completely hyalinized and acellular, whereas 10% may be small and sclerotic and contain only Sertoli cells. Other conditions in which this variable pattern can be observed include mumps and gonococcic orchitis, cryptorchidism, adult seminiferous tubule failure, and irradiation damage.

Treatment cannot correct the infertility, which is permanent, and hormone replacement therapy is not needed.

Reifenstein's Syndrome

This hereditary testicular disorder is characterized by hypospadias, postpuberal atrophy of the seminiferous tubules, azoöspermia, and varying degrees of eunuchoidism and gynecomastia (186). Evidence is accumulating that this entity is not based on a close genetic linkage to Xg^a (187). In contrast to patients with Klinefelter's syndrome, which this entity resembles, patients with Reifenstein's syndrome apparently have an XY sex chromosomal complement in all tissues. Therefore, the buccal smear pattern in these patients is chromatin-negative.

Urinary testosterone levels are generally decreased, whereas estrogen excretion titers are within normal limits. Total (or general) urinary gonadotropin levels have been found to be elevated or normal. Serum FSH and LH titers may be elevated.

The testicular histology reveals a picture of variable damage, i.e., from completely hyalinized tubules to tubules that contain all cellular elements in decreased numbers. This is particularly true for the more mature spermatids. Also, in contrast to Klinefelter's syndrome, elastic fibers are usually present in and around the hyalinized seminiferous tubules. This finding indicates that the seminiferous tubules have undergone some puberal development before the damage was manifest. Leydig cell hyperplasia is usually present.

Androgen replacement therapy is indicated for treatment of the Leydig cell deficiency. Although studies are incomplete, there appears to be no end-organ insensitivity to androgen administration in these patients. The hypospadias and gynecomastia should be corrected surgically, as indicated.

Functional Prepuberal Castrate Syndrome (Testicular "Agenesis," Anorchia)

In affected patients there is no recognizable functioning testicular tissue (188). The damage may occur during either the fetal or the prepuberal period of life. In some, there is a disturbance in embryologic development so that the fetal gonad atrophies, leaving behind wolffian duct derivatives which then usually descend into the scrotum. Whether vascular anomalies, infectious processes, or other factors are responsible is not known. Chromosomal studies are lacking; therefore the possibility that genetic abnormalities are involved in the pathogenesis of this entity has not been explored. Since these patients have male phenotypes, the failure of testicular tissue must occur sometime after the seventh to fourteenth week of fetal life. Failure of the male gonad prior to somatic differentiation would lead to a female phenotype, according to the work of Jost and others (189–191) (Ch. 8). In other patients, fetal development is apparently normal but damage to the testes occurs before puberty, resulting in complete atrophy. Surgical manipulations, such as bilateral herniorrhaphy or orchiopexy, trauma, and infections have been indicated as causal factors, but actually, in most instances, the etiology is obscure.

Somatic and visceral anomalies are not associated with the testicular disorder; thus these patients may readily be distinguished from those who have "male Turner's syndrome."

Since there is no gonadal tissue to respond to endogenous or exogenous stimulation, *puberty fails to occur*. Therefore, these patients are characterized by sexual infantilism and appear to have an

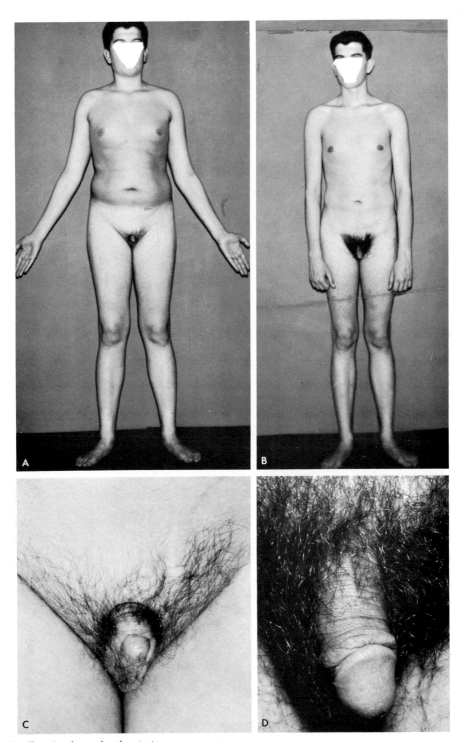

Figure 6-12. Functional prepuberal castrate.

A and *C*, Before treatment. Note the "empty" scrotum and eunuchoidal features. No testicular tissue was found at the time of surgical exploration. Note also the absence of somatic anomalies.

B and *D*, After 1½ years of testosterone therapy, scalp hair recession, penile development, and hair growth have occurred. The body habitus has attained masculine proportions, and muscle development is now that of a normal adult male.

"empty" scrotum (Fig. 6–12). This latter feature frequently leads to the mistaken diagnosis of the bilateral cryptorchidism with abdominal testes. However, on careful palpation, small ill-defined scrotal "masses" are usually encountered. Biopsy of these scrotal contents reveals remnants of wolffian duct derivatives or hyalinized prepuberal testes. These patients may be of short stature, in contrast to patients with forms of eunuchoidism, in which they are usually tall or of normal height.

Urinary 17-KS levels are low and urinary-estrogen excretion is low or absent. Urinary gonadotropin excretion becomes markedly elevated at the expected time of puberty. This includes both serum FSH and LH titers.

As an aid to diagnosis, hCG could be administered and serial measurements of serum testosterone titers performed. Winter et al. found a 3- to 12.5-fold increase in serum testosterone levels within 4 days following the administration of hCG, 2000 I.U./day, to 4 boys with bilateral cryptorchidism (192). However, since Santen did not observe such increases when bilateral cryptorchidism was associated with hypogonadotropic eunuchoidism (193), caution should be exercised in concluding that testes are absent if there is no rise in testosterone levels during hCG administration.

Androgen replacement therapy (p. 355) should be instituted to produce full sexual maturation.

Male Turner's Syndrome (Ullrich-Turner)

Patients who exhibit decreased testicular function coexistent with features similar to those encountered in phenotypic females who have Turner's syndrome (Ch. 8) are classified as having "male Turner's syndrome" (194–197). Characteristic findings include short stature, webbed neck, low-set ears, shieldlike chest, cryptorchidism, diminished spermatogenesis and usually decreased Leydig cell function, cubitus valgus, ocular anomalies such as ptosis, and cardiovascular anomalies. Mental retardation, gynecomastia, and persistent lymphedema of the hands and feet (dorsal aspect) may also be present.

In some, the testes fail to develop, and only fibrous remnants can be found communicating with the vas deferens. The majority demonstrate recognizable testes with abnormal spermatogenesis. The testicular biopsy specimen does not show a unique histologic pattern. Some tubules contain only Sertoli cells, whereas others have decreased numbers of germinal cells in various stages of maturation. Leydig cells may be increased in number but do not show the characteristic adenomatous clumping seen in Klinefelter's syndrome.

General gonadotropin excretion titers are elevated in patients who have reached the age of expected puberty. Although plasma or urinary testosterone levels have not been studied, the clinical status of these patients indicates that androgen production is usually decreased. End-organ insensitivity is not an issue, since virilization readily occurs with appropriate treatment.

The evidence for chromosomal changes was ex- amined in a review of 86 patients where peripheral blood cultures were performed in 34 (197). Twenty-seven were noted to have a normal XY, 46 pattern. In the remaining seven patients, various sex chromosomal abnormalities were detected (XO, XXY, XO/XY, XO/XY/XYY, XisoX/XXabnormalY). One patient was reported to have autosomal anomalies in addition to the sex chromosomal derangement (196). Thus the presence of the various congenital somatic and visceral anomalies plus the chromosomal changes indicate a pathogenesis distinct from Reifenstein's syndrome, Klinefelter's syndrome, functional prepuberal castrate syndrome, and uncomplicated cryptorchidism. The development of a male phenotype in these patients probably is related to the presence of a functional Y chromosome during the critical time of fetal gonadal development. Further study is required before definitive concepts of the entire clinical picture can be established. This is particularly true with regard to the origin of the webbed neck and cardiovascular anomalies.

Treatment is directed toward correcting the androgen deficiency. Orchiopexy will not rectify the inherent spermatogenic abnormality. However, this procedure may be indicated for psychologic reasons. Since testicular carcinoma appears to be less of a hazard than it is in the testicular feminizing syndrome, orchiectomy is not mandatory.

Adult Seminiferous Tubule Failure

Orchitis With Epidemic Parotitis. About 15–25% of males with epidemic parotitis develop acute orchitis. If this happens before puberty, most will recover completely, but when the puberal or adult testes are involved, permanent damage to the seminiferous tubules usually results (198). Even if only one testis is involved clinically, degenerative changes have been observed in the other.

During the acute phase, the pathologic findings vary from interstitial edema and cytoplasmic swelling of the germinal cells to complete sloughing of the germinal epithelium (199). Chronic changes involve progressive tubular sclerosis and hyalinization. Sometimes the histologic picture resembles that seen in Klinefelter's syndrome, including the Leydig cell "clumping" (Fig. 6–1, *D*). It has been emphasized that the full extent of the damage may not be evident until 10–20 years after the acute infection. Leydig cell function usually remains intact, but in severe cases complete loss of testicular function can develop.

Serum FSH titers may be normal or elevated, and there is oligospermia or azoöspermia. The testes are small and soft, and if androgen secretion is impaired, climacteric symptoms and a very slow regression of secondary sex characteristics will occur.

Administration of estrogens during the acute phase has been advocated as a means of preventing permanent damage (200). However, long-term studies are lacking to establish the effectiveness of this treatment. Supposedly estrogen therapy would be beneficial by suppressing spermatogenesis, thus making the germinal cells less vulnerable. But since it takes several weeks to significantly depress spermatogenesis and since the orchitis usually runs its course in 6–8 days, estrogen therapy does not appear logical. Prednisone treatment has not been uniformly effective during the acute phase, but observations on the chronic course are not available (201). Probably the best treatment is still the supportive measures of bed rest, scrotal support, and so forth.

Gonorrhea. Acute orchitis of a similar nature is seen associated with gonorrheal infections. The sequelae are essentially the same. Progressive sclerosis of the tubular membranes secondary to chronic orchitis occurs in patients having *leprosy*, and these also resemble the Klinefelter testis.

Irradiation. Exposure to x-rays, neutrons, and radioactive materials can cause germinal cell destruction (202–204). Under acute conditions of exposure, spermatogenesis may eventually recover, provided that the dose is not excessive. The maximum dose that permits full recovery is not known with certainty, but probably lies between 400 and 600 r. (204) for a radiation source consisting of 250-kv. x-ray energy.

Spermatogonia are quite sensitive to irradiation. Indeed, using 20 r. gamma irradiation (205), Oakberg found significant cell destruction in the mouse. Recent studies emphasize the sensitivity of the human testis to x-ray exposure. With 250-kv. x-rays, spermatogenesis is temporarily damaged by dose levels as low as 15 r. (204, 206). These studies demonstrate that both "cell kill" and "mitosis halting" mechanisms occur after radiation exposure. It has been determined that the ED_{50} estimates for "cell kill" and "mitosis halting" are 75 and 27 r., respectively (207). Histologic changes occur rapidly following exposure to radiation. As early as 27 days after 100 r. x-ray, the reduction in all but the mature spermatids is striking (Fig. 6–13).

In contrast, Leydig cell function is quite resistant to irradiation. The highest tolerated dose is not established, but it probably exceeds 800 r. x-rays.

Since Leydig cell function remains intact, testosterone levels as well as urinary LH excretion titers are normal (206). FSH levels increase as a reflection of the damaged spermatogenesis. These levels return to normal when the germinal epithelium is replenished.

Although the importance of protecting gonadal function from accidental radiation exposure is self-evident, no preventive means are presently available except appropriate external shielding.

Myotonia Dystrophica. The major clinical features of this disorder in males include not only myotonia but also lenticular opacities, frontal baldness, and testicular atrophy (208, 209). Hypogonadism is present in approximately 80% of these patients. Clinically the testes are small and softer than normal. Puberal development is usually normal, and the testicular damage occurs at varying times during adult life. Leydig cell function usually remains normal, and gynecomastia is *not* a characteristic finding.

Examination of the testicular biopsy specimen reveals damage ranging from complete hyalinization and fibrosis of the seminiferous tubules to moderate derangement of spermatogenesis. Drucker et al. concluded from their study that the hyalinized tubular membranes in these patients underwent more infolding than in Klinefelter's syndrome (208). This was believed to represent damage to previously normal seminiferous tubules. Leydig cells may tend to be clumped but this is not a characteristic finding.

Although the testicular changes resemble those encountered in Klinefelter's syndrome, X chromosomal abnormalities are not an integral factor in the pathogenesis of this disorder. In 18 cases studied by Drucker et al., only one patient manifested a positive chromatin pattern. In some patients with

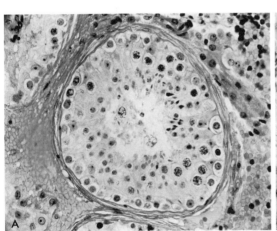 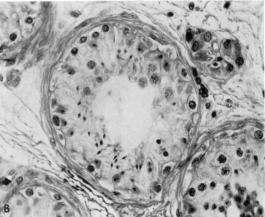

Figure 6–13. *A*, Testicular biopsy specimen (× 350) from normal adult. Spermatogenesis is active and all germ cell types are present in normal numbers. *B*, Biopsy specimen (× 350) from same patient 27 days following exposure to 100 r. x-ray. Only the mature spermatids are present in normal numbers. The progressive depletion of the germinal epithelium is due to lack of immature cell types undergoing maturation. The majority of spermatogonia were killed at the time of exposure. Note the absence of significant tubular membrane fibrosis. Leydig cells are normal.

myotonia, chromosomal gonadal dysgenesis may coexist (210).

Despite the primary nature of the gonadal disorder, urinary gonadotropin excretion titers have not been found to be uniformly elevated (208–210). This is due to the fact that general gonadotropin rather than specific FSH assays have usually been employed. For example, Harper et al. found serum FSH levels elevated (18.3–92.5 mI.U./ml.; their normal male range was 5.2–14.5) in all 33 afflicted males studied, aged 15–44 years (211).

There is no known treatment for the infertility. Testosterone administration is not indicated since androgen production is usually normal.

Adult Leydig Cell Failure ("Male Climacteric"). In contrast to ovarian function, spermatogenesis and testosterone production do not suddenly decline at a certain point in the life of the male unless a pathologic process intervenes. Spermatogenesis is more vulnerable to metabolic and systemic disorders but age per se does not appear to alter this process. This is supported in part by the presence of normal-sized testes in older men who have not sustained major disease (108). Furthermore, retention of fertility is not uncommon, although extensive seminal fluid studies are lacking in this age group.

As mentioned previously (p. 331), serum testosterone levels usually remain within the normal adult male range throughout old age. These are values for total testosterone levels and may be misleading since Vermeulen has suggested that the AFTC (apparent free testosterone concentration) is decreased due to an increase in testosterone binding by globulin (TBG). Production rate, as well as metabolic clearance rate, reveals a decline with increased age. The physiologic significance of these findings requires further clarification, since routine androgen therapy in older men is not accompanied by convincing results.

When Leydig cell function does decline with total serum testosterone levels below the normal male range, symptoms similar to those in postmenopausal women may appear; these are related to androgen withdrawal (212). In addition to experiencing the hot flashes, approximately half of these patients experience increased irritability, inability to concentrate, episodes of depression, etc., and libido and sexual potentia invariably decrease. This entity has been designated the "male climacteric" (213–215).

Causal factors include Klinefelter's syndrome, testicular atrophy (secondary to mumps orchitis or disruption of testicular blood supply during such procedures as bilateral herniorrhaphy), and idiopathic primary Leydig cell failure. In our experience, the most common etiologic factor is Klinefelter's syndrome. Idiopathic primary Leydig cell failure is rare.

The age of onset is variable and depends on the pathogenesis involved. In those patients with Klinefelter's syndrome who experienced reasonably good Leydig cell function earlier in life, androgen production may decline to lower than normal levels sometime after age 40. The same sequence is observed in men who have sustained severe mumps orchitis during early adult life. Although testicular blood supply can be interrupted at any age following surgery in that region, older men appear to be more vulnerable to this complication.

Establishing the correct diagnosis is less a problem when the aforementioned pathologic processes are responsible, since the clinician is alerted to the possibility of androgen failure by the presence of small, atrophic testes or testes that are at least smaller than normal. (The size of the testes does *not* diminish with just increasing age, *supra vide*.) Also, the secondary sex characteristics are more apt to have regressed because of the more severe and long-standing involvement of the Leydig cells. Ideally, the diagnosis can be confirmed by determining the level of circulating plasma testosterone. The presence of a value definitely below normal, e.g., <0.15 µg./100 ml., would be considered significant. If urinary testosterone assays are used, the value should probably be below 20 µg./24 hr. to be significant. The use of LH assays is *not* helpful, since serum LH titers increase in many men after age 45 despite normal testosterone levels. This finding probably reflects decreased steroidogenic efficiency. Thus more tropic hormone is needed.

Difficulty usually arises in attempting to differentiate idiopathic Leydig cell failure from psychogenic impotence, which is seen much more frequently. This is particularly true if specific laboratory tests for androgen production are not available. Each can present the same clinical picture of vasomotor symptoms, fatigability, and decreased libido and sexual potentia. In both, sperm counts (if seminal fluid examination is possible) and physical findings may be entirely normal. For this situation, the "testosterone therapeutic test" may be helpful. Testosterone enanthate or cypionate is administered weekly for 4 weeks, 200 mg./wk. This is followed by 4 weekly injections of placebo (sesame oil). One to two weeks after the cessation of the last injection, the patient is interviewed. The test is considered *positive* for Leydig cell failure if (1) amelioration of the "climacteric" symptoms occurred slowly, i.e., during the second week, and (2) relapse occurred gradually during the period of placebo injections. The test is *negative* if no benefit results from the administered androgen or if the symptoms rapidly ameliorate and promptly return, coincident with the initiation and cessation of the androgen plus the placebo injections. Further objectivity can be achieved by performing this test in a double blind fashion. The nurse decides whether the androgen injections precede or follow the 4-week course of placebo injections. After the patient interview, the physician is informed of the schedule.

Once the diagnosis is established, maintenance androgen replacement therapy is given (p. 355). In the older patients, improvement of sexual function may not be important, but treatment should still be instituted to correct the negative nitrogen balance that exists. This will improve muscle strength and stamina, as well as the osteoporosis which is usually present. In psychogenic impotence, emo-

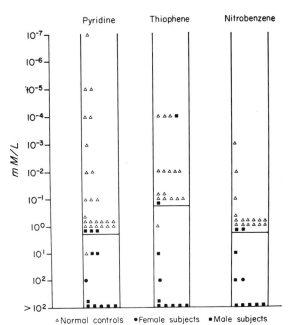

Figure 6–14. Olfactory threshold for normal adults and patients with hypogonadotropic eunuchoidism. (From Santen, R. J., et al.: *J. Clin. Endocr. 36*:47, 1973.) Testing performed according to procedures outlined by Henkin. (From Henkin, R. I., et al.: *J. Clin. Invest. 45*:1631, 1966.) Ordinate indicates molar concentration of reagents used for testing.

tional problems are usually involved, and the patient should have a psychiatric evaluation. The administration of a potent androgen may not be desirable in some patients. In this situation one of the anabolic agents that is somewhat weaker in androgenicity, such as methandrostenolone, may be substituted.

Other factors responsible for decreased sexual potentia should not be neglected. These include vascular disorders and neurogenic factors. Since the ability to have an erection depends on an adequate blood supply to the penis, arteriosclerotic changes such as are observed in Leriche's syndrome may result in decreased sexual potentia. The finding of diminished femoral arterial pulsations or the history of gluteal claudication suggests the diagnosis. Patients with diabetes mellitus frequently complain of diminished sexual ability. In addition to the vascular changes seen in these cases, sympathetic neuropathies occur frequently. Since the integrity of the sympathetic fibers is necessary for the sexual responses, such neurologic involvement may be responsible for the impotence seen in diabetics.

Androgen therapy does not improve the symptoms in the vascular or neurogenic disorders.

Hypogonadotropic Syndromes

Hypogonadotropic Eunuchoidism

By definition, the prepuberal boy is in a state of physiologic hypogonadotropic eunuchoidism (H.E.). If the unknown triggering mechanism responsible for initiating puberty fails to promote normal pituitary gonadotropin secretion, then the syndrome of hypogonadotropic eunuchoidism

ensues (43, 131, 216–218). This syndrome, therefore, represents an indefinite postponement of puberty, with a deficiency in testosterone secretion which results in failure of maturation. Occasionally puberty may not begin until age 18 or 19 (219). Thus at initial evaluation, only those patients who fit the picture and who are 20 years old or more can be considered to have the classic form of H.E.

The incidence of this disorder is not known with certainty, but it represents the most common form of hypogonadism aside from Klinefelter's syndrome and adult seminiferous tubular failure. Usually the disorder involves only a single member of a given family, but multiple cases may be present.

Data based on testing for the presence of anosmia, hyposmia, or normal sense of smell (Fig. 6–14) indicate that H.E. is inherited as an autosomal dominant disorder (Fig. 6–15). Examination of six kindred suggests that there is either incomplete expressivity or genetic heterogeneity (220). The various abnormalities detected in these kindred

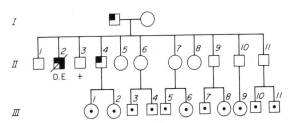

Figure 6–15. Kindred 1 studied for mechanism of genetic transmission of hypogonadotropic eunuchoidism. Opaque area upper left hand corner depicts anosmia. Note *male* to *male* transmission. Opaque area entire right side depicts hypogonadism. Diagonal line indicates cryptorchidism. Central dot indicates prepuberal age. (From Santen, R. J., et al.: *J. Clin Endocr. 36*: 47, 1973.)

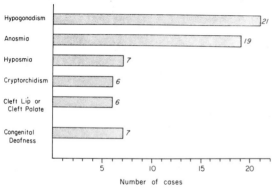

Hypogonadism — 21
Anosmia — 19
Hyposmia — 7
Cryptorchidism — 6
Cleft Lip or Cleft Palate — 6
Congenital Deafness — 7

Number of cases

Figure 6–16. Incidence of abnormalities in 97 adult family members from 6 kindred studied, who either had hypogonadotropic eunuchoidism or were at risk because they were born to an affected or carrier parent. (From Santen, R. J., et al.: *J. Clin. Endocr.* 36:47, 1973.)

and the frequency of each are depicted in Figure 6–16.

The basic defect in these patients is located in the hypothalamus rather than the pituitary. Although direct measurements of the releasing hormone levels are not possible as yet, the administration of LH releasing hormone (LHRH) to patients with H.E. produces a significant increase in LH and FSH levels (221–225)—hence, the consideration that the pituitary gland is normal.

The classification of this syndrome has been revised (Table 6–5) now that more precise information is available. In both the classic and the variant forms of hypogonadotropic eunuchoidism, the involved tropic hormones are completely deficient in terms of biologic effectiveness. Sometimes, the involved tropic hormones are secreted to some extent, but less than normal. When this occurs, the patients are considered incomplete examples of their respective categories.

Classic Form. Clinically these patients are usually tall or of normal stature and exhibit eunuchoidal features (Fig. 6–17). The testes are of prepuberal size and consistency. Gynecomastia, gross or microscopic, occurs very rarely in untreated patients. Since other facets of pituitary function are intact, secondary hypothyroidism and adrenal insufficiency do not occur (Fig. 6–18). Congenital anomalies commonly associated with H.E. include anosmia or hyposmia, harelip, and cleft

TABLE 6–5. CLASSIFICATION OF HYPOGONADOTROPIC EUNUCHOIDISM*

I. Hypogonadotropic Eunuchoidism

A. Classic Form
   Decreased FSH and LH

B. Variant Forms
   Isolated LH deficiency ("Fertile" Eunuch)
   Isolated FSH deficiency (?)
   Gonadotropin and growth hormone deficiency

*In any given category, the designated gonadotropin deficiency may not be complete.

palate. Also present, but to a lesser or more variable degree, are the following: congenital deafness, cryptorchidism, and craniofacial asymmetry. Indeed, the correlation between anosmia and eunuchoidism is such that, when the two defects are present together, the diagnosis of hypogonadotropic eunuchoidism is virtually assured. The presence of anosmia is not always appreciated by the physician. The reason for this is that most patients with an inadequate sense of smell do not volunteer this information to the physician. Hyposmia requires quantitative testing to be identified.

Microscopic examination of the testicular biopsy specimen reveals immature seminiferous tubules containing mainly undifferentiated germinal epithelial elements with an occasional early spermatogonium. Sertoli cells are not seen. There are no well-defined Leydig cells; the interstitial spaces contain mesenchymal precursors only (Fig. 6–1, F). The histologic pattern described is therefore that of the immature testis.

Urinary gonadotropins are usually absent, but if serial determinations are performed, an occasional low value may be obtained. Serum FSH and LH titers are usually below the normal male range in patients with the classic form of this syndrome (193, 226). When serum gonadotropin levels overlap with normal values and some puberal changes have occurred so that the diagnosis is uncertain, clomiphene citrate may be administered as a test of pituitary-hypothalamic responsiveness (124) (Figs. 6–19 and 6–20). Despite occasional reports to the contrary, patients with well-documented hypogonadotropic eunuchoidism do not respond to clomiphene, even when administered on a long-term basis. Plasma testosterone levels are low, being in the female range.

If untreated, these patients will remain in their prepuberal state indefinitely. Testicular biopsy specimens from hypogonadotropic eunuchoids in their sixth decade demonstrate the same histologic findings as are encountered in younger patients (Fig. 6–21).

Since the absence of LHRH synthesis appears to be the basic defect, the most logical form of therapy would be the administration of synthetic LHRH. Mancini et al. have reported on such treatment in one patient (227). Full spermatogenesis (histologic criteria) and early sexual development were achieved. LHRH is not yet available commercially but should be in the near future.

Although expensive, treatment with human gonadotropins is the next logical choice if fertility is to be attained (131, 193, 217, 228–232). Two commercial preparations are available. Purified from the urine of pregnant women, hCG behaves like LH in the male by stimulating Leydig cell function. Human menopausal gonadotropin (hMG), purified from the urine of postmenopausal women, is rich in FSH. It also contains LH; the marketed product contains 75 I.U. of FSH *and* LH/ampule.* Since the defect in these patients is

*The trade name is Pergonal (menotropins).

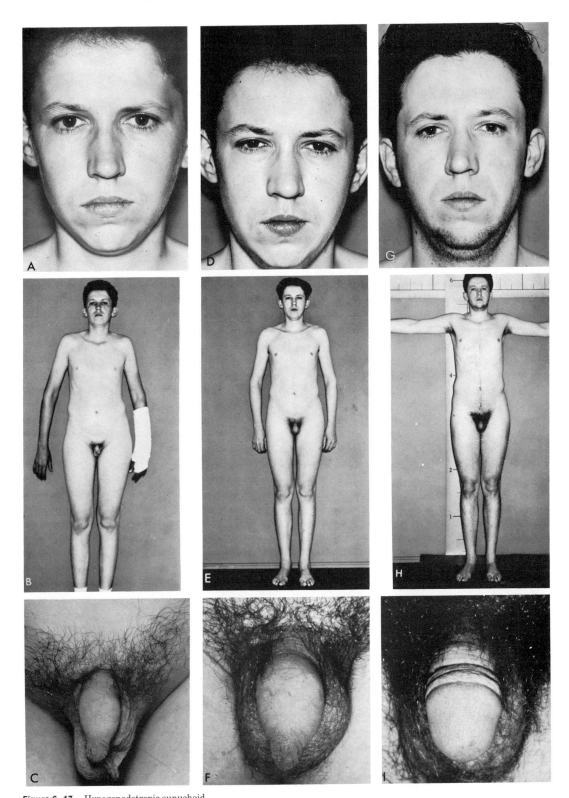

Figure 6–17. Hypogonadotropic eunuchoid.

A, B, and *C,* Puberal development had not progressed past minimal pubic hair growth by age 22.

D, E, and *F,* After 6 months of chorionic gonadotropic therapy, facial hair growth is evident on the upper lip and penile growth has occurred. Note the appearance of scrotal rugae.

G, H, and *I,* After 5 years of intermittent chorionic gonadotropin therapy, full sexual maturation has been achieved. Note the increase in testicular size to essentially normal dimensions.

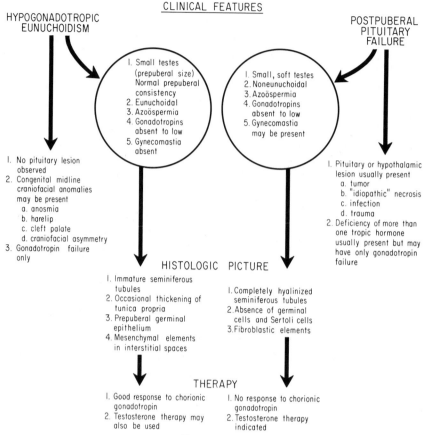

CLINICAL FEATURES

HYPOGONADOTROPIC EUNUCHOIDISM

1. Small testes (prepuberal size) Normal prepuberal consistency
2. Eunuchoidal
3. Azoöspermia
4. Gonadotropins absent to low
5. Gynecomastia absent

POSTPUBERAL PITUITARY FAILURE

1. Small, soft testes
2. Noneunuchoidal
3. Azoöspermia
4. Gonadotropins absent to low
5. Gynecomastia may be present

1. No pituitary lesion observed
2. Congenital midline craniofacial anomalies may be present
   a. anosmia
   b. harelip
   c. cleft palate
   d. craniofacial asymmetry
3. Gonadotropin failure only

1. Pituitary or hypothalamic lesion usually present
   a. tumor
   b. "idiopathic" necrosis
   c. infection
   d. trauma
2. Deficiency of more than one tropic hormone usually present but may have only gonadotropin failure

HISTOLOGIC PICTURE

1. Immature seminiferous tubules
2. Occasional thickening of tunica propria
3. Prepuberal germinal epithelium
4. Mesenchymal elements in interstitial spaces

1. Completely hyalinized seminiferous tubules
2. Absence of germinal cells and Sertoli cells
3. Fibroblastic elements

THERAPY

1. Good response to chorionic gonadotropin
2. Testosterone therapy may also be used

1. No response to chorionic gonadotropin
2. Testosterone therapy indicated

Figure 6–18.

permanent, treatment must continue for an extended period of time. For optimal results, the following regimen is suggested. HCG should be started initially, since hMG alone does not stimulate the immature testis, at least with reasonable dose schedules. Also due to its cost, hMG therapy is deferred until needed. The dosage of hCG is 2000–4000 I.U. three times weekly. Clinical evidence of sexual maturation or serial serum testosterone determinations dictates the dose level required. During hCG therapy, Leydig cells mature, seminiferous tubules enlarge, Sertoli cells differentiate, and spermatogenesis begins and proceeds to varying degrees of "completeness." These seminiferous tubule changes are considered to be primarily due to the direct action of endogenous androgens. With prolonged treatment, sexual maturation can be achieved (Fig. 6–17), and plasma testosterone levels rise to normal male levels (Fig. 6–23). Certain data had suggested that the testes of these patients do not respond adequately to exogenous gonadotropins (233). In our experience this is not the case, except when bilateral cryptorchidism is present (193).

Occasionally, hCG treatment by itself stimulates spermatogenesis sufficiently for sperm to appear in the ejaculate. However, most patients with the classic form of the syndrome require added FSH to achieve a more predictable testicular maturation. Therefore, when necessary, it is recommended to add hMG in doses of 150 I.U. three times weekly to the hCG regimen. HCG is still required since hMG by itself does not contain sufficient LH to maintain satisfactory Leydig cell function. Fertility has been documented using this general therapeutic plan. Because of the expense, it will be necessary to switch eventually to replacement testosterone therapy (p. 355). Even though there are two case reports (234, 235) which state that testosterone induced normal spermatogenesis by itself, the overall experience does not support this plan.

Variant Forms

Isolated LH Deficiency ("Fertile" Eunuch). This interesting group of patients is characterized by eunuchoidism and evidence of effective endogenous FSH secretion (193, 220, 236–238). This latter finding is variable, ranging from viable sperm in the ejaculate to azoöspermia but with spermatogenesis present in the testicular biopsy

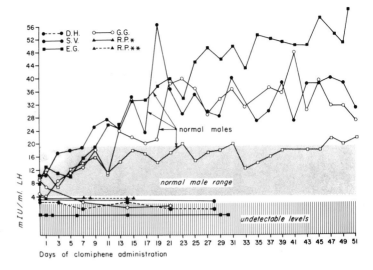

Figure 6–19. Serum LH titers during clomiphene citrate administration (50 mg. bid × 51 days) to 4 normal adult men, 4 patients (D. H., S. V., E. G., and G. G.) with hypogonadotropic eunuchoidism, and 1 patient (R. P.) with pituitary adenoma. The patient group received clomiphene 50 mg. bid for 14–31 days, and R. P. was tested before and after pituitary irradiation. Stippled area depicts normal adult male range in basal state. (From Santen, R. J., et al.: *J. Clin. Endocr. 33*:970, 1971.)

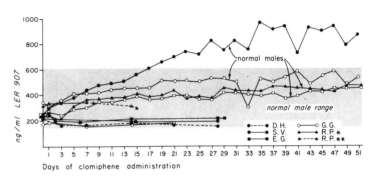

Figure 6–20. Serum FSH titers during clomiphene citrate administration to normal adult males and to patients with pituitary disease. Protocol and patients identical to that stated in legend for Figure 6–20. (From Santen, R. J., et al.: *J. Clin. Endocr. 33*:970, 1971.)

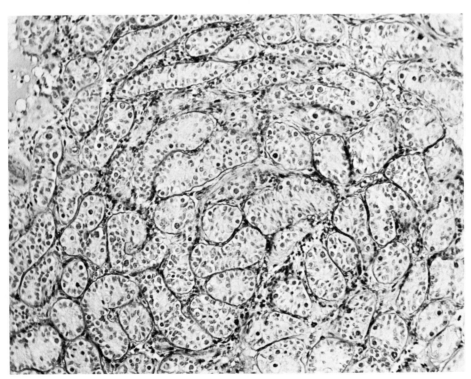

Figure 6–21. Hypogonadotropic eunuchoid testis. This patient was 52 years of age when studied. Note that the testicular histology of this biopsy specimen is similar to that of the prepuberal boy and hypogonadotropic eunuchoid of an earlier age (compare with Figure 6–1, *F*) (× 250).

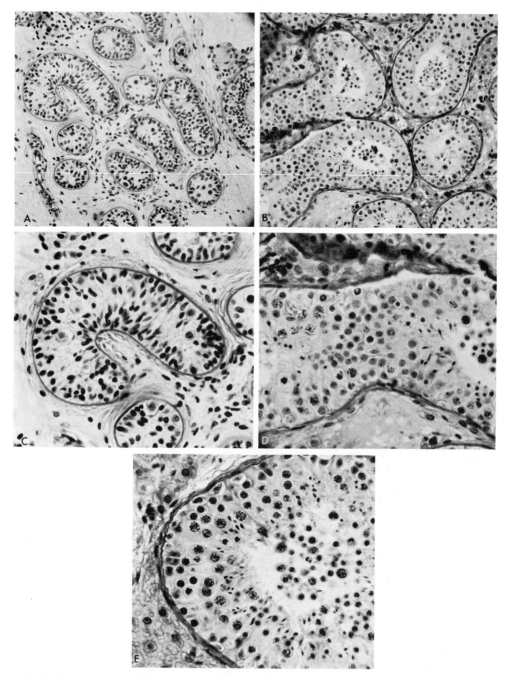

Figure 6–22. *A*, Biopsy specimen (× 250) from untreated 20-year-old hypogonadotropic eunuchoid patient. Note the immature germinal syncytium and interstitial mesenchymal cells. *B*, Specimen (× 150) from same patient 59 weeks after hCG therapy. Spermatogenesis is in progress, and all germ cell types can be detected up to mature spermatids. *C, D, E*, Biopsy specimens from same patient at higher magnification (× 300) to show the germinal epithelium in detail. *C*, Before treatment, immature syncytium. *D*, Fifty-nine weeks after hCG therapy was started. All germ cell types present. *E*, Thirty-one weeks after combined hCG-hMG therapy. Note the increased numbers of all germ cells. Sperm count at this time ranged from 10 to 13.6 m./ml.

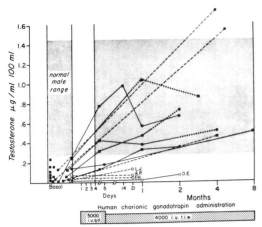

Figure 6–23. Plasma testosterone levels during acute and chronic hCG administration in 13 patients with hypogonadotropic eunuchoidism. Open circles denote 4 patients with bilateral cryptorchidism. Dashed lines refer to patients not tested acutely (e.g., 4-5 days). Dotted lines indicate nonconsecutive plasma sampling. Stippled area indicates normal basal levels for adult males.. Note all patients tested achieved normal testosterone levels within one month *except* those with bilateral cryptorchidism. Of 5 patients tested acutely, 3 achieved normal male levels. (From Santen, R. J., et al.: *J. Clin. Endocr.* 36:55, 1973.)

specimen. Gynecomastia is likely to be present in the fertile eunuch, in contrast to patients with the classic form of the syndrome. The reason for this is not known. Serum LH and testosterone levels are below normal, while serum FSH levels are normal

(193, 239). Of interest is the observation that despite these normal FSH titers, clomiphene administration does not elicit any rise (124).

The approach to treatment is similar to that in patients with the classic form. Treatment with hCG by itself is more apt to induce full testicular maturation in these patients than in patients of the other categories. This is undoubtedly due to the presence of endogenous FSH. The lesion is permanent so that either gonadotropin or androgen replacement therapy is required on a permanent basis.

Isolated FSH Deficiency (?).   No well-defined patient that fits this category has been documented for the male. A possible female example has been described in a single case report (240).

Decreased Gonadotropin and Growth Hormone Deficiency.   Combined FSH, LH, and hGH deficiencies without the presence of a lesion such as a tumor is uncommon but well-documented (238). These patients resemble patients with pituitary dwarfism (panhypopituitarism) except ACTH, TSH, and ADH secretion are intact. No unique feature characterizes these patients, aside from the sexual infantilism and short stature. It should be emphasized that, when the arginine or insulin-induced hypoglycemia test for hGH deficiency is employed, false-positive results may be obtained in any sexually immature male or female unless the clinician administers estrogen prior to the test. For this purpose, 0.5 mg. diethylstilbestrol b.i.d. for two days may be used. Treatment of the gonadotropin deficiency is the same as for all

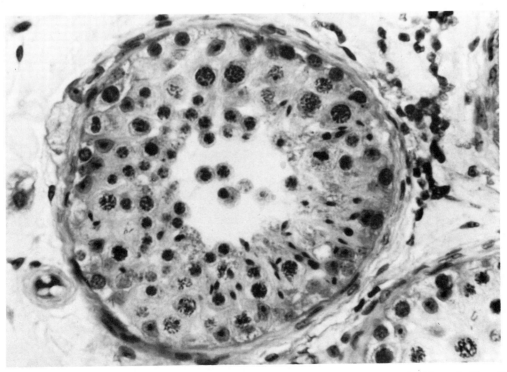

Figure 6–24.   Testicular biopsy specimen (× 270) from patient D. H., aged 28 years, who is an example of the variant form, "fertile eunuch." He had no previous treatment. His serum LH was <1.0–2.4 mI.U./ml.; serum FSH was 180–215 ng. LER 907/ml.; serum testosterone was 0.10 μg./100 ml. (see page 331 for normal adult values). Note that germ cells of each maturation phase are present, including Sc and Sd spermatids (Fig. 6–2). Maturing or mature Leydig cells could not be identified.

patients with H.E. Human GH is only available for investigational purposes.

Delayed Puberty. Puberty normally begins before age 15 years. When it is delayed beyond that time, the boy is classified as a "late" bloomer. The reason for the phenomenon is not clear, but a familial pattern sometimes exists. If delayed puberty is the correct diagnosis, the boy will eventually achieve sexual maturity, usually by age 20–22 years. The main problem with these patients is our inability to sort out and identify examples of delayed puberty separately from patients with hypogonadotropic eunuchoidism who do not have anosmia, hyposmia, or a clear-cut genetic history. There was hope that the clomiphene test might provide the physician with a means for correct diagnosis. Unfortunately, "prepuberal" patients *do not* respond to clomiphene regardless of whether they will be normal in the future. The reason for this is that intrinsic hypothalamic maturation has to occur. Decreased gonadotropin titers are seen during clomiphene administration (Ch. 8).

Treatment for delayed puberty is reserved for those boys who experience social and psychological problems related to their sexual underdevelopment. Therapy consists of a 12-week course of hCG, 4000 I.U. intramuscularly three times weekly. If the response is too sharp, the dosage should be reduced to 2000 I.U. at the same time intervals, and then therapy is discontinued for a period up to 12 weeks. During this "waiting" period, the condition follows one of three courses: maturation may progress, it may remain stationary, or it may regress. The status can usually be determined by interview; occasionally serial serum testosterone determinations are required. If maturation does not progress, an additional course of hCG is given, followed by another "waiting" period. In our experience, patients with delayed puberty do not require more than 3 or 4 such courses of hCG treatment. Patients who regress after multiple courses of hCG tend to be examples of hypogonadotropic eunuchoidism.

Prepuberal Panhypopituitarism (Pituitary Dwarfism)

Lesions involving anterior pituitary or hypothalamic function early in childhood result in this clinical syndrome. Lack of growth highlights the clinical picture but the presence of sexual infantilism and decreased thyroid and adrenal function should not be overlooked (Ch. 2). The testicular morphology resembles that of a normal prepuberal boy prior to age 6–8. Leydig cells and differentiated Sertoli cells are not seen.

Even though epiphysial closure is delayed, the skeletal measurements are not of eunuchoidal proportions. This is most likely due to the absence of growth hormone elaboration.

Since pituitary function is irreversibly damaged, chorionic gonadotropin stimulatory therapy is not practical. Therefore, androgen replacement therapy is indicated in addition to thyroid, corticoids, and if possible hGH.

Postpuberal Pituitary Failure

The testis is unable to maintain its germinal and hormonal function independently if pituitary gonadotropin secretion fails during adult life. Decreased libido, impotence, and a gradual regression of the secondary sex characteristics then follow. The testes become small and soft and, histologically, varying degrees of damage are noted. After normal puberty has been attained, the seminiferous tubules do not revert to a prepuberal state when pituitary failure occurs. Instead, partial or complete cellular "arrest" follows, in which hypoplasia, disorganization and sloughing, or total absence of the germinal epithelium may be seen. The tunica propria becomes thickened, and peritubular proliferation develops. In many instances the testes become completely hyalinized (Fig. 6–4). Leydig cells progressively decrease in number and show degenerative changes.

Although one tends to find the severest testicular damage in those patients having the longest history of involvement, duration of testicular damage alone apparently does not account for the variation observed. Gonadotropin secretion is probably maintained to a certain extent in some patients even though urinary gonadotropins are not detectable by assay. Serum FSH and LH levels may be in the low-normal male range or undetectable. Clomiphene administration may be helpful in difficult cases (p. 348).

Clinically, those patients having involvement of gonadotropin secretion may be divided into two major groups: selective pituitary failure and panhypopituitarism (241–245).

In selective pituitary failure, the gonadotropin deficiency may occur singly or in combination with impairment of adrenocorticotropin secretion.

The occurrence of isolated gonadotropin failure is relatively rare and is usually idiopathic and not related to tumor growth. Sometimes in the progression of such tumors as pituitary chromophobe adenomas, gonadotropin failure precedes TSH and ACTH failure by several months to years. However, in the category under discussion, progression beyond gonadotropin failure does not occur. Isolated gonadotropin "failure" may also be noted in patients receiving suppressive steroid therapy (e.g., androgen or estrogen), and in those suffering from a catabolic disease process. Since these are not examples of primary pituitary disease, they should not be considered as representative of this syndrome.

Another group of patients designated as having selective pituitary failure exhibit deficiency of adrenocorticotropin and gonadotropin secretion (242). Thyroid function remains normal as attested by clinical evidence of euthyroidism, normal radioactive iodine uptake, and normal protein-bound iodine values. Presumably, this means that TSH secretion is not significantly affected. However, because there is some evidence that at times the thyroid may be capable of maintaining autonomous function, TSH secretion may also be involved in these cases. Direct measurement of TSH levels will be necessary to clarify this point.

Finally, patients having panhypopituitarism will have hypogonadotropic hypogonadism in addition to their hypothyroidism and adrenal insufficiency (Ch. 2).

The treatment of hypogonadism is essentially the same for each group. In contrast to the patients having hypogonadotropic eunuchoidism, patients with postpuberal gonadotropin failure do not respond uniformly to chorionic gonadotropin therapy (Fig. 6–18). In fact, when the testis is completely hyalinized (Fig. 6–4), the interstitial fibroblastic elements are refractory to stimulation.

How the testis remains potentially responsive is not known with certainty. MacLeod et al. (246), Gemzell and Kjessler (247), Mancini et al. (248), and other workers (249) have demonstrated that hMG-hCG or hPG therapy may be effective in restoring spermatogenesis and Leydig cell function if treatment is instituted shortly after pituitary function is lost. We encountered a nonresponsive testis 5 years after development of panhypopituitarism. In this instance, a basal skull fracture pinpointed the onset of the lesion. For practical purposes, though, androgen replacement therapy is indicated unless fertility is an issue. This should be instituted as outlined here and maintained for life.

ANDROGEN REPLACEMENT THERAPY

When the testes are damaged primarily to the extent that male hormone production by the Leydig cells is not normal, androgen replacement therapy with one of the various testosterone preparations is indicated (Table 6–6). Furthermore, as mentioned in the discussion of hypogonadotropic eunuchoidism (p. 347), stimulatory therapy by means of chorionic gonadotropin may prove impractical, so that the physician must rely on androgen therapy instead. Likewise, androgens are employed in managing patients with postpuberal pituitary failure, since the response to gonadotropin administration is generally poor and since the defect is invariably permanent, requiring lifelong treatment.

TABLE 6–6. ANDROGEN PREPARATIONS

Medication	Dose, mg.	Route	Administration Schedule
Testosterone enanthate	200	IM	Every 1–2 weeks for full effectiveness,
Testosterone cyclopentylpropionate	200	IM	then every 2-3 weeks for maintenance
Testosterone propionate	50	IM	Three times weekly
Testosterone pellets* (unconjugated)	450	Subcutaneous	Every 4–6 months
Methyltestosterone† (linguets)	25–50	Buccal	Daily
Fluoxymesterone†	5–10	Oral	Daily

*Each pellet contains 75 mg. unconjugated testosterone.
†At these doses, which have been recommended by other authors, the clinical response is less than that obtained with the long-acting esters. It is of interest that, even when the dose of fluoxymesterone is increased five times, the patient's response is not optimal.

Eunuchoidal patients whose testicular disease has interfered with normal puberal development need somewhat higher doses of testosterone to obtain full sexual maturation than the doses needed to maintain a patient with postpuberal Leydig cell deficiency. The long-acting enanthate, or cyclopentylpropionate esters of testosterone are preferred because of their potency and the steady response obtained. The recommended dosage schedule is 200 mg. intramuscularly every 1–2 weeks for a period of 2–3 years, at which time full development is usually attained. Then 100–200 mg. is administered every 2–3 weeks for maintenance.

Unconjugated testosterone pellets may be used in place of the intramuscular injections. In this instance, six 75-mg. testosterone pellets are placed subcutaneously by means of a pellet injector* into the medial aspect of the thighs (three on each side). This procedure must be repeated every 4–6 months to maintain effective levels of androgen. The necessity of performing minor surgery and the cost factor are the major disadvantages of this form of therapy.

Intramuscular administration of an aqueous suspension of testosterone is not tolerated by the patient as well as the ester solutions in oil, and the clinical response is somewhat erratic. Testosterone propionate, a short-acting compound, is effective but not practical for long-term therapy. Oral medication in the form of methyltestosterone or fluoxymesterone elicits an androgenic response, but it does not approach the potency of testosterone enanthate or unconjugated testosterone pellets.

Androgen treatment is usually without complications, but several points should be kept in mind. Since testosterone may stimulate an *existing* prostatic carcinoma, the presence of such carcinoma is a contraindication to this therapy. Benign prostatic hyperplasia is not affected adversely (250). On occasion, however, in patients over age 50 who have had long-standing androgen deficiency, the prostate gland may be quite sensitive to testosterone.† In these men it is prudent to start with short-acting preparations, such as testosterone propionate, so that if bladder neck obstruction does occur, it will be only temporary. If this happens, then the physician has to weigh the benefits of hormonal therapy against the problems of prostatic surgery in such a patient.

Alterations in liver function may develop with methyltestosterone therapy and, to a much lesser extent, with fluoxymesterone therapy. The characteristic histologic abnormality is biliary capillary stasis with little if any parenchymal damage. Clinically, the findings are those of obstructive jaundice, and recovery is rapid and uneventful after steroid withdrawal (251, 252). This complication has not been reported with the use of the unconjugated or esterified forms of testosterone.

*Kerns Pellet Injector, H. Laurent & Co., Inc., 18 Columbia St., Newark, N.J.

†The increased sensitivity is probably related to preexisting prostatic hyperplasia which regressed because of the androgen deficiency.

An elevated hematocrit value due to stimulation of erythropoiesis is sometimes encountered in eunuchoidal males receiving testosterone. When this occurs the dose should be reduced. Elevated blood pressure, presumably secondary to salt retention, may also develop and require attention, e.g., also a reduction in dosage. For some individuals who are more sensitive to the administered testosterone, one may have to be satisfied with less than optimal androgen therapy.

Although priapism has been stated to interfere with treatment in some hypogonadal males, strictly speaking this is not the case. Frequent erections to the point of disturbance do occur, but such problems can be overcome by adjusting the level of medication and conferring with the patient at least weekly. It must be remembered that a eunuchoidal patient over 30 years of age, for example, may find even two erections per day troublesome, since he has had to compensate considerably for his abnormality. Thus the physician has to guide an individual of this type through his "induced" puberty carefully. As in normal puberty, the patient learns to control his libido and sexual potentia, and the number of erections and incidence of masturbation decrease with time. It should also be emphasized that males with severe androgen deficiency are quite passive, which leads to a somewhat ambivalent attitude toward treatment. Only by insisting on a definite therapeutic regimen and by making certain that the patient adheres to it will the physician ensure a successful result.

EFFECTS OF EXTRAGONADAL ENDOCRINE DISORDERS ON GONADAL FUNCTION

Addison's Disease

Impotence and decreased libido are commonly present in males having Addison's disease. This observation plus the very low 17-ketosteroid excretion encountered in these patients has suggested that primary adrenal insufficiency invariably leads to decreased testicular function. Whereas, as mentioned previously, catabolic conditions will inhibit pituitary gonadotropin secretion in many instances, some have postulated from animal studies that the loss of adrenal function directly affects the testis. Morales and Hotchkiss (253), however, demonstrated that normal spermatogenesis persisted after adrenalectomy in men maintained on cortisone. Our observations in men having Addison's disease were similar (254).

Therefore, when impaired testicular function develops in Addison's disease, it is most likely due to a nonspecific reduction in pituitary function. Even when gonadotropin secretion and, thus, testicular function remain normal, it is difficult to visualize the presence of normal libido and sexual potentia if one considers the degree of weakness occurring with adrenal insufficiency.

Myxedema

Most observations regarding spermatogenesis in myxedema have been made in elderly men, so that definite conclusions as to thyroid-gonadal interrelationships cannot be made. Myxedematous changes in the pituitary to the point of *panhypopituitarism* may occur, which would naturally lead to testicular atrophy. Beierwaltes (255) found that urinary gonadotropins were normal in men and young women having myxedema but lower than expected in myxedematous, postmenopausal women. Hellman and coworkers (256) demonstrated that the conversion of exogenous testosterone to androsterone was decreased in myxedema. Also, there was a reduction in the endogenous production of androsterone, which was returned to normal by the administration of triiodothyronine. Probably, most myxedematous males exhibit some abnormality in spermatogenesis, Leydig cell function, and/or seminal fluid characteristics before treatment (257).

Congenital Adrenal Hyperplasia

Testicular development is retarded in patients with this disorder. When cortisone therapy is instituted, normal testicular function, including spermatogenesis, ensues (258). If therapy is discontinued during adulthood, spermatogenesis may not be totally inhibited. For example, Prader et al. (259) examined four men, 3–12 years after cortisone therapy had been discontinued. Each patient was well-defined with respect to the correct diagnosis (i.e., elevated pregnanetriol and 17-KS excretion). Their sperm counts were 12–113 million/ml. Serum testosterone and LH titers were normal. These findings are interesting in light of the suggestion that minimal (congenital) or acquired adrenal hyperplasia plays a significant role in the pathogenesis of male infertility.

Feminizing Adrenocortical Carcinoma

Spermatogenesis and Leydig cell function are inhibited in this condition, characterized by increased estrogen production (260, 261). Surgical and chemotherapeutic palliation result in resumption of testicular function, including return to normal status. The increased estrogens inhibit pituitary-hypothalamic function, resulting in decreased gonadal function.

Liver Cirrhosis

Although this disease is not strictly an endocrine disorder, hypogonadism and gynecomastia (p. 358) are frequently present in patients with chronic liver disease. Traditionally, increased circulating estrogens have been considered responsible for the decreased testicular function, gynecomastia, palmar erythema, and spider angiomata. Sophisticated examination of steroid metabolism has produced conflicting data (262–264), but certain conclusions can be drawn. Testosterone production and metabolic clearance rates are reduced. Total serum estradiol levels are *not* uniformly elevated. Furthermore, the correlation between estradiol levels and the presence of gynecomastia is poor. The questions that remain unsettled include: (1) Does the presence of "normal" estradiol levels have a pathologic impact when the "free" and "bound" testosterone levels are reduced? (2) Are "free" estradiol levels uniformly elevated, or at least elevated in the majority of patients? (3) What are the mechanisms responsible for normal LH levels in the presence of reduced testosterone titers?

Acromegaly apparently does not alter the testis unless the eosinophilic adenoma interferes with anterior pituitary function by direct expansion (Ch. 2).

In *Cushing's syndrome,* there is a variable increase in production of androgens and estrogens by the adrenal cortex which may inhibit the testis. Also, nonspecific changes in pituitary function may occur, depending on the degree of catabolism. Thus, if testicular function is impaired in patients with Cushing's syndrome, hypercorticoidism is not directly responsible. For example, Maddock and associates (264a) observed no alteration in gonadal function in patients who received high doses of cortisone.

EFFECTS OF SPINAL CORD DAMAGE

Over 50% of males with paraplegia sustained by trauma exhibit decreased testicular function of varying degrees (265–269). The commonest defect encountered is spermatogenic arrest associated with generalized hypoplasia of the germinal epithelium. Leydig cells usually appear normal, but the presence of nodular hyperplasia has been reported (267, 268). Androgen production is considered to be essentially normal in paraplegic men.

Attempts have been made to correlate the level of the cord lesion with the incidence and extent of testicular damage. Although these studies have not indicated a precise relationship, the data suggest that in general when the lesion occurs in the lower cord segments less damage to the germinal epithelium is observed.

Impairment of gonadal temperature is probably the major factor in causing abnormal spermatogenesis in these patients. Studies in animals and humans have amply demonstrated the susceptibility of the germinal cells to increased temperatures. Scrotal skin temperatures increase when the lumbar sympathetics are interrupted. Furthermore, when the cremasteric reflex is absent, temperature regulation is hampered. The importance of the heat factor is emphasized by the observations of Bors and his associates (270), who noted a relationship between the segmental level of sweat impairment and the severity of seminiferous tubule damage. Moreover, they observed an improvement in the sperm counts of one patient after daily application of ice bags to his scrotum for a period of 3 months.

Urinary gonadotropin excretion has been found to be low or absent in the majority of paraplegic men so studied. This finding is likely related to the negative nitrogen balance commonly noted in these patients and may be partly responsible for the decreased seminiferous tubule function.

Even if spermatogenesis remains normal, paraplegic men may lose the ability to ejaculate and therefore are infertile. In 84 patients studied by Munro and co-workers (269), only 7% were able to have ejaculations. They concluded that the ability to ejaculate is most likely lost if the cord lesion is extensive and between D6 and L3.

Although paraplegia does not preclude normal fertility, in patients with impaired spermatogenesis or who have lost their sexual potentia, the outlook for correction of their infertility is dismal. Endocrine therapy is directed to correcting the nitrogen loss when present. For this purpose, testosterone or one of the synthetic anabolic steroids, such as methandrostenolone, may be used.

CRYPTORCHIDISM

At birth the incidence of undescended testes in all males is about 10%, but after the first year this figure drops spontaneously to approximately 1.7–3.0% (271, 272). During the prepuberal period, this number is further reduced by the "late" descending testes. Most common of these are the so-called *retractile* testes (pseudocryptorchidism), which migrate into the scrotum periodically until puberty. At this time, they usually remain in the scrotum and thus present no problem in medical management. Postpuberally about 0.3–0.4% of males have either unilateral or bilateral undescended testes. Failure of one testis to descend occurs four to five times as frequently as bilateral maldescent. The reader is referred to the works of Charny (271) and Scott (273) for detailed discussions of the mechanism involved in testicular descent.

Mention should be made at this point that some bilaterally "cryptorchid" patients are *functional prepuberal castrates* or patients with *"male Turner's syndrome."* Also, other examples of hypogonadism, such as Klinefelter's syndrome, male pseudohermaphrodism, Sertoli-cell-only syndrome, and hypogonadotropic eunuchoidism, are not infrequently encountered with cryptorchidism and therefore should be kept in mind when the patient with undescended testes is being evaluated. The following discussion assumes the diagnosis and exclusion of these conditions.

Ectopic testes, which represent a small proportion of the retained testes, apparently develop and travel through the inguinal canal normally, only to be diverted from their pathway before entering the scrotum. The mechanisms by which the testes are diverted are poorly understood. Ectopic testes are located and classified as follows: pubopenile, perineal, femoral (crural), and superficial inguinal (271, 273). Surgery is indicated when the diagnosis is established, since orchiopexy performed prior to puberty usually results in a normally functioning testis. This is probably due to the fact that the ectopic testis contains inherently normal germinal epithelium and, further, that the spermatic cord, including the spermatic artery, is of adequate length, which diminishes the likelihood of impairment to testicular blood supply after orchiopexy.

In *"true" cryptorchidism,* the testes are situated intra-abdominally or in the inguinal canal. A commonly encountered "etiologic" factor is the presence of a short spermatic artery, which Charny believes may be merely a manifestation of poor testicular development (dysgenesis). Others have advocated that most retained testes are essentially normal until puberty, when exposure to internal body temperatures damages the germinal epithelium (274, 275). However, the observations of Nelson (276) and Sohval (277) support the concept that testicular dysgenesis plays an important role in maldescent and also suggest that, even if embryogenesis has been normal, further testicular development may be retarded during the prepuberal years by virtue of the nonscrotal position. Mancini et al. (278), in a detailed extension of their earlier work (279), noted fewer immature spermatogonia in the cryptorchid testis prior to age 4 years. They compared the cytologic features of the cryptorchid testes with the contralateral scrotal testes and finally with the testes of a control population of similar age who did not exhibit cryptorchidism. Before puberty, the changes were slight, but as the puberal process progressed, the discrepancy in germinal cell maturation between the cryptorchid and scrotal testes widened precipitously. Nelson's studies indicate that age 6–7 may be the critical time for surgical intervention, whereas Mancini's study suggests that orchiopexy might be considered even earlier. However, it remains to be established whether early treatment will improve the "salvage" rate. In Charny's series of 61 patients with unilateral cryptorchidism subjected to orchiopexy at varying ages (either before or after puberty had started), not a single patient was observed to exhibit normal spermatogenesis in follow-up examination of testicular biopsy specimens (280). Others report greater success, but as a general rule critical histologic evaluation has been erratic (281). The situation with bilateral cryptorchidism appears to be different. For example, Gross and Jewett (282) report "acceptable" fertility in 79% of their 38 cases.

Whenever possible, unnecessary surgery on the migratory or pseudocryptorchid testes should be avoided. Therefore, until it is demonstrated that early treatment is more beneficial, surgical therapy should be delayed until the first signs of puberty. Sometimes an associated inguinal hernia will require correction prior to puberty. In this instance, orchiopexy can best be performed at the same time. The incidence of inguinal hernia in cases of cryptorchidism has been reported to range from 57 to 93%, but usually such hernias are of anatomic rather than clinical importance.

It may be desirable to prognosticate in the prepuberal patient whether orchiopexy will be required at puberty. This can be accomplished by administering chorionic gonadotropin at a dose of 4000 I.U. three times weekly for 3 weeks. Testicular descent will occur in the majority of patients during this test period. In some, the descent will be permanent, but in most, the testis or testes will return to a nonscrotal position. However, in these it can be predicted that at puberty permanent descent will occur and surgery will not be necessary. In patients who fail to respond, surgery will be indicated at the onset of puberty if spermatogenesis is to be preserved (provided that the potential is there). The dosage schedule as recommended above will not damage the testes, nor will undesirable androgenic effects occur.

When orchiopexy is performed, bilateral testicular biopsy specimens should be obtained, even if there is only unilateral involvement. Then 18 months to 2 years later, repeat biopsy specimens should be obtained for study. If the once-cryptorchid testis shows abnormal spermatogenesis at this time, it is unlikely that active spermatogenesis will ever develop. Leydig cell function is usually normal, provided the blood supply to the testis is reasonably adequate.

Another controversial point is the relative importance of malignant changes developing in cryptorchid testes. Carroll (283) suggests that the incidence is overrated, whereas others emphasize the danger. Campbell (284) stresses the point that 12% of the cases of primary testicular carcinoma occur in cryptorchid men, who make up less than 0.4% of the adult male population. Therefore he concludes that a cryptorchid testis is at least 40 times more likely to become malignant than is a scrotal testis. It should be pointed out that placing the testis into the scrotum does not guarantee against later development of cancer, for it seems that the "now-scrotal, once-cryptorchid" testis still has an increased chance of becoming malignant (285–287). With the low incidence (0.002% of all males) of testicular carcinoma, however, prophylactic orchiectomy in cryptorchidism does not appear to be justified.

GYNECOMASTIA

Gynecomastia, or "benign glandular" enlargement of the male breast, occurs in the majority of males at some time during their life span. It is usually grossly evident but can be limited to microscopic changes. Clinically, it should be differentiated from other causes of breast enlargement, which include such entities as lipoma, carcinoma, neurofibromatosis, and, in the obese patient, a diffuse increase in adipose tissue. Gynecomastia represents a *concentric* increase in glandular and stromal tissue. When the enlargement is grossly evident, it varies from a small "button" subareolar enlargement to that indistinguishable from the adult female breast (Fig. 6–25). Although more common bilaterally, unilateral gynecomastia also occurs.

Microscopically, the *normal* male breast consists

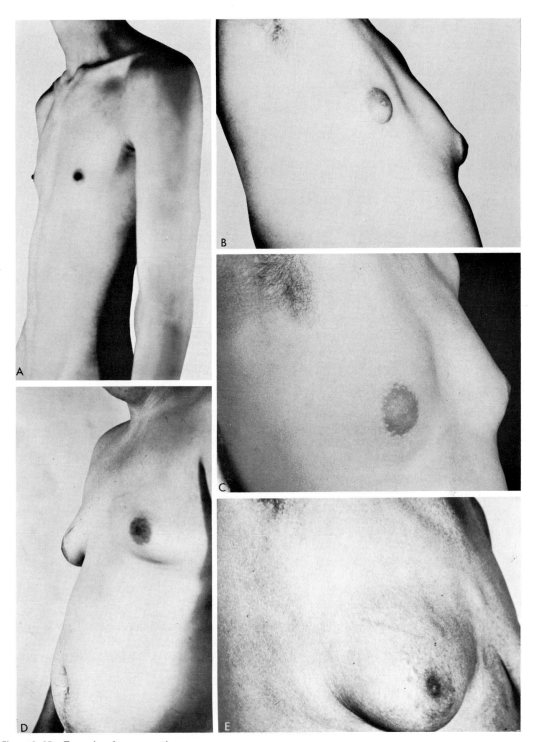

Figure 6–25. Examples of gynecomastia.
A, Puberal type. Note the plaque-like enlargement best seen in the lateral view of the right breast. *B*, *C*, *D*, and *E*, Gynecomastia of increasing severity in males with either Klinefelter's syndrome or the functional prepuberal castrate syndrome.

of a few scattered ducts containing low cuboidal epithelium. Strands of moderately dense collagenous tissue in the interlobular spaces support the ductal elements, and the periductal area is composed of scanty amounts of fiber-poor connective tissue. When gynecomastia is present, the histologic picture falls into two general patterns. In one, the major changes occur in the parenchymal elements, and thus ductal hyperplasia and lobular formation are the main features. In the other group, alterations in interlobular and periductal tissue predominate, with an increase in dense collagenous fibers and adipose tissue, although ductal proliferation is seen (288, 289).

Nicolis et al. (290) have interpreted the histologic pattern in a different manner. Their data, as well as the extensive studies by Bannayan et al. (291), indicate that the duration of the gynecomastia rather than etiologic factors dictates the histologic appearance. The exception to this thesis may be the development of acini that is associated with estrogen ingestion or elevated endogenous estrogens. The contention of Nicolis et al. and Bannayan et al. may be correct, but this author has encountered many adult patients who originally were considered to have had gynecomastia of short duration which subsequently proved to have been present for a longer time, although intermittent episodes of exacerbation had been experienced. The chart survey that Bannayan et al. conducted would therefore possess inherent deficiencies.

Therefore the two basic microscopic patterns could still imply different causal factors. The autopsy studies of Schwartz and Wilens support this contention (289). These investigators detected acinar or lobular development only in those patients with gynecomastia who had received estrogen therapy for palliation of prostatic carcinoma. In the remaining cases of gynecomastia, which were associated with either cirrhosis of the liver or systemic disorders, such as rheumatoid arthritis (on corticosteroid therapy), diabetes mellitus, chronic glomerulonephritis, or bronchogenic carcinoma, an increase in periductal connective tissue was the major feature. These observations agree with those of Morrione (292). Ductal proliferation was also noted. When parenchymal changes predominate, then, testosterone, estrogen, or adrenal steroids alone or in combination may be primarily responsible, with prolactin playing a permissive role. When stromal changes predominate, unknown factors may be primarily responsible. It is possible that end-organ (breast) tissue metabolism may be altered in certain patients, which predisposes the patient toward the development of gynecomastia, despite a normal hormonal environment. This latter possibility may be the basis for the genetic relationship observed in some otherwise healthy patients who have gynecomastia in the absence of gonadal disease (293).

One of the problems in evaluating the cause of gynecomastia is that enlargement of the male breast is found in many clinical conditions that seemingly have no common ground (294–299) (Table 6–7). Furthermore, since estrogens are con-

TABLE 6–7. CLINICAL CONDITIONS COMMONLY ASSOCIATED WITH GYNECOMASTIA

Normal puberty
Hypergonadotropic hypogonadism
  Klinefelter's syndrome
  Reifenstein's syndrome
Refeeding gynecomastia
  Recovery from generalized malnutrition or deranged
  metabolism associated with:
    Pulmonary tuberculosis
    Diabetes mellitus
    Liver cirrhosis
    Congestive heart failure—digitalis therapy
Drug exposure
  Estrogens
  Testosterone
  Chorionic gonadotropin
  Phenothiazines
  Meprobamate
  Hydroxyzine
  Reserpine
  Spironolactone
  Marihuana
Renal failure
  Chronic hemodialysis
Hyperthyroidism
Testicular tumors
  Choriocarcinoma
  Mixed cell, e.g., embryonal and trophoblastic elements
  Interstitial cell adenomas
Bronchogenic carcinoma (gonadotropin-like secretion)
Pituitary tumors
Adrenal cortical carcinoma (feminizing)
Hodgkin's disease
Hypothyroidism
Idiopathic factors

ventionally associated with breast development, the assumption has been either that estrogen secretion is increased or that estrogen degradation is impaired in *all* males developing gynecomastia. Only in those patients with "feminizing" adrenal carcinomas or estrogen-secreting interstitial cell adenomas or in those who have ingested estrogens has this relationship been convincing.

In patients with liver cirrhosis, the presence of "spider" angiomas and "liver" palms (incidence about 90%), combined with testicular atrophy and gynecomastia (incidence about 50%) or either separately, has been attributed to increased circulating estrogens (p. 356).

Androgens may also stimulate the male breast, but they differ from estrogens in their clinical effect. For example, gynecomastia commonly develops during the initial phase of testosterone therapy for hypogonadism, but instead of increasing with continued steroid administration, it usually recedes gradually. Although testosterone is converted *in vivo* to estrogens, methyltestosterone, which is not thus converted, also produces gynecomastia. It is possible that androgens and estrogens of testicular origin are responsible for the development of gynecomastia observed during puberty. This occurs normally in approximately 70% of puberal males and is usually transient and requires no treatment. Histologically, parenchymal stimulation is the major feature.

Shortly after World War II, a peculiar type of gynecomastia was documented (300–302). Many American soldiers were noted to have painful breast enlargement after their release from prisoner-of-war camps. These changes occurred while they were recovering from malnutrition and not during the period of inanition, when there might have been derangement in liver function, for instance (303)—hence the designation "refeeding" gynecomastia. Since pituitary gonadotropin secretion is quite sensitive to protein deprivation, testicular function in these men during their period of severe weight loss was undoubtedly quiescent because of pituitary "shutdown." When their diet improved and their metabolic processes returned to normal, pituitary gonadotropin secretion resumed, producing a "second puberty." This type of gynecomastia is probably more common than is appreciated and may explain the mechanism by which breast enlargement occurs in, for example, the initial phase of digitalis therapy in the patient with congestive heart failure. The gynecomastia that develops during chronic hemodialysis for renal failure may be another example of this type (304, 305). Hormonal studies have failed to find consistently elevated prolactin or estradiol levels. The same mechanism may also apply to the patient with liver disease, since the gynecomastia is commonly observed only after recovery from several episodes of decompensated liver function.

In hypogonadism, gynecomastia rarely develops when gonadotropin secretion is low or absent, as in the *classic* form, *hypogonadotropic eunuchoidism*. As stated previously, gynecomastia is seen frequently in the variant form, "fertile eunuchoidism." Furthermore, it is seen quite regularly in hypergonadotropic syndromes, such as Klinefelter's syndrome and functional prepuberal castration, in which estrogen excretion is low or absent. The histologic picture in these cases is characterized by stromal rather than parenchymal hyperplasia.

Another condition in which the pituitary has been implicated is the syndrome of precocious menstruation and galactorrhea in juvenile myxedema reported by Van Wyk and Grumbach (306). They postulated that there may be an increase of other anterior pituitary hormones in addition to the one expected, which in their cases of hypothyroidism would be thyroid-stimulating hormone. Moreover, since pituitary enlargement was observed in their patients, the hypothalamic-pituitary pathway which normally inhibits prolactin secretion might have been interrupted. Increased plasma prolactin levels have been observed in similar situations (307).

The widespread use of drugs that affect hypothalamic or midbrain function has been associated with development of gynecomastia or galactorrhea or both. Whether or not these agents act exclusively by releasing prolactin is not clear (307–311). Whether the gynecomastia associated with the intensive use of marihuana (312) falls into the CNS-affecting group of drugs or some other category remains to be determined.

Summary

It is quite apparent that the etiology of gynecomastia is not known in the majority of cases. Prolactin levels are uniformly elevated when galactorrhea is present (313, 314). The confusion with respect to estrogen levels and steroid metabolism in general may be due in part to methodologic difficulties. If so, improved technology will clarify the issues.

Regardless of the state of our knowledge, the clinician needs to proceed in detecting serious diseases. The following outline may be followed.
  I. Hormonal assays
     A. hCG: germinal cell, bronchogenic, mediastinal, and mesothelial carcinomas
     B. Serum estradiol: feminizing adrenocortical carcinoma, interstitial cell tumors
     C. Prolactin: pituitary tumors
 II. X-ray studies
     A. Skull: particularly in presence of galactorrhea
     B. Chest: bronchogenic and mediastinal carcinoma
III. Buccal smear: Klinefelter's syndrome (mosaic pattern)
 IV. Mammography or excision biopsy: mammary carcinoma is suspected
Finally, when the breast enlargement is sufficient to disturb the patient, surgical removal is the only means of treatment.

MALE INFERTILITY

Approximately 15% of married couples do not produce progeny (315). Naturally, with some, this is by their own design, but in the majority it is involuntary. Defects in the male partner's reproductive system are responsible in over 50% of the cases. Pathologic conditions, such as Klinefelter's syndrome, hypogonadotropic eunuchoidism, Sertoli-cell-only syndrome, cryptorchidism, and orchitis secondary to epidemic parotitis, have been discussed previously and therefore will be excluded from this section.

The majority of males seen at infertility clinics have no *endocrine* disease (132) and can be divided into two major groups: (1) those having oligospermia or azoöspermia, who constitute more than 90% of the cases, and (2) those having "normal" seminal fluid.

When azoöspermia is encountered, there may be a congenital or acquired obstruction to the egress of sperm in the ductal system (316), or severe defects in spermatogenesis may be present (317, 132). The finding of azoöspermia, normal FSH and LH titers, and normal spermatogenesis as ascertained by testicular biopsy clearly establishes the existence of complete ductal obstruction. This may be in the vas deferens or epididymis.

Abnormal spermatogenesis can be separated into the following histologic patterns: (1) germinal cell arrest, partial or complete; (2) hypoplasia, involving all cell types; and (3) disorganization and sloughing of the germinal epithelium. Peritubular fibrosis may be present in each instance. Improved means for quantitating the germinal epithelium should lead to a better classification of so-called adult seminiferous tubule failure (318–321). Since the etiologic mechanisms are usually not known, rational therapy is impossible. However, in studying the effects of testosterone administration on spermatogenesis in androgenically normal men, Heller and co-workers (322) found that, in some instances in which spermatogenesis was initially defective, histologic improvement followed the cessation of drug administration. With these observations in mind, Heckel treated oligospermic patients and observed in some a "rebound" increase in total sperm counts over pre-treatment values (323). Thus it seems that by temporarily suppressing spermatogenesis with testosterone and allowing the germinal epithelium to "rest," spermatogenesis may be improved, at least temporarily, after germinal cell activity has resumed. Unfortunately these reports were followed by indiscriminate use of this form of therapy in unselected cases with understandably poor results. Heller (324) and Charny (325) emphasize the need for proper selection of patients and conclude that when appreciable peritubular fibrosis and hyalinization are present testosterone therapy is not indicated. Heller compared the results obtained in 23 control patients who had received ascorbic acid therapy with results in 107 patients who had received testosterone: 10.6% of his control series impregnated their wives, whereas the incidence was 37.4% in the treated group. Pregnancies occurred from 7 to 16 months after the initial visit in the control series and from 3 to 48 months after therapy in the testosterone-treated patients (326). One mechanism by which this form of therapy works may be the depression of circulating sperm antibodies. This phenomenon is considered to be responsible for either disturbed spermatogenesis or sperm agglutination in certain men (327–329). Since antigenic material is present in the primary spermatocytes, testosterone administration would reduce the antigen-antibody complex and theoretically permit temporary improvement in spermatogenesis after treatment is discontinued. Even so, the overall experience with the testosterone rebound regimen has been disappointing.

No other form of medical therapy is presently available for infertile males not suitable for testosterone therapy or for those who fail to respond to testosterone. Theoretically, when spermatogenesis is impaired to a minor degree so that pituitary gonadotropin secretion is not elevated, it might prove beneficial to administer a preparation such as hMG. Although success with this agent has occasionally been reported, the role for this form of therapy has not been established (330). Similarly, the results with clomiphene therapy have not been promising (249). Vitamin or thyroid administration or both has been used empirically for some time without success.

One condition that deserves increased attention is the association of unilateral varicocele with impaired spermatogenesis. Histologically, the seminiferous tubules usually remain normal in size, and the peritubular membranes are free of hyalinization and fibrosis. Each germ cell type is reduced in numbers, but particularly so with regard to spermatocytes and spermatids. Seminal fluid sperm concentration ranges from oligospermic levels to azoöspermia. Sperm motility is depressed. However, the important clue to cause and effect relationship in this condition is the increased number of tapered sperms.

Originally it was considered that the presence of a varicocele interfered with scrotal temperature regulation, which resulted in higher than normal testicular temperatures (331). Recent studies have failed to substantiate this hypothesis (332). On the other hand, MacLeod has emphasized the pathologic importance of retrograde blood flow, which exists in the left spermatic vein involved with a varicocele (333, 334). Venographic studies have also demonstrated the presence of an anastomotic channel across the symphysis pubis which permits blood to reach the right testis from the left spermatic vein. Thus both testes may have abnormal venous drainage. Charny reported improved spermatogenesis in 23 of 36 men who underwent varicocelectomy (335). Similar results were reported by Scott and Young (336) and MacLeod (117).

It is beyond the scope of this chapter to detail the many studies underway that are designed to furnish more precise understanding of the pathophysiology in infertile males. Hopefully, the role of infections, autosomal disorders (e.g., D/D 13–15 translocation), and epididymal disorders that interfere with sperm maturation will be clarified.

HORMONAL ASPECTS OF TESTICULAR NEOPLASMS

In general, testicular malignancies are an uncommon problem; the incidence in the total male population is only 0.002%. However, in males aged 20–35 years, tumors of the testis constitute one of the most common forms of malignancy. Moreover, since they usually metastasize early, prompt recognition and treatment are important in obtaining good results.

Morphologically, testicular neoplasms are divided into two major categories: germinal and nongerminal. The germinal tumors, which comprise approximately 96% of the cases in most series, have been further classified by Dixon and Moore (338) as follows: (1) seminoma, pure; (2) embryonal carcinoma, pure or with seminoma; (3) teratoma, pure or with seminoma; (4) teratoma, with either embryonal carcinoma or choriocarcinoma or both and with or without seminoma; and (5) choriocarcinoma, pure or with either embryonal carcinoma or seminoma or both. In addition to the histologic differences, each group appears to follow a characteristic clinical course (337–339).

Clinically, in patients having germinal cell tumors, the most common initial symptoms are enlargement or hardness of the involved testes. Pain may be an associated finding at this time. Careful palpation of the scrotal contents, with proper identification of the intrascrotal parts, is very important in the diagnosis, since in one large series (338) the correct diagnosis was suspected in only 28% of the cases after the initial examination. Epididymitis was the most common incorrect diagnosis. Gynecomastia develops in approximately 30% of these patients and is usually, but not invariably, associated with choriocarcinomas. Breast enlargement may also occur in patients having Leydig cell tumors.

Therefore, in addition to careful palpation of the testes, assays for detecting hCG should be performed (Ch. 7). Although hCG is invariably secreted by testicular choriocarcinomas, germinal cell malignancies of other cell types may secrete hCG. When assays are positive for hCG (best method is radioimmunoassay utilizing β subunit antisera), the prognosis is very poor; the majority of patients die within 9–12 months.

The ability of these tumors to synthesize and secrete hCG would be comparable to oat cell carcinomas of the lung that secrete ACTH or other bronchogenic carcinomas that secrete hCG.

The measurement of alpha-fetoprotein, a normal alpha$_1$ globulin that usually disappears from the circulation about the time of birth, may also prove very useful in detecting germ cell malignancies (337). Experience with this procedure is required prior to assigning it an important role as a therapeutic monitor.

Treatment of testicular germinal cell tumors consists of orchiectomy followed by x-irradiation (337, 338, 340). In one series, the 5-year mortality after surgery for each group (see classification grouping, p. 362) was as follows: 10.5, 64.5, 29.2, 52.2, and 100%.

During the past two decades, the 5-year survival has improved from 50% to 65% for all cases and from 66% to 84% for localized disease. A large series of 700 patients revealed some improvement in treating testicular choriocarcinoma, namely a 5-year survival of 14%. The reader is referred to the review moderated by Rubin (342) for details of improved diagnosis, chemotherapy, etc.

Leydig cell tumors are the most important of the nongerminal testicular neoplasms. Functionally, these fall into two groups: those that are virilizing (342) and those that are feminizing (343). When the androgen-producing type develops in prepuberal boys, precocious development of the penis, beard, and muscles occurs. Linear growth is also accelerated. But when this type occurs in adult males, little change is noted, since excess androgen in the normal adult man does not alter the secondary sex characteristics or increase libido and sexual potentia. Gynecomastia, however, may develop.

Urinary 17-ketosteroid excretion is increased as well as urinary androgen excretion. Both values drop to normal after surgery if metastases are not present. Occasionally, in prepuberal boys, the diagnosis of Leydig cell tumor may be confused with congenital adrenal hyperplasia, since ectopic

adrenal cortical tissue may also be found along the spermatic cord. If there is any doubt, corticosteroid administration should be carried out to determine whether 17-ketosteroid excretion can be inhibited. If this occurs, then the correct diagnosis is congenital adrenal hyperplasia, and surgery would therefore not be indicated (Ch. 5).

Leydig cell tumors that produce estrogenic effects are found only in adult males. Here gynecomastia, impotence, and decreased hair growth result, and urinary estrogen excretion is high.

Surgery is indicated for both types, and, in contrast to the germinal cell tumors, Leydig cell tumors generally follow a more "benign" course, even though metastases may occur and recurrence may develop after surgical removal of the primary tumor.

HOMOSEXUALITY

Homosexuality and transvestism are psychiatric disorders and are not caused by disturbances in sex hormone production. While some have suggested that increased estrogen secretion is responsible for these aberrations in male sex behavior, this has not been borne out by fact. It should be emphasized that, if estrogen is administered to normal males, impotence and decreased sexual potentia result, but the direction of the sex drive remains unaltered.

The issue of a hormonal relationship in homosexual males has been reported. Kolodny et al. (345) point out that serum testosterone levels in a group of 30 homosexuals were significantly lower than in 50 heterosexual males. A later publication revealed elevated serum LH titers (346). Furthermore, many homosexual men studied demonstrated decreased sperm counts. Although these data are of interest, the gonadal aberrations so noted are probably secondary to the emotional conflicts in these men and the deviation in sexual activity (e.g., sodomy, increased incidence of genitourinary infection?). From a simplistic viewpoint, if testosterone levels are causally related to this problem, patients who occupy the "female" role should demonstrate lower testosterone levels than those patients who retain the "male" role.

While hypogonadism associated with alterations in development of the external genitalia or gynecomastia or both could conceivably confuse normal sex identification in some, it is uncommon for these individuals to become overtly homosexual. I found that most homosexuals have normal testicular function and sexual maturation. Careful psychiatric testing has demonstrated that many patients with Klinefelter's syndrome have subtle homosexual tendencies. Since it is beyond the scope of this discussion to deal with these findings, the reader is referred to the psychiatric literature for more details.

Attempts at psychiatric therapy are generally disappointing, since homosexual individuals usually do not desire treatment and profess to be satisfied with their status.

MALE CONTRACEPTION

Methods for male contraception have received relatively little attention in the past. Adverse social attitudes, suboptimal scientific expertise in male reproductive physiology, and the inherent prolonged period of spermatogenesis each contributed to this state. Recent shifts in social attitudes combined with improved scientific knowledge have provided renewed interest in this field (347). Undoubtedly the major force behind this change in focus was the fact that oral contraception for the female presented undesirable reactions in many women. Bilateral vasectomy was selected as a solution by many men. Since this procedure renders the male permanently infertile, for practical purposes other methods should be made available to assist the younger man in family planning (348). For example, it has been estimated that the average number of progeny for the men who selected vasectomy was 3.7.

The ideal method would act on the epididymis to interfere with sperm maturation. Basic studies are underway, but no nontoxic and effective compounds are presently available. If current knowledge is used, then the suppression of spermatogenesis by chemical means should be possible. Preliminary results suggest one approach that may be useful (349). Examination of additional approaches is underway, which should provide a greater selection of effective methods for male contraception.

REFERENCES

1. Smith, D. W.: *Recognizable Patterns of Human Malformations.* Philadelphia, W. B. Saunders, 1970.
2. Rimoin, D. L., and Schimke, R. N.: *Genetic Disorders of the Endocrine Glands.* St. Louis, C. V. Mosby, 1971.
3. Clermont, Y.: *Amer. J. Anat. 112:*35, 1963.
4. Heller, C. G., and Clermont, Y.: *Recent Progr. Hormone Res. 20:*545, 1964.
5. Barr, A. B.: *Fertil. Steril. 24:*381, 1973.
6. deKretser, D. M., and Burger, H. G., In *Gonadotropins.* Saxena, B. B., Beling, C. G., et al. (eds.). New York, John Wiley and Sons, 1972, p. 640.
7. Vilar, O., Perez del Cerro, M. I., et al., In *Human Testis.* Rosemberg, E., and Paulsen, C. A. (eds.), New York, Plenum Press, 1970, p. 63.
8. Rowley, M. J., Berlin, J. D., et al.: *Z. Zellforsch. 112:*139, 1971.
9. Fawcett, D. W., Long, J. A., et al.: *Recent Progr. Hormone Res. 25:*315, 1969.
10. Morse, H. C., Horike, N., et al.: *J. Clin. Endocr.,* 1973 (in press).
11. Setchell, B. P., In *The Testis.* Vol. 1. Johnson, A. D., Gomes, W. R., et al. (eds.), New York, Academic Press, 1970, p. 176.
12. Hudson, B., Coghlan, J. P., et al.: *Ciba Found. Colloq. Endocr.* Vol. 16. Boston, Little, Brown and Co., 1967, p. 140.
13. Paulsen, C. A., Gordon, D. L., et al.: *Recent Progr. Hormone Res. 24:*321, 1968.
14. van Wagenen, G., and Simpson, M. E.: *Embryology of the Ovary and Testis in Homo Sapiens and Macaca Mulatta.* New Haven, Yale University Press, 1965.
15. McArthur, J. W., In *Gonadotropins.* Saxena, B, B., Beling, C. G., et al. (eds.), New York, John Wiley and Sons, 1972, p. 487.
16. Blizzard, R. M., Penny, R., et al., In *Gonadotropins.* Saxena, B. B., Beling, C. G., et al. (eds.), New York, John Wiley and Sons, 1972, p. 502.
17. Kelch, R. P., In *Gonadotropins.* Saxena, B. B., Beling, C. G., et al. (eds.), New York, John Wiley and Sons, 1972, p. 524.
18. Swerdloff, R. S., Jacobs, H. S., et al., In *Gonadotropins.* Saxena, B. B., Beling, C. G., et al. (eds.), New York, John Wiley and Sons, 1972, p. 546.
19. Kulin, H. E., Grumbach, M. M., et al.: *Pediat. Res. 6:*162, 1972.
20. Crim, L. W., and Geschwind, I. I.: *Biol. Reprod. 7:*47, 1972.
21. Albert, A., Underdahl, L. O., et al.: *Proc. Mayo Clin. 28:*409, 1953.
22. Sniffen, R. C.: *Ann. N.Y. Acad. Sci. 55:*609, 1952.
23. Charny, C. A., Conston, A. S., et al.: *Ann. N.Y. Acad. Sci. 55:*597, 1952.
24. de Kretser, D. M., Catt, K. J., et al.: *Endocrinology 80:*332, 1971.
25. Means, A. R., and Vaitukaitus, J.: *Endocrinology 90:*39, 1972.
26. Mancini, R. E.: *J. Histochem. Cytochem. 15:*516, 1967.
27. Castro, A. E., Seiguer, A. C., et al.: *Proc. Soc. Exp. Biol. Med. 133:*582, 1970.
28. Murad, F., Strauch, S., et al.: *Biochim. Biophys. Acta 177:*591, 1969.
29. Kuehl, F. A., Patanelli, D. J., et al.: *Biol. Reprod. 2:*154, 1970.
30. Means, A. R., and Hall, P. F.: *Biochemistry 8:*4293, 1969.
31. Means, A. R., In *The Human Testis.* Rosemberg, E., and Paulsen, C. A. (eds.), New York, Plenum Press, 1970, p. 301.
32. Eik-Nes, K. B.: *Ciba Found. Colloq. Endocr.* Vol. 16. Boston, Little, Brown & Co., 1967, p. 120.
33. Lostroh, A. J.: *Endocrinology 76:*438, 1969.
34. Johnson, R. H., and Ewing, L. L.: *Science 173:*635, 1971.
35. Steinberger, E.: *Physiol. Rev. 51:*1, 1971.
36. Leonard, J. M., Flocks, R. H., et al.: Program of the Endocrine Society, 53rd Meeting. Abst. 113, 1971.
37. Kelch, R. P., Jenner, M. R., et al.: *J. Clin. Invest. 51:*824, 1972.
38. Longcope, C., Widrich, W., et al.: *Steroids 20:*439, 1972.
39. Maddock, W. O., and Nelson, W. O.: *J. Clin. Endocr. 12:*985, 1952.
40. Mottram, J. C., and Cramer, W.: *Quart. J. Exp. Physiol. 13:*209, 1923.
41. McCullagh, D. R.: *Science 76:*19, 1932.
42. del Castillo, E. B., Trabucco, A., et al.: *J. Clin. Endocr. 7:*493, 1947.
43. Howard, R. P., Sniffen, R. C., et al.: *J. Clin. Endocr. 10:*121, 1950.
44. Lacy, D., and Pettit, A. J.: *Brit. Med. Bull. 26:*87, 1970.
45. Johnsen, S. G.: *Acta Endocr.* (Kobenhavn) *45*(Suppl. 90):99, 1964.
46. Johnsen, S. G., In *The Human Testis.* Rosemberg, E., and Paulsen, C. A. (eds.), New York, Plenum Press, 1970.
47. Leonard, J. M., Leach, R. B., et al.: *J. Clin. Endocr. 34:*209, 1972.
48. de Kretser, D. M., Burger, H. G., et al.: *J. Clin. Endocr. 35:*392, 1972.
49. Franchimont, P., Millet, D., et al.: *J. Clin. Endocr. 34:*1003, 1972.
50. Heller, C. G., and Nelson, W. O.: *Recent Progr. Hormone Res. 3:*229, 1948.
51. Heller, C. G., Paulsen, C. A., et al.: *Ann. N.Y. Acad. Sci. 55:*685, 1952.
52. Naftolin, F., Espeland, E., et al., In *Gonadotropins.* Rosemberg, E. (ed.), Los Altos, Geron-X, 1968.
53. Llerena, L. A., Guevara, A., et al.: *J. Clin. Endocr. 29:*1083, 1969.
54. Sherins, R. J., and Loriaux, D. L.: *J. Clin. Endocr. 36:*886, 1973.
55. Capell, P. T., and Paulsen, C. A.: *Contraception 6:*135, 1972.
56. Lee, P. A., Jaffe, R. B., et al.: *J. Clin. Endocr. 35:*636, 1972.
57. Schally, A. V., Baba, Y., et al.: *Biochem. Biophys. Res. Commun. 42:*50, 1971.
58. Matsuo, H., Baba, Y., et al.: *Biochem. Biophys. Res. Commun. 43:*1334, 1971.
59. Matsuo, H., Arimura, A., et al.: *Biochem. Biophys. Res. Commun. 45:*822, 1971.
60. Kastin, A. J., Schally, A. V., et al.: *J. Clin. Endocr. 34:*753, 1972.
61. Lucas, W. M., Whitmore, W. F., Jr., et al.: *J. Clin. Endocr. 17:*465, 1957.
62. Bertel, G. W., and Eik-Nes, K. B.: *Proc. Soc. Exp. Biol. Med. 102:*553, 1959.
63. Slaunwhite, W. R., and Samuels, L. T.: *J. Biol. Chem. 220:*341, 1956.

64. Landau, R. L., and Laves, M. L.: *J. Clin. Endocr. 19*:1399, 1959.
65. Savard, K., and Goldzieher, J. W.: *Endocrinology 66*:617, 1960.
66. Kahnt, F. W., Neher, R., et al.: *Experientia 17*:19, 1961.
67. Klempien, E. J., Voight, K. D., et al.: *Acta Endocr. 36*:498, 1961.
68. Dorfman, R. I., Forchielli, E., et al.: *Recent Progr. Hormone Res. 19*:251, 1963.
69. Hall, P. F., Sozer, C. C., et al.: *Endocrinology 74*:35, 1964.
70. Eik-Nes, K.: *Physiol. Rev. 44*:609, 1964.
71. Christensen, A. K., In *The Human Testis.* Rosemberg, E., and Paulsen, C. A. (eds.), New York, Plenum Press, 1970, p. 75.
72. Pearlman, W. H., and Crépy, O.: *J. Biol. Chem. 242*:182, 1967.
73. Vermeulen, A., and Verdonck, L.: *Steroids 11*:609, 1968.
74. Rosner, W., and Beakins, S. M.: *J. Clin. Invest. 47*:109, 1968.
75. Wilson, J. D.: *New Eng. J. Med. 287*:1284, 1972.
76. O'Malley, B. W.: *New Eng. J. Med. 284*:370, 1971.
77. Lipsett, M. B., and Korenman, S. G.: *J.A.M.A. 190*:757, 1964.
78. Christensen, A. K., and Mason, N. R.: *Endocrinology 76*:646, 1965.
79. Rivarola, M. A., and Podesta, E. J.: *Endocrinology 90*:618, 1972.
80. Horton, R., and Tait, J. F.: *J. Clin. Invest. 45*:301, 1966.
81. Bullock, L. P., and Bardin, C. W.: *J. Clin. Endocr. 35*:935, 1972.
82. Biglieri, E. G., Herron, M. A., et al.: *J. Clin. Invest. 45*:1946, 1966.
83. Saez, J. M., de Peretti, E., et al.: *J. Clin. Endocr. 32*:604, 1971.
84. Goebelsmann, U., Horton, R., et al.: *J. Clin. Endocr. 36*:867, 1973.
85. Naftolin, F., Judd, H. L., et al.: *J. Clin. Endocr. 36*:285, 1973.
86. Kirshner, M. A., Lipsett, M. B., et al.: *J. Clin. Invest. 44*:657, 1965.
87. Resko, J. A., and Eik-Nes, K. B.: *J. Clin. Endocr. 26*:573, 1966.
88. Lipsett, M. B., Wilson, H., et al.: *Recent Progr. Hormone Res. 22*:245, 1961.
89. Vermeulen, A., Stoïca, T., et al.: *J. Clin. Endocr. 33*:759, 1971.
90. Kent, J. R., and Acone, A. B., In *Androgens in Normal and Pathologic Conditions.* Vermeulen, A., and Exley, D. (eds.), Amsterdam, Excerpta Medica Foundation Intern. Congr. Ser. *101*:31, 1966.
91. Lipsett, M. B., In *The Human Testis.* Rosemberg, E., and Paulsen, C. A. (eds.), New York, Plenum Press, 1970.
92. Kreuz, L. E., Rose, R. M., et al.: *Arch. Gen. Psychiat. 26*:479, 1972.
93. Rose, R. M., Gordon, T. P., et al.: *Science 178*:643, 1972.
94. Matsumoto, K., Takeyasu, K., et al.: *Acta Endocr. 65*:11, 1970.
95. Samuels, L. T.: *Recent Progr. Hormone Res. 4*:65, 1949.
96. West, C. D., Tyler, F. H., et al.: *J. Clin. Endocr. 11*:897, 1951.
97. Fukushima, D. K., Bradlow, H. L., et al.: *J. Biol. Chem. 206*:863, 1954.
98. Leach, R. B., Maddock, W. O., et al.: *Recent Progr. Hormone Res. 12*:377, 1956.
99. Dorfman, R. I., and Ungar, F.: *Metabolism of Steroid Hormones.* New York, Academic Press, 1965.
100. Sandberg, A. A., and Slaunwhite, W. R., Jr.: *J. Clin. Invest. 35*:1331, 1956.
101. Slaunwhite, W. R., Jr., and Sandberg, A. A.: *J. Clin. Endocr. 18*:1056, 1958.
102. Vande Wiele, R. L., MacDonald, P. C., et al.: *Recent Progr. Hormone Res. 19*:275, 1963.
103. MacDonald, P. C., Chapdilanie, A., et al.: *J. Clin. Endocr. 25*:1557, 1965.
104. Heard, R. D. H., Bligh, E. G., et al.: *Recent Progr. Hormone Res. 12*:45, 1956.
105. Nyman, M. A., Geiger, J., et al.: *J. Biol. Chem. 234*:16, 1959.
106. Schonfeld, W. A.: *Amer. J. Dis. Child. 65*:535, 1943.
107. Bartlett, P. D.: *Endocrinology 52*:272, 1953.
108. Lubs, H. A., Jr.: *New Eng. J. Med. 267*:326, 1962.
109. Bunge, R. G., and Sherman, J. K.: *Fertil. Steril. 5*:353, 1954.
110. Gassner, F. X., Goldzieher, J. W., et al.: *Fertil. Steril. 10*:488, 1959.
111. Falk, H. C., and Kaufman, S. A.: *Fertil. Steril. 1*:489, 1950.
112. MacLeod, J.: *Fertil. Steril. 1*:397, 1950.
113. MacLeod, J., and Gold, R. Z.: *Fertil. Steril. 4*:10, 1953.
114. MacLeod, J., and Gold, R. Z.: *Fertil. Steril. 4*:194, 1953.
115. Gordon, D. L., Moore, D. J., et al.: *J. Lab. Clin. Med. 65*:506, 1965.
116. Gordon, D. L., Herrigel, J. E., et al.: *Amer. J. Clin. Path. 47*:226, 1967.
117. MacLeod, J., In *The Human Testis.* Rosemberg, E., and Paulsen, C. A. (eds.), New York, Plenum Press, 1970, p. 481.
118. Steelman, S. L., and Pohley, F. M.: *Endocrinology 53*:604, 1953.
119. Albert, A.: *Recent Progr. Hormone Res. 12*:227, 1956.
120. Diczfalusy, E.: *Acta Endocr. 63*(Suppl. 142):1, 1969.
121. Morgan, C. R., and Lazarow, A.: *Diabetes 12*:115, 1963.
122. Midgley, A. R., Jr.: *Endocrinology 79*:10, 1966.
123. Midgley, A. R., Jr.: *J. Clin. Endocr. 27*:295, 1967.
124. Santen, R. J., Leonard, J. M., et al.: *J. Clin. Endocr. 33*:970, 1971.
125. Gandy, H. M., and Peterson, R. E.: *J. Clin. Endocr. 28*:949, 1968.
126. Mayes, D., and Nugent, C. A.: *J. Clin. Endocr. 28*:1169, 1968.
127. Nieschlag, E., and Loriaux, D. L.: *Z. Klin. Chem. Klin. Biochem. 4*:164, 1972.
128. Gordon, D. L., Barr, A. B., et al.: *Fertil. Steril. 16*:522, 1965.
129. Hotchkiss, R. S.: *N. Y. State J. Med. 41*:564, 1941.
130. Charny, C. W., In *Diagnosis in Sterility.* Engle, E. (ed.), Springfield, Ill., Charles C Thomas, 1941.
131. Heller, C. G., and Nelson, W. O.: *J. Clin. Endocr. 8*:345, 1948.
132. de Kretser, D. M., Burger, H. G., et al.: *J. Clin. Endocr. 35*:392, 1972.
133. Kjessler, B., and Wide, L.: *Acta Endocr. 72*:243, 1973.
134. Maclean, N., Harnden, D. G., et al.: *Lancet 1*:286, 1964.
135. Kaplan, N. M., and Norfleet, R. G.: *Ann. Intern. Med. 54*:461, 1961.
136. Paulsen, C. A., de Souza, A., et al.: *J. Clin. Endocr. 24*:1182, 1964.
137. Klinefelter, H. G., Jr., Reifenstein, E. C., Jr., et al.: *J. Clin. Endocr. 2*:615, 1942.
138. Heller, C. G., and Nelson, W. O.: *J. Clin. Endocr. 5*:1, 1945.
139. Becker, K. L., Hoffman, D. L., et al.: *Arch. Intern. Med. 118*:314, 1966.
140. Barr, M. L., Carr, D. H., et al.: *J. Ment. Defic. Res. 6*:65, 1962.
141. Day, R. W., Levinson, J., et al.: *J. Pediatrics 63*:589, 1963.
142. Stewart, J. S. S., Mack, W. S., et al.: *Quart. J. Med. 28*:561, 1959.
143. Nowakowski, H., and Lenz, W.: *Recent Progr. Hormone Res. 17*:53, 1961.
144. Ferguson-Smith, M. A.: *Lancet 1*:219, 1959.
145. de la Chapelle, A.: *J. Ment. Defic. Res. 7*:129, 1963.
146. Raboch, J.: *J. Clin. Endocr. 17*:1429, 1957.
147. Stewart, J. S. S.: *Lancet 1*:1176, 1959.
148. Tanner, J. M., Prader, A., et al.: *Lancet 2*:141, 1959.
149. Raboch, J., and Sipova, I.: *Acta Endocr. 36*:404, 1961.
150. Rohde, R. A.: *Lancet 2*:149, 1964.
151. Bomers-Marres, A. J. M. L.: *Lancet 2*:364, 1964.
152. Nielsen, J.: *Lancet 1*:1376, 1966.
153. Carr, D. H., Barr, M. L., et al.: *J. Clin. Endocr. 21*:491, 1961.
154. Ford, C. E.: *Brit. Med. Bull. 25*:104, 1969.
155. Gordon, D. L., Krmpotic, E., et al.: *Arch. Intern. Med. 130*:726, 1972.
156. Frøland, A.: *Danish Med. Bull. 16*(Suppl. 6):1, 1969.
157. Muldal, S., and Ockey, C. H.: *Lancet 2*:492, 1960.
158. Court Brown, W. M., Harnden, D. G., et al.: M.R.C. Special Report Series No. 305, London, Her Majesty's Stationery Office, 1964.
159. de la Chapelle, A.: *Amer. J. Hum. Genet. 24*:71, 1972.
160. Augustine, J. R., and Jaworski, Z. F.: *Arch. Path. 66*:159, 1958.
161. Ford, C. E., Jones, K. W., et al.: *Lancet 1*:709, 1959.
162. Nelson, W. O., and Heller, C. G.: *J. Clin. Endocr. 5*:13, 1945.
163. Sniffen, R. C., Howard, R. P., et al.: *Arch. Path. 51*:293, 1951.
164. de la Balze, A., Bur, G. E., et al.: *J. Clin. Endocr. 14*:626, 1954.
165. Warburg, E.: *Acta Endocr. 43*:12, 1963.
166. Court Brown, W. M., Mantle, D. J., et al.: *J. Med. Genet. 1*:35, 1964.
167. Plunkett, E. R., and Barr, M. L.: *J. Clin. Endocr. 16*:829, 1956.
168. Lipsett, M. B., David, T. E., et al.: *J. Clin. Endocr. 25*:1027, 1965.

169. Davis, T. E., Canfield, C. J., et al.: *New Eng. J. Med. 268*:178, 1963.
170. Caldwell, P. D., and Smith, D. W.: *J. Pediat. 80*:250, 1972.
171. Sergovich, F., Valentine, G. H., et al.: *New Eng. J. Med. 280*:171, 1969.
172. Ratcliffe, S. G., Stewart, A. L., et al.: *Lancet 1*:121, 1970.
173. Santen, R. J., de Kretser, D. M., et al.: *Lancet 2*:371, 1970.
174. Shakkebaek, N. E., Hultén, M., et al.: *J. Reprod. Fertil. 32*:391, 1973.
175. Melnyk, J., Thompson, H., et al.: *Lancet 2*:797, 1969.
176. Hudson, B., Burger, H., et al.: *Lancet 2*:699, 1969.
177. Vorhees, J. J., Hayes, E., et al.: *Ann. Intern. Med. 73*:271, 1970.
178. Price, W. H., Strong, J. A., et al.: *Lancet 1*:565, 1966.
179. Jacobs, P. A., Brunton, M., et al.: *Nature* (London) *208*:1351, 1966.
180. Hope, K., Philip, A. E., et al.: *Brit. J. Psychiat. 113*:495, 1967.
181. Jacobs, P. A., Price, W. H., et al.: *Ann. Hum. Genet. 31*:339, 1968.
182. Engle, E. T.: *J. Urol. 57*:789, 1947.
183. del Castillo, E. B., Trabucco, A., et al.: *J. Clin. Endocr. 7*:493, 1947.
184. Nelson, W. O., and Heller, C. G.: *Ann. Rev. Med. 2*:179, 1951.
185. Kjessler, B.: *Monographs in Human Genetics.* Vol. 2. Basel, S. Karger, 1966, p. 56.
186. Bowen, P., Lee, C. S. N., et al.: *Ann. Intern. Med. 62*:252, 1965.
187. Bremner, W. J., Ott, J., et al.: *Clin. Genet.* In press, 1974.
188. Heller, C. G., Nelson, W. O., et al.: *J. Clin. Endocr. 3*:573, 1943.
189. Jost, A.: *C. R. Ass. Anat. 34*:255, 1947.
190. Jose, A.: *Arch. Anat. Microscop. Morphol. Exp. 36*:271, 1947.
191. Raynaud, A., and Frilley, M.: *Ann. Endocr. 8*:400, 1947.
192. Winter, J. S. D., Taraska, S., et al.: *J. Clin. Endocr. 34*:348, 1972.
193. Santen, R. J., and Paulsen, C. A.: *J. Clin. Endocr. 36*:55, 1973.
194. Schoen, E. J.: *J. Clin. Endocr. 25*:101, 1965.
195. Heller, R. H.: *J. Pediat. 66*:48, 1965.
196. Urmenyi, A. M. C., Beattie, M. K., et al.: *J. Med. Genet. 3*:220, 1966.
197. Chaves-Carballo, E., and Hayles, A. B.: *Proc. Staff Meet. Mayo Clin. 41*:843, 1966.
198. Ballew, J. W., and Masters, W. H.: *Fertil. Steril. 5*:536, 1954.
199. Gall, E. A.: *Amer. J. Path. 23*:637, 1947.
200. Savran, J.: *Rhode Island Med. J. 29*:662, 1946.
201. Mongon, E. S.: *Amer. J. Med. Sci. 237*:749, 1959.
202. Oakberg, E. F., and Clark, E., In *Proceedings of the International Symposium on Effects of Ionizing Radiation in the Reproductive System.* Oxford, Pergamon Press, 1963, pp. 11–24.
203. Paulsen, C. A., In *Effects of Ionizing Radiation on the Reproductive System.* Carlson, W. D., and Gassner, F. X. (eds.), New York, Macmillan Co., 1964, pp. 305–307.
204. Heller, C. G., Wootton, P., et al.: Proc. 6th Pan-American Congress Endocrinol., Amsterdam, Excerpta Medica Foundation Intern. Cong. Ser. 112, 1966.
205. Oakberg, E. F.: *Radiat. Res. 11*:700, 1959.
206. Paulsen, C. A.: Final progress report of AEC contract AT(45–1)–2225, Task Agreement 6. RLO–2225–2, 1973.
207. Thorslund, T. W., and Paulsen, C. A., In *Proceedings of the National Symposium on Natural and Manmade Radiation in Space.* Warman, E. A. (ed.), NASA Document TM X-2440, 1972, pp. 229–232.
208. Drucker, W. D., Blanc, W. A., et al.: *J. Clin. Endocr. 23*:59, 1963.
209. Clarke, G. B., Shapiro, S., et al.: *J. Clin. Endocr. 16*:1235, 1956.
210. Bassöe, H. H.: *J. Clin. Endocr. 16*:1614, 1956.
211. Harper, P., Penny, R., et al.: *J. Clin. Endocr. 35*:852, 1972.
212. Heller, C. G., and Myers, G. B.: *J.A.M.A. 126*:472, 1944.
213. Werner, A. A.: *J.A.M.A. 112*:1441, 1939.
214. McCullagh, E. P.: *Cleveland Clin. Quart. 13*:166, 1946.
215. Werner, S. C.: *Amer. J. Med. 3*:52, 1947.
216. Albert, A., Underdahl, L. O., et al.: *Proc. Staff Meet. Mayo Clin. 29*:131, 1954.
217. Bartter, F. C., Sniffen, R. C., et al.: *J. Clin. Endocr. 12*:1532, 1952.
218. Kallman, F., Schonfeld, W. A., et al.: *Amer. J. Ment. Defic. 48*:203, 1944.

219. Greulich, W. W., Dorfman, R. I., et al.: Washington, D.C., Society for Research in Child Development, National Research Council 7:85, 1942.
220. Santen, R. J., and Paulsen, C. A.: *J. Clin. Endocr. 36*:47, 1973.
221. Naftolin, F., and Harris, G. W.: *Nature* (London) *232*:296, 1971.
222. Kastin, A. J., Gual, C., et al.: *Recent Progr. Hormone Res. 28*:201, 1972.
223. Job, J. C., Garneri, P. E., et al.: *J. Clin. Endocr. 35*:473, 1972.
224. Roth, J. C., Kelch, R. P., et al.: *J. Clin. Endocr. 35*:926, 1972.
225. Zarate, A., Kastin, A. J., et al.: *J. Clin. Endocr. 36*:612, 1973.
226. Boyar, R. M., Finkelstein, J. W., et al.: *J. Clin. Endocr. 36*:64, 1973.
227. Mancini, R. E., In *Hypothalamic Hypophysiotropic Hormones, Physiological and Clinical Studies.* Proceedings of the Serono Research Foundation Conference, Acapulco, Mexico, 1972. Amsterdam, Excerpta Medica Foundation, 1973.
228. Paulsen, C. A., In *Proceedings of the Sixth Pan American Congress of Endocrinology, Mexico City 1965.* Amsterdam, Excerpta Medica Foundation, 1966, pp. 398–407.
229. Paulsen, C. A., In *Gonadotropins.* Rosemberg, E. (ed.), Palo Alto, Geron-X, 1968, p. 491.
230. Paulsen, C. A., Espeland, D. H., et al., In *The Human Testis.* Rosemberg, E., and Paulsen, C. A. (eds.), New York, Plenum Press, 1970, p. 547.
231. Joel, C. A.: *Harefuah 71*:281, 1966.
232. Lunenfeld, B., Mar, A., et al.: *Fertil. Steril. 18*:581, 1967.
233. Bardin, C. W., Ross, G. T., et al.: *J. Clin. Invest. 48*:2046, 1969.
234. Hurxthal, L. M., Bruns, H. J., et al.: *J. Clin. Endocr. 9*:1245, 1949.
235. Werner, S. C.: *J. Clin. Endocr. 11*:612, 1951.
236. Pasqualini, R. Q., and Bur, G. E.: *Rev. Assoc. Med. Argent. 64*:6, 1950.
237. McCullagh, E. P., Beck, J. C., et al.: *J. Clin. Endocr. 13*:489, 1953.
238. Pasqualini, R. W., and Bur, G. E.: *Fertil. Steril. 6*:144, 1955.
239. Faiman, C., Hoffman, R. J., et al.: *Mayo Clin. Proc. 43*:661, 1968.
240. Robin, D., Spitz, I., et al.: *New Eng. J. Med. 287*:1314, 1972.
241. Paschkis, K. E., and Cantarow, A.: *Ann. Intern. Med. 34*:669, 1951.
242. Maddock, W. O., Leach, R. B., et al.: *Amer. J. Med. Sci. 226*:509, 1953.
243. McCullagh, E. P., Gold, A., et al.: *J. Clin. Endocr. 10*:871, 1950.
244. Albert, A., Underdahl, L. O., et al.: *Proc. Staff Meet. Mayo Clin. 29*:317, 1954.
245. Albert, A., Underdahl, L. O., et al.: *Proc. Staff Meet. Mayo Clin. 29*:368, 1954.
246. MacLeod, J., Pazianos, A., et al.: *Lancet 1*:1196, 1964.
247. Gemzell, C., and Kjessler, G.: *Lancet 1*:644, 1964.
248. Mancini, R. E., Vilar, O., et al.: *J. Clin. Endocr. 33*:888, 1971.
249. World Health Organization Technical Report Series No. 514: Agents Stimulating Gonadal Function in the Human. Geneva, World Health Organization, 1973.
250. Lesser, M. A., Vore, S. N., et al.: *J. Clin. Endocr. 15*:297, 1955.
251. Werner, S. C., Hanger, F. M., et al.: *Amer. J. Med. 8*:325, 1950.
252. Wood, J. C.: *J.A.M.A. 150*:1484, 1952.
253. Morales, P. A., and Hotchkiss, R. S.: *Fertil. Steril. 7*:487, 1956.
254. Maddock, W. O., Leach, R. B., et al.: Unpublished data.
255. Beierwaltes, W. H., and Bishop, R. C.: *J. Clin. Endocr. 14*:928, 1954.
256. Hellman, L., Bradlow, H. L., et al.: *J. Clin. Endocr. 19*:936, 1959.
257. Griboff, S. I.: *Fertil. Steril. 13*:436, 1962.
258. Wilkins, L., and Cara, J.: *J. Clin. Endocr. 14*:287, 1954.
259. Prader, A., Zachman, M., et al.: *Acta Endocr. 74* (Suppl. 177):57, 1973.
260. Sohval, A. R., and Gabrilove, J. L.: *J. Urol. 93*:711, 1965.
261. Solomon, S. S., Swersie, S. P., et al.: *J. Clin. Endocr. 28*:608, 1968.
262. Kent, J. R., Scaramuzzi, R. J., et al.: *Gastroenterology 64*:111, 1973.
263. Galvao-Teles, A., Anderson, D. C., et al.: *Lancet 1*:173, 1973.

264. Southren, A. L., Gordon, G. G., et al.: *Metabolism* 22:695, 1973.
264a. Maddock, W. O., Chase, J. D., et al.: *J. Lab. Clin. Med.* 41: 608, 1953.
265. Cooper, I. S., Rynearson, E. H., et al.: *J. Clin. Endocr.* 10:858, 1950.
266. Cooper, I. S., and Hoen, T. I.: *J. Clin. Endocr.* 9:457, 1949.
267. Horne, H. W., Paull, D. P., et al.: *New Eng. J. Med.* 239:959, 1958.
268. Stemmerman, G. H., Weiss, L., et al.: *Amer. J. Clin. Path.* 20:24, 1950.
269. Munro, D., Horne, H. W., Jr., et al.: *New Eng. J. Med.* 239:903, 1958.
270. Bors, E., Engle, E. T., et al.: *J. Clin. Endocr.* 9:457, 1949.
271. Charny, C. W., and Wolgen, W.: *Cryptorchidism.* New York, Paul B. Hoeber, 1957.
272. Bishop, P. M. F.: *Guy. Hosp. Rep.* 94:12, 1945.
273. Jones, H. W., Jr., and Scott, W. W.: *Hermaphroditism, Genital Anomalies and Related Endocrine Disorders.* Baltimore, Williams & Wilkins, 1958.
274. Anderson, H., Andreassen, M., et al.: *Acta Endocr.* 18:567, 1955.
275. Hand, J. R.: *Trans. Amer. Ass. Genitourin. Surg.* 47:9, 1955.
276. Nelson, W. O.: *Recent Progr. Hormone Res.* 6:29, 1951.
277. Sohval, A. R.: *Amer. J. Med.* 16:347, 1954.
278. Mancini, R. E., Rosemberg, E., et al.: *J. Clin. Endocr.* 25:927, 1965.
279. de la Balze, F. A., Mancini, R. A., et al.: *J. Clin. Endocr.* 20:286, 1960.
280. Charny, C. W.: *J. Urol.* 83:697, 1960.
281. Hortling, H., de la Chapelle, A., et al.: *J. Clin. Endocr.* 27: 120, 1967.
282. Gross, R. E., and Jewett, T. C.: *J.A.M.A.* 160:634, 1956.
283. Carroll, W. A.: *J. Urol.* 61:396, 1949.
284. Campbell, H. E.: *J. Urol.* 81:663, 1959.
285. Sumner, W. A.: *J. Urol.* 81:150, 1959.
286. Patton, J. F., and Mallis, N.: *J. Urol.* 81:457, 1959.
287. Linke, C. A., and Kiefer, J. H.: *J. Urol.* 82:347, 1959.
288. Nelson, W. O., and Heller, C. G.: *J. Clin. Endocr.* 5:13, 1945.
289. Schwartz, I. S., and Wilens, D. L.: *Amer. J. Path.* 43:797, 1963.
290. Nicolis, G. L., Modlinger, R. S., et al.: *J. Clin. Endocr.* 32:173, 1971.
291. Bannayan, G. A., and Hajdu, S. I.: *Amer. J. Clin. Path.* 57:431, 1972.
292. Morrione, T. G.: *Arch. Path.* 37:39, 1944.
293. Wallach, E. E., and Garcia, C. R.: *J. Clin. Endocr.* 22:1201, 1962.
294. Treves, N.: *Cancer* 11:1083, 1958.
295. Rosewater, S., Weinup, G., et al.: *Ann. Intern. Med.* 63:377, 1965.
296. Krant, M. J.: *Arch. Intern. Med.* 115:464, 1965.
297. Jull, J. W., and Dossett, J. A.: *Brit. Med. J.* 2:795, 1964.
298. Jull, J. W., Bonser, G. J., et al.: *Brit. Med. J.* 2:797, 1964.
299. Fusco, F. D., and Rosen, S. W.: *New Eng. J. Med.* 275:507, 1966.
300. Klatskin, G., Salter, W. T., et al.: *Amer. J. Med. Sci.* 213:19, 1947.
301. Hibbs, R. E.: *Amer. J. Med. Sci.* 213:176, 1947.
302. Jacobs, E. C.: *J. Clin. Endocr.* 8:227, 1948.
303. Shipley, R. A., and Gyorgy, P.: *Proc. Soc. Exp. Biol. Med.* 57:52, 1944.
304. Nagel, T. C., Freinkel, N., et al.: *J. Clin. Endocr.* 36:428, 1973.
305. Sawin, C. T., Longcope, C., et al.: *J. Clin. Endocr.* 36:988, 1973.
306. Van Wyk, J. J., and Grumbach, M. M.: *J. Pediat.* 57:416, 1960.

307. Canfield, C. J., and Bates, R. W.: *New Eng. J. Med.* 273:897, 1965.
308. Ayd, F. J., Jr.: *Amer. J. Psychiat.* 113:16, 1956.
309. Sulman, P. G., and Wennik, H. Z.: *Lancet* 1:161, 1950.
310. Pettinger, W. A., Horwitz, D., et al.: *Brit. Med. J.* 1:1460, 1963.
311. Robinson, B. A.: *Med. J. Aust.* 2:239, 1957.
312. Harmon, J., and Aliapoulios, M.: *New Eng. J. Med.* 287:936, 1972.
313. Frantz, A. G., Kleinberg, D. L., et al.: *Recent Progr. Hormone Res.* 28:527, 1972.
314. Volpe, R., Killinger, D., et al.: *J. Clin. Endocr.* 35:684, 1972.
315. Simmons, F. A.: *New Eng. J. Med.* 255:1140, 1186, 1956.
316. Sniffen, R. C., Howard, R. P., et al.: *Arch. Path.* 50:285, 1950.
317. Howard, R. P., Simmons, F. A., et al.: *Fertil. Steril.* 2:95, 1951.
318. Barr, A. B., Moore, D. J., et al.: *J. Reprod. Fertil.* 25:75, 1971.
319. Skakkebaek, N. E., and Heller, C. G.: *J. Reprod. Fertil.* 32:379, 1973.
320. Skakkebaek, N. E., Hammen, R., et al.: *Acta Path. Microbiol. Scand.* (A) 81:97, 1973.
321. Skakkebaek, N. E., Hulten, M., et al.: *Acta Path. Microbiol. Scand.* (A) 81:112, 1973.
322. Heller, C. G., Nelson, W. O., et al.: *Fertil. Steril.* 1:415, 1950.
323. Heckel, N. J., Rosso, W. A., et al.: *J. Clin. Endocr.* 11:235, 1951.
324. Heller, C. G., In *Report of the Thirty-fifth Ross Conference on Pediatric Research.* Fomon, S. J. (ed.), Columbus, Ohio, Ross Laboratories, 1961.
325. Charny, C. W.: *Fertil. Steril.* 10:557, 1959.
326. Rowley, M. J., and Heller, C. G.: *Fertil. Steril.* 23:498, 1972.
327. Shulman, S.: *CRC Crit. Rev. Clin. Lab. Sci.* 2:393, September, 1971.
328. Mancini, R. E., In *The Human Testis.* Rosemberg, E., and Paulsen, C. A. (eds.), New York, Plenum Press, 1970, p. 529.
329. Ansbacher, R., Keung-Yeung, K., et al.: *Fertil. Steril.* 24:305, 1973.
330. General Discussion: Treatment of male infertility, In *The Human Testis.* Rosemberg, E., and Paulsen, C. A. (eds.), New York, Plenum Press, 1970, p. 631.
331. Hanley, H. G., In Proc. 2nd World Congress on Fertility and Sterility, 1956.
332. Rivo, E., and Rock, J.: Presented at the 21st Annual Meeting of the American Society for the Study of Sterility, San Francisco, Calif., April, 1965.
333. MacLeod, J.: *Fertil. Steril.* 16:735, 1965.
334. Brown, J. S., Dubin, L., et al.: *Fertil. Steril.* 18:46, 1967.
335. Charney, C. W.: *Fertil. Steril.* 13:47, 1962.
336. Scott, L. S., and Young, D.: *Fertil. Steril.* 123:325, 1962.
337. Smith, J. B., and O'Neill, R. T.: *Amer. J. Med.* 51:767, 1971.
338. Dixon, F. J., and Moore, R. A.: *Cancer* 6:427, 1953.
339. Patton, J. F., Sutzman, D. N., et al.: *Amer. J. Surg.* 99:525, 1960.
340. Friedman, N. B., and Moore, R. A.: *Milit. Surg.* 99:573, 1946.
341. Parker, R. G., and Holyoke, J. B.: *Amer. J. Roentgen.* 83:43, 1960.
342. Current Concepts in Cancer, No. 29. *J.A.M.A.* 213:89, 1970.
343. Savard, K., Forman, R. I., et al.: *J. Clin. Invest.* 39:534, 1960.
344. Heideman, M. L., Jr.: *J. Clin. Endocr.* 19:1331, 1959.
345. Kolodny, R. C., Masters, W. H., et al.: *New Eng. J. Med.* 285:1170, 1971.
346. Kolodny, R. C., Jacobs, L. S., et al.: *Lancet* 2:18, 1972.
347. Marx, J. L.: *Science* 179:1222, 1973.
348. Johnson, D. S.: *Contraception* 5:327, 1972.
349. Skoglund, R. D., and Paulsen, C. A.: *Contraception* 7:357, 1973.

CHAPTER 7

The Ovaries

By Griff T. Ross and
    Raymond L. Vande Wiele

THE NORMAL OVARY

Morphology

Grossly the human ovary is a reniform structure attached to the posterior surface of the broad ligament by a peritoneal fold called the mesovarium. Nerves, blood vessels, and lymphatics transverse the mesovarium and penetrate the ovary at its hilum. In normal women, the combined weight of the ovaries during the reproductive years is 10–20 g., averaging 14 g.

Microscopic Anatomy

Microscopically the ovary consists of three distinct regions: an outer cortex, a central medulla, and an inner hilum around the point of attachment of the ovary to its mesentery. None of these areas is structurally homogeneous, and microscopic appearance varies with age, principally in terms of relative amounts of cellular constituents. The principal components consist of a covering by coelomic epithelium, follicles in varying stages of either maturation or degeneration, supportive tissues collectively referred to as stroma, and blood vessels and lymphatics. To appreciate changes occurring during fetal or postnatal development of the ovary, more detailed consideration must be given to cellular composition of follicles and stroma.

The Follicle

Maturation. Morphologically, the follicle changes as it matures. The most immature stage is referred to as a *primordial follicle* (Fig. 7–1, *A*). The primordial follicle, separated from surrounding stroma by an inconspicuous but definite basal lamina (basement membrane), contains a primary oocyte in attenuated prophase of the first meiotic division. The oocyte is surrounded by a single layer of spindle-shaped cells and protoplasmic processes which form a desmosomal union with the plasma membrane of the oocyte, providing a route for transfer of nutrients to the oocyte.

When the flat, spindle-shaped cells inside the basal lamina of a primordial follicle become cuboidal (Fig. 7–1, *A, B*), the term *primary follicle* is applied. Successive mitotic divisions of the cuboidal cells give rise to a multilayered stratum granulosum or zona granulosa, and a band of mucoid substance, secreted by the granulosa cells and called the zona pellucida, separates the cuboidal granulosa cells from the oocyte (Fig. 7–1, *B, C*). Protoplasmic processes from adjacent granulosa cells traverse the zona pellucida to establish contact with the plasma membrane of the oocyte. The contents of the follicle within the basal lamina remain avascular until after ovulation, and transfer of nutrients must occur by diffusion.

Coincident with proliferation of granulosa cells bounded by the basal lamina, adjacent stromal cells outside the basal lamina become arranged in concentric perifollicular layers, in which density of nuclei is less than that of stroma further removed

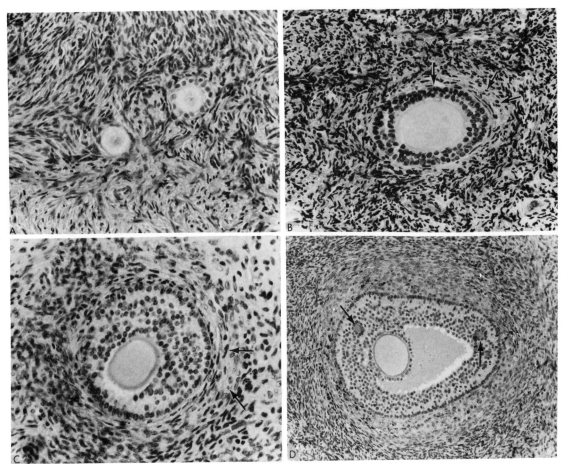

Figure 7–1. *A*, Primordial follicle (lower left) and primary follicle (upper right) in human ovary. *B*, Primary follicle with 3 layers of granulosa cells and incipient differentiation of theca (arrows) from surrounding stroma. *C*, Primary follicle with multiple layers of granulosa cells and beginning epithelioid transformation of the theca (arrows). *D*, Graafian follicle. Note the epithelioid character of theca cells and Call-Exner bodies (arrows) among granulosa cells.

from the follicle. This layer of differentiated and uniquely oriented cells constitutes the *theca* (Fig. 7–1, *B, C*). That portion of the theca adjacent to the basal lamina is called *theca interna*, while that portion merging with surrounding stroma is called *theca externa*. As numbers of granulosa cells continue to increase, some of the spindle-shaped cells in the theca interna acquire increased amounts of cytoplasm and appear rounded or epithelioid (Fig. 7–1, *C*). Capillaries and lymphatic spaces, which terminate at the basal lamina, appear among these cells.

Epithelioid transformation of the theca interna is followed by the appearance of cleftlike, fluid-filled spaces among the granulosa cells. These spaces become confluent to give rise to the fluid-filled *antrum*, the distinctive feature of a *graafian follicle* (Fig. 7–1, *D*). The fluid consists of a plasma transudate, the oncotic pressure of which is increased by mucoid substances secreted by granulosa cells. Some steroid hormones have been identified in the fluid in concentration orders of magnitude greater than those in peripheral blood.

The enlargement of the oocyte is completed about the time of appearance of the antrum. As

fluid accumulates in the antrum, the oocyte, surrounded by a small hillock of granulosa cells which are attached to its surface by the long cytoplasmic processes previously described, comes to occupy a polar, eccentric position within the follicle. This hillock of granulosa cells, called the *cumulus oophorus*, remains attached to the ovum for a few days after ovulation.

As the follicle develops from the primordial stage to maturity, the diameter of the follicle increases 200- to 400-fold, from 50 μ as a primordial follicle to 10,000–20,000 μ (10–20 mm.) as a mature follicle just prior to ovulation. Similarly, the diameter of the oocyte increases six- to tenfold from 15–20 μ in the primordial follicle to 150 μ in a mature preovulatory follicle.

Atresia. From the seventh month of fetal life until menarche, maturation terminates before the follicle reaches diameters equal to those required for ovulation, and the follicle degenerates. The degenerative process, called atresia, is characterized histologically by cessation of mitosis in the granulosa, separation of granulosa cells from the basal lamina, and death of the oocyte. All the constituent follicular cells undergo cytolysis, the basal lamina is penetrated by vessels from surrounding theca, and fibrous tissue replaces the granulosa cells, giving rise to a structure usually referred to as a *corpus candicans* or *corpus fibrosum.* Although this is the fate of more than 95% of follicles present at birth, the underlying causes for atresia remain to be determined.

Ovulation.   Beginning with the menarche and continuing until the menopause, one (or rarely more than one) of a cohort of maturing follicles will rapidly enlarge during the second half of the follicular phase of the cycle and rupture, extruding the oocyte surrounded by the cumulus oophorus. A number of hypotheses with supporting data have been advanced to account for ovulation. These include rupture secondary to increased intrafollicular oncotic pressure, enzymatic dissolution of the basal lamina, and mechanical rupture. In any event, a midcycle surge of human luteinizing hormone (hLH) or a surrogate, human chorionic gonadotropin (hCG), appears to be indispensable to the occurrence of rupture (see below).

About the time of rupture, the first meiotic division is resumed and completed with extrusion of the first polar body, leaving a secondary oocyte surrounded by granulosa cells of the cumulus oophorus. After the follicle has ruptured, vessels from the theca interna penetrate the basal lamina and form a *corpus luteum* (see below), which incorporates the granulosa cells remaining inside the collapsed postovulatory follicle and surrounding thecal cells. A new corpus luteum is formed in each menstrual cycle, and in subsequent cycles the epithelial cells of the older corpora lutea degenerate and are ultimately replaced by acellular, avascular connective tissue. The residual structure is called a *corpus albicans;* these structures accumulate in the medullary portion of the ovary.

The Stroma

The ovarian stroma contains ordinary connective tissue cells and some cells called *interstitial cells* thought to arise from undifferentiated theca interna of atretic follicles. Distinguishing between the two types of cells usually requires use of special connective tissue stains. The interstitial cells respond to stimulation with either hCG or hLH by undergoing morphologic changes suggestive of cells secreting steroid hormone. The large number of such cells in the stroma becomes apparent during pregnancy, when high levels of circulating hCG stimulate epithelioid transformation of interstitial cells, differentiating them from cells with a purely supportive function.

The Hilar Cells

The hilus of the ovary is the portal of entry and exit of blood and lymphatic vessels and of nerves. These structures and the supportive connective tissue are the most impressive components of the hilar region. However, careful examination of serial sections of the hilus of ovaries from sexually mature and postmenopausal women reveals the presence of another variety of cells, morphologically indistinguishable from Leydig cells, including crystalloids of Reinke, but are referred to as *hilar cells.* These cells are scattered around and sometimes among the fibers of nonmyelinated nerves which traverse the hilus of the ovary. Hilar cells are less conspicuous and more difficult to identify in ovaries examined from the first year of life until puberty. Occasionally, hyperplastic or neoplastic changes in these cells result in virilizing syndromes associated with production of excessive amounts of testosterone. Otherwise, the origin and function of these cells remains obscure.

Changes During Growth and Development and With Aging

The Fetal Ovary

An undifferentiated gonad, capable of giving rise to either ovary or testis, appears in the human embryo around the twenty-eighth to thirtieth postovulatory day and consists of a thickening of the coelomic epithelium overlying cells of the mesonephric blastema and primordial germ cells which have migrated into this region from the hindgut. The coelomic epithelium gives rise to the cortex, and the primitive urogenital mesenchyme to the medulla of the gonad. According to the inductor theory of gonadal differentiation (Ch. 8), cortical or medullary dominance of subsequent growth and development determines whether an ovary or a testis differentiates (Ch. 8). In the definitive ovary, granulosa cells are derived from the cortex while interstitial cells and theca cells are of medullary origin.

Successive mitotic divisions of primordial germ cells give rise to oogonia, the precursors of oocytes. Baker (1963) has estimated that there were 600,000 oogonia in the ovaries of fetuses he examined at two months of gestation. By five months he estimated that this number had increased to 6–7 million. Between the eighth and thirteenth week of gestation, some of the oogonia initiate meiosis, which proceeds to the diplotene stage of prophase of the first meiotic division. The nucleus remains in this condition until the first meiotic division is resumed and completed, with extrusion of the first polar body around the time of ovulation. Some oogonia undergo abnormal mitotic divisions and are eliminated before entering the first meiotic division.

Degeneration, occurring during both mitosis and meiosis, had reduced the number of oocytes to 2,000,000 at birth, after which the number declined further to 300,000 in ovaries from two 7-year-old girls. Virtually all oogonia have disappeared from the cortex of the ovary between the seventh month of gestation and term and have en-

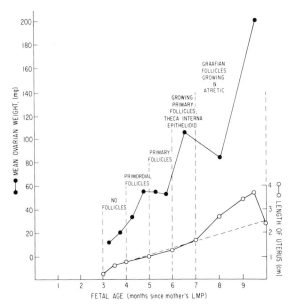

Figure 7–2. Changes in human fetal ovarian weight and morphology (adapted from data of Van Wagenen, G., and Simpson, M. E.: *Embryology of the Ovary and Testis — Homo Sapiens and Macaca Mulatta.* New Haven, Yale University Press, 1965) and human fetal uterine length (adapted from data of Scammon, R. E.: *Proc. Soc. Exp. Biol. Med.* 23:687, 1926) during gestation.

mone in response to gonadotropic stimulation of these cells. Since estrogen is a potent uterotropic agent, it is interesting to note that the slope of the line relating length of the fetal uterus to gestational age (Scammon, 1926) increases coincidentally with the appearance of epithelioid changes in the theca interna (Fig. 7–2).

The Premenarchal Ovary

Antral follicles with luteinized epithelioid theca interna cells are found on careful histologic study of ovaries obtained post mortem from neonates and prepubertal children. After they have been treated by traditional methods of fixation and staining, follicles in ovaries of neonates and premenarchal girls are morphologically identical to follicles of comparable size in the ovaries of normal women after the menarche. Increments in uterine weight, which begin around age 8, provide indirect evidence for estrogen production coincident with follicular maturation prepubertally. Large, benign, ovarian cysts are frequently found in premenarchal ovaries, and, rarely, these secrete sufficient estrogen to stimulate precocious development of secondary sexual changes (see below).

From birth to menarche, ovarian weight increases progressively with age so that a straight line describes mean ovarian weight changes as a function of age (Fig. 7–3). This increase in ovarian weight is the result of two processes. The first is accumulation of the stromal residue left after maturation and atresia of successive cohorts of follicles. The second is an increase in the volume achieved by maturing follicles before atresia. This latter increment parallels the increment in ovarian weight prior to puberty (Fig. 7–3).

Important changes occur in the ovarian stroma during the premenarchal years. Firstly, the medullary stroma increases as the residue of successive generations of atretic follicles accumulates. Secondly, as the ovary matures, the medullary stroma "invades" the cortex, resulting in wider separation of individual primordial follicles. Finally, the orientation of these stromal cells changes from one perpendicular to the long axis in immature ovaries to one parallel to the long axis in ovaries of sexually mature women.

The Postmenarchal Ovary: Morphologic Changes During the Menstrual Cycle

Around the time of the menarche, unknown factors result in the initiation of cyclic ovulation, while atresia continues. While follicle growth and maturation beyond the primary stage appears to be dependent upon gonadotropic stimulation, the period of time required for a primordial follicle to reach maturity once growth is initiated is not known for the human. However, women whose ovaries contain follicles not advanced beyond the primary stage can be made to ovulate with exogenous gonadotropins administered over a period

tered prophase of the first meiotic division to become primary oocytes incorporated into primordial follicles. Postnatally, there is no convincing evidence that additional oocytes are produced *de novo* from germinal epithelium in the human ovary.

Morphologic changes in the human ovary during fetal life, as recorded by Van Wagenen and Simpson (1965), are summarized in Figure 7–2. Primordial follicles first appear in the fetal ovary around the fifth month of gestation. Initially, these are found deep in the cortex, adjacent to the medulla, while oogonial divisions continue to occur in the outer cortex. These primordial follicles progressively increase in number and between the fifth and sixth month, some of them become transformed into primary follicles containing growing oocytes. Between the sixth and seventh months, the growing oocyte in some primary follicles is surrounded by several layers of cuboidal granulosa cells and epithelioid theca interna cells are first observed at this time. Concomitantly, atretic changes are noted in some primary follicles in the region of the corticomedullary junction.

Many developing primary follicles with epithelioid theca interna, a few graafian follicles, and follicles of both types undergoing atresia are characteristically found when serial sections of fetal ovaries are examined after the seventh month of gestation. The theca interna of fetal ovarian follicles gives a strong alkaline phosphatase reaction, which has been related directly to gonadotropic stimulation and steroidogenesis by these cells in ovaries of sexually mature women. The intensity of the alkaline phosphatase reaction in fetal ovarian theca interna may reflect the synthesis of this hor-

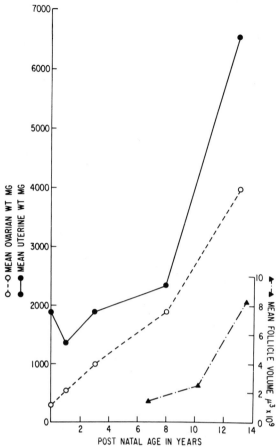

Figure 7–3. Increments in ovarian and uterine weights (adapted from data of Wehefritz, E.: *Z. Ges. Anat. 9*:161, 1923) and volumes of largest atretic follicle (adapted from data of Parini, F., and Molla, W.: *Ann. Obstet. Gynec. 62*:1629, 1940) in human ovaries from birth to 14 years.

of the largest normal antral follicles found early in the preovulatory phase of the cycle is smaller than that of normal antral follicles seen during the postovulatory phase (Fig. 7–5). In the light of this fact, it is reasonable to suppose that the cohort of graafian follicles developing during the luteal phase becomes atretic, perhaps as a result of declining amounts of circulating gonadotropins. As a result, follicles less than 1 mm. in diameter could be the "pool" from which the follicle destined to ovulate in the next cycle is chosen. The number of follicles equal to or greater than 100 μ in diameter present during the postovulatory phase of the cycle exceeds the number of such follicles seen during the preovulatory phase of the cycle. Maturation of these follicles may be initiated by estrogens secreted during the luteal phase; then antrum formation is stimulated by increasing concentrations of gonadotropins, initially follicle stimulating hormone (FSH) beginning 3–4 days prior to onset of menses and, subsequently, luteinizing hormone (LH) characteristically seen throughout the first half of the follicular phase of the cycle.

During the last half of the preovulatory phase of the cycle, the diameter of the largest follicle, presumably destined to ovulate, increases rapidly to values ranging from 10–20 mm. (Fig. 7–6). Coincident with this rapid increment, the concentration

not exceeding the follicular phase of the spontaneous ovulatory cycle. On the basis of such observations, it is reasonable to suppose that complete follicular maturation, beginning with a primary follicle, can be completed in 10–12 days.

The limited number of studies done provide evidence that the follicular apparatus undergoes cyclic changes during each menstrual cycle. The changes in follicular diameters during the menstrual cycle from the studies of Block (1951) have been replotted to coincide temporally with changes in pituitary gonadotropic hormone concentrations occurring during presumptive ovulatory cycles in normal young women in Figures 7–4, 7–5, and 7–6. There are two "peaks" in numbers of normal graafian follicles greater than 1 mm. in diameter, one occurring around the time of ovulation and the other in midluteal phase (Fig. 7–4). This latter peak of follicle growth during the luteal phase is coincident with declining concentrations of gonadotropins but increasing concentrations of estrogens (Fig. 7–4), suggesting that, in the human as in some other mammals, estrogens may stimulate preantral follicle growth. The mean diameter

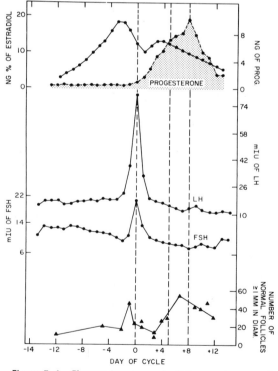

Figure 7–4. Changes in serum estradiol, progesterone, and LH and FSH concentrations (adapted from data of Ross, G. T., et al.: *Recent Progr. Hormone Res. 26*:1, 1970), and in the number of normal follicles equal to or greater than 1 mm. in diameter (adapted from data of Block, E.: *Acta Endocr. 8*:33, 1951). All data have been synchronized around the day of the LH peak.

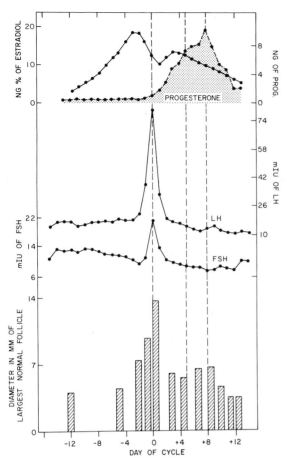

Figure 7–5. Diameters of the largest normal follicles in human ovaries (adapted from data of Block, E.: *Acta Endocr. 8:33, 1951*) and changes in serum hormone concentrations plotted as in Figure 7–4.

teum. In the formation of a corpus luteum, the succession of morphologic changes and the time required for completion of these is sufficiently characteristic that an experienced pathologist is able, by histologic criteria, to assign an age (in days of an idealized 28-day cycle) to the corpus luteum.

The Postmenopausal Ovary

Successive cycles of ovulation and atresia deplete what Hertig (1944) has called the "ovarian capital" of oocytes. One of the associated changes is a progressive decline in ovarian weight from an average of about 14 g. in the fourth decade to about 5 g. in the fifth, sixth, and seventh decades.

Grossly, the postmenopausal ovary is a yellowish, lusterless structure with a wrinkled surface. Microscopically, the wrinkled appearance is seen to be associated with undulating gyruslike formations in the cortex. The germinal epithelium persists and follows the undulations, in some of which connection of the epithelium with the surface is lost.

of FSH progressively declines, while the concentration of LH rises gradually. A dramatic increment in plasma LH, accompanied by a less impressive increment in plasma FSH, begins 24 hours prior to, and reaches a maximum about 16 hours prior to, ovulation.

After ovulation, one of the more dramatic ovarian morphologic changes occurring during the cycle relates to the formation of a corpus luteum. This structure arises by transformation of granulosa cells remaining behind after extrusion of the ovum and involves profound morphologic changes in cellular appearance as well as in the cytoplasmic organelles. The mitochondria, the endoplasmic reticulum, and the Golgi apparatus all acquire the properties of cells secreting steroid hormones. These intracellular changes are accompanied by vascularization of the corpus luteum with capillaries from the theca interna which penetrate the basal lamina. Cells, called K cells, morphologically distinct from the majority of granulosa cells, are thought by some to originate in the theca interna (White et al., 1951) and appear to be incorporated into the corpus lu-

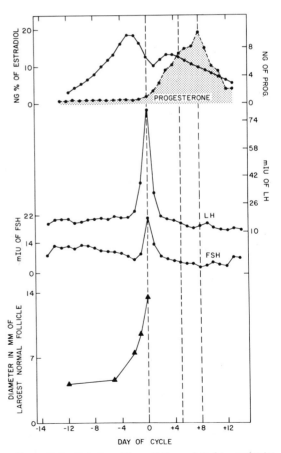

Figure 7–6. Data from Figure 7–5 are plotted to emphasize the rapid preovulatory follicular enlargement in the human ovary.

This phenomenon, coupled with epithelial metaplasia, gives rise to either inclusion cysts, lined with epithelium, or islands of metaplastic epithelium.

Primordial follicles have largely disappeared from the cortex of the postmenopausal ovary. Rarely, a few immature follicles undergoing maturation and atresia may be seen at the corticomedullary junction for up to five years after the last menses. Occasional, small follicular cysts not containing oocytes are also found.

Striking changes occur in the cortical stroma, which becomes hyperplastic in ovaries from women after the age of 40. The extent of the process may vary from multinodular proliferations in the periphery of the ovary, in its milder form, to an enlarged ovary consisting almost entirely of hyperplastic nodules in its most florid form.

Stromal hyperplasia and two other histologic lesions with which it is associated are of interest because of an increased frequency of these changes said to occur in ovaries from women with carcinomas of the endometrium or of the breast. The first of these other lesions consists of foci of cells containing lipid, referred to as "lutein cells," interspersed with areas of stromal hyperplasia. The second have been called cortical granulomas by Woll et al. (1948) and contain lipoids, lymphocytes, other mononuclear cells, and multinucleate giant cells arranged as in inflammatory tubercles. Whether cortical stromal hyperplasia can be equated with hormone synthesis by the postmenopausal ovary remains problematic since estrone, the principal estrogen produced after the menopause, has been shown to be derived from extraovarian, extra-adrenal aromatization of androstenedione (see below). Indeed, blood production rate of estrone remains unchanged after oophorectomy of some postmenopausal women, suggesting an adrenal origin of the precursor androgen.

Relative to the cortex, the medullary portion of the ovary, the repository of corpora albicantia and corpora candicantia, is proportionally larger in the postmenopausal ovary. As in the cortex, the stromal elements of the medulla become fibrotic, and blood vessels traversing this region become sclerotic and their lumens reduced.

Finally, hilar cells seem to be more readily apparent in ovaries from postmenopausal women. Indeed, virilizing syndromes secondary to hilar cell hyperplasia and neoplasia are more commonly seen in postmenopausal women (see below).

Function: The Hypothalamic-Pituitary-Ovarian Genital Axis

Introduction

In women, the reproductive process results from a complex series of interactions of hypothalamus, pituitary, ovary, and genital tract. The role of the ovary in coordinating interactions of these component organs must be understood prior to any logical consideration of the differential diagnosis of ovarian diseases. In the following section, both normal ovarian function and the response elicited in components will be considered.

Normal ovarian function results in two major classes of products: sex steroid hormones and ova. Both are products of the follicular apparatus interacting with surrounding stromal elements under the stimulus of hormones secreted by the pituitary, which is controlled, in turn, by hypophysiotropic hormones. Developmentally, the hormones, especially the estrogens, are produced long before ovulation occurs for the first time, and these substances play an important role in stimulating both somatic and genital growth prior to the menarche. During the reproductive epoch, as we shall see, the estrogens act locally to mediate some of the effects of gonadotropins in stimulating follicular maturation, and peripherally via the hypothalamus, to modulate anterior pituitary gonadotropin secretion. In addition to their role in modulating gonadotropin secretion, the sex steroid hormones play a fundamental role in gamete transport and thus in fertilization as well as in conditioning the uterus for implantation of the zygote.

Biochemical, Physiologic, and Clinical Manifestations of Normal Ovarian Function

Before the Menarche

Although a large body of indirect evidence suggests that gonadal steroid–hypothalamic-pituitary interactions occur before puberty, considerable contention still exists about the relationship of changes in sensitivity of the mechanism to pubescence. When serum and urinary gonadotropin concentrations among pre- and postpubertal girls are compared, mean levels are higher in specimens from postpubertal girls. However, there are no published accounts of long-term longitudinal studies of serum or urinary gonadotropin concentrations in specimens collected before, during, and after puberty in the same person. Here again, the role of alterations in pituitary gonadotropin secretion in producing pubertal changes in the individual is not defined and is still the subject of some controversy.

Recently, it has been found that the patterns differ when gonadotropin concentrations in blood collected from pre-, peri-, and postpubertal girls during sleep are compared. Perhaps this nocturnal variability will be shown to be an important factor in inducing pubertal changes.

Premenarchal ovarian function is manifest in accelerated linear growth (the pubertal growth "spurt") and by the appearance of the secondary sexual characteristics, including development of breasts, maturation of the genitalia, and the appearance of pubic and axillary hair. When the ovary is absent or functions inadequately, puberty

TABLE 7–1. CORRELATIONS OF DEVELOPMENT OF BREASTS AND PUBIC HAIR WITH EACH OTHER AND WITH MAXIMAL LINEAR GROWTH AND MENARCHE

Tanner Stage	Per Cent in Stage at Time of Maximal Linear Growth		Per Cent in Stage at Time of Menarche		Stage of Pubic Hair	Per Cent in Stage for Breasts			
	For Breasts	For Pubic Hair	For Breasts	For Pubic Hair		2	3	4	5
1	0	23 (23)*	0	1	1	61	22	4	0
2	26 (26)	28 (51)	1 (1)	4 (5)	2	29	28	10	2
3	51 (77)	36 (87)	26 (27)	19 (24)	3	8	33	24	7
4	23 (100)	13 (100)	62 (89)	63 (86)	4	2	16	51	36
5	0 (100)	0 (100)	11 (100)	14 (100)	5	0	1	11	56

*Cumulative percentage.
Adapted from Marshall, W. A., and Tanner, J. M.: *Arch. Dis. Child.* 44:291, 1969.

either fails to occur or progresses very slowly. Pubertal changes in these girls can be effectively reproduced by giving continuous estrogen alone, initially, followed by cyclic estrogen and progestogen treatment, indicating that sex steroid hormones mediate the role of the ovary (Ch. 8).

Age at onset of pubertal changes and their rates of progression are subject to a number of variables so that no universally applicable normative values exist. Ideally, the data should be derived from longitudinal studies of representative subjects in the population under evaluation. When such information is available, according to Marshall and Tanner (1969), it is helpful in answering three clinical questions.

1. Is a patient's pubertal development within normal limits for her age?

2. Once puberty has begun, are breasts and pubic hair developing at a normal rate?

3. Are breasts and pubic hair developing in unison and in the proper relation to the growth spurt and to menarche?

Marshall and Tanner (1969) have described the ages at onset of, and rates of progression of, development for breasts and pubic hair, the ages of achievement of maximal velocity in linear growth, and ages at menarche observed in longitudinal studies at three-month intervals of 192 English girls living in family groups in a children's home. While Marshall and Tanner have not regarded these as universally applicable, we have found ourselves returning to this paper again and again in relation to specific constellations seen in the clinic. We have found the relationships among different events and the probabilities of concomitance described to be helpful in deciding whether to temporize or to undertake a complicated and expensive series of studies. For this reason, in Tables 7–1 and 7–2 we have reorganized the data from Marshall and Tanner in the fashion in which they have been useful to us.

To use the tabulated information effectively, the clinician must be familiar with the stages 1–5 for development of breasts and pubic hair shown in Figures 7–7 and 7–8. While these were evaluated from photographs in the study of Marshall and Tanner (1969), they are easily applicable to the clinical examination. The criteria that we have found useful for breasts are modified from those described by Marshall and Tanner as follows:

Stage 1: No palpable glandular tissue; areola not pigmented. Except for nipple, breast does not project from anterior chest wall.

Stage 2: Glandular tissue is palpable at least coextensively with the diameter of the areola; nipple and breast project as a single mound from the anterior chest wall.

Stage 3: Increased glandular tissue to palpation; breasts enlarged; areola increasing in diameter and becoming more darkly pigmented, but contours of breast and areola remain in a single plane.

Stage 4: Further enlargement; increased areolar

TABLE 7–2. MEAN AGE ± STANDARD DEVIATIONS AT ACHIEVEMENT OF STAGE AND MEAN TIME ± STANDARD DEVIATIONS FOR COMPLETION OF INDICATED STAGES OF DEVELOPMENT OF BREASTS AND PUBIC HAIR

Tanner Stage	Mean Age ± S.D. in Years at Achievement of Stage		Mean Time (95th−5th Percentile) in Years for Completion of Stage	
	For Breasts	For Pubic Hair	For Breasts	For Pubic Hair
1	Prepubertal	Prepubertal	Prepubertal	Prepubertal
2	11.15 ± 1.10	11.69 ± 1.21	0.86 (1.03–0.21)	0.63 (1.27–0.16)
3	12.15 ± 1.09	12.36 ± 1.10	0.89 (2.19–0.13)	0.51 (0.93–0.18)
4	13.11 ± 1.15	12.95 ± 1.01	1.96 (6.82–0.12)	1.30 (2.37–0.57)
5	15.33 ± 1.74	14.41 ± 1.12	Mature	Mature

Adapted from Marshall, W. A., and Tanner, J. M.: *Arch. Dis. Child.* 44:291, 1969.

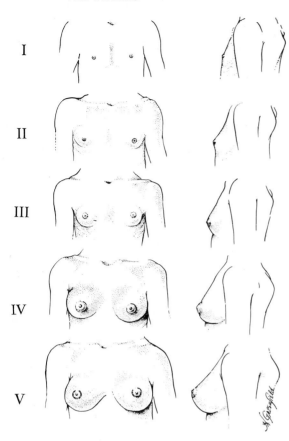

Figure 7–7. Diagrammatic representation of Tanner stages I to V of human breast maturation (adapted from Marshall, W. A., and Tanner, J. M.: *Arch. Dis. Child. 44*:291, 1969).

pigmentation; areola and nipple form a secondary mound above level of the breast.

Stage 5: Areola and nipple no longer project but have receded to make a smooth contour in profile view.

The stages for pubic hair related to change in quality, quantity, and distribution as follows:

Stage 1: None.

Stage 2: Occasional wispy strands, usually along the labia.

Stage 3: More, darker, coarser hair extending superiorly over the pubis.

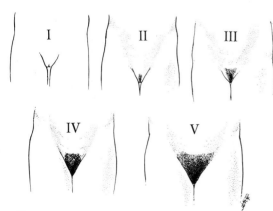

Figure 7–8. Diagrammatic representation of Tanner stages I to V for development of human pubic hair (adapted from Marshall, W. A., and Tanner, J. M.: *Arch. Dis. Child. 44*:291, 1969).

Stage 4: Dark, coarse, curly hair, covering the mons pubis in the adult pattern, but not extending to medial aspects of thighs.

Stage 5: Mature; extends to thighs but otherwise remains in female pattern.

In Tables 7–1 and 7–2, the significance of ages has been minimized, in view of the variability from population to population. Mean ages at achievement of Tanner stages 1–5 for development of breasts and pubic hair are included to indicate the following:

1. Breast changes usually constitute the first signs of puberty, becoming apparent earlier on the average than the appearance of pubic hair. However, once initiated, maturation of pubic hair progresses more rapidly.

2. The time required for completion of maturation averages approximately 4 years for breasts and approximately 3 years for pubic hair.

Rates of progression from one stage to another are very similar for breasts and pubic hair, averaging from 0.5 to 0.9 years from beginning through stage 4, but rate of advancement from stage 4 to 5 is more variable. In Table 7–1 it can be seen that appearance of breast changes heralds the onset of the pubertal growth spurt (maximal rate of linear growth). By the time breast development had reached stage 3, maximal rate of linear growth had been achieved by about 75% of girls.

Finally, in Table 7–2 it can be seen that completion of maturation of the breasts before the appearance of pubic hair is an uncommon event. Similarly, completion of the maturation of pubic hair before initiation of breast development is unusual. The former suggests a syndrome such as testicular feminization (Ch. 8), and the latter some virilizing syndrome.

It should be emphasized that wide individual differences are included within the spectrum of "normal" pubertal development. Further, evaluation of a number of indices has been shown to provide the most accurate measure of the progress of an individual in relation to others with respect to the chronology of maturation.

The Menarche

Zacharias and Wurtman (1969) have reviewed the literature concerning factors influencing age at menarche. They conclude that age at onset of menstruation is "not fixed, but varies from population to population, and changes with time," and is "susceptible to modification by certain socio-economic influences (such as nutrition and urban vs. rural living) and by specific disorders (for example, diabetes, obesity, and blindness)." In addition, Zacharias et al. (1970) studied retrospectively the influence of a number of factors on sexual maturation of 6217 students enrolled in 65 nursing schools in 35 states of the USA. Of these, 4844 were judged normal on the basis of health records. The results of their analysis of data are summarized in Table 7-3.

In this study, appearance of pubic hair either preceded or was coincident with breast development in groups from all geographic regions. Mean age at menarche for the entire group was 151.8 months (12.65 years), with a standard deviation of 14.1 months (1.17 years). The mean age at onset of menarche preceded the mean age at appearance of "regular" menses by about 14 months, and painful menses were noted at a mean interval of 10 months after menses became "regular." The standard deviations for the mean ages at appearance of both regular and painful menses were larger than those for mean age at menarche, indicating greater variability in ages for achievement of these two postmenarchal milestones. These data were used to produce a nomogram reproduced in Figure 7-9, from which it is possible to estimate a reasonable age for onset of menses when ages at appearance of pubic hair and breast budding are known.

A smaller number of women were excluded from the analysis of data for "normal" women by Zacharias et al. (1970) for medical reasons. All women excluded for the same reason were grouped, and when numbers of subjects in a category were 10 or more, data were analyzed. The only factor that was found to influence age at onset of menses significantly was obesity when weight exceeded normal weight by no more than 30%. Mean age at menarche for such women was significantly lower than that for girls with normal weights. In a series of retrospective studies done in the United States since 1932, mean age at menarche was noted to have declined from 13.5 to 12.6 years, so that a range of 9–16 years about this mean constitutes the period during which the onset of menstruation might be regarded as normal. Thus when menarche occurs before age 9 or is delayed beyond age 16, a pathophysiologic process should be suspected.

After the Menarche: The Menstrual Cycle

Length of the Normal Menstrual Cycle. Folklore associates the length of the menstrual cycle with the duration of a lunar cycle, but there is no evidence to support this association, and in

TABLE 7-3. AVERAGE AGES (MONTHS) FOR APPEARANCE OF SEVERAL SECONDARY SEXUAL CHARACTERISTICS AMONG PUBESCENT GIRLS FROM REGIONS INDICATED

Geographical Regions*	No.†	Pubic Hair	Breast Budding	Axillary Hair	Menarche	Regular Menses	Painful Menses
East Central	239	141.0	141.7	143.5	149.1	161.1	170.7
Middle Atlantic	1,265	141.4	142.2	144.1	151.0	164.7	173.1
New England	644	142.1	143.1	145.6	151.5	164.2	175.6
North Central	438	142.4	143.6	145.2	152.1	165.3	176.0
Southeast	579	143.4	143.4	144.7	152.3	166.3	176.3
Southwest	449	142.3	143.1	145.6	152.5	165.5	180.0
Midcentral	672	143.7	143.4	145.5	152.9	166.5	175.7
Northwest	558	143.9	143.7	145.4	153.0	165.6	177.5
Total Normal		142.5	143.0	144.9	151.8	165.2	175.4
Standard Deviation		13.9	14.5	15.1	14.1	24.2	29.8
Standard Error		0.21	0.21	0.23	0.20	0.39	0.65
Sample Size	4,844	4,390	4,683	4,395	4,844	3,830	2,072

*Geographical regions: East Central—Illinois, Kentucky, Ohio, West Virginia; Middle Atlantic—District of Columbia, Maryland, New Jersey, New York, Pennsylvania; New England—Connecticut, Massachusetts, New Hampshire, Rhode Island, Vermont; North Central—Michigan, Minnesota, Wisconsin; Southeast—Alabama, Florida, Louisiana, Mississippi, Tennessee, Virginia; Southwest—Arizona, Southern California, Oklahoma, Texas, Utah; Midcentral—Iowa, Kansas, Missouri, North Dakota; Northwest—Northern California, Montana, Oregon, Washington.

†No.—number of subjects.
From Zacharias, L. et al: *Amer. J. Obstet. Gynec. 108*:833, 1970.

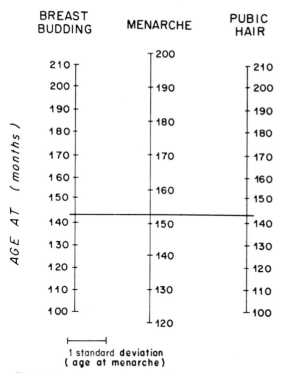

BREAST BUDDING   MENARCHE   PUBIC HAIR

Figure 7-9. Nomogram for estimating age at menarche when age at appearance of breast budding and pubic hair is known. (From Zacharias, L., et al.: *Amer. J. Obstet. Gynec. 108*:833, 1970.)

fact the woman with a 28-day cycle is the exception rather than the rule. There are numerous studies of the temporal aspects of the "normal" menstrual cycle, but as pointed out in a recent review the lack of uniformity in the criteria used in these studies makes it difficult to draw definitive conclusions. In one study, for instance, a mean cycle of 27.3 days was claimed, whereas another investigator calculated a mean value of 33.9. Similar discrepancies can be found in the extent of the variability between individual cycles in the same woman. The larger majority of the cycles falls between 25 and 30 days in length, although the distribution within this range is skewed toward cycles with 30 days. The greatest variability is found in the year following menarche and the years immediately preceding the menopause, during which the cycle length is greatly increased mainly because of the frequency of anovulation and of prolonged proliferative phases. The smallest variability is found between the ages of 20 and 30, but, interestingly enough, in all studies in which this factor was evaluated, there was a clear-cut decrease in the length of the cycle with increasing age. There have been several studies of the relative length of the proliferative and secretory phases, all of them indicating that the secretory phase is remarkably constant in duration and lasts approximately 13 days, while the length of the preovulatory phase is much more variable. In one study, 79.6% of the cycles have a preovulatory phase lasting 10–16 days, whereas 95% of the luteal phases fell within this range. There was a poor correlation of the length between

two consecutive cycles, but when a number of preceding cycles are known, the range of the subsequent cycles can be fairly well predicted. As an example, it has been calculated that the proportion of subsequent cycles that fell in the range of past cycles averaged 64% when based on the range of the past 3 cycles, but 90% when based on the range of the past 12 cycles.

Ovarian Steroid Hormone Secretion and Hormonal Changes

Ovarian Steroid Hormone Secretion. Until recently, most of our information about the secretion of the ovarian hormones was derived from studies of the excretion of their urinary metabolites. There are many limitations to this approach. Urinary metabolites represent only a small and often variable fraction of their secreted precursors. More importantly, they are often derived from more than one precursor, thereby making deductions about secretory processes hazardous, if not impossible. This situation is further complicated by the fact that most of the gonadal hormones are also secreted by the adrenal or may be derived from adrenal secretory products. Recent advances in analytic methods have made it possible to measure steroids in the blood directly, thereby overcoming some of the disadvantages of the urinary methods, but leaving unsolved several of the above-mentioned difficulties and in fact adding some new ones. Recently, for instance, it has been shown that steroids (and also gonadotropins) are secreted episodically, and consequently unless frequent sampling is carried out, this approach will yield erroneous results. In fact, increasing concern about this matter has given rise to a resurgent interest in the urinary methods, since total excretion of the metabolites in the urine should be a reflection of the integrated secretion of the hormone during the preceding 24 hours.

Theoretically at least, the most clear-cut way to determine what the ovary secretes would be by catheterization of the ovarian veins, either directly at the time of surgery or indirectly by fluoroscopically controlled catheterization via femoral veins. The existence of a concentration gradient for a hormone between the ovarian vein and a peripheral vein, in fact, constitutes the only unequivocal proof of the secretion of a hormone by the ovary. However, the information derived in this fashion is only qualitative, and to calculate secretory rates would require accurate information about blood flow which cannot be obtained. Furthermore, catheterization is not without hazard; it is technically difficult and obviously cannot be carried out repeatedly in the same individual.

More satisfactory solutions to the problem of the estimation of the rates of secretion of the ovarian hormones have come from advances in the use of isotopic methods. Besides offering quantitatively more reliable solutions, these methods have brought forward new insights into the complexity of the processes involved in the secretion and metabolism of the gonadal hormones. They also have led to the formulation of novel concepts, such as production rates, as distinct from secretory rates,

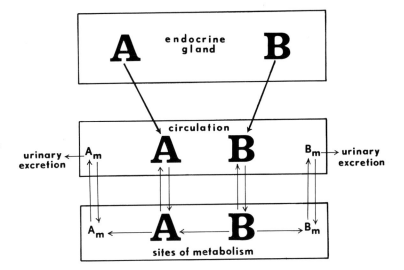

Figure 7–10. A or B may be secreted by the ovaries or adrenal. A_m and B_m represent inactive metabolites of A and B, respectively.

and metabolic clearance rates. Since familiarity with the concepts is of importance to the serious student of ovarian function, a short consideration of the definition of these new concepts is useful.

The *secretory rate* of hormone A (SR_A) is the amount of A released by the endocrine gland into the circulation per unit of time. Hormone A can, however, also be derived from the peripheral conversion of a second hormone, B [refer to Figure 7–10, in which the example of peripheral conversion of Δ_4-androstenedione (hormone B) to estrone (hormone A) has been depicted], secreted either by the same or by another endocrine gland. Hormone B, in this instance, is said to be a prohormone of A, and this pathway of formation of A will be referred to as the prohormone pathway.

The *production rate* in the blood of A (PR_A) is the total rate at which A enters *de novo* into the circulation; conversely, in a steady state, it can also be defined as the rate by which the hormone is irreversibly removed from the circulation. When a hormone derives exclusively from glandular secretion, the secretion rate and the production rate are obviously the same, but when the hormone originates from peripheral metabolism as well as from secretion, the production rate will be higher than the secretory rate.

The metabolic clearance rate (MCR) is a concept related to that of the blood production rate; it equals the volume of blood which, per unit of time, is irreversibly cleared of the hormone. It follows from this definition that the blood production rate will equal the MCR multiplied by the concentration of the hormone in the blood. For different hormones, the MCR may be very different, but it is relatively constant for individuals within a specific clinical group. Consequently, within such a group, production rates of a hormone may be assumed to vary as their concentrations.

The concepts of *secretory rate* versus *production rate* and also the concept of the prohormone are perhaps of more importance for the study of the ovarian hormones than for any other endocrine function. Menopausal women, for instance, excrete

significant amounts of estrogens, yet recent studies have shown that the secretory rate of estrogens in menopausal women is zero or very small, and that in these women most of the estrogen originates via the prohormone pathway, specifically via the peripheral conversion of androstenedione, secreted by the adrenal, to estrone (see below). A similar situation obtains in women with some forms of polycystic ovaries. These ovaries, while secreting large amounts of androstenedione, secrete only small amounts of estrogen, and most of the circulating estrogen is derived from the peripheral conversion of androstenedione to estrone.

In considering the prohormone concept, an additional complexity must be considered. Referring to Figure 7–10, it can be seen that, after the conversion of hormone B to hormone A, further metabolism of A may proceed via two pathways. In one instance, A enters into the circulation directly and in this case, in terms of its biologic effects, A produced via the prohormone pathway will have the same effect upon the target organ as if it had been directly secreted. Part or all of A originating from B in a site of metabolism may, however, be further metabolized in this same site and enter into the circulation only after such further metabolism (perhaps to an inactive form, such as one of the conjugates of A). Obviously in this case significant amounts of A metabolites may appear in the urine, but since A has never circulated as such in the blood, the production of even larger amounts of A via the prohormone pathway would have no biologic consequences. The hormones secreted by the normal ovary are listed in Table 7–4.

Hormonal Changes During the Normal Cycle

(1) *Estrogens:* Figure 7–11 illustrates the changes in plasma estradiol during the normal menstrual cycle. In the early period of follicular development, the levels of estradiol remain low. Approximately one week before the LH peak there is an initial slow and then a more rapid rise of estradiol reaching a maximum generally the day before the LH peak or coinciding with it. There is a sharp drop in the estrogens concomitant with the

TABLE 7-4. CONCENTRATION, METABOLIC CLEARANCE RATES, PRODUCTION RATES, AND OVARIAN SECRETION RATES OF STEROIDS IN BLOOD

Compound	"MCR"* of Compound in Peripheral Plasma, liters/day	Phase of Menstrual Cycle	Concentration in Plasma, μg/100 ml	PR** of Circulating Compound, mg/day	SR+ by Both Ovaries, mg/day
Estradiol	1,350	Early follicular	0.006	0.081	0.07
		Late follicular	0.033–0.070	0.445–0.945	0.4–0.8
		Midluteal	0.020	0.270	0.25
Estrone	2,210	Early follicular	0.005	0.110	0.08
		Late follicular	0.015–0.030	0.331–0.662	0.25–0.50
		Midluteal	0.011	0.243	0.16
Progesterone	2,200	Follicular	0.095	2.1	1.5
		Luteal	1.13	25.0	24.0
20α-hydroxyprogesterone	2,300	Follicular	0.05	1.1	0.8
		Luteal	0.25	5.8	3.3
17-hydroxyprogesterone	2,000	Early follicular	0.03	0.6	0–0.3
		Late follicular	0.20	4.0	3–4
		Midluteal	0.20	4.0	3–4
Androstenedione	2,010		0.159	3.2	0.8–1.6
Testosterone	690		0.038	0.26	
Dehydroisoandrosterone	1,640		0.490	8.0	0.3–3

*Metabolic clearance rate.
**Production rate.
+Secretion rate.
From Tagatz, G. E., and Gurpide, E.: Hormone secretion by the normal human ovary. In *Handbook of Physiology: The Female Reproductive System.* Sect. 7, Vol. II, Pt. 1. Bethesda, Maryland, American Physiological Society, 1973, pp. 603–613.

drop in LH, which in fact precedes the actual rupture of the follicle. During the luteal phase, estradiol rises again, reaching a maximum approximately 5–10 days after ovulation.

The changes in estrone are similar to those of estradiol but less marked (Fig. 7–12). Estrone is secreted directly by the ovary, but most of the estrone in the circulation is derived from the peripheral metabolism of other precursors. There is a small contribution from secreted estradiol to the levels of estrone, but the majority of the estrone in the circulation derives from the conversion of androstenedione to estrone. Since in women the production rate of androstenedione is approximately 3000 μg./day, and about 1% of androstenedione is converted to circulating estrone, 20–40 μg. of estrone are produced daily via this prohormone pathway. On the other hand, virtually all of the circulating estradiol comes from the direct secretion of estradiol, and the contribution from the peripheral conversion of testosterone to circulating estradiol is small.

Less than 0.2% of testosterone is converted to estradiol, and the production rate of testosterone in the normal female is less than one-tenth that of androstenedione. The relative contributions to the levels of estrone and estradiol at various times during the normal menstrual cycle have been calculated by Baird and are illustrated in Figure 7–13. Recent studies have shown that most of the estrone originating by the prohormone pathway enters di-

rectly into the circulation and therefore is available to the target organ. The significance of the circulating levels of estrone remains uncertain. Although, when measured by classic bioassay techniques, estrone has much less estrogenic activity than estradiol, biologic activities other than the growth-promoting activities on the uterus must be considered.

(2) *Progesterone and related substances:* The changes in progesterone during the normal menstrual cycle are illustrated in Figure 7–14. Since progesterone has been isolated from normal ovarian follicles, it is likely that the ovary secretes small amounts of progesterone during the follicular phase of the menstrual cycle. However, the bulk of progesterone in the circulation during the proliferative phase results from extraglandular conversion of adrenal pregnenolone and pregnenolone sulfate to progesterone. There is a small initial increase in the concentration of progesterone at the very beginning of the LH surge, followed by a second major increase, which parallels the increase in the estrogens during the luteal phase. The timing of the early rise in progesterone makes it likely that this rise is the result of a direct effect of the high levels of LH upon the unruptured ovarian follicles; the mechanism by which the progesterone secretion is turned on (and estrogen secretion is turned off) remains unknown.

The secretion by the ovary of *20α-dihydroprogesterone* has been clearly established, but the con-

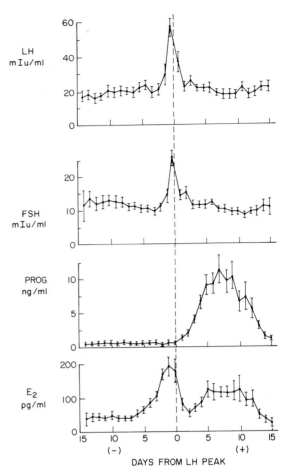

Figure 7–11. Mean LH, FSH, progesterone, and estradiol concentrations in serum specimens collected daily during presumptively ovulatory cycles from young women. (From Mishell, D. R., et al.: *Amer. J. Obstet. Gynec. 111*:60, 1971.)

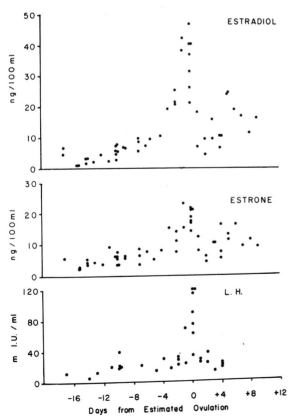

Figure 7–12. Concentration of luteinizing hormone (LH), unconjugated estrone, and estradiol-17β in peripheral plasma of women during the menstrual cycle (n = 51). Day 0 in the graph is the day of estimated ovulation. (From Baird, D. T.: *J. Clin. Endocr. 29*:149, 1969.)

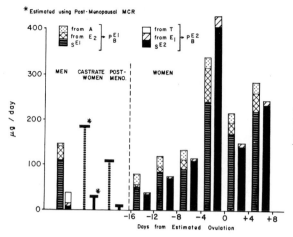

Figure 7-13. Metabolic clearance rates and blood production rates of estrone and estradiol, indicating relative amounts derived from ovarian secretion and from peripheral conversion of precursors. (From Baird, D. T., et al.: *Recent Progr. Hormone Res. 25*:611, 1969.)

tribution to the peripheral levels of secreted 20α-dihydroprogesterone relative to that of other precursors (mainly progesterone) is not known. There is no evidence that *20β-dihydroprogesterone* is secreted by the ovary, although significant amounts of this compound circulate during the luteal phase; it is assumed that this 20β-dihydroprogesterone is derived from secreted progesterone.

The changes in the concentration of *17α-hydroxyprogesterone* during the normal menstrual cycle are illustrated in Figure 7–14. There are two clearcut peaks, one corresponding to the phase of final follicular maturation, the other to the functioning corpus luteum.

Changes in serum concentrations of *Δ₅-pregnenolone* and of 17α-OH-Δ₅-pregnenolone throughout

the normal menstrual cycle have been described. Both compounds were found to be lower in the follicular phase than in the luteal phase. Maximal values did not exceed 4 ng./ml.

(3) *Androgens:* The most informative study comes from the work of Lloyd et al. (1971), who measured Δ₄-androstenedione, testosterone, and dehydroepiandrosterone simultaneously in the ovarian vein and peripheral blood. These studies are illustrated in Figure 7–15. Δ₄-Androstenedione is clearly the major androgen secreted by the ovary, but small amounts of testosterone appear to be secreted also at all times during the menstrual cycle. There is a need for more studies of the plasma levels of androgens during the normal menstrual cycle, but the evidence at hand indi-

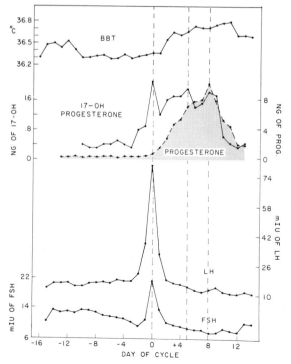

Figure 7-14. Mean daily plasma FSH, LH, progesterone, and 17α-OH progesterone concentrations and basal body temperatures during 16 presumptively ovulatory cycles from 15 young women. (Adapted from Ross, G. T., et al.: *Recent Progr. Hormone Res. 26*:1, 1970.)

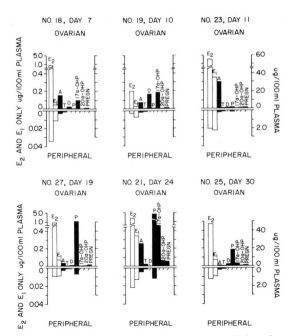

Figure 7–15. Concentrations of estrone, estradiol, androstenedione, testosterone, dehydroepiandrosterone, 17α-OH progesterone, 20α-OH progesterone, and pregnanediol in ovarian and peripheral venous blood samples collected on days of the menstrual cycle indicated. (From Lloyd, C. W., et al.: *J. Clin. Endocr.* 32:155, 1971.)

cates that the changes in the level of androstenedione parallel those of estradiol.

Most of the androstenedione in the circulation results from direct secretion. The relative contribution of the adrenal and of the ovary is unknown and obviously depends upon the stage of the menstrual cycle. The contribution of androstenedione to the circulating level of estrone has been discussed above. In addition, a fraction of the circulating testosterone is derived from the same source.

Although there is evidence that the ovary secretes small amounts of dehydroepiandrosterone and perhaps also of dehydroepiandrosterone sulfate, virtually all of the circulating dehydroepiandrosterone originates in the adrenal. Circulating dehydroepiandrosterone does not contribute significantly to the circulating levels of androstenedione and testosterone. Table 7–4 summarizes the concentrations, the metabolic clearance rates, the production rates, and ovarian secretion rates of steroids in normal women.

There are several hormonal changes during the normal menstrual cycle that are secondary to the effects of changes in ovarian secretion on other glands. During the luteal phase, there is an increase in aldosterone which probably is a compensatory mechanism to overcome the inhibitory effect of progesterone upon the sodium-retaining activity of aldosterone. Renin, on the other hand, has a midcycle maximum as well as a luteal maximum, and available evidence indicates that this is secondary to estrogen changes. There have been several studies of growth hormone in the course of the menstrual cycle, but definitive conclusions are

difficult, largely because of the extreme sensitivity of growth hormone to many other influences. Nevertheless, a pattern consisting of a midcycle peak as well as several elevations during the luteal phase seems to be emerging. Recently, it has become possible to measure the levels of prolactin, but, at least from available data, no characteristic pattern has emerged.

(4) *Relaxin:* Although relaxin was first described more than 40 years ago, its role in human physiology, or for that matter even its existence in man, remains in doubt. It was first isolated from sow corpora lutea and later from corpora lutea of other species. Relaxin increases in the tissues and blood of several animals during gestation. Human serum contains a substance that cross-reacts with antisera for porcine relaxin. The hormone has been purified to near homogeneity; it manifests itself as a polypeptide with a molecular weight of approximately 8000 and is capable of eliciting a specific immune response. In sensitive species, relaxin produces relaxation of the symphysis, inhibition of uterine contractility, and softening of the cervix. Although partly purified relaxin preparations have been extensively used in women with premature labor, the effectiveness of this treatment remains to be established.

Mechanisms Controlling the Normal Cycle. Although some of the aspects of the dynamic relationship between the gonadotropins and the gonadal hormones have been well understood for several decades, sufficient information to evolve a comprehensive theory about these relationships has been available only for the last few years. Until the advent of the radioligand methods, there were no analytic techniques of sufficient sensitivity to measure simultaneously, at daily or even more frequent intervals, the levels of FSH, LH, estradiol and estrone, progesterone, and androstenedione. Only when this could be done was it possible to analyze precisely the temporal and causal relationships between the fluctuations of these hormones. Much useful information also became available through the many studies in which purified FSH and LH have been administered to amenorrheic patients, studies which yielded necessary information about the quantitative relationship between the pituitary stimulus and the ovarian response.

In this section, for which we have relied heavily on an earlier article, we will describe in some detail a series of mechanisms that can account for the orderly sequence of events that constitutes the normal menstrual cycle. Some aspects of this theory—mainly quantitative—require additional experimental evidence, but the inclusion of these assumptions appears warranted. The reader is encouraged to familiarize himself with this concept of the menstrual cycle, since it offers a rational explanation for many types of ovarian disturbances that heretofore were difficult to explain.

As this chapter was being written, two new major developments in reproductive endocrinology emerged, which will have to be incorporated into this theory. The first was the observation that gonadotropins and steroid hormones are secreted in a pulsatile fashion, and the second was the identification and synthesis of gonadotropin releasing hormone (GnRH), which has made it possible to test precisely the responsiveness of the pituitary to hypothalamic inputs. These developments should add greatly to our understanding of the mechanisms controlling the menstrual cycle, but in any case available information is compatible with the concepts outlined here.

Feedback Systems. It has been generally thought that cyclic stimulation of the pituitary is inherent in the female hypothalamus, in contrast to the male hypothalamus in which stimulation is noncyclic. Although it remains possible and even likely that the response of the male and female hypothalamus to hormonal feedbacks is qualitatively similar but quantitatively different, it is increasingly evident that it is the changing input from the ovarian secretions that determines the cyclic secretion of the hypothalamus and the pituitary rather than a rhythm inherent in this axis.

Of the feedback mechanisms, the best known ones are obviously the negative feedback mechanisms of the steroids upon gonadotropin secretion. Both FSH and LH are subject to negative feedback mechanisms. This is evident from the well-known rise in FSH and LH after castration or during the menopause, and when these high levels are depressed after administration of estrogens. Although progesterone and androgens in large amounts will produce a negative feedback effect upon gonadotropic secretion, it is likely that estrogens are the most important components in the negative feedback effect of the ovarian secretion.

This feedback effect of estrogens is rapid and exerts its effect within hours. In addition, there is increasing evidence that the sensitivity of the hypothalamic pituitary axis to the inhibitory effect of estrogen changes with the changing levels of estrogens. At low levels of plasma estrogens, small increments in the concentration of estrogens produce major changes in the levels of FSH. Conversely, at higher estrogen levels (such as those observed during the late proliferative phase of the normal menstrual cycle), a large increment in estrogens will produce only small changes in the gonadotropins.

Positive Feedback. In addition to a negative feedback effect upon FSH and LH secretion, gonadal hormones also exert a positive effect on gonadotropin secretion, and it is this positive feedback effect that is the cardinal factor in the regulation of the menstrual cycle. Evidence in favor of a positive feedback effect of estrogens upon LH goes back as far as 1934, when Hohlweg reported that injection of estrogens induces ovulation in immature rats. Recent work has conclusively established this effect of estrogens upon LH secretion and has added much qualitative and quantitative information about the nature of this relationship. In contrast to their effect upon LH, estrogens appear not to have a positive feedback effect upon FSH secretion, while progesterone under appropriate experimental conditions has been shown to produce a rise

in both FSH and LH. It can be assumed that positive and negative mechanisms operate simultaneously, and that the net change in the secretion of the gonadotropins represents the algebraic sum of the positive and negative feedback inputs.

Follicle maturation is obviously dependent upon the stimulatory effect of FSH and LH in appropriate ratios. By their feedback effect upon the hypothalamic-pituitary axis, the gonadal hormones indirectly influence follicle maturation, but they also appear to modulate follicle growth by a direct intraovarian mechanism. Several studies in subprimate mammals have demonstrated that local applications of estrogens to the ovary produce increased responsiveness to both endogenous and exogenous gonadotropins, and that estrogens in the absence of pituitary function will actually induce follicular growth. Indirect evidence in women is consistent with this hypothesis. Androgens, on the other hand, appear to have an opposite activity and will inhibit the stimulatory effect of estrogens on follicular growth. In considering follicular growth, it is therefore necessary to take into account the stimulation not only of FSH (and LH) but also of the ratio of the stimulatory and inhibitory effect of the intraovarian concentrations of estrogens and androgens.

Schematic representation of the plasma levels of gonadotropins and of certain gonadal hormones are shown in Figures 7–16 and 7–17 as a background for the following discussion of the mechanism regulating the sequence of events during the normal menstrual cycle.

Sequential Pituitary-Ovarian Events During the Normal Cycle

Initial Follicle Growth. This phase begins in the late luteal phase of the preceding cycle and ends

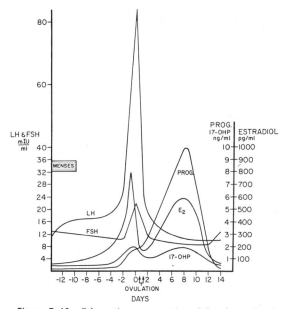

Figure 7–16. Schematic representation of the plasma levels of gonadotropins and gonadal steroids during the human menstrual cycle. The cycle is centered on day 0, the day of midcycle LH peak. (From Speroff, L., et al.: *Amer. J. Obstet. Gynec. 109*:234, 1971.)

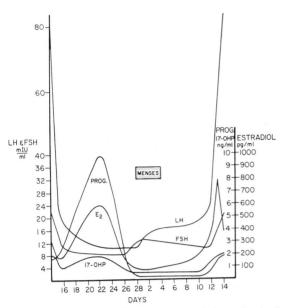

Figure 7-17. Schematic representation of plasma levels of gonadotropins and gonadal steroids during the human menstrual cycle. The changes during menses are emphasized by centering the cycle on day 28 and the beginning of menses. (From Speroff, L., et al.: *Amer. J. Obstet. Gynec.* 109:234, 1971.)

changes in LH and the direction of change will depend upon the relative importance of the two feedback mechanisms. Preliminary evidence indicates that the negative feedback mechanism of estrogens operates at lower levels for LH than for FSH and the positive feedback component therefore dominates.

The rapid growth of the follicle and the almost exponential rise of estrogens late in the proliferative phase, when FSH levels are actually decreasing, is consistent with the findings discussed above, indicating that as it matures the follicle becomes increasingly sensitive to gonadotropic stimulation as a result of the local effects of estrogens. While one follicle grows on to full maturity, other follicles of various sizes become atretic. As noted earlier, the mechanism that causes this atresia remains unclear, but preovulatory atresia may be caused by the decreasing levels of FSH. Such a decrease would not influence the "ovulatory" follicle, since it is protected by its own hormone production, resulting in high local concentrations of estrogens. The decrease in FSH would, however, be significant for the smaller follicles that have not reached a more advanced stage of development and thus produce less estrogen. Another possibility is that the atresia of the smaller follicles results from the local effect of the ovarian androgens.

The Ovulatory Period. During this period, a surgelike rise in the secretion of LH leads to the final steps in the maturation of the graafian follicle, follicle rupture, and expulsion of the oocyte. There is a concomitant but modest rise in FSH. Within hours after the beginning of the LH surge and before the rupture of the follicle, estrogens in the plasma drop, while progesterone increases slowly. The high levels of LH persist for approximately 24 hours and decrease in the early portion of the postovulatory period to values below the concentration in the proliferative period.

Available information strongly supports the theory that the rise in estrogens during the late proliferative phase is the trigger that sets off the preovulatory LH surge. It has been suggested that 17α-hydroxyprogesterone, which rises simultaneously, may also serve as a trigger for the LH surge, but direct experimental evidence for this suggestion is lacking. It is unlikely that progesterone plays a role in the initiation of the LH surge. As mentioned above, progesterone, under certain experimental conditions, will stimulate LH release, but careful analysis of the sequence of events during this period clearly indicates that the plasma levels of progesterone do not rise prior to the LH surge as do those of estrogens. The small increase in plasma progesterone concentration during the period of LH surge is therefore a consequence of, rather than the cause of, the surge. It is possible that this increase in progesterone during the ovulatory period has a central facilitative feedback effect that is of importance in maintaining and prolonging the surge of LH, but this remains to be established.

Originally it was thought that estrogen triggers

when a significant increase in estrogens is detectable, 6 or 7 days before the LH surge. Morphologically, this period is characterized by the growth of a new set of follicles, which can be identified already in the midluteal phase. It is assumed that this new wave of follicular growth results from the rise in estrogens at this stage of the cycle. The cardinal hormonal change during Phase One is the rise in the level of FSH, caused by the decrease in the level of estrogens concomitant with the waning activity of the corpus luteum—a rise which stimulates follicle growth. There is also a rise in LH, but it starts later than the increase in FSH. During this phase of early follicular growth, there is little change in the plasma levels of the gonadal hormones.

Follicular Maturation and Atresia; Steroidogenesis. During this phase, estrogens rise, first slowly and then more rapidly, reaching a peak just before ovulation. Concomitant with a rise in estrogens is a decrease in FSH, while, in contrast, LH increases slowly but steadily. A few days before ovulation, there is also an elevation of 17α-hydroxyprogesterone and of androstenedione. The relationship between the surge of the gonadotropins and the steroids is extremely complex and the dynamics are incompletely understood. Sufficient information is available, however, to allow an attempt to rationalize the interrelationship between the gonadotropins and steroids during this phase of the menstrual cycle.

As estrogens rise, there is a decrease in FSH because of a negative feedback effect of estrogens. An LH decrease, however, need not be expected since, in the case of LH, both positive and negative feedback mechanisms are in operation. The net the LH surge when the concentration reaches a critical level in the plasma. More recent evidence, however, suggests that this set point theory is incorrect and that it is the changing and rising titer of estrogen that stimulates the LH surge. It is not known whether the hypothalamus, once stimulated by the estrogen stimulus, reacts with an all-or-none response or releases GnRH at a rate proportionate to the stimulus.

The mechanisms that shut off the LH surge also remain unknown. Within hours of the rise in LH, there is a precipitous drop in the plasma estrogen, and it is likely that this removal of the stimulus that initiated the LH surge is an important controlling factor. Additional factors may be (1) the depletion of the LH stores in the pituitary, (2) a decrease in GnRH through the operation of a short feedback loop of LH, and (3) the rising concentration of progesterone.

Concomitant with the LH surge is a significant, although much smaller, FSH surge, which is to be expected in view of the fact that GnRH under all experimental conditions releases FSH as well as LH. The fall in plasma levels of estrogens occurs before the follicular rupture and probably reflects a morphologic change induced by LH, which is luteinization.

An adequate LH surge does not ensure ovulation. Ovulation occurs only if the follicle has reached a stage of maturity that allows a response to the luteinizing stimulus. In the normal cycle, LH release and final maturation of the follicle are coupled. Indeed, the time of the LH surge is controlled by the estrogen level, and since estrogen production is a function of follicular development, LH release and follicular maturity coincide.

The rupture of the follicle occurs 16–24 hours after the beginning of the LH surge. Weakening and disruption of the follicular wall are presumably effects of LH; however, the role of estrogens and progesterone in this process should be considered. The abrupt fall in estrogen production prior to ovulation may have a direct structural effect on the follicle. The low levels of progesterone present at this time may also have a cellular function in the process of follicular rupture. It has been suggested that the mechanical properties of the graafian follicle may provide a mechanism regulating the number of ova released in response to an ovulating stimulus. If only a few follicles satisfy the physical requirements for ovulation, multiple ovulation must be even further limited by the hormonal coordination required. The incidence of multiple ovulation may then reflect statistical chance of more than one follicle fulfilling all the requirements for ovulation.

Life and Death of the Corpus Luteum. Luteinization is initiated by LH, but recent studies have emphasized the role of follicular rupture and of the expulsion of the ovum on the process of luteinization. The luteal phase of the cycle is marked by an increase in the plasma levels of progesterone, of estradiol and estrone, and of 17α-hydroxyprogesterone. There is also a significant increase in the levels of androstenedione, but insufficient data are available to depict a curve of the changes in the androgens during the luteal phase. LH and FSH levels during this time are lower than during the preovulatory phase and are lowest when progesterone secretion is maximum.

According to both histologic and biochemical criteria, the human corpus luteum reaches full maturity 8 or 9 days after ovulation, following which regression begins unless pregnancy intervenes. A normal length of the luteal phase and hence the production of conditions allowing implantation of the fertilized ovum appears to be dependent on two sets of factors: complete maturation of the follicle before ovulation, and adequate LH levels during the luteal phase. Recent studies in hypophysectomized women have clearly shown that normal function of the corpus luteum is dependent on the continuing stimulation by LH. When ovulation was induced with LH in such patients, to ensure normal corpus luteum function, it was necessary for the ovulatory dose of LH to be followed by small "maintenance" doses of LH, approximating the secretory rate of LH during the normal luteal phase. To maintain the corpus luteum beyond the normal 14 days, increasing amounts of LH had to be injected, indicating that, as the corpus luteum grows old, it becomes less and less sensitive to the stimulatory effect of LH. Ross et al. (1970), in a study of women with short luteal phases, presented evidence that the length of the luteal phase may be already determined at the time of ovulation. They showed that, in women with short luteal phases, the ovulatory LH peak was perfectly normal, but the levels of FSH during the preovulatory phase were lower than in normal women, suggesting that incomplete maturation of the follicle was a cause of the short luteal phase.

Unless pregnancy intervenes and corpus luteum function is prolonged by the rapidly increasing levels of hCG, the levels of progesterone and estrogen start to drop 7–8 days after ovulation. The drop in estrogen level results in an increase of FSH and LH, and a new cycle starts.

This brief discussion of normal menstrual physiology immediately points to the many possible ways in which menstrual disturbances may originate even in the absence of true organic pathology, and it may be appropriate to elaborate on some of these possibilities. The onset of the new cycle is critically dependent upon the events in the late luteal phase of the preceding cycle. The precise quantitative relationship between the increments in the levels of estradiol and FSH at this time of the cycle will determine the magnitude in the rise of FSH that is necessary for new follicular growth, and any aberration in this relationship may result in either a delay or a failure to initiate a new cycle. During the early and midproliferative phase, there is need for a constant readjustment between the stimulatory effect of the gonadotropins and the ovarian hormonal output to ensure an orderly sequence of follicular growth. In the later stages of the proliferative phase, the follicle is dependent not only upon the stimulatory effect of the gonadotropin but also on an appropriate ratio of the stimulatory and inhibitory effects of the intra-ovarian estrogens and androgens. A premature rise of estrogen, or an increased sensitivity of the hypothalamic-pituitary axis to the positive feedback effect of estrogens, may set off an LH surge at the time when the mature follicle is not available or the pituitary stores of LH are not sufficient for an adequate LH surge. In both cases, one would expect luteinization of the maturing follicles to occur rather than ovulation. Similarly, a delayed rise in the estrogens or decreased sensitivity of the hypothalamic pituitary axis may delay the LH surge until the time when the follicles have matured beyond ideal size and are undergoing atretic changes.

Changes in Genital Tract Epithelium During the Normal Cycle. The cyclic changes in ovarian morphology and in gonadotropic and sex steroid hormone secretion having been described, consideration will now be given to the cyclic changes in the epithelia of the genital tract. These have been systematically studied and elegantly documented by Papanicolaou and his associates (1948). A schematic representation of their observations, coupled with measurements of pituitary and sex steroid hormones, is shown in Figure 7–18, which depicts the changes described below.

The Endometrium. The uterine mucosa consists of a surface layer of columnar epithelial cells and an underlying stroma composed of spindle-shaped cells permeated by blood vessels. The continuity of the surface layer is interrupted by crypts called "glands" lined by similar epithelial cells in a tubular arrangement that dip into the stromal layer. Some of the columnar epithelial cells are ciliated, while others are nonciliated and appear to be secretory cells. Normal cyclic changes affecting the morphology of epithelium, stroma, and blood vessels are sufficiently stereotyped to make microscopic evaluation of these valuable in diagnosing disorders of ovarian function (see below).

During the preovulatory phase of the cycle and under the influence of estrogenic substances secreted principally by the theca interna of developing follicles, the dominant changes are due to mitotic proliferation of the epithelium and the stroma. As a consequence, the mucosa thickens, and the tubular glands lengthen but remain straight. Nuclei of individual epithelial cells tend to be in a position midway between basal and luminal borders of the cell. Under the influence of progesterone produced by the corpus luteum, marked coiling of the glands, "loosening" suggestive of edema, and increased vascularity of the stroma are characteristic changes. These gross changes are accompanied by reduction in mitotic activity, vacuolization of the cytoplasm, and increase in glycogen content of the epithelial cells, the nuclei of which take up a more basal position. The most superficial stromal cells now come to resemble decidual cells characteristic of early pregnancy, while intermediate and deeper layers show no such changes. Coincident with declining function of the corpus luteum and reflected in decreasing plasma concentration of estrogens and progestogens, ne-

crotic changes occur in the mucosa, resulting in multifocal and progressive exfoliation of all save the cells lining the depths of the tubular glands. Necrosis of blood vessels opens vascular channels with resultant menstrual bleeding. After menstruation, the surface epithelium of the uterine mucosa is reconstituted by proliferation of epithelial cells in the depths of the glandular crypts and the cycle is repeated.

The Endocervical Glands. The epithelium of the endocervical glands undergoes cyclic changes more closely correlated with changes in the vaginal epithelium than with changes in the endometrium. Of greater interest and more easily evaluated, however, are the cyclic changes in both quantity and physical characteristics of the mucus secreted by these glands. During the first week after onset of the menses, small amounts of viscous mucus are produced. Coincident with rapid follicular growth and increasing plasma estrogen concentration in the second half of the follicular phase of the cycle, the quantity of mucus produced increases by up to thirty-fold. Qualitatively this mucus is more watery, more viscous, and more elastic. As progesterone secretion rises after ovulation, the quantity, the viscosity, and the elasticity of the cervical mucus decline. In castrate women, injections of estrogen reproduce the changes in cervical mucus seen in the second half of the follicular phase of a spontaneous menstrual cycle. Concomitant injections of progesterone reverse the estrogenic effects on cervical mucus. These changes in water content, viscosity, and elasticity secondary to changes in steroid hormone secretion provide the basis for simple effective indirect tests of ovarian function (see below).

The Vaginal Epithelium. The human vagina is lined by stratified squamous epithelium, which consists of superficial, intermediate, inner, parabasal, and basal layers. The morphologic properties of cells from each of these layers as seen in films of vaginal secretions stained with polychrome stains and in biopsies of vaginal mucosa were described by Papanicolaou and co-workers. More recently, uniform morphologic and tinctorial criteria for identification of cells from each of the five layers have been agreed upon by cytologists.

Proliferation and maturation of vaginal epithelium is influenced by estrogens and progestogens. When ovarian estrogen secretion is low, prepubertally and postmenopausally, vaginal epithelium is thin and susceptible to infection which may be accompanied by vaginal bleeding. Following either local application or systemic administration of estrogen, epithelial proliferation is stimulated, and the tinctorial and morphologic properties of the exfoliated cells change. Early in the follicular phase of the cycle, basophilic cells with vesicular nuclei predominate, but increasing ovarian estrogen secretion stimulates both proliferation and keratinization, and acidophilic cells with pycnotic nuclei come to predominate.

During the postovulatory phase of the cycle, regressive changes appear in both acidophilic and basophilic cells; the percentage of acidophilic cells

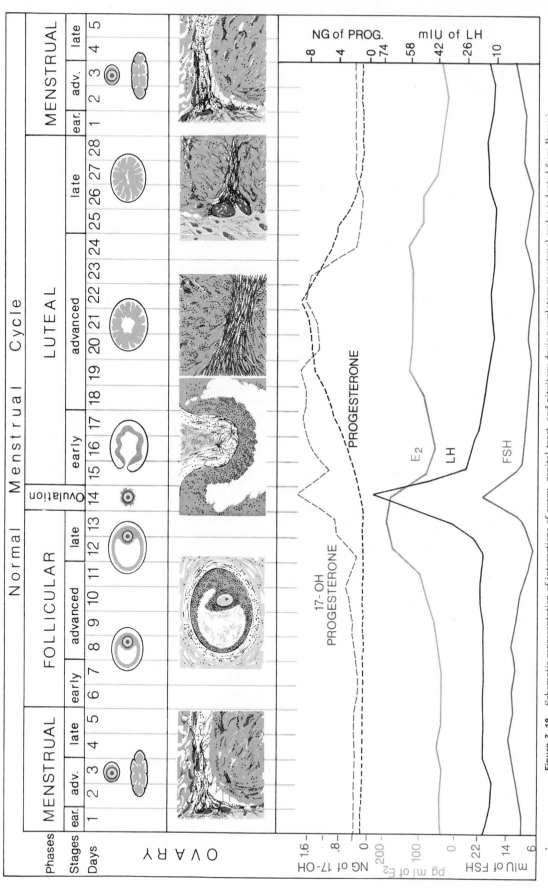

Figure 7–18. Schematic representation of interactions of ovary, genital tract, and pituitary during ovulatory menstrual cycles (adapted from Papanicolaou, G. N., et al.: *The Epithelia of Women's Reproductive Organs.* New York, Commonwealth, 1948, and Ross, G. T.: *Recent Progr. Hormone Res.* 26:1, 1970.)

(*Figure continued on opposite page.*)

Figure 7–18. *Continued.*

decreases, and increasing numbers of polymorphonuclear leukocytes appear.

The Urethral Epithelium. The character of cells exfoliated from the urethra changes with alterations in the sex steroid hormonal milieu. Properly prepared stained smears of epithelial cells in fresh urinary sediment reflect cyclic alterations in estrogen and progesterone levels in sexually mature women. These cells are more accessible than vaginal epithelial cells of infants and children and have been studied for diagnostic screening when excessive estrogen production is suspected.

Metabolic Effects of Sex Steroid Hormones. The use of estrogens and progestogens as contraceptive steroids has made us increasingly aware of the widespread effects of the gonadal hormones upon many metabolic processes. However, much confusion remains, and most of what we know relates to the synthetic rather than to the natural steroids. Since there are quantitative and qualitative differences between the physiologic effects of these two classes, evidence from studies in which synthetic steroids were used, often in unphysiologic doses, must be interpreted with caution. Even so, a number of facts appear to be well established. Estrogens enhance the insulin response to carbohydrate loads, but because of a concomitant increase in growth hormone and cortisol, the net effect may be a decrease in carbohydrate tolerance. This effect will obviously be more pronounced in women whose pancreas has a limited capacity to secrete insulin. Progesterone, at least in physiologic doses, appears to have little influence upon carbohydrate metabolism.

Estrogens augment plasma triglycerides mainly via an increase in the triglyceride-rich pre-β-lipoproteins. Lipoprotein lipase, as measured by postheparin lipolytic activity, is decreased. Progesterone has little effect, but some synthetic progestogens, such as norethindrone acetate, a progestogen with inherent androgenic activity, will decrease triglyceride levels in patients with hyperlipidemia.

Estrogens increase plasma proteins that bind steroids, such as cortisol, progesterone, and thyroxine, as well as plasma steroids that bind serum iron and copper. Recently, it has been established that, in addition to an increase in bound cortisol, estrogens produce also a moderate increase in unbound, and therefore physiologically active, cortisol. Estrogens reduce the secretory capacity of the liver for certain organic anions, such as bromsulfophthalein. Increases in liver enzymes and hyperbilirubinemia can occur, as well as idiosyncratic biliary secretory failure. If a disorder of biliary excretion is present, estrogens will aggravate the problem. Mention has already been made of the effect of estrogens upon plasma renin, angiotensin, and aldosterone and the resulting changes in the substance during the normal menstrual cycle. The role of estrogens in electrolyte regulation is complex, with an initial natriuresis followed by a period of sodium retention. Progesterone may also cause natriuresis, but its effects are transient.

The Menopause

The basic ovarian event in the menopause is the cessation of cyclic ovarian function. Although a few follicles, usually quiescent, have been shown to persist for as long as five years after the last menses (see above), functional changes can be attributed to depletion of follicles. Initially this is marked clinically by decreasing frequency of ovulation, sometimes associated with irregular menses or variable periods of amenorrhea and later by decreasing estrogen secretion. Thus ovulation and menses, last to appear at menarche, cease first, and estrogen production, first to appear at menarche, is last to decline at menopause.

Some years before the final cessation of menstruation, there is a decrease in the responsiveness of the ovary to gonadotropins. Recent studies indicate that, in women who are in the perimenopausal age group but who still have ovulatory periods, mean concentrations of FSH and LH are increased over levels seen in younger women, while the levels of estrogens and progesterone throughout the cycle are decreased.

Concentrations of estrogens in both ovarian venous blood and in peripheral blood decline to very low levels. There is increasing evidence to support the concept that after the menopause most of the estrogens are derived from peripheral conversion of androgenic precursors secreted principally by the adrenals (see above). Concentrations of androstenedione in ovarian venous blood from ovaries of some postmenopausal women are higher than are concentrations in samples of peripheral blood collected simultaneously. These observations allow for the possibility that the postmenopausal ovary may secrete small amounts of androgens which are aromatized and converted to estrogens peripherally. However, removal of the ovaries frequently fails to alter the quantities of estrogens excreted in the urine of postmenopausal women.

The declining estrogen secretion is accompanied by signs and symptoms of hormone deficits in the estrogen-dependent target organs, including pituitary, uterus, cervix, vagina, and breasts. Pituitary gonadotropin secretion rises and is reflected by increased quantities of gonadotropin in blood and urine; the endometrium becomes atrophic, myometrial mass decreases, and the vaginal epithelium becomes thin, deficient in glycogen, and fails to become keratinized.

Tests of Ovarian Function

Tests for Steroid Hormone Production

Indirect: Evaluation of Target Organ Responses. Some of the tissues and secretions that respond to steroid hormones produced by the ovary are easily accessible for examination. Studies of these tissues and secretions provide indirect evidence for the status of steroidogenic function of the organ both in the basal state and following perturbations of the hypothalamic-hypophysial-ovarian axis. These include the vaginal epithelium, the secretions of the endocervical glands, the epithelium of the urethra, and the endometrium.

Vaginal Epithelium. Steroid hormone–dependent cyclic changes in the morphology of the vaginal epithelium described earlier provide the basis for a reasonably accurate and rapid screening assessment of ovarian steroid hormone production. Studies of nuclear morphology, glycogen content, and extent of keratinization of vaginal epithelium, as well as of changes in numbers of polymorphonuclear leukocytes in properly prepared films of vaginal secretions provide rough indices of estrogenic and progestogenic activity in the absence of vaginal infections. Changes in appearance of smears taken at different times between two consecutive episodes of genital bleeding can provide indirect evidence of ovulation. The major usefulness of the vaginal smear for evaluation of ovarian function is when estrogens are low and routine assays are not sufficiently sensitive.

Endocervical Mucus. The mucoid secretions of the endocervical glands are qualitatively and quantitatively altered by estrogens and progestogens. As the quantity of estrogens elaborated during the preovulatory phase of the menstrual cycle increases, there is a ten- to thirtyfold increase in the quantity of endocervical mucus secreted. With increasing estrogen, the elasticity, usually referred to as "spinnbarkeit," of endocervical mucus increases, so that a long fine thread is generated by stretching a small drop of secretion. Stretching is maximal just before or when estrogen production is maximal. In addition, a characteristic ferning or palm leaf arborization is observed on microscopic examination when endocervical secretions aspirated with a clean pipette are spread as a thin film onto a clean glass slide and permitted to dry. This pattern is the result of crystallization of sodium chloride from dilute solutions containing proteins and polypeptides, but it is indicative of estrogen production when observed in secretions of endocervical glands. The pattern disappears coincident with maximal production of progesterone during the postovulatory phase of the menstrual cycle. Both the appearance and disappearance of ferning provide diagnostically useful information about ovarian steroid hormone production.

Urethral Epithelium. Examination of urinary tract epithelium in films prepared from sediment recovered by centrifugation of freshly voided urine samples has been said to be useful in infants and children under study for estrogenic stimulation. This has not been widely done, but recovery of the sample is without morbidity, an important consideration particularly in infants and children.

The Endometrium. As noted earlier, the morphologic changes in the endometrium throughout the menstrual cycle are sufficiently stereotyped to make microscopic examination of endometrial biopsies useful in studies of ovarian function. Criteria have been established for "dating" secretory endometrium, assuming that ovulation occurs on day 14 of a 28-day cycle.

A practical test of ovarian function based upon endometrial reactions is the progesterone withdrawal bleeding test, consisting of an intramuscular injection of 10–100 mg. of progesterone. If vaginal bleeding is observed within a week following the injection, it is reasonable to conclude that (1) the pituitary secretes FSH and LH; (2) the ovary has responded to these gonadotropins and secreted sufficient estrogen to stimulate the endometrium; (3) the endometrium responds to both estrogen and progesterone; (4) the hypothalamic-pituitary unit responds to changes in the sex steroid hormone milieu. Hence, in the evaluation of a patient with either primary or secondary amenorrhea, withdrawal bleeding following progesterone injection is indicative of hypothalamic-pituitary and utero-ovarian functional integrity. When the test is negative, additional studies are necessary to fix the locus of the abnormality.

The Basal Body Temperature. Perhaps the most widely used presumptive indicator of ovarian progesterone production is the so-called thermogenic shift detected by daily measurements of basal body temperatures. Thermometers especially designed for the purpose are used to measure either oral or (preferably) rectal temperatures daily before arising. Ovarian production of progesterone, presumably reflecting function of the corpus luteum, results in a "shift" of the basal body temperatures upward around the time of ovulation (Fig. 7–19). This thermogenic response results from a direct effect of progesterone upon the thermoregulatory center in the hypothalamus and can be shown in postmenopausal or castrate women and in men.

The thermogenic shift coincides with the rise in serum progesterone after the preovulatory LH surge in presumptive ovulatory cycles. Sufficient progesterone to induce an increase in basal body temperature may be inadequate to induce an appropriate secretory transformation of the endometrium.

Direct: Measurement of Gonadotropins and Steroids in Blood and Urine

Gonadotropins. As noted earlier, sex steroid hormones secreted by the ovary act on the hypothalamus to modulate pituitary gonadotropin secretion in sexually mature women. With rare exception, high levels of gonadotropins in serum and urine can be equated with states of primary gonadal failure in persons under evaluation for ovarian diseases after the age when puberty might have been expected to be completed.

Biologic assays are too insensitive to measure accurately the concentrations of FSH and LH in single, 24-hour urine specimens from sexually mature men and women. Since urine from prepubertal children contains less FSH and LH than does that of their postpubertal counterparts, biologic assay of a single, 24-hour urine specimen is virtually useless for diagnostic purposes. However, assays of multiple specimens have been shown to provide useful information.

Sensitive, precise radioimmunoassays have been developed and used to measure gonadotropin in serum and urine of men, women, and sexually immature boys and girls. A comprehensive review of the methodology involved in the measurement of gonadotropins in plasma was recently published (Vaitukaitis and Ross, 1973). Since concentrations of these hormones in serum are subject to significant circadian variations, comparisons of levels in randomly collected single specimens frequently fail to distinguish individual normal from individual pathophysiologic states of pituitary gonadotropin secretion. In contrast, similar assays of randomly collected, single, 24-hour urine specimens have been found to provide greater discrimination.

The Steroid Hormones. Methods for measurement of urinary metabolites of estrogen, progesterone, and androgen have been available for a number of years and were extensively used in the evaluation of ovarian function (Fig. 7–19). For estrogen and progesterone, the excretion of their urinary metabolites gives a fair estimate of secretory rate. For androgen, however, because of multiplicity of the precursors and contributions of the adrenal, the information acquired from their urinary metabolites is very limited (see above).

More recently, both radioligand binding and radioimmunoassays for estrogens, progesterone, and androgens have become available. A compre-

hensive review of the methods involved was recently published (Vande Wiele and Dyrenfurth, 1973).

THE ABNORMAL OVARY

Introduction

There is no completely satisfactory system for the etiologic classification of ovarian diseases. We have elected to base classification of ovarian diseases on the time in the life of the patient when signs and symptoms become apparent, with the exception of neoplastic diseases, among which we have elected to consider functioning ovarian neoplasms separately. All other varieties will be mentioned, as appropriate, in relation to the age of the patient.

Functioning Ovarian Tumors

Aberrant ovarian function has been associated with primary tumors arising in the ovary, with tumors metastasizing to the ovary from a primary site in another organ, and with tumors ectopically secreting gonadotropins. Both primary and secondary tumors, intrinsically without endocrine function, may alter ovarian function by mechanisms that remain to be elucidated. It is noteworthy that some of these tumors may influence ovarian function by producing gonadotropins. In the following discussion, emphasis will be placed on tumors that secrete androgens, estrogens, or, rarely, gonadotropins that stimulate steroid hormone secretion by the nontumorous portion of the ovaries. Attention is called to these tumors by signs and symptoms of estrogens and androgens produced either in excess or at such inappropriate times as prepubertally or postmenopausally.

In addition to gonadotropins, some ovarian tumors secrete other substances, such as serotonin and thyroxine, which are not usually regarded as secretory products of normal ovarian tissue, so that such tumors may be included among those associated with so-called "ectopic hormone production" (Ch. 30). Primary ovarian tumors that produce hormones and their important clinical features are listed in Table 7–5.

Tumors Producing Estrogens

Granulosa-Theca Cell Tumors

The most common functioning ovarian neoplasms are variously referred to as "granulosa-theca cell tumors," or, alternatively, as "feminizing mesenchymomas." These tumors collectively account for 15–20% of all solid ovarian neoplasms. Microscopically, these are composed of cells morphologically similar to granulosa and theca cells of

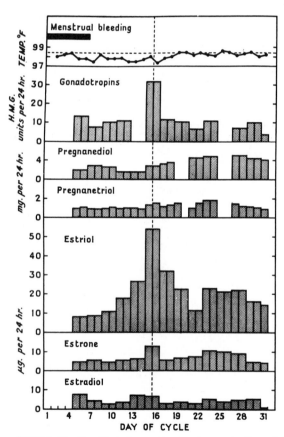

Figure 7–19. Basal body temperatures and concentrations of urinary gonadotropins, estrone, estradiol, estriol, pregnanediol, and pregnanetriol in urine specimens collected during a typical ovulatory cycle from a normal woman. (From Loraine, J. A., and Bell, E. T.: *Lancet* 1:1340, 1963.)

TABLE 7–5. CLINICAL FEATURES OF HORMONE-PRODUCING OVARIAN TUMORS

Tumor	Hormones Produced*	Incidence				Size Range in cm. (Per Cent Palpable)	Miscellaneous
		Age in Years		Malig-nancy	Bilater-ality		
		Peak	Range				
Arrhenoblastoma	Androgens, Estrogens	20–40	4–69	20%	rare	<5–>25 (85)	Most common viriliz-ing ovarian neo-plasm
Dysgerminoma	Androgens, Chorionic gonadotropin	10–30	6–76	100%	15%	3–50 (60)	
Gonadoblastoma	Androgens Estrogens	10–30	6–38	50%	40%	<1–>30 (?)	Usually occur in ge-netic males with fe-male external gentalia
Granulosa-Theca cell	Estrogens Androgens Progestogens	30–70	<1–92	5–20%	10–15%	<1–>30 (80–90)	Most common func-tioning ovarian neoplasm
Lipoid cell (Hilar cell type)	Androgens Estrogens	45–75	4–86	rare	rare	1–9 (50)	Hypertension in 50% Diabetes in 50%
Lipoid cell (adrenal-like)	Androgens Estrogens	20–50	6–78	20%	rare	0.5–30	Diabetes associated with lesion in 50%
Teratomas, benign cystic	Serotonin Thyroxine	10–40	<1–78	rare	10%	2–45 (90)	
Teratomas, malignant	Chorionic gonadotropin	6–15	6–42	100%	rare	>5 (100)	

*When more than one hormone is secreted, the major one is underlined.

normal follicles, sometimes arranged in folliculoid patterns and containing Call-Exner bodies. Care-ful microscopic examination of multiple sections reveals that these are rarely composed exclusively of either granulosa cells or theca cells, so that at-tempts to classify them separately have not seemed useful. Tumors consisting of theca cells only are called "thecomas" and are not discussed separately here.

Diddle (1952) collected a series of 926 putative granulosa cell tumors and 263 putative theca cell tumors from the literature. He found no thecomas in patients known to be premenarchal, but 6% of the granulosa cell tumors occurred in children 10 years of age or younger. However, in a review of the world literature on ovarian tumors associated with sexual precocity in girls 9 years of age or less, Serment et al. (1970) found 9 patients with the-comas.

Bleeding, manifest either as polymenorrhea or as irregular bleeding alternating with periods of amenorrhea, was the commonest presenting sign or symptom in all age groups in Diddle's study. Although these tumors are commonly thought of as producing signs and symptoms of estrogen excess, signs of virilism, including hirsutism, clitoromegaly, and increased libido, are found, particularly when the tumor is cystic and con-tains scattered foci of luteinized stromal cells. It should be noted that 80% or more of these tumors are palpable on bimanual abdominopelvic examination, so that signs of precocious puberty in children, menstrual irregularities in women during the reproductive years, and genital bleed-ing in postmenopausal women when associated with a palpable ovarian mass, should suggest the diagnosis of a granulosa-theca cell tumor prior to confirmatory laparotomy.

Miscellaneous Tumors Producing Estrogens

In addition to the granulosa-theca cell tumors, estrogen production has been attributed to lipoid cell ovarian neoplasms, which ordinarily secrete androgens (see below). Since these latter tumors are less frequently palpable, and since about 15% of granulosa-theca cell tumors are less than 6 cm. in diameter, failure to palpate an en-larged ovary does not eliminate the possibility of an ovarian tumor as the source of inappropriate estrogen secretion.

Tumors Producing Androgens

Secretion of androgens by ovarian neoplasms results in virilizing syndromes manifest by hetero-sexual pseudopuberty in prepubertal girls, and by hirsutism with or without other signs of virilism in premenopausal and postmenopausal women. Clinical characteristics of tumors that usually produce androgens are shown in Table 7–5. These include arrhenoblastomas, dysgerminomas, gonadoblastomas, lipoid cell tumors and adrenal-like and hilar cell tumors.

Arrhenoblastomas

Although arrhenoblastomas are the most common among the ovarian tumors secreting androgens, they occur rarely, accounting for less than 1% of the solid ovarian tumors. While arrhenoblastomas have been found in all age groups, about 70% occur in women less than 40 years of age. About 85% of arrhenoblastomas are large enough to be palpated on abdominopelvic examination – a percentage higher than that for any other ovarian neoplasm associated with virilism. Pedowitz and O'Brien (1960) found amenorrhea to be the commonest abnormality, occurring in 70% of 240 women with arrhenoblastomas. Hirsutism, present in 75% of cases, was associated with more advanced evidences of virilism, such as clitoromegaly and deepening of the voice in 50%. The insidious progression of changes was an impressive feature of the illness, with an average duration of more than one year prior to diagnosis. The virilizing effects have been shown to be related to production and secretion of testosterone by the tumors. Concentrations of testosterone have been elevated uniformly in urine and blood from women with virilizing neoplasms. Production of a few milligrams per day of testosterone is sufficient to virilize, but metabolism of this hormone gives rise to only very minimal amounts of androsterone and etiocholanolone, the principal urinary 17-ketosteroids (17-KS). It is not surprising that urinary 17-KS excretion has been found to be elevated in less than half the women with arrhenoblastomas with reported results.

Gonadoblastomas (Scully, 1970)

Among tumors secreting androgens, gonadoblastomas are unique in that these characteristically occur in genetic males with female external genitalia (male pseudohermaphrodites). In 40% of cases, the gonads were either undifferentiated streaks or intraabdominal testes, with approximately equal frequencies, but the nature of the gonad containing the tumor was indeterminate in 60% of cases. Rarely has a gonadoblastoma been identified in the ovary of a parous woman. About 40% of gonadoblastomas are bilateral – another unique feature. Appearance of virilizing signs in a phenotypic female with chromatin-negative nuclear sex should suggest the diagnosis.

Lipoid Cell Tumors

The term "lipoid cell tumor" has been used by Morris and Scully (1958) as a generic term to describe rare virilizing ovarian tumors of two kinds. The most commonly applied synonyms for the first of the two kinds are adrenal rest tumors or adrenal-like tumors, but the terms masculinovoblastoma, luteoma, hypernephroma, and androblastoma diffusum have also been used. Tumors of the second kind have been called hilar cell tumors and Leydig cell tumors. The variety of names is explained in part by the fact that tumors of the first group consist of cells reminiscent of adrenal cortical cells, luteinized ovarian stromal cells, or clear cells in hypernephromas, while those of the second group resemble hilar cells or Leydig cells.

The cells giving rise to these tumors have not been conclusively identified, and discussion of the controversy is not relevant here. However, for the clinician's purposes, there may be some virtue in maintaining the distinction between hilar cell and adrenal-like tumors for the following reasons:

1. The ages at maximum incidence of the two types of tumors are distinctly different, hilar cell tumors being more common among women over 50, while adrenal-like tumors are more common among women under 50.

2. The adrenal-like tumors more often tend to be malignant.

3. Urinary 17-KS excretion has been reported to be increased more often in patients with adrenal-like tumors.

4. Adrenal-like tumors are more often palpable.

Hughesden (1966) has critically evaluated the relevant literature and concluded that evidence of adrenal rests within the substance of the ovary is not convincing. He interpreted observations in serial sections of three lipoid cell tumors to indicate that the origins of these tumors lay in ovarian stromal cells "in a field of stromal hyperplasia" – juxtahilar in the case of hilar cell tumors.

Lipsett et al. (1970) critically evaluated the clinical and chemical evidence for the origin of lipoid cell tumors from adrenal rests. They pointed out that obesity, facial rounding, hypertension, acne, hirsutism, diabetes, and elevated urinary 17-KS, present in varying combinations in patients with both types of lipoid cell tumors, were inadequate to support a diagnosis of Cushing's syndrome. They pointed out that neither elevated plasma cortisol nor increased urinary free cortisol excretion had ever been reported for patients with lipoid cell tumors. Considering all the chemical evidence, they drew attention to the fact there was no firm evidence for the presence of 11- and 21-hydroxylating enzyme activities in lipoid cell tumors, and furthermore that there was no convincing evidence of lipoid cell tumor responsiveness to ACTH. Lastly, they noted that stimulation of steroidogenesis observed after administration of hCG to some patients with these tumors was consistent with an ovarian stromal cell origin. On the basis of all these facts, they rejected an adrenocortical cell origin of lipoid cell tumors.

Hypertension and either diabetic glucose tolerance curves or overt diabetes mellitus are found in about 50% of patients with lipoid cell tumors. Among patients with tumors categorized as adrenal-like, urinary 17-KS excretion is commonly elevated, more frequently than among patients with either arrhenoblastomas or hilar cell tumors. Both hilar cell tumors and adrenal-like tumors are less likely to be palpable than are arrhenoblastomas. Although both types of lipoid cell tumors have been reported in a wide range of patients, 50 hilar cell tumors (54%) found by Dunnihoo et al. (1966) were in women aged 50 or older, whereas only 58 adrenal-like tumors (20%) found by Pedowitz and Pomerance (1962) occurred in women over 50.

Miscellaneous Tumors Associated with Virilism

Signs and symptoms of virilism have been found to be associated with some dysgerminomas, occasionally with Brenner tumors, with some cystic granulosa-theca cell tumors, and with some tumors metastatic to ovary from primary sites in breast, stomach, and colon (Krukenberg's tumors). When any of these tumors are associated with virilizing syndromes, foci of luteinized cells, variable in extent, are observed in the stroma of the ovary bearing the tumor. While the basis for this change is unknown, recent observations that some gastrointestinal tumors secrete hCG provide a pathophysiologic basis for the stromal changes accompanying these tumors.

Tumors Producing Nonsteroidal Hormones

Tumors Producing Chorionic Gonadotropins

Occasionally a dysgerminoma and, more rarely, a malignant ovarian teratoma secrete a gonadotropin immunologically and biologically similar to hCG, produced by normal trophoblastic tissue. For the most part these have occurred in girls under 20 years of age (see below), but this type of tumor has occurred later.

Tumors Producing Serotonin and Thyroxine

Other teratoid tumors, the benign cystic teratomas or dermoids, have occasionally contained foci of chromaffin tissue producing serotonin, or consisted almost exclusively of thyroid tissue (struma ovarii) sufficiently differentiated to produce thyroxine. Production of serotonin has been sufficient to result in all the clinical manifestations of the carcinoid syndrome, including right heart failure. Evidence for thyrotoxicosis due to functioning of thyroid tissue in struma ovarii was found to be rare by Smith (1948) in his review of the literature. More recently Marcus and Marcus (1961), after reviewing the world literature, concluded that a diagnosis of thyrotoxicosis due to struma ovarii has been adequately established no more than 10 times.

Syndromes of Ovarian Dysfunction

In Infancy and Childhood

Two extremes of pubescence—precocious initiation and delayed achievement—provide the framework for discussion of syndromes of pathophysiologic ovarian function in infancy and childhood. It should be noted that these syndromes are encountered rarely outside of referral centers specializing in diagnosis and treatment of endocrine disorders in children. Nonetheless, when such problems arise, some understanding of their implications provides a basis for rational management by the physician who first sees the patient.

Precocious Puberty and Pseudopuberty

Introduction. Puberty is defined as the state of physical development when sexual reproduction first becomes possible, and in primate females, this is marked by the menarche. Normally, the acquisition of reproductive capability occurs *pari passu,* with development of estrogen-dependent secondary sexual characteristics, including maturation of the breasts, development of pubic and axillary hair, and accelerated linear skeletal growth. Pathophysiologically, however, development of secondary sexual characteristics may occur without concomitant maturation of the gametogenic function of the ovaries.

In either case, development of estrogen-dependent secondary sexual characteristics in girls under 9 years implies an aberration in mechanisms regulating sex steroid hormone secretion (Ch. 26). If the abnormality results from premature activation of cyclic hypothalamic-pituitary function, sex steroid hormone secretion is accompanied by follicular maturation and ovulation, and these processes appear to be regulated in a manner identical to that occurring in women during their reproductive years. Indeed, among such children ovulation with or without pregnancy has been demonstrated repeatedly, so that the syndromes are described appropriately as *precocious puberty,* or sometimes as *true precocious puberty.* In contrast, when the aberration consists in secretion of sex steroid hormones in the absence of pituitary gonadotropic stimulation and without ovulation, the syndrome should be referred to as *precocious pseudopuberty,* sometimes called *pseudoprecocious puberty,* since reproductive capability has not been attained. Though both are rare, precocious puberty is seen 5–6 times more frequently than precocious pseudopuberty.

Making the distinction between precocious puberty and precocious pseudopuberty is important clinically for two reasons, both of which relate to treatment. Firstly, while the cause of precocious puberty remains unknown in most instances, it is not regarded as primarily ovarian in origin, whereas primary ovarian abnormality is the basis for disease in most children with precocious pseudopuberty, with adrenal disease accounting for the remainder. Thus, making the distinction helps to establish the locus of disease. Secondly, the clinical course and consequences of the two processes differ. The clinical course is benign in most children with precocious puberty, but in about 10% of them, premature activation of cyclic hypothalamic-pituitary function can be shown to be associated with potentially life-threatening intracerebral diseases, including neoplasms. In contrast to the usually benign course of precocious puberty, precocious pseudopuberty is more frequently symptomatic of potentially life-threatening diseases, which may be curable if recognized early and treated appropriately. Failure to make the distinction between puberty and pseudopuberty may, then, result in delay of treatment, with important implications for survival of patients with pseudopuberty.

Making the distinction between puberty and pseudopuberty is complicated by the fact that the clinical signs of the two entities are similar in the absence of ovulation, which may not occur until late in the course of precocious puberty. Not uncommonly, screening diagnostic procedures fail to provide a definitive basis for making this distinction, so that the physician must decide whether to temporize or to pursue more complex diagnostic procedures; with either course, intrinsic morbidity and cost are significant. When the probability of a life-threatening disorder can be minimized simply, expectant waiting is justified and unlikely to increase morbidity significantly or to affect prognosis adversely.

Syndromes of Precocious Puberty. Syndromes of precocious puberty, both idiopathic and secondary to disease of the CNS, have been discussed in Chapter 12. Pseudopubertal variants, premature thelarche, and premature adrenarche have been discussed in Chapter 26. Some salient features, useful in differential diagnosis, are summarized in Table 7-6.

Syndromes of Precocious Pseudopuberty. When secondary sexual characteristics develop prematurely in the absence of maturation of the gametogenic function of the ovary, the syndrome is called *precocious pseudopuberty*. If secondary sexual changes seen in precocious pseudopuberty are consistent with those expected on the basis of the genetic sex of the child, the syndrome is referred to as *isosexual precocious pseudopuberty*. On the other hand, when virilizing signs characteristic of pubescent genetic males occur in girls, the syndrome is called *heterosexual precocious pseudopuberty*. Accelerated linear growth, breast development, appearance of pubic and axillary hair, genital maturation, and periodic vaginal bleeding, appearing in the same sequence as in normal puberty, have been observed in girls with isosexual precocious pseudopuberty. These changes may also occur in girls with heterosexual precocious pseudopuberty, but in addition, virilizing signs, such as acne, hirsutism, and clitoromegaly, may occur in children whose disease results from ovarian or adrenal neoplasms producing a combination of androgens and estrogens.

Precocious Pseudopuberty Due to Adrenal and Ovarian Disease. Adrenal tumors producing estrogens and androgens in children before the age of expected puberty are rare. Diagnostic procedures are discussed in detail in Chapter 5.

Primary ovarian lesions, including neoplasms and non-neoplastic cysts, though rare, are more commonly encountered than are adrenal neoplasms among children with isosexual and heterosexual precocious pseudopuberty. Granulosa cell tumors producing signs and symptoms of isosexual pseudopuberty account for about 60% of cases. The remainder are distributed approximately equally among arrhenoblastomas, lipoid cell tumors, chorioepitheliomas, and benign ovarian cysts.

In a recent comprehensive review of precocious pseudopuberty of ovarian origin, Serment et al. (1970) summarized findings in 234 cases of precocious pseudopuberty occurring in girls under 9 years of age. Among 148 patients with isosexual pseudopuberty secondary to granulosa cell tumors of the ovary for whom satisfactory data were available, enlargement of the breasts occurred in 138, pubic hair appeared in 131, and genital bleeding was noted in 120.

In 18 instances of arrhenoblastomas, Sertoli cell tumors, and lipoid cell tumors occurring in girls under 9 years old, breast enlargement was observed in 10, 8 of whom also had vaginal bleeding. Hirsutism and clitoromegaly were observed in about half of these girls.

For reasons that are not apparent, ectopic secretion of hCG by hepatoblastomas, which results in pseudopuberty in boys, has never been recognized in girls. In girls, then, pseudopuberty secondary to tumors producing hCG is limited to primary ovarian choriocarcinomas which, though rare, usually occur in children and young adolescents (Table 7-5). These tumors progress rapidly to a fatal issue, usually less than a year after onset of symptoms that lead to diagnosis. It is not surprising, therefore, that signs and symptoms of pseudopuberty frequently do not progress beyond minimal breast enlargement or the appearance of small amounts of pubic hair. While spotty bleeding has been observed, copious vaginal bleeding is unusual.

Benign ovarian cysts occur commonly in the ovaries of pre- and peripubertal girls. When these are of sufficient size to enlarge the ovary of a child with signs of precocious puberty, surgical exploration is required to distinguish a benign cyst from a malignant ovarian tumor. In a limited number of patients in whom a nonneoplastic cyst has been encountered at laparotomy, excision of the cyst has resulted in regression of secondary sexual characteristics until pubescence occurred at a normal age. More commonly, excision of these cysts has

TABLE 7–6. PHYSICAL FINDINGS AMONG PATIENTS WITH VARIOUS SYNDROMES OF PRECOCIOUS PUBERTY AND PSEUDOPUBERTY

Findings	Premature Thelarche	Premature Adrenarche	Precocious Puberty						Precocious Pseudopuberty					
									Isosexual			Heterosexual		
			Idiopathic	Central Nervous System Tumor	McCune-Albright Syndrome	Hypothyroid			Ovarian Tumors	Adrenal Tumors	Factitious	Ovarian Tumors	Adrenal Tumors	Adrenal Hyperplasia
Breast enlargement	Yes	No	Yes	Yes	Yes	Yes			Yes	Yes	Yes	Yes	Yes	Yes
Pubic hair	No	Yes	Yes	Yes	Yes	Unusual			Yes	Yes	Yes	Yes	Yes	Yes
Vaginal bleeding	No	No	Yes	Yes	Yes	Yes			Yes	Yes	Yes	Yes	Yes	Yes
Virilizing signs	No	No	No	No	No	No			No	Yes	No	Yes	Yes	Yes
Bone age	Normal	Normal to Minimally Advanced	Advanced	Advanced	Advanced	Normal or Retarded			Advanced	Advanced	Advanced	Advanced	Advanced	Advanced
Neurologic deficit	No	No	No	Yes	Yes	No			No	No	No	No	No	No
Abdomino-pelvic mass	No	No	Occ'l	No	No	Occ'l			Usually	No	No	Occ'l	No	No

failed to alter the course of pubertal change among girls with idiopathic precocious puberty. The virtue of the exploration, then, derives from eliminating the possibility that a resectable ovarian neoplasm underlies the precocious pseudopuberty rather than from the likelihood of altering the clinical course of pubertal changes.

There is a paucity of information about preoperative laboratory studies in children with precocious pseudopuberty due to ovarian tumors. Consequently, the usefulness of such studies in differentiating pseudopuberty from puberty remains to be established.

Urinary estrogen has been measured in 23 children with precocious pseudopuberty secondary to granulosa cell tumors. In 15 instances, values were equal to, or less than, those seen in sexually mature women during their reproductive years, while in eight, levels were markedly elevated to 60–720 μg./24 hr. In 22 of 24 patients studied, vaginal smears showed evidence of estrogenic effects. In all instances, urinary estrogen excretion ultimately declined after ablation of the tumor.

Urinary 17-KS excretion is not invariably elevated in girls with precocious pseudopuberty secondary to arrhenoblastomas and lipoid cell tumors of the ovary. In contrast, when heterosexual precocious pseudopuberty results from an adrenal tumor or from congenital adrenal hyperplasia, urinary 17-KS excretion has been found to be elevated in virtually 100% of cases. Thus normal 17-KS excretion suggests an ovarian tumor, but elevated values do not differentiate between ovarian and adrenal tumors in a child with heterosexual pseudopuberty. While determinations of plasma and urinary testosterone have been reported only rarely in children with such tumors, it is reasonable to suppose that values will be found to be elevated as they are in sexually mature women with similar tumors.

In view of the well-established negative feedback of estrogens on pituitary gonadotropin excretion in sexually mature women, it might be supposed that measurements of gonadotropins in urine or blood would be useful in distinguishing precocious pseudopuberty from precocious puberty in children. However, urinary gonadotropin excretion, usually the result of a single determination by bioassay, has been reported for very few children with granulosa cell tumors producing estrogen. In 13 of 14 patients in one series, values were 3–10 mouse uterine units/24 hr., while a value of 40 mouse uterine units was reported for a single patient, so that these determinations did not distinguish children with precocious pseudopuberty from those with precocious puberty. Urinary gonadotropin excretion in children with virilizing ovarian tumors has been studied too rarely to merit discussion. Urinary gonadotropins have been invariably markedly elevated in only one syndrome of precocious pseudopuberty—the syndrome secondary to ovarian tumors secreting chorionic gonadotropin.

Measurements of immunoreactive gonadotropins in a limited number of serum and urine specimens from girls with precocious pseudopuberty have not provided information useful in distinguishing these children from children with precocious puberty or from normal children.

Factitious Precocious Pseudopuberty. Very rarely, inadvertent ingestion of or topical application of estrogens has been reported to induce breast enlargement, appearance of pubic hair, and onset of vaginal bleeding in girls less than 8 years old. Sources of exogenous estrogens include foods, drugs, and cosmetics. Examples include ingestion of the hormone by a child playing with a jar of cleansing cream containing estrogen, topical application of creams marketed for control of "diaper rash," and use of vitamin preparations and a variety of other drugs contaminated with estrogen during manufacture. Identification of these sources of estrogens depends upon a carefully taken history, followed by either chemical or biologic detection of hormone in the suspected source. Laboratory studies reported have been too limited to be meaningful.

Clinical Evaluation of the Patient with Signs of Precocious Puberty and Pseudopuberty. Some of the diagnostic features of the syndromes of precocious puberty and pseudopuberty that can be determined by history and physical examination are summarized in Table 7–6. A scheme for further evaluation based upon findings at genital examination is shown in Figure 7–20. The objective of the scheme is to distinguish between pseudopuberty and puberty, and this distinction is based primarily on the presence or absence of virilizing signs and the presence or absence of an adnexal mass.

The History. A carefully taken history may provide diagnostically useful information. Firstly, one should inquire about possible inadvertent ingestion or topical application of estrogens. Mothers should be questioned carefully about medications taken and cosmetics, creams, and powders used for the child or by women with whom the child has repeated and frequent contact, including older siblings, maids, aunts, and grandmothers. It may be helpful to have the mother produce cosmetic containers, since laws in most countries require labeling of preparations containing hormones.

Secondly, mothers should be questioned carefully about behavioral changes or psychomotor equivalents of seizures. Evidence obtained in this way has led in our experience to identification of an intracerebral neoplasm underlying true precocious puberty.

Thirdly, when medical advice is sought late in the course of precocious puberty, careful dating of events may be helpful. Some authorities express the opinion that progression of changes from earliest evidence of breast maturation to onset of vaginal bleeding is more rapid when a tumor, secreting steroid hormones, is the basis of the process, but no firm data have been published to support this impression. If breast enlargement or appearance of pubic hair is to be followed by menarche, the rate of progression is similar to that

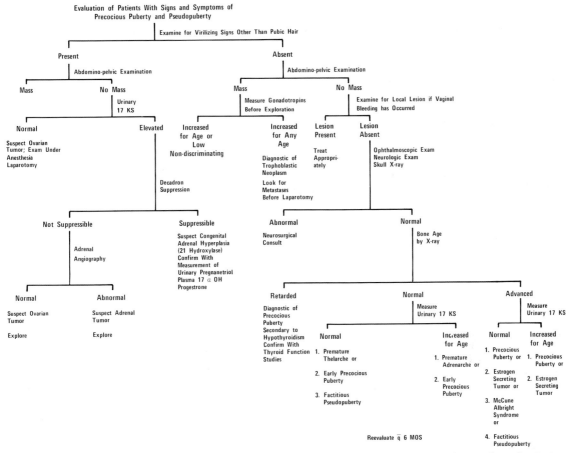

Figure 7–20. Outline for diagnostic evaluation of patients with signs and symptoms of precocious puberty and pseudopuberty.

seen in physiologic pubescence (see Tables 7–1 and 7–2). On the other hand, if the process represents premature thelarche or premature adrenarche, advancement will be delayed and menarche will occur at the expected age.

When vaginal bleeding occurs, a history of cyclicity suggests that the process may be under hypothalamic-pituitary control, leading to a diagnosis of precocious puberty. However, this is not definitive, since periodic genital bleeding has been observed in patients with pseudopuberty secondary to ovarian and adrenal neoplasms secreting sex steroid hormones.

The Extragenital Physical Examination. (a) The skin should be carefully inspected for café-au-lait spots. These lesions have been seen in instances of precocious puberty associated with phakomatosis and with the McCune-Albright syndrome. Cutaneous manifestations of hypothyroidism are suggestive of the syndrome of precocious puberty secondary to hypothyroidism. Excessive facial hirsutism and facial acne are suggestive of heterosexual precocious pseudopuberty. (b) Facial asymmetry or skeletal deformity are pathognomonic of the McCune-Albright syndrome. (c) Neurologic deficits are seen in precocious puberty due to disease of the CNS and may be seen in the

McCune-Albright syndrome as well. In the latter, these are more commonly cranial nerve deficits, thought to be secondary to sclerotic changes in the base of the skull.

The Genital Examination and Further Studies. Attention is directed to Figure 7–20. A careful search for evidence of virilization is an important part of the physical examination of children in whom appearance of pubic hair is the first sign of precocious puberty or pseudopuberty. One should look for acne, extragenital hirsutism, and clitoromegaly in these instances.

When virilizing signs are present, failure to palpate a pelvic or an abdominal mass after a satisfactory abdominorectal examination, under sedation or anesthesia if necessary, makes an ovarian source of the virilization an unlikely possibility, although rarely such tumors do not become palpable until late in the course of the disease. When no mass is palpated, urinary 17-KS excretion should be measured. If quantities are found to be normal in a 24-hour urine collection, an ovarian source of androgen is probable, even in the absence of a palpable mass, and abdominal exploration should be undertaken. In contrast, if urinary 17-KS excretion is elevated, a dexamethasone suppression test (Ch. 5) should be performed. If urinary 17-KS excretion is not suppressible, adrenal angiography, accompanied by measurement of dehydroepiandrosterone in adrenal venous effluent, may lead to a preoperative diagnosis of a unilateral adrenal neoplasm and obviate the need to explore both adrenals. If neither angiography nor adrenal venous hormonal concentration is abnormal, an ovarian tumor too small to be palpated should be suspected and sought at laparotomy. When elevated urinary 17-KS excretion is suppressible with dexamethasone, a diagnosis of congenital adrenal hyperplasia due to a 21-hydroxylase deficiency should be suspected. The finding of increases in either plasma 17-hydroxyprogesterone or its urinary metabolite, pregnanetriol, provides confirmatory evidence for the diagnosis.

When virilizing signs are absent in a girl under study for signs and symptoms of precocious puberty and pseudopuberty, an ovarian cause for the disease is rendered improbable but not excluded by failure to palpate an adnexal mass. On the other hand, palpating an adnexal mass does not establish an ovarian etiology of the disorder. When a mass is palpated, abdominal exploration is indicated, but results of measurements of gonadotropins in serum or urine should be obtained preoperatively. When gonadotropins are in excess of those attributable to pituitary secretion, a trophoblastic neoplasm should be suspected and appropriate studies for metastatic spread initiated before laparotomy. Gonadotropin levels that are minimally elevated, normal, or low for age provide no other discriminating diagnostic information, so that a functioning ovarian neoplasm should be suspected and the nature of the mass determined by laparotomy.

When vaginal bleeding has been observed in the absence of an ovarian or adrenal mass and in the absence of other signs and symptoms of precocious puberty or pseudopuberty, local lesions resulting in vaginal bleeding should be sought. These include vaginal infections, foreign bodies, and tumors. When no local lesion is found, ophthalmoscopic examination and neurologic examination and x-ray examination of the skull should be performed. When these are abnormal, further evaluation should be made under the supervision and direction of a neurosurgeon.

When no abnormalities are found by either skull x-ray or funduscopic or neurologic examination, x-ray determination of bone age will provide a useful basis for proceeding with further studies. If bone age is retarded, precocious puberty secondary to hypothyroidism should be suspected and confirmed by appropriate studies of thyroid function (Ch. 4).

When bone age is found to be normal or advanced for chronologic age, urinary 17-KS excretion should be measured. Among girls with *normal bone age and normal urinary 17-KS excretion*, diagnosis of premature thelarche, early precocious puberty, and factitious pseudopuberty should be considered if breast enlargement is the only sign of precocious maturation of secondary sexual characteristics. The diagnosis of premature thelarche can be eliminated if breast enlargement is accompanied by appearance of pubic hair or vaginal bleeding.

When *bone age is normal but urinary 17-KS excretion is increased for chronologic age*, findings are consistent with premature adrenarche if pubic hair is the sole evidence of precocious puberty. A diagnosis of early precocious puberty should be considered if breast enlargement accompanies the appearance of pubic hair.

When *bone age is advanced but urinary 17-KS excretion is normal or advanced for age*, precocious puberty is the most probable diagnosis. Rarely, factitious pseudopuberty or an ovarian tumor secreting estrogen, but not palpable, could be present. Reexamination at intervals of 3–6 months should make the distinction possible.

Delayed Menarche and Primary Amenorrhea

Introduction. Pathophysiologic ovarian function may manifest itself clinically as delayed development of secondary sexual characteristics and delayed menarche. As noted earlier, the range of ages at menarche extends from 9 to 16 years, normally. When menarche has not occurred by age 16, delayed menarche is an appropriate diagnosis. Since changes in vaginal smears, growth of breasts, and appearance of pubic hair usually precede first menses, the absence of these early signs of puberty at age 16 should suggest a tentative diagnosis of primary amenorrhea, as opposed to delayed menarche. Since primary amenorrhea is an objective manifestation of a pathophysiologic state, the underlying disorder must be identified.

Etiology. In a discussion directed primarily toward ovarian physiology and pathophysiology, the disorder may be considered to be either gonadal (ovarian) or extragonadal (extraovarian) in origin. A reliable estimate of the relative frequencies of these two etiologic groups is difficult to obtain from the literature, since patients described in all large series have been selected for a variety of reasons, not all of which are relevant to incidence. Despite the limitation, figures representing frequencies of occurrence have been derived from analysis of results from reports of more than 500 patients and summarized in Table 7–7.

Gonadal Abnormalities. The etiologic basis for amenorrhea appears to be gonadal in about half of the case reports summarized in Table 7–7. This results either from failure of gonadal differentiation per se, or from failure of the gonad to function appropriately either in fetal or postnatal life, with the result that the external genitalia were either inappropriate for the genetic sex of the patient or failed to mature. Collectively, the syndromes of gonadal dysgenesis and primary gonadal failure in phenotypic females who were genetic males accounted for about 40% of the patients with primary amenorrhea. These syndromes have been discussed in detail in Chapter 8.

Ovaries described as "polycystic" have been reported in about 10% of patients with primary

TABLE 7-7. ETIOLOGIC BASIS FOR PRIMARY AMENORRHEA IN 538 WOMEN

Series	Basis of Referral or Report	Number of Patients	Gonadal					Extragonadal			
			Genetic Males	Gonadal Dysgenesis	Polycystic Ovaries	Misc.	Hypogonado-tropic States	Dysgenesis of Müllerian Ducts	Delayed Menarche	Misc.	Unknown
Lewis	Cytogenetic	75	18	19	2	9	—	14	2	—	11
Shearman	Gynecologic	45	1	18	2	2	10	3	3	5	1
Black and Govan	Laparoscopy and gonadal biopsy	20	2	4	7	4	0	3	0	—	—
Reschini	Measurement of gonadotropins	35	0	16	0	—	11	8	0	—	—
Björo	Gynecologic	60	2	13	23	2	2	18	0	—	—
Jacobs et al.	Cytogenetic	56	2	16	5	1	0	3	19	5	5
Philip	Gynecologic	66	16	26	5	4	7	6	0	—	2
Henzl	Gynecologic	80	5	20	2	12	13	19	0	9	—
Hauser and Kumschick	Gynecologic	101	12	24	—	16	—	22	10	16	1
Total		538	58	156	46	50	43	96	34	35	20
Per Cent		100	11	29	8	9	8	18	6	6	4

TABLE 7–8. ETIOLOGIC BASIS OF PRIMARY AMENORRHEA IN 105 WOMEN LISTED UNDER MISCELLANEOUS OR UNKNOWN CATEGORIES IN TABLE 7–7

| Series | Total Number | Gonadal Number | Extragonadal | | | | Unknown |
			Number	Uterine or Endometrial	Adrenal	Cryptomenorrhea	
Lewis	20	9	–				11
Shearman	8	2	5		3	2	1
Black and Govan	4	4					
Björo	2	2					
Jacobs	11	1	5	4	1		5
Philip	6	4					2
Henzl	21	12	9	6	3		
Hauser and Kumschick	33	16	9	7		2	2
Total	105	50	28	17	7	4	21

amenorrhea. Since multiple cysts are commonly observed in ovaries from pre- and peripubertal girls, the significance of these polycystic ovaries remains unknown. This pathologic finding should not be equated with the Stein-Leventhal syndrome, a diagnosis made much less commonly among patients with primary amenorrhea.

Finally, there is a group of patients with primary amenorrhea in whom the evidence for a gonadal basis of the disorder is manifested by a paradoxical combination of small (hypoplastic) ovaries containing unstimulated follicles with increased gonadotropins in serum or urine. It seems improbable that the pathophysiologic basis of disease is identical for all such patients, and the term "resistant ovary syndrome" seems to be appropriate. Although the etiology of gonadal failure is not known, patients with this condition are included in the miscellaneous group of gonadal disorders in Table 7–8. Thus all gonadal causes together account for about 60% of women with primary amenorrhea.

Extragonadal Abnormalities. In about 40% of cases, the etiologic basis for primary amenorrhea can be shown to be extragonadal. Among the extragonadal causes for primary amenorrhea, aplasia or dysplasia of müllerian ducts is the most common and about twice as common as either hypogonadotropic states or delayed puberty. A miscellaneous group of diseases, including inflammatory disease of the pelvic peritoneum or endometrium, usually tuberculous, adrenal disease (congenital adrenal hyperplasia, most frequently), and cryptomenorrhea due to imperforate hymen account for the remainder of the extragonadal causes of primary amenorrhea (Table 7–8).

Finally, no etiologic basis, either gonadal or extragonadal, was established in about 4% of cases reported in these series.

Clinical Evaluation of the Patient with Primary Amenorrhea

The History. Information obtained from the history may be important in suggesting appropriate diagnostic studies. Among patients with the syndromes of gonadal dysgenesis, the following are useful clues:

(a) *Menstrual history of mother, aunts, sibling sisters:* Chromatin-positive gonadal dysgenesis (pure gonadal dysgenesis) may be familial.

(b) *History of mother's other pregnancies:* incidence of twin pregnancies and early abortions is increased among mothers of patients with chromatin-negative gonadal dysgenesis.

(c) *Patient's perinatal history:* infants with chromatin-negative gonadal dysgenesis frequently have edema of both upper and lower extremities during the neonatal period.

(d) *Age of initiation and rate of advancement in pubertal changes:* age at onset is delayed and rate of progression of changes is slower among patients with gonadal dysgenesis. Failure of appearance of, or failure of significant development of, axillary and pubic hair despite normal breast development is suggestive of testicular feminization. Normal times of appearance and rates of progression in secondary sexual changes are associated with aplasia or dysplasia of müllerian duct derivatives.

The Extragenital Physical Examination. A number of extragonadal features encountered on physical examination are suggestive of the syndromes of gonadal dysgenesis. These are summarized in Table 7–9.

The extent to which extragenital secondary sexual characteristics are developed provides an excellent basis for discriminating between gonadal

TABLE 7–9. EXTRAGENITAL PHYSICAL FEATURES SUGGESTIVE OF GONADAL DYSGENESIS

1. General
   A. Short stature
   B. Shield chest
   C. Widely spaced nipples
   D. Webbed neck
2. Skin
   A. Black freckles
   B. Café-au-lait spots
   C. Cutis laxa
   D. Abnormal dermatoglyphics
3. Musculoskeletal
   A. Short metacarpals or metatarsals
   B. Cubitus valgus
   C. Depressed medial tibial plateaus
   D. Hypoplasia, aplasia of muscles
4. Head and Neck
   A. Drooping eyelids
   B. Double eyelashes
   C. Receding chin
   D. Low-set ears
   E. Low-set hairline
   F. Narrow, high-arched, ogival palate

and extragonadal origins of primary amenorrhea. When the gonad has secreted sufficient sex steroid hormones to stimulate maturation of breasts and development of adult patterns of pubic and axillary hair, a gonadal basis for primary amenorrhea is unlikely. Furthermore, the same evidence is a reasonable basis for assuming that pituitary gonadotropin secretion is normal as well, so that an extragonadal, extrapituitary basis for the amenorrhea should be looked for in these instances. While sexual immaturity is not pathognomonic for gonadal disease, it is highly suggestive of this basis for the amenorrhea.

The genital features of differential diagnostic significance will be considered along with the other diagnostic maneuvers.

The Genital Examination and Further Studies. After the history and extragenital physical examination is completed, an outline for further evaluation of patients with primary amenorrhea is shown in Figure 7–21. Findings on examination of the genitalia serve as the basis for selection of additional tests in this schema. It is designed to be economical in both time and cost, as well as to be an adequate basis for diagnosis and rational therapy.

Among girls under evaluation for primary amenorrhea, external genitalia appear normal but sexually immature. A small number of these persons are observed at birth to have anomalous or ambiguous external genitalia, but they receive no treatment then despite the well-recognized importance of making appropriately timed plastic modifications consonant with the sex of rearing. Failure to appreciate the necessity for such modifications, or more tragically, failure to treat appropriately has been seen repeatedly in our experience. Patients with anomalous external genitalia will be considered separately from those with female external genitalia.

Patients with Female External Genitalia

Without a Vagina

When a vagina is lacking, if the external genitalia are female, particularly when secondary sexual characteristics are well developed, the most probable diagnosis is vaginal aplasia or atresia. For practical purposes, additional studies, such as determination of nuclear sex and measurements of urinary gonadotropins, are useful but not essential for appropriate therapy, including surgical construction of a vagina.

With a Vagina but Without a Cervix

Among patients with a vagina, presence or absence of a cervix is of differential diagnostic significance. In such patients, determination of nuclear sex in smears of buccal or vaginal epithelial cells is the first step in establishing the genetic (chromosomal) sex. Patients with a patent vagina, no cervix (or uterus), chromatin-positive nuclear sex, and

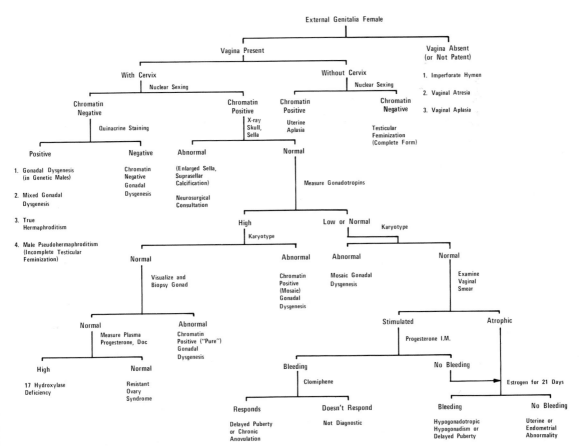

Figure 7–21. Outline for diagnostic evaluation of women with primary amenorrhea and female external genitalia.

normally developed extragenital secondary sexual characteristics are very rarely encountered and represent a variant of the syndrome of vaginal aplasia. In contrast, those with chromatin-negative nuclear sex are most likely genetic males and represent examples of the complete form of the syndrome of testicular feminization. Sparse to absent pubic and axillary hair but well developed breasts are characteristic findings. Occasionally inguinal masses, representing ectopic testes, and inguinal hernias will be found. Additional presumptive evidence for genetic maleness can be obtained by examining smears of peripheral blood stained with quinacrine mustard for a fluorescing chromocenter characteristic of a Y sex chromosome. This finding should be confirmed by study of the karyotype in metaphases from rapidly dividing cells. Excision of the gonadal tissue after puberty is indicated in these cases.

With a Vagina, a Cervix and Chromatin-Negative Nuclear Sex

Determination of the nuclear sex of patients with female external genitalia, a patent vagina, and a cervix provides the basis for ultimate exclusion of another significant population of patients with a diagnosis of primary amenorrhea. When nuclear sex is chromatin-negative, examination of smears of peripheral blood stained with quinacrine mustard should be useful in distinguishing genetic males with 46,XY karyotypes or mosaic variants thereof from persons with 45,X, 46,XXq− or 46,XXp−, or mosaic variants of these karyotypes associated with chromatin-negative nuclear sex. Presence of a Y chromosome is consistent with diagnosis of male pseudohermaphrodism with so-called "incomplete" forms of testicular feminization, and of genetic males with a variety of gonadal abnormalities, including undifferentiated streaks, undescended testes, and ovotestes. These are diagnosed as cases of gonadal dysgenesis, mixed gonadal dysgenesis, or true hermaphrodism, depending upon the gonadal morphology. Further diagnostic studies of these patients should be directed toward inspection, biopsy, and excision of the gonads of genetic males raised as females.

With a Vagina, a Cervix and Chromatin-Positive Nuclear Sex

For the patient with female external genitalia, a patent vagina, a cervix, and chromatin-positive nuclear sex, x-rays of the skull and sella turcica provide clues for a diagnosis of primary amenorrhea due to parapituitary or pituitary tumors. These are potentially life-threatening lesions for which the objective evidence may include delayed puberty and primary amenorrhea. For this group of patients, early neurosurgical consultation should be sought and additional diagnostic and therapeutic decisions based upon the recommendations of these consultants.

When skull x-rays reveal a normal sella turcica, measurements of gonadotropins in multiple specimens of serum or urine, coupled with a determination of the karyotype, should be undertaken. Increased urinary gonadotropin excretion and an abnormal karyotype are characteristic of most patients with chromatin-positive gonadal dysgenesis and mosaic variants of a 46,XX karyotype. Among patients with increased gonadotropin excretion, a normal karyotype in cells from a single tissue does not exclude the possibility of either sex chromosomal mosaicism or of gonadal dysgenesis. Final exclusion of gonadal dysgenesis requires inspection and biopsy of the gonad.

The finding of ovaries containing oocytes in patients with increased urinary gonadotropin excretion suggests a diagnosis of the so-called "resistant ovary syndrome," or more rarely of a congenital deficiency of the steroid 17-hydroxylase enzyme that results in failure of estrogen synthesis. Patients with this enzymatic deficit have markedly elevated plasma progesterone and plasma or urinary deoxycorticosterone concentrations, and some of them are hypertensive as well.

The constellation of female external genitalia, a patent vagina, a cervix, a normal sella turcica, chromatin-positive nuclear sex, and low or normal urinary gonadotropins does not exclude the diagnosis of gonadal dysgenesis. In such patients, the finding of mosaic karyotypes adds circumstantial evidence for a diagnosis of gonadal dysgenesis; but here again, inspection of the gonads is the only test by which the diagnosis can be firmly established. When the constellation includes a normal karyotype, so that after history-taking and physical examination, skull x-rays, measurement of gonadotropins, and determination of karyotype one is left with a sexually immature woman, further diagnostic evaluation is required. This necessitates provocative testing of the hypothalamic-hypophysial-gonadal-genital axis with sex steroid hormones and antagonists of these, coupled with measurements of gonadotropins.

A rational basis for planning these test procedures can be derived from results of an examination of smears of vaginal epithelial cells for evidence of estrogenic stimulation. When the vaginal epithelium has been stimulated by endogenous estrogen, testing should begin with an intramuscular injection of progesterone (50–100 mg.). As pointed out earlier, if vaginal bleeding is observed within a week following injection, it is reasonable to conclude that (1) the pituitary secretes FSH and LH; (2) the ovary has responded to these gonadotropins and secreted sufficient estrogen to stimulate the endometrium; (3) the endometrium responds to both estrogen and progesterone; and (4) the hypothalamic-pituitary unit responds to changes in the sex steroid hormone milieu. When all these are true, the most probable basis for the primary amenorrhea is either delayed puberty or chronic anovulation (sometimes referred to as polycystic ovaries). These diagnostic impressions are strengthened by further testing with clomiphene, an estrogen antagonist which will induce ovulation in about 80% of amenorrheic women who bleed after administration of progesterone. Clomiphene citrate (Clomid) is given in doses of 100 mg./day for 5 days. Response is monitored by indirect indicators of ovulation (see above) and by vaginal bleeding, occurring 20–30 days from the first day of treatment.

Persons with stimulated vaginal epithelium who fail to bleed in response to progesterone and persons with atrophic vaginal epithelium should be given 0.1 mg. of ethinyl estradiol daily for 21 days. Failure to bleed after the estrogen has been discontinued points to an endometrial abnormality. Alternatively, bleeding within a week after stopping the estrogen indicates that the endometrium is responsive to hormonal stimulation and that amenorrhea results from failure of ovarian estrogen production. In these patients, in whom urinary gonadotropin excretion is low or normal despite inadequate ovarian estrogen secretion, the most probable diagnoses are hypogonadotropic hypogonadism and idiopathic delayed puberty. Currently, the distinction between these two alternatives can be made only by the passage of time, unless hyposmia or other cranial nerve deficits characteristic of the syndrome of olfactogenital dysplasia, are present.

Patients with Ambiguous External Genitalia

In those rare instances when a patient with primary amenorrhea is found to have ambiguous external genitalia or female external genitalia with clitoromegaly, initial efforts should be directed toward establishing the nuclear sex of the patient (Fig. 7–22). When nuclear sex is chromatin-negative, smears of peripheral blood cells stained with quinacrine mustard should be examined for chromocenters suggestive of a Y sex chromosome. When evidence consistent with the presence of a Y chromosome is obtained, diagnoses of male pseudohermaphrodism, of mixed gonadal dysgenesis, and of true hermaphrodism should be considered. Distinction among these should be made by inspection and biopsy of gonadal tissue. The rare occurrence of virilism in patients with gonadal dysgenesis should be considered when there is no evidence suggestive of the presence of a Y sex chromosome.

When the nuclear sex of the patient with anomalous external genitalia is chromatin-positive, plasma DHA or urinary 17-KS and plasma testosterone should be measured. When these are elevated, congenital adrenal hyperplasia associated with an adrenal cortical 21-hydroxylase deficiency should be suspected. Increased concentrations of 17-OH progesterone in plasma or of pregnanetriol in urine, suppressible with dexamethasone (Ch. 5), confirm this diagnosis. Other diagnostic possibilities include chronic anovulation with polycystic ovaries and, very rarely, virilizing tumors of adrenal or ovary wherein a palpable adnexal mass may be a useful sign.

When nuclear sex is chromatin-positive and urinary 17-KS excretion and plasma dehydroandrosterone are within normal limits, gonadotropins in serum or urine should be measured. If gonadotropin secretion is increased, virilism associated with chromatin-positive gonadal dysgenesis should be suspected. Similar findings might be encountered among true hermaphrodites. The distinction depends upon inspection and biopsy of the gonads.

When nuclear sex is chromatin-positive, urinary 17-KS are within normal limits, and gonadotropins are not increased in serum or urine, diagnosis of an etiologic basis for primary amenorrhea depends upon inspection and biopsy of the gonads to distinguish chronic anovulation and a virilizing tumor from true hermaphrodism.

Treatment of Primary Amenorrhea. Since primary amenorrhea is a sign of an underlying dis-

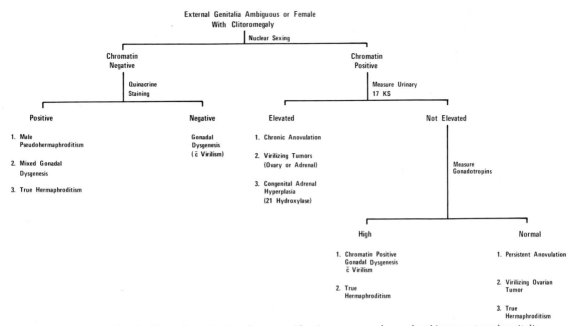

Figure 7–22. Outline for diagnostic evaluation of women with primary amenorrhea and ambiguous external genitalia.

order of the hypothalamic-hypophysial-gonadal-genital axis, rational therapy depends upon correct diagnosis of the pathophysiologic basis for the disorder. For those in whom the ovarian-genital portion of the axis is intact but the disorder is in the hypothalamic and pituitary unit, replacement therapy for maturation of secondary sexual characteristics consists in the use of sex steroid hormones as described in Chapter 8. When pregnancy is desired, ovulation induction with exogenous gonadotropins can be attempted (see below).

When the basis for the disorder is primarily gonadal or genital in origin, surgical correction should be undertaken when feasible, primarily to provide socially acceptable, functional genitals. Optimally, as noted earlier and discussed in Chapter 8, need for these procedures will have been recognized perinatally and their timing planned to conform with development of the peer group in the case of persons born with ambiguous genitalia. For the most part, fertility is an unrealistic goal for the majority of these patients, and the patient should be informed of this deficit as gently as possible.

After the Menarche: Secondary Amenorrhea

Secondary amenorrhea is defined as the absence of menses in a patient who previously has had normal menstrual function, while a patient with primary amenorrhea has never menstruated. To a large extent this distinction is artificial, since many conditions usually associated with primary amenorrhea will occasionally produce secondary amenorrhea. Even in congenital disorders, such as gonadal dysgenesis, the patient initially may have periods and in some cases even ovulate, and amenorrhea starts only after months of cyclic menstrual function. Conversely, a condition such as the polycystic ovary syndrome, which is almost always associated with secondary amenorrhea, may develop early enough to block cyclic ovarian function before the first menstrual bleeding. In fact, the occurrence of primary rather than secondary amenorrhea is often only a quantitative matter, the former occurring when estrogen levels remain below, the latter when estrogen levels exceed, at any one time, the threshold level for endometrial proliferation and subsequent necrosis. Even so, the distinction remains useful since the bulk of the congenital conditions will fall in the category of primary amenorrhea.

A completely consistent etiological classification is not possible at this time, but Table 7–10 illustrates an attempt to develop such a classification of the conditions associated with secondary amenorrhea. In this table we elected not to use the flow sheet approach as was done for primary amenorrhea because, in practice, we have found this approach to be less useful when dealing with secondary amenorrhea.

In discussing the various types of secondary amenorrhea and their causes, it is important to stress that amenorrhea is only the end point in a continuum of conditions that range from apparent normal function to total absence of ovarian func-

---

TABLE 7–10. CLASSIFICATION OF CAUSES OF SECONDARY AMENORRHEA

I. *With Normal Ovarian Function*
  A. Congenital
    1. Cryptomenorrhea
    2. Absence of uterus
  B. Acquired
    1. Intrauterine synechia (Asherman's syndrome)
    2. Hysterectomy
II. *With Decreased Ovarian Secretion of Estrogen, Progestogen or Androgen*
  A. With high gonadotropins (primary ovarian failure)
    1. Congenital
      A. Ovarian agenesis
      B. Gonadal dysgenesis
    2. Acquired
      A. Premature menopause
      B. Surgical oöphorectomy
      C. Radiation castration
      D. Ovarian destruction by infection (rarely)
  B. With low or normal gonadotropins (secondary ovarian failure)
    1. Feminizing ovarian tumor
    2. Hypothalamic-pituitary dysfunction
      A. Congenital deficiency of gonadotropin secretion
      B. Acquired
        I. Organic CNS disease
        II. Functional aberration of hypothalamic-pituitary axis
          Psychogenic
          Nutritional
          Intercurrent disease
          Extragenital endocrine disorders
          Pharmacologic – e.g., with tranquilizers or after prolonged use of antifertility hormones
          Unknown
III. *With Increased Ovarian Androgen Secretion*
  A. Masculinizing ovarian tumor
  B. Continuous estrus syndrome (polycystic ovary syndrome)

tion. In its milder form or in an early stage, the ovarian abnormality which later on will produce amenorrhea may manifest itself only by the presence of infertility while, at least by the usual criteria, the cycle is completely normal. In a more advanced form, the cycle remains ovulatory, but the luteal phase is more or less abnormal. Abnormal luteal function need not produce gross abnormalities in the length of the menstrual cycle. The basal body temperature chart may be normal, and only careful study of the endometrium and of the hormones secreted by the corpus luteum will bring the abnormality to light. As the condition progresses, the patient becomes anovulatory, but the ovary continues to secrete estrogens, occasionally cyclically, and the individual may still have fairly normal cycles. More often, however, there is oligomenorrhea, and, in this stage of ovarian dysfunction, excessive bleeding may alternate with episodes of amenorrhea. As the ovarian disturbance becomes more and more severe, the ovary secretes less and less estrogen until finally estrogen secretion ceases. The patient complains of amenorrhea and progressive symptoms of estrogenic deficiency with, in extreme cases, full atrophy of the vaginal mucosa. The differential diagnosis, shown in Table 7–10, applies to mild as well as to severe forms.

The first step in the diagnosis of secondary amenorrhea lies in a precise functional definition of the condition. The questions to ask and to answer are: (1) do the ovaries make progesterone, i.e., is the patient ovulatory? (2) do the ovaries secrete normal amounts of estrogens? and (3) do they secrete normal amounts of androgens? Approaches to these questions have been outlined in earlier sections of the chapter, and it must be stressed that, in almost all cases, the answer can be obtained easily by a simple evaluation of a few hormonal target organs: the vaginal smear, cervical mucus, endometrial biopsy, and the basal body temperature. Where there is evidence of a decrease in ovarian secretions, the second important step in the diagnosis requires the determination of the plasma gonadotropins. If the gonadotropins are in the menopausal range, one is dealing with primary ovarian failure; when they are low or in the normal pre- or postovulatory range, the patient has secondary ovarian failure. In some instances, a single determination of plasma gonadotropins will allow a distinction between these two categories. In general, repeated tests over a period of time are necessary to provide definitive information. The distinction between primary and secondary ovarian failure is critical, both in terms of etiology and in terms of prognosis and therapy. In primary ovarian failure, the etiology lies in the ovary, the condition is almost always irreversible, and there is little hope of successful therapy. On the other hand, in secondary ovarian failure, where the cause is to be found in the hypothalamic-pituitary axis, spontaneous reversal is frequent and therapy is successful in most cases.

Not included in Table 7–10 are the physiologic causes of secondary amenorrhea. It is important to stress that in patients with secondary amenorrhea the first diagnosis to be considered is pregnancy, and this diagnosis must be weighed until it can be ruled out. Too often in doing this one relies upon pregnancy tests or upon one of the classic signs of early pregnancy, such as uterine enlargement, bluish discoloration of the cervix, or softening of the isthmic part of the uterus — tests which all too often fail to yield a clear-cut answer. In most instances, an unequivocal answer can be obtained without delay by a simple examination of the cervix for mucus, since the presence of cervical mucus is incompatible with pregnancy. Absence of mucus obviously does not mean that the patient is necessarily pregnant, but it may mean that estrogens were absent, or present at a level below the threshold for the production of cervical mucus. This possibility can easily be ruled out by a vaginal smear. Additionally, in the majority of women with secondary amenorrhea, estrogen levels remain sufficiently high to produce significant amounts of cervical mucus. The two other major physiologic causes of secondary amenorrhea, puerperal amenorrhea and normal menopause, can be easily ruled out by history-taking.

With Normal Ovarian Function

Cryptomenorrhea and absence of the uterus have been discussed in connection with primary amenorrhea. In a few women with secondary amenorrhea, ovarian function is normal; although menses have been absent for a prolonged period, the presence of a biphasic temperature chart or of cyclic fluctuations in the secretion of ovarian hormone indicate that the ovaries are functioning normally. In most of these patients, the amenorrhea is due to the presence of intrauterine synechiae or adhesions, resulting in a more or less complete obliteration of the endometrial cavity. The diagnosis is easily made by history-taking and is confirmed by hysterosalpingography or hysteroscopy. It is interesting to note that complete absence of bleeding does not require complete obliteration of the endometrial cavity. In some patients with complete amenorrhea, the adhesions extend only over part of the cavity, and sufficient endometrium is present even to document cyclic changes by repeated endometrial biopsies; nevertheless, significant bleeding does not occur. In most instances, uterine synechiae result from a postabortal or postpartum endometritis. It has been thought by some that too vigorous curettage, with removal of most of the endometrium, causes amenorrhea, but the fact that lysis of the adhesions restores normal menstrual function demonstrates that this is not true. Tuberculous endometritis is another cause for the development of uterine synechiae, but this form of tuberculosis is infrequently seen in the United States of America.

Treatment of uterine synechiae consists of lysis of the adhesions, preferably under direct vision during hysteroscopy. In cases of advanced synechiae, recurrences are frequent, and the prognosis is poor. Figure 7–23, *A* and *B*, illustrates the

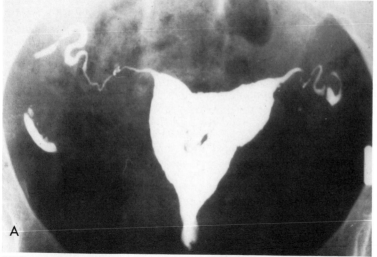

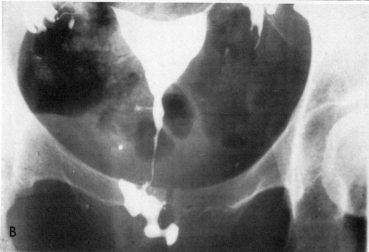

Figure 7–23. Hysterosalpingograms. *A*, Before and *B*, after lysis of synechiae.

radiologic findings before and after treatment of a case of uterine synechiae.

With Decreased Ovarian Secretion of Either Estrogens, Progesterone, or Androgens

With High Gonadotropins (Primary Ovarian Failure). Gonadal dysgenesis, commonly associated with primary amenorrhea, is included in this differential diagnosis, since occasionally this syndrome produces secondary amenorrhea. Gonadal dysgenesis is discussed in detail in Chapter 8.

Of the acquired forms of primary ovarian failure, premature menopause deserves further comment. Cessation of ovarian function due to exhaustion of the supply of oocytes normally occurs at approximately age 48 but can occur at an early age and has been reported in teen-age girls. The diagnosis is based on finding elevated gonadotropins and atrophy of the target organs of the estrogens. Since little is known about the factors controlling the rate of follicular atresia, the etiology of premature ovarian failure remains unknown.

Of great interest are recent studies implicating immunologic mechanisms in the pathogenesis of primary ovarian failure. Using an indirect immunofluorescent staining method, sera from a few women with primary ovarian failure and idiopathic Addison's disease have been shown to contain antibodies which react with cells from corpora lutea and theca interna in mature graafian follicles from human ovaries. These same sera contained antibodies that reacted with steroid hormone producing cells in all three layers of human adrenal cortex, and some but not all of them reacted with interstitial cells in human testis and with human trophoblastic epithelium. Absorption of any of these sera with extracts of human adrenal tissue and absorption of some of them with extracts of testis and placenta resulted in removal of these antibodies. Absorption with other human tissue extracts did not affect the immunoreactivity of any of these sera with adrenal, testis, ovary, or placenta, suggesting that the antibodies were directed toward antigenic determinants common to these steroid hormone-secreting tissues. Lack of uniformity in response to absorption was interpreted to indicate specificity of some sera for antigenic determinants characteristic of individual tissues that secrete steroid hormones.

When sera from many women with ovarian failure not associated with Addison's disease have been tested, antibodies have been found very rarely. It should be noted, however, that ovarian function was not always abnormal in women with Addison's disease whose sera gave positive tests for antibodies reacting with ovarian tissue.

In any event, it seems improbable that ovarian failure will be the sole clinical manifestation of a systemic autoimmune disease. Indeed, antibodies reacting with theca interna of antral follicles were found in only 8 of 16 women with premature menopause, complicating varying combinations of such autoimmune diseases as hypoparathyroidism, hypothyroidism, pernicious anemia, and idiopathic thrombocytopenic purpura. It is noteworthy that 7 of these 8 women also had idiopathic Addison's disease.

Recently several cases of premature menopause have been reported in which ovarian biopsies revealed the presence of morphologically normal oocytes. In some of the patients, treatment with high doses of gonadotropins overcame the relative insensitivity of the follicle and, in fact, induced ovulation.

With Low or Normal Gonadotropins. The signs and symptoms of feminizing ovarian tumors have been discussed earlier in this chapter.

In the vast majority of patients with hypothalamic-pituitary dysfunction, it has been impossible to distinguish between the hypothalamic and the pituitary origin of the amenorrhea. When gonadotropin releasing hormone (GnRH) became available, it was thought that finally it would become feasible to differentiate between pituitary and hypothalamic amenorrheas. The hypothesis was that patients having normal LH release following the administration of GnRH could be assumed to have hypothalamic amenorrhea and vice versa. Unfortunately, the situation does not seem to be that simple. For instance, sufficient evidence is already available to establish that in patients with pituitary tumors the response to GnRH may be perfectly normal. Furthermore, it is becoming increasingly evident that the dose of GnRH is not the only factor determining the release of LH, but that other variables, such as estrogens, modulate the stimulatory effect of GnRH upon LH release. Most recently, radioimmunoassays for GnRH have been developed which are sensitive enough to detect the GnRH in the peripheral circulation. It remains to be shown, however, (and current information makes it unlikely) that there is a correlation between levels of GnRH in the peripheral circulation and its concentration in the hypothalamic-pituitary portal system.

The CNS lesions most frequently associated with secondary amenorrhea are pituitary tumors, granulomas, and postpartum necrosis of the pituitary (Sheehan's syndrome). Galactorrhea is often seen in patients with pituitary tumors, but it is likely that in many cases the galactorrhea is secondary to compression by the expanding tumor upon the hypothalamus. As a result, there is a decrease in the release of the prolactin inhibitory factor (PIF) and a secondary increase of prolactin secretion. The association of galactorrhea and amenorrhea has been given several eponyms. Puerperal galactorrhea and amenorrhea is called the Chiari-Frommel syndrome, whereas nonpuerperal galactorrhea and amenorrhea is dubbed the Ahumada-Del Castillo syndrome when there is no pituitary tumor, and the Forbes-Albright syndrome when there is a tumor present. It is doubtful that these distinctions are worth making, since small, slow-growing pituitary tumors that do not enlarge the sella turcica may escape detection for many years. Lesions of the hypothalamus and intracranial lesions impinging upon the hypothalamus are less frequently the cause of secondary amenorrhea and, in most instances, the neurologic symptoms antedate the amenorrhea or dominate the clinical syndrome. Anosmia is often associated with secondary amenorrhea, but the precise anatomic or functional lesion responsible for this association is unknown.

In the vast majority of cases of secondary amenorrhea with low or normal gonadotropins, no organic disease can be found. Reference has already been made to the small size and slow growth of some pituitary tumors, but it is unlikely that this can account for a significant fraction of the secondary amenorrheas without known etiology. The condition of many patients has been followed over many years, and a number of autopsies performed decades after the onset of the secondary amenorrhea did not reveal an organic lesion to account for the amenorrhea. It is more likely that, in most patients, the cause of amenorrhea lies in a functional disarrangement of the control mechanisms that govern the relationship between the hypothalamic-pituitary axis and the ovary. These mechanisms have been discussed in detail in the section dealing with normal ovarian physiology, and several examples were then given, illustrating how "functional" alterations in the quantitative and temporal relationship between the ovarian and hypothalamic-pituitary signals may disrupt the cycle.

To study the dynamics of this relationship, we have recently constructed a mathematical model of the menstrual cycle. A number of algebraic and differential equations were developed to describe mathematically the morphologic and hormonal variables throughout the menstrual cycle. The model was then tested by computer simulations, and the effects of manipulations of one or more of the variables upon the performance of the other variables were analyzed. For example, we studied the influence of the introduction of small random fluctuations in the levels of FSH, LH, and estrogens. Such random fluctuations could be the result of changes during the day in activity, sleep, stress, and other variables. Surprisingly, these small, short-term variations occasionally produced important long-term changes in the simulated cycles, e.g., appreciable lengthening or shortening of the phases of the cycle and even periods of anovulation in some cases. It is likely that such mechanisms can account for a large number of menstrual abnormalities.

Obviously we know about a number of extragonadal influences that will disturb the normal hypothalamic-pituitary relationships. Psychologic reasons for amenorrhea are known to be quite frequent, but in most cases the diagnosis can only be made by exclusion since there is no characteristic pattern for this type of amenorrhea. The earlier assertion that low levels of LH in the presence of normal levels of FSH are diagnostic for psychogenic amenorrheas is no longer tenable, since this pattern is found in most cases of advanced secondary ovarian failure. The relation between obesity and secondary amenorrhea remains uncertain, but undernutrition is a frequent cause of amenorrhea. One interesting form is the amenorrhea seen in anorexia nervosa, a condition characterized by weight loss and amenorrhea, most frequently occurring in pubertal girls. A recent review of the clinical and biochemical features of anorexia nervosa reveals a very characteristic pattern.

In addition to emaciation and amenorrhea, hallmarks of this syndrome include severe constipation, bradycardia, and hypothermia. Endocrine findings include occasionally a low serum thyroxine level, low plasma LH and FSH, low urinary steroids, but consistently high plasma corticoids with reversal in the circadian rhythm and hyperresponsive ACTH tests. Leukopenia is common and more frequent than anemia. This characteristic combination of symptoms makes it easy to differentiate anorexia nervosa from other types of secondary amenorrhea.

Acute and chronic disease will often produce menstrual disturbances by central mechanisms and interference with the hypothalamic-pituitary axis. Acute infections (including infections of the reproductive tract, such as pelvic inflammatory disease) will rarely produce amenorrhea but in most cases merely postpone ovulation or cause irregular bleeding due to the occurrence of one or more anovulatory cycles. In contrast, chronic diseases, such as tuberculosis or cancer, will occasionally produce amenorrhea.

Diseases of the other endocrine glands, such as the thyroid, adrenal, and pancreas, are frequently the cause of secondary amenorrhea. Usually the symptoms of the primary disease will rapidly lead to the correct diagnosis, and, effective treatment will result in return of normal ovarian function.

Secondary amenorrhea (often associated with galactorrhea) is frequently seen during the administration of high doses of tranquilizers. Finally, there have been many case reports of amenorrhea following discontinuation of contraceptive steroids. There seems to be little doubt about this association, but the frequency with which it occurs is unknown.

With Increased Androgen Production

Masculinizing ovarian tumors that cause virilization and secondary amenorrhea have been discussed in an earlier part of this chapter. The polycystic ovary syndrome probably comprises a number of different syndromes. The symptom complex as reported in the literature is indeed too variable to assume that there is only one nosologic entity. Certain cases, however, have sufficient biochemical and pathologic features in common to constitute a specific clinical syndrome, and we should limit the diagnosis of polycystic ovary syndrome to these. A more appropriate name for the symptom complex would be the constant estrus syndrome, since the hallmark of the condition is anovulation and unopposed estrogen stimulation. The following features appear characteristic. The menstrual picture is variable, ranging from long-term amenorrhea to oligomenorrhea with episodes of menometrorrhagia, but the common denominator is anovulation, which is a *sine qua non* of the diagnosis. In most instances, the menstrual disturbance dates back to puberty. Essential also for the diagnosis is the uninterrupted production of estrogens as evidenced by the continuous formation of copious amounts of cervical mucus and the persistence of a well-developed proliferative endometrium. In a few cases, adenomatous hyperplasia of the endometrium has been reported, and in some of these the lesion had advanced to the point at which the diagnosis of adenocarcinoma *in situ* was warranted. The second cardinal symptom of the syndrome is the evidence of androgen overproduction. Virilization is not often seen, but hirsutism is frequent and appears to be more frequent with increased duration of the disease. In adequately studied cases, there is always biochemical evidence of androgen overproduction, even when clinical hirsutism is not present. Normal 17-KS levels are found, but when a group of patients with polycystic ovaries is compared with a group of normals, the mean level of 17-KS in the polycystic group is higher than that in the controls. Dexamethasone suppression will decrease the 17-KS, but the residual level remains clearly above the level seen in control patients, indicating the ovarian source of the excess 17-KS. Plasma levels of androstenedione, and to a lesser extent of testosterone, are increased, as are production rates of these steroids. In the ovarian veins, androstenedione levels are found to be greatly elevated, but estrogen levels are strikingly low. This finding is especially surprising in view of the above mentioned fact that these patients have continuously abundant cervical mucus and well-developed proliferative endometrium. The paradox has remained unresolved until recent studies determined that most of the circulating estrogens in patients with polycystic ovaries are not derived from ovarian secretions but from the peripheral conversion of androstenedione to estrone. Though the rate of conversion of androgens to estrogens in these patients is normal, the greatly increased production of androstenedione results in an overproduction of estrogens.

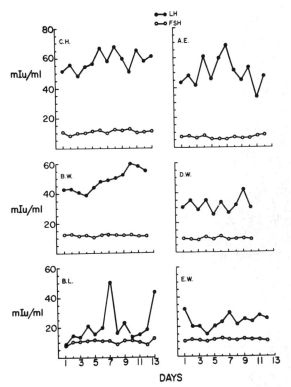

Figure 7-24. Serum LH and FSH levels in individual women with polycystic ovary syndrome. Note the "spiking" pattern of LH levels. (From Yen, S. S. C., et al.: *J. Clin. Endocr. 30*:435, 1970.)

FSH levels appear to be lower than normal, while LH levels are higher and characteristically show frequent peaks of low magnitude (Fig. 7–24).

In many but not all cases, the ovaries are en-larged to several times normal size. In typical cases, the ovary is globular with a thickened glistening capsule, often with characteristic telangiectasia (Fig. 7–25). Beneath the capsule there are many small follicular cysts in various stages of atresia, often with hyperplastic and luteinized thecal cells. Polycystic ovaries have been reported in association with Cushing's syndrome, congenital adrenal hyperplasia, and CNS pathology, but these are exceptions, and in virtually all cases there is no overt pathology outside the ovary. Claims have been made that the increased androgen secretion and the decreased estrogen secretion were due to deficient enzymatic conversion of androstenedione to estrone. Evidence in favor of this hypothesis came from experiments in which ovaries were incubated *in vitro* with various radioactive precursors. However, it was shown later that the conversion of androstenedione to estrone in such experiments was dependent more upon the conditions of the incubations than upon the source of the tissue. Also, the enzymatic hypothesis is incompatible with the fact that normal ovarian function can be restored by wedge resection and that ovulation can be induced by treatment with clomiphene or gonadotropins.

It is more likely that the pathogenesis of the polycystic ovary syndrome is to be found in a derangement of the relationship between the ovarian signal and the response of the hypothalamic-pituitary axis. There is an animal model that has many features in common with the human polycystic ovary syndrome; studies with this model have clarified the pathogenesis of the human syndrome. In rats (in which the hypothalamic-pituitary axis does not mature until several days after birth), the administration of testosterone to the newborn female rat permanently modifies the feedback relationships

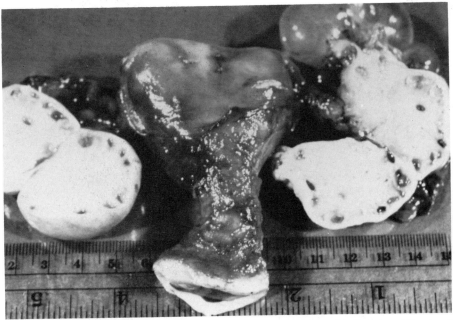

Figure 7-25. Uterus and ovaries removed from patient with polycystic ovaries. Note the glistening white color, the thickened capsule, and the multiple cortical cysts in the bivalved ovaries.

between the hypothalamic-pituitary axis and the ovary. At puberty, an animal so treated will not display cyclic ovarian function, but instead will enter into a state of continuous estrus; the ovaries contain many cystic follicles, and there is biologic evidence that production of estrogen and androgen is increased. The primary lesion lies not in the ovary but in the CNS, since transplantation of the cystic ovaries to an intact host is followed by resumption of normal cyclic function. In addition, the administration of LH induces ovulation as it does in the human female. From these and many other experiments, it has been assumed that in the rat the hypothalamus is undifferentiated at birth. In female rats, no further stimulus is necessary for later cyclic function. In male rats, testicular androgen "masculinizes" the hypothalamus, resulting in constant rather than cyclic secretion of LH. Although the analogy between this experimental model and the polycystic ovary syndrome is striking, caution must be exercised in translating data from the rodent to man, at least until the pathogenesis of the polycystic ovary syndrome is solved.

Treatment of Ovarian Dysfunction

Introduction

In the vast majority of patients with ovarian disturbances, therapy is related to the symptoms rather than to their causes. Such applies to the absence of sexual development in primary amenorrhea, hot flashes and vaginal atrophy of the menopausal patient, hirsutism, anovulation of infertile women, and many other symptoms associated with ovarian disturbances. Therapeutic advances, however, have been very rapid, and there is hardly a symptom of ovarian dysfunction that cannot be corrected by appropriate therapy, the only real exception being anovulation and infertility of the patient with primary ovarian failure.

Cases where therapy can remove the cause of the disturbance and restore cyclic ovarian function are, however, not infrequent. Removal of the cause is possible only among patients in whom the ovarian abnormality is secondary to a disturbance outside the reproductive axis, such as thyroid disease, adrenal disease, psychologic stress, and intercurrent nonendocrine disease. An exception applies to patients with polycystic ovarian disease, in whom wedge resection may restore cyclic function, occasionally for the rest of the patient's reproductive life, but the mechanism by which this occurs is unknown.

In considering therapy, it is essential to treat complaints rather than signs. For example, mere absence of menses is not necessarily a sufficient indication for treatment, and withdrawal bleeding need not be induced unless the amenorrhea is of concern to the patient because of fear of pregnancy or identification of menses as a sign of good health and femininity. Similarly, there is no reason to induce ovulation in an anovulatory patient unless she wants to conceive. Customarily, after finishing the work-up of a patient with ovarian dysfunction, we have a final conference with the patient (and her mother or husband, as appropriate) to discuss in some detail ovarian physiology and the degree to which her own ovarian function differs from the normal. If this is done intelligently, the problem of therapy can then be approached in a logical fashion by asking the patient what symptoms she wants to have corrected and treating only these symptoms. Such an approach very often will result in a final decision that no therapy is necessary and will assure that therapy will be adjusted to the real needs of the patient. In using this approach, it is essential that symptoms about which the patient may not be presently complaining, but which may develop in subsequent years, be discussed fully. As an example, in women whose ovaries are not secreting any estrogens, the problem of chronic calcium loss and the possibility of late development of osteoporosis as well as other metabolic consequences of estrogen deficiency must be discussed.

Varieties of Therapy

Therapy can be divided into two main categories:
1. Therapy of sex steroid hormone deficiency or excess
   - (a) *Substitution therapy:* In this type of therapy, hormones are administered to substitute for the failure of secretion of the gonadal hormones.
   - (b) *Inhibition therapy:* In this category, therapy aims at the inhibition of unwanted ovarian secretion.
2. Therapy of anovulation

Therapy of Sex Steroid Hormone Deficiency or Excess

Substitution Therapy

Estrogens. Although there is a large choice of estrogen preparations, we limit ourselves almost completely to the use of two: ethinyl estradiol (or its methyl ether), and conjugated estrogens (e.g., Premarin). Stilbestrol has the advantage of being much cheaper than the other estrogens, but it is to be avoided because equal doses produce more side effects and cause an unesthetic darkening of the nipples when given for prolonged periods. We do not use injectable and long-acting estrogens unless there is a contraindication for the use of oral preparations. Hormone creams have no place in the armamentarium of the gynecologic endocrinologist, with the possible exception of their topical use in patients with atrophic vaginitis.

In estimating the dose to be administered, it is useful to keep as a yardstick the rule that, in an average patient, 50-100 μg. of ethinyl estradiol, or 2-4 mg. of Premarin administered daily for 1-2 weeks produces well-developed proliferative endometrium and consequently produces withdrawal bleeding, even in the completely estrogen-deficient patient. In many instances (e.g., in castrate and menopausal patients), the dose can and should be maintained below the level that produces withdrawal bleeding. Hot flashes, for instance, can easily be controlled by the administration of 0.625 mg. of conjugated estrogens, a dose well below the threshold for endometrial stimulation. On the other hand, when estrogens are given for their hemostatic effects (e.g., in dysfunctional bleeding), it may be necessary to give much higher doses, and it is generally advantageous to combine estrogen treatment with one of the progestogens. When given for extended periods, they should always be administered in cyclic fashion. It is doubtful whether there is an advantage to administering progestogen together with estrogen as long-term therapy — for example, to produce sexual development in women with primary amenorrhea — although there is some evidence that progestogen may counteract some of the undesirable metabolic side effects of estrogen (e.g., alteration in carbohydrate and lipid metabolism).

Often the gynecologic endocrinologist will be consulted by women concerned about the small size of their breasts. When lack of breast development is due to a deficiency of estrogen secretion, such as in cases of primary or secondary amenorrhea, substitution therapy with estrogen will frequently (but not always) produce gratifying results. In women with normal ovarian function, estrogen therapy will only produce a transitory hypertrophy followed by a rapid regression as soon as the therapy is stopped. Furthermore, the dosage of estrogen required to produce hypertrophy is very high, exposing the patient to serious side effects, such as profuse or prolonged vaginal bleeding. In the very rare case in which there is a valid indication for breast enlargement in women with normal ovarian function, cosmetic surgery should be considered.

The long-term administration of estrogen to postmenopausal women remains controversial. There is a clear-cut indication for such therapy when hot flashes are a problem, when vaginal atrophy interferes with marital function, or in women with a tendency for osteoporosis. However, most of the other claims of the advocates of the "youth forever" approach are at best unconvincing, and there is increasing evidence that the long-term effects of estrogen (e.g., upon lipid metabolism), even in small doses, may be deleterious. A number of women taking estrogens during the perimenopausal period derive great psychological benefits from the knowledge that they are taking estrogen.

The use of estrogen to arrest growth in young girls in an effort to prevent excessive height remains controversial. The data in the literature are difficult to evaluate. The extent of inhibition achieved has to be judged on the basis of projected growth, estimated from standard tables of chronological and bone ages, or even less securely from the height of the mother and other siblings. A number of authors doubt that significant inhibition can be achieved. There is agreement that, if treatment is to be successful, estrogen must be started soon after the earliest signs of puberty, and that high doses (e.g., 10 mg. ± of conjugated estrogens) are necessary. Some authors object to this treatment, because they fear that the high doses of estrogen during this phase of development of the child may have long-term effects on subsequent menstrual function.

Progestogens. Some of the advantages of using progestogens have been mentioned in discussing indications for estrogen therapy. Progesterone, or some other progestogen, is mainly used to produce regular withdrawal bleeding in women with chronic anovulation. In these women, one frequently sees episodes of amenorrhea alternating with episodes of profuse or prolonged bleeding. Such forms of dysfunctional bleeding can easily be prevented by the administration of a progestogen every 4–6 weeks. The induction of withdrawal bleeding with progestogens has often been referred to as "medical curettage." The conditions necessary for progesterone withdrawal bleeding have been discussed above. To produce withdrawal bleeding, we administer 100 mg. of progesterone in oil, but one of the oral progestational agents may be used and is preferable in chronic conditions.

Androgens. There are only a few indications for the use of androgen in women with ovarian dysfunction. Occasionally in women with primary amenorrhea, androgen can be administered to induce linear growth or pubic and axillary hair growth.

In our opinion, androgens have no place in the treatment of dysfunctional bleeding or dysmenorrhea.

Earlier evidence derived from studies in which androgen was given to women with breast cancer clearly shows that large doses of androgen increase libido. It was, however, not clear in these studies whether the effect was due to direct action upon the CNS or to congestion of the external genitalia (more specifically of the clitoris). We are unaware of any "controlled" study in which the effect upon libido of nonvirilizing doses of androgen have been tested in normal women, and this indication for androgen remains controversial. There is no acceptable evidence that androgen is useful in women with fatigue, although claims for such effects have often been made.

Inhibition Therapy

Contraception. By far the most frequent indication for inhibition of ovarian function is contraception. Table 7–11 lists the composition of the oral contraceptives currently in use in the United States. The doses of estrogen and of progestogen now employed are much lower than those used when steroid contraceptives first became popular. The main pressure to reduce the dose of oral contraceptives was generated by a legitimate concern about the serious side effects occasionally described in women taking oral contraceptives. If this concern was and is legitimate, the present disenchantment of a significant fraction of the medical profession with steroid contraception ap-

TABLE 7–11.   ORAL CONTRACEPTIVES (U.S. 1973)*

Agent	Composition Estrogen	Composition Progestogen	Manufacturer	Type
Oracon	Ethinyl estradiol 0.100 mg.	Dimethisterone 25 mg.	Mead-Johnson	Sequential
Ortho-Novum 10	Mestranol 0.060 mg.	Norethindrone 10 mg.	Ortho	Combination
Ortho-Novum 2	Mestranol 0.100 mg.	Norethindrone 2 mg.	Ortho	Combination
Ortho-Novum 1/50	Mestranol 0.050 mg.	Norethindrone 1 mg.	Ortho	Combination
Ortho-Novum 1/80	Mestranol 0.080 mg.	Norethindrone 1 mg.	Ortho	Combination
Ortho-Novum SQ	Mestranol 0.080 mg.	Norethindrone 2 mg.	Ortho	Sequential
Micronor		Norethindrone 0.35 mg.	Ortho	Progestogen only
Norlestrin 2.5	Ethinyl estradiol 0.050 mg.	Norethindrone acetate 2.5 mg.	Parke-Davis	Combination
Norlestrin 1	Ethinyl estradiol 0.050 mg.	Norethindrone acetate 1 mg.	Parke-Davis	Combination
Demulen	Ethinyl estradiol 0.050 mg.	Ethynodiol diacetate 1 mg.	Searle	Combination
Enovid 5	Mestranol 0.075 mg.	Norethynodrel 5 mg.	Searle	Combination
Enovid-E	Mestranol 0.100 mg.	Norethynodrel 2.5 mg.	Searle	Combination
Ovulen	Mestranol 0.100 mg.	Ethynodiol diacetate 1 mg.	Searle	Combination
Norinyl 2	Mestranol 0.100 mg.	Norethindrone 2 mg.	Syntex	Combination
Norinyl 1/50	Mestranol 0.050 mg.	Norethindrone 1 mg.	Syntex	Combination
Norinyl 1/80	Mestranol 0.080 mg.	Norethindrone 1 mg.	Syntex	Combination
Norquen	Mestranol 0.080 mg.	Norethindrone 2 mg.	Syntex	Sequential
NOR-Q.D.		Norethindrone 0.35 mg.	Syntex	Progestogen only
Ovral	Ethinyl estradiol 0.050 mg.	Norgestrel 0.5 mg.	Wyeth	Combination

*Most contraceptive products now on the market belong to the combination type. In this type, estrogens and progestogens are combined and taken for a specified number of days of the cycle (20 or 21 days). In the sequential type of steroid contraception, an estrogen is taken during the first 14 or 16 days of the cycle, while for the subsequent 5 or 6 days, a combination of estrogen and progestogen is taken. In the progestogen-only type of contraceptive regimens, small amounts of a progestogen are taken continuously. The incidence of breakthrough bleeding in the latter type of contraception is much higher than in the combined or sequential types. The pregnancy rate is also much higher and presently is reported as 3 in 100 woman years. Recently, most contraceptive packages contain, in addition to the hormone-containing tablets, seven inert tablets. In this fashion, it is easier for the patient to keep track of her schedule, since she takes one tablet a day without interruption.

pears to be an overreaction, often based upon incomplete knowledge of the physiology and pathology of the gonadal hormones and other contraceptive steroids. Qualitatively, the metabolic effects of the synthetic contraceptive steroids are similar to those of the ovarian hormones' effects, which were briefly discussed in an earlier part of this chapter. There are some exceptions. The synthetic progestogens, particularly the 19-nor- derivatives, appear to have a more deleterious effect upon carbohydrate metabolism than does progesterone. On the other hand, in contrast to progesterone, they have the advantage of inhibiting the hyperlipidemic effect produced by estrogens. Although the side effects of the contraceptive steroids upon carbohydrate and lipid metabolism and other metabolic processes are significant, present evidence indicates that they are reversible. In addition, it is increasingly apparent that the fraction of the population at risk can be identified. Patients with various forms of hyperlipidemia seem to be peculiarly sensitive to the effects of estrogens and should not be given steroid contraception. Similarly, although there is a slight deterioration of carbohydrate metabolism in most women using oral contraceptives, the women most likely to develop significant changes are those with previously abnormal glucose values, a family history of diabetes mellitus, or a history of having excessively large infants. The most serious side effect of oral contraceptives is thrombosis, because embolism from it may be fatal. At this time, other than by a history of an earlier thrombosis, it is not possible to identify patients at risk, but some of the new methods (e.g., determination of fibrinogen split products) might help identify them. There has been increasing concern about the development of hypertension in patients on contraceptive steroids. Available evidence indicates that the incidence of hypertension is real but small; thus it is mandatory to check blood pressure in patients on contraceptive steroids. As pressure mounted to decrease the amount of steroids administered and as lower doses were tried, it became apparent that satisfactory contraception could be obtained, even at dose levels which were insufficient to inhibit ovulation. It is assumed that, in these cases, contraception results from interference with mechanisms such as the ones involved in tubal transport of the ova, implantation, sperm transport through the cervical mucus, and perhaps capacitation. In decreasing the amount of steroids administered, it was hoped that it would be possible to attain a level at which metabolic effects would become negligible while preserving an acceptably low pregnancy rate. This hope has not been completely fulfilled, and at those levels at which the metabolic effects of these steroids appear negligible, such as in the low-dose progestogen-only schedule, pregnancy rate rises sharply, and breakthrough bleeding becomes annoyingly frequent. Even so, it is imperative in choosing a contraceptive agent to choose the agent with the lowest level of estrogen compatible with an acceptable incidence of pregnancy and breakthrough bleeding.

Efforts are being made to optimize the ratio of side effects to contraception by changing the route of administration. It was thought that this might be possible by delivering the contraceptive mixture by subcutaneously implanted silastic capsules, through which small amounts of hormone would be released at a constant rate. The preliminary results of these attempts, however, are not encouraging. Most recently, plastic devices containing progestogen have been implanted in the uterus to deliver the hormone directly to one of its target sites, the endometrium, but insufficient information is available to judge the merit of this new approach.

Inhibition of Ovulation for Dysmenorrhea. The old dictum "nulla dysmenorrhea sine ovulatione" is still valid, and when dysmenorrhea becomes incapacitating, blocking of ovulation with estrogens or a combination of estrogens and progestogens is almost always successful. In patients with premenstrual tension, however, results are often disappointing.

Inhibition of Androgen Secretion. In women with hirsutism and other symptoms of virilization due to excessive androgen secretion of the ovaries, long-term ovarian suppression by estrogen, or preferably a combination of estrogen and progesterone, will prevent progressive virilization and often reverse the symptomatology. Prior to ovarian suppression, it is obviously necessary to rule out adrenal causes of virilization or the very rare functional ovarian tumor. Control determinations of androstenedione followed by repeated determinations during the ovarian suppression are useful guides in therapy and final proofs of the ovarian origin of the androgens. When acne is the predominant symptom of virilization, great improvement and, in many cases, cure can be expected within a few months, provided the initial diagnosis of an ovarian androgen excess was correct. It takes

many months of suppression before improvement in hirsutism is apparent, although objective measurements (such as regular shaving and weighing of the hair growth per unit of time over a marked area of the skin) will often show decreased hair growth within weeks after the onset of suppression. In most cases, a course of electrolysis at the end of suppression for 6–12 months will satisfactorily control the hirsutism. There is little solid information about the dose of estrogen and progestogen that is sufficient and necessary to inhibit the excessive androgen secretion by the ovary. We have had good results with combinations of norethynodrel (2.5 mg.) and mestranol (0.1 mg.) twice daily during the first 3–4 months; this dose is decreased to once daily in the subsequent months.

Therapy of Anovulation

Women who are anovulatory often revert spontaneously to ovulatory cycles, and the first evidence that they have returned to normal ovarian function may well be pregnancy. For a condition that has about a 20% tendency to resolve spontaneously, any treatment will have a significant chance of success, which may explain the transient popularity of such treatments as psychotherapy, thyroid hormone, corticosteroids, cyclic therapy with estrogen with or without progestogen, and many others. At the present time, there are three main ways to induce ovulation: ovarian wedge resection, clomiphene, and gonadotropins. The efficacy of these modes of therapy is very high, and it may be said that, provided patients with primary ovarian failure are excluded, ovulation can be induced in virtually all patients with anovulation. Evidently where anovulation is secondary to a disturbance with a known etiology (i.e., intercurrent disease), therapy must, if possible, be directed to the cause of the disturbance rather than to the symptoms.

Anovulatory patients fall into two categories: those who do and those who do not want to become pregnant. Although this should be unnecessary, it is worthwhile to stress that *there is no need to induce ovulation in a patient who is anovulatory unless she wants to become pregnant.*

Thyroid Hormones. Many women are still being treated with thyroid hormone merely because they are anovulatory. Although tests of thyroid function are normal, it has sometimes been assumed that certain patients have mild forms of hypothyroidism because of anovulation. This is not a reasonable assumption, and the diagnosis of hypothyroidism, and especially thyroid treatment, should not be based only on anovulation.

Glucocorticoids. In patients with biochemically proved forms of adrenal hyperplasia, anovulation is the rule, and treatment should obviously be directed to suppression of adrenal hyperactivity. In a few studies, glucocorticoids have also been administered with partial success in women with anovulation but in whom the adrenal origin of the abnormality could not be unequivocally established. In our hands, this treatment has met with very little success, and we believe that adrenal suppression with glucocorticoids should be limited to patients in whom there is a biochemical reason to suspect adrenal hyperplasia.

Clomiphene. Clomiphene, a nonsteroidal compound with weak estrogenic activity, is one of the most successful agents for inducing ovulation. Clomiphene has antiestrogenic activity, and probably acts by competing with circulating estrogen for estrogen receptor sites in the hypothalamus. In the presence of clomiphene, the negative feedback effect of the estrogens is blocked, and consequently the pituitary begins to secrete increased amounts of FSH and LH, thus initiating follicular maturation (Fig. 7–26). The resulting rise in circulating estrogen triggers an LH surge which induces ovulation. If this concept of the action of clomiphene is correct, it should be expected that clomiphene will be most effective in anovulatory women whose ovaries are still secreting estrogens and whose pituitary remains sensitive to the positive feedback effect of the estrogens. Extensive clinical experience has shown this to be true, and in only very exceptional cases will clomiphene treatment be successful in women with signs of estrogenic insufficiency. For these reasons, withdrawal bleeding that follows progesterone therapy is an excellent indication of an ovulatory response to clomiphene (see above).

Before starting treatment, it is important to ascertain that the ovaries are not enlarged and that the patient is not pregnant. Initially, treatment consists of one 50 mg. clomiphene tablet daily for 5 days, beginning on the fifth day of the menstrual cycle or at any time if the patient is amenorrheic. Patients are instructed to have intercourse between the fifth and ninth day after the last administration of clomiphene, since this is the period during which ovulation should be expected. If the patient does not ovulate, treatment can be repeated at the same dose level. If no response occurs after two 5-day courses of clomiphene, the dose is doubled (100 mg. daily for 5 days). In grossly obese women, it may be worthwhile to use a higher dose, but if an average patient does not ovulate after two or three courses at the 100-mg. level, it is unlikely that she will respond to a higher dose, and the risk of complications increases at higher dose levels. The major complication of both clomiphene and gonadotropin treatment is ovarian hyperstimulation. This complication is discussed below.

No serious toxic reactions have followed clomiphene therapy, but several side effects reminiscent of complications associated with its parent toxic compound, triparanol, have been reported. A few patients have experienced blurring of vision, but this is reversible, and no lens changes have been reported such as occurred with triparanol. Nevertheless, visual symptoms prompt immediate discontinuance of treatment. Abnormal sulfobromophthalein retention has also been observed in a few patients, and therefore liver damage is a contraindication to the use of clomiphene. The antiestrogenic effect of the drug probably accounts for the fairly common occurrence of hot flashes.

It is possible to induce ovulation in more than 70% of patients with anovulation despite their capacity to secrete estrogen. In our experience, 20–30% have become pregnant as a result of clomiphene therapy. About 10% of these pregnancies have resulted in multiple births, usually twins, in contrast to a general incidence of about 1%. Clomiphene has also been used in ovulatory patients who are having difficulties in conceiving. Rather than enhance fertility, clomiphene given to ovulatory women will often induce abnormal luteal phases, and its use is therefore contraindicated.

Gonadotropins. Gonadotropins are effective in inducing ovulation in many patients in whom clomiphene has failed. Since clomiphene has antiestrogenic activity, it is ineffective in patients with low estrogen levels, and it will obviously not work in patients whose pituitary has lost its secretory capacity. These patients are candidates for gonadotropin therapy. When human gonadotropins first became available for therapy, it was believed that they would be suitable only for anovulatory patients with low or undetectable levels of gonadotropins. This type of patient is an ideal candidate for gonadotropin therapy, but in our experience, treatment is as worthwhile in the anovulatory patient with "normal" gonadotropins. The only patient who obviously cannot be expected to respond to gonadotropins is the patient with primary ovarian failure; levels of gonadotropins in the menopausal range are therefore a contraindication to gonadotropin therapy.

Treatment with gonadotropin is a two-step treatment; in the first phase, follicular maturation is induced with a preparation having a high FSH-LH ratio. When sufficient follicular maturation is ob-

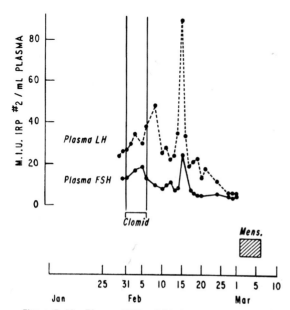

Figure 7–26. Plasma FSH and LH levels in a patient who ovulated in response to a 5-day course of clomiphene. (Adapted from Lipsett, M. B., et al.: *Ann. Intern. Med.* 72:933, 1970.)

tained, ovulation is induced with a luteinizing agent. For this purpose, hCG has been the agent of choice in most cases, but purified human LH of pituitary origin has also been used. FSH-LH is given intramuscularly, 75–150 I.U./day for 10–15 days. The patient must be examined frequently to determine the ovarian response.

This response is evaluated by observing changes in cervical mucus, vaginal cytologic changes, the size of the ovaries, and, most importantly, the level of urinary estrogens. When no response is obtained within 4–6 days, higher doses may be injected, but in these cases extreme caution should be exercised to avoid hyperstimulation. Human CG is withheld until there is evidence of complete follicular maturation and until adequacy of insemination is demonstrated by a postcoital test. When urinary estrogen excretion reaches 50–100 μg./day, a dose of 5000 to 10,000 I.U. of hCG is administered intramuscularly to induce ovulation (Fig. 7–27). Ovulation can be expected in almost 100% of patients treated in this manner, and pregnancy in about 60%, provided that there are no other causes of infertility.

While extremely effective in inducing ovulation, treatment with gonadotropins has a number of drawbacks. As with clomiphene, the risk of hyper-

stimulation is always present. In its mild form, hyperstimulation mainly produces abdominal pain and distention, nausea, and malaise. The full-blown syndrome, however, is manifested by massive enlargement of the ovaries, ascites, hydrothorax, and occasionally an ileus-like syndrome. Hyperstimulation is a complication of the second stage of the treatment with gonadotropins and will never occur until ovulation. Most cases of hyperstimulation can be avoided by judicious selection of patients and careful adjustment of the dose to the response. Urinary estrogens should be monitored throughout the last days of the FSH-LH treatment, and ovulation should not be induced in women whose urinary estrogens are excessive. In these cases, hCG is not administered, and after withdrawal bleeding treatment is started at a lower level.

If severe hyperstimulation develops, treatment is conservative and consists of bed rest and careful maintenance of the electrolyte balance. A laparotomy is not indicated unless there is evidence of intra-abdominal bleeding or of ovarian necrosis, which may be the result of twisting. Intra-abdominal bleeding appears to have been almost always a consequence of pelvic examination, which should be done with the utmost caution in patients with massively enlarged ovaries.

A second drawback in gonadotropin therapy lies in the frequency of multiple pregnancies, which is even higher than that seen in patients treated with clomiphene. Multiple pregnancies result in a higher abortion rate and, even more seriously, in a catastrophic fetal mortality due to prematurity in cases where there are more than two fetuses. While severe hyperstimulation can be avoided by careful monitoring of the treatment, multiple pregnancies cannot be completely avoided. Because timing is a critical factor in gonadotropin therapy, and treatment is expensive and time-consuming, it should not be undertaken unless laboratory facilities are available for determinations of estrogen levels and of the other parameters indicative of ovulation.

Ovarian Wedge Resection. Before clomiphene and gonadotropins were available, ovarian wedge resection was one of the few successful ways to induce ovulation in anovulatory women. This is still an acceptable form of therapy and, in our view, continues to be indicated occasionally. The major drawback of ovarian wedge resection is that it involves major surgery, but it has the significant advantage that, if successful, it will restore ovulation for years, if not for the rest of the patient's reproductive life. In contrast, treatment with clomiphene or with gonadotropins, even following a successful pregnancy, will rarely be followed by a resumption of spontaneous cycles.

Gonadotropin Releasing Hormone. With the recent availability of GnRH, it has become likely that ovulation can be induced by GnRH. However, it is too early to draw definite conclusions.

Estrogens. In the normal menstrual cycle, estrogens serve as the trigger for the preovulatory LH surge, and it should therefore be possible to in-

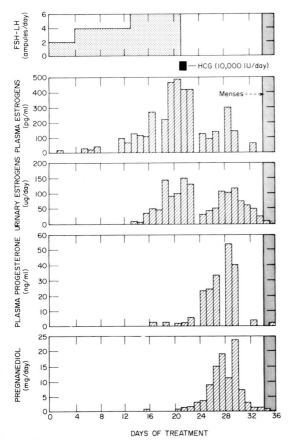

Figure 7–27. Plasma estrogens and progesterone and urinary estrogens and pregnanediol from a patient who ovulated following treatment with menopausal gonadotropins and hCG. (From Vande Wiele, R. L.: *Hospital Practice* 7:119, 1972.)

duce ovulation by the administration of estrogens. In anovulatory patients, estrogens will often induce a significant LH surge, but ovulation is only infrequently seen because the necessary sequence in follicular maturation → secretion of estrogens → LH surge has not been followed, and an immature follicle will not respond to LH.

X-ray Irradiation. This treatment was used until some years ago and was often considered as an alternative to wedge resection. With the availability of other methods to induce ovulation, it is no longer an acceptable treatment for infertility in view of the obvious genetic hazards.

REFERENCES

Morphology

Allen, E., Pratt, J. P., et al.: Human ova from large follicles; including a search for maturation divisions and observations on atresia. *Amer. J. Anat. 46*:1, 1930.

Baker, T. G.: A quantitative and cytological study of germ cells in human ovaries. *Proc. Roy. Soc.* (B) *158*:417, 1963.

Baker, T. G., and Franchi, L. L.: The fine structure of oogonia and oocytes in human ovaries. *J. Cell Sci. 2*:213, 1967.

Block, E.: Quantitative morphological investigations of follicular system in women; variations in different phases of sexual cycle. *Acta Endocr. 8*:33, 1951.

Boss, J. H., Scully, R. E., et al.: Structural variations in the adult ovary. Clinical significance. *Obstet. Gynec. 25*:747, 1965.

Brewer, J. I., and Jones, H. O.: Time of ovulation. *Amer. J. Obstet. Gynec. 53*:637, 1947.

Corner, G. W., Jr.: Histological dating of human corpus luteum of menstruation. *Amer. J. Anat. 98*:377, 1956.

Edwards, R. G., Steptoe, P. C., et al.: Steroid assays and preovulatory follicular development in human ovaries primed with gonadotropins. *Lancet 2*:611, 1972.

Gillman, J.: Development of the gonads in man, with consideration of the role of fetal endocrines and the histogenesis of ovarian tumors. *Contr. Embryol. Carneg. Instn.,* Pub. 210, *32*:81, 1948.

Hertig, A. T.: The aging ovary—a preliminary note. *J. Clin. Endocr. 4*:581, 1944.

Kraus, F. T., and Neubecker, R. D.: Luteinization of the ovarian theca in infants and children. *Amer. J. Clin. Path. 37*:389, 1962.

McKay, D. G., Pinkerton, J. H. M., et al.: The adult human ovary: a histochemical study. *Obstet. Gynec. 18*:13, 1961.

Manotaya, T., and Potter, E. L.: Oocytes in prophase of meiosis from squash preparation of human fetal ovaries. *Fertil. Steril. 14*:378, 1963.

Merrill, J. A.: Ovarian hilus cells. *Amer. J. Obstet. Gynec. 78*:1258, 1959.

Morris, J. M., and Scully, R. E.: *Endocrine Pathology of the Ovary.* St. Louis, C. V. Mosby, 1958.

Mossman, H. W., Koering, M. J., et al.: Cyclic changes of interstitial gland tissue of the human ovary. *Amer. J. Anat. 115*:235, 1964.

Ober, W. B., and Bernstein, J.: Observations on endometrium and ovary in the newborn. *Pediatrics 16*:445, 1955.

Parini, F., and Molla, W.: Contributo anatomo-istologico al significato biologico dell'atresia follicolare. *Ann. Obstet. Gynec. 62*:1629, 1940.

Polhemus, D. W.: Ovarian maturation and cyst formation in children. Pediatrics *11*:588, 1953.

Potter, E. L.: The ovary in infancy and childhood, In *The Ovary.* Grady, H. G., and Smith, D. E. (eds.), Baltimore, Williams & Wilkins, 1963, p. 11.

Ross, G. T., Vaitukaitis, J. L., et al.: Pituitary gonadotropins and preantral follicular maturation in women, In Excerpta Medica Intern. Congr. Ser. *273*, 1973.

Sauramo, H.: Histology, histopathology and function of the senile ovary. *Ann. Chir. Gynaec. Fenn. 41*(Suppl. 1):1, 1952.

Scammon, R. E.: The prenatal growth and natal involution of the human uterus. *Proc. Soc. Exp. Biol. Med. 23*:687, 1926.

Sternberg, W. H.: Morphology, androgenic function, hyper-

plasia and tumors of the human ovarian hilus cells. *Amer. J. Path. 25*:493, 1949.

Trevila, L.: The weight of ovaries after stress ending in death. *Ann. Chir. Gynaec. Fenn. 47*:232, 1958.

Valdes-Dapena, M. A.: The normal ovary of childhood. *Ann. N. Y. Acad. Sci. 142*:597, 1967.

Van Wagenen, G., and Simpson, M. E.: *Embryology of the Ovary and Testis: Homo Sapiens and Macaca mulatta.* New Haven, Yale University Press, 1965.

Wehefritz, E.: Systematische Geiwichtsuntersuchungen am Ovarien mit Beruecksichtigung anderer Druesen mit inner Sekretion. *Z. Ges. Anat. 9*:161, 1923.

Witschi, E.: Embryology of the ovary, In *The Ovary.* Grady, H. G., and Smith, D. E. (eds.), Baltimore, Williams & Wilkins, 1963, p. 1.

White, R. F., Hertig, A. T., et al.: Histological and histochemical observations on the corpus luteum of human pregnancy with special reference to corpora lutea associated with early normal and abnormal ova. *Contr. Embryol. Carneg. Instn.,* Pub. 592, *34*:55, 1951.

Woll, E., Hertig, A. M., et al.: Ovary in endometrial carcinoma, with notes on morphological history of aging ovary. *Amer. J. Obstet. Gynec. 56*:617, 1948.

Puberty

Blizzard, R. M., Johanson, A., et al.: Recent developments in the study of gonadotropin secretion in adolescence, In *Adolescent Endocrinology.* Heald, F., and Hung, W. (eds.), New York, Appleton-Century-Crofts, 1970.

Buckler, J. M. H., and Clayton, B. E.: Output of luteinizing hormone in the urine of normal children and those with advanced sexual development. *Arch. Dis. Child. 45*:478, 1970.

Marshall, W. A., and Tanner, J. M.: Variations in pattern of pubertal changes in girls. *Arch. Dis. Child. 44*:291, 1969.

Reiter, E. O., and Kulin, H. E.: Sexual maturation in the female. Normal development and precocious puberty. *Pediat. Clin. N. Amer. 19*:581, 1972.

Reynolds, E. L., and Wines, J. V.: Individual differences in physical changes associated with adolescence in girls. *Amer. J. Dis. Child. 75*:329, 1948.

Sizonenko, P. C., Burr, I. M., et al.: Hormonal changes in puberty. II. Correlation of serum luteinizing hormone and follicle stimulating hormone with stages of puberty and bone age in normal girls. *Pediat. Res. 4*:36, 1970.

Zacharias, L., and Wurtman, R. J.: Age at menarche, genetic and environmental influences. *New Eng. J. Med. 280*:868, 1969.

Zacharias, L., Wurtman, R. J., et al.: Sexual maturation in contemporary American girls. *Amer. J. Obstet. Gynec. 108*:833, 1970.

Cyclic Changes in Genital Tract Epithelium and Tests of Ovarian Function

Castellanos, H., and Sturgis, S. H.: Urinary cytology in the endocrine evaluation of the normal female. *Progr. Gynec. 4*:98, 1963.

Collett-Solberg, P. R., and Grumbach, M. M.: A simplified procedure for evaluating estrogenic effects and the sex chromatin pattern in exfoliated cells in urine: Studies in premature thelarche and gynecomastia of adolescence. *J. Pediat. 66*:883, 1965.

Davis, M. E., and Fugo, N. W.: Cause of physiologic basal temperature changes in women. *J. Clin. Endocr. 8*:550, 1948.

Gaudefroy, M.: Cytological criteria of estrogen effect. *Acta Cytol. 2*:347, 1958.

Goldenberg, R. L., Grodin, J. M., et al.: Withdrawal bleeding and luteinizing hormone secretion following progesterone in women with amenorrhea. *Amer. J. Obstet. Gynec. 115*:193, 1973.

Israel, S. L.: *Menstrual Disorders and Sterility.* 5th ed. New York, Hoeber Medical Division, Harper and Row, 1967.

Israel, S. L., and Schneller, O.: Thermogenic property of progesterone. *Fertil. Steril. 1*:53, 1950.

Noyes, R. W., Hertig, A. T., et al.: Dating endometrial biopsy. *Fertil. Steril. 1*:3, 1950.

Papanicolaou, G. N.: Sexual cycle in human female as revealed by vaginal smears. *Amer. J. Anat. 52*:519, 1933.

Papanicolaou, G. N., Traut, H. F., et al.: *The Epithelia of Women's Reproductive Organs.* New York, Commonwealth, 1948.

Preeyasombat, C., and Kenny, F. M.: Urocytograms in normal children and various abnormal conditions. *Pediatrics 38*:436, 1966.

Rock, J.: Medical Progress; Physiology of human conception. *New Eng. J. Med.* 240:804, 1949.

Silver, H. K.: Cytology of urinary sediment in childhood. *Pediatrics* 26:255, 1960.

Weid, G. L., and Keebler, C. M.: Vaginal cytology of female children. *Ann. N. Y. Acad. Sci.* 142:646, 1967.

Menopause

Bigelow, B.: Comparison of ovarian and endometrial morphology spanning the menopause. *Obstet. Gynec.* 11:487, 1958.

Grodin, J. M., Siiteri, P. K., et al.: Source of estrogen production in postmenopausal women. *J. Clin. Endocr.* 36:207, 1973.

Rogers, J.: Medical Progress; The menopause. *New Eng. J. Med.* 254:697, 750, 1956.

Measurement of Gonadotropins

Becker, K. L., and Albert, A.: Urinary excretion of follicle stimulating and luteinizing hormones. *J. Clin. Endocr.* 25:962, 1965.

Boyar, R., Finkelstein, J., et al.: Synchronization of augmented LH secretion with sleep during puberty. *New Eng. J. Med.* 287:582, 1972.

Franchimont, P.: *Sécrétion Normale et Pathologique de la Somatotropine et des Gonadotropines humaine.* Paris, Masson et Cie, 1971.

Jaffe, R. B., and Midgley, A. R., Jr.: Current status of human gonadotropin radioimmunoassay. *Obstet. Gynec. Surv.* 24:200, 1969.

Kulin, H. E., Rifkind, A. B., et al.: Total gonadotropin activity in the urine of prepubertal children. *J. Clin. Endocr.* 27:1123, 1967.

Midgley, A. R., Jr., and Jaffe, R. B.: Regulation of human gonadotropins. X. Episodic fluctuation of LH during the menstrual cycle. *J. Clin. Endocr.* 33:962, 1971.

Rifkind, A. B., Kulin, H. E., et al.: Follicle stimulating hormone (FSH) and luteinizing hormone (LH) in the urine of prepubertal children. *J. Clin. Invest.* 46:1925, 1967.

Rifkind, A. B., Kulin, H. E., et al.: Twenty-four hour luteinizing hormone (LH) and follicle stimulating hormone (FSH) excretion in normal children. *J. Clin. Endocr.* 31:517, 1970.

Rosenberg, E., and Keller, P. J.: Studies on urinary excretion of follicle stimulating and luteinizing hormone activity during the menstrual cycle. *J. Clin. Endocr.* 25:1262, 1965.

Ross, G. T., Cargille, C. M., et al.: Pituitary and gonadal hormones in women during spontaneous and induced ovulatory cycles. *Recent Progr. Hormone Res.* 26:1, 1970.

Vaitukaitis, J. L., and Ross, G. T.: Recent advances in evaluations of gonadotropic hormones. *Ann. Rev. Med.* 24:295, 1973.

Measurement of Steroid Hormones

Loraine, J. A., and Bell, E. T.: *Hormone Assays and Their Clinical Application.* 3rd ed. Baltimore, Williams & Wilkins, 1971, p. 684.

Vande Wiele, R. L., and Dyrenfurth, I.: Gonadotropin-steroid interrelationships. *Pharmacol. Rev.* 25:2, 1973.

Menstrual Cycle

Baird, D. T., Horton, R., et al.: Steroid prehormones. *Perspect. Biol. Med.* 3:384, 1968.

Baird, D. T., and Guevara, A.: Concentration of unconjugated estrone and estradiol in peripheral plasma in nonpregnant women throughout the menstrual cycle, castrate and postmenopausal women and in men. *J. Clin. Endocr.* 29:149, 1969.

Baird, D. T., Horton, R., et al.: Steroid dynamics under steady state conditions. *Recent Progr. Hormone Res.* 25:611, 1969.

Dyrenfurth, I., Jewelewicz, R., et al.: Temporal relationships of hormonal variables in the menstrual cycle, In *Biorhythms and Human Reproduction.* Ferin, M., Halberg, F., et al. (eds.), New York, John Wiley & Sons, 1973.

Grodin, J. M., Siiteri, P. K., et al.: Source of estrogen production in menopausal women. *J. Clin. Endocr.* 36:207, 1973.

Gurpide, E., and Gandy, H.: Dynamics of hormone production, In *Endocrinology of Pregnancy.* Fuchs, F., and Klopper, A. (eds.), New York, Harper and Row, 1971, p. 1.

Gurpide, E., and Mann, J.: Estimation of secretory rates of hormones from the specific activities of metabolites which have multiple secreted precursors. *Bull. Math. Biophys.* 27:389, 1965.

Hisaw, F. L., Jr., and Hisaw, F. L.: Effect of relaxin on the uterus

of monkeys *(Macaca mulatta)* with observations on the cervix and symphysis pubis. *Amer. J. Obstet. Gynec.* 89:141, 1964.

Johansson, E. D., Wide, L., et al.: Luteinizing hormone (LH) and progesterone in plasma and LH and oestrogens in urine during 42 normal menstrual cycles. *Acta Endocr.* 68:502, 1971.

Lloyd, C. W., Lobotsky, J., et al.: Concentration of unconjugated estrogens, androgens and gestagens in ovarian and peripheral venous plasma of women: the normal menstrual cycle. *J. Clin. Endocr.* 32:155, 1971.

MacDonald, P. C., Grodin, J. M., et al.: The utilization of plasma androstenedione for estrone production in women, In *Progress in Endocrinology.* Gual, C. (ed.), Amsterdam, Excerpta Medica Foundation, 1969, p. 770.

Mikhail, G.: Hormone secretion by the human ovaries. *Gynec. Invest.* 1:5, 1970.

Presser, H. B.: Temporal data relating to the human menstrual cycle, In *Biorhythms and Human Reproduction.* Ferin, M., Halberg, F., et al. (eds.), New York, John Wiley & Sons, 1973.

Ross, G. T., Cargille, C. M., et al.: Pituitary and gonadal hormones in women during spontaneous and induced ovulatory cycles. *Recent Progr. Hormone Res.* 26:1, 1970.

Salhanick, H. A., Vande Wiele, R. L., et al. (eds.), Metabolic effects of contraceptive steroids. *Proceedings of Conference on Metabolic Effects of Gonadal Hormones and Contraceptive Steroids, Boston, 1968.* New York, Plenum Press, 1969.

Schally, A. V., Arimura, A., et al.: Isolation and properties of the FSH and LH-releasing hormone. *Biochem. Biophys. Res. Commun.* 43:393, 1971.

Speroff, L., and Vande Wiele, R. L.: Regulation of the human menstrual cycle. *Amer. J. Obstet. Gynec.* 109:234, 1971.

Steinetz, B. G., Beach, V. L., et al.: Reactions of antisera to porcine relaxin with relaxin-containing tissues of other species in vivo and in vitro. *Acta Endocr.* 47:371, 1964.

Tagatz, G. E., and Gurpide, E.: Hormone secretion by the normal human ovary, In *Handbook of Physiology: The Female Reproductive System.* Greep, R., and Astwood, E. B. (eds.), Bethesda, Maryland, American Physiological Society, 1973.

Tait, J.: Review of the use of isotopic steroids for the measurement of production rates in vivo. *J. Clin. Endocr.* 23:1285, 1963.

Treloar, A. E., Boynton, R. E., et al.: Variation of the human menstrual cycle through reproductive life. *Intern. J. Fertil.* 12:77, 1967.

Vande Wiele, R. L., Bogumil, R. J., et al.: Mechanisms regulating the menstrual cycle in women. *Recent Progr. Hormone Res.* 26:63, 1970.

Vande Wiele, R. L., and Dyrenfurth, I.: Gonadotropin-steroid interrelationships. *Pharmacol. Rev.* 25:2, 1973.

Vande Wiele, R. L., Dyrenfurth, I., et al.: Estimation of the rates of secretion of the ovarian hormones by isotope dilution methods, In *Clinical Endocrinology II.* Astwood, E. G., and Cassidy, C. E. (eds.), New York, Grune & Stratton, 1968, p. 603.

Ware, D., and Haynes, D. M.: A study of relaxin in primagravidas. *Amer. J. Obstet. Gynec.* 83:792, 1962.

Warren, M. P.: Metabolic effects of contraceptive steroids. *Amer. J. Med. Sci.* 264:1, 1973.

Steroid Hormones

Brown, J. B., and Matthew, J. D.: The application of urinary estrogen measurements to problems in gynecology. *Recent Progr. Hormone Res.* 18:337, 1962.

Korenman, S. G., Perrin, L. E., et al.: A radio-ligand binding assay system for estradiol measurement in human plasma. *J. Clin. Endocr.* 29:879, 1969.

Loraine, J. A., and Bell, E. T.: Hormone excretion during the normal menstrual cycle. *Lancet* 1:1340, 1963.

Strott, C. A., and Lipsett, M. B.: Measurement of 17-hydroxyprogesterone in human plasma. *J. Clin. Endocr.* 28:1426, 1968.

Yoshimi, T., and Lipsett, M. B.: The measurement of plasma progesterone. *Steroids* 11:527, 1968.

Neoplastic Diseases

Allander, E., and Wagenmark, J.: Leydig cell tumors of the ovary. *Acta Obstet. Gynec. Scand.* 48:433, 1969.

Asadourian, L. A., and Taylor, H. B.: Dysgerminoma. An analysis of 105 cases. *Obstet. Gynec.* 33:370, 1969.

Audet-Lapointe, P., and Vauclair, R.: Les tumeurs de la granulosa. Revue de la littérature et présentation de 7 cas. *Bull. Cancer* 55:457, 1968.

Berge, T., and Borglin, N. E.: Brenner tumors. Histogenetic and clinical studies. *Cancer* 20:308, 1970.

Blanc, B.: Les gonadoblastomes. Revue Generale. *Rev. Franc. Endocr. Clin.* 11:529, 1970.

Boivin, Y., and Richart, R. M.: Hilus cell tumors of the ovary. A review with a report of 3 new cases. *Cancer* 18:231, 1965.

Breen, J. L., and Neubecker, R. D.: Ovarian malignancy in children with special reference to the germ-cell tumors. *Ann. N. Y. Acad. Sci.* 142:658, 1967.

Brown, P. A., and Richart, R. M.: Functioning ovarian carcinoid tumors. Case report and review of the literature. *Obstet. Gynec.* 34:390, 1969.

Burger, J. P., Schlaeder, G., et al.: Le chorioépithelioma primitif de l'ovaire. *Rev. Franc. Gynec.* 64:351, 1969.

Costin, M. E., Jr., and Kennedy, R. L. J.: Ovarian tumors in infants and in children. *Amer. J. Dis. Child.* 76:127, 1948.

Diddle, A. W.: Granulosa and theca cell ovarian tumors: Prognosis. *Cancer* 5:215, 1952.

Dockerty, M. B., and MacCarty, W. C.: Granulosa cell tumors, with report of 34 pound specimen and a review. *Amer. J. Obstet. Gynec.* 27:425, 1939.

Dunihoo, D. R., Grieme, D. L., et al.: Hilar cell tumors of the ovary. Report of 2 new cases and a review of the world literature. *Obstet. Gynec.* 27:703, 1966.

Eberlein, W. R., Bongiovanni, A. M., et al.: Ovarian tumors and cysts associated with sexual precocity. *J. Pediat.* 57:484, 1960.

Ein, S. H., Darte, J. M., et al.: Cystic and solid ovarian tumors in children: A 44-year review. *J. Pediat. Surg.* 5:148, 1970.

Fox, L. P., and Stamm, W. J.: Krukenberg tumor complicating pregnancy; report of a case with androgenic activity. *Amer. J. Obstet. Gynec.* 92:702, 1965.

Gross, R. E.: Neoplasms producing endocrine disturbances in childhood. *Amer. J. Dis. Child.* 59:579, 1940.

Hodgson, J. E., Dockerty, M. B., et al.: Granulosa cell tumor of ovary; a clinical and pathological review of 62 cases. *Surg. Gynec. Obstet.* 81:631, 1945.

Hughesdon, P. E.: Ovarian lipoid and theca cell tumors; their origins and interrelations. *Obstet. Gynec. Surv.* 21:245, 1966.

Lipsett, M. B., Kirschner, M. A., et al.: Malignant lipid cell tumor of the ovary: clinical, biochemical and etiologic considerations. *J. Clin. Endocr.* 30:336, 1970.

Malkasian, G. D., Jr., Dockerty, M. B., et al.: Functioning tumors of the ovary in women under 40. *Obstet. Gynec.* 26:669, 1965.

Marcus, C. C., and Marcus, S. L.: Struma ovarii. A report of 7 cases and a review of the subject. *Amer. J. Obstet. Gynec.* 81:752, 1961.

Mannubini, G.: Primary chorionepithelioma of the ovary. *Acta Obstet. Gynec. Scand.* 28:251, 1949.

Moore, J. G., Schifrin, B. S., et al.: Ovarian tumors in infancy, childhood, and adolescence. *Amer. J. Obstet. Gynec.* 99:913, 1967.

Norris, H. J., and Taylor, H. B.: Prognosis of granulosa-theca tumors of ovary. *Cancer* 21:255, 1968.

Norris, H. J., and Taylor, H. B.: Virilization associated with cystic granulosa tumors. *Obstet. Gynec.* 34:629, 1969.

Novak, E. R., Facog, J. K., et al.: Feminizing gonadal stromal tumors. *Obstet. Gynec.* 38:701, 1971.

Pedowitz, P., and Pomerance, W.: Adrenal-like tumors of the ovary. Review of the literature and report of two new cases. *Obstet. Gynec.* 19:183, 1962.

Peterson, W. F., Prevost, E. C., et al.: Benign cystic teratomas of ovary; clinico-statistical study of 1007 cases with a review of the literature. *Amer. J. Obstet. Gynec.* 70:368, 1955.

Taylor, H. B., and Norris, H. J.: Lipid cell tumors of the ovary. *Cancer* 20:1953, 1967.

Thompson, J. P., Dockerty, M. B., et al.: Ovarian and paraovarian tumors in infants and children. *Amer. J. Obstet. Gynec.* 97:1059, 1967.

Scully, R. E.: Gonadoblastoma. A review of 74 cases. *Cancer* 25:1340, 1970.

Shuster, M., Mendoza-Divino, E., et al.: Carcinoid tumor metastasizing to the ovaries. *Obstet. Gynec.* 36:515, 1970.

Smith, F. G.: Pathology and physiology of struma ovarii. *Arch. Surg.* 53:603, 1946.

Spadoni, L. R., Lindberg, M. C., et al.: Virilization coexisting with Krukenberg tumor during pregnancy. *Amer. J. Obstet. Gynec.* 92:981, 1965.

Zangeneh, F., and Kelley, V. C.: Granulosa-theca-cell tumor of the ovary in children. *Amer. J. Dis. Child.* 115:494, 1968.

Autoimmune Diseases

Irvine, W. J., Moira, M. W., et al.: The further characterization of autoantibodies reactive with extra-adrenal steroid-producing cells in patients with adrenal disorders. *Clin. Exp. Immunol.* 4:489, 1969.

Ruehsen, M., Blizzard, R. M., et al.: Autoimmunity and ovarian failure. *Amer. J. Obstet. Gynec.* 112:693, 1972.

Precocious Puberty and Pseudopuberty

Albright, F., Butler, A. M., et al.: Syndrome characterized by osteitis fibrosa disseminata, areas of pigmentation and endocrine dysfunction, with precocious puberty in females; report of 5 cases. *New Eng. J. Med.* 216:727, 1937.

Beas, F., Vargas, L., et al.: Pseudoprecocious puberty in infants caused by a dermal ointment containing estrogens. *J. Pediat.* 75:127, 1969.

Caparro, V. J., Bayonet-Rivera, N. P., et al.: Premature thelarche (review). *Obstet. Gynec. Surv.* 26:2, 1971.

Cloutier, M. D., and Hayles, A. B.: Precocious puberty. *Advances Pediat.* 17:125, 1970.

Dresch, C., Arnal, M., et al.: Étude de 22 cas de développement prémature isolé des seins ou "premature thelarche." *Helv. Paediat. Acta* 15:585, 1960.

Ferrier, P., Shephard, T. H., et al.: Growth disturbances and values for hormone excretion in various forms of precocious sexual development. *Pediatrics* 28:258, 1961.

Hall, R., and Warrick, C.: Hypersecretion of hypothalamic releasing hormones: a possible explanation of the endocrine manifestations of polyostotic fibrous dysplasia (Albright's syndrome). *Lancet* 1:1313, 1972.

Hertz, R.: Ingestion of estrogens by children. *Pediatrics* 21:203, 1958.

Jenner, M. R., Kelch, R. P., et al.: Hormonal changes in puberty. IV. Plasma estradiol, LH, and FSH in prepubertal children, pubertal females and in precocious puberty, premature thelarche, hypogonadism, and in a child with a feminizing ovarian tumor. *J. Clin. Endocr.* 34:521, 1972.

Kenney, F. M., Midgley, A. R., Jr., et al.: Radioimmunoassayable serum LH and FSH in girls with sexual precocity, premature thelarche and adrenarche. *J. Clin. Endocr.* 29:1272, 1969.

Liu, N., Grumbach, M. M., et al.: Prevalence of electroencephalographic abnormalities in idiopathic precocious puberty and premature pubarche: Bearing on pathogenesis and neuroendocrine regulation of puberty. *J. Clin. Endocr.* 25:1296, 1965.

McCune, D. J.: Osteitis fibrosa cystica: The case of a nine year old girl who also exhibits precocious puberty. *Amer. J. Dis. Child.* 52:743, 1936.

Ramos, A. S., and Bower, B. F.: Pseudoisosexual precocity due to cosmetic ingestion. *J.A.M.A.* 207:368, 1969.

Rosenfeld, R. L.: Plasma 17-ketosteroids and 17-beta hydroxysteroids in girls with premature development of sexual hair. *J. Pediat.* 79:260, 1971.

Royer, P.: La précocité-isoséxuelle. *Rev. Franc. Endocr. Clin.* 8:217, 1961.

Serment, H., Piana, L., et al.: Puberté précoce d'origine ovarienne. *Rev. Franc. Endocr. Clin.* 11:489, 1970.

Sigurjonsdottir, T. J., and Hayles, A. B.: Precocious puberty. A report of 96 cases. *Amer. J. Dis. Child.* 115:309, 1968.

Sigurjonsdottir, T. J., and Hayles, A. B.: Premature pubarche. *Clin. Pediat.* 7:29, 1968.

Silverman, S. H., Migeon, C., et al.: Precocious growth of sexual hair without other secondary sexual development; "premature pubarche," constitutional variation of adolescence. *Pediatrics* 10:426, 1952.

Steiner, M. M.: Enlargement of breasts during childhood. *Pediat. Clin. N. Amer.* 2:575, 1955.

Talbot, N. B., Sobel, E. H., et al.: *Functional Endocrinology from Birth through Adolescence.* Cambridge, Harvard University Press, 1952.

Thamdrup, E.: Precocious sexual development. A clinical study of 100 children. *Danish Med. Bull.* 8:140, 1961.

Van Wyk, J. J., and Grumbach, M. M.: Syndrome of precocious menstruation and galactorrhea in juvenile hypothyroidism: an example of hormonal overlap in pituitary feedback. *J. Pediat.* 57:416, 1960.

Wilkins, L.: *The Diagnosis and Treatment of Endocrine Disorders in Childhood and Adolescence.* 3rd ed. Baltimore, Williams & Wilkins, 1965.

Wood, L. C., Olichney, M., et al.: Syndrome of juvenile hypothyroidism associated with advanced sexual development: Report of two new cases and comment on the management of an associated ovarian mass. *J. Clin. Endocr.* 25:1289, 1965.

Zurbruegg, R. P., and Gardner, L. I.: Urinary C_{19} steroids in two girls with precocious sexual hair. *J. Clin. Endocr.* 23:704, 1963.

Delayed Menarche and Primary Amenorrhea

Black, W. P., and Govan, A. D. T.: Laparoscopy and gonadal biopsy for assessment of gonadal function in primary amenorrhea. *Brit. Med. J.* 1:672, 1972.

Bjoro, K.: Primary amenorrhea. A study with special reference to the morphology of the genital organs. *Acta Obstet. Gynec. Scand.* 44 (Suppl.):1, 1965.

Bjoro, K.: Amenorrhea. A study with particular attention to the problems of ovarian failure. *Acta Obstet. Gynec. Scand.* 45 (Suppl. 1):69, 1966.

Canales, E. S., and Zarate, A.: Primary amenorrhea associated with polycystic ovaries. Endocrine, cytogenetic and therapeutic considerations. *Obstet. Gynec.* 37:205, 1971.

Caspersson, T., Zech, L., et al.: Analysis of human metaphase chromosome set by aid of DNA-binding fluorescent agents. *Exp. Cell Res.* 62:490, 1970.

Counseller, V. S.: Congenital absence of vagina. *J.A.M.A.* 136:861, 1948.

Grover, S., Solanki, B. R., et al.: A clinicopathologic study of Müllerian duct aplasia with special reference to cytogenetic studies. *Amer. J. Obstet. Gynec.* 107:133, 1970.

Hauser, G. A., and Kumschick, F.: Die primare Amenorrheae. *Geburtshilfe Frauenheilkd.* 26:645, 1966.

Henzl, M., Presl, J., et al.: Practical possibilities for classification of primary amenorrhea with special reference to the use of pneumopelvigraphy. *Amer. J. Obstet. Gynec.*, 93:79, 1965.

Hertz, R., Odell, W. D., et al.: Diagnostic implications of primary amenorrhea. *Ann. Intern. Med.* 65:800, 1966.

Jacobs, P. A., Harnden, D. G., et al.: Cytogenetic studies in primary amenorrhea. *Lancet* 1:1183, 1961.

Jagiello, G. M., Kaminetsky, H. A., et al.: Primary amenorrhea. A cytogenetic and endocrinologic study of 18 cases. *J.A.M.A.* 198:30, 1966.

Jones, G. S., and de Moraes-Ruehsen, M.: A new syndrome of amenorrhea in association with hypergonadotropism and apparently normal ovarian follicular apparatus. *Amer. J. Obstet. Gynec.* 104:597, 1969.

Kadotani, T., Ohama, K., et al.: A preliminary cytogenetic survey in primary amenorrhea. *Jap. J. Hum. Genet.* 13:278, 1969.

Kinch, R. A. H., Plunkett, E. R., et al.: Primary ovarian failure; a clinicopathological and cytogenetic study. *Amer. J. Obstet. Gynec.* 91:630, 1965.

Lewis, A. C. W.: Chromosomal aspects of primary amenorrhea. *Proc. Roy. Soc. Med.* 63:297, 1970.

Morin, J. P., Sudan, J. P., et al.: Amenorrhees primaires par synechies uterines d'origine tuberculeuse. *Rev. Franc. Gynec. Obstet.* 64:539, 1969.

Pearson, P. L., Bobrow, M., et al.: Technique for identifying Y chromosomes in human interphase nuclei. *Nature* (London) 226:78, 1970.

Philip, J., Sele, V., et al.: Primary amenorrhea. A study of 101 cases. *Fertil. Steril.* 16:795, 1965.

Polishuk, W. Z., Sharf, M., et al.: Primary amenorrhea due to intrauterine adhesions. *Gynaecologia* (Basel) 154:181, 1962.

Reschini, E., Giestina, G., et al.: Radioimmunoassayable plasma luteinizing hormone in primary amenorrhea. *Amer. J. Obstet. Gynec.* 111:173, 1971.

Ross, G. T., and Tjio, J. H.: Cytogenetics in clinical endocrinology. *J.A.M.A.* 192:977, 1965.

Shearman, R. P.: A physiological approach to the differential diagnosis and treatment of primary amenorrhea. *J. Obstet. Gynaec. Brit. Emp.* 75:1101, 1968.

Starup, J., Sele, V., et al.: Amenorrhea associated with increased production of gonadotropins and a morphologically normal ovarian follicular apparatus. *Acta Endocr.* 66:248, 1971.

Steele, S. J., Beilby, J., et al.: Visualization and biopsy of the ovary in the investigation of amenorrhea. *Obstet. Gynec.* 36:899, 1970.

Turunen, A.: Ueber kongenitales Fehler der Scheide. *Ann. Chir. Gynaec. Fenn.* 46:125, 1957.

Weiser, P.: Beobachtungen bei Atresie von Uterus und Vagina. *Geburtshilfe Frauenheilkd.* 26:1388, 1966.

Zourlas, P. A., and Comninos, A. C.: Primary amenorrhea with normally developed secondary sex characteristics. *Obstet. Gynec.* 38:298, 1971.

Secondary Amenorrhea

Abraham, G. E., Marshall, J. R., et al.: Disorders of ovulation, In *Pathology of Gestation.* Assali, N. S. (ed.), New York, Academic Press, 1972.

Asherman, J. G.: Amenorrhoea traumatica (atretica). *J. Obstet. Gynec. Brit. Emp.* 55:23, 1948.

Bardin, C. W., and Lipsett, M. B.: Testosterone and androstenedione blood production rates in normal women and women with idiopathic hirsutism or polycystic ovaries. *J. Clin. Invest.* 46:891, 1967.

Bliss, E. A., and Branch, C. H.: *Anorexia Nervosa.* New York, Hocher, 1960.

Blizzard, R. M., Chee, D., et al.: The incidence of adrenal and other antibodies in the sera of patients with idiopathic adrenal insufficiency (Addison's disease). *Clin. Exp. Immun.* 1:119, 1966.

Bogumil, R. J., Ferin, M., et al.: Mathematical studies of the human menstrual cycle. I. Formulation of a mathematical model. *J. Clin. Endocr.* 35:126, 1972.

Bogumil, R. J., Ferin, M., et al.: Mathematical studies of the human menstrual cycle. II. Simulation performance of a model of the human menstrual cycle. *J. Clin. Endocr.* 35:144, 1972.

Goldzieher, J. W.: Polycystic ovarian disease, In *Progress in Infertility.* Behrman, S. J., and Kistner, R. W. (eds.), Boston, Little, Brown & Co., 1968, p. 351.

Irvine, W. J., Chan, M. M. W., et al.: Immunological aspects of premature ovarian failure associated with idiopathic Addison's disease. *Lancet* 2:883, 1968.

Jensen, P. A., and Stromme, W. B.: Amenorrhea secondary to puerperal curettage (Asherman's syndrome). *Amer. J. Obstet. Gynec.* 113:150, 1972.

Keys, A.: *The Biology of Human Starvation.* Minneapolis, University of Minnesota Press, 1950.

Kirschner, M. A., Bardin, C. W., et al.: Effect of estrogen administration on androgen production and plasma luteinizing hormone in hirsute women. *J. Clin. Endocr.* 30:727, 1970.

Kirschner, M. A., and Jacobs, J. B.: Combined ovarian and adrenal vein catheterization to determine the site(s) of androgen overproduction in hirsute women. *J. Clin. Endocr.* 33:199, 1971.

Klinefelter, H. F., Jr., Albright, F., et al.: Experience with quantitative test for normal or decreased amounts of follicle stimulating hormone in urine in endocrinological diagnosis. *J. Clin. Endocr.* 3:529, 1943.

Lipsett, M. B., Cargille, C. M., et al.: Reproductive endocrinology: Methodologic advances and clinical studies. *Ann. Intern. Med.* 72:933, 1970.

Lloyd, C. W., Lobotsky, J., et al.: Plasma testosterone and urinary 17-ketosteroids in women with hirsutism and polycystic ovaries. *J. Clin. Endocr.* 26:314, 1966.

De Moraes-Ruehsen, M., and Jones, G. E. S.: Premature ovarian failure. *Fertil. Steril.* 18:440, 1967.

Reifenstein, E. C., Jr.: Psychogenic or "hypothalamic" amenorrhea. *Med. Clin. N. Amer.* 30:1103, 1946.

Shearman, R. P., and Cox, R. I.: The enigmatic polycystic ovary. *Obstet. Gynec. Surv.* 21:1, 1966.

Tagatz, G., Fialkow, P. J., et al.: Hypogonadotropic hypogonadism associated with anosmia in the female. *New Eng. J. Med.* 283:1326, 1970.

Vallotton, M. B., and Forbes, A. P.: Distinction between idiopathic primary myxedema and secondary pituitary hypothyroidism by the presence of circulating thyroid antibodies. *J. Clin. Endocr.* 27:1, 1967.

Warren, M. P., and Vande Wiele, R. L.: Clinical and metabolic features of anorexia nervosa. *Amer. J. Obstet. Gynec.* 117:435, 1973.

Whitelaw, M. J., Nola, V. F., et al.: Irregular menses, amenorrhea, and infertility following synthetic progestational agents. *J.A.M.A.* 195:780, 1966.

Yen, S. S. C., Vela, P., et al.: Inappropriate secretion of follicle-stimulating hormone and luteinizing hormone in polycystic ovarian disease. *J. Clin. Endocr.* 30:435, 1970.

Treatment of Ovarian Dysfunction

Cullberg, J.: Mood changes and menstrual symptoms with different gestagen/estrogen combinations. A double blind comparison with a placebo. *Acta Psychiat. Scand.* 236 (Suppl.):1, 1972.

Engel, T., Jewelewicz, R., et al.: Ovarian hyperstimulation syndrome. Report of a case with notes on pathogenesis and treatment. *Amer. J. Obstet. Gynec. 112*:1052, 1972.

Gemzell, C. A.: Induction of ovulation with human gonadotropins. *Recent Progr. Hormone Res. 21*:179, 1965.

Greenblatt, R. B., McDonough, P. G., et al.: Estrogen therapy for the inhibition of linear growth. In *Clinical Endocrinology*. Astwood, E. B., and Cassidy, C. E. (eds.), New York, Grune & Stratton, 1968.

Kastin, A. J., Zarate, A., et al.: Ovulation confirmed by pregnancy after infusion of porcine LH-RH. *J. Clin. Endocr. 33*:980, 1971.

Kistner, R. W.: Induction of ovulation with clomiphene citrate, In *Progress in Infertility*. Behrman, S. J., and Kistner, R. W. (eds.), Boston, Little, Brown & Co., 1968.

Salhanick, H. A., Vande Wiele, R. L., et al. (eds.), *Metabolic Effects of Contraceptive Steroids*. New York, Plenum Press, 1968.

Taymor, M. L.: Human menopausal gonadotropin, In *Progress in Infertility*. Behrman, W. J., and Kistner, R. W. (eds.), Boston, Little, Brown & Co., 1968.

Vande Wiele, R. L.: Treatment of infertility due to ovulatory failure. *Hosp. Pract. 7*:119, 1973.

ACKNOWLEDGMENTS

The authors are grateful to Mesdames A. Ross, P. Summers, H. Chambers, T. Sellner, and L. Murtha for invaluable assistance in the preparation of the manuscript.

CHAPTER 8

Disorders of
Sex Differentiation

By Melvin M. Grumbach and
Judson J. Van Wyk

In our culture, the distinction between male and female is expected to be absolute, and these terms are often used to epitomize opposites. Usually the components of an individual's sexual makeup are indeed dominantly of one gender and conform to the chromosomal pattern established in the zygote at the time of fertilization. Most sexual characteristics, however, emerge from bipotential precursors in the embryo, and a spectrum of differentiation is possible at each level of sexual organization.

Advances in cytogenetics, experimental embryology, and steroid biochemistry have in recent years greatly clarified the determinants of many sex differences. In many instances, clinical abnormalities can now be interpreted as the counterpart of malformations that have been observed or experimentally induced in lower forms. It has become increasingly clear that failure at any of the stages of development to achieve full sexual differentiation may be responsible for either gross ambisexual development or less overt abnormalities in sexual function that first became apparent after sexual maturity.

NORMAL SEX DIFFERENTIATION

Sex-determining genes on the X and Y chromosomes make their impact on sexual development primarily by influencing the primitive bipotential gonad to develop either as a testis or as an ovary. Most of the other sexual characteristics are only secondarily influenced by the sex-determining genes and emerge from bipotential primordia that have an inherent tendency to feminize. Thus, female patterns of sexual development emerge in the course of development unless there is active intervention by some masculinizing influence. Since this masculinizing influence is normally conferred by the fetal testes, the sexual phenotype is usually predictable from the degree of testicular differentiation; only under pathologic circumstances do extragonadal factors influence this development in a contrary direction (Table 8–1).

Chromosomal Sex and X Chromatin (52, 53)

A systematized array of metaphase chromosomes from a single cell is known as a karyotype (36). The meaning of this term is usually extended

TABLE 8–1.   ONTOGENY OF SEXUAL CHARACTERISTICS

Characteristic	How Identified	Origin	Factors Determining Differentiation

Chromosomal sex	Karyotype analysis	Sex chromosomes of parental germ cells	Normal: chromosomal composition of sperm
			Abnormal:
			  Nondisjunction during meiotic divisions of parental germ cells
			  Nondisjunction or anaphase lag in early mitotic divisions of zygote
			  Structural errors due to chromosome breakage

X chromatin	Buccal smears; neutrophil spreads; smears or sections of other somatic tissues	Late replicating (heterochromatized) X chromosome	Partial inactivation and heterochromatization of all X chromosomes in excess of one
Y body	Same as for X chromatin; also seen in sperm	Y chromosome	Distal segment of long arm of Y
Gonadal sex	Histologic appearance	Testis Ovary	Testis: sex-determining genes on Y chromosome Ovary: sex-determining genes on two X chromosomes
Genital ducts	Pelvic examination; pelvic exploration	Müllerian and wolffian ducts	Intrinsic tendency to feminize; müllerian involution requires nonsteroidal macromolecular duct inhibitory factor from fetal seminiferous tubules; androgen stimulates male ducts

External genitalia	Inspection; investigation of urogenital sinus by urethroscopy and/or x-ray contrast study	Genital tubercle, urethral folds, labioscrotal folds, and urogenital sinus	Intrinsic tendency to feminize; masculinization requires androgenic stimulation before twelfth fetal week
			  Normal male: androgen from fetal testes
			  Virilized female: adrenal hyperplasia; maternal androgen
			  Incompletely differentiated male: insufficient testosterone secretion by fetal testes; end-organ refractoriness

Hormonal sex	*Secondary sex characteristics*
	  Male: sexual hair pattern; voice; muscularity; phallic size
	  Female: breast development; rounding of contours; growth of reproductive tract; menstruation; ovulation
	Hormonal patterns
	  Male: testosterone secretion from testes; tonic gonadotropin release
	  Female: cyclic secretion of gonadotropins, estrogen, and progesterone
		Hypothalamus and other neural centers;
		Pituitary gonadotropin;
		Secretory cells of testes, ovaries, and adrenals
			Hypothalamus and neural centers:
			  negative and positive feedback areas; gonadotropin releasing factor
			Pituitary: gonadotropin release governed by hypothalamic releasing factors and circulating levels of sex steroids
			Gonads: differentiation of secretory cells and biosynthetic enzymes; stimulation by pituitary gonadotropins
			Hormonal expression may be modified by end-organ sensitivity

Gender role	Social comportment; mannerisms and dress; direction of sex drive	Neuter at birth	Psychological environment during early years of paramount importance in establishing sexual identity:
			  Attitudes of parents
			  Interactions with both sexes
			  Conformity of genitalia to assigned sex
			Hormonal factors: adult sexual postures in lower species conditioned by hormonal factors in perinatal period

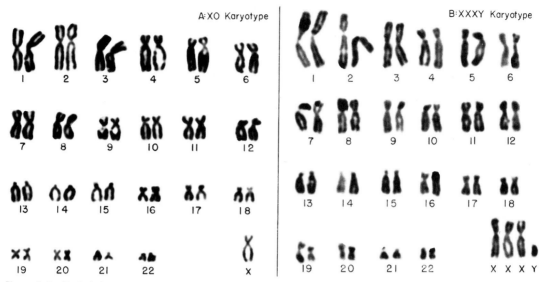

Figure 8–1. Typical chromosomal analyses from patients with abnormal gonadal differentiation. The XO karyotype on the left is from a patient with streak gonads, short stature, and the physical stigmata of Turner's syndrome. The XXXY karyotype on the right is from a phenotypic male with mental deficiency and seminiferous tubule dysgenesis (variant of chromatin-positive Klinefelter's syndrome).

to imply that the chromosomal pattern in that cell typifies all of the diploid cells of that individual or even of that species, although, as will be seen, this is by no means always true. When the 22 autosomes and two sex chromosomes (two X chromosomes or an X and a Y) are arrayed and serially numbered according to size, the X chromosome(s) are identified by their resemblance to the larger autosomes in the medium-sized group with submedian centromeres (group 6–12). The Y chromosome resembles the very short acrocentric autosomes in group 21–22 (36) (Fig. 8–1).

Positive identification of certain chromosomes can be made by pulse labeling cell cultures with tritiated thymidine and preparing autoradiographs of the chromosomal spreads. This technique is laborious but particularly useful in studying X chromosomal abnormalities. It was shown that one of two X chromosomes in the human female replicates late (107, 139), and that this characteristic is responsible for the distinctive X chromatin body seen in female somatic cells (*vide infra*).

Major advances in cytogenetics have recently come from the discovery of new chromosome staining techniques which differentially stain segments along the length of the chromosome. Caspersson and his associates (51, 53) introduced fluorescence staining with substances such as quinacrine mustard or quinacrine hydrochloride (Atabrine). Now referred to as the Q-staining method, this staining procedure gives a distinctive fluorescent banding pattern (Q bands) for each chromosome (Fig. 8–2) and for many of the arms of individual chromosomes (60). The distal portion of the Y chromosome is intensely fluorescent. Shortly thereafter, Pardue and Gall reported a Giemsa staining technique which preferentially stained only the centromeric regions of the chromosome.

These areas of constitutive (centromeric) heterochromatin are known as C bands (148). Stimulated by this finding, various workers modified the Giemsa staining technique (152), using a multitude of pretreatment procedures on fixed metaphase chromosomes (e.g., hypertonic saline, NaOH, variation of pH temperature, cation concentration, and proteolytic enzymes), which produced Giemsa-stained bands in human chromosomes identical (with minor exceptions) to the Q bands described by Caspersson (52); this method gives permanent preparations for conventional light microscopy (Fig. 8–2). The resulting bands are designated G bands (148). More recently, R-banding has been described (60, 148), which is a Giemsa staining method that produces a reverse pattern of chromosome banding to either the Q or G bands. The structural components of the chromosome that give rise to the banding patterns are currently under intensive study. There is evidence that the Q bands result from binding of quinacrine stains to adenine- and thymine (A-T)–rich regions of DNA; guanine- and cytosine (G-C)–rich regions of the chromosome quench the fluorescence. The G bands appear to be a consequence of differential dye binding by nonhistone protein (60) overlying the A-T–rich regions.

In any event, the chromosome banding procedures have provided precise methods for the identification of each chromosome and for the accurate analysis of chromosome abnormalities, including complex chromosome rearrangements (Fig. 8–2). The most recent recommendations for a standard nomenclature for the identification and designation of individual chromosomes, chromosome regions and bands, and structurally altered chromosomes are embodied in the report of the 1971 Paris Conference on Standardization in Human

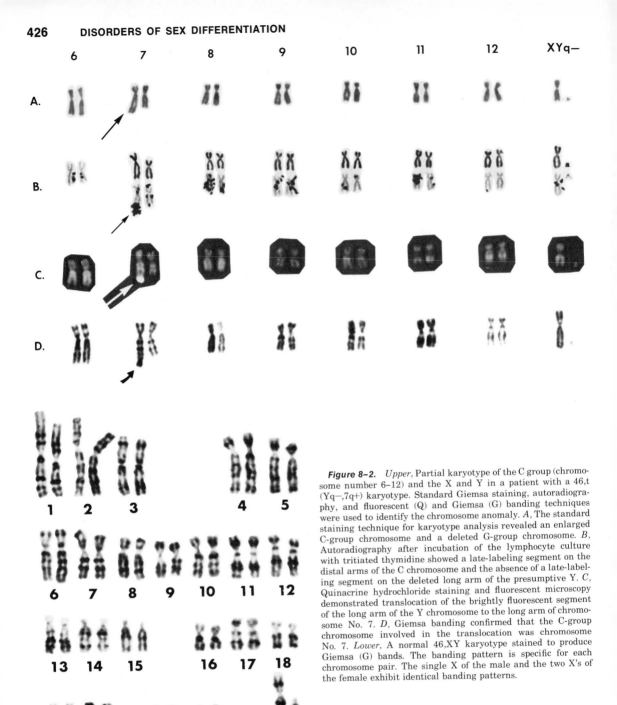

Figure 8–2. *Upper,* Partial karyotype of the C group (chromosome number 6–12) and the X and Y in a patient with a 46,t (Yq–,7q+) karyotype. Standard Giemsa staining, autoradiography, and fluorescent (Q) and Giemsa (G) banding techniques were used to identify the chromosome anomaly. *A,* The standard staining technique for karyotype analysis revealed an enlarged C-group chromosome and a deleted G-group chromosome. *B,* Autoradiography after incubation of the lymphocyte culture with tritiated thymidine showed a late-labeling segment on the distal arms of the C chromosome and the absence of a late-labeling segment on the deleted long arm of the presumptive Y. *C,* Quinacrine hydrochloride staining and fluorescent microscopy demonstrated translocation of the brightly fluorescent segment of the long arm of the Y chromosome to the long arm of chromosome No. 7. *D,* Giemsa banding confirmed that the C-group chromosome involved in the translocation was chromosome No. 7. *Lower,* A normal 46,XY karyotype stained to produce Giemsa (G) bands. The banding pattern is specific for each chromosome pair. The single X of the male and the two X's of the female exhibit identical banding patterns.

Cytogenetics (148). Table 8–2 summarizes the nomenclature applied to sex chromosome anomalies.

Within a short span of years, a vast literature has emerged, attempting to correlate sex chromosome abnormalities with both sexual and somatic abnormalities. It is becoming increasingly clear that anomalies in number and structure of sex chromosomes occur with far greater frequency than was previously suspected and that these anomalies are of such variety that they cannot be attributed to any single mechanism or stage of cellular replication. Although many confusing and contradictory findings have been reported, cytogenetic studies have shed considerable light on the biologic roles of the X and Y chromosomes.

Mechanisms of Chromosomal Anomalies

Chromosomal errors can arise from faulty replication of the germ cells during spermatogenesis or oögenesis, or they can arise from faulty mitotic

TABLE 8–2. NOMENCLATURE FOR DESCRIBING THE HUMAN KARYOTYPE PERTINENT TO DESIGNATING SEX CHROMOSOME ABNORMALITIES

Chicago and Paris Conferences	Description	Former Nomenclature
46,XX	Normal female karyotype	XX
46,XY	Normal male karyotype	XY
47,XXY	Karyotype with 47 chromosomes including an extra sex chromosome	XXY
45,X	One sex chromosome absent	XO
45,X/46,XY	Mosaic karyotype composed of 45,X and 46,XY cell lines	XO/XY
p	Short arm	S
q	Long arm	L
Xp−	Deletion of the short arm of the X	X^{DS}
Xq−	Deletion of the long arm of the X	X^{DL}
Xqi	Isochromosome of the long arm of X	X^I
Xpi	Isochromosome of the short arm of X	
Xr	Ring X chromosome	X^R
46,X,t (Xq−;9p+)	Translocation of the long arm of X onto the short arm of chromosome No. 9	X/9 translocation
Ydic	Dicentric Y chromosome	
Ypi	Isochromosome of the short arm of Y	
Yqi	Isochromosome of the long arm of Y	Y^I

division of cells in the zygote after fertilization. Aneuploid cells are those which contain a different number of chromosomes from that characteristic of the species.

Aneuploidy. One mechanism of producing aneuploidy is nondisjunction, a process which may occur during either mitotic or meiotic division. Nondisjunction is characterized by failure of either a pair of sister chromatids or members of a pair of homologous chromosomes to separate during anaphase. Thus one daughter cell receives an extra chromosome while the other remains one short (Fig. 8–3). Aneuploidy may also be caused by anaphase lag, in which there is simple loss of a chromosome from one or both of the two daughter cells. Presumably this is caused by failure of one chromosome to become properly oriented at the equatorial plate during metaphase. If both chromatids are extruded, both daughter cell lines will be lacking in this chromosome. If, however, only one member of the chromatid pair is subsequently lost, the descendants from one daughter cell will be normal, while the other will be one short (Fig. 8–3).

Mosaicism. Mosaicism is the term applied to individuals with two or more cell lines, differing in chromosomal constitutions but originating from a single zygote. Although this condition can arise only from errors in mitosis after fertilization has occurred, embryos derived from gametes of abnormal chromosomal makeup are prone to further errors of replication. Mosaicism has been found to be much more common than was first supposed from early karyotypic analysis, and many of the seeming paradoxes between genotype and phenotype are attributable to studies that have lacked sufficient data to exclude this explanation. The difficulties of detecting or, especially, excluding sex chromosome mosaicism are often formidable. When mosaicism is present, the sex chromosome constitution may vary in different tissues and even in different areas of the same tissue (140). For this reason, it may be necessary to examine cell lines from a variety of tissues. The following additional

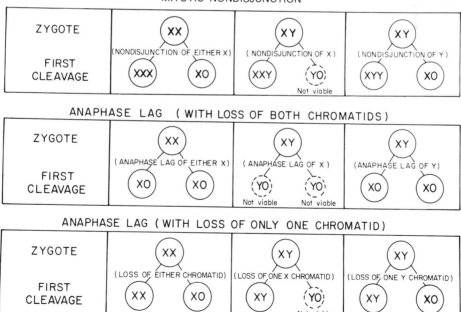

Figure 8–3. Daughter cell lines that can arise from mitotic nondisjunction or anaphase lag during the first mitotic division in the zygote. More complex mosaicism can result if the zygote is aneuploid or if replication errors arise beyond the one-cell stage. In females, nondisjunction or anaphase lag may involve either the maternal or paternal X chromosome. Deductions regarding the origin of X chromosomes in aneuploid patients can sometimes be made by correlating sex-linked traits with those in the parents.

factors must be considered when attempting to establish the presence of sex chromosome mosaicism:

1. Even in normal individuals, a small percentage of metaphase cells gain or lose chromosomes (usually the latter) for purely technical reasons.

2. A gradual and slight increase in the proportion of aneuploid cells with age, especially in females, has been observed by Jacobs et al. (120). In males, the aneuploidy is mainly due to the loss of the Y chromosome and in females to the loss of an X chromosome. By the age of 75 years this selective loss of a sex chromosome may involve as many as 5% of the metaphase figures in lymphocytes cultured from peripheral blood. This age-related aneuploidy is not a significant factor in assessing sex mosaicism before late adult life.

Chimerism. Chimerism is the term applied to individuals with more than one cell line, each of which has a different genetic origin. In the classic case of the freemartin, a common form of hermaphrodism in cattle, chimerism is derived by admixture of hemopoietic and primordial germ cells between biovular twins of opposite sex through anastomotic placental channels. Although it may be difficult to recognize the presence of chimerism if the separate cell lines have the same karyotype, the presence of cell lines of different sex will be marked by XX,XY mosaicism. Ford has discussed mechanisms by which XX,XY mosaicism could also result from (a) double fertilization (dispermy) of a binucleate ovum, (b) fusion of two complete zygotes or morulae before implantation, or (c) fertilization by separate sperms of an ovum and its polar body (90). It should be emphasized that the difference between mosaicism and chimerism depends solely on whether the different cell lines are of the same or different genetic origin.

Structural Errors. With increasing facility in identifying the morphologic characteristics of human chromosomes, abnormalities of structure as well as of number have been described. Structural errors are due to breakage or partial deletion, often followed by improper reunion of the fragments (Fig. 8–4). Most of the structural abnormalities that are sufficiently distinctive to be made visible by the light microscope are characterized by an abnormally long or short chromosome. Chromosomal fragments lacking a centromere or acquiring an additional centromere are usually eliminated from the cell. The nomenclature recommended by the Chicago and Paris Conferences for designating the human karyotype with reference to sex chromosome abnormalities is shown in Table 8–2 (36, 148). The following are the more common structural abnormalities:

Isochromosome formation is due to transverse rather than longitudinal division of the chromosome (Fig. 8–5), and the mutant chromosome may consist of either two long arms (e.g., Xqi) or two short arms (Xpi). *Deletion* is characterized by detachment and loss of a portion of a chromosome. The superscript q− refers to deletion of a portion of the long arm and p− to deletion of a portion of the short arm. *Duplication* occurs when a deleted seg-

PRODUCTION OF SOME STRUCTURAL ABNORMALITIES OF A CHROMOSOME

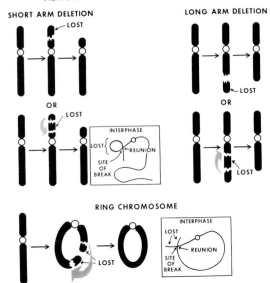

Figure 8–4. Diagram of chromosome breakage and recombination to form long- and short-arm deletions and ring chromosomes. The deleted segments also may be transposed to the terminal portions of other chromosomes as additions, or there may be reciprocal translocations of deleted segments with those from another chromosome.

ment is incorporated into another chromosome, usually the other member of a homologous pair. *Translocations* are characterized by exchanges of chromosomal segments between two chromosomes. *Ring chromosomes* (Xr) arise by deletions from the ends of a chromosome with reunion of the new distal portions to form a ring.

The larger the involved segment in structural errors, the more likely are polygenic abnormalities and resultant sterility. However, many visible chromosomal anomalies are compatible with fertility and are transmitted in a manner simulating mendelian laws of inheritance. Indeed, the distinction between congenital anomalies due to mutant genes and those due to chromosomal errors is based primarily on whether the disordered chromosomal structure is of sufficient size to be identified with current procedures for karyotype analysis.

Mutant genes or structural abnormalities of sex chromosomes, similar to those just described but involving chromosomal segments that are too short to be seen with the light microscope, may possibly account for certain discrepancies between the sex chromosomes and the gonadal morphology. It has been proposed but not established that an interchange of chromosomal segments between the X and Y chromosomes while they are aligned end to end (short arm to short arm) (152) during the first meiotic division of spermatogenesis (in the fathers) may explain the existence of both testes and ovaries in certain patients with true hermaphrodism as well as the development of testes in rare

ORIGIN OF ISOCHROMOSOME

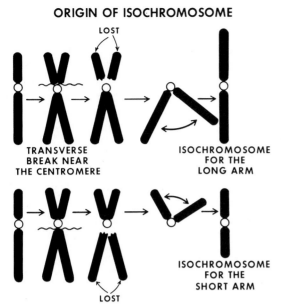

Figure 8–5. X Isochromosomes are thought to arise from transverse rather than longitudinal division of the centromere during the second meiotic division of germ cells in either parent or during mitosis in the zygote. Although two daughter cell lines might be expected, one with isochromosomes for the long arm and another for the short arm, this form of mosaicism has not been recognized. It is probable, however, that the break rarely occurs through the centromere, and the chromosomal segment which lacks a centromere is lost (see p. 428).

phenotypic males with an XX karyotype and no apparent mosaicism (85). In some of these cases, an autosomal gene mutation has been suggested, which leads to sex reversal and the development of XX phenotypic males, comparable to that found in other mammalian species (54).

Biologic Functions of the Y Chromosome

Until the advent of human chromosome analysis, it was believed by many that the Y chromosome was inert and that male determiners were carried on the autosomes. The finding of an XXY pattern in some patients with Klinefelter's syndrome has provided convincing demonstration that the Y chromosome carries powerful male-determining genes which can induce testicular development in the presence of two or more X chromosomes (5, 88, 190). Subsequent work has amply confirmed this conclusion. The presence of a Y chromosome leads to testicular differentiation even in individuals with an XXXXY sex chromosome constitution, whereas no testicular differentiation occurs in XO individuals (29). In addition to its role in gonadal differentiation, the Y has male germ-cell determinants and is essential to spermatogenesis.

The size of the human Y chromosome varies considerably—as much as threefold in length in normal men. The length and morphology of the Y is heritable, relatively constant in male relatives, and exhibits racial variation. Most of this variation is limited to the length of the long arm and its

distal brilliantly fluorescent segment in quinacrine(Q)-stained preparations (Fig. 8–6). As this polymorphism in the size of the fluorescent portion as well as a substantial part of the proximal nonfluorescent portion of the long arm is consistent with normal male sex differentiation and not associated with any specific phenotypic effects, it is quite likely that a large segment of the long arm of the Y is not engaged in gene transcription.

The number of genetic loci on the Y chromosome concerned with male sex determination is not known, but there must be more than one since partial deletion of the Y can result in incomplete male differentiation. Studies in patients with structural abnormalities of the Y are consistent with the localization of testis-determiners to the short arm of the Y close to the centromere (5, 84, 123, 140) and possibly the centromeric region of the long arm. It has also been adduced that the long arm of the Y contains loci homologous to those on the short arm of the X, since the presence of either of these segments of an X or Y chromosome with a normal X prevents the short stature and most of the somatic abnormalities found in Turner's syndrome (5, 84, 120, 123, 140). The presence of tall stature in XYY individuals suggests that this trait is transmitted through loci on the Y. The gene for hairy ears is thought to be carried on the Y chromosome (74).

Y Chromatin (Y Body) (151, 152).   The fluorescent end of the Y chromosome in human male metaphases, stained with the fluorochrome quinacrine hydrochloride or its mustard derivative, is represented as a small, brightly fluorescent body (Y body) in a high proportion of diploid interphase nuclei of the male, frequently located close to the nuclear membrane. The technique of fluorescence has been used to detect the Y body in interphase nuclei in a variety of tissue preparations, including buccal mucosal smears, lymphocytes and polymorphonuclear leukocytes in peripheral blood smears, hair root sheath cells, and cells grown in culture (152). In XY males, a single body, sometimes bipartite in structure, is present in interphase nuclei (Fig. 8–6), whereas two Y bodies are detectable in over 15% of nuclei in XYY and XXYY males (Table 8–3). Of interest are the reports of Pearson et al. (151) and others of the occurrence of a Y body in slightly less than 50% of mature sperms. In a small percentage of normal males (<0.05%) with small Y chromosomes that lack all or most of the distal fluorescent segment, a Y body is absent in somatic nuclei. Fluorescence of quinacrine-stained Barr bodies has been observed in cultured fibroblasts and certain other tissues from females, but the intensity of the fluorescent X body is less and the size 3–5 times larger than the Y body.

Biologic Functions of the X Chromosome (137)

The biologic functions of the large, paired X chromosomes are more complex. The requirement of a second X chromosome in man for the primitive

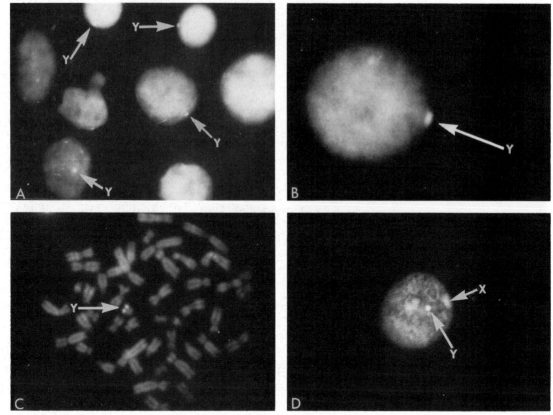

Figure 8-6. *A*, Quinacrine hydrochloride staining and fluorescent microscopy of interphase cells from a normal male, illustrating typical Y bodies. *B*, Enlarged photograph of one cell, showing the fluorescent Y body at the periphery of the nucleus. *C*, Metaphase chromosomes from a normal male, illustrating the brightly fluorescent distal segment of the long arm of the Y chromosome. *D*, An interphase nucleus in the buccal smear of a patient with a 47,XXY karyotype. A brightly fluorescent Y body, as well as an X chromatin body (which exhibits much weaker fluorescence) were identified by quinacrine staining and fluorescent microscopy.

gonad to differentiate into an ovary capable of oögenesis is suggested by the lack of normal ovarian differentiation in the XO individual. Studies of patients with various types of deletions

TABLE 8-3. SEX CHROMOSOME COMPLEMENT CORRELATED WITH X CHROMATIN AND Y BODIES IN SOMATIC INTERPHASE NUCLEI*

Sex Chromosomes	Maximum Number in Diploid Somatic Nuclei	
	X Bodies	Y Bodies
45,XO	0	0
46,XX	1	0
46,XY	0	1
47,XXX	2	0
47,XXY	1	1
47,XYY	0	2
48,XXXX	3	0
48,XXXY	2	1
48,XXYY	1	2
49,XXXXX	4	0
49,XXXXY	3	1
49,XXXYY	2	2

*The maximum number of X chromatin bodies in diploid somatic nuclei is one less than the number of X's, whereas the maximum number of Y fluorescent bodies is equivalent to the number of Y's in the chromosome constitution.

from one of the X chromosomes suggest further that there may be multiple loci involved in ovarian differentiation and that they are located on both the long and short arms (5, 84, 123, 140).

Whereas the Y chromosome is one of the smallest of human chromosomes and is mainly concerned with sex differentiation, the X chromosome is the eighth longest and contains about 5% of the total DNA content of a haploid set (X + 22 autosomes). Furthermore, the X chromosome contains genetic coding for functions involving every system in the body. Since females have twice the amount of this genetic material in their cells as do males, the biologic differences between the sexes should be far greater than is indeed the case. Recent theories that have been proposed to explain this paradox are an outgrowth of the pioneer observations of Barr of the X chromatin body in somatic cells of females.

X Chromatin (X or Barr Body) (12). In 1949, Barr and Bertram described the presence of a stainable chromatin mass at the periphery of the nucleus in resting ganglion cells of female cats but not of male cats (25). This distinguishing characteristic of the female sex was subsequently found to be present in the peripheral cells of most mammalian species. Since 1953, this nuclear difference has been used as a cytologic means of assessing the

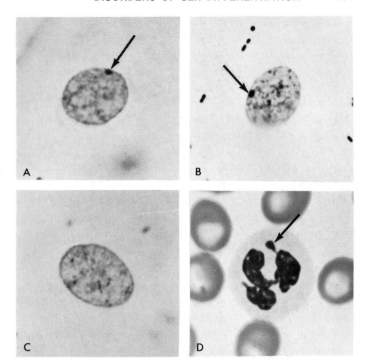

Figure 8-7. *A* and *B*, X chromatin body (Barr body) in nucleus of buccal mucosal cells obtained from normal female (thionine stain, × 2000). Such cells are found in about 25% of well-preserved nuclei. *C*, Buccal mucosal cell from normal male, illustrating absence of this body. *D*, A typical "drumstick" nuclear append-age found in a variable proportion of leukocytes of female subjects.

number of X chromosomes in humans with various errors of sex differentiation (Fig. 8–7) (12, 27).

The X chromatin body is usually planoconvex, with its flattened side in apposition to the inner surface of the nuclear membrane; in some nuclei, it has a bipartite structure. It measures about 1 μ in diameter and stains positively for DNA. In certain tissues, e.g., amniotic membrane, almost every interphase nucleus is chromatin-positive. In buccal mucosal smears, the most commonly used preparation for determining the X chromatin pattern, the proportion of X chromatin–positive nuclei in females may be lower than in other somatic tissues, but in most laboratories they are present in no less than 25% of well-preserved nuclei (12). A lower incidence of X chromatin–positive cells in the buccal epithelium of females during the first two days of life has been reported by Smith et al. (175). This difference has not been observed in our laboratory or that of Klinger (12) in which the thionine staining method is used.

The sexual dimorphism in polymorphonuclear leukocytes takes a different form; in females, 1–15% of neutrophils (mean 2.5%) have a drumstick-shaped, dense chromatin accessory nuclear appendage that is not found in normal males (Fig. 8–7, *D*). These appendages have the same significance as X chromatin in other somatic tissues (66).

In patients with more than two X chromosomes, the maximum number of X chromatin bodies in any diploid nucleus is one less than the total number of X chromosomes. In XXX females or XXXY males, for example, a maximum of two Barr bodies are present in diploid nuclei, whereas XY and XO individuals are X chromatin–negative (Table 8–3). Abnormalities in shape and size of the X chromatin body can often be correlated with

structural abnormalities of the X chromosome (Fig. 8–8). An abnormally small X chromatin body has been found in females with one normal X and one deleted X (XXp−) or with one ring X chromosome (XXr). A large X body is associated with a large X isochromosome (Xqi). When a structurally abnormal X is present, it is the aberrant X chromosome that replicates late and gives rise to the X chromatin (except in the rare X autosome translocations or when the sex chromosome complement consists of two structurally abnormal X chromosomes).

X Chromatin and Gene Expression. In 1959, Ohno reported the first evidence that X chromatin arises from only one of the two X chromosomes in the interphase nuclei of female somatic cells (145). The staining characteristics of such nuclei arise from the fact that a portion of one X chromosome is highly condensed (heteropycnotic); the other X does not contribute to the heterochromatic material since, like the autosomes, it is extended and filamentous (106). This difference in staining quality also betokens a striking difference in the functional roles of the two X chromosomes. By studying the sequence of incorporation of ^{3}H thymidine into replicating chromosomes, Morishima, Grumbach, and Taylor showed that the X that gives rise to X chromatin completes its DNA synthesis later than does any other chromosome in the cell and that the maximum number of X chromatin bodies in a single diploid nucleus is equal to the number of late-replicating X chromosomes (Fig. 8–9) (107, 139). These observations and the incisive genetic studies of Mary Lyon, Beutler, and other workers have led to the concept (Lyon hypothesis) that only one X chromosome per cell is genetically active during interphase; the other, which retains its het-

RELATION OF STRUCTURAL ABNORMALITIES
OF X CHROMATIN TO CONFIGURATION
OF X CHROMATIN MASS

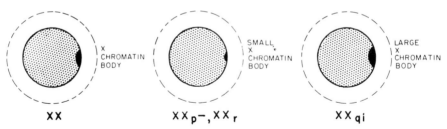

Figure 8–8. The relation of structural abnormalities of the X chromatin to the size of the X chromatin mass. The size of the X chromatin body in an XX individual (left) is compared with that found in individuals with a deleted X, ring X, or X isochromosome. (From Grumbach, M. M., In *Biologic Basis of Pediatric Practice.* Cooke, R. E. (ed.), New York, McGraw-Hill, 1967.)

erochromatic properties, is genetically inactive for many of its functions (37, 132). Lyon has recently critically and comprehensively reviewed X chromosome inactivation (133).

The change in state (heterochromatinization) of one of the X chromosomes in each female cell appears to be induced during the late blastocyst stage, between the twelfth and the eighteenth day in the human embryo (12, 106, 132, 280). The female germ cells beyond the stage of oögonia are the only cell lines known to be exempted from heterochromatinization, a finding in keeping with the requirement for a second X chromosome for normal ovarian differentiation to take place. Epstein has provided evidence that both X chromosomes in mouse oöcytes are active and code for the X-linked genes, glucose-6-phosphate dehydrogenase and hypoxanthine-guanine phosphoribosyl transferase (79, 80). In each of the other cells, it is by random chance whether the maternally or the paternally derived X chromosome becomes the inactive one. Once this transformation is established, however, the inactive state of that particular X chromosome is transmitted to all descendants of that cell. This control system appears to function as a mechanism of dosage compensation by which each female somatic cell functions as if it had virtually only one genetically active X chromosome (80, 133). The female, therefore, in effect, has no more active genetic material than does the male. This hypothesis is variously referred to as the "inactive X theory, " the "Lyon hypothesis," or the "fixed differentiation hypothesis of X chromosome behavior" (57, 106, 107, 133, 137, 139).

The implication that normal females function as genetic mosaics insofar as X-linked traits are concerned has found its strongest support in studies of the mouse (132) and in studies of X-linked traits in man (10, 133). Davidson, Nitowsky, and Childs demonstrated two populations of cells in females who were heterozygous for a mutant form of the X-linked gene, glucose-6-phosphate dehydrogenase, which has an electrophoretic mobility different from the normal form. Clones of cells grown in tissue culture from single cell precursors produced either the normal form of enzyme or the mutant form, but never both (Fig. 8–10) (65), whereas the uncloned cultured cells, which contained a mixture of cells in which either the normal or mutant forms of the enzyme were expressed, exhibited the electrophoretic bands of both forms. Heterochromatinization of all X chromosomes in excess of one also provides an explanation for the relatively minor phenotypic changes seen in women with more than two X chromosomes, since the supernumerary X chromosomes are also heterochromatinized and therefore relatively inactive (Fig. 8–11) (137). By way of contrast, strikingly severe changes are usually associated with trisomy for an autosome as small as chromosome No. 21, as in the case of mongolism. Little is known about the mechanism of X-chromosome inactivation (45, 107, 133). Brown and Chandra (45) have advanced a model in which a site on an autosome of maternal origin randomly activates one of the two X chromosomes in females and the single X in males.

It should be emphasized that in man, in contrast to the mouse, the inactivation of an X chromosome does not involve the entire chromosome or, alternatively, the heteropycnotic X is not completely inactive genetically. Individuals with XO or XXY constitutions, for example, have abnormalities both in their sexual development and in somatic features unrelated to sex. Further, recent evidence suggests that the X-linked blood group locus Xg is active on both X chromosomes in the female. This suggests that in normal individuals there are loci on both the heteropycnotic X and on the Y chromosome which are paired with a locus on the active X and which express a dosage effect.

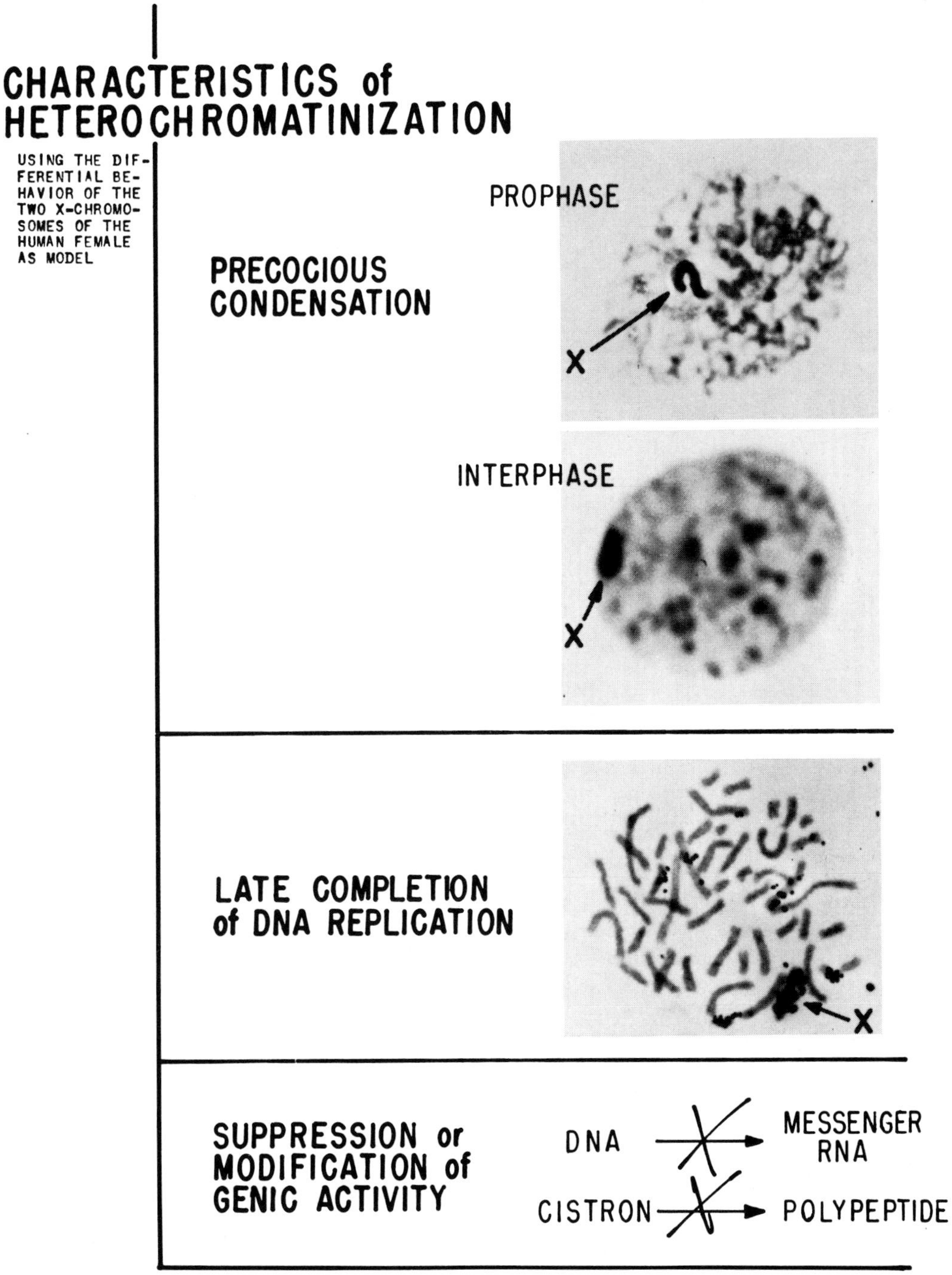

CHARACTERISTICS of HETEROCHROMATINIZATION

USING THE DIF-
FERENTIAL BE-
HAVIOR OF THE
TWO X-CHROMO-
SOMES OF THE
HUMAN FEMALE
AS MODEL

PRECOCIOUS
CONDENSATION

PROPHASE

INTERPHASE

LATE COMPLETION
of DNA REPLICATION

SUPPRESSION or
MODIFICATION of
GENIC ACTIVITY

DNA ⟶ MESSENGER RNA

CISTRON ⟶ POLYPEPTIDE

Figure 8–9. Characteristics of heterochromatinization as exemplified by the differential behavior of the two X chromosomes of the female in somatic cells. *1,* Precocious condensation of a large part of one of the two X chromosomes in prophase and the formation of the X chromatin body in interphase nuclei; *2,* delayed replication of DNA in one of the X chromosomes (the arrow indicates silver grains overlying one X chromosome in the autoradiogram of metaphase chromosomes from a normal female exposed to tritiated thymidine late in the synthetic period); *3,* suppression or modification of genic activity in the heterochromatinized portions of one X chromosome. (From Grumbach, M. M.: *Second International Conference on Congenital Malformations.* New York, International Congress, Ltd., 1963, p. 63.)

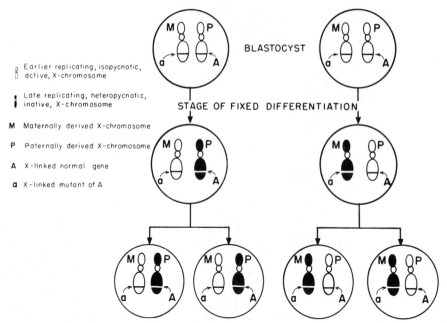

Figure 8–10.   Diagrammatic representation of the fixed differentiation or Lyon hypothesis of X chromosome behavior in somatic cells of the human female. At the late blastocyst stage (the time when X chromatin can first be identified), one of the two X chromosomes becomes heterochromatinized in each cell and gives rise to an X chromatin body; it is by random chance in each cell whether this differentiation involves the maternally derived X (X^M) or the paternally derived X (X^P). Once the differentiation has occurred, this characteristic is fixed in succeeding generations of somatic cells. The genes on the heterochromatinized portion of an X chromosome are suppressed or inactivated, thus serving as a means of "dosage compensation" for the increased number of X-linked genes in the female relative to the male. This mechanism has an important bearing on the expressivity and penetrance of an X-linked mutant gene in a heterozygous female. In the diagram, the maternally derived X carries a mutant gene (a) which is only expressed in cells in which this X is the isopycnotic, euchromatic active X (white X^M). Although the heterochromatinized X (black X) in this diagram is represented as being wholly inactive, it should be emphasized that some loci on the heterochromatinized X do remain active and exert genetic effects. It should also be noted that the female germ-cell line beyond the oögonia stage is exempted from heterochromatinization. (From Grumbach, M. M., In *Biologic Basis of Pediatric Practice.* Cooke, R. E. (ed.), New York, McGraw-Hill, 1967.)

In summary, it has been proposed that there are three kinds of genes on the sex chromosomes (5, 84, 122, 140).

1. *Sex-determining genes.* These are obviously not paired between the X and Y. Multiple sex-determining loci on both the long and short arms of two X chromosomes seem necessary for normal ovarian differentiation and oögenesis. Multiple loci on the Y chromosomes also are apparently required for full testicular differentiation and spermatogenesis; these appear to be located on the pericentromeric region of the short arm of the Y.

2. *"Paired" somatic genes.* Genes which are paired between the X and Y chromosome (in the sense that they express similar effects) are thought to be located on the short arm of the X and the longer of the arms of the Y. These loci on the heterochromatinized X are thought to be genetically

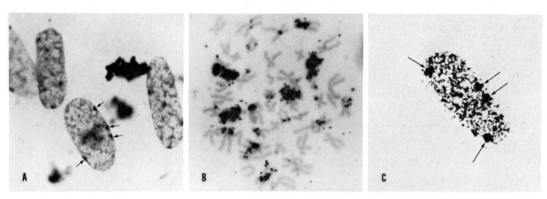

Figure 8–11.   Diploid somatic cells from a girl with a 49, XXXXX karyotype. *A,* Four X chromatin bodies in an interphase nucleus from a culture of skin fibroblasts. *B,* Autoradiogram of metaphase chromosomes, illustrating four areas of high grain density overlying four of the five X chromosomes. *C,* Autoradiogram of an interphase nucleus in a culture of skin fibroblasts; the four peripheral "hot" areas (indicated by arrows) of high grain density overlie four X chromatin bodies and provide direct evidence that each X chromatin body is derived from one late-labeling X chromosome. (From Grumbach, M. M., Morishima, A., et al.: *Proc. Nat. Acad. Sci. USA 49:*581, 1963, and Grumbach, M. M.: *Second International Conference on Congenital Malformations.* New York, International Congress, Ltd., 1963, p. 63.)

active, since lack of either a second X or a Y chromosome, or of their respective segments containing these genetic loci, leads to the short stature and many of the somatic abnormalities found in the syndrome of gonadal dysgenesis.

3. *Unpaired genes for biochemical and somatic traits.* On the Y chromosome the only trait for which there is firm evidence is the gene for hairy ears and determiners that lead to tall stature. On the X there are a large number of unpaired genes, missing on the Y, that are responsible for a wide variety of sex-linked traits. About 150 loci on the X chromosome of man are known. Using the technique of somatic-cell hybridization, recent studies have localized the loci for hypoxanthine-guanine phosphoribosyl transferase, phosphoglycerate kinase, glucose-6-phosphate dehydrogenase, and probably hemophilia A and color blindness, to the long arm of the X chromosome. Since the heterochromatinized X chromosomes are inactive for these genes, the unpaired genes on the active X chromosome act in each cell as if they were monosomic, no matter how many additional X chromosomes are actually present. Thus mutant sex-linked genes on the X chromosome are fully expressed in the male but to a much lesser extent in the female, unless she is homozygous for that trait. These genes play no role in producing the characteristic gonadal or somatic anomalies which typify XO individuals.

The foregoing hypotheses are based to a large extent on the cytogenetic findings in patients with anomalous sex chromosomes. Mapping of human chromosomes is yet in its infancy, and considerable elaboration and revision of these current hypotheses will undoubtedly take place when tested under further clinical circumstances and for other sex-linked traits.

Gonadal Sex Differentiation

Gametogenesis

Origin of Primordial Germ Cells. Primordial germ cells have been identified in the human in the 24-day embryo, at which time they are located in the dorsal endoderm of yolk sac close to the allantoic evagination. From this site, the germ cells, increasing in number by mitosis, migrate during the fourth and fifth weeks to the hindgut wall and then through the dorsal mesentery to the primordial gonad in the urogenital ridge (278, 282). In the complete absence of gonocytes, sterile gonadal ridges develop (5, 226, 227).

Spermatogenesis. During early testicular differentiation, the primordial germ cells become distributed throughout the primitive seminiferous tubules as progenitors of spermatogonia (263). During childhood the primordial germ cells remain quiescent and do not differentiate further until late in the prepubescent period. With the onset of adolescence, the basement membrane becomes lined by proliferating spermatogonia which have arisen by the mitotic division of primitive germ cells (244). The spermatogonia in turn give rise by mitotic division to primary spermatocytes.

The formation of haploid secondary spermatocytes from the euploid primary spermatocytes is accomplished by a special form of cell division known as meiosis. Whereas in mitotic division both daughter cells receive duplicates of each of the 46 parental chromosomes, in the first meiotic division each daughter cell receives only 23 chromosomes, one from each of the homologous pairs (Fig. 8–12). Thus half of the secondary spermatocytes contain 22 autosomes and an X chromosome, and the other half 22 autosomes and a Y chromosome. Each haploid daughter cell receives by random chance either the maternally or paternally derived chromosomes of each homologous pair, but not both. This process ensures great diversity in the genetic composition of the gametes, since by independent assortment and recombination of the paternal and maternal chromosomes constituting the 23 pairs it is possible to obtain 2^{23} different kinds of gametes (36). This is not the only mechanism for ensuring genetic variation, however, since the special nature of the prophase during this reduction division facilitates exchanges of DNA (crossing over) between homologous chromosomes. The details of this complex process are recounted in standard genetics texts.

Secondary spermatocytes give rise to spermatids by a second meiotic division, but this division is more analogous to mitosis than to the first meiotic division, since daughter cells are again produced by a longitudinal split of the two chromatid filaments comprising each of the unpaired chromosomes (Fig. 8–12). Thus the haploid number is not altered.

Spermatids do not undergo further division but rather develop into spermatozoa by a complex process of metamorphosis. Germ cells in the adult male are continually being renewed and undergoing maturation. Heller and Clermont have shown by labeling studies with tritiated thymidine that in adult males the complete cycle from spermatogonium to mature sperm requires about 74 ± 5 days (225).

Oögenesis. Female germ cells pursue a considerably different course from that of the male. During ovarian differentiation, the primary germ cells undergo vigorous replication and successive differentiation into oögonia and primary oöcytes. The period of oögonial proliferation results in a peak population of about 6–7 million germ cells in the two ovaries at 5 months, including oögonia, oöcytes in various stages of prophase, and degenerating germ cells (202). Formation of oögonia from primary germ cells has ceased by the seventh month of gestation and is never again resumed. Some of the oöcytes remain in undifferentiated nests, whereas others stimulate the formation of primordial follicles (282). The number of primordial follicles in the ovary is greatest at the time of birth, and from then on the number rapidly diminishes (261). In the germ cells that survive, the oöcyte is arrested at late prophase of its first meiotic division (diplotene state) and remains in this state from before birth until ovulation occurs many years later. The long life span of female germ cells,

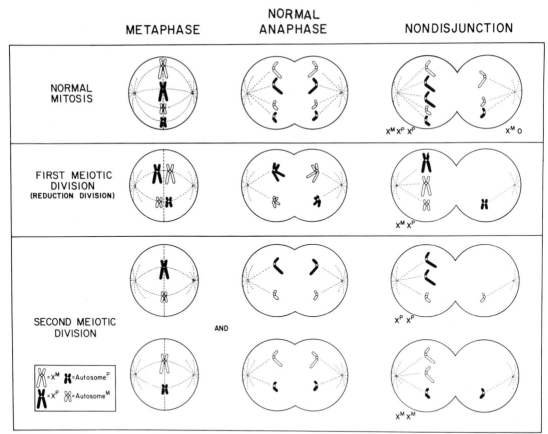

Figure 8–12. *Mitosis,* Diagram of female somatic cell undergoing mitosis. Represented at the metaphase plate are the two homologous C chromosomes and two homologous autosomes of the group 21–22. Division occurs through the centromere, giving two daughter cells of identical chromosomal composition. Replication of each arm into two chromatids takes place while the chromosomes are extended and prior to the next metaphase. *First Meiotic Division,* The first meiotic division involves pairing of homologous chromosomes. The centromere does not divide in this cell division. It is by random chance whether the maternal or the paternal member of each pair goes to the respective daughter cells. During the complex prophase of the first meiotic division (not shown), multiple chiasmata are formed between the chromosomes of each pair, thus facilitating exchanges of chromosomal segments (crossing over) between them. These peculiarities of the first meiotic division result in gametes with an almost infinite number of combinations of maternal and paternal genes. *Second Meiotic Division,* During the second meiotic division, the centromere again divides, giving daughter cells identical with the parent cell. This division more nearly resembles mitosis than the first meiotic division. *Nondisjunction,* Nondisjunction can take place either in mitosis or in the first or second meiotic division. Representative examples are illustrated.

as contrasted with those of the male, may have an important bearing on the increased prevalence of certain chromosomal anomalies with advanced maternal age.

Just before ovulation, the first polar body is extruded, thus completing the first meiotic division. The haploid secondary oöcyte immediately begins its second meiotic division but remains in metaphase and does not extrude the second polar body until the ovum is penetrated by a sperm cell. The frequent finding of triploidy in spontaneously aborted fetuses can be explained by either failure of the second polar body to be extruded (polygyny) or by double fertilization (polyspermy).

Differentiation of the Testis and Ovary (124, 234, 237, 272)

The gonads of both sexes develop from anlagen located on the medioventral border of the urogenital ridge, adjacent to the kidney and primitive adrenal (Fig. 8–13). Until the 12-mm. stage (approximately 42 days of gestation), the gonads of the male and female are indistinguishable on morphologic grounds and, indeed, could potentially differentiate either as a testis or as an ovary. The close ontogenic relationship between gonadal and adrenal cells at this early stage is noteworthy since, as differentiation proceeds, nests of adrenal cells frequently separate off with the gonad and are found as adrenal rests in the hilum of the mature ovary or testis (210). Such rests may become a problem in patients with long-standing untreated adrenal hyperplasia. Testicular rests, in particular, may later enlarge under persistent ACTH stimulation and be mistaken for tumors or true testicular enlargement.

The primitive undifferentiated gonad is derived from proliferation of the mesodermal coelomic epithelium, the mesenchymal cell mass on the urogenital ridge, and probably from mesonephric

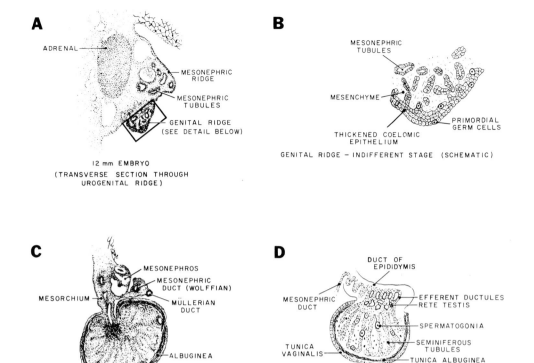

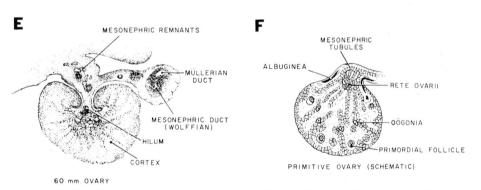

Figure 8–13. Anatomic and schematic representations of gonadal differentiation. *A* and *B,* Transverse section through urogenital ridge at stage of indifferent gonad. Note proximity of large fetal adrenal to hilar portion of gonad. *C* and *D,* Transverse section through fetal testis at 56-mm. stage. *E* and *F,* Transverse section through fetal ovary at 60-mm. stage. In ovarian development, the coelomic epithelium continues to proliferate for a much longer period. (Redrawn from Arey[199] and Witschi.[279])

elements (124, 235, 272). Also in the primitive gonad are found the large alkaline phosphatase–containing primordial germ cells which have migrated from the posterior endoderm of the yolk sac through the mesenchyme of the mesentery to the gonad (272, 278). By about 42 days, 300–1300 primordial germ cells have seeded the undifferentiated gonad. These large cells will later become either oögonia or spermatogonia. Lack of these germ cells is apparently incompatible with further gona-

dal differentiation. The coelomic epithelium is the primordium of the Sertoli cell in the testis and of the granulosa cell in the ovary.

Until recently, some embryologists believed that the testis is derived primarily from the medullary portion of the primitive gonad, whereas the ovary is derived primarily from the cortical portion (279, 281). According to this concept, the testis and ovary are not strictly homologous, since they differentiate from different primordial structures. Witschi (281) suggested that in genetic males the medullary portion secretes an inductor substance that stimulates development of seminiferous tubules and inhibits cortical development; conversely, the cortex of genetic females was thought to secrete an inductor substance that inhibited testicular development and resulted in ovarian dominance.

Jost (237), Jirósek (124), and van Wagenen and Simpson (272), among others, have recently called into question the older histologic descriptions of gonadal differentiation that served as the basis for these theories. After carefully examining numerous early embryos, Jost (237) and Jirósek (124) concluded that it was impossible to identify primary sex cords as such prior to the 15-mm. stage (about 45 days), when epithelial cords derived from the coelomic epithelium and the germ cells, antecedents of the seminiferous tubules, are already apparent in the male. With the onset of testicular differentiation and the incorporation of the germ cells into the primitive seminiferous cords, proliferation of the germ cells is suppressed, and differentiation beyond the primitive spermatogonial stage is arrested. After testicular differentiation (43–50 days gestational age) occurs (124), the male could also be recognized by beginning atrophy of the primitive müllerian ducts (30-mm. stage, about 60 days) and the differentiation of male external genitalia (40-mm. stage, 65–77 days). Leydig cells are first found in 32- to 35-mm. fetuses (about 60 days) and rapidly proliferate during the third month and the first half of the fourth month (124, 272); during this period the interstitial spaces between the seminiferous tubules are conspicuously crowded with Leydig cells.

In the gonad destined to be an ovary, the lack of differentiation persists; there is, however, continued proliferation of the coelomic epithelium and the primordial germ cells which gradually enlarge and become oögonia (Fig. 8–13). About the eleventh to twelfth week (80-mm. stage), long after differentiation of the testis in the male fetus, a significant number of germ cells begin to enter meiotic prophase, which characterizes the transition of oögonia into oöcytes; this event, the emergence of oöcytes, marks the onset of ovarian differentiation from the undifferentiated gonad. The formation of primordial follicles (in which the oöcyte is enveloped by a single layer of flat granulosa cells), reaches a maximum during the twentieth to the twenty-fifth week of gestation (202, 272); it is during this period that some of the primordial follicles mature to primary follicles. Hence, by the twentieth to the twenty-fifth week, the gonad has the morphologic characteristics of a definitive ovary.

The main events in gonadal differentiation, the timing of gonadal differentiation, and the relationship to the development of other male or female sexual characteristics is shown in Fig. 8–14.

Mechanisms of Gonadal Differentiation

In patients with an XO chromosomal constitution, neither testicular nor ovarian development takes place, and the postnatal gonad is represented

HUMAN SEX DIFFERENTIATION

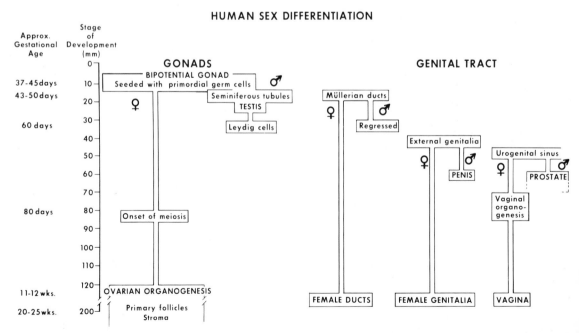

Figure 8–14. The sequence of sexual differentiation in the human fetus, as schematically depicted here, emphasizes that testicular development in the male fetus precedes all other forms of sexual dimorphism. There is an inherent propensity of the gonads, genital ducts, and external genitalia to feminize, whereas masculinization requires Y chromosome–mediated differentiation of the fetal testes. (Modified from Jost.[235])

by a long, pale streak of connective tissue in the mesosalpinx. Although the dense fibrous tissue is reminiscent of ovarian stroma, it is devoid of germ cells, primordial follicles, and seminiferous tubules. From this it may be concluded that the sex-determining genes on the Y chromosome are required for the undifferentiated gonad to develop into a testis, and a second X chromosome for differentiation into a normal ovary. Although there is abundant reason to presume a direct causal relationship between the presence of a Y chromosome and differentiation of the primitive gonad into a testis, the role of the second X chromosome in ovarian differentiation appears to be less direct. Female XO mice regularly have fertile ovaries, and fertility has also been reported in a rare human female with an apparently pure XO karyotype. The explanation may lie in the fact that germ cells are necessary for ovarian differentiation to take place and that, in contrast to the XO mouse, few germ cells in most human XO patients survive until this period of fetal life (see p. 458). Stated more succinctly, there is an inherent tendency for the primitive gonad to develop into an ovary, provided that germ cells are present and persist, unless prior testicular differentiation has occurred (233) (Fig. 8–14). The latter event is mediated in the male fetus by the testis determiners on the Y chromosome.

Many of our concepts of how sex-determining genes influence gonadal differentiation have been derived from studies in freemartins (124, 237). These are twin calf fetuses of opposite sex which share a common intrauterine circulation. The male twin develops normally, whereas the ovaries in the female twin are poorly developed and often contain sterile seminiferous tubules. Similarly, the müllerian ducts of the female twin undergo regression, and the external genitalia become masculinized. Jost and his associates have shown by studying freemartins at different stages of embryogenesis that development of seminiferous tubules in the female gonad occurs during the period in which the ovary normally differentiates and much later than in the normal male (233). These observations are compatible with the humoral transmission of a male inductor substance secreted by the fetal testes of the male twin (182). Since these changes cannot be reproduced with androgen, it may be inferred that testicular differentiation (and possibly inhibition of ovarian differentiation) may be attributed to a nonsteroidal humoral influence. It is conceivable that this hypothetical testicular inductor substance is related to, or promotes, the synthesis of the nonsteroidal testicular factor which causes involution of the müllerian ducts since the induction of seminiferous tubules in the "ovary" of the freemartin occurs concurrently with the involution of the müllerian ducts.

Regardless of the nature of the male inductor substance, the long period of latency before ovarian development can take place provides a rational explanation of why individuals with an XXY chromosomal constitution always develop testes, albeit defective ones, rather than ovaries. Prior differentiation of testes as a consequence of the action of the genes on the Y chromosome appears to preclude later differentiation as an ovary. Similarly, true hermaphrodism is less common in XY individuals than in XX individuals, because once testicular differentiation has occurred, ovarian differentiation is precluded.

In most clinical syndromes associated with anomalous sex chromosomal patterns, there is a high degree of correlation between testicular development and the presence of a Y chromosome, specifically the short arm of the Y. Conspicuous exceptions to this correlation are true hermaphrodites, who have both testicular and ovarian tissue. These individuals are usually found to have either a 46,XX or 46,XY karyotype. Further, phenotypic males have been reported with a 46,XX chromosomal constitution, and exhaustive tests have failed to reveal any evidence of mosaicism or translocation of the Y chromosome (70). Various theories have been advanced that might explain gonadal differentiation that is discordant with the apparent karyotype (70). Gene-linkage studies suggest that the most probable explanation is an undetected or extremely circumscribed mosaic cell line with a Y chromosome. A variant of this hypothesis is that an earlier existing line with a Y chromosome may have been completely eliminated. An alternative mechanism, which cannot be firmly excluded, is the X-Y interchange theory proposed by Ferguson-Smith (85). According to this hypothesis, interchange of sex-determining genes between the Y and X chromosomes might occur by translocation or crossing over during the first meiotic division of spermatogenesis in the father. None of these possibilities would be inconsistent with the decisive role of the Y chromosome in testicular development. As in lower species, gonadal differentiation also is influenced by autosomal and possibly X-borne genes [as evidenced by the occurrence of familial XX and XY gonadal dysgenesis (see pp. 468, 469) and by adverse intrauterine factors, e.g., in congenital anorchia].

Differentiation of the Genital Ducts

At the seventh week of intrauterine life, the fetus is equipped with primordia of both male and female genital ducts. The müllerian ducts serve as the anlagen of the uterus and fallopian tubes, whereas the mesonephric or wolffian ducts have the potentiality of differentiating further into the epididymis, vas deferens, seminal vesicles, and the ejaculatory duct of the male. During the third fetal month either the müllerian or wolffian ducts complete their development while involution occurs simultaneously in the opposite structures (Fig. 8–15).

It has been clearly demonstrated by Alfred Jost and other experimental embryologists that secretions from the fetal testis play a decisive role in determining the direction of genital duct development (234, 236). In the presence of functional

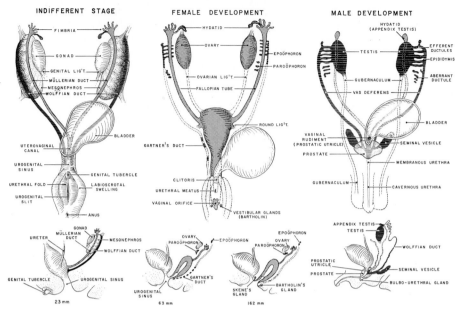

Figure 8–15. Embryonic differentiation of male and female genital ducts from wolffian and müllerian primordia. *A,* Indifferent stage showing large mesonephric body. *B,* Female ducts. Remnants of the mesonephros and wolffian ducts are now termed the epoöphoron, paraoöphoron, and Gärtner's duct. *C,* Male ducts before descent into scrotum. The only müllerian remnant is the testicular appendix. The prostatic utricle (vagina masculinus) is derived from the urogenital sinus. (Redrawn from Corning[209] and Wilkins.[16])

testes, the müllerian structures involute while the wolffian ducts complete their development, whereas in the absence of testes the wolffian ducts are resorbed and the müllerian structures mature (Fig. 8–16). Female development is not contingent on the presence of an ovary, since equally good development of the uterus and tubes will take place if no gonad is present.

The influence of a fetal testis on duct development is exerted locally and unilaterally since, if one testis is removed at an early stage of development, the oviduct will develop normally on that side, whereas müllerian regression will occur on the side with the intact testis (102).

The systemic administration of androgen to an early embryo has under no conditions been ob-

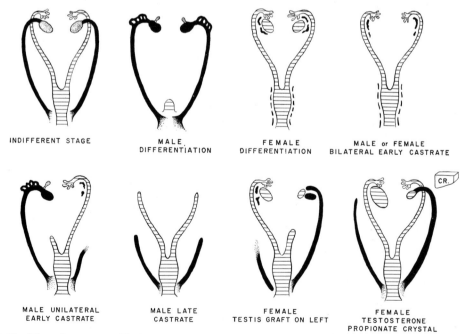

Figure 8–16. Schematic summary of Jost's experiments with rabbit embryos.[234, 236] The fetal testis plays a decisive role in determining the differentiation of genital ducts. Testosterone stimulates wolffian development but fails to effect involution of müllerian structures.

served to cause regression of müllerian structures. Even when high doses of androgen have been implanted locally in the gonadal region of female fetuses, the müllerian ducts have undergone no atrophy, although the wolffian ducts showed signs of stimulation (234, 236). On the other hand, if a testis is grafted onto an ovary, müllerian regression occurs on that side (Fig. 8–16). For these reasons, it has been proposed that the fetal testis secretes a müllerian duct–inhibiting substance that is distinct from ordinary androgens and is more likely a polypeptide or nucleic acid than a steroid.

Nathalie Josso has studied the influence of the fetal testis on müllerian duct inhibition in organ culture (231, 232, 233). Direct contact between the testis and the müllerian anlage was not necessary to bring about this inhibition. By separating the testis from the müllerian ducts by dialysis membranes, she concluded that the material secreted from the testis was macromolecular and not a steroid (231, 233). She also demonstrated that the human fetal testis, irrespective of its age, inhibits the müllerian ducts of 14.5-day-old fetal rats in similar organ culture studies, whereas the human postnatal testis has no müllerian duct–inhibiting activity (233). Using bovine fetal testes in which the tubules and interstitial tissue were isolated and assayed separately, she showed that müllerian duct–inhibiting activity was largely derived from the fetal seminiferous tubules rather than from the Leydig cells (232). Recently Josso reported that this substance is probably secreted by the fetal Sertoli cell.

Studies of humans with various forms of hermaphrodism have abundantly confirmed that a nonsteroidal substance secreted locally by the fetal testis is the decisive factor in causing regression of the müllerian ducts. In patients with rudimentary gonads, the uterus and fallopian tubes develop normally regardless of the chromosomal sex. In true hermaphrodites who have a testis on one side and an ovary on the other, regression of the müllerian ducts is most marked on the side of the testis (4,102). Similarly, müllerian derivatives are notably absent in males with the syndrome of testicular feminization, a condition characterized by unresponsiveness of peripheral tissues to the action of androgenic hormones. Conversely, early intrauterine exposure of human female fetuses to high levels of androgenic hormones (as in the adrenogenital syndrome) fails to hinder normal development of the uterus and fallopian tubes.

Although müllerian involution does not appear to be an androgen-dependent process, the stimulation of primitive wolffian ducts to differentiate into epididymis, vas deferens, and seminal vesicles appears to require androgen, at least in experimental animals. Congenitally androgen-insensitive male rats or rats treated with cyproterone acetate (an agent which blocks androgen action) show the expected regression of the müllerian ducts, but structures derived from wolffian ducts remain vestigial (257). Jost showed that the implantation of a crystal of testosterone adjacent to the fetal rabbit ovary stimulated the differentiation of male ducts on that side, but to a much lesser extent on the contralateral side; similar results were observed by grafting a fetal testis adjacent to the ovary (102) (Fig. 8–16).

The lateralization of these effects suggests that higher local concentrations of androgen are required for male duct stimulation than are required for masculinization of the external genitalia and derivatives of the urogenital sinus. In postnatal life, the testis possesses a gonadotropin-dependent mechanism for concentrating androgens within the seminiferous tubules and ejaculatory ducts. Working with postnatal rats, French and Ritzén showed that a high-affinity androgen-binding protein, which appears to be synthesized in Sertoli cells, is secreted into the lumen of the seminiferous tubules and flows outward in the seminal fluid through the rete testes and epididymides (216). The formation of this binding protein is apparently the mechanism by which androgen dependent germ cells and ejaculatory ducts are kept exposed to very high local concentrations of testosterone. The synthesis of the testicular androgen-binding protein is stimulated by FSH and abolished by hypophysectomy.

If a similar mechanism exists during embryonic life, it would adequately satisfy the experimental observations that male duct differentiation is androgen-dependent and requires the local presence of a testis. Wilson has shown in fetal rabbits that before and during the critical period of male duct differentiation, the wolffian ducts and their derivatives contain a specific testosterone-binding protein, whereas following this stage of development testosterone binding could no longer be demonstrated (275). Further studies will be required to determine whether this binding protein is a carrier protein secreted by the testis, as described by French et al., or whether it is an intracellular receptor similar to that found in all androgen responsive tissues. Conceivably, the binding of testosterone observed in these tissues might be due to a unique embryonic binding protein which functions transiently during the process of differentiation.

A further feature of male duct differentiation is that during organogenesis these tissues lack the 5α-reductase which converts testosterone to dihydrotestosterone. This is in striking contrast to the urogenital sinus and genital tubercle, which acquire this enzyme even before the testis has developed the capacity to synthesize testosterone (276). This difference may explain why the latter tissues are sensitive to systemic androgen, whereas this is not true for wolffian derivatives.

In human patients with ambiguous genitalia, well-differentiated male genital ducts are seen only in those patients who have testes. Female patients with congenital adrenal hyperplasia do not display this development, even though their external genitalia may be highly virilized *in utero*. Patients with asymmetric gonadal differentiation likewise have asymmetric male duct development which correlates very well with the degree of testicular differentiation on that side (67).

If the critical role of the testis in male duct development is to provide a mechanism whereby high levels of testosterone are concentrated locally at their site of action, it would be anticipated that male duct development would be deficient, even though testes are present, in patients with absolute defects in steroid biosynthesis (type VI congenital adrenal hyperplasia, pp. 478 and 481) or in XY patients whose tissues are highly unresponsive to testosterone (complete syndrome of testicular feminization, p. 485). Although the epididymides and vasa deferentia of these patients do indeed tend to be hypoplastic, the development of these structures is often better than that in experimental animals with corresponding defects. The reason for this species difference is not apparent.

Differentiation of External Genitalia

Origin of the External Genitalia

At the eighth fetal week the external genitalia of both sexes are identical and have the capacity to differentiate in either direction. They consist of a urogenital slit that is bounded by paired urethral folds, and, more laterally, by labioscrotal swellings. The urogenital slit is surmounted by a genital tubercle consisting of corpora cavernosa and glans (Fig. 8–17). The mucosa-lined urethral folds may remain separate, in which case they are called labia minora, or they may fuse to form a corpus spongiosum enclosing a phallic urethra. The fleshy labioscrotal swellings may remain separate to form labia majora, or they may fuse in the midline to form a scrotum and the ventral epidermal covering of the penis. The distinction between a clitoris

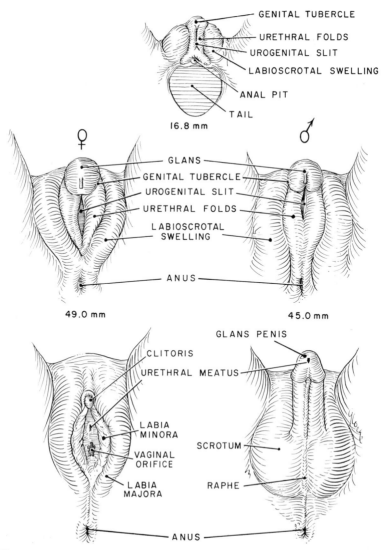

Figure 8–17.   Differentiation of male and female external genitalia from indifferent primordia. Male development will occur only in the presence of androgenic stimulation during the first 12 fetal weeks. (Redrawn after Spaulding.[268])

and penis is based primarily on size and whether or not the labia minora have fused to form a corpus spongiosum.

Origin of the Vagina

The urogenital sinus separates from a common cloaca in very early fetal life. The lower portion of the vagina initially develops as an outpouching of the urogenital sinus, whereas the upper portion is derived from the fused müllerian ducts. In normal female development, proliferation of the vesicovaginal septum pushes the vaginal orifice posteriorly so that it acquires a separate external opening; thus no urogenital sinus as such is preserved. In male development the vaginal pouch is usually obliterated when the müllerian ducts are resorbed, although by appropriate techniques a blind vaginal pouch known as the prostatic utricle can sometimes be demonstrated.

The prostate gland and bulbourethral glands of Cowper in the male are outgrowths of the urogenital sinus; their differentiation appears to be mediated by dihydrotestosterone and requires the presence of cytosol androgen receptors. In the female, the paraurethral glands of Skene and the vestibular glands of Bartholin have homologous origins (Table 8–4).

Role of Androgens in the Differentiation of External Genitalia

Testosterone and other androgenic hormones play the decisive role in the differentiation of external genitalia; testosterone is converted to dihydrotestosterone which binds to cytosol androgen receptors (binding protein) in the target cells. As in the case of the genital ducts, there is an inherent tendency for the external genitalia to feminize, and this requires no hormonal stimulant. Differentiation of these structures along male lines will occur only if androgenic stimulation is received during early fetal life. Androgenic hormones stimulate growth of the genital tubercle and induce fusion of the urethral folds and labioscrotal swellings. They also inhibit growth of the vesicovaginal septum, thereby preventing the separation of the vagina from the urogenital sinus. After the twelfth fetal week, when the vagina has already separated from the urogenital sinus, fusion of the labioscrotal folds will not occur, even under an intense androgenic stimulus (295). Androgenic stimulation will cause clitoral hypertrophy, however, at any time during intrauterine existence as well as after birth.

The fetal testicular Leydig cells begin to proliferate at about 60 days after conception (124), and in normal male fetuses androgens secreted by these

TABLE 8–4.   HOMOLOGIES BETWEEN MALE AND FEMALE SEXUAL STRUCTURES

Male Derivative	Primordial Structure	Female Derivative
	Gonad	
Seminiferous Tubules Leydig Cells Rete Testes Septa and Tunica Albuginea Tunica Vaginalis	Indifferent Gonad derived from Coelomic Epithelium Mesenchymal Cell Mass Mesonephric Elements	Graafian Follicles Granulosa Cells Theca Cells Interstitial Cells Rete Ovarii
Spermatogonia→Sperm	Primordial Germ Cells	Oögonia→Ova
	Genital Ducts	
Epididymis Aberrant Ductules	Mesonephric Tubules	Epoöphoron Paraoöphoron
Vas Deferens Seminal Vesicles	Mesonephric (Wolffian) Ducts	Gartner's Ducts
Appendix Testis (hydatid)	Müllerian Ducts	Fallopian Tubes Uterus Upper 1/3 Vagina
	External Genitalia	

Penis
  Corpora Cavernosa
  Glans Penis
	Genital Tubercle	Clitoris
		  Corpora Cavernosa
		  Glans Clitoris

Corpus Spongiosum (enclosing penile urethra)	Urethral Folds	Labia Minora
Scrotum & Ventral Epidermis of Penis	Labio Scrotal Swellings	Labia Majora
Prostate Bulbo-Urethral Glands (of Cowper) Prostatic Utricle (vagina masculinus)	Urogenital Sinus	Para-Urethral Glands (of Skene) Bartholin's Glands Vagina (lower 2/3)

cells account for masculinization of the genitalia. Acevedo et al. have shown that fetal testes are able to synthesize testosterone *in vitro* from labeled precursors (196). Wilson and Siiteri (276) found a precise correlation between the capacity of the rabbit fetal testis to synthesize testosterone, coincident with the appearance of the 3β-hydroxysteroid dehydrogenase-Δ^5-isomerase complex and the initiation of male sex differentiation of the somatic sex structures. Whereas in lower species fetal pituitary gonadotropins are required to initiate this prenatal testicular activity, in the human placenta chorionic gonadotropin also stimulates Leydig cell development. This probably explains why the external genitalia of male babies with anencephaly and presumptive pituitary gonadotropin deficiency usually differentiate normally in contrast to those of lower vertebrates hypophysectomized *in utero* (4, 234). Incomplete fusion of the labial folds and retention of the vaginal pouch in male infants may therefore be attributed to a primary testicular defect leading to deficient androgen secretion or failure of the target tissues to respond to androgenic stimulation. Conversely, if female infants are subjected *in utero* to androgenic stimulation from some extragonadal source, their ex-

ternal genitalia can exhibit any degree of masculinization, ranging from simple clitoral hypertrophy to the formation of a normal-appearing penis. Thus identical external abnormalities can be produced in the male by androgen deficiency (or failure of the target tissues to respond) or in the female by exposure to androgen from some pathologic source in the fetus or mother.

Hormonal Sex Differentiation (212)

Sex differentiation is not completed until the secondary sexual characteristics have developed and the ultimate goal, procreation, becomes possible. These developments as well as their timing are the culmination of less overt gonadal functions prior to this time (Fig. 8–18).

Maturation of Testicular Secretory Function

After the fetal Leydig cells have completed their intrauterine functions, they again revert into mesenchymal cells. Beginning about the eighteenth

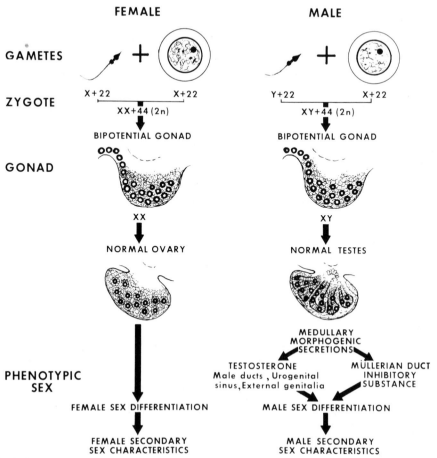

Figure 8–18. A diagrammatic representation of human sex determination and differentiation. Intrinsic or extrinsic factors adversely affecting any stage of these processes can lead to anomalies of sex. (Modified from Grumbach, M. M.[5])

to twentieth week there is a rapid decline in size and number, and at term they are sparse. There is a sharp peak in the concentration of plasma and testicular testosterone in the male fetus at 12 weeks, followed by a gradual decline to low levels by 24 weeks gestational age. Higher mean levels of serum testosterone are found in the male than in the female for the first six months after birth, after which there is no sex difference in testosterone values until the onset of puberty in the male. During childhood, the interstitial tissue gives little morphologic evidence of functional activity. At about the age of 11–12 years, following an increase in the secretion of LH, the mesenchymal cells again differentiate into mature Leydig cells and proliferate in nests between seminiferous tubules. There is a progressive increase in the concentration of plasma testosterone, beginning with the onset of puberty, which continues into late adolescence (201, 241). In some species, the major steroid product of the prepubescent testis is Δ^4-androstenedione rather than testosterone, and puberty is marked by a sharp reversal of this ratio in spermatic vein blood (212, 243). A similar reversal of the androstenedione:testosterone ratio in peripheral plasma, primarily due to a rise in testosterone, has recently been observed at puberty in human males (216). Testosterone is necessary for full maturation of the seminiferous tubules as well as for increase in muscle mass, deepening of the voice, a male pattern of sexual hair, and growth of the penis, prostate, and seminal vesicles.

Maturation of Ovarian Secretory Function (230, 261)

Since ovarian secretions play little or no role in the differentiation of either genital ducts or external genitalia, less is known about prenatal ovarian secretions than is the case with the testes. Winter and Faiman failed to detect either a higher concentration of estradiol in the fetal ovary than in fetal serum or a sex difference in the concentration of serum estradiol in male and female fetuses between the twelfth and twenty-fourth week of gestation. Postnatally, however, infantile mammary enlargement is more pronounced and often persists longer than in the male. During childhood, ovarian follicles exhibit irregular ripening and involution, and follicular cysts are not uncommon in sexually immature girls (260, 261). Nevertheless, before the ninth or tenth year, the ovary usually secretes too little estrogen to bring about cornification of the vaginal mucosa.

With the approach of adolescence, the cyclic ripening and involution of ovarian follicles is intensified, the fibrous stroma becomes more abundant, and there is an exaggerated tendency toward the development of ovarian cysts and hyperthecosis (248, 261). Rising estradiol levels (230) bring about development of nipples and mammary ducts, enlargement of the uterus, rounding of the body contours, and cornification of the vulvar and vaginal epithelium. Menarche signifies that sufficient estrogen has been secreted to elicit the requisite degree of endometrial proliferation.

There is now considerable evidence that an antecedent rise in the ovarian secretion of estradiol initiates the sharp preovulatory surge in LH and FSH. If the ovarian secretion is insufficient to raise and maintain the level of serum estradiol to a critical level for a sufficient period, the discharge of LH either does not occur or is insufficient to induce ovulation (242, 267) (see Ch. 7).

Ovulation and secretion of progesterone by corpora lutea do not usually occur until a number of anovulatory menstrual cycles have occurred. After ovulatory cycles are established, the proliferative endometrium is transformed into a secretory type, and the breasts become further rounded as alveoli are stimulated to develop. Although the period of physiologic sterility in adolescence is highly variable, studies of cultures in which adolescent sexual promiscuity is common suggests that ovulation does not usually occur until several years after the menarche (200).

Role of the Adrenal in Sex Differentiation

The capacity to secrete both androgens and estrogens is inherent in the adrenal glands as well as in the gonads of both sexes. During fetal life, the adrenal cortex is remarkably enlarged, primarily because of hyperplasia of the reticular zone. This fetal zone produces dehydroepiandrosterone sulfate in large quantity, and this substance in turn serves as the major precursor for estrogen synthesis by the placenta (213). Apparently the fetal pituitary is required for this enlargement of the adrenal, since babies with anencephaly lack this "fetal cortex" and the normal rise of estrogens in the mother during pregnancy does not take place (215). The contributions of the fetal zone of the adrenal to the hormonal environment of the fetus and mother in pregnancy are described more fully elsewhere.

Postnatally, remarkable involution of the fetal cortex occurs, and the adrenal secretion of androgens, which is relatively high at birth, falls off sharply. The urinary excretion of estrogen by the newborn also declines rapidly during the first few days of life (271). With the onset of adolescence, the adrenal again undergoes enlargement, largely because of proliferation of the zona reticularis, and the production of androgens and estrogens increases concomitantly (256, 265). In both sexes, androgenic hormones from both the adrenals and the gonads increase the growth rate and contribute to the development of increased muscle mass, sexual hair, and seborrhea. There is convincing evidence that the development of libido in women is primarily dependent upon adrenal androgens.

The changes in adrenal function at adolescence cannot be accounted for by increased secretion of ACTH, since there is no proportional increase in the secretion of 17-hydroxycorticoids (17-OHCS). The administration of estrogen to a prepubescent child stimulates both enlargement of the reticular zone and an increase in urinary 17-ketosteroids (17-KS). This effect is probably mediated through the pituitary, since it does not occur in hypopituitarism. Albright suggested that the "adrenarche" might be due to the secretion of luteinizing hormone (198).

The principal 17-KS secreted by the adrenal cortex are dehydroepiandrosterone (D), dehydroepiandrosterone sulfate (DS), and androstenedione (A). Although testosterone is also secreted in children with certain forms of congenital adrenal hyperplasia, most of the urinary testosterone of adrenal origin is formed by peripheral conversion of the other 17-KS. Elevations of A, D, and DS herald the onset of "adrenarche" and are also seen in both male and female children who develop pubic hair precociously (premature adrenarche) before other signs of sexual maturation appear (265).

Timing of Adolescence

Puberty is characterized by the development of secondary sex characteristics and the occurrence of the adolescent growth spurt, changes in body composition and behavior, an increase in strength, and the attainment of fertility. All of these developments derive from the maturation of the sex organs and the concomitant surge in secretion of sex hormones.

The time of onset of puberty and its course are variable. Marshall and Tanner have reviewed the pattern of pubertal changes in boys and girls (245, 246, 270) (see Chs. 6 & 7). Among the factors that affect the timing of puberty are inheritance and the genotype; socioeconomic factors, especially as they affect nutrition and general well-being; geography, including altitude; chronic disease; and light perception. The worldwide trend toward an earlier onset of physical maturity and toward an increase in adult height, e.g., the 3–4 month per decade advancement in age at menarche since 1830, seems mainly attributable to improved nutrition and general health and the concomitant earlier attainment of "critical weights."

Frisch and Revelle (217) have proposed the critical weight hypothesis derived from observations that the initiation of the weight growth spurt, the maximum rate of weight gain, and, in girls, menarche all occur at an "invariant mean weight" (about 47 kg. for menarche). The mean weight at menarche has not changed significantly in the United States and Western Europe over the past 125 years, but the age at which that weight is attained has decreased from 16.5 to 12.5 years (218). It has been suggested that the attainment of a critical body weight, representing a critical body composition, and the change to a critical metabolic rate is associated with a decrease in sensitivity of the hypothalamus to the negative feedback effect of sex steroids.

There is evidence that the hypothalamic-pituitary-gonadal circuit is operative in the human fetus, in whom pituitary and serum FSH and LH are present and appear to influence gonadal development and the growth of the external genitalia in the male fetus. Anencephalic, apituitary, and gonadotropin-deficient male fetuses have male differentiation, but have small testes, often undescended, and hypoplastic male external genitalia (241). By two years of age, the urinary excretion and concentration of serum FSH and LH are indistinguishable in males and females, but the mean values are higher than in children with multiple pituitary hormone deficiencies.

In normal prepubertal children between age 2 years and adolescence, small amounts of gonadotropins, mainly FSH, are excreted in the urine. The concentration of serum testosterone and estradiol is low, and there is no sex difference before the onset of puberty. That the hypothalamic-pituitary-gonadotropin-gonadal negative feedback mechanism is functional in prepubertal children is supported by a growing body of evidence (241). "Compensatory hypertrophy" has been described in the descended testis of prepubertal boys with unilateral cryptorchidism. Agonadal prepubertal children (e.g., as in the syndrome of gonadal dysgenesis) have elevated serum gonadotropins (mainly FSH). Small amounts of androgens or estrogens suppress urinary and plasma gonadotropins in prepubertal children (241). Hence the prepubertal gonads exert a restraining influence upon the hypothalamic "gonadostat" and the secretion of pituitary gonadotropins.

Present evidence suggests that at the onset of puberty the hypothalamic "gonadostat" exhibits decreased sensitivity to circulating sex steroids; this results in increasing release of gonadotropin releasing factor(s), LRF, and an orderly and sequential increase in the secretion of pituitary gonadotropins, followed by increased secretion of sex steroids by the testis and ovary (266). This change in hypothalamic sensitivity to sex steroids and the establishment of a new feedback setpoint at a higher level correlates with the general level of somatic maturity, as evidenced by skeletal age and with "critical weight." Young children have been observed to enter true puberty prematurely after exposure to exogenous sex hormones or after the removal of either virilizing or feminizing tumors. Similar observations have been recorded after the administration of sex steroids to rats (262). The development of true puberty under these circumstances correlates well with the degree of skeletal advancement.

Both sexual precocity and persistent sexual infantilism can be produced by diencephalic lesions, although little is known of the nature and precise loci of the controlling neural areas. The role of the pineal body and the secretion of melatonin (144), a pineal hormone, in primate puberty is not known.

Unlike the negative or inhibitory feedback mechanism that appears to differentiate in the fetus (222), the positive or stimulatory feedback mechanism responsible for the midcycle preovulatory surge of LH and FSH matures much later during midpuberty in human females.

Abundant data indicate that a critical concentration of plasma estrogen must be attained and maintained during the last part of the follicular phase to induce the ovulatory surge. The capacity of the cyclic system (positive feedback mechanism) to respond to the stimulatory action of estrogen is not elicitable before puberty is well advanced in the female (241). The administration of estrogen in such a manner as to produce the typical preovulatory rise in estrogen does not evoke a discharge of LH and FSH in individuals who are prepubertal or in early puberty, but it is effective at later stages of puberty and in adults. In addition to these two hypothalamic control mechanisms which undergo maturational changes with the onset of, and during, puberty, Boyar et al. (205) reported episodic secretion of LH during sleep in pubertal but not prepubertal children. The occurrence of periodic bursts of secretion of gonadotropins, which is superimposed on tonic secretion, is mediated by intrinsic CNS influences and is largely independent of the concentration of circulating sex steroids. Episodic secretion of gonadotropins first becomes apparent at puberty, at which time the discharge of gonadotropins is related to sleep; in the adult, there is no difference in the frequency or magnitude of episodic secretion of LH and FSH when awake or asleep. Recent studies have described the pattern of secretion during puberty of pituitary FSH and LH, testosterone, and estradiol in relation to skeletal age and the development of secondary sex characteristics (201, 230, 277) (Chs. 6 & 7).

The female skeleton is normally at all ages somewhat advanced beyond that of the male, and pubescence likewise occurs earlier in girls than in boys. These physiologic differences in timing are frequently exaggerated, since true sexual precocity occurs more commonly in females, whereas a physiologic delay in the onset of adolescence is predominantly a disorder of the male. Of interest is the greater FSH response to synthetic LRF in girls than in boys, which suggests that the pituitary of prepubertal girls contains more releasable FSH. Although studies of serum testosterone and estradiol in prepubertal children fail to reveal significant sexual differences until pubescence, ovaries undergo greater enlargement and exhibit far more histologic activity during childhood than do testes; these histologic differences suggest that the prepubescent ovary also has secretory activity. Thus the secretion of small amounts of estrogen or the conversion in extragonadal tissues of C-19 steroids to estrogens throughout the prepubescent years could at least in part explain both the more rapid skeletal maturation and the earlier onset of pubescence in the female.

Sexual Differentiation in the Hypothalamus and Pituitary (221)

Although in both sexes the control of gonadal function is mediated by both FSH and LH, the secretory patterns of the gonadotropins are very different in males and females. In man and many other species, the male pituitary gland characteristically secretes both FSH and LH in a relatively constant and sustained manner—so-called tonic release, whereas in the adult female, secretion of FSH and LH is cyclic and is characterized by a preovulatory surge which leads to ovulation.

In 1936, Pfeiffer reported studies in the rat suggesting that during the early postnatal period the pituitary becomes differentiated according to the nature of the gonads present in the individual (259). Subsequently it was shown, however, that the cyclic secretory pattern characteristic of the female pituitary is not an innate property of the pituitary itself. The pituitary of a male animal, when grafted under the hypothalamus of an adult female, is fully able to sustain the rhythm of repeated estrus cycles. When the male pituitary is grafted elsewhere in the recipient, ovulation fails to occur. Observations such as these suggest that the hypothalamus or higher neural centers function differently in the two sexes (212, 221, 224). It is now clear from the contributions of many workers that in the rat, mouse, hamster, and guinea pig there is an apparently inherent tendency toward the development of a female neurohypophysial pattern of gonadotropin release and that this pattern is converted to a male pattern if the newborn animal is exposed to androgens or estrogens during the neonatal period (204, 212, 221, 224); in the guinea pig, the androgen must be administered prenatally. Once the male pattern has been imprinted on the hypothalamus (usually by testicular androgens), the potential for cyclic activity on the part of the hypophysis is irrevocably lost. In the rat, the critical period is the first 10 days of life. Female rats given as little as 1 μg. of testosterone during this period develop permanent sterility, since gonadotropin secretion at maturity is sustained rather than cyclic, and ovulation does not occur. The ovaries of these rats develop multiple follicular cysts and no corpora lutea. Similarly, if male rats are castrated during the first few days of life, later ovarian implants form corpora lutea in a normal female manner.

In contrast, in man and subhuman primates, sex differentiation of the CNS mechanism mediating gonadotropin secretion has not been confirmed, even though testosterone has been administered to pregnant monkeys beginning early in gestation. Further evidence in support of species differences is the observation that most females with congenital virilizing adrenal hyperplasia, or females who have been exposed to androgens in utero, later develop normal ovulatory cycles, although cystic ovaries have been reported in rare patients (269). Moreover, in both men and male monkeys (240), the acute rise in concentration of serum estradiol following estrogen administration has elicited a surge in LH secretion; this suggests that in primates the potential for cyclic gonadotropin secretion is intact and that androgen-induced differentiation of the gonadotropin regulatory mechanism comparable to that described in rodents is not applicable to man.

Psychosexual Differentiation
(Gender Role)

By gender role is implied not only a person's legal and social designation of sex but also his psychosexual identification of himself in relation to other members of his own and the opposite sex. Outward manifestations of gender role are the dress, mannerisms, social comportment, and orientation of sexual impulses.

In lower species, the sexual role adopted at maturity is determined by the hormonal environment in early life (11, 211, 277). As is the case with other forms of sex differentiation, there appears to be an innate tendency toward the development of female sexual postures. Eventual development of male patterns of sexual behavior, on the other hand, is influenced to a large extent by whether there has been exposure to androgen in the prenatal period. This organizing capacity of certain androgens administered at a "critical stage" of development has been localized to specific areas in the brain. Once this has occurred, later castration of the male or exposure of the female to androgens may modify the intensity of the sexual drive but may not alter its pattern.

Studies of humans who have been reared in a sex opposite to their chromosomal or gonadal sex provide strong evidence that the gender role is not itself coded on the sex chromosomes, nor need it necessarily be concordant with the gonadal or hormonal sex (11, 238, 251, 253). Social and environmental influences during the early years of life exert such a strong impact on subsequent gender identity that some authors have discounted the importance of organic or hormonal influences. According to this concept, a newborn infant is neuter at birth, and the gender role is learned through early childhood experiences. A child is continually reminded of his sexual identification by the words and attitudes of those around him, by the clothes he wears, and by comparison of his own genitalia with those of others. In the absence of ambiguous attitudes on the part of the parents, sexual identity is well established by 18–30 months of age, even though there may exist some external genital discrepancy. Even the subsequent development of paradoxical secondary sexual characteristics and hormonal patterns characteristic of the opposite sex may not shake this conviction of sexual identity if it has been fixed with sufficient strength early in life. These considerations have an important bearing on the management of children born with ambiguous sexual characteristics.

In recent years, there has been a tendency to give stronger credence to the role of early hormonal influences on the patterning of adult sexual behavior in the human. Diamond (211) has reexamined the "neutrality at birth" hypothesis and presented arguments that humans, like other species, are already at birth, or very soon thereafter, predisposed to a male or female gender orientation, depending on whether or not an androgenic imprint has been left on the critical neural centers.

Most observers have failed to detect any evidence of hypogonadism or diminished virility in the majority of male homosexuals (11). This conclusion has recently been challenged by several studies which suggest that a substantial number of male homosexuals have abnormally low plasma testosterone levels. In 1971, Kolodny et al. (242a) reported that, among a population of normal and homosexual college men, approximately 25% of the latter group had plasma testosterone levels below the lowest recorded values in a normal control group. Similarly, the group with the lowest testosterone levels ranked among the most extreme on Kinsey's 6-point rating scale for homosexuality. Many of these men had low sperm counts as well. These findings might possibly be attributable to some poorly classified form of congenital hypogonadism resulting in incomplete masculinization of the neural centers controlling sexual behavior. Other explanations, however, are equally plausible. Psychologic factors exercise an important influence on both sperm counts and testosterone levels. Both fall markedly during depressive episodes, and conceivably homosexuality per se or some consequence of homosexuality could be responsible for the diminished gonadal function observed in these patients, rather than the reverse.

If prenatal exposure to androgen predisposes to a male gender role in humans, it might be expected that female infants who were virilized *in utero* might display male sexual attitudes and postures in later life. Ehrhardt et al. (213a) have found that prenatal virilization due to adrenal hyperplasia or maternal ingestion of progestogens does indeed influence the subsequent development of behavior, although to a limited extent. Such girls display tomboy behavior and greater interest in competitive sports than is usually expected of girls. They are often more interested in careers than romance and lack a strong interest in maternal doll play. However, they do not display lesbianism or loss of feminine gender identity, and most of them eventually achieve a satisfactory female sexual role in marriage.

The eventual outcome of this "nature" versus "nurture" controversy is of practical importance, since it might possibly alter the attitude of society towards transvestism and homosexuality. The evidence obtained in both hypogonadal males, the syndrome of feminizing testes, and prenatally virilized girls supports the thesis that exposure to androgens before birth does play a role in programming a male gender role in later life. In both groups, however, there is abundant evidence that these hormonal factors are rarely decisive and that the most important element in the development of gender role is the assigned sex of rearing and the reinforcement that this receives during the period of infancy and early childhood. If this reinforcement is weak because of ambiguous attitudes in the parents, the outlook for attaining a normal gender identity in adult life is greatly diminished. These interpretations are strongly supported by the empirical evidence obtained from the use of a pragmatic approach to the assignment of sex in patients with ambiguous genitalia. This approach, as outlined on page 491, has proven to be eminently successful and should not be lightly discarded.

CLASSIFICATION OF ERRORS IN SEX DIFFERENTIATION

Classification of individuals with hermaphroditic development according to their gonadal morphology has been the practice for many years and still has great usefulness. In the terminology introduced by Klebs, a *true hermaphrodite* is a person who possesses both ovarian and testicular tissue. A *male pseudohermaphrodite* is one whose gonads are exclusively testes but whose genital ducts or external genitalia or both exhibit in one or more respects the phenotypic characteristics of a female. A *female pseudohermaphrodite* is a person with exclusively ovarian gonadal structures, but whose genital development exhibits some masculine characteristics. This system of classification completely ignores the genetic sex of such hermaphroditic individuals and fails to include major errors of sex differentiation in which the genital structures are not ambiguous.

More recent attempts at classification have incorporated the rapidly advancing knowledge of chromosomal errors and other etiologic mechanisms into the old Klebs classification. This has been only partly successful, since clinically similar disorders may arise from widely divergent mechanisms, and the same mechanisms may cause a spectrum of disorders ranging from sexual ambiguity in some patients to only mild hypogonadism in others. The problem is further complicated by the many terms used to designate the same entity and by the propensity of each author to attach a different scope to each of his nosologic categories.

From a pragmatic standpoint, it has seemed advisable to group together sexual disorders due to abnormal gonadogenesis with or without chromosomal errors involving the X and Y chromosomes and to separate these disorders from forms of male and female pseudohermaphrodism due to other mechanisms (Table 8–5). Despite the convenience of this nosology, however, dysgenetic male pseudohermaphrodism (in which there is a defect in gonadogenesis) must be considered in the differential diagnosis of male pseudohermaphrodism and accordingly is listed in both categories.

Faulty gonadal differentiation often can be attributed to abnormalities of the sex chromosomes, and less commonly to a mutant gene. In these patients, the rest of the sexual phenotype correlates quite well with the structural differentiation of the gonad. Male or female pseudohermaphrodism arising in patients with fully differentiated gonads, on the other hand, is usually due to either a mutant gene or exposure to some abnormal hormonal influence. In these patients, the sexual karyotype is usually normal, and some aspect of the sexual phenotype is paradoxical to the gonadal morphology. Lastly, it has seemed advisable to treat separately an assorted group of sexual anomalies in which the etiology is unknown and in which there is little or no sexual ambiguity. The main feature that these disorders have in common is that they would confuse an otherwise tidy scheme if included elsewhere.

SEX CHROMOSOME ANOMALIES AND DISORDERS OF GONADAL DIFFERENTIATION

Not all patients with anomalies of their sex chromosomes have abnormal gonads and, conversely, congenital defects in gonadal differentiation cannot always be ascribed to detectable chromosomal errors. The association is so frequent, however, that these topics are now inseparable. Exceptions to this association are often of special importance in defining the chromosomal requirements for normal gonadogenesis.

Seminiferous Tubule Dysgenesis; Klinefelter's Syndrome and its Variants

XXY Seminiferous Tubule Dysgenesis (Typical Klinefelter's Syndrome)

Seminiferous tubule dysgenesis is one of the most common forms of primary hypogonadism and infertility in the male, with an increased prevalence in mentally retarded males. Concepts of this syndrome have been modified considerably since 1942, when it was first defined as a clinical entity by Klinefelter, Reifenstein, and Albright. As originally described, the characteristic features, which first become manifest during adolescence, were gynecomastia, a variable degree of eunuchoidism, small atrophic testes with hyalinization of the seminiferous tubules and aggregation of Leydig cells, aspermatogenesis, and increased urinary excretion of gonadotropin. In 1956, several groups found that a high proportion of patients with this syndrome were X chromatin-positive in contrast to their phenotypic male appearance. Soon thereafter, the syndrome was separated into a chromatin-positive form and a less common chromatin-negative form. Although the clinical features of the two groups were similar, subtle differences were found in the histologic structure of the testes in the two forms. Mental retardation is associated primarily with the chromatin-positive group. The chromatin-negative group of patients usually have a normal XY karyotype (Ch. 6). The present discussion is concerned primarily with the chromatin-positive group.

In 1959, Jacobs and Strong (119) and Ford et al. (88) first reported an XXY sex chromosome constitution in patients with this disorder, thus explaining the positive chromatin pattern. More recently, a variety of other sex chromosome complexes, including mosaicism, have been described. Virtually all these variants have in common the presence of

TABLE 8–5.   CLASSIFICATION OF ANOMALOUS SEXUAL DEVELOPMENT

Condition	Distinguishing Features

I. Disorders of gonadal differentiation
  A. Seminiferous tubular dysgenesis (Klinefelter's syndrome)
  B. Syndrome of gonadal dysgenesis and its variants (Turner's syndrome)
  C. True hermaphrodism
  D. Familial and sporadic XX and XY gonadal dysgenesis and their variants
  E. Other forms
	1. Usually attributable to anomalous sex chromosomes: karyotype, X chromatin and Y bodies variable
	2. Differentiation of genital ducts, external genitalia, and hormonal sex concordant with gonadal histology
	3. Frequently associated with mental retardation and somatic abnormalities

II. Female pseudohermaphrodism
  A. Congenital virilizing adrenal hyperplasia
  B. Androgens and synthetic progestogens transferred from maternal circulation
  C. Malformations of intestine and urinary tract
  D. Other teratologic factors
	1. X chromatin–positive: XX karyotype
	2. Ovaries and internal ducts normal female
	3. External genitalia may range from mild clitoral hypertrophy to simulant cryptorchid male

III. Male pseudohermaphrodism
  A. Inborn errors of testosterone biosynthesis
    1. Errors affecting synthesis of both corticosteroids and testosterone (variants of congenital adrenal hyperplasia)
      (a) Cholesterol 20α-hydroxylase deficiency (congenital lipoid adrenal hyperplasia)
      (b) 3β-hydroxysteroid dehydrogenase deficiency
      (c) 17α-hydroxylase deficiency
    2. Errors primarily affecting testosterone biosynthesis
      (a) 17,20-desmolase (lyase) deficiency
      (b) 17β-hydroxysteroid oxidoreductase deficiency (Reifenstein's syndrome?)
  B. End-organ insensitivity to androgenic hormones
    1. Complete syndrome of testicular feminization
    2. Incomplete syndrome of testicular feminization
  C. Male pseudohermaphrodism with normal virilization at puberty (Delay of onset of Leydig cell function, or transient fetal Leydig cell insufficiency)
    1. Familial perineal hypospadias with ambiguous development of urogenital sinus and male puberty (pseudovaginal perineoscrotal hypospadias)
    2. Less severe forms of hypospadias
  D. Ambiguous genitalia due to dysgenetic male pseudohermaphrodism
    1. X chromatin–negative variants of the syndrome of gonadal dysgenesis (e.g., XO,XY; XYp–)
    2. Incomplete form of XY gonadal dysgenesis
  E. Associated with degenerative renal disease
  F. Female genital ducts in otherwise normal men (uteri herniae inguinale)
  G. Maternal ingestion of estrogens or progestogens
  H. Other forms
	1. X chromatin–negative; XY karyotype
	2. Testes only; some authors exclude dysgenetic testes due to chromosomal anomalies from this group, but for clinical considerations this category is listed in D
	3. Genital ducts usually male
	4. External genitalia from mild hypospadias to simulant female attributable to:
	  (a) insufficient production of testosterone by fetal testes during period of sex differentiation
	  (b) defect in response of target tissues to androgen

IV. Unclassified forms of abnormal sexual development
  A. In males
    1. Cryptorchidism
    2. Anorchia (the "vanishing testes" syndrome)
    3. Familial forms of primary hypogonadism and gynecomastia (Rosewater syndrome)
  B. In females
    1. Absence or anomalous development of uterus and fallopian tubes
    2. Congenital absence of the vagina
	Heterogeneous group of disorders in which the etiology is uncertain. Some may be variants of other forms of intersexuality. Sex chromosomes, however, are presumptively normal, and ambiguity of genitalia is not usually a prominent feature.

at least two X chromosomes and a Y chromosome, except for the rare group with only an XX constitution.

The differentiation of testes and lack of ovarian differentiation in patients with an XXY, and more strikingly an XXXXY complement, indicates that the male-determining genes on a single Y chromosome are sufficient to bring about male sex differentiation in the presence of as many as four X chromosomes. This may be explained by the fact that the testis-determining genes on the Y cause testes to differentiate earlier in fetal life than do ovaries. Thus the direction of differentiation may have already been fixed before ovarian differen-

tiation could be initiated, a possibility that is consistent with Jost's interpretation of gonadogenesis.

Clinical Features (93, 149).   The only constant clinical features of chromatin-positive seminiferous tubule dysgenesis are small, usually firm testes that measure less than 3 cm. in length (and often less than 1.5 cm.), sterility, and a male phenotype (Fig. 8–19). The disorder should be suspected in prepubertal males with abnormally small testes (length, volume) and in boys who have personality and behavioral disorders with or without intellectual subnormality, relatively long legs, and small external genitalia (46). Detection of X

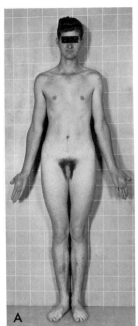
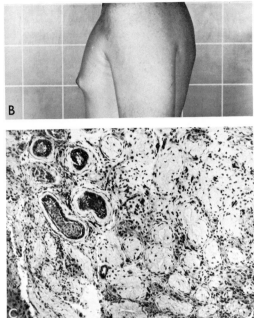
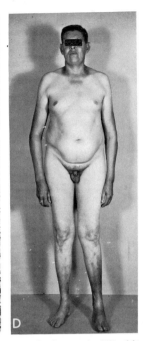

Figure 8-19. A, Typical 19-year-old phenotypic male with chromatin-positive seminiferous tubule dysgenesis (Klinefelter's syndrome). This patient had a positive X chromatin pattern and an XXY karyotype. His 17-ketosteroid excretion was 11.2 mg./24 hr. and urinary gonadotropin excretion > 100 m.u. These patients vary widely in their habitus and degree of virilization. B, This patient was well virilized but had long extremities with eunuchoidal proportions and exhibited gynecomastia. The testes measured 1.8 × 0.9 cm. and were small and firm. Testicular biopsy, C, revealed a severe degree of hyalinization of his seminiferous tubules and Leydig cell hyperplasia. D, Forty-eight-year-old man with chromatin-positive Klinefelter's syndrome who came to medical attention only because his severe leg varicosities were thought to reveal a "female trait."

chromatin in buccal mucosal nuclei of such boys supports the diagnosis; karyotype analysis can then be performed in the Barr body–positive patients. Gynecomastia and signs of androgen deficiency occur in more than half of the cases and usually become evident during puberty, which may be delayed. Hypospadias and true cryptorchidism are rare. Patients with this syndrome tend to be taller than average, mainly because of the disproportionate length of their legs (93,149). This finding is often present before clinical signs of puberty are evident and may not be accompanied by a proportional increase in span (46). The eunuchoidal proportions cannot be attributed to delayed epiphyseal fusion, since skeletal maturation follows a normal male pattern (181). Prominent gynecomastia seems more common in patients with normal stature and body proportions. The excretion of urinary FSH and LH and the concentration of plasma FSH and LH are increased, while the concentration of plasma testosterone is often less than the normal range for men and shows decreased response to the administration of chorionic gonadotropin (149). Urinary estrogen values and the secretion of estrogen are usually within the range for normal men. Diminished potency is common in the adult patient. These findings are consistent with impaired Leydig cell function. Gynecomastia and eunuchoidal proportions correlate better with gonadotropin levels in the urine than with estrogen excretion (Ch. 6).

About one in four XXY patients is mentally retarded (63). There is an increased frequency of psychopathology, including antisocial behavior and delinquency.

Associated Abnormalities. Plunkett et al. and others have reported abnormalities of thyroid function, such as decreased uptake of radioactive iodine and a poor response to thyroid stimulating hormone (TSH) (154). Although it has been suggested that thyroid disease may be more frequent in these patients, there is as yet insufficient information on this matter. Ferguson-Smith et al. did not find an increased incidence of thyroid antibodies in this disorder, in contrast to these findings in the syndrome of gonadal dysgenesis.

The frequency of mild diabetes mellitus is increased. Nielsen et al. reported that, in a group of 31 patients, in 39% the glucose tolerance test indicated diabetes; 19% of their mothers had diabetes mellitus (143).

Jackson et al. suggested that XXY patients with gynecomastia have an increased predisposition for cancer of the breast (118), and this has been confirmed by Harnden (110). In a survey of 187 males with breast cancer, 8 patients with chromatin-positive seminiferous tubule dysgenesis were detected, about 18 times the expected prevalence (110). There is some evidence to suggest that chronic pulmonary disease and varicose veins may also be more prevalent in adults with Klinefelter's syndrome. Although statistical studies are lacking, it is the impression of some observers that these patients are uncommonly prone to ill health from a variety of somatic ailments.

Frequency. Surveys of the prevalence of a positive X chromatin pattern among phenotypic males in newborn nurseries have disclosed an incidence of about one in 500. Among 14,526 infants studied in the three largest series, there were 30 who were chromatin-positive (135). The karyotypes of 18 chromatin-positive male infants included 12 XXY, one XXYY, and five XY,XXY mosaics. Since an XY cell line may modify the clinical syndrome and even lead to the development of fertile testes, XXY patients with XY mosaicism may not exhibit the clinical features of the syndrome. The frequency of chromatin-positive males in institutions for the mentally retarded is about one in 100 (134). Concurrent trisomy 21 and XXY seminiferous tubule dysgenesis have also been described in mentally retarded patients, but it is not known whether this is a significant association or a chance occurrence.

Whereas an XO constitution has a highly unfavorable effect on survival of the embryo and young fetus, decreased intrauterine viability has not been evident in XXY embryos and fetuses.

Testicular Lesion. The changes in the histologic structure of the testis which occur with age in XXY individuals are noteworthy (82, 104, 180). Blanc and Grumbach studied the testes of a chromatin-positive premature male infant, weighing 1700 g. and found that the histology was normal, including the complement of germ cells and the appearance of the seminiferous tubules and Leydig cells (5). Subtle changes were detected in the testes of other XXY patients in later infancy and childhood. The main feature at this stage of development is a diminished number of spermatogonia (182). In considering the pathogenesis of the testicular lesion in XXY seminiferous tubule dysgenesis, it seems that a normal or near-normal complement of spermatogonia is present until late in fetal life. During the late prenatal period and early infancy, a drastic loss of germ cells apparently occurs. This reduction in the germ cell complement in XXY individuals may represent an exaggeration of the normal degeneration of spermatogonia that occurs in the perinatal period. Excessive germ cell loss could occur either because of defective maturation or from failure of the germ cells to migrate to the periphery of the tubule and to align themselves in apposition to the basement membrane (Fig. 8–26, p. 437) (5).

With the approach of adolescence, and even before pubertal signs are well advanced, the action of pituitary gonadotropins on the intrinsically defective testis induces progressive hyalinization of the seminiferous tubules and pseudoadenomatous clumping of Leydig cells. However, the mean volume of Leydig cells is usually normal. After pubescence, the testes are characterized by small dysgenetic tubules which have undergone arrested development and often early fibrosis and hyalinization (180). Peritubular elastic tissue is usually absent in the small dysgenetic tubules and diminished in the others (82). That gonadotropin secretion plays a direct or indirect role in bringing about this change was illustrated in a 7-year-old XXXY male with precocious puberty and elevated urinary gonadotropins. Unlike the relatively nor-

mal architecture that is found in most boys of this age with Klinefelter's syndrome, the testes of this boy exhibited extensive hyalinization and fibrosis of the tubules and clumping of Leydig cells (Fig. 8–20).

Hyalinization of the tubules is usually extensive but varies considerably in degree from patient to patient and even between the testes of the same patient. The fibrosis tends to progress with age, and in some older patients few tubules can be identified. Conversely, in an occasional patient, the tubules are lined by Sertoli cells, tubular fibrosis is relatively slight, and the histologic appearance closely resembles that of germinal cell aplasia. Rarely, spermatogenesis is found in isolated tubules, and there have been sporadic reports of alleged paternity; most of these cases have proved to have had sex chromosome mosaicism; in others acceptable documentation of paternity has not been provided. Those fertile patients who were proven to have XY,XXY mosaicism often lacked features that otherwise distinguished them from typical Klinefelter's syndrome. The XY,XXXY patient of Barr et al. who was detected in a survey of mentally retarded males had normal-sized testes with active spermatogenesis (28). Cultures of the peripheral blood lymphocytes grew out only an XY cell line, but cultures of the skin and testes revealed the mosaicism.

Origin of XXY Constitution. XXY males may develop from nondisjunction of the sex chromosomes during either the first or second meiotic division in either parent or from mitotic nondisjunction in the zygote at the time of or following fertilization (Figs. 8–3 and 8–12). The evidence suggests that both meiotic and mitotic errors occur (Fig. 8–21). Fertilization of either an XX ovum by a Y-bearing sperm or of an X-ovum by an XY-bearing sperm would yield an XXY zygote. Mitotic nondisjunction of the sex chromosomes in an XY zygote could yield an XXY and a YO daughter cell (Fig. 8–21). Since the YO cell line is nonviable, only the XXY cell line would survive.

The abnormalities of meiosis just discussed almost always occur in a parent with a normal sex chromosome constitution. However, Rosenkranz has described two XXY patients, one of whose mothers was XXX and the other an XX,XXX mosaic (164). Whether an XXY karyotype is derived from a polysomic X constitution in the mother more frequently than previously suspected remains to be determined.

Pedigree studies using X-linked markers, such as color vision, Xg blood group, serum Xm group, and G-6-PD have disclosed that, in informative pedigrees, both X's are of maternal origin ($X^M X^M Y$) in 72.5% of cases and one X is paternal ($X^M X^P Y$) in 27.5% (70, 160). Similar observations have been made in mice (166).

Ferguson-Smith et al. (83) and others (93) have reported a positive association with advanced maternal age in XXY patients, although this association is less marked than in mongolism. These data suggest that a high proportion of $X^M M^M Y$ cases may result from nondisjunction during oögenesis

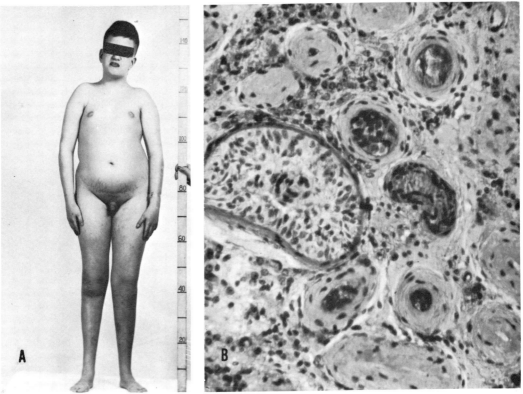

Figure 8–20. *A,* An 8 8/12-year-old boy with an XXXY sex chromosome constitution, mental retardation, precocious sexual development, and accelerated growth. Appearance of pubic hair noted at age 6. By 8 years acne, a deep voice, tall stature, and axillary hair were present. Height 148 cm. (+2.9 SD); weight 47.7 kg. (+3.9 SD); span 140 cm.; upper segment/lower segment = 0.87. Testes measured 2.1 × 1.3 cm. Note long legs, prognathism, small hands and feet, and the gynecomastia and secondary sexual characteristics. IQ 62. Urinary 17-KS 3.2 mg./day; urinary gonadotropins > 10 m.u., < 50 m.u./day. Bone age 13½ years. Buccal smear contained diploid nuclei with a maximum of two X chromatin bodies. Karyotype of cells derived from skin and blood was 48, XXXY. *B,* Testicular biopsy showed hyalinized tubules and clumping of Leydig cells; germ cells were absent. The findings suggest that the precocious puberty, with stimulation of the juvenile testes by pituitary gonadotropin, led to the premature appearance of the typical histologic changes of seminiferous tubule dysgenesis. (From Grumbach, M. M., Morishima, A., et al.: Unpublished data.)

rather than from mitotic nondisjunction in the first cell division of an XY zygote. Data in the $X^M X^P Y$ group suggest that paternal nondisjunction is not dependent on age (83), a finding also reminiscent of autosomal trisomies.

Etiologic Factors. The most important factor so far imputed in the etiology of an XXY sex chromosome constitution is advanced maternal age (83, 93). As discussed on page 435, the maternal age effect in chromosome abnormalities may be a consequence of the long diplotene stage of human ova. They remain suspended in prophase of the

Figure 8–21. The origin of an XXY sex chromosome constitution. The superscripts M and P designate respective matriclinous and patriclinous X chromosome. The interrupted circle indicates a nonviable cell line. (From Grumbach, M. M., In *Cecil-Loeb Textbook of Medicine.* 13th ed. Beeson, P. B., and McDermott, W. (eds.), Philadelphia, W. B. Saunders Company, 1971, p. 1811.)

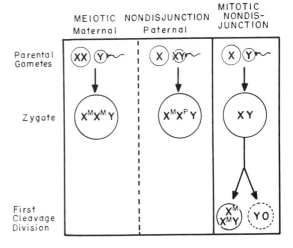

first meiotic division from birth to ovulation, which may not occur for 40 years or longer. The defective segregation of the two X chromosomes could be caused, at least in part, by reduction of the chiasma between certain chromosomes as the length of the diplotene stage increases. As in gonadal dysgenesis, there is also suggestive evidence that the prevalence of twinning in sibships of XXY individuals is increased (180).

Genetic factors that predispose to nondisjunction may also be important and have been demonstrated in lower species. While chromosome abnormalities are usually sporadic, a number of pedigrees have been reported in which leukemia and different chromosome abnormalities have occurred in siblings and relatives. In addition, patients with two coexisting forms of trisomy seem to be found more frequently than expected by chance alone. The role of radiation and viruses as predisposing factors is not known.

Other Sex Chromosome Abnormalities and the Clinical Variants of X Chromatin — Positive Seminiferous Tubule Dysgenesis

Sex chromosome aberrations other than XXY have been associated less commonly with this syndrome. These patients have tended to show more severe defects than have the XXY cases.

XXYY. This group of patients not only have the typical features of the syndrome but also may exhibit several additional characteristics (30, 95, 95a). They comprise about 3% of chromatin-positive phenotypic males. Almost all of the reported patients have been mentally retarded. The XXYY karyotype is usually associated with tall stature (the mean height of 26 patients is 181 cm. compared with 172 cm. for XXY males), disproportionately long lower extremities, often delinquent behavior, and unusual dermatoglyphic patterns. Peripheral vascular disease, especially varicose veins, and stasis dermatitis are prevalent in this group. The X chromatin pattern is indistinguishable from that of the XXY group; however, two Y bodies are present in a high proportion of somatic nuclei. In two informative pedigrees, the Xg blood groups indicated that the father contributed an X as well as the two Ys, which suggests that fertilization of an X ovum by an XYY sperm (arising by successive nondisjunction in the first and second meiotic divisions) is the usual origin of XXYY individuals.

XXXY and XXXYY. All of the reported patients with an XXXY karyotype have been mentally retarded, usually to a more severe degree than in the XXY group (49). A few patients have had minor skeletal anomalies (Fig. 8–20), including radio-ulnar synostosis in about 10% of patients. The XXXYY patient reported had a prominent jaw and was 76 inches tall. Duplicate X chromatin bodies are present in a variable proportion of diploid nuclei.

XXXXY. More than 35 subjects with this karyotype have been described (195) since the first report of Fraccaro et al. in 1960 (91). The diagnosis may be suspected before puberty from the clinical picture. In addition to mental deficiency, often of a severe degree, these patients tend to exhibit certain phenotypic similarities including (a) a variety of skeletal abnormalities, especially radio-ulnar synostosis, and (b) hypoplastic external genitalia with a small penis, underdeveloped scrotum, and very small and frequently undescended testes; the appearance of the external genitalia may be ambiguous, owing to hypospadias, bifid scrotum, hypoplastic phallus, and cryptorchidism. In adult patients, gynecomastia is absent and androgen deficiency is severe. Before puberty, the testes often contain hypoplastic seminiferous tubules. Other described anomalies include congenital heart disease, cleft palate, strabismus, and microcephaly. The facies not infrequently has a characteristic appearance: mandibular prognathism, hypertelorism, strabismus, and myopia. These patients have three chromatin bodies in a proportion of their diploid nuclei.

XX. De la Chapelle has analyzed 45 cases of phenotypic males (70). In general, the clinical features and hormone values were similar to those of X chromatin–positive Klinefelter's syndrome. However, XX males were shorter (mean height 168 cm.) than XXY or normal males but taller than normal females, and their skeletal proportions were usually normal. Intellectual subnormality, behavioral disorders, and mental illness seemed to occur less frequently than with XXY seminiferous tubule dysgenesis. Mean maternal age was not advanced. The histology of the testes was usually indistinguishable from that of XXY males but, in some cases, the morphology was that of the syndrome of germinal cell aplasia or intermediate between the two. Although evidence of sex chromosome mosaicism was extensively sought, no evidence of Y-bearing cell lines was detected in the multiple tissues examined, including the testes. Barr body, Y body, autoradiography, and G-band studies were all consistent with an XX karyotype. No evidence of a brightly fluorescent segment comparable to all or a part of the distal long arm of the Y chromosome has been found on any of the X chromosomes or on an autosome; this, however, is not the portion of the Y that contains testes determiners.

Three theories have been advanced to explain this rare but interesting example of sex reversal: a mutant autosomal gene that leads to testicular differentiation in an XX fetus, as described in the goat and mouse; X-Y interchange at paternal meiosis, with translocation or insertion of male determiners into the X (or an autosome); and mosaicism with an undetected Y-containing cell line or one that has been lost. The distribution of blood group Xg^a positive and negative individuals in 33 cases appeared more likely to represent an XXY than an XY distribution, as do the Xm serum group phenotypes, observations which are consistent with the maternal origin of both X's in these patients. De la Chapelle has reviewed the evidence for each of the three hypotheses and none can be definitely excluded. Although the origin of these XX males may be heterogeneous, he favored the possibility that at least some cases arise as a consequence of mosaicism in which an XY or XXY cell line has either been lost or remains undetected.

XY,XXY and Other Mosaics. Second only to the XXY constitution, XY,XXY mosaicism is the most frequent karyotype encountered in phenotypic males with positive X chromatin patterns. As in the syndrome of gonadal dysgenesis, the normal cell line may have a beneficial effect in preventing manifestations of the syndrome (99, 136). Patients with well-documented fertility have been described in this group (62).

Origin of Other Sex Chromosome Abnormalities. The other karyotypes described in this syndrome may arise by single or successive disjunctional errors during meiosis in one or both parents or during mitosis after fertilization. Some of the errors may be due to a combination of meiotic and mitotic nondisjunction. The XX,XXY and XY,XXY mosaics may be explained by chromosome loss due to anaphase lag in an XXY zygote.

Pedigree studies using marker genes on the X chromosome revealed that all the X chromosomes were of maternal origin in two XXXXY individuals ($X^MX^MX^MX^MY$) and in two XXXY patients. In one XXYY patient, the X as well as the two Y chromosomes were of paternal origin (X^MX^PYY) (160). In other than the XXY group, late maternal age has not been an apparent etiologic factor.

The Syndrome of Gonadal Dysgenesis; Turner's Syndrome and its Variants (5, 15, 61, 78, 84, 130, 140, 156, 185)

In 1938, Turner described seven phenotypic females who exhibited dwarfism, sexual infantilism, webbing of the neck, and cubitus valgus. Subsequent studies of this intriguing syndrome and its variants have contributed more to the evolution of our current concepts of sex differentiation than have studies in any other group of patients.

In the early 1940's Albright et al. and Varney and associates found that the excretion of urinary gonadotropin was increased in affected adolescents and adults. Wilkins and Fleischmann soon thereafter described the gonads as bilateral, pale "streaks" of connective tissue situated in the mesosalpinges and devoid of any germ cells (191). In 1950, Wilkins proposed, in the light of Jost's fetal castration experiments in the rabbit, that some of these functionally agonadal patients might be genetic males, since fetal castration of either sex invariably leads to a female phenotype (16). The discovery in 1954 that many of these patients, contrary to their phenotype, were X chromatin-negative seemed initially to confirm the hypothesis that some of these patients were indeed genetic males (67, 155, 192). However, in 1959, soon after techniques became available to determine the actual chromosome constitution, Ford et al. reported that the sex chromosome constitution in a 14-year-old phenotypic female with this syndrome was XO rather than XY (89). Work in many

laboratories has now defined more precisely the chromosomal basis of this and related disorders (61, 84, 130, 140).

The absence of a second sex chromosome (X chromosome monosomy) is associated with four cardinal features: (1) female phenotype, (2) short stature, (3) sexual infantilism owing to rudimentary gonads, and (4) a variety of associated somatic abnormalities. Any or all of these features may be modified by the presence of lesser degrees of sex chromosome deficiency. It is therefore useful to consider the syndrome of gonadal dysgenesis and its variants as a continuum of clinical features ranging from those of the typical XO phenotype to a normal female or male. The functional importance of chromosomal additions to the basic XO pattern can be deduced from the extent to which they modify toward normal, in at least some cases, the dwarfism, sexual infantilism, and somatic anomalies that typify the patient with complete sex chromosome monosomy.

Partial sex chromosome monosomy may be attributed to a structurally abnormal second sex chromosome (X or Y), sex chromosome mosaicism involving an XO cell line, or both a structural abnormality and mosaicism.* It is important to emphasize, however, that even though the modified clinical forms are almost invariably associated with partial sex chromosome monosomy, the contrary is not necessarily true; apparently identical partial sex chromosome monosomies in other patients may be associated with the typical clinical picture found in XO patients. For this reason, classifications of these variants based solely on sex chromosome constitution tend to be confusing. Subdivision of these variants according to their X chromatin pattern, however, is helpful, since this test is readily available and immediately discloses the presence or absence of X chromosome additions to the monosomic X. X chromatin-positive patients tend to fall within the clinical spectrum ranging from sexually infantile females to normal females, whereas X chromatin-negative patients usually range between sexually infantile females and hypogonadal males. There are numerous exceptions to these generalizations, however, most of which may be explained by sex chromosome mosaicism.

Typical Turner's Syndrome (XO Gonadal Dysgenesis) (7, 84, 136)

Of those cases displaying all the cardinal features that typify sex chromosome monosomy, the X chromatin pattern is negative in about 80% (4); most of these have an XO sex chromosome constitution. The remainder of the chromatin-negative cases with other sex chromosome patterns and all the chromatin-positive cases represent instances

---

*The term "partial monosomy" is usually limited to deletion or deficiency of one chromosome in a homologous pair. In this section, the authors have included mosaicism in this definition.

in which the additional sex chromosomal material fails to be clinically manifested.

Associated Somatic Stigmata. The typical patient (Fig. 8–22) is often recognizable by her distinctive facies in which micrognathia, epicanthal folds, prominent, low-set or deformed ears or both, a fishlike mouth, and ptosis are present with varying degrees of frequency. The chest is usually square and shieldlike with microthelia. The neck is short and often broad with a low hairline in back. Webbing of the neck is present in 40% of the patients and coarctation of the aorta in 10–20%. Those with coarctation almost universally also have webbing of the neck. Additional anomalies include cubitus valgus, congenital lymphedema of the feet and hands (30%) (Fig. 8–23) or, more fre-

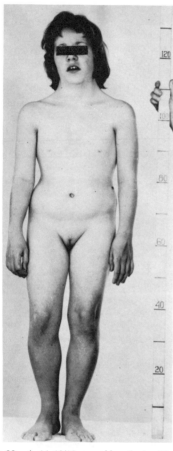

Figure 8–22. A 14 10/12-year-old patient with the typical form of the syndrome of gonadal dysgenesis (Turner's syndrome). The X chromatin pattern is negative and the karyotype 45, XO. She is short (height 134.5 cm.; height age 9 5/12 years), sexually infantile except for the appearance of sparse pubic hair, and exhibits characteristic stigmata of the syndrome. There is a short webbed neck, shield-like chest with widely separated nipples, bilateral metacarpal signs, puffiness over the dorsum of the fingers, cubitus valgus, and increased number of pigmented nevi. The facies is characteristic and the ears are low set. The bone age is 13 6/12 years; urinary 17-KS 5.1 mg/day; urinary gonadotropin > 100 m.u./day. Vaginal smears and the urocytogram showed an immature pattern in which cornified squamous cells were absent. With estrogen therapy, female secondary sex characteristics were induced; the cyclic administration resulted in periodic estrogen-withdrawal bleeding.

quently, puffiness of the dorsum of the fingers, short fourth metacarpal (50%), renal abnormalities (60%), high-arched palate, a variety of skeletal anomalies, an excessive number of pigmented nevi, tendency to keloid formation, hypoplastic nails, recurrent otitis media, perceptive hearing loss, unexplained hypertension (15%), and, rarely, gastrointestinal bleeding secondary to intestinal telangiectasia. The incidence of mental retardation is not increased. Money (251) has reported that impairment of directional sense and space-form recognition is a common occurrence; this cognitive disability results in a lower mean performance IQ than is found in the general population, whereas verbal ability is not affected. Severe psychopathic manifestations are uncommon, in contrast to the XXY individuals who also exhibit an increased frequency of mental retardation.

The eponym "Bonnevie-Ullrich syndrome" has been applied to phenotypic female infants who have lymphedema of the distal extremities and loose folds of skin over the back of the neck in addition to the other classic features of gonadal dysgenesis (Fig. 8–24) (102). Pleural effusions and ascites that clear spontaneously are not uncommon (100), and, rarely, pericardial effusion has been reported. The serous effusions, as well as the lymphedema, are attributable to defects in the lymphatic system. XO abortuses commonly exhibit generalized edema and a large hygroma of the neck (173). The latter abnormality results in webbing of the neck postnatally.

In addition to coarctation of the aorta, the commonest cardiovascular abnormalities, aortic stenosis and bicuspid aortic valve, may occur as conjoint or separate defects. Coarctation and cystic medial necrosis of the aorta may lead to dissecting aneurysm. Other cardiovascular anomalies are uncommon, in contrast to the situation in pseudo-Turner's syndrome (p. 470).

The most common renal abnormalities are rotation of the kidney, horseshoe kidney, duplication of the renal pelvis and ureter, and hydronephrosis secondary to ureteropelvic obstruction. Abnormal differentiation of the kidneys and upper collecting system is found so commonly in this syndrome that routine intravenous urography is warranted.

Skeletal maturation is normal or only slightly delayed in childhood but lags in adolescence (181). In most cases, the skeleton exhibits localized areas of rarefaction, especially of the hands and feet, elbow, and upper femur (158). Adults who are not treated with estrogen often develop a severe form of the postmenopausal type of osteoporosis and may suffer from collapse of vertebrae. Osteochondrosis-like changes in the spine are commonly seen (158). In addition to the metacarpal sign (shortening of the fourth metacarpal), Kosowicz described a "carpal sign" characterized by a more acute angular configuration of the proximal row of carpal bones (127). The knee may show deformities of the medial tibial epicondyles, with obliquely tipped tibial epiphyses and medial projections of the tibial metaphyses. The pelvis tends to have a male-type inlet.

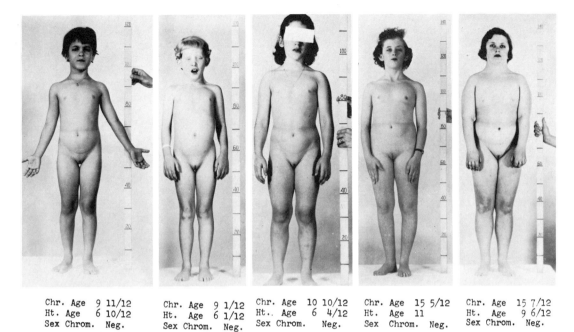

Chr. Age 9 11/12	Chr. Age 9 1/12	Chr. Age 10 10/12	Chr. Age 15 5/12	Chr. Age 15 7/12
Ht. Age 6 10/12	Ht. Age 6 1/12	Ht.. Age 6 4/12	Ht. Age 11	Ht. Age 9 6/12
Sex Chrom. Neg.	Sex Chrom. Neg.	Sex Chrom. Neg.	Sex Chrom. Neg.	Sex Chrom. Neg.

Figure 8-23. Variation in physical appearance in five patients with typical form of the syndrome of gonadal dysgenesis (Turner's syndrome). All these patients had an XO karyotype, and all had differences between their height age and chronological age of 3 years or more. (From Grumbach, M. M., In *Clinical Endocrinology, I.* Astwood, E. B. (ed.), New York, Grune & Stratton, 1960, p. 407.)

Short Stature. This feature is invariably present in XO individuals. The average height attained is 55 in., with a range of 48–58 in. The concentration of fasting serum immunoreactive GH and the response to insulin-induced hypoglycemia

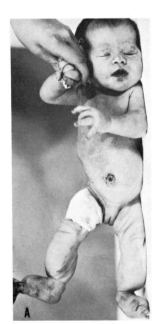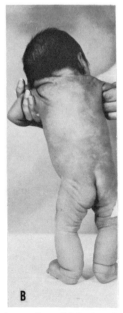

Figure 8-24. Infant with the syndrome of gonadal dysgenesis (karyotype XO) and associated lymphedema of the extremities. The term Bonnevie-Ullrich's syndrome is applied when this characteristic swelling of the feet or hands, or both is associated with other features of Turner's syndrome. (From Grumbach, M. M., and Barr, M. L.: *Recent Progr. Hormone Res. 14:*335, 1958.)

and arginine are normal. On the other hand, Almqvist et al. have reported elevated levels of serum sulfation factor (18). Although the administration of exogenous human growth hormone produces nitrogen retention, the response in terms of linear growth is usually modest, but high doses have accelerated growth in a few patients. Acromegaly has been described by Willemse in a woman with the typical syndrome; her height increased from 139 cm. to 154 cm. between the ages of 18 and 28 (193).

Intrauterine growth retardation is not uncommon in XO infants, and their mean birth weight is significantly below the mean weight for normal newborns of comparable gestational age (102, 130). The postnatal growth pattern of affected children is variable. Whereas some are retarded from birth, others grow at a relatively normal rate (within two standard deviations of the mean value for height) for the first 5 years of life. All the 62 XO children studied by Morishima and Grumbach were short at the time that they reached school age, however (140). The expected growth spurt at adolescence does not occur, irrespective of estrogen therapy.

Sexual Infantilism. The genital ducts and external genitalia in this syndrome are entirely female in character but immature. Located in the mesosalpinges parallel to the fallopian tubes are long, attenuated, pale, fibrous streaks of connective tissue. Typically, these streak-like or spindle-shaped structures consist of fibrous stroma arranged in whorls similar to those found in ovarian stroma, but they lack primordial follicles or seminiferous tubules. Vestigial medullary elements and rudimentary mesonephric tubules like those found deep in the primitive genital ridge are common at the hilus. After puberty, aggregates of epithelioid cells resembling Leydig or hilus cells are found in variable quantity.

Except for the development of sparse pubic and axillary hair, maturation of female secondary sex characteristics does not occur, and these patients remain sexually infantile and amenorrheic. The concentration of immunoreactive serum FSH and the excretion of urinary FSH is usually elevated beginning in infancy; it tends to fall in mid childhood, rising again to castrate levels after the age of 9 or 10 years. On the other hand, immunoreactive LH commonly is not increased until 10 years of age.

While the findings just described are the rule, exceptions have been well documented. Primordial follicles that contain oöcytes have been found in the ridge in some individuals (95, 189), and correlate with the rare occurrence of menarche and a variable but usually attenuated period of regular menses (5). Court Brown et al. described a woman with an XO karyotype who menstruated for 13 years (61). The most striking exception is in the report by Bahner and associates of a 32-year-old woman who gave birth to a normal son (21). Extensive search of the mother, including karyotype studies on fibroblasts cultured from her ovary, failed to show sex chromosome mosaicism.

Singh and Carr studied the gonadal ridges of eight spontaneously aborted embryos and fetuses ranging in gestational age from 5 weeks to 4 months (173). Primordial germ cells were observed in all eight specimens. Until the third month of gestation, no appreciable differences were noted between these gonads and those from XX fetuses; after that, an increase in connective tissue stroma and impaired formation of primordial follicles were found. These observations suggest that primordial germ cells seed the primitive gonad in XO gonadal dysgenesis but usually fail to mature into oöcytes and, quite likely, degenerate at an accelerated rate (Fig. 8–26) (140, 189). Apparently, two active X chromosomes are required in the human for oögonia to develop. The presence of some germ cells in the gonadal streak of XO infants is probably not unusual at birth, although it is an uncommon finding by later childhood. An alternative possibility that might explain the viability of oöcytes in some XO individuals is that a certain number of XO germ cells undergo mitotic nondisjunction with the formation of XX oögonia. This process normally occurs in the female creeping vole and serves as a sex-determining mechanism.

Clitoral enlargement is another rare finding in patients with an XO karyotype. Grumbach and Morishima studied one such case. The enlargement of the clitoris may be present at birth or first become manifest at puberty. Secretion of androgen by "Leydig cells" in the gonadal streak is a likely explanation of this.

Incidence in Abortuses, Newborns, and Twins. The frequency of a negative X chromatin pattern in live, newborn, phenotypic females is 0.37/1000, or 1/2700 (5 in a total of 13,642 female infants) (135). There is, however, a considerable loss of XO

embryos and fetuses. Carr found an XO karyotype in 5% of spontaneous abortuses (49, 50). It is estimated that the frequency of XO zygotes is 0.8%, probably the commonest chromosome anomaly in man, but less than 3% of XO conceptuses survive to term (50). Not only is an XO constitution associated with a high risk of intrauterine death; it also is accompanied by a higher mortality rate in infancy.

There is some evidence that the prevalence of monozygotic twinning in affected sibships is increased. Four pairs of XO monozygotic twins have been described, but mosaicism with an XO cell line appears to occur more frequently in monozygotic twins (161). Turpin described a pair of monozygotic twins, one of whom was an XO phenotypic female with gonadal dysgenesis and the other an XY male. Dent and Edwards reported monozygotic twins of opposite phenotypic sex, both of whom were XO,XY mosaics on lymphocyte culture; in this instance, however, chimerism with exchange of migrating cells via intrauterine vascular channels may have occurred.

Associated Disorders. Engel and Forbes studied the association between gonadal dysgenesis and other selected clinical disorders in 48 adult patients (mean age 42 years) (78). Positive associations were found with obesity, hypertension due to causes other than coarctation of the aorta, diabetes mellitus, Hashimoto's thyroiditis, precocious aging, achlorhydria, cataracts, and corneal opacity or scarring. There is an increased prevalence of thyroid antibodies (78, 86); decreased glucose tolerance is common in patients over the age of 16 years. IgG levels are reported to be lower than in normal males and females (19).

Origin of XO Constitution. An XO chromosome constitution may arise by a variety of chromosome errors (Figs. 8–3 and 8–12). It may be a consequence of nondisjunction or chromosome loss during gametogenesis in either parent, resulting in a sperm or ovum lacking any sex chromosome. Although errors of mitosis in a normal zygote often lead to mosaicism, a purely XO constitution may arise at the first cleavage division from anaphase lag with loss of a sex chromosome or, less likely, mitotic nondisjunction with failure of the complementary XXX or XYY cell line to survive (Fig. 8–3). There is indirect evidence to suggest that loss of one X or a Y chromosome between fertilization and the first cleavage division may be a frequent but not the only cause of the XO embryo (140).

Several lines of evidence support a mitotic error in this syndrome: (1) the lack of association with advanced maternal age, in contrast to chromatin-positive Klinefelter's syndrome (6, 42, 130); (2) the prevalence of sex chromosome mosaicism; (3) the increased frequency of twinning in sibships with an XO individual (142, 185); and (4) the occurrence of an XY monozygotic co-twin of an XO individual.

Family studies of such X-linked traits as color blindness and the Xg blood group indicate that loss of the paternally derived sex chromosome is more common than would be expected if either the maternally or paternally derived sex chromosome were lost randomly (160). An excess of X^MO over X^PO in mice has been found by Russell and Chu, who considered sex chromosome loss as the most likely mechanism for this chromosomal error (166).

The underlying cause of the sex chromosome abnormality is not known. An increased incidence of XO mice was noted by Russell following irradiation of the mother soon after mating (166). Recent observations of Williams et al. (194) and of Engel and Forbes (78) point to an increased frequency of thyroid autoimmunity in patients with the syndrome of gonadal dysgenesis and in their parents (86). Their observations and those of others suggest that the genetic predisposition to develop autoantibodies in one or both parents is associated with an increased prevalence of an XO constitution and certain other chromosomal abnormalities in their offspring.

The familial occurrence of XO gonadal dysgenesis is very rare (75).

Partial Sex Chromosome Monosomy and Clinical Variants of the Syndrome of Gonadal Dysgenesis

Sex chromosome abnormalities that can be regarded as examples of partial sex chromosome monosomy may or may not modify the expression of the classic XO phenotype (5, 84, 138, 140). Approximately 20% of patients with the typical syndrome of gonadal dysgenesis are X chromatin-positive. This group usually has a structurally abnormal X chromosome or, more commonly, sex chromosome mosaicism involving an XO cell line. Chromatin-positive and chromatin-negative clinical variants of the syndrome of gonadal dysgenesis will be discussed in relation to the more usual types of sex chromosome aberrations with which they may be associated. A diagrammatic scheme interrelating the variable effect of partial sex chromosome monosomy on the cardinal clinical features of the syndrome is shown in Figure 8-25.

In patients with sex chromosome mosaicism, the ratio in each gonad of XO primordial germ cells or blastemal components or both to those with a normal XX or XY constitution is probably the major determinant of whether the ultimate gonadal structure will be a streak, a hypoplastic ovary or testis, or a relatively normal gonad (5, 84, 140). The weight of evidence supports the notion that, after migration into the primitive gonad, primordial cells that bear an XO constitution degenerate more rapidly than do XX or XY germ cells. If germ cells fail to survive in the gonad, ovarian development will not occur (5, 6, 104, 170); if the gonadal blastemal components do not contain an appropriate number of XY cells, testicular development will not take place (Fig. 8-26).

The quantitative relation in peripheral tissues between XO cell lines and those with an XX or XY pattern may also be responsible for the variable effect of mosaicism on stature and associated somatic stigmata (5, 140).

In patients with single-cell lines of structurally abnormal sex chromosomes, the somatic and gonadal consequences appear to be related to the extent of the short- or long-arm deficiency of the second X or the Y chromosome (84, 140). Table 8-6 summarizes the correlation between structural abnormalities of the X and Y chromosome and the clinical manifestations. As yet, only a small number of cases have been studied by the new techniques for G and Q bands in order to establish better the structure of the abnormal sex chromosome. Structural abnormalities often result in mosaicism, owing to loss of the structurally abnormal chromosome from the stem-cell line.

X Chromatin--Positive Variants of Gonadal Dysgenesis (7, 84, 136, 140) (Fig. 8--27)

XO,XX; XO,XXX; and XO,XX,XXX Mosaicism. XO,XX mosaicism is the most common finding in patients with chromatin-positive gonadal dysgenesis and is second in frequency only to XO. Patients with these forms of mosaicism usually exhibit fewer of the associated somatic anomalies, are not invariably short, and may menstruate and even be fertile (7, 84, 136, 140). One gonad may be of the streak type and the contralateral gonad either a hypoplastic or normal ovary, or both ovaries may be either normal or hypoplastic. During a family survey for a leukocyte anomaly, Briggs et al. discovered fortuitously a normal grandmother with XO,XX,XXX mosaicism. Some appreciation of the variable clinical features may be gleaned from nine patients with these forms of mosaicism studied by Morishima and Grumbach (140). All had female external genitalia. Of seven who attained pubertal age, four showed some development of female secondary sex characteristics, and two menstruated regularly. One of these two has had three pregnancies. In some, no important somatic abnormalities were detected, and two were of normal stature. One of the XO,XX patients had a webbed neck, coarctation of the aorta, and a variety of other stigmata but was of normal stature and has menstruated regularly since puberty. A 12-year-old XO,XX,XXX patient had hypothyroidism and Hashimoto's thyroiditis.

The X chromatin pattern may provide clues to the presence of mosaicism. The proportion of X chromatin-positive cells often is less than in normal females, although this is not a consistent finding. The buccal smear, as well as smears from other tissues, may vary from chromatin-negative to a normal proportion of X chromatin-positive nuclei. If the patient harbors an XXX cell line, nuclei with duplicate X chromatin bodies may be found (Fig. 8-8).

XXqi and XO,XXqi. Patients with an Xqi structural abnormality (presumptive isochromosome for the long arm of the X) have an X chromosome that consists of two long arms but lacks a short arm (Fig. 8-27). All patients with XXqi and XO,XXqi

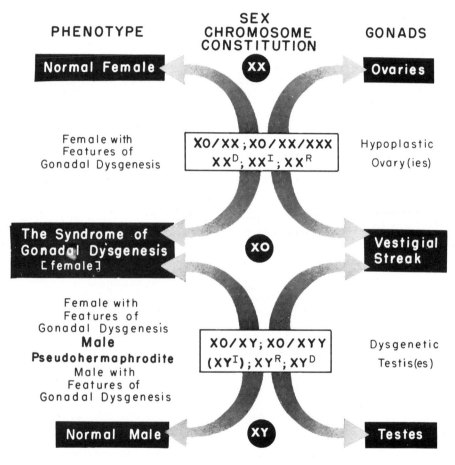

THE RELATIONSHIP OF PHENOTYPE & GONADS TO THE SEX CHROMOSOME CONSTITUTION IN THE SYNDROME OF GONADAL DYSGENESIS & ITS VARIANTS

X^D = Deleted X, X^I = Isochromosome X, X^R = Ring X

Figure 8–25.   Range of phenotypic and gonadal expression, which occurs in the variants of the syndrome of gonadal dysgenesis, and its relationship to the sex chromosome constitution. The typical phenotypic and gonadal findings in monosomic XO gonadal dysgenesis may be modified by the presence of a mosaic chromosomal constitution or by the presence of a structurally abnormal second sex chromosome. For example, XO/XX, XO/XXX mosaicism may be associated on the one hand with normal stature, minimal somatic features of Turner's syndrome, and some degree of ovarian differentiation, or on the other hand with a clinical picture indistinguishable from classic XO gonadal dysgenesis. The phenotype and gonadal differentiation apparently depend upon the proportion of XO to XX or XXX cell lines in the somatic and germ cells during differentiation. Similarly, the presence of a structurally abnormal X chromosome frequently alleviates some features of the classic syndrome. When XO,XY mosaicism or a structurally abnormal Y chromosome is present, varying degrees of testicular differentiation may be found. The spectrum of clinical findings may thus extend from that of a phenotypic male through pseudohermaphrodism to a phenotypic female, depending upon the degree of fetal testicular insufficiency. In addition, the beneficial effects of the normal XY cell line or the presence of some part of a Y chromosome may lead to normal stature and a modification of somatic defects associated with XO monosomy. (From Grumbach, M. M., In *Biologic Basis of Pediatric Practice.* Cooke, R. E. (ed.), New York, McGraw-Hill, 1967.)

THE PRIMORDIAL GERM CELLS,
THE SEX CHROMOSOMES
AND GONADOGENESIS

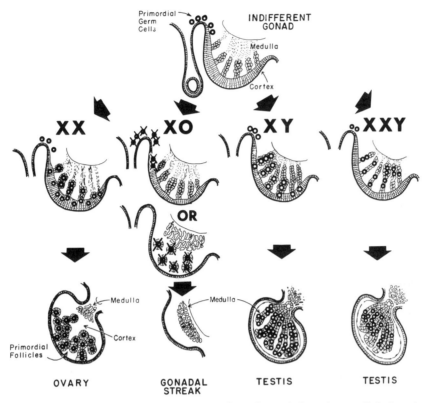

Figure 8-26. The primordial germ cells, the sex chromosomes, and gonadogenesis. Loss of germ cells during migration to or after seeding of the indifferent gonad in an XO individual would give rise to a gonadal streak, as germ cells are necessary for ovarian development of the indifferent gonad; recent evidence suggests that the loss occurs after the germ cells implant. In the presence of XO,XX mosaicism, gonadal differentiation may vary from that of an ovary to that of a gonadal streak. Similarly in XO,XY mosaics, depending on the sex chromosome constitution of the germ cells and of the gonadal blastema, gonadal differentiation may vary from that of a testis to that of a gonadal streak. In XXY individuals, germ cells become implanted in the primitive testis, but a marked loss of spermatogonia seems to occur in the perinatal period. (From Grumbach, M. M., In *Biologic Basis of Pediatric Practice*. Cooke, R. E. (ed.), New York, McGraw-Hill, 1967.)

TABLE 8-6. RELATIONSHIP OF STRUCTURAL ABNORMALITIES OF THE X AND Y TO CLINICAL MANIFESTATIONS OF THE SYNDROME OF GONADAL DYSGENESIS

Type of Sex Chromosome Abnormality	Karyotypes	Phenotype	Sexual Infantilism	Shortness of Stature	Somatic Anomalies of Turner's Syndrome
Loss of an X or Y	XO	Female	+	+	+
*Deletion of short arm of an X	XXqi	Female	+(occ.±)	+	+
	XXp−	Female	+, ±, or −	+	+
*Deletion of long arm of an X	XXpi	Female	+	−	− or (±)
	XXq−	Female	+	−(+)	− or (±)
Deletion of ends of both arms of an X	XO,XXr	Female	− or +	+	+ or (±)
Loss of short arm of Y	XYqi	Female	+	−	−

*In Xp− and Xq−, the extent and site of the deleted segment is variable.

Xqi = isochromosome for long arm of an X; Xp− = deletion of short arm of an X; Xpi = isochromosome for short arm of an X; Xq− = deletion of long arm of an X; Xr = ring chromosome derived from an X; Yqi = isochromosome for long arm of a Y.

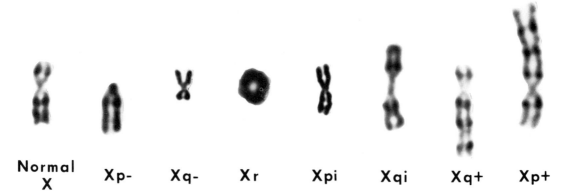

| Normal X | Xp- | Xq- | Xr | Xpi | Xqi | Xq+ | Xp+ |

Figure 8–27. Some structural anomalies of the X chromosome. The normal X is on the left and is "G"-banded; there is a dark band on the short arm and two bands on the long arm. The Xq–, Xr, and Xpi are not banded. These structural anomalies were ascertained to be X chromosomes by their late-replicating patterns by using tritiated thymidine. The Xqi is "G"-banded. Note that the G-banding pattern on both arms is identical. The Xq+ is G-banded, and an extra band is noted on the long arms of the X. The Xp+ chromosome has 6 bands (the normal 3 plus 3 more on the p arm of the X). This entire chromosome replicates late: it forms equal-size bipartite X chromatin bodies, and by C-banding exhibits two centromeric bands—over the centromere and on the p+ arm. This chromosome presumably arose as a consequence of an X-X translocation with telomeric fusion of two X chromosomes, short arm to short arm; despite the extra "C band" (centromeric chromatin), the second centromere is suppressed.

mosaicism so far reported were short; minimal breast development was not infrequent, but menstruation was rare (84, 130, 140, 334). Coarctation of the aorta and lymphedema of the hands and feet were not present in the XXqi cases. Other somatic abnormalities were diminished in frequency, and if webbing of the neck was present, it was rarely more than slight. These findings suggest that absence of a short arm on the second X, even in the presence of an X chromosome composed of two long arms, leads to shortness of stature, failure of ovarian development, and some somatic stigmata of Turner's syndrome. The prevalence of Hashimoto's thyroiditis and diabetes mellitus is higher in patients with structural abnormalities of the X chromosome, especially XXqi (194).

X chromatin bodies are larger than normal in patients with an XXqi constitution (Fig. 8–8), but their increased size may be less evident in buccal smears than in other tissues. The structurally abnormal X is always the late replicating X chromosome, not the normal X, and gives rise to the X chromatin body (107, 140).

The formation of isochromosomes is thought to be due to a transverse rather than a longitudinal division of the centromere during the second meiotic division of germ cells in either parent or during mitosis in the zygote (Fig. 8–5). It would be expected that when this occurs, two daughter-cell lines would be formed, one with isochromosomes for the long arm and another with isochromosomes for the short arm. De la Chapelle et al. have found dicentric centromeres in the cells of some patients with long-arm isochromosome X, suggesting that the short-arm isochromosome frequently lacks a centromere and is thus incapable of further division (69). Derivatives of this cell would either be propagated as an XO cell line or be lost entirely. Informative pedigrees, using X-linked traits as markers, suggest that the Xqi is derived more commonly from the paternal X chromosome (161).

Structurally abnormal X chromosomes are predisposed to loss at mitosis. Morishima and Grumbach studied two patients with gonadal dysgenesis and complex forms of mosaicism that involve an XXqi cell line (140). In one patient, the mosaicism consisted of six cell lines: XO,XqiO,XX,XXqi,XXX,XXXqi; in the second, five cell lines were found: XO,XqiO,XX,XXqi, XXXqi. The clinical features were similar to those observed in patients with an XXqi constitution.

XXpi. A few patients have been reported with this structural abnormality of the X chromosome (short-arm isochromosome X) (71). All were sexually infantile, of normal or near-normal height, and had few and minor somatic stigmata of Turner's syndrome (Fig. 8–28). The X chromatin body was slightly smaller than normal. In the patient reported by de la Chapelle et al., and in the one shown in Figure 8–28, the identity of the structural abnormality was supported by autoradiography, quinacrine fluorescence, and G-band studies. These patients are of especial interest because they support the hypothesis that genes located on both the long and short arms of the X affect gonadogenesis, while loci that influence stature and prevent the expression of the major somatic abnormalities appear to be situated mainly on the short arm of the X.

XO,XXr. A ring X chromosome (Xr) has been described in several patients as part of XO,XXr mosaicism or a more complex mosaicism involving these cell lines (Fig. 8–27) (130, 140). The two patients with XO,XXr mosaicism studied by Grumbach and Morishima were short. The prepubertal girl had a moderate number of associated somatic abnormalities but no webbed neck or coarctation of the aorta. She also had thyrotoxicosis and documented Hashimoto's thyroiditis. The other, who had mild features of the syndrome, developed female secondary sex characteristics at puberty and suffered from dysfunctional bleeding. At least

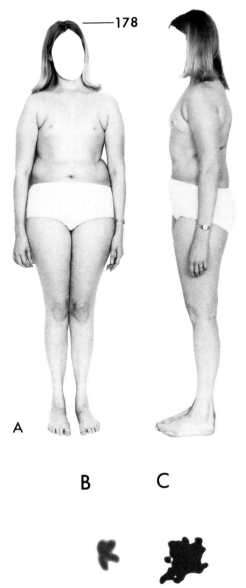

—178

A

B   C

Figure 8–28. *A,* A 22-year-old tall female with the chief complaint of primary amenorrhea, who has an XXpi sex chromosome constitution. At 12 years of age, she developed pubic hair that remained sparse. Breast development did not occur, and she remained sexually infantile. Height 178 cm. (+2.6 SD); weight 70 kg. (+1.2 SD). No somatic stigmata of the "syndrome of gonadal dysgenesis" were noted. Plasma gonadotropins were elevated; LH 5.6 ng./ml. (LER-960), and FSH 36.5 ng./ml. (LER-869). The buccal smear showed a normal proportion of X chromatin bodies that were slightly smaller than usual. Karyotype analysis (46,XXpi). A Giemsa-stained Xpi (*B*) is shown, which exhibited the late-labeling pattern characteristic of an X chromosome (*C*).

three additional patients who had XXr and XO cell lines have been reported, two of whom harbored additional cell lines (XX or XXrXr). All were short and exhibited some of the associated somatic stigmata of the syndrome of gonadal dysgenesis, although two of them have menstruated.

The proportion of X chromatin–positive cells is decreased in patients with a ring X chromosome, and the X chromatin bodies are small. The ring X

chromosome consistently exhibits late DNA replication, except for the case of a very small ring (140).

The ring X chromosome arises by loss of both ends of a chromosome with union of the proximal breaks; as a consequence, a variable amount of chromatin material is lost from each arm (Fig. 8–4). Ring chromosomes are especially unstable, and there is, commonly, a considerable variability in the size of the ring chromosome in different cells. In relation to the syndrome of gonadal dysgenesis, patients with ring X chromosome provide evidence that loss of both terminal ends of an X chromosome need not lead to the development of streak gonads.

XXp– and XO,XXp–. About 12 patients with an XXp–(Xp–=deletion of short arm of an X chromosome) constitution have been described; the abnormal X is acrocentric and similar in size to a D-group chromosome (61, 84, 140). The clinical findings in these patients, with or without an XO cell line, are comparable to those observed with an XO karyotype; all had short stature; some exhibited webbed neck, and many had other somatic features of the XO syndrome. One XXp– patient had a small remnant of the short arm of the X and differed from the other cases in that she had well-developed female secondary sex characteristics and bilateral ovaries and menstruated regularly prior to the occurrence of dysfunctional bleeding (Fig. 8–29) (140).

The heteromorphic X chromosome in these patients is the late DNA-replicating X chromosome and is the origin of the small X chromatin body in interphase nuclei (Figs. 8–4 and 8–8).

XXq– and XO,XXqi–. Less than a dozen patients with XXq– (Xq– = deletion of the long arm of the X chromosome) have been described (61, 84). The X chromatin mass is diminished in size, and the abnormal X exhibits late DNA replication. Most patients with XXq– are of normal stature and have only a few of the somatic anomalies of Turner's syndrome (61, 84, 111). It is therefore striking that all had streak gonads, primary amenorrhea, and sexual infantilism. Exceptions to the generalization that XXq– patients are usually of normal stature and have fewer of the somatic stigmata and to the implication that gene loci that affect these features are mainly clustered on the short arm of the X have been reported (111). It is possible that at least some of these exceptional cases may represent a more complex X chromosome abnormality or harbor an undetected XO cell line; moreover, it is likely that the site and extent of the deleted segment on the long arm varies. The application of the G- or Q-band technique for the analysis of the chromosome anomaly should serve to clarify this matter. The clinical manifestations in the XXq– patients together with those in XXp– and isochromosome X (XXqi, XXpi) individuals, strongly suggest that genes on both the short and the long arms of the X are involved in ovarian differentiation (84, 130, 140).

X Autosome Translocations and X,Giant X Chromosome Karyotypes. Cohen et al. (59) reviewed the findings in 11 patients with X autosome translocations, of which four were analyzed by Q or

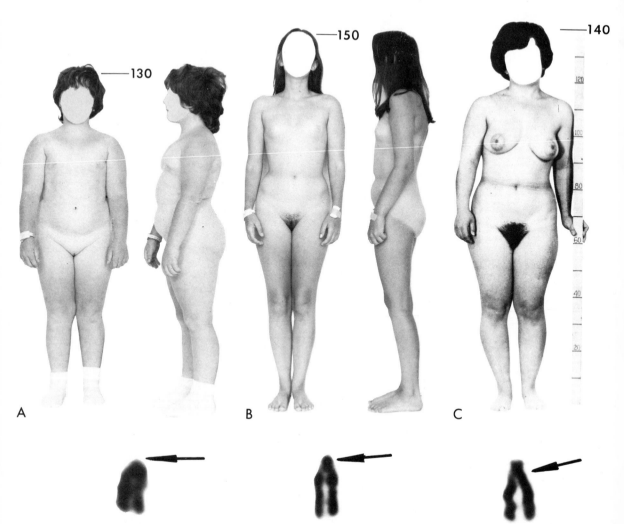

Figure 8–29. The variable gonadal function and phenotypic stigmata in three patients with a deletion of the short arm of the X chromosome (XXp−) of differing degree. *A*, A 13-year-old phenotypic female of short stature (−3.5 SD), with low-set ears, a high-arched palate, a low hair line, a broad chest with wide-spaced areolae, cubitus valgus, puffy hands and feet, and short 4th meta-carpals. There was no evidence of secondary sexual characteristics at 13 years of age. Plasma gonadotropins were elevated; LH 1.6 ng./ml. (LER–960), and FSH 26 ng./ml. (LER–869). Plasma estradiol was less than 6 pg./ml. The buccal smear contained a nor-mal proportion of X chromatin bodies in the interphase nuclei which were conspicuously small. Karyotype analysis and autoradiog-raphy revealed a 46,XXp− karyotype. The abnormal X chromosome appeared to lack the entire short arm. *B*, A 17 4/12-year-old pheno-typic female with stigmata of the syndrome of gonadal dysgenesis. Her height was 151 cm. (−3 SD), and she had multiple nevi, cubitus valgus, and a short 4th metacarpal on the right hand. At age 13, the patient noted the spontaneous onset of breast development which did not progress. Plasma gonadotropins were elevated; LH 7.3 ng./ml. (LER–960), and FSH 53 ng./ml. (LER–869). The concentra-tion of plasma estradiol was 19 pg./ml. On buccal smear the cells had a normal proportion of X chromatin bodies which appeared small. Karyotype analysis and autoradiography indicated a 46,XXp− chromosome had been deleted close to the centromere, but a small segment of the short arm is visible distal to the centromere. *C*, A 20-year-old phenotypic female with a chief complaint of dysfunctional uterine bleeding. She had short stature, slight puffiness of her hands and feet, and short 4th metacarpals. Female secondary sexual characteristics appeared at 11 years of age, and menarche at 13 years was followed by regular menses which later became irregular. The buccal smear exhibited nuclei with a normal proportion of small sex chromatin bodies. Bilateral ovaries were identified grossly and histologically during an appendectomy. The karyotype was 46,XXp−. The extent of deletion of the short arm of the abnormal X chromosome in this patient is less than that seen in patients A and B. A segment of the short arm is readily discernible above the centromere.

It appears that, in these three patients with XXp- karyotypes, the somatic and gonadal manifestations of the "syndrome of gonadal dysgenesis" correlated with the magnitude of the deletion of the short arm of the X chromosome.

G banding and autoradiography. Two of the patients had primary amenorrhea. In some, the normal X and not the translocated X chromosome segment exhibited late DNA replication, whereas in other cases the translocated X chromosome was late-replicating, in some instances with and in some without the autosomal segment. Hence, some X autosome translocations are exceptions to the virtually invariable pattern of late DNA replication of a structurally abnormal X chromosome.

Four cases of an X,giant X chromosome complement are known, and we have studied 2 additional cases; in 5 of the 6 cases, an XO cell line was present also. All 6 patients had many of the clinical features of the syndrome of gonadal dysgenesis, including short stature, sexual infantilism, and some somatic abnormalities. The X chromatin body in interphase nuclei of these patients is the largest so far described and often bipartite in appearance. In the patient studied by Distèche et al. (73) and in two unreported cases of Conte and Grumbach, the G- and Q-band and autoradio-

graphic analyses are consistent with fusion of two X chromosomes to form a giant X (Fig. 8–27).

X Chromatin–Negative Variants of the Syndrome of Gonadal Dysgenesis

The pattern of sex chromosome mosaicism and structural abnormalities of the Y chromosome is similar to that described for the X chromosome, although the chromatin–negative variants are less common. Usually as a consequence of its effect on gonadal differentiation, a Y-bearing cell line modifies the classic female phenotype of the syndrome by leading to a variable degree of masculine differentiation of the genital tract.

XO, XY; XO,XYY; XO,XY,XYY, and Related Abnormalities. A highly diverse phenotype is encountered in these forms of mosaicism (2, 140, 153). Such individuals may appear as phenotypic females, as individuals with ambiguous external genitalia, or as phenotypic males (Fig. 8–30). As

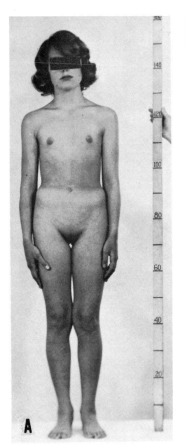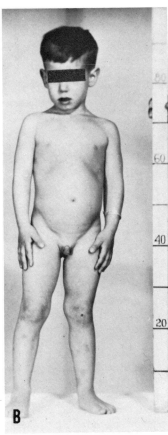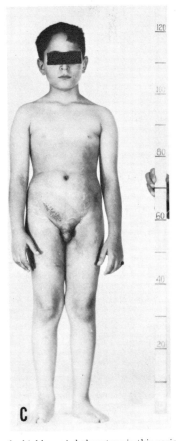

Figure 8–30. Three patients with XO,XY sex chromosome mosaicism who illustrate the highly varied phenotype in this variant of the syndrome of gonadal dysgenesis. (Patient numbers refer to designation in Table 8–7.) *A*, Patient 1, a phenotypic female, was 15 4/12 years of age. She had shortness of stature (−3.1 SD), increased number of pigmented nevi, puffiness over the dorsum of the fingers, and broad and short hands, and was sexually infantile (the breast development seen in the photograph followed estrogen therapy), except for sparse pubic and axillary hair. The titer of urinary gonadotropin was > 80 m.u./day. *B*, Patient 3, a 3 1/12-year-old child, had ambiguous external genitalia, a perineal hypospadias, and undescended gonads. He was of average height and had a broad chest and a duplication of the left kidney. *C*, Patient 9, an 8 1/12-year-old phenotypic male with a penile urethra and unilateral undescended gonad, was of average height and had cubitus valgus, short fourth metacarpals, and puffiness of the dorsum of the fingers. By 15 years of age, male secondary sexual characteristics were well advanced, and the scrotal testis, which was normal in histologic appearance, measured 4.0 × 2.4 cm.

TABLE 8-7. GENITAL STRUCTURES IN NINE PATIENTS WITH XO,XY SEX CHROMOSOME MOSAICISM*

Case	External Genitalia	Uro-genital Sinus	Phallic Enlarge-ment	Gonads	Genital Ducts		
					Female		Male
1	Female	−	−	Rt. streak?	Rt. fallopian tube?	uterus	Rt. −
				Lt. streak?	Lt. fallopian tube?		Lt. −
2	Ambiguous	+	+	Rt. testis	Rt. fallopian tube	uterus	Rt. vas deferens
				Lt. streak	Lt. fallopian tube		Lt. −
3	Ambiguous	+	+	Rt. not found	Rt. fallopian tube	uterus	Rt. −
				Lt. streak	Lt. fallopian tube		Lt. −
4	Ambiguous	+	+	Rt. dysgenetic testis	Rt. fallopian tube	vestigial uterus	Rt. vas deferens
				Lt. dysgenetic testis	Lt. fallopian tube		Lt. −
5	Ambiguous	+	+	Rt. dysgenetic testis	Rt. fallopian tube	uterus	Rt. vas deferens
				Lt. dysgenetic testis	Lt. fallopian tube		Lt. vas deferens
6	Ambiguous	+	+	Rt. dysgenetic testis	Rt. fallopian tube	uterus	Rt. −
				Lt. dysgenetic testis	Lt. fallopian tube		Lt. −
7	Ambiguous	+	+	Rt. dysgenetic testis	Rt. −		Rt. vas deferens
				Lt. dysgenetic testis	Lt. −		Lt. vas deferens
8	Ambiguous	+	+	Rt. dysgenetic testis	Rt. fallopian tube	uterus	Rt. vas deferens
				Lt. streak	Lt. fallopian tube		Lt. −
9	Male	−	Normal penis	Rt. streak	Rt. fallopian tube	vestigial uterus	Rt. −
				Lt. testis	Lt. −		Lt. vas deferens

*From Morishima, A., and Grumbach, M. M.: *Ann. N.Y. Acad. Sci. 155*:695, 1968.

in XO,XX mosaicism, short stature and the associated somatic abnormalities are inconstant features, and they may vary independently of each other and of gonadal differentiation.

Of nine patients with XO,XY or XO,XY,XYY mosaicism studied by Morishima and Grumbach (140), one was a phenotypic female, one was a phenotypic male, and seven had ambiguous external genitalia (Table 8-7). The differentiation of the gonads varied from presumed bilateral streaks in the phenotypic female to bilateral dysgenetic testes. In others the development was asymmetric: one patient had a streak in one mesosalpinx and a rudimentary testis on the contralateral side, and another patient had a normal testis in the scrotum and a herniated streak, fallopian tube, and a vestigial uterus (hernia uteri inguinale) in the contralateral inguinal region. In at least one reported case, the streak gonad contained a few primordial follicles. The development of the genital ducts, urogenital sinus, and external genitalia usually correlates well with the extent of testicular differentiation.

The restricted local action of the testes on the differentiation of genital ducts is well demonstrated in patients with asymmetric gonadal development. In such patients, the development of

male ducts and involution of the müllerian structures are also asymmetric and parallel the degree of testicular development on each side. As discussed on page 440, local action of the testis on müllerian regression is mediated through a nonsteroidal müllerian duct-inhibiting substance, whereas unilateral stimulation of male ducts is probably through mechanisms which serve to concentrate high local levels of testosterone in the wolffian ducts and their derivatives. Male differentiation of the external genitalia, however, would be brought about by testicular tissue in either fetal gonad, as masculinization of these structures is responsive to systemic androgens, and these may be secreted by either testis. The external appearance may range from simulant female with only slight clitoral hypertrophy to a completely male configuration. XO,XY mosaicism has been reported in a few patients with the phenotype of the "male Turner's syndrome" (165, 169). Although in most patients the secretion of androgenic hormones at adolescence is predictable from the extent to which the external genitalia were masculinized *in utero*, virilization has occurred at puberty in some patients with a predominantly female phenotype. Feminization at or after the age of puberty is rare, and when it occurs, a gonadal tumor should be suspected. We have studied one XO,XY patient who exhibited breast development and had a pubertal level of serum estradiol; at laparotomy a gonadoblastoma was found that apparently secreted small amounts of estradiol (Fig. 8–33). The propensity of patients with XO,XY mosaicism to develop gonadal tumors is much increased, and prophylactic removal of the streak gonads or dysgenetic undescended testes is warranted (see p. 475). A useful clue to the presence of functional testicular elements before puberty is the detection of a rise in the concentration of serum testosterone above prepubertal values following a course of human chorionic gonadotropin, e.g., 4000 U./day for four days (255, 340).

The spectrum of findings in patients with these karyotypes provides a link between the syndrome of gonadal dysgenesis and male pseudohermaphrodism (6, 103, 134). However, although many of these patients fulfill the criteria for male pseudohermaphrodism as defined by Klebs (p. 449) and thus present clinically, some authors now restrict this term to exclude patients with chromosomal errors or those whose testes are not fully differentiated. Familial cases of XO,XY mosaicism are rare (117).

Caspersson et al. (52) studied the fluorescent pattern of the Y chromosome in 7 patients with XO,XY mosaicism. The brightly fluorescent distal portion of the Y was absent in 4 of the cases; the 3 fathers who were studied all had a longer Y chromosome that exhibited the normal fluorescent pattern. These findings suggest that a Y chromosomal rearrangement during paternal gametogenesis, possibly translocation, may be a factor in the origin of some XO,XY mosaics. On the other hand, Conte and Grumbach found a normal Y fluorescent pattern in 12 of 13 XO,XY patients.

Mixed, asymmetric, or *atypical gonadal dysgenesis* is a term that has sometimes been used to describe patients with a streak gonad on one side and a testis on the other (176). It is important to emphasize that, while this association is not uncommon in XO,XY mosaicism, these gonadal findings are not specific for XO,XY mosaicism, as they may occur with an XY karyotype. Even an XX,XY karyotype has been found in one patient (23).

Warkany, Chu, and Kauder reported a phenotypic male with XO,XXXY mosaicism who had a small proportion of chromatin-positive nuclei and some double-positive nuclei in buccal smears (188). He had a penis that was bound down, a partially bifid scrotum, and bilateral inguinal herniae. The right inguinal hernia contained a fallopian tube, vestigial uterus, and what was probably a vestigial streak gonad; a testis and vas deferens were found in the hernia on the left side. This patient had some somatic stigmata of Turner's syndrome and thus could be classified as a variant.

Structural Abnormalities of the Y Chromosome. Structural abnormalities of the Y chromosome, which are of clinical significance in regard to sex differentiation and the syndrome of gonadal dysgenesis, are much rarer than those involving an X chromosome. This may be because a deleted Y chromosome, being much smaller than most abnormal portions of the X, is more readily lost from the cell during mitosis. Hence, some XO individuals may arise as a consequence of a structural abnormality of the Y that is lost at an early cleavage division.

Two patients with isochromosomes of the long arms of the Y (XYqi) have been reported by Jacobs and Ross (122). Both were phenotypic females who had primary amenorrhea, sexual infantilism, and bilateral streak gonads, but they were of normal stature, and the somatic stigmata of the syndrome of gonadal dysgenesis were absent or minimal. Dzarlieva and Van Wyk studied a similar XYqi patient who in addition to sexual infantilism had severe generalized lymphedema, including massive pleural infusions requiring frequent thoracocenteses. Both XYqi patients described by Jacobs likewise had histories of lymphedema. Recently, Robinson and Buckton (162) studied the quinacrine fluorescent patterns of interphase and metaphase cells from these patients and positively identified the Yqi that exhibited intense fluorescence of both arms; most of the Y bodies in buccal mucosal cells had a double structure. These observations and those of others imply that the testicular determinants are located on the short arm of the Y, and that loci on the long arm prevent development of the short stature and many of the associated somatic abnormalities of gonadal dysgenesis (84, 162). However, the occurrence of clitoral enlargement and of a rudimentary epididymis in the XO,XYqi patient with the syndrome of gonadal dysgenesis reported by Ferguson-Smith et al. suggests that factors on the long arm of the Y may have some modifying effect on the development of streak gonads.

Nine patients with an XYqdic (a dicentric chromosome for the long arm of the Y) karyotype have been reported; in 8 patients, the structural abnormality of the Y chromosome was associated with mosaicism and an XO cell line (XO,XYqdic) (20, 162). The phenotype was highly variable and exhibited the spectrum extending from a normal adult male through individuals with ambiguous genitalia and male pseudohermaphrodism to a short phenotypic female with bilateral streak gonads and the somatic features of Turner's syndrome. In two patients (20, 162), the Yqdic was confirmed by fluorescent microscopy of interphase cells and metaphase figures; a proportion of interphase nuclei in buccal smears contained a Y body with a double structure. The variation in clinical findings is best explained by the effect of the XO cell line and the extent of loss of the short arm of the Y. The Yqdic is presumed to arise from a break in the short arm with loss of the short arm distal to the break and sister chromatid reunion of the proximal portion. This yields a Y chromosome with two centromeres in close approximation, two long arms and a small but variable pericentric part of two short arms. The error could occur during paternal meiosis or at an early division of the zygote, with loss of the mutant Y from some cells.

The 3 sexually infantile phenotypic females with XO,XYpdic (a dicentric chromosome of the short arm of the Y) mosaicism had the clinical features of the syndrome of gonadal dysgenesis, except that one patient had a height of 150 cm. (162). An XO,XYr individual was a male with azoöspermia (162), suggesting that the testicular determiners on the short arm of the Y are located close to the centromere.

Pericentric inversions of the Y chromosome and deletions of the distal fluorescent portion of the long arm of the Y have been reported in normal men (162).

A minute presumptive sex chromosome, with or without an XO cell line, has been described in some patients with features of the syndrome of gonadal dysgenesis. In many, it was uncertain whether the small chromosome was derived from an X or a Y chromosome. However, in some, the presence of clitoral enlargement or ambiguous external genitalia and unilateral or bilateral dysgenetic testes, strongly suggested that the minute chromosomal fragment was a deleted chromosome.

Various mosaic patterns have been reported with XO cell lines found in combination with others containing different combinations of normal or mutant Y chromosomes. In most of these cases, there were ambiguous genitalia, dysgenetic testes, or a testis and a gonadal streak (84, 138, 140).

Several instances of Y autosome translocations are known: usually there is translocation of the distal fluorescent portion of the long arm of an autosome, and male sex differentiation is normal (Fig. 8-2).

Pure Gonadal Dysgenesis

This term has been applied to a group of phenotypic females who have bilateral rudimentary streak gonads and remain sexually infantile, but who are of normal or tall stature and lack the somatic stigmata of Turner's syndrome (177). At puberty, they exhibit the usual effects of prepubertal castration, and the excretion of urinary gonadotropin is increased. The X chromatin pattern may be either positive or negative. The X chromatin–negative patients occasionally have clitoral enlargement, which may be present at birth or first become manifest at puberty; clitoral enlargement is rarely present in X chromatin–positive patients.

The designation "pure gonadal dysgenesis" was introduced by Harnden and Stewart in 1959 in their report of a 19-year-old phenotypic female with the described features who had an XY sex chromosome constitution (109). This represented an elaboration of the concept of gonadal dysgenesis in normal-appearing females which had been propounded earlier by Hoffenberg et al. (114). It is now appreciated, however, that a variety of etiologic factors may lead to the development of this clinical picture. The karyotype has been variable in the reported patients (40, 44). Commonly, a normal XX or XY sex chromosome constitution has been described; however, sex chromosome mosaicism has not been infrequent, and XO,XY and XO,XY,XYY karyotypes have been detected in the X chromatin–negative and XO,XX mosaicism in X chromatin–positive patients. In addition, patients with a structural abnormality of the second X or Y may have the same clinical features; XY,XX chimerism was found in one patient. We have chosen to classify patients with the clinical features of "pure gonadal dysgenesis" as variants of the syndrome of gonadal dysgenesis if they have partial sex chromosome monosomy (p. 455) and restrict the term "pure gonadal dysgenesis" for those with XX or XY gonadal dysgenesis.

Familial XX Gonadal Dysgenesis and its Incomplete Forms. More than 60 phenotypic female patients have been described who had normal stature, sexual infantilism, bilateral streak gonads (similar in structure to those of XO gonadal dysgenesis), normal female internal and external genitalia, primary amenorrhea, elevated gonadotropins, low values of serum and urinary estrogens, and a 46,XX karyotype (172). The habitus was often eunuchoid. Rare cases had a few somatic abnormalities, including cubitus valgus but not the phenotypic manifestations of Turner's syndrome. Occasionally clitoral enlargement, hirsutism, and other signs of virilization were present; the concentration of serum testosterone was modestly increased above the range for normal women in one such patient studied by Judd et al. (126). The streak gonads secreted testosterone, presumably from the nests of hilus cells which were found on histologic examination. Quite likely, the high concentration of gonadotropins led to hilus cell hyperplasia and a modest increase in testosterone secretion which, in the presence of meager estrogen production, had more potent biologic action.

In the absence of familial cases, the syndrome is rarely recognized before the age of puberty. The buccal smear is X chromatin–positive, but variant forms of the syndrome of gonadal dysgenesis, such as XO,XX mosaicism, or certain structural abnormalities of the X chromosome (e.g., XXpi and XXq−) can be excluded only by chromosome analysis.

Families in which multiple siblings are affected are not uncommon (172), and in 4 instances the parents were consanguineous. These findings are consistent with autosomal recessive inheritance. No families are reported in which both XX and XY gonadal dysgenesis occurred in the same sibship or among relatives. In three families, all the affected sisters had deaf mutism of the sensorineural type (172). It is uncertain whether most of the sporadic cases, in which an X chromosome abnormality has been reasonably excluded, are a consequence of this rare autosomal recessive gene. Genetic heterogeneity is suggested by concordance of the gonadal defect with deaf mutism in some families.* In any

---

*Impaired hearing is not uncommon in XO gonadal dysgenesis, owing to recurrent episodes of otitis media which lead to conductive hearing loss.

event, autosomal recessive XX gonadal dysgenesis provides evidence that a mutant gene on a pair of autosomes can lead to a profound disturbance of ovarian differentiation; the abnormal gonadogenesis may be a consequence of the effect of the mutant gene on the primordial germ cell and its descendants.

In a few of the familial cases, an affected sibling has exhibited a varying degree of ovarian function, including breast development and spontaneous menses followed by secondary amenorrhea. In at least one case, a unilateral gonadal streak was found in one adnexa, and severe ovarian hypoplasia in the other. Further, a number of sporadic cases of a similar type are reported (174). We believe that at least some of the patients represent a less severe or incomplete form of XX gonadal dysgenesis in which there is some ovarian differentiation, usually unilateral, and function. This notion is supported by the occurrence of the incomplete form and the severe form of XX gonadal dysgenesis in the same sibship.

In contrast to XY gonadal dysgenesis, gonadal neoplasms are rare in XX gonadal dysgenesis (167).

Familial XY Gonadal Dysgenesis and its Incomplete Forms. Over 90 patients with XY gonadal dysgenesis have been described. This syndrome in its complete form is characterized by a female phenotype, normal to tall stature, bilateral streak gonads, sexual infantilism with primary amenorrhea, eunuchoid habitus, and a 46,XY karyotype. Somatic features of Turner's syndrome are inconspicuous or absent. Their internal genital structures are female, with bilateral tubes, a uterus, and a vagina. Clitoral enlargement is not uncommon, and the frequency of gonadal neoplasms, especially gonadoblastoma and dysgerminoma, is high. Rare patients may exhibit some breast development. The concentration of plasma gonadotropins and the urinary excretion of gonadotropins is increased. In some patients, the level of serum testosterone is increased above prepubertal and normal female values, because of secretion of androgens by the hilus cell in the streak gonads. A male proportion of single Y bodies is present in interphase nuclei. Excluded from this syndrome are patients with variants of the syndrome of gonadal dysgenesis, such as XO,XY mosaicism and structural abnormalities of the Y chromosome (e.g., XYqi). The Y chromosome in the XY complement exhibits a normal fluorescent pattern.

Familial aggregations are well described (55, 81, 172). They include instances in which multiple siblings are affected and in which the disorder is transmitted in different sibships within a family through unaffected females (81). Concordant monozygotic twins, but not parental consanguinity, have been reported. These observations are consistent with the transmission of XY gonadal dysgenesis as an X-linked recessive or as a male-limited autosomal dominant trait. Thus the action of an unpaired mutant gene located on an autosome or an X chromosome in an XY individual can drastically modify testicular differentiation. XX gonadal dysgenesis and XY gonadal dysgenesis have not been reported in the same family; each of these forms is a distinct entity with a different pattern of inheritance and a different propensity for the development of gonadal neoplasms.

In 3 families in which at least one sibling had XY gonadal dysgenesis, another had ambiguous external genitalia. The sibship described by Chemke et al. (55) had 2 affected siblings with the typical features who were raised as females and a "brother" with a well developed hypospadiac phallus, bound-down penis (chordee), and a bifid scrotum. At operation, a urogenital sinus, bilateral fallopian tubes, a small uterus, and bilateral dysgenetic testes were found in this "brother." The dysgenetic testis located in an inguinal hernia sac had an epididymis and a vas deferens. Thus the common genetic defect may only be partly expressed in some affected individuals.

It is quite likely that when the spectrum of clinical features in the *incomplete form of familial XY gonadal dysgenesis* is better defined it will exhibit the same gamut of variations found in XO,XY gonadal dysgenesis, with varying degrees of ambiguity of differentiation of the external genitalia and genital ducts, and either bilateral dysgenetic testes or a dysgenetic testis on one side and a gonadal streak on the other (24). Some of the reported cases of sporadic male pseudohermaphrodism with an XY karyotype and dysgenetic testes (or a testis and a streak gonad on opposite sides, so-called "mixed gonadal dysgenesis"), in which an XO cell line and a structurally abnormal Y chromosome were sought but not found, are probably examples of the incomplete form of XY gonadal dysgenesis (31).

There is a high prevalence of gonadal tumors, usually gonadoblastoma or dysgerminoma, in this syndrome. The tumors may be bilateral and can occur in more than one affected sibling. Further transformation may occur of a gonadoblastoma into the metastasizing dysgerminoma, or the dysgerminoma may be coincidental. Hence, bilateral prophylactic gonadectomy is indicated and can be performed when the diagnosis is established. In the first affected member of a family, this is usually at the age of puberty in the complete form and in infancy in patients with ambiguous external genitalia.

So-Called "Male Turner's Syndrome"

Over 150 phenotypic males have been reported with short stature, webbed neck, and other somatic abnormalities associated with the syndrome of gonadal dysgenesis in whom the testes were hypoplastic and frequently undescended (92, 112, 178). The resemblance of these males to phenotypic females with XO gonadal dysgenesis suggested a pathogenetic parallelism between Turner's syndrome in the male and the female. However, with rare exceptions (165, 169), this interrelationship is no longer tenable (5). A few patients with the phenotypic features of male Turner's syndrome have had a sex chromosome abnormality, such as XO,XY mosaicism (165, 169), and they represent a partial sex chromosome monosomy variant of Turner's syndrome. In all the other karyotypic studies of these patients, the sex chromosome constitution was XY. The XY cases form a heterogeneous clinical group in which there may be multiple causes. Unless partial sex chromosome monosomy can be demonstrated, these patients ought not to be considered as the clinical parallel in the male of Turner's syndrome in phenotypic females. Many of the cases previously categorized as "male Turner's syndrome" are examples of the syndrome of webbed neck, ptosis, hypogonadism, and short stature usually associated with congenital heart disease and mental retardation (5, 108, 144).

Syndrome of Webbed Neck, Ptosis, Hypogonadism, Congenital Heart Disease, and Short Stature (XX and XY Turner Phenotype, Pseudo-Turner's Syndrome, Noonan's Syndrome, Ullrich's Syndrome)

Among the group of phenotypic males previously classified as "male Turner's syndrome," a distinctive clinical entity was identified which led to the identification of its counterpart in the female and its distinction from the syndrome of gonadal dysgenesis (5, 76, 108, 129, 144). A variety of eponyms has been applied to this syndrome, but while at present there is no consensus, we prefer to exclude Turner from the designation in order to avoid confusion with Turner's syndrome, which is a consequence of partial or complete sex chromosome monosomy. It is of interest that in 1938, the year Henry Turner's paper appeared, Bizarro reported a female with the features of the syndrome described therein. Table 8–8 lists the clinical features in 2 phenotypic males and 12 phenotypic females with this entity. These patients have a characteristic facies and, frequently, a webbed neck and short stature (Fig. 8–31); in 12 of 14 cases, congenital heart disease was present. The most common cardiac malformations have been pulmonic stenosis and atrial septal defect or both; ventricular septal defect, patent ductus arteriosus, and eccentric ventricular hypertrophy also may be found (76). Coarctation of the aorta and aortic stenosis, the most common cardiovascular anomalies in the syndrome of gonadal dysgenesis, have occurred but are infrequent findings. Pectus excavatum, cubitus valgus, and impaired mental development are often present. In both sexes, the sex

TABLE 8–8. SUMMARY OF CLINICAL FINDINGS IN 14 PATIENTS WITH THE SYNDROME OF WEBBED NECK, PTOSIS, HYPOGONADISM, CONGENITAL HEART DISEASE, AND SHORT STATURE*

Clinical Characteristics	Males	Females	Clinical Characteristics	Males	Females
Short stature (> 2 sd below mean)	2/2	8/12	Both PS and ASD	2/2	3/10
			Patent ductus arteriosus (PDA)	0/2	2/10
Typical facies	2/2	12/12	Undiagnosed heart disease	0/2	2/10
Triangular shape of face	2/2	7/12	Incompletely evaluated	0/2	2/12
Prominent brow	2/2	12/12			
Hypertelorism	2/2	12/12	Extremities		
Epicanthus	2/2	9/12	Cubitus valgus	2/2	9/12
Antimongoloid palpebral slant	2/2	10/12	Gracile fingers	1/2	8/12
Ptosis	2/2	12/12	Short stubby fingers	1/2	2/12
Depressed nasal bridge	1/2	2/12	Lymphedema	0/2	3/12
Broad apex nasi	2/2	11/12	Dystrophic nails	2/2	2/12
			Shortened fourth metacarpal(s)	0/2	3/12
Low-set and/or malformed ears	2/2	8/12	Clinodactyly of fifth finger(s)	1/2	2/12
			Palmar simian crease	1/2	1/12
High-arched palate	2/2	8/12			
			Undescended testes	2/2	–
Neck					
Short	2/2	10/12	Delayed puberty	1/1	3/3
Webbing	2/2	10/12			
Low hairline	2/2	10/12	Skeletal retardation	2/2	8/10
Chest			Mental development		
Shieldlike	1/2	11/12	Retarded	2/2	4/12
Wide-spaced nipples	2/2	11/11	Borderline	0/2	5/12
Pectus excavatum	2/2	5/12	Normal	0/2	3/12
Cardiac abnormalities	2/2	11/12	Intrauterine growth retardation	1/2	4/12
Pulmonic stenosis (PS)	2/2	5/10			
PS and ventricular septal defect	0/2	1/10	Renal collecting system		
Atrial septal defect (ASD)	2/2	6/10	Normal	2/2	7/8
ASD with anomalous pulmonary			Abnormal	0/2	1/8
venous return	0/2	1/10			
Endocardial cushion defect (ECD)	0/2	2/10	Normal karyotype	2/2	12/12
ECD + patent ductus arteriosus and mitral insufficiency	0/2	1/10			

*After Grumbach, Morishima, and Liu (108).

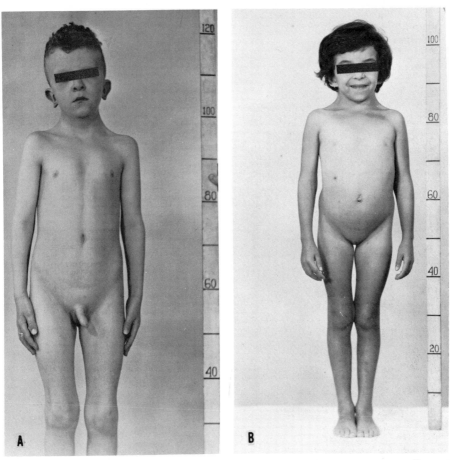

Figure 8–31. A phenotypic male and female with the syndrome of webbed neck, ptosis, congenital heart disease, short stature, and hypogonadism (Pseudo-Turner's syndrome; Noonan's syndrome). *A,* A 9 7/12-year-old boy who exhibited the characteristic abnormalities: triangular facies, prominent brow, hypertelorism, ptosis, antimongoloid slant of palpebral fissures, broad apex nasi, low set ears, webbed neck, pectus excavatum, pulmonic stenosis and atrial septal defect, short stature (−3.5 SD), bilateral undescended testes, and high grade mental retardation. At 18 years of age, he was 154.0 cm. in height (height age: 12 5/12 years); the boy had Leydig cell hypofunction. Biopsy of the testes showed germinal aplasia. 46,XY chromosome constitution with a normal karyotype. (From Grumbach, M. M., and Barr, M. L.: *Recent Progr. Hormone Res. 14*:335, 1958.) *B,* An 8-year-old girl with similar features. Height 106.2 cm. (height age 4 4/12 years). Pulmonic stenosis was present. 46,XX karyotype.

chromosome constitution is normal, and the direction of gonadal differentiation is appropriate for the phenotypic and chromosomal sex. In males, cryptorchidism is common, and the testes are usually hypoplastic and exhibit germinal aplasia. Androgen deficiency is not uncommon at puberty. However, some affected males have normal testicular function, including fertility. At present we prefer to limit this diagnosis to patients with four or more of the cardinal features of the syndrome and a normal chromosome constitution. The females have functioning ovaries, and although the onset of puberty may be delayed, female secondary sexual characteristics eventually emerge.

While the majority of cases are sporadic, familial aggregation has been described (76, 129), including parent-to-child transmission consistent with autosomal dominant inheritance and pedigrees that suggest an autosomal recessive trait. However, in addition to the possibilities of genetic hetero-

geneity and phenocopy, an undetected chromosomal abnormality has not been excluded. In an affected father and daughter studied by Conte and Grumbach, the G- and Q-banding patterns appeared normal.

True Hermaphrodism (8, 14)

Definition

The diagnosis of true hermaphrodism requires the presence of both ovarian and testicular tissue in either the same or opposite gonads. Failure to adhere to this definition has led to considerable confusion. Gonadal stroma arranged in whorls, similar to that found in the ovary but lacking oöcytes, should not be considered as sufficient evidence to regard the rudimentary gonad as an ovary. Similarly, when testicular tissue is present in the contralateral gonad, the presence of a few oöcytes in a streak gonad is not considered by the authors as adequate evidence for the diagnosis of true hermaphrodism. Since rare female-type germ cells may be found in patients with XO gonadal dysgenesis, it seems of little value from the clinical, cytogenetic, embryologic, or nosologic standpoint to classify as true hermaphrodites those XO,XY mosaics in whom a dysgenetic testis is present with exceedingly rare oöcytes. Similarly, the status of the internal and external genitalia, while invariably exhibiting some degree of ambisexual development, should not be used as a criterion for the classification of an individual as a true hermaphrodite.

Classification

This syndrome is probably more common than is supposed. In a study of 1525 human embryos whose gestational age was estimated to be 6–7 weeks, Lee (128) found 16 who had both testicular and "ovarian" tissue. Since the ovary differentiates later than the testis, it is possible that the "ovarian" element may represent delayed differentiation of testicular tissue rather than the progenitor of an ovary or ovotestis. Overzier collected 171 reported cases up to 1962, and in 1969 Polani (157) reviewed 310 cases; chromosome studies were performed on 108. Patients with this syndrome may be subclassified clinically according to the type of gonads.

Lateral. A testis on one side and an ovary on the other—this arrangement occurs in about one-third of patients. The ovary is found more frequently on the left side.

Bilateral. Testicular and ovarian tissue is found bilaterally, usually as ovotestes; this disposition occurs in about one-fifth of patients.

Unilateral. Testicular and ovarian tissue on one side and a testis or ovary on the other; this occurs in slightly less than one-half of the cases. A testis or ovotestis may be situated anywhere along the normal pathway of descent of a testis, but an ovary lies almost invariably in its normal position.

Clinical Features

The differentiation of the genital tract and the development of secondary sexual characteristics are highly variable (Fig. 8–32). The external genitalia may simulate those of either a male or a female. Often they are ambiguous, and three-fourths of the patients have been reared as males because of the size of their phallus. Almost all the subjects have hypospadias, which varies in extent from perineal to penile, with incomplete fusion of the labioscrotal folds. In rare cases a penile urethra is present. Cryptorchidism is common, and an inguinal hernia, which may contain a gonad or uterus, is present in about one-half of the cases. In virtually all cases there is a uterus. The differentiation of the genital ducts usually follows that of the gonads (102). In the patients with a testis on

one side and an ovary on the other, the development of the homolateral duct is usually consistent with that of the gonad, despite the varied appearance of the external genitalia. Most patients with an ovotestis have predominantly female development of the genital ducts. The relationship between gonadal structure and differentiation of the genital tract in true hermaphrodism provides added evidence for the essentially local effect of the müllerian duct inhibitor secreted by the fetal testis (102).

About two-thirds of the patients have appreciable breast development, and about the same proportion menstruate; however, menstruation has not been noted in X chromatin–negative cases. Periodic hematuria due to menstruation is a late clue to the diagnosis. Ovulation is not uncommon, but spermatogenesis is rare, and, as yet, no true hermaphrodite has begotten a child. Some degree of virilization is often found at puberty.

Chromosomal Findings

About 70% of true hermaphrodites are X chromatin–positive (6). Benirschke et al. analyzed the cytogenetic findings in 108 patients: 61 patients were 46,XX, 23 had a 46,XY karyotype, and 35 were mosaics or chimeras, including 10 XX,XY chimeras and 6 cases of XY,XXY mosaicism (35).

Polani (157) noted that, in XX true hermaphrodites (including X chromatin–positive cases who did not have chromosome analysis), an ovary was found more frequently on the left side and the inappropriate gonad, either a testis or ovotestis, on the right, whereas in XY and X chromatin–negative cases, the reverse situation occurred more often — a testis on the right side and an ovary or ovotestis on the left.

The absence of a Y chromosome in patients with testicular tissue seems at first to be contrary to current concepts of sex determination. Undetected mosaicism with a Y-bearing cell line is undoubtedly present in some of the reported XX cases. In support of this contention are the various types of sex chromosome mosaicism with a Y-bearing cell line that have been described in true hermaphrodites (7, 35, 157).

Origin of True Hermaphrodism

The XX,XXY mosaicism may arise by loss of a Y chromosome at an early cleavage division of an XXY zygote, whereas the XX,XXYY and XX,XXY,XXYYY patterns could be a consequence of mitotic nondisjunction in an XXY zygote. However, chimerism (7, 90) arising as a consequence of double fertilization or possible fusion of two normally fertilized ova is the more likely cause of XX,XY mosaicism, and this has been demonstrated by genetic studies in some cases. The first case of XX,XY chimerism, a 2 1/2-year-old true hermaphrodite with an ovary and ovotestis and

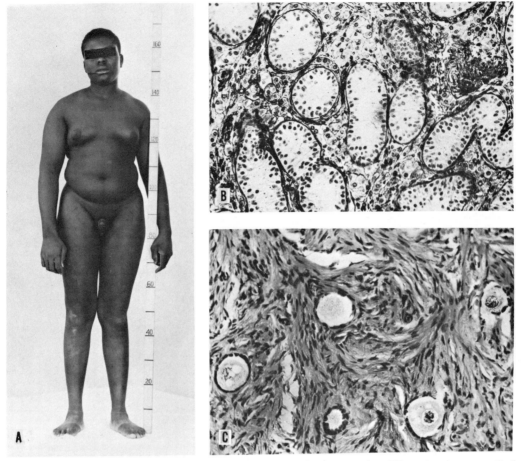

Figure 8-32. *A*, A 17-year-old true hermaphrodite with bilateral scrotal ovotestes and an XX sex chromosome constitution in cultures of the peripheral blood and skin, a perineal hypospadias (partially repaired in the photograph), moderate bilateral gynecomastia and pubic hair (recently shaved in the picture), sparse axillary hair, a high-pitched voice, and absent facial hair. Height 66 inches. Urinary 17-KS 1.3 mg./day; urinary gonadotropin > 10 m.u., < 80 m.u./day. At operation there was a male type of urethra, bilateral scrotal fallopian tubes and ovotestes, and a rudimentary bicornate uterus and vagina attached to the posterior urethra.

Photomicrograph showing histopathology of the demarcated ovarian and testicular portion of one ovotestis: *B*, immature seminiferous tubules lined with Sertoli cells and spermatogonia and Leydig cells; *C*, ova and follicles. (From Grumbach, M. M., and Barr, M. L.: *Recent Progr. Hormone Res.* 14:335, 1958.)

iris heterochromia, was reported by Gartler et al. (94). The patient had two populations of red blood cells with multiple blood group antigenic differences. The father, who was heterozygous at two loci (MNSs and Rh), contributed both alleles to the patient, whereas inheritance of these loci from the mother was the same in each of the two red cell populations. These observations provided evidence for the fertilization of a binucleate ovum by two sperms, one bearing an X and the other a Y. The segregation of the haptoglobin phenotype in the XX,XY true hermaphrodite of Josso et al. leads to a similar interpretation (125). The XX,XY patient described by Zuelzer et al. was a phenotypic male without evidence of true hermaphrodism; a likely mechanism for the mosaicism in this case, based on the blood group studies and other findings, is fusion of two zygotes or fertilization of an ovum and its polar body.

In addition to true hermaphrodism and the patient of Zuelzer who had a normal male phenotype,

XX,XY chimerism has been associated with (1) a female phenotype with female secondary sexual characteristics but primary amenorrhea, female duct development, a dysgerminoma replacing the left gonad, and a streak gonad on the right side (23); and (2) ambiguous external genitalia with a dysgenetic testis containing a gonadoblastoma (147).

The problem of excluding mosaicism in karyotype studies is a formidable one, especially in true hermaphrodites in whom only X-bearing cell lines are detected. However, even though there may be good reason to suspect that many of the XX true hermaphrodites may harbor an XY or other Y-bearing cell line, especially in the testicular tissue, mosaicism need not be invoked to explain all instances in which testicular tissue has formed in a patient lacking a Y chromosome. Three siblings with XX true hermaphrodism have been reported by Clayton et al. (58, 163) and two chromatin-negative siblings by Milner et al. These familial cases suggest that a recessive gene may be the cause in some cases (6), comparable to the mutant gene which has been implicated in certain forms of intersexuality in mice, goats, and pigs (7, 54).

Other hypotheses may be advanced to account for XX or XY true hermaphrodites and especially for the preponderance of isolated XX cases. Transfer of male-determining genes from a Y to an X chromosome during the prophase of the first meiotic division in the father could lead to a sperm-bearing male determiners on its X chromosome. During this step the X and Y chromosomes are normally aligned end to end, and it is not difficult to visualize how small translocations of genetic material could occur from the minute short arms of the Y to the X. Ferguson-Smith developed this notion further, and suggested that gonadal differentiation could be determined by which one of the X chromosomes is inactivated in a given cell at an early embryonic stage, the normal X or the X-bearing translocated male-determining loci (X^y) (85). To simplify this theory: if the X^y chromosome is inactivated predominantly in the cells that give rise to the gonadal primordia, these cells would lack the male-determining genes; therefore, ovarian and not testicular development would ensue. Contrariwise, if the normal X is inactivated predominantly in the same primordial cells, these cells would contain an active X^y and promote testicular differentiation. Variations in the proportions of cells with an active or inactive X^y in the gonadal primordia would determine whether the gonad ultimately differentiated into a testis, ovary, or ovotestis. In the few cases in which the fluorescence technique was used, no evidence of the insertion of the fluorescent portion of the Y into an X chromosome was observed nor was there an abnormality of the G-band pattern of the X.

In addition to genetic factors, a deleterious environmental factor acting locally could modify gonadal development, as in experimentally produced, true hermaphrodism in lower species (206).

Some Sex Chromosome Abnormalities Unassociated with Gonadal Defects

Four sex chromosome abnormalities that are not accompanied by a typical gonadal defect but in which mental retardation is frequent will be discussed.

XXX. This is the third most common sex chromosome abnormality, following XXY and XYY in frequency. It is usually detected by finding two X chromatin bodies in peripheral cells. A frequency of 0.56/1000 newborn female infants was reported by Barr et al. from a review of surveys in newborns (32) and 0.8/1000 in females of all ages in a general hospital population (22). Although the first subject reported by Jacobs et al. had premature menopause, mental deficiency has been the only frequent feature, and even this has not been invariable (7, 32). The prevalence of XXX individuals in institutions for the mentally retarded is 4.3/1000 (32). While a few patients have had menstrual abnormalities, most XXX women are completely normal. Of 33 children born to 13 XXX women, only one had a sex chromosome abnormality, an XXY phenotypic male (164). In addition, a mother with XX,XXX mosaicism had an XXY son (164). The reason that chromosomal errors are not detected more frequently in the offspring of these mothers is not known; about half of the offspring of mothers with mongolism are affected.

XXXX. Sixteen females with an XXXX have been described; all but one were mentally retarded, usually severely; no distinctive clinical features were present; all beyond pubertal age had normal female secondary sexual characteristics and menstruated regularly (7, 37). Three X chromatin bodies were detected in some diploid nuclei.

XXXXX. Two such cases have been described in mentally defective females with patent ductus arteriosus, minor somatic abnormalities, and intrauterine growth retardation. A proportion of diploid nuclei contained four X chromatin bodies.

XYY. The first patient reported with an XYY constitution by Sandberg et al. was an essentially normal fertile man of average intelligence. He was detected only because he had a daughter with mongolism. Much publicity was focused on the XYY syndrome when surveys in penal and mental institutions disclosed a reputed increase in prevalence in these settings, especially in prisoners over 6 feet tall; this gave rise to an undeserved stereotype. As one of the more common sex chromosome abnormalities, it is estimated to occur in from 1/500 to 1/1000 male births. Ratcliffe et al. detected five XYY male infants in a survey of 3500 consecutive liveborn males in two Edinburgh hospitals; all had a normal male phenotype. Among the features that have been associated with an XYY karyotype are tall stature, deviant and antisocial behavior, nodulocystic acne, and skeletal anomalies (especially radio-ulnar synostosis) (7, 63, 115). The frequency of these features in noninstitutionalized XYY individuals is not known. Even though the prevalence of XYY's in prisons and institutions for the criminally insane is significantly greater than in the general population, it is not as high as was inferred in the early reports. Recent data suggest that only a small percentage of XYY's manifest antisocial behavior (115). Secretion of testosterone and gonadotropins is normal. A few reports have described hypogonadism, ambiguous genitalia, and nonspecific somatic abnormalities in XYY's.

Two fluorescent Y bodies are found in somatic interphase nuclei stained with quinacrine dyes. Surveys of the prevalence in an unselected population of males of individuals with YY bodies in the nuclei in oral mucosal, or blood smears should serve to clarify many of the disquieting questions about this syndrome. Hook has provided a thoughtful discussion of its behavioral implications and the clinical dilemma it may pose (115). XYY males have fathered XY males, but no XYY or XXY sons have been reported.

XYYY. This karyotype has been described by Townes et al. in a 5-year-old boy who was mildly retarded in psychomotor development; his phenotypic appearance was unremarkable (184). He was of average stature but had undescended testes, inguinal hernia, pulmonic stenosis, simian lines, and defective teeth. A similar case was reported in a 9-year-old boy who had three fluorescent Y chromosomes in metaphase preparations and three Y bodies in a proportion of interphase nuclei.

Gonadal Neoplasms in Dysgenetic Gonads (115, 168, 182, 365, 373)

The prevalence of gonadal neoplasms is greatly increased in patients with certain types of dysgenetic gonads (182, 342, 373, 379). Dysgerminoma, seminoma, teratoma, and gonadoblastoma have been found most commonly. In 1959, Melicow and Uson reviewed 140 cases of gonadal neoplasms in patients with ambiguous sexual development and added five additional cases (373). Although they did not include cases of cryptorchidism not associated with intersexuality, it is well established that undescended testes are also more prone to malignant change than are scrotal testes. The relative risk of these specific abnormalities is difficult to assess, since such cases are more apt to be reported than are cases of either gonadal tumors in normal individuals or gonadal defects not associated with tumors. Nevertheless, some provisional judgments are warranted by the frequency with which neoplasms have been reported in certain types of patients.

Gonadal neoplasms are apparently quite rare in patients with XXY seminiferous tubule dysgenesis and in the streak gonads of patients with XO gonadal dysgenesis. The prevalence is increased in patients with (1) XO,XY mosaicism and other variants of the syndrome of gonadal dysgenesis in which there is a Y-containing cell line (either with a normal Y or a structurally abnormal Y chromosome) and (2) XY gonadal dysgenesis [including the complete (pure gonadal dysgenesis) and the incomplete forms (ambiguous genitalia, dysgenetic male pseudohermaphrodism)] (Fig. 8–33) (40, 168, 182, 373, 379, 384).

Malignant transformation of a gonad has been reported in at least five cases of true hermaphrodism, although the true frequency is unknown. In a survey of 24 reported cases of gonadal malignancy in phenotypic females with gonadal dysgenesis, Goldberg et al. (98) found only six cases (including her study) with the somatic stigmata of Turner's syndrome. Of these, three had clitoromegaly. XO,XY mosaicism was demonstrated in one of these patients and XO,XX mosaicism in her own patient who lacked clitoromegaly. This patient had a papillary pseudomucinous cystadenocarcinoma replacing gonadal structures on one side and a streak gonad on the other (364). Warren et al. reported a hilus cell adenoma with signs of virilization in an XO,XX patient with bilateral streak gonads (384).

The most comprehensive review of gonadoblastoma to date has been published by Scully (379) (Fig. 8–33). In 27 of his 74 cases, a tumor was found in both gonads. Thirty patients were under age 15 when the tumor was first diagnosed, and 10 patients were less than age 10. A third of these tumors were diagnosed only after microscopic sections were prepared of dysgenetic gonads removed for other purposes. In patients in whom chromosomal studies had been carried out, the predominant pattern was either XO,XY or XY. Although 80% of these patients had been reared as females, most of them displayed some degree of clitoromegaly or hirsutism; rarely, these tumors may secrete enough estrogen to induce breast development (Fig. 8–33). Even though the gonadoblastoma itself is rarely if ever malignant, these tumors frequently contain dysgerminomas or other malignant tumors that can metastasize and cause death. Teter and Boczkowski (41, 182) have emphasized the increased risk of gonadal neoplasms in dysgenetic gonads and reviewed its familial occurrence in patients with XY gonadal dysgenesis.

In view of the now well-documented malignant potential of dysgenetic gonads, the question of prophylactic gonadectomy merits serious attention. The neoplasms are infrequently detected in childhood, but the risk rises appreciably in young adults. It is possible that high gonadotropin levels play a role in their growth, and that substitution therapy with sex steroids might afford some protection. A prudent course is to advise laparotomy and castration of all patients with XY gonadal dysgenesis (complete and incomplete forms) and in patients with the syndrome of gonadal dysgenesis who are found to have a cell line with a normal or a structurally abnormal Y chromosome, or exhibit some degree of virilization regardless of the apparent karyotype. Patients with XO Turner's syndrome who have no suggestion of clitoromegaly are not at risk. The risk of gonadal tumors in patients with only X chromosome abnormalities, such as XO,XX, XXr, and XXq−, is low; these patients, however, should be examined at regular intervals for signs of gonadal neoplasm. Further, only one case of XX gonadal dysgenesis with a neoplasm − a gonadoblastoma − has been described. The strikingly disparate propensity for neoplastic transformation in the streak or dysgenetic gonads of patients with XY gonadal dysgenesis in contrast to XX gonadal dysgenesis must be emphasized. Similarly, in patients with variants of the syndrome of XO gonadal dysgenesis in whom there is a cell line containing a Y or a mutant Y chromosome, the risk of gonadal tumor is significantly increased, in contrast to XO patients and patients with XO,XX mosaicism or a structural abnormality of an X chromosome in whom a higher frequency of gonadal tumors has not been established.

The gonad should be preserved in a patient who has been raised as a male only if it is represented by a relatively normal testis that can be relocated in the scrotum. The fact that a gonad is palpable does not guarantee against a disastrous result, however, since seminomas tend to metastasize at an early stage before a local mass is obvious.

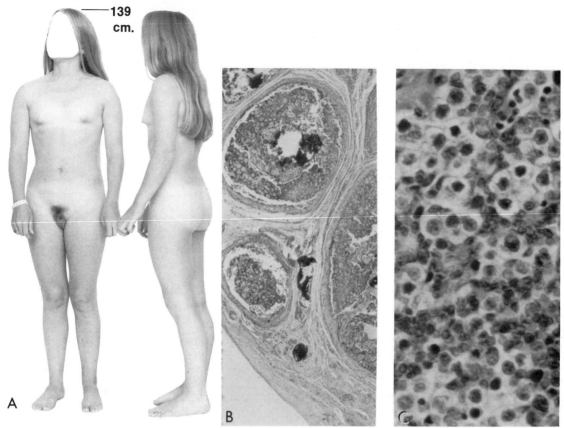

Figure 8–33.   XO,XY mosaicism with a feminizing gonadoblastoma. *A,* A 20-year-old female with many of the stigmata of the syndrome of gonadal dysgenesis, including short stature, multiple nevi, cubitus valgus, and hyperconvex, small nails. The buccal smear was X chromatin–negative; on fluorescent microscopy, 30% of the interphase nuclei had a single Y body. The karyotype was XO,XY. The patient had spontaneous development of pubic and axillary hair at 12 years of age. At 18 years of age, breast development was noted. Her height was 139 cm. (−5.1 SD) and weight 39 kg. (−2.5 SD). The bone age was 17 years; an intravenous pyelogram was normal. The concentration of plasma gonadotropins at 20 years of age was elevated; plasma LH 8 ng./ml. (LER–960), and FSH 50 ng./ml. (LER–869). A urocytogram showed a "moderate" estrogen effect. The concentration of plasma estradiol was 26 pg./ml. and of estrone 32 pg./ml.; plasma testosterone was less than 20 ng./100 ml. On exploratory laparotomy, normal-appearing Fallopian tubes and uterus were found. The right gonad was a typical "streak," with whorls of fibrous connective tissue. *B,* The left gonad was replaced by a 1.3 × 1 × 1-cm. tumor mass which, on histologic section, revealed well-defined nests and islands of Sertoli-Leydig–like cells and germ cells, as well as calcification consistent with the diagnosis of "gonadoblastoma." *C,* Higher magnification illustrates the aggregates of germ cells and smaller epithelial cells resembling immature Sertoli cells, as well as cells indistinguishable from Leydig cells.

FEMALE PSEUDOHERMAPHRODISM

Female pseudohermaphrodism is the easiest of the sexual anomalies to comprehend, as the ovaries and müllerian derivatives are normally developed and anatomical ambisexuality is limited to the external genitalia (p. 443). Since in the absence of testes there is an inherent tendency for the external genitalia to feminize, a female fetus will be masculinized only if subjected to an environment of androgens from some extragonadal source (295). The degree of fetal masculinization is determined by the stage of differentiation at the time of exposure. Once the vagina has separated from the urogenital sinus (about the twelfth fetal week), androgens will cause only clitoral hypertrophy (Fig. 8–34). Even with severe masculinization of the external genitalia, the uterus and fallopian tubes remain normal since the regression of the primordia for these structures, the müllerian duct, requires the secretion of the müllerian duct–inhibiting substance by fetal testes, and this action cannot be mimicked by androgenic steroids. Although the presence of virilized genitalia usually provides *prima facie* evidence of an androgenic influence during early gestation, ambiguous genitalia, superficially resembling those produced by androgen, are an occasional feature of other more generalized teratologic malformations.

Congenital Virilizing Adrenal Hyperplasia (20, 286, 288, 303)

Congenital virilizing adrenal hyperplasia accounts for most of the cases of female pseudohermaphrodism and approximately half of all patients with ambiguous external genitalia (20).

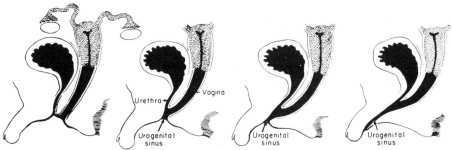

Figure 8–34. Female pseudohermaphrodism induced by prenatal exposure to androgens. Exposure after the twelfth fetal week leads only to clitoral hypertrophy (diagram on left). Exposure at progressively earlier stages of differentiation (depicted from left to right in drawings) leads to retention of the urogenital sinus and labioscrotal fusion. If exposure occurs sufficiently early, the labia will fuse to form a penile urethra. (From Grumbach, M. M., and Ducharme, J. R.: *Fertil. Steril. 11*:157, 1960.)

Biochemical Variants of Congenital Adrenal Hyperplasia

Six major types of congenital adrenal hyperplasia have been described, each with its distinctive clinical picture and specific biochemical lesion (286, 288, 303). All are transmitted as an autosomal recessive trait. (See Ch. 5, pages 276, 277, and 278.) The common denominator in all six biochemical types is impaired cortisol formation with consequent hyperplasia of the adrenal cortex due to hypersecretion of ACTH through the negative feedback mechanism. Only types I, II, and III, however, are predominantly virilizing disorders. In these types, the most striking abnormality of the sexual phenotypes is prenatal masculinization of the female fetus due to overproduction of adrenal androgens. The male is also affected, but this is not a prominent feature at birth. Hence these disorders will be discussed in this chapter as causes of female pseudohermaphrodism.

Biochemical types IV, V, and VI have in common defects in steroid hormone synthesis, which not only block cortisol synthesis but also impair the production of sex steroids by the gonads as well as by the adrenal glands. Hence affected males exhibit varying degrees of male pseudohermaphrodism due to deficient androgen production by the fetal Leydig cells, whereas affected females may or may not exhibit virilization. If present, virilization in females is usually considerably less than in types I, II, and III. These forms of adrenal hyperplasia will accordingly be discussed in a later section as causes of male pseudohermaphrodism. The administration to the pregnant rat of selective synthetic inhibitors of the enzymes involved in adrenal and testicular steroid biogenesis has produced abnormalities of sex differentiation in the offspring which are the counterparts of congenital adrenal hyperplasia in man and has served to clarify further the role of steroidogenic enzymes in the control of fetal sex differentiation (220).

Type I: Partial C_{21} Hydroxylase Defect (Simple Virilization).

A partial defect in C_{21} hydroxylation leads to simple virilism. These patients conserve sodium normally, since aldosterone secretion is normal or increased.

Type II: Complete C_{21} Defect (Virilization with Salt-Losing Tendency).

The salt-losing variant is due to a more absolute block in C_{21} hydroxylation; in these patients aldosterone secretion is likewise impaired, although not totally lacking. Such patients are prone to severe salt-losing crises and often die in the early weeks of life unless they are properly diagnosed and adequately treated. It is possible that certain of the intermediary compounds that are greatly elevated in the untreated patient potentiate the addisonian state by blocking the action of aldosterone at the renal tubular level. It has been suggested that the difference in clinical expression of types I and II, both of which are a consequence of 21-hydroxylase deficiency, is related to the existence of multiple alleles for the gene that regulates this enzyme (290, 292).

Types I and II account for over 90% of the patients with congenital adrenal hyperplasia.

Type III: C_{11} Hydroxylase Defect (Virilization with Hypertension).

A defect in hydroxylation at C_{11} leads to the hypersecretion of 11-deoxycorticosterone (DOC) and 11-deoxycortisol (Compound S) in addition to adrenal androgens. Such patients exhibit hypertension in addition to virilization.

Type IV: 3β-Hydroxysteroid Dehydrogenase Defect (Male or Female Pseudohermaphrodism and Adrenal Insufficiency).

This disorder is due to a deficiency of the enzyme in 3β-hydroxysteroid dehydrogenase (287). This enzyme acts at a more primitive stage in steroid biosynthesis and is required by both the adrenal and the gonads for the synthesis of their respective biologically active hormones. Females exhibit less masculinization than is the case with types I, II, and III, whereas affected males exhibit varying degrees of male pseudohermaphrodism due to defective secretion of androgen by the fetal Leydig cells. Most patients with this disorder also exhibit a salt-losing tendency, and the mortality in early life is exceedingly high.

Type V: 17 α-Hydroxylase Defect (Male Pseudohermaphrodism, Sexual Infantilism, Hypertension, and Hypokalemic Alkalosis) (314).

These patients are unable to make derivatives of 17α-hydroxyprogesterone, such as androgens, estrogens, and cortisol. The secretion of large quantities of corticosterone and 11-deoxycorticosterone leads to hypertension and hypokalemic alkalosis. Affected males are male pseudohermaphrodites.

Type VI: Cholesterol Desmolase Complex Defect; ?Cholesterol 20α-Hydroxylase Deficiency (Male Pseudohermaphrodism, Sexual Infantilism, and Adrenal Insufficiency). These patients have congenital lipoid adrenal hyperplasia and a primitive biosynthetic defect that interferes with the conversion of cholesterol into any biologically active steroid. Degenhart et al. (292) studied adrenal tissue from these patients and found evidence of impaired 20α-hydroxylation of cholesterol. Males exhibit pseudohermaphrodism, and few affected children have survived early infancy owing to the severe cortisol and aldosterone deficiency (337, 345).

The clinical manifestations of each of these forms of congenital adrenal hyperplasia are summarized in Table 8–9.

Effect of Virilizing Forms of Congenital Adrenal Hyperplasia on Female Sexual Development

The first three and most common types of congenital adrenal hyperplasia have in common a defect beyond the 17α-hydroxyprogesterone stage of steroid biosynthesis. Thus cortisol synthesis is impaired and, as a consequence of compensatory hypersecretion of ACTH, the adrenal is stimulated to manufacture excessive quantities of androgens and other steroids proximal to the block in the biosynthetic pathway. Affected children of both sexes may exhibit addisonian-like pigmentation at birth, a reflection of high ACTH levels. The finding of elevated levels of 17-KS and 3α-, 17α-, 20α-pregnanetriol in the urine and of plasma 17α-hydroxyprogesterone is almost pathognomonic of these disorders. Unless appropriate treatment is instituted, the secretion of androgens continues postnatally, leading to early and severe virilism

(Fig. 8–35, B). Although growth is accelerated during childhood, the bone age advances disproportionately, and premature closure of the epiphyses leads to shortened adult stature.

The genitalia of females with virilizing forms of hyperplasia may exhibit any degree of masculinization from simple enlargement of the clitoris to complete labioscrotal fusion with a normal appearing penis (Fig. 8–35, A). In most cases the urogenital sinus is preserved and serves as a common outlet for both the urethra and the vagina. It may thus be presumed that hypersecretion of androgens begins well before the twelfth fetal week (Fig. 8–35, A). The uterus, tubes, and ovaries are, however, always normal in these patients, no matter how severely the external genitalia are masculinized (p. 439). The more severely masculinized females are frequently mistaken for boys at birth and raised in this sex until the mistake is discovered. In the era before effective therapy was available, rearing in the male sex was often preferable because of the severe virilism that developed early and persisted throughout adult life. The high levels of adrenal steroids maintained a positive inhibition on gonadotropin secretion, and the gonads consequently remained in their prepubescent state (Fig. 8–35, B).

The spectrum of masculinization in the three forms of adrenal hyperplasia causing female pseudohermaphrodism varies with the nature of the biochemical defect. Girls with the C_{21}-hydroxylase deficiency who are severe salt-losers are likewise the most severely masculinized (304) and are often mistakenly diagnosed as males. Next in severity are the patients with the non-salt-losing form of adrenal hyperplasia. Patients with the 11β-hydroxylase deficiency may exhibit only equivocal clitoral enlargement at birth, and postnatal virilization may be delayed and of mild degree.

In 1950, Wilkins demonstrated that by providing adequate substitution therapy with cortisone the adrenal can be kept well suppressed and further virilization prevented (Ch. 5) (20, 36). With the ad-

TABLE 8–9. CLINICAL MANIFESTATIONS OF VARIOUS TYPES OF CONGENITAL ADRENAL HYPERPLASIA

Enzymatic Defect	Cholesterol Desmolase System (Cholesterol 20α-Hydroxylase)		3β-Hydroxysteroid Dehydrogenase		17α-Hydroxylase		11β-Hydroxylase		21α-Hydroxylase	
Type	VI		V		IV		III		II & I	
Chromosomal Sex	XX	XY	XX	XY	XX	XY	XX	XY	XX	XY
External Genitalia	Female	Female	Female (Clitoromegaly)	Ambiguous	Female	Female or ambiguous	Ambiguous	Male	Ambiguous	Male
Postnatal Virilization	— (Sexual infantilism at puberty)		±	Mild to moderate	— (Sexual infantilism at puberty)		+		+	
Addisonian Crises	+		+		—		—		+ in 40% (type II)	
Hypertension	—		—		+		+		—	

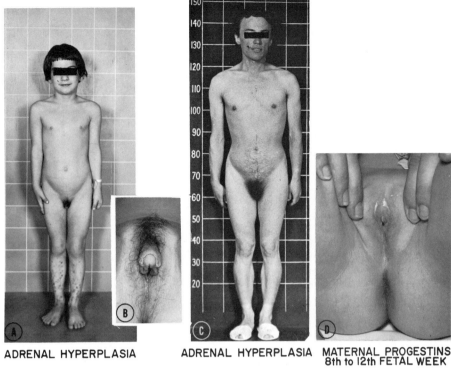

	ADRENAL HYPERPLASIA	ADRENAL HYPERPLASIA	MATERNAL PROGESTINS 8th to 12th FETAL WEEK
	FEMALE PSEUDOHERMAPHRODITISM		
AGE - - - - - -	4 4/12 yrs.	23 yrs.	8 yrs.
HT. AGE - - - -	5 yrs.	I I yrs.	8 yrs.
BONE AGE- -	9 yrs.	ADULT	8 1/2 yrs.
I7 K.S.- - - -	6.0 mgm / 24 hrs.	50 mgm / 24 hrs	1.8 mgm / 24 hrs.
Pregnanetriol	13.6 mgm / 24 hrs.	—	<0.5 mgm / 24 hrs.

Figure 8–35. *A* and *B*, Untreated girl with relatively mild form of congenital adrenal hyperplasia. Androgens caused disproportionate acceleration of bone maturation as compared with stature. *C*, Virilized adult female with adrenal hyperplasia. Patient had deep voice, shaved daily, and wore a toupee for baldness. After treatment with cortisone her 17-KS fell to normal levels, her breasts enlarged, she underwent a normal menarche, and hair regrew on her head. Note short stature and short extremities. (From Wilkins, L.: *The Diagnosis and Treatment of Endocrine Disorders in Childhood and Adolescence.* 3rd ed. Courtesy of Charles C Thomas, Publisher, 1965.) *D*, Female pseudohermaphrodism due to maternal ingestion of oral progestational compound from eighth to twelfth week of pregnancy. Labioscrotal fusion is sufficient to obscure vaginal orifice and create urogenital sinus. The clitoris is enlarged. There is no progressive virilizing tendency, and adolescent normal female development and fertility can be expected.

vent of effective therapy, it has become mandatory that affected females all be reared as girls. Feminization and menstruation can be expected after adolescence, and many of these patients have given birth to normal babies (309). Polycystic ovaries and sterility have been reported in certain forms of adrenal hyperplasia, although the frequency of this finding is not known (269).

Effect of Virilizing Forms of Congenital Adrenal Hyperplasia on Male Sexual Development

Males with the first three forms of adrenal hyperplasia have normal differentiation of their sexual organs. At birth, the penis is often slightly larger and more erectile than normal and the scro-

tum abnormally pigmented. Pronounced virilism appears at an early age unless the condition is recognized and treated. As long as the adrenal remains unsuppressed, the high levels of adrenal steroids suppress the release of gonadotropic hormones, and the testes consequently remain infantile. With adequate adrenal suppression with cortisone or other glucocorticoid preparations, adult testicular maturation and spermatogenesis will occur if or when the appropriate degree of physical maturation has been achieved. The age at which adolescence occurs in these patients corresponds more nearly with their skeletal age than with their chronologic age (307). Those with an accelerated bone age may enter true adolescence prematurely after adrenal suppression is achieved.

Aberrant adrenal rests are common in boys with adrenal hyperplasia and may be mistaken for either adult testicular maturation or testicular neoplasms (210, 301). These adrenal rests, which are often bilateral, arise by the incorporation of hyperplastic nests of adrenal cells into the hilum of the primitive gonad before the gonad separates from the urogenital ridge (Fig. 8–13). Histologically, these aberrant adrenal cells are often indistinguishable from Leydig cells, and the erroneous diagnosis of "sexual precocity due to a Leydig cell adenoma" is not uncommon in boys who are later proven to have the adrenogenital syndrome (301). If the adrenal is adequately suppressed with cortisol, these nests may remain inconspicuous throughout life, and the testes will undergo normal maturation at adolescence.

Maternal Androgens and Progestogens

Masculinization of the external genitalia of female babies has been frequently observed following the maternal ingestion of testosterone or synthetic progestational agents during the first trimester of pregnancy (294, 295, 308). If the exposure occurs after the twelfth week of gestation, fusion of the labioscrotal folds does not occur, although there may be clitoral enlargement (295). Severe virilization may be caused by methyltestosterone in dosages as small as 3 mg. daily, even though androgenic effects are not noticeable in the mother.

Since progesterone itself is only very slightly active when administered orally, various synthetic derivatives which may be taken by mouth have frequently been prescribed for women with habitual or threatened abortion. Most of these compounds are intrinsically androgenic to some degree and regularly produce virilization of female fetuses in experimental animals. Before this potential complication was publicized, norethindrone (Norlutin) and various commercial forms of ethisterone (Pranone, Lutocylol, Progestoral) have been responsible for most cases, but female pseudohermaphrodism also has been induced by norethynodrel and medroxyprogesterone acetate (308).

Bongiovanni, Di George, and Grumbach collected four similar cases of female pseudohermaphrodism in which the mother had received only stilbestrol in large dosage (285). The mechanism of virilization in these cases is obscure, but it may be related to inhibition of adrenal 3β-hydroxysteroid dehydrogenase by this compound. Recently (228), maternal ingestion of stilbestrol and other chemically related nonsteroidal synthetic estrogens during pregnancy has been associated with an increased prevalence of clear-cell adenocarcinoma of the vagina and cervix in adolescent and young adult females. Transplacental carcinogenesis by stilbestrol was implicated in at least 46 of 66 cases of this rare tumor by Herbst et al. (228); in light of these findings, stilbestrol and related analogues should not be given to pregnant women.

In rare instances, masculinization of the female fetus may occur if the mother is suffering from a virilizing ovarian or adrenal tumor (usually an ovarian arrhenoblastoma or Krukenberg tumor) or if she develops virilism from some other cause during the course of her pregnancy (295, 298, 299). Occasionally a child with female pseudohermaphrodism is encountered in whom no source of prenatal androgen exposure can be identified (8, 16, 295). The absence of virilism in the mother does not exclude a maternal source of androgens in these children, however, since the quantities required to masculinize the external genitalia of an early female fetus may be less than those which cause overt manifestations in the mother (295).

Female pseudohermaphrodism arising from fortuitous early exposure to androgens is the most easily treated of all types of ambisexual development. No hormonal therapy is necessary, postnatal virilism does not occur, and female secondary sexual characteristics can be expected to emerge at the usual age of adolescence. Surgical correction of the external genitalia restores feminine appearance and permits normal sexual function.

Van Wyk has studied two female cretins who had marked clitoromegaly. One of these infants had been given a boy's name on the advice of the referring physician. The karyotype was XX and there was no evidence of adrenal hyperplasia. It was considered possible that prenatal virilization had occurred as a consequence of impaired conjugation of androgens *in utero*.

Malformations of the Intestine and Urinary Tract

Genital abnormalities are frequently associated with imperforate anus, renal agenesis, and other congenital malformations of the lower intestine and urinary tract (4, 14, 300). Carpentier and Potter have reviewed the findings in such infants and have suggested the term "nonspecific female pseudohermaphroditism" (289). Some, but not all, of these anomalies are incompatible with life. Pyelonephritis is frequently present and may confuse the picture with that of salt-losing congenital adrenal hyperplasia. In contrast with other forms of female pseudohermaphrodism, the internal genital ducts may also be malformed. The findings in these patients may be quite bizarre, and persistence of the primitive cloaca is not infrequent. The pathogenesis of these anomalies is different from other types of ambisexual development and should be considered in the context of other forms of teratology. Fraser has reported a familial occurrence of nonadrenal female pseudohermaphrodism with multiple congenital anomalies (293).

MALE PSEUDOHERMAPHRODISM

Definition

Male pseudohermaphrodism is a condition in which the gonads are exclusively testes but in which either the genital ducts or external genitalia lack full masculinization and display to some degree the phenotypic characteristics of a female. The clinical spectrum may thus range from an individual simulating a female to a male with only mild hypospadias or cryptorchidism.

With the elucidation of etiologic mechanisms, systems of nomenclature based on phenotype are becoming of diminished importance. It is convenient to categorize separately male pseudohermaphrodites who are incompletely masculinized because of an initial defect in testicular differentiation — so-called dysgenetic male pseudohermaphrodism; in such patients the gonadal defect is most commonly due to some anomaly of their sex chromosomes and less frequently to a mutant gene that leads to defective gonadogenesis. In these and other patients with dysgenetic testes, the failure of the internal genital ducts and external genitalia to undergo full male differentiation correlates quite well with the incompleteness of testicular differentiation. These patients are discussed in the section dealing with disorders of gonadal differentiation.

In this section, the forms of "male pseudohermaphrodism" in XY individuals with relatively normal embryonic differentiation of their testes will be discussed. In such patients, defective male development must be ascribed to a more specific failure of the fetal testes to overcome the inherent tendency to feminize the somatic sex structures. This failure may stem either from a secretory failure of the testes themselves during the critical period of sex differentiation or from a failure of the target tissues to respond normally to androgen stimulation. The classification of male pseudohermaphrodism outlined in Table 8–5 reflects an attempt to classify the many forms of male pseudohermaphrodism on the basis of etiology, insofar as this is known. This outline will be followed in the sections that follow.

The ability of the testes to virilize the patient at adolescence is frequently a recapitulation of their performance in masculinizing the external genitalia *in utero*. The greater the development of the phallus, the greater likelihood that male secondary sex characteristics will emerge. Individuals with ambiguous genitalia may remain eunuchoid, exhibit mild virilism, or develop breast enlargement and other feminine secondary sex characteristics. Those with an external female phenotype will usually either feminize or remain sexually infantile. These are only approximate guides, however, and the paradoxical development of sexual characteristics at adolescence is sometimes encountered.

Inborn Errors of Testosterone Biosynthesis (Fig. 8–36)

Errors Affecting Synthesis of Both Corticosteroids and Testosterone (Variants of Congenital Adrenal Hyperplasia)

Cholesterol Desmolase Complex Deficiency (?Cholesterol 20α-Hydroxylase Deficiency). Prader has described a group of infants with severe adrenal insufficiency, enormous accumulations of lipid in the cells of both the adrenal cortex and gonads, and, in affected males, female external genitalia with male genital ducts (336, 337). 17-KS were totally lacking in the urine, and the genitalia of affected female children were normal. Few of

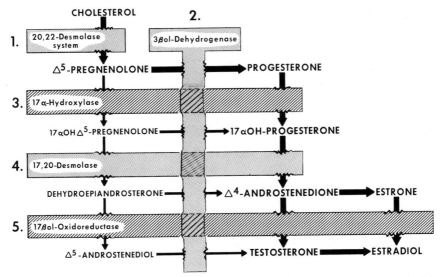

Figure 8-36. Enzymatic defects in the biosynthetic pathway for testosterone. All five of the enzymatic defects cause male pseudohermaphrodism in affected males. Even though all of the blocks affect both gonadal and adrenal cortical steriodogenesis, those at steps 1, 2, and 3 are associated with major abnormalities in the biosynthesis of glucocorticoids and mineralocorticoids.

these patients survived infancy. This disorder is usually called congenital lipoid adrenal hyperplasia.

A chromatin-negative XY phenotypic female patient with a similar disorder, who is now 7 years old, has been studied by Grumbach and co-workers. The external genitalia were female, but the genital ducts were male. Bilateral testes were palpable in the inguinal region. The infant had an addisonian-like electrolyte disorder. Plasma cortisol was not detected, and the urine did not contain aldosterone, 17-KS, 17-OHCS, pregnanediol, pregnanetriol, or the 3β-hydroxy analogues of these compounds. Recently, Kirkland et al. (296) reported a similar case in an 8-year-old phenotypic female with testes and an XY sex chromosome constitution who had severe adrenal insufficiency. The testes were deficient in spermatogonia, and the basement membrane of the seminiferous tubules was thickened.

Degenhart et al. (292) incubated adrenal tissue obtained at autopsy from patients with this disorder and found deficient 20α-hydroxylation of cholesterol, a critical step in the conversion of cholesterol to Δ^5-pregnenolone (Fig. 8–36). The deficiency in cholesterol 20α-hydroxylase leads to adrenal insufficiency, with defective cortisol and aldosterone biosynthesis and, because of deficient testosterone synthesis by the testis, lack of or impaired masculinization of the external genitalia and urogenital sinus. This disorder is transmitted as an autosomal recessive trait.

3β-Hydroxysteroid Dehydrogenase Deficiency. Male pseudohermaphrodism is a usual finding in affected males with the rare variant of the adrenogenital syndrome due to 3β-hydroxysteroid dehy-

drogenase deficiency (287, 288). Since the block occurs at an early stage of steroid biosynthesis (Fig. 8–36), both adrenal steroidogenesis and testosterone production by the fetal Leydig cells are impaired. Thus, affected males exhibit incomplete masculinization of their external genitalia (Fig. 8–37). The presence of normal male genital ducts and the absence of müllerian structures in those males who have come to autopsy provide further evidence that the testicular duct–organizing substance is not a steroid. Although most of the reported cases have died in infancy, a few patients with this enzymatic defect have survived and entered puberty (332). At this time, the testes secreted excessive amounts of 3β-hydroxy precursors of testosterone but were able to produce normal amounts of testosterone, although adrenal insufficiency persisted. The male pseudohermaphrodite described by Parks et al. (333) developed gynecomastia at puberty as well as male secondary sex characteristics.

17α-Hydroxylase Deficiency. Biglieri, Herron, and Brust described the first clinical example of C_{17}-hydroxylase deficiency (Fig. 8–36) (314). Their patient was a 35-year-old female with no C_{21} steroids derived from 17α-hydroxyprogesterone, and minimal quantities of C_{19} steroids derived from 17α-hydroxyprogesterone and 17α-hydroxypregnenolone. She was sexually infantile, and negligible estrogen production could be demonstrated. Secretory rates of steroids not dependent on 17-hydroxy precursors were greatly elevated. These included progesterone, 11-deoxycorticosterone, and corticosterone. These steroids permitted survival of the patient but led to hypertension and hypokalemic alkalosis. Suppression of the adrenal

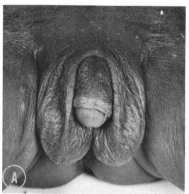

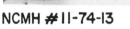

NCMH #11-74-13   3 MO. MALE   KARYOTYPE: XY

CONGENITAL ADRENAL HYPERPLASIA DUE TO 3-β HYDROXY-STEROID DEHYDROGENASE DEFICIENCY
17 KS : 3.2 mgm / 24 hrs
"pregnanetriol": 1.4 mgm / 24 hrs.

Figure 8–37.   Genitalia of male infant with congenital adrenal hyperplasia due to 3 β-hydroxysteroid dehydrogenase deficiency. This boy was admitted at 9 days of age in a salt-losing crisis and died at 3 months of unexplained muscular paralysis. Paresis, resembling that of the Werdnig-Hoffmann syndrome, became progressively more severe even though adrenal replacement therapy was adequate and blood electrolytes were normal. The biochemical findings revealed a severe block in the conversion of Δ-5,3 β-hydroxy-steroids to Δ-4,3 ketones. The findings in this boy were reported by Bongiovanni (Case IV).[287]

with cortisone reversed the hypertension and electrolyte abnormality, but the formation of sex steroids was not enhanced.

In the previous edition of this textbook, it was predicted that, should a male with this enzymatic defect come to light, he would display male pseudohermaphrodism in addition to the metabolic abnormalities described by Biglieri. New (328) subsequently described a 24-year-old male pseudohermaphrodite with deficiency in secondary sexual characteristics and gynecomastia. Detailed studies confirmed the presence of partial 17α-hydroxylase deficiency. Hayles studied two brothers who were phenotypic females with testes, hypertension, female external genitalia, a vagina, male duct development, and absence of secondary sex characteristics.

Errors Primarily Affecting Synthesis of Testosterone

17, 20-Desmolase (Lyase) Deficiency. Zachmann et al. (346) studied 3 patients—two first cousins and a maternal aunt—with a familial form of male pseudohermaphrodism which they ascribed to a partial defect in the conversion of 17α-hydroxyprogesterone and 17α-hydroxypregnenolone to C_{19} steroids by the testes and adrenal glands. The patients had ambiguous external genitalia, inguinal or intra-abdominal testes, and an XY sex chromosome constitution. Both first cousins had severe hypospadias but a male-type urethra and male duct development. The aunt who was sexually infantile had a laparotomy and bilateral orchidectomy previously and was reputed to have a vagina and some rudimentary müllerian derivatives in addition to a vas deferens and epididymis. The cousins who were studied at 1.8 and 2.2 years of age excreted appropriate amounts of 17-KS and 17-OHCS for their age. The excretion of urinary pregnanetriol was normal, but pregnenetriol and 11-ketopregnanetriol were increased. Following the administration of hCG, urinary testosterone glucuronide was unchanged in contrast to age-matched normal males, but there was a striking increase in 11-ketopregnanetriol. After ACTH administration, the excretion of dehydroepiandrosterone remained undetectable, but 11-ketopregnanetriol increased fourfold and 17-OHCS rose normally. A sample of testicular tissue from one patient was studied *in vitro* with appropriate C_{21} steroid precursors, and a defect in the conversion to testosterone was demonstrated. These results are consistent with a deficiency of adrenal and testicular 17,20-desmolase (Fig. 8-36). In this family, the first described, the familial aggregation suggests male-limited autosomal dominant or X-linked recessive inheritance.

The incomplete masculinization and the steroid studies suggest that the defect was partial. Unlike patients with 17-oxidoreductase deficiency, gynecomastia should not occur at puberty. The disorder must be distinguished from the incomplete form of testicular feminization and familial male pseudo-

hermaphrodism with virilization at puberty, from a persistent urogenital sinus (pseudovaginal perineoscrotal hypospadias), and, before puberty, from 17-oxidoreductase deficiency. If the diagnosis is established in infancy, these patients can be reared as males and treated with testosterone to induce male secondary sex characteristics and adequate growth of the phallus.

17β-Hydroxysteroid Oxidoreductase (17β-Hydroxysteroid Dehydrogenase) Defect. Saez et al. described a familial form of male pseudohermaphrodism which they attributed to a partial block in the reduction of 17-KS to 17β-hydroxysteroids (339, 341) (Fig. 8-36). At birth these patients have female or ambiguous external genitalia, testes (usually located in the inguinal canal) and, in the patient reported by Saez et al., a blind vaginal pouch. Puberty was characterized by progressive clitoral enlargement and virilism, failure to menstruate, and simultaneous enlargement of the breasts. At puberty the concentration of testosterone is low for a male and does not rise above the levels found in early male puberty, but the plasma androstenedione and estrone are strikingly elevated and fall after gonadectomy or testicular suppression with synthetic androgens. Knorr et al. (297) demonstrated impaired conversion of androstenedione to testosterone by testicular tissue in their patient. The karyotype is XY, and only male genital ducts are present. Histologic examination of the testes reveals marked Leydig cell hyperplasia and usually absent or deficient germinal elements. A well-studied 46-year-old patient was reported recently by Goebelsmann et al. (346a).

The clinical picture of these patients conforms precisely to what uncritically might be expected in the incomplete form of testicular feminization. The differential point in the present syndrome is that the testosterone levels are considerably lower, and that there is a reversal between the usual testosterone-to-androstenedione ratio and the estradiol-to-estrone ratio in serum. This reversal is particularly marked in the testicular venous effluent. Further, these patients respond to the administration of testosterone by normal retention of nitrogen.

This defect in testicular biosynthesis can be detected even in infancy by the response to the administration of chorionic gonadotropin (hCG), three injections (2000 U.) given every other day over a 6-day period. The concentration of serum androstenedione and estrone exhibits a much greater rise than that of testosterone and estradiol.

The familial cases of ambiguous external genitalia, male genital ducts, gynecomastia, and virilization at puberty described by Witschi and Mengert (1942), Gilbert-Dreyfus et al. (1957), and Lubs et al. (1959) have been regarded by some as examples of the incomplete form of the feminizing testes syndrome. However, the clinical manifestations seem more consistent with a partial block in testosterone biosynthesis of the 17β-hydroxysteroid oxidoreductase type (Fig. 8-36). Similarly, we now include Reifenstein's syndrome (see below) in this category, based on indirect evidence of a deficiency of this enzyme; this possibility remains to be ex-

plored with appropriate studies. If this hypothesis is correct, then the 17-oxidoreductase deficiency may be inherited as a male-limited autosomal dominant or an X-linked recessive trait and not as an autosomal recessive.

In patients with this syndrome reared as females, the proper treatment is castration followed by estrogen substitution. If they have been reared as males, they will require supplemental testosterone therapy to achieve full masculinity. A plausible explanation for the absence of spermatogenesis in these patients is the elevated level of plasma estrone and the well-known dependence of the tubular epithelium on testosterone to provide the environment required for germ cell maturation. It is conceivable that the provision of appropriate dosages of exogenous testosterone at the onset of puberty might have a beneficial effect on fertility as well as on male secondary sexual characteristics and sexual potency.

Reifenstein's Syndrome (Hypospadias, Hypogonadism, and Gynecomastia). This hereditary form of male pseudohermaphrodism is characterized by hypospadias, postpubertal testicular atrophy with azoöspermia, and signs of androgen deficiency usually accompanied by gynecomastia (Fig. 8–38) (316). The concentration of serum testosterone is low, and the excretion of urinary gonadotropin may be normal or increased. The testicular histology differs from that in XXY seminiferous tubule dysgenesis and resembles most closely the changes seen in myotonic dystrophy: a variable degree of postpubertal tubular fibrosis, defective maturation of spermatogonia and, inconstantly, Leydig cell hyperplasia. The sex chromosome constitution is XY.

This disorder is limited to males and, like the syndrome of feminizing testes, is transmitted either as an X-linked recessive trait or as a male-limited autosomal dominant. It is unlikely that the findings in this syndrome can be attributed to target organ resistance, since these patients apparently respond to exogenous androgen in an appropriate manner. The defective differentiation of the external genitalia, the gynecomastia, and impaired testosterone secretion at puberty can be explained by a deficiency of 17β-hydroxysteroid oxidoreductase (Fig. 8–36); we have tentatively classified these patients under this defect in testicular biosynthesis.

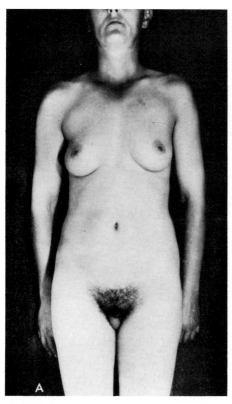 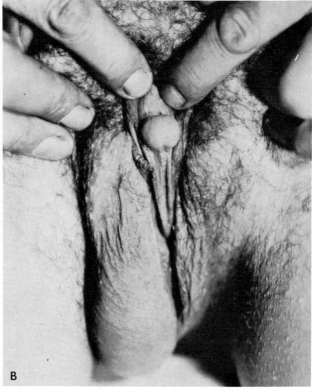

Figure 8–38. Patient with Reifenstein's syndrome. Both this patient and a brother had gynecomastia and a comparable degree of hypospadias. The internal genital ducts were male. Both had a normal karyotype. The testes of the patient illustrated tubular fibrosis and no germinal elements beyond the secondary spermatocyte stage. At age 33, this man had elevated gonadotropin hormone excretion (> 100 m. u.) and 17-KS of 15.6 mg./24 hrs. At age 53 he had decreased excretion of testosterone glucuronide and "normal" urinary estrogens (24 μg. total estrogens/24 hrs). The findings can be explained by a defect in testicular 17-oxidoreductase that leads to impaired synthesis of testosterone and overproduction of androstenedione and estrone. (From Bowen, P., Lee, C. S. N.: *Ann. Intern. Med. 62*:252, 1965. Courtesy of Dr. E. C. Reifenstein, Jr.)

End-Organ Insensitivity to Androgenic Hormones

Complete Syndrome of Testicular Feminization, Feminizing Testes (Simulant Female)

Clinical Features. The term "testicular feminization" has been applied to a highly distinctive hereditary disorder in which half of the genotypic males within an affected family may be expected to resemble females (325, 342). That they are indeed genetic males is attested to by chromatin-negative somatic cells and an XY karyotype. The testes may be located in the labia majora or inguinal canals or intra-abdominally. The seminiferous tubules are usually immature and fetal in appearance, contain primitive spermatogonia and Sertoli cells, and usually do not exhibit peritubular fibrosis, even when the testes are undescended (318). The Leydig cells become hyperplastic after adolescence and tend to form adenomas. These testes are predisposed to malignant degeneration, and Morris reported seven malignant cases among the 82 that he reviewed (325). The internal ducts are predominantly male but hypoplastic on microscopic examination, and spermatoceles of the epididymis or paratesticular structures are common. The external genitalia resemble those of a female, although the vagina is shallow and ends blindly in a pouch (Fig. 8–39). At adolescence, female secondary sexual characteristics develop, notably well-developed breasts and rounding of the body contours. Menstruation, of course, does not occur. Pubic and axillary hair is scanty in most patients, and in approximately one-third of them sexual hair is completely lacking.

The mode of inheritance is consistent with either an X-linked recessive or a male-limited autosomal dominant trait (4, 137, 334, 342, 355). Thus, in an affected sibship, one could expect all the females to be normal and half the males to be affected and reared as females. It has been reported that the mothers of some of these patients are deficient in axillary hair, suggesting that they are heterozygous for the mutant gene (355).

Etiology and Pathophysiology. The etiology and pathophysiologic mechanisms that produce the various clinical features of this disorder have been greatly clarified in recent years. Although it was formerly believed that the genetic abnormality was due to some biosynthetic defect in the testes, this has not been found to be the case, and all the clinical features can now be attributed to androgen resistance on the part of the target tissues (319, 320). Incubation of these testes with labeled precursors *in vitro* reveals substantial conversions to testosterone. In young adults with this syndrome, the levels of testosterone in plasma, urine, and spermatic venous plasma are well within the range for normal adult males and much higher than in females (320, 322, 326, 343, 344). The 17-KS excretion is normal or slightly elevated. Estrogen levels in plasma and in urine are in the lower range of normal for females; the concentration of estradiol in spermatic venous plasma is elevated above the range for normal men (322). Peripheral conversion of testosterone to estrogen has been excluded as a pathogenic mechanism (319). The concentration of serum LH is increased, but the level of FSH is usually normal (320a, 322). After castration, testosterone levels fall precipitously, and estrogen levels fall somewhat less dramatically. The excretion of both FSH and LH rises to postmenopausal levels. Hot flushes are experienced by some patients after castration unless substitution therapy is provided.

Wilkins first suggested that the failure of androgen-sensitive target tissues to masculinize *in utero* as well as the failure of male secondary sexual characteristics to emerge at adolescence could be explained by end-organ resistance to androgen stimulation. He observed that the administration of large dosages of testosterone to a woman with this syndrome failed to produce clitoral enlargement, voice changes, or growth of sexual hair (16). This observation, amply confirmed by subsequent workers, was extended by Bahner and Schwarz (311) and by French et al. (319), who found that the administration of large dosages of testosterone failed to stimulate the retention of nitrogen, phosphorus, or citric acid (320). Thus the failure of the end organs to respond to androgen stimulation encompasses both the protein anabolic effects of testosterone as well as the responses of the sexual targets. Absence of spermatogenesis may likewise be explained by the dependence of germ cell maturation on an androgenic environment. The complete involution of müllerian ducts in this syndrome provides additional confirmatory evidence that the müllerian inhibiting substance (see p. 440) is not an androgenic steroid. The male genital ducts in this syndrome, although often hypoplastic, are usually better developed than those in androgen-insensitive male rates (p. 441) (312). This species difference suggests either that the androgen dependency of the male genital ducts may be less stringent in the human or that these structures may have some unique mechanism in uterine life (216a, 275) which renders them less vulnerable to the biochemical lesion causing androgen insensitivity in other structures.

French et al. proposed that the hypothalamic feedback mechanism similarly lacks normal sensitivity to testosterone and that hypersecretion of gonadotropic hormones is responsible for the adenomatous Leydig cell hyperplasia (Fig. 8–39) (320). Feminization was explained by the fact that estrogen levels as well as testosterone levels normally rise in response to LH stimulation. Female secondary sexual characteristics develop as a consequence of this stimulation, particularly in the absence of any androgenic antagonism at the cellular level. As long as the gonads remain *in situ*, gonadotropin levels fail to reach the greatly elevated levels found after castration, since the gonadotropin receptors in the hypothalamus and pituitary are normally sensitive to estrogen (320a, 322). Thus a new equilibrium is reached at a high level of testicular stimulation.

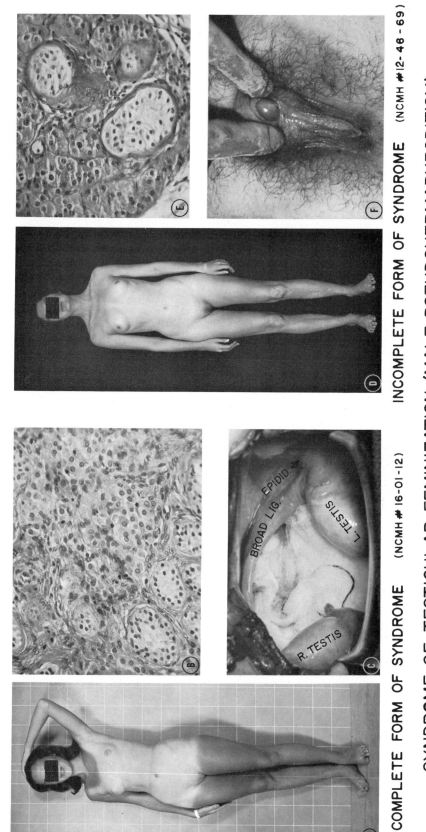

COMPLETE FORM OF SYNDROME   (NCMH # 16-01-12)   INCOMPLETE FORM OF SYNDROME   (NCMH #12-46-69)

SYNDROME OF TESTICULAR FEMINIZATION (MALE PSEUDOHERMAPHRODITISM)

Figure 8–39. Syndrome of testicular feminization (male pseudohermaphrodism). *A*, Seventeen-year-old patient with complete syndrome. This girl is chromatin-negative and has total absence of sexual hair with feminine secondary sexual development. A small vagina ends blindly. *B*, The testes exhibit Leydig cell hyperplasia, and the seminiferous tubules lack germinal elements (× 440). *C*, At laparotomy abdominal testes and male genital ducts were found. The structure resembling a broad ligament contained no identifiable müllerian derivatives. The epididymes connect with normal vasa deferentia. *D*, Incomplete form of syndrome in 25-year-old girl. Proportions are eunuchoidal. Sexual hair is present, though scanty. *E*, The testes exhibit extreme Leydig cell hyperplasia, and the seminiferous tubular membranes are thickened (× 560). *F*, The clitoris is hypertrophied, but there is no labial fusion. A shallow vagina ends blindly. Findings at laparotomy were similar to those in patient in *A*.

Although most, if not all, of the clinical findings in the syndrome of testicular feminization can be satisfactorily explained on the basis of a single biochemical lesion that prevents the action of testosterone at the cellular level, the nature of the cellular defect remains obscure. For a time it was suspected that the biochemical lesion was a deficiency in the 5α-reductase enzyme which converts testosterone to its active form, dihydrotestosterone, in target tissues (330). Strickland and French, however, showed that the low levels of this enzyme represent a consequence of androgen insensitivity rather than the cause of the syndrome (345).

A genetic model for studying the syndrome of testicular feminization has been found in mutant strains of various species, most notably the mouse and rat, in which half the male offspring display pseudohermaphrodism as a consequence of androgen insensitivity (312); the defect in these species is transmitted as an X-linked recessive trait. In these animals, the defect appears to lie in the mechanism by which androgens are transported to the nucleus (312, 338). This deficient nuclear binding of testosterone appears to be a consequence of a deficiency or abnormality of the specific cytoplasmic androgen receptor. The studies of Gehring, Tomkins, and Ohno, and Bardin et al. in the genetic androgen-insensitive male pseudohermaphroditic mouse and rat strongly suggest that lack of cytosol receptors for androgen provide an adequate explanation of the genetic defect in this animal model (312). Although not yet shown, similarities between the human syndrome and these animal models make it likely that the disorder in man is due to the genetically determined absence of, or defective, cytosol androgen receptors (274).

Incomplete Syndrome of Testicular Feminization (Genitalia Ambiguous)

A variant of the syndrome of testicular feminization is one in which affected individuals exhibit some phallic enlargement and labioscrotal fusion (Fig. 8–39). Often the fusion is sufficient to obscure the vaginal orifice, thus preserving the urogenital sinus. Although breast development occurs in these patients at adolescence, feminization is less complete than in the typical syndrome, and hirsutism or true virilism may emerge in addition to the female sexual characteristics (14, 342, 378). This disorder must be distinguished from male pseudohermaphrodism caused by a defect in 17-oxidoreductase (p. 483).

Although it is reasonable to presume that incomplete variants of the syndrome of feminizing testes may be explained on the basis of lesser degrees of insensitivity to androgens, practical considerations make this hypothesis difficult to test. Conclusive evidence would require the demonstration of a shift in the dose-response curve to testosterone rather than total insensitivity to high dosages. By measuring nitrogen, phosphorus, and citric acid excretion under metabolic ward conditions, French has accumulated suggestive data that this may indeed be so in a few children with presumptively incomplete forms of this syndrome; final proof, however, requires the performance of age- and sex-matched control studies in a normal population. Rosenfield has provided evidence for a partial degree of androgen insensitivity in a 13-year-old girl (378).

Male Pseudohermaphrodism With Normal Virilization at Puberty

Whereas the preceding categories of male pseudohermaphrodism can be attributed to defective androgen biosynthesis or defective end-organ response, there are other familial forms of male pseudohermaphrodism in which no such abnormality has been demonstrated. In these patients both the secretion of testosterone and the response of androgen-responsive target organs appear to be entirely normal, since full virilization occurs at puberty (340). The karyotype is uniformly XY, and only male internal genital ducts are present. As with other forms of male pseudohermaphrodism, these patients encompass the full range of external sexual ambiguity, extending from those with only mild hypospadias and a normal-size phallus to individuals more closely resembling females with minimal clitoral enlargement and incomplete masculinization of the urogenital sinus. The more severe familial forms constitute a clinically distinctive entity and therefore should be differentiated from the milder forms.

All of the findings in these patients could be explained on the basis of a partial intrauterine deficiency of testosterone production during the first 12 weeks of fetal life, when male differentiation of the external genitalia takes place, or be related to a period of transient end-organ hyporesponsiveness. The former could involve a transient deficiency of one or more enzymes in the biosynthesis of testosterone; the latter, delayed maturation of the Δ⁴-5α-reductase enzyme which converts testosterone to dihydrotestosterone, or of the intracellular androgen receptor in the external genitalia and urogenital sinus.

Familial Perineal Hypospadias With Ambiguous Development of Urogenital Sinus and Male Puberty (Pseudovaginal Perineoscrotal Hypospadias)

These patients resemble those with other forms of male pseudohermaphrodism by having an XY karyotype, normally differentiated testes, male internal genital ducts, and ambiguous external genitalia. Opitz et al. (332) have provided detailed descriptions of 10 affected individuals in 5 kindreds. Clitoromegaly at birth usually was of mild degree, and all but 3 of them had been assigned a female sex of rearing. The testes resided inside the abdomen, in the inguinal region, or in the bifid labioscrotal folds. At adolescence the size of the clitoris increased markedly as virilization took place. The incomplete degree of prenatal masculinization was also reflected by bifid labioscrotal folds and, in some, by persistence of the urogenital sinus. In several of the patients, there was a single perineal opening, and roentgenographic studies or endoscopy or both was necessary to demonstrate the blind vaginal pouch. In the others, the distal portion of the vagina had migrated posteriorly and acquired a perineal outlet separate from the urethra. Since the upper portion of the vagina, derived from the müllerian tract, was absent, the vaginal pouch ended blindly, as in patients with the complete form of the syndrome of feminizing testes or with enzyme defects in testosterone biosynthesis. This finding led them to propose the name of pseudovaginal perineoscrotal hypospadias. Fertility has not been reported in affected patients.

The differential point between this syndrome and other forms of male pseudohermaphrodism is that marked virilization takes place at adolescence and that breast enlargement does not take place or is minimal in degree. Many pedigrees resembling those of Opitz et al. (332) have been described (8, 335), and such patients are classified as having forms of "masculinizing male hermaphrodism" by Jones and Scott (8). The occurrence of consanguinity and the familial aggregation are consistent with an autosomal recessive mode of inheritance, in which the trait is expressed only in homozygous males.

This syndrome can be distinguished in prepubertal patients from other forms of male pseudohermaphrodism with similar anatomic findings owing to enzymatic defects in testosterone biosynthesis by the hCG test with the determination of plasma sex steroids (see pp. 483, 484). However, differentiation from the incomplete form of testicular feminization is more difficult. This may be possible by studying the metabolic response to a trial administration of testosterone and its effect on the size of the phallus.

The syndrome of familial perineal hypospadias with ambiguous development of the urogenital sinus and male puberty serves to emphasize the importance of determining the X chromatin pattern and carrying out selective roentgenographic studies in patients with hypospadias and unilateral or bilateral cryptorchidism early in infancy.

Dysgenetic Male Pseudohermaphrodism (Ambiguous Genitalia Due to Dysgenetic Gonads)

Ambiguous development of the genital ducts, urogenital sinus, and external genitalia as a consequence of defective testicular gonadogenesis occurs in patients with X chromatin–negative variants of the syndrome of gonadal dysgenesis, e.g., XO,XY mosaicism or certain structural abnor-

malities of the Y chromosome (see pp. 450, 455, and 459), and in patients with the incomplete form of familial XY gonadal dysgenesis (see p. 468). These disorders are classified as disorders of gonadal differentiation but are also included as a subgroup of male pseudohermaphrodism. Patients with faulty testicular differentiation are found with the clinical syndrome of male pseudohermaphrodism, and it must be considered in the differential diagnosis. We have used the designation "dysgenetic male pseudohermaphrodism," a term suggested by Federman, to describe this group of patients whose gonadal development is often asymmetric and on any one side varies from gonadal streak to dysgenetic testis to a normal testis. The prevalence of malignant gonadal tumors in dysgenetic male pseudohermaphrodism is strikingly increased (p. 475).

Associated with Degenerative Renal Disease

Several cases are recorded of male pseudohermaphrodism associated with the early onset of severe primary degenerative renal disease and hypertension. The two well-studied XY patients described by Drash et al. (317) had a Wilms' tumor, an association noted previously. In this syndrome, there appears to be defective development of the kidney and testes and a predisposition for malignant renal neoplasms. In addition to incomplete masculinization of the external genitalia, the development of the genital ducts is variable; the genital ducts may exhibit male, female, or ambiguous differentiation, or they may be absent.

Female Genital Ducts in Otherwise Normal Men (Herniae Uteri Inguinale)

A number of men and boys have been described with a relatively well-developed testicular morphology and male external genitalia who possess well-developed müllerian structures in addition to their male ducts (8, 316a, 320). The diagnosis is often unsuspected until the uterus prolapses through an inguinal hernia, or is encountered in the course of abdominal surgery. Retention of the müllerian structures in these cases may be thought of as a specific failure of the fetal testes to elaborate the müllerian duct–inhibiting substance, or failure of the müllerian structures to involute in response to it (p. 441). Unilateral or bilateral cryptorchidism is a common finding. The testes are usually hypoplastic, and there is a propensity for malignant transformation. These patients virilize well at adolescence, and fertile patients have been reported. Van Wyk found an XY karyotype in a 16-year-old, well-virilized male with this disorder. The presence of a uterus was discovered in the course of surgery to transfer inguinal gonads into the scrotum. Testicular biopsy revealed normally structured testes with active spermatogenesis. Several instances of affected brothers are known, including two studied by the authors. The pedigrees suggest that this disorder is inherited as an autosomal recessive trait, but an X-linked trait has not been excluded. Although transitional forms with other types of male pseudohermaphrodism may have features of this disorder, the group is sufficiently distinctive to be considered an entity.

Maternal Ingestion of Estrogens and Progestogens

In his series of 100 patients with hypospadias, Aarskog encountered 9 boys whose mothers had received synthetic progestogens during the first trimester of their pregnancy. Hypospadias occurred anywhere from a subcoronal location to the base of the penile shaft, the location correlating well with the precise week in gestation that exposure occurred (310). Although an etiologic relationship between progestogen ingestion and hypospadias has not been proven in man and the evidence is no more than suggestive, Neumann et al. (257) observed that relatively high doses of progesterone or 19-nor, 17α-hydroxyprogesterone can interfere with urethral groove fusion in a low percentage of fetal male rats. Aarskog postulated that maternal progestogens might impair testosterone production by the fetal testes by inhibiting 3β-hydroxysteroid dehydrogenase. Goldman and Bongiovanni have provided some experimental support for this mechanism of action (219, 220). Alternatively, synthetic progestational compounds might exercise a direct teratogenic effect on the primordia of the external genitalia.

Although apparently less common, Kaplan (321) has described male pseudohermaphrodism in a boy whose mother received large doses of diethylstilbestrol during early pregnancy (205). This may not have been the result of high estrogen levels per se and inhibition of testosterone secretion but rather a direct teratogenic effect of synthetic nonsteroidal estrogens. A recent striking increase in the incidence of adenocarcinoma of the vagina and cervix in adolescent girls and young women (228) and its association with treatment of their mothers with diethylstilbestrol, dienestrol, or hexestrol (all nonsteroidal estrogens) during the first trimester of pregnancy is discussed on page 480. The findings in the patients reported by Herbst et al. (228) suggest that these nonsteroidal estrogens cause a disturbance in the interplay between müllerian and urogenital sinus epithelium early in intrauterine life when the lower urogenital tract is being formed. Such a mechanism could explain the development of male pseudohermaphrodism in males exposed prenatally to stilbestrol and possibly to synthetic progestational agents.

Unclassified Forms of Male Pseudohermaphrodism

A significant advance in our understanding of male pseudohermaphrodism and its heterogeneity

has occurred since the fourth edition of this book. The major subgroups are now defined, including recognition of enzyme defects in testosterone biosynthesis not associated with clinical abnormalities of adrenocortical functions. Nonetheless, there are forms of male pseudohermaphrodism that are not readily categorized and others in which the pathogenesis is obscure.

SEXUAL ABNORMALITIES OF UNKNOWN CAUSE (NOT USUALLY ASSOCIATED WITH INTERSEXUALITY)

Many of the known causes of hermaphrodism produce a spectrum of sexual anomalies ranging from the more classic forms of intersexuality to normal-appearing individuals with adequate sexual function in adult life. There remains a large variegated group of congenital sexual abnormalities in which sexual ambiguity is not a prominent feature and in which the mechanism is as yet unknown. Many of these disorders are familial and probably due to the inheritance of a rare mutant gene or chromosomal anomaly. It is also possible that further study of the pathogenesis in these disorders will disclose presently unrecognized requirements for normal sexual differentiation.

Sexual Abnormalities of Unknown Cause in Males

Hypospadias

When hypospadias occurs as an isolated finding (about 1 in 700 newborn males), it is, by definition a mild form of male pseudohermaphrodism; however, this is an impractical and unfortunate designation for those individuals who ultimately masculinize fully and achieve fertility. Although, on theoretical grounds, deficient virilization of the external genitalia implies subnormal Leydig cell function *in utero* or refractoriness of the end organ, in most patients there are few grounds in adult life for suspecting either mechanism, and nonendocrine factors which affect differentiation of the primordia may be responsible for the anomaly. Hypospadias as an isolated anomaly is occasionally observed in multiple members of families. Sörenson found familial occurrence in 38% of cases and a concordance rate in twins of about 50% (357). In addition, it occurs in a wide variety of genetic syndromes (15).

Aarskog (310) has carried out a careful prospective study of 100 consecutive patients with hypospadias without other somatic anomalies, the majority of whom were referred from a plastic and reconstructive surgery clinic. No familial cases were encountered. One patient was a genetic female with congenital virilizing adrenal hyperplasia; 5 patients had sex chromosomal abnormalities (XO,XY or XX,XY mosaicism); one had the incomplete form of XY gonadal dysgenesis; and 9 were from pregnancies during which the mother had taken exogenous progestational compounds during the first trimester (see p. 489). Hence, in 15% of these patients, a pathogenic mechanism was found or suspected.

Cryptorchidism

Although normal testes may fail to descend into the scrotum because of coincidental anatomical abnormalities, in many instances cryptorchidism is due to faulty testicular differentiation. It is the view of Charny and of Sohval that many cases of true testicular maldescent may be explained by testicular dysgenesis (207, 348, 358). Cryptorchidism is considered in greater detail in Chapter 6.

Anorchia (the "Vanishing Testes" Syndrome)

Occasionally cryptorchid boys are encountered in whom no gonadal tissue is discovered after careful exploration (2, 4, 14, 16). The ducts are male but end blindly. The penis is usually small, and virilization does not occur at the usual age of adolescence. The chromosomal pattern is XY. Since there can be little doubt that testes were present in fetal life to initiate male development, resorption must have occurred after that period. No other satisfactory explanation has been advanced to explain anorchia in such boys.

More rarely, bilateral anorchia is associated with incomplete differentiation of the male genitalia. In some instances, not only the gonad but also the internal genital structure has been absent or rudimentary; this suggests that the abnormality that resulted in loss of the fetal testes may have also involved the primordia of the genital ducts. The chromosomal pattern in three such cases was XY. The abnormal genitalia suggest that fetal testes were present to initiate male sex development but vanished before differentiation was finished. It is not known whether the fetal testes are inherently dysgenetic and undergo regression or are normal and disappear as a result of some untoward event, such as bilateral torsion and infarction; either factor may be operative in this heterogeneous syndrome.

Kirschner et al. investigated the problem of anorchia by retrograde catheterization of the spermatic veins in two 19-year-old males with male external genitalia, absent testes, and eunuchoidism (352). With retrograde dye injection, they found it possible to identify the site of the missing testes and at the same time to obtain spermatic venous blood for testosterone measurements; although higher levels of testosterone were found in the spermatic vein than in the peripheral blood in the two patients, no recognizable testicular tissue was identified at surgery. The low levels of testosterone in the peripheral plasma rose after the administration of hCG. It was thought that only Leydig cells had persisted after the initial differentiation of the fetal testis that had induced development of a male genital tract and that these were the source of testosterone. Although no Leydig cells were actually identified, the designation "Leydig-cell-only syndrome" was proposed. In rare patients, masses of Leydig cells were present along the distal portion of the vas deferens. Testosterone levels are usually subnormal in patients with anorchia and fail to respond to stimulation with exogenous gonadotropins.

Familial Forms of Hypogonadism and Gynecomastia (Rosewater Syndrome)

Many forms of familial hypogonadism have been described, often affecting male but not female members in one or more generations (351, 355, 358). In these families, a mutant gene is strongly suspected, but the pattern of transmission has not been worked out. Gynecomastia is a variable feature. Increased excretion of estrogen, decreased excretion of urinary gonadotropins, gynecomastia, and arrested germinal maturation were found in the cases described by Rosewater et al. (Rosewater syndrome) (356). Conversion of C-19 steroids to estrogens has not been studied in these patients to exclude the possibility of excessive transformation of androgens to estrogens by peripheral tissues, nor has a defect in testosterone biosynthesis been ruled out. In other pedigrees, the gonadotropin excretion has been elevated, and the hypogonadism has been more clearly due to faulty testicular embryogenesis (358).

In yet other families, deficient secretion of gonadotropic hormones appears to be the pathophysiologic mechanism. The association of anosmia, due to agenesis of the olfactory lobes, and secondary hypogonadism is known as Kallmann's disease.

Sexual Disorders of Unknown Cause in Females

Absence of or Anomalous Development of Uterus and Fallopian Tubes

Absence of or anomalous development of müllerian derivatives in genetic females cannot be explained on the basis of defective gonadogenesis, since the conversion of müllerian primordia into uterus and fallopian tubes requires no gonadal mediating factor. The karyotype in these patients has been uniformly XX. An abnormal hormonal environment in the fetus is also an unlikely explanation, since the testicular factor that inhibits müllerian development in males is not believed to be one of the known steroid hormones. Although women with this syndrome do not menstruate and are incapable of bearing children, several hormonal studies show that their ovarian function follows the normal female cyclic pattern and that ovulation probably occurs (362).

The fact that bicornuate or unicornuate uterus

or congenital absence of the uterus often occurs in association with anomalies of the urinary tract suggests that these malformations stem from anomalous development of the urogenital ridge in the early weeks of fetal life (360). The incidence of renal anomalies has been as high as 25-50% in such patients (368). In addition, there is a high incidence of skeletal anomalies, particularly midline anomalies of the vertebral column, scapulae (Sprengel's deformity), and pelvis (359).

Congenital Absence of the Vagina

Failure of the vagina to descend normally in genetic females is usually due to androgenic exposure; in such patients, absence of an external vaginal orifice is usually accompanied by labioscrotal fusion and clitoral hypertrophy. In patients with congenital absence of the vagina, the normal opening of the vagina is represented by only a dimple, and there is neither labial fusion nor any other manifestations of virilization. In most of these patients, the uterus is also lacking or rudimentary, and the vaginal hypoplasia is secondary to anomalous müllerian development. Familial occurrence has been reported but is rare. Any phenotypic female with vaginal atresia and absence of müllerian structures should be examined for the possible presence of testes and a negative X chromatin pattern to distinguish this subject from genetic males with the syndrome of feminizing testes. Concomitant anomalies of the urinary tract should be sought in chromatin-positive patients (360).

MANAGEMENT OF PATIENTS EXHIBITING AMBISEXUAL DEVELOPMENT

Considerations Governing Choice of Sex for Rearing

With proper assignment of sex for rearing and appropriate subsequent management, individuals with ambiguities in their sexual makeup should be able to lead well-adjusted lives and ultimately attain the goal of a satisfactory marriage. To obtain this favorable result, it is incumbent upon the attending physician to make a correct diagnosis as early as possible and reach a firm decision on the sex for rearing. Once the sex for rearing is assigned, the gender role is thereafter reinforced by the appropriate employment of whatever surgical, hormonal, and psychologic measures are indicated.

Deeply ingrained in our culture is the concept that some innate biologic difference between males and females is responsible for the behavioral differences between boys and girls as well as the sexual orientation of adults. Studies of patients reared in a sex discordant with their chromosomal sex, gonadal sex, hormonal sex, and even external genital organs have clearly shown, however, that no one parameter can be used infallibly as a basis upon which to assign sex for rearing (364). This choice should therefore be governed principally by the possibilities that exist for achieving unambiguous and sexually useful genital structures.

The hormonal sex expected at maturity and the possibilities for fertility are of secondary importance and decisive only in the case of female pseudohermaphrodites, in whom the abnormality is limited to the external genitalia and in whom fertility is often achieved. Such patients should all be reared as females, since ambiguity can be removed by appropriate surgery of the external genitalia. In the case of congenital adrenal hyperplasia, further masculinization is prevented by the provision of adrenal substitution therapy.

Except in female pseudohermaphrodites, ambiguities of the external genitalia are caused by lesions that almost invariably render the patient sterile. The major consideration in these patients, therefore, should be the possibilities for surgical reconstruction of the external genitalia. In considering a decision to recommend a male sex for rearing, it is our belief that greater attention should be directed to the size of the shaft and glans than to the degree of labioscrotal fusion. Boys with a microphallus rarely develop an adequately sized penis, even after intensive treatment with testosterone. It has been our experience that virtually all the tragic outcomes in later life have resulted from an early unwise assignment of a male sex for rearing to a child whose phallus, for whatever reason, held little promise of developing into an organ adequate for normal sexual function and masculine self-esteem. Therefore, unless it is reasonable to expect that the hypospadias can be satisfactorily corrected and that the adult phallus will be of adequate size, it is far better to rear the child as a female. Principles governing the differential diagnosis and the surgical, hormonal, and psychological management of patients with genital ambiguity are treated more extensively in the following sections.

Differential Diagnosis of Ambisexual Development in Infancy

Abnormalities of sex differentiation should be suspected not only in infants with grossly ambiguous genitalia but also in apparent females with inguinal masses, inguinal herniae, or slight clitoral enlargement. Apparent males with cryptorchidism, hypospadias, or unusually small genitalia or gonads likewise deserve close scrutiny. Sufficient investigation should be carried out in the newborn period to permit the assignment of sex with enough firmness to preclude future uncertainty. An accurate determination of the X chromatin pattern is an imperative first step in all such newborns since the presence of X chromatin bodies in the nuclei of mucosal cells should suggest the need for additional studies to determine whether or not female pseudohermaphrodism is present (Table 8-10). Karyotype analysis is, of course, a better means of determining the chromosomal sex.

TABLE 8–10.   STEPS IN THE DIAGNOSIS OF INTERSEXUALITY IN INFANCY AND CHILDHOOD*

History: family history, pregnancy (hormones), "crises," virilization
Inspection
Palpation of inguinal region and labioscrotal folds and rectal examination
Oral mucosal smear—X chromatin pattern; karyotype—sex chromosome constitution
Excretion of 17-ketosteroids and pregnanetriol; serum 17-hydroxyprogesterone
Serum electrolytes and urea nitrogen
Provisional diagnosis

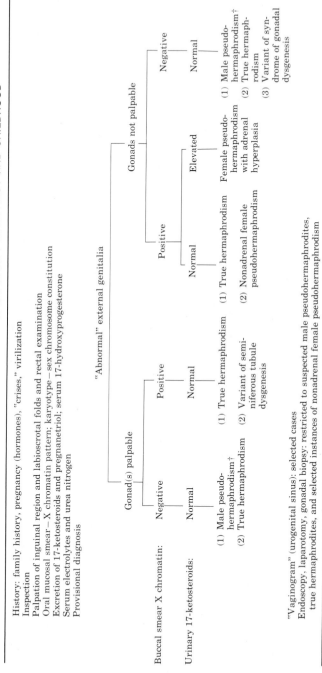

"Abnormal" external genitalia

	Gonad(s) palpable		Gonads not palpable		
Buccal smear X chromatin:	Negative	Positive	Positive		Negative
Urinary 17-ketosteroids:	Normal	Normal	Normal	Elevated	Normal
	(1) Male pseudo-hermaphrodism†	(1) True hermaphrodism	(1) True hermaphrodism	Female pseudo-hermaphrodism with adrenal hyperplasia	(1) Male pseudo-hermaphrodism†
	(2) True hermaphrodism	(2) Variant of semi-niferous tubule dysgenesis	(2) Nonadrenal female pseudohermaphrodism		(2) True hermaph-rodism
					(3) Variant of syn-drome of gonadal dysgenesis

"Vaginogram" (urogenital sinus): selected cases
Endoscopy, laparotomy, gonadal biopsy: restricted to suspected male pseudohermaphrodites, true hermaphrodites, and selected instances of nonadrenal female pseudohermaphrodism

*From Grumbach, M. M., In *Pediatrics*. 13th ed. Holt, L. E., Jr., McIntosh, R., and Barnett, H. L. (eds.), New York, Appleton-Century-Crofts, 1962.
†Excretion of 17-ketosteroids is increased in male pseudohermaphrodites who have congenital adrenal hyperplasia due to a defect in 3β-hydroxysteroid dehydrogenase.

Infants with X Chromatin–Positive Nuclear Patterns

All infants with sexual ambiguity and a positive X chromatin pattern should receive sufficient study in the neonatal period to differentiate the various forms of female pseudohermaphrodism, on the one hand, from true hermaphrodism or variants of gonadal dysgenesis, on the other.

Congenital Adrenal Hyperplasia. If female pseudohermaphrodism is secondary to congenital adrenal hyperplasia, the excretion of 17-KS should be elevated. During the first three weeks of life, the values of normal infants may be as high as 4 mg./24 hr. (16). If the 17-KS values are equivocal, the finding of significant quantities of pregnanetriol (Ch. 5) may settle the diagnosis; however, the excretion of urinary pregnanetriol glucuronide usually is not increased during the first few weeks of life. Recently, a strikingly increased concentration of plasma 17-hydroxyprogesterone has been demonstrated in patients with defective 21-hydroxylation; values over 1 μg./100 ml. in an infant with ambiguous genitalia who is 18 hours of age or older is virtually diagnostic of the type I and II forms. Any infant with ambiguous external genitalia who fails to thrive or who develops vomiting and dehydration during the first few weeks of life should be suspected of the salt-losing type of adrenal hyperplasia. If such an infant is found to have hyperkalemia associated with acidosis or hyponatremia, the diagnosis is virtually assured, and vigorous therapy with cortisone, salt, and salt-retaining steroids should be instituted on an urgent basis to prevent collapse and sudden death. Once the diagnosis of adrenal hyperplasia is established, cortisone therapy should be instituted and continued for life.

Other Forms of Female Pseudohermaphrodism. X chromatin–positive infants may be presumed to have simple female pseudohermaphrodism if adrenal hyperplasia has been excluded and if there is a reliable history that the mother received androgens or progestational hormones during pregnancy or if she developed some virilizing tendency. These children will require no further hormonal medication during childhood and will feminize normally at adolescence. The diagnosis of female pseudohermaphrodism can likewise be made with some confidence in X chromatin–positive infants if gross anomalies of the lower intestine or urinary tract are present. Such children should be studied for the presence of pyelonephritis and anomalies in other systems. Patients with female pseudohermaphrodism usually have a normal uterus and fallopian tubes with ovaries situated in the normal location. For this reason, the diagnosis should be viewed with suspicion if there is an inguinal hernia or if the gonads are palpable in the groin. Such patients more frequently have testes. The presence of a uterus can often be detected in the newborn period by digital examination via the rectum. It is often possible to confirm the presence of endometrial tissue by cytologic means after expressing mucoid secretions from a urogenital sinus by bimanual manipulation of the suspected uterus. Once the physiologic hyperplasia that exists at birth has regressed, the interpretation of a rectal examination may be inconclusive.

True Hermaphrodism. Seventy per cent of patients with true hermaphrodism are X chromatin–positive (6), and it may be difficult to distinguish some of them from the rare idiopathic cases of female pseudohermaphrodism. True hermaphrodites, however, often have gonads located in their labia or inguinal canals. In all of these cases, the assignment of sex should be deferred until the nature of the internal genital structures and gonads can be determined by urethroscopy, radiologic study with contrast media (383), or pelvic exploration. Karyotype analysis is necessary for the detection of those patients with sex chromosome abnormalities. The assignment of sex to a true hermaphrodite should be based on the possibilities for surgical correction of the external genitalia. It is often possible to remove the heterologous gonadal tissue in these patients. The risk of malignant degeneration in gonads that are retained (p. 475) should be carefully weighed before arriving at a final decision.

X Chromatin–Positive Seminiferous Tubule Dysgenesis (Klinefelter's Syndrome). A positive X chromatin pattern is found in approximately one of every 500 newborn phenotypic males (135). Most of these infants will have an XXY karyotype and will not come to attention during infancy because their external genitalia exhibit normal male development and only rarely hypospadias.

Infants with X Chromatin–Negative Patterns

A negative X chromatin pattern is found in all patients with male pseudohermaphrodism (by current definition), in approximately 80% of those with the syndrome of gonadal dysgenesis, and in 30% of true hermaphrodites. In many of these patients, the phenotype will be so clearly male or female that the sex for rearing will not be in question. Nonetheless, efforts should be made, insofar as possible, to establish an etiologic diagnosis, since this may have an important bearing on subsequent management (372). A detailed family history with construction of a pedigree should not be neglected, since many sexual abnormalities are hereditary in nature, and this type of historical information is not readily volunteered. For example, a history of "aunts" who have never menstruated or of an inguinal hernia or labial mass in a phenotypic female may suggest the diagnosis of the syndrome of testicular feminization. The mother, likewise, should be queried about drugs or hormones that she may have received during the early part of pregnancy.

Studies during the newborn period should always include an examination of the karyotype. A sufficient number of metaphase plates should be examined to reduce the possibility of overlooking mosaicism. The morphology of the Y chromosome should be examined with the Giemsa and quinacrine-banding techniques.

Roentgenologic studies of the urogenital sinus following the injection of contrast media (370, 383) and possibly endoscopic examination may aid in this initial evaluation. Laparotomy is usually not necessary during the neonatal period since, in choosing the sex for rearing, primary emphasis should be placed on the external genitalia and the possibilities for ultimately obtaining adequate sexual function.

Except in patients with congenital adrenal hyperplasia, steroid excretion studies during early infancy have, in our hands, proven of little value in differentiating the various causes of sexual ambiguity. Of greater value has been the determination of the response to human chorionic gonadotropin (hCG). This hormone is given daily in a dosage of 500-1000 I.U. for 7–10 days, with frequent monitoring of plasma testosterone levels. This treatment will usually result in significant enlargement of the phallus. Thus, in addition to providing objective information on the functional capacity of the Leydig cells to secrete testosterone, it provides evidence of the capacity of androgen-sensitive target tissues to respond to this stimulus. Although such minimal endocrine studies may help to decide the appropriate sex for rearing in borderline cases, they usually fall short of defining a precise biochemical lesion in patients with hereditary errors in testosterone biosynthesis. More sophisticated studies to define such lesions are much more likely to be productive if carried out at a later age under metabolic ward conditions.

The problem of sex assignment in boys with a micropenis is particularly vexing. Boys with congenital hypopituitarism frequently have diminutive genitalia, and this diagnosis should be excluded by appropriate pituitary function studies before considering the possibility of sex reassignment. It is our belief that male infants with microphallus should also be given trial administrations of adequate doses of exogenous testosterone before concluding that their phallus lacks the capacity for growth. The administration of a dose of 50 mg. testosterone enanthate intramuscularly every two weeks for about eight weeks should provide ample stimulus to make this assessment. This treatment admittedly may cause undesirable advancement of the skeletal age, but this consideration is trivial when weighed against the more momentous question of deciding the child's sexual destiny.

Once the decision is made, on the basis of the criteria stated above, to rear the infant as a boy or girl, there should be no further indecision in the minds of either the physician or parents. It is nevertheless required in most patients to carry out surgical exploration at some later date to determine the structure of the internal genital ducts and gonads. This pelvic exploration can be deferred until such time that plastic procedures on the external genitalia are undertaken (369).

Reassignment of Sex After the Newborn Period

Frequently, children are assigned to a totally inappropriate sex because of errors in diagnosis or because of ignorance of the principles that should properly govern this choice. In such patients, the knotty decision to change the sex for rearing or to leave matters undisturbed is largely dependent upon the age of the child and the degree to which the gender role has been established. Money and the Hampsons have shown that a change in the sex for rearing is feasible until the age of $1\frac{1}{2}$ years and is sometimes successful until $2\frac{1}{2}$ years, but thereafter serious psychiatric consequences may be anticipated (374). A change of sex after 18 months should be undertaken only after a most painstaking review of possible alternatives and only if provision has been made for close supervision and long-term counseling.

After adolescence, the patient himself may reach the decision that he or she has been reared in the wrong sex and may request assistance in changing his or her sex of assignment. If there are sufficient anatomical grounds for this belief, the request should be seriously considered and honored if possible. Such patients usually have serious psychiatric disturbances, and both psychiatric and legal counsel should be sought.

Reconstructive Surgery

Since the presence of ambiguous external genitalia is apt to reinforce doubt regarding the sexual identity, it is desirable to initiate reconstructive surgery as early as is surgically feasible. For psychological reasons, it is highly desirable that surgery on the external genitalia be completed prior to 18 months of age. Jones and Verkauf (369) reviewed the results of surgical correction of the ambiguous genitalia of 84 female pseudohermaphrodites with congenital adrenal hyperplasia. Satisfactory results from initial reconstructive surgery were achieved in 80% of the patients. Accordingly, they recommend repair of the external genitalia as soon after 2 months of age as is convenient. Money's group (374) has stressed the importance of both early genital operation and psychological support for the family in ensuring a successful psychological outcome. In a child reared as a female, it may be better to sacrifice a conspicuous clitoris than to leave a large erectile organ which may later be the source and focus of extreme psychological turmoil (367). Although the patient may be partly handicapped in her later sexual experiences, it has been demonstrated that erotic responses and orgasm can be achieved after clitoridectomy (375). If the clitoris is only moderately enlarged, it may be rendered less conspicuous by the clitoral recession procedure of Lattimer (Fig. 8–40) (371). In our hands, however, this procedure has proven unsatisfactory in patients with marked clitoromegaly, and in some patients it has been necessary to carry out a secondary clitoral amputation with plastic reconstruction of a nonfunctional "cosmetic clitoris."

Reconstruction of a vagina, if necessary, should be deferred until requested by the patient. A small vaginal pouch can sometimes be adequately enlarged by daily manipulations with a test tube or other suitable mold (8, 361). Even if the vagina re-

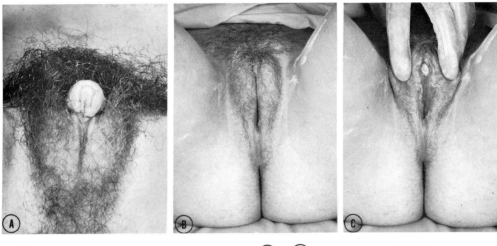

Ⓐ **PRE-OPERATIVE**   Ⓑ & Ⓒ **POSTOPERATIVE**

NCMH # 15-89-01

CLITORAL RECESSION AND SURGICAL REPAIR OF UROGENITAL SINUS IN 8 YR. OLD FEMALE PSEUDOHERMAPHRODITE WITH UNTREATED ADRENOGENITAL SYNDROME

Figure 8-40. Clitoral recession operation in 8-year-old female with previously untreated congenital adrenal hyperplasia. *A,* Preoperatively there was almost complete posterior fusion of the labia with a single, funnellike urogenital sinus at the base of a large erectile phallus. *B* and *C, A* satisfactory cosmetic appearance was achieved without sacrificing the glans or corpora cavernosa. Posterior incision of fused labia has eliminated the urogenital sinus, thus providing a separate external opening for the vagina.

mains too shallow for satisfactory sexual relations, manipulations of this sort make it easier to carry out subsequent surgical correction. A comprehensive discussion of the surgical management of these procedures can be found in the text of Jones and Scott (8).

A male with hypospadias usually requires multiple operations to create a phallic urethra. Circumcision should be avoided in order to preserve as much tissue as possible. Pelvic exploration can be undertaken simultaneously with the initial operation to correct chordee. It is often desirable to insert prosthetic testes to give the scrotum dependency and to improve the cosmetic appearance; these may be exchanged for adult-sized prostheses in adolescence.

Removal of the Gonads

A high incidence of gonadal tumors in patients with certain forms of gonadal dysgenesis and various other forms of hermaphrodism makes it mandatory that an evaluation of this risk be given priority over other considerations in deciding if and when the gonads should be removed. Currently available information on the incidence of tumors in the various forms of gonadal dysgenesis is reviewed on pp. 475, 476. Although the incidence of gonadoblastomas, seminomas, or dysgerminomas increases near the normal time of adolescence, a significant number of these tumors have been discovered during the first decade. Since temporization serves no useful purpose and may expose the child to hormone secretions inappropriate to the chosen sex for rearing (374), it is advisable to pro-

ceed with gonadectomy concurrently with the initial repair of the external genitalia in patients who are at risk. Similarly, gonadectomy and removal of the uterus should be carried out as early as possible in the rare cases of female pseudohermaphrodism who have been mistakenly reared as boys and in whom change of sex is inadvisable.

Although Morris reported a 9% incidence of gonadal tumors in his 1953 review of 82 cases of testicular feminization, it is quite possible that some of these patients who developed tumors actually had atypical forms of gonadal dysgenesis. Recent reports of gonadal tumors arising in patients with the complete syndrome of testicular feminization have been rare. Although gonadectomy should ultimately be carried out in these patients, it is often desirable to leave the gonads *in situ* until late in the second decade, in the hope that testicular estrogens will bring about the development of normal feminine sexual characteristics. This greatly reinforces the patient's own concept of her sexual identity, and prophylactic castration to prevent malignancy is then more easily explained and readily accepted.

In patients with the incomplete form of this syndrome and with other forms of male pseudohermaphrodism in which a female sex for rearing has been assigned, there is a high risk of masculinization at the time of puberty, and castration should be carried out in early childhood. In less severe forms of male pseudohermaphrodism in which a male sex for rearing has been chosen, it can be anticipated that at least some degree of virilism will occur with the onset of puberty. Providing that the testes are not dysgenetic and are sufficiently descended to permit ready palpation, it is probably safe to leave the testes *in situ*. Such patients should be carefully examined at frequent intervals for the presence of a tumor.

Hormonal Substitution Therapy

Hormonal substitution therapy in hypogonadal patients should be prescribed in such a way that secondary sexual characteristics emerge appropriately in both timing and sequence. The goal of therapy should be to approximate normal adolescent development as closely as possible.

If the patient is dwarfed, it is advisable to defer treatment for as long as possible to achieve maximal stature. Usually, however, psychological considerations dictate that treatment be started by the fourteenth or fifteenth year. Patients with short stature associated with gonadal dysgenesis have normal GH levels, and no more than a modest increase in stature, if any, can be induced by the administration of exogenous GH in the doses used for the treatment of hypopituitary dwarfism. The value of synthetic, weakly androgenic hormones (so-called "protein anabolic agents") to stimulate a growth spurt in these patients remains highly controversial; some authors have reported highly significant acceleration of growth rates (366), whereas other observers have not had this experience and believe that the final stature is either relatively unaffected or compromised by disproportionate advancement in the skeletal age (264). A therapeutic trial with oxandrolone in a dose of 0.25 mg./kg. daily is unlikely to be harmful, provided that the patient is observed for early signs of virilization and the duration of treatment is not overly prolonged. It is particularly important in short-statured patients that substitution therapy with estrogens be initiated at a very low dosage, since higher dosages bring about rapid cessation of growth.

Hormonal substitution treatment in females is initiated by continuous estrogen treatment for a period of time to bring about breast enlargement and growth of the uterus. Cyclic therapy with estrogen and an oral progestogen is begun after about 6 months of continuous estrogen therapy or after menstrual bleeding occurs. Cyclic therapy is more easily remembered if it is related to the calendar rather than to the lunar month. Certain of the contraceptive drugs now offer conveniently packaged sequential estrogen-progestin combinations that introduce hormones in a sequence that closely resembles the normal menstrual cycle. Nonsteroidal estrogens such as stilbestrol are contraindicated because of their suspected carcinogenicity. In one series, three cases of endometrial carcinoma developed among a group of 24 patients with gonadal dysgenesis treated five or more years with stilbestrol (64, 228).

In males, more adequate virilization is usually obtained by repository injections of testosterone cyclopentylpropionate or testosterone enanthate than by methyltestosterone. Methyltestosterone has the added disadvantage of predisposing to biliary stasis and jaundice. However, sudden virili-

zation is often inadvisable, and it is preferable to bring about adolescent changes gradually over a period of many months in a manner similar to that in normal boys. Due regard should be given to the fact that the effect of sex steroids on skeletal maturation is dosage-related, whereas the effect on linear growth is less so. Thus, at the inception of therapy, the relation between attained stature and skeletal maturation as well as the dosage of androgen prescribed will determine the ultimate effect of this therapy on the adult height. An initial dose of 5 mg. methyltestosterone daily by the oral or buccal route often can be appropriately initiated at 12 or 13 years of age, with increments up to a total of 25 mg. daily as the boy grows older. When greater virilization or more sexual potency is desired, it is often necessary to switch to intramuscular injections of one of the repository testosterone preparations (Ch. 6).

Psychological Management

Few people are sufficiently sophisticated to accept a sex for rearing discordant with their chromosomal or gonadal sex. For this reason, it is advisable to avoid such a disclosure from the beginning and to present the issues in more readily comprehended terms. There should never be any doubt in the mind of parent or patient that a child is being reared in his own "true sex," although it is best to admit uncertainty regarding the "true sex" until sufficient studies have been completed. This approach is completely honest if the physician himself fully recognizes that sex is not a single biologic entity with one decisive parameter but rather the net expression of many morphologic characteristics and functional potentialities. Thus, in the strictest sense, an infant's "true sex" is in fact the one to which he is assigned after these many factors have been thoroughly evaluated. A simple embryologic explanation of the double set of sexual organs present in early life is useful, since it lays the groundwork for the concept that sex differentiation is often not completed *in utero*. An analogy to other congenital malformations such as cleft lip or congenital heart disease is accurate and easily understood. The parents should be reassured that their child does not have a "reversed sex" nor is he "half boy and half girl." It should be clearly stated that the anatomical abnormalities in sexual development do not predispose to homosexual drives.

Children reared in an atmosphere in which their sex for rearing is accepted with conviction need not have catastrophic psychological problems. With proper surgical reconstruction and hormonal substitution, when required, most individuals with ambisexual development should reach adulthood as well-virilized men or as feminine women capable of achieving satisfactory sexual relationships, although usually unproductive of issue.

Dr. Van Wyk is USPHS Career Research Awardee (5K6 AM–14, 115–05).

REFERENCES

General

1. Armstrong, C. N., and Marshall, A. J. (eds.): *Intersexuality in Vertebrates Including Man.* New York, Academic Press, 1964.
2. Federman, D. D.: *Abnormal Sexual Development.* Philadelphia, W. B. Saunders Company, 1967.
3. Gardner, L. I. (ed.): *Endocrine and Genetic Diseases of Childhood.* Philadelphia, W. B. Saunders Company, 1969.
4. Grumbach, M. M., and Barr, M. L.: *Recent Progr. Hormone Res.* 14:335, 1958.
5. Grumbach, M. M.: In *Biologic Basis of Pediatric Practice.* Cooke, R. E. (ed.), New York, McGraw-Hill, 1967.
6. Hamerton, J. L.: *Human Cytogenetics, General Cytogenetics.* Vol. 1. New York, Academic Press, 1970.
7. Hamerton, J. L.: *Human Cytogenetics, Clinical Cytogenetics.* Vol. II. New York, Academic Press, 1971.
8. Jones, H. W., and Scott, W. W.: *Hermaphroditism, Genital Anomalies and Related Endocrine Disorders.* 2nd ed. Baltimore, Williams & Wilkins Company, 1971.
9. Levine, H.: *Clinical Cytogenetics.* Boston, Little Brown & Company, 1971.
10. McKusick, V. A.: *Mendelian Inheritance in Man.* 3rd ed. Baltimore, Johns Hopkins University Press, 1971.
11. Money, J., and Ehrhardt, A. A.: *Man and Woman, Boy and Girl: The Differentiation and Dimorphism of Gender Identity from Conception to Maturity.* Baltimore, Johns Hopkins University Press, 1972.
12. Moore, K. L. (ed.): *The Sex Chromatin.* Philadelphia, W. B. Saunders Company, 1966.
13. Odell, W. D., and Moyer, D. L.: *Physiology of Reproduction.* St. Louis, C. V. Mosby Company, 1971.
14. Overzier, C. (ed.): *Intersexuality.* New York, Academic Press, 1963.
15. Rimoin, D. L., and Schimke, R. N.: *Genetic Disorders of the Endocrine Glands.* St. Louis, C. V. Mosby Company, 1971.
16. Wilkins, L.: *The Diagnosis and Treatment of Endocrine Disorders in Childhood and Adolescence.* 3rd ed. Springfield, Ill., Charles C Thomas, 1965.
17. Young, W. C. (ed.): *Sex and Internal Secretions.* 3rd ed. Baltimore, Williams & Wilkins Company, 1961.

Biology of the Sex Chromosomes and Errors in Gonadal Differentiation

18. Almqvist, S., Hall, K., et al.: *Acta Endocr.* 46:451, 1964.
19. Almqvist, S., Lindsten, J., et al.: *Acta Endocr.* 42:168, 1963.
20. Armendares, S., Buentello, L., et al.: *J. Med. Genet.* 9:96, 1972.
21. Bahner, F., Schwarz, G., et al.: *Acta Endocr.* 35:397, 1960.
22. Baikie, A. G., Garson, O. M., et al.: *Lancet* 1:398, 1966.
23. Bain, A. D., and Scott, J. S.: *Lancet* 1:1035, 1965.
24. Baron, J., Rucki, T., et al.: *Gynaecologia* (Basel) 153:298, 1962.
25. Barr, M. L., and Bertram, E. G.: *Nature* (London) 163:676, 1949.
26. Barr, M. L.: In *Second International Conference on Congenital Malformations.* New York, International Medical Congress, Ltd., 1964, p. 11.
27. Barr, M. L., and Carr, D. H.: *Acta Cytol.* (Baltimore) 6:34, 1962.
28. Barr, M. L., Carr, D. H., et al.: *J. Ment. Defic. Res.* 6:65, 1962.
29. Barr, M. L., Carr, D. H., et al.: *Canad. Med. Ass. J.* 87:891, 1963.
30. Barr, M. L., Carr, D. H., et al.: *Canad. Med. Ass. J.* 90:575, 1964.
31. Barr, M. L., Carr, D. H., et al.: *Amer. J. Obstet. Gynec.* 99:1047, 1967.
32. Barr, M. L., Sergovich, F. R., et al.: *Canad. Med. Ass. J.* 101:247, 1969.
33. Beatty, R. A.: *Cambridge Monographs in Experimental Biology,* No. 7, 1957.
34. Becker, K. L., Hoffman, D. L., et al.: *Arch. Intern. Med.* 118:314, 1966.
35. Benirschke, K., Naftolin, F., et al.: *J. Obstet. Gynec.* 113:449, 1972.
36. Bergsma, D., Hamerton, J. L., et al. (eds.): Chicago Conference: Standardization in human cytogenetics. *Birth Defects: Orig. Art. Ser.* 2(2):1966.

37. Beutler, E., Yeh, M., et al.: *Proc. Nat. Acad. Sci. USA* 48:9, 1962.
38. Bieger, R. C., Passarge, E., et al.: *J. Clin. Endocr.* 25:1340, 1965.
39. Blackston, R. O., and Chen, A. T. L.: *J. Med. Genet.* 9:230, 1972.
40. Boczkowski, K., and Teter, J.: *Acta Endocr.* 51:497, 1966.
41. Boczkowski, K., Teter, J., et al.: *Amer. J. Obstet. Gynec.* 113:952, 1972.
42. Boyer, S. H., Ferguson-Smith, M. A., et al.: *Ann. Hum. Genet.* 25:215, 1961.
43. Bray, P., and Sr. Ann Josephine: *J.A.M.A.* 184:179, 1963.
44. Brøgger, A., and Strand, A.: *Acta Endocr.* 48:490, 1965.
45. Brown, S. W., and Chandra, H. S.: *Proc. Nat. Acad. Sci. USA* 70:195, 1973.
46. Caldwell, P. D., and Smith, D. W.: *J. Pediat.* 80:250, 1972.
47. Carr, D. H., Barr, M. L., et al.: *J. Clin. Endocr.* 21:491, 1961.
48. Carr, D. H., Morishima, A., et al.: *J. Clin. Endocr.* 22:671, 1962.
49. Carr, D. H.: *Obstet. Gynec.* 26:308, 1964.
50. Carr, D. H.: *Advance Hum. Genet.* 2:401, 1971.
51. Caspersson, T., Zech, L., et al.: *Chromosoma* 30:215, 1970.
52. Caspersson, T., Hulten, M., et al.: *Hereditas* 68:317, 1971.
53. Caspersson, T., and Zech, L.: *Hospital Practice* 7:51, 1972.
54. Cattanach, B. M., Pollard, C. E., et al.: *Cytogenetics* 10:318, 1971.
55. Chemke, J., Carmichael, R., et al.: *J. Med. Genet.* 7:105, 1970.
56. Chen, A. T. L., and Falek, A.: *Amer. J. Hum. Genet.* 22:45a, 1970.
57. Childs, B.: *Pediatrics* 35:798, 1965.
58. Clayton, G. W., Smith, J. D., et al.: *J. Clin. Endocr.* 18:1349, 1958.
59. Cohen, M. M., Lin, C-C., et al.: *Amer. J. Hum. Genet.* 24:583, 1972.
60. Comings, D. E.: *Advances Hum. Genet.* 3:237, 1972.
61. Court Brown, W. M., Harnden, D. G., et al.: *Med. Res. Council Spec. Rept. Ser.,* No. 305, 1964.
62. Court-Brown, W. M., Mantle, D. J., et al.: *J. Med. Genet.* 1:35, 1964.
63. Court Brown, W. M.: *Int. Rev. Exp. Path.* 7:31, 1969.
64. Cutler, B. S., Forbes, A. P., et al.: *New Eng. J. Med.* 287:628, 1972.
65. Davidson, R. G., Nitowsky, H. M., et al.: *Proc. Nat. Acad. Sci. USA* 50:481, 1963.
66. Davidson, W. M.: *Intersexuality.* Overzier, C. (ed.), New York, Academic Press, 1963, p. 72.
67. Decourt, L., Sasso, W. daS., et al.: *Rev. Ass. Med. Brasil* 1:203, 1954.
68. de la Chapelle, A., and Hortling, H.: *Acta Endocr.* 44:165, 1963.
69. de la Chapelle, A., Wennström, J., et al.: *Hereditas* 54:260, 1966.
70. de la Chapelle, A.: *Amer. J. Hum. Genet.* 24:71, 1972.
71. de la Chapelle, A., Schröder, J., et al.: *Ann. Hum. Genet.* 36:79, 1972.
72. del Castillo, E. B., Trabucco, A., et al.: *J. Clin. Endocr.* 7:493, 1947.
73. Distèche, C., Hagemaijer, A., et al.: *Clin. Genet.* 3:388, 1972.
74. Dronamraju, K. R.: *Nature* (London) 201:424, 1964.
75. Dunlap, D. B., Aubry, R., et al.: *J. Clin. Endocr.* 34:491, 1972.
76. Ehlers, K. H., Engle, M. A., et al.: *Circulation* 45:639, 1972.
77. Elliott, G. A., Sandler, A., et al.: *J. Clin. Endocr.* 19:995, 1959.
78. Engel, E., and Forbes, A. P.: *Medicine* 44:135, 1965.
79. Epstein, C. J.: *Science* 163:1078, 1969.
80. Epstein, C. J.: *Science* 175:1467, 1972.
81. Espiner, E. A., Veale, A. M. O., et al.: *New Eng. J. Med.* 283:6, 1970.
82. Ferguson-Smith, M. A.: *Lancet* 1:219, 1959.
83. Ferguson-Smith, M. A., Mack, W. S., et al.: *Lancet* 1:46, 1964.
84. Ferguson-Smith, M. A.: *J. Med. Genet.* 2:142, 1965.
85. Ferguson-Smith, M. A.: *Lancet* 2:475, 1966.
86. Fialkow, P. J., Uchida, I. A.: *Ann. N.Y. Acad. Sci.* 155:759, 1968.
87. Ford, C. E., and Hamerton, J. L.: *Nature* (London) 178:1020, 1956.
88. Ford, C. E., Jones, K. W., et al.: *Lancet* 1:709, 1959.
89. Ford, C. E., Jones, K. W., et al.: *Lancet* 2:711, 1959.

90. Ford, C. E.: *Brit. Med. Bull. 25*:104, 1969.
91. Fraccaro, M., Kaijser, K., et al.: *Lancet 2*:899, 1960.
92. Fraccaro, M., Ikkos, D., et al.: *Acta Endocr. 36*:98, 1961.
93. Frøland, A.: *Danish Med. Bull. 16*(Suppl. 6):1, 1969.
94. Gartler, S. M., Waxman, S. H., et al.: *Proc. Nat. Acad. Sci. USA 48*:332, 1962.
95. German, J.: *Clin. Genet. 1*:15, 1970.
96. German, J.: In *Proceedings Third International Congress Hum. Genetics.* Crow, J. F., and Neel, J. V. (eds.), Baltimore, Johns Hopkins University Press, 1967, p. 123.
97. Giorgi, E. P., and Sommerville, I. F.: *J. Clin. Endocr. 23*:197, 1963.
98. Goldberg, M. B., Scully, A. L., et al.: *Amer. J. Med. 45*:529, 1968.
99. Gordon, D. L., Krmpotic, E., et al.: *Arch. Intern. Med. 130*:726, 1972.
100. Gordon, R. R., and O'Neill, E. M.: *Brit. Med. J. 1*:483, 1969.
101. Greenblatt, R. B.: *Recent Progr. Hormone Res. 14*:335, 1958.
102. Grumbach, M. M., Van Wyk, J. J., et al.: *J. Clin. Endocr. 15*:1161, 1955.
103. Grumbach, M. M., In *Clinical Endocrinology.* Astwood, E. B. (ed.), New York, Grune & Stratton, 1960, p. 407.
104. Grumbach, M. M., Blanc, W. A., et al.: *J. Clin. Endocr. 17*:703, 1957.
105. Grumbach, M. M., Marks, P. A., et al.: *Lancet 1*:1330, 1962.
106. Grumbach, M. M., and Morishima, A.: *Acta Cytol. 6*:46, 1962.
107. Grumbach, M. M., Morishima, A., et al.: *Proc. Nat. Acad. Sci. USA 49*:581, 1963.
108. Grumbach, M. M., Morishima, A., et al.: *J. Pediat. 67*:966, 1965 (abstract).
109. Harnden, D. G., and Stewart, J. S. S.: *Brit. Med. J. 2*:1285, 1959.
110. Harnden, D. G., Maclean, N., et al.: *J. Med. Genet. 8*:460, 1971.
111. Hecht, F., Jones, D. L., et al.: *J. Med. Genet. 7*:1, 1970.
112. Heller, R. H.: *J. Pediat. 66*:48, 1965.
113. Hirschhorn, K., Decker, W. H., et al.: *New Eng. J. Med. 263*:1044, 1960.
114. Hoffenberg, R., Jackson, W. P. U., et al.: *J. Clin. Endocr. 17*:902, 1957.
115. Hook, E. B.: *Science 179*:139, 1973.
116. Hsu, L. Y. F., Geller, J., et al.: *J. Clin. Endocr. 26*:104, 1966.
117. Hsu, L. Y. F., Hirschhorn, K., et al.: *Ann. Hum. Genet. 33*:343, 1970.
118. Jackson, A. W., Muldal, S., et al.: *Brit. Med. J. 1*:223, 1965.
119. Jacobs, P. A., and Strong, J. A.: *Nature* (London) *183*:302, 1959.
120. Jacobs, P. A., Brunton, M., et al.: *Nature* (London) *197*:1080, 1963.
121. Jacobs, P. A., Brunton, M. M., et al.: *Nature* (London) *208*:1351, 1965.
122. Jacobs, P. A., and Ross, A.: *Nature* (London) *210*:352, 1966.
123. Jacobs, P. A.: *Brit. Med. Bull. 25*:94, 1969.
124. Jirósek, J. E.: *Development of the Genital System and Male Pseudohermaphroditism.* Baltimore, Johns Hopkins University Press, 1971.
125. Josso, N., de Grouchy, J., et al.: *J. Clin. Endocr. 25*:114, 1965.
126. Judd, H. L., Scully, R. E., et al.: *New Eng. J. Med. 282*:881, 1970.
127. Kosowicz, J.: *Amer. J. Roentgen. 93*:354, 1965.
128. Lee, S.: *Biol. Neonate 18*:418, 1971.
129. Levy, E. P., Pashayan, H., et al.: *Amer. J. Dis. Child. 120*:36, 1970.
130. Lindsten, J.: *The Nature and Origin of X Chromosome Aberrations in Turner's Syndrome. A Cytogenetical and Clinical Study of 57 Patients.* Stockholm, Almqvist & Wiksell, 1963.
131. Lipsett, M. B.: *J. Clin. Endocr. 22*:119, 1962.
132. Lyon, M. F.: *Amer. J. Hum. Genet. 14*:135, 1962.
133. Lyon, M. F.: *Biol. Rev. 47*:1, 1972.
134. Maclean, N., Mitchell, J. M., et al.: *Lancet 1*:293, 1962.
135. Maclean, N., Harnden, D. G., et al.: *Lancet 1*:286, 1964.
136. Mattevi, M. S., Wolff, H., et al.: *Humangenetik 13*:126, 1971.
137. McKusick, V. A.: *On the X Chromosome of Man.* Washington, D. C.: American Institute of Biological Sciences, 1964.
138. Miller, O. J.: *Amer. J. Obstet. Gynec. 90*:1078, 1964.

139. Morishima, A., Grumbach, M. M., et al.: *Proc. Nat. Acad. Sci. USA 48*:756, 1962.
140. Morishima, A., and Grumbach, M. M.: *Ann. N.Y. Acad. Sci. 155*:695, 1968.
141. Muldal, S., Ockey, C. H., et al.: *Acta Endocr. 39*:183, 1962.
142. Nance, W. E., and Uchida, I.: *Amer. J. Hum. Genet. 16*: 380, 1964.
143. Nielsen, J., Johansen, K., et al.: *J. Clin. Endocr. 29*:1062, 1969.
144. Noonan, J. A.: *Amer. J. Dis. Child. 116*:373, 1968.
145. Ohno, S., Kaplan, W. D., et al.: *Exp. Cell Res. 18*:415, 1959.
146. Ohno, S., Beçak, W., et al.: *Chromosoma 15*:14, 1964.
147. Overzier, C.: *Klin. Wschr. 42*:1052, 1964.
148. Paris Conference (1971): Standardization in human cytogenetics. *Birth Defects: Orig. Art. Ser. 8*(7): 1972.
149. Paulsen, C. A., Gordon, D. L., et al.: *Recent Progr. Hormone Res. 24*:321, 1968.
150. Paulsen, C. A., de Souza, A., et al.: *J. Clin. Endocr. 24*:1182, 1964.
151. Pearson, P. L., Bobrow, M., et al.: *Nature* (London) *226*:78, 1970.
152. Pearson, P.: *J. Med. Genet. 9*:264, 1972.
153. Pfeiffer, R. A., Lambert, B., et al.: *Arch. Gynaekol. 206*:369, 1968.
154. Plunkett, E. P., Rangecroft, G., et al.: *J. Ment. Defic. Res. 8*:25, 1964.
155. Polani, P. E., Hunter, W. F., et al.: *Lancet 1*:120, 1954.
156. Polani, P. E.: *Brit. Med. Bull. 17*:200, 1961.
157. Polani, P. E.: *Proc. Roy. Soc. Med.* (Ser. B) *259*:187, 1969.
158. Preger, L., Howard, M. B., et al.: *Amer. J. Roentgen. 104*: 899, 1968.
159. Price, W. H., Strong, J. A., et al.: *Lancet 1*:565, 1966.
160. Race, R. R., and Sanger, R.: *Brit. Med. Bull. 25*:99, 1969.
161. Riekhof, P. L., Horton, W. A., et al.: *Amer. J. Obstet. Gynec. 112*:59, 1972.
162. Robinson, J. A., and Buckton, K. E.: *Chromosoma 35*:342, 1971.
163. Rosenberg, H. S., Clayton, G. W., et al.: *J. Clin. Endocr. 23*:203, 1963.
164. Rosenkranz, W.: *Helv. Paediat. Acta 20*:359, 1965.
165. Ross, G. T., Holland, J. M., et al.: *J. Clin. Endocr. 25*:141, 1965.
166. Russell, L. B.: In *Progress in Medical Genetics.* Steinberg, A. G., and Bearn, A. G. (eds.), New York, Grune & Stratton, 1962, p. 230.
167. Salet, J., DeGennes, J. L., et al.: *Ann. Endocr.* (Paris) *31*:927, 1970.
168. Schellhas, H. F., Trujillo, J. M., et al.: *Amer. J. Obstet. Gynec. 109*:1197, 1971.
169. Schoen, E. J.: *J. Clin. Endocr. 25*:101, 1965.
170. Segal, S. J., and Nelson, W. O.: *J. Clin. Endocr. 17*:676, 1957.
171. Simpson, J. L., Christakos, A. C., et al.: *Birth Defects: Orig. Art. Ser. 7*(6):215, 1971.
172. Simpson, J. L.: *Clin. Obstet. Gynec. 15*:157, 1972.
173. Singh, R. F., and Carr, D. H.: *Anat. Rec. 155*:369, 1966.
174. Slotnick, E. A., and Goldfarb, A. F.: *Obstet. Gynec. 39*:269, 1972.
175. Smith, D. W., Marden, P. M., et al.: *Pediatrics 30*:707, 1962.
176. Sohval, A. R.: *Physiol. Rev. 43*:306, 1963.
177. Sohval, A. R.: *Amer. J. Med. 38*:615, 1965.
178. Steiker, D. D., Meillman, W. J., et al.: *J. Pediat. 58*:321, 1961.
179. Stern, C.: *Amer. J. Med. 34*:715, 1963.
180. Stewart, J. S. S., Mack, W. S., et al.: *Quart. J. Med. 28*: 561, 1959.
181. Tanner, J. M., Prader, A., et al.: *Lancet 2*:141, 1959.
182. Teter, J., and Boczkowski, K.: *Cancer 20*:1301, 1967.
183. Tjio, J. H., and Levan, A.: *Hereditas 42*:1, 1956.
184. Townes, P. L., Ziegler, N. A., et al.: *Lancet 1*:1041, 1965.
185. Turner, H. H., and Zanartu, J.: *J. Clin. Endocr. 22*:660, 1962.
186. Uchida, I. A., Miller, J. R., et al.: *Amer. J. Hum. Genet. 16*:284, 1964.
187. Van Den Berghe, H., Steeno, I., et al.: *J. Clin. Endocr. 25*:1246, 1965.
188. Warkany, J., Chu, E. H. Y., et al.: *Amer. J. Dis. Child. 104*:172, 1963.
189. Weiss, L.: *J. Med. Genet. 8*:540, 1971.
190. Welshons, W. J., and Russell, L. B.: *Proc. Nat. Acad. Sci. USA 45*:560, 1959.

191. Wilkins, L., and Fleischmann, W.: *J. Clin. Endocr. 4*:357, 1944.

192. Wilkins, L., Grumbach, M. M., et al.: *J. Clin. Endocr. 14*:1270, 1954.

193. Willemse, C. H.: *Acta Endocr. 39*:204, 1962.

194. Williams, E. D., Engel, E., et al.: *New Eng. J. Med. 270*:805, 1964.

195. Zaleski, W. A., Houston, C. S., et al.: *Canad. Med. Ass. J. 94*:1143, 1966.

**Gonadogenesis and the Differentiation of Sex
Structures and Characteristics**

196. Acevedo, H. F., Axelrod, L. R., et al.: *J. Clin. Endocr. 23*:885, 1963.

197. Albert, A.: In *Sex and Internal Secretions, 1.* Young, W. C. (ed.), Baltimore, Williams & Wilkins Company, 1963, p. 305.

198. Albright, F., Forbes, A. P., et al.: Josiah Macy Conf. Metab. Aspects Conval. Trans. *17*:139, 1948.

199. Arey, L. B.: *Developmental Anatomy.* 7th ed. Philadelphia, W. B. Saunders Company, 1965.

200. Ashley-Montagu, M. F.: *Quart. Rev. Biol. 14*:13, 1939.

201. August, G. P., Grumbach, M. M., et al.: *J. Clin. Endocr. 34*:319, 1972.

202. Baker, T. G.: *Proc. Roy. Soc.* (B) *148*:417, 1963.

203. Barr, M., Diczfalusy, E., et al.: *Acta Endocr. 37*:241, 1961.

204. Barraclough, C. A.: *Recent Progr. Hormone Res. 22*:503, 1966.

205. Boyar, R., Finkelstein, J., et al.: *New Eng. J. Med. 287*:582, 1972.

206. Burns, R. K.: *Amer. J. Anat. 98*:35, 1956.

207. Charny, C. W., Conston, A. S., et al.: *Ann. N.Y. Acad. Sci. 55*:597, 1952.

208. Cohen, R. A., Wurtman, R. J., et al.: *Ann. Intern. Med. 61*:1144, 1964.

209. Corning, H. K.: *Lehrbuch det Entwicklungsgeschichte des Menschen.* Munich, J. F. Bergmann, 1921.

210. Dahl, E. V., and Bahn, R. C.: *Amer. J. Path. 40*:587, 1962.

211. Diamond, M.: *Quart. Rev. Biol. 40*:147, 1965.

212. Donovan, B. T., and Van Der Werff Ten Bosch, J. J.: *Physiology of Puberty,* Baltimore, Williams & Wilkins Company, 1965.

213. Easterling, W. E., Jr., Simmer, H. H., et al.: *Steroids 8*:157, 1966.

213a. Ehrhardt, A. A., Epstein, R., et al.: *Johns Hopkins Med. J. 122*:165, 1968.

214. Fitschen, W., and Clayton, B. E.: *Arch. Dis. Child. 40*:16, 1965.

215. Fraandsen, V. A., and Stakemann, G.: *Acta Endocr. 47*:265, 1964.

216. Frasier, S. D., and Horton, R.: *Steroids 8*:777, 1966.

216a. French, F. S., and Ritzén, E. M.: *Endocrinology. 93*:88, 1973.

217. Frisch, R. E., and Revelle, R.: *Science 169*:397, 1970.

218. Frisch, R. E.: *Pediatrics 50*:445, 1972.

219. Goldman, A. S., and Bongiovanni, A. M.: *Ann. N.Y. Acad. Sci. 142*:755, 1967.

220. Goldman, A. S.: In *Colloq. Biol. Chem., Sect. 2. Reproduction.* Gibian, H., and Plotz, E. J. (eds.), 1970, p. 389.

221. Gorski, R. A.: In *Frontiers in Neuroendocrinology.* Martini, L., and Ganong, W. F. (eds.), London, Oxford University Press, 1971, p. 237.

222. Grumbach, M. M., and Kaplan, S. L.: In *Foetal and Neonatal Physiology.* Cross, K. W., and Nathanielez, P. (eds.), Cambridge, Cambridge University Press, 1973, p. 462.

223. Hampson, J. L., and Hampson, J. G.: In *Sex and Internal Secretions, 2.* Young, W. C. (ed.), Baltimore, Williams & Wilkins Company, 1961, p. 1401.

224. Harris, G. W.: *Endocrinology 75*:627, 1964.

225. Heller, C. G., and Clermont, Y.: *Recent Progr. Hormone Res. 20*:545, 1964.

226. Hemsworth, B. N., and Jackson, H.: *J. Reprod. Fertil. 5*:187, 1963.

227. Hemsworth, B. N., and Jackson, H.: *J. Reprod. Fertil. 6*:229, 1963.

228. Herbst, A. L., Kurman, R. J., et al.: *New Eng. J. Med. 287*:1259, 1972.

229. Jacobs, P. A.: *Brit. Med. Bull. 25*:94, 1969.

230. Jenner, M. R., Kelch, R. P., et al: *J. Clin. Endocr. 34*:521, 1972.

231. Josso, N.: *J. Clin. Endocr. 32*:404, 1971.

232. Josso, N.: *C. R. Acad. Sci.* (Paris) *274*:3573, 1972.

233. Josso, N.: *J. Clin. Endocr. 34*:265, 1972.

234. Jost, A.: *Recent Progr. Hormone Res. 8*:379, 1953.

235. Jost, A.: *Trans. Roy. Soc.* (B) *259*:119, 1970.

236. Jost, A.: In *Hermaphroditism, Genital Anomalies and Related Endocrine Disorders.* 2nd ed. Jones, H. W., and Scott, W. W. (eds.), Baltimore, Williams & Wilkins Company, 1971, p. 16.

237. Jost, A.: *Johns Hopkins Med. J. 130*:38, 1972.

238. Jost, A., Vigier, B., et al.: *Recent Progr. Hormone Res. 29*:1, 1973.

239. Junkmann, K., and Neumann, F.: *Acta Endocr. 45*(Suppl. 90):139, 1964.

240. Karsch, F. J., Dierschke, D. J., et al.: *Science 179*:484, 1973.

241. Kelch, R. P., Grumbach, M. M., et al.: In *Gonadotropins.* Saxena, B. B., Beling, C. G., et al. (eds.), New York, John Wiley & Sons, 1972, p. 524.

242. Knobil, E., Dierschke, D. J., et al.: In *Gonadotropins.* Saxena, B. B., Beling, C. G., et al. (eds.), New York, John Wiley & Sons, 1972, p. 72.

242a. Kolodny, R. C., Masters, W. H., et al.: *New Eng. J. Med. 285*:1170, 1971.

243. Lindner, H. R.: *J. Endocr. 23*:139, 1961.

244. Mancini, R. E., Narbaitz, R., et al.: *Anat. Rec. 136*:477, 1960.

245. Marshall, W. A., and Tanner, J. M.: *Arch. Dis. Child. 44*:291, 1969.

246. Marshall, W. A., and Tanner, J. M.: *Arch. Dis. Child. 45*:13, 1970.

247. McCann, S. M., and Ramirez, V. D.: *Recent Progr. Hormone Res. 20*:131, 1964.

248. Merrill, J. A.: *Southern Med. J. 56*:225, 1963.

249. Mills, I. H., Brooks, R. V., et al.: In *The Human Adrenal Cortex.* Currie, A. R., Symington, T., et al. (eds.), Baltimore, Williams & Wilkins, 1962, p. 204.

250. Mintz, B.: *J. Embryol. Exp. Morph. 5*:396, 1957.

251. Money, J., Hampson, J. G., et al.: *Bull. Johns Hopkins Hosp. 97*:301, 1955.

252. Money, J., and Ehrhardt, A. A.: *Recent Progr. Hormone Res. 28*:735, 1972.

253. Money, J., Alexander, D., et al.: *J. Pediat. 69*:126, 1966.

254. Moore, C. R.: *J. Clin. Endocr. 4*:135, 1944.

255. Moshang, T., Jr., Vallet, H. L., et al.: *J. Pediat. 80*:460, 1972.

256. Nathanson, I. T., Towne, L. E., et al.: *Endocrinology 28*:851, 1941.

257. Neumann, F., von Berswordt-Wallrabe, R., et al.: *Recent Progr. Hormone Res. 26*:337, 1970.

258. Odell, W. D., Ross, G. T., et al.: *J. Clin. Invest. 46*:248, 1967.

259. Pfeiffer, C. A.: *Amer. J. Anat. 58*:195, 1936.

260. Polhemus, D. W.: *Pediatrics 11*:588, 1953.

261. Potter, E. L.: In *The Ovary.* Grady, H. G., and Smith, D. E. (eds.), Baltimore, Williams & Wilkins Company, 1963, p. 11.

262. Ramirez, V. D., and Sawyer, C. H.: *Endocrinology 76*:1158, 1965.

263. Roosen-Runge, E. C.: In *Second International Conference on Congenital Malformations.* New York, International Medical Congress, Ltd., 1964, p. 32.

264. Rosenbloom, A. L., and Frias, J. L.: *Amer. J. Dis. Child. 125*:385, 1973.

265. Rosenfield, R. L.: *J. Pediat. 79*:260, 1971.

266. Roth, J. C., Kelch, R. P., et al.: *J. Clin. Endocr. 35*:926, 1972.

267. Schwartz, N. B., and McCormack, C. E.: *Ann. Rev. Physiol. 34*:425, 1972.

268. Spaulding, M. H.: *Carnegie Inst. Contrib. Embryol. 13*(61):69, 1921.

269. Sizonenko, P. C., Schindler, A. M., et al.: *Acta Endocr. 71*:539, 1972.

270. Tanner, J. M.: *Growth at Adolescence.* 2nd ed. Springfield, Ill., Charles C Thomas, 1962.

271. Troen, P., Nilsson, B., et al.: *Acta Endocr. 38*:361, 1961.

272. van Wagenen, G., and Simpson, M. E.: *Embryology of the Ovary and Testis, Homo Sapiens and Macaca Mulatta.* New Haven, Yale University Press, 1965.

273. Vestergaard, P., Raabo, E., et al.: *Clin. Chim. Acta 14*:540, 1966.

274. Wilson, J. D.: *New Eng. J. Med. 287*:1284, 1972.

275. Wilson, J. D.: *Endocrinology 92*:1192, 1973.

276. Wilson, J. D., and Siiteri, P. K.: *Endocrinology 92*:1182, 1973.

277. Winter, J. S. D., and Faiman, C.: *Pediat. Res.* 6:126, 1972.
278. Witschi, E.: *Carnegie Inst. Contrib. Embryol.* 32:67, 1948.
279. Witschi, E.: *Development of Vertebrates.* Philadelphia, W. B. Saunders Company, 1956.
280. Witschi, E.: *Science* 126:1288, 1957.
281. Witschi, E., Nelson, W. O., et al.: *J. Clin. Endocr.* 17:737, 1957.
282. Witschi, E.: In *The Ovary.* Grady, H. G., and Smith, D. E. (eds.), Baltimore, Williams & Wilkins Company, 1963, p. 1.
283. Young, W. C.: In *Sex and Internal Secretions, 2.* Young, W. C. (ed.), Baltimore, Williams & Wilkins Company, 1961, p. 1173.

Female Pseudohermaphrodism

284. Bergman, P., Sjögren, B., et al.: *Acta. Endocr.* 40:555, 1962.
285. Bongiovanni, A. M., Di George, A. M., et al.: *J. Clin. Endocr.* 19:1004, 1959.
286. Bongiovanni, A. M., and Root, A. W.: *New Eng. J. Med.* 268:1283;1342;1391, 1963.
287. Bongiovanni, A. M.: *J. Clin. Invest.* 41:2086, 1964.
288. Bongiovanni, A. M.: In *Metabolic Basis of Inherited Disease.* 3rd ed. Stanbury, J. B., Wyngaarden, J. B., et al. (eds.), New York, McGraw Hill, 1972, p. 587.
289. Carpentier, P. J., and Potter, E. L.: *Amer. J. Obstet. Gynec.* 78:235, 1959.
290. Childs, B., Grumbach, M. M., et al.: *J. Clin. Invest.* 35:213, 1956.
291. Degenhart, H. J., Visser, H. K. A., et al.: *Acta Endocr.* 48:587, 1965.
292. Degenhart, H. J., Visser, H. K. A., et al.: *Acta Endocr.* 71:512, 1972.
293. Fraser, G. R.: *Ann. Hum. Genet.* 25:387, 1962.
294. Grumbach, M. M., Ducharme, J. R., et al.: *J. Clin. Endocr.* 19:1369, 1959.
295. Grumbach, M. M., and Ducharme, J. R.: *Fertil. Steril.* 11:157, 1960.
296. Kirkland, R. T., Kirkland, J. L., et al.: *J. Clin. Endocr.* 36:488, 1973.
297. Knorr, D., Bidlingmaier, F., et al.: *Acta Endocr.* (Suppl. 173):37, 1973.
298. Murset, G., Zachmann, M., et al.: *Acta Endocr.* 65:627, 1970.
299. Novak, D. J., Lauchlan, S. C., et al.: *Amer. J. Med.* 49:281, 1970.
300. Park, I. J., Johanson, A., et al.: *Obstet. Gynec.* 39:100, 1972.
301. Schoen, E. J., DiRaimondo, V., et al.: *J. Clin. Endocr.* 21:518, 1961.
302. Sizonenko, P. C., Schindler, A. M., et al.: *Acta Endocr.* 71:539, 1972.
303. Stempfel, R. S., and Tomkins, G. M.: In *The Metabolic Basis of Inherited Disease.* 3rd ed. Stanbury, J. B., Wyngaarden, J. B., et al. (eds.), New York, McGraw Hill, 1966.
304. Verkauf, B. S., and Jones, H. W.: *South. Med. J.* 63:634, 1970.
305. Whalen, R. E., Peck, C. K., et al.: *Endocrinology* 78:965, 1966.
306. Wilkins, L.: *J. Pediat.* 41:860, 1952.
307. Wilkins, L., and Cara, J.: *J. Clin. Endocr.* 14:287, 1954.
308. Wilkins, L.: *J.A.M.A.* 172:1028, 1960.
309. Wilson, R. B., and Keating, F. R.: *Amer. J. Obstet. Gynec.* 76:388, 1958.

Male Pseudohermaphrodism

310. Aarskog, D.: *Acta Paediat. Scand.* (Suppl. 203):1, 1970.
311. Bahner, F., and Schwarz, G.: In *Physiologie des Melanophanelhormons.* Nowakowski, H. (ed.), Berlin, Springer-Verlag, 1962, p. 314.
312. Bardin, C. W., Bullock, L. P., et al.: *Recent Progr. Hormone Res.* 29:65, 1973.
313. Bergada, C., Cleveland, W. W., et al.: *Acta Endocr.* 40:493, 1962.
314. Biglieri, E. G., Herron, M. A., et al.: *J. Clin. Invest.* 45:1946, 1966.
315. Boczkowski, K., and Teter, J.: *Acta Endocr.* 49:497, 1965.
316. Bowen, P., Lee, C. S. N., et al.: *Ann. Intern. Med.* 62:252, 1965.
316a. David, L., Saez, J. M., et al.: *Acta Paediat. Scand.* 61:249, 1972.
317. Drash, A., Sherman, F., et al.: *J. Pediat.* 76:585, 1970.

318. Ferenczy, A., and Richart, R.: *Amer. J. Obstet. Gynec.* 113:399, 1972.
319. French, F. S., Baggett, B., et al.: *J. Clin. Endocr.* 25:661, 1965.
320. French, F. S., Van Wyk, J. J., et al.: *J. Clin. Endocr.* 26:493, 1966.
320a. Judd, H. L., Hamilton, C. R., et al.: *J. Clin. Endocr.* 34:229, 1972.
321. Kaplan, N. M.: *New Eng. J. Med.* 261:641, 1959.
322. Kelch, R. P., Jenner, M. R., et al.: *J. Clin. Invest.* 51:824, 1972.
323. Lubs, H. A., Jr., Vilar, O., et al.: *J. Clin. Endocr.* 19:1110, 1959.
324. Mauvais-Jarvis, P., Bercovici, J. P., et al.: *J. Clin. Invest.* 49:31, 1970.
325. Morris, J. M.: *Amer. J. Obstet. Gynec.* 65:1192, 1953.
326. Morris, J. M., and Mahesh, V. B.: *Amer. J. Obstet. Gynec.* 87:731, 1963.
327. Neumann, F., Elger, W., et al.: *Endocrinology* 78:628, 1966.
328. New, M. I.: *J. Clin. Invest.* 49:1930, 1970.
329. Nilson, O.: *Acta Chir. Scand.* 83:221, 1939.
330. Northcutt, R. C., Island, D. P., et al.: *J. Clin. Endocr.* 29:422, 1969.
331. Nowakowski, H., and Lenz, W.: *Recent Progr. Hormone Res.* 17:53, 1961.
332. Opitz, J. M., Simpson, J. L., et al.: *Clin. Genet.* 3:1, 1972.
333. Parks, G. S., Bermudez, J. A., et al.: *J. Clin. Endocr.* 33:269, 1971.
334. Philip, J., and Sele, V.: *Acta Endocr.* 48:297, 1965.
335. Philip, J., and Trolle, D.: *Amer. J. Obstet. Gynec.* 93:1076, 1965.
336. Prader, A., and Gurtner, H. P.: *Helvet. Paediat. Acta* 10:397, 1955.
337. Prader, A., and Anders, G. J.: *Helvet. Paediat. Acta* 17:285, 1962.
338. Ritzén, E. M., Nayfeh, S. N., et al.: *Endocrinology* 91:116, 1972.
339. Saez, J. M., dePeretti, E. M., et al.: *J. Clin. Endocr.* 32:604, 1971.
340. Saez, J. M., Frederich, A., et al.: *J. Clin. Endocr.* 32:611, 1971.
341. Saez, J. M., Morera, A. M., et al.: *J. Clin. Endocr.* 34:598, 1972.
342. Simmer, H., Pion, R. J., et al.: *Testicular Feminization.* Springfield, Ill., Charles C Thomas, 1965.
343. Southren, A. L., Tochimoto, S., et al.: *J. Clin. Endocr.* 25:1441, 1965.
344. Southren, A. L., Ross, H., et al.: *J. Clin. Endocr.* 25:518, 1965.
345. Strickland, A. L., and French, F. S.: *J. Clin. Endocr.* 29:1284, 1969.
346. Zachmann, M., Völlmin, J. A., et al.: *Clin. Endocr.* 1:369, 1972.
346a. Goebelsmann, U., Horton, R., et al.: *J. Clin. Endocr.* 36:867, 1973.

Other Sexual Anomalies

347. Bergada, C., Cleveland, W. W., et al.: *Acta Endocr.* 40:521, 1962.
348. Charny, C. W., and Wolgin, W.: *Cryptorchidism.* New York, Hoeber, 1957.
349. Drucker, W. D., Blanc, W. A., et al.: *J. Clin. Endocr.* 23:59, 1963.
350. Herbst, A. L., Kurman, R. J., et al.: *New Eng. J. Med.* 287:1259, 1972.
351. Kallmann, F. J., Schoenfeld, W. A., et al.: *Amer. J. Ment. Defic.* 48:203, 1944.
352. Kirschner, M. A., Jacobs, J. B., et al.: *New Eng. J. Med.* 282:240, 1970.
353. Mack, W. S., Scott, L. S., et al.: *J. Path. Bact.* 82:439, 1961.
354. Muldal, S., and Ockey, C. H.: *Lancet* 2:601, 1961.
355. Nowakowski, H., and Lenz, W.: *Recent Progr. Hormone Res.* 17:53, 1961.
356. Rosewater, S., Gwinup, G., et al.: *Ann. Intern. Med.* 63:377, 1965.
357. Sörenson, H. R.: *Hypospadias, with Special Reference to Aetiology.* Copenhagen, Munksgaard, 1953.
358. Sohval, A. R., and Soffer, L. J.: *Amer. J. Med.* 14:328, 1953.
359. Turunen, A., and Unnérus, C. E.: *Acta Obstet. Gynec. Scand.* 46:99, 1967.
360. Woolf, R. B., and Allen, W. M.: *Obstet. Gynec.* 2:236, 1953.

Management

361. Frank, R. T.: *Amer. J. Obstet. Gynec. 35*:1053, 1938.
362. Fraser, I. D., Baird, D. T., et al.: *J. Clin. Endocr. 36*:634, 1973.
363. Frasier, S. D., Bashore, R. A., et al.: *J. Pediat. 64*:740, 1964.
364. Goldberg, M. B., and Scully, A. L.: *J. Clin. Endocr. 27*:341, 1967.
365. Hughesdon, P. E., and Kumarasamy, T.: *Virchows Arch. Path. Anat. 349*:258, 1970.
366. Johanson, A. J., Brasel, J. A., et al.: *J. Pediat. 75*:1015, 1969.
367. Jones, H. W., Jr., and Wilkins, L.: *Amer. J. Obstet. Gynec. 82*:1142, 1961.
368. Jones, H. W., Jr., and Wheeles, C. R.: *Amer. J. Obstet. Gynec. 104*:348, 1969.
369. Jones, H. W., Jr., and Verkauf, B. S.: *Obstet. Gynec. 36*: 1, 1970.
370. Josso, N., Fortier-Beaulieu, M., et al.: *Acta Endocr. 62*:168, 1969.
371. Lattimer, J. K.: *J. Urol. 86*:113, 1961.

372. Lewis, V. G., Ehrhardt, A. A., et al.: *Obstet. Gynec. 36*:11, 1970.
373. Melicow, M. M., and Uson, A. C.: *Cancer 12*:552, 1959.
374. Money, J., Hampson, J. G., et al.: *Bull. Johns Hopkins Hosp. 97*:284, 1955.
375. Money, J.: *J. Nerv. Ment. Dis. 132*:289, 1961.
376. Robinson, A., Priest, R. E., et al.: *Lancet 1*:111, 1964.
377. Rosenbloom, A. L., and Frias, J. L.: *Amer. J. Dis. Child. 125*:385, 1973.
378. Rosenfield, R. L., Lawrence, A. M., et al.: *J. Clin. Endocr. 32*:625, 1972.
379. Scully, R. E.: *Cancer 25*:1340, 1970.
380. Teter, J., and Tarlowski, R.: *Amer. J. Obstet. Gynec. 79*: 321, 1960.
381. Teter, J., Philip, J., et al.: *Acta Endocr. 46*:1, 1964.
382. Teter, J., and Boczkowski, K.: *Amer. J. Obstet. Gynec. 93*:1084, 1965.
383. Tristan, T. A., Eberlein, W. R., et al.: *Amer. J. Roentgen. 76*:562, 1956.
384. Warren, J. C., Erkman, B., et al.: *Lancet 1*:141, 1964.

CHAPTER 9

The Pancreas

By Robert H. Williams and
Daniel Porte, Jr.*

---

*It is not possible in this brief review of extensive literature to
include more than a small portion of the references. Moreover, in
the text only the name of the first of coauthors is usually mentioned. Sometimes we have referred to reviews rather than original reports.

The pancreas plays an important role in the digestion and assimilation of food. Almost all its structure plays an active role in gastrointestinal function, but its islets markedly influence metabolism throughout the body, mainly through the actions of insulin and glucagon. Too much insulin causes hypoglycemia, and too little produces diabetes mellitus. Too much glucagon causes diabetes, and too little permits hypoglycemia. Too much gastrin produces gastrointestinal ulcer, diarrhea, malabsorption, and the Zollinger-Ellison syndrome (Ch. 14).

Diabetes is the commonest disease associated with the pancreatic islets; presumably more than 10 million people in the United States are so afflicted. The highest incidence has been reported in Pima Indians; 50 per cent of that group were found by Bennett to have diabetes. This disorder is the eighth leading health-related cause of death. More than 50 per cent of diabetics die because of coronary disease; renal failure is the cause of death of most juvenile-onset diabetics. Diabetes is the second commonest cause of blindness. It frequently causes cerebral vascular disorders, gangrene of the legs, and neuropathy. The total annual costs for the disease in the United States are estimated to be at least 2 billion dollars, including medical care and loss of compensation for work. Much remains to be learned with respect to the etiology. There is a strong need for much earlier diagnosis and better treatment.

The endocrine role of the pancreas was recognized in 1886 when Minkowski and Von Mering produced diabetes by total pancreatectomy in the dog. This was about thirty-five years before Banting and Best isolated insulin and over 70 years before Sanger demonstrated its amino acid sequence.

The chemical synthesis of insulin was reported by Meienhofer in 1963 and Katsoyannis in 1964. Steiner (1967) discovered that proinsulin was the biosynthetic precursor of insulin. Hodgkin recently reported the three-dimensional structure of insulin.

CHEMISTRY OF INSULIN, PROINSULIN, AND GLUCAGON

Chemistry of Insulin

Extraction of Insulin from the Pancreas

Almost all of the insulin supplied is extracted from the pancreas, usually with acid-ethanol, followed by ether-ethanol precipitation. Further purification is obtained by various methods, particularly by Sephadex and DEAE ion-exchange chromatography. The manner in which insulin is extracted doubtless changes many of its chemical properties. For example, insulin migrates electrophoretically to the cathode, but increasingly strong treatment with acid removes an increasing number of amino groups, eventually causing it to migrate to the anode.

Some Physical and Chemical Properties of Insulin

Crystallization of insulin by Abel (1926) led to studies dealing with its chemical nature. The three-dimensional structure of insulin crystals has been demonstrated by x-ray analysis (Hodgkin). Two atoms of zinc were found to be present with six molecules of insulin in a spheroid unit. The A chain rested in a pocket made by three main sections of the B chain. The covalent bonding of the two chains, through the disulfide residues, was observed to be reinforced by van der Waals' interactions between residues belonging to strategically placed nonpolar groups. The surface of the molecule exposed the polar groups, together with a few nonpolar residues. Insulin dimers were found to be compact, cylindrical structures with largely exposed hydrophilic residues and a few hydrophobic residues.

The connecting peptide of proinsulin (discussed later) directs and holds the A and B chains in a conformation favorable for correct and efficient pairing of cysteinyl residues as proinsulin is released from ribosomal units. Sanger demonstrated the amino acid sequence of insulin. This was the first protein whose structure was elucidated, and the accomplishment led to the analysis of many other biologically active polypeptides and proteins. He found insulin to be composed of two long polypeptide chains with a specific amino acid sequence bound together by two disulfide bridges at positions 7 and 20 in the A chain and 7 and 19 in the B chain (Fig. 9–1). The A chain has 21 amino acids and is acidic. The B chain has 30 amino acids and

is basic. Also, there is an intrachain disulfide bridge linking positions 6 and 11 in the A chain.

The series of 6 amino acids in the S-S ring of chain A is of special interest. The peptides oxytocin and vasopressin also contain 6 amino acids in an S-S bridge, and this configuration has been found to be significant in the interaction of the peptides and the hormone-sensitive cell. It has been suggested that this portion of insulin is one of the more exposed parts and may be the site of binding to muscle and other tissues. The threonine, serine, and isoleucine in positions A-8, 9, and 10 and the threonine in position B-30 are the amino acids that differ most in common species of animals (Fig. 9–1).

There can be considerable species-specific variations in amino acid sequence; indeed, as many as 29 of the 51 positions can be replaced. The amino acids in the internal ring of the A chain and those immediately adjacent to it on its C-terminal side (positions 12 to 14), as well as the N- and C-terminal parts of the B chain, are most frequently involved in molecular differentiation between species. These areas exert important antigenic responses in heterologous species. Human insulin differs from porcine insulin by a single amino acid; in the B-30 position, human insulin has threonine rather than alanine (Fig. 9–1). The carboxyl terminal octapeptide from the porcine B chain can be replaced simply by an analogous synthetic human octapeptide (Ruttenberg). This preparation is useful for preparing specifically labeled human insulin. Whether practical therapeutic advantage will result from this remains to be determined.

Modification of insulin by esterification of carboxyl groups causes a loss of activity, as does altering the phenolic hydroxyl and iminazolyl groups. When insulin in solution is heated at a pH below 3.5, molecules aggregate to form fibers which once formed are stable at pH values from 0 to 10. Small fibril fragments formed and placed in acid solutions of insulin will initiate further fibril formation

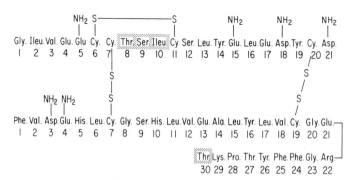

Figure 9–1.   Structure of human insulin. The structures of insulin from certain animal spaces differ only as follows:

	Chain A			Chain B
	8	9	10	30
Man	Thr	Ser	Ileu	Thr
Pig	Thr	Ser	Ileu	Ala
Rabbit	Thr	Ser	Ileu	Ser
Beef	Ala	Ser	Val	Ala

without heating. The fibril formation is inhibited by disruption of the disulfide bonds and by removal of the carboxy-terminal amino acid of the B chain. Fibrous insulin formed in aqueous solutions returns to soluble insulin with full biologic activity in highly alkaline solutions, but when formed in phenol it will not revert to soluble form.

The extent of aggregation of insulin molecules varies with many factors, including temperature, pH, and zinc content. Zinc, especially, promotes aggregation, possibly through bonding of histidine at B-10. The acid used to extract insulin from the pancreas removes zinc. To crystallize the hormone it is necessary to add zinc or other metal ions such as nickel, cobalt, or cadmium. Crystalline insulin usually contains from 0.3 to 0.6 per cent zinc. Dimers and hexamers are sometimes formed. The molecular weight of zinc-free insulin has been found to be 12,000 in an acid pH and 6000 in a basic pH. Insulin is relatively insoluble within the pH range of 4 to 7 (isoelectric point, pH 5.3). Molecular dissociation is favored by extremes of pH and by low ionic strength; concentrated solutions of guanidine hydrochloride also have this effect.

Insulin readily adsorbs loosely to many substances, including cellulose, agar, glassware, and certain serum proteins. Specific insulin antibodies bind it much more strongly than do any of the foregoing compounds and pull the insulin from them. When dealing quantitatively with minute amounts of insulin, as in experimental studies, it is important to avoid binding to glassware, paper, etc. Many proteins inhibit the adsorption, but albumin and casein are two of the better compounds for preventing this.

For investigative studies, insulin has been labeled in a great variety of ways, but the commonest label used now is I^{125}. The tyrosyl hydroxyl groups exchange with I^{125}. More than 75 per cent of the I^{125} usually is fixed to the A chain, although the B chain also has two tyrosyl groups. Under carefully controlled conditions, it has been possible to label only the A chain, apparently because it is more exposed than the B chain. With heavy radioiodination there is loss of biologic activity as well as alteration in physical-chemical activity of many of the insulin molecules. "Pure" insulin-I^{125}

can be removed from degradation products by permitting adsorption of the former to cellulose. This process also removes free insulin from antibody-bound insulin, which does not adhere to the cellulose.

Chemistry of Proinsulin

On the basis of physical-chemical principles, it was predicted about a decade ago that the disulfide bonds of insulin could form more efficiently by synthesizing chains A and B as integral parts of one long chain than by synthesizing the chains separately and then combining them. In 1967, Steiner and colleagues showed that insulin was formed from a large molecular weight, single-chain precursor, which they named proinsulin (Fig. 9–2). Subsequently, hormones of the pancreatic alpha cells, parathyroid glands, and pituitary gland have also been found to be formed from larger, biologically less active precursors by limited intracellular proteolysis. They are apparently synthesized in this manner.

Proinsulin is extracted from pancreas by acid-ethanol and by some other solvents used to extract insulin. Indeed, proinsulin and proinsulin-related intermediates account for 3–6 per cent of protein in commercial insulin preparations. Proinsulin and various related proteins have been isolated by DEAE-cellulose chromatography and urea-containing buffer. Other methods used for isolating proinsulin from plasma and tissues include chromatography on Sephadex G-50 or Biogel P-30, paper chromatography, and starch and polyacrylamide gel electrophoresis. However, none of these procedures completely separates the various intermediate forms of proinsulin from proinsulin itself.

Proinsulin has a molecular weight of about 9000. It reacts with zinc to form a hexamer with a molecular weight of 55,000. This material can be crystallized under a variety of conditions in the presence or absence of zinc. After complete reduction of proinsulin in 8 M urea, reoxidation in dilute alkali buffer results in recovering 70–80 per cent of proinsulin, but reduction-reoxidation of insulin permits recovery of only 1 per cent of insulin.

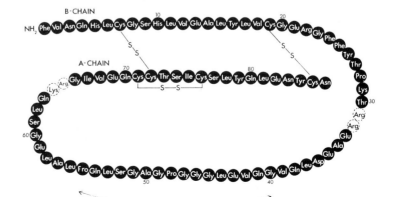

Figure 9–2. Proposed primary structure of human proinsulin. Residues in dotted circles have not yet been demonstrated by direct sequence analysis; the order shown is that known to occur in bovine and porcine proinsulin. [From Steiner, D. F., et al., In *Diabetes.* Proc. Seventh Cong. Int. Diab. Fed. Rodriguez, R. R., and Vallance-Owen, J. (eds.), Amsterdam, Excerpta Medica Foundation, 1971, p. 281.]

PROINSULIN C - PEPTIDES

	1	2	3	4	5	6	7	8	9	10	11	12	13	14	15	16
HUMAN:	Glu	Ala	Glu	Asp	Leu	Gln	Val	Gly	Gln	Val	Glu	Leu	Gly	Gly	Gly	Pro
MONKEY:	Glu	Ala	Glu	Asp	Pro	Gln	Val	Gly	Glx	Val	(Glx	Leu	Gly	Gly	Gly	Pro
PORCINE:	Glu	Ala	Glu	Asn	Pro	Gln	Ala	Gly	Ala	Val	Glu	Leu	Gly	Gly	Gly	Leu
BOVINE:	Glu	Val	Glu	Gly	Pro	Gln	Val	Gly	Ala	Leu	Glu	Leu	Ala	Gly	Gly	Pro

	17	18	19	20	21	22	23	24	25	26	27	28	29	30	31
HUMAN:	Gly	Ala	Gly	Ser	Leu	Gln	Pro	Leu	Ala	Leu	Glu	Gly	Ser	Leu	Gln
MONKEY:	Gly	Ala	Gly	Ser	Leu	Gln	Pro	Leu	Ala	Leu	Glu	Gly	Ser	Leu	Gln
PORCINE:	Gly	—	Gly	—	Leu	Gln	Ala	Leu	Ala	Leu	Glu	Gly	Pro	Pro	Gln
BOVINE:	Gly	Ala	Gly	—	—	—	—	—	Gly	Leu	Glu	Gly	Pro	Pro	Gln

Figure 9–3. Amino acid sequence of C-peptide from four species. [From Steiner, D. F., et al., In *Diabetes.* Proc. Seventh Cong. Int. Diab. Fed. Rodriguez, R. R., and Vallance-Owen, J. (eds.), Amsterdam, Excerpta Medica Foundation, 1971, p. 281.]

The complete structures for porcine and bovine proinsulins are known, and the structure for the nearly intact human connecting peptide segment is known. In these three species, approximately 50 per cent of the connecting peptide (C-peptide) residues are variant (Fig. 9–3), in contrast to the low degree of variance in insulins. The connecting peptide of porcine proinsulin differs from bovine and human by 12 and 10 residues, respectively. Bovine C-peptide has 26, porcine C-peptide 29, and human C-peptide 31 residues. All three peptides have two glutamic acids very near the amino-terminal region, one glutamic acid located four residues from the carboxyl end, and an additional glutamic acid residue located about a third of the way along the peptide chain. This distribution suggests that these residues may interact with specific side chains in the insulin portion of the proinsulin molecule to direct the folding of the peptide chain in a specific manner. Preliminary studies of the monkey C-peptide indicate that it is identical to the human C-peptide except for a single substitution of Pro for Leu at position 5.

Human proinsulin contains four additional basic residues (1 Lys, 3 Arg) not accounted for by the composition of either the insulin or the C-peptide portions of the molecule. It is probable that these residues are arranged in human proinsulin, as they are in bovine and porcine proinsulin, at either end of the C-peptide, linking this peptide to the insulin region. Thus human proinsulin consists of an 86-residue single-chain polypeptide having the B chain of insulin at its N-terminus linked by two basic residues to the 31-residue C-peptide, which in turn is linked through a second pair of basic residues to the A chain of insulin (Fig. 9–2). Therefore, this one chain of proinsulin consists of NH_2–B chain–Arg–Arg–C–peptide–Lys–Arg–A chain–COOH.

The C-peptide portion of the connecting polypeptide contains acidic residues, proline, lysine, alanine, valine, and leucine but no aromatic residues, histidine, basic amino acids, or sulfur-containing acids. Clearly, this must indicate the existence of some specific requirements with regard to the properties of the side-chain groups in this portion of molecule, perhaps with respect to the maintenance of the appropriate balance between hydrophilic and hydrophobic components in the molecule as a whole. The polar and nonpolar characteristics of the amino acid side chains of C-peptides of different species are preserved when interspecies amino acid substitutions occur. At either end of the C-peptide are regions having a high proportion of polar residues, and just beyond these regions in intact proinsulin there are two additional polar basic residues. These regions of the proinsulin molecule are quite hydrophilic. However, the central portion of the connecting peptide contains a high concentration of glycine residues surrounded by residues that are essentially all nonpolar. This composition indicates that the central part of the molecule is more flexible and may, in fact, be bent back upon itself through interactions of the nonpolar side chains to produce a hydrophobic micelle, which may interact with some hydrophobic area on the surface of the insulin molecule during peptide folding. This distribution may help to maintain these hydrophilic regions on the outside of the molecule where they will be readily accessible to the proteolytic cleavage enzymes that convert proinsulin to insulin.

Some of the immunologic properties of proinsulin are similar to those of insulin. Proinsulin and split proinsulin are about 45 per cent as reactive with insulin antibodies as is insulin, on an equimolar basis. Arginine insulins were found to be about 75 per cent as reactive with insulin antibodies as is insulin. Thus the presence of one or two arginine residues on the COOH terminus of the B chain may also interfere with antibody binding sites. The antiserum which is used routinely for the immunoassay of insulin cross-reacts with proinsulin to the extent of 25–50 per cent or even more, depending upon what antiserum is used. The lesser reactivity of the proinsulin is most likely due to some of the antibody binding sites on the insulin portion of proinsulin being masked by the connecting peptide. Because the amino acid composition of insulin of different species varies relatively little, the antiserum directed against insulin of one species usually cross-reacts with insulin of other species. Moreover, since proinsulin of different species contains the same antigenic determinants in the insulin portion of the molecule, anti-insulin serum generally cross-reacts with heterologous proinsulin. Thus human, bovine, or porcine proinsulin, like insulin of these species, interacts with porcine insulin antiserum. C-peptides have no immunoreactivity against insulin antiserum.

Proinsulin antiserum reacts with both insulin and proinsulin of different species. The cross-reactivity is presumably due to antibodies directed against the antigenic determinants in the insulin portion of the molecule. However, as discussed above, there are many species differences in the composition of the C-peptides. Immunoadsorbance with insulin-Sephadex preparations results in a highly specific antiserum which, unlike insulin antiserum, is species specific and does not cross-react significantly with proinsulin or C-peptide of other species. Proinsulin antiserum which has not been adsorbed by insulin does react with the proinsulin of other species. Since all of the proinsulin-like fragments of the connecting peptides containing sequence B_{33-54} react similarly with porcine proinsulin antiserum, it seems clear that the determinant of reactivity resides in the sequence B_{33-54}, especially B_{41-54}. This sequence is an unusually hydrophobic region and has great variability in the amino acids between species. Leu_{54} is specifically important for immunoreactivity, since a removal of this amino acid causes a loss of cross-reactivity.

Human C-peptide coupled to rabbit serum albumin, using a water-soluble carbodiimide, has been found to produce antibodies sufficient to give a sensitivity in immunoassay procedures between 0.05 and 0.1 ng./ml, using a final antiserum dilution 1:1000. However, such an assay probably does not distinguish between intact proinsulin and various partly cleaved intermediate forms that might still have most of the C-peptide portion of the molecule attached to one of the insulin chains. Thus the plasma proinsulin fraction may be a mixture of both intact proinsulin and various intermediate species. Separation of these forms by polyacrylamide gel electrophoresis appears to offer a good approach in separating these immunoreactive substances.

C-peptide does not react with insulin antibodies, but it does combine with proinsulin antibodies that are produced by the antigenic determinants in the connecting peptide of proinsulin. Therefore, to measure C-peptide, it is desirable to separate it from proinsulin by means of gel filtration prior to immunoassay.

C-peptide has not been found to have a specific action. Moreover, it does not antagonize or potentiate the effects of insulin, proinsulin, or their intermediates. C-peptide has not been shown to serve beneficial effects once it has been removed from proinsulin, although it has been suggested that it

aids in the proper reformation of insulin that has been reduced and then reoxidized in the presence of glutathione-insulin-transhydrogenase.

Presumably, many intermediates of proinsulin and insulin could be produced in the body. Among those that have been more commonly found when bovine proinsulin has been subjected to the action of trypsin and carboxypeptidase B are proinsulin without Lys_{59}-Arg_{60} and proinsulin without Arg_{31}-Arg_{32}. Comparable desdipeptides have been derived from porcine proinsulin. Other porcine proinsulin-insulin intermediates produced by trypsin are diarginine insulin and monoarginine insulin.

As measured by the mouse convulsion assay, proinsulin and split proinsulin are about 20 per cent as active as insulin, whereas both desdipeptide proinsulin (Lys_{62}-Arg_{63} absent) and desnonapeptide proinsulin (B_{55-63} absent) and both arginine insulins are about 65 per cent as active (Chance). A free NH_2-terminal glycine on the A chain is associated with greater activity, and the same applies to the presence of free COOH-terminal alanine on the B chain. Using inhibition of epinephrine-stimulated lipolysis in fat cells for assay, porcine proinsulin, or split proinsulin, has about 3 per cent the activity of insulin, but desnonapeptide proinsulin and arginine insulins are about 75 per cent as active.

Chemistry of Glucagon

It is difficult to isolate glucagon and insulin from the pancreas separately. Many commercial insulin preparations contain glucagon. When the acetone precipitate from pancreas is dissolved in acid and repeatedly dialyzed against dilute sodium acetate and sodium phosphate buffers, glucagon precipitates and is readily crystallized from mild alkaline solution. Traces of zinc and other metals are associated with glucagon, but these metals do not form an integral part of the crystal as they do in insulin. Glucagon is relatively insoluble in water, particularly in the pH range from 3 to 9; its isoelectric point is between pH 7.5 and 8.5. Electrolytes decrease its solubility, but mildly acidic and basic conditions increase it. Alkaline conditions are more favorable than acid since insoluble fibrils form with the latter. Moreover, the alkaline stability of glucagon permits inactivation of trace amounts of insulin.

Glucagon has a molecular weight of 3485. Bromer has shown that the amino acid composition of glucagon is quite different from that of insulin (Fig. 9–4). Glucagon is composed of one long chain. All of its amino acids are of the L-configuration, connected by peptide bonds. Tryptophan and methionine are constituents of glucagon but not of insulin, while cystine, isoleucine, and proline are components of insulin but not of glucagon. Glucagon is cleaved by carboxypeptidase, trypsin, leucine aminopeptidase, dipeptidyl aminopeptidase I (Fig. 9–4), and chymotrypsin. Since none of the degradation products of glucagon retains hyperglycemic activity, the integrity of most of the molecule seems to be required for physiologic activity.

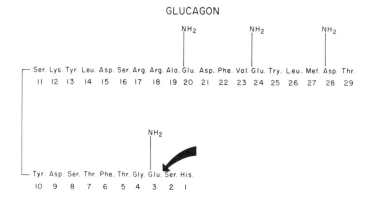

Figure 9–4. Amino acid sequence of glucagon, showing the site of cleavage by dipeptidyl aminopeptidase I.

Although native glucagon contains no metals or prosthetic groups, metal-glucagon complexes are readily prepared; one example is zinc-glucagon. It is less soluble than glucagon and has a prolonged biologic action. In acidic aqueous solutions, glucagon readily forms fibrils and gels that redissolve at pH 11. Glucagon is stable in aqueous solutions for 3 months when kept at 4° C and at pH 2.5–3.0. Molecules of glucagon apparently bind together strongly in solution. Glucagon is capable of conformational alterations, changing from a random coil in aqueous solution to either a beta structure in acidic gels or alpha-helix in the crystal state. Under physiologic conditions, the random coil probably predominates (Bromer).

Many reports of plasma immunoreactive glucagon levels have not indicated correctly the amounts of pancreatic glucagon secretion, because varying amounts of glucagon-like material from the gut have reacted with the antibody used for assay. Recently, Unger has partially clarified this. Extracts of gastrointestinal tissue contain glucagon-like biologic activity and glucagon-like immunoreactivity (GLI), which are separable by gel infiltration into two fractions. The similar molecular size, glycogenolytic activity, and electrophoretic behavior of peak 2 GLI and pancreatic glucagon indicate that the two substances are closely related, yet peak 2 GLI differs from the pancreatic

glucagon with respect to its reactivity with certain antisera, suggesting that its molecular structure differs in some way from that of glucagon. Certain hexoses (e.g., fructose, glucose) given intravenously increase GLI but decrease pancreatic glucagon. After amino acid infusion, the pancreaticoduodenal vein plasma shows a large peak of immunoreactivity in the glucagon-I[131] zone and a very small peak before the insulin-I[131] zone. Both peaks were readily measured in the glucagon-specific assay system, suggesting their pancreatic origin. GLI differs from glucagon in that it causes only slight or no (a) liver glycogenolysis, (b) hyperglycemia, and (c) insulin release. Moreover, its plasma levels are not influenced by amino acids, starvation or pancreozymin.

SYNTHESIS, STORAGE, AND RELEASE OF INSULIN AND GLUCAGON

Islet Anatomy and Histology

For an understanding of the pancreatic secretory mechanisms, a few anatomic features must be considered. Both the exocrine and endocrine portions of the pancreas develop as dorsal and ventral buds from cells of the duodenal and hepatic diverticulum (Fig. 9–5). The islets are formed from these

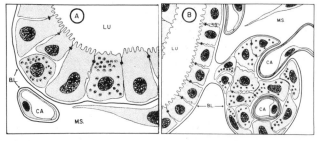

Figure 9–5. Hypothesis for the histiogenesis of the endocrine pancreas. It is suggested that islets are formed by an inversion of the polarity of the axis of cell division. *A,* The axis of division is parallel to the apical-basal cell axis. The consequence of this division is that one of the two daughter cells is no longer joined to its neighbors by junctional complexes. The presence of a few cells containing endocrine gland granules and still facing a lumen indicates that the position is not a regulation in itself. *B,* Repetition of this process leads to an accumulation of endocrine cells between the exocrine cells in the basal lamina. The basal lamina surrounding the newly formed islet can eventually fuse at the origin of the outpocketing, thus separating the intercellular spaces of the endocrine and exocrine cells. At the same time, islets are penetrated by lumen (LU), capillaries (CA), mesenchymal spaces (M.S.), and basal lamina (B.L.). (From Pictet, R. L., In *Handbook of Physiology,* Section 7: Endocrinology, Vol. 1: *Endocrine Pancreas.* American Physiological Society, Field, John (ed.), Baltimore, Williams and Wilkins, 1972, p. 41.)

pancreatic elements but lose most of their connections with the duct system after the third month in utero, when insulin and glucagon production begins. The arterial supply of the pancreas arises from the splenic, hepatic, and superior mesenteric arteries and the venous drainage is into the splenic and superior mesenteric veins. Insulin is demonstrable in the pancreas of human fetuses at about the fiftieth day of pregnancy (Steinke, Williams). The endocrine portion of the pancreas, the islets of Langerhans, constitutes only about 1 per cent of the weight of this organ, but there are up to 2 million islets, 20–300 μ in diameter. In normal man the islets are composed of at least three types of cells: A, B, and D cells (Figs. 9–6 and 9–7). A cells secrete glucagon, and B cells secrete insulin. D cells contain secretory granules, but the product is unknown. One cell type probably contains gastrin, but as reviewed by Munger, it is not clear whether this is the "F" cell, the "fourth" cell, or the D cell. Other cell types have been reported, but if present, they are few in number (< 2 per cent). The cytoplasm of all of these cells contains granular endoplasmic reticulum, ribosomes, polysomes, mito-

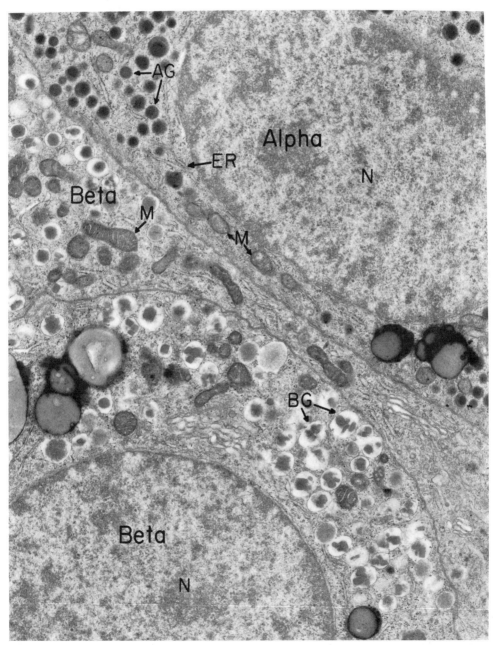

Figure 9–6.   Electron micrographs of islets from a man aged 25. Portions of two β-cells are seen, with their characteristic granules (BG), formed by 1–4 rhomboid crystals enclosed by a limiting membrane. In the α-cells are round granules (AG) with dense center and pale periphery. Nuclei (N), mitochondria (M), and endoplasmic reticulum (ER) are noted (× 17,000).

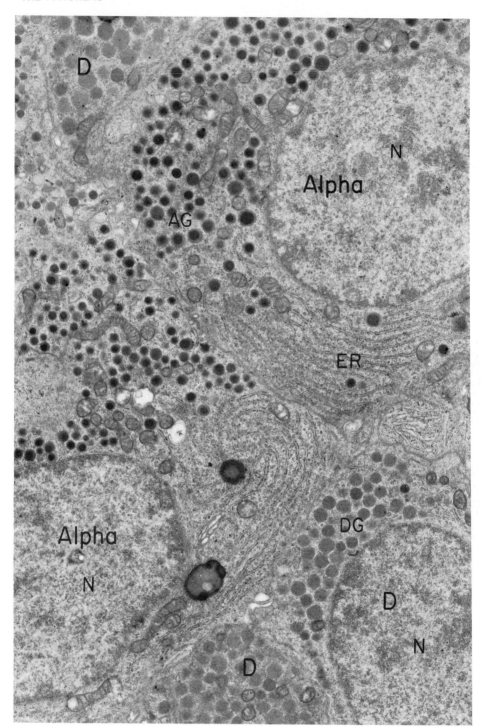

Figure 9–7. Another part of the same islet shows two α-cells and part of three D-cells. The D-cells contain numerous closely packed homogeneous granules (DG) of less density than the α-cell granules. A limiting membrane is closely applied to all the granules (× 14,000). (Figs. 9–6 and 9–7 were kindly supplied by Dr. Felice Caramia.)

chondria, Golgi complex, secretion granules, microtubules, and cytosol.

The detailed fine structure of B cells varies somewhat in the guinea pig, rabbit, rat, and dog, but the A cells have a relatively uniform appearance in all of these species. A cells differ from B cells in that the concentration and density of the A granules are greater and the Golgi complex is smaller. The A cells have smaller granules and a more ovoid nucleus. The granules of the D cells are less dense and more homogeneous than are the A and B granules.

Nerve fibers and their terminations on islet cells are observed by light microscopy, and electron microscopy shows unmyelinated fibers closely applied to plasma membranes of islet cells. Both sympathetic and parasympathetic nerve endings have been identified. These nerve endings are in close association (?synaptic) with A, B, and D cells. The function of these nerves has just recently been appreciated as part of the insulin and glucagon control system.

The islets are surrounded by a basement membrane which encloses all three cell types. It is separate from the capillary basement membrane, and therefore, hormones must cross two basement membranes before they enter the blood stream. There is an elaborate labyrinth of anastomosing capillaries in islets, providing a very rich vascular supply. Electron microscopic studies have shown that the endothelial cells of the capillaries are fenestrated, partly accounting for the rapid appearance of insulin in the circulation after islet stimulation.

Insulin Synthesis and Storage

There is considerable evidence that the synthesis of insulin begins on ribosomes on the surface of the rough endoplasmic reticulum (RER). Insulin is formed as a single polypeptide chain, proinsulin, containing from 81–86 residues, depending on the species. The amino acids are so arranged that there is spontaneous folding of this molecule into a form in which the disulfide bonds characteristic of insulin are easily made. The conversion of proinsulin to insulin occurs by proteolytic cleavage, which reduces the molecular weight of the protein from 9000 (proinsulin) to one of 6000 (insulin) and one of 3000 (C-peptide). This conversion occurs at the time of, or soon after, the transport of proinsulin to the Golgi complex, where it is apparently packaged into granules. Since the granules contain insulin and C-peptide in equimolar amounts, it seems likely that the packaging occurs first and is followed by cleavage within the granule. Insulin is complexed with zinc and stored. The B-cell granule also contains lipids and, in some species, monoamines. The complete structure of the B-cell granule is not yet known.

By electron microscopy, insulin granules vary considerably in their staining properties. Since there is some evidence that the oldest granules are released first, it appears that these different staining granules represent stages in the maturing process, but since no more than 2–5 per cent of the total content of the insulin-like materials in pancreas is proinsulin, it is unlikely that these changes represent alterations in the relative contents of proinsulin and insulin. The number of B-cell granules is a good indication of the amount of insulin present; however, it does not reflect the synthesis rate or release rate of insulin, but simply the balance between them at any one time. A large quantity of insulin is stored in the pancreas, e.g., in man, about 4 U./g. or 200 U. In general, when there is a prolonged decrease in the insulin synthesis and secretion rate, a number of changes in the

B cells are observed, including a decrease in the size of the nuclei, decreased granulation, decreased prominence of the Golgi apparatus, and fewer ribosomes. On the other hand, with an increase in the activity of the B cells due to continuous glucose stimulation, there is an increase in the size of the nucleus, the granulation tends to diminish, and the Golgi apparatus becomes spread out and more prominent; the RER increases in amount and in the number of prominent ribosome clusters and may become dilated (Fig. 9–8). With continued stimulation of the B cells by glucose, infiltration with glycogen may be observed. With prolonged marked stimulation, there may be hydropic changes.

Proinsulin synthesis and cleavage and insulin storage are not directly coupled to release; these processes appear to be separately regulated. Insulin synthesis is sensitive to glucose. An increase in synthesis due to glucose can be shown to occur in the absence of insulin secretion, for example, by incubation in a low-calcium medium (Steiner). This effect cannot be reproduced by pyruvate, indicating the specificity of the response by its lack of a relationship to the general availability of energy. Sulfonylurea drugs, which are known to cause release of insulin, have not been shown to increase synthesis. The conversion of proinsulin to insulin is known to be an energy-dependent step. A trypsin-like enzyme is believed to be involved but has not been identified certainly.

Insulin Release

B granules are stored until a stimulus for insulin secretion is applied, such as glucose, glucagon, or tolbutamide. The early change in the release process is a margination of the beta granules to the plasma membrane of the B cell (Fig. 9–9). The walls of these sacs fuse with the plasma membrane of the cell and rupture, and granules are then liberated into the extracellular space. They then rapidly disappear from the extracellular space, as viewed by electron microscopy, apparently undergoing rapid dissolution. Lacy has called this process of granule ejection into the extracellular fluid *emiocytosis*. With the disappearance of the granule, cytoplasmic projections called microvilli remain. These extend from the surface of the B cell into the intercellular space. These microvilli have been counted by Lacy and shown to increase in number in proportion to the rate of release of the beta granules by emiocytosis.

The insulin release process from beta cells has been shown to require extracellular calcium. The rate of its release following glucose stimulation is correlated with the rate of calcium uptake by the islet; this has led to the concept that there is a coupling of the stimulus to secretion by calcium in a manner analogous to the stimulus/contraction coupling in muscle. Lacy has also presented evidence for the existence of microtubules in B cells and for their participation in intracellular transport of the secretory granules to the plasma mem-

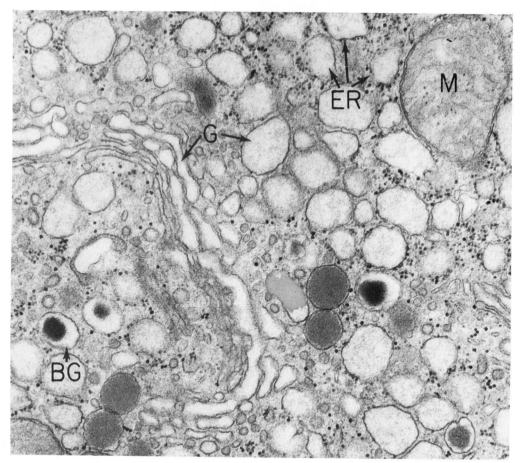

Figure 9–8.   Mouse β-cell stimulated by repeated (21 days) administration of insulin antibody, showing almost total disappearance of β-granules (BG). Endoplasmic reticulum (ER), and Golgi apparatus (G) are very prominent (× 48,000). (Courtesy of J. Lobothetopoulos.)

branes. His working hypothesis is that calcium triggers a contractile process in which the microtubules facilitate the movement of the granules from the interior of the cell to the cell surface. Adenosine 3'5'-monophosphate (cAMP) presumably has an important role in the release process. Cerasi and Luft postulated that cAMP was the direct effector for insulin secretion, but this now seems unlikely; instead, it appears that cAMP is an important intracellular regulator of insulin secretion rate and that it modulates the islet response to some other primary stimulant or depressant. This modulation appears to be independent of calcium uptake by the cell, but there may be an internal rearrangement or alteration in calcium-binding intracellularly which mediates the cAMP effect.

The importance of ionic fluxes in the release of the granules has been recently underscored by the demonstration that islet cells are electrically active. Dean and Matthews were able to record miniature action potentials in cells exposed to glucose, and the number of cells firing was dependent upon glucose concentration. They concluded that the action potential activity was due predominantly to calcium entry and that extracellular sodium ions

tend normally to repress this calcium influx. Other sugars that increase insulin secretion also produce action potentials; inhibitors of insulin secretion such as epinephrine block the development of action potentials. Thus transport and membrane phenomena are critical determinants of insulin secretory rates.

This current view of the synthesis, storage, and release of insulin is schematically depicted in Figure 9–10. Although quantitatively *emiocytosis* is possibly the most important mechanism of B-granule release, it may not be the only mechanism. For example, it may be that some insulin remains in soluble form and is not incorporated into a recognized granule, that granules dissolve in the cell, releasing insulin to the interior of the cell, or that some granules are released directly from synthetic sites by separate release mechanisms without prolonged storage.

Physiology of Insulin Secretion

Insulin, proinsulin and C-peptide circulate freely in the plasma. Measurement of insulin is now made by insulin immunoassay. A noninsulin

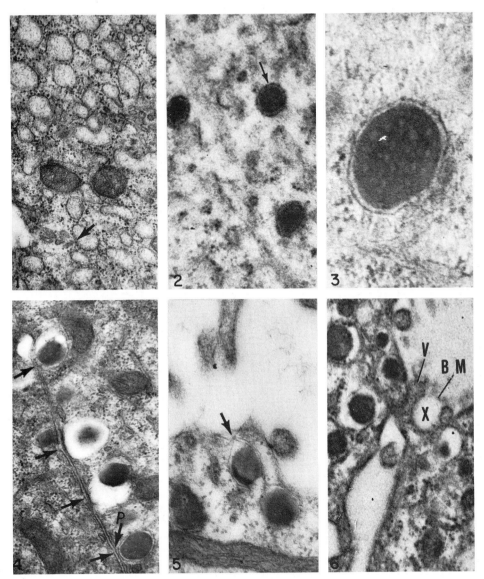

Figure 9–9. Sequential changes in insulin secretion in rats. *1*, Pale, amorphous material in vesicles of RER (↑) (× 34,000). *2*, β-granule with ribonucleoprotein granules attached to the outer surface of its sac (× 45,000). *3*, High magnification of β-granule (× 100,000). *4*, β-granules lining the cell membrane (↑); membranous sac of the granule in the right lower corner is separated from the plasma membrane (× 36,000). *5*, Fusion of the membranous sac of granule with the plasma membrane (P) shown at the arrow (× 55,000). *6*, Space (X) previously occupied by a β-granule. Basement membrane (BM) overlying the opening of the sac is slightly bulged. The cytoplasm to the left of this protrudes, forming a microvillus (V) (× 35,000). (From Williamson, J. R., et al.: *Diabetes* *10*:460, 1961.)

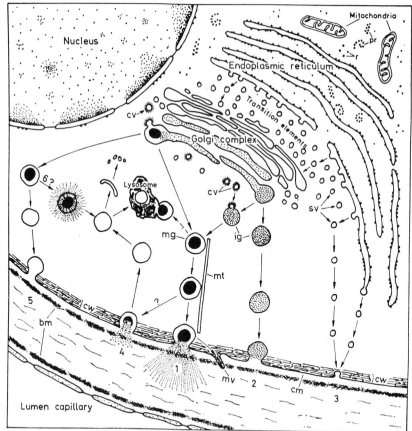

Figure 9–10. Diagrammatic representation of the morphologic events of the secretory process in an insulin-producing cell. Proinsulin is synthesized on the membrane-associated ribosomes of the endoplasmic reticulum and transferred to the Golgi complex by way of transition elements where the granules are formed. (Pro)insulin-containing granules which bud from the Golgi cisternae can be hypothesized to be released by one or more of six possible processes: (1) conventional emiocytosis of mature secretory granules in conjunction with contractile microtubular elements; (2) emiocytosis of immature secretory granules; (3) release of microvesicles independent of the Golgi apparatus; (4) release of insulin from the granule as a result of increased permeability of the granular membrane with retention of the membrane after evacuation of its contents; (5) emiocytosis of granules having previously undergone physical and chemical alteration of granule content; (6) physicochemical change in granule content followed by its passage into the cytoplasm. Although the majority of insulin is probably released by process (1), other methods have not been adequately explored.

Abbreviations: r = free ribosome; pr = polyribosomes; sv = smooth vesicles; cv = coated vesicles; ig = immature granules; mg = mature granules; mt = microtubules; cw = cell web; bm = basement membrane; mv = microvillus; cm = cell membrane. (From Renold, A., et al.: *Diabetes* 21:622, 1971).

compound with insulin-like biologic activity circulates in plasma in a concentration ten times higher than that of insulin, as measured by bioassay, but its activity is not suppressible by insulin antibody. This substance with nonsuppressible insulin-like activity (NSILA) is not derived from the pancreas. A discussion of its characteristics is presented later. In presently available immunoassays, both proinsulin and insulin interact with the same antibody, and therefore both are measured unless plasma is pretreated in some way. Clearly both peptides contain common immunologic determinants, and therefore it will be impossible to develop direct immunoassays for insulin which do not measure some proinsulin. On the other hand, the three-dimensional structure of proinsulin appears to be sufficiently different from insulin that proinsulin does not react well with insulin antibodies.

In the basal state (after a 16-hour fast) of a normal non-obese man, between 5–15 μU. of immunoreactive "insulin" (IRI) circulates in plasma; 5–30 per cent of this is proinsulin. Insulin antibodies bind about one-half of the proinsulin present, and therefore only a small percentage (about 15 per cent) of what is measured as insulin by immunoassay is proinsulin. Turner and Genuth have both estimated posthepatic basal insulin secretory rates of about 0.5 U./hour. Since the methods of estimation were different, these may be reasonably reliable. If the liver extracts about 50 per cent of the insulin delivered to it in a single passage, we estimate basal pancreatic insulin output to be about 1 U./hour. After intravenous glucose challenge, peak peripheral insulin concentration occurs in 3–5 min., and with a maximal 20-g. stimulus it is 8–10 times the baseline concentration. After 100 g. of oral glucose, the peak peripheral IRI concentration occurs in 30–60 min. and is 6–8 times the baseline level. No reliable estimates of true secretion rates after glucose are available.

Kinetics of Release

Since insulin is the most important storage or anabolic hormone, it is not surprising that its secretion is carefully regulated. Many substrates and hormones seem to participate in this regulation. The relationship between individual controllers and insulin secretion is a complex function. First, the duration of the stimulus, as well as its strength, determines insulin secretion rate. In addition, a stimulus of variable strength, but of constant duration, produces a sigmoid dose-response curve of insulin output. To illustrate these concepts, we will examine the kinetics of the process before evaluating the primary substrate controllers and the secondary hormonal and neural controllers.

The best studied and probably most important stimulus for insulin secretion is glucose. When glucose is presented to the islet as a sudden increase in concentration and held constant above 100 mg./100 ml., there is an immediate islet response (30 sec. - 1 min.), which peaks within a few minutes. Thereafter the secretion rate falls, and then gradually rises to reach another steady level (Fig. 9-11). The magnitude of the initial, or first-phase, response depends upon the previous history or "set" of the islet, the glucose concentration, and the species involved. The second phase appears to depend on the metabolism of glucose. This biphasic pattern of insulin secretion has been studied primarily in the rat but is known to occur in man. When glucose infusion is stopped, insulin secretion quickly returns to control values. In order to explain this biphasic pattern, mathematical models have been developed which generally suggest compartmentation of the stored insulin, such that only a small portion of it is immediately available for release (Fig. 9-12). The second phase of secretion involves provision of additional insulin to this compartment or delayed release from a second, much larger, compartment. The dose-response relationships for both phases of release appear to be sigmoidal in nature, with a very slow rise in secretion rate up to 100 mg./100 ml., followed by a sharp rise

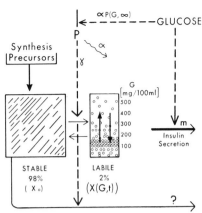

Figure 9-12. A two-compartment model for insulin secretion. This model has been utilized to explain the biphasic insulin release observed in the isolated perfused rat pancreas. Insulin is distributed in units or packets in a labile pool which are released when their glucose threshold is reached. Glucose also controls the provision of insulin to this small compartment through a hypothetical intermediate substance, P. This model can be defined in quantitative terms and has been simulated on a digital computer. (From Grodsky, G. M.: *J. Clin. Invest. 51*:2050, 1972.)

in insulin secretory rate up to 200 mg./100 ml., and maximum output at above 300 mg./100 ml.

Insulin is also secreted in the intact animal in the basal state without an exogenous glucose stimulus. Glucose also appears to be a part controller of this level of insulin secretion, but this control appears to differ from either the first or second phases of exogenous glucose-stimulated insulin release. For this reason, basal insulin secretion is considered separately from stimulated insulin secretion. This basal insulin secretion rate can be used to predict insulin responses to challenge. The reason for this predictability is not completely understood but has been interpreted to mean that basal insulin secretion reflects the "set" of the islet, and that this "set" is one of the determinants of the magnitude of stimulated insulin release. This system appears to permit the islet to make long-term feedback adjustments, which can then modulate the response to a sudden challenge to the B cell. The basal insulin secretion can be used as an index of that "set." It is presumed that many of the substrate and hormonal controllers which have been used to demonstrate stimulated insulin release also participate *in vivo* in the regulation of basal insulin secretion, but since the basal and stimulated secretory functions are separate, the quantitative interaction between any of these substances and the basal secretory outputs is unknown.

In summary, insulin secretion is considered to be a nonlinear function of substrates and hormonal controller concentrations. It has been subdivided into two broad categories—insulin release in response to external stimulus, and insulin release in the basal state in the absence of an external stimulus. Basal insulin secretion is a reflection of the long-term set of the islet. The insulin release in response to external stimulus has been further subdivided into first-phase insulin release and second-phase insulin release, because the duration of

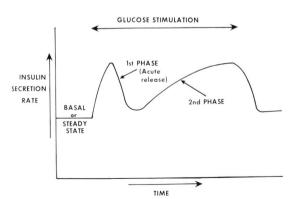

Figure 9-11. The effect of constant glucose stimulation on insulin secretion. Note the two phases of insulin release and their separation from a basal or steady state prior to glucose stimulation.

the stimulus partly determines the response. First-phase insulin release clearly involves only the release of stored hormone. It has the sigmoid dose-response curve characteristic of a saturable system. Second-phase insulin release, stimulated by glucose, involves predominantly the release of stored hormone, but becomes more and more dependent upon protein synthesis as its duration persists. Some stimuli, such as glucose, interact with this system by influencing all three types of insulin secretion, but other stimuli interact with only one or two types. With this complexity, it is not surprising that interpreting and predicting insulin responses to challenge has been difficult.

Clinical Physiology

Clinical tests have been designed using glucose to evaluate insulin secretory response in man. Most of the early data were confusing because the complex way in which glucose regulates insulin secretion was not appreciated, and therefore there was no separation of the various phases of insulin response to glucose, nor was there separation of basal insulin secretion from insulin secreted in response to a challenge. When the nonlinear nature of the glucose-induced insulin response was defined, it was possible to develop models for man which could be used to interpret the clinical tests. They are very similar to the models that have been developed for the perfused rat pancreas. The model that we have used is shown in Figure 9–13. It consists of two pools (or compartments) – a small pool available for immediate release comparable to that responsible for first-phase insulin secretion, and a much larger pool responsible for second-phase insulin release, which occurs either directly or via the small storage compartment. Insulin synthesis is responsible for refilling the large storage pool and is also a major contributor to insulin secretion in the basal state or after prolonged administration of glucose (several hours). In clinical testing

with oral glucose, the early phases of the test (0–30 min.) are dominated by the sensitivity of release of the small storage pool, the size of the small storage pool, and the rate of rise of glucose concentration, i.e., the magnitude of the challenge. The intermediate period (30–90 min.) is dominated by the sensitivity of the large storage pool to release insulin, and the later phases by the rate of insulin synthesis. When glucose is given intravenously and instantaneously and there is no further glucose input during the remainder of the test, the two phases tend to become a little better separated. The immediate response from the small storage pool is observed for the first 10 min., whereas the second-phase insulin release assumes dominance between 10–45 min. Then there is a gradual increase in synthesis-related release after 45–90 min. The "set" of the islet is reflected in insulin secreted in the basal state prior to the stimulus. This output appears to give an index of the size and sensitivity of the storage pools. Thus, in normal subjects, one expects that a greater secretion rate in the basal state will be reflected by greater release from both the small and large storage pools after a challenge. Deviations from this expected response will be discussed in the section on the Pathophysiology of Insulin Secretion.

Substrate-Induced Insulin Secretion

Substrates are the primary regulators of insulin secretion, and all three major classes—carbohydrates, fats, and proteins—have been shown to influence insulin output. Little progress has been made in delineating the control of basal insulin secretion, and therefore this section will be focused predominantly on stimulated insulin release. Glucose and fructose are the only important sugars in the regulation of insulin secretion. Since fructose is largely converted to glucose during absorption and is a relatively weak stimulus, glucose becomes the dominant carbohydrate regulator.

The mechanism by which glucose regulates insulin secretion has been of intense interest. Both D-*manno*-heptulose and 2-deoxyglucose inhibit phosphorylation of glucose and inhibit insulin secretion. Xylitol, a sugar alcohol metabolized by the hexose monophosphate shunt pathway, stimulates insulin secretion. Therefore, from two points of view, glucose metabolism has been correlated with insulin secretion. It was therefore concluded that the metabolism of glucose was essential for insulin release. Recently, however, Matchinsky showed that insulin secretion occurs in an intact animal without an increase in the concentration of the metabolic intermediates of glucose. From these studies he has concluded that early or first-phase insulin secretion is the direct result of the recognition of glucose as a molecule by a "glucoreceptor." It seems likely that these concepts are compatible, and that glucose stimulates the release of insulin as a result of its metabolism and its recognition as glucose. Since glucose clearly stimulates the synthesis of insulin as well, it seems likely that glu-

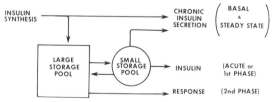

Figure 9–13. Schematic representation of a two-pool model for insulin secretion in man. Glucose is believed to regulate insulin output in three separate ways: (1) as a direct controller of the small storage pool, responding to a rate of change in glucose concentration to produce the rapid or first phase insulin release; (2) by its metabolism as a controller of the large storage pool to produce a delayed response and a second phase of challenge; and (3) by production of an intermediate which regulates insulin synthesis producing a very delayed response, labeled here "chronic insulin secretion." This delayed response controls insulin secretion in the basal state as well. (From Cook, D.: A systems model study of blood glucose homeostasis. Master's thesis, University of Washington, Seattle, 1969.)

cose interacts with islet cells in three separate ways—recognition as a molecule, metabolism of glucose specifically, and as a general energy substrate. This is fortunate for the physiologists who model insulin secretion, since almost all the models require more than one controller to explain the complex nonlinear process by which glucose regulates insulin output.

Amino Acids. Although leucine was first shown to release insulin in pathologic states, it now seems that most, if not all, amino acids increase insulin release (Fig. 9–14). Of those tested, arginine is the most potent. There is a wide range of potency of the other amino acids, perhaps related to the simultaneous stimulation of glucagon and growth hormone, which also affect insulin secretion. Little is known about the mechanism of action, but since a nonmetabolizable amino acid can also induce insulin release, metabolism of the amino acid is not required. Arginine-induced insulin secretion has been shown to be multiphasic, indicating that the duration of this stimulus is also a variable which is important to the amino acid control of insulin secretion. Superimposed upon a primary effect of individual substrates is an interaction between them. For example, synergistic effects have been reported between glucose and protein or amino acids.

Fatty Acids. Fatty acids and ketone bodies have also been reported to increase insulin levels; however, this appears to be predominantly in animals, particularly in dogs. In man, the effect is either not obtained at all or is extremely weak, and therefore does not seem to be important to the control of human metabolism.

Hormones

Gastrointestinal Hormones. The intestinal absorption of foods releases several gastrointes-

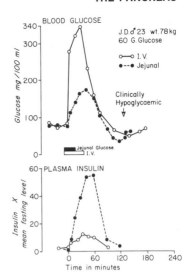

Figure 9–15. Despite the much smaller rise in plasma glucose level following its intrajejunal administration, compared with its intravenous administration, there is a far greater increment in the plasma insulin with the intrajejunal route (>50 × fasting). (From McIntyre, N., et al.: *J. Clin. Endocr.* 25:1317, 1965.)

tinal hormones—gastrin, secretin, cholecystokinin-pancreozymin, and enteroglucagon. Insulin secretion has been reported to result from release of each of these hormones. Augmentation of the primary response to a substrate has also been found after the simultaneous administration of these hormones and glucose or of amino acids. The discovery of this augmentation effect has in large part explained the observation that any substrate given orally produces a larger effect on insulin output than does the same amount of substrate infused intravenously (Fig. 9–15). Physiologically, the release of these augmenting hormones at the beginning of absorption appears to be useful in that the subsequent nutrient load will be anticipated by the pancreas to give a much larger response. On the other hand, in the absence of simultaneously administered substrates, these hormones have relatively weak effects on islets, and predominantly only stimulate acute or first-phase insulin release. The vagus nerve probably also participates in this gastrointestinal anticipation phenomenon by controlling gastrointestinal hormone release and by a direct stimulating effect on B cells.

Glucagon. Glucagon also increases insulin secretion, even in very small amounts, as a direct B-cell effect. Although glucose regulates insulin and glucagon reciprocally, so that as one rises the other tends to fall, amino acids stimulate both simultaneously. Therefore, there are circumstances in which glucagon may be expected to potentiate the insulin-stimulatory properties of amino acids. In addition, of course, glucagon tends to mobilize liver glycogen and prevent the uptake and storage of glucose by the liver during absorption. Presumably, this would allow for the storage of amino acids in peripheral muscles in response to secreted insulin, while at the same time glucagon protects the cerebral cortex from hypoglycemia.

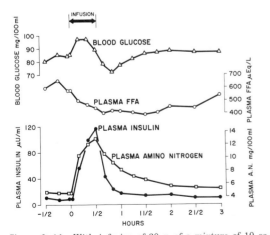

Figure 9–14. With infusion of 30 g. of a mixture of 10 essential amino acids in 35 healthy subjects tested 51 times, there is an immediate rise in plasma IRI, correlating with a rise in amino nitrogen. There was only a slight and transient rise in blood glucose but a progressive decline in plasma FFA. (From Floyd, J. C., et al.: *J. Clin. Invest.* 45:1487, 1966.)

Other Hormones. Several other hormones increase insulin levels and the peripheral tissue resistance to insulin. These are growth hormone, glucosteroids, and the sex steroids—progesterone and estrogen. Whether the hyperinsulinism observed is a compensation for the insulin resistance feeding back through glucose or one of the other substrates or hormones, or whether this is a direct effect upon islet function is unknown; however, most likely it is an indirect effect upon the islet. The presence of increased levels of these hormones is reflected as an increase in basal insulin secretion and, in compensated normal subjects, as an increased insulin response to challenge. The question remains, how does the islet know when the peripheral tissue is insulin-resistant? The same question can be asked concerning several patho-logic states associated with insulin resistance, such as obesity and uremia. This is an important unanswered question in the field of diabetes. The insulin-resistant states are discussed later.

Neural Regulation

The neurotransmitters, acetylcholine and nor-epinephrine, have been shown to influence directly insulin secretion. Epinephrine and norepinephrine are the *only endogenous* substances known to inhibit insulin release (Fig. 9–16). They share this property by stimulating the alpha adrenergic receptor. Each also simultaneously stimulates the beta adrenergic receptor, which tends to increase insulin secretion. This provides a push-pull control

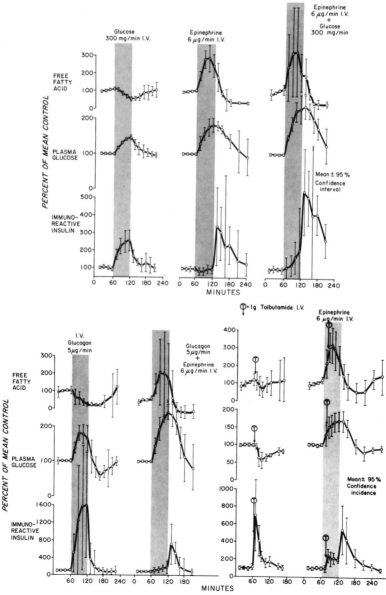

Figure 9–16. Demonstration that epinephrine inhibits the insulin-releasing effect of glucose, glucagon, and tolbutamide. (From Porte, D., et al.: *J. Clin. Invest.* 45:228, 1966).

of islet function, such that when catechols are present, the net effect of these hormones is to inhibit the secretion of insulin by the alpha receptor effect, but when catechols are removed, the islet remains in a supersensitive, hyperresponsive state because of previous beta receptor stimulation (Fig. 9–17). Although many stimuli to secretion are inhibited by catechols, secretin and arginine are not. The physiologic significance of this difference is not known. Although catecholamine regulation may take place primarily via circulating catecholamines released from the adrenal medulla, there has long been known to be autonomic innervation of pancreatic islets. The recent rediscovery of this fact has focused attention on the central nervous system as a regulator of carbohydrate metabolism. Sympathetic nerves to the pancreas have been stimulated in the dog, and when this is done, glucose-stimulated insulin release is diminished. All mammalian species examined have autonomic nerve endings in pancreatic islets, although there has been little systematic evaluation in man. The importance of the sympathetic nervous system to stress hyperglycemia will be discussed later, but there is now evidence in man that there is probably continuous modulation of basal insulin secretion by the sympathetic nervous system. Alpha blocking agents can increase basal insulin secretion, and beta blocking agents lower it (Fig. 9–18). Several sites within the brain have been implicated in this control, including the hypothalamus, floor of the fourth ventricle, and lower cervical spinal cord. The ventromedial nucleus of the hypothalamus has been of particular interest, because it contains a group of neurons that respond to changes in blood-glucose concentration by altering their electrical activity. Stimulation of this region has resulted in increased glucose and glucagon levels and in suppression of insulin release.

As might be expected, to provide balanced autonomic control of the pancreas, acetylcholine, the parasympathetic transmitter, stimulates insulin secretion. Stimulation of the vagus or the pancrea-

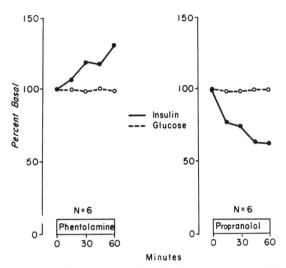

Figure 9–18. A demonstration of tonic adrenergic control of insulin secretion in man. α-Adrenergic blockade with phentolamine and β-adrenergic blockade with propranolol result in either an increase or a decrease in basal insulin secretion (o--o, control; •—•, experimental). (From Robertson, R. P., and Porte, D., Jr.: Diabetes 22:1, 1973.)

tic nerve in the dog increases insulin output, which is blocked by atropine. Insulin secretion and hypoglycemia can be conditioned in rats, and the conditioning reversed by atropine or vagotomy. The administration of atropine to man has not been associated with any change in basal insulin secretion, and therefore it is presumed that, during fasting, sympathetic nervous system activity predominates, but one expects increased vagal activity and insulin secretion during feeding. In the dog, a clear-cut "cephalic" insulin response can be demonstrated simply by introducing food into the esophagus.

Pathophysiology of Insulin Secretion

Diabetes — Relative Insulin Deficiency

Diabetes is characterized by a deficient insulin response to glucose. For this conclusion, it is necessary to segregate abnormalities in circulating insulin levels into two components, a basal component and a stimulated component. It has been found that non-obese patients with fasting hyperglycemia have normal levels of circulating insulin in the basal state and that obese patients with fasting hyperglycemia have elevated levels of circulating insulin which are proportional to their obesity. If the fasting state plasma glucose is greater than 115-120 mg./100 ml., these types of patients lose the ability to respond rapidly to intravenous glucose challenge and show no acute or first-phase increase in insulin levels during an intravenous glucose tolerance test (Fig. 9–19). If fasting plasma glucose levels are below this range, there is a linear relation between carbohydrate tolerance (glucose disappearance rate, K_g) and acute insulin

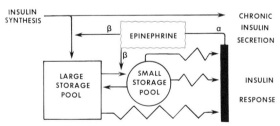

Figure 9–17. A schematic representation of the α- and β-adrenergic effects of epinephrine. Alpha inhibits the entire insulin response, both first and second phase from both storage pools and that portion of the basal state derived from the small storage pool. At the same time, epinephrine activates the β-adrenergic receptor which increases provision to the small storage pool from either the large storage pool or via insulin synthesis. Chronic insulin secretion is partially inhibited by the α-adrenergic effect but stimulated by the β-adrenergic effect. Prolonged epinephrine stimulation, therefore, results in enlargement of the small storage pool, inhibition of insulin output from the small storage pool, and stimulation of β-adrenergic–mediated insulin secretion.

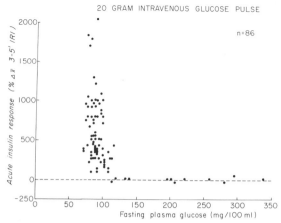

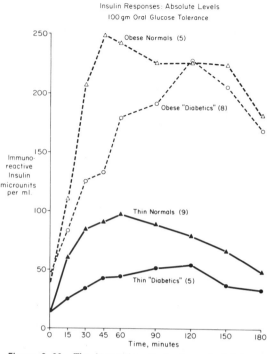

Figure 9–19. The relation of acute or first-phase insulin secretion to a 20-g. glucose challenge and fasting plasma glucose. Note the lack of any rapid insulin response when fasting plasma glucose exceeds 115 mg./100 ml. (Courtesy of Brunzell et al.)

release. This is independent of the later second-phase increment in circulating insulin, which occurs approximately 10–15 min. after the glucose challenge. If obese subjects are included in this group with mild carbohydrate intolerance, absolute insulin responses may, in fact, exceed normal. This is due to the higher islet "set." It is reflected in increased insulin secretion in the basal state of such subjects and can be corrected by calculating the relative insulin response; that is, the insulin response in proportion to the basal insulin level. When insulin responses are calculated in this way, all subjects with carbohydrate intolerance demonstrate progressive decreases in the relative acute insulin response.

Oral glucose tolerance tests show the same relation between insulin secretion and performance. However, many patients with fasting hyperglycemia who do not respond to intravenous glucose will secrete insulin during the oral test. The explanation for this difference is probably related to the (GI) hormonal augmentation of glucose-stimulated insulin release. Even in the oral test, however, by either using suitably matched control groups, with equal degrees of obesity (Fig. 9–20), or by calculating the relative insulin response, there is a relative deficiency of insulin release in response to challenge with declining glucose tolerance.

There has been a variety of theories to explain the loss of first-phase or acute insulin release in diabetes. Several agents, i.e., secretin and isoproterenol, are capable of stimulating acute insulin secretion in diabetic patients who cannot secrete insulin after intravenous glucose. Thus it seems likely that the defect within the diabetic islet accounting for the lack of response to glucose is specific for this molecule. This finding has given rise to the concept of a defect in a specific glucose receptor. Although Cerasi and Luft have hypothesized that this inability of the pancreatic islet to secrete insulin to glucose is caused by defects within the beta adrenergic receptors related to cAMP and

Figure 9–20. The interaction of obesity and diabetes on insulin responses during oral glucose (100 g.) tolerance test. Note that obese diabetics secrete more insulin than thin normal subjects, but less insulin than obese normals. Both obese groups and both thin groups start with the same basal insulin levels, despite the difference in carbohydrate tolerance. (From Bagdade, J. D., et al.: *J. Clin. Invest. 46*:1553, 1967.)

adenyl cyclase activity, the normal response to the beta adrenergic stimulator, isoproterenol, in diabetic subjects with no insulin response to intravenous glucose, as shown by Robertson and Porte (Fig. 9–21), indicates that beta adrenergic receptor abnormalities are not likely to explain a defective insulin response to glucose in diabetes.

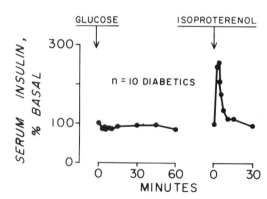

Figure 9–21. The β-adrenergic receptor in diabetes. Ten diabetic subjects with fasting plasma glucose greater than 115 mg./100 ml. were studied. Note the total absence of an insulin response to glucose with a brisk response to β-adrenergic stimulation (isoproterenol). These findings have been interpreted to indicate a selective defect in the insulin response to glucose in diabetes. (From Robertson, R. P., and Porte, D., Jr.: *J. Clin. Invest. 52*:870, 1973.)

Insulin-Resistant States

The "set" of the islets is reflected in the basal insulin level. One important factor that regulates this "set" is the peripheral sensitivity to insulin. Basal insulin levels, therefore, are elevated in clinical states of insulin resistance. Such resistance to the peripheral action of insulin has been associated with obesity, glucocorticoid therapy, Cushing's syndrome, estrogen therapy, uremia, acromegaly, and pregnancy. Of these clinical states, the best studied has been obesity. It has been found that obese subjects have a significant linear relationship between per cent ideal body weight and the basal level of circulating insulin. Moreover, the higher the level of circulating basal insulin (increased "set"), the greater the magnitude of the insulin response after glucose. Hence, when comparing insulin responses among individuals with different basal insulin levels, it is essential to express the responses as percentages of the individual's basal level. This relative insulin response correlates well with carbohydrate tolerance in such conditions as obesity and uremia.

Stress

Stress plays an extremely important role in the regulation of insulin secretion. Stress accompanies a variety of common clinical illnesses and has been shown to be associated with elevation of basal glucose levels, glucose intolerance, and inhibition of the acute insulin response following intravenous glucose or tolbutamide. Since catecholamines inhibit the acute insulin response by stimulating the alpha adrenergic receptor, the stress effect is probably an index of sympathetic nervous system overactivity. Several studies have shown that abnormally inhibited acute insulin secretion during stress can be improved by alpha blockade and have supported the concept that inhibition of insulin secretion during stress is attributable to overactivity of the adrenergic nerves. Responses are similar in a variety of clinical illnesses, including burns, anesthesia, hypothermia, exploratory laparotomy, cardiovascular shock, and pheochromocytoma. Perhaps the most common clinical area studied has been that of myocardial stress. Reports by Taylor and by Allison have demonstrated that fasting hyperglycemia and inhibited acute insulin response in patients with myocardial infarction and congestive heart failure can be reversed by alpha adrenergic blockade. Activation of this system by myocardial stress has been recently confirmed by Lukomsky and Oganov, who have shown that during the first several days after an acute myocardial infarction both plasma and urinary circulating catecholamine levels are elevated. Whether stress or abnormal adrenergic nerve activity can be related to the diabetic syndrome has not been fully determined, but recently Robertson has suggested that abnormal alpha adrenergic mechanisms may be operative during abnormal insulin secretion in some nonstressed patients with hyperglycemia and clinical diabetes mellitus.

Glucagon Storage and Synthesis

Although the existence of glucagon has been known almost as long as insulin, and although it has been known that it is clearly located in the A cells of the pancreas, detailed knowledge of A-cell function is lacking. A-cell granules show less species variation than does insulin, presumably because of the great similarity, if not identity, of the primary amino acid sequence among species. A granular endoplasmic reticulum is abundant, as are the typical secretory granules, which are symmetrically round, electron-dense, and surrounded by a limiting membrane. There is a prominent Golgi complex with granules within the complex, and therefore, it is believed that the same synthetic sequence occurs in the A cell as in the B cell—that is, synthesis in the endoplasmic reticulum, transport to the Golgi complex, and packaging for export as granules. There is also some inconclusive evidence for a larger molecular weight precursor (?proglucagon). Pancreatic glucagon content in most species reported is approximately 5–10 μg./g. wet weight. Although some authors, such as Lazarus, have produced evidence that emiocytosis is the method of glucagon secretion, this has not been universally agreed upon (see, for example, Munger). Details of the synthesis of glucagon are completely unknown. Nor is there any conclusive information on such fine details of secretory release mechanisms as their possible control by ions or substrates or the effect of metabolic inhibitors. The recent interest in the physiologic control of glucagon secretion will, it is hoped, stimulate a more complete and penetrating biochemical evaluation of the A cell.

Physiology of Glucagon Secretion

The measurement of glucagon in plasma has been considerably more difficult than that of insulin, primarily because of circulating materials, arising from the GI tract, with a larger molecular weight but immunologic determinants quite similar to glucagon. Since 1969, however, several antibodies which are almost specific for pancreatic glucagon have been developed. The use of these antibodies has allowed at least a beginning to be made into the physiology of glucagon secretion, but there is uncertainty about the correctness of the absolute concentrations of glucagon that are reported. The other major technological problem has been the finding that plasma contains an enzyme-degrading system which rapidly inactivates glucagon. Presumably, this system exists *in vivo* and contributes to the turnover of the hormone. In addition, glucagon, like insulin, is taken up by the liver and rapidly removed. However, the fractional extraction, i.e., the proportion taken out by the liver in a single passage, is unknown, but very likely is more than 50 per cent. Peripheral plasma levels are now reported to be approximately 100 pg./ml. This is lower than once thought, as investigators have discovered various artifacts in plasma which tend to increase the level. Even now, it appears from some bioassay experiments that there may be as much as a 100 per cent error and that the normal basal concentrations are probably around 50 pg./ml. The kinetics of release have not been evaluated; however, in general terms, it is known that certain substrates, hormones, and the neural system interact to determine the final secretory rate from the pancreas.

The concept has been proposed by Unger that glucagon and insulin form a regulatory couple. Each is controlled by factors that regulate its effects on the same peripheral tissues. The net effect on any tissue then depends on the relative concentrations of the two hormones. This implies that prediction of the state of activity of any tissue depends on the concentrations and effects of at least insulin and glucagon. In addition, it may be that the extracellular concentration in the pancreas of each influences the secretion rate of the other. This gives a more important role to glucagon as a regulator of metabolism and provides a very sophisticated interactive regulatory system for metabolic processes.

Substrate Controls

Under normal conditions, there is an inverse relationship between glucagon output and glucose concentration, such that hyperglycemia suppresses glucagon secretion (Fig. 9–22) and hypoglycemia augments it. Some have hypothesized that this is mediated in part by changes in insulin secretion, whereas others have concluded that it is primarily related to the concentration and uptake of glucose. Evidence can be marshaled on both sides of the argument. As will be reviewed later, diabetic sub-

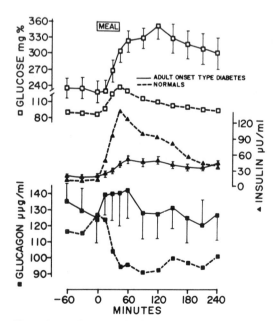

Figure 9–22. The effect of a carbohydrate meal on plasma glucose, insulin, and glucagon. Note the poor insulin response and the lack of glucagon suppression in the diabetic subjects. (From Müller, D., et al.: *New Eng. J. Med. 283*:109, 1970.)

jects with fasting hyperglycemia have normal basal glucagon levels despite the hyperglycemia and may respond with a hypernormal glucagon response to amino acid challenge. If ketoacidosis is present, the levels are greatly elevated and these elevations can be reversed by insulin therapy. Such findings support the idea that insulin controls glucagon output directly. On the other hand, blocking of glucose metabolism by mannoheptulose also elevates glucagon levels, but this is not reversed by insulin treatment. In addition, although glucagon can be shown to be suppressed by glucose administration in normal subjects and very poorly suppressed in diabetic subjects who have insufficient insulin response to glucose, injecting insulin at the time of the glucose challenge does not restore the suppressivity of the diabetic A-cell to normal. One cannot, therefore, conclude at present whether it is glucose, insulin or both which tends to suppress glucagon output. The glucose (?insulin) effect can be shown *in vitro*, and therefore does not require active participation of the neuroendocrine system. However, the magnitude of the changes *in vitro* is small, suggesting that physiologically there may be interactions with the neuroendocrine system that are important to the magnitude of the response.

Amino Acids. Intravenous amino acid and oral protein have been shown to stimulate glucagon secretion (Fig. 9–23). There are major differences in the potency of amino acids in stimulating glucagon release unrelated to their potency in stimulating insulin secretion. Arginine is the most potent for both, but leucine, another good insulin stimulant, does not stimulate glucagon secretion. In general, it appears that most glucogenic amino acids increase glucagon output. Some, such as alanine, probably only increase glucagon and not insulin directly. The physiologic importance of these interactions is presumably to prevent hypoglycemia when protein is ingested and to maximize amino acid storage in peripheral tissues; i.e., if protein stimulated only insulin release, the subject would tend to develop hypoglycemia. The hypoglycemia is prevented, however, by the simultaneous release of glucagon, which activates liver glycogenolysis. Glucagon also tends to augment insulin secretion, which further accelerates amino acid uptake by muscle.

Fat Metabolism. Glucagon is known to activate adipose-tissue adenyl cyclase and therefore is a lipolytic hormone. In some species, it is liberated in sufficient quantities to play a role in the acceleration of lipolysis. Therefore, studies have been performed to determine whether fatty acids play a role in the regulation of glucagon secretion. In dogs, elevated fatty-acid levels suppress glucagon secretion, whereas lowered fatty-acid levels increase glucagon output. However, there is no evidence for this feedback system in man.

Neuroendocrine Control

In animals and man, pancreozymin has been found to be a potent stimulator of glucagon secre-

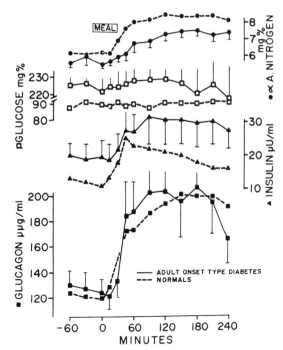

Figure 9-23. The effect of a protein meal on plasma glucose, glucagon, and insulin. Note the prompt rise in glucagon to this mixed amino acid meal. The rise in glucagon in the diabetic subjects has been interpreted to be inappropriate, in view of the severe degree of hyperglycemia. (From Müller, D., et al.: *New Eng. J. Med. 283*:109, 1970.)

tion. Since this hormone is released during the absorption of protein, the consequent glucagon stimulation is believed to play an important role in communicating information from the GI tract to the islets. Pancreozymin also stimulates insulin release, thus synergizing storage of amino acids with their absorption. Evidence for other hormonal controllers is more controversial and less readily available. It has been suggested that secretin inhibits the release of glucagon when stimulated by amino acids in the dog, but this has not been confirmed in man.

An interaction between the sympathetic nervous system and glucagon release has been suspected and postulated for a number of years by Sokal. This has now been confirmed. Glucagon release has been shown to occur during hypoglycemia, and this secretion is partially blocked by adrenergic blocking agents. Stimulation of the lateral hypothalamus has been shown to increase glucagon output in the rat by activation of sympathetic nerves, and glucagon secretion in dogs occurs after direct stimulation of the autonomic nerve to the pancreas. The nature of the adrenergic receptor for these effects is under intense investigation, but the type has not been conclusively defined. Increased glucagon secretion has also been found during exercise in the dog and in man, and therefore the concept is developing that activation of the sympathetic nervous system tends to increase glucagon output while it simultaneously inhibits in-

sulin secretion. No definitive studies of the effects of acetylcholine or of stimulation of the vagus nerve are available, but it would not be surprising if the entire autonomic nervous system were shown to be a modifier of glucagon secretion, as it has been demonstrated for insulin.

Pathophysiology of Glucagon Secretion

Studies of pathophysiology have been focused almost entirely upon the regulation of glucagon secretion in diabetes mellitus. There is no doubt that pancreatic glucagon secretion is abnormal in this syndrome; this is most easily shown in ketoacidosis in which very high levels are present. Basal glucagon levels are normal in diabetic subjects with a milder metabolic abnormality and fasting hyperglycemia. Unger has argued, however, that these are inappropriate for the level of hyperglycemia, since similar hyperglycemia in a normal subject would suppress glucagon concentration. Furthermore, Unger has shown that diabetic subjects, when given glucose, show suppression of glucagon secretion much more slowly than do normal subjects (Fig. 9-22). Glucagon levels are normal, even in insulin-dependent diabetics, indicating that alpha-cell function is maintained despite severe loss of beta-cell function. Only with pancreatitis or pancreatectomy have glucagon levels been shown to be low in diabetics. Glucagon responses to protein ingestion have also been shown to be normal in diabetics (Fig. 9-23), but again Unger argues that this is inappropriate, since in these subjects who do not secrete insulin, prevention of hypoglycemia is unnecessary. He has also found greater than normal glucagon responses to arginine infusion in insulin-dependent diabetics (Fig. 9-24) and therefore has marshaled impressive evidence that glucagon secretion is usually inappropriately controlled in the diabetic syndrome. The material is biologically active and therefore presumably contributes to the hyperglycemia observed.

Hyperglucagonemia has also been reported in patients with acromegaly, pheochromocytoma, and pancreatic tumors that primarily produce glucagon. A discussion of the role of glucagon in syndromes with hypoglycemia is given in Chapter 10.

DISTRIBUTION OF INSULIN AND PROINSULIN

In the majority of studies on the distribution of insulin and proinsulin, these hormones have been labeled with radioactive iodine (I^{131}), which in some instances has changed the biochemical reactions of the hormones. However, data suggest that with only one iodine atom per molecule of hormone the reactions are not changed significantly.

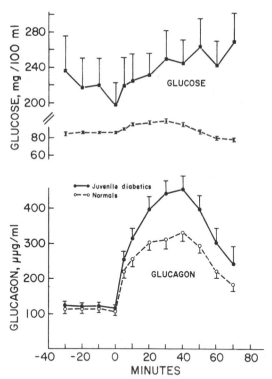

Figure 9-24. Glucagon responses to intravenous arginine in normal and insulin-dependent diabetic subjects. Note the inordinately great and statistically significant higher glucagon response to this intravenous amino acid challenge in the diabetic subjects. (From Unger, J., et al.: *J. Clin. Invest.* 49:837, 1970.)

Insulin Distribution

There are many factors that influence the distribution of insulin, including especially its rate of degradation in different tissues. When insulin-I[131] is injected into normal man, less than 15 per cent is present in the plasma after 1 hour. Grodsky, on administering 10 units of crystalline insulin intravenously to a normal subject, found that 90 per cent had disappeared in 20 minutes and all in 60 minutes. In other studies, crystalline porcine insulin in diabetics and normal men was found to have a half-life of less than 5 minutes. Insulin is found concentrated in bile with a peak level reached about 45 minutes after glucose ingestion. Insulin is filtered through the glomerulus but usually is almost completely reabsorbed from the proximal tubule. The reabsorbed insulin is apparently utilized in renal metabolism as well as being reabsorbed into the general circulation for use elsewhere.

Once insulin has crossed the capillary membrane, entering the extracellular fluid, it remains in this lymph fluid much longer than in the blood vascular system. For example, after intravenous glucose administration, lymph insulin was found to peak at about 1 hour, whereas in blood the peak was reached in 5 minutes. The lymph insulin levels were observed to correlate better with glucose assimilation rates than did serum insulin levels.

Elgee's studies with rats showed that almost all tissues accumulate some insulin but in markedly different concentrations. Brain and red blood cells took up essentially no hormone, while the greatest concentrations were seen in the kidney and liver, which, together with skeletal muscle and plasma, accounted for 61 per cent of the insulin-I[131]. The liver normally removes far more insulin than does any other organ, chiefly because insulin secreted by the pancreas must traverse the liver before reaching the peripheral circulation. Field estimates that approximately 40–50 per cent of the portal vein insulin is removed by the liver in a single transhepatic passage. Thus the liver plays an important role in regulating peripheral insulin levels. The kidney extracts about 40 per cent of the insulin delivered to it by the systemic circulation in a single passage. The renal medullas extract very little hormone, whereas the cortices, and particularly the proximal convoluted tubules, trap large quantities. In patients with severe renal disease, there is a twofold decrease in the rate of disappearance of I[125]-insulin from plasma, presumably due chiefly to an associated decrease in rate of insulin degradation by kidney. Small amounts of insulin and proinsulin have been found in human urine.

The amount of insulin removed by different organs depends upon its concentration in plasma and the number of free specific insulin receptors in cell plasma membranes; this is discussed in detail later. Some investigators have reported certain concentrations of insulin in the cytosol and intracellular particles, whereas others maintain that no insulin penetrates the plasma membrane. Using special methods for the preparation of the sarcolemma and muscle-cell nuclei after incubation of rat striated muscle with I[131]-insulin, Edelman reported that the sarcolemma bound 40 per cent of the radioactivity, and the soluble cell fraction bound 50 per cent. The sarcolemma (myocellular membrane) constitutes less than 2 per cent of the cell mass. The transverse tubules (T-system) (Fig. 9–25) which are lined by invaginations of the sarcolemma are continuous with the extracellular space, thus constituting a channel for direct passage of electrolytes and other substances. The insulin is bound to the sarcolemma by electrovalent and covalent (disulfide) bonds, the latter involving the 6 or 11 position or both in the A chain. In the light of the T system as seen in Figure 9–25, it is conceivable that, in a number of reports of subcellular distributions of insulin, the hormone in the microtubular system has been regarded as being in the cytosol. On the other hand, with the techniques used it might be possible to conclude erroneously that no insulin had penetrated the plasma membrane. This is because some of the insulin not bound to the specific receptor may be degraded, despite the low temperatures used during most of the procedure, as a result of the relatively long intervals required for preparation of the subcellular components.

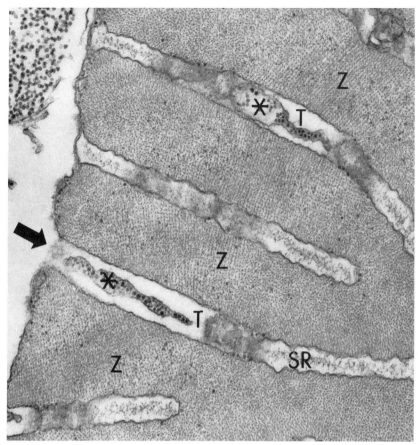

Figure 9-25. Section of muscle fiber, cutting across the Z line (Z), showing the middle of the T system (T) cisternae. The opening to extracellular space is shown by the arrow. Strands of sarcoplasm (*) penetrate the T system from neighboring fibers. The sarcoplasmic reticulum (SR) is observed. (Original magnification, × 38,000.) The tubules apparently supply good conduits for insulin, and the sarcolemma may constitute an important site of insulin action. (From Franzini-Armstrong, C., and Porter, K. R.: *J. Cell Biol.* 22:675, 1964.)

Proinsulin Distribution

Using an insulin-specific protease obtained from muscle for assaying for immunoreactive proinsulin (IRP), Duckworth measured, by immunoassay, IRP and total immunoreactive insulin (TIR) levels in plasma from subjects fasted overnight and at intervals during 3 hours after the oral administration of 100 g. glucose. The TIR levels represented the total amount of material bound to pork insulin antiserum. This consisted of insulin + proinsulin + proinsulin-like components (PLC). IRP consisted of the components bound to the insulin antiserum after incubation with insulin specific protease. This enzyme promoted degradation of most of the insulin, but of only a small amount of proinsulin and PLC. Other investigators have used other methods for gaining an index of proinsulin levels. Because a specific human proinsulin antiserum has not been available, serum proinsulin and PLC have been measured with an insulin or C-peptide antiserum and a human proinsulin standard after separation of insulin and C-peptide by gel filtration. Assays of unextracted serum with these two immunoassay systems meas-

ure total insulin immunoreactivity (insulin plus PLC) and C-peptide immunoreactivity (C-peptide plus PLC), respectively. In a severely hypoinsulinemic patient, the percentage of PLC increases, regardless of the etiology of the hypoinsulinemia (Gorden et al.). In normal subjects and patients whose concentrations of total plasma insulin are normally increased, the percentage of PLC in the basal state or following glucose stimulation usually does not exceed 30 per cent of the total circulating insulin. These investigators found reasonably good agreement between the gel filtration method and the insulin-specific protease techniques, but the finding of up to 75 per cent PLC in the basal state in normal subjects is considerably greater with the enzyme method than with the gel filtration techniques. Equimolar amounts of C-peptide and insulin were found in the serum of subjects over a wide range of insulin values.

Tissues degrade insulin much more rapidly than they degrade PLC. With the rapid disappearance from the plasma of insulin and the much slower disappearance of PLC, the ratio becomes basal. The immunologic half-time of porcine proinsulin has been found to be 20 min. in swine and 18 min.

in baboons (Stoll). In contrast to insulin, porcine proinsulin and C-peptide were not cleared by isolated perfused rat liver. Dog kidney has been found to extract an amount of proinsulin equivalent to the quantity of insulin extracted.

Since the liver extracts such a large quantity of insulin and little, if any, proinsulin, this could account for a considerable proportion of the difference in the plasma levels of the two hormonal components following glucose administration. When proinsulin was injected intravenously into rats, no evidence of conversion of proinsulin to insulin was found one hour later. Nevertheless, injection of proinsulin can produce marked hypoglycemia, suggesting that proinsulin exerts insulin-like effect without being converted to insulin. As discussed earlier, apparently all the insulin derived from the pancreas results from transformation of proinsulin to insulin induced by a specific enzyme system involving proteolysis. This enzyme system has not been demonstrated in other tissues. Kidney and pancreas have higher ratios of PLC:insulin than do other tissues. The reason that the kidney extracts relatively so much proinsulin has not been established. Little is known about the fate of the C-peptide.

DEGRADATION OF INSULIN AND PROINSULIN

Insulin is degraded by essentially all tissues of the body. Little or none is resynthesized from the degraded products. Results of the amount of degradation vary with the techniques used for study. The total degradation by liver and kidney greatly exceeds that of other organs. Presumably, they can remove 80 per cent of the total amount secreted. Most of the insulin removed by the kidneys is degraded rather than excreted. The liver is the first organ through which insulin passes after its secretion, and it is a big organ and one with a very active insulin-degrading system. Kitabchi reported that degradation of insulin and proinsulin appeared to be in the soluble portion of the liver cells, with the particulate fraction having less than 10 per cent of the total degradative activity, and that the proinsulin degrading activity was considerably less than that degrading insulin. Degradation of insulin presumably occurs by means of glutathione-insulin transhydrogenase and by proteolysis. The extent to which the two mechanisms are involved under normal conditions in the body is not known. Insulin can be degraded also by reduced glutathione and related substances as follows: $GSSG + TPNH + H^+ \rightarrow 2GSH + TPN$, catalyzed by glutathione reductase. Then glutathione-insulin transhydrogenase catalyzes the reductive cleavage of the insulin disulfide bonds by GSH, with liberation of chains A and B in reduced form. These chains undergo rapid proteolytic degradation, yielding small molecular weight components. In the presence of glutathione, insulin-degrading activity was reported present in all tissues tested (Chandler). The relative degrading activity (per mg. of tissue protein) was as follows: pancreas > liver > intestines > spleen > kidney, testes, thymus, fat, lung > brain > heart > diaphragm, skeletal muscle. The degradation was blocked by the addition of N-ethylmaleimide. Almost no degradation occurred with omission of reduced glutathione from the assay mixture. Moreover, the reaction was dependent upon the concentration of this reducing agent over a wide range.

Kitabchi, using different techniques, found that approximately 90 per cent of the degradative activity for immunoreactive insulin and immunoreactive proinsulin was located in the supernatant fraction from each of many tissues studied. The amount of insulin destroyed/min./tissue was in the following decreasing order: liver, pancreas, kidney, testis, adrenal, spleen, ovary, lung, heart, muscle, brain, and fat. With the exception of the pancreas and kidney, no organ extract exhibited degradative activity of immunoreactive proinsulin greater than 10 per cent of that for immunoreactive insulin. The degradation of proinsulin by the different supernatant organ fractions was in the following decreasing order: liver, pancreas, kidney, adrenal, testis, spleen, ovary, lung, heart, muscle, brain, and fat. Thus the rates of degradation of insulin and proinsulin were in essentially the same decreasing order in the different organs. Studies of a freshly purified insulin protease of kidney showed there was a tenfold greater rate of degradation of insulin than proinsulin (Kitabchi). Addition of other hormones, such as ACTH, glucagon, and growth hormone, did not affect the rate of degradation of insulin. Using a limited amount of insulin and I^{125}-insulin, the addition of more insulin is several times more effective in decreasing the amount of degradation of I^{125}-insulin than are equimolar quantities of proinsulin. There was inhibition of insulin-degrading enzyme activity by sulfhydryl-group inhibitors but a lack of effect of glutathione or aprotinin (Trasylol). Comparison of the properties of partially purified insulin-degrading enzyme from liver, muscle, and kidney suggested that the enzyme preparation from each organ had similar biochemical properties with high specificity for insulin. A single enzyme that proteolytically degraded insulin was isolated from rat skeletal muscle and purified a thousandfold (Duckworth). Insulin linked to agarose at the B-29 lysine residue did not bind the insulin-specific protease. With this linkage, the protease did not degrade it, but degradation occurred when it was linked at the phenylalanine residue. The purified enzyme degraded insulin but not proinsulin. This enzyme was found to be sulfhydryl-dependent, with a physiologic pH optimum (7.4). Insulin-specific protease is not dependent on glutathione for activity.

Freychet et al. showed that insulin was rapidly degraded by liver-cell membranes. After 90 min. of incubation of these membranes at 30° C, less than 10 per cent of the insulin was intact when measured by its capacity to bind specifically to other liver-cell membranes. They found that binding by anti-insulin antibody, precipitation by trichloroacetic acid, and adsorption by talc were less sensitive methods for measuring insulin degradation. They also found that insulin degradation was independent of its binding to its specific receptor. For example, desalanine-desasparagine insulin, which had an affinity for receptor that was only 2 per cent that of insulin, was degraded to the same extent as insulin. There was no relationship between the bioactivity of an insulin analogue and its ability to prevent degradation of insulin. Moreover, the K_m for insulin degradation was 40 times greater than the concentration of insulin that produced half-maximal inhibition of specific binding of I^{125}-insulin to receptors in liver-cell membrane. Insulin that was recovered from membranes upon the dissociation of the hormone receptor complex had not been degraded. While insulin was bound to a specific receptor, it was protected from degradation. Whereas proinsulin was very slowly degraded by the liver-cell membrane, it acted as a competitive inhibitor of insulin degradation. Proinsulin was also found to exert this inhibitory effect when insulin-specific protease of muscle and liver were tested. Freychet et al. could not detect in purified liver-cell membrane a significant amount of glutathione-insulin transhydrogenase activity. They found a marked similarity between the insulin-degrading system of the purified liver-cell membrane and the partially purified soluble enzyme from rat muscle and liver described by Kitabchi. Moreover, both systems showed a relative specificity for insulin. Sulfhydryl inhibitors inhibited the degradation of insulin, whereas reduced glutathione stimulated degradation. A significant amount of insulin degradation was observed at concentrations close to those in hepatic portal blood. The liver plasma membranes were found to be rich in protease activity.

Degradation of proinsulin by liver insulin-specific protease is less than 10 per cent of the rate of degradation of insulin (Kitabchi). The rate of degradation of proinsulin by glutathione-insulin transhydrogenase is far slower than the degradation of insulin. However, insulin and proinsulin degradation occurs at a comparable rate when incubated with fat cells for two hours. With whole pieces of fat, the degradation rate of insulin is about twice that of proinsulin. Both insulin and proinsulin are degraded at a much more rapid rate by homogenates of pieces of fat tissue than by homogenates of fat cells. The plasma membrane from fat cells and the soluble extract from the plasma membrane of the cells contain a highly active insulin-degrading system. The insulin-degrading system of the plasma membrane may be one of the physiologic mechanisms by which the response of fat cells to insulin is terminated. Whereas a pancreatic trypsin inhibitor (Kunitz) inhibits proinsulin degradation, it does not decrease insulin degradation. It is suggested that proinsulin degradation initially involves a trypsin-like activity with subsequent degradation by a system similar to that affecting insulin degradation. Although studies with tissue homogenates have shown cleavage of insulin into chains A and B, careful immunoassays for these chains in plasma have not definitely demonstrated their presence (a) during fasting, (b) after oral glucose, or (c) after intravenous insulin administration (Touber).

Insulin obtained from the plasma or the pancreas of some diabetics has been found to be more resistant than normal to degradation by insulinase (O'Brien). The amino acid content of pancreatic insulin obtained from the diabetics was normal, but there possibly could be an abnormality in the amino acid sequence.

ACTIONS OF INSULIN

Insulin is a powerful hormone with broad influences. Directly or indirectly, it affects the structure and function of every organ in the body — indeed, of every biochemical constituent.

The amount of insulin action depends at least on the (a) amount of insulin secretion, (b) insulin distribution, (c) type of tissue, (d) amount of insulin binding to its specific receptor, (e) types and amounts of nutrients inside and outside the cells, (f) types of ions and their concentrations, and (g) amounts and types of other hormones.

Some of the tissues that insulin has been shown to affect are listed in Table 9–1; adipose tissue, muscle, and liver have been studied most (Fig. 9–26).

Insulin's main functions are to stimulate anabolic reactions involving carbohydrates, fats, proteins, and nucleic acids. It catalyzes the formation of macromolecules in cells, which then are used in cell structure, energy stores, and regulation of many cell functions. Insulin stimulates the synthesis of protein from amino acids, nucleic acids from mononucleotides, polysaccharides from monosaccharides, and lipids from fatty acids.

The following are some of the specific actions of insulin. Insulin increases (a) plasma membrane transfer of glucose and certain other monosaccharides, some amino acids, some fatty acids, K^+, and Mg^{++}; (b) Mg^{++}-activated $(Na^+ + K^+)$ ATPase activity; (c) glucose oxidation; (d) glycogenesis; (e) lipogenesis; (f) proteogenesis; and (g) formation of ATP, DNA, and RNA. Insulin decreases (a) glycogenolysis, (b) lipolysis, (c) proteolysis, (d) gluconeogenesis, (e) ureogenesis, and (f) ketogenesis. Some of the activities of insulin result from its inhibition of the supply of cAMP, causing less activity of protein kinase. This is associated with less phosphorylation of enzymes, but an increase in ac-

TABLE 9–1. TISSUES RESPONSIVE TO INSULIN

Muscle (skeletal and heart)	Cartilage and bone
Adipose tissue	Skin
Liver	Lens
Leukocytes	Pituitary
Mammary glands	Peripheral nerve
Seminal vesicles	Aorta
Fibroblasts	Thymocytes
Smooth muscle cells	

Liver Cell   Muscle Cell

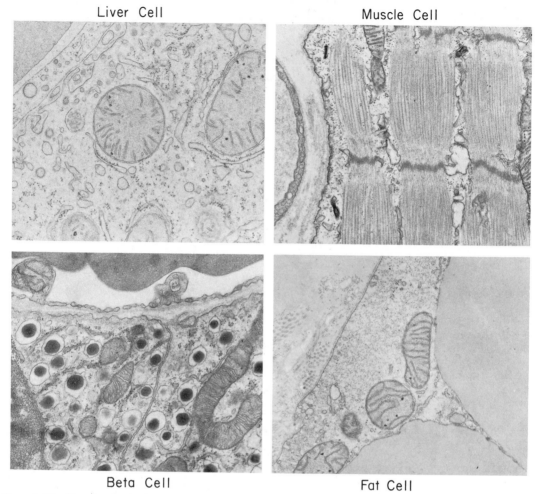

Beta Cell   Fat Cell

Figure 9-26.   Site of synthesis of insulin and the three tissue sites of action that have been studied most extensively. Insulin promotes protein synthesis in each of these tissues. In adipose tissue, its major function consists of synthesis and storage of fat. In muscle, its chief function is to stimulate energy utilization. It inhibits gluconeogenesis and ketogenesis in the liver (× 36,000). (Photomicrographs kindly supplied by J. Luft and J. Logothetopoulos.)

tivity of some nonphosphorylated enzymes. The latter enzymes tend to promote anabolism: glycogenesis, proteogenesis, lipogenesis, increased levels of nucleic acids, and mitogenesis. Insulin does not stimulate glucose transport in red blood cells or in the brain, nor does it promote tubular reabsorption of glucose by the kidney or glucose absorption by the intestinal mucosa.

Mechanisms of Insulin Action

There is considerable evidence for the existence of insulin-sensitive sugar transport systems in skeletal muscle, cardiac muscle, adipose tissue, fibroblasts, and other cells. It is believed that penetration of the cell membranes of such tissues is prevented in some way by a specific material which is either temporarily removed or altered in the presence of insulin. Some of the key points relative to the specificity of this system are as follows:

1. It exhibits stereospecificity, being receptive to sugars, such as galactose, D-xylose, and L-arabinose, but not to D-arabinose, rhamnose, gluconate, or glucuronate.

2. It demonstrates saturation kinetics, indicating a limited availability of a specific carrier.

3. The rate of entry of the sugars into the cell interior is relatively slow compared with their diffusion into the extracellular fluid.

4. The insulin-responding sugars compete with each other for transportation.

5. In rat diaphragm the insulin effect is more temperature-sensitive than would be expected by simple diffusion.

6. During cell entry the responsive sugars are not phosphorylated.

It seems that enhancing sugar entry in the absence of insulin, as for example by increasing the extracellular glucose concentration, should result in the same metabolic changes as follow addition of insulin in the presence of a lower concentration of glucose. However, there are a number of differences, one being that insulin promotes greater usage of glucose for the formation of glycogen than for other pathways. This has been attributed by certain investigators to the capacity of insulin to stimulate glycogen synthetase. Anoxia and certain inhibitors of oxidative phosphorylation greatly augment the entry of glucose into cells, but many of the metabolic consequences differ considerably from those of insulin; for example, the amount of glycogenesis is greatly decreased.

Insulin Receptor

A series of excellent studies by Cuatrecasas, Freychet, and others have shown that insulin must become bound to a specific protein in the plasma membrane in order for it to exert its action. Most of such studies have been performed with membranes of adipose tissue or liver, and the binding characteristics of these two tissues have been remarkably similar. Insulin binding is limited almost entirely to the plasma membrane, with none attached to nuclei, microsomes, mitochondria, or other cytoplasmic components, whether the insulin is added to intact or homogenized liver or to adipose tissue cells. Insulin covalently hooked to agarose beads that are much larger than fat cells stimulates glucose transport and inhibits lipolysis. This suggests that the insulin receptor is on the surface of the cell membrane. The receptor has a high degree of specificity for binding insulin and insulin derivatives.

The amount of binding of each constituent is proportional to its amount of insulin-type biologic activity. Various insulin derivatives displace one another and insulin in proportion to the total biologic potency of each. For example, the maximal action of insulin can be attained with a concentration of proinsulin 20 times greater than that of insulin. Displacement of insulin by proinsulin similarly requires a twenty times greater concentration of proinsulin, indicating a twentyfold greater affinity of the receptors for insulin. Bound insulin is not displaced by noninsulin peptides such as GH, ACTH, and glucagon, even when each hormone is added in very high concentration. There are a limited number of insulin-binding sites in each cell; about 11,000 molecules of insulin can be bound per cell.

The binding of insulin to its receptor presumably does not result in inactivation or other chemical changes in insulin or its receptor; no stable covalent forces or disulfide interchange between insulin and its receptor is involved in the binding. Tyrosyl and possibly histidyl, components of the membrane, may be important in the binding interaction, but sulfhydryl, tryptophanyl, and carboxyl groups do not seem to be involved. The insulin-cell receptor complex appears to be a simple dissociable combination. Homogenization of fat cells does not change the total insulin-binding capacities.

Physiologic changes that decrease insulin action, produced by hydrocortisone or fasting, do not alter insulin binding.

Results of some studies indicate that the insulin receptor may be a glycoprotein with surface sialopeptides, which may not be essential for insulin binding but are important for transmitting signals from the receptor site to other parts of the cell. Removal of cell membrane phospholipids can increase insulin binding, but it also increases the sensitivity of the residual membrane to protease action, and this can lead to destruction of the insulin-binding capacity. Ordinarily, the amount of insulin function parallels the amount of insulin binding, but under certain conditions, for example, with neuraminidase digestion, it is possible to abolish the biologic activity without affecting insulin binding. Neuraminidase removes sialic acid, which is one component of the lipoprotein complex on the outer part of the plasma membrane. Neuraminidase in small doses increases glucose uptake, whereas large doses decrease it, and abolishes insulin action on glucose transport and lipolysis, but does not change insulin binding. Phospholipase C or A, when incubated with the membrane of fat cells or liver cells, can markedly increase binding yet decrease the insulin effect on glucose uptake and on lipolysis. Following incubation with phospholipase C, the addition of phosphatidyl ethanolamine or phosphatidyl serine to the incubated membrane residue restores the insulin effect.

The insulin receptor has been extracted quantitatively from liver and fat cell membranes in water-soluble form. It appears to be an asymmetric protein (not lipoprotein) with a molecular weight of about 300,000 (Cuatrecasas). Insulin bound to agarose or to glass beads extracts particles that contain specific insulin receptors from a suspension of cell membrane.

Leukocytes, erythrocytes, and fibroblasts contain specific insulin-binding receptors (Gavin). The binding sites in white blood cells seem similar to those in the plasma membranes of liver and fat cells.

Much remains to be elucidated concerning the ways in which insulin promotes biochemical changes. Many of its effects result from changes in plasma membrane permeability, and others seem to result from certain changes in the plasma membrane, which relay messages for biochemical changes in interior portions of the cell. Insulin promotes permeation of the plasma membrane by certain sugars, amino acids, and ions but not others. In vitro, insulin has been found, as recently reviewed by Manchester, to increase protein synthesis in adipose tissue cells in the absence of amino acids or glucose in the incubation media. It enhances the incorporation of amino acids into proteins synthesized in the cell. It increases the attachment of monoribosomes to RNA and the ratio of polysomes to monoribosomes. These effects of insulin apparently result from an increase in the supply of a small molecular weight material in the cytosol that catalyzes the foregoing reactions. Numerous changes in the metabolism of carbohydrate, fat, protein, nucleotides, and other constituents occur. In order to gain a clearer picture of the effects of insulin on them, it is desirable to review some aspects of the metabolism of these compounds. This will be followed by a discussion of many actions of insulin on adipose tissue, liver, and muscle, and of certain interrelationships of metabolic activities in these tissues.

Carbohydrate Metabolism

Carbohydrates constitute about 50 per cent of the total caloric intake in the United States. Much of this carbohydrate is either ingested as glucose or transformed into it. A considerable amount of glucose can be utilized in the absence of insulin, but it is necessary for the blood glucose level to rise significantly in order for this to happen. In normal persons, the tissue threshold to glucose is approximately 70–90 mg./100 m., while in those with untreated diabetes it increases to 400 or more; sufficient insulin returns the threshold to normal. Tolbutamide or phenethylbiguanide also lowers the threshold.

Muscle, including the heart, is the greatest consumer of glucose, but as the availability of this nutrient decreases, a considerable amount of fat can be used; indeed, more than 90 per cent of the energy can be derived from fat. No gluconeogenesis takes place in muscle.

Immediately after entrance into the cell, glucose is phosphorylated at position 6 by adenosine triphosphate (ATP) in the presence of hexokinase and Mg^{++}. This reaction is irreversible and exergonic. Moreover, since the cell membrane is impervious to phosphoric acid esters, phosphorylation of glucose traps the sugar intracellularly. At least five fates are available for glucose 6-phosphate (G-6-P) (Fig. 9–27): (1) glycolysis, (2) phosphogluconate-oxidative pathway, (3) glucuronic acid pathway, (4) glycogenesis, and (5) conversion to glucose by glucose-6-phosphatase. Certain tissues lack the enzymes for some of these pathways.

Glycolysis

This pathway has also been called the Embden-Meyerhof pathway. G-6-P may be metabolized by enzymes in intracellular water to lactic acid via anaerobic glycolysis, yielding two moles of ATP per mole of glucose glycolyzed; an additional six moles are generated through the oxidation of DPNH. G-6-P is isomerized to fructose-6-phosphate (F-6-P), which is further phosphorylated to form F-1,6-P in the presence of 6-phosphofructokinase. This phosphorylation requires high-energy phosphate (ATP) to form a low-energy ester; the reaction is largely one-way. The reverse reaction requires the conversion of F-1,6-P to F-6-P and inorganic phosphate, catalyzed by 1,6-diphosphatase (very important in gluconeogenesis). F-1,6-P is split in the presence of aldolase, with the upper three carbons forming dihydroxyacetone phosphate and the lower three forming glyceraldehyde-3-phosphate;

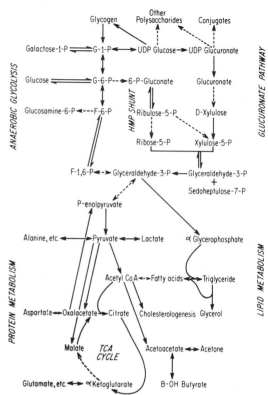

Figure 9–27. Some key aspects of glycogenesis, glycogenolysis, oxidative pathway, glucuronate pathway, anaerobic glycolysis, lipogenesis, lipolysis, ketogenesis, cholesterologenesis, and gluconeogenesis. (See also Fig. 10–3, Ch. 10.)

these two compounds are interconvertible in the presence of triose phosphate isomerase. Glyceraldehyde-3-phosphate, in the presence of phosphoglyceraldehyde dehydrogenase DPN and inorganic phosphate, is converted to 1,3-diphosphoglycerate, which in the presence of ADP forms 3-phosphoglycerate and ATP. The phosphorus is transferred to the 2 position and then phosphoenolpyruvate (PEP) is formed, with the loss of one molecule of water. PEP, with ADP, is converted to pyruvate and ATP. This entire glycolytic pathway can proceed anaerobically (anaerobic glycolysis). The DPNH formed can be converted to DPN by forming lactate from pyruvate, in the presence of lactic dehydrogenase. For each mole of glucose metabolized by glycolysis, two moles of ATP are generated.

Phosphogluconate-Oxidative Pathway

This pathway has also been designated hexose monophosphate, pentose-phosphate, and direct oxidative pathway. In this pathway the G-6-P undergoes dehydrogenation to form 6-phosphogluconolactone, a cyclic ester which is enzymatically hydrolyzed to 6-phosphogluconate. The latter is dehydrogenated and decarboxylated, producing ribulose-5-phosphate. The first two reactions of this pathway lead to the removal of carbon dioxide and four hydrogens, TPN serving as the receptor. Several additional biochemical reactions occur, leading to the formation of fructose-6-phosphate and glyceraldehyde-3-phosphate. The initial oxidative steps are in essence irreversible; however, the other changes in the "shunt" reaction are reversible. Thus, in tissues such as muscle lacking the enzymes necessary for the dehydrogenation of G-6-P, ribose synthesis can occur from fructose-6-phosphate by transketolation and transaldolation. The phosphogluconate-oxidative pathway differs particularly from the glycolytic pathway in that (1) CO_2 is produced, (2) oxygen is consumed, (3) ATP is not required for oxidation of G-6-P, and (4) phosphorylation is not coupled to oxidation. The glycolytic pathway involves DPN, whereas the phosphogluconate-oxidative pathway involves TPN. The TPNH formed is a very important cofactor in lipogenesis as will be discussed subsequently; a deficiency in TPNH contributes to ketoacidosis.

Glucuronic Acid Pathway

After conversion of G-6-P to G-1-P, the latter reacts with uridine-triphosphate (UTP) to form uridine-diphosphoglucose (UDPG) and pyrophosphate. The UDPG then can undergo several changes, including the formation of glycogen, the formation of uridine-diphosphogalactose, and possibly also epimerization and metabolism in other positions to form sugars such as mannose or galactosamine. It may also follow the glucuronic acid pathway associated with oxidation at the sixth carbon of glucose to form uridine-diphosphoglucuronic acid (UDPGA) and DPNH by the diphosphoglucuronic acid pathway. The UDPGA may be used in the synthesis of polysaccharides and mucopolysaccharides, or it may contribute the glucuronic acid utilized in the conjugation of many substances such as bilirubin and steroids. The glucuronate may be transformed further to L-gulonate, 3-ketogulonate, L-xylulose, xylitol, D-xylulose, and D-xylulose 5-phosphate, and it is used in the hexose monophosphate shunt. Winegrad has reported an increase in the quantity of L-xylulose in diabetics. He concluded that increased production, as the result of hyperactivity of the glucuronic acid pathway, was the most likely cause of the increased L-xylulose. Insulin decreased the level of L-xylulose, while growth hormone or epinephrine increases it. There probably are a number of other alterations in the glucuronic acid pathway in diabetes.

Glycogenesis

The UDPG formed in the manner described in the previous section is stimulated by glycogen synthetase to form glycogen. The amount of G-6-P

has been shown to enhance markedly the glycogen synthetase reaction by accelerating condensation of UDPG with preformed glycogen.

The carbohydrate storage form of glucose is chiefly glycogen. This polysaccharide consists of numerous glucose residues linked to each other by glucosidic bonds, rendering a tree-like branching pattern, with a molecular weight as high as 200,000,000. Most glycogenesis presumably proceeds through a route stimulated by glycogen synthetase, rather than by phosphorylase, as follows:

$$\text{UDP-glucose} + (\text{glucose})_n \longrightarrow \text{UDP} + (\text{glucose})_{n+1}$$

Glycogen synthetase stimulates the removal of glucosyl units from uridine-diphosphate glucose (UDPG) for incorporation into glycogen (Fig. 9–28). Steiner found that synthetase activity was stimulated by glucose-6-P, glucosamine-6-P, and fructose-6-P but inhibited by 2-deoxyglucose-6-P. Hepatic synthetase activity was markedly subnormal, unless G-6-P was added. With excess of this cofactor, synthetase activity was hypernormal. Treatment of diabetic rats with insulin resulted in a rapid (within 2 hours) rise in hepatic synthetase activity, coincident with increased glycogen deposition; insulin added *in vitro* was without effect. Injection of prednisolone into fasted normal rats 5 hours before sacrifice resulted in a marked rise in hepatic glycogen and G-6-P but no change in synthetase. Cortisone or glucagon injections in rats for several days caused a slight increase in synthetase. As will be discussed later, phosphorylase is the main enzyme promoting glycogenolysis.

Precursors of G-6-P include not only recently entered glucose but also amino acids that have been transformed into α-ketoacids: oxaloacetic, pyruvic, and α-ketoglutaric acid. The liver has the capacity to transform fructose, galactose, sorbitol, glucose, and other sugars into one another. However, a number of genetic disorders are characterized by enzyme deficiencies which impair the sugar transformations. Galactosemia results from the inability to form UDP-galactose from galactose-1-P. UDPG is the immediate precursor of glucuronides, but there is a deficiency in this reaction in dia-

GLYCOGENESIS and GLYCOGENOLYSIS

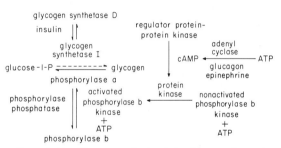

Figure 9–28. Glucagon and epinephrine, by promoting an increase in cAMP, lead to increased glycogenolysis. By decreasing cAMP and increasing glycogen synthetase activity, insulin decreases glycogenolysis and increases glycogenesis.

betes, in certain types of constitutional hepatic dysfunction, and in other disorders. In congenital pentosuria, the enzyme TPN-xylitol dehydrogenase is lacking, so that accumulated L-xylulose is excreted (pentosuria). In the glycogenoses, several enzymes have been found deficient, including a glycogen-debranching enzyme and glucose-6-phosphatase (von Gierke's disease).

Conversion to Glucose by Glucose-6-Phosphatase

This reaction constitutes the major source for nonalimentary glucose. Thus it is particularly important during carbohydrate deprivation in the diet. The liver and the kidney are the only two organs that contain significant amounts of glucose-6-phosphatase, the liver exerting more than 10 times the action of the kidney. A small amount of this enzyme is in intestinal mucosa, the placenta, and the islets of Langerhans, as well as certain other tissues. Whereas the other enzymes reacting with G-6-P are all found in the soluble portion of the cell, glucose-6-phosphatase is found in the microsomes. This enzyme dephosphorylates G-6-P, permitting free glucose to enter the blood. Its activity is inhibited by insulin and stimulated by gluconeogenesis; thus, in diabetes, starvation, and hyperglucosteroidism, there is an increase in its activities.

Pyruvate Metabolism

Aerobically pyruvate may undergo oxidative decarboxylation to acetyl coenzyme A (acetyl CoA), DPNH, and oxaloacetate (Fig. 9–27). Thus pyruvate serves as a precursor to both of the ingredients necessary for the tricarboxylic acid (TCA) cycle (Krebs). Acetyl CoA may proceed in several pathways but particularly in four: (1) oxidation in the tricarboxylic acid cycle, (2) incorporation into long-chain fatty acids, (3) incorporation into cholesterol, and (4) metabolism to acetoacetate and β-hydroxybutyrate. The lipid changes are discussed in a subsequent section.

Tricarboxylic Acid Cycle

More than 90 per cent of the energy of glucose is derived from the further metabolism of pyruvate by the TCA cycle. Acetyl CoA condenses with oxaloacetate to form citric acid, which is then metabolized further in the presence of specific enzymes for the TCA cycle (citric acid cycle). With each revolution of the cycle, one molecule of acetate is incorporated and two molecules of carbon dioxide are given off, while two molecules of DPNH, one molecule of TPNH, and one high-energy phosphate bond are generated. The enzymes for this cycle are in the mitochondria, as are the oxidation-reduction enzymes of the electron transport system: flavoproteins, cytochromes, and cytochrome oxidase. The TCA cycle is a major source of carbon dioxide. Phosphorylation is coupled with oxidation of glucose via the glycolytic and TCA pathways. This high-energy phosphate (ATP), along with the other polyphosphates of nucleotides (uridine triphosphate, cytidine triphosphate, guanosine triphosphate, etc.), creatine phosphate, and others, supplies the immediate energy for most endergonic processes in the body, including such important functions as muscle contraction, nerve conduction, secretory mechanisms, and synthesis of macromolecules. The dependence of both the glycolytic and the TCA cycles upon a supply of inorganic phosphate (Pi) and ADP is important in the suppression of glycolysis by oxygen (Pasteur effect). During anaerobiosis, all of the Pi and ADP is available for the glycolytic steps requiring these reagents, but when oxygen is abundant the competition is established for these two compounds between the substrate-coupled processes in glycolysis and the oxidative processes of the TCA cycle. The purpose of this chemoregulatory system is to conserve glucose. When total oxidation of glucose is possible, a smaller amount of glucose is needed to supply the energy requirements than when anaerobic glycolysis alone is proceeding. Compounds that uncouple oxidative phosphorylation, such as thyroxin, abolish the Pasteur effect, thereby making glycolysis uninfluenced by the presence of oxygen.

Dicarboxylic Acid Cycle

Since the direct conversion of pyruvate to phosphoenolpyruvate is difficult, another route for this conversion exists, at least in certain tissues which synthesize glucose, for example the liver and placenta. This pathway is sometimes designated the dicarboxylic acid shuttle. There may occur either a reductive carboxylation of pyruvate to malate in the presence of TPNH, followed by oxidation to oxaloacetate, or a direct carboxylation to oxaloacetate. The oxaloacetate then is decarboxylated and phosphorylated in the presence of inosine or guanosine triphosphate to form phosphoenolpyruvate. The TCA cycle supplies carbon atoms for various synthetic processes in the cell. In normal animals, the four carbon compounds so used are replaced by resynthesized oxaloacetate, produced by carbon dioxide fixation by phosphoenolpyruvate or via malate from pyruvate (Fig. 9–27). The deficiency of these substrates in diabetes has been stated by some investigators to cause decreased oxaloacetate. Oxaloacetate is needed to combine with acetyl CoA to form citric acid, which is then oxidized in the citric acid cycle, contributing significant energy. Acetyl CoA tends to pile up when there is (1) an increased amount formed from lipolysis, (2) decreased oxaloacetate to conjugate it for citric acid oxidation, and (3) decreased lipogenesis. As acetyl CoA increases, it tends by mass action to promote normal or increased carbon dioxide production by the TCA cycle.

Comments Concerning Energy Supply

The amount of energy produced by the glycolytic pathway is relatively small, but the reactions are quite important. This pathway, as well as the direct oxidative (through the hexosemonophosphate shunt), leads to the development of pyruvic acid, which to some extent may be regarded as a major crossroad for pathways. The TPNH formed through the shunt is very important in fat and cholesterol synthesis. About 90 per cent of the original energy of glucose is derived through the metabolism of the two pyruvate molecules. Most of the energy is provided by the exchange of hydrogen ions; DPN and TPN play a highly important role in this regard. The conversion of acetoacetate to fatty acids by one of the major pathways requires both DPNH and TPNH, while the malonyl pathway requires chiefly TPNH. DPNH seems to be readily available through a number of sources, but TPNH is derived chiefly by two routes: (1) from the oxidative decarboxylation of glucose-6-phosphate, which occurs in the first two steps of the hexose monophosphate shunt, and (2) from the isocitric dehydrogenase reaction in the TCA cycle. The second supplier is possibly not so readily available for reductive synthetic mechanism, since it is generated in the mitochondria, whereas the first reaction takes place in the soluble portion of the cell. TPNH is converted to DPNH in the metabolism of hexosephosphate to pentosephosphate and also by the fixation of carbon dioxide by pyruvate in the dicarboxylic acid shuttle to form malate. This last process generates DPNH from TPNH during the oxidation of malate to oxaloacetate. Several tissues have the capacity to bring about an enzymatic interconversion of DPNH and TPNH. The transhydrogenase involved is affected by a number of hormones. Lipogenesis and gluconeogenesis do not tend to proceed simultaneously in the same tissue to a significant degree. Indeed, the two processes tend to be reciprocal in the liver. TPNH is required for lipogenesis and DPNH for gluconeogenesis.

Lipid Metabolism

In the absence of insulin, there is a tremendous decrease in lipogenesis and increase in lipolysis, with a marked increase in energy derived from fat. A normal adult rat stores only about 3 per cent of ingested glucose as liver and muscle glycogen and 30 per cent as fat. Thus about 90 per cent of the glucose stored is deposited as fat, which, although reconvertible to acetyl CoA, cannot be reconverted to glucose, except from glycerol. Lipogenesis occurs predominantly in adipose tissue and liver. Most of the supply of fatty acids is from adipose tissue, but most of the ketogenesis and gluconeogenesis occurs in the liver.

Fatty Acid Synthesis

With minor exceptions, fatty acids synthesized in the cell derive their carbon from acetyl CoA.

Condensation of two molecules of acetyl CoA forms acetoacetyl CoA, which in turn is reduced by DPNH to yield β-hydroxybutyryl CoA. Dehydration of the latter forms crotonyl CoA and then butyryl CoA, if sufficient TPNH is present. With subsequent repeated condensations with acetyl CoA and reductions by DPNH or TPNH, there is formed the CoA derivative of the β-keto acid with two more carbon atoms, with subsequent reductions to the β-hydroxy acid, dehydration to the unsaturated acid, and then reduction to the saturated fatty acid. After a predetermined chain length has been obtained from the repeated elongations, free CoA is regenerated. The long-chain fatty acid is then esterified with L-α-glycerophosphate, leading to the formation of phosphatidic acids and then triglycerides or phospholipids. In like manner, there may also be esterification of the fatty acid with other alcohols such as cholesterol. The classic pattern for fatty acid synthesis apparently is operative chiefly in the mitochondria. In the cytoplasm, however, the synthesis proceeds with acetyl CoA in the presence of carbon dioxide, forming malonyl CoA, which then condenses with acetyl CoA or acyl CoA to form branched chain α-carboxyl, β-keto fatty acid, and then reduction of the keto group, dehydration and reduction of the double bond, and cleavage to carbon dioxide of the same carboxyl formerly derived from carbon dioxide. Thus the total reaction leads to elongation of the acyl residue by two carbons, without evident carbon dioxide in the end product. It is thought likely that in the catabolism of the fatty acids the classic process is most likely the one involved.

Even in normal individuals, oxidation of fatty acids to carbon dioxide is the major source of energy. About 40 per cent of the calories of the average American diet are derived from fat, and, in addition, a significant quantity of carbohydrate is converted to fat. Untreated diabetics oxidize much more fat than do normal persons. Oxidation of fatty acids requires flavin adenine dinucleotide (FAD) as a cofactor. Oxidation of fat occurs in mitochondria, as do glycolysis and proteolysis, while lipogenesis takes place in the soluble supernatant fraction of the cell and in the mitochondria. The first step in the oxidation of fatty acid consists of its activation by ATP and coenzyme A to form the fatty acid CoA derivative. In each stage of oxidation, one molecule of DPNH and one of FADH are produced, and a molecule of acetyl CoA is split off. The eight molecules of acetyl CoA resulting from palmitate oxidation can enter the TCA cycle for further oxidation to carbon dioxide and water, yielding the equivalent of 96 molecules of ATP. The DPNH and FADH can lead to ATP production through subsequent oxidation.

Cholesterol Synthesis

Every organ in the body, with the possible exception of the adult brain, can synthesize cholesterol, but the liver is the major site. Cholesterologenesis and lipogenesis follow the same path up to the formation of acetoacetyl CoA (Fig. 9–29). In cholesterologenesis, a third acetyl CoA is added, yielding

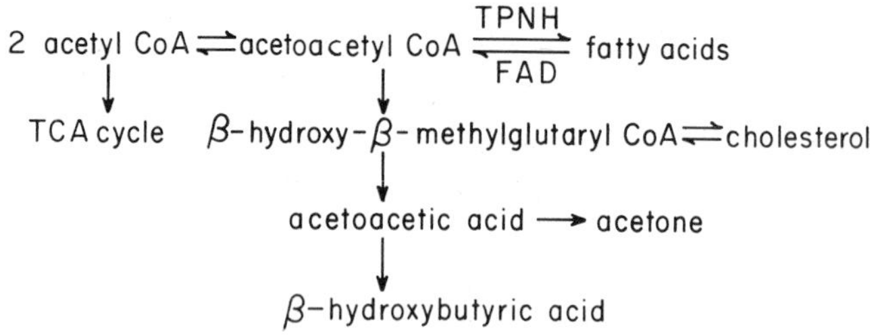

$$2 \text{ acetyl CoA} \rightleftharpoons \text{acetoacetyl CoA} \xrightarrow[\text{FAD}]{\text{TPNH}} \text{fatty acids}$$

TCA cycle β-hydroxy-β-methylglutaryl CoA $\rightleftharpoons$ cholesterol

acetoacetic acid $\longrightarrow$ acetone

β-hydroxybutyric acid

Figure 9–29. Some key steps in lipid metabolism. Note that acetyl CoA is an important constituent for (a) the TCA cycle, (b) lipogenesis, and (c) ketogenesis. TPNH is needed in fatty acid synthesis and flavine adenine dinucleotide in lipolysis. Through hydroxymethylglutaryl CoA are formed cholesterol and ketones. A large proportion of fatty acids are formed from citrate. See Figure 9–27 for more details.

β-hydroxy-β-methylglutaryl CoA (HMG CoA). From this intermediate, both cholesterol and ketone bodies are formed. HMG CoA then loses the CoA and is reduced by TPNH to form mevalonic acid. The mevalonic acid is decarboxylated to form an isopentenyl derivative similar in structure to isoprene. Three isoprenoid units condense to form a 15-carbon compound of which two condense, end-to-end, to form squalene, which folds, condenses, splits off three methyl groups, and then after a single reduction in the side chain forms cholesterol. Diabetes has been reported variously to be associated with both increases and decreases in cholesterologenesis. In severe diabetes a decrease has definitely been found.

Ketogenesis

Circulating ketone bodies are derived almost exclusively from liver, and they increase in the body when their production exceeds their utilization. Most of the oxidation of ketone bodies occurs in extrahepatic tissue. The greater the supply of fatty acids to the liver, the more ketones are formed. The ketone bodies consist of β-hydroxybutyric acid, acetoacetic acid, and acetone. Some of the factors that increase lipolysis and, hence, ketosis, are epinephrine, norepinephrine, GH, ACTH, glucosteroids (in diabetics), thyroxin, starvation, and diabetes.

The following substances decrease lipolysis and are therefore antiketogenic: glucose, protein, and insulin. Lipogenesis is stimulated by insulin, glucose, fat, protein, rest, dehydrocorticosterone, and prolactin. Acetoacetyl CoA and β-hydroxybutyryl CoA may lead to the formation of long-chain fatty acids, cholesterol, or acetoacetate and β-hydroxybutyrate, the two principal ketones. The ketones may result after the synthesis of β-hydroxy-β-methylglutaryl CoA with subsequent liberation of the acetoacetate and with acetoacetyl CoA again engaging in the acetyl CoA pool. The acetoacetyl CoA can also be deacylated, resulting in the formation of acetoacetate. The acetoacetate is carried to all tissues, but before being utilized for oxidation or synthetic reactions it has to be reactivated by CoA in the presence of ATP, or by transfer of CoA from succinyl CoA formed in the TCA cycle. Both of these reactions occur especially in muscle.

A Few Changes in Lipid Metabolism in Diabetes

The factors producing ketoacidosis in diabetes may be recapitulated as follows: decreased glucose uptake causes increased fat oxidation, and decreased lipogenesis results from the inadequate supply of TPNH. A deficiency of pyruvate and phosphoenolpyruvate causes decreased concentrations of oxaloacetate. This decrease tends to inhibit the TCA cycle, but accumulation of excess acetyl CoA stimulates the TCA cycle and also produces excess HMG CoA. Excess ketones and, under certain conditions, excess cholesterol are formed from HMG CoA. With a decrease in glucose utilization, as in starvation or diabetes, an increase in plasma free fatty acid (FFA) is found. Presumably, most of the FFA is derived from triglyceride of adipose tissue. The extent to which the release of FFA is dependent upon increased lipase activity and upon decreased triglyceride synthesis is unknown. When ketones are produced by the liver faster than the entire body can utilize them, ketoacidosis occurs. When glucose utilization is decreased even slightly, there is an excess plasma level of FFA, triglyceride, and other components, which is discussed later.

Protein Metabolism

Proteins serve important functions in body structure, muscle contraction, and enzyme reactions. When the supply of glucose, stored as glycogen, declines significantly, protein is converted to glucose and used as energy.

Insulin deficiency leads to decreased protein synthesis and increased protein catabolism. This defective protein metabolism is associated with impaired growth in young animals and with a negative nitrogen balance. It presumably also contributes to the delayed healing of wounds seen in diabetes. Extracellular proteins and peptides cannot pass through cell membrane. They must first be hydrolyzed to amino acids. There are eight amino acids that must be supplied in the diet because the body cannot synthesize them: isoleucine, leucine, lysine, methionine, phenylalanine, threonine, tryptophan, and valine. The others can by synthesized by the following reactions:

Reductive Amination. α-Ketoglutaric acid, from the TCA cycle (Fig. 9–27), is converted to L-glutamic acid:

$$\text{HOOCCH}_2\text{CH}_2\text{COCOOH} + \text{NH}_3 + \text{DPNH (or}$$
$$\text{TPNH)} + \text{H}^- \rightleftharpoons \text{HOOCCH}_2\text{CH}_2\text{CHNH}_2\text{COOH} +$$
$$\text{DPN (or TPN)} + \text{H}_2\text{O}$$

Transamination. Pyruvic acid, from the glycolytic cycle, can react with L-glutamic acid to yield L-alanine. L-Aspartic acid is synthesized from oxaloacetic acid in this manner.

Peptide Synthesis. Peptide synthesis can be coupled with the liberation of inorganic phosphate from high-energy phosphate compounds, e.g.:

$$\text{Glutamic acid} + NH_3 + ATP \rightleftharpoons$$
$$\text{glutamine} + ADP + \text{phosphate ion}$$

Apparently, every tissue incorporates into its proteins every common L-amino acid, and the incorporation of a single amino acid is largely independent of others present. Inhibitors of respiration and phosphorylation inhibit amino acid and protein synthesis. A few details involved in protein synthesis are presented now; there is additional coverage in other chapters.

There are five important stages in protein synthesis:

1. Amino acids are transported into the cell.

2. They may be formed within the cell by a combination of ammonia and α-ketoglutarate to form glutamic acid which, in turn, can undergo transamination to form any of the nonessential amino acids.

3. Intracellular amino acids are activated by ATP to form amino acid adenylates.

4. These are bound to soluble RNA, forming sRNA–amino acid complexes (there is a separate, specific form of sRNA for each amino acid).

5. sRNA amino acids are transferred into the ribosomes of the microsomes for peptide bonding. The completed protein is then released from the ribosomal particle into the soluble portion of the cell.

Insulin both stimulates the transport of amino acids into the cell and independently catalyzes the incorporation of the amino acids into protein. Both of these actions are independent of insulin's effect on the transport of glucose. This hormone accelerates the incorporation of acetate or pyruvate into protein; this has been demonstrated in both diaphragm and adipose tissue. Oxidative phosphorylation, as a source of energy, is necessary for protein synthesis in the mitochondria. Oxidative phosphorylation is markedly impaired in diabetes. Insulin stimulates the formation of messenger RNA, which, of course, is needed to transmit the polypeptide code from DNA to the ribosomes. Insulin may also influence the synthesis of sRNA and ribosomal RNA. Insulin exerts an especially prominent effect on the formation of the polypeptides which takes place in the microsomes. It also significantly influences the release of the protein, particularly from RNA, a process which requires ATP and probably a special type of releasing enzyme activity.

Insulin influences protein anabolism at two principal cellular sites, mitochondria and microsomes. Its intracellular effects related to protein synthesis consist chiefly of (a) its stimulation of oxidative phosphorylation, which occurs in mitochondria, (b) peptide bonding, which occurs in microsomes, and (c) synthesis of RNA, particularly mRNA. It has been shown to stimulate protein metabolism in the diaphragm, liver, adipose tissue, heart, bone marrow, and other tissues, although most of the studies have been conducted with muscle, liver, and adipose tissue; this will be presented in greater detail in the discussions of those tissues.

The 20 amino acids are metabolized differently. They ultimately converge to some common pathways leading to the TCA cycle. The carbon atoms of amino acids enter this cycle by (a) acetyl CoA→ citrate (alanine, cysteine, glycine, serine, threonine, isoleucine, leucine, tryptophan, phenylalanine, tyrosine, lysine), (b) oxaloacetate (aspartate, asparagine), (c) fumarate (tyrosine, phenylalanine), (d) succinyl CoA (isoleucine, methionine, valine), and (e) glutamate → α-ketoglutarate (arginine, histidine, glutamine and proline).

Certain amino acids can form glucose. The glucogenic amino acids are alanine, aspartic, arginine, citrulline, glutamic, glycine, histidine, norleucine, lysine, serine, threonine, and valine. To be converted to glucose, protein is broken down to amino acids, then to keto acids via oxidation or transamination and then to pyruvate, oxaloacetate, or α-ketoglutarate. After the glycolytic pathway is traversed in reverse order, G-6-P is formed. Glucose is liberated from this only in cells containing glucose-6-phosphatase — chiefly in liver, kidney, and intestinal mucosal cells (Fig. 9–27). With the excess protein degradation, there is an increase of plasma amino acids and nonprotein nitrogen. In diabetes, starvation, and other conditions in which there is an increase in gluconeogenesis, there is a very significant increase in the activity of transaminases, phosphopyruvic carboxykinase, fructose-1,6-diphosphatase, and glucose-6-phosphatase. At the same time, there is a decrease in certain enzymatic activities such as glucokinase and hexokinase.

The effect of growth hormone on nitrogen retention is markedly reduced in diabetes and can be restored with insulin. Insulin appears to have an independent anabolic effect as well. For example, it can promote increased growth and nitrogen retention to a significant degree in hypophysectomized rats. The anabolic effects of testosterone are also much greater in the presence of insulin.

The negative nitrogen balance of diabetes is greatly diminished after adrenalectomy or hypophysectomy. The negative nitrogen balance produced by large doses of corticosteroids is not reversed by insulin.

Glycoproteins

Most of the carbohydrate in animal tissues is conjugated to either proteins (glycoproteins) or lipids (glycolipids). Presumably, the only carbohydrate polymers in animal tissues without this association are glycogen and hyaluronic acid. Glycoproteins are diverse groups of compounds; a number of different carbohydrates may associate with a wide range of protein types. The sugars most commonly involved are D-galactose, D-mannose, D-glucose, L-fucose, D-xylose, N-acetyl-D-glucosamine, N-acetyl-D-galactosamine, and various derivatives of neuraminic acid (sialic acids). The carbohydrate content of glycoprotein varies from about 1–80 per cent of the weight of the molecule, with as few as two or as many as seven sugar types in a given protein. The glycoproteins as a group have the carbohydrate covalently attached to the protein and require some enzymatic mechanism for assembly and degradation.

Collagen is one of the most abundant of the glycoproteins and is a major component of basement membrane. Of course, thickening of the basement membrane of capillaries constitutes one of the major pathologic changes in the microangiopathies of diabetes. Synthesis from glucose of the carbohydrate components of glycoprotein is not under the metabolic regulation of insulin, and since some cells do not require insulin for marked glucose utilization, with hyperglycemia there are increases in sugar nucleotides and glycoproteins in glomeruli and other tissues of diabetics. With experimentally induced insulin deficiency, there is an increase in glucosyl transferase, which is important in the assembly of hydroxylysine-linked carbohydrate units of the basement membrane. This enzyme activity can be decreased to normal with insulin injection in experimental animals.

Response to Insulin by Individual Tissues

Adipose Tissue

The main function of adipose tissue is to serve as a reservoir of energy. It has the highest concentration of calories of any tissue in the body. The average normal-weight man has about 15 kg. of adipose tissue, 90 per cent of which is triglyceride (approximately 120,000 calories). The water content is about 15 μL./100 mg., whereas muscle has five times this level. The concentrations of free fatty acids (FFA), glucose, and single amino acids are relatively low. Adipose tissue does not liberate glucose but releases large quantities of FFA and some amino acids. Insulin is the principal hormone that promotes storage of nutrients in adipose and other tissues. There are numerous hormones that produce catabolic changes. Insulin binds to a specific protein receptor in the plasma membrane of adipose tissue cells, and produces changes in the membrane and probably other parts of the cell that increase the transport of some sugars, some amino acids, K^+, and Mg^{++}. Insulin activates ($Na^+ + K^+$) ATPase. In some manner, insulin presumably promotes the release from the membrane of a compound (not cAMP) into the cytosol that stimulates synthesis of glycogen, fat, protein, and nucleic acids (Fig. 9–30). Insulin increases glucose oxidation. It markedly increases formation of triglyceride by (a) increasing formation of fatty acid in the fat cells, and (b) increasing the uptake of glucose, the immediate precursor of α-glycerol phosphate. α-Glycerol phosphate is conjugated with FFA to form triglyceride. Insulin stimulates increased formation of ATP, DNA, RNA, and mRNA. There is also an increase in the attach-

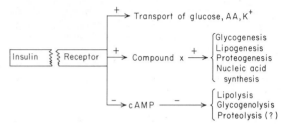

Figure 9–30. Insulin becomes attached to a specific receptor on the plasma membrane. It then initiates changes in the membrane which affect transportation of specific compounds and affects functions of the nucleus, polysomes, and other subcellular components. (+ signifies increase; − signifies decrease.)

ment of monoribosomes to mRNA. The ratio of polyribosomes to monoribosomes is increased. Insulin seems to increase the rate of translation of the message transmitted by RNA. Increased protein synthesis follows increase in uptake of amino acids, and increased transamination of carbohydrate to amino acids.

Insulin decreases glycogenolysis, lipolysis, and proteolysis. As indicated in Table 9–2, there are many compounds that affect lipolysis. Glucosteroids and GH promote induction of lipase. These hormones and thyroid hormones markedly augment the lipolytic effect of catecholamines. Most compounds that increase lipolysis have been demonstrated to increase the level of cAMP, and the reverse applies to those that reduce lipolysis. Presumably, an increase in cAMP causes the regulator protein to release protein kinase (PK), which then stimulates the phosphorylation of lipase, thereby promoting an increase in the rate of hydrolysis of triglyceride to FFA and glycerol.

In summary: lipolytic hormone $\overset{+}{\to}$ cAMP $\overset{+}{\to}$ unbound PK $\overset{+}{\to}$ lipase $\overset{+}{\to}$ triglyceride hydrolysis $\overset{+}{\to}$ FFA and glycerol. Under some conditions, insulin apparently decreases the level of cAMP and decreases activation of protein kinase. Much less insulin is needed to inhibit lipolysis than to affect glucose uptake, glucose oxidation, cAMP level, or blood glucose level.

FFA are liberated from cells when there is insufficient α-glycerolphosphate to produce reesterification. Lipolysis decreases when α-glycerolphosphate or β-hydroxybutyrate increases. Lactate inhibits lipase activity and glycolysis. This may partly

TABLE 9–2. COMPOUNDS THAT AFFECT LIPOLYSIS IN ADIPOSE TISSUE

Increase Lipolysis:	
Catecholamines	Chorionic somatomammotropin
Serotonin	ACTH
Thyroid hormones	MSH, α and β
Glucagon	TSH
Secretin	LH
Glucosteroids	Vasopressin (arginine)
GH	Methyl xanthines
Decrease Lipolysis:	
Insulin	Nicotinic acid
Prostaglandin E	β-adrenergic blockers

account for the decrease in ketoacidosis as lactic acidosis develops. Compounds that promote lipolysis tend to increase the efflux of K^+ from cells and decrease both glucose oxidation and protein synthesis.

Some hormones have actions on fat cells in addition to their lipolytic effects: glucosteroids decrease glucose uptake; soon after administration, GH exerts an insulin-like action, whereas a few hours later it promotes counter-insulin actions. Bornstein has shown that hydrolysis of GH by pituitary polypeptidase yields two polypeptides, one of which has an anti-insulin effect on glucose uptake, glucose oxidation, pyruvate oxidation, fatty acid synthesis, and lipolysis; the other one has insulin-like effects. Growth hormone increases protein synthesis.

Catecholamines stimulate glycogenolysis, lipolysis, glucose uptake, and glucose oxidation. Large adipocytes from obese subjects have been shown to be somewhat insulin-insensitive. Presumably this is due in part to subnormal binding capacity for insulin. Also, the insulin resistance may be due to changes in the biochemical sequence of insulin actions that are subsequent to its binding, possibly involving the transmissions of signals from the insulin receptor, since insensitivity may occur even when glucose transport and oxidative processes are presumably unimpaired (Livingston). Likewise, the diminished response to insulin exhibited by isolated fat cells from rats that have been either starved, treated with prednisone, or made diabetic with streptozotocin is due neither to changes in the quantity of insulin receptor in fat cells nor to the affinity of those receptors for insulin (Bennett).

The Glucose–Fatty Acid Cycle

It has long been recognized that with increased ketogenesis there is some resistance to insulin action. In this connection, many investigators have studied the relationship of fatty acid metabolism to the metabolism of glucose. Randle, in particular, has been a leader in this field and has described what is spoken of as the "glucose–fatty acid cycle." The main principle of this is that there is a reciprocal relationship between the oxidation of fatty acids and the metabolism of glucose by glycolysis and oxidation. With glucose less available for oxidation, as for example during fasting, there is an increased release of fatty acid from the triglycerides of muscle and adipose tissue. The muscle then depends chiefly on the oxidation of the fatty acids for its supply of energy. Conversely, when the supply of carbohydrate is increased, there is a decrease in fatty acid liberation and in its oxidation, and there is an increase in glucose utilization prompted by the increased release of insulin from the pancreas. However, in alloxan-diabetes, the cycle is disturbed in such a way that the oxidation of fatty acids in muscles continues at an accelerated rate for some time after the provision of adequate glucose and insulin. This accelerated rate of fatty acid oxidation in the muscles leads to a decrease in their uptake and oxidation of glucose even in the presence of insulin, thus producing insulin insensitivity or antagonism.

Randle has listed some of the disturbances in glucose metabolism of rat heart and diaphragm that might be attributed to augmented release and oxidation of fatty acids in alloxan-diabetic animals: (1) decreased glucose transport rate at low insulin concentrations, (2) decreased phosphorylation of glucose, (3) decreased phosphorylation of F-6-P, (4) decreased glycolysis, (5) decreased pyruvate oxidation, (6) increased intracellular concentration of FFA, (7) increased intracellular concentration of long-chain fatty acyl CoA, (8) increased liberation of glycerol, (9) increased ratio of acetyl CoA to CoA, and (10) increased citrate concentration. The decrease in glucose transfer may, of course, be due to alteration in the membrane of the cell, or it may be due to certain enzyme changes discussed later. The decreased phosphorylation of glucose by hexokinase could be due among other things to a decrease in available glucose, to a decrease in the hexokinase induction, or to inhibition of the action of hexokinase. The decreased rate of glycolysis is attributable to a decrease in phosphofructokinase activity. The diminished rate of pyruvate oxidation is attributed to a decrease in pyruvate dehydrogenase activity, which in turn can be caused in a number of ways. However, each of these last four abnormalities of glucose metabolism can be induced in normal muscles *in vitro* by the addition of fatty acids to the medium.

Irrespective of the detailed factors involved, the overall oxidation of glucose is decreased by diabetes and by fatty acid and ketone bodies, partly because of impaired uptake of glucose, partly because of decreased glycolysis, and partly because of decreased pyruvate oxidation. A marked increase in FFA and long-chain fatty acyl CoA is readily demonstrable in diabetic muscle. Indeed, this can also be shown in perfused rat hearts, in which the tissues are removed from circulating fatty acids, and consequently the fatty acids within the tissue apparently result from lipolysis. Moreover, there is an increase in the rate of liberation of glycerol from heart and diaphragm of diabetic rats. The liberation of the FFA can be greatly decreased by the decrease in the concentration of lipolytic substances, glucosteroids, growth hormone, catecholamines, and other hormones, as discussed in a subsequent section.

It is interesting that the inhibitory effects both of diabetes and of fatty acids on normal tissue may be corrected by anaerobiosis or by sodium salicylate. With diabetes or with other conditions associated with an increase in fatty acids, there are pronounced decreases in (a) pyruvate dehydrogenase, (b) phosphofructokinase, and (c) hexokinase (Fig. 9–31). With the increase in the ratio of the concentration of acetyl CoA to CoA, pyruvate dehydrogenase is inhibited, and there is thus a decrease in the conversion of pyruvate to acetyl CoA. An increase in this ratio also leads through the citrate synthetase reaction to an increase in the concen-

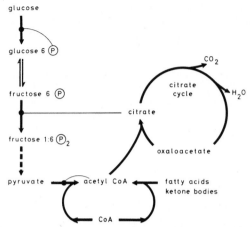

Figure 9-31. Control of glucose metabolism in muscle by fatty acid metabolism. Bold arrows signify an enzyme-catalyzed reaction or reactions. (—• indicates feedback inhibition of a particular enzyme-catalyzed reaction by the metabolite shown.) (From Randle, P. J., In *On the Nature and Treatment of Diabetes.* Leibel, B. S., and Wrenshall, G. A. (eds.), Amsterdam, Excerpta Medica Foundation, 1965, p. 364.)

tration of citrate. This rise, in turn, inhibits phosphofructokinase, and hence glycolysis decreases. With the inhibition of phosphofructokinase, there is a piling up of G-6-P, which in turn is known to inhibit hexokinase. In diabetes there is a significant increase in plasma FFA and in ketones, each of which inhibits glucose uptake and oxidation. After the administration of a glucose load to diabetics, there is a slower than normal fall of plasma FFA despite demonstrable normal or high plasma concentrations of glucose and insulin, which indicates that the FFA are suppressing insulin action. As the FFA return to normal, the effectiveness of insulin in decreasing the blood sugar increases. Randle has suggested that the delay in the hypoglycemic action of insulin may be due to the fact that the hormone has first to correct the accelerated release of fatty acid from glyceride, and that this delay is sometimes longer than is necessary to correct the plasma FFA, because FFA may continue to be released for a while from muscle glycerides.

Study of arteriovenous glucose, FFA, and K^+ differences in the forearms of a group of subjects with maturity-onset diabetes demonstrated that even though the basal glucose uptake was normal and the arterial FFA was in the range of the control values, insulin infusions increased the glucose uptake of both muscle and adipose tissue only half as much as in normal subjects. The insulin-induced effects on potassium uptake and FFA release were slower to appear and about half as great as in normals.

Muscle

After the transport of glucose into the muscle cells, hexokinase catalyzes its phosphorylation. As G-6-P accumulates, it exerts an allosteric effect in its inhibition of hexokinase activity, and, in so doing, it is competing with one of the substrates, ATP. Thus the inhibitory effect depends upon the ratio of G-6-P to ATP. The entry of glucose into the cell is the main limiting step as long as insulin is not present, but when it is present, G-6-P is the main limiting factor, adjusting the rate of glucose phosphorylation to that of overall utilization of the hexose monophosphate pool in resting muscle. Adipose tissue is similar in these regards.

Hexokinase and glycogen synthetase are present in muscle in much smaller quantities than are phosphorylase, phosphofructokinase, and other glycolytic enzymes. Thus, for net synthesis of glycogen, it is necessary to have efficient control of the activity of phosphorylase and phosphofructokinase. The main purpose of the potent glycolytic chain in muscle is to make ATP from ADP-AMP. Both glycolysis and glycogenesis involve a key enzyme which is sensitive to allosteric regulation either by end-product inhibition or by initial substrate activation. In aerobiosis, the regulation of glucose metabolism also involves allosteric regulatory mechanisms. When oxygen is present to reoxidize mitochondrial DPNH, glycolysis produces citrate. Oxidation of citrate, the major ATP-producing pathway, is controlled by the first irreversible step, the DPNH-dependent action of isocitrate dehydrogenase, by the allosteric dependence of this enzyme on ADP as activator. Aerobic accumulation of citrate increases the feedback inhibition of phosphofructokinase. The feedback effects on this enzyme of the two end products of glycolysis, ATP and citrate, apparently are the key mechanisms for exerting the Pasteur effect. Muscle lacks the dehydrogenases involved in the first two oxidative steps of the hexose monophosphate shunt, although it does have other phases of the shunt and probably synthesizes pentoses by means of the transaldolase and transketolase reactions. Lack of these dehydrogenase activities leads to a deficiency in TPNH, and this in turn leads to relatively little lipogenesis. Muscle also seems to lack the dicarboxylic acid shuttle. Since muscle also lacks glucose-6-phosphatase, it cannot liberate sugar into the bloodstream. It can, however, liberate lactate and pyruvate, which can then journey to the liver and be converted to glucose and glycogen. Muscle uses glucose, ketone bodies, and fatty acids for energy. Indeed, under certain conditions, as for example during marked starvation or diabetic acidosis, it can derive essentially all its energy from nonglucose sources. With an increase in ketones and FFA in muscle, there is a decrease in entry of glucose into muscle cells and, in addition, apparently a decrease in glycolysis.

Many of insulin's actions on muscle are similar to those on adipose tissue, but in muscle it causes much more synthesis of protein, nucleotides and glycogen, and much less synthesis of triglyceride. Relatively little energy is stored in the form of triglyceride, and the total amount of energy stored in the form of glycogen is not very great despite the large muscle mass. Insulin increases glycolysis and the oxidation of glucose and pyruvate. Muscle is the main source of alanine, glutamine, pyruvate, and lactate, which in turn are used in gluconeogenesis (discussed later).

Insulin action on muscle is mainly anabolic. Insulin decreases fatty acid oxidation, glycogenolysis, proteolysis, and lipolysis. In muscle cells, as in adipocytes, insulin promotes increased transport through the plasma membrane of certain sugars, some amino acids, K^+, and Mg^{++} (Fig. 9–30). It also apparently causes the release from the plasma membrane of a messenger which catalyzes the synthesis of glycogen, protein, fat, and nucleic acid (Manchester). Insulin increases protein synthesis *in vitro* in the absence of added amino acid or of glucose and stimulates formation of certain amino acids from carbohydrates. It increases the attachment of monoribosomes to mRNA and increases the ratio of polyribosomes to monoribosomes. It increases the total levels of RNA, mRNA, and DNA.

Within about the first half-hour after GH is added to muscle, glucose uptake actually increases, but thereafter it decreases. This hormone also decreases glycolysis but increases protein synthesis. Glucosteroids decrease glucose utilization and hexokinase activity, leading to a net decrease in G-6-P. Glucosteroids promote proteolysis of muscle. Catecholamines decrease glucose utilization but increase glycogenolysis and proteolysis. Catecholamines cause an increase in the formation of cAMP which then releases protein kinase from its regulator protein. Protein kinase catalyzes the formation of activated phosphorylase b kinase (Fig. 9–28), which leads to the formation of activated phosphorylase a, which then catalyzes glycogenolysis. As insulin activity increases sufficiently to suppress cAMP levels, glycogenolysis results, and glycogenolysis declines. Thyroid hormones cause proteolysis and glycogenolysis. Some of these changes are discussed below.

Zierler has studied extensively the influence of insulin on the electrical potential of muscle. There is a difference in electrical potential between extracellular fluid and the inside of muscle fibers. Insulin affects the flux of a number of ions. It leads to a net increase in intracellular K^+ and decrease in Na^+. The effect on K^+ is highly sensitive, requiring only minute amounts of insulin; hyperpolarization of the membrane occurs with increased intracellular K^+ and also with increased permeability to Cl^{2-}. These electrolyte shifts appear very important in determining the amount of polarization produced by insulin. It is suggested that the changes in the membrane potential may play an important role in many of the transport functions of the cell wall.

Liver

The liver plays an important role in the synthesis of glycogen, lipids, and proteins (Table 9–3). The total amount of glycogen in the liver at any one time is far less than in the muscle, and the total synthesis of fatty acids is considerably less

TABLE 9–3. ACTIONS OF INSULIN IN LIVER*

Increase	Decrease
Glucose phosphorylation	Glycogenolysis
Glycogenesis	Lipolysis
Glycolysis	Gluconeogenesis
Pentose phosphate shunt	Proteolysis
Proteogenesis	Fatty acid oxidation
Lipogenesis	Ketogenesis
ATP	Ureogenesis
DNA	Uptake of alanine & other
RNA	glucogenic substrates
Mg^{++}, K^+ uptake	cAMP
	Protein kinase activity

*The extent to which these actions are subsidiary is unknown. The activities of numerous enzymes are altered by insulin, most of them presumably by subsidiary reactions. Some of them involved are:

A. *Increased activity:* glucokinase, glycogen synthetase, glycolytic enzymes (phosphofructokinase and pyruvate kinase), TCA cycle enzymes (pyruvate dehydrogenase, citrate synthetase), lipogenic enzymes, proteogenic enzymes, DNA polymerase, RNA polymerase.

B. *Decreased activity:* glycogen phosphorylase, glucose-6-phosphatase, gluconeogenetic enzymes (pyruvate carboxylase, phosphoenolpyruvate carboxykinase, fructose-1,6-diphosphatase), fatty acid oxidizing enzymes, and ketogenesis enzymes.

than in the adipose tissue, but the synthesis of protein is relatively large. Liver can also readily degrade glycogen, lipids, and proteins and provide energy in the form of glucose, ketones, and other substances. All of these reactions are significantly influenced by insulin, directly or indirectly, and are now considered in some detail.

Unlike muscle and adipose tissue, where a specific transport system is involved, catalyzed by insulin, liver cells are freely permeable to glucose. Within them the initial reaction is phosphorylation, with the formation of G-6-P, which is catalyzed by hexokinase and a unique enzyme, glucokinase. The key ways in which glucokinase differs from hexokinase are as follows (Sols):

1. Its K_m for glucose is 100 times greater.

2. There is no allosteric inhibition by G-6-P (there is with hexokinase).

3. Phosphorylation of fructose and glucosamine is poor (good with hexokinase).

4. There is strong competitive inhibition by *N*-acetylglucosamine.

5. There is only slight stability *in vitro*.

6. The content in starved animals is markedly decreased (hexokinase is normal).

7. It is absent in diabetic animals (hexokinase is normal).

Both of these enzymes, however, are soluble, require ATP-Mg as phosphoryl donors, yield 6-phosphate as the primary product, and are moderately sensitive to inhibition by ADP-Mg. There is evidence that glucokinase is an inducible enzyme, with insulin rather than glucose serving as the inducer. Insulin exerts long-term control of the amount of enzyme present, but short-term regulation is based on the sensitivity of the enzyme to changes in glucose concentrations within the physiologic range.

The amount of glucokinase is greatly decreased

in diabetics and during starvation. It increases within a few hours after the administration of insulin. However, its reappearance is blocked by inhibitors of protein synthesis or of RNA synthesis. Two other enzymes involved in glycolysis that are very much stimulated by insulin are phosphofructokinase and pyruvate kinase, as discussed in more detail later. Insulin exerts a marked stimulating effect on glycogen synthetase, which is a key enzyme in the synthesis of glycogen. Insulin increases the activities of glucose-6-phosphate dehydrogenase and 6-phosphogluconate dehydrogenase. With increased activities in the hexose monophosphate shunt, TPNH is produced which is utilized in lipid synthesis.

Synthesis of fatty acids in the liver in diabetes may be reduced by more than 90 per cent. Once pyruvate is formed, it may be oxidatively decarboxylated to form acetyl CoA and DPNH. There are many pathways leading from the acetyl CoA, but four of the major ones are: oxidation in the tricarboxylic acid cycle, incorporation into long-chain fatty acid, incorporation into cholesterol, and metabolism to acetoacetate and β-hydroxybutyrate. With a decrease in the supply of glucose to various tissues of the body or a decrease in its utilization or both, a number of tissues are called upon to release certain compounds that can serve for energy. The processes involved are chiefly lipolysis, glycogenolysis, and proteolysis. Several hormones stimulate these degrading reactions. Since the brain uses chiefly glucose for energy, it requires emergency supplies. These are available in the form of glycogen, which can be rapidly cleaved to liberate glucose.

Glycogenolysis in the liver is stimulated by catecholamines and by glucagon (Fig. 9–28). These hormones stimulate the adenyl cyclase system to form cAMP, which with protein kinase leads to the formation of active phosphorylase from inactive phosphorylase. Consequently, G-1-P is formed and then G-6-P, which in the presence of glucose phosphatase is dephosphorylated, and free glucose enters the bloodstream. Normally, as the blood sugar level rises above approximately 120 mg./100 ml., release of glucose from the liver is markedly inhibited, and the glucose uptake by the liver increases. These changes are catalyzed by insulin. In diabetes, however, the blood sugar level may be as high as 900 mg./100 ml. without a decrease in hepatic glucose output (Madison). As the blood sugar level progresses below 120 mg./100 ml., there is correspondingly less output and intake of glucose by the liver. As the blood sugar attains progressively lower levels, or with decreased insulin effect, increasing amounts of lipolysis and gluconeogenesis are stimulated. These processes are stimulated particularly by diabetes, starvation, and increases of GH, glucosteroids, epinephrine, glucagon, and other lipolytic hormones.

As the FFA supply builds up, the conversion of acetyl CoA to long-chain fatty acids is inhibited. The liver uses considerable energy from the oxidation of fatty acids, leading to the formation of ketones. The accumulation of acetyl CoA inhibits pyruvate dehydrogenase, thereby reducing the quantity of pyruvate which is converted to acetyl CoA. There is also a marked inhibition of the citric acid cycle as well as of glycolysis. There also tends to be relatively less phosphofructokinase in the liver than in muscle and brain, where glycolysis is prominent; this favors greater utilization of G-6-P in other pathways in the liver. In diabetes, there is a decrease in lactic dehydrogenase and malate dehydrogenase activities. Direct carboxylation of pyruvate to oxaloacetate is markedly stimulated by the increased quantity of acetyl CoA, consequently greatly increasing the amount of gluconeogenesis.

In the absence of glucosteroids, relatively little gluconeogenesis occurs, even after the administration of glucagon (Exton). Endogenous glucose is formed from amino acids, glycerol, lactate, pyruvate, and a few other such compounds. After lactate enters the cell, it is converted to pyruvate, which enters the mitochondrion, where it, and also ketoglutarate, is carboxylated to oxaloacetate. Oxaloacetate cannot leave the mitochondrion as such (Fig. 9–32) but is converted to malate, fumarate, and aspartate, which pass into the cytoplasm and are then reconverted to oxaloacetate (Exton), which is then decarboxylated and phosphorylated to phosphoenolpyruvate. Phosphoenolpyruvate generates glucose by reversal of the Embden-Meyerhof pathway, except that two energetically unfavorable kinase activities are bypassed through two special enzymes, fructose diphosphatase and glucose-6-phosphatase. Fructose on entering the liver is phosphorylated and split into 3-carbon compounds which enter the gluconeogenetic pathway at several points. Fructose promotes gluconeogenesis faster than lactate, suggesting that steps prior to the formation of 2-phosphoglycerate must limit gluconeogenesis from lactate. With the accumulation of G-6-P, G-6-phosphatase is stimulated and glucose is released into the bloodstream. Glucagon has essentially no effect on gluconeogenesis from fructose, but it stimulates that from pyruvate, suggesting that the glucagon-sensitive step lies prior to the formation of the 3-carbon in-

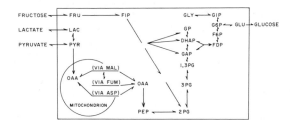

Figure 9–32. Pathways of gluconeogenesis from lactate and fructose in the liver cell. The rectangle represents the plasma membrane of the cell, and the circle represents a mitochondrion. Abbreviations: OAA (oxaloacetate), MAL (malate), FUM (fumarate), ASP (aspartate), PEP (phosphoenolpyruvate), F1P (fructose-1-phosphate), PG (phosphoglycerate), GAP (glyceraldehyde-3-phosphate), DHAP (dihydroxyacetone phosphate), GP (α-glycerophosphate), GLY (glycerol), FDP (fructose diphosphate), F6P (fructose-6-phosphate), G6P (glucose-6-phosphate), G1P (glucose-1-phosphate). (From Exton, J. H., et al.: *Amer. J. Med.* 40:709, 1966 [slightly modified].)

termediates. There is evidence that the principal site of action of epinephrine and glucagon in gluconeogenesis resides between pyruvate and phosphoenolpyruvate and that their action is mediated by means of cAMP.

Insulin antagonizes the action of cAMP-stimulated glycogenolysis, gluconeogenesis, potassium loss, and phosphoenolypyruvate carboxykinase activity. However, a number of the effects insulin has on the liver are apparently not activated through its influence on cAMP concentration. A substantial quantity of cAMP is compartmentalized and is physiologically inactive. Insulin presumably does not affect this but tends to decrease the "free cAMP," which seems to be important in the minute-to-minute output of glucose, K^+ fluxes, and other processes in liver (Park). Insulin depresses the activity of adenyl cyclase stimulated by glucagon or epinephrine (Illiano).

The glucagon receptor in liver cells differs from the catecholamine receptor. Indeed, catecholamines have two receptors: (a) the beta type which activates adenyl cyclase, and (b) the alpha type which seems to lower cAMP levels. The amount of insulin required for affecting the cAMP-mediated processes in the liver is apparently higher than the amount needed to decrease hepatic release of glucose or to decrease hepatic uptake of amino acids. However, the liver is exposed to much higher concentrations of insulin than are the other tissues, since the hormone leaving the pancreas must first go through it, and more than half of the insulin in the plasma is removed with each passage.

Steiner has reviewed much of his work and others' relative to the action of insulin in the liver. He used particularly rats with alloxan-diabetes for studying sequential changes after the administration of insulin. The earliest enzymatic change that apparently has been observed so far is an increase in glycogen synthetase, which is noted within 40 min. after insulin administration and long before there is an increase in G-6-P. No increase is found generally in the enzymes involved in lipogenesis until approximately 24 hours have elapsed. During the first 12 hours, the liver more than doubles in wet weight; much of this increase is due to increased glycogen and water. There is a significant increase in DNA polymerase within 24 hours and in DNA specific activity between 24 and 36 hours. There is no measurable increase in DNA until approximately 36 hours after the initiation of insulin therapy, but within 72 hours the total amount has almost doubled. By this time there is massive proliferation of the liver cells and the appearance of many mitotic figures. Within 30–60 min. after insulin therapy has been initiated, there is an increase in the specific activity of liver RNA, most of it being in the nuclear fraction. Insulin presumably does not increase the transfer of RNA to cytoplasm. There is a notable increase in the RNA polymerase in 2 hours and almost a doubling within 12 hours. There is an increase in the total RNA in the liver, the peak level being obtained at about 36 hours. Increases in rRNA and tRNA follow the increase in mRNA.

With untreated diabetes, there is a marked decrease in protein synthesis. This apparently results from a decreased ability of the ribosomes to incorporate amino acids into protein rather than a lack of the soluble factor. During the early action of insulin on liver, there is an increase in glycogen and RNA synthesis before there is a detectable increase in the total protein. The inhibitory effect of actinomycin on insulin-stimulated glycogen and protein synthesis suggests that mRNA is involved.

FFA are taken up by the liver in proportion to their plasma concentration. They are then metabolized completely to CO_2, or partially to ketone bodies, or esterified with glycerol phosphate to form triglyceride (TG). The newly synthesized TG is largely secreted into the plasma as very-low-density lipoprotein. The balance between oxidation and ketogenesis and TG synthesis appears to be regulated by insulin.

The amount of fatty acid synthesized by the liver is small compared with that taken up from the plasma (Woodside). Insulin increases fatty acid synthesis, partly because of its stimulation of fatty acid synthetase (Laksmanan).

In the intact animal, increasing the delivery of FFA and amino acids to the liver may result in a decrease rather than an increase in hepatic glucose output (Madison). This decrease results from the augmented secretion of endogenous insulin that is stimulated by the elevated levels of FFA and amino acids. However, with diabetic ketoacidosis, the increased plasma levels of FFA to the liver accelerate hepatic gluconeogenesis because of the lack of available insulin.

In stress associated with anoxia and lactic acidosis, gluconeogenesis plays an important role in limiting the amount of lactic acidosis by converting the lactate to glucose. Lactate formed by glycolysis in blood cells, brain, and other tissues also contributes to glucose recycling, which may represent as much as 30 per cent of the glucose turnover in normal man (Exton).

Action of Insulin on Other Cell Types

Insulin produces *in vitro* certain biochemical changes in fibroblasts, smooth muscle cells, lymphocytes, thymocytes, and many other cell types (Table 9–1). Directly or indirectly, insulin affects the chemical composition of all cells and body fluids. It influences the amounts and types of various components of protein, lipid, carbohydrates, and nucleotides, and amounts of water and electrolytes.

Role of Insulin and Other Factors in the Integration of Nutrient Metabolism

As indicated earlier, the major nutrients ingested are carbohydrate, fat, and protein. Within two or three hours after a meal, most of the energy supplied to the body is from glucose delivered to the bloodstream by the GI mucosa. Glucose is taken up by cells of various parts of the body, with muscle, liver, and adipose tissue acquiring most of what leaves the circulation (see recent reviews by Cahill, Felig, Ensinck, Exton, and Levine). In muscle and liver, the glucose not used at the time is converted to glycogen and stored as such. In adipose tissue, the major portion is converted to triglyceride and the energy is stored in this form. The brain takes chiefly glucose from the plasma for its supply of energy (with ketoacidosis it can use a significant quantity of acetoacetate and hydroxybutyrate). After an overnight fast, the approximate amount of glucose used in a day by a normal adult man is 150 g. by the brain, 50 g. by blood cells, and 50 g. by muscles and other tissues (Felig); small amounts are also used by the peripheral nerves and adrenal medullas. The plasma level of glucose is carefully controlled within a relatively narrow range (approximately 60–100 mg./100 ml.). It is important that there be the most appropriate type and amount of metabolism of carbohydrate, fat, and protein for different body needs. There are many factors concerned with this metabolic regulation, including especially certain hormonal activities and the autonomic nervous system. Insulin is the main hormone concerned with the storage of nutrients. Glucagon, catecholamines, gluco-

steroids, and GH are the principal hormones that break down the macromolecular energy stores for more appropriate transport and use for energy. Some metabolic regulations that occur with feeding, fasting, and diabetes are now presented.

One Hour After Glucose Ingestion

Immediately after glucose ingestion, the plasma insulin level is significantly increased, whereas the levels of glucagon and GH decrease; presumably, catecholamines also decrease. The increase in insulin causes an increase in the uptake, oxidation, and conversion of glucose to its storage forms — glycogen in muscle and liver, and TG in adipose tissue. There is a decrease in the release of FFA from adipose tissue, of glucose from liver, and of lactate and pyruvate from blood cells and muscle. Other changes are shown in Table 9-4.

Only a relatively small amount of insulin is usually required to decrease hepatic glucose release, lipolysis, and release of amino acids from muscle, but a much larger quantity is needed to stimulate glucose uptake by adipose tissue, muscle, and other tissues and to increase amino acid uptake by muscle. Therefore, much more insulin is

TABLE 9-4. CHANGES IN HORMONE AND NUTRIENT LEVELS WITH FASTING OR DIABETES*

Nutrients	Adipose Tissue In	Adipose Tissue Out	Muscle In	Muscle Out	Liver In	Liver Out	Plasma	Hormone Secretion
One Hour After Glucose								
Glucose	++	0	++	0	++	--	+++	Insulin +++
Alanine	+	-	+	+	-	0	++	Glucagon -
FFA	++	--	+	-	--	-	--	Catecholamines -
Ketones	-	0	-	0	-	--	-	Glucosteroids ±
								GH --
After Overnight Fast								
Glucose	--	0	--	0	--	+	-	Insulin -
Alanine	±	±	-	+	++	0	-	Glucagon +
FFA	-	++	++	+	++	+	+	Catecholamines +
Ketones	+	0	+	0	+	+	+	Glucosteroids ±
								GH +
After One-Week Fast								
Glucose	---	0	---	0	---	++	-	Insulin --
Alanine	-	±	--	--	+++	0	--	Glucagon ++
FFA	--	+++	+++	+	+++	+	+++	Catecholamines +
Ketones	++	0	+++	0	++	++	+++	Glucosteroids ±
								GH ±
Diabetic Ketoacidosis								
Glucose	---	0	---	0	---	+++	+++	Insulin ---
Alanine	-	+	--	+	+++	0	---	Glucagon +++
FFA	---	+++	+++	++	+++	+	+++	Catecholamines ++
Ketones	+++	0	++	0	++	+++	+++	Glucosteroids ++
								GH ++

*The reference standard for the values is about 4 hours after a normal meal. Plus marks indicate the relative amount of increase in levels, and minus signs signify decline. Total net changes are signified. Many factors influence the levels of these parameters, in some instances even changing an increase to a decrease in level. (Many of the evaluations are based upon studies by Felig and Cahill. This table and Table 9-5 were kindly reviewed by Dr. Felig.)

required to promote storage of nutrients than to prevent catabolism and tissue release of nutrients.

Overnight Fast

Within a few hours after completion of the evening meal, the supply of glucose tends to be significantly decreased, including what has been converted to glycogen. This necessitates an increase in supply of FFA from adipose tissue and of glucose precursors (predominantly from muscle). There is a significant decrease in the plasma level of insulin but increases in glucagon and GH; catecholamines presumably increase (Table 9-4). The lipolytic hormones cause increased lipolysis in several tissues, but adipose tissue is distinctly the most important one. As much as 85 per cent of body energy may be derived from this mechanism, with most of the remainder supplied by amino acids from muscle and by lactate and pyruvate from blood cells and muscle. A small amount of energy is derived from glycogenolysis from the liver.

Since the brain demands chiefly glucose and the supply derived from the intestinal tract has either been used or converted to other constituents, the liver has the main responsibility overnight for manufacturing glucose from glucogenic amino acids, glycerol, lactate, and pyruvate, using considerable amounts of energy from carnitine-mediated oxidation of FFA. During these periods of conservation of glucose, skeletal muscle, heart, renal cortices, and a number of other tissues utilize chiefly FFA and ketones (acetoacetate and β-hydroxybutyrate) for energy. Muscle and liver use most of the FFA liberated from adipose tissue. With progressive decrease in glucose utilization by the fat cells, there is a concomitant decrease in formation of glycerol phosphate and an increase in the liberation of FFA. The amount of glycerol phosphate formed is dependent on the supply of glucose. As discussed earlier, FFA and ketone bodies depress glucose uptake and oxidation in muscle. Accumulation of FFA in the fat cells also inhibits pyruvate oxidation, glycolysis, and glucose transport. These changes apparently result chiefly from the accumulation of acetyl CoA. With accumulation in the cells of phosphorylated intermediates, there is a decrease in hexokinase activity and consequently a decrease in glucose utilization. Further consequences of the increase in FFA are described in an earlier section, Glucose–Fatty Acid Cycle.

Protein cannot freely pass in or out of cells without being degraded to individual amino acids. There is a significant difference in the role of the different amino acids. They vary in their effect on hormone secretion and action and vice versa. For example, some amino acids exert little or no influence upon the release of insulin, glucagon, or growth hormone, but others have major actions (Fajans). Insulin does not affect the amount of transport of some of the amino acids through the cell wall but has a marked effect on others (Manchester). Insulin also exerts a much greater effect on the release of certain amino acids than on that of others. It is especially effective in decreasing the release from muscle of branched-chain amino acids (leucine, isoleucine, valine), tyrosine, phenylalanine, and threonine, but it does not decrease the release of alanine, glutamine, or some other amino acids. Insulin decreases significantly the liver uptake of alanine, glutamine, lactate, pyruvate, and glycine.

With fasting, there is a pronounced difference in the release of various amino acids from muscle. Alanine and glutamine are released in far greater quantities than any of the others (Felig, Ruderman). Moreover, the liver extracts much more of these amino acids than others. Much of the alanine that muscle releases is not derived from protein but is synthesized by transamination of pyruvate. The rate of alanine formation is determined to a considerable extent by the rate of peripheral glucose utilization and pyruvate formation. The pyruvate is derived through glycogenolysis and glycolysis (discussed further in the next section). Glycogenolysis in muscle is stimulated especially by catecholamine activity. The amount of this activity depends not only upon the catecholamine level but also on the quantity of glycogen stores and on the plasma levels of insulin and glucose. The glucose-alanine cycle becomes prominent during fasting. The recycling of glucose carbon skeletons through the glucose-alanine cycle can occur at approximately 50 per cent the rate of the Cori cycle (muscle glycogen⟶lactate⟶liver glycogen⟶ blood glucose ⟶ muscle glycogen). In muscle, the glucose is changed to pyruvate and then to alanine, which then is transported to the liver where it is deaminated and converted to glucose. The glucose then returns to muscle and is again submitted to glycolysis. Pyruvate is formed and may again be converted to alanine. After the plasma glucose and insulin levels rise sufficiently, there is decreased glycogenolysis, lipolysis, and proteolysis; storage of carbohydrate, fat, and protein proceed.

One-Week Fast

Changes in plasma hormone levels during one week of fasting include decreased insulin and increased glucagon, glucosteroids, and catecholamines; most of these changes occur with one day of fasting. GH levels are essentially normal. The body makes a greater effort than after the overnight fast to conserve glucose for those tissues that require it. With progression of fasting, there is an increasing utilization of fatty acids and ketones for energy by muscle, heart, liver, and many other tissues (Table 9-4). With fasting, a marked increase in the release of amino acids from muscle occurs (Felig, Ruderman). Glutamine and alanine constitute about 50 per cent of the amino acids released into plasma, although their concentration in muscle is far less than this. In diabetics, there is an even greater release of amino acids, principally glutamine and alanine. Alanine and glutamine not only are present in the blood in highest concentra-

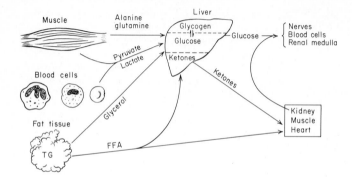

Figure 9–33. During fasting, adipose tissue is the major supplier of energy. Much of its liberated FFA is used directly by heart muscle and other tissues, but some of it is first converted (by liver) to ketones. The brain derives most of its energy from glucose, formed chiefly from liver and kidney, with the dominant precursors consisting of alanine, glutamine, pyruvate, and lactate—supplied chiefly by skeletal muscle.

tion during fasting and with diabetes, but also are proportionately used the most for glucose synthesis by the liver (Fig. 9–33). Some alanine and glutamine are derived by proteolysis, but the largest proportion results from their synthesis in muscle. Synthesis of alanine is catalyzed by glutamate-pyruvate aminotransferase, and that of glutamine by glutamine synthetase. The α-amino nitrogen for alanine and glutamine is derived chiefly from branched-chain amino acids (leucine, isoleucine, valine), which are deaminated and oxidized in muscle. Some contribution is also made by lysine and histidine, which are deaminated in muscle and then oxidized in liver. The carbon skeleton for alanine synthesis is derived from pyruvate. The carbon chain for glutamine is probably glutamate and aspartate, derived from proteolysis. The amount of glutamine synthesized depends upon the amount of α-ketoglutarate formed.

After 48 hours of fasting, liver and muscle glycogen supplies are largely depleted, and amino acids constitute the prime precursors for glucose formation. At this stage, however, most of the amino acids must come from protein that is serving an important role in cell structure, enzyme activities, and other areas. No longer can a significant amount of alanine be derived from pyruvate, because much less of it is formed. After prolonged starvation, gluconeogenesis decreases and the plasma alanine level is less than after an overnight fast. That this is a limiting factor in the amount of glucose produced by the liver is indicated by the observation that infusion of alanine promptly increases the blood glucose level (Felig). During prolonged starvation, gluconeogenesis increases in kidney and decreases in liver; eventually the amount of gluconeogenesis in the two organs may become about equal (Exton). With ketoacidosis, ammonia is very much needed to neutralize acids in the urine, and the ammonia is extracted from glutamine; the liver not only rejects glutamine released from muscle but also may even produce some glutamine to provide the kidney with an appropriate amount of substrate for ammonia synthesis. However, alanine continues to be used by the liver in large amounts for gluconeogenesis, but in time its decreased levels in blood prevent this; eventually hypoglycemia may occur. At the same time, glutamine continues to serve a

glucogenic role, with the kidney supplying most of the gluconeogenic action on it during the acidotic state. Thus glutamine serves a dual purpose, supplying ammonia for neutralization of the acid and glucose for the benefit of the brain and other tissues.

Diabetic Ketoacidosis

Many hormonal and nutrient changes that occur during the one-week fast are observed in diabetic ketoacidosis but are more marked. With severe diabetes, there is a marked decrease in insulin but an increase in glucagon, catecholamines, glucosteroids, and growth hormone. Glycogenesis, lipogenesis, and proteogenesis are decreased, and glycogenolysis, lipolysis, and proteolysis are increased (Table 9–4). Some of the effects of diabetes on nutrient changes may be summarized as follows: diabetes $\overset{+}{\to}$ lipolysis $\to$ FFA $\overset{+}{\to}$ acetyl CoA $\overset{+}{\to}$ citrate $\to$ phosphofructokinase $\overset{-}{\to}$ F-6-P and G-6-P $\to$ hexokinase activity $\to$ glucose utilization. Diabetes $\overset{+}{\to}$ release from muscle of pyruvate, lactate, amino acids $\overset{+}{\to}$ plasma levels of glucogenic substrate $\overset{+}{\to}$ their uptake by liver $\overset{+}{\to}$ gluconeogenesis $\overset{+}{\to}$ plasma glucose; insulin reverses these changes. There is a manifold increase in plasma levels of valine, leucine, isoleucine, and α-aminobutyrate—the amino acids whose peripheral release is inhibited by insulin. Moreover, leucine and isoleucine are ketogenic and therefore contribute to hepatic ketogenesis. However, there is a decrease in plasma alanine, glycine, threonine, and serine. Thus augmentation of gluconeogenesis occurs with insulin lack, yet there is a decrease in circulating glucogenic substrates. These observations suggest stimulation of hepatic uptake of glucose precursors in the absence of adequate insulin. The amount of alanine extracted by the livers of diabetics may be more than twice that extracted by nondiabetics.

In normals, with feeding there is an increase in the rate of conversion of glucose to pyruvate (glycolysis), whereas with diabetes, fasting, exercise, protein feeding, or various stresses, there is a reversal of substrate flow, with pyruvate going to glucose (gluconeogenesis). When there is excess glucosteroid, there is a tendency for decreased ketone production.

Correlations of Amount of Insulin Activity with Insulin Structure

The amount of insulin activity, determined by bioassay, varies considerably with the conditions of the assay procedure and is discussed in detail in subsequent sections. The assays are usually conducted *in vitro* but sometimes *in vivo*. *In vitro*, most of the assays are performed with isolated adipose tissue cells or with rat diaphragm. There are distinct differences in the results, depending upon the following conditions: constituency of the incubation medium, including the amount and types of ions, proteins, carbohydrates, other hormones, amount of oxygen supply, temperature, pH, incubation interval, parameter tested, and duration of incubation. *In vivo*, assays are usually tested by measuring the amount of blood sugar–lowering activity or the amount of glucose oxidation.

No definite part of the insulin molecule can be designated as the active center. Addition of one arginine residue to Ala-30 (B chain) decreases biologic activity about 30 per cent. A strong effect on the properties of insulin is exerted by spatial fixation of the N-terminals (Brandenburg). An important structural component of insulin for biologic activity is the spatial relationship of the three disulfide bridges (Carpenter). Split of the A7-B7 disulfide bond does not decrease biologic activity very much. Cleavage of both disulfide bridges between the chains causes total loss of insulin activity; oxidation or reduction of the disulfide groups inactivates insulin. Some investigators have thought that insulin becomes bound to tissue via sulfur linkages; however, insulin can bind to adipose tissue and diaphragm *in vitro*, despite the blockage of sulfhydryl groups, but sulfhydryl-blocking agents inhibit insulin action.

The amount of insulin activity depends not only upon the specific types and placing of the individual amino acids but also on the configuration of the insulin molecule (Chance, Hodgkin). A free NH_2-terminal glycine on the A chain is needed for full biologic activity. Very little demonstrable insulin activity is found when there is removal of glycine, removal of C-terminal octapeptide from the B chain, or reduction or photo-oxidation of histidine, or when insulin is split into two chains.

The amount of insulin activity is distinctly subnormal when there is (a) removal of the carboxyl-terminal asparagine or aspartic acid from the A chain, (b) removal of part of the heptapeptide sequence of the B chain of bovine insulin, (c) insulin in dimer form, (d) splitting of A7-B7 disulfide bond, (e) addition of one arginine or other components, or (f) addition of more than one iodine atom per insulin molecule.

There is little, if any, decrease in insulin activity produced by (a) removal of the carboxyl-terminal alanine of B chain of bovine insulin, or the amide group on the carboxyl-terminal asparagine of A

chain, (b) removal of the Phe residue from the B chain, or (c) removal of B30 alanine (porcine).

As stated earlier, the amount of biologic activity of proinsulin is about 10 per cent that of insulin, depending upon the assay method used. With the mouse convulsion assay procedure, Chance found that an equimolar amount of proinsulin had 18 per cent of the action of insulin; proinsulin with Leu_{54} - Ala_{55} bond split, 20 per cent; desdipeptide proinsulin (Lys_{62}-Arg_{63} absent), 58 per cent; diarginine insulin (Arg_{31}-Arg_{32} attached to Ala_{30}), 62 per cent; monoarginine insulin (Arg_{31} attached to Ala_{30}), 66 per cent. Thus the mere persistence of attachment of one or more amino acids to the end of insulin can very significantly decrease its biologic activity.

Factors of Noninsulin Origin with Insulin-like Activities

There are a number of factors that can simulate one or more actions of insulin, including GH, anoxia, chymotrypsin, and a protein in plasma with insulin-like activities (ILA). Unlike insulin, the actions of this protein are not influenced by the addition of insulin antibodies (Poffenbarger). Thus this substance has been designated as nonsuppressible ILA or NSILA. This factor has also been called "atypical" insulin and is possibly the same as "protein-bound insulin" and "complex insulin." It is possible that each of these plasma factors, as well as others discussed below, is derived from a product from GH or from a compound produced directly or indirectly from it. It is conceivable that various chemical manifestations of plasma account for varying results of investigators.

Serum ILA was found to be decreased when the serum was first passed through a cation exchange resin. The ILA bound to the resin could be eluted and exerted an insulin-like response on rat fat pads but showed no activity with rat diaphragm. What became bound to the resin was designated "bound insulin," and the part that passed through the resin readily was designated "free insulin." The bound insulin was considered to be converted to the free insulin by purified adipose tissue extract. "Atypical insulin" was that part of ILA which could not be measured by rat diaphragm or immunoassay but could be demonstrated by fat pad bioassay in serum depleted of "typical insulin" by treatment with excess antibody.

NSILA was shown to have many insulin-like actions on adipose tissue and skeletal muscle. It lowers blood sugar but is much more active *in vitro* than *in vivo*. NSILA does not disappear from the plasma after pancreatectomy but partly disappears after hypophysectomy. Under some circumstances, as much as 90 per cent of ILA in serum is NSILA. It is extractable by acid-ethanol, electrophoresis, and column chromatography. It is destroyed by alkali, reduced glutathione, performic acid, oxidation, and sulfitolysis. Its physical-chemical characteristics differ depending upon methods for extraction and isolation. Its molecular weight was reported to be 45,000 (Poffenbarger), but in human serum NSILA has been found to consist of two components (Humbel). Most of the biologic activity measured by adipose tissue assay in native serum was exerted by a fraction with a molecular weight over 100,000, which was precipitated by acid-ethanol and was not retained on Dowex resin. A smaller fraction (NSILA-S), corresponding to about 5–15 per cent of the total NSILA, had a molecular weight of 6000–10,000. This material was soluble in acid-ethanol and had physical-chemical characteristics of what had been attributed to "bound insulin." These two molecular weight compounds are not interconvertible (Humbel). NSILA has been found in most tissues of the body. Under certain circumstances, it decreases the action of insulin.

There are now considerable data to indicate that NSILA-S is somatomedin. Somatomedin has long been called the "sulfation factor" (Hintz, Hall), and is formed through interaction of GH and the liver (Hall). Among its insulin-like effects are (a) incorporation of amino acids into rat diaphragm, (b) glucose oxidation by fat pads, (c) antilipolytic action in epinephrine-stimulated epididymal fat pads, and (d) stimulation of protein synthesis in cell replication. Somatomedin has a molecular weight of about 7000. Sulfation factor and thymidine factor activities cannot be dissociated after purification of somatomedin to about 25,000-fold (Hintz). Somatomedin, at physiologic concentrations, competes with I^{125}-insulin for receptor sites in plasma membrane of adipocytes, hepatocytes, liver membranes, and isolated chondrocytes. *In vitro*, the relative binding affinities of insulin and somatomedin reflect biologic potency of the two hormones in tissues. Somatomedin is the only peptide other than insulin, proinsulin, or derivatives of insulin that competes for insulin-binding sites; this signifies structural as well as functional similarity between somatomedin and insulin.

It remains to be determined to what extent somatomedin is important in the pathogenesis of diabetes. Levels of serum NSILA (100–200 μU./ml.) were found to be similar in normal subjects and in patients with diabetes under various metabolic conditions. Diabetic patients, including those in diabetic ketoacidosis, and patients with insulinoma have been found to have similar levels of NSILA. No correlations have been found in the levels of NSILA and of insulin.

showed a component residing with plasma albumin that inhibited insulin action on rat diaphragm but not on adipocytes. The antagonism was greatest in fractionated diabetic plasma. This type of antagonism was observed when reduced chain B was bound to albumin. There was a suggestion that chain B became bound to albumin and accounted for antagonism to insulin. Hence this material was spoken of as having synalbumin-insulin activity (SIA), and it was thought to be a polypeptide of low molecular weight. Conflicting results, some due to methodologic artifacts, have been obtained by different investigators. Because of the high plasma level of SIA in diabetic patients (50-60 per cent of relatives), Vallance-Owen proposed that the SIA is transmitted as an autosomal dominant and constitutes a biochemical marker of diabetes. SIA was found in higher levels in extracts of serum from diabetics and prediabetics than in normal serums or serums of pancreatectomized patients with or without diabetes, but it was not found in the absence of adrenal cortical steroids. Elevated SIA levels were found in about 75 per cent of patients with myocardial disease, in more than 66 per cent of mothers with congenitally defective babies, and in 50 per cent of women in their third trimester with stillborn fetuses. When injected into rats intraperitoneally or intravenously, SIA either decreased or did not alter glucose disposal. In man, SIA levels tend to fall after oral or intravenous glucose administration, thus implying a role for SIA in glucose regulation. Considering all the factors at hand, it is difficult to assign SIA an important role in the pathogenesis of diabetes. Not all diabetics have increased levels of SIA, and the reproducibility and specificity of SIA for human diabetes can be questioned because of methodologic artifacts; serum antagonism can be demonstrated with porcine, bovine, rat and egg albumin, and gelatin. Synalbumin antagonism is frequently manifested when the whole plasma is free of antagonistic activity. The mechanisms of action, structure, and physiologic role of SIA are unclear. Since extracts of human plasma contain not only albumin but also insulin, ILA, and other substances, the combined effect of these factors in SIA is difficult to interpret. Apparently, some of these extracts irreversibly inhibit oxygen consumption, sugar and amino acid transport, and protein synthesis in isolated muscles, suggesting a toxic effect.

Synalbumin-Insulin Antagonism

The many studies of Vallance-Owen and of others on a reported insulin-antagonistic factor in plasma, synalbumin, have recently been reviewed (Berson, Ensinck, Davidson). Vallance-Owen and colleagues, using rat diaphragm for assay, found that insulin added to plasma from insulin-dependent, uncontrolled diabetics did not demonstrate full activity. After adequate treatment, insulin added to the plasma of normal and diabetic subjects was recovered quantitatively. Later studies

Antagonism to Insulin Action by Antibodies

As recently reviewed by Lazarus and Berson, commercial insulin preparations contain proinsulin, proinsulin intermediates, and insulin dimers, as well as insulin. Some information suggests that many more antibodies are produced by the contaminating substances than by insulin. However, these antibodies that are produced by the noninsulin compounds can also bind insulin and interfere with its usual biologic activities. Commercial beef insulin produces more insulin antagonism than does commercial pork insulin. When the insulin preparation is purified by removal of insulin-related products, repeated injections of the residue, monocomponent insulin, produce relatively few antibodies. However, monocomponent insulin combines with antibodies produced by proinsulin, proinsulin intermediates, and related products. ACTH and glucosteroids have been reported to reduce insulin requirements without reducing antibody levels. Patients who exhibit high insulin antibody levels after therapy with the common insulin preparations have shown a decrease in IgG antibodies to insulin when switched to monocomponent insulin preparations. There is considerable variation in antibody production among individual patients. There is a relationship between antibody affinity and instability in diabetic control. There have been occasional reports of insulin antibodies in the plasma of patients who have never had insulin injections.

Other Plasma Factors Influencing Insulin Action

There have been reports of various plasma factors that influence the action of insulin. Antagonism to insulin action has been described (Berson, Lazarus) for certain plasma fractions composed chiefly of α_2 and β globulins, lipoprotein fractions, nonlipoproteins, components of α_1 globulin, and other fractions. However, further studies are needed to clarify the origin of such components and whether in some instances they have been created by the method of chemical treatment of the plasma. Their physiologic significance must also be investigated further.

PROINSULIN ACTION

Proinsulin appears to resemble insulin in all its biologic actions in liver, muscle, and adipose tissue, but the relative potency of proinsulin in stimulating various metabolic reactions *in vivo* and *in vitro* has not been clearly elucidated. Compared with insulin, highly purified porcine or bovine proinsulin has a relatively low level of activity on rat muscle and adipose tissue (20–30 per cent) and even lower activity on isolated fat cells (2–3 per cent). Some studies indicate that the molecules of proinsulin that become bound to a specific plasma membrane receptor are as active as an equivalent number of molecules of insulin that become bound, but some tissues bind only about 10 per cent as much proinsulin as insulin. Proinsulin can produce hypoglycemia, but on an equimolar basis this action is only about 10 per cent that of insulin. The C-peptide from proinsulin has not been shown to have any biologic effects that either resemble or antagonize those of insulin, but more work is needed in this area.

OTHER HORMONES INFLUENCING INSULIN ACTION

There are many hormones that in one way or another act on carbohydrate, fat, and protein metabolism differently from insulin (Table 9–5). Some of these act like insulin in certain ways, but in most instances the action is contrary to that of insulin. These are now discussed, but some are presented more fully in Chapter 10.

Glucagon

Glucagon exerts a marked effect on carbohydrate, fat, and lipid metabolism. It has the capacity to stimulate glycogenolysis from the liver, *in vitro* and *in vivo*. It also promotes proteolysis and lipolysis. The lipolysis occurs not only in adipose tissue, but also in the liver. With the increase in lipolysis, there is an increase in ketogenesis and gluconeogenesis. Glucagon increases cAMP in the liver, heart, skeletal muscle, and adipose tissue.

As evidence of the potency of glucagon, 0.7 μg./kg. is sufficient to produce a 50 per cent increase in blood sugar. Approximately 25 times this amount of insulin on a molar basis is required to produce a fall in blood sugar of the same magnitude.

Distribution and Degradation of Glucagon

Earlier studies on the distribution and degradation of glucagon need to be repeated using newer

TABLE 9–5.   EFFECTS OF HORMONES ON INSULIN SECRETION AND ON NUTRIENT EXCHANGE IN TISSUES

	Insulin Secretion	Liver Release		Muscle		Adipose Tissue	
		Glucose	Ketones	Glucose Uptake	Supply for Gluconeo-genesis	Glucose Uptake	Lipolysis
Epinephrine	D*	I	I	D	I	I or D†	I
Glucagon	I	I	I	0	?	I or D†	I
Glucosteroid	I	I	I	D	I	D	I
GH	I	I	I	D	D	I & D	I
Insulin	D	D	D	I	D	I	D

*D = decrease; I = increase.

†Small amounts cause increase; large amounts cause decrease, especially in diabetes.

techniques. Elgee found that I^{131}-glucagon disappeared from the plasma much faster than did I^{131}-insulin. Essentially all tissues took up some I^{131}-glucagon but in markedly different concentrations. The relative concentrations of I^{131}-insulin and glucagon in various tissues were similar. Liver degraded a higher percentage of glucagon than insulin. Glucagon injected into the general circulation has been reported to have a half-life of 5–10 min.

Studies with unlabeled glucagon in human subjects (Assan) showed that no glucagon was present in urine of normal subjects but that glucagonuria appeared after intravenous injection of glucagon in patients with proximal tubule deficiency. Glucagon (or GLI material) was found in bile, and there was an increased amount after administration of exogenous glucagon.

I^{131}-glucagon has been shown to be degraded by many tissues, especially liver and kidney. The greatest degrading activity in liver was found in the residual supernatant fraction after ultracentrifugation of homogenate. The degradation occurred after cleavage of peptide linkages of the hormone. Glucagon degradation by liver preparations has been found to be inhibited by the addition of insulin, cysteine-inactivated insulin, A or B chain of insulin, ACTH, and GH. Although earlier it was believed that a glucagonase was a specific enzyme for the degradation of glucagon, recent information suggests that dipeptidyl aminopeptidase I has characteristics that were attributed to glucagonase. Dipeptidyl aminopeptidase I also has been found to degrade β-corticotropin, B chain of oxidized insulin, angiotensin II amide, COOH-terminal tetrapeptide of gastrin, secretin, and a wide variety of peptides. Chloride and sulfhydryl activators are essential for the degradation of glucagon by this aminopeptidase (MacDonald). This enzyme removes the NH_2-terminal His-Ser (Fig. 9–4), thereby producing a loss of biologic activity of glucagon.

As discussed in other sections, in measuring glucagon levels in tissues and body fluids, it is very important to prevent glucagon degradation. Aprotinin (Trasylol) has been used most often to protect against the degradation of glucagon in human plasma specimens, but it is very expensive. Recently, benzamidine has proven to be very effective in preventing the degradation of glucagon, and its cost is only about 1 per cent of that of aprotinin (Ensinck).

Glucagon Actions in Liver

Many of the changes that are found to follow glucagon administration in normal animals have been found in untreated diabetic animals (Table 9–4). Glucagon has a noncovalent binding to a specific receptor in the liver plasma membrane (Rodbell). This binding is not influenced significantly by other polypeptide hormones. The receptor site presumably is a lipoprotein that includes lysolecithin. GTP and GDP bind to the plasma membrane at sites close to the glucagon receptor. These nucleotides increase the turnover of glucagon and increase the activation of adenyl cyclase by the hormone. Binding of glucagon and its effect on adenyl cyclase tend to run parallel. Glucagon increases the liver uptake of amino acids, especially alanine (Mallette), that depend upon the Na^+ transport system. The increase in cAMP produced by glucagon increases Na^+ transport. Pyrophosphate increases the stimulating effect of glucagon on adenyl cyclase activity. In liver, glucagon increases glycogenolysis, gluconeogenesis, and catabolism of protein (Sokal, Marks). Glucagon increases gluconeogenesis from amino acids, pyruvate, and lactate. It increases ureogenesis, ketogenesis, and fatty acid oxidation but decreases glucose oxidation. Glucagon decreases the liver output of glycine, glutamate, and phenylalanine but increases the liver output of leucine, isoleucine, valine, and tyrosine. It increases slightly the output of lysine and histidine. It presumably stimulates the intracellular utilization of glycine, alanine, glutamate, and phenylalanine and the intracellular production of leucine, isoleucine, and valine. Glucagon increases glycogenolysis by increasing adenyl cyclase activity (Fig. 9–28). The resulting increase in cAMP stimulates protein kinase activity, which activates inactive phosphorylase, thereby inducing glycogenolysis. The increase in cAMP levels increases alanine transferase and other gluconeogenic enzymes. Maximal gluconeogenesis occurs only in the presence of an adequate supply of fatty acids. Glucagon and catecholamines can increase this supply by stimulating lipolysis in liver and adipose tissue. At physiologic concentrations, glucagon increases liver glycogenolysis and gluconeogenesis. It does not produce gluconeogenesis in kidney. Glucosteroids produce an increase in gluconeogenesis, chiefly by means of their extrahepatic actions. They do not increase glucose and urea production by isolated perfused liver, but by stimulating induction of some enzymes in liver, they augment the actions of glucagon.

Glucagon-like immunoreactive material (GLI), also called enteroglucagon, is secreted from the intestinal tract by endocrine cells that resemble α_2 cells. GLI increases slightly insulin secretion. It also increases glycogenolysis and lipolysis in liver.

Actions of Glucagon on Other Tissues

Glucagon decreases the following activities in the GI tract: (a) gastric and intestinal motility, (b) gastric and pancreatic exocrine secretion, and (c) actions of gastrin and pancreozymin. Glucagon increases markedly the volume of secretion by the small intestinal mucosa.

Glucagon binds to a specific receptor in the plasma membrane of beta cells, and then increases the activity of adenyl cyclase. Glucagon increases the release of insulin; the greater the glucose utilization by the beta cells, the greater is the insulin-releasing activity of a given amount of glucagon.

Glucagon increases adenyl cyclase activity in adipose tissue, resulting in increased lipolysis. In rats, the lipolytic effects of glucagon decreases with age (Manganiello). Glucagon tends to decrease hypercalcemia and hyperphosphatemia, presumably by increasing the secretion of thyrocalcitonin. Glucagon promotes cellular release of potassium, calcium, and inorganic phosphate (Wieland). Glucagon has an inotropic effect on the heart and increases the force of myocardial contraction, cardiac output, and arterial pressure. After a myocardial preparation is solubilized by a nonionic detergent (Lubrol-PX), its adenyl cyclase activity is unresponsive to glucagon and norepinephrine. The addition of phosphatidylserine restores the responsiveness of glucagon but not of norepinephrine (Levey). This demonstrates that a specific type of lipoprotein complex is important in the action of glucagon.

Summary of Actions of Glucagon in Relation to Other Hormone Activities

Glucagon is one of the most important hormones involved in the mobilization of energy (Fig. 9–28; Tables 9–4 and 9–5). It is assisted in this function by other hormones, particularly by catecholamines, glucosteroids, and GH. Glucagon's actions are antagonized by insulin; the latter promotes energy storage.

For maximal storage of energy, there should be very little glucagon present but much insulin. An increase in concentration of fatty acid or glucose tends to increase insulin and decrease glucagon. An increase in amino acids increases the levels of insulin and glucagon, but increases in both glucose and amino acids tend to increase insulin levels sufficiently to decrease glucagon secretion. The insulin:glucagon molar ratio is very important in determining the balance of energy storage and energy mobilization (Unger). After an overnight fast, the molar ratio of insulin to glucagon is > 3:1, but after fasting for three days it is < 1:1; after a carbohydrate meal, it is approximately 70:1. The activities of glucagon are largely nullified when the insulin:glucagon ratio is in the range between 3:1 and 70:1. This range is considered by Unger to represent a state of "biologic equality." In plasma of diabetic patients, there is a decrease in the level of insulin and an increase of glucagon.

Most of the extrahepatic activities of glucagon require doses of glucagon beyond the usual physiologic level. Glucagon is used pharmacologically under the following circumstances: (a) in hypoglycemia and when the administration of glucose is difficult; (b) in the diagnosis of pheochromocytoma; (c) in testing pituitary function, with measurement of GH release; (d) in acute hypercalcemia, in the absence of a supply of thyrocalcitonin; (e) in the diagnosis of insulinoma; (f) in the diagnosis of glycogenosis of the liver; (g) in the treatment of acute pancreatitis; and (h) in the treatment of refractory heart failure.

Correlation of Glucagon Structure with Biologic Activity

Deshistidine glucagon does not activate the glucagon-sensitive adenyl cyclase system in the plasma membrane of either hepatocytes or adipocytes. The amino-terminal histidine residue of glucagon is essential for biologic activity, and the hydrophobic near-carboxyl-terminal region (residues 22–27) is essential for the binding of glucagon to its specific receptor in the plasma membrane (Assan). The binding has characteristics of hydrophobic bonding and seems to be of lipophilic type. The structure of glucagon that is responsible for lipolysis is contained inside the 19–22 amino acid sequence, while the structure necessary for glycogenolysis and insulinogenesis is located in the 24–29 segment. There are two antigenic sites inside the glucagon molecule, and one (N-terminal + central portion) is also present in some catabolic fragments of glucagon circulating in the blood; it also appears to be present in enteroglucagon. This site appears to be the one most often bound by glucagon antibodies.

None of the peptides resulting from proteolytic actions of trypsin, chymotrypsin, or subtilisin retains hyperglycemic activity; neither does glucagon 1–18, resulting from carboxypeptidase digestion. Biologic activity is not destroyed by cleavage of the carboxyl-terminal tetrapeptide. Loss of histidine-1 leads to loss of hormone function. Apparently, residues 1, 2, and 19–24 play important roles in the biologic activity of glucagon.

Epinephrine and Norepinephrine

Epinephrine and norepinephrine stimulate glycogenolysis (Fig. 9–28; Tables 9–4 and 9–5), lipolysis, proteolysis, and gluconeogenesis. They increase plasma Na^+ concentration and decrease plasma K^+ concentration. They stimulate glucose uptake and utilization in adipose tissue but decrease glucose uptake in muscle; this could be because of an increase in G-6-P, which in turn inhibits hexokinase, consequently reducing glucose uptake. They increase cAMP in adipose tissue, muscle, liver, and heart, but insulin antagonizes these changes. Other actions of catecholamines are presented in Chapters 5 and 10.

Corticosteroids

Cortisol inhibits epinephrine-induced glycogenolysis in muscle. Of course, the amount of glycogenolysis caused by catecholamines and glucagon depends upon the amount of glycogen available. Consequently, glycogenolysis decreases with liver disease, starvation, diabetes, adrenal insufficiency, and pituitary deficiency. Adrenalectomy greatly ameliorates diabetes produced by pancreatectomy. Adrenalectomized nondiabetic animals, when fasted, develop hypoglycemia and a decrease in muscle and liver glycogen; glucosteroids reverse these changes. The main endogenous corticosteroids with glucosteroid action are cortisol and cortisone. They stimulate gluconeogenesis, chiefly in the liver, with resulting increased storage of glycogen in liver and muscle. They also increase G-6-P activity and glucose output by the liver, causing hyperglycemia (Figs. 9–27 and 10–3).

In livers of diabetic animals, there is a marked decrease in glucose phosphorylation and a pronounced increase in gluconeogenesis. However, adrenalectomy in diabetic animals almost normalizes the gluconeogenesis and ameliorates the diabetes. Neither adrenalectomy nor cortisone treatment influences glucose phosphorylation in liver slices from normal or diabetic rats pretreated with insulin. Glucosteroids inhibit glucose phosphorylation in muscle (Fig. 9–31) and adipose tissue as well as in liver but do not decrease permeability of cell membranes to glucose.

Cortisone can markedly increase liver G-6-P and glycogen without increasing glycogen synthetase activity. The increase in liver glycogen and blood glucose occurs before there is demonstrable increase in glucose-6-phosphatase. Cortisol injection decreases glucose uptake by adipose tissue but not by muscle.

Glucosteroids markedly inhibit lipogenesis in liver, but this probably is secondary to inhibition of glycolysis. In diabetic rats these steroids promote marked lipolysis, lipemia, and ketogenesis. Adrenalectomized rats do not respond to epinephrine with lipolysis unless glucosteroids are given also. Indeed, none of the hormones produce much lipolysis in the absence of glucosteroids.

Glucosteroids have a marked effect on protein metabolism. They (a) stimulate protein catabolism, (b) increase plasma amino acid (in hepatectomized as well as intact animals), (c) increase hepatic capture of amino acids, (d) increase gluconeogenesis (Fig. 9–32), (e) inhibit growth, (f) induce a negative nitrogen balance, (g) cause atrophy of many tissues (skin, blood vessels, muscle, bone, lymph nodes), and (h) increase liver tryptophan peroxidase and transaminase. In diabetes, as in Cushing's disease, there may be a marked increase in gluconeogenesis. In the former, protein catabolism may greatly exceed gluconeogenesis. Patients with Cushing's disease may have a markedly negative nitrogen balance and marked catabolic changes in skin, muscle, and bone yet have no hyperglycemia or glycosuria. These facts and others suggest that a major action of glucosteroids may be to supply products of protein degradation; the degraded protein may be converted to carbohydrate, thereby supplying energy, or it may serve as a building block for tissue resynthesis (Fig. 9–33).

Disturbances in carbohydrate metabolism following adrenalectomy resemble those after hypophysectomy (discussed below) but are not as marked; a similar though less marked effect on diabetes is also observed. The diabetes is intensified by glucosteroid treatment, which increases liver glycogen, muscle glycogen (in nonfasting states), and blood sugar. Prolonged treatment with large doses of glucosteroids has produced diabetes in certain animals and in man has changed occult diabetes to overt diabetes; it does not produce permanent diabetes in man when the diabetes trait does not exist. When the adrenals are intact, the effects of ACTH are comparable to those of glucosteroids. In some species, glucosteroids produce hypertrophy and hyperplasia of the β-cells, reversible degranulation, and irreversible vacuolation.

Houssay found that in subtotally depancreatized rats, different glucosteroids increased the incidence of diabetes, but when glucosteroid administration was continued for several months some of the animals initially diabetic reverted to normal carbohydrate metabolism.

A decrease in glucose tolerance may be found with either primary or secondary aldosteronism. Indeed, there is a decrease in glucose tolerance in about 50 per cent of patients with primary aldosteronism. The plasma insulin curve associated with glucose tolerance tests is somewhat similar to that found with maturity-onset diabetes. The carbohydrate defect and the defect in plasma insulin response can be changed toward normal by potassium loading. Potassium does not decrease aldosterone production; on the contrary, it tends to increase it. With a decrease in the potassium concentration in the cells and in the plasma, there is a decrease in insulin released into the plasma. Consequently, increasing the potassium stores by administering potassium corrects the defects of carbohydrate tolerance and insulin secretion.

Pituitary Hormones

Each of the anterior pituitary hormones, as well as vasopressin, can influence carbohydrate, fat, protein, electrolyte, and water metabolism directly or indirectly. Some of these hormones have a marked effect. Although ACTH can directly promote lipolysis, most of its activities are through the adrenal glands. In the same way, TSH acts chiefly through the thyroid and gonadotropin through the gonads. As discussed in other portions of the book, ACTH secretion is significantly increased by hypoglycemia and other factors that decrease carbohydrate utilization. ACTH secretion is increased by a large variety of stress reactions, including those produced by a loss of body fluid and hypotension. Vasopressin increases ACTH release. Glucosteroids are the main hormones that decrease ACTH secretion. GH secretion is increased by a decrease in glucose utilization. This applies especially to the amount of glucose utilized by the hypothalamus (chiefly the median eminence). There is a significant increase in GH release with fasting (Table 9–4), hypoglycemia, and rapid decrease in plasma glucose, or by factors that inhibit glucose utilization, such as deoxyglucose. The secretion of GH is also increased by the ingestion of protein and by amino acids, especially arginine.

FFA decrease GH release. It is increased by a large variety of physical or emotional stresses or both. Exercise or vasopressin also promotes its secretion (Yalow). The main function of GH is to promote growth of most of the tissues of the body. In doing this, it markedly stimulates the synthesis and utilization of protein. It has a net effect of decreasing glucose utilization, but it can markedly increase fat utilization.

Growth hormone promotes the deposition of protein, carbohydrate, and water and loss of fat (Table 9-5). The increase in protein apparently results from increased protein synthesis, while the increased carbohydrate appears to be due to decreased carbohydrate oxidation. GH promotes lipolysis in fat depots, increased plasma FFA, increased liver fat, increased ketone production, increased fat oxidation, and decreased fat synthesis. It promotes a relative increase in metabolism of glucose through the anaerobic glycolytic pathway and through the uronic pathway; the latter utilizes TPNH, and consequently GH depletes TPNH, while insulin increases it. On the basis of Randle's studies dealing with the glucose-fatty acid cycle, it is quite likely that some of the decrease in insulin activity induced by GH results from its lipolytic action. In muscle, in contrast to adipose tissue, GH produces a decrease in the phosphorylation of glucose and a decrease in glucose uptake, possibly resulting from an increase in fatty acids and ketones produced by the GH. They lead to a decrease in glycolysis at the level of phosphofructokinase, which in turn causes an increase in G-6-P. This tends to inhibit hexokinase and consequently to decrease glucose utilization.

Houssay showed, as discussed later, that hypophysectomy increases the hypoglycemic response to insulin and alleviates the severity of diabetes in depancreatized animals; for example, it markedly decreases glycosuria, ketonuria, and nitrogen balance. Luft has shown that human GH causes a marked exacerbation in the diabetes of hypophysectomized patients. Although many investigators have shown that excess GH causes a decrease in glucose tolerance despite hypernormal plasma insulin levels, the plasma insulin level may be many times normal without a decrease in glucose tolerance.

Insulin stimulates protein synthesis in the absence of GH, but GH promotes only slight protein synthesis in the absence of insulin; its effects are considerably greater in the presence of insulin. GH alone produces very little growth in depancreatized animals; insulin injections markedly augment the growth produced by GH. These hormones have opposite effects with response to fat: insulin markedly stimulates lipogenesis; GH stimulates lipolysis.

GH exerts innumerable effects, chiefly indirect, upon carbohydrate, fat, and protein metabolism which may be summarized in large part as follows: It decreases blood glucose by (a) directly stimulating glucose uptake by muscle, (b) increasing insulin secretion (early), and (c) decreasing insulin degradation. It may increase blood glucose by (a) promoting β-cell "exhaustion," (b) increasing hepatic glucogenesis, (c) decreasing insulin fixation to tissue, (d) increasing release from the pancreas of glucagon, and (e) decreasing responsiveness of certain tissues to insulin.

As discussed in another section of this chapter, a portion of GH is converted in the liver to somatomedin (Hintz). There is much to indicate that somatomedin and NSILA are the same compound. As discussed earlier, NSILA exerts an insulin-like action. However, another component of the GH exerts an anti-insulin effect in various ways, including antagonism to glucose uptake, glucose oxidation, fatty acid synthesis, pyruvate oxidation, and lipogenesis (Bornstein). The discovery (Brazeau) of a somatotropin-release inhibiting factor provides a possible approach for significantly influencing the course of diabetes.

The following changes in carbohydrate metabolism result from hypophysectomy or pituitary destruction:

1. There is a decrease in the rate of absorption of sugar from the GI tract and an increase in glucose tolerance.

2. Within a few hours after a meal, there may be subnormal concentrations of glycogen in the liver and muscles, hypoglycemia, and convulsions.

3. There is a marked increase in sensitivity to insulin—greater than that following adrenalectomy. Hypoglycemia may occur approximately 2 hours or more after the administration of glucose or epinephrine. This is corrected by GH or glucosteroids or both.

4. The hyperglycemic response to epinephrine and glucagon is decreased.

5. In diabetic animals or patients there is an amelioration of the diabetic state, including the following changes:

   (a) less hyperglycemia and glycosuria— even a tendency to hypoglycemia during fasting;
   (b) marked sensitivity to insulin; the diabetes may be controlled with 20 per cent or less of the preoperative dose;
   (c) increased capacity for glucose utilization;
   (d) decreased fat and protein catabolism—hence, less ketonuria and azoturia;
   (e) decreased glucose:nitrogen; and
   (f) fewer clinical manifestations of diabetes.

Hypophysectomy does not cause atrophy of the islets, but it does cause some atrophy of acinar tissue.

As discussed earlier, permanent diabetes has been induced in some species by injections of GH, and it has also been induced with prolactin. It is produced by ACTH when the adrenals are present. Hypophysial diabetes is intensified by ACTH or glucosteroids. Moreover, GH restores to normal insulin resistance that has been decreased by adrenalectomy. Thus glucosteroids and hypophysial extracts each augment the diabetogenic effect of the other.

In adipose tissue from normal rats, prolactin stimulates increased glucose uptake, increases glucose oxidation (especially through the hexose monophosphate shunt), and increases lipogenesis.

Thyroid Hormones

The rate of absorption of glucose from the intestine is increased in hyperthyroidism and decreased in hypothyroidism. In some patients with hypothyroidism, there is increased sensitivity to insulin and, indeed, spontaneous hypoglycemia may occur. This is due to decreased adrenal and pituitary function along with decreased insulin degradation. The necessary dose of insulin for glucose regulation is significantly decreased in most patients with myxedema and increased in those with thyrotoxicosis.

The administration of large doses of thyroid hormone (TH) for several months to certain species, when the animals have been rendered subdiabetic by subtotal pancreatectomy or mild alloxanization, will produce a permanent state of diabetes, which is designated as metathyroid diabetes. The TH produces an increase in hepatic glucogenesis. In the rat it also produces hypertrophy and hyperplasia of the β-cells. There is an increased incidence of diabetes in thyrotoxicosis, but the reverse does not apply. However, each disease makes management of the other more difficult. Thyroxine is important in promoting lipid synthesis from carbohydrate in adipose tissue and liver; however, it conditions lipolysis. It increases gluconeogenesis, proteolysis, glycogenolysis, and insulin secretion. It also increases glucose uptake by peripheral tissues.

Sex Hormones and Chorionic Somatomammotropin

The incidence of diabetes is greater in offspring of diabetic mothers than in those of diabetic fathers, but the exact reasons for this have not been elucidated. Most of the effects of sex hormones on diabetes have been demonstrated in rats. Diabetes appears one or two months after ablation of about 95 per cent of the pancreas; in one series, 89 per cent of the males and 27 per cent of the females were diabetic at the end of six months. Removal of the testes decreases the incidence of diabetes, and removal of the ovaries increases it. Androgen causes an earlier appearance, increased incidence, and increased severity of diabetes in subtotally depancreatized rats. The insulin content of the pancreas is similar in both sexes in rats, but females have more islet tissue. Among humans, diabetes is more common in women than in men, but during childhood there is no difference.

With an increase in the duration of pregnancy, the placenta produces a large amount of hormone that has many chemical, biologic, and immunologic characteristics of human growth hormone. Indeed, 86 per cent of the 190 amino acid residues of the 2 hormones are identically placed. Sometimes this hormone has been designated as growth hormone–like substance, or chorionic somatomammotropin, which in the past was called placental lactogen. It, like growth hormone, has growth-promoting and lactogenic properties. Moreover, it exerts a strong antagonistic action to insulin.

Pregnancy in nondiabetics is associated with a normal glucose tolerance test, but in order to maintain the normal tolerance, more insulin must be secreted than is necessary in the same subject after delivery. Diabetics, when pregnant, have much poorer glucose tolerance than when they are not pregnant, despite the fact that plasma insulin levels are far higher. These changes begin to regress within a few hours after delivery. Moreover, within one week after delivery, less than one-fourth of the amount of insulin secreted during pregnancy is sufficient to maintain essentially normal glucose tolerance. Chorionic somatomammotropin does not cross the placenta.

Contraceptive steroids produce an abnormal glucose tolerance in some normal women tested, and this increases with the duration of use (Adams). Some steroids are more diabetogenic than others, and some women are more subject to the changes than others.

Mestranol increases the plasma insulin response to oral glucose and promotes deterioration of carbohydrate tolerance in some subjects; ethinyl estradiol produces less of this effect. There is a higher incidence of abnormal glucose tolerance found in women who have taken mestranol plus norethindrone or mestranol plus ethynodiol than in those taking mestranol alone. These hormones cause greater alteration in carbohydrate tolerance in diabetics than in nondiabetics.

The mechanism by which oral contraceptives alter carbohydrate metabolism has not been clearly established, but it appears that much of the effect is associated with increased secretion of glucosteroids and some increased GH secretion.

There is no definite evidence that the oral contraceptives produce an increase in atherosclerosis, but they sometimes promote reversible increases in blood pressure, presumably in part because of increased angiotensin formation. They do increase the incidence of thromboembolic disease. Since much more information is needed to clarify the ill-effects of contraceptive steroids, other methods of contraception (intrauterine devices, diaphragms) should be used by diabetics, or one member of the couple eventually should be sterilized.

Progesterone alone does not appear to change carbohydrate metabolism significantly, but it does increase the plasma insulin response to glucose and tolbutamide and impairs the hypoglycemic response to injected insulin. Estrogen effects in diabetic animals vary with the species, amounts and duration of administration, and other factors.

Nerve Growth Factor

A nerve growth factor (NGF), recently discovered, has many chemical and functional activities similar to those of insulin (Frazier). It enhances the growth of sympathetic ganglia and stimulates many metabolic processes in embryonic sympathetic and sensory neurons. It promotes the synthesis of RNA, protein, and lipid; it increases glucose uptake and utilization. In high concentration insulin exerts some similar actions on the same neurons as NGF. For example, each of these hormones increases glucose utilization, synthesis of RNA and protein, and polyribosome formation.

NGF is widely distributed throughout the tissues and body fluids of all mammals. It occurs in high concentration in the submaxillary glands. It is of interest that the major sources of NGF (submaxillary gland) and of insulin (pancreas) both originate in the entoderm of the embryonic gut. Each has acinar structures and secretes enzymes and other materials into the GI tract. Each hormone is secreted into the bloodstream and is widely distributed throughout the body.

Because of the aforementioned similarities in NGF and insulin, interest in the possible role of submaxillary gland function in glucose metabolism and in diabetes is active. In investigating this specific subject, no significant differences in plasma glucose and insulin responses were observed in dogs before and after total bilateral extirpation of submaxillary glands (Steinberg). Although these glands show pathologic changes with increased frequency in diabetics, the significance of this relationship has not been established.

NGF from mice is composed of two identical polypeptide chains associated by noncovalent forces. Each chain has 118 amino acids. There are 3 intrachain disulfide bonds. The molecular weight of NGF is 13,259.

Antibodies to NGF cause marked destruction of sympathetic nerve fibers. Indeed, this has served as a very useful tool for effecting sympathectomy. It is possible that insulin antibodies produced in diabetic patients treated over long intervals with insulin contribute to the observed degeneration of glial and Schwann cells, retinal mural cells, bone pericytes, and kidney mesenchymal cells, but it has not been shown that insulin antibodies produce the nerve changes or whether a deficiency in NGF or NGF antibodies is responsible for the nerve degenerative reactions in diabetes.

Despite many similarities in the chemical structure and function of NGF and insulin, there are also many differences. The main actions of NGF are to stimulate the early development of the sympathetic nervous system and later to play a part in its maturation.

DIABETES IN LABORATORY ANIMALS

Methods of producing diabetes-like states, which may persist temporarily or in some instances permanently, are listed in Table 9-6. The causative agent may act only temporarily to produce permanent diabetes. The pancreas normally has a reserve capacity to secrete much more insulin than is usually required.

Since some phases of diabetes cannot be studied in detail in man, most investigations are carried out with animals (Table 9-7). Spontaneous diabetes occurs in many species, and diabetes can be produced in normal animals by various chemical and physical means. Although numerous characteristics of diabetes in animals simulate those in man, we cannot be certain of the extent to which

TABLE 9-6. SOME DIABETOGENETIC FACTORS

Genetic

Dietary
  High caloric intake, particularly carbohydrate, for frequent and long intervals
  Starvation (diabetes-like)

Hormonal
  Frequent administration of:
    Somatotropin
    Prolactin
    Adrenocorticotropin
    Glucosteroid
    Glucagon
    Epinephrine
    Vasopressin
    Estrogen
    Insulin (pancreatitis)

β-Cell Destruction or Removal
  Pancreatectomy
  Chemicals—alloxan, streptozotocin, dehydroascorbate, and many others
  Pancreatitis
  Neoplasm

Other
  Insulin antibodies or other antagonists
  Piqûre
  Liver disease

(The diabetic status is transient in some instances.)

there are differences. Today most of the diabetic animal models have spontaneous diabetes, or are made diabetic by streptozotocin or alloxan. In some studies of the acute phases of diabetes, the intravenous administration of insulin antibodies has been valuable.

Spontaneous Diabetes in Animals

As recently reviewed by Renold, the variety of animal species with temporary or permanent diabetes used for research is growing rapidly (Table 9-7). The frequency and intensity of diabetes can be increased by selective breeding, by certain environmental factors, and particularly by using high-carbohydrate diets. The Egyptian sand rat is a species that develops diabetes on a high-caloric diet. Restricted caloric intake appears to alleviate the diabetic condition. The KK mouse is a genetically defective species in which the pancreas has no primary abnormality but peripheral tissues appear to be insensitive to insulin. This insensitivity is partly compensated for by increased insulin production. Obese hyperglycemic mice (ob) and diabetic mice (db) have genetic predisposition for the disease, but diabetes is greatly intensified by high caloric intake. In some instances, the mode of inheritance is autosomal recessive, in others autosomal dominant, and in some multifactorial. In the spiny mouse and the sand rat, the genetic pattern is unknown. The tendency to develop a diabetes-like picture is inherited as a dominant trait in yellow (A^y) obese mice and as a recessive trait in diabetic (db), obese (ob), and adipose (ad) mice, while the transmission presumably is multifac-

TABLE 9–7. DIABETIC-LIKE SYNDROMES IN SMALL RODENTS

Species*	Some Diabetic-Like Characteristics
Type A Yellow (A^y) Obese (ob) Adipose (ad) New Zealand obese (NZO) KK (Japan) C$_3$HfXl, F$_1$ (Wellesley) "Fatty" rats	This group is characterized by obesity, modest hyperglycemia, absence of ketoacidosis, prominent hyperplasia of betacytes, hypernormal levels of immunoreactive insulin in plasma. It simulates humans with obesity and very mild diabetes.
Type B Diabetic (db) Spiny mouse (Acomys cahirinus) Sand rat (Psammomys obesus)	The course of the disease in this group is initially similar to that in type A, but eventually the net amount of insulin action is insufficient. Severe hyperglycemia and ketoacidosis develop; death may occur.
Type C Chinese hamster (Cricetulus griseus)	This group differs from the others in that no obesity occurs. The clinical course varies from mild intermittent glucosuria to severe ketoacidosis and death. Hyperplasia of betacytes and elevated immunoreactive insulin levels are transient.

*All nondesignated species are mice.

torial in the inbred KK and NZO strains of mice. It is multifactorial in Wellesley hybrids and Chinese hamsters. In any single species, the abnormality appears to result from several distinct mutations, some of which may be transmitted as dominant and others as recessive traits.

In all animals shown in Table 9–7, there is at one time or another, even though transiently, increased pancreatic and circulating immunoreactive insulin. There follows a severe decrease in insulin only in those syndromes that terminate in progressively pronounced hyperglycemia and ketoacidosis. In each of the species, except for the Chinese hamster, obesity is common. All of them, at least in the early phases, have demonstrable islet hyperplasia.

High caloric intake has been shown to be important in most all of the animal types of diabetes listed in Table 9–7. The syndrome in these animals extends from diabetes without obesity (Chinese hamster) to varying degrees of hyperglycemia and obesity and to "fatty" rats with obesity associated with hyperlipemia and hypercholesterolemia but not carbohydrate intolerance (Renold). Presumably in many instances the diabetes-like syndrome begins with decreased responsiveness to insulin as a primary event, appearing spontaneously or provoked by diet (sand rats). Striated muscle appears to be particularly resistant to insulin in the hyperglycemic obese mice and the NZO mice, whereas the liver is a site for decreased insulin effectiveness in the diabetic (db) mice. Decreased effectiveness of insulin action usually is associated with hyperinsulinemia, which may be transient (Chinese hamsters) or persistent (obese mice). The insulin resistance tends to be most pronounced in adult or middle-aged animals and decreases later. Both hypertrophy and hyperplasia of the β-cells are present during some portion of the spectrum of the syndrome for most of the animals, with the exception of the Chinese hamsters and the diabetic (db) mice. In some instances, however, hypertrophy and hyperplasia can no longer compensate for the demand for insulin, so that diabetes progresses and frank decompensation may occur. Heavy caloric intake hastens this decompensation.

In spiny mice, release of IRI in response to glucose, arginine, glucagon, isoproterenol, aminophylline, and dibutyryl cAMP is delayed (Cameron). The defect in IRI release apparently involves transport of insulin out of the β-cell.

As shown in Table 9–7, some characteristics of the animal diabetes-like syndrome are similar to those in man, but there are distinct differences among the various animal species. Despite the fact that none of the animal syndromes may exactly duplicate diabetes in man, pathophysiologically there are many very interesting corollaries. Some of the animals develop ketoacidosis and changes related to microvascular abnormalities: retinopathy and glomerulosclerosis.

When refed after prolonged fasting, animals and man may have glycosuria; this has been demonstrated in fasted rats given a high-carbohydrate intake, even when the total calories were subnormal. With the refeeding there is a subnormal insulin release. The administration of insulin improves the carbohydrate tolerance. When rats maintained on a high-fat diet are suddenly shifted to an isocaloric high-carbohydrate diet, they develop glycosuria that is only partly controlled by insulin.

Pancreatectomy or β-Cell Damage

The amount of pancreas that must be removed in order to produce glycosuria depends upon the species and the load of carbohydrate. In most animal species, more than 80 per cent of the pancreas must be removed in order to produce permanent diabetes. The secretory activity of a pancreatic remnant can become exhausted in some species, particularly with a high-carbohydrate diet, and degenerative changes in the β-cells may occur.

Alloxan and streptozotocin produce diabetes by selectively destroying the β-cells; with large doses, it is possible to destroy essentially all these cells. A large dose may damage the liver and kidney, but if the acute effects are survived, the animal makes a good recovery except that it is diabetic. Pancreatectomy of an alloxanized or streptozotocinized diabetic animal decreases the insulin requirement, supposedly because the source of glucagon has been removed, and also because removal of the source of pancreatic enzymes results in poor absorption of food. Alloxan and streptozotocin cause triphasic changes in the blood glucose level: (a) immediate hyperglycemia, probably resulting from hepatic glycogenolysis; (b) hypoglycemia due to excess insulin release from damaged β-cells; and (c) hyperglycemia resulting from insulin deficiency.

There is a relatively large amount of easily ionizable zinc in β-cells, and alloxan has an affinity to combine with it. In this manner, alloxan is concentrated in β-cells and is toxic to them.

The diabetogenic effects of alloxan can be avoided in some species if certain compounds are administered immediately before the alloxan is given. These compounds include nicotinic acid, pyridine, dicarboxylic acid, sodium bisulfite, glutathione, cysteine, British anti-lewisite, and methylene blue.

Nearly complete protection against the diabetogenic effect of streptozotocin is effected by the administration of nicotinamide given sometime between 30 min. before and 10 min. after streptozotocin injection. When nicotinamide is administered at other times, it does not prevent diabetes. Streptozotocin produces a marked depletion of nicotinamide adenine dinucleotides (NAD and NADH) in the islets, but nicotinamide prevents this. Nicotinic acid does not exert antidiabetic effect. Streptozotocin tends to be less damaging than alloxan to structures other than β-cells. Therefore, it is a commonly used method for producing diabetes.

Insulin Antibodies

Administration of anti-insulin serum to rats produces severe degranulation of the β-cells and may be associated with interstitial edema and leukocytic infiltration by eosinophils, lymphocytes, and neutrophils (Lacy). Similar changes may be observed after the injection of insulin from a different species.

Hyperglycemia, glycosuria, ketonuria, polyuria, and polydipsia are produced in rats by intravenous infusion of large amounts of insulin antibodies. Severe diabetes and ketoacidosis can be produced in this manner. The severity of the diabetes depends upon the amount of antibodies administered and the duration of their administration. Glycosuria appeared within 1–2 hours of the initiation of the infusion and ketonuria within 4–8 hours. The diabetic state results from binding of endogenous insulin to the injected antibodies. This procedure constitutes a useful method for producing diabetes, because it is not associated with the side effects of streptozotocin, alloxan, or pancreatectomy.

DIABETES MELLITUS

General Principles

Diabetes mellitus is not a disease in the classic sense, i.e., it has no distinct and definable pathogenesis, etiology, invariable set of clinical findings, specific laboratory tests, and definitive and curative therapy. Rather, it should be viewed as a syndrome—a clinical entity which can involve any or all of a long list of symptoms and clinical laboratory findings—which shows a variable response to therapy. The term diabetes mellitus, then, is one of convenience for the physician, rather than one that conveys definite pathologic meaning for the patient. Because it has been easiest to measure and was the first discovered abnormality, the major focus has been to define the disease by glucose measurement, and various commissions and committees have periodically attempted to define the normal limits of glucose metabolism. Yet there are no standards of normal limits upon which all agree. This is largely because carbohydrate tolerance is distributed as a continuous function. This may be owing to the distance of the measurement from the underlying genetic abnormality, a series of genes regulating carbohydrate metabolism, or to the variable interaction of hereditary with environmental factors or to both. Therefore, in the absence of a genetic factor which can be measured, the presence or absence of diabetes mellitus can only be imprecisely assigned. Nevertheless, most clinicians can make a pragmatic diagnosis most of the time. In doing so, we consider that four general areas are affected in the complete clinical syndrome and that these should be considered in making a clinical diagnosis.

1. *Hyperglycemia.* There is an abnormality of carbohydrate metabolism resulting in hyperglycemia and often associated with accelerated fat and protein catabolism. It may contribute to the other features but seems unlikely to be their sole cause.

2. *Large vessel disease.* There is accelerated atherosclerosis and medial calcification.

3. *Microvascular disease.* There is an abnormality of capillary basement membranes characterized by thickness and abnormal function. These capillary-related lesions are often termed the microvascular or small-vessel concomitants of diabetes.

4. *Neuropathy.* There are peripheral sensory-motor defects, segmental demyelination, and abnormalities of Schwann cells.

None of these findings is specific for diabetes, as each is also found in other diseases and syndromes. It is likely that more than one mechanism can produce each of these four abnormal findings. Since the primary defect in diabetes is unknown, a patient with any one or all of these abnormalities must be considered as a possible diabetic. The final decision is based on clinical and laboratory observations and depends largely on the particular frame of reference and concept of the term "diabetes mellitus" for each clinician. Therefore, for purposes of discussions to follow, we shall use the term "diabetes" in reference to the sum total of all clinical and laboratory observations, and such terms as hyperglycemia and thickened basement membrane to describe specific measured or observed findings. Because plasma glucose can be measured simply and accurately, it remains the standard most often used, but better parameters in the future are hoped for.

Classification

Because one or more hereditary factors are believed to be essential parts of the disease in most cases and therefore present at birth, an attempt has been made to separate the syndrome into the clinical phases as they present themselves to the physician.

These classifications are based upon the presence or absence of hyperglycemia or the degree of measurable carbohydrate tolerance. Several such classifications are shown in Table 9–8 and discussed below, using the American Diabetes Association terminology. This approach ignores the other three facets of the disease. The separation between categories is arbitrary, and such a classification does not mean to infer that an individual necessarily progresses from one stage of carbohydrate abnormality to the next, or that there is any specific order in the various categories that have been proposed. They are simply definitions which are used in communication between clinicians. Thus, in the natural history of carbohydrate intolerance, progression or regression from one stage to the next (1) may never occur, (2) may occur very slowly over many years, or (3) may be rapid and even explosive. Carbohydrate metabolism appears to fluctuate from time to time in many individuals, and this appears to be particularly true in persons with diabetes mellitus.

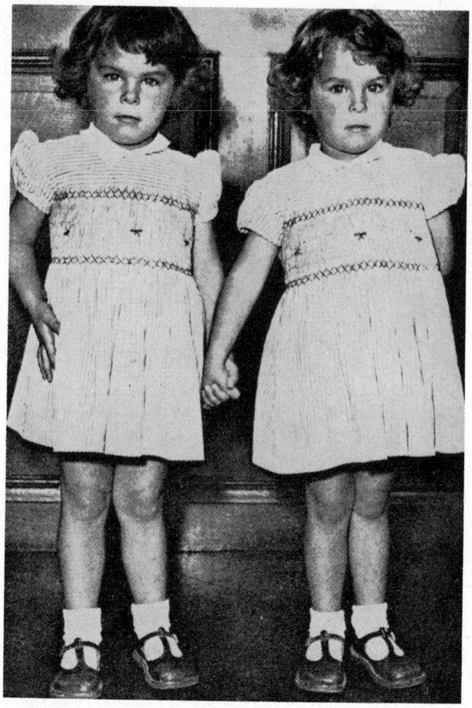

Figure 9–34. Identical twins with acute onset of diabetes appearing simultaneously at age 2½ years. (From Lister, J.: *The Clinical Syndrome of Diabetes Mellitus.* London, H. K. Lewis and Co., 1959.)

Prediabetes

This category is essentially theoretical in that it designates individuals who have the diabetic gene or genes but in whom there is no measurable carbohydrate abnormality. It covers the interval between conception and the time when abnormalities in glucose metabolism can be identified. This stage is likely to be realized with high certainty in the nondiabetic identical twin of a diabetic patient (Fig. 9–34) and with less certainty in the offspring of two diabetic parents. However, since the specific genetic abnormality of the disease has not yet been determined, this diagnosis cannot be made with certainty, and the designation "potential diabetes" may be better. The glucose metabolism of groups of individuals with high genetic risk have been studied. In general, subnormal plasma insulin re-

TABLE 9–8.   STAGES IN THE NATURAL HISTORY OF DIABETES MELLITUS

	Predia-betes*	Subclinical Diabetes	Latent Diabetes	Overt Diabetes
Fasting blood sugar	Normal	Normal	Normal or ↑	↑
Glucose tolerance test	Normal	Normal; abnormal during pregnancy, stress	Abnormal	Not necessary for diagnosis
Cortisone-glucose tolerance test	Normal	Abnormal	Not necessary	—
Delayed and/or decreased insulin response to glucose	+	++	+++	++++
Terminology employed by:				
American Diabetes Association	Prediabetes	Suspected diabetes	Chemical or latent diabetes	Overt diabetes
British Diabetes Association	Potential diabetes	Latent diabetes	Asymptomatic diabetes (subclinical or chemical)	Clinical diabetes

*Can be suspected in the "nondiabetic" identical twin of a known diabetic or in the nondiabetic offspring of two diabetic parents. (From Fajans, S.: *Med. Clin. N. Amer. 55*:794, 1971.)

sponses to glucose, amino acid, and tolbutamide administration have been found in these genetically high-risk individuals. Microvascular thickening of the capillary basement membrane of the quadriceps muscles has been reported in more than 50 per cent of these subjects by Siperstein.

Suspected Diabetes

This has also been called subclinical diabetes or latent diabetes. The fasting blood sugar and the glucose tolerance test is normal. Diabetes is suspected because of decreased glucose tolerance after cortisone administration or after certain other types of drug therapy, during pregnancy, or with stressful illnesses such as myocardial infarction or surgery. Since few long-term follow-ups of such patients have been made, the percentage of genetically abnormal persons uncovered by stress hyperglycemia is unknown.

Chemical Diabetes

This has also been variously described as latent diabetes or asymptomatic diabetes. Since this terminology overlaps with the previous category, there has been quite a bit of confusion. The fasting blood sugar is normal, but the glucose tolerance test is abnormal. Normal performance usually includes 95 per cent of an age-corrected population as normal. However, this cut-off point has been quite variable and is responsible for most of the controversy in defining this group. Appropriate standards are discussed in the section on Carbohydrate Tolerance Testing.

Overt Diabetes

This has also been termed clinical diabetes and is the symptomatic form of the disease that has been familiar to medical practitioners for 2000 years. Fasting blood sugar is *always* elevated, and the most severely affected patients have classic signs and symptoms of the disease. In severe failure of carbohydrate metabolism, ketoacidosis and death will occur without insulin therapy. Patients with similar degrees of hyperglycemia (e.g., Cushing's syndrome or pheochromocytoma) of nongenetic cause are not considered by some physicians to have diabetes, simply because this scheme is based upon the concept that diabetes by definition includes a genetic component.

Genetic Factors

It is generally agreed that diabetes is often a familial disease. Although the degree of heritability of the syndrome varies widely in published reports, positive family histories in diabetic patients are somewhere between 25 and 50 per cent. Perhaps the best evidence for clear-cut genetic factors are the studies of diabetes in monozygotic and dizygotic twins and in the children of diabetic parents (conjugal diabetes). The reported incidence of diabetes is much higher in the children of diabetic parents and in the monozygotic twins (Fig. 9–34) than in fraternal twins or in the control population. In some studies the concordance has been high enough to suggest that diabetes was inherited as a simple recessive trait. However, these findings are in the minority, and generally it appears that no more than 50 per cent of these groups are identified as being abnormal by any of the sophisticated tolerance tests now being performed. This suggests that either the simple recessive hypothesis is incorrect, or that environmental factors play a significant role in the phenotypic expression of the diabetic genotype. To explain these discrepancies, a variety of alternative genetic hypotheses have been proposed, including one major gene plus nonallelic modifiers, polyallelic inheritance, two or more independent genes, and genetic heterogeneity. Thus all possible modes of inheritance have been proposed for diabetes mellitus, but none of them explains all available data. One of the great problems is that blood glucose concentration in a population consists of a continuous rather than a bimodal distribution. That is, there is no clear-cut distinction between normal and abnormal glucose tolerance tests, as would be expected if diabetes were due to a single-gene mutation and the tests were a direct measurement of this mutant gene. This has led to the concept that either inheritance is multifactorial (polygenic) or the frequency of the gene has been low enough to be obscured in a test in which there are many other influencing factors. However, it has been recently reported (Rushforth) that the Pima Indians demonstrate clear-cut bimodality in glucose tolerance tests. Investigation of such a unique population will clearly contribute to our ability to test the various genetic hypotheses proposed to explain the inheritance of the diabetes-related gene.

Genetic Risk.   Since the mode of inheritance of diabetes is still in question, accurate genetic counseling is impossible. The best approach would be a simple table to delineate for the clinician the statistics of inheriting a diabetic genotype. Perhaps a more practical approach is the assessment of risk based upon clinical diabetes rather than upon the presence of the diabetic gene or an abnormality of glucose tolerance. Such a practical approach and a discussion of its uses and limitations are given in Chapter 25.

ENVIRONMENTAL FACTORS AND DIABETES MELLITUS

Obesity

The most commonly associated physical finding in a patient with diabetes is obesity. In the hyperglycemic population aged over 20, approximately 80–90 per cent are more than 10 per cent overweight. When such individuals lose weight permanently, there may be complete regression of glycosuria, and in many instances carbohydrate metabolism may become completely normal. This prompts the question of whether or not hyperglycemia in an obese person is a manifestation of the diabetic syndrome or is primarily related to the obesity. Since many obese hyperglycemic subjects demonstrate other features of the diabetic syndrome, including accelerated atherogenesis, microvascular disease, neuropathy, and even ketoacidosis, it has been impossible to segregate these syndromes. However, the minority of obese subjects have hyperglycemia or other cardinal characteristics of the diabetes syndrome. Moreover, there has been no consistent relationship between the degree of obesity and abnormality of carbohydrate tolerance. A significant influence of obesity per se on carbohydrate metabolism has been demonstrated, however, as there is a clear-cut decrease in sensitivity to insulin action in peripheral tissues. As a result, obese people need to secrete more insulin to maintain normal carbohydrate metabolic homeostasis, and more insulin to maintain fat and protein metabolism comparable to that of non-obese subjects. This has led to the concept that obesity represents an environmental factor which imposes a continuous stress on the mechanisms for the synthesis and secretion of insulin. In the genetically susceptible individual, this stress may eventually lead to relative insulin deficiency and carbohydrate intolerance. It is not clear whether these genetically susceptible individuals will always develop other aspects of the diabetic syndrome in the absence of obesity, or whether obesity and the hyperglycemia eventually associated with it prompt the development of the vascular and neuropathic abnormalities in diabetes. In the great majority of experimental models for diabetes in genetically abnormal animals, the same strong association between obesity and carbohydrate intolerance has been found. Therefore, it is possible that this apparent environmental factor may be partly genetic, as obesity has often been found to be familial.

Drugs

Other environmental influences that may produce carbohydrate intolerance or overt hyperglycemia include a number of drugs. Among the more common drugs are the glucocorticoids and the estrogen component of the birth control pills. Both appear to induce a state of insulin resistance. At reasonable dose levels, most normal people compensate by the secretion of additional amounts of insulin. Certain individuals appear unable to maintain this response, and hyperglycemia appears. In most instances, when these hormones are withdrawn carbohydrate tolerance reverts to normal. In some cases ketoacidosis has been precipitated, but this is unusual. However, even in these instances, there is a marked improvement in carbohydrate metabolism after the removal of the offending drug. It is not clear whether these are true expressions of the diabetic syndrome precipitated by these drugs (they usually have not been given long enough or to large enough groups for any effect on the vascular or neural components of the diabetic syndrome to have been observed) or manifestations of some unusual sensitivity to the side effects of the drugs. Experiences with the cortisone glucose tolerance test indicate that individuals who react abnormally to this test subsequently have a distinctly higher incidence of overt diabetes than do those with a normal response. Thus at least some of the individuals who develop drug-induced hyperglycemia seem to have the genetic abnormality of the diabetic syndrome. Other drugs affecting carbohydrate tolerance testing are discussed later.

Stress

A variety of severe stress states have been associated with carbohydrate intolerance or symptomatic glycosuria or both. Pregnancy, with its increased estrogen and chorionic somatomammotropin concentrations, produces resistance to the action of insulin and is one example of stress to carbohydrate tolerance. Other examples are those related to injury or illness, associated with increased secretion of four other glucose-regulatory hormones: (a) glucocorticoid, (b) glucagon, (c) catecholamines, and (d) growth hormone. The clinical importance of this stress-related hyperglycemia and its interaction with carbohydrate tolerance is discussed elsewhere.

Not uncommonly, medical-legal problems arise with respect to stress (e.g., the trauma of automobile accidents, including cerebral trauma, or other trauma related to emotional and neurologic illnesses). Hyperglycemia is often observed in conjunction with the stress of any acute illness and will disappear entirely during the recovery phase. The question arises periodically as to whether diabetes can be produced by trauma in a normal person (no genetic abnormality). The authors are inclined to believe that there is not sufficient evidence that stress per se can produce a permanent diabetic syndrome in a genetically normal individual. Since more than 80 per cent of the pancreas must be removed to produce diabetes by surgery, for trauma to produce diabetes most of the pancreas presumably must be destroyed. We know of no patient who has developed a chronic diabetic status on this basis.

FREQUENCY OF DIABETES

Because a specific method of identifying the diabetic subject is lacking, the prevalence (percentage of population affected) and the incidence (number of new cases per year) have been approximate at best. It is clear, however, that diabetes is one of the most common chronic diseases, affecting 1–5 per cent of the total population. The prevalence of diabetes appears to increase in populations which are (a) older, (b) obese, (c) female, (d) Jewish, and (e) well supplied with physicians. Approximately 10 times as many cases of diabetes are diagnosed in people over the age of 45 as in those under 45. The incidence in females is approximately 25 per cent higher than in males. A positive family history increases the frequency 2–4 times. The incidence of diabetes can only be estimated from data from the annual number of newly diagnosed cases, because information of the true appearance of new disease is lacking. Even here, data are scanty but have been estimated at 5–10 per cent of the total number/year, making about 200,000 new cases/year in the United States.

DIAGNOSIS AND DETECTION

Despite the importance of neuropathy, microangiopathy, and large vessel disease to the diabetic syndrome, they are rarely useful in the diagnosis, because the diagnosis has been almost wholly based upon hyperglycemia. This is partly because of the lack of quantitative methods for evaluating the degree of importance of these other findings and partly because none is specific for the diabetic syndrome. However, as mentioned elsewhere, Siperstein measured the basement membrane in biopsy specimens of human muscle and found increased thickness in 97 per cent of overt diabetics. Other investigators have observed these changes less frequently. Futhermore, some consider these abnormalities to be "complications" of the disease, in view of the fact that hyperglycemia usually precedes their diagnosis. The degree of hyperglycemia in some individuals with neuropathy or microvascular disease is so slight that it cannot be clearly distinguished from that of the aging American population, and therefore controversy persists as to whether or not hyperglycemia causes the "complications," or whether they are separate abnormalities in the same syndrome. Our bias is to consider them concomitants.

Carbohydrate Metabolism

Since plasma glucose levels are regulated by many endocrine systems, hyperglycemia may indicate a variety of changes in body metabolism. In carbohydrate tolerance tests of normal populations, therefore, some of the hyperglycemia may be due to physiologically normal states usually related to stress. Thus, in general, tests that are the least sensitive in showing hyperglycemia tend to be the most specific for the diabetic syndrome. To establish a sure diagnosis, it is therefore best to start with the most specific and least sensitive tests and probably to limit the testing to studies which are necessary to make a therapeutic decision. Since at present there is considerable controversy as to which level of blood sugar should induce the physician to treat the patient, the number and type of tests will depend on the willingness of any individual physician to treat the disorder. The tests most generally used are, in order of decreasing specificity, (1) urine glucose plus acetone; (2) fasting plasma glucose; and (3) glucose tolerance test, either oral or intravenous.

Methodology

Urine. Since the major purpose of all of these tests is to estimate abnormalities in glucose metabolism, it is desirable to use routinely only those methods that measure glucose specifically. The most specific method available involves glucose oxidase, which oxidizes glucose to gluconic acid and liberates hydrogen peroxide, which is measured. This is applied to either the blood or the urine. Strips impregnated with the enzyme are available which can quite easily detect 125 mg./100 ml. of glucose in the urine. However, for daily follow-up, the color changes are relatively small, and it may be difficult for a patient to detect accurately the amount of glucose present. Furthermore, some drugs, such as Mercuhydrin and ascorbic acid, may interfere with the detection of glucose by this method. Copper sulfate solutions or Clinitest tablets are the alternative method, but these will also detect other sugars, such as fructose, lactose, galactose, and pentoses; large quantities of drugs, such as salicylates, aminopyrine, para-aminobenzoic acid, chloral hydrate, and ascorbic acid; or normal metabolites, such as uric acid and creatinine. Therefore, there is no ideal urine test. If glucose is present, ketone bodies should also be determined. In general, this is most quickly and conveniently done by use of specially prepared nitroprusside reagent in tablet, stick, or powder form: Acetest tablet, Ketostix, or Labstix (Ames Company, Elkhart, Indiana); Denco Acetone Test Powder (Denver Chemical Manufacturing Company, New York, New York). In either case, the reaction color is much more sensitive to acetoacetic acid than to acetone and, therefore, is only a qualitative evaluation of ketone body excretion. Phthalein, or the urine preservative, 8-hydroxyquinoline, may give false-positive results. In ketoacidosis, the same reagents may be used to semiquantitate, by serial dilution, the extent of ketone body accumulation in serum or plasma.

Blood. Blood analysis of glucose may also rely on glucose oxidase; however, the autoanalyzer is more commonly used with a ferricyanide reagent. This reagent is sensitive to certain nonsugar reducing substances, such as creatinine and bilirubin, the levels of which may be high with uremia and jaundice. A more reliable method, which is specific for hexoses, is the Somogyi-Nelson method, but it is not adaptable to automated analysis. Venous blood glucose has been used for most standard tests, but it is important to remember that arterial or capillary blood values may be considerably higher, particularly during glucose tolerance testing. Furthermore, there is a growing trend to use plasma or serum rather than whole blood in the determination of glucose. This eliminates the complicating factor of anemia as a cause of increased blood glucose values, but in comparing whole blood and plasma, one must remember to make a 14–15 per cent correction. This is due to the lower glucose concentration of the red cells in relationship to their volume. The correction can be calculated using the formula: whole blood glucose = plasma glucose $\times$ [1 minus (0.3 $\times$ hct.)], as described by Dillon. This correction allows one to measure plasma glucose and compare it with published standards based upon whole-blood glucose.

Melituria

Melituria, sugar in the urine, should always make one strongly suspicious of diabetes under any circumstance. However, glycosuria may occur in normal individuals sufficiently to cause a positive reaction in one of the more sensitive glucose oxidase tapes. In addition, some rare individuals have a low renal threshold, which leads to glycosuria at normal blood glucose concentrations (renal glycosuria). During pregnancy, a lower threshold is common and must be distinguished from pathologic hyperglycemia. Certain hexoses and pentoses may cause a positive copper reduction test, such as the Benedict's Test or Clinitest, whereas the more specific glucose oxidase tests are negative, indicating nonglucose melituria. Repeated gross glycosuria without any other underlying cause should be sufficient to make the diagnosis of diabetes. In the fasting state, there will be a gross abnormality of fasting plasma glucose, since glycosuria does not ordinarily occur unless the plasma glucose level exceeds 180–200 mg./100 ml.

Renal Glycosuria

The maximal renal tubular transport rate for glucose is approximately 300–350 mg./min. Thus the presence of glucose in the urine will depend not only on the concentration of arterial glucose but also on the dynamics of glomerular perfusion, filtration rate, individual nephron reabsorption rate, and urine flow. Since these vary considerably from person to person, glucose may appear in the urine at widely varying arterial glucose levels. Most physicians will, therefore, not consider a diagnosis of renal glycosuria unless there is a significant amount of glucose in the urine after an overnight fast. Using this criterion, the syndrome is very rare and probably consists of several related familial genetic defects. In the Joslin Clinic Series reported by Marble, only 85 patients out of 50,000 cases of renal melituria were found. The renal threshold for glucose in this syndrome is altered in two ways: either there is a low tubular transport maximum (low Tm glucose), or there is a change in the relationship between the glucose load and the reabsorbed glucose, such that the maximum is not changed but the efficiency of reabsorption is reduced for any glucose load (increased glucose splay). Some families have one of these abnormalities, but other families have both of the abnormalities, indicating some degree of genetic heterogeneity. Some families demonstrate an autosomal dominant pattern; others suggest an autosomal recessive. Most of the patients do not have an associated abnormality of the GI tract, but a series of patients has been described with both glucose and galactose malabsorption along with renal glycosuria. Aside from this group, the rest of the patients are not ill, absorb and metabolize glucose normally, and are generally asymptomatic.

Fanconi Syndrome

A heterogeneous group of patients with a common defect in tubular reabsorption of a variety of substances can be considered to have the "Fanconi syndrome." Glycosuria is common but is probably one of the least important aspects of the syndrome. This is because of the impairment in the reabsorption of water, PO_4^{3-}, Na^{1+}, HCO_3^{1-}, amino acids and other organic acids. Although cystinosis is one of the more common causes of this syndrome, a wide variety of conditions in which this syndrome occurs are listed Table 9–9. Total glucose loss is small and does not contribute in any significant way to the symptomatology but may alert the clinician to the possibility of primary renal disease.

Nonglucose Melituria

Fructose, galactose, lactose, maltose, mannoheptulose, and L-xylulose have been found in the urine, usually in conjunction with a familial metabolic disorder. All these sugars give a positive copper reduction test but do not react with glucose oxidase. Fructose appears readily in the urine, as

TABLE 9–9. CAUSES OF CYSTINOSIS AND THE FANCONI SYNDROME*

I. Metabolic defect with Fanconi syndrome as a major finding
   A. Cystinosis
   B. Idiopathic
   C. Lowe's syndrome
   D. Tyrosinemia
II. Metabolic defect with Fanconi syndrome not a major finding
   A. Galactosemia
   B. Glycogen storage disease (glucose-6-phosphatase deficiency)
   C. Hereditary fructose intolerance
   D. Wilson's disease
III. Other conditions
   A. Human kidney transplantation
   B. Multiple myeloma
IV. Exogenous toxins
   A. Heavy metals
   B. Lysol (cresol) burn
   C. Maleic acid (in rats)
   D. Methyl-c-chromone
   E. Degraded tetracycline

*From Schneider, J. A., and Seegmiller, J. E., In *The Metabolic Basis of Inherited Disease.* 3rd ed. Stanbury, J. B., Wyngaarden, J. B., et al. (eds.), New York, McGraw-Hill, 1972, p. 1581.

there is no tubular reabsorption of this sugar, and it does not compete with glucose or galactose for absorption or reabsorption. Three separate familial disorders with fructosuria have been described. *Essential fructosuria* is an asymptomatic disorder due to a defect in fructokinase activity, which is inherited as an autosomal recessive trait. This enzyme phosphorylates fructose in the liver, and therefore fructose appears in the urine after an oral load, as it is metabolized more slowly by the nonspecific phosphorylating hexokinases. Approximately 10–20 per cent of the amount of fructose ingested is excreted. It is a benign asymptomatic condition and requires no treatment. A more serious condition, *hereditary fructose intolerance*, is characterized by hypoglycemia (see Ch. 10), nausea, and vomiting following a fructose load, which leads to hepatomegaly, jaundice, Fanconi syndrome, and fructosuria. It is due to a deficiency of fructose-l-phosphate aldolase. There is complete inhibition of glucose output by the liver after fructose ingestion in this disease by a mechanism not completely understood. Most family studies indicate that an autosomal recessive gene is responsible. A similar syndrome with hypoglycemia and fructosuria but without liver disease has been described, called *familial galactose and fructose intolerance* (see Ch. 10), since both sugars produce hypoglycemia. The biochemical and genetic abnormality is completely unknown.

Galactosemia and galactosuria resulting from hereditary defects in the metabolism of galactose have been described as a result of two separate biochemical abnormalities. First, a defect in galactose-1-phosphate-uridyltransferase is found in children and results in nutritional failure, liver disease, cataracts, and mental retardation. This *transferase deficiency galactosemia* is present in a variety of tissues, including the liver and RBC's, and leads to the accumulation of galactose-1-phosphate, which appears to be toxic. The second syndrome, due to *galactokinase deficiency*, is seen in older subjects and leads primarily to cataracts by accumulation of galactitol via an alternative metabolic pathway in the lens. These are both autosomal recessive disorders in which galactosuria is only present after galactose ingestion.

The presence of L-xylulose in the urine has been termed *chronic essential pentosuria*. In contrast to the other syndromes, the sugar is found in the urine regardless of dietary ingestion. This is because there is a block in the metabolism of glucuronic acid at the step in which xylulose is dehydrogenated to xylitol. It is a benign disorder, again due to autosomal recessive gene, primarily restricted to Jews and estimated at 1:40,000 to 1:50,000 in the American population.

Lactosuria occurs physiologically during the period of postpartum lactation. Occasionally lactose may also be found in the urine during the last few days of a normal pregnancy. In the more severe cases of intestinal lactase deficiency, lactose may also appear in the urine, but this is not common in the milder forms of the syndrome.

Fasting Plasma Glucose

Normal fasting plasma glucose in venous plasma is between 60–100 mg./100 ml. Values above 120 mg./100 ml., when confirmed, are usually considered diagnostic of overt diabetes. There is reasonable agreement that fasting hyperglycemia in the absence of complicating illness is sufficient to diagnose diabetes. A substantial number of individuals with apparently abnormal glucose tolerance tests may have normal fasting plasma glucose values. In some clinics, these individuals are considered chemical diabetics, while in others an abnormality of carbohydrate tolerance is recorded but the term "diabetes" is not used. Since no long-term study has been completed, it is not clear what percentage of these people will eventually develop overt diabetes mellitus, nor is it known what may be the relationship between development of other concomitants of the diabetic syndrome and the blood glucose level. In population studies of large vessel disease, there is a linear relationship between blood glucose and atherosclerotic complications. Reliance on the fasting glucose for diagnostic purposes has the advantage that most other metabolic disorders interfering with carbohydrate metabolism do not usually produce fasting hyperglycemia in otherwise normal individuals.

Carbohydrate Tolerance Testing

In order to detect the diabetic syndrome at an earlier stage, carbohydrate tolerance testing has been used extensively in the hope of detecting affected individuals prior to the development of vascular and neurologic problems. It is by far the most sensitive detection device available but suffers from lack of specificity. It is abnormal in a wide variety of diseases and is influenced by dietary and other variables which are often not controlled. In order to use the test accurately, it is essential that it be performed under *standardized* test conditions. Standardized procedures for drawing blood samples should be followed at precise times, and other causes of carbohydrate intolerance should be considered in evaluating the results. Because of the importance of all these variables and the frequency with which one is misled, the authors feel that a random measurement of postprandial blood sugar is unsatisfactory in the diagnosis of the diabetes syndrome and often is misleading when used as a screening or detection test. Since the concentration of the plasma glucose during oral glucose testing depends on (a) the fasting plasma glucose level, i.e., the point of starting, (b) the rate of absorption of glucose, and (c) its uptake by tissues and excretion in urine, it is obvious that the glucose values during the test are only partly related to the utilization of glucose by tissues.

Indications for Oral Glucose Tolerance Test (OGTT)

The following may be used as indications for the OGTT: (a) family history of diabetes; (b) symptoms or signs compatible with diabetes with or without its concomitants (retinopathy, neuropathy, nephropathy, hypercholesterolemia, hypertriglyceridemia, coronary disease, peripheral vascular disease, or cerebrovascular disease, particularly when these are apparent before the age of 50); (c) glucosuria (fasting plasma glucose normal); (d) borderline or abnormal postprandial plasma glucose level (this applies whether the patient is pregnant, sick, or receiving drug treatment at the time of the test); (e) history of spontaneous abortion, premature labor, stillbirth, neonatal death, large baby, hydramnios, or toxemia; (f) high birth weight of the individual to be tested; (g) reactive hypoglycemia, particularly 3 hours or longer after food intake (see Ch. 10).

Conditioning of Subjects for OGTT

It is important to prepare the patient psychologically and physically for the OGTT. Not uncommonly, the patient is told that he will have "a test for diabetes." Since there is great fear and distress in the minds of some patients about the possibility of being labeled diabetic, this can lead to a false-positive result. We strongly emphasize the importance of each subject who is to receive an OGTT having the proper diet preparation for at least 3 days before the test. If he has been on a weight reduction regimen, he should have this dietary preparation for at least 5 days. Each day he should receive a standard diet with maintenance calories, adequate protein, and a minimum of 300 g./day of carbohydrate. Some clinicians state that 150 g./day of carbohydrate is sufficient. However, as emphasized by Seltzer, there are times when this can be inadequate. It is desirable for the subject to fast for 10–12 hours before the test. On the day of the test, he must not have even black coffee or tea and should not smoke. On that day, he should have relatively little exercise and should rest for 30 minutes before the test is started, between 7 and 9 A.M. In every way he should be put at ease mentally and physically before and during the test. If he has an acute illness, the test should be postponed. It is especially important that he not be receiving drugs that influence the test. Indeed, since there are so many that affect it, all of them should be omitted for 3 days prior to the test. Table 9–10 lists some of the many compounds and other conditions that may influence the results of the OGTT.

Glucose Administration and Collection of Plasma Specimens

Venous blood is preferable to capillary specimens (finger-prick or ear-prick), but in infants and

TABLE 9–10. AGENTS AFFECTING GLUCOSE TOLERANCE

Associated with Hyperglycemia		Associated with Hypoglycemia
ACTH	Glucagon	Ethanol
Aldosterone	GH	INH
Caffeine	Indomethacin	MAO inhibitors
Catecholamines	Nicotine	Methimazole
Chlorpromazine	Nicotinic acid	Oxyphenbutazone
Corticosteroids	Oral contraceptives	PAS
Diphenylhydantoin	Chorionic	Probenecid
Ethacrynic acid	somatomammotropin	Propranolol
Furosemide	Thiazides	Salicylates
		Sulfonamide

others offering difficulties with venipuncture, capillary blood can be used. (Capillary blood glucose values are closer to arterial than to venous levels.) After an overnight fast the capillary values are only 2–3 mg. higher than the venous, but after carbohydrate loading in normal subjects, the capillary level may be 20–30 mg./100 ml. higher than venous and remain much higher for more than an hour after glucose ingestion. Capillary glucose levels are distinctly more variable than venous; the flow is often less dependable and may be mixed with lymph. Plasma specimens are more satisfactory than whole blood for glucose analysis. Plasma reflects more accurately the absorption, production, and tissue uptake of glucose. Plasma values are independent of the hematocrit level; variations in hematocrit can account for distinct differences in whole blood glucose levels, since glucose levels in plasma are about 15 per cent higher than those in whole blood. Serum glucose values are about the same as plasma values, but if 2–3 hours are allowed for the blood to clot at room temperature, as much as 40 mg. glucose/100 ml. can disappear from normal blood by means of glycolysis. Therefore, specimens of blood should be refrigerated until clotted, and then serum is separated from clot.

In preparing plasma specimens, an anticoagulant of some type is used—usually oxalate, heparinate, or EDTA. Heparinate is one of the most useful anticoagulants. When measurements of Na^+, K^+, or BUN (urease method) are included, it is desirable to use lithium heparinate rather than the Na^+, K^+, or NH_4^+ derivative. Sodium EDTA (1 mg./ml. blood) can be used as an anticoagulant, but it interferes with various enzyme tests on blood. Blood at room temperature loses ±7mg. glucose/100 ml. per hour; at 4°C. the loss is ±2 mg./100 ml. Fluoride preserves glucose in whole blood when there is 1–2 mg. NaF/ml. blood. This amount of fluoride does not inhibit glucose oxidase activity but prevents significant glycolysis for 8 hours at room temperature and for 48+ hours at 4°C. Fluoride does not inhibit hexokinase activity, which can be used for glucose assay. Even with the use of fluoride, it is desirable to centrifuge the blood within an hour or so and then to refrigerate the plasma. Instead of heparinate, oxalate may be used. Two mg. oxalate powder and 2 mg. fluoride/1 ml. blood are used.

As a challenge, glucose is preferable to a meal, because meals vary in content and in absorption. For example, West reported in middle-aged and older subjects that the 2-hour blood glucose level was 21 mg./100 ml. higher after 75 g. of oral glucose than after breakfast containing 75 g. of carbohydrate. One hour after glucose, it was 49 mg./ml. higher than after the test breakfast. Glucose is preferred to Glucola, but the latter is a satisfactory substitute in some instances when nausea and other GI symptoms are associated with glucose administration, because sometimes it is more palatable. It consists of corn syrup in carbonated water flavored with cola or cherry; 7 oz. contain the equivalent of 75 g. of glucose. False-negative results are sometimes obtained with Glucola.

Glucose, 1.75 g./kg. ideal body weight, is given orally as a 25 per cent solution, permitting up to 5 min. for ingestion. Most normal adults can be given a standard 100 g. of glucose; however, recently some groups have used 40 g./m². Within limits, the amount of glucose makes only a small difference in the type of response.

Urine should be collected hourly throughout the test and glucose measured. Sometimes it is worthwhile also to evaluate the creatinine clearance. Blood specimens are acquired at 0, 1, 1.5, 2, and 3 hours. They are also collected at 4 and 5 hours if a reactive hypoglycemia is suspected. The times for the collection of the specimens are related to the beginning of the swallowing of the glucose solution. In collecting the venous specimens, undue stasis of the blood should be avoided.

Results and Their Interpretation

Ages 15 to 50. As discussed in other parts of this chapter, many factors influence the level of plasma glucose. Thus it is not uncommon that one glucose tolerance test will be inadequate for determining whether a given subject has chemical diabetes. In ascertaining amounts of variation in the results of OGTT in individuals, MacDonald found in 400 male volunteers that, in a series of 6 tests on each individual over a period of 1 year, some had plasma glucose levels that were interpreted as borderline or diagnostic for chemical diabetes, but at other times the tests were normal. On the other hand, there were many who consistently had the same range of plasma glucose values with the OGTT performed 6 times during a year. Since we know that during the early stages of diabetes some patients show marked fluctuations in their diabetic manifestations, we must be cautious in concluding on the basis of a single negative result that a person is free of diabetes, or on the basis of a positive result that he has the disease.

A flat glucose curve is seen occasionally. It may or may not be due to faulty intestinal abosrption; a similar curve is observed occasionally after the intravenous administration of glucose. The most characteristic alterations in the glucose tolerance

curves are (a) increased apogee, (b) delayed return to normal, and (c) late hypoglycemia (3–5 hour interval).

The delay in return of plasma glucose to normal is the most helpful factor in the diagnosis of chemical diabetes; the fasting level is normal in this stage. The apogee tends to be found in the ½-hour specimen; it is quite variable in amount. During OGTT, Conn and colleagues observed hypoglycemia accompanied by symptoms in 110 diabetics, 44 per cent of whom had a family history of diabetes. This usually occurs between 2.5 and 5 hours after glucose ingestion. Table 9–11 gives the upper limit of normal for *plasma* glucose under a variety of circumstances. To consider all the glucose levels collectively has more value and reliability than to consider any one individually. As seen by the Fajans-Conn criteria, chemical diabetes is diagnosed when all 3 values equal or exceed those given. With the criteria of Remein-Wilkerson,

TABLE 9–11. CRITERIA FOR DIAGNOSIS OF CHEMICAL DIABETES BY ORAL GLUCOSE TOLERANCE (ADJUSTED FOR PLASMA GLUCOSE)

	Criteria Based on Plasma Glucose (mg./100 ml.)
Fajans and Conn* 1.75 g./kg. of ideal weight	1 hr. — >185 1½ hr.— >160 2 hr. — >140 All three values abnormal for diagnosis
USPHS — Wilkerson** 100 g. to all subjects	Fasting — >130 = 1 point 1 hr. — >195 = ½ point 2 hr. — >140 = ½ point 3 hr. — >130 = 1 point Points for abnormal values; 2 points for diagnosis
ADA† 40 g./m.²	Fasting — >115 1 hr. — >185 1½ hr.— >165 2 hr. — >140 Elevated fasting or all three values abnormal for diagnosis
Pregnancy — O'Sullivan‡ 100 g. to all subjects	Fasting — >105 1 hr. — >190 2 hr. — >165 3 hr. — >145 Two or three values abnormal for diagnosis
Children — Seltzer§ 1.75 g./kg.	Capillary whole blood Fasting — >115 1 hr. — >175 2 hr. — >140 3 hr. — >125 Elevated fasting or two of three post-test values abnormal for diagnosis

*Ann. N.Y. Acad. Sci. 82:208, 1959.
**J. Chronic Dis. 13:6, 1961.
†Diabetes 18:299, 1969.
‡Diabetes 13:278, 1964.
§Diabetes Mellitus: Theory and Practice. Ellenberg, M., and Rifkin, H. (eds.), New York, McGraw-Hill, 1970, p. 480.

chemical diabetes is indicated if 3 values exceed or equal the 4 values given; with the point system, it is diagnosed when the values equal or exceed 2 points. Some investigators claim that when the sum of the 0-, 1-, 2-, and 3-hour specimens equals or exceeds 600, chemical diabetes is present.

Diabetes in Children

Normal children have a better OGTT than active young adults. Moreover, the curves are slightly lower in children below the age of 6 than in those from 6–13; 25 per cent of these young children have flat OGTT curves (all values less than 110 mg./100 ml.). Thus chemical diabetes using adult standards in children indicates a greater loss of physiologic carbohydrate tolerance than does the same stage in adults (Seltzer). A test with at least 2 values, at 1, 2, and 3 hours above 175, 140, and 125 mg./100 ml. capillary blood, respectively, can be considered as diagnostic of "chemical diabetes."

Diabetes in the Aged

It often is difficult to diagnose diabetes in the elderly group. With the usual OGTT, so many of them are found to have a decreased tolerance that some diabetologists regard this as a normal physiologic change in the aged. However, an important question pertains to whether this change is contributing to the aging process. Andres has recently reviewed the problem of changes in glucose responses with aging. According to a National Health Survey, using oral glucose (50 g.), males showed increase in the 1-hour blood glucose concentration of 10 mg./100 ml./decade; the increase in females was 13 mg./100 ml./decade. The percentage of male subjects with 1-hour values > 160 mg./100 ml. was 1 per cent in the 18–24 year group, 15 per cent in the middle-aged group, and 25 per cent in the 75–79 year group. Females had the values of 5, 25 and 58 per cent, respectively. With a 50 g. dose of glucose, there was a greater deviation from normal after 1 hour than after 2 hours, but the reverse was true with 100 g. On the basis of a series of OGTTs, using 1.75 g. glucose/kg., Andres constructed a nomogram which correlated glucose levels with age (Fig. 9–35). This allows one to compare the ranking of an individual test to an age-matched cohort. Jackson found, in studying 144 healthy, active, elderly subjects living in homes for the aged, none who had previously been designated as having diabetes and 48 per cent who were hyperglycemic with OGTT using conventional criteria. Half of the patients in this initial hyperglycemia group subsequently had symptoms of diabetes within 5 years, whereas most of the control group did so only after 10–20 years. Many other investigators have reported on the increase in blood sugar with advancing age.

Seltzer has suggested that much of the decrease in glucose tolerance observed in the aged groups is due to their relatively low intake of carbohydrate. When two groups of elderly nondiabetics were given glucose (100 g.) before and after high-carbohydrate intake for 3 days, the 2-hour blood sugar level was less in more than 90 per cent of the subjects prepared with extra carbohydrates. Thus almost all the groups studied not given a high-carbohydrate diet had false-positive glucose intolerance. These observations could be of great significance; others should pursue similar investigations.

Intravenous Glucose Tolerance Test (IVGTT)

For satisfactory results with the IVGTT, the same precautions that were emphasized in performing the OGTT must be followed. It is generally used in patients with significant GI disturbances (for example, after stomach operations) and whenever there might be unduly rapid or slow absorption of glucose. It has advantages in that it can be performed within 1 hour, and the results are expressed as a single number. The oral test is more physiologic in that this is the usual mechanism for ingress of food. It stimulates the secretion of several GI hormones, which in turn have a highly significant effect on the secretion and action of insulin.

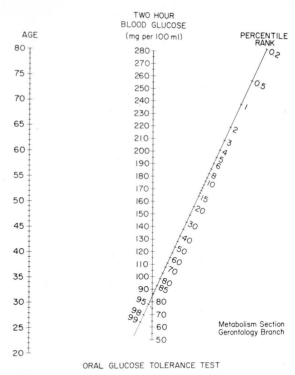

ORAL GLUCOSE TOLERANCE TEST

Figure 9–35.   A nomogram for the determination of percentile performance two hours after an oral glucose load (1.75 g./kg. ideal body weight), showing age corrections. This study is based upon free-living adults with no apparent disease eating their usual diet. (From Andres, R.: *Med. Clin. N. Amer. 55*:841, 1971.)

In most instances, the dose of glucose selected for IVGTT has been 25 g.; more recently the dose of 50 g./1.73 m.[2] body surface area has been employed, or 0.5 g./kg. of body weight. Glucose is usually administered as a 25 or 50 per cent solution, and the infusion is completed within 2–4 min.

The results are expressed by the so-called k value, which signifies the decrease in blood glucose in %/min. The curve forms a straight line on semilogarithmic paper, indicating that the decrease is exponential. When one selects on the abscissa the time interval during which the blood glucose has fallen from a certain value to half that value ("half-time"), the k value can be simply calculated as follows:

$$k = \frac{0.693}{t_{1/2}} \times 100\%/\text{min.}$$

Lundbaek found the average figure for nondiabetic patients to be 1.72. This value declines with age to approximately 1.3. Between 0.9 and 1.1 is a borderline zone. Overt diabetics have k values below this level. The k value is influenced significantly by the effect of insulin on hepatic glucose output and peripheral glucose removal.

Cortisone – Oral Glucose Tolerance Test

The administration of cortisone or other drugs that diminish the peripheral sensitivity to injected insulin may in susceptible subjects impair performance on a carbohydrate tolerance test and, after prolonged administration of large doses, may even lead under certain conditions to the appearance of clinical diabetes mellitus. The long-term follow-up of subjects who demonstrate less than average performance after cortisone trial is unknown, and therefore, at the present time this test often serves only a research function. Subjects receive 50–62.5 mg. of cortisone acetate, 8.5 and 2 hours before an OGTT. A positive test under age 50 consists of plasma glucose values exceeding 185 at 1 hour, 170 at 1.5 hours, and 160 at 2 hours. The finding that subjects with diabetic family histories perform less well than those without such histories has been the greatest stimulus to its use as a diagnostic test. Fajans and Conn reported that only 3 per cent of a control group performed as poorly as 28 per cent of a group of diabetic relatives, with a substantial portion of these individuals eventually receiving a diagnosis of overt diabetes. Performance in this test is also worse in older subjects; therefore, the age of the subject must be taken into account in interpreting the result of the test. Since glucocorticoid administration is known to be followed by increased insulin output in normal subjects, this test appears to determine the ability of the pancreas to augment its insulin secretion.

Intravenous Tolbutamide Tolerance Test

The rapid injection of tolbutamide (1.0 g.) is one of the more reliable tests for insulinoma. It is used less frequently as a diagnostic test for diabetes, although the blood glucose level falls slower and the insulin responses are often less in diabetic subjects. This is not invariably true, and individuals with relatively poor performance on glucose tolerance tests may do reasonably well after intravenous tolbutamide. Again, performance declines with age, and a nomogram has been constructed by Swerdloff. Samples are usually drawn before and at 20 and 30 min. after tolbutamide, and either of these points, or the sum of the two, is used for diagnostic purposes. Best data on performance are available from the nomogram, but at the present time this test is much less sensitive and reliable than the OGTT. For the differential diagnosis of hypoglycemia, the test must be performed over a longer period (see Ch. 10).

Clinical Signs and Symptoms of Diabetes

Signs and symptoms in diabetes may be related solely to the poor metabolism of carbohydrate and overmobilization of fat in this syndrome or result from large and small vessel disease or neuropathy or both. Patients with cardinal clinical signs related to poor carbohydrate metabolism complain of polyuria, polydipsia, polyphagia, weight loss, and loss of strength. Less common are repeated skin infections, particularly vulvar, with or without pruritus, refractive changes with blurring of vision, anorexia, headache, and drowsiness. Such symptoms may be explosive in their onset and are usually related to a coincident infection or some other stress which may simultaneously increase the need for insulin and decrease the ability to secrete it. Sudden onset of symptomatic hyperglycemia is more common in younger subjects but may occur at any age. Milder forms are more stable and appear to develop more slowly and are therefore more common in older age groups. However, it has become clear in screening surveys of high-risk families that many young patients have gross abnormalities of carbohydrate metabolism with minimal symptoms, which can be relatively stable over many years.

Some patients will come to the physician with symptoms related only to atherosclerotic complications, such as myocardial infarction or peripheral vascular disease, or with chronic renal failure secondary to microvascular disease. In others, neuropathy may be the chief complaint, usually a polyneuropathy with pain and numbness as the initiating symptom. A mononeuritis is not unusual, however, and any peripheral nerve may be involved. Here, loss of motor function may be more common. Autonomic insufficiency may be manifested as nocturnal diarrhea, incontinence, nausea, orthostatic hypotension, or impotence. However, complaints related to large vessel disease, microangiopathies and neuropathy increase with duration of known carbohydrate abnormalities and are therefore less likely to be initial complaints. Their listing here emphasizes the basic problem that early diabetes detection is difficult, because often this has been an asymptomatic disease for many years. This fact has led to great emphasis on carbohydrate-tolerance testing as a method of early case-finding. In view of the fact that treatment of chemical diabetes is controversial, except for weight reduction of overweight individuals, the validity and usefulness of carbohydrate testing remains unproven.

PATHOLOGY

Pancreas

The pathology of the pancreas varies greatly in diabetes. Moreover, relatively little is known about the type and quantity of changes that exist before diabetes develops and the extent to which such changes account for the diabetic process. Four types of lesions have been observed: (1) glycogen infiltration of β-cells, (2) hydropic degeneration of the β-cells, (3) hyalinization of the islets, and (4) lymphocytic infiltration of the islets (Fig. 9-36). Despite these findings, as indicated earlier, more than 80 per cent of the pancreas must be removed for frank and permanent hyperglycemia to be produced. This degree of destruction is rarely observed in the average case of diabetes mellitus; however, there is an increased incidence of hyperglycemia in chronic pancreatitis, occasional cases are associated with carcinoma, and there is a definite association between hyperglycemia and hemochromatosis. A decrease in the number of granules in β-cells is common and is accompanied by a decrease in insulin content. Wrenshall found that in normal individuals the amount of insulin extractable from the pancreas correlates best with the body surface area and is greatest in the most obese individuals. The amount of extractable insulin and the number of β-cells increase with age from early childhood until they reach the adult level at age 12–16. In general, diabetic subjects had lesser amounts of insulin than nondiabetic controls. This reduction averaged 40 per cent, but most of the difference was in subjects under the age of 20. It also is important to point out that patients in this study with hypoglycemia rather than hyperglycemia also had very low levels of pancreatic insulin. Thus low extractable insulin levels did not necessarily correlate with a decreased insulin secretion. In animals, low granulation states have been observed under conditions of very large insulin secretion, presumably depleting stores, and in conditions where insulin secretion has been very low for long periods, presumably due to atrophy of stores.

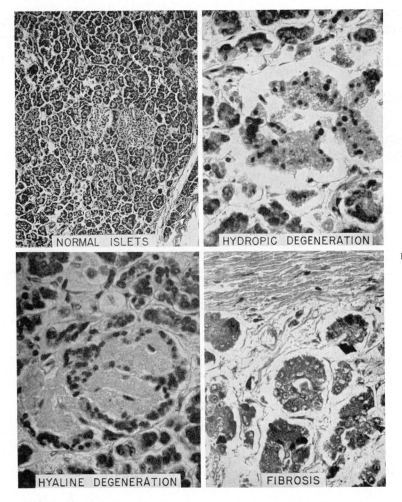

Figure 9-36. Islet changes found in patients with diabetes mellitus.

Among other pancreatic pathologic changes associated with diabetes, the most common is vacuolation of the β-cells. These vacuoles give a positive PAS reaction, suggesting glycogen within them. Such alterations are usually only found at autopsy when there has been consistent untreated hyperglycemia, and they do not occur in the treated diabetic syndrome. Similar findings are observed in untreated experimental diabetes, in which there may also be an increase in glycogen of the ductular epithelium. Occasionally, these vacuoles become complex and contain lipids as well as carbohydrates. Such lesions have been called "hydropic degeneration" and have been considered by some to be precursors to β-cell death.

Hyalinization of the islets is relatively common, occurring in approximately 30–40 per cent of diabetics examined. This hyaline material consists of deposits of a homogeneous, subendothelial, acidophilic substance. A similar material may be found in nondiabetic subjects. There is a better correlation between the amount of hyaline and the age of the patient than between the former and the duration of severity of the carbohydrate abnormality. There is considerable evidence that this hyaline material is, or closely resembles, amyloid, which has raised questions regarding autoimmunity in the causation of diabetes mellitus. Such suppositions have been somewhat strengthened by the lymphocytic infiltrations observed in the absence of generalized pancreatic inflammatory disease in young diabetics examined soon after the onset of diabetes. This finding has been termed "insulitis" and is of interest since similar inflammatory changes have been found in the islets of cows and rabbits immunized with homologous insulin. However, any association between diabetes and immunologic abnormalities remains speculative.

The Cardiovascular System

Morphologic aberrations involving the entire vascular system are seen. Those in the larger arteries and coronary circulation can appear in nondiabetic subjects but seem to be more frequent and to occur at an earlier age in the diabetic population. There appears to be no specific morphologic lesion related to diabetes, however; rather, the atherosclerotic process appears to be accelerated (Strandness). The capillaries are also involved with a pathologic process which leads to thickening of the basal lamina or basement membrane. Although this may be seen occasionally in other conditions, the lesion is often so characteristic that in the kidney it is termed diabetic nephropathy, in the eye, diabetic retinopathy, and in the muscle, diabetic basement membrane thickening. Cardiovascular lesions account for 75–80 per cent of the total mortality in diabetes and have therefore assumed great importance as the cause of premature death in this syndrome. The degree of vascular disease does not appear to be proportional to the alterations in carbohydrate metabolism but rather correlates best with the duration of the disease and the age of the patient. White, for example, found that there was a 92 per cent incidence of vascular disease in juvenile diabetics studied for more than 20 years. This acceleration of the vascular process greatly reduces the differences between the sexes. Therefore, the presence of diabetes in females aged 20–50 years is likely to increase the frequency of cardiovascular disease eight- to tenfold.

Large Vessel Arterial Disease

This has been termed arteriosclerosis and consists of two independent but related processes—atherosclerosis and medial calcification. Atherosclerosis consists of the accumulation of lipids in the subintimal tissues of arteries to form lipid-filled plaques or atheromas. The lipid appears to be deposited or synthesized in smooth muscle cells that proliferate and migrate from the media into the intima and become transformed into foamy cells. These cells eventually rupture, leading to the noncellular deposition of lipid (Fig. 9–37). The fatty plaques then can undergo further changes, such as fibrosis, calcification, and ulceration, eventually leading to thrombosis and arterial occlusion.

For reasons that are not completely clear, advanced vascular disease in the lower legs is common in diabetics and particularly severe, leading to gangrene or death of the affected extremity. Diabetics also develop atherosclerotic complications in the cerebral circulation and in the renal and mesenteric circulations, leading to occlusive disease and complications in these organs as well. It has been suggested that the concomitant neuropathy and loss of pain and touch sensation may explain the high frequency of lower-leg vascular disease seen in the diabetic population; however, there may be an interaction between capillary microangiopathy and arteriosclerosis which is also important.

Medial calcification or Mönckeberg's calcific medial sclerosis may also lead to an increased firmness in the arterial wall and thus can contribute to arteriosclerosis. The process by which calcium is deposited in the muscular wall is unknown; however, it is independent of atherosclerosis and ordinarily does not lead to vascular occlusion. It may occur in nondiabetic individuals, but in patients below the age of 40, diabetes is almost always present. Since calcification also occurs in the complicated atherosclerotic lesion, it is not possible to determine from a roentgenogram whether one is dealing with atherosclerosis or medial calcification. It has been reported by Lindbum that there is a tendency for medial calcification and atherosclerosis not to affect simultaneously the same portions of the artery.

Arteriolosclerosis

This appears to be an entirely separate pathologic process which is prominent in diabetics but

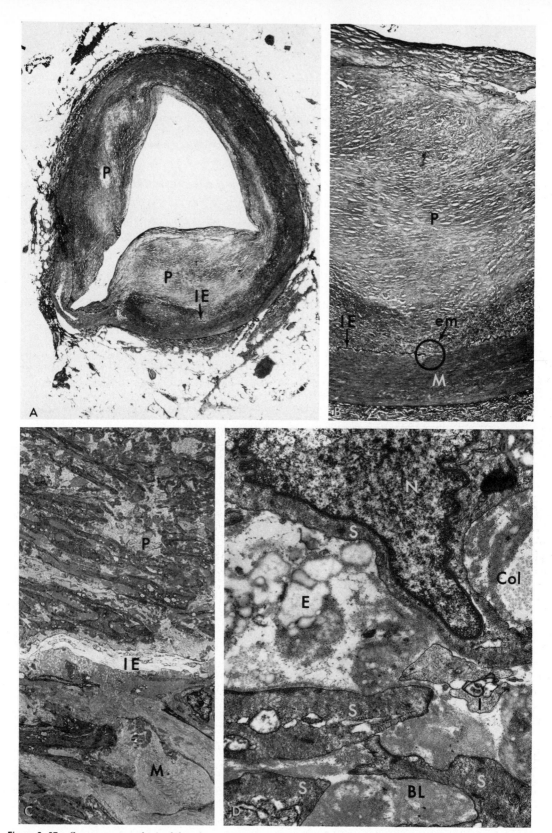

Figure 9–37. Coronary artery obtained three hours post mortem from male, aged 52, with atherosclerosis. *A*, Cross section of artery near branch point (× 20). P indicates each of two fibrous plaques; IE is internal elastic membrane delimiting plaque from arterial media. *B*, Magnification (× 63) of portion of lower plaque seen in *A* compared with media (M). Lighter color of plaque (P) shows presence of abundant collagen and basement lamina material surrounding cells. *C*, Electron micrograph (× 1800) of region indicated in *B* at base of plaque. Cells in plaque region (P) are somewhat distorted smooth muscle cells. Larger smooth muscle cells in more regular arrays appear under the internal elastic membrane (IE) in the media (M). *D*, Electron micrograph (× 14,500) showing portions of four smooth muscle cells (S) forming the plaque. N is a portion of nucleus of one cell. Collagen (Col), some elastic (E), and much basal lamina (BL) type material are irregularly distributed between the cells. Lipid present but not evident is *not* a prominent feature of this plaque, as is frequently the case with other plaques. (Courtesy of Dr. Earl P. Benditt and Dr. Ned Moss.)

indistinguishable from that found in essential hypertension. It appears as a concentric hyaline thickening of the arterioles, widening of the endothelium, and eventual encroachment on the vascular lumen by a plaque which stains with PAS. There is some evidence that this material is related to, or resembles, basement membrane, since it is PAS-positive and presumably contains glycoprotein. However, the exact nature of the deposit is unknown. Prevalent sites in the diabetic are the kidney, particularly if the individual has had clinical nephropathy, but other organs, including the pancreas, are frequently involved.

Capillary Microangiopathy

Although arterioles and venules may be similarly affected, the morphologic feature which best characterizes diabetic microangiopathy is a thickened capillary basement membrane. This thickening has been reported in practically every capillary bed, including skin, skeletal muscle, adipose tissue, kidney, pancreas, and peripheral nerves; however, it has been best documented and studied in skeletal muscle capillaries and kidney. The involvement is not global, however, and even within the various skeletal muscles some areas may be thicker than others. The lesion has been reported by Siperstein to occur in a significant number of in-

dividuals with prediabetes (potential diabetes). These observations have given greater support to the concept that the vascular lesions of diabetes are concomitants of the disease. Although some have suggested that this lesion is specific for diabetes, recent evidence suggests that it occurs in other disease, although rather rarely, and is then usually associated with some type of inflammatory process.

Recently it has been suggested by Vracko that basal lamina provides a microskeleton for cellular regeneration and that its apparent thickening may be related to cell turnover. According to this concept, the "thickening" is due to accumulation of abnormally large numbers of normally thick layers of basal lamina, each layer being deposited by a cell generation replication. This intriguing idea, which indicates that accumulated layers of basal lamina reflect an accelerated cell turnover in the diabetic population, requires further evaluation. Examples of a normal-appearing basal lamina in skeletal muscle capillary and accumulation of multiple layers as the process occurs with advancing age in a nondiabetic subject and in diabetes mellitus are shown in Figure 9–38. All investigators agree that long-term diabetics, regardless of treatment, have thickened basement membranes in comparison with suitably matched control subjects; however, Williamson found that this is an age-related phenomenon; that is, the basement

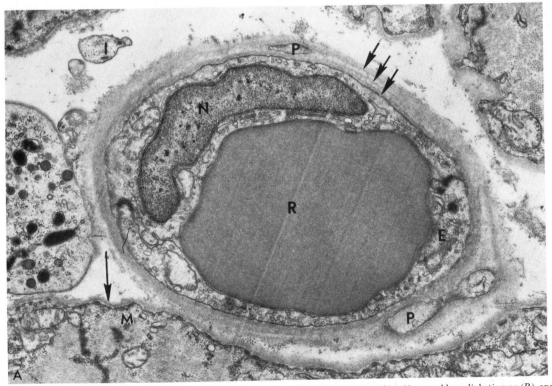

Figure 9–38. Cross sections of tibial skeletal muscle from a 9-year-old nondiabetic boy (*A*), a 69-year-old nondiabetic man (*B*), and a 68-year-old diabetic man (*C*), showing portions of muscle fibers (M), their basal lamina (long arrows), interstitial cells (I) and capillaries composed of basal lamina (short arrows), pericytes (P), endothelium (E), endothelial nuclei (N), and red blood cells (R). *A* shows structures as they normally occur in a young individual. In *B* and *C*, the basal lamina investment is "thickened" because of the accumulation of abnormal numbers of basal lamina layers (short arrows).

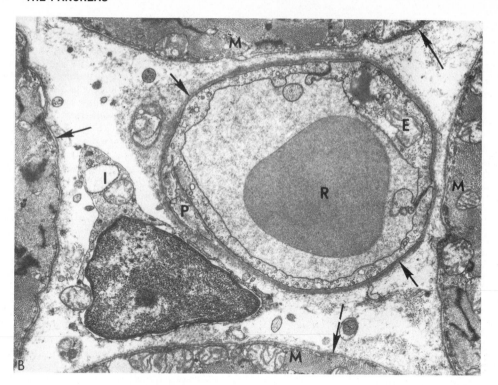

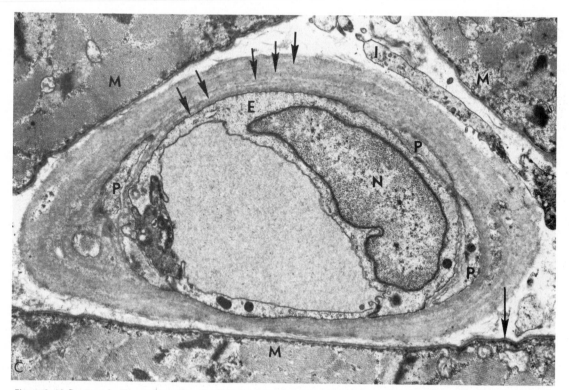

Figure 9–38 *Continued.* The capillary from the diabetic (*C*) has accumulated at least five layers, while that from the aged nondiabetic has three layers. Cell debris, which is present between the layers of basal lamina in diabetic capillaries, indicates that cell death has occurred. That basal lamina layers have not been produced by the same cell generation is suggested by the presence of a single layer of basal lamina between pericytes and endothelial cells. Layering of basal lamina identical to that seen in *B* and *C* can be produced in nondiabetic animals by alternating cycles of endothelial cell death and regeneration. All electron micrographs are shown at approximately the same magnification (× 14,700). (Electron micrographs and their interpretation have been provided by Dr. Rudolf Vracko.)

membrane gets thicker normally with aging, and this age-effect is a critical factor in estimating the degree of thickening. Siperstein did not find an age-related effect, nor did he find the duration or degree of carbohydrate intolerance important in its intensity. It seems likely that further investigation will demonstrate that both groups of investigators are correct; that is, basement membrane thickening does occur as part of the aging process, and this is exaggerated in diabetes. It may occur prior to, or independently of, the carbohydrate abnormality as an integral part of the diabetic syndrome, but the duration of carbohydrate intolerance increases the chance of finding such a lesion.

Despite the use of muscle capillary basement membranes to investigate this lesion, the primary clinical importance of microangiopathy is related to chronic renal disease and blindness due to retinal involvement, the kidney and the eye being the two organs most clearly associated with severe functional deterioration. The cause of this basement membrane thickening is unclear, largely because there is little known about the normal composition, origin, and function of the basement membrane. Recent studies by Spiro have greatly expanded our knowledge of the glycoprotein contained within this structure. His analysis has been based upon the glomerular basement membrane, in which carbohydrates comprise about 10 per cent of the glycoprotein as glucose, galactose, mannose, hexosamines, sialic acids, and fucose. It is of interest that this is one of the few glycoproteins that has been shown to contain glucose. There are unusually large amounts of hydroxyproline and hydroxylysine. This hydroxylysine content is of importance, because a large number of these residues are involved in the linkages to a disaccharide unit containing glucose and galactose (Fig. 9–39). In his studies of the diabetic basement membrane, a normal composition was found, except for an increased amount of hydroxylysine residues and an increase in the hydroxylysine-linked disaccharide units. From these findings, he has postulated the increased availability of glucose for glycoprotein synthesis as being in part responsible for the chemical abnormality described. The finding in experimental diabetes of increased glucosyltransferase activity, an enzyme responsible for the assembly of the hydroxylysine-linked disaccharide units of the glomerular basement membrane, which is reversed by insulin, has suggested to him that this enzymatic activity may be involved in the abnormal production of glycoproteins in diabetes mellitus. Spiro's postulate is that the hyperglycemia of diabetes causes excessive basement membrane synthesis, because the kidney is an organ which utilizes glucose without insulin being present. This of course conflicts with the evidence that the degree of hyperglycemia, or even its presence, does not correlate well with basement membrane thickening and the finding by Siperstein that individuals without carbohydrate intolerance may have thickened basement membranes. Resolution of these conflicts awaits further research.

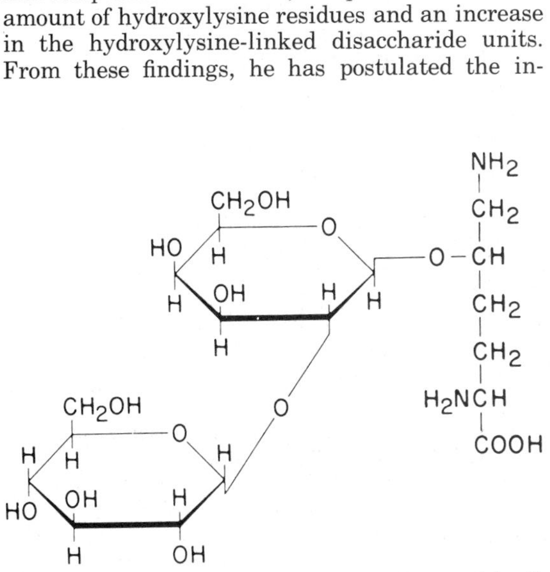

The Nervous System

Dysfunction of the brain, spinal cord, and peripheral nerves appears to be an integral part of the diabetic syndrome. It had been claimed, particularly by Fagerberg from vascular performance studies in diabetes, that there is a vascular cause for the peripheral neuropathy, partly because the two lesions appear to progress simultaneously in many diabetic subjects. However, since both the vascular abnormality and the peripheral neuropathy are dependent upon time and duration of illness, one does not necessarily cause the other. More recent evidence obtained by electron microscopic examination of nerves suggests that the early lesion is a thickening of the Schwann cell basement membrane and a segmental demyelinization as described by Thomas and Lascelles. Eventually, however, one may find marked degeneration of the dorsal root ganglia and associated axons. These observations of morphologic changes in the nerves have been partly substantiated by biochemical analysis of nerve biopsy specimens, which show changes in the lipid composition. The pathology of any changes occasionally found in the spinal cord and central nervous system is obscure.

Although the autonomic nervous system (ANS) is frequently involved, the mechanism by which these abnormalities occur appears to be very poorly studied except for one investigation which showed dendrite degeneration in the peripheral sympathetic ganglia. An abnormality of afferent input into the autonomic nervous system has been primarily implicated by Whalen in the gastrointestinal tract since jejunal dilation is not followed by pain. This has been reinforced by studies showing that postganglionic efferent autonomic pathways remain intact, because transmitter drugs produce normal reactions.

Despite the evidence for permanent structural damage to the nerves, clinical neuropathy varies greatly from time to time, suggesting either that

Figure 9–39. Structure and peptide attachment of the disaccharide unit of the glomerular basement membrane (2-*O* α-D-glucopyranosyl-*O*-β-D-galactopyranosylhydroxylysine). (From Spiro, R. G.: *J. Biol. Chem.* 242:4813, 1967.)

these lesions can be repaired or that the function of these nerves is also dependent upon metabolic or functional changes that are in part reversible.

SPECIFIC ORGAN INVOLVEMENT

Heart

Atherosclerotic coronary heart disease is the commonest cause of death in diabetics (Fig. 9–40). Partamian found that coronary heart disease accounted for 53.3 per cent of the deaths in diabetics. Within 2 months of the initial myocardial infarction, 38 per cent had died; 54.7 per cent of those with a subsequent myocardial infarct died. Only 37.8 per cent of those with a subsequent infarct survived more than 5 years. Other reports indicate that among nondiabetics with myocardial infarctions 49–83 per cent survive more than 5 years. In diabetic subjects, females experienced infarcts somewhat more frequently than males. Those with myocardial infarcts frequently had other vascular concomitants, such as retinopathy and glomerulosclerosis or peripheral vascular disease or both. The incidence of coronary disease is dependent to some extent on the duration of the diabetes, the degree of hyperglycemia, the age of the patient, and the presence of other complicating illnesses, such as hypertension and obesity. The presence of ketoacidosis during acute myocardial infarction worsens the prognosis. Population studies have shown a relationship between atherosclerotic complications and blood sugar. Therefore the question arises whether some atherosclerosis has as its basis, at least in part, a subnormal glucose utilization which in turn affects lipid and protein metabolism, or whether some common underlying abnormality leads to both hyperglycemia and atherosclerosis.

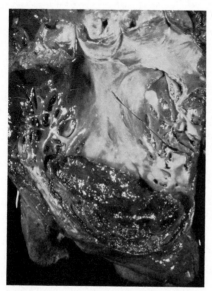

Figure 9–40. Myocardial infarction resulting from coronary atherosclerosis, the commonest cause of death in diabetics.

Treatment

Glycosuria tends to get worse when diabetic patients have myocardial infarction. If the patient's illness is particularly unstable, it may be advisable to follow a treatment program suitable for mild ketoacidosis, in which insulin and fluid therapy are evaluated every 6 hours. Anticoagulants and other treatments usually used in myocardial infarction without diabetes are administered. It is important to avoid hypoglycemia, because this has been known to induce a coronary occlusion. For this reason, the insulin therapy should not be quite as vigorous as it might be otherwise. On the other hand, one must control the glycosuria to prevent excessive fluid and electrolyte loss. Obese adult subjects will require more insulin than thin subjects to lower the blood sugar.

A high proportion of individuals who previously have not been regarded as having diabetes are noted to have glycosuria and hyperglycemia at the time of an acute myocardial infarction. Thus the question is raised whether such individuals have diabetes. When the hyperglycemia and glycosuria last 2 weeks or longer, the diagnosis of diabetes is likely. When they last only a few days, diagnosis is uncertain but this is likely to be stress hyperglycemia. Diabetes should be suspected and the patient checked with respect to its possible progression. Treatment during the acute phase depends on the degree of carbohydrate imbalance regardless of the diagnosis.

Prevention

An effort should be made to reduce risk factors for atherosclerosis. Weight reduction is instituted when there is obesity. Hypertension is lowered when present. Regular exercise of moderate degree is encouraged. Smoking should be omitted. Control of the carbohydrate abnormalities is discussed elsewhere. Hyperlipidemia should be considered and treated as indicated.

Peripheral Vessels

Peripheral occlusive vascular disease is primarily due to atherosclerosis and is not related to medial calcification, which is also common in diabetes. Although all the larger arteries may be involved to varying degrees with atherosclerosis, it is more common and severe in the arteries of the legs.

Symptoms of peripheral vascular disease are rare before the age of 50. They are most typically those of intermittent claudication, with coldness of the feet, pain, and various parasthesias — burning, tingling, and numbness. The numbness may be due either to vascular narrowing or to an associated neuropathy. On physical examination the skin of the lower legs and feet appears atrophic, shiny, and cool, with marked redness in the dependent position and a waxy pallor on elevation of the legs. A dependent rubor is a sign of arterial insufficiency when there is no venous stasis. The volume of pulsation of the posterior tibial artery and the dorsalis pedis artery of the foot varies markedly. At times pulsations may be normal, but sometimes they may be reduced or imperceptible.

Although hypertension contributes to atherosclerosis in some instances, one third of the diabetics with gangrene are found not to have hypertension. Gangrene develops as rapidly in diabetics with mild carbohydrate abnormalities as in diabetics with severe carbohydrate intolerance. In some patients with gangrene, a carbohydrate abnormality is not apparent until later. Bartels, for example, studied 100 consecutive patients with peripheral vascular disease of the lower extremities; the patients were unselected except that all those who had a history of diabetes or glycosuria were eliminated. There was some evidence of abnormal glucose tolerance in 59 per cent. Only 23 per cent of the entire group had entirely normal results. Thus, in patients with peripheral vascular disease, carbohydrate intolerance appears to be unusually common.

Goldner reported on the natural history of diabetes in 71 patients with amputation of one limb. Other concomitants were common: 8 per cent had retinitis, 36 per cent nephropathy, and 63 per cent neuropathy. However, in more than 50 per cent, the carbohydrate metabolism had been under fair control. Twenty-nine of the 41 patients studied within 2 years of amputation had lesions of the second leg, and 47 of the 71 studied had involvement of the second leg within 5 years after involvement of the first. Thirty-two of these 47 subsequently had to have the other leg amputated. These observations emphasize the progressive nature of the disease.

Vasodilators are not of much help, possibly because they dilate the more healthy blood vessels and probably draw blood away from the sclerotic ones. Exercise is good, and walking to the point of claudication should be encouraged. Buerger's exercises or some modifications are also indicated. Tobacco should be avoided. Endarterectomy is rarely indicated, and bypass operations are not often of much help. Alcohol injection into the nerve fibers and sympathectomy rarely prove to be of any significant value.

Gangrene

Complete occlusion of a major vessel may lead to gangrene. An occasional instance of gangrene of the upper extremities has been reported, and the mesenteric arteries may be involved sufficiently to produce abdominal angina and mesenteric infarction. In diabetics, the frequency and the degree of involvement of the lower extremities are the same for both sexes; in nondiabetics such gangrene is distinctly more common in males. Bell found that gangrene was 156 times more frequent in diabetics than in nondiabetics in the fifth decade, and 85 times more common in the seventh. An important but often overlooked factor is the concomitant peripheral neuropathy which may contribute to this high incidence of gangrene by lack of recognition of leg trauma.

Gangrene may involve small areas or an entire foot or leg (Fig. 9–41). In one study, the gangrene extended above the ankle in only 7 per cent of diabetics compared with 50 per cent of nondiabetics. This is probably because atherosclerosis in the smaller arteries is more common in diabetics than in nondiabetics and possibly because of microangiopathy. When the larger arteries are occluded, the gangrene tends to be massive, whereas it tends to be spotty with occlusions of the smaller arteries and arterioles. Spotty distribution is found in 70 per cent of diabetics. Fifteen to 25 per cent of diabetics with gangrene have been reported to have normal or only slightly decreased pulsations in the corresponding dorsalis pedis artery. There is a better opportunity for developing a collateral circulation with atherosclerotic occlusion when only the larger vessels are involved, possibly because the smaller blood vessels that will participate in the collateral circulation are available. Therefore, gangrene results from an occlusion more often in diabetics with frequent smaller artery involvement.

The major goal is prevention of gangrene by avoiding trauma and infection and by not restricting blood flow. The patient can accomplish this to some extent by keeping the feet clean, applying lanolin or some other bland ointment to hard, dry areas on the feet, wearing clean footwear, avoiding garters, wearing only properly fitting shoes, avoiding undue exposure to cold and heat, trimming the toenails carefully and inserting a wedge of cotton under ingrowing toenails, removing calluses by soaking in warm water and rubbing off the surplus skin with a coarse towel, avoiding the use of adhesive on the skin, and treating associated epidermophytoses. Despite these measures, gangrene may still occur. When present, it may be wet or dry. Since the pathology and clinical picture of these two types differ, they are discussed separately.

Dry Gangrene

This can be defined as tissue necrosis resulting from arterial occlusion. It often starts in association with trauma of a mechanical, thermal, or chemical type. The swelling induced by the injury further impairs an already poor circulation, and consequently the tissue dies. Corns and calluses are frequently the sites at which gangrene begins. When dry gangrene appears, the patient should be kept in bed and the gangrenous area exposed to air free of dressings, antiseptics, or ointments. It is advisable to cover the foot with a cradle which will prevent pressure from the covers. The leg should be placed so that pressure to the heel is avoided. Heat should not be used because this increases the oxygen demand and thereby makes the gangrene worse. The head of the bed should be elevated slightly so that the feet are about 8 inches below

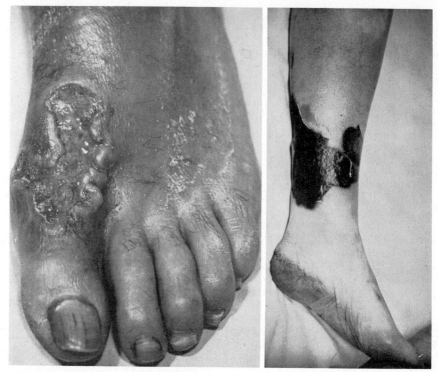

Figure 9–41. Gangrene in diabetics, produced by two different mechanisms. Left, the more common type of gangrene is due to diabetic angiopathy; only part of the foot is involved. Right, gangrene is due to atherosclerosis of the large arteries of the leg, involving the entire lower leg; this type of gangrene occurs in nondiabetics as well as in diabetics. Gangrene is over 40 times more common in diabetics than nondiabetics.

the level of the heart. Buerger's exercises may be used. Salicylates or Butazolidin are given for pain. Every effort is made to control carbohydrate metabolism. The aim in the treatment of dry gangrene is to promote mummification and a sharp line of demarcation between the dead and the viable tissue. This is then followed by a conservative amputation.

Wet Gangrene

This can be defined as tissue death complicated by infection. The outcome depends on whether the trouble is caused predominantly by vascular insufficiency or by infection. Surgical drainage, antibiotics, and intermittent use of wet dressings are often employed for wet gangrene, but amputation is indicated unless the process largely clears in a couple of weeks. Roentgenograms should be taken to determine whether osteomyelitis is present. Either type of gangrene commonly requires eventual amputation.

Kidney

Two nephropathies occur almost exclusively in diabetes: nodular glomerulosclerosis and tubular nephrosis. There are, in addition, several other renal lesions that are less specific for diabetes but that occur with increased frequency: diffuse glo-

merulosclerosis, atherosclerosis, arteriosclerosis, pyelonephritis, necrotizing papillitis, acute tubular necrosis, and toxemia of pregnancy.

Glomerulosclerosis (GS)

On the basis of the differences in the pathologic appearance, there are three types of GS: nodular, diffuse, and exudative.

Nodular Glomerulosclerosis

This lesion is found in about one quarter of diabetic patients dying in hospitals. It is characterized by spherical nodules 20–100 μ in diameter situated at the periphery of the glomerular capillary tufts (Fig. 9–42). They appear laminated and have one or more layers of nuclei embedded around the circumference. There are prominent reticulin fibers and deposition of significant quantities of PAS-positive glycoproteins as well as of other carbohydrates and lipids. This material by electron microscopy appears as nodular accumulations of "basement membrane" in the mesangium. This is the most specific glomerular lesion of diabetes and has also been called Kimmelstiel-Wilson syndrome or nodular intercapillary GS. Kimmelstiel and Wilson (1936) concentrated on the nodular form, but the more common and less specific diffuse lesion was described by Bell. It is this type of

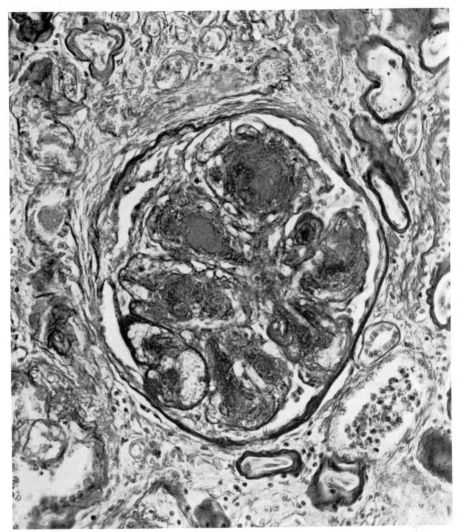

Figure 9–42. Nodular glomerulosclerosis. A considerable amount of PAS-positive material is present. Since the changes involve essentially all glomeruli, it is easy to see how the nephrotic syndrome and uremia are produced. This patient also had chronic and acute pyelonephritis, arteriosclerosis, retinopathy, neuropathy, and a small myocardial infarction. (Alcian blue PAS stain.) (Courtesy of Dr. Karl Mottet.)

lesion, however, that accounts for uremia in most insulin-dependent diabetes. It is desirable to drop the "intercapillary" terminology in relation to this syndrome, because the changes are primarily in the mesangium.

Diffuse Glomerulosclerosis

This condition consists of thickening of the capillary basement membrane. Except in the early stages, all the loops of the glomerular tufts are involved, though not to the same degree. The capillary lumens are reduced in size and eventually become occluded. The thickened basement membrane, which is PAS-positive, then spreads to involve the endothelial cells, leading eventually to extensive diffuse deposits. In contrast to nodular GS, however, reticulin fibers are not demonstrable.

This lesion is more common in diabetics than in nondiabetics, but it is less specific for diabetes than is nodular GS. In diabetics, it is believed that the diffuse lesion is the precursor of the nodular lesion.

Exudative Glomerulosclerosis

This is the least common of the three lesions and the least specific for diabetes. Its mechanism and pathology appear to be entirely different. Part of the deposit is seen as a clear, intensely eosinophilic substance within Bowman's space but attached to the capsular surface of the glomerular tuft. It shows staining characteristics of fibrinoid. It does not contain collagen but does contain triglyceride, cholesterol, and PAS-positive polysaccharides. A lesion similar to the exudative type has been produced in animals by cortisone administration.

Clinical Considerations

The ability to diagnose diabetic nephropathy can be improved by frequent consideration of the relatively large proportion of the diabetics who eventually develop it. For example, renal biopsies of 51 diabetics—half without clinically diagnosed renal disease—were reported by Salomon. He concluded that "all patients with diabetes had some glomerular alterations." The major lesion was diffuse GS due to thickening of the capillary basement membrane and prominence of the intercapillary space or mesangium. In the more severe cases, the same material accumulated to produce nodules. He found no correlation between the degree of diabetic nephropathy and the degree of systemic involvement of the cardiovascular or nervous system. It may be expected clinically in 50 per cent of diabetics who survive more than 20 years; it is present in essentially all insulin-dependent diabetics who survive for 20 years. Consequently, the physician must look every 1–2 years for decreased creatinine clearance in all diabetics and later for azotemia. The urine characteristically shows proteinuria, white blood cells, and casts. These alterations increase in intensity as the process becomes advanced, and hypoalbuminemia with the nephrotic syndrome, nitrogen retention, and hypertension may be observed. The degree of these changes is an indication, at least partial, of the intensity of the GS. As renal impairment becomes severe, a decrease in glycosuria may be noted. This is due partly to the decrease in glomerular filtration and to the relatively greater impairment of glomerular function than of tubular function, permitting reabsorption of a relatively greater proportion of the filtered glucose. This decrease in glycosuria may also be due to the fact that the degradation of insulin, which normally occurs to a significant extent in the kidneys, is reduced, so that a given amount of insulin is more effective.

The alterations of renal function occurring with GS are not pathognomonic of this condition; therefore, it is important to be sure that this is of diabetic etiology if only minimal hyperglycemia is present. One should (1) ascertain whether other microangiopathies are present, and (2) attempt to eliminate other nephropathies that might account for the renal changes under observation. Evidence for renal infection should also be sought. It should be emphasized, however, that pyelonephritis is very commonly associated with diabetes and, indeed, often coexists with GS. Occasionally, a renal biopsy is indicated, since it is usually not difficult to establish the diagnosis when opportunity is afforded to study the tissue. Some studies have suggested that the more poorly controlled the carbohydrate metabolism, the greater the incidence and severity of GS. However, it may be that the poor control is not due to lack of proper effort or ability on the part of either the patients or the physician; it may simply be that the diabetic process is more intense in these subjects. Moreover, the severity of the GS is not well correlated with the intensity of the carbohydrate abnormality. Sometimes GS is observed even before there is evidence of hyperglycemia and glycosuria. At the other extreme, severe alterations in carbohydrate metabolism may exist over many years with no clinical or microscopic evidence of GS. In the absence of a prospective study, the relation between control of carbohydrate metabolism and nephropathy remains unclear.

As the GS progresses, the physician has the problem of dealing with the nephrotic syndrome, uremia, cardiac failure, and other manifestations of microangiopathy, such as retinopathy and blindness. Numerous symptomatic measures may be employed. Nevertheless, the disease process tends to be progressive and irreversible once it has become advanced. In a few instances chronic renal dialysis has been performed. Diabetic patients have not fared well, and therefore this must still be considered an experimental procedure.

Tubular Nephrosis

In tubular nephrosis, tubular epithelial cells show vacuoles containing glycogen. These are especially common in the proximal tubules. Their presence is well-correlated with the degree of hyperglycemia and is probably reversible. There does not appear to be an associated tubular functional abnormality. When GS is present, a similar peritubular PAS-positive polysaccharide is often found, possibly related to similar basement membrane thickening.

Arteriolosclerosis and Atherosclerosis

Bell found severe atherosclerosis in the small renal arteries in 83 per cent of diabetics aged over 50 examined post mortem. Hyalinization of the arterioles (arteriolosclerosis) was equally common and tended to involve both the efferent and the afferent juxtaglomerular arterioles. The efferent arteriolar involvement is almost pathognomonic for diabetes. The renal involvement from atherosclerosis and hyaline arteriolosclerosis does not appear different from this type of vascular disease seen in other organs and tissues.

Infections of the Kidney and Urinary Tract

Frequently infection develops in the kidney or urinary tract or both. It is important to detect such developments promptly and to eliminate them. The infection intensifies the manifestations of the diabetes and may also eventually lead to significant impairment in kidney function. The most important considerations are to look for and correct obstructions and to select the most appropriate antibacterial compound and give it in sufficiently large doses to eliminate the infection completely. Catheterization in general should be avoided as much as possible, and this applies all the more to the diabetic. Carefully collected, clean, voided specimens can be used both for immediate direct examination and for urine cultures.

Pyelonephritis

As mentioned earlier, pyelonephritis is frequent in diabetics. When glucose is present in the urine, it may be more difficult to eradicate the infection. Under such conditions, improved carbohydrate regulation should be combined with antimicrobial therapy.

Necrotizing Renal Papillitis

This is a very acute, relatively rare form of pyelonephritis associated with severe infection, which produces ischemic necrosis of the renal papillae (Fig. 9–43). It occurs in diabetics much more often than in nondiabetics. It is characterized by fever, hematuria, renal colic, and rapidly advancing azotemia. Characteristic pyelographic changes are observed, and sloughed portions of the renal papillae may be found in the urine. The bacteria involved should be identified and treatment based upon their drug sensitivity.

Acute Tubular Necrosis

Acute tubular necrosis occasionally occurs as a complication of diabetic coma, usually when there are prolonged periods of hypotension and shock.

Toxemias of Pregnancy

There is an increased incidence of preeclampsia and eclampsia in diabetes. The glomeruli may become enlarged and ischemic. There is swelling of the epithelial cells, basement membrane, and endothelial cells. The major clinical changes are hypertension, proteinuria, and edema, sometimes with intermittent retinal vascular spasm. Convulsions may also develop.

The Eye

Retina

Changes in the retinas of diabetics are common and among the most characteristic findings in the syndrome. Because of the opportunity for direct observation, the changes in the eyes may be followed more accurately than those in the kidneys and other tissues. The earliest change may be a functional abnormality of the blood vessels. The capillary patterns are distorted, and the veins appear distended, tortuous, and sacculated. The presence of severe varicose venous changes in the retinas in young individuals is almost pathognomonic for diabetes. The pathologic retinal alterations may be classified as three types: microaneurysms, exudates and hemorrhages, and retinitis proliferans. Diabetic retinopathy can usually be distinguished from other types (Table 9–12).

Microaneurysms

Microaneurysms tend to be among the earliest and most specific lesions in the retina (Fig. 9–44). Minute aneurysmal dilation of the capillaries, arterioles, or occasionally the venules occurs. These aneurysms average 30–90 μ in diameter. The exact mechanism for their production is not known. They progress to a thick-walled sack, which stains densely with PAS. Infiltration with lipids may be observed early in their development, and eventu-

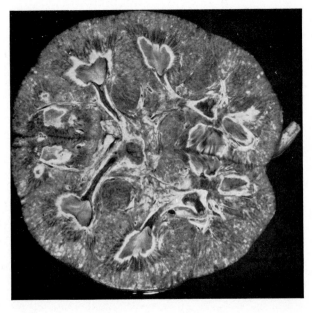

Figure 9–43. Extensive acute necrotizing renal papillitis in a diabetic. Massive infarction involves the renal papillae.

TABLE 9–12.   CLINICAL PATHOLOGY OF DIABETIC RETINOPATHY

Stage	Pathologic Lesion	Source	Ophthalmoscopic Recognition
I. Diagnostic of diabetes	Central microaneurysms Central waxy exudates	Capillaries (venous), especially at bifurcations	*Punctate* lesions resembling round, dotted hemorrhages and white dots of hyalinized lesions respectively around the macula and the optic disk; a few halo hemorrhages around the microaneurysms
II. Suggestive of diabetes	Patchy hyaline exudates and confluent, round hemorrhages still mostly in the central area	Capillaries	*Confluent* patchy central lesions, including smooth, waxy, lipid exudates and hemorrhages
III. End-stage of a number of conditions other than diabetes	Venous thromboses; widespread, massive exudates; retinal and vitreous hemorrhages; new vessels arising from the disk area; retinitis proliferans; retinal detachment	Capillaries and veins	Diffuse thickening and tortuosity of retinal veins; diffuse yellow to gray exudates and circinate hemorrhages; new vessels and fibrous tissue arising from the optic disk and invading the vitreous humor; gray areas of retinal detachment and vitreous hemorrhages
Mixed stages	All of above or in varying combinations, with (I) always present	Capillaries and veins	Findings as above singly or in combination with those of Stage I present, unless obscured by subsequent changes
Associated changes: Hypertensive Renal Arteriosclerotic May occur at any time	Exudates and hemorrhages Arteriolosclerosis Arteriosclerosis	Capillaries, veins, arteries	A-V nicking; spasms of vessels; woolly exudates; striate or flame-shaped hemorrhages A-V nicking; widened light reflex

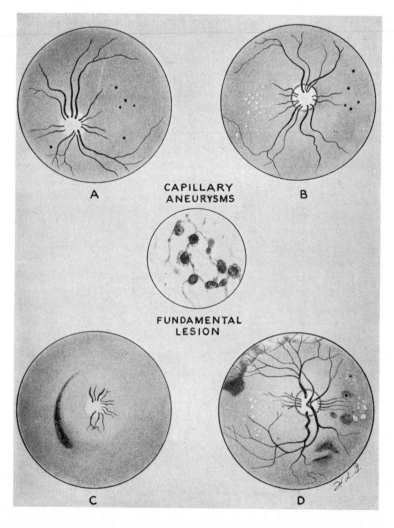

Figure 9–44. Characteristic eyeground changes in diabetic retinopathy as seen by ophthalmoscopic examination. Early punctate hemorrhages, *A* and *B* (right), with waxy, round exudates, *B*, (left). *C*, Vitreous hemorrhage obscuring all but the nerve head. *D*, Retinitis proliferans with fibrosis emanating from the nerve head; retinal detachment (top); flame-shaped hemorrhage and tortuosity of the retinal venules (below the center). The fundamental capillary lesions, the "microaneurysms," are shown in the center as they appear in a high-power microscopic view.

ally thrombosis, as well as leakage and rupture, may occur. Many hypotheses have been advanced to explain this lesion, including venous stasis, hyaline deposition, capillary basement membrane thickening, a disorder of polysaccharide metabolism, and loss of mural pericytes; none has been established as the sole etiologic agent. However, pathologically there are several definitely associated features: (1) increased basement membrane width, (2) loss of mural cells or pericytes, and (3) arteriolosclerosis, which is similar to that found in the kidney and elsewhere. Microaneurysms appear through the ophthalmoscope as small, round, red dots along the course of the capillaries. They tend to be most numerous in the perimacular region. Such aneurysms may occasionally occur with conditions other than diabetes, such as malignant hypertension, pernicious anemia, obstruction of the central vein, sickle cell anemia, and hypercorticosteroidism (iatrogenic or endogenous). However, they tend to be much more numerous and to occur with much greater frequency in diabetes, and they are almost always bilateral.

Exudates and Hemorrhages

In time, the microaneurysms become more numerous and coalesce. After they have been present for several months, they may even seem to be disappearing. This may be due to rupture, hemorrhage, or leakage of plasma proteins. Eventually these proteins are organized into deposits which consist chiefly of hyalinized material and lipids that stain heavily with PAS. The exudates are close to the microaneurysms, beginning on the vitreous side of the retina but eventually including all layers.

Particularly in the early stages of the retinitis, there may be a considerable number of remissions and exacerbations. The course is variable, but hemorrhages and exudates are never permanent lesions. Spontaneous improvement is common; thus the evaluation of various treatment programs has been particularly difficult.

Retinitis Proliferans

In approximately 25 per cent of diabetics with retinopathy, a proliferative change occurs. Usually such patients have microaneurysms, hemorrhage, and exudates, but it is not clear whether these are causative or associated lesions. Retinitis proliferans has been assumed to begin with retinal hemorrhage into the vitreous, although recent evidence suggests the vessel growth precedes such an event. Whatever the initial event, it is followed by an ingrowth of blood vessels and invasion with fibrous tissue. With contraction of the resulting scar tissue, separation of the retina and hemorrhage may occur. The hemorrhages and the neovascularization may occur anywhere in the retina but tend to be more numerous in the vicinity of the optic disk. A decrease in, or total loss of, vision may result. The proliferative changes tend to be more frequent in the younger diabetics, but this may be related to the length of time required for the changes in the retina to develop. On the average, retinitis proliferans is found 15 years from the time of the diagnosis in younger diabetics, as opposed to only about 6–10 years in older diabetics. It therefore tends to develop in individuals with diabetes of long duration. Although it is particularly likely to be associated with GS and other chronic manifestations of diabetes, in one-third of the patients albuminuria and hypertension are absent. Retinitis proliferans is not absolutely specific for diabetes. It is found occasionally with retinal vein occlusion and sickle cell anemia.

Conjunctival Alterations

The dilation of venules in the retinas seen in diabetic subjects has been observed in the conjunctival vessels as well by Ditzel. In contrast to normal subjects, venule diameter may vary in the course of one day (Fig. 9–45). Ditzel found that the early conjunctival changes consisted of elongation and distention of the venular end of the capillary. This dilation becomes more fixed as the duration of

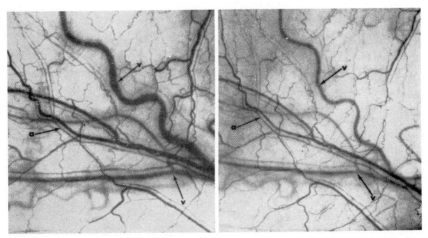

Figure 9–45.   Reversibility of venular dilation and congestion between 8:00 A.M. (left) and 4:00 P.M. (right) in an insulin-treated female diabetic aged 22 (× 48). (From Ditzel, J., Beaven, D. W., et al.: *Metabolism 9*:400, 1960.)

diabetes increases and tends to become irreversible in most subjects with diabetes of over 15 years duration. At this time, there tends to be sausage-shaped sacculation and actual evidence of exudation. However, the dilation is not specific for diabetes and has been observed in patients with infections of various types.

Iridopathy

In untreated diabetes, an excess of glycogen is deposited in the pigment epithelium of the posterior surface of the iris, leading to depigmentation of that layer. This process can be seen externally and gives the iris a moth-eaten appearance. Sometimes, neovascularization of the anterior surface of the iris and the anterior chamber results in a hemorrhagic glaucoma (rubeosis iridis). These changes are usually associated with proliferative retinopathy, but they are sometimes seen with central vein occlusion.

Cataracts

Cataracts in diabetics are considered to be of two types, metabolic or snowflake, and senile. The metabolic type tends to occur particularly in the insulin-treated diabetic and may be related to the degree of glucose control. These cataracts have a snowflake appearance and start in the subcapsular region of the lens. The senile type appears more often in the elderly patient and is similar to the cataracts in other elderly subjects. The presence of this type of cataract appears to be no more frequent in the diabetic than in the nondiabetic population, but they are said to mature more rapidly in the diabetic and lead to an increase in cataract extraction rate. Experimentally, hyperglycemia alone can induce cataracts in animals which are probably similar to the metabolic cataracts of the diabetic. This is one of the few instances in which a pathologic change can apparently be directly related to the carbohydrate abnormality.

The mechanism by which this occurs has been clarified recently by studies of lens metabolism that indicate that the relatively poorly transported sugar alcohol, sorbitol, is present in high concentrations when cataracts have been induced by high extracellular glucose levels. Aldose reductase is the enzyme responsible for the reduction of glucose to sorbitol and is known to be present in lens tissue. It is apparently the presence of the same enzyme that is responsible for the reduction of galactose to its polyol and which in turn may be responsible for cataract formation in galactosemia. In euglycemic individuals there is no buildup of the polyol, because the production of sorbitol is limited, and there is time for its further oxidation to fructose by the enzyme, sorbitol dehydrogenase. Thus, in the hyperglycemic state, intracellular glucose levels increase in insulin-independent tissues and increase the production of sorbitol. This increase in production raises tissue levels mark-edly, apparently because of the relatively slow further metabolism to fructose, and the two factors combined are responsible for the high sorbitol levels. It has been hypothesized that sorbitol increases intracellular osmolarity and subsequent water uptake, which directly or via changes in myoinositol metabolism promotes cataract formation. A similar metabolic pathway (the polyol pathway) has been described by Gabbay in peripheral nerves and may contribute to some of the neural abnormalities found in diabetes.

Not uncommonly, alterations in accommodation and in refraction are observed, particularly in insulin-treated diabetics. These changes are most likely related to osmotic changes in the lens, but some of them are possibly due to metabolic alterations in the ciliary body. Myopia may suddenly appear, as may other refractive alterations. These changes in accommodation and in refraction tend to be corrected rapidly by an improvement in the carbohydrate abnormality. For this reason, changes in the patient's glasses should not be prescribed until a steady state of regulation of the carbohydrate metabolism has been attained.

Treatment of Retinopathy

The treatment of ocular concomitants of diabetes is a major therapeutic problem. Retinopathy now stands as the fourth leading cause of blindness. Although there are a number of discrepancies in the correlation of the carbohydrate regulation and the ocular changes, there are reports that there is a significantly higher incidence of retinopathy in patients judged to have been under poor control than in those with better control. Moreover, some have found that patients under poor control have a higher incidence of the more severe forms of diabetic retinopathy. In evaluating this kind of retrospective data, the problem is that control may have been poorer in some subjects because the disease was more fulminant. Caird has reviewed some studies conducted in London and Boston. He reports that, among patients with retinopathy who had initially good vision in both eyes, visual deterioration sufficient to cause difficulty with employment develops in both eyes at the rate of (a) 5 per cent/yr. when the retinopathy is restricted to hemorrhage and exudates, (b) 11 per cent when there is proliferative retinopathy in younger diabetics, and (c) 25–30 per cent in older diabetics. The comparable rates when there is gross visual deterioration are (a) 2.5 per cent, (b) 7–9 per cent, and (c) 10–15 per cent/yr. Berkow in retrospective studies in 180 blind diabetic patients found that the average age at onset of diabetes in the entire group was 14.6 years, and the mean age at onset of severe blindness was 31.4 years. Among 85 diabetics, the average lifespan, after the onset of severe blindness due to diabetic retinopathy, was 5.8 years. Thus the life expectancy of a diabetic is very poor after the onset of blindness due to retinopathy. This, of course, is important in weighing the recommendation of major therapeutic procedures such as pituitary ablation.

Pituitary Ablation

The chance observation by Poulsen of significant improvement in diabetic retinopathy of a woman who developed postpartum hypopituitarism led to the introduction of the therapeutic induction of hypopituitarism as a treatment for diabetic retinopathy. The value of this treatment has been highly controversial, but after 10 years of experience, certain generalizations seem to hold true. First, retinopathy often progresses after complete pituitary removal, and therefore this form of therapy can only be considered as a temporary expedient. Second, there is some alleviation of the retinopathy in a substantial number of individuals in whom the procedure is performed, but this usually means no progression rather than reversal of the process. Third, there are many complications associated with the induction of hypopituitarism in a diabetic patient, and therefore the treatment itself is very hazardous. Fourth, although there may be improvement of the retinopathy or lack of progression, other areas of microangiopathy, as in the kidney, or neuropathy are not beneficially influenced by hypophysectomy. Therefore, in individuals who have severe atherosclerosis, neuropathy, or nephropathy, operative intervention is probably contraindicated.

The total explanation for the reported beneficial effects is unknown, but reduction of growth hormone secretion is believed to be the most important factor. The type of procedure used to produce the hypopituitarism appears to be of lesser importance than the operator's skill and experience with any specific technique. Therefore, benefits have been reported with surgical ablation, stalk section, and pituitary irradiation. Unfortunately, control studies of the effectiveness of this procedure are very few, and the authors are only aware of one study in which patients were chosen randomly for follow-up or treatment, and this study only involved 12 patients (Lundbaek). Total surgical mortality has been less than 10 per cent, and stabilization or improvement has been reported in 50–80 per cent of subjects so treated, the variability depending primarily on the patients selected for this approach. Since stabilization or improvement in untreated patients approaches 30 per cent, experience with hypophysectomy is not very encouraging. Patient selection is fairly critical, and most groups find that 4 out of 5 patients referred for such treatment are considered unsuitable. The general criteria in many clinics include a 3 months' trial of maximal diabetic therapy before surgery to determine whether the retinal lesions are stable or still progressing, preferably documented by fundus photographs. It should be determined that useful vision of at least one eye could be attained, assuming that the hemorrhagic tendency and further fibrosis will not recur as a result of pituitary ablation. If macular vision is destroyed or deteriorated to the point where it cannot likely be restored, or if massive vitreous hemorrhage precludes adequate observation, the patient should not be so treated. Contraindications for this therapy are significant nephropathy (markedly reduced creatinine clearance or excessive proteinuria), atherosclerotic heart failure, and severe microangiopathy or neuropathy. The patient must be a well-educated individual with a good family environment, as diabetic treatment will be much more complex after pituitary ablation. Retinal photocoagulation, which appears to be a much simpler procedure, has drastically reduced the number of pituitary ablations being performed. As far as the procedure to produce hypopituitarism is concerned, there is only one important difference among the various therapies. Proton beam irradiation of the pituitary, performed in two centers in the United States, produces hypopituitarism very slowly, usually requiring 3–12 months, whereas with the surgical or local radiation implantation techniques, hypopituitarism develops rapidly.

Photocoagulation

In the past several years, the availability of photocoagulation has largely displaced and superceded pituitary ablation. The light energy of xenon, and more recently that of ruby or argon lasers, has been used to produce first a burn and then a scar in the retina by absorption of light energy by the retinal pigment epithelium. At first, photocoagulation was directed toward specific abnormal areas of neovascularization and suspected bleeding sites, and later it was directed toward microaneurysms, hemorrhages, and exudates. In a symposium on photocoagulation, stabilization of angiopathy was claimed to occur in 65 per cent of the treated eyes. Although it would be relatively easy to plan a prospective study of the effectiveness of technique, none is available. Most recently, retinal lesions have not been treated directly, but rather 300–1100 small retinal scars have been made throughout the retina in an attempt to alter the course of the retinopathy. The mechanism by which such scars should reduce proliferation is unknown, but preliminary results have been encouraging. The procedure is not without its hazards, however, as complex lesions may bleed as a result of the treatment, leading to retinal detachment and vitreous hemorrhage. Nevertheless, it is a relatively simple procedure in expert hands and has excited much enthusiasm.

Nervous System

The neuropathic disturbances can be classified into five groups: radiculopathy, mononeuropathy, polyneuropathy, amyotrophy, and autonomic neuropathy (Fig. 9–46).

Radiculopathy

Diabetic radiculopathy is an infrequent form of peripheral neuropathy. The disorder is character-

CLASSIFICATION OF DIABETIC PERIPHERAL NEUROPATHY ON AN ANATOMICAL BASIS

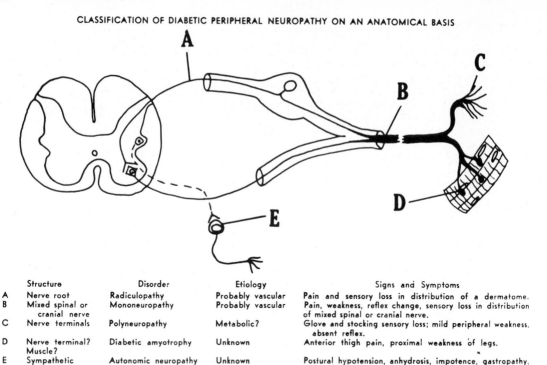

	Structure	Disorder	Etiology	Signs and Symptoms
A	Nerve root	Radiculopathy	Probably vascular	Pain and sensory loss in distribution of a dermatome.
B	Mixed spinal or cranial nerve	Mononeuropathy	Probably vascular	Pain, weakness, reflex change, sensory loss in distribution of mixed spinal or cranial nerve.
C	Nerve terminals	Polyneuropathy	Metabolic?	Glove and stocking sensory loss; mild peripheral weakness, absent reflex.
D	Nerve terminal? Muscle?	Diabetic amyotrophy	Unknown	Anterior thigh pain, proximal weakness of legs.
E	Sympathetic ganglion	Autonomic neuropathy	Unknown	Postural hypotension, anhydrosis, impotence, gastropathy, vesical atony.

Figure 9–46. Diabetic peripheral neuropathy. (From Locke, S.: *Diabetes 13*:307, 1964.)

ized by lancinating pain in the distribution of a single dermatome. When it involves a root of brachial or lumbar distribution, distinction from a herniated nucleus pulposus is sometimes difficult. When nerve roots are affected near the dorsal root ganglion, proximal degeneration may ensue. This results in a loss of myelin and axis cylinders in the posterior columns of the spinal cord and is associated with impairment of position sense, positive Romberg's sign, and loss of deep tendon reflexes. When pupillary abnormalities are noted in association with this disorder, the patient with lancinating pain may be diagnosed as diabetic pseudotabes.

Mononeuropathy

Mononeuropathy, in contrast to radiculopathy, affects a major nerve trunk. It has often been assumed that the lesion involves a larger vessel than in the radicular syndrome, but a vascular basis for this lesion has never been proven. Pain may be prominent; sensory loss, motor weakness, and deprivation of sympathetic innervation in the distribution of a major spinal or cranial nerve contribute to the symptomatology. Clinically, there is acute onset of weakness or sensory loss in an arm or leg. Corresponding to this there is an absence of the appropriate reflex. Palpation of the nerve may disclose striking tenderness. The spinal fluid appears unremarkable. Spontaneous recovery is the rule. Cranial nerve palsies belong to this group. Involvement of the third, fifth, sixth, seventh, eighth,

tenth, and twelfth cranial nerves has been reported, but rarely are any of the nerves affected except those influencing facial contractions and extraocular movements. The third and the sixth nerves are most often involved. Paralysis of the extraocular movements occurs in approximately 1 per cent of the diabetics and is in large part confined to patients over age 50 with long-standing diabetes. Diplopia and ptosis are two common manifestations (Fig. 9–47). The paralysis is associated with retrobulbar pain and pain in the forehead on the affected side. The prognosis is good, with most patients recovering in 2–3 months.

Polyneuropathy

The most frequent form of diabetic neuropathy is the distal, bilateral comparatively symmetrical polyneuropathy, which is predominantly sensory. The sensory loss and associated motor weakness do not conform to the distribution of a single nerve root or peripheral nerve but involve the distribution of overlapping peripheral terminals of many segmental nerves. Since the longest nerves are affected first, symptoms appear earlier and more severely in the feet. The sensory loss is greatest in the most peripheral portion and less proximally. This produces the so-called *"glove and stocking"* loss of sensation which characterizes the disorder. Symptoms are scarce, and many patients are unaware of the sensory disturbance until their attention is called to it by the examiner. There is a

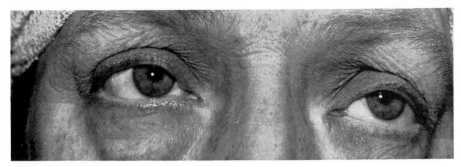

Figure 9–47. Paresis of external rotation of the left eye of a patient, aged 55, with diabetes of 20 years' duration. Function is usually regained within a few months.

demonstrable reduction in nerve conduction velocity in affected patients, but nerve conduction may be reduced in patients without obvious evidence of neuropathy. Trophic changes of the extremities may be associated with a distal polyneuropathy. The feet are often cold and blue. There may be hyperhidrosis or anhidrosis associated with shiny, thin skin and loss of hair. Perforating ulcers and Charcot's joints are frequently related to the lack of sensation (Fig. 9–48).

Amyotrophy

The syndrome of diabetic amyotrophy is found characteristically in elderly men with mild abnormalities of glucose metabolism. With this syndrome, a prominent muscle weakness of the iliopsoas, quadriceps, gluteal, and hamstring muscles, with muscle wasting, fasciculation, weight loss, and myalgia, are associated with dysesthesias of the anterior thigh and extensor plantar responses

and an ill-defined sensory loss to pin prick. This disease may be difficult to distinguish from a number of other neuropathies and myopathies. With diabetic amyotrophy, the spinal fluid protein may reach levels as high as 200 mg./100 ml. The electromyogram suggests primary muscle disease as well as a neurogenic lesion. Muscle biopsy reveals a characteristic pattern of single-fiber atrophy. The symptoms often improve within 18–24 months.

Autonomic Neuropathy

It is now becoming apparent that the autonomic nervous system is involved diffusely, and often early, in the course of the disease, although in general there is a relationship between the duration of the disease and the severity of the autonomic neuropathy. When the viscera are involved, it may be difficult to distinguish such a syndrome clinically from an intrinsic lesion of the organ.

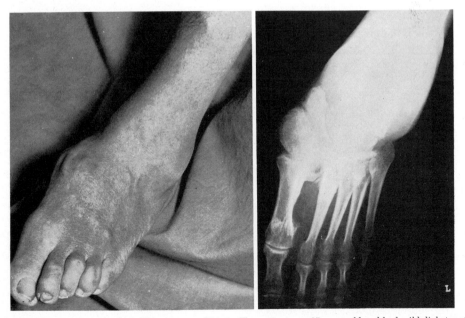

Figure 9–48. Diabetic neuropathy with Charcot type of joints. The patient was 65 years old and had mild diabetes of unknown duration—probably many years. In diabetes, contrary to syphilis, the Charcot type of joint change is much commoner in distal joints than in proximal.

Gastrointestinal

Gastroparesis has been observed similar to that found after vagotomy, which is followed by a dilated stomach and slow peristalsis. Gallbladder dysfunction has also been attributed to a neuropathy, but lacking any way of specifically delineating the neurologic lesion, it is difficult to determine whether such a lesion exists in any single patient. Nocturnal diarrhea is common and is sometimes associated with steatorrhea. Because jejunal biopsy usually reveals normal mucosa, it is assumed that nocturnal diarrhea is related to an associated neurologic abnormality.

Urogenital

Urinary retention due to an atonic bladder is common and may contribute to the urinary tract infections found so commonly in the older diabetic. Sexual impotence in the male is now recognized as perhaps the *most common* symptom of neuropathy in diabetes. It has been partly overlooked in the past, mainly because of poor history taking. Recent studies have reported impotence in as many as 60 per cent of patients within five years of diagnosis of diabetes.

Vasomotor

Other autonomic control systems are frequently abnormal; sweating disturbances with or without an accompanying polyneuropathy may be observed, or orthostatic hypotension, often with significant symptomatology, may be found. The vasomotor reactions in peripheral neuropathy are similar to those found following sympathectomy, and the absence of circulatory reflexes in such patients is common.

The pathology of the lesion is unknown; however, it has been alleged to be distal to the spinal cord since the symptoms are so similar to those of postganglionic nerve section.

Spinal Fluid Changes

Approximately 70 per cent of patients with diabetic neuropathy have an increase in spinal fluid protein (50–100 mg./100 ml.). This protein presumably arises from the damage to the nerve root adjacent to the spinal fluid protein.

Spinal Cord Disease

Diabetic myelopathy is rare, but it has been found occasionally. The spinal cord may show segmentally localized degeneration in the posterior column and localized necrosis and degenerative changes in the lateral columns as well. Thickening and hyalinization of the arterioles in the involved areas have been observed. The symptomatology is determined by the site and extent of involvement.

Skin

Three types of skin lesions have been found with a high degree of frequency in diabetes mellitus and have at one time or another been considered specific for it; hence the names diabetic dermopathy, necrobiosis lipoidica diabeticorum, and xanthoma diabeticorum. None of these lesions is absolutely specific for diabetes, and at times questions have been raised whether they are even more frequent in the diabetic population. Most studies seem to show that they are, but it is unlikely that any of these lesions can be considered specific for the syndrome.

Diabetic Dermopathy

The lesion has been described by Binkley to consist of red or red-brown papules that evolve into sharply circumscribed atrophic patches, usually located in the pretibial area (Fig. 9–49). They are often hyperpigmented and scaly. It was thought the skin lesions were similar to other microangiopathic changes in diabetes mellitus; however, Danowski has been unable to confirm this, and he reports finding similar lesions in a fair number of normal individuals and in subjects with a variety of other endocrine disorders with no abnormality of glucose tolerance.

Necrobiosis Lipoidica Diabeticorum

This lesion occurs in the same location and is described as a sharply bordered, plaquelike lesion,

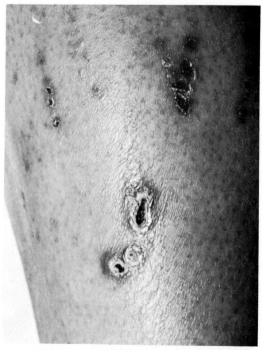

Figure 9–49. Early lesions of dermopathy showing central crusting; in this patient the lesions appear in a somewhat linear arrangement. (From Binkley, G. W.: *Arch Derm.* 92:625, 1965.)

beginning as a red or red-brown lesion, which eventually expands to form a shiny atrophic plaque (Fig. 9–50). Dermal vessels become sclerotic, and an obliterative endarteritis occurs.

Xanthoma Diabeticorum

This term is used to describe typical eruptive xanthomas which arise whenever chylomicronemia occurs in the presence of uncontrolled diabetes mellitus (Fig. 9–51). These lesions are seen in the syndrome of diabetic lipemia and are identical to those found whenever chylomicrons are present and circulating in very high concentrations from any cause; therefore, they are not specific for diabetes mellitus. Physically they are small red-yellow papules that arise in crops and have an erythematous base. They develop primarily on the buttocks, elbows, and backs of the thighs—the so-called extensor surfaces. Chemical analysis has revealed typical chylomicron triglyceride fatty acids.

Skin Infection

It is not clear whether patients with diabetes mellitus have a more likely predisposition to bacterial or mycotic infections, but it is generally agreed that, when such infections occur, they are more difficult to control than in nonhyperglycemic individuals. Perineal pruritus in a diabetic is almost always associated with *Candida albicans* and occurs in both the pregnant and nonpregnant female. Glycosuria seems to be an important factor in the maintenance of the lesion; however, Candida may occur on other areas of the body, most usually in the intertriginous regions.

The occurrence of a fungal infection of the interdigital areas in the diabetic can be a problem because the epidermal fissures and erosions serve as portals of entry for other organisms which can lead to cellulitis and gangrene. Prophylaxis should be used in all diabetics and prompt treatment started to eradicate the fungus, either with local agents if the infection is minor or with systemic antifungal agents with well-entrenched, long-standing problems.

PREGNANCY AND DIABETES

Pregnancy is a clear example of the effects of stress on carbohydrate metabolism. In a susceptible individual, clinical diabetes may become manifest. In the normal individual, compensation maintains glucose concentration with only slight changes; however, this is only at the expense of a total reorganization of many of the hormonal factors that impinge upon carbohydrate, fat, and protein metabolism. Pregnancy tends not only to place stress on carbohydrate metabolism in a diabetic but may also influence adversely the vascular concomitants of the disease. Furthermore, although

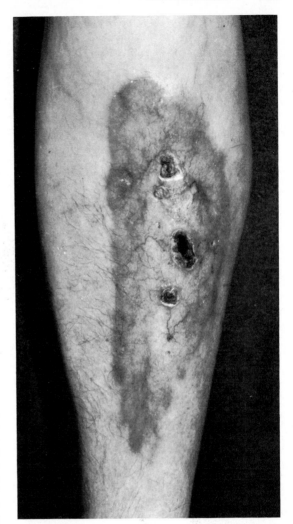

Figure 9–50. Extensive dry ulcerative plaque of necrobiosis lipoidica diabeticorum. (Courtesy of Dr. George Odland.)

fertility in the diabetic female is only slightly subnormal, the chance of a diabetic mother producing a live child is decreased, and the number of surviving children is also decreased. The diagnosis of diabetes is more difficult, and treatment of carbohydrate metabolism in the pregnant diabetic must be changed as the pregnancy progresses. In contrast to the controversy that surrounds close blood sugar management in other aspects of the diabetic syndrome, this is not the case in the pregnant diabetic, since the outcome of the pregnancy may depend in part upon the degree of carbohydrate control.

Pregnancy and Carbohydrate Tolerance

The predominant effect of pregnancy on carbohydrate metabolism is related to the hormonal changes induced by the pregnancy and to the presence of the fetus, which depends upon the mother for its entire fuel (mostly glucose) and nutrient supply. All the hormones whose secretion is increased during pregnancy (including estrogen,

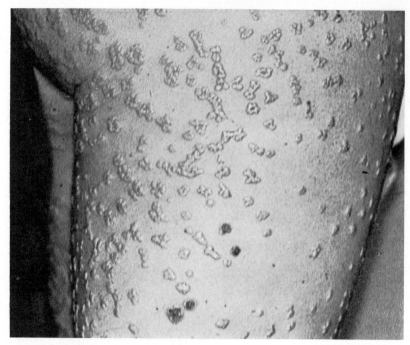

Figure 9–51. Xanthoma diabeticorum. These eruptive xanthomas, composed chiefly of lipid deposits, are not confined to diabetics.

progesterone, chorionic somatomammotropin, and corticosteroids) antagonize the effects of insulin on carbohydrate uptake and utilization, thus inducing a state of peripheral insulin resistance. At the same time, there is an accelerated utilization of stored nutrients and glucose to feed the fetus overnight and between meals, so that in the morning the pregnant woman often has a lower fasting blood glucose level, elevated FFA levels, and mild ketonuria. Furthermore, there is evidence that destruction of insulin occurs in the placenta, thus accelerating the peripheral turnover of this hormone. This requires more insulin secretion to maintain adequate plasma levels. The effect of an uncomplicated pregnancy in producing a minimal change in glucose tolerance but markedly higher insulin levels is shown at the top of Figure 9–52. This insulin-resistant state is reversed immediately after delivery.

Diagnosis of Diabetes

Standards for the diagnosis of diabetes by carbohydrate tolerance testing are clearly altered by the pregnant state. In general, the upper limit of normal for a fasting blood sugar is usually reduced approximately 10 mg./100 ml. because of the accelerated utilization of glucose during fasting; however, the values after challenge are raised 20–25 mg./100 ml. because of the insulin antagonism (Table 9–5). The use of urine glucose excretion as an index of diabetes is not advisable, since the normal pregnancy reduces the apparent threshold for glucose, and a significant number of normal women have glycosuria during pregnancy. Treatment during pregnancy usually means insulin

therapy. Therefore, the determination of carbohydrate tolerance may not be useful during pregnancy, as the therapeutic decision to use insulin usually rests upon finding a significant elevation of fasting blood glucose.

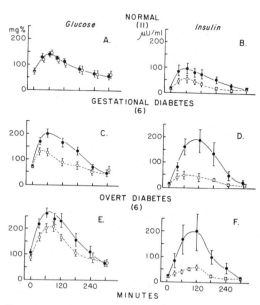

Figure 9–52. The effect of pregnancy on glucose and insulin. Note that with nondiabetic pregnancy, the glucose tolerance tests were the same as they were post partum, but much higher levels of plasma immunoassayable insulin were attained than in the postpartum period. The glucose levels in diabetics were higher during pregnancy than following delivery, despite far greater plasma insulin levels. (From Kalkhoff, R., et al.: *Trans. Ass. Amer. Physicians* 77:270, 1964.)

Interaction of Diabetes and Pregnancy

Recognizing that pregnancy is a stress to carbohydrate metabolism, it is logical to expect that the patient with clinical diabetes, whether treated with insulin or oral agents, will experience a change in the need for insulin. Because of the numerous factors influenced by the pregnancy, it is impossible to predict exactly the net effect in every patient; however, in general terms, insulin requirement or the need to begin insulin therapy in an asymptomatic patient will increase during the second half of the pregnancy. Note, for example, the further deterioriation in glucose tolerance of subjects with mild prepartum carbohydrate intolerance in Figure 9-52. Most clinics, therefore, will switch patients who are on oral agents to insulin, at least for the duration of the pregnancy. During the first half of the pregnancy, the increased utilization of glucose by the fetus may balance the contrainsulin hormones that have been secreted, and the insulin requirement may not change; in fact, in some cases, it may decrease. This depends in part upon the nutrition of the pregnant woman, as her food intake may fluctuate widely during the first trimester. The greater the food intake, the greater the need for insulin. In the second and third trimesters, insulin requirements will always increase because of the insulin antagonistic hormones.

Ketoacidosis is associated with a marked increase in fetal death rate. In general, most pregnant diabetics are seen more frequently and managed more closely to prevent this complication, as the fetal death rate may increase to 30 per cent or more. On the other hand, accelerated fasting or starvation ketosis is common in normal pregnancies and must be distinguished from ketoacidosis. In general, this is fairly straightforward, since starvation ketosis is not associated with significant hyperglycemia. The use of carbohydrate-restricted diets may accelerate this possibility in the diabetic population and is therefore definitely contraindicated during pregnancy. In general, it is probably preferable to increase the carbohydrate content of the diet in the pregnant diabetic. Should starvation ketosis develop, it can be treated quite easily by the use of glucose solution, usually oral. Management of ketoacidosis in the pregnant diabetic is no different from that of the nonpregnant diabetic.

The more challenging problem is to determine whether pregnancy has adverse effects on the vascular concomitants of diabetes in addition to its effects on carbohydrate metabolism. There seems to be no doubt that pre-eclampsia is more common in diabetic patients. In the presence of severe renal disease or rapidly accelerating renal disease, termination of the pregnancy is usually indicated. It is not clear whether the retinopathy, neuropathy, and large vessel disease are compromised by pregnancy, but it is the general feeling of most clinicians that there is some acceleration of these processes; however, no incontrovertible evidence has been forthcoming. The presence of vascular disease considerably reduces the possibility of a live baby, and it is generally felt, therefore, that pregnancy is contraindicated in such a patient.

Infant of the Diabetic Mother

Excessive body weight and size, and neonatal hypoglycemia are well-recognized fetal complications of a diabetic pregnancy. Fetal hyperinsulinemia has been documented and, since insulin does not pass the placental barrier, it is believed due to the hyperglycemia of the mother. It seems likely that it is this increased insulin output which acts as a growth factor and leads to the increased body fat and visceromegaly. The postpartum hypoglycemia probably results from continued insulin secretion in the absence of glucose supplied by the placenta. There is true hypertrophy and hyperplasia of the pancreas in these infants. Most authors find an increase in congenital anomalies in infants of diabetic mothers, but this is a controversial point. Fetal loss is high in the diabetic pregnancy, and intrauterine death increases after the thirty-seventh week of pregnancy. This fact has led to the development of criteria for accelerating delivery. On the other hand, premature removal of the fetus leads to an increased incidence of the fetal respiratory distress syndrome, also a major problem. The problem of picking an optimal delivery time is illustrated in Figure 9-53. According to White, 80 per cent of diabetic pregnancies result in a live birth, compared with 90 per cent in the general population; perinatal mortality occurs in about 10 per cent of deliveries, compared with 3 per cent of nondiabetics.

Management of the Pregnant Diabetic

There are three major goals in the treatment of the pregnant diabetic. The first is to prevent ketosis, the second is to minimize glycosuria, and the

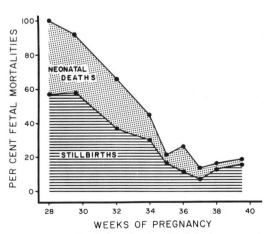

Figure 9-53. Fetal mortality in 705 diabetic pregnancies according to duration. (From Miller, M., In *On the Nature and Treatment of Diabetes*. Leibel, B. S., and Wrenshall, G. A. (eds.), Amsterdam, Excerpta Medica Foundation, 1965.)

third is to optimize the length of gestation. Diet in the pregnant diabetic is essentially unchanged, except for an increase in total calories to allow a weight gain of approximately 20–25 pounds per pregnancy. Carbohydrates should not be restricted, in view of the rapid switch from the fed to the fasting state, which takes place during the normal pregnancy. This will ordinarily require somewhere between 35–40 cal./kg. of *ideal* body weight, with 45 per cent of calories as carbohydrate. Since this is the same proportion of carbohydrate calories as in an average American diet, it can be approached usually by self-selection. As in other patients with the diabetic syndrome, regularity of diet and total daily caloric intake are probably the most important features, along with intermittent snacks (4–6 feedings daily) to minimize wide swings in blood glucose. Glycosuria will occur in almost all diabetic patients on such a regimen because of the low renal threshold of pregnancy. It may be necessary to determine the renal threshold in each patient in order to assess properly the degree of insulin control that is achievable without risking serious hypoglycemia. All authors agree that frequent clinic visits are absolutely essential to maximize fetal salvage rate.

The major problem in diabetic pregnancy is to determine the optimal time for delivery. The general goal is to allow the pregnancy to go at least 35 weeks and then to check the patient carefully until the thirty-seventh or thirty-eighth week, if possible. It is probably advisable to hospitalize her at the thirty-fifth week so that determinations of fetal status and maturity can be made frequently. This is partly related to estimation of uterine size and fetal weight but more usually dependent upon endocrine testing. Estriol and pregnanediol can be used to get an estimate of fetal-placental mass. More recently, tests of fetal maturity using amniotic fluid have been recommended. These employ the bilirubin content, creatinine concentration, phospholipid content, and the cytology of the desquamated fetal cells. The evaluation of these procedures has been discussed by Tyson. All are aimed at determining as precisely as possible whether there is sufficient fetal maturity for survival. Induction of labor occurs when the maximum chance of the fetus living has been realized, and, if unsuccessful, cesarean section is performed. Estriol assays, by reflecting fetoplacental function, suggest optimal time for delivery (Rivlin et al.; Beischer and Brown). Some clinics perform cesarean section on all such patients, whereas others attempt a vaginal delivery first, usually with 30–50 per cent success. After delivery, there is a rapid reduction in insulin resistance, which should be anticipated by decreasing insulin dosage to prepregnancy levels or lower (2/3 the third trimester dosage).

Contraception and Sterilization

Both estrogen and progestogen, as already mentioned, clearly promote insulin resistance and may cause frankly abnormal glucose tolerance tests in a significant number of women taking these hormones. Thus diabetic patients are likely to find the same changes occurring while taking these pills that occur normally during pregnancy. If the patient already has carbohydrate intolerance, the pills may precipitate overt clinical diabetes and are therefore clearly contraindicated. In the insulin-treated diabetic, there will be a small increase in insulin requirement, but it is not known whether this increase in any way alters the vascular concomitants of the syndrome. Lacking this information, it has been generally recommended that the oral contraceptives not be used by diabetic patients; however, the physician must weigh the risks of a possible pregnancy against the risk of unknown effects of oral contraceptives in a patient who is unwilling to be sterilized or to use other methods of contraception. In general, pregnancy is ill-advised in the presence of significant large vessel disease, microvascular disease, or neuropathy, as fetal salvage rate is low, and the likelihood of long-term survival of the mother is reduced.

TREATMENT OF DIABETES

General Principles

Treatment in diabetes has been generally related to control of the glucose level in the hope of preventing or treating the microvascular, atherosclerotic, and neuropathic concomitants of diabetes mellitus. Despite several decades of experience and a great number of retrospective analyses, it is still not clear whether this goal has been achieved. There is general agreement that treatment of overt diabetes should be directed toward a control of the measured metabolic abnormalities so as to normalize fat, protein, and daily carbohydrate metabolism. To what extent this can be achieved without eliminating all hyperglycemia is unknown. One usually sets a series of priorities in relation to the known metabolic effects of relative or absolute insulin deficiency present in overt diabetes: *first,* control of excessive fatty acid mobilization and oxidation (i.e., treatment and prevention of ketoacidosis); *second,* control of excessive protein catabolism and muscle wasting, carbohydrate wastage, and urinary caloric loss (overt diabetes). After these two major problems have been treated, we are often still left with hyperglycemia and must consider the treatment of chemical diabetes. Treatment of overt diabetes to the point of eliminating ketosis and glycosuria may restore total daily carbohydrate, protein, and fat turnover to normal. Quantitatively, these are not abnormal in chemical diabetes, but two unanswered questions remain: (1) does further control of hyperglycemia per se provide any benefit to the patient? and (2) is it possible to achieve normal control of mild hyperglycemia with the therapeutic modalities presently available?

The description of a number of insulin independent pathways such as those leading to the synthesis of polyols, and basement membrane glycoproteins which may have increased activity in hyperglycemic subjects have raised the possibility that hyperglycemia per se is deleterious to health. Because it is currently impossible to simulate the complexities of normal insulin secretion and thereby achieve normal glucose homeostasis, tests of the hypothesis that control of hyperglycemia would improve all aspects of the diabetic syndrome have not been possible. The tests that have been done with current therapeutic modalities have suggested that treatment of hyperglycemia does not per se improve the mortality rate in adult diabetics. The authors feel that convincing evidence for or against the hypothesis that treatment delays or prevents the chronic concomitants of diabetes is not yet available. On this basis we would suggest that at the moment it is reasonable to attempt to limit excessive excursions of blood glucose, particularly avoiding symptomatic glycosuria and hypoglycemia, while at the same time permitting the patient to live a comfortable life.

Dietary Therapy

The inability to provide insulin in a truly physiologic manner requires that diet be an *essential* part of all therapeutic programs. Since the fundamental physiologic abnormality in diabetes is the inability to store calories properly for later use, dietary therapy should stress caloric control and regularity. In general, sufficient calories are provided to achieve and maintain ideal body weight (in children and adolescents, this includes normal growth and development). Thus, if the patient is malnourished and underweight, he must be provided with additional calories to restore weight. If he is overnourished or obese, caloric restriction must be prescribed. In general terms, an average non-obese adult uses 30–50 cal./kg./day for weight maintenance, while an obese individual may use 20–30 cal./kg./day. From many metabolic studies, we have found that weight maintenance in a metabolic ward, i.e., that of sedentary activity in adults, can be calculated from the following formula: cal./kg./day $= 52.2 - [15.5 \times \%$ ideal weight (kg. actual weight/kg. ideal weight)]. Clt is valid up to 250 per cent of ideal weight, by the Metropolitan Life tables for medium frame. Increased activity increases caloric need.

Younger individuals require more calories on a weight basis, and this may reach as high as 50–60 cal./kg./day in children. Just as important are the size and distribution of the individual caloric loads. It is quite clear that insulin secretion in response to food stimulation is defective in diabetes mellitus and that this defect is most obvious when very large caloric loads are given, which probably explains the greater diagnostic discrimination for both the 100 g. OGTT compared with the 50 g. test, and the 20–40 g. IVGTT compared with the 5–10 g. test. Thus, even in the noninsulin-treated diabetic, large caloric loads should be avoided. Most such patients should eat at least four meals a day,

children perhaps six. This type of meal spacing also requires caloric regularity from day to day. Although normal individuals can cope with caloric intakes that vary widely from day to day, i.e., 5000 cal. one day and 1000 cal. the next, the diabetic does poorly under such circumstances. It is this inability to handle large caloric loads that is probably responsible for the clinical observation that "cheating" on diabetic diets results in prompt glycosuria. It is the inappropriately large caloric load rather than the type of foodstuffs eaten that leads to hyperglycemia and glycosuria.

Although in the past major emphasis has been placed on the proportion of carbohydrate, fat, and protein calories in the diet, recent evidence (Brunzell) suggests that this is of less importance. In fact, clinicians over the years have prescribed diets varying from 10 to 65 per cent carbohydrate, and all have been claimed therapeutic successes. As far as glucose control is concerned, the per cent carbohydrate content of the diet does not usually seem to have much influence on hyperglycemia and glycosuria, provided that calories remain constant and caloric distribution is unchanged. As stated by Albrink and Davidson, perhaps the most that can be concluded is that diabetics tolerate an amazingly wide range of dietary carbohydrate intake, and there is very little firm evidence either for or against any diet in respect to its long-range effect on the progress of diabetes. For this reason, the American Diabetes Association presently recommends a diet that contains roughly normal proportions of carbohydrate, protein, and fat (somewhere between 45 and 50 per cent carbohydrate and 15 per cent protein). This freedom to prescribe carbohydrate calories is particularly important in view of the recent desire of many physicians to use low-animal-fat and low-cholesterol diets to prevent atherosclerosis. It appears that such a diet, inherently high in carbohydrate content, is suitable for the diabetic population.

Having decided on the total caloric content, distribution, and type of diet to be prescribed, the physician is faced with the necessity of educating the patient to achieve these therapeutic goals. The further the diet prescribed deviates from the average American diet, the greater the need for precise and careful dietary instruction. In the past, the use of carbohydrate-restricted diets has required either weighing the diet on small home-kept scales or using the food exchange system developed by the American Diabetes Association in association with the American Dietetic Association. This was developed to simplify dietary prescription by segregating foods into exchange lists, each food group on the list containing about the same amount of carbohydrate, protein, and fat as any other food on the list. It allows for reasonable variety in the meals and yet does not require the accurate weighing of food prior to preparation. Without carbohydrate restriction, however, the need for such complex dietary plans has been drastically reduced. Although it is still essential for the patient to be aware of the caloric value of foods, random selection will usually lead to a diet containing approximately 45 per cent of calories as carbohydrate. An example of this approach is the use of the unmeasured diet in diabetic subjects of normal body weight. The patient is instructed to eat food that is balanced in composition, but the quantity ingested is regulated by his needs and his appetite rather than by prescription. Such an individual, however, is encouraged to eat approximately the same amount of foods each day at each meal; in the studies performed by Knowles and colleagues, four to six meals per day were prescribed. This plan is in general only applicable to insulin-dependent diabetics, since it is this group that is usually of normal body weight. In most subjects with milder degrees of carbohydrate intolerance, obesity is a constant problem, and therefore caloric control must be instituted. Again, a balanced diet is explained and provided, but the total number of calories made available is reduced. Because caloric restriction reduces even further the ability to respond to nutrient ingestion, it is even more important that dietary regularity be instituted in such patients and that intermittent periods of fasting and feasting are avoided in the obese diabetic subject as he attempts to regulate body weight. Since this group may respond to caloric restriction alone with significant improvement in glycosuria and hyperglycemia, insulin and oral therapeutic agents are not given until the effectiveness of dietary control can be evaluated. At the present time, it is our practice to instruct patients in the caloric value of foods, to prescribe total caloric levels to be adhered to by each patient, and to attempt to achieve this without complex dietary programs. In subjects unable to achieve weight maintenance satisfactorily, we often use the exchange list as a means to educate the patient to the caloric value of a wide variety of foods. This list is then used to maintain a desired caloric intake until ideal weight is achieved. Actually, only a few of the obese subjects ever attain ideal weight.

Exercise

Exercise increases glucose utilization by a mechanism which does not depend upon increased secretion of insulin. In normal individuals, this increased utilization is balanced by an increased output of glucose by the liver. Therefore, plasma glucose levels are not changed. This is because normal individuals inhibit insulin secretion during the exercise period by activation of the sympathetic nervous system. In insulin-treated diabetics, this compensation cannot occur. Since the exercise-induced increase in glucose utilization is not compensated for by any alteration in hepatic output, blood glucose levels decline. This problem can be overcome by ingestion of food immediately before the exercise or by instituting a plan that will include regular amounts of exercise at specified times. In the noninsulin-treated diabetic, insulin secretion can be inhibited normally, and therefore hypoglycemia during exercise is a rather unusual occurrence.

Education

The diabetic must substitute external control of diet and insulin, for which he is responsible, for internal control of insulin which in the normal individual keeps plasma glucose levels relatively constant. Therefore, education in normal metabolism and in the external controls that will be prescribed by the physician is an essential part of the treatment program. In general, it is probably best to think of the diabetic as caring for his own disease with the advice and consultation of the physician rather than as a patient for whom all the therapeutic decisions are made by the physician. The diabetic should be aware of the effects of diet and exercise on metabolic control and be cognizant of methods of measuring the degree of metabolic control as reflected in the urine and blood. He also should be able to make adjustments in his treatment program, depending upon his physiologic and pathophysiologic state, as it changes from day to day. Much of this information can be imparted through formal classwork, but the physician should use the routine clinic visit for continuing education of the diabetic. In general, it is preferable for the formal educational programs to be coordinated in a community or area, so that there may be interaction between the patient, other diabetics, and the instructor. There is a growing tendency for this work to be done by paramedical personnel as part of a teaching unit.

The following areas should be part of any teaching program: (1) the clinical signs and symptoms and genetic aspects of the disease and the general nature of the disordered pathophysiology; (2) discussion of diet, including a general discussion of the metabolism of various foodstuffs, the need for regularity in diet, specific nature of the dietary program recommended for the individual patient, and the importance of interaction between diet, insulin, and exercise on metabolic control; (3) insulin—every patient should be capable of injecting himself with insulin, whether or not the therapeutic program requires this form of therapy at the moment. The nature and source of insulin, types and action of insulin, method of injection, and side-effects of insulin therapy should be covered; (4) oral hypoglycemic agents, with a general discussion of the differences between insulin and the oral agents, the nature of the oral agents available, and a frank discussion of their uses and limitations; (5) methodology for urine and blood testing, with specific instruction on urine glycosuria and ketonuria; and (6) general health care, which needs to be emphasized particularly for the diabetic, such as care of the lower extremities, handling of minor infections and illnesses, diagnosis and therapy of dermatophytoses, and some discussion of the concomitants of diabetes, particularly the microangiopathy, neuropathy, and large vessel disease.

Insulin Treatment

When the ability to secrete insulin in response to a challenge diminishes sufficiently, the patient with diabetes mellitus begins to lose significant portions of his daily calories as glycosuria. With this there is increased gluconeogenesis to maintain carbohydrate-metabolism and wastage of body protein. At this point, a severe complication of insulin deficiency, ketoacidosis, occurs. Such individuals require exogenous insulin in order to maintain weight without caloric excess. In the normal individual, insulin secretion is regulated by the nature and amount of exogenous foodstuffs in order to maintain normal metabolism of ingested carbohydrate, fat, and protein. The patient with insulin-dependent diabetes mellitus differs from a normal individual in that he receives a fixed dose of insulin to which he must match his food intake, as there will not be normal peaks of insulin in association with food ingestion. Therefore, even with insulin therapy, diabetic patients are unable to store foodstuffs as efficiently as a normal individual, who responds to the challenge by suddenly secreting insulin. Since exogenous insulin treatment is an inadequate physiologic replacement, the attainment of reasonable metabolic control requires an understanding of the properties of the various insulin preparations, the nature of the interaction of injected insulin with basic metabolic processes, and the potential complications of insulin therapy.

Insulin Preparations

Data on a variety of insulin preparations are given in Table 9-13. Essentially, they all consist of extracts of either beef or pork pancreases which have been commercially purified to approximately 95 per cent insulin. The 5 per cent contamination consists partially of insulin polymers, proinsulin intermediates, and degradation products. There has been continued improvement in purifying the product, with great progress made recently by using Sephadex chromatography to exclude the larger molecular weight aggregates. This more pure material (99 per cent) is now termed "single peak" insulin and is available for use. Within the near future, a "single component" insulin, 100 per cent insulin (6000 molecular weight), should be available commercially.

Crystalline Zinc Insulin (CZI)

Crystalline zinc insulin, semilente insulin, and regular insulin are in forms that are most rapidly acting and metabolized. The other preparations have been modified so as to prolong the effect of injected insulin. Regular, crystalline zinc insulin, and semilente insulin are the only forms which can be given intravenously. They may also be injected subcutaneously 15-30 minutes before a meal, so that the concentration will parallel that produced by meal-eating.

Protamine Zinc Insulin (PZI)

The initial modification of insulin to prolong its duration of action was made by Hagedorn and co-workers, who found that a properly buffered solution containing protamine would produce a precipitate with poor solubility and slow absorption. Prior to its introduction as a therapeutic agent in the 1930's, regular insulin alone was insufficient to prevent protein loss and dwarfism. The introduction (1936) of the first long-acting insulin prevented these disabling consequences. The problem with this material was that its excess content of protamine became bound to insulin when it was put into the same syringe, thereby making it also long-acting. This led to development of neutral protamine Hagedorn (NPH) insulin. It is injected subcutaneously only.

Neutral Protamine Hagedorn (NPH) Insulin

Partly because of the difficulty in mixing crystalline zinc insulin and protamine zinc insulin and partly because of the very long duration of action of PZI, a near stoichiometric mixture of protamine, and insulin with a shorter duration of action and compatibility with crystalline zinc insulin, was rapidly adopted world-wide in the 1930's. Available for subcutaneous injection, its pattern of action was more closely related to normal meal-eating patterns than that of any of the other insulins available at that time.

TABLE 9-13. AMERICAN PREPARATIONS OF INSULIN

Type of Insulin	Buffer	pH	Suspension	Zinc mg./100 U.	Interval of Maximum Action (hrs.)	Total Duration of Action (hrs.)
Lente series						
Semilente	Acetate	7.1–7.5	Amorphous	0.2 –0.25	4–6	12–16
Lente	Acetate	7.1–7.5	(30% Amor. 70% Cry.)	0.2 –0.25	8–12	18–24
Ultralente	Acetate	7.1–7.5	Crystalline	0.2 –0.25	16–18	30–36
Crystalline zinc	None	2.5–3.5	(Solution)	0.01–0.04	4–6	6–8
NPH (isophane)	Phosphate	7.1–7.4	Crystalline	0.01–0.04	8–12	18–24
Protamine zinc	Phosphate	7.1–7.4	Amorphous	0.2 –0.25	14–20	24–36
Globin	None	3.4–3.8	(Solution)	0.25–0.35	6–10	12–18

Lente Insulins

In the 1950's, a series of insulins was described in which zinc insulin crystals of two types could be produced, and which in acetate buffer yielded a very long-acting form similar to PZI and a very short-acting form similar to crystalline zinc insulin. The advantage of this material was that it permitted the patient to mix the long- and short-acting insulins in any combination desired, and its lack of an extra protein, such as protamine or globin, reduced allergic reactions. A mixture of 70 per cent of the long-acting form (ultralente) and 30 per cent of the short-acting form (semilente) gave a time course of action very similar to NPH insulin and was marketed as lente insulin. With this series of insulins, any combination of long- and short-acting insulin could be prescribed in a compatible form by the physician, making it very popular. Some idealized curves for the various types of insulin are given in Figure 9–54.

Clinical Pharmacology

Insulin injected subcutaneously is absorbed directly into the bloodstream, but differences in the rates of absorption from different sites contribute to variations in response. In general, all types of commercial insulin are stable, even when stored for moderate intervals at room temperature. Although it is desirable to keep insulin refrigerated so as to maintain full potency for two years, during periods of traveling – even up to a month – there is no appreciable loss of activity at room temperature. Insulin put into intravenous fluid, such as has occurred during surgery, has caused problems, not the least of which is the binding of insulin. As much as 50 per cent of the insulin can bind to glass and plastic surfaces when the fluid contains no protein. Moreover, since there is no fixed ratio between insulin and glucose administration in any individual case, hyperglycemia or hypoglycemia may result.

Physicians and patients should be aware of factors that determine responses to insulin. In general, the larger the dose of any insulin, the longer is its duration of action and the later is its maximal effect. Therefore, in an insulin-resistant patient who requires more than 200 U. of insulin a day, regular crystalline zinc insulin may be effective for as long as NPH or lente insulin. Important factors that are determinants of the insulin "requirement" are hormones that antagonize insulin actions, insulin-resistant states, and especially the amount of circulating insulin antibodies. Estrogen, growth hormone, chorionic somatomammotropin, and corticosteroid induce insulin resistance. Therefore, with all other factors remaining equal, excess of any of these hormones decreases the effectiveness of insulin. Certain physiologic and pathophysiologic states will have the same effect. The most important of these, obesity, always induces insulin-resistance in proportion to the degree of adiposity and necessitates larger amounts of insulin for maintaining metabolic control. Chronic liver disease and uremia also produce insulin-resistant states.

Insulin Antibodies

Insulin antibodies are produced in significant amounts in any diabetic patient treated with non-purified insulin for more than 30 days. The levels have not been accurately quantified, but in some patients they are high enough to impair markedly insulin action. High levels of insulin antibodies and periodic variations in their amounts may cause difficulty in the regulation of insulin therapy. In most patients who require more than 200 U. of insulin per day, a high antibody titer is present. Whenever more than average insulin dosage is required or there is significant problem in regulation, it is desirable to consider the use of insulins that are less immunogenic or to consider modifying the antibody response in some fashion. Since most commercial insulin is a beef-pork mixture and the antibody titers are higher to beef insulin, switching to pure pork insulin may result in a lessening of insulin requirement. There is recent evidence that the immunogenic component of commercial

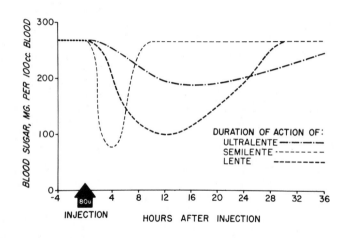

Figure 9–54. The extremes in rates and degrees of hypoglycemic effects are demonstrated by ultralente and semilente insulin preparations after subcutaneous injection. Intermediate types of responses result from mixtures of these solutions, as illustrated by lente insulin, which is composed of 70 parts of ultralente and 30 parts of semilente.

insulin preparations is only in small part due to the single component (6000 molecular weight) hormone and to a greater extent due to some form of molecular aggregate. It has been found that the use of insulin more purified than the present commercial supply causes less antibody production. The level of antibody itself and its amount of insulin-binding may be reduced by the administration of glucosteroids. Usually, fairly high doses of a potent glucosteroid such as prednisone, 40–60 mg./day, must be given. Although glucosteroids induce peripheral insulin resistance, this effect may be outweighed by reduction in antibody production in patients with very high insulin antibody titers and may be sufficient to markedly reduce insulin requirements.

Allergic Reactions

Local reactions to the injection of insulin are not unusual, but their true incidence is unknown. The range in published studies has varied from 1–56 per cent. This variability is probably because the majority are mild and remain unreported. The presence of such a side-effect appears to be unrelated to the development of circulating IgG and IgM insulin antibodies, which neutralize the effects of the injected hormone; that is, there appears to be no tendency for those with high circulating antibody titers to develop allergy more frequently than those with low titers. Recent reevaluation of commercial insulin preparations and the development of purified insulin have revealed that the antigenic component consists of higher molecular weight substances. The use of purified insulin preparations is said not to be associated with the development of circulating anti-insulin IgG antibodies. Whether such insulin will reduce the incidence of local allergic responses is unknown, but since these local allergic responses are probably related to IgE insulin antibodies, it is not certain they will disappear altogether.

The most common local reactions are relatively mild and include stinging or itching at the injection site, which may or may not be followed by heat, induration, erythema, and an urticarial reaction. Some patients develop generalized urticaria accompanied by nausea, vomiting, diarrhea, or, in rare instances, angioneurotic edema and serum sickness. Occasionally, reports have been made of anaphylactic shock and, in a few instances, purpura as well. The incidence of these allergic reactions appears to be decreasing, perhaps because of the increased purity of insulin preparations, indicating that some of them are due to the contaminants. Some authors have concluded that the added protamine has produced some of these allergic reactions, and that the use of non–protamine-containing insulin preparations may be beneficial. Since insulin is often a necessary treatment regardless of the hypersensitive state, treatment of the allergy is usually necessary. Fortunately, over 95 per cent of the reactions are local and mild. Usually, the patients are treated systemically with antihistaminic compounds, and the type of insulin is changed. In some instances, it has been claimed that boiling the insulin in the closed vial reduces the number of local reactions, but most of the reactions diminish in time regardless of the treatment. Occasionally, glucosteroids must be given; epinephrine is injected in an emergency.

Lipodystrophy

The subcutaneous injection of insulin in certain susceptible patients may result in either hypertrophy or atrophy of the local adipose tissue mass (Fig. 9–55). The hypertrophy is easily explainable by insulin's known action on the synthesis of lipids by the fat cells. The cause of the atrophy is completely unknown but appears not to be related to inflammatory changes or trauma imposed by the injection. Either event is benign and potentially reversible if the site is avoided. No specific treatment is effective. The best way of preventing it is by careful rotation of injection sites. The patient should use the abdomen or other area where subcutaneous atrophy or hypertrophy is less of a cosmetic problem.

Clinical Insulin Use

Although many physicians have believed that patients who cannot be managed without ex-

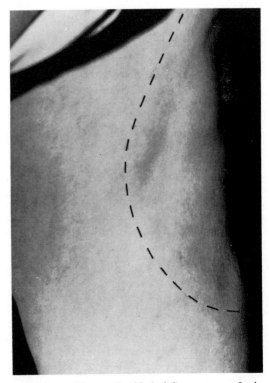

Figure 9–55. Lipoatrophy. Marked disappearance of subcutaneous fat in localized area of thigh (to right of broken line), leaving prominent depression. This was the site of frequent insulin injections. Atrophy sometimes also occurs in areas not injected.

ogenous insulin secrete no endogenous insulin, recent studies by Rubinstein and collaborators indicate that a fair number of insulin-treated patients do have the capacity to synthesize and secrete small amounts of insulin. In fact, the ability of many patients to be treated with one dose of long-acting insulin per day may be dependent upon this small residual insulin secretion. In difficult cases, including totally pancreatectomized individuals, it is often desirable to prescribe insulin in more than one dose per day. Generally, it is the authors' practice to begin with an intermediate-acting insulin and to increase its dose until glycosuria is no longer present in the late afternoon specimen. If glycosuria is still significant before the morning or noon meal, crystalline insulin is added until glycosuria is ameliorated or clinical hypoglycemia occurs. Under these conditions, if the patient is still hyperglycemic before breakfast or has frequent irregular episodes of hypo- and hyperglycemia, we usually prescribe two doses of insulin per day, with the bulk of the intermediate acting insulin injected 20 minutes before breakfast and 1/6 to 1/3 of the total dose before dinner. The two most important modifiers of patient response are the pattern of meal-eating and the degree of exercise. If exercise is intermittent and irregular, it is our habit to add calories in the form of a snack just prior to exercise rather than to manipulate the insulin dosage. Even though the expected exercise may be quite vigorous, food ingestion has not hampered the patients' ability to perform, even in competitive sports. All patients who are treated with insulin of intermediate or prolonged action should have food snacks in midmorning, midafternoon and at bed time.

Patient Instruction

The patient, or in some instances a relative or friend, must be given instruction regarding the use of insulin therapy. During recent years insulin has been available as 40 U./ml. and 80 U./ml., which has led to confusion in dosage. The American Diabetes Association has recently recommended that only one strength of insulin, 100 U./ml., be supplied. Whichever concentration is adopted, a syringe should be prescribed with only one set of units on the barrel. A metric system in which 100 U./ml. of solution is available is a simple and convenient pattern. This requires syringes that are as accurately calibrated as the standard 1-ml. tuberculin syringe. There has been a growing use of disposable syringes and needles for the diabetic population, and it has been found that one such syringe and needle may last up to a week with safety, thus markedly reducing the cost. The advantage of disposable needles is their consistently sharp point. Either a 24- or 26-gauge needle of 1/2-inch length is satisfactory. Patients should be instructed in a method of injection which uses a different site each time, preferably moving up one thigh and down the other, but the abdominal wall or arms may be used if necessary. It is desirable for the physician to induce a minor hypoglycemic reaction so that the patient will be acquainted with its manifestations and its relief by carbohydrate-containing liquids. The patient should have a card or a "medic-alert" tag to indicate that he is a diabetic and is taking insulin.

Oral Hypoglycemic Agents

There are two groups of oral drugs which effectively lower the blood sugar. In one group, the active portion in each compound is a sulfonylurea radical, so that drugs in this group are called sulfonylureas (Fig. 9–56). They are derivatives of sulfur-containing antibiotics which are ineffective as antimicrobial agents. Although their potency, metabolism, and side-effects differ, their major mechanism of action is believed to be the same, and therefore they are discussed together. The other class of compounds consists of biguanides, which have an entirely different mode of action. They depend on the presence of the biguanide radical, which is a complex linear grouping of nitrogen, carbon, and hydrogen (Fig. 9–56).

When these oral agents were first described, there was much hope that their use in chemical or mild overt diabetic subjects would improve longevity by inhibiting progression of atherosclerosis, microvascular disease, and nephropathy. However, the report of the University Group Diabetes Program in 1971 and 1972 indicated that patients treated with tolbutamide for eight years had a higher incidence of death from cardiovascular dis-

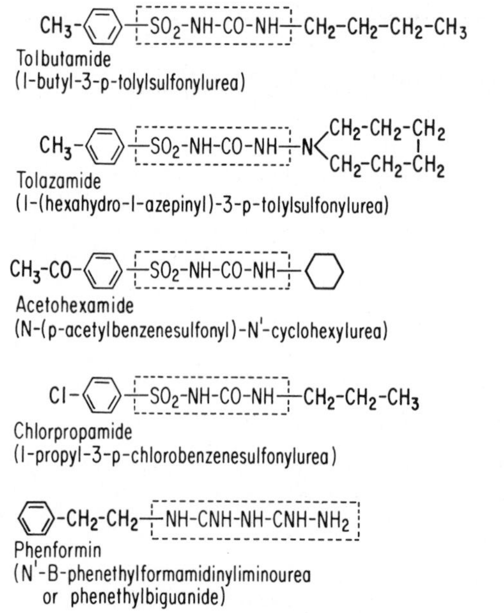

Figure 9–56. The five oral antidiabetic compounds that are most often used. The component of the first four that is active in lowering blood glucose is the rectangular portion (−SO2−NH−CO−NH−), sulfonylurea radical. The active portion of the fifth compound is the biguanide radical (−NH−CNH−NH−CNH−NH₂).

ease than did control patients. Subsequently, phenformin (phenethylbiguanide) has also been reported to be associated with an increased incidence of cardiovascular deaths. Some other investigators have reported net benefits from these drugs, but their observations have been less extensive. This has created a massive and persistent controversy, concerning not only the use of tolbutamide and phenformin but also the use of other sulfonylureas. We do not yet know to what extent the long-range advantage of these other sulfonylureas outweighs their disadvantages. Therefore, at the present time, a number of factors must be considered in deciding between insulin and oral hypoglycemic therapy. The patient should share in the decision, if possible, and be aware of the inherent risks of both forms of treatment of altered carbohydrate metabolism.

Insulin therapy requires meticulous attention. Dosage must be adjusted in relation to exercise and meals, and hypoglycemia is a fairly frequent complication in cases of severe diabetes. Effective self-administration of insulin requires more patient education and greater visual acuity than does oral therapy. Oral hypoglycemic agents are rarely associated with hypoglycemia but may interact with other drugs ingested by the patient; occasionally they may be associated with unwanted side-effects or may have their effectiveness altered by changes in hepatic metabolism or renal excretion. Some may increase the risk of cardiovascular death. Therefore, no hard and fast rules can be made, and each patient's problem must be approached individually. Insulin and the oral agents are compared in Table 9–14.

Sulfonylureas

Mechanism of Action

In general, it appears that the mechanism of action of each sulfonylurea is similar, but the strength and duration of action differ considerably. The presence of responsive islets is necessary for these compounds to lower blood sugar. Since they can all be shown to increase acutely the secretion of insulin, it is generally believed that this is the primary mechanism of action; however, under certain circumstances, it is possible to demonstrate some increase in the sensitivity of peripheral tissues and liver to the effects of insulin, and, therefore, it may be that some blood sugar–lowering is related to an interaction of sulfonylurea with organs other than the pancreas. In clinical studies, one can demonstrate increased basal insulin secretion and insulin output in response to challenge for several weeks after starting sulfonylurea. However, long-term administration of these compounds is generally associated with a sustained blood sugar–lowering action and the return of insulin to pretreatment levels.

Such findings have been interpreted in two ways: either the initial effect is due to increased insulin secretion and the delayed effect is to improve insulin-stimulated glucose uptake so that no increase in insulin secretion is necessary, or the chronic effects are related to an increased sensitivity of the pancreatic response to the same glucose challenge, so that the same insulin levels are achieved after glucose administration but with less absolute hyperglycemia needed. The authors are inclined to favor a primary pancreatic mechanism. In fact, the primary effect of the drugs is on the fasting glucose level, with little alteration in postglucose increments in long-term sulfonylurea-treated patients. Thus, over a period of time, fasting blood sugar decreases while insulin output, which can be related to this fasting blood sugar, remains the same, suggesting that in the basal state the sulfonylurea itself is now partly responsible for the insulin secreted. After challenge, the deficient insulin response remains about the same, and blood sugar levels are only lower because of the lowered fasting blood glucose. Thus the deficient insulin response and impaired carbohydrate tolerance in diabetic subjects is not really improved by these agents. Rather, it is the fasting blood glucose that is lowered and the insulin output in the fasting state that is increased by sulfonylurea administration. Physiologically, the patient remains abnormal, even though he is treated with a sulfonylurea agent.

The nature and mechanism of the B-cell response to these compounds is largely unknown. In general, it is believed that there is no increase in B-cell size or number with the most commonly used compounds. However, some authors have suggested that the more potent compounds may actually increase the number of B-cells. The specific details of the mechanism by which sulfonylureas increase insulin release is unknown, but studies *in vitro* suggest that it is quite different from that of glucose or other substrates. In particular, it appears that insulin synthesis, which is definitely stimulated by glucose, is not increased by sulfonylureas.

Metabolism and Excretion

Although the sulfonylureas probably interact with the B cell by a common mechanism, there are

TABLE 9–14. COMPARISONS OF SOME ACTIONS OF INSULIN, SULFONYLUREAS, AND PHENFORMIN

	Insulin	Sulfonylureas	Phenformin
Insulin secretion	Decreased	Increased	Decreased
Glucose uptake by peripheral tissues	Increased	Increased	Increased
Hepatic glucogenesis	Decreased	Decreased	Unknown
Gluconeogenesis	Decreased	Decreased	Unknown
Liver glycogen	Increased	Increased	Unknown
Blood sugar–lowering effect			
Normal subjects	Marked	Moderate	Slight
Depancreatized subjects	Marked	None	Significant
Marked hypoglycemia	Common	Occasional	Rare
Lactate production	Unchanged	Unchanged	Increased

major differences in their degradation, rates of absorption, and methods of excretion. In general, the compounds with short action are metabolized in the liver to inactive forms which are then excreted in the urine. The longer acting compounds are metabolized poorly, if at all, by the liver, and are excreted unchanged in the urine. They or their metabolites may induce hypoglycemia. In the case of a completely nonmetabolized drug, binding to plasma protein plays an important role in duration of action.

Tolbutamide is carboxylated in the liver to an inactive compound, carboxytolbutamide, which is excreted in the urine. When given orally, the biologic half-life is about 3–5 hours. Therefore, the duration of action is short and not dependent upon renal function. *Acetohexamide* is also rapidly metabolized by the liver to form hydroxyhexamide. However, in this case, the metabolic product is definitely hypoglycemic and believed to be somewhat more potent than the parent compound. Approximately 75 per cent of acetohexamide is excreted in this more active form. Since the liver does not diminish the hypoglycemic potency of the compound, the material has an intermediate duration of action which is dependent upon renal excretion and plasma protein binding, which is relatively weak. *Tolazamide* is also rapidly metabolized to at least six metabolic products, but many of them induce hypoglycemia. This leads to an intermediate duration of action very similar to acetohexamide, but at a somewhat lower dose. *Chlorpropamide,* the longest acting compound of the group, is very poorly metabolized. It is tightly bound to protein and is therefore active for long periods. It is dependent upon renal excretion for the termination of its activity and is therefore contraindicated for individuals with significantly reduced renal function.

Side Effects

Many of these compounds have effects on metabolism independent of their hypoglycemic properties. The magnitude of the effect may vary considerably, depending upon the specific drug, but, in general, differences in their effects are quantitative and not qualitative.

Thyroid Gland.   Many reports indicate that sulfonylureas, particularly tolbutamide, decrease I^{131} uptake, but this change appears to be transient and can be reversed by iodide administration. Since only an occasional patient with goiter and myxedema apparently related to sulfonylurea therapy has been reported, it seems likely that some underlying abnormality of thyroid function must be present for the drug to cause hypothyroidism.

Antidiuretic Hormone–Like Effect.   Some patients treated with chlorpropamide have developed symptomatic hyponatremia and water intoxication. Chlorpropamide appears to have an effect on renal tubules similar to that of antidiuretic hormone (ADH) and has even been used to treat patients with ADH insufficiency. Some ADH seems to be necessary for this effect to occur. ADH exerts its antidiuretic action by stimulating adenyl cyclase activity; chlorpropamide presumably augments this enzyme reaction in some manner. No other sulfonylurea has been reported to potentiate ADH action.

Drug Interactions.   The potency of any sulfonylurea may be altered by other drugs. One of the most common effects reported consists of augmentation of the hypoglycemic potency of the sulfonylureas. This is probably observed more frequently because hypoglycemia is clinically obvious and important, whereas a diminution in the potency of the agent and hyperglycemia may erroneously be attributed to some other factor. Drugs such as sulphaphenazole, phenylbutazone, probenecid, salicylate, bishydroxycoumarin, alcohol, sulfisoxazole, and monoamine oxidase inhibitors have been implicated in severe hypoglycemia associated with sulfonylurea administration. It is likely that these compounds either decrease sulfonylurea excretion or reduce its binding to plasma proteins. Some of the foregoing drugs may produce only subclinical hypoglycemia when given alone yet significantly augment the hypoglycemic action of sulfonylureas. Because of the prolonged hypoglycemic activity of sulfonylurea in these clinical settings, observation and treatment may be required for more than 24 hours (Seltzer).

Hypoglycemia.   With moderate doses of sulfonylureas given to patients in relatively good health, and particularly without significant impairment of renal or liver function, hypoglycemia is rare. However, sulfonylurea-induced hypoglycemia may occur without any other drug therapy. This is not really a side-effect, but it is either a manifestation of overdosage with sulfonylurea or, more likely, the result of dosages that are clinically inappropriate. Thus more than 90 per cent of reported episodes of severe sulfonylurea-induced hypoglycemia have occurred in acutely or chronically starved patients or in patients who had demonstrable hepatic or renal impairment or both. This is often compounded by the intake of alcohol, which by itself causes hypoglycemia in the starved individual.

Toxic Side Effects

Gastrointestinal Tract.   Toxic reactions to the sulfonylureas are similar to those of the sulfonamides, from which they are derived. Intestinal symptoms such as anorexia, nausea, vomiting, diarrhea, and abdominal pain are observed in about 5 per cent of patients treated with sulfonylurea, but this incidence is not much higher than that associated with placebo ingestion. A reaction to alcohol similar to that seen after disulfiram, with a clinical syndrome of headache, flushing, and tachycardia, may be seen in a number of patients treated with sulfonylurea, particularly chlorpropamide. The mechanism is unknown but is of sufficient importance and magnitude to make patients aware of such a possibility when beginning treatment with a sulfonylurea. Hepatic reactions to the drug are less frequent, but mild to severe cholestatic jaundice has been reported. In general, the more the hypoglycemic potency, the more likely it is to cause liver impairment. This toxic effect is dose related, especially with chlorpropamide. Hepatocellular damage has been suggested at times, but liver biopsies usually have shown only canalicular bile stasis, similar to that reported for chlorpromazine.

Skin. Maculopapular eruptions have been reported, often with pruritus, and are probably symptoms of allergic hypersensitivity.

Hematopoietic System. Hematologic toxicity has been reported rarely; it includes agranulocytosis and pancytopenia.

Cardiovascular System. The sulfonylurea compounds have been used not only for control of symptomatic hyperglycemia but also to reduce diabetic concomitants such as microvascular disease, atherosclerosis, and neuropathy. Many of these patients have elevated blood sugars but only minimal to moderate glycosuria. To determine the true efficacy of this therapy, the National Institutes of Health sponsored observations of mild diabetics throughout 8 years. They were divided into 5 groups to receive either (a) placebo administration, (b) tolbutamide, (d) phenformin, (d) a fixed dose of insulin, or (e) a variable dose of insulin. The study was started in 1961, and the results caused a furor in 1970, when it was reported that, compared with placebo or insulin groups, there was an increase in cardiovascular deaths in a group of over 200 patients treated with tolbutamide in a fixed dose. As a result, the Food and Drug Administration recommended that oral hypoglycemic agents should be used only when diet alone is ineffective and insulin impractical or unacceptable. The data (Table 9–15) showed an increase in cardiovascular-related deaths for the tolbutamide group (Fig. 9–57) and later an increase in cardiovascular deaths for the phenformin-treated group. Although both tolbutamide and phenformin groups had an in-

TABLE 9–15. NUMBER OF DEATHS OF DIABETIC PATIENTS TREATED WITH TOLBUTAMIDE, INSULIN, OR PHENFORMIN*

	Tolbutamide	Insulin** Standard	Insulin† Variable	Placebo	Phenformin‡
Total Deaths	30	20	18	21	31
CV-Related Deaths	26	13	12	10	26

*UGDP Study—823 patients, *Diabetes* 19:747, 1970.
**10–16 U., depending on body surface area.
†Dosage varied to lower blood sugar.
‡Added and reported later.

crease in total mortality, this was not statistically different from the other groups. The increasing percentage of death related to cardiovascular disease became apparent between the third and fifth year of the study. Because of this increase, the study was discontinued in the eighth year and the recommendations referred to above made.

Many criticisms of this study are available, perhaps the best of which are summarized by Feinstein and Cornfield. These two authors suggest that a difference in cardiovascular mortality was not established by the study. The study investigators thought this unlikely but possible. On the other hand, no critic has suggested that a beneficial effect of the drugs is likely to have been overlooked. Therefore, there is no evidence that these oral compounds prevent the cardiovascular and neuropathic abnormalities of diabetes. It is hoped that these studies will lead to more research into the basic nature of the diabetic defect and to better therapy for all aspects of the disease. Comparable observations of the results of prolonged use of chlorpropamide, acetohexamide, tolazamide, and

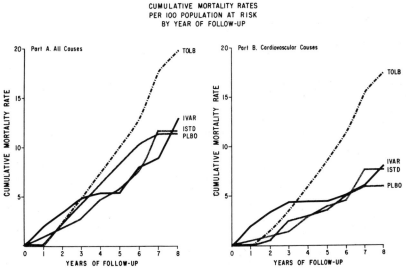

Figure 9–57. Results of the cumulative mortality statistics for the 8-year University Group Diabetes Program (UGDP) Study. Rates are given per 100 population at risk by year of follow-up. TOLB = tolbutamide, 1.5 g./day; IVAR = insulin, enough to keep blood sugar normal; ISTD = insulin, 10–16 units based on surface area; PLBO = placebo. (From Meinert, C. L., et al.: *Diabetes* 19:789, 1970.)

other sulfonylureas have not been reported, but there are many similarities in chemical characteristics and biologic activity.

Dosage and Practical Use

The choice of sulfonylurea depends on its potency, biologic half-life, cost, and side-effects. In general, the most potent compounds are those most slowly metabolized and therefore the most likely to produce unwanted hypoglycemia. In a diabetic taking insulin, it is not possible to predict with certainty whether a sulfonylurea can be used satisfactorily as a substitute. Since the reports of the University Group Diabetes Program (UGDP) studies, this substitution has become much less frequent. In general, individuals who have had episodes of ketoacidosis or who use more than 40 units of insulin per day are unlikely to be responsive to sulfonylureas. The dosage used is that necessary to maintain blood sugar at the desired level up to the maximum indicated for each compound (Table 9–16). The incidence of secondary failures is not established but appears to be about 5 per cent/yr. Sulfonylureas are rarely used for pregnant women in the United States, but in some investigations in Scotland and South Africa, no ill-effects were reported. During elective surgery, minor infections, and other minor illnesses, it is not necessary to substitute insulin unless ketosis appears. In emergency surgery or severe infections, it is best to substitute insulin. It is of some interest that studies of apparently well-selected patients have indicated that approximately 30 per cent could be maintained without sulfonylurea therapy when pills were withdrawn from all subjects randomly in an outpatient diabetic clinic. This suggests that the disease may fluctuate from time to time and has raised consideration of the desirability of intermittent rather than continuous treatment of symptomatic hyperglycemia and glycosuria.

Biguanides

Mechanism of Action

Guanidine and many of its derivatives long have been known to produce hypoglycemia, but interest has been centered predominantly on the condensed diguanidine, phenethylbiguanide (phenformin). Since this material is derived from a very toxic compound, it affects many metabolic processes *in vitro*. Despite numerous investigations, the mechanism for its plasma glucose lowering effect *in vivo* remains uncertain. It does not depend on insulin for its actions. Three attractive hypotheses concerning its actions are:

1. Phenformin increases peripheral glucose utilization by interfering with oxidative metabolism of glucose, thereby accelerating anaerobic glycolysis and the uptake of glucose by peripheral cells. This hypothesis has been supported by direct observations of such effects *in vitro* and by the increase in plasma lactate which it produces.

2. It decreases glucose output by the liver, particularly when this output is increased by accelerated gluconeogenesis which may be present in diabetic subjects. Evidence for inhibition of gluconeogenesis has been primarily derived from studies in the guinea pig. It has been considered unlikely to occur in the rat and has never been demonstrated conclusively in man; results of radioisotopic studies (see the following) in fact suggest an increase in glucose turnover during phenformin therapy. Therefore, this appears to be a species-specific effect.

3. Phenformin decreases absorption or delays the absorption of glucose from the GI tract. Several groups have reported that the oral glucose tolerance test is improved by phenformin, but the intravenous glucose tolerance test is not, and that the oral test is associated with lower insulin levels, indicating that improvement cannot be related to increased insulin secretion. Kruger and associates have also demonstrated some inhibition of active transport in everted sacs of rat intestine, and Cgyzyk and associates have shown a decreased uptake of glucose from dog intestinal segments *in vivo*. Nonetheless, in intact man, glucose turnover and recycling, as estimated from C^{14} glucose studies by Searle, show increased glucose turnover and increased glucose recycling from lactate.

The general conclusion to be drawn seems to be that guanidine derivatives are toxic to many tissues. Studies performed *in vitro* are therefore difficult to interpret. From studies *in vivo*, it appears that increased glucose uptake in peripheral tissues and the decreased rate of absorption from the small intestine are the two major effects of the biguanide. It seems likely that normal compensatory mecha-

TABLE 9–16.   DOSAGE OF ORAL COMPOUNDS

Generic Names	Trade Names	Total Daily Doses (g.)		Doses Per Day	Approx. Duration of Action (hr.)
		Common	*Range**		
Tolbutamide	Orinase	1.5	0.5 –3.0	2–3	6–10
Acetohexamide	Dymelor	0.7	0.25–1.25	1–2	10–16
Tolazamide	Tolinase	0.25	0.1 –0.75	1	10–16
Chlorpropamide	Diabinese	0.25	0.1 –0.5	1	40–72
Phenformin	DBI–TD	0.1	0.05–0.15	2	6–10

*The authors rarely use the highest level of these ranges. The increase in the antidiabetic effect must be weighed against a possible increase in side-effects.

nisms prevent these effects from being reflected in significant hypoglycemia in normal man, and probably the therapeutic effects in diabetic patients are due to these two mechanisms, which vary quantitatively from patient to patient. Increased production of lactate accompanies use of the compound, but in most circumstances it is metabolized or recycled. Thus, although lactic acidosis is a potential complication of the drug, it seems to require a predisposing abnormality.

Metabolism and Excretion

Studies with C^{14}-labeled phenformin indicate that the material is primarily concentrated in the liver and GI tract, with eventual recovery of all of the C^{14} in the urine. Thus, although the product may be metabolized, it is not associated with oxidation of the carbon structure. It has been estimated that approximately one-third is excreted as a metabolite and two-thirds as the unchanged compound. Biologic half-life is not known precisely but is estimated to be approximately 3 hours.

Drug Interactions

No drugs are known to increase or decrease the therapeutic potency of phenformin. However, since its mechanism of action is different from that of the sulfonylureas, the two may be used together with additive results. Similarly, other hypoglycemic agents, such as salicylates, may be expected to potentiate the effects of phenformin. Hypoglycemia is rare.

Side Effects

Side effects are very common with the biguanides, and the line that divides a therapeutically effective dosage from that causing annoying side effects is very thin in many patients. The side effects are mostly gastrointestinal and include a metallic taste in the mouth, various degrees of anorexia, nausea, vomiting, and occasional diarrhea. They are less common with the sustained-release form of the drug, which is used almost invariably now, and are definitely dose-related, as they often disappear when the dosage is reduced. Allergic reactions appear to be very unusual, although transient erythema with pruritus and urticaria has been reported.

Toxicity to the liver and kidney has been essentially nonexistent, despite the known toxicity of this class of compounds. The major problem has been the relationship of phenformin to the development of lactic acidosis in the diabetic subject and the recent evidence for vascular effects in the UGDP study.

Lactic Acidosis. Lactic acidosis is a rare complication of diabetes mellitus which seems to occur with somewhat greater frequency in patients taking phenformin. It significantly increases lactic acid production. Whether or not there is a concomi-

tant increase in lactate levels depends upon the compensatory increase in lactate uptake and metabolism by the liver and other tissues. It seems unlikely that the drug could cause this complication alone. It is more likely that it requires the presence of some predisposing factor, such as chronic renal or hepatic failure, hypovolemic shock, myocardial or mesenteric infarction, peripheral gangrene, or severe congestive heart failure. It is also possible that large quantities of alcohol contribute to the development of hyperlactic acidemia and lactic acidosis; if so, patients should be warned of the dangers of excessive alcoholic intake.

Cardiovascular Effects. Phenformin was one of the study compounds included in the UGDP study of vascular complications in patients with mild carbohydrate intolerance. As with tolbutamide, an approximate twofold increase in mortality from cardiovascular diseases was observed at the end of eight years. The drug was therefore discontinued and the conclusion drawn that phenformin was no more effective than diet alone and may be potentially hazardous to this group of patients.

Dosage and Practical Use

The sustained-release form of phenformin is virtually the only one used at the present time, since it greatly minimizes side-effeects. Very few patients will benefit from as little as 50 mg./day, and very few will be able to tolerate more than 150 mg./day. Thus almost all patients are treated with 50 mg. twice daily. As is the case with the administration of sulfonylureas, it is generally recommended that any severe illness should be treated with insulin, but any minor illness can be managed without insulin therapy. Phenformin may be combined with sulfonylurea, since the effects are additive. Although some have suggested that it may be useful in insulin-treated patients, there is no good evidence to support benefit. It is not the authors' practice to use either of the oral agents in combination with insulin therapy. Very careful clinical trials have shown in double-blind fashion that phenformin leads to more weight loss than does placebo. However, this effect is very small (in the range of one to five pounds per year) and therefore is not a very compelling reason to use the drug for obese subjects.

For practical purposes then, phenformin has been used predominantly in younger, otherwise healthy obese subjects with glycosuria and rather severe hyperglycemia who will not restrict calories or take insulin. Phenformin can maintain plasma glucose lowering in diabetic patients, even in the presence of moderate to severe ketosis. Therefore, glycosuria may be minimal because of the drug's ability to lower the blood sugar in a patient with insufficient insulin to prevent ketoacidosis. It is important, therefore, not to overlook ketoacidosis in phenformin-treated patients who are not well but have minimal glycosuria. The authors use this drug very little.

Recapitulation and Conclusions Concerning Diet, Drug, and Insulin Therapy in Diabetes

Despite major scientific advances in the last 50 years, there is little knowledge of the basic etiology and pathogenesis of diabetes, and, therefore, treatment directed toward the vascular and neuropathic concomitants of the disease has been inadequate. Insulin treatment for severe insulin deficiency is obvious. Treatment for milder carbohydrate abnormalities is more complex. Obese, overt diabetics with hyperglycemia and glycosuria should begin with caloric restriction; oral drugs or insulin treatment is to be started whenever there are indications that diet (caloric control) cannot achieve or is not achieving control of the glycosuria. The choice of therapy between insulin and the oral antidiabetic agents in this group can be made only after the possible problems and benefits from both forms of therapy are considered and discussed with the patient. A long-term program *must* be developed. The therapy of asymptomatic hyperglycemia (chemical diabetes) remains a very controversial issue. In view of the difficulties with insulin therapy and the potential hazards of the oral antidiabetic agents, many physicians at the present time are inclined to treat such patients only with diet (caloric restriction).

COMPLICATIONS OF DIABETES

The so-called complications of diabetes all seem to be related chiefly to insufficient glucose utilization, with resultant abnormalities in carbohydrate, fat, protein, nucleotide, mineral, and vitamin metabolism. Changes in these constituents are probably also important in the production of the so-called chronic manifestations of diabetes, including cardiovascular, renal, retinal, neural, and dermal abnormalities. However, we consider that these phases are not complications of diabetes but diabetic *concomitants;* that is, they are really part of the disease process. The important acute complications include ketoacidosis, hyperosmolar coma, lactic acidosis, and infections of the skin and other parts of the body.

Ketoacidosis

Ketoacidosis is a manifestation of diabetes which must be given immediate and very careful attention, or dire consequences may result (Danowski, Hockaday). For example, mortality has been found to occur in from 5–15 per cent of patients in a number of large centers. The rate of death from diabetic coma reduces the duration of life by 21 years on the average. The factors that seem to be most important in prognostication are age, hypotension, "associated conditions," high blood urea, and the degree and duration of coma. Of these factors, "associated conditions" (e.g., infection, cardiac disease), degree of unconsciousness, duration of coma, and hypotension appear to have the following ratios of frequency in promoting death: 140:67:10:3.

Pathogenesis

The most important pathogenic element in the production of ketoacidosis is usually a marked reduction in insulin action, but also there commonly are increases in glucagon, catecholamines, glucosteroids, and GH (Table 9–5). As discussed earlier, these last four hormones antagonize, in one way or another, all the actions of insulin. Among the changes resulting from too little insulin action are the release of FFA, followed by accumulation of large quantities of ketone bodies, particularly acetoacetic acid and β-hydroxybutyric acid, thereby producing acidosis (Fig. 9–58).

Adipose Tissue

In an analysis of sequential changes producing ketoacidosis, attention must first be given to adipose tissue, since it supplies most of the ketone precursors. As discussed earlier, insulin markedly stimulates synthesis of fatty acids, leading to the

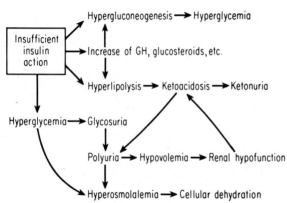

Figure 9–58. With marked insufficiency in insulin action, there are increases in gluconeogenesis, ketogenesis, glycogenolysis, hyperglycemia, hyperosmolalemia, excessive loss of water and electrolytes, acidosis, and many additional sequelae.

formation and storage of triglycerides, chiefly in adipose tissue. Insulin also exerts a potent action in keeping triglycerides stored. In rats, production of diabetes by infusion of insulin antibodies is associated with increased FFA within 1 hour. This loss of the antilipolytic action of insulin apparently precedes evidence for decrease in glucose uptake by adipose tissue. In long-standing diabetes, impaired reesterification of fatty acids plays an important role in causing persistent elevation of plasma FFA levels. However, there are many hormones that prompt lipolysis, and they may override insulin's action; this occurs with a decrease in the supply of insulin or an increase in the supply of lipolytic agents. Among the lipolytic hormones are epinephrine, norepinephrine, glucagon, glucosteroids, thyroxine, triiodothyronine, TSH, ACTH, MSH, GH, vasopressin, and chorionic somatomammotropin. Lipolytic hormones stimulate lipolysis in adipose tissue, and glucosteroids, in the presence of insulin deficiency, decrease reesterification of fatty acids by suppressing the metabolism of glucose. The highly significant role of the adrenal hormones and pituitary hormones in ketogenesis has been demonstrated by removing the respective glands and by administering the various hormones.

GH, glucagon, catecholamines, and glucosteroids have been found in increased quantities in ketoacidosis. Of course, there are many life situations that increase the supply of one or more of these hormones; among them are emotional disturbances, a vast number of disease processes (infections, injuries, thyrotoxicosis), and many physiologic changes (pregnancy, lactation, starvation). When normal rats are fasted for about one week and the pancreas removed, no significant ketoacidosis is produced, apparently because the precursor for the ketones (triglycerides) has been greatly depleted during the starvation. Such a phenomenon probably accounts for the benefits of marked food restriction in the preinsulin era. Conversely, a diet composed chiefly of fat contributes to ketogenesis.

Muscle

Skeletal muscle and heart can derive almost all their energy from FFA and ketones; indeed, these substances are used preferentially. Some of the hormones that promote lipolysis in adipose tissue also lead to protein breakdown in muscle, but glucosteroids have the strongest effect. In ketoacidosis, there generally is a decrease in uptake by muscle of glucose and amino acids.

Liver

In the liver, ketoacidosis is associated with (a) an increase in uptake of fatty acids and amino acids but a decrease in glucose uptake, (b) a decrease in lipogenesis, (c) an increase in ketogenesis, (d) an increase in gluconeogenesis, (e) an increase in glycogenolysis, and (f) an increase in intravascular release of glucose and ketones (Fig. 9–33, Table 9–4, Fig. 9–58).

Acetyl CoA is in the center of several of the foregoing reactions, since it is a common intermediate in the metabolism of fatty acids, glucose, and amino acids. There are three main pathways for its disposal: (a) condensation with oxaloacetate to form citrate, and oxidation in the Krebs cycle, (b) condensation of two acetyl CoA molecules to form acetoacetyl CoA, the precursor of acetoacetate, and (c) fatty acid synthesis from acetyl CoA via malonyl CoA. In ketoacidosis there is an increase in the acetyl CoA converted to acetoacetate, attributable partially to (a) inhibition of fatty acid synthesis by inhibition of acetyl CoA–carboxylase by acyl CoA–thioesters, and (b) inhibition of citrate synthetase by these thioesters, causing a decrease in oxidation in the Krebs cycle.

Most of the energy derived from glucose is obtained from its oxidation via the TCA cycle. With an increase in fatty acid oxidation in the liver, there is an increase in DPNH and a decrease in the ratio of ATP to ADP formed. The increase to DPNH is highly important in the gluconeogenesis that commonly accompanies ketoacidosis because it is the major supply of H^+ (Fig. 9–59). The increase in DPNH inhibits the oxidation of malate to oxaloacetate. Wieland found a marked increase in the malate:oxaloacetate ratio in livers of ketoacidotic rats. With inhibition of citrate synthetase by acyl CoA and with a decrease in oxaloacetate, there is a decrease in citrate formed in the liver. However, since in subjects with ketoacidosis there is an increase in citrate concentration in the systemic circulation, there is an increased supply of citrate from certain sources, including muscle and bone. With the decrease in citrate formed in the liver, there is a decrease in lipogenesis; this ordinarily is a major route for synthesis of fatty acids.

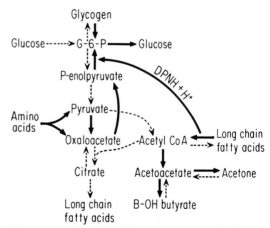

Figure 9–59. Some key biochemical changes in the liver during ketoacidosis. With increase in lipolysis and increase in fatty acids, lipogenesis is inhibited and acetyl CoA accumulates. There is inhibition of citrate synthetase and decrease in citrate oxidation, but an increase in ketogenesis and gluconeogenesis.

The increase in acetyl CoA stimulates direct carboxylation of pyruvate to oxaloacetate, and the oxaloacetate, since its oxidation in the Krebs cycle is inhibited, is more available for utilization in gluconeogenesis. In this process the liver derives energy from production of ketones by partial oxidation of long-chain fatty acids. In gluconeogenesis, the fatty acids supply most of the hydrogen atoms for reduction of pyruvate toward the formation of glucose, and amino acids supply most of the carbon atoms required, i.e., via pyruvate, directly or indirectly; fatty acids are unable to contribute carbon for gluconeogenesis. The synthesis of one molecule of glucose from two molecules of pyruvate is expected to be associated with the accumulation of one half-molecule of acetoacetate and one molecule of urea when the pyruvate is derived from amino acids. Under certain experimental conditions, fructose, glycerol, and propionate have each been demonstrated to exert significant antiketogenic effects. However, clinically these compounds have not proved efficacious in the treatment of ketoacidosis.

When insulin deficiency is mild, the extra ketones, hyperglycemia, and glycosuria are not excessive. Formation of large amounts of glucose is accompanied by the formation of large quantities of ketones. Up to about 1500 cal./day can be consumed in the form of ketones. However, the surplus acetoacetate and β-hydroxbutyrate are excreted in the urine predominantly as anions in conjunction with cations, thereby significantly depleting Na^+ and K^+ and abetting the osmotic diuresis and dehydration produced by glucosuria; these changes increase the metabolic acidosis.

Kidneys

The kidneys play a highly important role in ketoacidosis, not only from the point of view of water and electrolyte balance, but also in the elimination of the increased nitrogenous products, glucose and other elements. With marked ketoacidosis, the amount of gluconeogenesis is decreased in the liver but increased in the kidneys. Indeed, the kidneys can probably produce as much as 50 per cent of the total supply of glucose under these circumstances. However, gluconeogenesis in the kidneys serves a more useful purpose by producing ammonia (important in the regulation of acid-base balance) than by producing glucose.

Hyperglycemia

Hyperglycemia results from excess production of glucose, chiefly by the liver, and from a decrease in its utilization by various tissues. With the decrease in glucose uptake by cells, there is a net decrease in intracellular electrolytes, water, and other elements (Fig. 9–58). The hyperosmolality of the plasma produces an osmotic diuresis, with loss of water in excess of electrolytes, although there is also a marked loss of the electrolytes, including Na^+, K^+, Cl^-, PO_4, Mg^{++}, Ca^{++}, H^+, and other ions.

Increasing osmolality of the plasma occurs, leading to more cellular dehydration and eventually to extracellular dehydration and hypovolemia. With marked reduction in plasma volume, the renal function becomes impaired, permitting intensification of the acidosis, greater disturbances in electrolyte equilibria, and azotemia. The blood sugar may attain levels in excess of 1000 mg./100 ml., whereas with normal renal function it usually does not exceed 500. With severe impairment of renal function, there may be less glucose and ketones in the urine than with less severe diabetes; thus the urinary findings sometimes are misleading.

Hyperketonemia

Werk has found that many "controlled" diabetics, in either a fasting or a postprandial state, had hyperketonemia. Many also had increased plasma levels during fasting, though not postprandially. The ketone values increased with blood glucose concentration. It appears that the level of plasma ketones sometimes more satisfactorily reflects the adequacy of diabetic control than do the levels of blood sugar or FFA. The metabolic consequence of the accumulation of acetoacetate and β-hydroxybutyric acid is a decrease in pH. This increase in H^+ ions from the organic acids shifts the bicarbonate system to the left, resulting in more H_2CO_3 and CO_2. The decrease in pH stimulates the respiratory center to increase activity, characterized by very deep and rapid Kussmaul respiration. Kussmaul breathing does not occur at pH above 7.2 (Fig. 9–60). As the pH is lowered below 7.0, the respiratory effort may decrease because of muscular

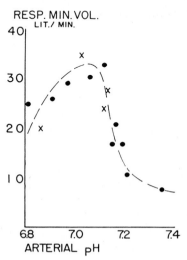

Figure 9–60. With decrease in plasma pH, the pulmonary ventilation increases, reaching a maximum at about pH 7.1; with further decrease in pH, the ventilation decreases. Thus, with decreasing rate of ventilation, the patient may be changing for either the better or the worse. The circles consist of data from patients who ultimately recovered and the crosses from those who succumbed. (From Kety, S. S., et al.: *J. Clin. Invest.* 27:500, 1948.)

fatigue and respiratory center narcosis. With this there is a further decrease in pH and a grave prognosis. The buffering effect of the bicarbonate system and the hyperventilation lower the CO_2 but do not rid the body of excess H^+. The ultimate correction of this depends upon the oxidation of the ketones or renal excretion of H^+. The latter is accomplished by either (a) the preferential exchange of H^+ for Na^+ by the renal tubules, or (b) the excretion by the renal tubules of ammonia, which reacts with H^+ to form NH_4^+. Therefore, the kidney is very important in preventing the accumulation of H^+; renal impairment permits intensification of ketosis. Decreases in extracellular volume secondary to sodium losses diminish renal plasma flow and glomerular filtration. Moreover, renal impairment decreases ammonia production, not only because of decreased renal cellular activity but also because of decreased delivery of ammonia precursors (glutamine and amino acids) to the kidneys. In diabetic acidosis there is not as much lowering of the urinary pH as in comparable degrees of acidosis of other types, because of depletion of renal cellular potassium in the former. There develops a vicious circle in which ketoacidosis promotes Na^+ and K^+ depletion and, in turn, an increase in H^+. The increase in H^+ causes not only hyperventilation but also mobilization of bone minerals. The ketosis may be compensated for weeks, but decompensation readily occurs with nausea and vomiting, because dehydration decreases renal blood flow and renal function.

Serum Lipid Changes

With decreased glucose utilization there is an increase in serum levels of FFA, followed by an increase in triglyceride, phospholipid and cholesterol. The changes in FFA are very labile and are good indicators of glucose utilization.

Lipoproteins accumulate because of a decrease in the ability of peripheral tissues to utilize their triglyceride. Fredrickson has emphasized that, when a patient goes from a state of severe ketoacidosis to a level of good control, the associated increase in peripheral utilization may prompt serial manifestation of 4 of the 5 major abnormal lipoprotein patterns. With severe acidosis, the plasma is often creamy; in some instances lipid may occupy as much as 48 per cent of the plasma. There is a great excess of very-low-density lipoprotein (VLDL), accompanied by marked chylomicronemia. This type V pattern indicates dissociation between the rate of entry of plasma triglycerides and their removal from the circulation due to an insulin-dependent deficiency in the lipoprotein lipase system. With improved control of diabetes, the lipoprotein pattern shifts to a pattern dominated by certain LDL, which have a great excess of glyceride in relation to their usual complement of protein. The density of these LDL is much lower than that of normal LDL, and "floating-β" lipoproteins appear in the ultracentrifuge fraction in which normally only VLDL appears; this is a type III lipoprotein pattern. With further improvement, the type IV pattern appears, with a simple increase in VLDL. As the acidosis becomes fully controlled, all the excess triglycerides and lipoproteins disappear, leaving a transient wake of LDL, normal in composition but excessive in concentration (type II). This pattern is short-lived. With excellent control of the diabetes, a normal lipoprotein pattern may be regained (Ch. 18).

Protein and Amino Acid Changes

With ketoacidosis, there is a marked increase in the breakdown of proteins and many changes in amino acid metabolism, particularly in muscle and liver, as discussed earlier (Table 9-4). There are marked decreases in plasma levels of glucogenic amino acids: glycine, threonine, serine, alanine, and glutamine. There are increases in the ketogenic amino acids: leucine, isoleucine, and valine. There is an increase in mobilization of amino acids from muscle, with increased hepatic extraction of the glucogenic amino acids.

Changes in Oxidative Processes

The level of lactic acid is usually increased in ketoacidosis. Indeed, as discussed later, some of the patients with ketoacidosis also have lactic acidosis. There is some increase in pyruvate in ketoacidosis, but the increase in lactate is proportionately greater. About one-third of diabetic coma patients have been found to have decreased pO_2, and 2,3-diphosphoglycerate (DPG). Increased conversion of glucose to sorbitol, acidosis, and low phosphate tend to reduce DPG, while increased pyruvate tends to elevate it. There is defective oxygen release from hemoglobin, presumably related to the decrease in DPG related to acidosis. The decrease in oxidative reactions very likely plays an important role in the course of the ketoacidosis. The reduced blood volume, poor cardiac output, and hypotension that commonly are found with ketoacidosis all contribute to the diminished oxygen supply.

Alterations in Functions of Central Nervous System

Depression in nervous system activities occurs with ketoacidosis, and eventually coma may occur. With coma there is a significant decrease in cerebral oxygen consumption without a decrease in cerebral blood flow or arterial oxygen saturation. All the factors contributing to the coma are not clear, but the following three are important: (a) increased acetoacetate, (b) increased H^+, (c) dehydration, and (d) hyperosmolarity.

Clinical Considerations

Contributing Factors. Diabetic coma occurs chiefly in the juvenile-onset, insulin-dependent type; it infrequently occurs in the adult-onset type and usually does not develop in patients with Cushing's disease. It is much commoner in females than males. It usually occurs in patients in whom diabetes has been diagnosed previously.

As shown in Figure 9–58, ketoacidosis results from a decrease in glucose utilization. This may be caused by a decreased glucose intake, insufficient insulin, hyperadrenocorticism, and many other factors. It apparently is not due to excess carbohydrate intake; on the contrary, within certain limits, this helps to decrease ketosis. Under certain conditions, an increase in the blood glucose concentration increases hepatic glucogenesis rather than decreases it as in normal persons. Often the patient, because he does not "feel well," decreases his food intake and simultaneously decreases his dose of insulin. Each of these promotes ketogenesis. Moreover, the complaint of "not feeling well" may be due to an infection or some other illness associated with increased adrenal activity, and the latter will contribute to ketosis. Concomitant diseases and psychologic problems are apparently the commonest contributors to ketoacidosis. Children sometimes omit or decrease the insulin dosage as part of a revolt against parental authority. Repeated episodes of ketosis in association with emotional upheavals should prompt psychiatric attention. Surgical stress, acromegaly, thyrotoxicosis, pregnancy, hyperadrenocorticism, and the accumulation of a large supply of insulin antibodies also contribute to ketosis.

Symptoms and Signs. The early phases of ketoacidosis are characterized by intensification of diabetic symptoms, polyuria and polydipsia in particular. Anorexia, followed by nausea and vomiting, commonly develops, along with weakness, malaise, and muscle aches. Abdominal pain is frequent in children but not in adults; pleural pain is occasionally present. The conjunctival, oral, and nasopharyngeal mucous membranes are dry and covered with inspissated secretions. The skin is dry and inelastic. The eyeballs appear sunken and are softer than normal. There are tachycardia and hypotension. With reduction of the plasma pH to 7.2 or below, hyperpnea is prominent, but there is no subjective dyspnea; cyanosis occurs with circulatory collapse.

Depression of the central nervous system is manifested by headache, drowsiness, stupor and coma. Muscle tone decreases and the reflexes are symmetrically depressed. The eyes roll in an uncoordinated manner; the pupils are dilated and equal.

Differential Diagnosis

Diabetic ketoacidosis must be distinguished from a large number of other conditions, especially when diabetes has never been diagnosed before, or when the examining physician does not know that the patient had been diagnosed as having diabetes. However, even when the physician involved has been the patient's physician for many years and knows that he has severe diabetes, many possible problems may need consideration. For example, a diabetic patient may have a cerebrovascular accident, or may have taken sedatives, or one or more of a large number of other drugs that produce features of diabetic ketoacidosis. Many diabetics are victims of different cardiovascular disorders and also of renal acidosis. Initially, the question is often whether the subject is suffering from ketoacidosis or from hypoglycemia. Table 9–17 shows some of the differences in results of laboratory tests with ketoacidosis, lactic acidosis, renal acidosis, plasma hyperosmolarity, and hypoglycemia. In addition to ketoacidosis, many subjects simultaneously suffer from renal acidosis and hyperosmolarity. It is common for diabetic patients with ketoacidosis to have excess lactate and occasionally a number of other features of lactic acidosis. At any one time, the same patient may have diabetic ketoacidosis, renal acidosis, lactic acidosis, and hyperosmolarity. However, as the hyperosmolarity becomes severe, the hyperketonemia tends to subside somewhat.

Distinctly the commonest problem is to distinguish coma due to ketoacidosis from that due to an excess of injected insulin. Diabetic ketoacidosis is always associated with increased glucose and ketones in the blood and usually in the urine. A patient may experience such a severe hypoglycemic reaction as to die subsequently, yet when seen by the physician he may show hyperglycemia and ketonemia. In this instance, the subject has mobilized his homeostatic mechanisms by increasing hepatic glucogenesis and decreasing glucose utilization. In most cases of insulin coma, the urine shows no sugar, particularly when the bladder is emptied and a new specimen is obtained; moreover, the blood sugar level is low and the urine is free of ketones. Hypoglycemic coma has a much more rapid onset than does ketoacidotic coma. Anorexia, nausea, and vomiting occur with ketoacidosis, but not with hyperinsulinism. Respirations are deep and rapid with ketoacidosis, but normal or shallow with hyperinsulinism. Dehydration occurs with

TABLE 9–17. PLASMA CHANGES WITH STUPOR AND COMA IN DIABETICS

Serum	Glucose	Ketones	pH	Na	Urea	"Excess" Lactate	Volume
Ketoacidosis	+++	+++	---	- to N	+++	+	---
Lactic acidosis	N to +++	0 to +	---	- to N	N to +++	+++	-- to N
Renal acidosis	N to +	0 to +	---	- to N	++++	0	N to +
Hyperosmolarity	++++	0 to +	- to N	N to +++	+ to +++	0	---
Hypoglycemia	---	0 to +	N	N	N	0	N

N = normal; + = above normal; − = below normal; 0 = negative. Many exceptions to the above occur.

the former but not with the latter. With ketoacidosis there are decreased reflexes and no increased sympathetic reaction. With hyperinsulinism there are sweating, nervousness, tachycardia, and other features of an overactive sympathetic nervous system. Hypoglycemia ordinarily responds rapidly to glucose administration, but after severe brain damage there may be no observable response.

Salicylate poisoning is associated with hyperventilation, positive urine reduction test, and mild ketonuria. However, the blood sugar level is not increased, and the glucose oxidase test of the urine is negative. Early in salicylate poisoning the hyperventilation causes alkalosis; acidosis may supervene later.

Laboratory Findings

There is marked glycosuria and ketonuria in most cases; with severe impairment of glomerular function, very little sugar and ketones may be present. Acetest tablets or Ketostix have been used for roughly quantitating the amount of ketones in plasma. Ketostix reacts with acetone, but it has only about one-seventh as much sensitivity in its reaction with acetoacetate; it does not react with 3-hydroxybutyrate. The last compound is normally present in twice the concentration of acetoacetate, but with ketoacidosis the ratio often increases to 30:1. When there is a discrepancy between pH and the Ketostix reaction, lactic acidosis should be suspected.

Four-plus reactions are seen only in ketoacidosis. The plasma may be diluted to varying degrees for measuring the ketosis. However, methods are available for the exact measurement of ketones, and one of these is preferable when the opportunity exists. Sometimes more than 300 mg. ketones/100 ml. plasma is present. In most patients hospitalized for ketoacidosis, the blood sugar level is between 400 and 800 mg./100 ml. The CO_2-combining power may be as low as 2 mEq./liter in profound acidosis and below 15 in moderately severe acidosis. The plasma pH is a better indicator of the degree of acidosis than is the carbon dioxide–combining power; the pH is significantly lowered, sometimes to as low as 7.0. Hyperventilation with a low pCO_2 may persist in spite of a rising plasma bicarbonate level, and mild respiratory alkalosis may succeed metabolic acidosis. The plasma is essentially always hyperosmolal. Normally its osmolality is approximately 300 mOsm./liter, accounted for as follows: Na^+, 140; Cl^-, 100; HCO_3^-, 28; K^+, 4; urea, 10; glucose, 5; other, 13±. Since the serum osmolality is of great importance in the pathogenesis of certain aspects of the ketoacidosis syndrome, careful efforts are made to determine its amount and to correct it completely. Estimations can be made quickly with an osmometer, but it is often more convenient and more informative to apply the following formula:

$$2 \times [Na + K \,(mEq./liter)] + \frac{\text{blood glucose (mg./100 ml.)}}{18} = \text{serum osmolality} \,(\pm5\%)$$

Each 100 mg./100 ml. of blood glucose has osmotic effects comparable to 2 mEq./liter of serum sodium. Despite the markedly negative Na^+ balance (often > 40 g.), the plasma concentration of Na^+ may be hypernormal, normal, or subnormal. Additional information about water and saline status can be obtained from the hematocrit and weight of the patient, when previous values are known. These are of some aid in evaluating therapeutic changes. Measurements of plasma volume and of extracellular fluid volume are helpful, but usually these are not conveniently obtained.

Despite the markedly negative K^+ balance, hyperkalemia is often present because the acidosis causes the K^+ to shift from inside the cell to the extracellular space. This contributes to a decrease in glucose uptake and utilization. As a general index in severe ketoacidosis, the following approximations are helpful in determining the level of intracellular (IC) K^+ from the serum K^+ values: high K^+ = normal ICK^+, normal K^+ = low ICK^+, low K^+ = very low ICK^+. However, a nomogram is superior (Fig. 9–61). Many other factors such as the metabolic state of the cells and renal function also must be considered. The serum K^+ level will always fall with therapy because of (1) correction of acidosis and (2) intracellular transfer as insulin promotes glucose utilization. Initially, there usually is hyperphosphatemia, but with treatment with insulin and fluids, this often changes to hypophosphatemia.

Leukocytosis is common; values between 15,000 and 30,000 are obtained even in the absence of infection. Therefore, the leukocyte count frequently is not of assistance in diagnosing infection in the presence of ketoacidosis.

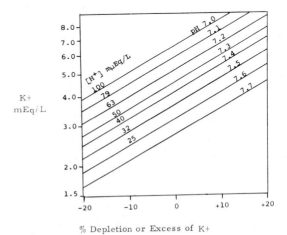

Figure 9–61. Using this nomogram, when a line parallel to the baseline is drawn from the level of serum K^+ found, the point at which it crosses the line showing either the pH or carbon dioxide combining power of the plasma at that time indicates the extent of abnormal deviation of the body K^+. Therefore, this nomogram can be used to signify therapeutic needs in correcting the level of the body K^+. (From the Division of Nephrology, University of Washington, Seattle.)

Treatment

General Plans

Because an insufficient net effect of insulin is the prime cause of ketoacidosis, we make a great effort to begin insulin treatment as rapidly as possible as patients may die before the insulin reverses the changes. This can occur despite large doses of insulin. Even with what we consider to be very good treatment of diabetic ketoacidosis, several days are required for some of the changes to be reversed, especially some in the CNS. The patient may die because of complications not directly due to the diabetes (e.g., from infection). Many die from abnormalities in water and electrolyte balance. Death in these instances is due to the combination of many factors, including hypovolemia, acidosis, ketosis, and impairment of function of many organs, especially the brain, heart, or kidneys.

After injecting what is considered to be an appropriate amount of insulin and awaiting its effect, using a direct approach we attempt to correct the complications, such as infection and abnormalities in water and electrolyte balance. On the basis of several studies, we know that while developing ketoacidosis many patients develop deficiencies to the following extent, expressed as changes per kg. of body weight: 100 ml. water; 7 mEq. Na^+; 5 mEq. K^+; 5 mEq. Cl^-; 0.5 mEq. Mg^{++}; 1 millimole PO_4^{---}. Generally, there is also a marked deficiency in the total carbohydrate content of the body, and significant losses of protein and fat.

In dealing with ketoacidosis, aside from administering insulin, physicians concentrate most of their attention on water and electrolyte changes, especially the acidosis. Sometimes the therapy produces such marked and rapid changes in some elements of the plasma and extracellular fluid that the intracellular concentration of some components is worsened, particularly in the brain. For example, periodically one sees patients admitted to the hospital who do not appear to be dangerously ill and are not comatose. After vigorous treatment for decreasing plasma glucose, metabolic acidosis, and hypotension, the patient may rapidly lapse into coma and show signs of increased intracranial pressure. Autopsy shows cerebral edema and changes similar to those of hypoxia. Increasing information suggests that some of these changes may result from increased polyol pathway activity in the brain (Clements). Hyperglycemia stimulates the activity of this pathway in tissues containing aldose reductase and in which the intracellular transport of glucose is not regulated by insulin, such as in the CNS. The higher the glucose level, the more this enzyme activity is stimulated, resulting in a considerable amount of glucose conversion to sorbitol and other polyols. Polyols are relatively slowly metabolized and released from cells. As they accumulate, they apparently increase intracellular osmolarity. The effects of the intracellular hyperosmolarity are intensified by an abrupt fall in extracellular glucose, Na^+, and other extracellular constituents. Increased intracellular osmotic pressure can eventually produce a marked increase in intracranial pressure. Presumably hypoosmolarity of the plasma can promote relative hyperosmolarity within the brain cells.

In rabbits it has been shown (Arieff) that 2 hours after hyperglycemia induced by infusion of 50 per cent glucose, brain and muscle lost about 10 per cent of water content. After hyperglycemia for 4 hours, the water content of muscle remained low, but it was normal in brain. Yet osmolarity in brain and cerebrospinal fluid was equally hypernormal. Increases in the concentrations of Na^+, K^+, Cl^-, glucose, sorbitol, lactate, urea, myoinositol, and amino acids accounted for only one-half of the increase; the unidentified solute was called "idiogenic osmoles." With rapid decrease of plasma glucose produced by insulin there was (a) gross brain edema, (b) increase in brain content of water, Na^+, K^+, Cl^-, and idiogenic osmoles, and (c) hyperosmolality in brain, but normal osmolality in plasma. It was concluded that (a) during extracellular hyperosmolality there was an increase in idiogenic osmoles in brain cells rather than a loss of water or gain in solute, and (b) despite the brain-to-plasma osmotic gradient, there was no net movement of water into brain until plasma glucose fell below 225 mg./100 ml., and then cerebral edema occurred.

In patients with diabetic ketoacidosis, rapid correction of extracellular acidosis by the intravenous infusion of large quantities of sodium bicarbonate may actually promote more acidosis in the CNS, with resulting impairment in consciousness. In other words, in rapidly correcting a number of the abnormalities in plasma, death can be promoted. It is important to bear in mind the thesis that, if we permit nothing to get worse, the patient will not die.

We have a number of excellent parameters for evaluating the status of extracellular fluid, but it is very difficult to appraise the intracellular status. These considerations suggest that we may be wise to exercise conservatism in the rapidity with which we reverse some of the extracellular abnormalities. Because of the large variation in the characteristics of each patient with diabetic ketoacidosis, we cannot satisfactorily apply many rigid routines in treatment. We give therapies of different types in a guarded manner, reevaluate the situation, give more treatment, again evaluate the results and so forth. Proper treatment of ketoacidosis demands continuing attention to the clinical status of the patient and frequent repetition of measurements of some biochemical components.

Prompt and coordinated attention by a well-trained team is important and can make the difference between life and death. Moreover, intense attention to the patient may be required for many hours. Ketoacidosis and the many problems which may or may not be related to it demand great competence in both the art and science of medicine. Only a few of the detailed steps indicated in diagnosis and treatment are presented here. Special attention should be devoted to the state of hydration and to complications in the nervous, respiratory, or circulatory systems, as well as elsewhere. When venipunctures offer great difficulty, it is advisable to insert a polyethylene catheter. The patient should be kept warm. Gastric lavage should be performed when there is gastric dilation or persistence of vomiting.

A careful record should be kept of the various diagnostic and therapeutic procedures and the results. Urine sugar and ketones should be measured at hourly intervals. Initial blood measurements should be made of the glucose, acetone, CO_2, pH, Na^+, K^+, urea, and hematocrit. Certain of these tests should be repeated at 2- to 6-hour intervals as indicated. Systematic measurements of the blood pressure, pulse, respirations, mental state, and water balance should be made and recorded frequently.

Insulin Administration

In ketoacidosis, there always appears to be a deficiency, relative or absolute, in the amount of insulin. The sooner this is corrected, the sooner the patient will progress toward recovery. However, it is important to recall that some of the biochemical abnormalities resulting from insulin deficiency require many hours to change. Moreover, the more pronounced the severity and duration of the insulin deficiency, the longer the interval required to produce significant changes. When there is insufficient insulin for long intervals, these enzyme systems may be considered to have undergone "repression," and before insulin can exert its full effectiveness, these systems must "be induced."

It is not possible to predict accurately the amount of insulin required, because there are numerous factors which influence this. The most important principle is to start administering insulin as soon as possible, continuing at frequent intervals and giving it in excess but not inducing hypoglycemia. Short-acting insulin is always used. The use of monocomponent insulin when it is marketed may prove to be advantageous. The duration of coma and the time required for the blood sugar to fall to 300 mg./100 ml. have been found to be the same in patients receiving 80, 160, or 240 U. every 2 hours. However, there are unquestionably some patients who require massive doses, particularly those who have accumulated large quantities of insulin antibodies in the plasma. The antibodies must be saturated with insulin before much insulin can remain unbound and exert its action. In addition to decreased insulin action caused by antibodies, there are a number of hormonal, electrolytic, nutritional, and other changes that decrease insulin's effectiveness. In 123 cases of coma treated successfully at the Joslin Clinic, the average total dose of insulin in the first 3 hours was 126 U.

Sometimes the patient's life may be saved by the administration of 50 to 100 U. of insulin before he is brought to the hospital. However, in this case it is very important for the physician to feel confident about the diagnosis. Soon after arrival at the hospital, 100 U. of insulin or 1.5 U./kg. is given intravenously or subcutaneously; the former is particularly important when the circulation is poor. Only crystalline zinc insulin or amorphous (regular) insulin is used for intravenous therapy. From 50–100 U. (sometimes 200) is given hourly until a significant decrease in blood sugar and ketones occurs. Once the blood sugar level falls to approximately 300 mg./100 ml. or less, the insulin dosage is significantly reduced. When the blood sugar level has not fallen within a few hours, the insulin dosage should be significantly increased, because the patient may have marked insulin resistance. Rarely, a patient may require several thousand units during the first day. It is highly important in severe cases that definite insulin action be apparent within the first few hours of therapy. When marked insulin resistance becomes apparent, it may be useful to institute glucosteroid therapy immediately, using 100–200 mg. of hydrocortisone hemisuccinate, or a comparable preparation, intravenously. Subsequent administrations are given as indicated. Although the glucosteroid hinders insulin's actions in certain ways, this hindrance is overbalanced by the steroid's effectiveness in decreasing the antibody action. After the first few doses of insulin, some physicians follow a "rule of thumb" regimen such as the one that follows: 50 U. for 4+ glycosuria (red), 20 for 3+ (orange), 15 for 2+ (yellow), and 10 for 1+ (green). Such a regimen must be weighed in connection with careful evaluation of the pathophysiologic changes in each patient. We prefer to be guided predominantly by blood levels of glucose, ketones, and electrolytes, and to follow with additional therapy as needed to get the pH elevated to at least 7.2. The deeper the coma and the longer its duration, the larger is the amount of insulin required. As already indicated, infections and other stresses increase the insulin requirements. Since, however, hypoglycemic reactions are most apt to appear after 6–12 hours, efforts must be made to avoid them and to detect early any that develop.

Properly measured, the ketone values are better guides than the glucose values, but both are helpful. Ketones can be measured accurately in the blood or semiquantitatively by serial dilution of plasma. As mentioned earlier, the Acetest tablets do not react with β-hydroxybutyric acid, which, like acetone, is a metabolic product of acetoacetic acid. β-Hydroxybutyric acid is more plentiful than acetone. Patients with mild acidosis do not require such vigorous treatment. Lente insulin is used along with semilente insulin after the ketosis has largely cleared; subsequently, it is used alone for most patients.

Fluid and Electrolyte Therapy

Although there is a deficiency of fluid and some electrolytes in each of the three major compartments—vascular, extracellular, and intracellular—more urgent attention is required for restoration in the first two in order to promote proper function of many vital organs, particularly the brain and kidneys. Marked acidosis is harmful and should be decreased soon. The following mixture can be used for marked acidosis: 0.9 per cent saline, 500 ml.; distilled water, 400 ml.; 7.5 g. $NaHCO_3$, 100 ml. This mixture is infused over the first 2 hours. During the third to the fifth hour, normal saline or the following mixture may be indicated: 0.9 per cent saline, 600 ml.; distilled water, 400 ml.; 50 mEq. K^+ phosphate (2 g. $K_2HPO_4 + 0.4$ g. KH_2PO_4). In the first 2 hours, the plasma K^+ and PO_4^- tend to be hypernormal, but cells are deficient in these components. Each one serves an important function. It is desirable, however, not to infuse them until their extracellular levels become near normal. With marked impairment of renal function, they must be administered with special caution.

The amount of alkali to be used varies with the severity of acidosis and with the adequacy of renal function. A rough guide to the total deficit is provided by multiplying by 3 the amount required to return the extracellular fluid HCO_3^- system to normal. This permits restoration of other body buffers to normal. Example: in a 70-kg. man, initial $HCO_3^- = 5$ mEq./liter. To change this to a normal of 25 mEq./liter would require $25 - 5$ (20 mEq.) $\times$ 15 (extracellular volume) $\times$ 3, or 900 mEq. alkali. In practice, much less is desirable, because complete correction is not the goal, and because any renal H^+ excretion should be subtracted from this amount, and alkalosis with hypokalemia may result.

Extremes in K^+ concentration are very important; they can occur quickly and cause death. A rapid fall in serum K^+ occurs with insulin and alkali therapy, necessitating K^+ administration. Consequently, the patient must be evaluated clinically with electrocardiograms and with K^+ determinations on several occasions, especially in the first 12 hours. There is a marked net loss of K^+ in all cases of severe ketoacidosis. However, death can be inflicted by K^+ therapy, even while a net deficiency persists, if the K^+ is given too rapidly. Conversely, death from hypokalemia can occur a few hours after initial hyperkalemia. The decrease in K^+ is due to urinary loss, to dilution of extracellular fluids by various infusions, and to reentry of K^+ into the cells with the increase in pH and glucose utilization.

The serum K^+ values must be considered in conjunction with the serum pH, since they tend to vary inversely. A K^+ value that would ordinarily be normal is abnormal if the pH is abnormal (Fig. 9-61). Potassium therapy should be given 3-4 hours after insulin and fluid therapy has been initiated; occasionally it is started immediately. One should hesitate to give K^+ therapy with marked renal impairment, but sometimes it is necessary under these circumstances. Greater care than usual must be exercised in monitoring the patient; less K^+ than usual is required, because there tends to be less deficiency, and repletion occurs more rapidly. In the ordinary patient with pronounced ketoaci-

dosis, K^+ is given at the rate of 20 mEq./hr., preferably as K_2HPO_4 and KH_2PO_4 in a ratio of 4:1. Quite often 100–200 mEq. K^+ is given in the first 12 hours. Potassium-containing foods, such as beef broth, are then prescribed. The electrocardiogram gives useful information relative to potassium. Hyperkalemia is suggested by all peaked T waves, while hypokalemia is indicated by prolongation of the Q-T interval, depression of the ST segment, low and inverted P waves, depressed T waves, and prominent U waves. However, the electrocardiographic tracings can be influenced by a number of factors other than plasma K^+.

Carbohydrate Administration

Glucose is rarely given initially because hyperglycemia is usually marked, and giving more glucose would intensify the hyperosmolarity and interfere with the use of glucose measurements as a guide to insulin therapy. However, glucose should be given after a few hours, since it will be needed for energy and because it helps prevent ketoacidosis. Even with a blood sugar value of 1000 mg./100 ml., less than 600 cal. may be provided. Even though the plasma contains an increased food supply, tissues contain subnormal amounts of carbohydrate. Glucose is infused with other intravenous fluids when the blood glucose level has declined below 300 mg./100 ml. Ordinarily it is given as a 5 per cent solution. Fructose has not proved superior to glucose; in ketoacidosis most of it is converted to glucose in any case.

Other Measures

The circulatory complications of ketoacidosis are responsible for most of the therapeutic failures. Hypotension is often present initially or up to several days after hospitalization. There is decreased blood flow peripherally as well as in the kidneys. The hypotension usually responds to the administration of NaCl solutions. In some severe cases, 1 or 2 units of plasma is helpful. Catecholamines should be avoided as much as possible, because they promote lactic acidosis in states of shock and inhibit insulin's action on muscles. All associated disorders should be sought and corrected as rapidly as possible. Special attention should be devoted to the brain, heart, lungs, and kidneys. Infections should be rapidly identified and treated as specifically as possible. When anemia is present, transfusion may be indicated. In severe cases, anoxia of tissues is often present. Part of this is due to hypotension and poor perfusion, but some of it is due to an increased binding of oxygen by hemoglobin. Sometimes oxygen therapy is indicated.

When GI disturbances, circulatory problems, and cerebral difficulties have abated, it is desirable to start the patient on frequent liquid feedings, including meat broths in particular. Changes should be made rapidly in order to institute the diet that is to become standard. Efforts toward regulation with insulin are then made using lente insulin predominantly. An exercise program should also be initiated. Attempts should be made to ascertain the major factors contributing to the ketoacidosis and to avoid them in the future.

Response to Therapy

Prevention of marked hypokalemia forestalls the development of a number of complications, such as ascending muscular paralysis, cardiac arrhythmias, digitalis toxicity, gastric atony, intestinal ileus, and alkalosis. Carbohydrate administration has reduced hypoglycemic reactions.

With the therapy described above, most patients show progressive improvement. The blood sugar tends to fall below 300 mg./100 ml. within 6 hours or soon thereafter. Ketonuria persists for 8–12 hours. Recovery of extracellular fluid occurs in 24–48 hours, but complete restitution of intracellular fluid and electrolytes may require as long as 10 days. An even longer interval may be required for attaining a normal nitrogen storage and for regaining the former status of carbohydrate tolerance and of insulin requirements.

Improvement in CNS function occurs rapidly in younger subjects, but in older patients coma may last 24 hours or longer and be followed by some mental confusion for several days.

The mortality has been found to range from 1.5–15 per cent. It depends very much upon the amount and duration of CNS dysfunction, circulatory status, age of the patient, degree of biochemical abnormalities, and complicating illnesses.

Prevention of Ketoacidosis

In all severe cases of diabetes, we are continually attempting to avoid development of ketoacidosis. Even with our best efforts with severe diabetes, there are intervals each day when the control is not fully effective. These patients generally have some hyperketonemia. However, most of the time we prevent this from becoming significantly marked. The following situation is one that frequently confronts us, even in dealing with very intelligent and very cooperative patients. As a result of "the flu" or some other illness, the patient may not feel very well in general and may experience anorexia, nausea, and vomiting. He eats little or no food and reasons that he probably should take no insulin. This pattern does not persist more than a few hours before ketoacidosis is evolving at a rapid rate, although it did not exist at the time that the aforementioned symptoms began. With inadequate metabolism of glucose, fatty acids and ketones accumulate in order to supply energy. To avoid this in excess, insulin and glucose must be provided. In this situation, it is desirable for the patient to come to the Emergency Room in order to receive attention along whatever lines may be indicated. "The flu" may in reality not have existed as such, the symptoms having been produced by some other disorder. Indeed, they should be attributed to ketoacidosis until proven otherwise. But even when such is not the case, it often is desirable to administer insulin and to infuse 5 or 10 per cent glucose in 0.9 per cent saline. Other steps may also need to be taken. In this manner, it is possible to prevent the development of fulminant ketoacidosis, which will prompt hospitalization for several days.

Hyperosmolar (Nonketotic) Coma

The syndrome of hyperosmolar (nonketotic) coma has been observed largely in individuals over age 60, either with a history or mild diabetes or with no history of diabetes (Matz, Schwartz). This syndrome has been reported only rarely in juvenile-onset diabetics.

Associated Factors

In most instances, the subjects have not previously had an episode of this type, and many of them have not been known to have diabetes. Indeed, in some instances, diabetes is never proven to be present. Many of the patients have some other disease process at the time that the syndrome develops. Among the factors possibly contributing to the development of the syndrome are the following: diphenylhydantoin, thiazide diuresis, glucosteroid treatment, peritoneal dialysis or hemodialysis (using hyperosmolar dialysates), hypothermia, hyperthyroidism, diabetes insipidus, severe burns treated with solutions containing high concentrations of glucose, CNS disorders, mannitol diuresis, dehydration, and acute pancreatitis.

Symptoms and Signs

Relatively few individuals below the age of 60 have developed this syndrome. Some of the subjects have a history of polyphagia, prompting a relatively heavy intake of carbohydrates. Polydipsia and polyuria are often present, but later polyuria changes to oliguria. Vomiting and diarrhea are present in many of the subjects, although to less of an extent than with ketoacidosis. The patient rapidly becomes stuporous and comatose. On examination, in addition to the dull sensorium or coma, there may be other manifestations of dysfunction of the CNS, including areflexia, vestibular dysfunction, focal neurologic disturbances, and hallucinatory behavior. There are many manifestations of marked dehydration: dry skin and mucous membranes, hypotension, and soft eyeballs. Fever, tachycardia, and rapid respiration (not Kussmaul) are often present. Occasionally there is abdominal tenderness, but it tends to be less frequent and severe than with ketoacidosis. There may be associated a cerebral vascular accident, myocardial infarction, or other type of disorder.

Laboratory Findings

Laboratory findings are as follows: plasma glucose, 1000 ± mg./100 ml. (may be 2500 or higher); plasma osmolarity, > 350 mOsm./kg. water; azotemia (essentially always present); high hematocrit; Na$^+$, 100–180 mEq./L.; K$^+$, low, normal, or high; pH tends to be normal but may be low. There usually is no ketonemia in the classic cases, but there can be a moderate amount. Compared with ketoacidosis, there is less elevation of the plasma FFA, GH, and cortisol. In the one patient reported with measurement of plasma insulin, the level was found to be low normal. Leukocytosis is marked. In cerebrospinal fluid, there is hyperosmolarity, before and after treatment with insulin and hypotonic salt solution (Carroll), comparable to that of plasma.

Pathophysiology

There is considerable uncertainty about the pathogenesis of this syndrome (Arieff, Clements). Because of insulin deficiency, hyperglycemia develops, and several factors can contribute to it and to other aspects of the syndrome. Concomitantly, there also is an increase in concentration of Na$^+$ and rapid loss of water, leading to general dehydration and hyperosmolarity of the plasma. Presumably, as the hyperglycemia becomes marked, there is increased conversion of glucose to sorbitol and other polyols in brain cells, and, as discussed earlier, with their increase there is an increase in osmotic action. These changes lead to the various CNS symptoms and signs described above. Of course marked renal insufficiency is present in all of these cases; otherwise the high glucose levels would not be attained. Much of the renal insufficiency is a result of the decreased plasma volume and renal blood flow. However, many of these subjects had preexisting renal disorder.

It is somewhat puzzling why the patients show no ketonuria or significant amount of ketonemia. The following factors seemingly are at work: hyperglycemia and dehydration each have been shown to exert an antiketogenic effect; the amount of insulin deficiency is presumably relatively little. Since insulin has approximately a ten times greater effect in inhibiting lipolysis than in promoting glucose uptake by tissues, one can visualize that there is enough insulin present to prevent any significant amount of lipolysis and ketogenesis, but insufficient insulin to prevent hyperglucosemia. The lesser elevation of plasma growth hormone and cortisol than that found with ketoacidosis could be associated with less lipolysis and ketogenesis. It is possible that the marked hyperglucosemia might inhibit glucagon and catecholamine secretion, but adequate data along these lines are not available.

Treatment

Insulin should be given immediately after the diagnosis is made. Less total insulin is required than with ketoacidosis; rarely is it necessary to use more than 100 U. on the first day. Although the plasma shows marked hyperosmolarity and decreased volume (many of the adults are deficient by as much as 15–20 liters), it presumably is wise not to attempt to correct these abnormalities too rapidly because of the supposed marked increase in polyols and fluid in brain cells. A very rapid reduction in the osmolarity extracellularly may produce excessive water retention intracellularly. It has been common custom to give 10–20 liters of fluid on the first two days, using chiefly 0.45 per cent saline. However, we prefer using 0.6 per cent NaCl and not infusing more than 5–10 liters on the first day. The rate of administration depends upon the cerebrovascular and general circulatory status, including the amount of hypotension, dehydration, mental status, amount of diuresis and rate of changes in plasma glucose, electrolytes, and other changes.

Prognosis and Subsequent Course

The mortality from hyperosmolar coma has generally been reported to be between 40 and 50 per cent. Those who recover subsequently do not offer much difficulty in diabetes control. Indeed, either diet alone or sulfonylurea treatment has usually controlled plasma glucose levels reasonably well.

Lactic Acidosis

Lactic acidosis occurs in nondiabetics as well as in diabetics (Danowski, Huckabee). It is of grave consequence, with a death rate > 80 per cent in some series. It tends to occur in the advanced stages of a variety of disorders, particularly uremia, diabetes, bacterial infection, arteriosclerotic heart disease, pneumonia, acute pancreatitis, and chronic alcoholism. However, a vast number of other conditions have been found to predispose to lactic acidosis. In order to identify some of the mechanisms involved, a few basic considerations are now reviewed.

Normally, a large amount of pyruvate may be converted to lactate in the presence of lactic acid dehydrogenase and DPNH. With an appropriate supply of DPN, the lactate is readily reconverted to pyruvate; but when oxygen is lacking, the supply of DPN is inadequate, and consequently lactic acid accumulates. Huckabee has shed considerable light on mechanisms involved in lactate metabolism and lactate acidosis. He divides lactate acidosis into several classes as follows:

Type I. In this group the lactic acid (L) is slightly increased above basal values of approximately 1 mmole/liter in venous blood, with a proportionate increase in pyruvic acid (P) to maintain the usual L:P ratio of 10:1. This is observed quite often in patients who are hospitalized with any of a variety of diseases. It occurs also with muscular tension, exercise, hyperventilation, or infusions of pyruvate, bicarbonate, saline, glucose, insulin, or epinephrine. It is important that in this group there is no excess lactate (XL). Moreover, there is usually no decrease in pH, but there may be some decrease in carbon dioxide. Occasionally alkalosis (pH 7.6) may exist, with a pCO_2 as low as 20 mm. Hg. On the other hand, there may be a slight acidosis. Normally the body is capable of removing a large quantity of lactate very readily. All tissues except red blood cells produce and remove lactate.

Type II. In this type, lactic acid is increased without a proportionate increase in pyruvic acid, resulting in an L:P ratio in excess of 10. This tends to be found with conditions that produce hypoxia or circulatory failure or both. It is produced experimentally by prolonged slow bleeding, by circulatory shock, and by injection of cyanide, epinephrine, and a number of other substances.

Type IIA is found in patients with obvious or presumed tissue anoxia, as in those with a history of hemorrhage, or in the presence of hypotension, low arterial blood oxygen saturation, or primary carbon dioxide retention. Blood transfusions and other mechanisms for correcting the hypoxia or the circulatory collapse of both tend to reduce the lactic acid level and bring about recovery.

Type IIB occurs in patients who have no evidence of disorders which produce tissue hypoxia and no clinical evidence of circulatory failure. However, it is assumed that tissue hypoxia is present and marked. The prognosis in this group is very grave.

Factors that Contribute to Lactic Acidosis

Many of the conditions in which lactic acidosis is found are associated with some degree of shock. To compensate for this, the blood flow to the visceral organs, particularly the kidneys, liver, spleen, and intestines, is reduced, with the objective of maintaining as well as possible the blood supply to the brain and the heart. Vasoconstrictor compounds reduce further the blood flow to the abdominal viscera. The hepatic blood flow is markedly reduced when epinephrine or norepinephrine is administered. Indeed, norepinephrine administered over a long interval can decrease the plasma volume by as much as 25 per cent. With continuation of marked vasoconstriction over a number of hours, necrosis is observed in the liver, the GI mucosa, and many other tissues. With this, hemorrhage may recur, contributing further to the shock, as does the release into the bloodstream of certain toxic materials.

As mentioned, some of the disorders most often associated with lactic acidosis are cardiovascular disorders, pulmonary disease, infections, kidney disorders, diabetes, pancreatitis, alcoholism, and acute blood loss. In addition, a number of compounds inhibit tissue respiration and consequently could contribute in varying degrees to lactic acidemia. Among this group are *p*-aminophenol, barbiturates, diethylstilbestrol, sulfonamides, salicylates, disulfiram (Antabuse), antihistaminics, certain adrenergic blocking agents, chlorpromazine, ethanol, and phenformin. The last two of these compounds need brief discussion.

Ethanol inhibits lactic acid clearance, and con-sequently ethanol intoxication, associated with other etiologic factors, can contribute to lactic acidosis. As for phenformin, a considerable amount has been written about its possible role in lactic acidosis. Although, as discussed earlier, a number of basic studies have demonstrated that phenformin produces a state of mild anaerobiosis, evidence thus far tends to indicate that the usual dosage of this compound per se does not produce lactic acidosis. It generally does not increase the plasma lactate level very much in normal individuals.

Clinically, the picture of lactic acidosis is quite variegated, because of a marked difference in the factors that contribute to its development. Moreover, the manifestations of the acidosis per se vary with its magnitude. In general, however, the onset of this disorder is relatively acute. The patients rapidly develop stupor progressing to coma and exhibit Kussmaul respirations within a few hours. Clinical manifestations of anoxia may or may not be present. The same is true with regard to hypotension. The main point in the diagnosis of lactic acidosis is familiarity with the conditions under which it occurs, especially when acidosis is present; whether or not there are other factors that could be blamed for the acidosis, the possibility of excess lactate should be investigated.

The normal level of lactate under fasting resting conditions is 0.4–1.4 mmole/liter and of pyruvate, 0.07–0.14 mmole/liter. Excess lactate is present when L:P is greater than 10:1. Tranquada diagnoses lactic acidosis when the level is 7 mmole/liter. However, in view of the many factors that increase lactate, at least temporarily, and do not cause lactic acidosis, it is desirable to show an excess of lactate over pyruvate or a persisting high level of lactate. In Tranquada's series, the average lactate level was 17.5 mmole/liter. The pH and the carbon dioxide–combining power are subnormal. The Na^+ level is usually normal but may be high or low. The K^+ tends to be high or normal. The glucose level may be normal, high, or low. Of course, in diabetics it is consistently elevated, sometimes markedly so. Ketones in the plasma and the urine are often only slightly elevated. Indeed, many patients give negative tests for ketones. Excess lactate inhibits lipolysis, and this can result in decreased ketogenesis. Excess lactate can also decrease glycolysis, thereby decreasing alanine and pyruvate, causing a decrease in gluconeogenesis. The pCO_2 tends to be subnormal. The HCO_3^- level is generally low, since it tends to be the reciprocal of the lactate level. The Cl^- level tends to be normal or low. Chemical evidence of impaired liver function was found in 20 of 64 cases analyzed by Tranquada. Frequently, the serum levels of lactic dehydrogenase, transaminases, and amylase are increased. The blood urea nitrogen and the creatinine are often increased. The serum inorganic phosphate was elevated in most of the patients in whom this was measured; the reason for the increase is not known.

In the light of present information, it appears that marked increases in the lactic acid content of the blood, and even marked excesses of lactate over pyruvate, are not of primary importance, since the acidosis, which causes most of the damage, can be corrected very rapidly. The important point seems to be that a marked excess of lactate is an index of grave underlying problems. Experimentally, however, the level of the excess lactate has shown a reasonably good correlation with respect to the prognosis. Since anoxia seems to be one of the most important causes of the syndrome, it is important to concentrate on discerning the major underlying problems and to attempt to correct them as quickly as possible. Thus, when there is shock in association with a decrease in blood or plasma volume or both, these volumes should be restituted as quickly as possible. Cardiac and respiratory insufficiencies should likewise be dealt with immediately. Glucosteroids and fludrocortisone should be administered in certain disorders as indicated. Vasoconstrictors should be avoided as much as possible because, as discussed earlier, they often intensify the process. When diabetes is associated with the lactic acidosis, it should be treated immediately by the principles that have been described previously for the treatment of diabetic ketoacidosis. Thus appropriate amounts of insulin, water, and alkali (preferably sodium bicarbonate) should be given immediately and continued as indicated. Some subjects apparently have benefited from the intravenous administration of methylene blue (5 mg./kg.) in the effort to convert the lactate to pyruvate.

Other Forms of Coma in Diabetes

For purposes of discussion, hyperosmolar coma, lactic acidosis coma, and ketoacidosis coma have been separated; however, there are various gradations of these disorders and, indeed, sometimes the picture of one of these can be transformed into another. The authors have seen in the same patient classic ketoacidosis followed by a dominant picture of hyperosmolar coma, succeeded chiefly by lactic acidosis. In addition to these types of coma, one naturally must watch carefully for hypoglycemic coma, as well as for coma from a large variety of medical disorders, such as cerebrovascular stroke, uremia, hepatic coma, and drug intoxication.

Table 9–17 shows relative amounts of change in some laboratory findings in several types of stupor and coma in diabetics. One variant in the picture of hyperosmolar coma consists of patients who have marked hypernatremia with little or no hyperglycemia. Most of the clinical manifestations are quite similar to those in subjects with marked hyperglucosemia. The ones with the hypernatremic syndrome are treated with several liters of 2.5 per cent glucose. No insulin treatment is needed as long as there is no hyperglucosemia.

RECIPROCAL INFLUENCES OF CERTAIN CONDITIONS AND DIABETES

Diabetes is a metabolic disorder associated with a large number of biochemical derangements in the body, as discussed earlier. It can and does affect numerous functions throughout the body. In turn, the functions of the various systems of the body can markedly influence the course of diabetes. Some of the more important of these are now considered.

Brain Status

Influence of the Brain on Diabetes

There is no question that certain types of emotional reaction intensify the diabetic status. Indeed, sometimes the first frank manifestation of the disease occurs at the time of such reactions. Some subjects manifest emotional conflict years before the development of frank diabetes; in children there may be frequent temper tantrums, phobias, nightmares, and anxieties, and in later life nervous breakdowns, family struggles, sexual conflicts, dietary indiscretions, indecisiveness, vacillation, nervousness, depression, and suspicions. Diabetics subjected to threatening situations develop diuresis and have a decrease in the concentration of glucose but an increase in the total amount excreted. A *stress diuresis* occurs during acute interpersonal conflict and may be intense and of long duration. The marked loss of fluid and glucose as well as other biochemical alterations may actually precipitate ketosis. No single pattern of mood, thought, behavior, or personality disturbance is consistently present in diabetics. The subjects, however, tend to become discouraged, particularly after the onset of the diabetes, because it is not uncommonly first manifested when a person finds himself coping with a difficult life situation. Such patients find it difficult to follow a rigid regimen meticulously over many years and at times feel set apart from their fellow men. The constant daily attention to the many aspects of their disease keeps it ever at the front of their minds. Children periodically may rebel against their parents and physician. Moreover, a number of adults may periodically show indications of rebellion, particularly if the regimen is highly strict. As discussed earlier, such emotional disturbances markedly alter the course of diabetes. There are many endocrine and metabolic changes accompanying the emotional changes.

The autonomic nervous system greatly influences the metabolic state, including carbohydrate, fat, protein, water, and electrolyte metabolism. Emotional reactions can, within a few minutes, markedly elevate the FFA content of the plasma and, as indicated earlier, can induce ketosis. They can also elevate the blood sugar very rapidly or in other instances lower it. Increases in catecholamines markedly inhibit insulin action (Fig. 9–16). The sympathetic nervous system, which is involved particularly with increasing the blood sugar, is stimulated by a decrease in blood sugar. With hypoglycemia, impulses are set up in the hypothalamus and pass through the pontine and bulbar centers, the lateral horns of the spinal cord, the lateral ganglia, and the splanchnic nerve to the liver and adrenal medullas. In this manner, hypoglycemia promotes secretion of epinephrine and hepatic glycogenolysis. With the development of hyperglycemia, the parasympathetic centers, located in the hypothalamus and the bulb, are stimulated and impulses go through the vagus to the pancreas and promote insulin secretion. Both the liver and the pancreas have the capacity to respond directly to changes in the glucose concentration of the plasma which bathes them, but the autonomic nervous system probably is more sensitive to slight changes. Claude Bernard showed that a puncture of the floor of the fourth ventricle produced hyperglycemia and glycosuria. This presumably resulted from stimulation of the sympathetic nervous system. Since then, hyperglycemia has been found to be associated with a number of different types of cerebral pathology—for example, hemorrhage into the subarachnoid space or the brainstem, tumors at the base of the brain, and injury or stimulation of the hypothalamus. The cerebral lesions cause only transient alterations in the carbohydrate metabolism. When diabetes is already present, it temporarily is greatly intensified.

Influence of Diabetes on the Brain

As previously discussed, emotional disturbances tend to intensify diabetic manifestations and, conversely, diabetes produces emotional disturbances.

Both severe hypoglycemia and ketoacidosis impair mentation and, indeed, may lead to deep coma and death or permanent brain damage. In each instance, there is a decrease in oxygen consumption by the brain. Various investigators have shown that roughly 60 per cent of persons with unstable diabetes who experience infrequent hypoglycemic reactions have permanent alterations in the electroencephalogram; this incidence is 5–10 times that found in normal subjects (abnormalities are found in some "normal" persons). There is a significant increase in the incidence of abnormal electroencephalographic records, even in patients with mild stable diabetes receiving no insulin. Although there is a high percentage of abnormal records in those receiving insulin, there is no difference discernible between the patients with stable and unstable diabetes on insulin therapy. With the increase of cerebral arteriosclerosis in diabetes, there is an increased impairment of mental function. There is also an increase in the incidence of cerebral vascular accidents.

Reske-Nielsen studied clinical observations and neuropathologic findings in the brains of 16 juvenile-onset diabetics dying of diabetic angiopathy after many years of diabetes. A characteristic histologic pattern was observed in all of the cases, consisting of diffuse degenerative abnormalities of the brain tissue, often with severe pseudocalcinosis or with atrophy of the dentate nucleus, demyelinization of the cranial nerves, fibrosis of the leptomeninges, and angiopathy. The degenerative changes were so pronounced that a dual pathogenesis was considered likely, consisting of ischemia produced by the angiopathy and a primary diabetic abnormality of the brain tissue. The clinical symptoms varied from insignificant to pronounced. A correlation was found between the symptoms and the number of areas of softening of the brain. The histologic pattern was regarded as different from that of other clinical conditions, and it was thought that the term *diabetic encephalopathy* was justified.

Gastrointestinal Status

As stated earlier, there are several GI hormones that influence significantly the secretion of insulin and glucagon.

There does not seem to be any increased incidence of dental caries in diabetes, but there is a significant increase in periodontal disorders. These consist of gingivitis, pyorrhea, deposits of tartar, and dental root abscesses. These are more prominent in poorly controlled diabetes.

In untreated diabetics there is a markedly subnormal incidence of peptic ulcer. Diabetes may lead to anorexia, nausea, vomiting, and abdominal pain, particularly during ketoacidosis. Nausea, vomiting, and abdominal distention are sometimes related to autonomic neuropathy involving the upper GI tract. In these instances there may be roentgenographically demonstrable atony of the tract with puddling such as is found in certain nutritional disorders; these roentgenographic changes may also be found without symptoms. A few instances of steatorrhea associated with diabetes are reported, but the frequency with which this occurs is not known. Certain studies indicate that normal pancreatic enzymes are secreted into the intestinal tract, except in instances of pancreatic calcinosis. Diarrhea, occurring especially at night, is sometimes very troublesome and apparently is due to autonomic neuropathy involving the colon. Since there is an increased incidence of anacidity in diabetes, this may also contribute to diarrhea.

Of course, the diabetic may periodically become the victim of a large variety of GI disturbances which are not induced by diabetes. Anorexia, nausea, vomiting, and diarrhea all can contribute markedly to the development of ketoacidosis. Moreover, fever and a decrease in food and water intake also promote ketoacidosis. When the patient takes his usual dose of insulin at the time of a marked decrease in food intake, hypoglycemia may result, but if he omits insulin, ketoacidosis may develop. Ordinarily, he should take about one-half to two-thirds the usual dosage and make an effort to take a number of sugar-containing drinks, soft foods, etc. When significant difficulties seem imminent, he should contact his physician.

Liver Status

The net effect of liver disease on the blood glucose concentration is highly variable and depends

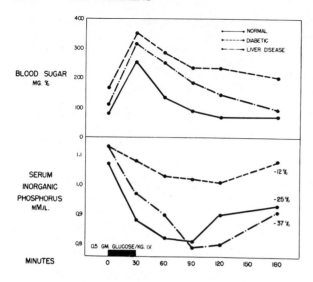

Figure 9–62. Characteristic changes in serum inorganic phosphorus during the intravenous glucose tolerance test. (N. B.: Such striking changes are not always found in practice.)

upon a number of factors. The fasting blood sugar concentration may be normal, subnormal, or slightly increased. A significant hypoglycemia during fasting is not common, except with a hepatic carcinoma. With a glucose tolerance test, the apogee tends to occur between 30 and 60 minutes and is higher than normal (Fig. 9–62). Sometimes severe liver disease is associated with a high plateauing, as is seen in diabetes. Between 2 and 4 hours after administration of glucose, the blood sugar may remain elevated or become normal or occasionally actually subnormal. Hypoglycemia in association with liver disease could be related to a decrease in insulin degradation and a decrease in hepatic glucogenesis. The decrease in hepatic glucogenesis may be due to a decrease in gluconeogenesis (deficiency in the pituitary or adrenals or both), to a genetic deficiency in certain enzymes (as in galactosemia and von Gierke's disease), or to hepatocellular degeneration. The liver's capacity to respond to hypoglycemia with glucogenesis can be tested by a combined epinephrine and glucagon test. A large variety of diseases involving the liver may influence its role in carbohydrate metabolism. Included in this group are diseases that affect hepatic blood flow, e.g., congestive heart failure.

Sometimes it is difficult to differentiate blood sugar changes due to liver disease from those related to a decrease in insulin secretion. One of the studies that can be of some aid in this differentiation is the measurement of the plasma phosphate concentration after glucose administration. A fall in serum phosphorus level is related to the active entry of glucose into the glycolytic cycle of the peripheral tissues, especially the muscle; relatively much less glucose is utilized for liver glycogenesis. Forsham found in normal persons a 25 per cent fall in serum inorganic phosphorus 60–90 min. after infusion of glucose was started (Fig. 9–62). Patients with absolute or relative insulin lack showed only a 12 per cent fall, while patients with various types of liver disease experienced a 37 per cent fall.

After long intervals of poorly controlled diabetes, the liver tends to be somewhat enlarged, chiefly as a result of fat infiltration. In most diabetics the liver function, as measured by the usual tests, is not significantly impaired.

Thyroid Status

Disturbances in carbohydrate metabolism are common in thyrotoxicosis, but the incidence of frank diabetes persisting after cure of the thyrotoxicosis is not much above average. Joslin found that 30 per cent of patients with toxic diffuse goiter had glycosuria. The glycosuria was more frequent with toxic diffuse goiter than with toxic nodular goiter. About 1 per cent of those patients had frank diabetes. Joslin also found glycosuria in 14 per cent of patients with nontoxic nodular goiters. At the Mayo Clinic, 5.7 per cent of patients with toxic nodular goiter and 1.7 per cent of those with toxic diffuse goiter were found to have diabetes. More than 50 per cent of thyrotoxic patients have been reported to have a decreased glucose tolerance, but the changes are transient and related to the poor nutritional status, other hormone changes, emotional instability, and other factors. It seems probable that thyrotoxicosis does not induce diabetes unless the subject is predisposed to it. In animals that have been subtotally depancreatized, the administration of large doses of thyroid can induce a diabetic state, the so-called metathyroid diabetes. Presumably thyrotoxicosis can change occult diabetes into a frank form. It can induce not only hyperglycemia but also ketosis. In general, thyrotoxicosis promotes hypernormal utilization of glucose by extrahepatic and hepatic tissue and decreases liver glycogen, presumably by increasing hepatic glucose utilization and glycogenolysis. The glycogenolysis can be brought about by various factors, including a state of relative anoxia in the liver as well as by increased sympathetic activity and hyperepinephrinemia. The increased metabolic rate produces an increased requirement for insulin and an increase in its rate of degradation. Concomitant diabetes tends to be more brittle. Even in the absence of diabetes, the fasting blood sugar level in thyrotoxicosis may be normal or slightly increased. With a glucose tolerance test, the apogee is higher than normal, but after 2 or 3 hours, the blood glucose value is normal or below. The higher apogee is probably related to an increased rate of absorption of glucose from the GI tract, increased hepatic glycogenolysis, and poor nutritional status.

In myxedema there tends to be a decrease in the severity of diabetes, particularly the adult-onset type. The fasting blood sugar value may be normal or subnormal. The rate of removal of glucose by various tissues tends to be subnormal, and there is a decrease in the rate of absorption of glucose from the GI tract. There is also a decrease in hepatic glucogenesis, which most likely is due to decreased adrenocortical and medullary activity as well as to decreased sympathetic action. As a result of the factors mentioned, the glucose tolerance curve may be flat. Since there is a decreased rate of insulin degradation, the response to a given dose of insulin may be normal or increased. The insulin requirements in diabetics with myxedema tend to be less than when these subjects are in a euthyroid state. In myxedema as well as in untreated diabetes, the plasma lipoprotein lipase activity is subnormal; hyperlipemia and hypercholesterolemia are common.

Infections

Infections, especially in the skin and the urinary tract, are more common in diabetics, particularly when the diabetes is uncontrolled. The infections clear up more slowly as long as the diabetes remains uncontrolled. The increased predisposition to infections and the decreased defense are related to circulatory impairments, alterations in polysaccharide metabolism, increase in glucose concentration, altered nutritional states, abnormalities in the immunologic responses, and other factors. The skin is prone to attack, especially by staphylococci, β-hemolytic streptococci, and fungi. Furuncles and carbuncles are more common and troublesome in diabetics (Fig. 9–63). When they occur, the increased requirement for insulin is sometimes manifold. The organism should be identified quickly and the appropriate antibiotic administered.

The urinary tract is involved particularly by the colon bacilli and the staphylococci. Severe infections may make apparent an occult state of diabetes, and when diabetes is already present, the infection may greatly increase its intensity and render its control more difficult. Occasionally with infections, enormous insulin resistance may develop as a result of a great increase in the quantity of insulin antibodies due to an anamnestic reaction. The hyperadrenocorticism developing in association with the infection tends to increase other insulin antagonistic factors as well. With infection,

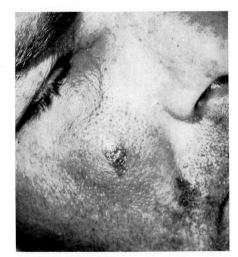

Figure 9–63. Lesion common in diabetics – furuncle; even such a small infection sometimes necessitates an increase in the dose of insulin.

particularly when associated with fever and leukocytosis, the hypermetabolism and increase in insulin degradation increase the requirements for insulin. Viral infections and tuberculosis cause less increase in the insulin needs in general than do pyogenic infections. Both the patient and his physician should be constantly on the alert to detect infection and make a vigorous effort to control or eliminate it as rapidly as possible. Moreover, great emphasis should be placed on prevention as well as therapy.

Pulmonary tuberculosis has been said to be approximately twice as common in diabetics as in nondiabetics and actually three times as common in those taking more than 40 U. of insulin daily. It is about twice as common in diabetics below standard weight as in those obese and tends to be more fulminant in diabetics than in nondiabetics. Repeated attacks of ketoacidosis are especially conducive to the development of active tuberculosis. Tuberculosis, when active, tends to intensify the diabetes but not as much as many other infections. These two diseases constitute a bad combination, and an effort should be made to attack tuberculosis in its early phases and control it as soon as possible.

Cancer

Alteration in carbohydrate tolerance, particularly decreased tolerance, is frequently found in patients with cancer. It is difficult, however, to determine accurately the contribution of each to the other. Abnormal glucose tolerance tests have been found in > 30 per cent of cancer patients, but it is difficult to properly assess the results of these tests because of associated anxieties. Joslin did not find the incidence of cancer in diabetics to be different from that in nondiabetics. Some observers have reported that in individuals over the age of 40 cancer of the pancreas occurs twice as frequently in diabetics as in nondiabetics. Cancer of the pancreas apparently can produce diabetes, but it tends to be mild and is often overlooked. The islets are not extensively invaded.

As discussed in Chapter 10, cancer sometimes may produce severe hypoglycemia; large abdominal fibrosarcoma and hepatoma are some common offenders.

PROGNOSIS

Diabetes ranks approximately eighth among the major causes of death in the United States, accounting for about 2 per cent. The death rate rises sharply in the sixth decade and is somewhat higher in females than in males (Fig. 9–64). For the last four decades, there has been a progressive decrease in the incidence of death from this disease, but in the last few years it has not changed very much, there being about 16 deaths per 100,000 per year. Joslin and colleagues investigated the cause of death in 5016 diabetics. The following major causes of death were found:

	Per cent
Vascular disease	76
Cancer	7
Infections	5
Coma	1
Other	11

Coronary disease was distinctly the major cause of death, but in the juvenile-onset diabetics, particularly those living more than 15 years, nephropathy was the most common cause of death. The life expectancy of the diabetic, aged 10, is 17 years less than that of the general population. With increasing age, the disparity decreases until, at the age of 70, the difference is only 3.7 years; in terms of percentage, this is a highly significant difference. In males the death rate in diabetics is three times that of nondiabetics up to age 50, and thereafter it

is twice as great. In females the death rate is four times as great in diabetics as in nondiabetics.

In general, juvenile-onset diabetes is regarded as a much more severe type than the adult-onset variety. The juvenile-onset type, as discussed earlier, is much more unstable and is more prone to be associated with ketoacidosis; among those who have had the disease for over 20 years, over 90 per cent have major vascular alterations such as retinitis and nephropathy. The adult-onset type is much easier to control from the point of view of maintaining a nearly normal blood sugar concentration and preventing ketoacidosis. However, the good carbohydrate control can be misleading, since 20 years later a significant number of these individuals may reveal marked vascular alterations. Indeed, this group accounts for most of the cases of diabetic gangrene. Many of them also reveal retinitis and other vascular abnormalities. Conversely, many studies indicate that the frequency and intensity of the complications correlate more with poor control than with the duration of the diabetes; this applies especially to the juvenile-onset variety.

Obesity is an important factor in the prognosis. For example, insurance statistics show that among obese individuals aged 45 years or over, the mortality rate from diabetes is at least six times greater than that of subjects of normal weight; the mortality in underweight individuals is less than 5 per cent that of the obese group. Weight reduction alone restores to normal the impaired glucose tolerance of approximately 75 per cent of obese diabetics, but in the majority, marked weight loss is not accomplished.

It appears that the greatest progress in dealing with diabetes will consist of early detection and early and continued therapy. For early detection, it seems important not only to carry out extensive screening programs, probably much more intensive than have been conducted thus far, but also to conduct specific studies of close relatives of known diabetics. A cortisone-glucose tolerance test may be included when other measures do not show abnormalities.

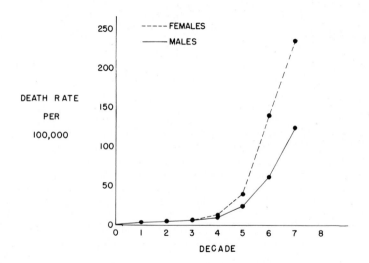

Figure 9–64. Sex-based difference in death rate from diabetes mellitus.

Transient remissions of diabetes occur not uncommonly soon after the diagnosis and institution of treatment in juvenile diabetics. However, most patients subsequently relapse and develop a severe form of the disease. Actual cure of diabetes, particularly the idiopathic variety, is indeed rare. Cure does occur in some individuals whose diabetes is the result of Cushing's disease, pheochromocytoma, and other causes which can be removed. Partial remissions may be obtained in some instances when stressful factors such as infections and emotional disturbances are eliminated. Indeed, diabetes may not be recognizable in certain instances unless special stressing tests are performed. The following brief case résumé is presented to indicate the large number of problems that may develop in diabetes in spite of conscientious efforts by the patient and a competent diabetologist:

Case Abstract

A housewife, aged 41, was recently admitted (terminal) to the University Hospital stating that diabetes had been diagnosed 20 years previously. The disease was definitely unstable at times, and on several occasions the patient was hospitalized for ketoacidosis and at other times had major hypoglycemic reactions. Three years before death she was observed to have hypertension and the onset of a nephrotic syndrome. During the last few years of her life she developed marked diabetic retinopathy and finally a few manifestations of neuropathy. She also developed a urinary tract infection which was resistant to treatment.

At necropsy she was found to have extensive diffuse and nodular glomerulosclerosis, chronic pyelonephritis, arteriosclerotic heart disease with microscopic infarction of the left ventricle, atherosclerosis of many of the larger, medium-sized, and smaller blood vessels, and calcification of the media of a number of the arteries (Fig. 9–65). In summary, despite good efforts for control on her part and that of her physician, this patient developed repeated episodes of ketoacidosis and eventually generalized arteriosclerosis at a relatively young age, with coronary arteriosclerosis, myocardial infarction, retinopathy, diffuse and nodular type of glomerulosclerosis, acute and chronic pyelonephritis, severe renal failure, and neuropathy.

UNUSUAL ETIOLOGIES OF DIABETES

Pancreatectomy

At least 90–95 per cent of the pancreas must be removed in man before clinical diabetes develops. Such an operation is ordinarily not performed except for an occasional instance of insulinoma or cancer of the pancreas. Pancreatectomy for cancer is largely being abandoned because of the high morbidity and the failure to cure the carcinoma. With subtotal pancreatectomy, the diabetes tends to be mild and stable, requiring very little insulin. After total pancreatectomy, the diabetes is very labile and difficult to control. Ketoacidosis may develop frequently at one extreme and hypoglycemia at the other. The daily dosage of insulin usually does not exceed 50 U. and averages about 25 U. An occasional instance of diabetic retinopathy has been reported to develop several years after the production of diabetes by pancreatectomy.

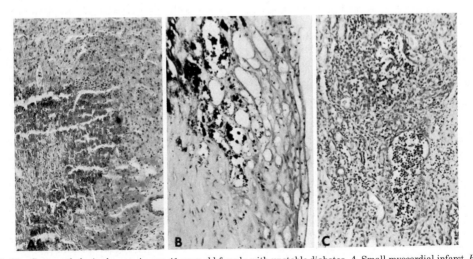

Figure 9–65. Some pathologic changes in one 41-year-old female with unstable diabetes. *A*, Small myocardial infarct. *B*, Atherosclerosis of aorta, showing hyalinization, lipid infiltration, and calcium deposition. *C*, Acute and chronic pyelonephritis. Other pathologic changes found related to the diabetes consisted of nodular and diffuse glomerulosclerosis (Fig. 9–42), retinopathy, and neuropathy. She had had several severe attacks of ketoacidosis and hypoglycemic reactions, despite persistently good efforts by the patient and her competent diabetologist. Thus she was the victim of most of the major acute and chronic problems in diabetes.

Trauma

We are consulted frequently regarding lawsuits in which claims are made that diabetes had been produced by trauma to the pancreas. However, we know of no instance where it has been shown definitely that a chronic status of diabetes has so resulted. Whereas one can visualize a crushing injury of a type that would totally destroy the pancreas, when such occurs the patient apparently does not survive. Although parts of the pancreas can be destroyed by trauma, not enough is destroyed to produce a picture of chronic diabetes. Diabetes sometimes becomes demonstrable by a positive glucose tolerance test following a trauma, the test having been normal only a few months previously. In this situation, trauma should be regarded as serving the role of cortisone in a cortisone-glucose tolerance test. In other words, an underlying diabetic process pre-existed, and the trauma brought it to a recognizable level. However, this occurrence can be advantageous to the patient in that the process is recognized earlier than otherwise and prompts earlier initiation of treatment.

Pancreatitis

Glycosuria is found in about 11 per cent of the patients with acute pancreatitis; it is found in 35 per cent of those to whom the pancreatitis proves fatal. Hyperglycemia is observed in one-quarter to one-half of the patients. An impaired glucose tolerance test is predictable in almost every patient with acute pancreatitis. The disturbances in the carbohydrate metabolism tend to be only transient. Only 2 per cent develop permanent diabetes. The hyperglycemia associated with acute pancreatitis is probably due to several factors, including increased amylase activity, which promotes glycogenolysis, the general body reaction to stress, and perhaps an increase in insulin degradation.

Diabetes has been reported in 13 per cent of the patients with chronic pancreatitis without pancreatic calcinosis and in 45 per cent of those with it. The diabetes becomes apparent only after several attacks of pancreatitis, and in most instances it is relatively mild, but occasionally it is severe and labile. During remissions from the pancreatitis, the average insulin requirement is about 30–40 U. daily. About one-third of the patients do not require insulin. Steatorrhea may be present. An occasional patient subsequently develops diabetic retinopathy and diabetic glomerulosclerosis.

Great interest has centered recently on the possible viral etiology of diabetes in man because it has been observed on repeated occasions in animals. There have been many instances of diabetes in man where examination of the pancreas has demonstrated lymphocytic infiltration characteristic of a toxic, viral, or autoimmune response in the islets. There are some cases of frank diabetes that have been immediately preceded by apparent pancreatitis. Several viruses have recently been found which affect the pancreas. Among the commoner ones are (a) mumps, (b) certain strains of encephalomyocarditis virus (EMC), and (c) virus associated with foot-and-mouth disease in cattle. Although pancreatitis occurs with mumps, the incidence of diabetes following mumps is low. However, with foot-and-mouth disease, there is a more frequent association of histologic changes in the islets and diabetes. The EMC virus seems to attack the islets in preference to the acinar tissue. Hyperinsulinemia has been observed in animals in association with this isletitis, and later there is insulin deficiency and diabetes. Thus far, the EMC virus has not been demonstrated to be diabetogenic in man. However, in a study by Taylor of 114 subjects with newly diagnosed severe diabetes, 46 per cent had complement fixation tests that were positive for antibodies against Coxsackie V viruses, compared with 21 per cent in the control. More studies are necessary to determine to what extent the Coxsackie virus, or other viruses, may be important in producing diabetes in man.

Many reports of the histologic examination of the islets in diabetics reveal sclerosis, hyalinization, and lymphocytic infiltration. The total β-cell mass and pancreatic insulin content are markedly reduced in patients who have manifested juvenile-onset diabetes for more than 2 years. However, in patients with this disorder who die from other causes within a few weeks after the diabetes is manifested, a normal β-cell mass and a relatively good supply of pancreatic insulin are found. There is much uncertainty about the pathophysiology involved here. It is possible that, after initial insult from a viral infection or through some other mechanism, an autoimmune disease is established. A specific immune isletitis has been experimentally produced and in some instances has been shown to be associated with a decrease in glucose tolerance. Eosinophil infiltration has been found in the islets of about 30 per cent of newborn infants of diabetic mothers (Renold), and a striking lymphocytic infiltration was observed in a large proportion of the youth-onset diabetics who were autopsied within the first few weeks of life, following the onset of symptoms of diabetes. Circulating antibodies to insulin have ordinarily not been found in previously untreated diabetics, but there have been a few reports of this as well as the binding of insulin to the basement membrane in diabetic vascular lesions. There is an increased incidence of thyroid and gastric autoantibodies in diabetics and a frequent association of diabetes with idiopathic adrenocortical insufficiency. In the last instance, an autoimmune mechanism has been claimed as the basis for the disorder as well as for some cases of primary myxedema.

Hemochromatosis

Hemochromatosis is characterized by an excessive accumulation of iron in the body. There is excessive iron absorption from the GI tract, which causes excessive serum iron and an increase in saturation of the iron-binding protein of the serum. There may be an excessive deposit of iron throughout the body, particularly in the form of hemosiderin, involving especially the pancreas, the liver, and the skin. Severe cirrhosis and diabetes may develop. In addition, there may be skin pigmentation consisting of both melanin and hemosiderin. There may be loss of hair, testicular atrophy, impotence, and congestive heart failure. Males acquire hemochromatosis 13 times as often as females, who lose much of the extra iron at the time of menstruation and during pregnancy. The basis for the diabetes in hemochromatosis is not known exactly, but it has been attributed to excessive iron deposit in the β-cells. The diabetes usually is not difficult to control, although an occasional patient may show marked insulin resistance and highly unstable diabetes. Diabetics with hemochromatosis usually do not respond to sulfonylurea treatment. Ketoacidosis is a common cause of death. Treatment of the diabetes in hemochromatosis consists of diet and insulin therapy, along with repeated phlebotomies.

Recent studies of 115 patients with idiopathic hemochromatosis demonstrated that 63 per cent had diabetes (Dymock). Nephropathy, neuropathy, and peripheral vascular disease, singly or together, were found in 22 per cent of the patients. Approximately the same percentage was found to have mild retinopathy with microaneurysms or exudates or both. Five of the patients showed insulin resistance shortly after diagnosis, and there was a high incidence of fat atrophy. In the individuals with diabetes and hemochromatosis, it was found that 25 per cent had a first-degree relative with diabetes, compared with 4 per cent in the nondiabetic group. However, an abnormal glucose tolerance test was found in one-third of the patients who did not have clinical diabetes. Some of the individuals in this group were found to have elevated serum insulin levels in association with intravenous glucose tolerance tests. Forty per cent of the patients with diabetes experienced improvement in carbohydrate tolerance following venesection. The basis for this change has not been established.

Acromegaly

Approximately 25 per cent of patients with acromegaly have been found to have definite diabetes. An additional 25 per cent have a decrease in glucose tolerance. In general, the diabetes is mild and stable, but occasionally it may be very severe and insulin-resistant. The insulin requirements sometimes wax and wane. As the acromegaly becomes quiescent, so does the diabetes. Diabetic retinopathy is occasionally found in acromegalic patients with diabetes. Assays of the plasma for insulin have been conducted in a number of these subjects, and the level has been found to be several times normal; the rise following a glucose load is especially marked. Moreover, there is a decrease in the insulin binding to tissues of acromegalics. As discussed earlier, there is also decreased effectiveness of a given amount of insulin because of formation of antagonistic factors in the plasma.

Cushing's Syndrome

The various ways in which glucosteroids influence the actions of insulin have been discussed previously. When glucosteroids have been administered to normal persons for several days and a glucose load is then given, plasma insulin levels reach several times normal, but there is a resistance to the actions of insulin.

Frank diabetes is found in about 25 per cent of patients with Cushing's syndrome, and in more than 50 per cent of the others impaired glucose tolerance tests have been reported. Thus only one-fifth had normal glucose tolerance tests. Clinically, the diabetes tends to be stable, usually mild, relatively insensitive to insulin, and associated with a negative nitrogen balance which is not completely corrected by insulin administration. Ketoacidosis rarely appears, and when it does it is mild. Many of the patients seem to get along essentially as well without insulin as with it. Presumably, most of them secrete hypernormal quantities of insulin themselves. After the administration of a large dose of glucose to normal persons, there is a rise in the blood pyruvate and lactate concentrations. In non-obese diabetics without Cushing's syndrome, there is either no increase in these constituents or a delay and a slight rise. In Cushing's syndrome, the fasting levels of pyruvate and lactate are elevated, and after a glucose load the pyruvate and lactate levels both rise to hypernormal levels. It is also of interest that obese diabetics tend to have an elevated fasting pyruvate level and tend to have a higher rise following glucose administration than is found with the thin diabetic. With steroid diabetes, the α-ketoglutarate level tends to be elevated in the fasting state, whereas in thin juvenile diabetics it tends to be low.

Diabetic retinopathy is found in less than 5 per cent of patients with Cushing's syndrome. No cases of diabetic glomerulosclerosis in association with Cushing's disease have been reported, but studies along this line have not been very extensive. Adrenalectomy usually causes disappearance of the diabetes in the majority of patients with Cushing's disorder.

While there is a high incidence of abnormal glucose tolerance tests in patients with endogenous Cushing's syndrome, they are relatively infrequent in those subjects treated over long intervals with ACTH or corticosteroids. Indeed, only 1 per cent show it, and even these usually have a personal or a family history of diabetes. In most instances, although not in all, the diabetes disappears with cessation of corticosteroid therapy. This diabetes tends to be insensitive to insulin, shows a striking decrease in glycosuria with fasting even in the absence of insulin, and is associated with a negative nitrogen balance. Even in patients with known diabetes, glucosteroids may be used when the indications are great and when appropriate precautionary measures are taken, such as the institution of a diabetic type of diet and the administration of insulin. Great care must be exercised upon withdrawing glucosteroid therapy in insulin-treated diabetics, because the adrenals tend to be inactive and severe hypoglycemic reactions may develop.

Pheochromocytoma

Some patients with a pheochromocytoma develop the clinical picture of diabetes. This usually disappears with removal of the tumor. The diabetes ordinarily is not severe. The marked influences of catecholamines upon insulin secretion and actions have been discussed earlier.

Glucagonoma

An occasional instance of diabetes has been associated with pancreatic islet tumor. McGavran reported a patient with a glucagon-secreting α-cell carcinoma and diabetes, but the latter disappeared after removal of the neoplasm.

Lipoatrophic Diabetes

Lipoatrophic diabetes is characterized by (a) generalized complete lipoatrophy involving subcutaneous fat as well as other fat depots throughout the body, (b) diabetes which tends to be resistant to insulin but does not tend to lead to ketoacidosis, (c) intensive hyperlipemia with the development of subcutaneous xanthomas, (d) hepatomegaly, and (e) increased basal metabolic rate but a euthyroid status.

Podolsky has recently summarized many additional aspects. The disorder is present at birth or manifested at a relatively young age. Parental consanguinity is relatively common; frequently siblings are involved. Muscular development often appears to be greater than normal, and subcutaneous veins are prominent. Hepatosplenomegaly is often observed, and impaired liver function is usually demonstrable. Mental retardation is seen occasionally. Females are involved about twice as often as males. There is accelerated linear growth, and advanced bone age is demonstrated frequently. Sometimes there is mild prognathism and some other features simulating acromegaly. The adult patients have hyperglycemia, which is commonly insulin-resistant, but some of the children are insulin-sensitive; indeed, some of the latter are prone to have hypoglycemia. The absence of ketosis is striking. Enlargement of external genitalia is common as is general hirsutism. There is abundant curly hair. The basal metabolic rate may be very high, but the serologic tests for thyroid hormone are normal, and the radioiodine uptake by the thyroid is normal. Hyperlipemia is common, with most of the increase in fat being triglyceride, although some elevation of cholesterol is also frequently found. The rate of CO_2 production from nonglucose sources is hypernormal, but the production from glucose may be subnormal. There is a hypernormal conversion of acetate to triglycerides and cholesterol. Radioimmunoassayable insulin levels of the plasma are hypernormal, but there is a suboptimal response in glucose disappearance to the administration of insulin. GH levels are normal. Lipoprotein lipase activity has been found to be normal. X-rays show an increase in density of the long bones.

The pathogenesis of the disorder is not clear. Some cases, but not all, are due to genetic disorders. Although there is no absence of fat depots, there is a defect in the deposition of fat in most of the fat depots. Therefore, a large proportion of the ingested carbohydrate that is converted to fat remains in the blood stream or is deposited in liver and in some other organs, including arterial walls. This promotes atherosclerosis. The diabetes differs from the usual type of juvenile-onset diabetes in that there is extreme resistance to insulin, hypernormal levels of plasma immunoreactive insulin, absence of ketosis, and a normal pancreas. However, a number of these patients have been found to have microangiopathic changes, simulating those in the usual type of diabetes, including glomerulosclerosis. Hepatic insufficiency is a common cause of death. In some of these patients, a polypeptide hormone has been demonstrated which is adipokinetic and diabetogenic, and shows anti-insulin properties. This compound decreases glucose tolerance when injected into healthy dogs. The diabetes is treated with insulin; sometimes as much as 2000 U. of insulin are given daily because of marked insulin resistance. Steroids potentiate the action of insulin and accelerate clearing of lipemia. Prolonged use of insulin and prednisone has lowered plasma glucose but elevated all blood lipid fractions. Lowering the dietary fat intake has not been found to decrease the lipemia. Clearing of xanthomata and decrease in hepatosplenomegaly have occurred following the combined use of large doses of insulin plus prednisone.

Partial Lipodystrophy

Partial lipodystrophy occurs, usually in females between the ages of 5–15. Patients with this disorder have characteristics of lipoatrophic diabetes in parts of their body. They may have complete absence of subcutaneous fat above the waist but a normal or excessive amount below the waist. Sometimes the lipodystrophy is below the waist without involvement of the tissue above the waist. They have insulin-resistant diabetes, hepatomegaly, and hypermetabolism. About 40 per cent have emotional disturbances. There is a high incidence of renal disease, including glomerulonephritis and hydronephrosis.

Leprechaunism

This is a rare, lethal syndrome of infancy. The facies supposedly simulates that of leprechauns of Irish mythology. Children with this disorder have a complete absence of subcutaneous fat, wide-set eyes, low-set ears, very hairy heads, and lanugo-like hair on the face. Females have an enlarged clitoris. At autopsy, marked hyperplasia of the islets is found. A number of other features in leprechaunism and congenital total lipodystrophy are similar.

Other Etiologies

An increased incidence of diabetes has been reported to occur with Friedreich's ataxia, Klinefelter's syndrome, Turner's syndrome, optic atrophy, Refsum's syndrome, Laurence-Biedl syndrome, gout, pernicious anemia, and hypothyroidism.

There are additional etiologies of diabetes. For example, subjects have been observed who secrete a markedly hypernormal quantity of insulin. Indeed, in some instances the blood level may be more than a thousand times greater than normal, yet persistent glycosuria, hyperglycemia, and frequently ketonemia and ketonuria are present. The primary difficulty in such instances seems to be a defect in the end-organs such that they do not respond to insulin. It is possible that in certain instances diabetes could be due to excessive insulin degradation in the body, although this point has not been elucidated.

Prader-Willi Syndrome

This syndrome is characterized by obesity, characteristic facies, hypotonia, mental retardation, and mild diabetes appearing before age 20.

Werner's Syndrome

Werner's syndrome is characterized by progeria, baldness, premature atherosclerosis, cataracts, and characteristic skin changes. Diabetes is present in about 50 per cent of the patients; insulin resistance is present. There seems to be some deficiency in adipose tissue. This disorder is probably inherited as an autosomal recessive trait.

Alström's Syndrome

There is an increased incidence of diabetes with Alström's syndrome. This is a genetic disorder characterized by childhood blindness due to retinal degeneration, infantile obesity, deafness, diabetes, and slowly progressive chronic nephropathy. These patients also have the following characteristics: acanthosis nigricans, baldness, hyperuricemia, hypertriglyceridemia, scoliosis, and hyperostosis frontalis interna. There is insulin resistance in these subjects. They have an autosomal recessive mode of inheritance.

Congenital Temporary Diabetes

This disorder is characterized by a severe acute diabetic syndrome which manifests itself at the time of birth or shortly thereafter. It occurs frequently without ketosis and is unassociated with a family history of diabetes. The hyperglycemia disappears permanently after a few months. Possibly this syndrome is related to a poor capacity of the islet cells to secrete an adequate supply of insulin during infancy, but adequate function is subsequently attained.

D-Cell Disorder

Thus far the only known function of the D cells is to secrete gastrin. The Zollinger-Ellison syndrome is associated with neoplasms of these cells. The major clinical manifestations are gastric hyperacidity and severe peptic ulceration with or without diarrhea; there is at least one gastrin-secreting neoplasm, and there may be more. To what extent gastrin influences the secretion of glucagon or vice versa needs further study; it causes some increase in insulin secretion. Thus far, there is no evidence that disease of D cells causes diabetes.

REFERENCES

General

Bondy, P. K., and Felig, P. (eds.): Symposium on diabetes mellitus. *Med. Clin. N. Amer.* 55:791, 1971.
Danowski, T. (ed.): *Diabetes Mellitus: Diagnosis and Treatment.* Vol. I. New York, American Diabetes Association, 1964.
Danowski, T., and Hamwi, G. J. (eds.): *Diabetes Mellitus: Diagnosis and Treatment.* Vol. II. New York, American Diabetes Association, 1967.
Ellenberg, M., and Rifkin, H. (eds.): *Diabetes Mellitus: Theory and Practice.* New York, McGraw-Hill, 1970.
Fajans, S. S., and Sussman, K. E. (eds.): *Diabetes Mellitus: Diagnosis and Treatment.* Vol. III. New York, American Diabetes Association, 1971.
Knowles, H. C. (ed.): *Diabetes.* Proc. Fiftieth Anniv. Insulin Symp., Indianapolis, American Diabetes Association, 1971.
Lefebvre, P., and Unger, R. H. (eds.): *Glucagon, Molecular Physiology, Clinical and Therapeutic Implications.* Oxford, Pergamon Press, 1972.
Luft, R., and Randle, P. J. (eds.): *On the Pathogenesis of Diabetes Mellitus.* Fourth Capri Conference, Milan, Il Ponte, 1970.
Marble, A., White, P., et al. (eds.): *Joslin's Diabetes Mellitus.* Philadelphia, Lea & Febiger, 1971.
Ostman, J., and Milner, R. D. G. (eds.): *Diabetes.* Proc. Sixth Intern. Diabetes Fed., Amsterdam, Excerpta Medica Foundation, 1969.
Pfeiffer, E. F. (ed.): *Handbook of Diabetes Mellitus.* Vol. I. Munchen, J. F. Lehmanns Verlag, 1969.
Porte, D., Jr., and Bagdade, J. D.: Human insulin secretion: An integrated approach. *Ann. Rev. Med.* 21:219, 1970.
Pyke, D. A. (ed.): *Clinics in Endocrinology and Metabolism. I. Diabetes and Related Disorders.* London, W. B. Saunders Co., 1972.
Renold, A. E., Stauffacher, W., et al., In *The Metabolic Basis of Inherited Disease.* Stanbury, J. B., Wyngaarden, J. B., et al. (eds.), New York, McGraw-Hill, 1966.
Robison, G. A., Butcher, R. W., et al.: *Cyclic AMP.* New York, Academic Press, 1971.
Rodriguez, R. R., and Vallance-Owen, J. (eds.): *Diabetes.* Proc.

Seventh Cong. Intern. Diabetes Fed., Buenos Aires, Excerpta Medica Foundation, 1971.

Shafrir, E. (ed.): Impact of insulin on metabolic pathways. Intern. Symp. Fiftieth Anniv. Insulin, Jerusalem. *Israel J. Med. Sci.* 8:271, 1972.

Stanbury, J. B., Wyngaarden, J. B., et al. (eds.): *The Metabolic Basis of Inherited Disease.* 3rd ed. New York, McGraw-Hill, 1972.

Steiner, D. F., and Freinkel, N. (eds.): *Handbook of Physiology. I. Endocrinology.* Washington, D.C., American Physiological Society, 1972.

Sussman, K. E. (ed.): *Juvenile-type Diabetes and Its Complications: Theoretical and Practical Considerations.* Springfield, Illinois, Charles C Thomas, 1971.

Williams, R. H. (ed.): *Diabetes.* New York, Paul B. Hoeber Co., 1960.

Williams, R. H., and Ensinck, J. W.: The Banting Memorial Lecture. Secretion, fats, and actions of insulin and related products. *Diabetes* 15:623, 1966.

Williams, R. H., and Ensinck, J. W.: Current studies regarding diabetes. *Arch. Intern. Med.* 128:820, 1971.

Chemistry and Metabolism of Insulin, Proinsulin, and Glucagon

Brandenburg, D., Gattner, H. G., et al., In *Diabetes. The Biochemistry of Insulin* Rodriguez, R. R., and Vallance-Owen, J. (eds.), Proc. Seventh Cong. Intern. Diabetes Fed., Amsterdam, Excerpta Medica Foundation, 1971.

Bromer, W. W.: Chemistry of glucagon and gastrin, In *Handbook of Physiology.* Steiner, D. F., and Freinkel, N. (eds.), Washington, D.C., American Physiological Society, 1972.

Chance, R. E.: Amino acid sequences of proinsulins and intermediates. *Diabetes* 21(Suppl. 2):461, 1972.

Chandler, M. L., and Varandani, P. T.: Insulin degradation. II. The widespread distribution of glutathione-insulin transhydrogenase in the tissues of the rat. *Biochim. Biophys. Acta* 286:136, 1972.

Chance, R. E.: Chemical, physical, biological, and immunological studies on porcine proinsulin and related polypeptides, In *Diabetes.* Rodriguez, R. R., and Vallance-Owen, J. (eds.), Proc. Seventh Cong. Intern. Diabetes Fed., Buenos Aires, Excerpta Medica Foundation, 1971.

Crofford, O. B., Rogers, N. L., et al.: The effect of insulin on fat cells. An insulin degrading system extracted from plasma membranes of insulin responsive cells. *Diabetes* 21(Suppl. 2):403, 1972.

Duckworth, W. C., Heinemann, M. A., et al.: Purification of insulin-specific protease by affinity chromatography. *Proc. Nat. Acad. Sci. USA* 69:3698, 1972.

Duckworth, W. C., Kitabchi, A. E., et al.: Direct measurement of plasma proinsulin in normal and diabetic subjects. *Amer. J. Med.* 53:418, 1972.

Elgee, N. J., Williams, R. H., et al.: Distribution and degradation studies with insulin-I[131]. *J. Clin. Invest.* 33:1252, 1954.

Field, J. B.: Insulin extraction by the liver, In *Handbook of Physiology.* Steiner, D. F., and Freinkel, N. (eds.), Washington, D.C., American Physiological Society, 1972.

Freychet, P., Kahn, R., et al.: Insulin interactions with liver plasma membranes. Independence of binding of the hormone and its degradation. *J. Biol. Chem.* 12:3953, 1972.

Gorden, P., Roth, J., et al.: The circulating proinsulin-like components. *Diabetes* 21:673, 1972.

Grodsky, G. M., and Forsham, P. H.: Insulin and the pancreas. *Ann. Rev. Physiol.* 28:347, 1966.

Hodgkin, D. C.: The structure of insulin. *Diabetes* 21:1131, 1972.

Humbel, R. E., Bosshard, H. R., et al.: Chemistry of insulin, In *Handbook of Physiology.* Steiner, D. F., and Freinkel, N. (eds.), Washington, D.C., American Physiological Society, 1972.

Katzen, H. M., and Tietze, F.: Studies on the specificity and mechanism of action of hepatic glutathione-insulin transhydrogenase. *J. Biol. Chem.* 241:3561, 1966.

Kitabchi, A. E., Duckworth, W. C., et al.: Direct measurement of proinsulin in human plasma by the use of an insulin-degrading enzyme. *J. Clin. Invest.* 50:1792, 1971.

Kitabchi, A. E., Duckworth, W. C., et al.: Properties of proinsulin and related polypeptides. *CRC Crit. Rev. Biochem.* February, 1972.

Kitabchi, A. E., and Stentz, F. B.: Degradation of insulin and proinsulin by various organ homogenates of rat. *Diabetes* 21:1091, 1972.

Mirsky, I. A.: The metabolism of insulin. *Diabetes* 13:225, 1964.

Mirsky, I. A., Jinks, R., et al.: The isolation and crystallization of human insulin. *J. Clin. Invest.* 42:1869, 1963.

O'Brien, D.: The biochemistry of insulin, In *Diabetes.* Rodriguez, R. R., and Vallance-Owen, J. (eds.), Proc. Seventh Cong. Intern. Diabetes Fed., Amsterdam, Excerpta Medica Foundation, 1971.

Oyer, P., Cho, S., et al.: Studies on human proinsulin. Isolation and amino acid sequence of the human pancreatic c-peptide. *J. Biol. Chem.* 246:1375, 1971.

Rubenstein, A. H., Block, M. B., et al.: Proinsulin and c-peptide in blood. *Diabetes* 21(Suppl. 2):661, 1972.

Rubenstein, A. H., and Steiner, D. F.: Proinsulin. *Ann. Rev. Med.* 22:1, 1971.

Rudman, D., Garcia, L. A., et al.: Cleavage of insulin by mammalian adipose tissue: release of a biologically active peptide from the hormone molecule. *J. Clin. Invest.* 44:1093, 1965.

Ruttenberg, M. A.: Human insulin: facile synthesis by modification of porcine insulin. *Science* 177:623, 1972.

Sanger, F.: Chemistry of insulin. *Science* 129:1340, 1959.

Smith, L. F.: Amino acid sequences of insulins. *Diabetes* 21:457, 1972.

Steiner, D. F., Oyer, P., et al.: Structural and immunological studies on human proinsulin, In *Diabetes.* Rodriguez, R. R., and Vallance-Owen, J. (eds.), Proc. Seventh Cong. Intern. Diabetes Fed., Buenos Aires, Excerpta Medica Foundation, 1971.

Stoll, R. W., Touber, J. L., et al.: Hypoglycemic activity and immunological half-life of porcine insulin and proinsulin in baboons and swine. *Endocrinology* 88:714, 1971.

Tomizawa, H. H.: Mode of action of an insulin-degrading enzyme from beef liver. *J. Biol. Chem.* 237:428, 1962.

Touber, J. L., Stoll, R. W., et al.: Immunological studies of the A and B chains of insulin. *Diabetes* 19:409, 1970.

Synthesis and Release of Insulin, Proinsulin, and Glucagon

Allison, S. P., Chamberlain, M. J., et al.: Intravenous glucose tolerance, insulin, glucose, and free fatty acid levels after myocardial infarction. *Brit. Med. J.* 4:776, 1969.

Bagdade, J. D., Bierman, E. L., et al.: The significance of basal insulin levels in the evaluation of the insulin response to glucose in diabetic and nondiabetic subjects. *J. Clin. Invest.* 46:1549, 1967.

Cerasi, E., and Luft, R.: Diabetes mellitus: a disorder of cellular information transmission? In *The Pathogenesis of Diabetes Mellitus.* Cerasi, E., and Luft, R. (eds.), Thirteenth Nobel Symposium, Stockholm, Almqvist & Wiksell, 1970.

Cerasi, E., and Luft, R.: The plasma insulin response to glucose infusion in healthy subjects and in diabetes mellitus. *Acta Endocr.* 55:278, 1967.

Crockford, P. M., Porte, D., Jr., et al.: Effect of glucagon on serum insulin, plasma glucose, and free fatty acids in man. *Metabolism* 15:114, 1966.

Dean, P. M., and Matthews, E. K.: Electrical activity in pancreatic islet cells: effect of ions. *J. Physiol. (London)* 210:265, 1970.

Dean, P. M., and Matthews, E. K.: Glucose induced electrical activity in pancreatic islet cells. *J. Physiol. (London)* 210:255, 1970.

Dupre, J., and Beck, J. C.: Effect of an intestinal mucosal extract on glucose disposal and serum insulin-like activity in man. *Diabetes* 15:555, 1966.

Fajans, S. S., Floyd, J. C., Jr., et al.: Effect of amino acids and proteins on insulin secretion in man. *Recent Progr. Hormone Res.* 23:617, 1967.

Frohman, L. A., and Bernardis, L. L.: Effect of hypothalamic stimulation on plasma glucose, insulin, and glucagon levels. *Amer. J. Physiol.* 221:1596, 1971.

Genuth, S. M.: Metabolic clearance of insulin in man. *Diabetes* 21:1003, 1972.

Goodner, C. J., and Porte, D., Jr.: Determinants of basal islet secretion in man, In *Handbook of Physiology. I. Endocrinology. Endocrine Pancreas.* Steiner, D. F., and Freinkel, N. (eds.), Washington, D.C., American Physiological Society, 1972.

Grodsky, G. M.: A threshold distribution hypothesis for packet storage of insulin and its mathematical modeling. *J. Clin. Invest.* 51:2047, 1972.

Grodsky, G. M., and Bennett, L. L.: Effect of glucose "pulse," glucagon, and the cations Ca^{++}, Mg$^+$, and K$^+$ on insulin secretion *in vitro. J. Clin. Invest.* 45:1018, 1966.

Lacy, P.: Beta cell secretion—from the standpoint of a pathobiologist. *Diabetes* 19:895, 1970.

Lacy, P., and Greider, M. H.: Ultrastructural organization of mammalian pancreatic islets, In *Handbook of Physiology. I. Endocrinology*. Steiner, D. F., and Freinkel, N. (eds.), Washington, D.C., American Physiological Society, 1972.

Lazarus, S. S., Shapiro, S., et al.: Secretory granule formation and release in rabbit pancreatic A-cells. *Diabetes* 17:152, 1968.

Like, A., and Orci, L.: Embryogenesis of the human pancreatic islets: a light and electron microscopic study. *Diabetes* 21:511, 1972.

Logothetopoulos, J., and Bell, E. G.: Histological and autoradiographic studies of the islets of mice injected with insulin antibody. *Diabetes* 15:205, 1966.

Logothetopoulos, J., Davidson, J. K., et al.: Degranulation of beta cells and loss of pancreatic insulin after infusions of insulin antibody or glucose. *Diabetes* 14:493, 1965.

Lukomsky, P. E., and Oganov, R. G.: Blood plasma catecholamines and their urinary excretion in patients with myocardial infarction. *Amer. Heart J.* 83:182, 1972.

Matschinsky, F. M., Landgraf, R., et al.: Glucoreceptor mechanisms in islets of Langerhans. *Diabetes* 21:555, 1972.

McIntyre, N., Holdsworth, C. D., et al.: Intestinal factors in the control of insulin secretion. *J. Clin. Endocr.* 25:1317, 1965.

Munge, B.: The histology, cytochemistry and ultrastructure of pancreatic islet A-cells, In *Glucagon, Molecular Physiology, Clinical and Therapeutic Implications*. Lefebvre, P. J., and Unger, R. H. (eds.), Oxford, Pergamon Press, 1972.

Munger, B. L.: The biology of secretory tumors of the pancreatic islets, In *Handbook of Physiology. I. Endocrinology*. Steiner, D. F., and Freinkel, N. (eds.), Washington, D.C., American Physiological Society, 1972.

Pictet, R. L., Clark, W. R., et al.: An ultrastructural analysis of the developing embryonic pancreas. *Develop. Biol.* 29:436, 1972.

Porte, D., Jr.: A receptor mechanism for the inhibition of insulin release by epinephrine in man. *J. Clin. Invest.* 46:86, 1967.

Porte, D., Jr., Girardier, L., et al.: Neural regulation of insulin secretion in the dog. *J. Clin. Invest.* 52:210, 1973.

Porte, D., Jr., Graber, A. L., et al.: The effect of epinephrine on immunoreactive insulin levels in man. *J. Clin. Invest.* 45:228, 1966.

Porte, D., Jr., and Robertson, R. P.: Regulation of insulin secretion by catecholamines, stress and the sympathetic nervous system. *Fed. Proc.* 32:1792, 1973.

Rabinowitz, D., and Zierler, K. L.: Forearm metabolism in obesity and its response to intraarterial insulin. Characterization of insulin resistance evidence for adaptive hyperinsulinism. *J. Clin. Invest.* 41:2173, 1962.

Rall, L. B., Pictet, R. L., et al.: Is glucagon a developmental hormone? *Proc. Nat. Acad. Sci. USA*, 1973 (in press).

Robertson, R. P., Brunzell, J. D., et al.: Paradoxical hypoinsulinemia: an alpha adrenergic-mediated response to glucose. *Lancet* 2:787, 1972.

Robertson, R. P., and Porte, D., Jr.: The glucose receptor: a defective mechanism in diabetes mellitus distinct from the β-adrenergic receptor. *J. Clin. Invest.* 52:870, 1973.

Robertson, R. P., and Porte, D., Jr.: Adrenergic modulation of basal insulin secretion in man. *Diabetes* 22:1, 1973.

Rocha, D. M., Faloona, G., et al.: Glucagon-stimulating activity of 20 amino acids in dogs. *J. Clin. Invest.* 51:2346, 1972.

Samols, E., Marri, G., et al.: Promotion of insulin secretion by glucagon. *Lancet* 2:415, 1965.

Sokal, J. E.: Glucagon—an essential hormone. *Amer. J. Med.* 41:331, 1966.

Steiner, D. F., Kemmler, J. L., et al.: The biosynthesis of insulin, In *Handbook of Physiology. I. Endocrinology*. Steiner, D. F., and Freinkel, N. (eds.), Washington, D.C., American Physiological Society, 1972.

Steinke, J., and Driscoll, S. G.: The extractable insulin content of pancreas from fetuses and infants of diabetic and control mothers. *Diabetes* 14:573, 1965.

Taylor, S. H., and Majid, P. A.: Insulin and the heart. *J. Mol. Cell. Cardiol.* 2:293, 1971.

Turner, R. C., Grayburn, J. A., et al.: Measurement of the insulin delivery rate in man. *J. Clin. Endocr.* 33:279, 1971.

Unger, R. H.: Circulating pancreatic glucagon and extrapancreatic glucagon-like materials, In *Handbook of Physiology. I. Endocrinology*. Steiner, D. F., and Freinkel, N. (eds.), Washington, D.C., American Physiological Society, 1972.

Yalow, R. S., and Berson, S. A.: Immunoassay of endogenous plasma insulin in man. *J. Clin. Invest.* 39:1157, 1960.

Actions of Insulin, Proinsulin, and Related Compounds

Aoki, T. T., Brennan, M. F., et al.: Effect of insulin on muscle glutamate uptake. *J. Clin. Invest.* 51:2889, 1972.

Bennett, P. H., Burch, T. A., et al.: Hyperglycemia in North American (Pima) Indians: Diabetes mellitus or not? Read before the International Diabetes Federation, Buenos Aires, 1970.

Berson, S. A., and Yalow, R. S.: Insulin "antagonists" and insulin resistance, In *Diabetes Mellitus: Theory and Practice*. Ellenberg, M., and Rifkin, H. (eds.), New York, McGraw-Hill, 1970.

Bierman, E. L.: Insulin and hypertriglyceridemia. *Israel J. Med. Sci.* 8:303, 1972.

Cahill, G. F., Jr.: Physiology of insulin in man. *Diabetes* 20:785, 1971.

Carpenter, F. H.: Relationship of structure to biological activity of insulin as revealed by degradative studies. *Amer. J. Med.* 40:750, 1966.

Cuatrecasas, P.: The insulin receptor. *Diabetes* 21(Suppl. 2):396, 1972.

Davidson, M. B., and Poffenbarger, P. L.: Role of synalbumin insulin antagonist in the pathogenesis of diabetes mellitus. *Metabolism* 19:668, 1970.

Edelman, P. M., Edelman, J. C., et al.: Insulin-like effects of adenosine 3',5'-monophosphate (cyclic AMP) on rat striated muscle. *Fed. Proc.* 25:442, 1966.

Ensinck, J. W., and Williams, R. H.: Hormonal and nonhormonal factors modifying man's response to insulin, In *Handbook of Physiology. I. Endocrinology*. Steiner, D. F., and Freinkel, N. (eds.), Washington, D.C., American Physiological Society, 1972.

Fain, J. N., and Rosenberg, L.: Antilipolytic action of insulin on fat cells. *Diabetes* 21(Suppl. 2):414, 1972.

Felig, P.: The glucose-alanine cycle. *Metabolism* 22:179, 1973.

Felig, P.: Interaction of insulin and amino acid metabolism in the regulation of gluconeogenesis. *Israel J. Med. Sci.* 8:262, 1972.

Felig, P., and Wahren, J.: Amino acid metabolism in exercising man. *J. Clin. Invest.* 50:2703, 1971.

Fredrickson, D. S.: Hyperlipoproteinemia with carbohydrate intolerance, In *Diabetes Mellitus: Diagnosis and Treatment*. Vol. III. Fajans, S. S., and Sussman, K. E. (eds.), New York, American Diabetes Association, 1971.

Freychet, P., Roth, J., et al.: Insulin receptors in the liver: specific binding of [I-125] insulin to the plasma membrane and its relation to insulin bioactivity. *Proc. Nat. Acad. Sci. USA* 68:1833, 1971.

Gavin, J. R., III, Roth, J., et al.: Insulin receptors in human circulating cells and fibroblasts (lymphocytes/monoiodoinsulin/glucose oxidation). *Proc. Nat. Acad. Sci. USA* 69:747, 1972.

Hall, K., and Uthne, K.: Some biological properties of purified sulfation factor (SF) from human plasma. *Acta Med. Scand.* 190:137, 1971.

Hintz, R. L., Clemmons, D. R., et al.: Competitive binding of somatomedin to the insulin receptors of adipocytes, chondrocytes, and liver membranes. *Proc. Nat. Acad. Sci. USA* 69:2351, 1972.

Humbel, R. E., Bunzli, H., et al.: Insulin-like substances: the insulin dimer, and non-suppressible insulin-like activity, In *Diabetes*. Rodriguez, R. R., and Vallance-Owen, J. (eds.), Proc. Seventh Intern. Cong. Diabetes Fed., Amsterdam, Excerpta Medica Foundation, 1971.

Illiano, G., and Cuatrecasas, P.: Modulation of adenylate cyclase activity in liver and fat cell membranes by insulin. *Science* 175:906, 1972.

Kitabchi, A. E.: The biological and immunological properties of pork and beef insulin, proinsulin, and connecting peptides. *J. Clin. Invest.* 49:979, 1970.

Krahl, M. E.: Insulin action at the molecular level: facts and speculations. *Diabetes* 21(Suppl. 2):695, 1972.

Lakshmanan, M. R., Nepokroeff, C. M., et al.: Control of the synthesis of fatty-acid synthetase in rat liver by insulin, glucagon, and adenosine 3',5' cyclic monophosphate. *Proc. Nat. Acad. Sci. USA* 69:3516, 1972.

Lazarus, N. R.: Insulin and insulin-like substances in the circulation, In *Clinics in Endocrinology and Metabolism*. Vol. I. Pyke, D. A. (ed.), London, W. B. Saunders Co., 1972.

Levine, R.: Action of insulin: an attempt at a summary. *Diabetes* 21(Suppl. 2):454, 1972.

Levine, R., and Haft, D. E.: Carbohydrate homeostasis. *New Eng. J. Med.* 283:175, 1970.

Livingston, J. N., Cuatrecasas, P., et al.: Insulin insensitivity of large fat cells. *Science* 177:626, 1972.

Madison, L. L.: Role of insulin in the hepatic handling of glucose. *Arch. Intern. Med.* 123:284, 1969.

Manchester, K. L.: Effect of insulin on protein synthesis. *Diabetes* 21(Suppl. 2):447, 1972.

Mortimore, G. E.: Influence of insulin on the hepatic uptake and release of glucose and amino acids, In *Handbook of Physiology. I. Endocrinology.* Steiner, D. F., and Freinkel, N. (eds.), Washington, D.C., American Physiological Society, 1972.

Park, C. R., Lewis, S. B., et al.: Relationship of some hepatic actions of insulin to the intracellular level of cyclic adenylate. *Diabetes* 21(Suppl. 2):439, 1972.

Poffenbarger, P. L., Ensinck, J. W., et al.: The nature of human serum insulin-like activity (ILA): Characterization of ILA in serum and serum fractions obtained by acid-ethanol extraction and adsorption chromatography. *J. Clin. Invest.* 47:301, 1968.

Randle, P. J., Garland, P. B., et al.: The glucose fatty acid cycle and diabetes mellitus. *Ciba Foundation Colloq. Endocr.* 15:192, 1964a.

Rubenstein, A. H., Melani, F., et al.: Circulating proinsulin: immunology, measurement and biological activity, In *Handbook of Physiology. I. Endocrinology.* Steiner, D. F., and Freinkel, N. (eds.), Washington, D.C., American Physiological Society, 1972.

Ruderman, N. B., and Lund, P.: Amino acid metabolism in skeletal muscle. Regulation of glutamine and alanine release in the perfused rat hindquarter. *Israel J. Med. Sci.* 8:295, 1972.

Sherman, B. M., Pek, S., et al.: Plasma proinsulin in patients with functioning pancreatic islet cell tumors. *J. Clin. Endocr.* 35:271, 1972.

Sols, A.: Regulation of liver glucokinase and muscle hexokinase, In *On the Nature and Treatment of Diabetes.* Leibel, B. S., and Wrenshall, G. A. (eds.), Amsterdam, Excerpta Medica Foundation, 1965.

Spiro, R. G.: Glycoproteins: their biochemistry, biology and role in human disease (Part I). *New Eng. J. Med.* 281:991, 1969.

Steiner, D. F.: Insulin and the regulation of hepatic biosynthetic activity. *Vitam. Horm.* 24:1, 1966.

Vallance-Owen, J.: Insulin antagonists, In *On the Nature and Treatment of Diabetes.* Leibel, B. S., and Wrenshall, G. A. (eds.), Amsterdam, Excerpta Medica Foundation, 1965.

Walaas, O., Walaas, E., et al.: Effect of insulin and epinephrine on cyclic AMP-dependent protein kinase in rat diaphragm. *Israel J. Med. Sci.* 8:353, 1972.

Weber, G., Singhal, R. L., et al.: Synchronous behavior pattern of key glycolytic enzymes: glucokinase, phosphofructokinase, and pyruvate kinase. *Advances Enzyme Reg.* 4:59, 1966.

Werk, E. E., and Knowles, H. C.: The blood ketone and plasma free fatty acid concentration in diabetic and normal subjects. *Diabetes* 10:22, 1961.

Winegrad, A. I., and Burden, C. L.: L-xylulose metabolism in diabetes mellitus. *New Eng. J. Med.* 274:298, 1966.

Woodside, W. F., and Heimberg, M.: Hepatic metabolism of free fatty acids in experimental diabetes. *Israel J. Med. Sci.* 8:309, 1972.

Vann Bennett, G., and Cuatrecasas, P.: Insulin receptor of fat cells in insulin-resistant metabolic states. *Science* 176:805, 1972.

Zierler, K. L.: Possible mechanisms of insulin action on membrane potential and ion fluxes. *Amer. J. Med.* 40:735, 1966.

Other Hormones Influencing Insulin Actions

Adams, P. W., and Oakley, N. W.: Oral contraceptives and carbohydrate metabolism. In *Clinics in Endocrinology and Metabolism.* Vol. I. Pyke, D. A. (ed.), London, W. B. Saunders Co., 1972.

Assan, R., and Slusher, N.: Structure/function and structure/immunoreactivity relationships of the glucagon molecule and related synthetic peptides. *Diabetes* 21:843, 1972.

Assan, R., Tchobroutsky, G., et al.: Intervention of kidney and liver in glucagon catabolism and clearance from plasma, In *Current Topics on Glucagon.* Austoni, M., Scandellari, C., et al. (eds.), Padova, Cedam, 1971.

Bornstein, J.: A proposed mechanism of the diabetogenic action of growth hormone and its relation to the action of insulin. *Israel J. Med. Sci.* 8:407, 1972.

Brazeau, P., Vale, W., et al.: Hypothalamic polypeptide that inhibits the secretion of immunoreactive pituitary growth hormone. *Science* 179:77, 1973.

Ensinck, J. W., Shepard, C., et al.: Use of benzamidine as a proteolytic inhibitor in the radioimmunoassay of glucagon in plasma. *J. Clin. Endocr.* 35:463, 1972.

Exton, J. H.: Gluconeogenesis. *Metabolism* 21:945, 1972.

Exton, J. H., Jefferson, L. S., Jr., et al.: Gluconeogenesis in the perfused liver. *Amer. J. Med.* 40:709, 1966.

Frazier, W. A., Angeletti, R. H., et al.: Nerve growth factor and insulin. *Science* 176:482, 1972.

Houssay, B. A., and Penhos, J. C.: Diabetogenic action of pituitary hormones on adrenalectomized hypophysectomized dogs. *Endocrinology* 61:774, 1957.

Levey, G. S.: Restoration of glucagon responsiveness of solubilized myocardial adenyl cyclase by phosphatidylserine. *Biochem. Biophys. Res. Commun.* 43:108, 1971.

Luft, E., and Cerasi, E.: Effect of human growth hormone on insulin production in panhypopituitarism. *Lancet* 2:124, 1964.

Mallette, L. E., Exton, J. H., et al.: Effects of glucagon on amino acid transport and utilization in the perfused rat liver. *J. Biol. Chem.* 244:5724, 1969.

Manganiello, V., and Vaughan, M.: Selective loss of adipose cell responsiveness to glucagon with growth in the rat. *J. Lipid Res.* 13:12, 1972.

Marks, V.: Glucagon, In *Clinics in Endocrinology and Metabolism.* Pyke, D. A. (ed.), London, W. B. Saunders Co., 1972.

McDonald, J. K., Callahan, P. X., et al.: Inactivation and degradation of glucagon by dipeptidyl aminopeptidase I (Cathepsin C) of rat liver. *J. Biol. Chem.* 244:6199, 1969.

Rodbell, M., Birnbaumer, L., et al.: The reaction of glucagon with its receptor: evidence for discrete regions of activity and binding in the glucagon molecule. *Proc. Nat. Acad. Sci. USA* 68:909, 1971.

Rodbell, M., Birnbaumer, L., et al.: Properties of the adenyl cyclase systems in liver and adipose cells: the mode of action of hormones. *Acta Diabetol. Lat.* 7(Suppl. 1):9, 1970.

Sokal, J. E.: Glucagon, In *Diabetes Mellitus: Theory and Practice.* Ellenberg, M., and Rifkin, H. (eds.), New York, McGraw-Hill, 1970.

Steinberg, T., Passy, V., et al.: Effect of submaxillary gland extirpation on glucose and insulin tolerance in dogs. *Diabetes* 21:722, 1972.

Wieland, O.: Hormonal regulation of carbohydrate and lipid metabolism in liver. In *Diabetes.* Rodriguez, R. R., and Vallance-Owen, J. (eds.), Proc. Seventh Cong. Intern. Diabetes Fed., Amsterdam, Excerpta Medica Foundation, 1971.

Yalow, R. S., and Berson, S. A.: Secretory responses of HGH and ACTH in diabetic and nondiabetic subjects, In *Diabetes.* Rodriguez, R. R., and Vallance-Owen, J. (eds.), Proc. Seventh Intern. Diabetes Fed., Amsterdam, Excerpta Medica Foundation, 1971.

Diabetes in Laboratory Animals

Cameron, D. P., Stauffacher, W., et al.: Defective immunoreactive insulin secretion in the acomys cahirinus. *Diabetes* 21:1060, 1972.

Renold, A. E., Cameron, D. P., et al.: Endocrine-metabolic anomalies in rodents with hyperglycemic syndromes of hereditary and/or environmental origin. *Israel J. Med. Sci.* 8:189, 1972.

Clinical Diabetes

Bierman, E. L., Bagdade, J. D., et al.: Obesity and diabetes: the odd couple. *Amer. J. Clin. Nutr.* 21:1434, 1968.

Edwards, J. H.: Should diabetics marry? *Lancet* 1:1045, 1969.

Fajans, S. S.: What is diabetes. Definition, diagnosis, and course. *Med. Clin. N. Amer.* 55:793, 1971.

Joslin, E. P.: The prevention of diabetes mellitus. *J.A.M.A.* 76:79, 1921.

Pyke, D. A.: Glucose tolerance and serum insulin in identical twins of diabetics. *Brit. Med. J.* 4:649, 1970.

Rimoin, D. L.: Inheritance in diabetes mellitus. *Med. Clin. N. Amer.* 55:807, 1971.

Rushforth, N. B., Bennett, P. H., et al.: Diabetes in the Pima Indians. *Diabetes* 20:756, 1971.

Simpson, N. E.: Diabetes in the families of diabetics. *Canad. Med. Ass. J.* 98:427, 1968.

Diagnosis of Diabetes

Andres, R.: Effect of age in interpretation of glucose and tolbutamide tolerance tests, In *Diabetes Mellitus: Diagnosis and*

Treatment. Fajans, S. S., and Sussman, K. E. (eds.), New York, American Diabetes Association, 1971.

Cerasi, E., and Luft, R.: The prediabetic state, its nature and consequences—a look toward the future. *Diabetes 21*(Suppl. 2):685, 1972.

Dillon, R. S.: Importance of the hematocrit in interpretation of blood sugar. *Diabetes 14*:672, 1965.

Fajans, S. S., and Conn, J. W.: Prediabetes, subclinical diabetes, and latent clinical diabetes: interpretation, diagnosis and treatment, In *On the Nature and Treatment of Diabetes.* Leibel, B. S., and Wrenshall, G. A. (eds.), Amsterdam, Excerpta Medica Foundation, 1965.

Field, R. A., and Skyler, J. S.: Nonglucose melliturias, In *Diabetes Mellitus: Theory and Practice.* Ellenberg, M., and Rifkin, H. (eds.), New York, McGraw-Hill, 1970.

Hayner, N. S., Kjelsberg, M. O., et al.: Carbohydrate tolerance and diabetes in a total community, Tecumseh, Michigan. *Diabetes 14*:413, 1965.

Jackson, W. P. U., and Vinik, A. I.: Hyperglycemia and diabetes in the elderly, In *Diabetes Mellitus: Theory and Practice.* Ellenberg, M., and Rifkin, H. (eds.), New York, McGraw-Hill, 1970.

Krane, S.: Renal glycosuria, In *The Metabolic Basis of Inherited Disease.* Stanbury, J. B., Wyngaarden, J. B., et al. (eds.), New York, McGraw-Hill, 1972.

Lundbaek, K.: Intravenous glucose tolerance as a tool in definition and diagnosis of diabetes mellitus. *Brit. Med. J. 1*:1507, 1962.

Marble, A.: Laboratory procedures useful in diagnosis and treatment, In *Joslin's Diabetes Mellitus.* Marble, A., White, P., et al. (eds.), Philadelphia, Lea & Febiger, 1971.

Marble, A.: Nondiabetic melituria, In *Joslin's Diabetes Mellitus.* Marble, A., White, P., et al. (eds.), Philadelphia, Lea & Febiger, 1971.

McDonald, G. W.: *Diabetes Source Book.* U.S. Department of Health, Education and Welfare, Public Health Service, Division of Chronic Diseases, #1168, 1964 (Revised 1968).

McDonald, G. W., Fisher, G. F., et al.: Reproducibility of the oral glucose tolerance test. *Diabetes 14*:473, 1965.

McDonald, G. W., and O'Sullivan, J. B.: Screening for diabetes mellitus, In *Diabetes Mellitus: Diagnosis and Treatment,* Vol. III. Fajans, S. S., and Sussman, K. E. (eds.), New York, American Diabetes Association, 1971.

O'Sullivan, J. S., and Mahan, C. M.: Criteria for the oral glucose tolerance test in pregnancy. *Diabetes 13*:278, 1964.

Remein, R. R., and Wilkerson, H. L. C.: The efficiency of screening tests for diabetes. *J. Chronic Dis. 13*:6, 1961.

Rull, J. A., Conn, J. W., et al.: Levels of plasma insulin during cortisone glucose tolerance tests in "nondiabetic" relatives of diabetic patients. *Diabetes 19*:1, 1970.

Seltzer, H. S.: Diagnosis of diabetes, In *Diabetes Mellitus: Theory and Practice.* Ellenberg, M., and Rifkin, H. (eds.), New York, McGraw-Hill, 1970.

Seltzer, H. S., Fajans, S. S., et al.: Spontaneous hypoglycemia as an early manifestation of diabetes mellitus. *Diabetes 5*:437, 1956.

Service, F. J., Molnar, G. D., et al.: Urine glucose analyses during continuous blood glucose monitoring. *J.A.M.A. 222*:294, 1972.

Soeldner, J. S.: The intravenous glucose tolerance test, In *Diabetes Mellitus: Diagnosis and Treatment.* Fajans, S. S., and Sussman, K. E. (eds.), New York, American Diabetes Association, 1971.

Streeten, D. H. P., Gerstein, M. D., et al.: Reduced glucose tolerance in elderly human subjects. *Diabetes 14*:579, 1965.

Swerdloff, R. S., Pozefsky, T., et al.: Influence of age on the intravenous tolbutamide response test. *Diabetes 16*:161, 1967.

Pathology of Diabetes

Bartels, C. C., and Rullo, F. R.: Unsuspected diabetes mellitus in peripheral vascular disease. *New Eng. J. Med. 259*:633, 1958.

Beisswenger, P. J., and Spiro, R. G.: Human glomerular basement membrane: chemical alteration in diabetes mellitus. *Science 168*:596, 1970.

Bell, E. T.: *Diabetes Mellitus.* Springfield, Illinois, Charles C Thomas, 1960.

Berkow, J. W., Sugarman, R. G., et al.: A retrospective study of blind diabetic patients. *J.A.M.A. 193*:867, 1965.

Binkley, G. W.: Dermopathy in the diabetic syndrome. *Arch. Derm. 92*:625, 1965.

Caird, F. I., Pirie, A., et al.: *Diabetes and the Aged.* Oxford, Blackwell, 1969.

Danowski, T. S., Sabeh, G., et al.: Skin spots and diabetes mellitus. *Brit. J. Derm. 80*:275, 1968.

Ditzel, J., Beaven, D. W., et al.: Early vascular changes in diabetes mellitus. *Metabolism 9*:400, 1960.

Fagerberg, S. E.: Recent advances in diabetic neuropathy, In *On the Nature and Treatment of Diabetes.* Leibel, B. S., and Wrenshall, G. A. (eds.), Amsterdam, Excerpta Medica Foundation, 1965.

Gabbay, K. H., Merola, L. O., et al.: Sorbitol pathway: presence in nerve and cord with substrate accumulation in diabetes. *Science 151*:209, 1966.

Gabbay, K. H., and O'Sullivan, J. B.: The sorbitol pathway. Enzyme localization and content in normal and diabetic nerve and cord. *Diabetes 17*:239, 1968.

Gamstorp, I., Shelburne, S. A., Jr., et al.: Peripheral neuropathy in juvenile diabetes. *Diabetes 15*:411, 1966.

Gellman, D. D., Pirani, C. L., et al.: Diabetic nephropathy: a clinical and pathologic study based on renal biopsies. *Medicine 38*:321, 1959.

Goldberg, M. F., and Fine, S. L. (eds.): *Symposium on the Treatment of Diabetic Retinopathy.* Washington, D.C., U.S. Public Health Service Publication, #1890, 1969.

Goldner, M. G.: The fate of the second leg in the diabetic amputee. *Diabetes 9*:100, 1960.

Jordan, W. R.: Neuritic manifestations in diabetes mellitus. *Arch. Intern. Med. 57*:307, 1936.

Lindbom, A.: Arteriosclerosis and arterial thrombosis in the lower limb. *Acta Radiologica* (Suppl. 80):1, 1950.

Locke, S.: The peripheral nervous system in diabetes mellitus. *Diabetes 13*:307, 1964.

Lundbaek, K., Malmros, R., et al.: Hypophysectomy for diabetic angiopathy. A controlled clinical trial, In *Symposium on Treatment of Diabetic Retinopathy.* Goldberg, M. F., and Fine, S. L. (eds.), Washington, D.C., U.S. Public Health Service Publication, 1968.

Ostrander, L. D., Jr., Francis, T., Jr., et al.: The relationship of cardiovascular disease to hyperglycemia. *Ann. Intern. Med. 62*:1188, 1965.

Parker, F.: An electron microscopic study of experimental atherosclerosis. *Amer. J. Path. 36*:19, 1960.

Partamian, J. O., and Bradley, R. F.: Acute myocardial infarction in 258 cases of diabetes. *New Eng. J. Med. 273*:455, 1965.

Poulsen, J. F.: Houssay phenomenon in man: recovery from retinopathy in a case of diabetes with Simond's disease. *Diabetes 2*:7, 1953.

Reske-Nielsen, E., Lundbaek, K., et al.: Pathological changes in the central and peripheral nervous system of young long-term diabetes. *Diabetologia 1*:233, 1965.

Salomon, M. I.: Diabetic nephropathy: clinicopathologic correlation. A study based on renal biopsies. *Metabolism 12*:687, 1963.

Siperstein, M. D., Unger, R. H., et al.: Studies of muscle capillary basement membranes in normal subjects, diabetic, and prediabetic patients. *J. Clin. Invest. 47*:1973, 1968.

Spiro, R. G.: Glycoproteins and diabetic microangiopathy, In *Joslin's Diabetes Mellitus.* Marble, A., White, P., et al. (eds.), Philadelphia, Lea & Febiger, 1971.

Spiro, R. G.: Glycoproteins: Their biochemistry, biology and role in human disease. *New Eng. J. Med. 281*:991, 1969.

Strandness, D. E., Jr., Priest, R. E., et al.: Combined clinical and pathologic study of diabetic and nondiabetic peripheral arterial disease. *Diabetes 12*:366, 1964.

Thomas, P. K., and Rascelles, R. G.: The pathology of diabetic neuropathy. *Quart. J. Med. 35*:489, 1966.

Vracko, R., and Benditt, E. P.: Basal lamina: The scaffold for orderly cell replacement. *J. Cell. Biol. 55*:406, 1972.

Vracko, R., and Benditt, E. P.: Capillary basal lamina thickening. Its relationship to endothelial cell death and replacement. *J. Cell. Biol. 47*:281, 1970.

White, P.: Childhood diabetes. Its course and influence on the second and third generations. *Diabetes 9*:345, 1960.

Williamson, J. R., Vogler, N. J., et al.: Microvascular disease in diabetes. *Med. Clin. N. Amer. 55*:847, 1971.

Wrenshall, G. A., and Best, C. H.: Extractable insulin of the pancreas and effectiveness of oral hypoglycemic sulfonylureas in the treatment of diabetes in man—a comparison. *Canad. Med. Ass. J. 74*:968, 1956.

Pregnancy and Diabetes

Beck, P., Parker, M. L., et al.: Radioimmunologic measurement of human placental lactogen in plasma by a double antibody method during normal and diabetic pregnancies. *J. Clin. Endocr. 25*:1457, 1965.

Beischer, N. A., and Brown, J. B.: Current status of estrogen assays in obstetrics and gynecology. Part 2: Estrogen assays in late pregnancy. *Obstet. Gynec. Surv. 27*:303, 1972.

Freinkel, N.: The effect of pregnancy on insulin homeostasis. *Diabetes 13*:260, 1964.

Kalkhoff, R., Schalch, D. S., et al.: Diabetogenic factors associated with pregnancy. *Trans. Ass. Amer. Physicians 77*:270, 1964.

Rivlin, M. E., Mestman, J. H., et al.: Value of estriol estimations in the management of diabetic pregnancy. *Amer. J. Obstet. Gynec. 106*:875, 1970.

Tyson, J. E.: Obstetrical management of the pregnant diabetic. *Med. Clin. N. Amer. 55*:961, 1971.

White, P.: Pregnancy and diabetes, In *Joslin's Diabetes Mellitus.* Marble, A., White, P., et al. (eds.), Philadelphia, Lea & Febiger, 1971.

Treatment of Diabetes

Albrink, M. J., and Davidson, P. C.: Dietary therapy and prophylaxis of vascular disease in diabetics. *Med. Clin. N. Amer. 55*:877, 1971.

Arky, R. A., and Abramson, E. A.: Insulin response to glucose in presence of oral hypoglycemics. *Ann. N.Y. Acad. Sci. 148*:768, 1968.

Brunzell, J. D., Lerner, R. L., et al.: Improved glucose tolerance with high carbohydrate feeding in mild diabetes. *New Eng. J. Med. 284*:521, 1971.

Butterfield, J., Fry, I. K., et al.: Effects of insulin, tolbutamide and phenethyldiguanidine on peripheral glucose uptake in man. *Diabetes 7*:449, 1958.

Chu, P. C., Conway, M. J., et al.: The pattern of response of plasma insulin and glucose to meals and fasting during chlorpropamide therapy. *Ann. Intern. Med. 68*:757, 1968.

Committee on Nutrition of the American Diabetes Association: Principles of nutrition and dietary recommendations for patients with diabetes mellitus. *Diabetes 20*:633, 1971.

Cornfield, J.: The University Group Diabetes Program. A further statistical analysis of the mortality findings. *J.A.M.A. 217*:1676, 1971.

Czyzyk, A., Tawecki, J., et al.: Effect of biguanides on intestinal absorption of glucose. *Diabetes 17*:492, 1968.

Feinstein, A. R.: Clinical Biostatistics—VIII. An analytic appraisal of the University Group Diabetes Program (UGDP) study. *Clin. Pharmacol. Ther. 12*:167, 1971.

Galloway, J. A.: New forms of insulin. *Diabetes 21*:637, 1972.

Garcia, M., Miller, M., et al.: Chlorpropamide-induced water retention in patients with diabetes mellitus. *Ann. Intern. Med. 75*:549, 1971.

Knowles, H. C., Jr., Guest, G. M., et al.: The course of juvenile diabetes treated with unmeasured diet. *Diabetes 14*:239, 1965.

Krall, L. P.: The oral hypoglycemic agents, In *Joslin's Diabetes Mellitus.* Marble, A., White, P., et al. (eds.), Philadelphia, Lea & Febiger, 1971.

Kruger, F. A., Altschuld, R. A., et al.: Studies on the site and mechanism of action of phenformin. II. Phenformin inhibition of glucose transport by rat intestine. *Diabetes 19*:50, 1970.

Schlichtkrull, J., Brange, J., et al.: Clinical aspects of insulin-antigenicity. *Diabetes 21*:649, 1972.

Searle, G. L., Schilling, S., et al.: Body glucose kinetics in nondiabetic human subjects after phenethylbiguanide. *Diabetes 15*:173, 1966.

Seltzer, S., and Holbrooke, S.: Drug-induced hypoglycemia. *Diabetes 21*:955, 1972.

Stone, D. B., and Conner, W. E.: The prolonged effects of a low cholesterol, high carbohydrate diet upon the serum lipids in diabetic patients. *Diabetes 12*:127, 1963.

University Group Diabetes Program. A study of the effects of hypoglycemic agents on vascular complications in patients with adult-onset diabetes: I. Design. II. Mortality Results. *Diabetes 19*(Suppl. 2):747, 1970.

Weissman, P. N., Shenkman, L., et al.: Chlorpropamide hyponatremia. *New Eng. J. Med. 284*:65, 1971.

Williams, R. H., and Steiner, D. F.: Summarization of studies relative to the mechanism of phenethylbiguanide hypoglycemia. *Metabolism 8*:548, 1959.

Acute Complications

Arieff, A. I., and Kleeman, C. R.: Studies on mechanisms of cerebral edema in diabetic comas. Effects of hyperglycemia and rapid lowering of plasma glucose in normal rabbits. *J. Clin. Invest. 52*:571, 1973.

Carroll, H. J., and Arieff, A. I.: Osmotic equilibrium between extracellular fluid and cerebrospinal fluid during treatment of hyperglycemic, hyperosmolar, nonketotic coma. *Trans. Ass. Amer. Physicians 84*:113, 1971.

Clements, R. S., Jr., Blumenthal, S. A., et al.: Increased cerebrospinal-fluid pressure during treatment of diabetic ketosis. *Lancet 1*:671, 1971.

Committee Report, Danowski, T. S., Chairman: Lactic acidosis in diabetes mellitus. *J.A.M.A. 184*:47, 1963.

Danowski, T. S.: Diabetic acidosis and coma, In *Diabetes Mellitus: Theory and Practice.* Ellenberg, M., and Rifkin, H. (eds.), New York, McGraw-Hill, 1970.

Hockaday, T. D. R., and Alberti, K. G. M. M.: Diabetic coma, In *Clinics in Endocrinology and Metabolism. I. Diabetes and Related Disorders.* Pyke, D. A. (ed.), London, W. B. Saunders Co., 1972.

Matz, R.: Coma in the nonketotic diabetic, In *Diabetes Mellitus: Theory and Practice.* Ellenberg, M., and Rifkin, H. (eds.), New York, McGraw-Hill, 1970.

Huckabee, W. E.: Abnormal resting blood lactate: I. Significance of hyperlactatemia in hospitalized patients. *Amer. J. Med. 30*:833, 1961.

Schwartz, T. B.: Nonketotic coma, In *Diabetes Mellitus: Diagnosis and Treatment.* Fajans, S. S., and Sussman, K. E. (eds.), New York, American Diabetes Association, 1971.

Reciprocal Influences of Certain Conditions and Diabetes

Reske-Nielsen, E.. Lundbaek, K., et al.: Pathological changes in the central and peripheral nervous system of young long-term diabetes. *Diabetologia 1*:233, 1965.

Rare Etiologies of Diabetes

Dymock, I. W., Cassar, J., et al.: Observations on the pathogenesis, complications and treatment of diabetes in 115 cases of haemochromatosis. *Amer. J. Med. 52*:203, 1972.

McGavran, M. H., Unger, R. H., et al.: A glucagon-secreting alpha-cell carcinoma of the pancreas. *New Eng. J. Med. 274*:1408, 1966.

Podolsky, S.: Lipoatrophic diabetes and miscellaneous conditions related to diabetes mellitus, In *Joslin's Diabetes Mellitus.* Marble, A., White, P., et al. (eds.), Philadelphia, Lea & Febiger, 1971.

Taylor, K. W., and Gamble, D. R.: Viruses and other toxic factors in the aetiology of diabetes mellitus. *Acta Diabetol. Lat. 7*(Suppl. 1):397, 1970.

CHAPTER 10

Disorders Causing Hypoglycemia

By John W. Ensinck and
Robert H. Williams

Man expends energy continuously, yet he ingests food intermittently; hence, he must store fuels for consumption between feedings and as a contingency for prolonged fasting. The major endogenous fuel repositories are in the form of triglyceride in adipose tissue, protein in muscle, and glycogen in muscle and liver. Most tissues can use either glucose, derived from liver glycogen, or free fatty acids (FFA), originating from triglyceride, whereas the central nervous system and, to a lesser extent, some other specialized organs depend almost exclusively upon glucose as their energy substrate. Therefore, a highly integrated system for assimilation and *de novo* generation of glucose is required. The remarkable constancy of circulating plasma glucose, ranging from 60–160 mg./100 ml. in normal man during fasting and fed states, is a result of a complex, synchronized interaction between neural and hormonal factors. Hypoglycemia is an abnormal depression of the extracellular glucose concentration reflected in plasma, which is manifested by a characteristic symptom complex initiated when the nervous system is deprived of glucose. Symptomatic hypoglycemia usually occurs when plasma glucose levels fall below 55 mg./100 ml. (blood glucose levels less than 45 mg./100 ml.). Since hypoglycemia is not a disease but rather represents a perturbation of normal glucose homeostasis by diverse causes, the diagnosis and rational treatment of glucopenia require an understanding of the mechanisms of normal glucose regulation. These are detailed in Chapter 9 and are recapitulated briefly in the following sections.

GLUCOSE HOMEOSTASIS IN THE FED STATE

The diet of the average adult in the Western world consists of approximately 45% each of carbohydrate and fat and 10% protein. After food ingestion, a rise in the plasma glucose concentration occurs, which primarily reflects sugar that is absorbed from the intestinal tract. Of the 350 g. of carbohydrate eaten daily, 60% is starch, 30% is sucrose, and the remainder is milk lactose. Within the gut lumen and intestinal brush border, the complex carbohydrates are hydrolyzed to monosaccharides—glucose (80%), fructose (15%), and galactose (5%)—which, with the exception of fructose, subsequently are actively transported to the blood by a carrier-mediated system within intestinal cells. Similarly, protein and fat are cleaved enzymatically within the gut and transported as amino acids and mono- and diglycerides, respectively, by energy requiring carrier systems (41). The rates of gastrointestinal transit, digestion, and absorption of these various nutrients vary; thus plasma glucose is usually returned to preprandial levels within 2 to 3 hours after carbohydrate intake, whereas amino-acidemia and lipemia may persist for 8 hours.

During alimentation, a series of factors which promote secretion of insulin coincide with the passage and absorption of fuels (Ch. 9). Intracellular glucose is the major substrate causing the release of insulin by the pancreatic beta cell, although a number of amino acids, notably arginine, lysine, and leucine, act synergistically with glucose to stimulate insulin secretion (34). Furthermore, several ancillary hormonal factors, originating within the gastrointestinal mucosa, potentiate the insulin-secreting actions of glucose and amino acids. Gastrointestinal hormones, such as gastrin, pancreozymin-cholecystokinin, enteric glucagon-like substances ("gut glucagon"), and secretin, have been proposed as factors responsible for the greater insulin levels achieved when glucose is given orally as compared with the intravenous route. With the exception of "gut glucagon," each of these hormones has been shown to elicit a rapid and transitory increase in plasma insulin when given intravenously in pharmacologic amounts (34). Thus it has been postulated that a sequential cascade of these intestinal hormones, which act primarily to stimulate digestive processes, may operate secondarily to anticipate or facilitate the insulinogenic effects of glucose and amino acids. Nevertheless, for a number of reasons cited by Creutzfeldt (23), none of the known intestinal hormones fulfills all of the criteria for the hypothetical enteric insulinogenic hormone. Recently, Turner and colleagues (95) have isolated a factor from intestinal extracts which may be the enteric insulin secretogogue. The mechanism of the insulinogenic action of this enteric factor is not clear. It may enhance insulin release by augmenting pancreatic blood flow, through potentiation of glucose-mediated insulin secretion, or by exerting a direct effect on a readily accessible compartment of insulin within the beta cell. In addition, the increased cholinergic activity occurring during alimentation may enhance the secretion of insulin by direct vagal innervation of islet tissue. Consequently, following the ingestion of a mixed meal, a number of signals may contribute to the release of insulin, which has a predominant anabolic action on fuel utilization and storage (38).

In order to simulate the plasma glucose patterns occurring during the fed state, glucose (50–100 g.) is usually given orally after an overnight fast, and the alterations in plasma (or blood) glucose levels

TABLE 10–1. FACTORS INVOLVED IN GLUCOSE DISPOSITION AFTER ORAL CARBOHYDRATE

Ascent of Plasma Glucose
1. Gastric transit time and rate of intestinal absorption
2. Release of insulin [glucose and enteric factor(s)]
3. Inhibition of glucose efflux from liver
4. Distribution in glucose compartments

Zenith
    Outflow equals inflow

Descent of Plasma Glucose
1. Persistent glucose absorption
2. Decline in insulin release
3. Resumption of hepatic glucose efflux
4. Glucopenia with counter-regulation

are monitored for the ensuing 5 hours. Because glucose homeostasis may be disturbed postprandially, it is helpful to categorize the dynamic events contributing to the rise and decline in plasma glucose as described by Freinkel (38) (Table 10–1). The rising limb of the plasma sugar level coincides with the delivery of glucose from the gastrointestinal tract at a rate which is determined by gastric emptying and intestinal absorption. Glucose transit through the stomach is intermittent and is determined by the waves of gastric motility and pyloric relaxation, which are reflexly governed through complex neural and hormonal pathways mediated through [H$^+$] and osmotic receptors in the stomach and upper intestine. Normally, the stomach empties approximately one-third of a 750-ml. volume of 10% glucose within 30 minutes. When gastric emptying time is decreased by operative procedures, such as gastrectomy or pyloroplasty, glucose delivery to the intestine and thereafter to the blood will be accelerated. The increased glucose concentrations, abetted by one or more gastrointestinal factors, evoke insulin secretion, and elevated insulin levels are usually demonstrable in the peripheral blood within 20 minutes after carbohydrate ingestion (Fig. 10–1). The released insulin immediately decreases hepatic glucose output by inhibition of glycogenolysis and gluconeogenesis through mechanisms that probably involve a decline in intracellular concentrations of cyclic nucleotides (cAMP and cGMP) (15, 31). The liver, which is freely permeable to glucose, extracts approximately 50% of the carbohydrate load; this glucose is then phosphorylated through the action of glucokinase (type IV hexokinase). On the basis of studies in lower species, it appears that in man this reaction may be controlled by insulin. Most of the carbohydrate assimilated by the liver is converted to glycogen, catalyzed by a cascade of enzyme reactions, including glycogen synthetase, an enzyme regulated by insulin (Fig. 9–28). Consequently, in the fed state, the liver, in the presence of insulin, functions as an important organ for glucose storage.

Sugar, which is not sequestered in the liver, eventually is distributed within the extracellular space, accounting for the increasing plasma glucose levels. Hyperglycemia stimulates additional

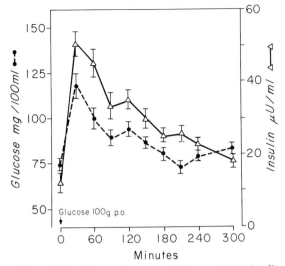

Figure 10–1. Plasma glucose and immunoreactive insulin levels in 16 healthy young men who ingested 100 gm. of glucose. (I = ± SEM.) (From Ensinck, J. W., Dudl, R. J., et al.: Unpublished.)

GLUCOSE HOMEOSTASIS IN THE FASTED STATE

In the postabsorptive phase, which gradually evolves within 3 to 4 hours after eating and eventually extends into protracted periods of fasting, glucose production is maintained at the expenditure of other fuel sources, as summarized by Cahill (16). In the normal 70-kg. man, caloric reserves reside in adipose tissue triglyceride (85%), muscle protein (15%), and muscle and liver glycogen (<1%). During fasting, glycogen is only a transient source of energy for emergent situations, and the body attempts to conserve protein for mechanical and catalytic processes within the cell; consequently, FFA are the major fuels used by most tissues. Throughout a 24-hour fast, a normal man who expends 1800 calories uses about 75 g. of protein and 160 g. of triglyceride to generate about 180 g. of glucose by means of glycogenolysis and hepatic gluconeogenesis (Fig. 10–2). Of the glucose formed, 70% is diverted to brain and the remainder to skeletal muscle and the cellular elements of the blood, peripheral nerves, and renal medullae, where it is utilized through glycolytic pathways. Free glucose is virtually confined to the extracellular compartments and the intracellular water of the liver, nervous system, and erythron, to which it is freely permeable (equivalent to 50% of body weight). In the average person, the glucose pool in the postabsorptive period approximates 10–20 g. at plasma glucose concentrations ranging from 50–70 mg./100 ml., and the glucose turnover approximates 180 g./day, 50% of which is oxidized to CO_2 and water.

When the glucose pool is abruptly depleted, the major source of replacement is from hepatic gly-

release of insulin, which operates to translocate extracellular glucose primarily into muscle and fat. In these tissues, insulin also enhances glucose oxidation, glycogen synthesis, potassium influx, amino acid transport, and protein synthesis (15). In addition, in man, insulin inhibits the release of amino acids from muscle, and in adipose cells, it restrains lipolysis and enhances lipogenesis. These anabolic effects are most readily demonstrated by a decrease in circulating FFA derived from triglyceride, associated with the ascending plasma sugar concentration due to continued absorption from the intestine. Under normal circumstances, the utilization of glucose by insulin-sensitive tissue increases in conjunction with the rising level of insulin. Most commonly, the plasma glucose peaks within 1 hour and seldom exceeds 160 mg./100 ml., which coincides with a transitory steady state; thereafter, the plasma sugar declines, reflecting both the enhanced utilization of glucose and its smaller supply from intestinal absorption. Although plasma sugar levels are most often displayed as smooth curves, more frequent analyses reveal a number of peaks with parallel fluctuations in insulin concentrations (Fig. 10–1). Nonetheless, a direct correlation between glucose and insulin concentrations has not been demonstrated, and the eventual return to preprandial levels of glucose, insulin, and FFA cannot be attributed solely to a nonregulated gradual diminution in insulin actions as a result of degradation of this hormone. Since no intrinsic hepatic mechanisms exist for automatic resumption of glucose production by the liver, a number of factors that counter-regulate the action of insulin, operating both on hepatic glucose output and on glucose uptake by peripheral tissues, prevent a continued drop in plasma sugar during the postabsorptive state (30).

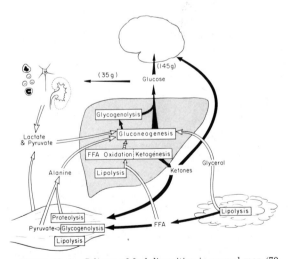

Figure 10–2. Scheme of fuel disposition in normal man (70 kg.), fasted for 24 hr. and consuming 1800 cal. Glucose directed primarily for cerebral consumption is released from hepatic glycogen, and new glucose is generated from precursors derived from fat, muscle, blood cells, nerve, and renal medullae. Free fatty acids (FFA) from triglyceride hydrolysis and ketones from hepatic ketogenesis are oxidized in muscle and brain as alternate energy sources.

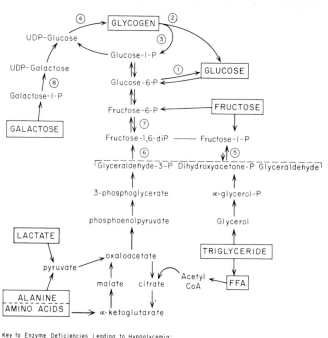

Figure 10–3. Pathways of gluconeogenesis, glycogenesis, and glycogenolysis within the liver.

Key to Enzyme Deficiencies Leading to Hypoglycemia:

1. Glucose-6-phosphatase
2. Amylo-1,6-glucosidase
3. Phosphorylase
4. Glycogen synthetase
5. Fructose-1-phosphate aldolase
6. Fructose-1,6-diphosphate aldolase
7. Fructose-1,6-diphosphatase
8. Galactose-1-phosphate uridyl transferase

cogen. Although 500 g. of carbohydrate is stored as this complex glucose polymer in both muscle and liver, only the latter (and to an insignificant extent the renal cortex) is capable of rapid conversion of glycogen to free glucose. The average hepatic glycogen content is 75 g. Through the mediation of a complex cascade of enzymatic reactions, glycogen is reduced to glucose-6-phosphate and then to free glucose by the action of glucose-6-phosphatase (Figs. 9–27 and 10–3). Under physiologic conditions, glycogenolysis in the liver is stimulated by glucagon and possibly catecholamines which activate phosphorylase (Fig. 9–28). In the immediate postabsorptive period, 75–85% of net glucose balance originates from glycogen, but usually by 24–48 hours, glycogen reserves are dissipated, and the glucose pool must be replenished by synthesis of glucose from other fuels.

The site of gluconeogenesis and sources of precursors depend upon the duration of caloric deprivation. Although the kidney assumes importance as a source of new glucose during protracted starvation, 90% of total gluconeogenesis occurs in the liver during brief fasting (16). Of the several gluconeogenic precursors in man, glycerol is only a minor contributor. Resynthesis of glucose from pyruvate and lactate represents a major route of disposal of lactate, and in sedentary man, 10–30% of glucose is recycled from lactate originating from glycolytic processes in blood cells and nervous tissue. However, with exercise, anaerobic glycolytic catabolism in muscle is increased, with enhanced production of lactate, which is used in gluconeogenesis.

Since neither glycerol nor lactate generation is adequate to meet the needs for gluconeogenesis, amino acids derived from proteolysis in muscle are the most important substrate. All amino acids except leucine are potential glucogenic precursors in man; however, alanine, synthesized from pyruvate, and, to a lesser extent, glutamine, have been shown by Felig (35) to be the preferential glucogenic amino acids utilized during the immediate postabsorptive period and during exercise (Ch. 9).

The sequence of major reactions by which substrates are converted to glucose and glycogen in the hepatic cell is shown schematically in Figures 9–28 and 10–3. The multiple factors regulating these complex processes have been reviewed extensively by Exton (31). In brief, they include (1) determinants influencing the provision of substrates, such as diet, fasting, obesity, and hormones; (2) substrate uptake by the liver. Among the potential gluconeogenic precursors, only amino acids are hormonally dependent with regard to hepatic influx. Splanchnic uptake of alanine and other glucogenic amino acids is diminished by insulin and increased by glucagon, cortisol, and growth hormone, by mechanisms as yet undefined; (3) mitochondrial metabolite transport, which is probably carrier-mediated and may be regulated by epinephrine, glucagon, and cortisol; (4) enzymatic control points as indicated in Figures 9–27 and 10–3. The unidirectional series of synthetic reactions leading to new glucose are catalyzed sequentially by enzymes which are complexly regulated. The diversion of the 3-carbon skeleton of pyruvate to oxaloacetate, which is ultimately synthesized to

GLUCOSE CONSUMPTION

(Brain)

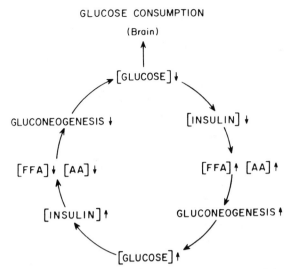

Figure 10-4. Cycle of glucose homeostasis in fasting. Substrates or hormones in brackets refer to plasma concentrations. (From Cahill, G. F., Jr.: *New Eng. J. Med.* 282:669, 1970.)

glucose, involves a number of reactions, one or more of which may be the major sites of regulation by cortisol, glucagon, and insulin. The high Km glucokinase is important in hepatic glucose release, because it provides adaptation to glucose levels perfusing liver and is decreased during starvation and insulin deprivation, ultimately increasing glucose efflux. Within the period extending from the postabsorptive phase through brief fasting, it is likely that the gradual decline in insulin and the rise in glucagon are the major determinants favoring augmented hepatic glycogenolysis and gluconeogenesis. In addition, the lowered insulin concentration leads to diminished glucose uptake in muscle and adipose tissue with concomitant increased lipolysis and proteolysis, thereby providing a flow of glucogenic precursors (Fig. 10-4).

After extended periods of food deprivation, there is a gradual fall in glucose output (about 90 g./day), with a simultaneous decline in protein catabolism manifested by a marked decrease in alanine levels. Associated with the increased contribution of the kidney to gluconeogenesis (sometimes as much as 50% of total glucose generated), there is an enhanced tubular secretion of ammonia, which neutralizes the excreted ketoacids (35).

Although it has long been recognized that fat is a major source of energy, it has been appreciated only recently that FFA are transported to and assimilated by a variety of tissues. In the immediate postprandial period in an environment of excess glucose, lipogenesis and re-esterification in fat cells are catalyzed by insulin, whereas in the postabsorptive phase and during protracted fasting, lipolysis is augmented as a function of the reduced availability of insulin and coincident increased activity of counter-regulatory hormones (30). After an overnight fast, plasma concentrations of FFA approximate 600 μEq./L. (15 mg./100 ml.), and

they have rapid half-lives (2–4 minutes). In the period extending from the immediate postabsorptive phase into early and late starvation, FFA influx into the plasma is doubled.

From studies in isolated systems and under pharmacologic conditions in man, it has been inferred that FFA may also be glucogenic precursors; yet it has not been proven that, physiologically, they are transmuted directly to glucose within the liver. Nonetheless, they have been shown to influence gluconeogenic processes indirectly through the provision of energy derived from carnitine-mediated oxidation within hepatic mitochondria. During the postabsorptive period, 40% of FFA (3 g./hr.) is taken up by the liver and (1) oxidized via acetyl CoA to ketoacids, (2) metabolized to CO_2 and water, or (3) re-esterified to form triglyceride which is stored within hepatic cells. Although ketoacids are minor metabolic fuels during the early postabsorptive state, in later stages of fasting, ketogenesis is doubled, and the ketoacids assume major importance as energy sources. These adaptive processes, whereby fat substitutes for glucose in muscle, are also applicable to the central nervous system. In the past, the brain was considered to have a chronic obligate requirement for glucose; now, ketoacids are recognized as the principal fuels utilized by the brain during protracted fasting and in the early neonatal period (16). Hence, during food deprivation, the adaptation of virtually all tissues to fat as energy sources, concurrent with restriction in gluconeogenesis, may be explained teleologically as a compensatory mechanism to minimize protein breakdown. Plasma glucose concentrations gradually decline by 20–30% within 3–4 days of fasting to 60–65 mg./100 ml., and this nadir is maintained for long periods (Fig. 10–5)

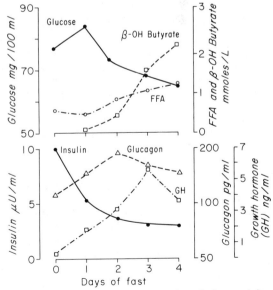

Days of fast

Figure 10-5. Alterations in key fuels and glucoregulatory hormones in man during fasting. Average values are reported in composite. (Modified from studies by Cahill, G. F., Jr., Herrera, M. G., et al.: *J. Clin. Invest.* 45:1751, 1966, and Aguilar-Parada, E., Eisentraut, A. M., et al.: *Diabetes* 18:717, 1969.)

(17). Coincident with the drop in blood glucose there is a fall in circulating insulin to 40–50% of basal level and activation of neuroendocrine systems which have a primary catabolic role.

HORMONES COUNTERACTING INSULIN

In order to protect the brain against abrupt diversion of glucose to subsidiary organs during insulin excess and to provide a mechanism for mobilization of alternative fuels during fasting, a complex neuroendcrine control system has been evolved which, for the most part, opposes the anabolic actions of insulin (25). Hormones exerting anti-insulin effects at physiologic levels include glucagon, catecholamines, growth hormone, and glucocorticoids (30). Several humoral and cellular factors which also impede insulin action have been described; however, since they have not been identified nor their physiologic roles ascertained, they will not be discussed.

Glucagon

Long neglected because of lack of identifiable disorders due to its deficiency or excess, pancreatic glucagon has now achieved recognition as a major factor in glucose homeostasis (97). As a result of the common embryonic origin of the gut and pancreas, substances with some of the immunochemical and biologic properties of glucagon occur in the mammalian intestinal tract ("gut glucagon"). Two species of "gut glucagon" with different physical and biologic properties have been described. The most prominent action of pancreatic glucagon (glucagon), and perhaps its major physiologic role, is to cause a rapid elevation in blood glucose through hepatic glycogenolytic and gluconeogenic pathways. In the isolated, perfused, rat liver preparation, glycogenolysis is both rapid in onset and transient with physiologic amounts of glucagon. Dramatic increases in hepatic glucose output also are demonstrable within seconds after small amounts of glucagon are infused into man (2 μg./min.). Normally, in the postprandial state, when hepatic glucose is augmented, an increase in glucagon secretion is coordinated with the decline in insulin output. To meet emergency fuel requirements during strenuous exercise and various clinical conditions of "stress," glucagon is also increased, thereby promoting glycogenolysis. Since hepatic cAMP levels are increased by glucagon and decreased by insulin, the mechanism of the rapid effects of these hormones on glycogen breakdown or storage is explained, at least in part, by the reciprocal actions on phosphorylase and glycogen synthetase activities (Fig. 9–28). At physiologic concentrations in rat liver preparations, glucagon also promptly stimulates gluconeogenesis, mediated through cAMP and possibly modulated by guanosine nucleotides. In contrast to the short duration of action on glycogenolysis, the gluco-

neogenic effects of glucagon *in vitro* persist for several hours. The mechanisms by which glucagon induces gluconeogenesis is still unsettled. It has been proposed that the increased cAMP levels activate a hepatic lipase, with liberation of FFA from triglyceride with partial oxidation to acetyl CoA, which in turn results in allosteric activation of pyruvate carboxylase and depression of pyruvate kinase and phosphofructokinase, thereby switching the setting from glycolysis to gluconeogenesis. An alternate hypothesis states that cAMP might alter the mitochondrial efflux of calcium with inhibition of pyruvic carboxylase (31).

Other hormones have been shown to modify the glycogenolytic and gluconeogenic actions of glucagon. Catecholamines augment these processes by acting on separate membrane receptors to perturb adenyl cyclase. However, relative to glucagon, the catecholamine-induced rise in cyclic nucleotides is less, and, at physiologic concentrations of epinephrine infused through the isolated rat liver or by portal vein in intact animals, hepatic glucose release is not altered. The dependence of glucagon-induced gluconeogenesis on glucocorticoids has been firmly established; adrenalectomy prevents the gluconeogenic response to glucagon, and treatment with glucocorticoids restores this activity. The term "permissive" has been used to describe the mechanisms by which adrenal steroids influence a variety of metabolic events (7). It has been proposed that a part of the function of steroids is to maintain normal sensitivity of these processes to cAMP, which may be mediated through alterations in levels of intracellular ions, such as calcium (31). Viewed physiologically, the balance between the effects of glucagon and insulin may be the most important factor influencing hepatic glucose output, and the bihormonal ratio, which is altered during feeding and fasting, has been cited as the crucial control for glucose release by the liver.

It is now clear that glucagon can promote insulin release when injected into man with amounts that are undetectable in the peripheral blood (80). Whether "gut glucagon" or pancreatic glucagon is of importance in the regulation of insulin secretion is unresolved. Because "gut glucagon" levels rise in plasma corresponding with increased insulin secretion after oral glucose, it has been suggested that "gut glucagon" is a betasecretogogue; yet recent reports, indicating a temporal discrepancy between levels of "gut glucagon" and insulin after oral hexose loading, do not support this notion. To what extent glucagon released locally within the islet plays a physiologic role in insulin secretion during nutrient absorption is conjectural. Glucagon release is inhibited by glucose; therefore, it seems unlikely to be a significant factor in insulin secretion after carbohydrate feeding. However, since glucagon secretion is increased by amino acids, it may exert an insulinotropic effect with ingestion of protein in a mixed meal.

When given in supraphysiologic doses *in vivo*, glucagon has several extrahepatic effects. In certain species, particularly avian, it is lipolytic both *in vitro* and *in vivo*. In man, after glucagon administration, there occur lower levels of amino acids, and elevations of plasma ketones and FFA, with negative nitrogen balance, which indicate that glucagon has catabolic effects on adipose tissue and muscle. Despite these pharmacologic actions, a physiologic role for glucagon as a lipolytic substance in man is equivocal. After 3 days of fasting, glucagon infusions (0.1 mg./min.) cause an immediate and sustained rise in plasma FFA; however, this has not been confirmed in protracted fasting. A direct effect of glucagon on skeletal muscle of man has not been substantiated, and unlike the adenyl cyclase system of cardiac muscle, skeletal muscle enzyme is insensitive to glucagon yet responds to catecholamines. Although amino acid precursors for gluconeogenesis are highest during early fasting, it is not certain if glucagon exerts a regulatory influence on peripheral proteolysis. In addition, with pharmacologic doses of glucagon, miscellaneous effects on a variety of systems have been observed, including changes in vascular tone, myocardial contractility, gastric secretion, enteric motility, thyroid and pituitary functions, sympathetic nervous activity, renal excretion of sodium, and calcium metabolism. All presumably reflect the action of glucagon on adenyl cyclase in the respective tissues. Nevertheless, since these systems have other primary controls, these diverse actions of glucagon are unlikely to be physiologically important, and the major site of action of glucagon would appear to be confined to the liver.

Factors regulating glucagon secretion have been only partly elucidated because of methodologic difficulties in differentiating pancreatic glucagon from "gut glucagon." The latter comprises up to 80% of circulating immunoreactive glucagon-like substances, and the two forms of "gut glucagon" are released into the blood from the intestinal mucosa during hexose absorption. Recently, by the use of more specific immunologic assay techniques, a number of stimuli and inhibitors of pancreatic glucagon secretion have been described, using as models *in vitro* pancreatic systems and subprimate species. Nevertheless, it is uncertain whether all exert physiologic control. Of the various factors so far studied in man, the most profound increases (five- to tenfold) in plasma glucagon levels are achieved by parenteral amino acids, notably arginine and alanine, or following the ingestion of protein. Consequently, it has been implied that circulating amino acids, specifically alanine, may be an important alpha cell stimulus, particularly during fasting. Glucagon secretion is also stimulated by hypoglycemia, as shown in Figure 10–6. Conversely, glucose has been shown to markedly suppress basal plasma glucagon levels. In men, glucagon levels in plasma gradually rise to a peak of 150% of basal by the third to fourth day of fasting. In contrast, women tend to have greater increases in plasma glucagon, associated with lower plasma glucose levels during fasting. By indirect studies in diabetic patients, Unger (97) has proposed that the alpha cell senses intracellular glucose concentration by an insulin-dependent mechanism, which determines the rate of release of glucagon. In addition, a role for the sympathetic nervous system in glucagon release has been postulated. In situations where catecholamine secretion is markedly augmented, such as in patients with pheochromocytoma, in severe exercise, infection, trauma, or in diabetic ketoacidosis, elevated glucagon levels have been found. Although Sokal (30) first suggested that the hyperglycemia following epinephrine was due to a catecholamine-induced release of glucagon, it has been difficult to demonstrate uniformly a direct glucagonotropic effect of catecholamines in isolated rat islets or by infusion in various species, including man. Under conditions where activation of the sympathetic nervous system occurs, such as in acute hypoglycemia and in protracted starvation, no consistent inhibition of hyperglucagonemia has been

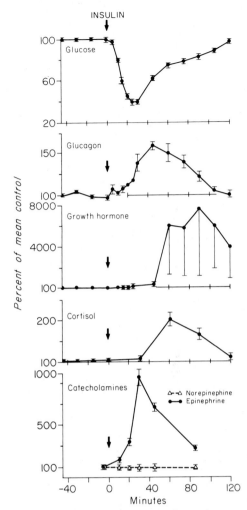

Figure 10–6. Changes in glucoregulatory hormones in healthy young men after administration of insulin (0.1 U./kg.). The results in five subjects are expressed as per cent of mean control because of intersubject variation. (I = ± SEM.) (From Walter, R. M., and Ensinck, J. W.: Unpublished.) For convenience, the data on catecholamine release have also been included. (From Vendsalu, A.: *Acta Physiol. Scand. 49*(Suppl. 173):1, 1960.)

shown by either alpha or beta adrenergic blockade, from which one may infer that the sympathetic nervous system is not a primary regulator of glucagon release in man. In the dog, pancreozymin and secretin have been reported to stimulate and inhibit glucagon release respectively; however, in man, secretin has no apparent effect. At present, it is uncertain which is the primary stimulus to the alpha cell during conditions of physiologic need. It is conceivable that during acute stress, such as hypoglycemia and exercise, glucagon is released as a consequence of intra-alpha cell glucopenia, whereas during fasting, multiple signals, including low blood glucose and elevated amino acids, act in conjunction to effect a sustained hypersecretion of glucagon to meet gluconeogenic requirements.

Catecholamines

Epinephrine and norepinephrine have major effects on fuel disposition by influencing glucose generation, lipolysis, and the release and action of insulin (Ch. 9). Hyperglycemia results from epinephrine infusion, which has been ascribed to the effects of this catecholamine on hepatic glycogenolysis and gluconeogenesis with decreased glucose utilization in muscle (46). Whether or not catecholamines have a direct effect on glucose output by the liver is controversial, since in isolated liver systems, epinephrine does not evoke glycogenolysis at levels achieved in the circulation of man during stress. As alluded to previously, the possibility that catecholamines directly stimulate glucagon release in subprimate species has been raised; however, this remains to be confirmed in man. Judging from studies in lower species, it is conceivable that activation of the splanchnic sympathetic nerves may also induce hepatic glycogenolysis in the human. At physiologic concentration of epinephrine, glycogen breakdown in muscle with resultant increased plasma lactate may be a source of precursors for gluconeogenesis. With supraphysiologic doses, epinephrine inhibits insulin-mediated glucose transport in muscle, possibly by blocking glucose phosphorylation; however, when epinephrine is infused into the human forearm at concentrations achieved during stress, glucose uptake is not diminished, despite increased blood flow and concurrent glycogenolysis. In addition, the prompt restoration to euglycemia following insulin-induced glucopenia in cortisol-treated, adrenalectomized patients suggests that epinephrine is not a significant determinant of this counter-regulatory response. However, activation of the sympathetic nervous system to secrete norepinephrine and thereby promote glycogenolysis cannot be discounted. A prominent physiologic effect of catecholamines on fuel metabolism relates to their role in enhancing lipolysis with provision of FFA and glycerol. An additional major indirect control on glucose homeostasis exerted by the sympathetic nervous system is through the regulation of insulin release. Both epinephrine and norepinephrine inhibit insulin secretion in man, despite concurrent hyperglycemia. With fasting, profound exercise, and orthostatic changes, norepinephrine secretion is enhanced, whereas following insulin-induced hypoglycemia, no alteration in plasma levels can be ascertained, which contrasts with the marked increases in circulating levels of epinephrine (Fig. 10–6). Since sympathetic nerve endings have been shown to ramify extensively around islets, it seems possible that norepinephrine released locally also modulates insulin secretion. Thus, during hypoglycemia and fasting, the combined effect of activation of the sympathetic nervous system is to decrease insulin release and enhance hepatic glucose output (30).

Growth Hormone

For many years, growth hormone (GH) has been recognized as integral to glucose homeostasis, yet despite its ability to modify the hypoglycemic action of insulin, a function for GH unique in the human adult has been elusive. GH serves an anabolic role in promoting protein synthesis; yet conversely, it exerts a catabolic or antianabolic effect on fat and carbohydrate metabolism (73). In animals, GH causes mineral and nitrogen retention reflected by increased amino acid uptake. From studies *in vitro* it has been concluded that GH stimulates protein synthesis which requires the presence of insulin. An effect of GH on carbohydrate tolerance in man is supported by a number of clinical observations, such as the high incidence of diabetes in acromegaly and the exacerbation of hyperglycemia by GH in hypophysectomized, diabetic patients (62). Nonetheless, in normal man, large parenteral doses of GH over long periods do not significantly perturb fasting blood sugar levels. This is explained by the hyperinsulinism produced in normal persons, which overcomes the diabetogenic actions of GH. This hormone profoundly influences human fat metabolism. After a delay of 30–120 minutes following GH administration, lipolysis is observed (30). Before lipolysis is manifest, GH increases FFA uptake and oxidation in skeletal muscle and impedes insulin-mediated glucose assimilation. The lipolytic activity of GH is potentiated by glucocorticoids, presumably by mechanisms different from those of catecholamines. These may involve an indirect modulation of cAMP activity, leading to induction of messenger RNA synthesis.

Disappearance rate of glucose, after its oral or parenteral administration, is diminished by supraphysiologic amounts of GH. Thus glucose utilization is impaired despite concurrent hyperinsulinism; yet, in acromegalic patients, FFA release is appropriately inhibited by insulin and glucose. These seemingly paradoxical responses of insulin and GH have been attributed to a dissociation of their actions on muscle and fat. The diminished responsiveness of muscle to insulin has been considered to be due to defective phosphorylation resulting from feedback inhibition by glycolytic intermediates derived from elevated FFA and ketoacids. Since GH does not have these anti-insulin effects when tested directly *in vitro*, it has been inferred that, in the liver, this hormone either is transformed into or induces the synthesis of an active product which has been equated with the "sulfation factor" (somatomedin). Recently, somatomedin has been postulated to be one of the three components constituting nonsuppressible insulin-like activity with anabolic properties similar to insulin. Moreover, Bornstein has shown that GH can be cleaved into components that have differential actions on tissues (73). In addition, GH may have an indirect influence on insulin secretion by potentiating the normal physiologic stimuli which modulate insulin release.

Extensive studies of factors regulating GH secretion in man have not added significantly to our understanding of the specific role of this hormone in fuel regulation. Plasma levels are extremely labile and fluctuate spontaneously. GH is most consistently released by onset of deep sleep; however, a relationship exists between levels of hormone and exercise, fasting, stress, and adipose mass, and its secretion is modulated by polypeptides originating in the hypothalamus termed "GH releasing factor" (GHRF) and "GH inhibitory factor" (73). Other hormones influence GH release, as indicated by increased plasma levels with elevation of thyroid hormones, estrogens, and testosterone, and low levels of GH when glucocorticoids and progestogens are excessive. GH secretion is also stimulated by amino acids. After a meal containing carbohydrate and protein, plasma levels of insulin, glucagon, and GH all rise, from which it has been inferred that insulin and GH direct amino acids to protein, while GH and glucagon oppose insulin action on glucose disposal.

A major factor controlling GH secretion is the plasma glucose level, presumably monitored by the hypothalamus. GH release is accentuated by hypoglycemia (Fig. 10–6), whereas hyperglycemia tends to inhibit its secretion except during sleep. Four to six hours after glucose ingestion, GH levels increase, coinciding with a secondary rise in plasma FFA. This may be due to a decline in plasma glucose and activation of the sympathetic nervous system. It is not certain whether GH is involved as an anti-insulin substance in acute regulation of glucose. In fasted man, individual levels of GH are variable and do not correlate with circulating fuels. However, in ateliotic dwarfs lacking GH, profound falls in plasma sugar with high levels of FFA and ketoacids have been observed, attesting to a glucoregulatory role for GH in the fasting state. It has also been suggested that the FFA levels elevated during fasting tend, in turn, to inhibit GH release.

Glucocorticoids

Glucocorticoids, represented mainly by cortisol, have diverse effects on fuel metabolism which, in general, are opposite to those of insulin and tend to elevate plasma sugar concentrations (10). Thus chronic excessive glucocorticoid levels increase total body carbohydrate, and fasting plasma glucose concentrations are frequently elevated, associated with impaired glucose tolerance. Conversely, adrenalectomized animals have decreased glycogen in liver and muscle; therefore, the hypoglycemia in patients with Addison's disease induced by fasting, and the attenuated posthypoglycemia rebound after insulin are due to decreased hepatic sugar output with augmented peripheral glucose uptake (25). Impairment of peripheral glucose utilization with chronic steroid administration has not been confirmed in man; however, insulin sensitivity has been found in isolated muscle from adrenalectomized animals. This is reversed by corticosterone treatment, and a block in glucose phosphorylation in muscle has been proposed as a site of steroid action. That glucocorticoids have catabolic effects on fat and muscle is well documented. They inhibit glucose utilization and esterification in adipose tissue, and, after a time lag, lipolysis is enhanced. Because their lipolytic action differs from that of catecholamines and glucagon, it has been proposed that glucosteroids exert an indirect effect, possibly by modification of cAMP metabolism through induction of protein synthesis. In addition, chronic steroid excess eventuates in augmented protein catabolism with increased amino acid levels and urinary nitrogen excretion. After adrenalectomy, the main effects on muscle and fat are the depletion of glycogen stores and of amino acids and products of lipolysis. Thus glucocorticoids influence predominantly the pathways leading to glucose formation by mechanisms which are uncertain and designated as "permissive," since they permit other hormones to produce normal responses (7). Within a few hours after steroid administration, free amino acids and RNA activity within the liver are increased. Glucocorticoid treatment is associated with activation of glycogen synthetase by glucose-6-phosphate and pyruvate carboxylase by acetyl CoA accompanied by saturation of gluconeogenic enzymes by precursors and indirect inhibition of glycolysis by FFA, resulting in increased glycogenesis (31). Adaptation to chronic steroid administration is reflected by *de novo* formation of gluconeogenic enzymes, presumably through actions on nuclear DNA-dependent RNA synthesis. Therefore, a lack of steroids eventually results in deficient gluconeogenesis.

Regulation of glucocorticoid secretion occurs through the hypothalamic-hypophysial axis, which is detailed in Chapters 5 and 12. Cortisol release is enhanced with the stress of hypoglycemia (Fig. 10–6) but probably does not play an acute role in glucose rebound and is unlikely to contribute to the moment-to-moment control of glucose levels. In summary, it appears that, through adaptive mechanisms in gluconeogenesis, glucocorticoids play primarily a "permissive" role in glucose homeostasis.

Thyroid and Gonadal Hormones

That thyroid hormones influence fuel regulation is indicated by the general hypercatabolic state associated with thyroid excess in man. They cause increased oxygen consumption, glucose oxidation, glycogen depletion, gluconeogenesis, ketogenesis, lipolysis, and proteolysis (92). Thyroid hormones markedly potentiate the catabolic activities of catecholamines, lower plasma glucose levels, and impede glucose disposal (25). Since thyroid hormones have long biologic half-lives and are not altered acutely, they are not involved in moment-to-moment regulation of plasma glucose.

Estrogens and progestogens increase plasma sugar levels in humans, and elevated insulin levels have been reported (90). It is uncertain, however, whether the gonadal hormones have a direct effect on the beta cell or act indirectly by induction of peripheral insulin resistance, leading to compensatory insulin release. Recently, it has been proposed that the insulin resistance is the consequence of estrogen-enhanced secretion of GH. In most instances, glucose homeostasis is not altered consistently throughout the menstrual cycle or after gonadal failure. Hyperglycemia may occur under conditions of excessive circulating gonadal hormones (oral contraceptives and pregnancy); however, neither estrogens nor progestogens would seem to play a primary glucoregulatory role under normal circumstances. During pregnancy, plasma sugar levels are ordinarily increased, with concurrent hyperinsulinism which is presumed to reflect the actions of chorionic somatomammotropin (placental lactogen) released into the maternal circulation in large amounts in the last trimester (53). This placental hormone is without apparent feedback regulation and resembles GH in its several anabolic, catabolic, and immunologic properties.

Summary of Actions of Anti-Insulin Hormones

In Table 10–2 the major actions of hormones which oppose insulin and tend to replenish the glucose pool during fasting and hypoglycemia are summarized. In general, they do so by (1) augmentation of hepatic glucose output through glycogenolysis and gluconeogenesis, (2) hindrance of glucose uptake in insulin-sensitive tissues, (3) provision of glucogenic precursors, (4) inhibition of insulin release, and (5) mobilization of alternative fuel sources.

THE NERVOUS SYSTEM IN FUEL HOMEOSTASIS

Because the brain relies primarily on glucose for its energy, particularly during the early postabsorptive phases of fasting, an autonomic nervous system is necessary to enable analysis of circulating glucose levels and rapid transmission of signals to the periphery for the mobilization of appropriate hormones and substrates (30). Although not established in man, evidence in lower species favors the inclusion of the limbic system and hypothalamus as the "visceral brain" which regulates autonomic neural responses. The mechanisms whereby the brain monitors the flow of fuels involve (1) the sympathetic nervous fibers ramifying in vascular walls and around parenchymal cells of adipose tissue, muscle, liver, pancreatic islets, and adrenal medulla; (2) parasympathetic innervation of the pancreas; and (3) a portal system serving as a conduit for transmission of specific peptide releasing and inhibitory factors, which modulate the secretion of hypophysial polypeptide hormones.

Based upon studies in several lower species, the ventromedial (VMH) and lateral hypothalamic (LH) nuclei have been postulated as mutually interacting centers in the neural regulation of carbohydrate and lipid metabolism (8). In the cat, there is a reciprocal relationship between the VMH (satiety center) and LH (hunger center). It is thought that substrate-sensitive receptors in these areas modulate the signals to the periphery. Thus, in the cat, LH units increase and VMH units decrease firing rates during food deprivation or insulin injection, with converse results during glucose infusions or eating. In the rat and rabbit, stimulation of the VMH is followed by hyperglycemia, which is considered to be due to sympathetic activation with concomitant hyperglucagonemia. There is mounting evidence in favor of glucoreceptors, which "sense" intracellular glucose levels in both VMH and LH with reciprocal firing of the sympathetic and parasympathetic nervous systems during fasting and feeding. In man, stimulation of the adrenergic system relates to the rate of decline and degree of reduction of blood glucose attained during hypoglycemia (Fig. 10–6). By extrapolation,

TABLE 10–2. PROBABLE PHYSIOLOGIC ACTIONS OF INSULIN-COUNTERACTING HORMONES IN NORMAL MAN

	Insulin Release	Muscle Glucose Uptake	Hepatic Glucogenesis	Lipolysis	Proteolysis
Catecholamines	↓	↓	↑	↑	↑
Glucagon	—	—	↑	—	—
Growth hormone	—	↓	—	↑	—
Glucocorticoids	—	↓	↑	↑	↓ ↑

↑ = Increase; ↓ = decrease; — = no significant primary effect.

centers sensitive to high and low concentrations of glucose probably exist in the human "visceral brain," and it is likely that cells within the hypothalamic ventromedial nucleus monitor plasma glucose levels and, through tonic activity of the autonomic nervous system, exert a control on fuel mobilization. Indirect evidence in lower mammals also favors the suggestion by Mayer (8) that cells in this region may be dependent upon insulin for glucose transport. In addition, there is a circadian periodicity in hormonal release, as well as substrate mobilization and utilization, which presumably reflects cyclic activity of the nervous system. Thus, in briefly fasted humans, plasma glucose and insulin levels peak in the early morning hours and reach an ebb in the late afternoon, whereas the converse temporal relationships apply to FFA and amino acids. Cortisol, which is intermittently released from the adrenal cortex throughout the day, reaches a maximum level between 4 and 8 A.M., correlating with increased ACTH secretion. In contrast, GH concentrations are highest with the onset of deep sleep. Since the polypeptide hormones from the pituitary are regulated by hypothalamic factors, their periodicity is probably governed by the "visceral brain." It seems likely, therefore, that superimposed upon the stimuli evoked by feeding or fasting, the rhythmic waxing and waning of the autonomic nervous system regulates substrate flow and hormonal release, which act conjointly to control plasma glucose levels.

CLINICAL AND PATHOLOGIC FEATURES OF HYPOGLYCEMIA

Since glucose is the major energy source for the brain and cerebral cells have limited stores of glycogen, circulating glucose is the reservoir for this substrate. Most of the intracellular glucose enters an amino acid pool, and the remainder (30%) is oxidized to CO_2 and water by glycolytic processes. In general, glucose oxidation correlates closely with cerebral oxygen uptake; however, the brain tolerates anoxia for only short periods, while glucose deprivation is associated with longer survival, presumably because the brain metabolizes additional substrates derived from amino acid pools, glycogen, ketoacids, and protein. Cerebral impairment may also reflect the decline in energy-rich phosphorylated compounds, such as ATP, because of diminished glucose oxidation. Recent studies in the rabbit suggest differences between hypoglycemia and anoxia in that glucopenia is associated with increased intracellular electrolytes (Na^+, K^+) and edema, which are not found in hypoxic states (5). The degree to which a given area of the brain is affected by glucopenia depends upon the order of its phylogenetic evolution. Thus, in descending order, the areas with the greatest glucose dependence and oxygen consumption are the neocortex and the various anatomic areas of the primitive brain which regulate cardiorespiratory activities (Table 10–3) (47). It is to be emphasized that cerebral dysfunction is related to intracellular glucopenia rather than extracellular hypoglycemia. Although the neuroglucopenic effects and the plasma sugar level are generally well-correlated, occasionally there is a discrepancy between them. In contrast to muscle or fat, glucose extraction by the cerebral cortex is relatively constant, and, therefore, uptake does not correlate with plasma glucose concentration. The manifestations of hypoglycemia are usually not apparent until the plasma glucose has fallen below 55 mg./100 ml. (blood glucose of 45 mg./100 ml.). Since the clinical features of hypoglycemia simulate those of hypoxia, symptoms may occur at higher plasma sugar levels in patients with compromised cerebral circulation, exemplified by atherosclerosis in the elderly. Hence, it is to be stressed that no absolute correlation exists between symptomatology and level of circulating glucose.

Although the clinical manifestations of neuroglucopenia may be protean, two distinct clinical patterns predominate, depending upon (1) the rate of fall in plasma glucose, and (2) the level of plasma sugar attained and duration of hypoglycemia (82). With a rapid fall in circulating glucose, as seen after acute insulin injections, the constellations of symptoms include faintness, weakness, tremu-

TABLE 10–3. SYMPTOMS AND SIGNS OF DIFFERENT PHASES OF HYPOGLYCEMIA*

Phases	A-V O_2 Diff.	Symptoms and Signs
Cortical	6.8	Somnolence, perspiration, hypotonia, tremor.
Subcortico-diencephalic		Loss of consciousness; primitive movements (sucking, grasping, grimacing), twitches, restlessness, clonic spasms, hyper-responsiveness to pain, sympathicotonia (tachycardia, erythema, perspiration, mydriasis).
Mesencephalic	2.6	Tonic spasms, inconjugate ocular deviation, Babinski sign.
Premyencephalic		Extensor spasms. Rotation of head causes extensor spasm of extremities on the side toward which the chin points and flexor spasm on the opposite side.
Myencephalic	1.8	Deep coma, shallow respiration, bradycardia, miosis, no pupillary reaction to light, hypothermia, atonia, hyporeflexia, absent corneal reflex.

*After Himwich, H. E.: *Brain Metabolism and Cerebral Disorders.* Baltimore, Waverly Press, 1951.

lousness, nervousness, anxiety, hunger, palpitation, tachycardia, and diaphoresis. This symptom complex is attributable to activation of the sympathetic nervous system, resulting in augmented hepatic glycogenolysis and inhibition of insulin release. Cerebral manifestations of abrupt hypoglycemia may also consist of headache, blurred vision, diplopia, lethargy, confusion, inappropriate affect, and motor incoordination. If counter-regulatory mechanisms fail and the plasma sugar falls to persistently low levels, more primitive parts of the brain are depressed. A wide array of neurologic and psychiatric disorders may be mimicked, including losses of sensory and motor function with paralysis and bizarre behavior patterns. With protracted hypoglycemia, neurologic dysfunction may progress to coma and death from failure of the medullary centers controlling cardiorespiratory function. Although the clinical presentation of hypoglycemia may vary from individual to individual, the sequential manifestations and patterns of recurrence tend to be repetitive in any one person. Unless glucose levels have been persistently low, resulting in cell death, restoration to euglycemia usually reverses the symptoms and signs of hypoglycemia. Depending upon the duration and degree of glucopenia, recovery may be immediate or prolonged over days. Irreversible damage to neural cells may permanently impair mental function, personality, and peripheral motor and sensory nerve function. Fever (38-39° C) may occur, attributable to cerebral edema. The evolution from coma to death may range from minutes to months. Both electroencephalographic and histologic changes from severe neuroglucopenia resemble those of anoxia. Beta and delta waves replace the dominant alpha waves; these changes may be permanent with severe injury. In patients who die from hypoglycemia, the brain shows spotty ischemic necrosis, which is most marked in the cerebral cortex, basal ganglia, hippocampus, and vasomotor centers. Acute alterations include scattered petechiae, congestion, and nerve swelling (Fig. 10–7), with ultimate loss of cells with glial reaction and demyelination (47). Most of the damage due to hypoglycemia occurs in the brain, but peripheral nerve degeneration is sometimes encountered.

The wide spectrum of clinical manifestations of hypoglycemia may be mimicked by a diversity of other disorders. The most common are psychiatric and neurologic syndromes in which vasomotor and behavioral disturbances predominate. Patients with hypoglycemia are frequently misdiagnosed as being neurotic or as having nonmetabolic organic brain syndromes. Psychotic behavior and dementia due to chronic hypoglycemia may be difficult to differentiate from other causes. Among the neurologic diseases, various types of epilepsy, particularly in children, must be ruled out. Patients with ischemic vascular disease involving the brain or heart may have complaints which are difficult to distinguish from those of hypoglycemia and, correspondingly, are at greater risk for infarction if hypoglycemia should occur. Intoxication from amphetamines, ethanol, barbiturates, or other drugs may simulate the catecholamine actions and cerebral depressive phases of neuroglucopenia (37, 82).

Conversely, the public has been led to believe that hypoglycemia is a widespread and unrecognized condition manifested as depression, chronic fatigue, allergies, nervous breakdown, alcoholism, juvenile delinquency, childhood behavior problems, drug addiction, and inadequate sexual performance. These concerns have no valid support. After appropriate examination and tests necessary to exclude other diseases, the patients should be reassured that hypoglycemia does not underlie their symptoms.

CLASSIFICATION OF DISORDERS CAUSING HYPOGLYCEMIA

Since a low plasma sugar level by itself does not provide a diagnosis, appropriate treatment requires establishment of the etiology of the hypoglycemia. A number of categories have been proposed on the basis of physiologic mechanisms, organic systems involved, and clinical presentations [Conn and Seltzer (20), Marks and Rose (64)]. Each of these classifications has some merit; however, we favor the categorization outlined in Table 10–4, in which spontaneous hypoglycemia is classified by causes related to fed and fasting states and those due to pharmacologic and toxic agents. This format has the advantage of relative simplicity based upon known mechanisms of fuel regulation and thereby facilitates a logical approach to diagnosis and treatment.

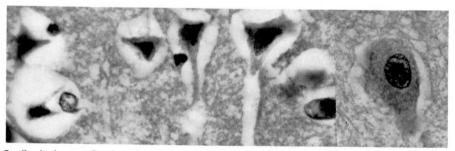

Figure 10–7.   Cerebral cortex. Cytodegenerative changes in neurons resulting from severe hypoglycemia; shrunken neurons with pyknotic nuclei and enlarged perineuronal spaces. Inset shows normal neuron. (Hematoxylin and eosin, × 640.) (Modified from Williams, R. H. (ed.): *Diabetes.* New York, Paul B. Hoeber, Inc., 1960.)

TABLE 10-4. CLASSIFICATION OF
CAUSES OF HYPOGLYCEMIA

I. Spontaneous Hypoglycemia
  A. "Reactive" (postabsorptive) hypoglycemia
    1. Induced by glucose
      a. Early phase
        (1) Postgastric surgery
        (2) Functional (essential, idiopathic)
      b. Late phase
        (1) Diabetes mellitus (chemical stage)
      c. Variable
        (1) Pancreatic beta cell tumor
    2. Induced by galactose (galactosemia)
    3. Induced by fructose (hereditary fructose intolerance)
    4. Induced by leucine (leucine hypersensitivity; branched-
       chain ketonuria)
  B. Fasting hypoglycemia
    1. Deficient glucose production
      a. Hepatic dysfunction
        (1) Inborn errors of glucogenesis
          (a) Glycogen storage disease (glycogenosis)
          (b) Deficient gluconeogenesis (ketotic hypogly-
              cemia)
        (2) Acquired liver disease
          (a) Inflammation, infarction, neoplasia
      b. Endocrine organ hypofunction
        (a) Deficiency of glucocorticoids, glucagon, and
            catecholamines
      c. Extrapancreatic neoplasms (mesotheliomas and car-
         cinomas)
    2. Overutilization of glucose
      a. Pancreatic beta cell hyperfunction (insulinoma)
      b. Growth hormone deficiency
      c. Neonatal hypoglycemia (diabetic mothers)
      d. Erythroblastosis fetalis
      e. Idiopathic hypoglycemia of childhood
      f. Miscellaneous
II. Pharmacogenic and Toxic Causes of Hypoglycemia
  A. Exogenous insulin administration (factitious, iatrogenic)
  B. Sulfonylureas
  C. Ethanol
  D. Miscellaneous compounds

DIAGNOSTIC APPROACHES IN THE EVALUATION OF HYPOGLYCEMIA

Although the astute clinician may frequently suspect the presence of hypoglycemia from the history and occasional appearance of a unique constellation of physical signs in an infant or adult, frequently the symptoms are subtle and intermittent and attributed to psychosomatic disorders. Hypoglycemia is documented when plasma glucose is below 55 mg./100 ml. (true blood glucose below 45 mg./100 ml.). In such an instance, the following questions should be asked: (1) Is the patient taking parenteral or oral medications which might cause hypoglycemia? (2) Does hypoglycemia occur only within the immediate postabsorptive period (within 5 hours of eating)? (3) Is hypoglycemia manifested during periods of fasting (in excess of 6 hours postprandially)? Plasma sugar levels obtained sporadically when the patient has symptoms suggesting neuroglucopenia may often be within normal limits or elevated because of counter-regulation. Therefore, a systematic approach to the work-up of a patient will depend upon the relationship of the symptom-complex to the fed and fasted state.

Since dietary restrictions may alter the secretory reserve of endocrine organs involved in glu-

cose homeostasis, in order to allow meaningful interpretation of tests, the adult patient should ingest 300 g. of carbohydrate daily for a minimum of 3 days before testing (Ch. 9).

Evaluation of Fasting Blood Sugar in Response to Oral and Intravenous Glucose

Food is restricted after 6 P.M. the preceding night, and a venous sample for plasma or blood sugar is obtained at 9 A.M. Values for fasting plasma sugar in excess of 60 mg./100 ml. usually exclude intrinsic disorders involving glycogenolysis and gluconeogenesis; however, 20% of insulin-producing tumors may not lower the plasma sugar concentration to hypoglycemic ranges.

Oral Glucose Tolerance Test (OGTT). After an overnight fast, the patient ingests within 5 minutes 100 g. (60 g./square meter body surface) of a standardized glucose solution (e.g., Glucola), and plasma is sampled at 0, 30, 60, 90, 120, 180, 240, and 300 minutes after glucose intake. In addition, plasma specimens should be obtained when the patient reports symptoms. This test is indispensable in the differentiation of the causes of the postabsorptive or "reactive" hypoglycemias.

Intravenous Glucose Tolerance Test (IVGTT). Occasionally, in patients with hypoglycemia occurring during an OGTT, it may be helpful to assess both the plasma sugar and insulin responses to glucose by a route independent of its rate of absorption from the gut. Glucose, 0.5 g./kg. body weight, is injected within 1 minute, and plasma sugar loads are obtained beforehand and at 10-minute intervals for 60 minutes afterwards and the log rate of disappearance of glucose (Kg) calculated. In contrast to patients with diabetes mellitus, normal values for Kg are found in individuals with early-phase "reactive" hypoglycemia.

Provocative Tests For Insulin Hypersecretion. In patients with hypoglycemia due to abnormal patterns of insulin secretion, the following tests have been devised to accentuate the release of insulin from the abnormal beta cell. (1) *Intravenous tolbutamide test.* After an overnight fast, tolbutamide (1 g.) is infused within 30 seconds, and plasma is obtained for glucose and insulin levels at 0, 2, 5, 15, 30, 45, 60, 90, 120, 150, and 180 minutes. It is to be emphasized that in normal individuals the peak level of insulin occurs within 5 minutes, whereas the nadir for plasma glucose is within 15–30 minutes and is normally 50% of basal level. There is usually a gradual return to original levels by 90 to 120 minutes. In contrast, profound and protracted hypoglycemia associated with an inordinate release of insulin may occur after tolbutamide administration in patients with hyperfunctioning islet tissue, and parenteral glucose should be given to abort a severe reaction (36). An exaggerated insulin response is also found in patients with obesity, acromegaly, Cushing's syndrome, and after anabolic steroid treatment; however, pronounced hypoglycemia is not found in these clinical states of insulin resistance. (2) *Intravenous glucagon test.* After an overnight fast, glucagon (1 mg.) is infused within 30 seconds (or injected i.m.) and samples obtained for glucose and insulin at 0, 2, 5, 10, 15, 30, 45, 60, 90, and 120 minutes. As glucagon promotes acute insulin release and hepatic glycogenolysis, it has a twofold advantage in assessing patients with hypoglycemia. If excessive insulin responses are found within the first few minutes after parenteral glucagon, islet cell hyperfunction is probable (56). In contrast, blunted glucose responses with normal insulin rises implicate hepatic or other endocrine organ dysfunction in the genesis of the hypoglycemia.

Oral Leucine Test. L-leucine (200 mg./kg. body weight) in tomato juice is given by mouth and plasma concentrations of glucose and insulin measured beforehand and at 10-minute intervals for 1 hour. Leucine stimulates an acute and marked release of insulin in children with symptomatic hypoglycemia due to leucine hypersensitivity and in 70% of patients with insulin-producing tumors. Between 30 and 45 minutes after intake of leucine, a plasma sugar value below 50 mg./100 ml. is suggestive of one of these disorders (36, 70).

Prolonged Fast. In order to test the integrity of regulation of glucogenesis during fasting as well as the possibility of sporadic hypersecretion of insulin, subjects may be fasted up to 72 hours, with periodic moderate exercise. Plasma samples for glucose and insulin are obtained at 6-hour intervals or when the patient has symptoms suggesting hypoglycemia. Close monitoring of the patients within a hospital environment is imperative. Symptoms of neuroglucopenia coupled with plasma glucose levels below 50 mg./100 ml. are strongly suggestive of an organic cause of hypoglycemia. An inappropriately elevated plasma insulin level in the presence of fasting hypoglycemia is virtually diagnostic of islet cell hyperfunction.

Insulin Tolerance Test. In order to determine whether fasting hypoglycemia might be the consequence of a deficiency of GH or a failure in the hypothalamic-pituitary adrenal axis, glucopenia is induced by insulin (0.1 U./kg. body weight), with plasma samples taken beforehand and at intervals of 10 minutes for 2 hours, with analyses of glucose, GH, and cortisol (Fig. 10–6). In patients with spontaneous hypoglycemia who may have impaired glucogenesis, this test is potentially hazardous, particularly in the elderly with advanced atherosclerosis. Therefore, it should be used with caution and may be supplanted by other stimuli of the hypothalamic-pituitary axis, such as glucagon, arginine, metyrapone, vasopressin, or specific pituitary releasing factors (Ch. 2).

Measurement of Plasma Insulin and Proinsulin Levels. The measurement of insulin concentrations in plasma is of great value in discriminating states of insulin hypersecretion from other causes of hypoglycemia and is universally available through commercial laboratories. As previously indicated, a number of values should be obtained at short intervals after specific provocative tests and during protracted periods of fasting. In contrast, insulin levels are virtually of no assistance in the diagnosis of "reactive" hypoglycemia and are mainly obtained to exclude insulin-producing tumors. Recently, proinsulin has been shown to be markedly increased in patients with insulinomas and may prove to be the most sensitive technique for distinguishing hyperfunctioning pancreatic tumors. However, the currently available methods for measurement of proinsulin are cumbersome and restricted to research laboratories.

Circulating Insulin Antibodies. In a patient in whom hypoglycemia is suspected to be self-induced, the detection of titers of insulin antibody in the plasma will justify more intensive efforts to ascertain whether insulin has been administered surreptitiously.

SPONTANEOUS DISORDERS CAUSING HYPOGLYCEMIA

"Reactive" (Postabsorptive) Hypoglycemia

Most causes of hypoglycemia are directly related to food ingestion, with symptoms appearing at varying intervals within 5 hours postprandially. The "reactive" hypoglycemias reflect disorders evoked by one or more of the dietary constituents and can be classified on the basis of their induction by (1) glucose, (2) galactose, (3) fructose, and (4) leucine. In general, the glucopenic syndromes induced by galactose, fructose, and leucine are genetically transmitted and first appear in infancy and childhood, whereas those caused by glucose occur most frequently in adults. With the exception of those with pancreatic beta cell tumors, patients with glucose-induced "reactive" hypoglycemias are characterized by normal fasting plasma glucose levels, and within 5 hours after food intake, they sustain an abrupt decline in circulating glucose followed by a rapid rebound. The hypoglycemia pattern is determined by the rate of plasma sugar ascent and the level and duration of the plasma sugar zenith. The symptoms coinciding with the rapid fall in plasma sugar are primarily those of hyperepinephrinemia, and they usually subside within 15–20 minutes. Although disorientation may occur, loss of consciousness and convulsions are rare. The glucose-induced hypoglycemias are usually attributed to one or more of the following defects: (1) hypersecretion of insulin, (2) hypersensitivity of peripheral tissues to insulin, or (3) deficiency of counter-regulatory mechanisms (2). Following an OGTT, these syndromes can be recognized from the configuration of the plasma glucose profile and the temporal onset of hypoglycemia (38). From patterns of glucose and insulin responses, segregation into early- and late-onset hypoglycemias has provided partial insight into their etiology and has been of particular help in distinguishing some of the disorders previously classified as functional or idiopathic (55). In general, however, the diagnosis can be established from the postabsorptive glucose profile alone, and measurements of insulin levels or provocative tests are not necessary.

Hypoglycemia Induced by Glucose

Early-Phase "Reactive" Hypoglycemia

Postgastric Surgery. In 5–10% of patients who have undergone gastrointestinal surgery (partial or total gastrectomy, gastrojejunostomy, or pyloroplasty, with or without vagotomy), symptomatic hypoglycemia occurs from 90–180 minutes after meals. Symptoms vary from a vague feeling of uneasiness to marked manifestations of hyperepinephrinemia. Characteristically, these patients have a rapid ascending limb of plasma glucose, achieving a peak usually exceeding 200 mg./100 ml., followed by an abrupt descent to hypoglycemia. Exaggerated insulin responses are usually, but not invariably, demonstrated (Fig. 10–8). Since the Kg following intravenous glucose and insulin release after provocative tests are normal, it has been postulated that the elevated insulin responses after oral glucose are appropriate to the level of blood sugar attained. The rapid ascent and high blood glucose levels have been attributed to the increased delivery of hypertonic glucose into the small bowel as a consequence of the elimination of the gastric reservoir or impaired pyloric sphincter ("tachyalimentation"). It is conjectural whether there is also an increase in activity of the enteric insulinotropic factors in such patients. Although "gut glucagon" has been found to rise inordinately after oral glucose in gastrectomized patients, it is unlikely to be responsible for the excessive insulin secretion for reasons previously

cited. Since gastrectomized patients have higher plasma sugar and lower insulin levels than do individuals after pyloroplasty, Breuer (14) has proposed that the gastric antrum provides a signal, possibly mediated through secretin, which acts synergistically with glucose to stimulate insulin secretion. It is inferred that the combined effects of the hyperglycemia and enteric insulinotropic activity induce hyper-responsivity of the beta cell, with exaggerated insulin release leading to glucopenia (88).

The clinical presentation of "tachyalimentary" hypoglycemia should be distinguished from that of the "dumping" syndrome found in patients after surgical procedures which increase gastric emptying. The "dumping" syndrome usually occurs within 60 minutes after food ingestion and is associated with epigastric discomfort, fullness, nausea, weakness, and palpitations. These symptoms have been ascribed to distention of the jejunum, due to a rapid increase in osmolality within the jejunal lumen, resulting in enhanced transfer of fluids from the blood into the gut. Vasoactive factors, such as serotonin and kininlike activities, have also been implicated in the hyperperistalsis and in the vasomotor hyperactivity that are characteristic of this disorder. Rarely, both the "dumping" syndrome and the later manifestations of hypoglycemia may occur in the same patient.

Early "reactive" hypoglycemia with a nadir of blood sugar around 3 hours also occurs in 20–60% of patients with peptic ulcers in whom insulin levels tend to be elevated (101). It is conceivable that the hyperinsulinemia is due to enhanced gastric motility and accelerated glucose absorption in these tense, apprehensive patients with an ulcer diathesis. It is also possible that increased gastric acidity may stimulate excessive secretion of secretin, which augments the glucose-induced release of insulin. In most patients, the hypoglycemia abates with the healing of the peptic ulcer. During the acute phases of the ulcer disease, in which symptomatic hypoglycemia is also a feature, restriction of dietary carbohydrate is recommended in conjunction with frequent anticholinergic and antacid therapy.

Functional (Vagotonic) Hypoglycemia. A low plasma sugar level 2–4 hours after food intake in apparently healthy young adults without previous gastric surgery or history of diabetes mellitus is the most common hypoglycemic syndrome (70%) (20, 55). These individuals tend to be of thin habitus, emotionally unstable, tense, anxious, and compulsive in personality. Somatic manifestations of a hyperactive autonomic nervous system are reflected by gastric hypermotility, excessive gastric acid, nausea, vomiting, and an irritable colon. Anderson (2) has claimed that such patients release more catecholamines than do normal persons. Some of these persons with functional hypoglycemia show postprandial plasma glucose profiles and insulin responses with rapid gastric emptying resembling the findings in patients after gastric surgery. However, as shown in Figure 10–8, the majority of these individuals

LATE HYPOGLYCEMIA FOLLOWING ORAL GLUCOSE LOAD (100gm)

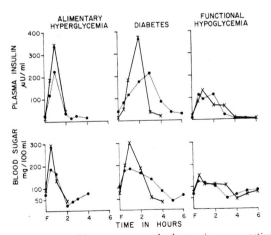

Figure 10–8. Plasma sugar and plasma immunoreactive insulin concentrations during an OGTT in patients with reactive hypoglycemia. Two patients, *each* with (1) early-onset (alimentary) hypoglycemia, (2) late-onset hypoglycemia (early diabetes mellitus), or (3) functional hypoglycemia are shown. (From Yalow, R. S., and Berson, S. A.: *Diabetes 14*:341, 1965.)

have a normal ascent rate and apogee of plasma sugar yet may have an early onset of hypoglycemia without apparent insulin excess (63, 91). As in patients with "tachyalimentary" hypoglycemia, it has been proposed that an enteric insulinogenic factor may be operative and, indeed, "gut glucagon" has been found to be elevated in a few patients (75). For reasons previously cited, this may not be primary but may rather reflect increased glucose absorption; this has been demonstrated in 3 patients. Although a parasympathetic influence on insulin release is suspected in these emotionally labile patients, the inability to document inappropriately elevated insulin levels may alternatively be explained by the possibility of enhanced insulin sensitivity or sluggish counter-regulatory mechanisms or both. At present, these speculations have not been substantiated, and, in the absence of systematic studies of the mechanisms involved in this group, they must be currently included in an idiopathic category.

Late-Phase "Reactive" Hypoglycemia

Early-Onset Diabetes Mellitus. Spontaneous attacks of low plasma glucose, occurring 3–5 hours after meals, are not infrequently documented in association with early phases of the development of diabetes mellitus in adults (20). These individuals have normal or slightly elevated fasting plasma glucose levels, with a slow ascent and high zenith (exceeding 160 mg./100 ml.) and a persistence of hyperglycemia, followed by a gradual fall to hypoglycemic levels. In contrast to the lean, hyperkinetic patients with early-phase hypoglycemia, these patients have a tendency to be more phlegmatic and have a higher incidence of obesity and family histories of diabetes mellitus (63). The rise in plasma insulin is sluggish, but excessive concentrations are achieved by 2–4 hours, and the decline in plasma glucose has been considered to be due to inappropriately high insulin levels (Fig. 10–8). Both the glucose and insulin responses to a variety of intravenous stimuli are usually attenuated in these patients, and a fall in plasma glucose is usually less precipitous than in other causes of "reactive" hypoglycemia (55). Thus, a defect in beta cell release of insulin is inferred. In contrast to adults, "reactive" hypoglycemia is uncommon in diabetic children. With time, the adult may progress into more advanced stages of diabetes mellitus, and as pancreatic beta cell reserve is further compromised, the hypoglycemic manifestations disappear. In obese subjects without a family history of diabetes or apparent hyperglycemia, insulin levels have been found to rise rapidly after oral glucose and to be sustained, eventuating in glucopenia. It is not yet known whether such patients are also potentially diabetic. The hypoglycemia has been attributed to the hyperinsulinemia, which is linked to the insulin resistance associated with the increased adipose mass. It should be emphasized, however, that "reactive" hypoglycemia is uncom-

mon in obese subjects and, when present, tends to be more frequently seen in the younger age group.

Treatment of Glucose-Induced "Reactive" Hypoglycemias

Since patients with the early- and late-onset "reactive" hypoglycemias tend to have in common an exaggerated insulin response to ingested glucose, the principle of treatment is to minimize the aberrant insulin release by dietary manipulation (38). Specific therapies are also based on the pattern of the "reactive" hypoglycemia. For the most part, restriction of carbohydrate has proven impractical on a long-term basis. High-protein intake has been advocated, based upon the rationale that amino acids stimulate insulin release to a lesser extent than does glucose, which is also more rapidly absorbed. In patients with early-phase hypoglycemia (postsurgical and idiopathic), rapid excursions of blood glucose are often dampened by small, high-protein feedings taken frequently. It is possible that the concomitant increased secretion of glucagon counterbalances the action of insulin. Decreased intake of sugar-containing foods, frequent high-protein feedings, and caloric restriction for weight reduction have also been found to be effective in patients with late-onset hypoglycemia due to diabetes mellitus and associated with obesity. In patients with accelerated glucose absorption, anticholinergic drugs have been employed to inhibit vagal action and delay gastric emptying. In the anxious, hyperkinetic patient, avoidance of caffeine-containing beverages and cigarettes should be urged, and sedatives, such as phenobarbital (30 mg. 2–3 times daily) or diazepam (5 mg. 2 times daily), may be efficacious in alleviating symptoms. A variety of pharmacologic agents has also been recommended based upon their different mechanisms of action. Phenformin hydrochloride has been reported to alleviate the hypoglycemia in obese subjects by inhibition of intestinal glucose absorption, thereby leading to diminished insulin release (48). Compounds such as diazoxide, diphenylhydantoin, and propranolol have been proposed for treatment because they inhibit the secretion of insulin. As yet, evaluation of the efficacy of these drugs has been inadequate to justify their use. In subjects with hypoglycemia associated with early-onset diabetes, a beneficial effect has been reported with the use of sulfonylureas (3), possibly through partial restoration of the sensitivity of the beta cell to respond to normal physiologic signals.

Hypoglycemia Induced by Galactose (Galactosemia)

The term "galactosemia" describes a rare, hereditary syndrome resulting from the inability to metabolize galactose, the major constituent of milk lactose. Galactosemia is now known to encompass two disorders of galactose metabolism due to specific enzymatic defects involved in the conversion of galactose to glucose (85). The constellation of nutritional failure, liver disease, cataracts and mental retardation occurring in infants after galactose ingestion results from a deficiency in galactose-1-phosphate uridyl transferase (transferase deficiency galactosemia) (Fig. 10–3). Another syndrome with hypergalactosemia and galactosuria associated with cataracts has recently been ascribed to a deficiency of galactokinase (galactokinase deficiency galactosemia). Patients with either disease cannot adequately utilize ingested galactose, and the clinical manifestations are related to galactose administration. Transferase deficiency galactosemia presents most commonly in the newborn as failure to thrive, with vomiting or diarrhea or both after milk ingestion. Within a few days, jaundice, hepatomegaly, and cataracts ensue, and hemolysis may also be apparent. With time, growth and development are impaired, and mental retardation is often observed after the first few months of life. Liver function tests are usually deranged, and hyperchloremic acidosis, albuminuria, and aminoaciduria are characteristic features. Glucopenia usually coincides with hypergalactosemia but is not an invariable consequence of lactose ingestion. Although the relative contribution of the low plasma sugar to the initial symptom complex is uncertain, it seems likely that persistent neuroglucopenia is a major factor in the evolution of the mental deterioration. As a result of the transferase enzymatic deficiency, galactose-1-phosphate accumulates in many tissues, and the occasional severe hypoglycemic episodes have been attributed to decreased hepatic gluconeogenesis because of inhibition of phosphoglucomutase, which catalyzes the conversion of glucose-1-phosphate to glucose-6-phosphate. In addition, galactose-1-phosphate may interfere with renal tubular resorption of amino acids, leading to diminished circulating gluconeogenic precursors. Both glycogen formation and glycogenolytic responses to glucagon are impaired. Unless galactose is eliminated from the diet, death occurs from inanition and multiorgan injury, possibly as a result of the toxicity of galactitol, which accumulates along with galactose-1-phosphate.

The disease, transmitted by an autosomal recessive gene, may be suspected on clinical grounds and demonstration of galactosemia and galactosuria. Lactosuria may occur in intestinal lactase deficiency, and defective galactose metabolism is found in severe liver disease. Because a galactose tolerance test is hazardous, it should be avoided. The diagnosis is confirmed by direct assay of red cell transferase activity, which is low or absent. Management of these patients is dependent upon the elimination of dietary galactose, which, if accomplished, results in striking regression of all symptoms and signs. Despite apparent improvement in galactose tolerance with age, leading to the interpretation that alternative pathways for galactose metabolism develop with maturity, strict adherence to a galactose-free diet has been advocated throughout adulthood.

Galactokinase deficiency galactosemia has only recently been described in seven patients. Deficiency of this enzyme limits conversion of galactose to galactose-1-phosphate. Although the patients developed lenticular cataracts, they have not been found to have hepatic or renal disease, and hypoglycemia is not a feature of the syndrome.

Hypoglycemia Induced by Fructose (Hereditary Fructose Intolerance)

Fructose is an important source of dietary carbohydrate, which is passively absorbed by the gut and normally converted to glucose by liver, kidney, and intestine. The disorder of fructose metabolism termed "hereditary fructose intolerance" is characterized by severe hypoglycemia and vomiting shortly after the intake of fructose. The disease, transmitted through an autosomal recessive gene, is due to a deficiency of hepatic fructose-1-phosphate aldolase, resulting in the accumulation of fructose-1-phosphate with abnormally high plasma fructose levels and fructosuria after oral or intravenous fructose (39). Infant and adult patients with this abnormality are healthy and asymptomatic unless they eat fructose-containing food. The clinical picture of chronic fructose poisoning in small children consists of failure to thrive, vomiting, jaundice, and hepatomegaly, with albuminuria and aminoaciduria. The children characteristically develop a strong aversion to fructose-containing food and sweets, which probably explains why the characteristic clinical patterns are not usually found in adults. Clinical manifestations can be evoked by intravenous fructose administration. The smallest dose which always produces hypoglycemic symptoms without causing nausea and vomiting is 0.25 g./kg. body weight in adults or 3 g./m.² body area in children. Levels of plasma glucose and phosphorus fall gradually and remain low for several hours. Hypophosphatemia precedes hypoglycemia and may be the only abnormal finding when a very small amount of fructose is given. Glucopenia, which may be profound, is neither associated with hyperinsulinism nor corrected by glucagon, implicating a defect in glycogenolysis. Although the precise mechanism for the hypoglycemia is still uncertain, Froesch (39) has suggested that it is due to fructose-1-phosphate aldolase deficiency (Fig. 10–3), resulting in accumulation of fructose-1-phosphate; the latter competitively inhibits fructose-1,6-diphosphate aldolase, thereby interfering with substrate flow in hepatic gluconeogenesis. The therapeutic approach to this disorder is the avoidance of fructose in the diet.

Hereditary fructose intolerance should not be confused with essential fructosuria, which is a rare, harmless abnormality characterized by fructosemia and fructosuria, reflecting a failure of conversion to fructose-1-phosphate due to a deficiency of hepatic fructokinase. Hypoglycemia has never been found with this benign condition. In two sisters, plasma glucose levels of 20 mg./100 ml. after the oral intake of both fructose and galactose have been reported. Although fasting insulin levels were allegedly elevated in these patients, red cell galactose-1-phosphate uridyl transferase was normal, and a relationship to galactosemia or to hereditary fructose intolerance has not been established.

Hypoglycemia Induced by Amino Acids (Leucine Hypersensitivity of Infancy and Childhood; Branched-Chain Ketonuria)

In a study of children presenting with hypoglycemia previously designated as idiopathic familial hypoglycemia of childhood, Cochrane and associates (18) reported that approximately 30% of infants in this group were distinguished by the onset of hypoglycemia following the ingestion of L-leucine. The clinical syndrome is usually apparent within the first 2 years of life, affecting both sexes equally and appearing as both severe fasting glucopenia and profound "reactive" hypoglycemia after the intake of dietary protein with a high leucine content. Seizures may occur with prolonged fasting, and permanent neurologic damage with mental retardation are common sequelae. In most instances, by the time the patients reach the age of 5 to 6 years, plasma sugar levels have spontaneously returned to normal. There is a high family incidence of leucine hypersensitivity; however, spontaneous leucine-induced hypoglycemia in adults is extremely rare and is usually demonstrable only postprandially (21). There are no pathognomonic signs or symptoms of this disease, and it may be difficult to distinguish these patients from individuals with functioning beta cell tumors, two-thirds of whom release inordinate amounts of insulin after leucine intake.

Although a number of amino acids are insulinogenic in normal man, the provocation of hypoglycemia in these affected children is almost exclusively found after L-leucine or closely related metabolites (α-ketoisocaproic acid and isoleucine) (72). It is now established that leucine evokes hypoglycemia by augmentation of insulin release in susceptible children. The plasma sugar concentration usually reaches its lowest point within 30–60 minutes after leucine intake. Fajans and colleagues (33) have shown that, in healthy individuals, leucine administered either orally or intravenously causes moderate rises in insulin levels, which become more pronounced with concurrent administration of sulfonylureas. Thus it has been inferred that leucine-induced hypoglycemia in these children represents a marked exaggeration of physiologic responses to this amino acid. The reason for the beta cell sensitivity to leucine is unclear. Postmortem examination in several of these patients has revealed islet cell hyperplasia, yet the pancreatic insulin content has been within normal limits. The high frequency of fasting hypoglycemia in the face of normal plasma insulin levels suggests that additional factors involved in glucogenesis are impaired.

The diagnosis is established by demonstration of a decrease in plasma glucose in excess of 20 mg./100 ml. after oral leucine or 25 mg./100 ml. after its intravenous administration (150–250 mg./kg. body weight). This challenge usually results in a two- to threefold rise in plasma insulin levels above basal. Although severe hypoglycemia can be exacerbated in patients with insulin-producing tumors as well as in leucine-sensitive patients, the former are uncommon in childhood, and fasting hypoglycemia in the latter is more severe with higher levels of insulin. Insulin responses to tolbutamide in subjects with leucine hypersensitivity tend to be within normal limits (27). The management of patients with this disorder is similar in principle to that for patients with "idiopathic hypoglycemia of childhood" (see below). It has been suggested, but not proved, that restriction of the leucine content in the diet is beneficial. Glucocorticoids, such as prednisone, usually cause amelioration of the hypoglycemia (21); however, adverse effects, particularly growth retardation, may preclude the use of steroids. Diazoxide, in oral doses of 10–15 mg./kg. body weight/day, may be effective in control of the hypoglycemic attacks (40). Subtotal pancreatectomy, although once recommended, is not justifiable in most cases since the disease is self-limited.

Hypoglycemia has been described in newborns as one of the metabolic anomalies associated with the defects occurring in the degradative steps of the three-branched chain amino acids—leucine, valine, and isoleucine. This autosomal recessive disease termed "branched-chain ketonuria" or "maple syrup urine disease" is a consequence of a block in oxidative decarboxylation of α-ketoisocaproic acid and α-keto-β-methyl-valeric acid, resulting in accumulation of their branched-chain amino acid precursors (24). The affected infants are normal at birth but fail to thrive, become lethargic, and have muscle hypotonicity and convulsions. Approximately 50% develop symptomatic hypoglycemia. Death usually is caused by intercurrent infection. Mental retardation and neurologic deficits are stigmata in longer survivors. The only distinctive clinical feature is the odor of the urine, which resembles that of burnt sugar. The diagnosis is confirmed by measurement of elevated branched-chain ketoacids or amino acids in blood and urine and demonstration of the enzyme defect in peripheral leukocytes. The pathogenesis of the hypoglycemia is uncertain; however, as it is demonstrable only in the fed state, it has been assumed that it may be related to the accumulation of certain amino acids, particularly leucine, which induces increased insulin secretion; this hypothesis remains to be substantiated. Branched-chain amino acids are preferentially catabolized in muscle and serve as a source of nitrogen and indirectly as glucose precursors. Whether gluconeogenesis is impaired indirectly by their loss in the urine has not been established. Although a diet with reduced amounts of branched-chain amino acids apparently tends to prevent the serious complications of the disease, the severe restrictions in food selection imposed by this dietary regimen may be impractical.

Fasting Hypoglycemia

As outlined in preceding sections, during the transition from the fed to the fasting state a number of factors operate normally to regulate the provision of fuels for the maintenance of glucose homeostasis. Five to six hours postprandially the stabilization of blood glucose levels reflects increased hepatic glucose output, coincident with a rise in circulating gluconeogenic precursors. Hypoglycemia in the fasted state can be conveniently categorized into disorders in which there is an underproduction of glucose and, conversely, those in which this sugar is excessively utilized (6). In some children with both fasting and "reactive" types of hypoglycemia, the mechanism is uncertain and therefore classified as "idiopathic." Frequently, glucopenia during fasting tends to be profound and protracted and, hence, accompanied by clinical manifestations of cerebral depression.

Deficient Glucose Production

Hepatic Dysfunction

Inborn Errors of Glucogenesis

Glycogen Storage Diseases. A number of disorders involving glycogen synthesis or breakdown in various tissues because of specific enzyme deficiencies have been recognized, and their clinical features are distinctive. The clinical manifestations appear early in infancy and childhood, and their severity is related to the degree of enzyme impairment affecting glycogen metabolism and whether alternative substrates are available. A classification of the types of glycogenosis with major organ involvement and specific enzyme abnormalities is given in Table 10–5. Patients with each type have in common excessive deposition of glycogen in various organs, and in most the en-

zyme defects are transmitted as autosomal recessive traits (50). Of the eight inherited diseases of glycogen metabolism, types II, IV, V, VII, and VIII do not have hypoglycemia as a feature of the clinical syndrome and will not be considered further.

Glycogen storage diseases types I, III, and VI have several clinical features in common; however, the course of the latter two abnormalities is milder than that of type I. Children with type I glycogenosis usually are short in stature with normal proportions. Hypotonia and a tendency to obesity are also frequent. Massive hepatomegaly, the most striking and common physical finding, persists throughout life, while the kidneys, which are also enlarged, may require radiographic confirmation because of the prominence of the liver. Most of these patients also have xanthomas located characteristically over the extensor surfaces of the extremities. Fasting hypoglycemia occurs shortly after birth and may be variable in severity, with plasma sugar concentrations ranging as low as 10 mg./100 ml., often without symptoms. The glucopenia is accompanied by striking increases in plasma levels of lactate, pyruvate, triglycerides, phospholipids, cholesterol, ketones, and uric acid. Clinical gout may occur in early adulthood as a manifestation of the hyperuricemia, which is due to both increased production of uric acid and the competitive inhibition of its renal elimination by the elevated ketoacids. The high lactic acid levels and hyperlipidemia with evidence of excess lipid deposition in skin and liver reflect the excessive mobilization of gluconeogenic precursors in response to hypoglycemia.

Individuals with type I glycogenosis characteristically have minimal or absent hyperglycemic responses to epinephrine, glucagon, galactose, or fructose. Oral glucose tolerance tests often resemble those seen in patients with diabetes mellitus and insulin responses are usually blunted. The extraordinary accumulation of glycogen with normal structure, in liver and kidney, is due to a lack of the enzyme glucose-6-phosphatase, which normally leads to the hydrolysis of glucose-6-

TABLE 10–5. GLYCOGEN STORAGE DISEASES

Type	Eponym	Organs	Enzyme Defect	Glycogen Structure	Fasting Hypo- glycemia	Clinical Features
I	Von Gierke's disease	Liver, kidney	Glucose-6-phosphatase	Normal	++	Early onset, hepatomegaly, xanthomatosis
II	Pompe's disease	Generalized	α-1,4-glucosidase	Normal	0	Hypotonia, cardiomegaly, death from cardiorespiratory failure
III	Cori's disease	Liver, muscle, heart, erythrocytes	Amylo,1,6-glucosidase	Abnormal	++	Similar to type I but less severe
IV	Andersen's disease	Liver, leukocytes	α-1,4-glucan: 1,4-glucan-6-glucosyl transferase	Abnormal	0	Hypotonia, hepatosplenomegaly, death due to progressive cirrhosis
V	McArdle's disease	Muscle	Phosphorylase	Normal	0	Muscle cramping with exercise, myoglobinuria
VI	Her's disease	Liver, leukocytes	Phosphorylase	Normal	+	Similar to type I but less severe
VII	—	Muscle, erythrocytes	Phosphofructokinase	Normal	0	Muscle cramping with exercise, myoglobinuria
VIII	—	Liver, leukocytes	Phosphorylase b kinase	Normal	0	Hepatomegaly

phosphate to glucose (Fig. 10–3). Despite this defect in a key enzyme, a number of patients survive into adulthood, and therefore glucose must be made available through hydrolysis of glucose-6-phosphate by nonspecific phosphatases. The biochemical diagnosis is made by demonstration of increased amounts of normal glycogen by histochemical staining and absence of glucose-6-phosphatase by enzyme analysis of freshly frozen liver, which is best obtained by open biopsy.

Patients with type III glycogen storage disease cannot be distinguished by physical examination from those with type I (72). However, their clinical course tends to be less severe, although occasionally marked hypoglycemia and convulsions may occur. The hepatomegaly seen in childhood inexplicably tends to diminish at puberty, and renal enlargement is not found. Hyperglycemia after epinephrine and glucagon is variable, and lactose and fructose are readily converted to glucose. Because of the deficiency of amylo-1,6-glucosidase or "debrancher enzyme" (Fig. 10–3), abnormal forms of glycogen accumulate in large amounts in the liver. The diagnosis is confirmed by histologic evidence of abnormally short outer branches of glycogen in erythrocytes, muscle, or liver.

Hers has described a heterogeneous group of patients with clinical features analogous to mild forms of type I glycogenosis (50). The increased hepatic glycogen is associated with a 25% reduction of hepatic phosphorylase activity, eventuating in impaired generation of glucose-1-phosphate (Fig. 10–3). At this time, however, there is controversy over the validity of inclusion of these patients as a separate entity, because of the problem in assaying total liver phosphorylase activity.

Since there are no specific means of rectifying the enzyme abnormalities in the glycogen storage diseases, therapy is directed toward preventing hypoglycemia by frequent intake of food high in protein content. Experience with the use of repository forms of glucagon or infusions of catecholamines has been unsatisfactory. Diazoxide, which has been tried in a few patients with type I glycogen storage disease, offers some promise, and portacaval transposition has been associated with growth spurts and reduction of liver size in some patients; nevertheless, the procedure remains experimental.

Ketotic Hypoglycemia of Childhood. In 1964, Colle and Ulstrom (19) described the clinical features of "ketotic hypoglycemia," which is the most common form of glucopenia in children. The patients are usually hyperactive males of short stature and low weight, and hypoglycemia is most frequently encountered after 18 months of age. Low plasma glucose is episodically found in the morning after carbohydrate deprivation and is accompanied by vomiting and ketonuria. Symptoms are promptly reverted by parenteral glucose, and between attacks the patients are normoglycemic and have no abnormalities in plasma sugar or insulin responses to parenteral glucose, tolbutamide, L-leucine, glucagon, and epinephrine. Symptomatic hypoglycemia in these patients is invariably provoked by a hypocaloric, low carbohydrate diet high in fat content. However, ketonuria is not a constant feature. Most of these children are of normal intelligence, and good health is restored by a balanced dietary intake; after the age of 6 years, hypoglycemia can no longer be elicited. The pathogenesis of this disorder is uncertain. Insulin levels are appropriate for the blood glucose concentration. During hypoglycemic episodes provoked by ketogenic diets or after brief caloric restriction, glucagon administration fails to elevate blood glucose, thereby suggesting an impairment in glycogenesis. Pagliarra (72) has presented evidence that a deficiency in gluconeogenic precursors, notably alanine, rather than a defective hepatic gluconeogenic apparatus per se is responsible for the impaired glucose homeostasis. On the other hand, in four children with fasting hypoglycemia and ketosis provoked by a ketogenic diet, a lower activity in hepatic fructose-1,6-diphosphatase (Fig. 10–3) has been documented associated with impaired glycogen synthetase activity, which has been considered to be a secondary defect. Hypoglycemia in these patients may be precipitated by both glycerol and fructose, possibly through intracellular phosphorus depletion.

At this time, it is not clear whether all patients with "ketotic hypoglycemia" have similar enzyme deficiencies or whether this disorder may constitute a spectrum of inherited abnormalities of gluconeogenesis (4, 72). It has been postulated that the perturbed glucose homeostasis may represent an extreme degree of normal responsiveness to deprivation of carbohydrate and calories. Clinical management is empirical and primarily prophylactic since the hypoglycemic attacks gradually decrease with age. It is desirable to maintain adequate caloric intake high in carbohydrate content during periods when acetonuria is demonstrable. In one patient with hepatic fructose-1,6-diphosphatase deficiency, folic acid resulted in symptomatic improvement and increased enzyme activity. Ephedrine sulfate eliminated the hypoglycemic episodes in one of two patients. In general, dietary manipulations suffice, but glucocorticoids may occasionally be required in patients with severe hypoglycemia.

Acquired Liver Disease. In view of the central role of the liver in glucogenesis and the evidence that hepatectomy in experimental animals causes sustained glucopenia, hypoglycemia would be expected to be a common complication of severe liver disease. Yet the functional reserve of the liver is such that more than 80% of its mass may be removed without disturbance of glucose homeostasis. Hence, fasting hypoglycemia is evident only when there is widespread injury or replacement of the liver parenchyma. Moreover, there is no correlation between the development of hypoglycemia and severity of hepatic disease as measured by conventional liver function tests. A wide spectrum of diseases of the liver has been implicated as causes of fasting hypoglycemia; but the incidence is small in patients with cirrhosis, metastatic carcinoma, or hepatitis (102). Rarely, patients with fulminant hepatitis have marked hypoglycemia, and deranged glucose metabolism may occasionally be associated with diseases such as ascending cholangitis, hepatic abscesses, and empyema of the gallbladder. Hypoglycemia is infrequently observed, even in the terminal phases of Laennec's cirrhosis; yet alcoholics who have impaired liver function varying from massive hepatic fatty infiltration to cirrhosis may also have hypoglycemia because of excessive ethanol ingestion and inadequate caloric intake (described below). Fasting glucopenia has been documented in severely malnourished children; in adolescents deprived of protein (kwashiorkor) who have fatty infiltration of the liver as a complication, sudden death after refeeding has been attributed to hypoglycemia. In some patients with severe congestive heart failure, passive congestion of the liver may disrupt glucogenesis, resulting in hypoglycemia. Occasionally, in the third trimester of pregnancy, women may develop acute fulminant hepatitis and yellow atrophy of the liver with marked hypoglycemia. Continuous intravenous glucose infusion is necessary and mortality is high. A variety of hepatotoxins, notably phosphorus, chloroform, carbon tetrachloride, glycol, and halothane, may cause massive necrosis with attendant hypoglycemia. Hepatic infiltration by metastatic carcinoma is rarely extensive enough to diminish the glucogenic capacity of the liver. Primary tumors of the liver are not infrequently associated with hypoglycemia for reasons other than the destruction of hepatic cells (see the following).

The hypoglycemia ensuing from hepatocellular dysfunction is explained by deficient gluconeogenesis and glycogenolysis resulting in reduced hepatic glucose output. The impaired capability of the liver to form glycogen or release glucose is reflected by the fasting hypoglycemia with elevated postprandial plasma glucose levels which gradually decline to low levels within 4–5 hours. The diagnosis of liver disease is usually evident from other clinical features of hepatocellular failure. Treatment of acute fulminant hepatic disease entails the maintenance of plasma sugar levels with parenteral glucose administration, and restoration of glucose homeostasis occurs with liver regeneration. In patients with marginal residual function of the liver, frequent feedings high in carbohydrate may be necessary to minimize glucopenic episodes.

Endocrine Organ Hypofunction

As summarized previously (Table 10–2), glucocorticoids, GH, glucagon, and catecholamines operate in concert to counter the action of insulin during the transition from the fed to the fasting state and provide signals for *de novo* glucose formation. Although each hormone may act by several mechanisms, deficiencies in secretion of glucagon, catecholamines, and glucocorticoids result primarily in impaired hepatic glucogenesis. Despite its lipolytic activity leading to glucogenic precursors, GH would appear to exert its major effect on glucose homeostasis by impeding insulin action in peripheral tissues; therefore, GH insufficiency is discussed under hypoglycemia due to ex-

cessive utilization of glucose. Since both ACTH and GH are produced in the anterior pituitary, destruction of this organ may cause glucopenia through combined bihormonal failure.

Glucocorticoid Deficiency. Diseases of the adrenal cortex with impaired secretion of glucocorticoids are commonly associated with plasma glucose levels of less than 60 mg./100 ml., which may fall further to symptomatic ranges with food deprivation (99). Since cortisol influences glucose homeostasis through "permissive" actions on hepatic gluconeogenesis and possibly anti-insulin effects on peripheral tissues, patients with inadequate glucocorticoid production are vulnerable to intermittent fasting hypoglycemia and sensitive to insulin administered exogenously (10). Spontaneous glucocorticoid insufficiency may be due to (1) primary adrenal failure (Addison's disease), (2) congenital enzymatic defects in the pathways of cortisol synthesis (adrenogenital syndrome), and (3) defective ACTH secretion (panhypopituitarism, solitary ACTH deficiency, or diminished CRF release). Glucopenia may also be encountered in patients after bilateral adrenalectomy if steroid replacement is inadequate. The clinical features and procedures used to establish the diagnosis of these disorders are detailed in Chapter 5. Adrenocortical hypofunction can occur secondary to a solitary defect in ACTH secretion, and several reported cases have presented with fasting hypoglycemia. The diagnosis is confirmed by failure to demonstrate adequate ACTH levels following provocative challenges, such as insulin-induced glucopenia, pyrogen, or metyrapone. Hypoglycemia due to glucocorticoid lack is rectified completely by administration of one of several available naturally occurring or synthetic glucocorticoids (e.g., cortisol, 20-30 mg. daily, or prednisone, 5–7.5 mg. daily).

Glucagon Insufficiency. McQuarrie (70) and Grollman (44) independently reported fasting hypoglycemia in a few infants and adults who, by histologic evaluation at autopsy, had marked reduction of pancreatic alpha cells relative to beta cells. These findings led them to conjecture that the relative lack of glucagon might explain the hypoglycemia on the basis of impaired hepatic gluconeogenesis; however, no measurements of plasma glucagon levels were performed. In 1969, Bleicher (11) described a man believed to have hypoglycemia as a consequence of glucagon deficiency. The patient had recurrent glucopenia induced by both fasting and ingestion of protein. Plasma sugar responses to oral glucose resembled those seen in diabetic patients. With extended fasting, insulin and glucagon levels were very low. After arginine infusions, plasma glucagon concentrations remained virtually unmeasurable. Following treatment with a high carbohydrate diet, glucopenic symptoms were alleviated. Thus isolated alpha cell insufficiency may be a distinct entity; however, it appears to be a rare cause of hypoglycemia in the adult. Recently, a blunted glucagon response to severe glucopenia has been observed in infants of diabetic mothers, and a transitory lack of glucagon has been implicated in this form of neonatal hypoglycemia (see the following).

Disorders of the Sympathetic Nervous System.

Although catecholamines antagonize actions of insulin in glucose homeostasis, it is conjectural whether spontaneous hypoglycemia can be ascribed to deficiency states of the sympathetic nervous system. Among children with fasting hypoglycemia of undetermined etiology (idiopathic hypoglycemia of childhood), a subgroup without elevated circulating insulin levels, leucine hypersensitivity, or "ketogenic hypoglycemia" has been found to have diminished urinary excretion of epinephrine under basal conditions (72). Moreover, following insulin-induced hypoglycemia the affected children have little or no increment in epinephrine excretion, whereas normal children respond with a five- to twentyfold increase. The quantitative defect in adrenal medullary secretion is in keeping with the clinical evidence of lack of catecholamine effects, e.g., vasoconstriction and tachycardia, when profound hypoglycemia is manifested as a convulsive seizure. These patients show an increased sensitivity to insulin, with a prolonged fall in plasma glucose levels. Nonetheless, they have normal hyperglycemic responses to exogenously administered epinephrine. Since norepinephrine metabolism in these children is apparently unaltered, it has been proposed that the pathogenesis is related to the inability to synthesize epinephrine within the adrenal medulla. Recently, Tietze (93) has demonstrated that some of these children have impaired release of cortisol as well as catecholamines. Because glucocorticoids promote synthesis of epinephrine by activation of phenylethanolamine-N-methyl transferase, it is possible that adrenocortical dysfunction contributes to decreased epinephrine production. That the hypoglycemia cannot be attributed solely to a deficiency of epinephrine is further substantiated by the well-known experience that hypoglycemia does not occur in patients following bilateral adrenalectomy when they have received adequate replacement therapy with glucocorticoids. Furthermore, adults with familial dysautonomia or patients with sympathetic denervation rarely have spontaneous fasting hypoglycemia. Thus it is unlikely that catecholamine deficiency is the sole determinant of the glucopenia in the patients described by McQuarrie.

Extrapancreatic Neoplasms

As reviewed by Laurent (58), a relationship has been established between hypoglycemia and tumors which do not have an endocrine origin. Although this association is infrequent (approximately 220 reported cases), the clinical manifestations may be indistinguishable from those observed in patients with insulin-producing pancreatic tumors. As indicated in Table 10–6, these nonendocrine neoplasms are heterogeneous in composition and location. While some of the tumors derived from epithelial anlage originate in a number of different organs, most of the neoplasms evolve from mesoderm and are situated within the thoracic and peritoneal cavities, with the highest frequency in the retroperitoneal space.

TABLE 10–6. DISTRIBUTION OF EXTRAPANCREATIC (NON–BETA CELL) TUMORS ASSOCIATED WITH HYPOGLYCEMIA*

Origin	Distribution (%)
Mesenchymal	45
Hepatoma	23
Adrenocortical carcinoma	10
Gastrointestinal carcinoma	8
Lymphoma	6
Miscellaneous (ovary, lung, kidney)	8
	100

*After Laurent, J., et al.: *Hypoglycaemic Tumours*. Amsterdam, Excerpta Medica Foundation, 1971.

The mesenchymal tumors are diverse histologically but most commonly are classified as fibrosarcomas, rhabdomyosarcomas, leiomyosarcomas, or fibromas. They are usually of low-grade malignancy, enlarge slowly, and are frequently of extraordinary size (2–4 kg. and occasionally > 20 kg.). They are most commonly encountered in older individuals, with equal sex distribution. The initial symptoms are most frequently related to glucopenia, and the patient may be unaware of the large tumor, which is detected by physical signs or radiologic examination. Fasting plasma glucose levels may be extremely low without activation of the sympathetic nervous system, and the clinical manifestations are primarily those of depressed cerebral function. Extrapancreatic neoplasms of epithelial origin, accompanied by glucopenia, also tend to be large and generally slow-growing. Among Chinese subjects with hepatocellular carcinoma, McFadzean and Yeung (68) have characterized a group with poorly differentiated tumors with accelerated growth, accompanied by rapid and continuous depletion of the extracellular glucose pool. Gigantic size is also a common feature of neoplasms derived from gastrointestinal cells, as well as those located in miscellaneous sites.

The pathogenesis of the hypoglycemia associated with these massive tumors remains speculative. Recent studies of the glucose kinetics in some of these patients have suggested a multifactorial etiology. Thus, in any individual, increased glucose utilization, decreased glucose production, defective glycogen synthesis and release, and impaired mobilization of alternate metabolic substrates may coexist, thereby causing profound hypoglycemia (57). In only a few instances has there been adequate documentation of increased glucose consumption by these gigantic tumors. In these patients, glucose turnover rates have been shown to be elevated, with excessive diversion of blood glucose to the neoplastic tissue and eventual conversion to lactic acid through anaerobic glycolysis. Although augmented assimilation of sugar may contribute, in part, to the glucopenia, considerable data indicate that these tumors release a factor influencing glucose homeostasis. There is no reliable evidence that these tumors are able to synthesize and store insulin or its precursors. Circulating levels of immunoreactive insulin are very low, and little or no rise is obtained after various stimuli

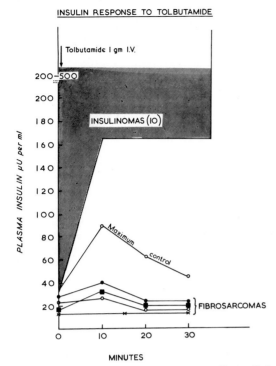

INSULIN RESPONSE TO TOLBUTAMIDE

Tolbutamide I gm I.V.

INSULINOMAS (IO)

Maximum

control

} FIBROSARCOMAS

PLASMA INSULIN µU per ml

MINUTES

Figure 10–9. Insulin response to intravenous tolbutamide in patients with insulinoma and fibrosarcoma associated with hypoglycemia. (From Samols, E.: *Postgrad. Med. J.* 39:634, 1963.)

amined; hence the identity of the hypoglycemic factors has not been established. Although an antigluconeogenic humoral factor has yet to be repetitively demonstrated in these patients, the preliminary data suggest that a tumor-elaborated substance may be important in the pathogenesis of the hypoglycemia.

A large intrathoracic or intra-abdominal mass, in conjunction with hypoglycemia and low levels of circulating immunoreactive insulin and relative hyporesponsiveness to insulinotropic stimuli, distinguish patients with nonpancreatic neoplasms from those with insulin-producing (beta cell) tumors. Treatment is directed primarily to maintenance of tolerable plasma glucose levels, since the size and location of the tumors usually preclude surgical resection and, in general, they are resistant to irradiation or chemotherapy. Frequent intake of food high in carbohydrate may sustain plasma sugar levels, and glucocorticoids in pharmacologic doses occasionally provide some benefit. In a few reported cases, diazoxide has been ineffectual.

Overutilization of Glucose

Functioning Beta Cell Tumors of the Pancreas (Insulinoma)

A relationship between hypoglycemia and pancreatic beta cell tumors was established in 1927, and since then, the natural history of this disease has been summarized in various series (49, 58, 84). Although the prevalence of functioning islet cell neoplasms has not been ascertained, it is relatively uncommon. At routine autopsy, the incidence of islet cell tumors has been reported to vary from 1 in 8000 to 1 in 63. In a survey at the Mayo Clinic, in 10,314 autopsies, 44 islet cell tumors were found, 8 of which were functional (60). In most series, adenomas are multiple in less than 8%, and microadenomatosis (hyperplasia) is extremely rare. Amyloid deposits within the tumor are frequently found. The majority of the tumors measure 10–50 mm. (75% < 30 mm.) in diameter, with an occasional adenoma under 1 mm. Thus, their small size may preclude radiographic demonstration or palpation at operation. Ectopic sites of the tumors are also rare and located along the gastrointestinal tract. Single adenomata have a comparable frequency of distribution in the head, body, and tail of the pancreas. Approximately 10% of all insulinomas are malignant and metastasize most frequently to the liver and regional lymph nodes. Histologic differentiation between adenoma and carcinoma in pancreatic masses may be difficult without evidence of capsular invasion or extrapancreatic extension.

The clinical manifestations due to hyperfunctioning beta cell tumors are most common in persons 30–60 years of age, with equal sex distribution. Functional tumors are rare in the newborn (15 cases) and in adolescents (< 60 cases) (94). The clinical characteristics mimic a wide variety of neuropsychiatric disorders (Table 10–7), and the diagnosis may be unsuspected for many years (22).

such as tolbutamide (Fig. 10–9); thus, a causal relationship between insulin and the tumor hypoglycemic factor is untenable (79). In a few patients, elevated levels of insulin-like activity (ILA, also denoted nonsuppressible ILA), measured by adipose tissue or diaphragm bioassays, have been reported both in plasma and tumor extracts, which has led to the supposition that this ill-defined substance(s) is responsible for the hypoglycemia. Despite many similarities between ILA and insulin in isolated assay systems, a biologic role for ILA in man has yet to be established, and the data implicating ILA in the pathogenesis of tumor-related hypoglycemia are not well-founded. Since in *in vitro* systems ILA promotes glucose transport, it would be predicted that, if in excess in patients with tumors, ILA should enhance glucose utilization, an event which is infrequently found.

Much of the current data has pointed to a substance(s), produced by the neoplasm, which inhibits hepatic gluconeogenesis. By isotopic techniques, diminished glucose production by the liver has been found in some of these patients and, in one person with a mesenchymal tumor, a factor of low molecular weight extracted from the tumor has been reported to inhibit the conversion of lactate to glucose in an isolated liver perfusion system. Since tryptophan has been shown to interfere with gluconeogenesis and has been found in elevated amounts in plasma of a few patients with malignancy, this amino acid or its metabolites have been proposed as the inhibitory substance (89). Nevertheless, tryptophan or its metabolites have not been found to be increased in all patients ex-

TABLE 10–7. SIGNS AND SYMPTOMS EXHIBITED BY 193 PATIENTS WITH INSULINOMAS*

	Per Cent		Per Cent
Loss of consciousness	58	Noisy behavior	20
Confusional state	54	Headache	20
Weakness and fatigue	41	Tremor	18
Deep coma	40	Hunger	14
Sweating	36	Positive Babinski sign	13
Drowsiness and stupor	35	Paresthesias	13
Lightheadedness	30	Irritability	11
Visual disturbances	30	Transient hemiplegia	10
Amnesia	28	Abdominal pain	8
Clonic convulsions	24	Palpitation	3

*After Crain, E. L., and Thorn, G. W.: *Medicine* 28:427, 1949.

Aberrant behavior patterns and disturbances in consciousness are the most common features. Although symptoms may occur sporadically, they usually appear before breakfast and are ameliorated shortly after eating. They are often exacerbated by protracted fasting or vigorous physical exercise. Because of the gradual decline in plasma sugar, excessive catecholamine release may be inconsequential, and loss of consciousness and depression of vasomotor function may be the initial manifestations. Hunger is an uncommon symptom and obesity is not a distinguishing feature of this disorder. Between attacks there are no distinctive physical findings; nevertheless, there may be insidious intellectual deterioration depending upon the duration and degree of hypoglycemia. The clinical picture associated with malignant beta cell tumors may be indistinguishable from that of the benign islet cell neoplasm; however, the severity of the hypoglycemic episodes is usually more intense, and an enlarged, hard liver may be a clue to the cancer. Although occasionally indolent, functioning islet cell carcinomas usually grow rapidly, and death ensues 2–3 years after the diagnosis has been established. In contrast, patients with benign insulinomas may have neuroglucopenic symptoms which have been recurrent for many years and attributed to other causes of organic brain syndrome.

It is obvious that hypoglycemia in this setting is the direct consequence of the actions of excessive circulating levels of insulin and its precursors released by the neoplastic beta cell. The combined actions of insulin, including inhibition of hepatic glucose output and diminished flow of gluconeogenic precursors, with concomitant augmented glucose translocation into peripheral tissues deplete the extracellular glucose pool. Despite the release of several counter-regulatory hormones, their actions are overwhelmed by the inordinate amounts of circulating insulin.

Although insulinomas are comprised entirely of islet tissue, beta granules are infrequently found by microscopy, suggesting abnormalities in storage and release of insulin. This is corroborated by the aberrant control of insulin secretion in these autonomously functioning neoplasms. Normally, granular discharge of insulin is linked to the ambient glucose level, whereas in insulinomas, insulin may be discharged episodically or continuously at inappropriately low blood sugar concentrations.

A further index of the abnormal secretory apparatus is provided by the reversal of the relative responsiveness to factors that stimulate beta cells. Thus the normal beta cell responds to glucose > tolbutamide > glucagon > leucine; whereas the neoplastic beta cell responds to glucagon > tolbutamide > leucine > glucose (36). This reversal of responsiveness forms the basis for the provocative tests of insulin hypersecretion in insulinomas. Additional support for deranged synthesis and release of insulin is provided by the studies of Melani (71), who has demonstrated excessively high levels of proinsulin and related insulin precursors in plasma of patients with insulinomas. In one series, 9 of 11 subjects had elevations of proinsulin ranging from 28–91% of total immunoreactive insulin levels. Of interest is the extraordinarily high percentage of proinsulin-like substances found in plasma of patients with islet cell carcinoma.

An insulinoma may be suspected in a patient who fulfills the triad described by Whipple (symptomatic fasting hypoglycemia reversed by glucose) (20). Nevertheless, since these criteria are nonspecific, confirmation of the diagnosis depends upon (1) documentation of inappropriately elevated levels of insulin, and (2) identification of the pancreatic tumor. The following procedures are helpful in substantiating the diagnosis.

Fasting Blood Sugar and Insulin Levels. After fasting for 12–14 hours, 80% of patients with islet cell tumors will have abnormally low levels of plasma glucose with inappropriately high insulin concentrations. This abnormal reciprocal relationship is unique to patients with insulinoma (Fig. 10–10) (96). However, since the secretion from these tumors may be sporadic, it may be necessary to repeat these analyses on several mornings. With more prolonged periods of food deprivation, there is an increased likelihood of demonstrating inappropriate levels of glucose and insulin. Consequently, hospitalized patients may be subjected to fasting up to 72 hours under close supervision with periodic blood sampling, particularly at times when they become symptomatic. Moderate exercise may be superimposed to accentuate a hypoglycemic episode. The intravenous infusion of ethanol, which inhibits gluconeogenesis and thereby enhances the probability of developing hypoglycemia, has also been proposed as a test for patients with insulinoma. In the series reported by Scholz (84), 75% of patients had glucopenic reactions within 24 hours

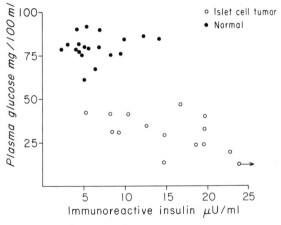

Figure 10–10. Plasma glucose and immunoreactive insulin levels in healthy control subjects and patients with insulinoma after an overnight fast. (Modified from Turner, R. C., Oakley, N. W., et al.: *Brit. Med. J.* 2:132, 1971.)

of fast and in only two was it necessary to continue food deprivation beyond 48 hours. Patients with islet cell carcinoma usually develop profound hypoglycemia with markedly elevated immunoreactive insulin levels within 24 hours. Although still only available in a research environment, the measurement of circulating proinsulin-like substances, if elevated, favors the diagnosis of insulinoma.

After oral glucose loading, plasma sugar levels are frequently difficult to interpret in patients with insulinoma. Typically, the profile of blood glucose responses tends to be considerably lower than normal throughout a 5-hour test period; however, not infrequently, they may paradoxically resemble the patterns characteristic of diabetes mellitus (64). This widely variable response reflects the autonomous nature of the tumor and thereby limits the value of the OGTT in diagnosis of this disease.

Intravenous and Oral Provocative Tests. Techniques to evoke an excessive release of insulin which distinguishes patients with islet cell neoplasms include (1) intravenous tolbutamide, (2) intravenous glucagon, and (3) oral leucine. The experiences with the diagnostic precision of these procedures have been independently reviewed by Marks and Samols (66), Floyd (36) and Khurana (56). With islet cell tumors, the tolbutamide response is characterized by an acute decline in plasma glucose with an attenuated rebound during 120–150 minutes (Fig. 10–11). Plasma insulin usually rises rapidly to very high levels, which are sustained for 40–90 minutes (Fig. 10–9) (79). In some series, 90% of patients have an abnormal response, yet a number of false-negative and false-positive results have also been reported (Fig. 10–13) (56). Tolbutamide should not be administered to patients with fasting plasma glucose below 45 mg./100 ml., and the test should be terminated with parenteral glucose if the patient becomes unconscious or disoriented. The use of rapid blood glucose sampling with glucose oxidase strips (Dextrostix) and quantification by a reflectance meter may be helpful. Similarly, intravenous glucagon causes an inordinate release of insulin in patients

with insulinoma (Fig. 10–12) (56), and, because it induces glycogenolysis with hyperglycemia, it is safer than tolbutamide and may be advantageous in evaluation of older subjects. Furthermore, fewer false-negative results have been reported with glucagon (Fig. 10–13). Leucine, administered orally (or occasionally intravenously), elicits an excessive insulin response in patients with islet cell tumors, as well as in children with leucine hypersensitivity (52). However, as with tolbutamide and glucagon, leucine testing may not separate patients with an insulinoma from normal individuals (Fig. 10–13). Thus, from the accumulated experience, it would appear that no single provocative test will establish the diagnosis of insulinoma. Based upon our own experience, we recommend that, in patients suspected of harboring a functional islet cell tumor, the use of the glucagon and tolbutamide tolerance tests on successive days, followed by a protracted period of fasting with measurement of plasma glucose and immunoreactive insulin levels, will have the greatest likelihood of documentation of inappropriate insulin secretion. Once the diagnosis of hyperinsulinism has been confirmed, the localization of an intrapancreatic mass may be aided preoperatively by angiographic techniques by means of selective catheterization of the celiac and superior mesenteric arteries. The success of positive radiographic identification ranges from 20–80% (mean 63%), and the variation in accuracy probably reflects the dimensions and vascularity of the tumor and the experience of the radiologist (42). Malignant transformation may be suspected if the tumor margins are not well circumscribed. Although this procedure may occasionally be of assistance in guiding the surgeon, ultimately the tumor must be palpated at laparotomy or located in serial frozen sections.

Treatment of Insulinomas. In patients in whom there are no medical contraindications to a laparotomy, surgical resection of the functional benign islet cell tumor is the preferred treatment,

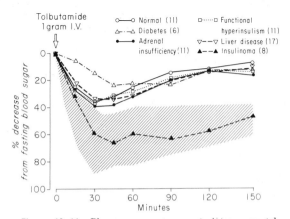

Figure 10–11. Plasma sugar responses to intravenous tolbutamide in patients with various types of hypoglycemia. The results are expressed as per cent decrease from fasting blood sugar. The hatched zone represents the range of responses for patients with insulinomas; number of patients is shown in parentheses. (Modified from the data of Fajans, S. S., Schneider, J. M., et al.: *J. Clin. Endocr.* 21:371, 1961.)

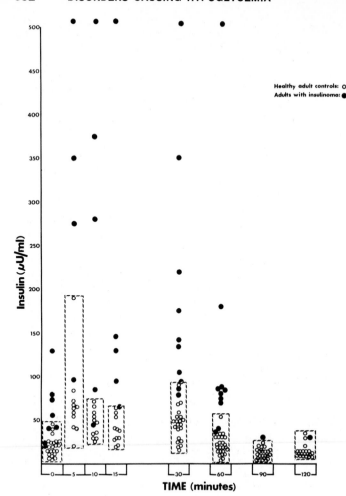

Figure 10–12. Plasma insulin levels in healthy controls and patients with insulinoma after glucagon administration (1 mg. I.M.). The ranges of normal responses are indicated in columns. (From Khurana, R. C., Nolan, S., et al.: *Amer. J. Med. Sci.* 262:123, 1971.)

since it usually effects a cure. Because of the threat of sporadic, sustained hypoglycemia during the operation, the anesthesiologist should be alerted to the need for the infusion of 5 or 10% glucose. Preoperative administration of glucose, with or without intramuscular or intravenous glucocorticoids, has been advocated routinely as preoperative prophylaxis against hypoglycemia and occasional high postoperative fever encountered in these patients. Alternatively, the medical consultative team may elect not to infuse glucose, since a small adenoma may not be palpated or may be overlooked on pancreatic sections, and serial plasma glucose levels, which rise after resection of a segment, may serve as an indication to cease the search (83). In all cases, low plasma sugar concen-

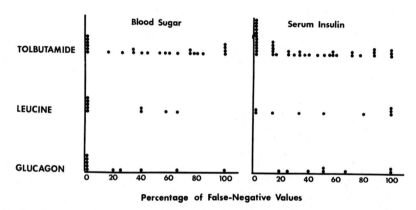

Figure 10–13. Percentage frequency of false-negative glucose or insulin values in patients with insulinoma based upon all of the sampling points of each tolbutamide, leucine, and glucagon test. (From Khurana, R. C., Nolan, S., et al.: *Amer. J. Med. Sci.* 262:124, 1971.)

trations should be assiduously avoided because of the potential for cerebral damage. If the tumor is not discovered within the pancreas or along the sites of ectopic rest formation, progressive sectioning of the pancreas from tail to head is undertaken, with examination of the specimens by the pathologist as well as frequent monitoring of plasma glucose. At the University of Washington, our surgical colleagues usually do not exceed a 90% pancreatectomy as a primary procedure (54). Failure to find tumors or persistent postoperative hypoglycemia may require reoperation or, alternatively, long-term medical management. When metastatic lesions are found on laparotomy, resection of the malignancy in the pancreas is normally not performed. Diabetes may appear following subtotal pancreatectomy but is transient and usually disappears within 6–8 weeks. Recently, however, in 5 of 11 patients who had benign insulinomas resected, an abnormal OGTT with low insulin response has persisted (26).

In patients in whom surgery may be delayed, refused, or deemed inappropriate, pharmacologic management must be provided with the object of maintaining normal or moderately elevated plasma glucose. Occasionally, treatment may require only dietary manipulation by frequent intake of foods high in carbohydrate, since in these patients, unlike in those with "reactive" hypoglycemia, insulin release is usually not linked to carbohydrate administration. With profound unremitting hypoglycemia, continuous infusions of 10 or 20% glucose may be needed. In addition, a number of hormones and pharmacologic agents have been used to maintain plasma sugar with varying success. Zinc glucagon (1–5 mg.) administered subcutaneously may elevate plasma sugar for several hours. Epinephrine also increases plasma glucose, but it requires intravenous administration and may have adverse cardiovascular effects. Glucocorticoids, administered intramuscularly as cortisone acetate (100–200 mg.) or intravenously as hydrocortisone hemisuccinate (100 mg.), may blunt the glucopenic manifestations. In most instances, all of these hormones, given singularly or in combination, are temporarily palliative and often have undesirable side effects.

In recent years, diazoxide, a nondiuretic benzothiadiazene, has been found to be beneficial in treating patients with hypoglycemia of diverse etiology, notably those with hyperinsulinism (65). Diazoxide has raised plasma glucose in a few patients with "idiopathic hypoglycemia of childhood" and occasionally in individuals with type I glycogen storage disease. Although the mechanism of its hyperglycemic action has not been completely resolved, diazoxide presumably has a direct effect on the beta cell to inhibit insulin release and enhances the secretion of epinephrine, which also impedes insulin output (61). Recent studies in lower species suggest that diazoxide increases hepatic glycogenolysis and glucose uptake by muscle by inhibiting phosphodiesterases. Therapeutic oral doses of diazoxide vary between 300 and 800 mg./day in patients with insulinoma. Major adverse effects include fluid retention, gastrointestinal irritation, hypertrichosis, and agranulocytosis. Intravenous diazoxide may rarely cause hypotension. Thus this drug provides an important adjunct in therapy of patients with intractable hypoglycemia (33). Nevertheless, in some patients with islet cell carcinoma and in most with hypoglycemia due to extrapancreatic neoplasms, this agent is ineffectual.

In subjects with metastatic islet cell carcinoma, alloxan, 5-fluorouracil, and nitrogen mustard have been used with little success because of tumor refractoriness and host toxicity. Recently, streptozotocin (an N-methyl-nitroso-urea-glucosamine antibiotic) has been shown to be cytotoxic to pancreatic beta cells. Fifty-two patients treated with this drug have been reported to experience remission of symptomatic hypoglycemia along with objective evidence of tumor regression lasting for several months (81). This diabetogenic compound has been administered by peripheral vein or into the celiac artery to maximize concentrations within the pancreas and liver. Current recommended intravenous dosage is 1 g./m.² body surface area/week. Adverse sequelae from this agent include nausea and vomiting, reversible hepatitis, and, of greatest concern, progressive azotemia due to renal tubular toxicity, which may limit its recurrent administration. Diphenylhydantoin, which causes hyperglycemia in man through inhibition of insulin release, has been reported to raise plasma glucose in a patient with an insulinoma; and recently, in a subject with an insulinoma that was unresponsive to streptozotocin, plasma glucose was maintained after treatment with L-asparaginase.

Insulinoma Associated with Other Endocrine Syndromes. Functioning beta cell tumors may coexist with other primary endocrine abnormalities. The syndrome of multiple endocrine adenomatosis (MEA) is characterized by the appearance of several tumors or hyperplasia involving diverse endocrine organs (59). Although these constellations are characteristically familial, the abnormalities in endocrine organs tend to cluster into two major groups. In the first, termed "multiple endocrine neoplasia type I," there is a grouping of tumors or hyperplasia of the parathyroids, pancreatic islets, and pituitary, frequently accompanied by a fulminant peptic ulcer diathesis (Zollinger-Ellison syndrome). The second association, "multiple endocrine neoplasia type II," is characterized by a common occurrence of pheochromocytoma, medullary thyroid carcinoma, and less frequently, parathyroid adenomata. In one extensive review of MEA, pancreatic islet cell involvement was found in 69 of 85 cases, with hypoglycemia in 36%. Thus, in "multiple endocrine neoplasia type I" in addition to glucopenia, clinical manifestations of hyperparathyroidism, hyper- or hypofunction of the pituitary, and intractable ulcer disease may appear in various combinations. Patients with the Zollinger-Ellison syndrome have severe peptic ulcer disease, diarrhea, and steatorrhea. Elevated basal acid secretion, the hallmark of this disorder, is due to excessive gastrin production from one or more islet cell tumors consisting histologically of alpha$_1$ or delta cells. In 260 patients with gastrin-secreting adenomas, Ellison and Wilson (29) found that 10 had coexisting insulinomas.

The common denominator in the etiology of the diverse endocrine organ involvement in MEA remains speculative. It has been postulated that the primary defect originates from a proliferation of the pancreatic ductal cell, leading to an excessive production of insulin, glucagon, or gastrin, which in turn chronically stimulate other endocrine organs, ultimately resulting in autonomous function. Since the endocrine organs involved are derived from neuroectoderm, it is also possible that the abnormality resides in informational coding in all affected tissues. Practically, in a setting of hypoglycemia compatible with a pancreatic islet cell tumor, the clinician should be alerted to a possible family history of endocrine dysfunction or ulcer diathesis and exclude other endocrine abnormalities in such patients.

Sporadic reports have appeared describing patients with islet cell tumors in whom gastrin, insulin, and glucagon have all been excessively produced, reflecting autonomous hyperfunction of the three major cell types normally residing in the islets of Langerhans. In addition, in a few patients with islet cell carcinoma, the ectopic manufacture of polypeptide hormones, including ACTH, MSH, vasopressin, and parathyroid hormone in one or more combinations, has been documented. Thus manifestations of hypoglycemia may coexist with the clinical picture of other endocrine abnormalities because of hormones elaborated by neoplastic pancreatic tissue. The aberrant production of hormones normally not manufactured by islet cells has been attributed to activation of genetic structural information which is derepressed by the neoplastic transformation. Conversely, in a few cases, heterotopic pancreatic tumors associated with hypoglycemia have been found in the duodenum and lung, which appear histologically as carcinoids and secrete excessive amounts of 5-hydroxytryptophan. Another group of patients has been described in whom massive watery diarrhea is the predominant clinical feature associated with hypokalemia and achlorhydria (WDHA syndrome). In 40 of these cases reported up to 1970, islet cell tumors without detectable gastrin or insulin have been found. Hypoglycemia is not a manifestation of the WDHA syndrome. Brown has isolated a 43-amino acid polypeptide from pork intestine, termed "gastric inhibitory peptide," which stimulates intestinal secretion, as well as enhancing insulin release, and indirect evidence by immunofluorescent techniques has implicated this substance as the cause of the WDHA syndrome (28). In patients with multiple endocrine dysfunction, the diagnostic approaches and treatment of the insulin-secreting pancreatic tumors are similar to those cited above.

Growth Hormone Deficiency

Symptomatic fasting hypoglycemia is found in approximately 10% of patients with panhypopituitarism maintained on glucocorticoids (12). Although protracted fasting may aggravate the glucopenia, neuroglucopenic manifestations are uncommon symptoms of pituitary failure. That GH modifies the action of insulin has been established in hypophysectomized humans by the marked attenuation of the rebound of plasma sugar after insulin, which is rectified by GH administration (62). These data suggest that, in the absence of GH, peripheral glucose utilization is increased, due to the unopposed action of insulin. Both fasting and "reactive" hypoglycemia may be present in patients with GH deficiency. A variety of lesions leading to total or partial pituitary insufficiency may result in hypoglycemia. These include chromophobe adenomas, craniopharyngiomas, and, more rarely, granulomatous infiltrations and acute pituitary necrosis due to postpartum hemorrhage, carotid aneurysms, or thrombosis. Following hypophysectomy for treatment of retinopathy, insulin-dependent diabetics are frequently more difficult to manage because of hypoglycemic episodes.

Low blood sugar may accompany pituitary dwarfism, which describes forms of short stature due to genetically transmitted defects in GH secretion. It is now recognized that absence of GH may occur as an isolated phenomenon or in combination with deficiencies of one or more other trophic hormones. Six distinct forms of hereditary pituitary dwarfism have been reviewed by Rimoin and Schimke (77). They include congenital absence of the pituitary, familial panhypopituitarism, isolated GH deficiency I, isolated GH deficiency II, Laron-type dwarfism, and pygmies. They have many clinical features in common, including a normal appearance at birth with a gradual growth retardation. Each of the different categories may have characteristic physical findings. Hypoglycemic attacks occur in all forms, except those with isolated GH deficiency II and pygmies. With the exceptions of the Laron-type dwarf and the pygmy, GH levels are diminished, both in fasting and in response to various stimuli. The measurement of normal or elevated levels of immunoreactive GH in the former two syndromes has led to the speculation that these dwarfs have either a circulating hormone that is biologically inert or that their tissues are insensitive to normal GH. The procedures to establish the diagnosis of GH deficiency in states of pituitary hypofunction are detailed in Chapter 2. Because of its scarcity, hGH is reserved primarily for treatment of short stature; hence, therapy of hypoglycemic episodes requires dietary manipulation by frequent feedings high in protein and occasionally the use of oral glucocorticoids.

Neonatal Hypoglycemia in Infants of Diabetic Mothers

During the first 48 hours of life, infants born to diabetic mothers may have sustained hypoglycemia with plasma sugars below 15 mg./100 ml. The degree of glucopenia in these infants has been shown to correlate with maternal carbohydrate tolerance (72). It is now established that affected neonates have elevated circulating insulin levels with increased pancreatic insulin content and beta cell hyperplasia. The most plausible explanation for this transitory hyperinsulinemia is that the fetus is exposed to chronic hyperglycemia originating from the maternal circulation, thereby inducing beta cell hyperfunction. At birth, gluconeogenic mechanisms are inhibited by high levels of plasma insulin, leading to hypoglycemia. This effect may be aggravated by temporary glucagon insufficiency. In most patients, frequent feedings suffice to revert plasma glucose to normal within a few days; however, parenteral glucose is required occasionally. McCann (67) has reported that the neonatal hypoglycemia may be mitigated by intravenous infusion of fructose to the mother for 2–3 hours prior to delivery, and to the infant immediately after parturition. The rationale for this proposed treatment is that fructose does not stimulate insulin release and may be gradually converted to glucose.

Erythroblastosis Fetalis

In infants who sustain hemolysis because of Rh immunization (erythroblastosis fetalis), hypoglycemia may occur during the first 3 days of life. The severity of the glucopenia is correlated with the cord blood hemoglobin concentration. Plasma insulin levels in cord blood have been shown to be elevated during the first 24 hours of life, and pancreatic islet cell hyperplasia with increased insulin content has been documented. During exchange transfusion, plasma insulin levels have been noted to rise markedly (74). Although the mechanism is uncertain, it has been proposed that insulin in the fetus is rapidly destroyed by the hemolyzed red cells, leading to a compensatory islet cell hyperplasia. Thus, in the newborn, the increased hyperinsulinemia occurring during exchange transfusion may be explained by the diminished insulin degradation after replacement with nonhemolyzed cells. Treatment is primarily supportive, with parenteral glucose, and if the child survives the hemolytic crisis, glucopenia remits spontaneously.

Idiopathic Hypoglycemia of Infancy and Childhood

A number of hypoglycemic disorders occurring in the newborn and extending into adolescence have been characterized clinically and the pathogenesis explained in part, so that they are no longer classified as idiopathic. In spite of advances in our understanding of the mechanisms underlying several of these hypoglycemic syndromes, there remains a group of children with causes of low plasma sugar that are unresolved and, therefore, are retained under this ill-defined category.

In the newborn with idiopathic transient hypoglycemia, plasma glucose levels of less than 20 mg./100 ml. are frequently seen. The susceptible infants are usually males and of low birth weight

for the period of gestation, with a tendency to polycythemia, primary nervous system damage or anomalies, and hypocalcemia (87). Clinical manifestations occur within 72 hours and usually include apnea, tremor, apathy, cyanosis, limpness, and convulsions. In association with glucopenia, impaired responses to glucagon and epinephrine have been observed, and isolated insulin levels have been reported to be high, with diminished cortisol production rates. Hence, the pathogenesis is probably multifactorial, and it has been suggested that, during intrauterine life, the fetus is malnourished, with inadequate compensatory mechanisms for gluconeogenesis. Treatment consists of parenteral glucose administration, and within a few days, plasma sugars return to normal.

Of the cases of hypoglycemia developing in children before the age of 2 years, the majority have been shown to be related to hypersensitivity to leucine or have been inducible by a ketogenic diet; however, a small group remains without a well-defined mechanism for the hypoglycemia. Low blood sugars may be continuous or intermittent, and symptoms are variable in severity. Eventually the hypoglycemia undergoes spontaneous remission over a period of months or years. Although a familial tendency was originally stressed, this has not been invariable. Of possible significance is the fact that five of seven affected children reported by Rosenbloom and Sherman (78) ultimately developed diabetes mellitus, and a high proportion of close relatives of these children had abnormal carbohydrate tolerance. Although high insulin levels were not found during episodic hypoglycemia in these children, it is possible that an abnormality in insulin release may have been a factor in the glucopenic phases of this disorder.

Beckwith and Widemann initially drew attention to a syndrome in neonates consisting of hypoglycemia with macroglossia, omphalocele, postnatal gigantism, visceromegaly, and various other defects which are inherited as an autosomal recessive trait (77). Islet cell hyperplasia has been reported in a few patients, but no consistent changes in pancreatic insulin content have been measured. Treatment has involved the use of glucocorticoids up to the age of 4–5 months, and diazoxide has been claimed to be effective.

Donohue first described an infant with elfinlike facial features, hirsutism, and multiple endocrine abnormalities, including hypoglycemia; this syndrome has been called leprechaunism (77). Glucopenia occurs during fasting, and islet cell hyperplasia has been noted in some autopsied cases; nonetheless, there is no proof that hyperinsulinism is linked to the hypoglycemic episodes.

Miscellaneous

Spontaneous hypoglycemia has been reported sporadically in individuals who have been chronically deprived of calories during famines. It is rarely a feature of protracted fasting for weight reduction and has only been adequately documented in patients with extreme inanition. Presumably, the diminished blood glucose reflects lack of gluconeogenic precursors from muscle and fat. During strenuous work, peripheral demand for glucose is increased. Yet even in conditioned athletes, after completion of an exhausting marathon race, plasma sugar levels usually do not decline below 45 mg./100 ml., and it is unlikely that this contributes significantly to fatigue. Excessive elimination of glucose from the intestinal tract, kidneys, or breasts has never been documented adequately as a cause of symptomatic hypoglycemia in man, although it is subject to conjecture on the basis of such occurrences in lower species.

PHARMACOGENIC AND TOXIC CAUSES OF HYPOGLYCEMIA

Exogenous Insulin Administration

Self-administration of insulin is the most common form of spontaneous hypoglycemia in clinical practice. In almost all instances, the patients are diabetic; however, occasionally, for bizarre psychological reasons, individuals may inject themselves surreptitiously with insulin to simulate organic disease. This so-called "factitious" cause of hypoglycemia is most commonly found in younger women with some exposure to medical practice, e.g., nurse's aides. The clandestine use of insulin results in symptoms mimicking those of an insulinoma and may lead to an extensive and enthusiastic work-up for an insulin-producing tumor. Factitious hypoglycemia should be suspected in a patient with an inconsistent history and numerous hospitalizations, usually resulting in laparotomy for a variety of abdominal complaints. Such patients have been described as having Munchausen's syndrome ("problem peregrinating patients," since they wander from hospital to hospital) (51). The psychopathology of this condition is uncertain and is usually resistant to therapy. In all young women with this background who appear with fasting hypoglycemia, examination of plasma for insulin antibodies should be made and an intensive search for an insulin ampule or syringe should be undertaken. Addition of ^{131}I to the ampule with detection of radioisotope in the patient's thyroid or urine confirms the diagnosis. Occasionally, depressed patients have self-injected insulin as a means for committing suicide.

Hypoglycemic episodes among insulin-dependent diabetics are the rule rather than the exception, and the ill consequences are far more common and serious than are generally appreciated. Abnormal electroencephalograms have been found in 50% of diabetics with frequent severe insulin reactions (43). Insulin reactions are correlated with the severity and instability of the diabetes. Although the symptoms vary from individual to individual, they tend to have a characteristic pattern for each subject. Rapid decline in plasma sugar usually triggers the sympathetic nervous system with symptoms characteristic of autonomic nervous system discharge. This constellation is most frequently seen in patients receiving short-acting insulin. Convulsions are more common in children than in adults, and most attacks are reverted spontaneously by endogenous counter-regulation or are aborted by food intake before marked cerebral cortical depression occurs. With intermediate and long-acting insulins, notably protamine zinc insulin, plasma sugar levels may decline more gradually without activating the sympathetic nervous system, resulting in depression of higher cortical centers and eventuating in convulsions or coma or both. Because of these adverse effects, many of the long-acting insulins have found disfavor among clinicians. A cardinal point to be emphasized in the management of such patients is the early recognition and prompt treatment of hypoglycemia. In the insulin-dependent diabetic who is first seen in an emergency room in a comatose state, it is obviously important to distinguish iatrogenic hypoglycemia from ketoacidosis. The major clinical and laboratory findings which differentiate these disorders are outlined in Table 10–8. If the physician is uncertain as to which is the cause of coma, it is wise to administer parenteral glucose promptly after obtaining a sample for glucose analysis, since in this instance, less cerebral damage results from an error of commission than from one of omission.

Sulfonylureas

Seltzer (86), in a recent review of the published cases of severe drug-induced hypoglycemia, found 220 of 473 cases attributable to sulfonylureas, with the greatest number due to chlorpropamide. The incidence of hypoglycemia with sulfonylureas is doubtless greater than is documented in the literature. It has been estimated that about 5% of individuals receiving oral hypoglycemic agents have glucopenic reactions. The proposed mechanisms of actions of sulfonylureas are discussed in Chapter 9. It is not known how these agents produce sustained hypoglycemia in susceptible subjects; however, it has been assumed that their major actions are to promote excessive insulin release and also to have a direct inhibitory effect on hepatic glucose output. Although the development of hypoglycemia after sulfonylureas may be idiosyncratic, there are a number of factors that predispose to the drug-induced glucopenia: (1) decreased food intake or chronic malnutrition, (2) age, particularly early youth or old age, (3) abnormality in hepatic and renal function, and (4) adrenal cortical insufficiency. Thus the adverse effects are most likely to be encountered in the older diabetic who is undernourished with impaired liver or renal function or both, leading to decreased metabolism and excretion of the drug. In addition, sulfonylurea-induced hypoglycemia may be potentiated by ethanol, salicylates, sulfonamides, bishydroxycoumarin, and phenylbutazone. Glucopenic reactions may be profound and last for many hours or days. Since it cannot be predicted in advance who may be sensitive to the sulfonylureas, it is important to avoid large doses in elderly subjects with abnormal liver or kidney function and to eliminate potentiating drugs. Phenethylbiguanide (phenformin) has been implicated in severe hypoglycemia in only two diabetic patients; one had lactic acidosis and coma,

TABLE 10-8. DIFFERENTIAL DIAGNOSIS IN COMA OF KNOWN DIABETIC

	Hypoglycemia	Ketoacidosis
History	Insufficient food, excess insulin, excess exercise.	Insufficient insulin, infection, gastrointestinal upset.
Onset	Following *short-acting insulin:* Suddenly, a few hours after injection. Following *long-acting insulin:* relatively slower, many hours after injection.	Gradual over many hours.
Course	Anxiety, sweating, hunger, headache, diplopia, incoordination, twitching, convulsions, coma. (Headache, nausea, and haziness especially following long-acting insulin.)	Polyuria, polydipsia, anorexia, nausea, vomiting, labored deep breathing, weakness, drowsiness, possible fever and abdominal pain, coma.
Physical findings	Pale moist skin, full rapid pulse, dilated pupils, normal breathing, blood pressure normal or elevated, overactive reflexes, positive Babinski sign.	Florid, dry skin, Kussmaul breathing with acetone odor, decreased blood pressure, weak rapid pulse, soft eyeballs.
Laboratory findings	Second urine specimen sugar- and ketone-free, low blood sugar, normal serum CO_2.	Urine contains sugar and ketone bodies, high blood sugar, low serum CO_2.

and the other attempted suicide unsuccessfully. Treatment of patients with severe protracted hypoglycemia from these agents requires hospitalization and parenteral glucose administration until the drug has been eliminated.

Ethanol

A diverse array of disturbances of mental function, disorders of personality, convulsions, and neurologic manifestations are sequelae of the chronic abuse of ethanol. Although this picture may occur in alcoholics with normal plasma sugar levels, it is now recognized that hypoglycemia may be a feature of ethyl alcohol ingestion and simulate the clinical presentation of acute alcoholic intoxication. The clinical and biochemical characteristics of ethanol-induced hypoglycemia have been extensively investigated by Freinkel (37), and the toxic effects on multiple biologic systems have been reviewed by Hawkins and Kalant (45). Alcoholic hypoglycemia is most frequently seen in a setting of chronic ethanol intake in an adult; however, a profound drop in plasma sugar may occur in binge-drinkers and also in adolescents during their first encounter with alcohol. In general, the typical alcoholic who develops hypoglycemia will be malnourished and will have been without food for some time prior to the onset of glucopenia. He may be brought to the emergency room either confused or comatose, with physical findings that are indistinguishable from those of acute alcoholic stupor. The unsuspecting physician may ascribe these features to intoxication rather than to neuroglucopenia, because of the odor of alcohol on the breath. Plasma glucose is usually below 45 mg./100 ml. and may be less than 10 mg./100 ml. Coincidently there is ketonuria with diminished plasma CO_2 content. Hepatic function, measured by conventional laboratory tests, may be marginally abnormal. Glycogenolytic responses to glucagon are markedly attenuated, and plasma insulin levels are low, with enhanced sensitivity to exogenously administered insulin and tolbutamide. The OGTT often reveals a diabetic type of configuration. In

animal models as well as in humans who have received sufficient intravenous ethanol to simulate intake to the level of mild intoxication, hypoglycemia is evoked during relatively short periods of fasting (within 72 hours); this suggests that alcohol interferes with gluconeogenesis. In healthy volunteers, the induction of ethanol glucopenia requires several days of preliminary fasting, whereas in chronic alcoholics, this occurs within a shorter period. Within the hepatic cytoplasm, alcohol is oxidized to acetate with simultaneous reduction of diphosphopyridine nucleotide (NAD to $NADH_2$). The increase in the $NADH_2:NAD$ ratio leads to a diversion of NAD from normal substrate oxidation required for gluconeogenesis. Gluconeogenic precursors, such as lactate and glutamate, which normally enter pathways via pyruvate or α-ketoglutarate, accumulate in the unfavorable redox environment. The net effect is to inhibit substrate flow, with eventual suppression of gluconeogenesis. Thus, in a setting of decreased glycogen reserves as in fasting, alcohol makes the recipient vulnerable to hypoglycemia. It is to be emphasized that glucopenia occurs not only in malnourished chronic alcoholics but also in weekend spree-drinkers and may be a potentiating factor in hypoglycemia in insulin-requiring diabetics and patients taking oral sulfonylureas. In most instances, the intravenous administration of glucose results in a prompt and dramatic cessation of all neurologic manifestations of hypoglycemia. Nevertheless, mortality in adults from ingestion of toxic amounts of alcohol is about 11% and in children, it has been reported as high as 25%. Prophylactically, susceptible alcoholics should be persuaded, if possible, to diminish ethanol intake and to eat more regularly.

Miscellaneous Compounds

A variety of pharmacologic agents and toxins have been implicated as causal agents of glucopenia in man. These substances either have an independent effect or potentiate the actions of previously described hypoglycemic drugs. In isolated case reports, salicylate, para-aminobenzoic acid, haloperidol, propoxyphene, and chlorpromazine have been incriminated as causes of profound hypoglycemia by mechanisms which presumably interfere with gluconeogenesis. Propranolol, a beta adrenergic blocker, may cause hypoglycemia in susceptible individuals who are (1) severely ill and undernourished, (2) diabetics on insulin or receiving sulfonylureas, (3) on a weight reduction program, (4) undergoing vigorous exercise, and (5) ingesting excessive amounts of alcohol. The mechanism is obscure; presumably, it is related to the adrenergic blocking activity of propranolol (76).

In Jamaica, profound hypoglycemia in association with protracted vomiting has been observed in individuals who have inadvertently eaten the unripened fruit of the tropical plant, *Blighia sapida* (ackee fruit). The amino acid L-α-amino-β-methylenecycloproprionic acid (hypoglycin) contained in the ackee fruit is converted to its acetic acid derivative in the liver, where it interferes with carnitine-dependent oxidation of long-chained fatty acids, thus limiting energy for generation of new glucose (13). Impaired fatty acid oxidation in muscle may also divert glucose to this tissue, thereby accentuating hypoglycemia. Treatment of these drug- or toxin-induced hypoglycemic episodes is by parenteral glucose administration and discontinuance of the intake of the offending substance.

REFERENCES

1. Anand, B. K., In *Handbook of Physiology. Alimentary Canal.* Code, C. F., and Heidel, W. (eds.), Washington, D. C., American Physiological Society, 1967, p. 249.
2. Anderson, J. W., and Herman, R. H.: Classification of reactive hypoglycemia. *Amer. J. Clin. Nutr.* 22:646, 1969.
3. Anderson, J. W., and Herman, R. H.: Treatment of reactive hypoglycemia with sulfonylureas. *Amer. J. Med. Sci.* 261:16, 1971.
4. Antony, G. J., Underwood, L. E., et al.: Studies in hypoglycemia of infancy and childhood. Diagnosis and treatment. *Amer. J. Dis. Child.* 114:345, 1967.
5. Arieff, A. I., Doerner, T., et al.: Studies on the mechanisms of hypoglycemic coma: Evidence for a direct effect of insulin on electrolyte transport in brain. *Clin. Res.* 21:615, 1973.
6. Arky, R. A.: Pathophysiology and therapy of the fasting hypoglycemias. *Disease-A-Month* (Chicago) 1–47, Feb., 1968.
7. Ashmore, J., and Weber, G.: Hormonal control of carbohydrate metabolism in liver, In *Carbohydrate Metabolism and Its Disorders.* Vol. 1. Dickens, F., Randle, P. J., et al. (eds.), New York, Academic Press, 1968, p. 354.
8. Balagura, S.: Neurophysiologic aspects: Hypothalamic factors in the control of eating behavior. *Advances Psychosom. Med.* 7:25, 1972
9. Bauer, H.: Severe and prolonged hypoglycemic shock during sulfonylurea treatment. *Metabolism* 14:220, 1965.
10. Baxter, J. D., and Forsham, P. H.: Tissue effects of glucocorticoids. *Amer. J. Med.* 53:573, 1972.
11. Bleicher, S. J., Levy, L. J., et al.: Glucagon-deficiency hypoglycemia: A new syndrome. *Clin. Res.* 18:355, 1970.
12. Brasel, J. A., Wright, J. C., et al.: An evaluation of seventy-five patients with hypopituitarism beginning in childhood. *Amer. J. Med.* 38:484, 1965.
13. Bressler, R., Corredor, C., et al.: Hypoglycin and hypoglycin-like compounds. *Pharmacol. Rev.* 21:105, 1969.
14. Breuer, R. I., Moses, H., et al.: Gastric operations and glucose homeostasis. *Gastroenterology* 62:1105, 1972.
15. Cahill, J. F., Jr.: Physiology of insulin in man. *Diabetes* 20:785, 1971.
16. Cahill, J. F., Jr.: Starvation in man. *New Eng. J. Med.* 282:668, 1970.
17. Cahill, J. F., Jr., Herrera, M. G., et al.: Hormone-fuel interrelationships during fasting. *J. Clin. Invest.* 45:1751, 1966.
18. Cochrane, W. A., Payne, W. W., et al.: Familial hypoglycemia precipitated by amino acids. *J. Clin. Invest.* 35:411, 1956.
19. Colle, E., and Ulstrom, R. A.: Ketotic hypoglycemia. *J. Pediat.* 64:632, 1964.
20. Conn, J. W., and Seltzer, H. S.: Spontaneous hypoglycemia. *Amer. J. Med.* 19:460, 1955.
21. Cornblath, M.: Hypoglycemia, In *Carbohydrate Metabolism and Its Disorders.* Vol. 2. Dickens, F., Randle, P. J., et al. (eds.), New York, Academic Press, 1967, p. 51.
22. Crain, E. L., Jr., and Thorn, G. W.: Functional pancreatic islet cell adenomas. *Medicine* 28:427, 1949.
23. Creutzfeldt, W., Feurle, G., et al.: Effect of gastrointestinal hormones on insulin and glucagon secretion. *New Eng. J. Med.* 282:1139, 1970.
24. Dancis, J., and Levitz, M.: Abnormalities of branched-chain amino acid metabolism, In *The Metabolic Basis of Inherited Disease.* 3rd ed. Stanbury, J. B., Wyngaarden, J. B., et al. (eds.), New York, McGraw-Hill, 1972, p. 426.
25. DeBodo, R. C., and Altszuler, N.: Insulin hypersensitivity and physiological insulin antagonists. *Physiol. Rev.* 38:389, 1958.
26. Dunn, D. C.: Diabetes after removal of insulin tumors of pancreas. A long-term follow-up survey of 11 patients. *Brit. Med. J.* 1:84, 1971.
27. Ehrlich, R. M., and Martin, J. M.: Tolbutamide tolerance test and plasma insulin response in children with idiopathic hypoglycemia. *J. Pediat.* 71:485, 1967.
28. Elias, E., Polak, J. M., et al.: Pancreatic cholera due to production of gastric inhibitory polypeptide. *Lancet* 2:791, 1972.
29. Ellison, E. H., and Wilson, S. D.: Ulcerogenic tumor of the pancreas, In *Progress in Clinical Cancer.* Vol. 3. Ariel, I. M. (ed.), New York, Grune & Stratton, 1967, p. 225.
30. Ensinck, J. W., and Williams, R. H.: Hormonal and nonhormonal factors modifying man's response to insulin, In *Handbook of Physiology. Endocrine Pancreas.* Steiner, D. S., and Freinkel, N. (eds.), Washington, D. C., American Physiological Society, 1972, p. 665.
31. Exton, J. H.: Gluconeogenesis. *Metabolism* 21:945, 1972.
32. Fajans, S. S., Schneider, J. M., et al.: The diagnostic value of sodium tolbutamide in hypoglycemic states. *J. Clin. Endocr.* 21:371, 1961.
33. Fajans, S. S., Floyd, J. C., Jr., et al.: Mechanisms involved in the hyperglycemic action of diazoxide. Usefulness in the treatment of patients with functioning pancreatic islet cell tumors, In *Diabetes.* Östman, J. (ed.), Amsterdam, Excerpta Medica Foundation, 1969, p. 887.
34. Fajans, S. S., and Floyd, J. C., Jr.: Stimulation of islet cell secretion by nutrients and by gastrointestinal hormones released during digestion, In *Handbook of Physiology. Endocrine Pancreas.* Steiner, D. S., and Freinkel, N. (eds.), Washington, D. C., American Physiological Society, 1972, p. 473.
35. Felig, P.: Interaction of insulin and amino acid metabolism in the regulation of gluconeogenesis. *Israel J. Med. Sci.* 8:262, 1972.
36. Floyd, J. C., Jr., Fajans, S. S., et al.: Plasma insulin in organic hyperinsulinism: Comparative effects of tolbutamide, leucine, and glucose. *J. Clin. Endocr.* 24:747, 1964.
37. Freinkel, N., Cohn, A. K., et al.: Alcohol hypoglycemia: A prototype of the hypoglycemias induced in the fasting state, In *Diabetes.* Östman, J. (ed.), Amsterdam, Excerpta Medica Foundation, 1969, p. 873.
38. Freinkel, N., and Metzger, B. E.: Oral glucose tolerance curve and hypoglycemia in the fed state. *New Eng. J. Med.* 28:820, 1969.
39. Froesch, E. R.: Essential fructosuria and hereditary fructose intolerance, In *The Metabolic Basis of Inherited Disease.* 3rd ed. Stanbury, J. B., Wyngaarden, J. B., et al. (eds.), New York, McGraw-Hill, 1972, p. 131.
40. Goodman, H. G., Morishima, A., et al.: The use of diazoxide in hypoglycemia in childhood. *Ann. N. Y. Acad. Sci.* 150:367, 1968.

41. Gray, G. M.: Intestinal digestion and maldigestion of dietary carbohydrates. *Amer. Rev. Med. 22*:391, 1971.

42. Gray, R. K., Rösch, J., et al.: Arteriography in the diagnosis of islet-cell tumors. *Radiology 97*:39, 1970.

43. Greenblatt, M., Murray, J., et al.: Electroencephalographic studies in diabetes mellitus. *New Eng. J. Med. 234*:119, 1946.

44. Grollman, A., McCaleb, W. E., et al.: Glucagon deficiency as a cause of hypoglycemia. *Metabolism 13*:686, 1964.

45. Hawkins, R. D., and Kalant, H.: The metabolism of ethanol and its metabolic effects. *Pharmacol. Rev. 24*:67, 1972.

46. Himms-Hagen, J.: Sympathetic regulation of metabolism. *Pharmacol. Rev. 19*:367, 1967.

47. Himwich, H. E.: *Brain Metabolism and Cerebral Disorders.* Baltimore, Williams and Wilkins Co., 1951.

48. Hollobaugh, S. L., Rao, M. B., et al.: Studies on the site and mechanism of action of phenformin. *Diabetes 19*:45, 1970.

49. Howard, J. M., Moss, N. H., et al.: Collective review: Hyperinsulinism and islet cell tumors of the pancreas. *Int. Abstr. Surg. 90*:417, 1950.

50. Howell, R. R.: The glycogen storage diseases, In *The Metabolic Basis of Inherited Disease.* 3rd ed. Stanbury, J. B., Wyngaarden, J. B., et al. (eds.), New York, McGraw-Hill, 1972, p. 149.

51. Ireland, P., Sapira, J. D., et al.: Munchausen's syndrome. *Amer. J. Med. 43*:579, 1967.

52. Javier, A., and Gershberg, H.: Leucine-sensitive hypoglycemia. *Amer. J. Med. 41*:638, 1966.

53. Kalkhoff, R. K., Richardson, B. L., et al.: Relative effects of pregnancy, human placental lactogen and prednisolone on carbohydrate tolerance in normal and subclinical diabetic subjects. *Diabetes 18*:153, 1969.

54. Kavlie, H., and White, T. T.: Pancreatic islet beta cell tumors and hyperplasia. *Ann. Surg. 175*:326, 1972.

55. Khurana, R. C., Dhawer, V. P. S., et al.: Glucose, tolbutamide and leucine tolerances in hypoglycemia. Reactive hypoglycemia as a variant of normal or chemical diabetes mellitus. *Postgrad. Med. 53*:118, 1973.

56. Khurana, R. C., Nolan, S., et al.: Insulin and glucose patterns in control subjects and in proven insulinoma. *Amer. J. Med. Sci. 262*:115, 1971.

57. Kreisberg, R. A., and Pennington, L. F.: Tumor hypoglycemia: A heterogeneous disorder. *Metabolism 19*:445, 1970.

58. Laurent, J., Debry, G., et al.: *Hypoglycemic Tumors.* Amsterdam, Excerpta Medica Foundation, 1971.

59. Levin, M. E.: Endocrine syndromes associated with pancreatic islet cell tumors. *Med. Clin. N. Amer. 52*:295, 1968.

60. Lopez-Kruger, R., and Dockerty, M. B.: Tumors of the islets of Langerhans. *Surg. Gynec. Obstet. 85*:495, 1947.

61. Loubatière, A.: Therapeutic modification of islet function, In *Handbook of Physiology. Endocrine Pancreas.* Steiner, D. S., and Freinkel, N. (eds.), Washington, D. C., American Physiological Society, 1972, p. 660.

62. Luft, R., and Cerasi, E.: Human growth hormone as a regulator of blood glucose concentration and as a diabetogenic substance. *Diabetologia 4*:1, 1968.

63. Luyckx, A. S., and Lefebvre, P. J.: Plasma insulin in reactive hypoglycemia. *Diabetes 20*:435, 1971.

64. Marks, V., and Rose, F. C.: *Hypoglycaemia.* Oxford, Blackwell, 1965.

65. Marks, V., and Samols, E.: Diazoxide therapy of intractable hypoglycemia. *Ann. N. Y. Acad. Sci. 150*:442, 1968.

66. Marks, V., and Samols, E.: Diagnostic tests for evaluating hypoglycemia, In *Diabetes.* Östman, J. (ed.), Amsterdam, Excerpta Medica Foundation, 1969, p. 864.

67. McCann, M. L., Chen, C. H., et al.: Prevention of hypoglycemia by fructose in infants of diabetic mothers. *New Eng. J. Med. 275*:1, 1966.

68. McFadzean, A. J. S., and Yeung, R. T. T.: Further observations on hypoglycemia in hepatocellular carcinoma. *Amer. J. Med. 47*:220, 1969.

69. McIlwain, H.: *Biochemistry of the Central Nervous System.* London, J. & A. Churchill, 1966, p.13.

70. McQuarrie, I.: Idiopathic spontaneously occurring hypoglycemia in infants. *Amer. J. Dis. Child. 87*:399, 1954.

71. Melani, F., and Steiner, D. F.: On the pathogenesis of diabetes mellitus. *Acta Diabet. Lat. 7*(Suppl. 1):107, 1970.

72. Pagliara, A. S., Karl, I. E., et al.: Hypoglycemia in infancy and childhood. Parts I and II. *J. Pediat. 82*:365 & 558, 1973.

73. Pecile, A., and Müller, E. E. (eds.), *Growth and Growth Hor-*mone. Amsterdam, Excerpta Medica Foundation, 1971.

74. Raivio, K. O., and Oesterlund, K.: Hypoglycemia and hyperinsulinemia associated with erythroblastosis fetalis. *Pediatrics 43*:217, 1969.

75. Rehfeld, J., Heding, L. G., et al.: Increased gut glucagon release as pathogenetic factor in reactive hypoglycemia. *Lancet 1*:116, 1973.

76. Reveno, W. S., and Rosenbaum, H.: Propranolol and hypoglycaemia. *Lancet 1*:920, 1968.

77. Rimoin, D. L., and Schimke, R. N.: *Genetic Disorders of the Endocrine Glands.* St. Louis, C. V. Mosby Co., 1971.

78. Rosenbloom, A. L., and Sherman, L.: The natural history of idiopathic hypoglycemia of infancy and its relation to diabetes mellitus. *New Eng. J. Med. 274*:815, 1966.

79. Samols, E.: Hypoglycemia in neoplasia. *Postgrad. Med. J. 39*:634, 1963.

80. Samols, E., Tyler, J., et al.: Glucagon-insulin interrelationships, In *Glucagon. Molecular Physiology, Clinical and Therapeutic Implications.* Lefebvre, J., and Unger, R. H. (eds.), New York, Pergamon Press, 1972, p. 151.

81. Schein, P.S.: Chemotherapeutic management of the hormone-secreting endocrine malignancies. *Cancer 30*:1616, 1972.

82. Scheinberg, P.: Observations on cerebral carbohydrate metabolism in man. *Ann. Intern Med. 62*:367, 1966.

83. Schnelle, N., Molnar, J. D., et al.: Circulating glucose and insulin in surgery for insulinomas. *J.A.M.A. 217*:1072, 1971.

84. Scholz, D. A., ReMine, W. H., et al.: Clinics on endocrine and metabolic diseases. Hyperinsulinism: review of 95 cases of functioning pancreatic islet cell tumors. *Proc. Staff Meet. Mayo Clin. 35*:545, 1960.

85. Segal, S.: Disorders of galactose metabolism, In *The Metabolic Basis of Inherited Disease.* 3rd ed. Stanbury, J. B., Wyngaarden, J. B., et al. (eds.), New York, McGraw-Hill, 1972, p. 174.

86. Seltzer, H. S.: Drug-induced hypoglycemia. *Diabetes 21*:955, 1972.

87. Shelley, H. J., and Neligan, G. A.: Neonatal hypoglycemia. *Brit. Med. Bull. 22*:34, 1966.

88. Shultz, K. T., Neelon, F. A., et al.: Mechanism of postgastrectomy hypoglycemia. *Arch. Intern. Med. 128*:240, 1971.

89. Silverstein, M. N., Wakim, K. G., et al.: Role of tryptophan metabolites in the hypoglycemia associated with neoplasia. *Cancer 19*:127, 1966.

90. Spellacy, W. N.: A review of carbohydrate metabolism and the oral contraceptives. *Amer. J. Obstet. Gynec. 104*:448, 1969.

91. Sussman, K. E., Stimmler, L., et al.: Plasma insulin levels during reactive hypoglycemia. *Diabetes 15*:1, 1966.

92. Tata, J. R.: Biological action of thyroid hormones at the cellular and molecular level, In *Actions of Hormones on Molecular Processes.* Litwak, G., and Kritchevsky, D. (eds.), New York, Wiley, 1964, p. 58.

93. Tietze, H. U., Zurbrügg, R. P., et al.: Occurrence of impaired cortisol regulation in children with hypoglycemia associated with adrenal medullary hyporesponsiveness. *J. Clin. Endocr. 34*:948, 1972.

94. Todd, R. M., Rickham, P. P., et al.: Islet cell tumor of the newborn. *Helv. Paediat. Acta 27*:131, 1972.

95. Turner, D. S., and Marks, V.: Enhancement of glucose-stimulated insulin release by an intestinal polypeptide in rats. *Lancet 1*:1095, 1972.

96. Turner, R. C., Oakley, N. W., et al.: Control of basal insulin secretion with special reference to the diagnosis of insulinomas. *Brit. Med. J. 2*:132, 1971.

97. Unger, R. H., and Lefebvre, P.: Glucagon physiology, In *Glucagon. Molecular Physiology, Clinical and Therapeutic Implications.* Lefebvre, J., and Unger, R. H. (eds.), New York, Pergamon Press, 1972, p. 213.

98. Vendsalu, A.: Studies on adrenaline and nor-adrenaline in human plasma. *Acta Physiol. Scand. 49*(Suppl. 173):1, 1960.

99. Wajchenberg, B. L., Pereira, A. A., et al.: On the mechanism of insulin hypersensitivity in adrenocortical insufficiency. *Diabetes 13*:170, 1964

100. Yalow, R. S., and Berson, S. A.: Dynamics of insulin secretion in hypoglycemia. *Diabetes 14*:341, 1965.

101. Zieve, L., Jones, D. G., et al.: Functional hypoglycemia and peptic ulcer. *Postgrad Med. J. 40*:159, 1966.

102. Zimmerman, H. J., Thomas, L. J., et al.: Fasting blood sugar in hepatic disease with reference to infrequency of hypoglycemia. *Arch Intern. Med. 91*:577, 1953.

CHAPTER 11

Parathyroid Hormone, Calcitonin, and the Calciferols*

By Howard Rasmussen

*The writing of this chapter has been greatly aided by the help of numerous colleagues: Drs. Claude and Sara Arnaud, Dr. Ralph Goldsmith, Dr. Larry Riggs, and Dr. Lynwood Smith, all of the Mayo Clinic; Dr. John Haddad of Washington University; Dr. Bryan Brewer of the National Institutes of Health; Dr. Olav Bijvoet of the University of Leiden; Dr. Stanley Garn of the University of Michigan; Dr. Hector DeLuca of the University of Wisconsin; and Dr. Constantine Anast of the University of Missouri. I am particularly indebted to Dr. Philippe Bordier of Paris for the entire discussion of bone remodeling concepts, and to Dr. Daniel Bikle, Dr. Ralph Goldsmith, and Dr. David Baylink, who have served as critical reviewers of this chapter. No effort has been made within these pages to give specific credit to individuals for the recent developments in this field. To name them all is impossible, but I have included a list of selected references.

660

INTRODUCTION

As well as being an essential structural component of the skeleton, calcium plays a key role in many fundamental biologic processes. Its concentration in cellular and extracellular fluids is constant, in spite of marked variations in intake and excretion. The highly developed multicellular organism has a complex system of controls to ensure this constancy. These controls are predominantly hormonal in nature. Three hormones are of most immediate importance: vitamin D, parathyroid hormone, and calcitonin.

The history of these agents began with the recognition of rickets nearly three centuries ago, but our understanding of the nature of these controls began to develop in the latter part of the last century. At this time, Sandstrom, Gley, and others made the anatomical distinction between the parathyroid and the thyroid glands. A few years later, in 1898, Vassale and Generali established the relationship between parathyroidectomy and the onset of severe and fatal tetany. Simultaneously, Welsh reported the first adequate histologic description of these organs, and Groschuff and Kurtsteiner described their embryologic origin. Shortly thereafter, in 1903, Erdheim noted the relationship of these glands to bone diseases. These investigations initiated an intensive study of the histology of the parathyroids. As early as 1904, Askanazy suggested, on the basis of postmortem findings, an association between tumors of the parathyroid glands and the fibrocystic disease of bone which had been described by von Recklinghausen in 1891. In 1906, Erdheim observed that the parathyroid glands were enlarged in a patient with osteomalacia and correctly surmised that the osseous changes were primary and that the parathyroid enlargement was a secondary manifestation. From these and similar observations, the concept emerged that enlargement of the parathyroid glands was a secondary consequence of bone disease. However, Schlangenhaufer in 1915 and Maresch in 1916 proposed that in some instances enlargement of the parathyroids was the cause rather than the result of bone disease and recommended parathyroidectomy as the rational treatment. This was not adopted until 1926 when Mandl in Vienna reported the first successful removal of a parathyroid adenoma from a patient with bone disease.

Across the Atlantic, American physiologists had begun work in a seemingly unrelated field of study. Loeb in 1901 reported that muscular twitching could be produced by the injection of a variety of agents, all of which were capable of precipitating calcium *in vitro*. This was followed by the demonstration that the calcium content of the blood was less than normal in patients with tetany. Shortly thereafter, Netter observed clinical improvement in three cases of tetany following the oral administration of calcium salts. In 1908 MacCallum and Voegtlin were able to relieve the tetany induced by complete parathyroidectomy by administering calcium salts and proposed that the function of the parathyroid glands was to regulate calcium exchange. This report was followed by the observations of Greenwald that, in addition to changes in calcium metabolism, there was, following parathyroidectomy, a decrease in the excretion of phosphate in the urine and an elevation in the concentration of this ion in the blood. Greenwald concluded that the retention of phosphate was an important factor in the pathogenesis of tetany. In spite of these chemical correlations and reasonable deductions, there continued to be a widespread belief that the parathyroids played a predominantly antitoxic or detoxifying function in the body. This belief persisted for nearly ten years. In 1921, however, Kramer and Tisdall devised a method for measuring microscopic quantities of calcium in small samples of blood plasma. The introduction of this method led to a reinvestigation of the relationship between the parathyroid glands and calcium metabolism. Collip and his associates then confirmed the endocrine nature of the parathyroid glands and their role in the regulation of calcium and phosphate metabolism. In 1925 they, along with Hanson, announced the preparation of a stable acid extract of these glands which was capable of relieving tetany in thyroparathyroidectomized dogs and of elevating the plasma calcium concentration in normal or thyroparathyroidectomized animals. Shortly thereafter, Aub and Bauer demonstrated the effectiveness of this agent in man. These physiologic data led DuBois to the diagnosis of the first case of hyperparathyroidism in America, unaware that a few months earlier Mandl in Europe had successfully removed a parathyroid adenoma from such a patient. Within a few years, a number of cases of hyperparathyroidism had been described, and Albright had begun his classic studies on the physiology of these organs in man and their relationship to a variety of metabolic bone diseases.

Together with these developments came the understanding of the relationship between rickets and vitamin D. About 1920 Mellanby discerned an association between rickets and the presence in the diet of a fat-soluble substance capable of preventing or curing this disease. This was followed by Steenbock's description of a routine method for the preparation of this vitamin and its addition to foodstuffs. Shortly thereafter, in 1931, Angus and his associates described the isolation and characterization of this vitamin. At approximately the same time, Albright demonstrated its usefulness in the treatment of hypoparathyroidism. Shortly thereafter, McLean and Hastings published their nomogram concerning the relationship between tetany and the ionized calcium concentration of plasma.

Interest waned over the next 15 to 20 years, but the past 25 years have seen an explosive increase in our knowledge of the hormonal control of both calcium and phosphate homeostasis, and of skeletal remodeling. Parathyroid hormone (PTH) has been isolated, characterized, and synthesized. Calcitonin (CT) has been discovered, isolated, characterized, and synthesized. The complex sequence of cholecalciferol (vitamin D_3) metabolism has been elucidated. The biologically active metabolites of vitamin D_3 have been identified as 25-hydroxycholecalciferol [25(OH)D_3] and 1,25-dihydroxycholecalciferol [1,25(OH)$_2D_3$]. Great progress has been made toward elucidating the mode of action of all three major hormones [PTH, CT, and 1,25(OH)$_2D_3$], and new insights have been gained into the nature of mineral homeostasis, skeletal remodeling, and metabolic bone diseases by the application of quantitative microradiographic and histologic techniques to the study of bone cells and bone structure.

MINERAL METABOLISM

A discussion of the endocrine control of mineral metabolism and bone remodeling divides itself naturally in several ways. A fundamental division, the distinction between mineral homeostasis and skeletal remodeling, depends upon the fact that the endoskeleton of higher organisms serves two important functions: a mechanical supportive, locomotive, and protective function; and a metabolic function in the maintenance of a dynamic steady state of ionic constituents of the body's extracellular fluids. To best serve the first of these functions, the skeleton normally undergoes a process of continual remodeling throughout life. This remodeling is responsive to changes in the mechanical stresses placed upon the skeleton. It is also responsive to, and regulated in part by, the concentrations of many of the hormones of the body: parathyroid hormone, calcitonin, 1,25-dihydroxycholecalciferol, thyroxine, growth hormone, gonadal hormones, and adrenal glucocorticoids, to mention the most important.

All these hormones also influence bodily mineral homeostasis, but the three of major importance are PTH, CT, and 1,25(OH)$_2D_3$. In maintaining mineral homeostasis, these three hormones act not only upon the skeleton but also upon the intestine and kidney. Because of the common participation of bone cells in both skeletal remodeling and mineral homeostasis, these two processes are interrelated. It is possible, however, to have conditions in which skeletal remodeling is greatly increased (e.g., Paget's disease) or decreased without significant derangement of plasma mineral homeostasis. Likewise, it is possible to have disorders of calcium homeostasis (e.g., hypercalcemia) with either high or low rates of skeletal remodeling. Finally, in many conditions, a derangement of mineral homeostasis will lead to an alteration in skeletal remodeling (e.g., vitamin D deficiency).

A second natural division is that between events at the subcellular and cellular levels of biologic organization, on the one hand, and the extracellular level on the other. Of greatest interest is the fact that it has become possible to relate the behavior of the homeostatic system of the organism directly to the behavior of isolated cellular systems and to the adaptation and extension of systems developed early in cellular evolution to maintain intracellular calcium homeostasis. For this reason, discussion will begin with a consideration of the cellular metabolism of calcium, phosphate, hydrogen ion, and to a lesser extent magnesium, because these form within the cells the basic ionic net upon which the extracellular controls operate.

Cellular Mineral Metabolism

The relationship between Ca^{2+}, HPO_4^{2-} and H^+ in an idealized mammalian cell is shown in Figure 11–1 and Table 11–1. In the case of Ca^{2+}, its concentration in the extracellular fluid is normally approximately 10^{-3} M, in the cell cytosol 10^{-6} to 10^{-7} M, and in the mitochondria 10^{-4} M. In the mitochondria, however, there is an additional large pool of complexed calcium (as its phosphate salt). Moreover, as shown in Figure 11–1 and Table 11–1, phosphate and hydrogen ions are asymmetrically distributed among the three compartments. These ionic asymmetries are maintained by the expenditure of metabolic energy by the cell. There is either a calcium pump or a Na^+ gradient-mediated calcium efflux across the cell membrane, and a primary H^+ pump at the mitochondrial membrane, which leads to an energy-dependent Ca^{2+}-H^+ exchange across this membrane. Phosphate exchanges appear to be passive. Because the intrami-

TABLE 11–1. ESTIMATED ION ACTIVITIES IN THE VARIOUS FLUID PHASES OF A TYPICAL MAMMALIAN CELL

Fluid Phase	H^+	Ca^{2+}	HPO_4^{2-}
ECF	4×10^{-8}M	5×10^{-4}	2×10^{-4}
Cytosol	1.5×10^{-7}	2.5×10^{-7}	1×10^{-4}
Mitochondria-S	1.2×10^{-8}	0.2×10^{-4}	5×10^{-4}
Mitochondria-I*	—	1.6×10^{-3}	1.1×10^{-3}

*All values for phases are given as ion activities except the values of insoluble mitochondrial phase (mitochondria-I), which are given as moles per liter of mitochondrial H_2O.

tochondrial pH is maintained higher than that in the cytosol, Ca^{2+} taken up by the mitochondria interacts with phosphate to form a complex, with the release of H^+. This large pool of non-ionic calcium and phosphate within the mitochondria serves as a buffer for all three ions: Ca^{2+}, HPO_4^{2-} and H^+. It is one of the fundamental cell buffer systems. If, for example, the phosphate concentration in the extracellular fluids is increased, the cytosolic phosphate concentration rises, and the phosphate concentration in the mitochondrial ionic compartment increases. This leads to the formation of $Ca_3(PO_4)_2$ within the mitochondria, to a fall in cytosolic $[Ca^{2+}]$, to a rise in cytosolic $[H^+]$, and eventually to an increased uptake of Ca^{2+} by the cell. On the other hand, an increase in extracellular $[H^+]$ will lead eventually to a liberation of some of the complexed calcium and phosphate within the mitochondria and an increase in the concentration of both Ca^{2+} and HPO_4^{2-} within the cell cytosol.

This basic net is also clearly coupled to the other major cellular and extracellular buffer system: the CO_2/HCO_3^- system. This in turn is linked directly to cell metabolism, because CO_2 is one of the major end products of cellular metabolism. One of the most primitive controls of this complex system is exerted by H^+. When intracellular pH falls, glycolysis is inhibited at the phosphofructokinase

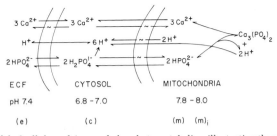

Figure 11–1. A schematic model of cellular calcium and phosphate metabolism illustrating the relationship between the activities of these two ions and H^+ in the extracellular fluids, the cell cytosol, and the mitochondrial matrix space (see also Table 11–1). Of major importance is the fact that there is an asymmetric distribution of these ions between the various fluid compartments (Table 11–1) which is maintained by the metabolic activity of the cell. In addition, the calcium and phosphate within the mitochondrial matrix space exist in two forms, as separate soluble ions and as an un-ionized complex $[Ca_3(PO_4)_2]$. When the complex is formed, H^+ is released. This means that the entire system operates as a major cell buffer system for Ca^{2+}, HPO_4^{2-}, and H^+. Moreover, because the Ca^{2+} distribution across the cell membrane is determined in part by the Na^+ gradient, the $[Na^+]$ on the two sides of this membrane influences Ca^{2+} permeability. Thus the system controlling calcium and phosphate distribution is coupled to that controlling monovalent cation distribution. Finally, because of the relationship between H^+ and the calcium phosphate system, this latter system is coupled to the cellular and extracellular bicarbonate/CO_2 buffer system. The whole forms an ionic net within the cellular and extracellular fluids which forms an important regulatory system in cell function and response. The symbols (e), (c), (m), and $(m)_i$ represent the extracellular space, the cytosolic space, the mitochondrial matrix space, and the insoluble calcium phosphate pool within the mitochondria, respectively.

step, but isocitrate dehydrogenase is activated, leading to a decrease in fixed acids (lactate, citrate, and isocitrate) within the cell and an increase in the production of the weak acid, CO_2, so that the change in pH is limited by the substitution of a weak volatile acid for strong nonvolatile ones.

In most cells the absolute rates (per unit surface area) of calcium flux across cellular and mitochondrial membranes are of the same order of magnitude. However, the total extent of the surface area of the inner mitochondrial membrane is 100 to 10,000 times greater than that of the plasma membrane. For this reason, it is evident that changes in calcium flux across the mitochondrial membrane are of key importance in the control of the $[Ca^{2+}]_c$ of the cell cytosol.

Control of Cell Calcium Metabolism

Control of the $[Ca^{2+}]$ of the cell cytosol is of key importance in the regulation of metabolic events in a wide variety of cell types. Changes in the $[Ca^{2+}]$ of the cell cytosol regulate muscle contraction, exocrine and endocrine secretion, neurotransmitter secretion, hormone action, and energy metabolism in a wide variety of cells. Two basic mechanisms have evolved to regulate the $[Ca^{2+}]$ in the cell cytosol.

The first mechanism operates in various types of muscle cells and probably in many secretory cells. It involves the release of calcium which is bound either to that membrane or to a specialized extension of that membrane, the sarcoplasmic reticulum. Depolarization of the plasma membrane leads to a release of bound Ca^{2+} and an increase in the permeability of the membrane to calcium, so that the rate of flux of Ca^{2+} from extracellular fluids to cell cytosol increases. Within the cytosol Ca^{2+} ions act as second or intracellular messengers, and in skeletal muscle as a "trigger" initiating the release of the Ca^{2+} stored in the sarcoplasmic reticulum.

The second mechanism involves a coupling between events at the cell surface with those at the mitochondrial membrane. It is most clearly illustrated by the action of a number of peptide hormones (including PTH) upon their respective target tissues. In this mechanism, interaction of a first messenger (hormone) with its receptor site on the cell surface leads to two events: an activation of the enzyme, adenyl cyclase, and an increase in Ca^{2+} permeability of the cell membrane. The resulting increase in C-AMP within the cell has at least two actions: an activation of a class of enzymes, protein kinases, and an increase in the efflux of Ca^{2+} from the mitochondria. This latter action may be mediated by a C-AMP-dependent phosphorylation of the mitochondrial membrane by a kinase, but this remains to be established. The combined effect of the first messenger on calcium entry from the ECF and of C-AMP on calcium entry from the mitochondrial pool leads to a rise in cytosolic $[Ca^{2+}]$, which has at least three important effects: (1) activation or inhibition of enzymes, some of which are the phosphoprotein products of C-AMP-dependent protein kinases; (2) inhibition of adenyl cyclase, i.e., a negative feedback loop in this basic cellular control system; and (3) changes in the permeability of the cell membrane to monovalent cations.

This model accounts for many aspects of the action of parathyroid hormone upon bone and kidney cells and forms the basis for considering the actions of CT and $1,25(OH)_2D_3$ on these cells. The mode of action of these hormones is discussed on page 692. The remaining considerations to be discussed at this juncture are the relationship of Mg^{2+} and the monovalent cations to the cellular ionic net.

The regulation of cellular Mg^{2+} homeostasis is poorly understood. Magnesium deprivation in humans or experimental animals leads to a fall in plasma Mg^{2+} concentration before there is any evident change in cell Mg^{2+} concentration. Nearly 60 per cent of the total cellular Mg^{2+} is within the mitochondrial compartment of the cell, and at least part of this fraction exists as a phosphate salt (similar to calcium). The cytosolic Mg^{2+} concentration has been estimated to be approximately 0.5 mM, and that within the mitochondrial matrix space 1.0 mM. These figures mean that Mg^{2+}, much like Ca^{2+}, is distributed asymmetrically within the body fluid compartments. Magnesium ions may share some common transport systems with Ca^{2+}. It is clear, however, that cellular Mg^{2+} and Ca^{2+} metabolism are regulated by independent factors, because the transport and metabolism of these ions differ in different hormonal states.

One of the most intriguing relationships, which remains to be fully explored, is that between thyroxine and cellular Mg^{2+}. Changes in the thyroid status of man or other mammals lead to changes in Mg^{2+} distribution between cellular and extracellular fluid compartments. Hyperthyroidism is characterized by a decrease in plasma Mg^{2+}, an increase in total cellular Mg^{2+}, and an increase in the rate of cellular Mg^{2+} and Ca^{2+} exchange. The converse is seen in hypothyroidism. The physiologic significance of these shifts is not known.

The relationship between Ca^{2+} and monovalent cations in cell function is complex. At the level of the cell membrane, Ca^{2+} acts as a stabilizing agent in the sense that the higher the extracellular $[Ca^{2+}]$, the less permeable the membrane to Na^+, K^+, and other ions. Conversely, in many cells, one of the determinants of the Ca^{2+} distribution across the cell membrane is the Na^+ gradient which, in turn, is maintained by the activity of the Na^+-K^+-activated ATPase. When intracellular $[Na^{2+}]$ increases, the cytosolic $[Ca^{2+}]$ also increases. Finally, changes in $[Ca^{2+}]$ within the cell cytosol influence the permeability properties of the cell membrane in a different way than do changes in extracellular $[Ca^{2+}]$. A rise of cytosolic $[Ca^{2+}]$ within the range of 10^{-7} to 10^{-5} M leads to an increase in K^+ permeability and, in some cells at least, to an increase in Na^+ permeability as well. These very complex interrelationships mean that whenever the concentration of one ion, e.g., Ca^{2+}, changes within the cytosolic compartment of the cell, the concentrations of the others, including H^+, HPO_4^{2-}, Mg^{2+}, Na^+, and K^+, also change. This ionic net operating within the cell acts as a complex buffer system maintaining ionic homeostasis. It also acts as an amplifying system for the signal initiated by first messenger-receptor interaction at the cell surface.

Extracellular Mineral Metabolism

The homeostatic mechanisms responsible for the control of extracellular mineral metabolism are dependent upon organ autoregulation and hormonal control. The hormones of greatest importance are PTH, CT, and $1,25(OH)_2D_3$. The ions of greatest interest are calcium, phosphate, pyrophosphate, hydrogen, and magnesium. Before the nature and mechanism of action of the three hormones are considered, current knowledge about extracellular mineral metabolism will be reviewed.

Calcium

The average adult human body contains approximately 1,000 to 1,200 g. of calcium. Nearly 99 per cent of this resides in the hydroxyapatite crystals of bone. Approximately 1 g. exists in the extracellular fluids. With this enormous reservoir of bone mineral, the concentration of ionized calcium in plasma is maintained constant in the face of wide variations in intake and excretion. This is brought about by a highly complex system of controls. The main organs involved in this control are the intestine, kidney, bone, and, during lactation, the mammary gland. There are small losses in sweat.

State of Calcium in Extracellular Fluids

The calcium in plasma exists in three forms (Table 11–2): ionized, complexed to organic anions, and protein-bound. The total concentration is normally 2.45 mM or 10 mg. per 100 ml. Of the total, 46 per cent is protein-bound (primarily to serum albumin), and 54 per cent is ultrafilterable. Of the latter, 1.18 mM exists as ionized calcium, and the remainder, 0.16 mM, is complexed with phosphate, citrate, and other anions. The importance of these different forms is that the ionized calcium concentration is the important biologic variable that is controlled and that in turn regulates a variety of biologic processes. Hence an increase in plasma protein concentration may lead to a rise in total plasma calcium without a change in calcium ion concentration. Changes of this type do not represent fundamentsl disorders of calcium homeostasis, but a change in ionized calcium concentration usually does. The measurement of calcium ion concentration is not easily carried out, even though a new method using a calcium-sensitive

TABLE 11–2. FORMS OF CALCIUM AND PHOSPHATE IN NORMAL PLASMA*

	mmoles/L	% Total
Calcium		
Free ions	1.16	47.5
Protein-bound	1.14	46.0
CaHPO$_4$	0.04	1.6
CaCit$^-$	0.04	1.7
Unidentified complexes	0.07	3.2
Total	2.45	100.0
Phosphate		
Free HPO$_4^-$	0.50	43.0
Free H$_2$PO$_4^-$	0.11	10.0
Protein-bound	0.14	12.0
NaHPO$_4^-$	0.33	29.0
CaHPO$_4^-$	0.04	3.0
MgHPO$_4^-$	0.03	3.0
Total	1.15	100.0

*From Walser, M.: *J. Clin. Invest.* 40:723, 1961.

electrode has recently been developed. Because of this, it is customary to measure total plasma calcium and assume a normal distribution between the free and bound forms.

Both hypo- and hypercalcemia are commonly seen in metabolic bone diseases and disorders of calcium homeostasis. Their causes and treatments are discussed in later sections of this chapter.

It is worth noting at this point, however, that calcium is a coupling factor between excitation and secretion in a variety of endocrine organs, e.g., in the response of the beta cells of pancreatic islets to glucose and the cells of the adrenal cortex to ACTH. As a consequence, hypo- and hypercalcemia alter the responses of these cells to their normal stimuli. This means that the homeostatic system which operates to maintain plasma calcium homeostasis influences the responses of many of the other endocrine control systems.

Metabolism in Man

A schematic model of calcium metabolism in a normal adult human having a calcium intake of 1 g. per day is presented in Figure 11–2.

Calcium is absorbed primarily in the duodenum and upper jejunum. Its absorption is increased by hypocalcemia, vitamin D, parathyroid hormone, lactose, an acid environment in the intestine, growth hormone, and a proper amount and form of dietary phosphate. Its absorption is decreased by cortisol, excess unabsorbed fatty acids in the intestinal contents, excess inorganic phosphate, undigestible organic phosphates, and the ingestion of alkali.

In addition to the calcium ingested in the diet, some 600 mg. is added to the intestinal contents in the various intestinal secretions. Of the total of 1,600 mg., 700 mg. is reabsorbed, and 900 mg. appears in the feces.

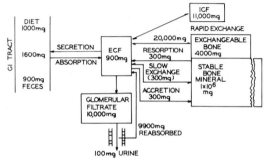

Figure 11–2. A schematic model of calcium metabolism in an adult human having a calcium intake of 1 g. per day. The net absorption of dietary calcium is 100 mg. per day. Secretion into the intestine is 300 mg. This is mixed with the 1000 mg. from the diet, and 400 mg. is absorbed. The 900 mg. of calcium in the extracellular fluids (ECF) exchanges with that in bone by three mechanisms: (1) rapid exchange; (2) slow exchange; and (3) accretion and resorption. Only the last processes lead to net movements of calcium into and out of bone. Extracellular fluid calcium also exchanges with that in the intracellular fluids (ICF). Approximately 10,000 mg. of calcium is filtered by the renal glomeruli, but nearly all is reabsorbed by the renal tubule; only 100 mg. is excreted in the urine.

Once absorbed, the calcium enters the extracellular pool. The calcium in this pool is being exchanged constantly with that in the intracellular fluids, the glomerular filtrate, and the bone. The entire extracellular pool exchanges 40 to 50 times each 24 hours. The two major pools with which it is in rapid exchange are the glomerular filtrate and the so-called exchangeable compartment of bone mineral.

The glomerular filtrate contains 10,000 mg. of calcium, but the renal tubular conservation of this ion is normally so complete that only 100 mg. appears in the urine each day. If hypercalcemia exists, the urinary excretion of calcium rises, but it rarely exceeds 500 mg. per day, even in situations of marked hypercalcemia. Because of the inability of the kidney to rid the body of excess calcium, hypercalcemia is often seen in metabolic bone diseases characterized by rapid bone destruction. Renal tubular reabsorption of calcium is increased by parathyroid hormone, by benzothiadiazine diuretics, by a fall in plasma calcium, and possibly by vitamin D. Calcium excretion is increased by saline diuresis, phosphate deprivation, acidosis, adrenal steroids, excess parathyroid hormone or vitamin D (in which case it results from the hypercalcemia), and excess thyroid hormone, even when no hypercalcemia is present.

The exact size and anatomical location of the pool of exchangeable bone mineral is not known. The term is derived from the behavior of radioactive calcium (Ca^{47}) injected intravenously into a normal human or animal. If the concentration of isotope in plasma is followed as a function of time, initially it is found to disappear very rapidly (within minutes), then at a less rapid but still significant rate (hours), and eventually more slowly, with a turnover time of days. The initial very rapid phase is due to mixing of Ca^{2+} in plasma and extracellular fluids; the next two phases are considered to represent an exchange of isotope between the calcium on the surface of bone crystals and that in plasma, and the fourth is presumed to represent the accretion of calcium into new bone mineral. The limitations of this technique are discussed on page 715. For the present, it is necessary only to indicate that part of the second phase probably represents an exchange between the calcium in the intracellular fluids of many tissues and that in plasma, and that the anatomical site of this exchangeable compartment in bone is not established.

In addition to short-term rapid exchange, the calcium in body fluids is slowly but constantly exchanging with that in the stable bone mineral. The magnitude of this exchange is difficult to estimate, but by all indications it is significant.

Aside from these isotopic exchanges, in which there is no net movement of calcium to or from the extracellular fluids, there are two processes, *bone resorption* and *bone formation* (or more correctly *mineral accretion*), which involve the net movement of calcium out of and into bone, respectively. In a normal young adult, these two processes are in balance, i.e., skeletal homeostasis is maintained.

One additional excretory route of calcium, not shown in Figure 11–2, is through the skin. Calcium ions are a normal component of sweat, and 30 to 120 mg. of calcium are excreted in this manner each day.

Plasma Calcium Homeostasis

The concentration of ionized calcium in the blood plasma is normally maintained within narrow limits. When this concentration is changed suddenly, either by the infusion of calcium or of a calcium chelating agent such as ethylenediamine tetraacetate (Fig. 11–3), the homeostatic system rapidly adjusts to meet this perturbation. Within 3

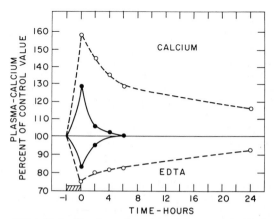

Figure 11–3. The change in plasma calcium concentration induced by calcium or EDTA infusions into dogs before (●———●) and several months after (○-----○) thyroparathyroidectomy. Note that the normal animal is able to respond quickly to either hypo- or hypercalcemia and the plasma calcium concentration is rapidly restored to the control value, but the thyroparathyroidectomized animal is unable to compensate quickly to either hypo- or hypercalcemia. (From Sanderson, P. H., Marshall, F., et al.: *J. Clin. Invest. 39*:661, 1960.)

to 4 hours after cessation of the infusion of sufficient agent to cause a significant change in ionized calcium, the value of plasma inonized calcium has normally returned to the initial concentration. As shown in Figure 11–3, however, if the thyroid and parathyroid glands are experimentally removed and the animal is maintained upon physiologic amounts of thyroxine, then the animal's response is quite different. Infusion of the same amount of calcium or calcium chelator leads, respectively, to a much greater rise or fall in plasma calcium concentration, and the original concentration is not reestablished, even 24 hours after the infusion has been terminated.

As will be discussed below (p. 695), the mammalian thyroid gland is the source of calcitonin, a peptide hormone that is secreted in response to an increase in plasma calcium concentration, which calcitonin lowers. The parathyroid glands are the source of the peptide hormone, parathyroid hormone, which is secreted in response to a fall in plasma calcium concentration, which parathyroid hormone increases. In the absence of both the thyroid and parathyroid glands, neither hormone is secreted in response to changes in plasma calcium concentration. As a consequence, the normal hormonal control of plasma calcium concentration does not take place. Eventually, however, the plasma calcium concentration will return to its initial concentration after such a perturbation, illustrating the principle that hormones generally do not initiate new reactions or processes but rather control the rates of existing physiologic processes.

In considering calcium homeostasis, three additional factors are of significance: (1) there is a circadian variation in plasma calcium concentration; (2) the age of the organism influences the response of the homeostatic system; and (3) the presence of the proper amount of vitamin D, or more accurately its active metabolite, $1,25(OH)_2D_3$, is necessary for the system to respond properly. The last two points will be discussed more fully subsequently.

A variation in the concentrations of plasma PTH, calcium, protein, phosphate, and growth hormone is seen in normal subjects throughout a 24-hour period. There is an early morning (4:00 A.M.) rise in both PTH and phosphate concentrations, preceded by a rise in growth hormone and accompanied by a fall in plasma albumin and calcium. There is probably a fall in plasma ionized calcium as well.

Inorganic Phosphate

The adult human body contains 500 to 600 g. of phosphate (measured as inorganic phosphorus), 85 per cent of which is in the skeleton. The remainder is located primarily in the organic and inorganic pools of intracellular phosphates.

State in Extracellular Fluids

In contrast to calcium, the concentration of plasma phosphate varies with age, diet, and hormonal status. In the human adult (Table 11–2), the range of values is 2.5 to 4.3 mg. per 100 ml. or a mean of 1.2 mM; in the rat, however, the values are 10 ± 1 mg. per 100 ml. The values in male children are slightly lower than female children. In younger children, the normal range is 5.0 to 6.0 mg. per 100 ml. The value is also high in cases of acromegaly. The state of ionization of uncomplexed phosphate in biologic fluids at physiologic pH has been calculated to be: (1) $HPO_4^{2-} - 0.50$ mM; (2) $H_2PO_4^- - 0.11$ mM and (3) $PO_4^{3-} - 8 \times 10^{-5}$ mM. Between 12 and 20 per cent of the phosphate is normally protein-bound, and a significant amount exists in the form of complexes with mono- or divalent cations. There is not universal agreement upon this point, but it is of considerable importance in any consideration of the manner in which the renal tubule handles phosphate.

The concentration of phosphate in plasma can be altered by changes in diet. In animals placed on low phosphate diets, the level may fall to values of 1.0 mg. per 100 ml. or less, with little change in the intracellular content of organic or inorganic phosphate. Some metabolic disorders lead to changes in plasma phosphate concentration, many of which are discussed in a later section of this chapter.

In addition to playing a key role in the initiation of mineral accretion, phosphate is of central importance to cellular economy. The ribonucleic acids are polyphosphate polymers; the major lipid constituents of cellular membranes are phospholipids; the major sources of chemical energy for intracellular work are the phosphorylated adenine and guanine nucleotides; and inorganic phosphate is of central importance in the regulation of glycolysis and energy metabolism. In spite of this great importance, very little is known about the mechanism whereby the cells assure themselves of an adequate supply of phosphate.

Metabolism in Man

More than 70 per cent of ingested phosphate is absorbed from the intestinal tract. In the rat, the site of maximal absorption of phosphate is the midgut, in contrast to that for calcium, the duodenum. Absorption depends upon the presence of both sodium and calcium ions as well as metabolic energy. Absorption is increased by a low calcium diet, growth hormone, vitamin D, parathyroid hormone, and acids; it is decreased by a high calcium intake, beryllium poisoning, aluminum hydroxide ingestion, and greatly diminished calcium absorption.

The major excretory route for phosphate is the kidney. A 70-kg. man on a diet containing 900 mg. of phosphate per day will excrete 600 mg. in the urine. The renal handling of phosphate involves glomerular filtration, tubular reabsorption, and possibly tubular secretion. The latter is a point of continuing debate. The evidence in favor of tubular secretion is this: (1) net secretion is observed routinely in birds, reptiles, and amphibians; (2) net secretion is not commonly seen in mammals, but it is seen under certain experimental conditions, particularly if Walser's statement is correct that 10 to 20 per cent of the plasma phosphate does not appear in the glomerular filtrate; (3) lesions of the distal tubule may lead to a decreased response to parathyroid hormone, i.e., a lack of phosphaturia after hormone administration; and (4) the parathyroid hormone–induced phosphaturia is associated with an increased uptake or turnover or both of labeled phosphate (P^{32}) in various phosphate pools in the kidney cells.

The urinary excretion of inorganic phosphate is decreased by dietary phosphate deficiency, azotemic renal disease, growth or growth hormone administration, lactation, osteopetrosis, hypoparathyroidism, Addison's disease, and metastatic neoplasia of bone. Its excretion is increased in vitamin D excess, vitamin D deficiency with secondary hyperparathyroidism, hyperparathyroidism, acute osteoporosis of disuse, neoplasia of bone, acidosis, sarcoidosis, and a variety of renal tubular disorders.

Plasma Phosphate Homeostasis

When an animal is placed on a severely restricted intake of phosphate but a normal intake of vitamin D, the plasma phosphate falls sharply, phosphate disappears from the urine, and the animal develops rickets. In spite of these dramatic changes, there is very little change in total, acidsoluble, or inorganic phosphate in the cells. Either normal or increased levels of plasma calcium are observed, associated with increased intestinal absorption and urinary excretion of calcium as well as a negative calcium balance. Neither parathyroidectomy nor parathyroid hormone administration leads to any change in plasma calcium or phosphate in phosphate-deficient rats. However, starvation leads to a prompt rise in plasma phosphate and a fall in plasma calcium which are uninfluenced by parathyroid hormone. This situation may represent a mobilization of intracellular phosphate with a consequent deposition of calcium and phosphate into bone.

A major mechanism of phosphate conservation in states of phosphate deficiency is that of cessation of bone mineral deposition at specific sites on the bone matrix. Bone mineral formation may begin by the phosphorylation of specific sites on the bone matrix. This initial step is critically dependent upon the concentration in plasma of inorganic phosphate Hence, in states of phosphate deficiency, bone matrix (collagen) formation continues, but mineral accretion ceases, leading to rickets or osteomalacia. There is also evidence that bone resorption increases in severe phosphate deficiency, even though the PTH concentration in plasma is lower than normal.

Phosphate is also important in regulating bone formation and bone resorption, even that induced by PTH. In patients or experimental animals having increased rates of bone resorption, the administration of phosphate by mouth or vein leads to a marked decrease in urinary calcium excretion (see Figure 11–54). This effect has been known for nearly 30 years and has generally been attributed to an increased deposition (accretion) of mineral due to the elevation of the ion product (calcium × phosphate) in plasma. However, this decrease may also reflect a direct effect of phosphate upon the resorption process, because excretion of hydroxyproline may decrease in this circumstance, and the former is considered an independent indicator of the rate of bone resorption (cf. p. 673). In addition to enhancing bone mineral accretion, an increase in phosphate concentration in the extracellular fluids stimulates the formation of new bone matrix. These local effects of phosphate upon bone resorption and formation are also seen in studies of bone fragments grown in tissue culture (p. 690). Their importance lies in the fact that regulation of the complex processes of formation and resorption are brought about by changes both in hormonal concentrations and in the local ionic environment. The mechanism by which phosphate exerts these effects may be related to its effect upon cellular calcium metabolism (see Fig. 11–1). If, as discussed subsequently, the concentration of Ca^{2+} in the cytosol of bone cells is an important second messenger regulating both the activity and the proliferation of bone-forming and bone-resorbing cells, then an increase in phosphate concentration could cause a shift of Ca^{2+} from cytosol to mitochondria and inhibit these calcium-dependent processes.

A major effect of plasma phosphate deficiency is related to its effects upon red cell metabolism, oxygen affinity, and tissue respiration. Hypophosphatemia leads to a fall in 2,3-diphosphoglycerate and ATP concentrations in circulating red cells. Both of these metabolic products bind to hemoglobin, and both bind more strongly to deoxyhemoglobin than to oxyhemoglobin. Thus they serve as important components of the physiologic mechanisms involved in the release of oxygen from red cells in the peripheral tissue. A fall in their concentrations leads to an increased hemoglobin-oxygen affinity, which in turn impairs the delivery of oxygen to the peripheral tissues. It has been proposed that, in children with familial hypophosphatemia (p. 761), an alteration in tissue-oxygen delivery might well be a component of the observed decrease in growth rate. However, it is also possible that in other tissues such as bone, which depends upon high rates of aerobic glycolysis, phosphate deficiency can lead directly to changes in energy balance and the cellular ability to maintain high ATP concentrations.

Inorganic Pyrophosphate

The total body content of pyrophosphate is not known, but pyrophosphate is present in all cells and in bone and is excreted in the urine. The total content in bone is 50 to 80 mmoles (3 to 5 g. measured as phosphorus). The major route of formation of pyrophosphate is by reactions of the general type

$$AMP \sim PP + X \longrightarrow AMP \sim X + PP$$

Pyrophosphate is broken down by the enzyme pyrophosphatase, which catalyzes the reaction

$$PP \longrightarrow 2Pi$$

It is found in all tissues, including bone.

Pyrophosphate is excreted in the urine of the adult at a rate of approximately 30 μmoles per day. The rate is higher in young children. Practically nothing is known about the factors regulating the urinary excretion of this anion. Its rate of excretion is increased in women at the time of menopause, in hypophosphatasia, and by the administration of inorganic phosphate. It is decreased in certain patients with urolithiasis.

The importance of pyrophosphate lies in its ability to inhibit precipitation of calcium and phosphate from metastable solutions of these salts *in vitro* and to inhibit as well the dissolution of hydroxyapatite crystals. It may play a similar role *in vivo*, i.e., preventing formation and dissolution of hydroxyapatite. In this view, hydroxyapatite forms in bone, because the pyrophosphatase in this tissue is sufficient to hydrolyze the pyrophosphate and thus overcome the natural inhibition; the hydroxyapatite crystals in bone dissolve during resorption by similar lowering of pyrophosphatase concentrations. Much further work is necessary before this hypothesis can be accepted, but it is of interest that alkaline phosphatase is also a pyrophosphatase and there is evidence that the activity of this enzyme is increased at the sites of bone formation. Another possible role of pyrophosphate is that of keeping the calcium and phosphate in urine from forming crystals, i.e., preventing renal calcification and stone formation. Some patients with recurrent calculi have a diminished excretion of this anion.

The most recent data concerning bone mineralization have led to the conclusion that it is directly controlled by osteoid osteocytes and chrondrocytes that release membrane-bound vesicles into the extracellular space at sites of bone mineralization. These vesicles contain calcium and phosphate ions and are rich in pyrophosphatase activity. Addition of pyrophosphate to isolated vesicles increases their uptake of calcium. It is assumed that, as the vesicle ages, its membrane disappears and the mineral deposits that have formed within it now act as sites of extracellular mineral crystal growth. In this view, pyrophosphate and the enzyme pyrophosphatase are critically important in the initial formation of bone mineral (probably amorphous calcium phosphate) within these matrix-calcifying vesicles.

Structural analogues of pyrophosphate, known as diphosphonates and having the general formula,

$$\begin{array}{ccccc} & O & x_1 & O & \\ & \| & | & \| & \\ {}^-O & {-}P{-} & C{-} & P{-} & O^- \\ & | & | & | & \\ & OH & x_2 & OH & \end{array}$$

have been introduced on an experimental basis in the treatment of certain metabolic bone diseases. The rationale for their use has been that they inhibit bone mineral crystal formation and dissolution *in vitro* and PTH-induced bone resorption *in vitro*. They have also been shown to inhibit experimental aortic calcification *in vivo*. The most widely used of these compounds, ethane-1-hydroxy-1,1 diphosphonate, in which x_1 and x_2 are a hydroxyl and a methyl group, respectively, has been used in patients with osteoporosis. Its major effect has been that of producing osteomalacia and secondary hyperparathyroidism. Similar observations have been made in experimental animals. These results are consistent with pyrophosphate having a role in the initiation of bone mineralization.

Magnesium

The total body content of magnesium is 200 mmoles (in a 70-kg. man). Half of this total is in the skeleton. The other half is nearly all found within cells. Only 1 per cent is contained in the extracellular fluids. The plasma magnesium concentration is 1.66 $\pm$ 0.009 mEq. per liter in the adult human. This concentration is maintained constant except in severe magnesium restriction. The average adult ingests roughly 25 mmoles per day. About 8 to 10 mmoles is absorbed and appears in the urine. Very little is known about the specific factors involved in magnesium homeostasis, although there is increasing evidence that at least one of these is parathyroid hormone. The evidence is this: (1) hypomagnesemia may occur in hyperparathyroidism, and a negative magnesium balance is common; (2) parathyroid hormone increases the renal tubular reabsorption of magnesium; (3) parathyroid hormone increases the fractional rate of exchange of tissue magnesium; (4) parathyroid hormone specifically alters the magnesium permeability of the mitochondrial membrane. However, the situation is complex and other factors must certainly be involved.

The total concentrations of Mg^{2+} and K^+ in intracellular fluids are nearly identical to the supposed ionic composition of the pre-Cambrian oceans. Thus it appears that the present-day intracellular environment is strikingly similar to that in which life apparently originated. Because of this it is not surprising that both Mg^{2+} and K^+ are important regulators of many enzymes as well as of protein biosynthesis. In particular, the following types of enzymatic reactions are affected by Mg^{2+}: (1) enzymes with thiamine diphosphate as cofactor, e.g., carboxylase and pyruvate oxidase; (2) enolase; (3) certain peptidases; (4) all reactions involving ATP synthesis and hydrolysis; (5) alkaline phosphatase and pyrophosphatases; (6) isocitric dehydrogenase; and (7) the complex reactions involved in ribosomal protein synthesis.

The rate of exchange of intracellular magnesium is extremely rapid in cardiac muscle, rapid in liver, slow in brain, and very slow in bone and skeletal muscle.

Absorption

Little is known of the factors that control the gastrointestinal absorption of magnesium. Calcium seems to inhibit magnesium absorption and large doses of vitamin D to enhance it. However, in contrast to calcium, magnesium absorption is normal in vitamin D–deficient animals and is uninfluenced by physiologic doses of vitamin D.

Renal Excretion

Just as in the intestine, so in the renal tubule there appears at first glance to be a common transport mechanism for calcium and magnesium because (1) the reabsorption of both is increased by parathyroid hormone; (2) hypocalciuria is present in magnesium deficient rats; (3) the two ions appear together and before inulin in stop-flow experiments; and (4) calcium infusion leads to increased magnesium excretion. However, other experiments employing long-term perfusions in rats indicate that the renal excretion of these two ions can vary independently.

Magnesium in Bone

Magnesium appears to be stored in bone, possibly on the surfaces of the hydroxyapatite crystal lattice. However, when radioactive magnesium is injected into experimental animals, the exchangeable compartment of bone magnesium is considerably less than that predicted from measurements of bone mineral exchange by calcium kinetics.

BONE

On a dry-weight basis, bone consists of approximately 65 to 70 per cent inorganic crystals of *hydroxyapatite* and 30 to 35 per cent organic matrix (osteoid), of which collagen is the major constituent (95 to 99 per cent).

Chemistry of Bone

Inorganic Phase of Bone

It is now generally accepted that the bone mineral is a single crystal type giving the x-ray diffraction pattern that is characteristic of the apatite lattice and more specifically of the *hydroxyapatites*

$$[Ca^{2+}_{10-x} (H_3O^+)_{2x} \cdot (PO_4^{3-})_6 (OH^-)_2].$$

This lattice structure is common to an entire series of solid calcium phosphates whose molar ratio, Ca/P, varies from 1.3 to 2.0; thus the Ca/P ratio may vary from bone mineral to bone mineral while the lattice structure is retained. The hydronium ions (H_3O^+) can replace the Ca^{2+} in the crystal lattice. In addition, the lack of stoichiometry is attributed to the extremely small size of the crystals of bone mineral.

The best estimates are that the crystals are no larger than $500 \times 250 \times 100$ angstroms. Because of their relatively large surface area, the crystals absorb excess phosphate, thereby lowering the Ca/P ratio. The chemisorption in turn leads to the binding of water, which produces the so-called hydration shell of water on the crystal surface. Throughout the life of the crystal, all of its reactions involve the transfer of ions across this crystal-solution interface. It also seems likely that certain ions, such as Na^+, can replace Ca^{2+} on the surface of the crystal but not in its interior. Such a phenomenon could account for the sodium content of bone. In the living organism, the crystals are exposed to a solution of many different ions. Some of these can penetrate only the hydration shell, others can penetrate to the ion layer on the crystal surface, and others can replace ions in the interior of the crystal. These ion-exchange reactions help to account for the observed variability in the composition of the bone mineral and explain the fact that changes in the concentration of the hydrogen ions, the bicarbonate ions, or the sodium ions in the extracellular fluid are buffered by exchanges with the bone crystals.

In addition to hydroxyapatite, bone contains a variable amount of amorphous calcium phosphate $(Ca_3 (PO_4)_2)$. The amount of this amorphous material is greater in young than in older bone. It seems even likely that the initial bone mineral formed (first within the matrix vesicles) is this amorphous material, and that as the bone ages this material is gradually converted into the final solid phase, hydroxyapatite, by a dissolution and recrystallization process.

Organic Phase of Bone

Although on a weight basis the mineral component is by far the largest constituent of bone, it is the production of a calcifiable matrix that determines the size and the shape of a given bone. This matrix is primarily collagen, a fibrous protein which is rich in glycine, proline, and hydroxyproline, but which also contains small amounts of methionine, lysine, hydroxylysine, and tyrosine. The bone collagen appears to be structurally similar to that found in other connective tissues. The other components of the organic matrix include a number of poorly defined proteins and a group of acid mucopolysaccharides and mucoproteins. These constitute the "ground substances." Their exact location has not been established, and their state of aggregation in different states of bone metabolism is not known. However, at sites of calcification, both at the calcification front on membranous bone and in the endochondrial plate, the concentrations of these mucoproteins decrease as calcification proceeds. Their possible function in the calcification process is not clear.

The basic structural component of the extracellular collagen matrix of all connective tissues is

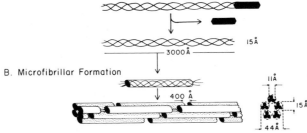

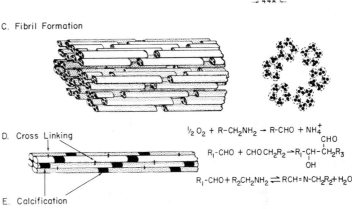

A. Procollagen to tropocollagen

B. Microfibrillar Formation

C. Fibril Formation

D. Cross Linking

$$\tfrac{1}{2} O_2 + R-CH_2NH_2 \rightarrow R-CHO + NH_4^+$$

$$R_1-CHO + CHOCH_2R_2 \rightarrow R_1-\overset{\overset{\displaystyle CHO}{|}}{C}H-\overset{\overset{\displaystyle |}{OH}}{C}H_2R_3$$

$$R_1-CHO + R_2CH_2NH_2 \rightleftharpoons RCH=N-CH_2R_2 + H_2O$$

E. Calcification

Figure 11-4. The extracellular events in bone collagen synthesis, maturation and mineralization.

the tropocollagen molecule. This is a long rodlike cylinder, $3,000 \times 15$ Å., with an approximate molecular weight of 300,000. It is composed of three separate monomer units called alpha chains, which exist in a triple coil or helix wound around each other, much like three strands of a cable (Fig. 11–4), and are held together by weak intermolecular linkages. Typically, two of the alpha chains are identical in amino acid sequence, and the third is slightly different. All contain approximately 100 proline, 100 hydroxyproline, 330 glycine, and 30 lysine and hydroxylysine residues, with lesser amounts of the other amino acids, but no cysteine or cystine.

Relationship Between Organic and Inorganic Phases of Bone

The feature of bone mineral that most distinguishes it from hydroxyapatites formed *in vitro* is its close and ordered association with the collagenous matrix (Fig. 11–4). When bone is examined by electron microscopy or x-ray diffraction, the increased electron density of the bone mineral is found at regular intervals along the longitudinal axis of the collagen fibrils. The period of these intervals is approximately 640 Å. and is identical to the normal periodicity of unmineralized collagen.

Another feature of this association is that the mineral crystals do not grow progressively but reach a maximum size of approximately 400 Å. by 30 Å. Moreover, during the process of bone matrix mineralization, the forming crystals displace an equal volume of water. Finally, if collagen from a variety of sources is dissolved and then reprecipi-

tated into its native configuration with the 640 Å. axial repeat pattern, it can serve as a template to initiate mineral crystal formation *in vitro* from a metastable solution of calcium and phosphate. On the other hand, if the collagen is precipitated out of solution in a variety of other non-natural configurations, it will not serve as a template in this way.

This all suggests that, in bone, the mineral is deposited on or within specific regions of the supramolecular collagenous matrix, i.e., that there are holes in the collagen matrix that are sites of mineral deposition.

To account for the structural features, the axial repeat pattern, and the presence of holes, it was originally proposed that the holes were formed by a two-dimensional staggered array of tropocollagen molecules, in which in any row of tropocollagen molecules there is a gap of 400 Å. between the end of one tropocollagen molecule and the beginning of the next; because the sites of these gaps in adjacent rows are staggered, however, the whole exists as a stable structure. More recent evidence indicates, though, that the more likely structure is one in which the staggered rows of tropocollagen molecules are arranged in pentagonal array, forming a five-stranded microfibril (Fig. 11–4).

In this model, in addition to the gaps, there is a central core or cavity within the microfibril. The combined volumes of this cavity and of the gaps in the five-stranded microfibril are sufficient to account for over 90 per cent of the volume of mineral crystals found in fully calcified bone. It is thought at present that these represent the sites within bone matrix where mineral is deposited. If so, it is clear that the relationship between the organic and inorganic phases of bone is intimate and accounts for the unique mechanical properties of bone and its ability to generate piezoelectricity (see p. 680). It is also clear why bone resorption must of necessity involve both the destruction of matrix and the dissolution of bone mineral. As bone becomes fully mineralized, the water previously occupying the intrafibrillar spaces is displaced, and the rate of exchange of mineral ions between the lattice sites on the bone mineral crystals and the surrounding ground substance becomes too slow to be physiologically important.

Metabolism of Bone Matrix

As part of the general process of skeletal remodeling, bone matrix is being continually synthesized, secreted, organized, mineralized, and finally destroyed. It is the rates of these processes which determine the overall rate of bone remodeling and the net skeletal balance.

The synthesis of the extracellular bone collagen matrix is a complex process, which can be conveniently divided into intra- and extracellular phases.

The first event in the intracellular synthesis of collagen (Fig. 11–5) is the ribosomal synthesis of the protocollagen molecule in the classical sequence, which leads eventually to the formation of a three-stranded triple helix. Each strand is of a separate type of protocollagen monomer. Once formed, the protocollagen contains approximately 20 per cent proline and 33 per cent glycine, with the sequence -gly-x-pro- appearing repeatedly. The protocollagen serves as a substrate for the enzyme protocollagen hydroxylase, which uses O_2, Fe^{2+}, and α-ketoglutarate as substrates and cofactors, and catalyzes the hydroxylation of specific proline residues. Approximately half the proline residues become hydroxylated. A second enzyme catalyzes

the hydroxylation of a few of the lysine residues in the molecule, and these then are substrates for the final step in synthesis, glycosylation.

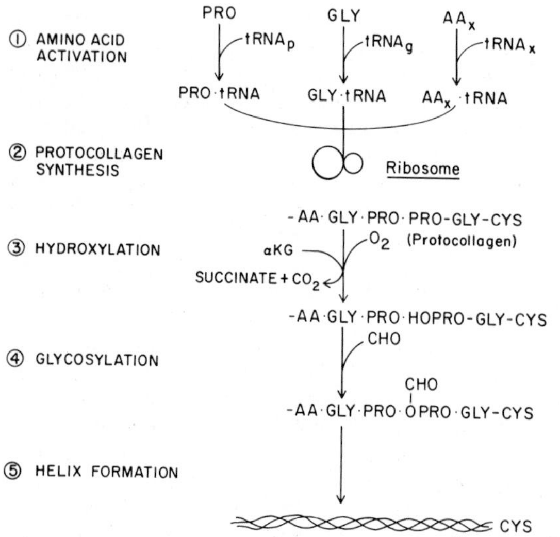

The hydroxylated, glycosylated protocollagen, now known as procollagen, is then secreted into the extracellular space. Either at the time of secretion or shortly thereafter, it undergoes conversion to tropocollagen. Procollagen is a triple helix having a molecular weight of approximately 360,000 (Fig. 11–4). It is acted upon by a specific enzyme which cleaves a fragment of approximately 20,000 M.W. from the NH_2–terminal end of each of its three chains, leaving a tropocollagen molecule consisting of three chains, each having a molecular weight of approximately 100,000. This conversion is necessary for fibril formation to take place. After proteolysis, the tropocollagen molecules, 3000 Å. by 15 Å., polymerize into microfibrils of considerable length, centimeters or more, but of 5 units in diameter (44 Å.). These microfibrillar pentameters then polymerize further to form collagen fibrils ranging in diameter from 150 to 1300 Å.

Polymerization is a spontaneous process that involves specific interactions of the amino acid side chains of the tropocollagen subunits. These are primarily hydrophobic interactions between adjacent chains.

Polymerization is followed by the three-dimensional distribution of the collagen fibrils. This is a highly ordered process, particularly in lamellar bone, in which successive bundles or layers of collagen fibrils are arranged in distinct layers or lamellae, each of which is oriented in a specific radial pattern. The control of this long-range, three-dimensional patterning is not well understood.

Even after this patterning has taken place, there are continuing changes in collagen structure. The most important is the formation of covalent chemical bonds, either by the formation of Schiff bases and their subsequent reduction or by aldol condensation. Both processes require the formation of aldehyde groups on the collagen molecule. Their formation is catalyzed by the enzyme, amine oxidase,

$$R{-}CH_2{-}NH_3^+ \xrightarrow{\frac{1}{2}O_2} RCHO + NH_4^+$$

acting primarily on the amine groups of lysine and hydroxylysine residues.

The formation of these intermolecular covalent bonds takes place slowly over a matter of days or weeks. Their formation changes greatly the solubility of extracellular collagen. Freshly synthesized collagen is soluble in 0.14 M NaCl (Fig. 11–6) but older collagen is not. In Marfan's syndrome, formation of these covalent bonds is deficient. Their formation is also blocked in lathyrism. Both conditions are characterized by disorders of connective tissues, including bone. In both conditions, however, the mineralization of the bone collagen is normal. This signifies that formation of these covalent bonds is not a necessary component of the "maturation" of bone matrix which precedes its mineralization.

In the normal process of membranous bone for-

Figure 11–5. The intracellular events in procollagen synthesis.

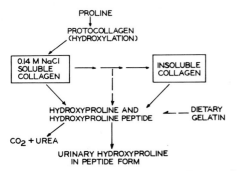

PROLINE

PROTOCOLLAGEN
(HYDROXYLATION)

0.14 M NaCl
SOLUBLE
COLLAGEN → INSOLUBLE
COLLAGEN

HYDROXYPROLINE AND
HYDROXYPROLINE PEPTIDE ← DIETARY
GELATIN

CO_2 + UREA

URINARY HYDROXYPROLINE
IN PEPTIDE FORM

Figure 11–6. The metabolism of proline, collagen, and hydroxyproline. (Based upon information obtained from Dr. D. Prockop.)

mation, there is a delay of 5 to 10 days between the synthesis of an extracellular matrix and its subsequent mineralization. The reason for this delay is not clear. It has generally been assumed that it represents a maturation of the matrix, i.e., its transformation from a noncalcifiable to a calcifiable substrate. In view of the recent hypothesis that the initial formation of bone mineral takes place in membrane-bound vesicles that are secreted by bone cells, however, it seems possible that the delay is a reflection of the transition of a cell (osteoblast) from one synthesizing collagen and other matrix constituents to one (osteoid osteocyte) involved in the synthesis and secretion of the matrix calcification vesicles.

The final phase of collagen turnover is its destruction. The resorption of bone requires the dissolution of the bone mineral crystals and the proteolytic digestion of the underlying collagenous matrix. In this process, a key component of skeletal remodeling, osteocytes and osteoclasts are responsible. Bone resorption by osteoclasts depends upon the prior mineralization of collagen. Osteoclasts appear incapable of bringing about the resorption of uncalcified bone matrix but can destroy previously calcified matrix.

Urinary Hydroxyproline

When collagen is destroyed, most of it is hydrolyzed to its constituent amino acids, which are then reused or degraded further to carbon dioxide and urea. However, 5 to 8 per cent of the collagen is only partially degraded into soluble hydroxyproline-containing peptides which circulate in the bloodstream and are excreted in the urine. This means that urinary hydroxyproline can serve as a natural label for the study of collagen metabolism. Unfortunately, the situation is such that it is not possible to ascribe changes in excretion only to changes in bone resorption, although this is frequently done. The difficulties are these: (1) not all collagen is in bone; and there is no convincing evidence that bone collagen is the sole source of urinary hydroxyproline; (2) there are several pools or types of collagen that can serve as the immediate

precursor for urinary hydroxyproline; (3) the size of these pools can vary independently; and (4) dietary gelatin can serve as a source of urinary hydroxyproline. In order to provide a better understanding of the complexities involved, the relationship between collagen and hydroxyproline metabolism is depicted in Figure 11–6.

Either the soluble or the insoluble collagen can serve as the precursor of urinary and plasma hydroxyproline, as can dietary gelatin. At any given time, there is a spectrum of extracellular collagen aggregates, which have been classified according to their solubilities. Soluble collagen is that which is soluble in cold 0.14 M NaCl. Moreover, when young animals are injected with C^{14}-proline, the labeled hydroxyproline which appears in the urine is derived from at least three pools, with half-lives of 1 day, 5 days, or 50 to 100 days. Collagens from pools one and two are thought to be soluble, and from pool three, insoluble. In older animals, there is normally only one major pool, presumably of insoluble collagen, with a half-life of 300 days. The studies correlating collagen pools and hydroxyproline excretion have usually involved skin collagen, and the assumption is that the situation in bone is similar. Because of technical difficulties, however, very few direct measurements of collagen pools in bone have been made.

Theoretically, urinary hydroxyproline excretion can be increased by the following: (1) increased rates of collagen synthesis, with a concomitant increase in the soluble collagen pool; (2) a decreased rate of conversion of soluble to insoluble collagen (or an increased rate in the opposite sense) leading again to an increase in the soluble collagen pool; (3) an increased rate of degradation of insoluble or soluble collagen or both; (4) a decreased rate of the terminal degradation of hydroxyproline to carbon dioxide and urea; and (5) the presence or absence of normal mineralization in bone. Several of these possibilities have been noted from experiments on animals. These are summarized in Table 11–3.

Parathyroid hormone and calcitonin are thought to alter hydroxyproline excretion exclusively by their effects upon bone. There are few experimental data to rule out effects upon other tissues, however. In the case of these two hormones, the generally accepted conclusion, which is based on their effects on hydroxyproline excretion, is that both agents predominantly influence bone resorption.

The measurement of urinary hydroxyproline has been used in the study of various metabolic bone diseases. If done with the proper precautions, this measurement has turned out to be useful in determining the degree of bone resorption. In addition, it has been found that the hydroxyproline-containing peptides in human urine can be divided into two broad classes on the basis of their molecular weights. The class with the larger molecular weight normally represents only 5 to 10 per cent of the total but appears to reflect predominantly changes in rate of bone collagen synthesis, i.e., the peptides appear to be derived from the saline-soluble collagen pool, whereas the smaller peptides ap-

TABLE 11-3. INFLUENCE OF VARIOUS AGENTS UPON COLLAGEN METABOLISM AND URINARY HYDROXYPROLINE EXCRETION

Agent	Collagen Synthesis	Collagen Soluble	Collagen Degrad.	Collagen Insol.	HOP†
Growth hormone	↑	↑	↑	↑	↑
Ascorbic acid def.	↓	↓	↓	↓	↓
Cortisol	↓	↓	n	↓	↓
Thyroxine	↑ n, ↓	↓	↑		↑
Lathyrogens*	n or ↑	↑	n	↓	↑
PTH	↓	n or ↓	↑	↓	↑
CT	?	?	↓	?	↓

*β-amino propionitrile.
†Urinary hydroxyproline.

pear to reflect the breakdown of older collagen molecules. At least in Paget's disease and in primary hyperparathyroidism, a reasonable correlation has been found between the rate of excretion of the larger peptides and the rate of bone formation.

Metabolism of Bone Mineral

During the process of skeletal remodeling, bone mineral must also turn over. As indicated above, mineral deposition follows, in time, the elaboration of a suitable organic matrix. The process, whether taking place at the epiphyseal plate or at sites of primary membranous bone formation, is under cellular control. It is dependent principally upon the presence of appropriate amounts of one or more active metabolites of vitamin D and upon the presence of sufficient amounts of calcium and phosphate in the extracellular fluids. In both vitamin D and phosphate deficiency, mineralization of bone matrix fails to take place. As a consequence, increased amounts of uncalcified matrix or osteoid are seen in the bones of such animals or humans.

During the normal process of mineralization, it is now believed that the mineral ions are accumulated within membrane-bound vesicles which are derived either from the Golgi region of the cell or directly from processes of the cell membrane.

In the absence of vitamin D, these matrix vesicles are still present but contain little or no mineral. It is possible that the concentration of bone alkaline phosphatase, or more correctly pyrophosphatase, measured in blood plasma is an indirect measure of the number of these vesicles, because they have been found to contain considerable amounts of this enzyme.

Structure of Bone

Macroscopic Structure of Bone

Macroscopically, adult bone can be divided into two types: (1) the spongiosa, which occurs in the metaphysial portion of the long bones and is composed of delicate spicules of bone called trabeculae; and (2) the compact or cortical bone, which is found in the cortex and the diaphysis of the long bones. The size, the number, and the disposition of the trabeculae of the spongiosa change in response to atered mechanical demands. This part of bone is the most active metabolically and is the first portion (along with the endosteal surfaces of the cortex) to respond to changes in the amount of parathyroid hormone or to other stimuli.

Microscopic Structure of Bone

Microscopically, bone exhibits two orders of structure. The first level of organization is the basic distribution of collagen fibers, and the second is the way these fibers are built into a three-dimensional pattern.

At the first level, two types of bone can be distinguished: woven and lamellar. Woven bone is composed of loosely and randomly arranged collagen bundles. The collagen fiber bundles vary considerably in size, some reaching 13 microns in diameter. This type of bone contains large numbers of osteocytes per unit volume. These vary in size and shape and lie in lacunae which vary in size and orientation. Woven bone is found in both the cortical and cancellous bone of young growing animals. During the normal process of skeletal maturation, it is progressively replaced by lamellar bone so that, in man, by the age of 14 or 15 years, no woven bone remains. However, it reappears both as the first bone made at fracture sites and in certain metabolic bone diseases, most notably Paget's disease, osteitis fibrosa cystica secondary to primary hyperparathyroidism, and renal osteodystrophy. In the adult, the presence of woven bone in the skeleton is nearly always indicative of high rates of bone turnover. However, in the case of hyperthyroidism, woven bone does not appear, even though bone turnover rates are high.

Lamellar bone is composed of highly ordered, uniform bundles of collagen fibers, approximately 2 to 4 microns in diameter, arranged in successive distinct layers. Between these layers, the osteocytes are uniformly arranged with their long axes parallel to the long axis of the collagen bundle. This type of bone is characteristic of the normal adult skeleton. It is the type of bone normally formed during primary membranous bone formation. In contrast, at the epiphyseal plate, the normal sequence of events is: (1) the formation of a cartilaginous matrix; (2) its transformation into a calcifiable substrate; (3) its mineralization; (4) its partial resorption; (5) synthesis of woven bone at sites of resorption; (6) resorption of woven bone; and (7) replacement with lamellar bone.

During the production of lamellar bone, the sequence of events is: (1) secretion of collagen by a layer of uniform osteoblasts; (2) lamellar organization of secreted collagen bundles; (3) incorporation of the osteoblasts into bone as osteocytes as the next wave of osteoblasts secretes collagen; (4) transformation of these *osteoid osteocytes* from cells capable of collagen synthesis to cells capable of secreting matrix calcification granules; (5) secretion of such granules; (6) extracellular accumulation of calcium and phosphate by these granules; (7) disappearance of the granule membrane; and (8) recrystallization of the amorphous calcium phosphate into hydroxyapatite crystals located within the collagen fibrils. There is normally a delay of several days (8 to 10 in human bone) between the production of the matrix and its subsequent mineralization. Thus at sites of active new bone growth, there is normally a small amount of uncalcified matrix or *osteoid;* because the onset of its calcification is quite uniform, a sharp line or *calcification front* is evident if undecalcified bone sections are stained with a variety of dyes *in vitro* or if the animal is injected with tetracycline *in vivo.*

This normal coupling, in time, between matrix formation and its mineralization depends upon the presence of vitamin D metabolites. One of the most characteristic features of vitamin D deficiencies is a marked prolongation of this time, *mineralization lag time,* with the consequent appearance of increased amounts of osteoid.

Increased amounts of osteoid in undecalcified sections of bone are also seen in osteitis fibrosa cystica and Paget's disease. They may also be seen in hyperthyroidism, in patients treated with fluoride or diphosphonates, and in patients treated for long periods with calcitonin. The possible reasons for these observations are discussed in a later section of this chapter. In general, an increase in the amount of osteoid is due either to an increase in rate of new bone formation or to an increase in the lag time between collagen formation and its subsequent mineralization.

At the second level of organization, adult bone is organized either as trabecular or haversian bone (Fig. 11-7), both of which are lamellar in structure. In the first, which is synonymous with cancellous bone, there are no blood vessels within the bone substance. The bone is built in a pattern of interlacing trabeculae. Remodeling takes place upon the surfaces, which are perfused by blood from the medullary cavity of the bone. The surface-to-volume ratio is relatively large. In cellular terms, the mesenchymal cells of the lining cell envelope are relatively numerous in relation to the osteocytes within the bone substance. It is these mesenchymal bone cells that, upon appropriate signals, become active bone cells. Because of its relatively

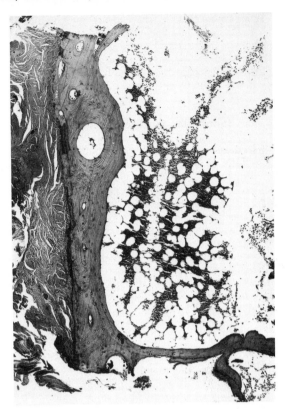

Figure 11-7. A section of undecalcified human bone illustrating, along the left, cortical lamellar bone composed of a haversian system, and across the bottom, a spicule of trabecular lamellar bone. (Figure kindly supplied by Dr. Philippe Bordier.)

cellular makeup, trabecular bone is remodeled at a considerably higher rate than is haversian bone. As a consequence, the first reflections of metabolic bone diseases are seen in the cancellous bone.

Haversian bone develops as a consequence of the remodeling of cortical bone. It is normally the predominant type of bone in the cortices of the bone of the adult organism. Its organization is determined by the distribution of the bone microcirculation. A haversian system forms as a result of a vascular invasion of bone. The vessels responsible for this invasion are always derived from those on the endosteal surface. Invasion is characterized by osteoclastic resorption of a cone of bone, with the long axis of the cone running parallel to the long axis of the bone. The resulting resorption cavities, approximately 0.1 mm. in diameter, may run for several millimeters along the long axis of the bone. After a short period of time, formation of new (haversian) bone follows this resorptive phase. Formation consists of the laying down of successive layers of lamellar bone oriented as concentric rings around the walls of the cylindrical resorption cavity. As these are laid down, there is a progressive reduction in cylinder diameter, until only a central canal containing a small arteriole and venule remain—the haversian canal. These vessels are separated from direct contact with the bone surfaces by a surrounding layer of endothelial cells and a layer of bone mesenchymal cells.

In this type of bone, the ratio of surface mesenchymal cells to internal osteocytes is quite small, so that the major determinant of the metabolism of a haversian unit or osteon is the metabolism of the internal osteocytes. In general, haversian remodeling is less rapid than that seen in trabecular bone.

Bone Cells: Surface Remodeling

In order to understand bone structure and physiology fully, it is necessary to comprehend the relationships that exist between the various types of bone cell. Four general cell types are recognizable: mesenchymal or osteoprogenitor cells, osteoclasts, osteoblasts, and osteocytes.

Bone as an organ system, in terms of its cellular organization, can be considered as a triple-surface system in which there are three anatomically distinct bone cell envelopes: periosteal, endosteal, and haversian. The term "cell envelope" emphasizes that all three surfaces of a normal bone are completely covered by an envelope of *mesenchymal* cells or *osteoprogenitor* cells (Fig. 11–8), which gives rise to osteoclasts, osteoblasts, and osteocytes, but which also functions as the surface layer of a cell syncytium involving all the osteocytes in a particular functional unit of bone.

The periosteal envelope participates in both the transverse and longitudinal growth modeling and remodeling during the growth of the organism. At this surface, growth remodeling requires both resorption and formation. When skeletal maturation is achieved, longitudinal growth ceases, and transverse growth is greatly slowed. Remodeling and growth do continue at a slow rate throughout adult life, however. The balance of remodeling activities on this surface is in favor of formation, so that there is a small but perceptible increase, with age, in the transverse diameter of the long bones in normal humans (Fig. 11–9).

During skeletal growth and maturation, the endosteal bone cell envelope is coupled to events at the epiphyseal plate as well as to the medullary remodeling which is a component of the transverse growth of long bones. The endosteal bone cell

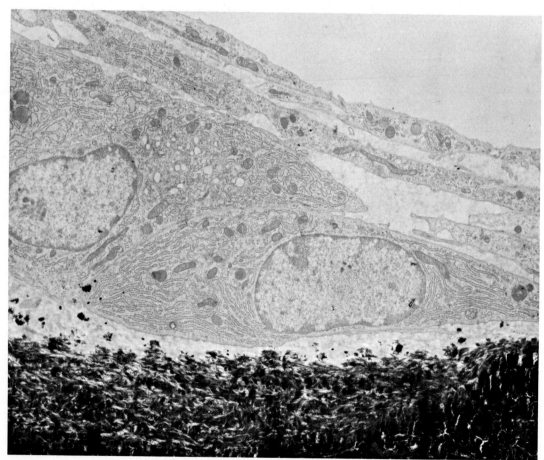

Figure 11–8.   An electron micrograph of the normal trabecular surface. The dark material at the bottom of the picture is calcified collagen. Immediately above it are uncalcified collagen fibrils covered by osteoblasts. The two osteoblasts are apposed, and both contain extensive, rough endoplasmic reticulum. Above the osteoblasts is a layer of elongated cells, of which one is seen stretching across the entire picture. This is an osteoprogenitor cell which lies in the mesenchymal cell envelope covering the entire bone surface. At the top right is the lumen of a small blood vessel surrounded by endothelial cells. (Kindly supplied by Drs. D. A. Cameron and R. H. Robinson.)

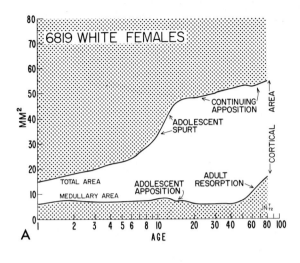

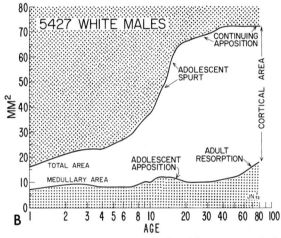

Figure 11–9. *A,* Plot of the size of total bone area, cortical bone area, and medullary bone area according to age in standard bone samples from white American females. Note the marked increase in total bone area with adolescent growth and the slowly continuing apposition of cortical area throughout life. Note also the striking increase in medullary area beginning after age 40, which leads to a definite decrease in cortical thickness in later life. *B,* A similar plot from bone of white American males. (Both figures kindly supplied by Dr. Stanley Garn.)

envelope also participates in active bone remodeling throughout life. It covers the surface of both trabecular and cortical bone. The rate of remodeling on these surfaces is considerably greater than the rate upon periosteal surfaces. Thus, in most metabolic bone diseases, the earliest and most-pronounced changes in bone structure and bone cell dynamics are observed on the endosteal bone surfaces. If this results in a net skeletal loss, this loss is reflected radiologically as an increase in the size of the medullary cavity (Fig. 11–9).

A second distinctive feature of endosteal bone remodeling is that, in the normal human adult from approximately age 35 onward, the balance of formation versus resorption is in favor of resorption. This leads to a net loss of skeletal mass which is greater than the much smaller gain in skeletal mass at periosteal surfaces, so that total skeletal mass normally decreases with age (Fig. 11–9).

The haversian bone cell envelope is an extension of the endosteal cell envelope. Haversian bone remodeling is initiated by a vascular invasion from the endosteal surface vessels. Haversian remodeling is less rapid than trabecular remodeling of cancellous bone, but in a variety of metabolic bone diseases, the changes in haversian and endosteal bone remodeling are qualitatively similar. Also with age, haversian remodeling becomes less complete, so that new resorption cones are not completely reossified, resulting in a more porous cortical bone in older individuals.

In the adult, the function of all three envelopes is that of controlling mineral and nutritional exchange between the extracellular fluids and the bone cells, i.e., the osteocytes. In addition, all three participate in the continuing process of skeletal remodeling. However, as noted above, the rates of remodeling and the net balance, formation versus resorption, of the remodeling events differ on the different bone surfaces. In spite of these local differences, the cellular basis of remodeling in the adult skeleton is the same on all surfaces.

The most distinctive feature of bone remodeling is that it is a quantized process which has a distinctive life cycle. The initial event is the *activation* of a group of mesenchymal, or osteoprogenitor, cells, in one of the bone cell envelopes. These cells undergo one, or perhaps several, successive mitoses, being converted in the process to daughter cells which have been variously identified as preosteoclasts, preosteoblasts, or a pluripotential cell that can give rise to both osteoclasts and osteoblasts. This phase lasts from a few hours to a few days. It has been designated *differentiation* by some and *modulation* by others.

The next phase is a *resorptive* one. Multinucleated osteoclasts appear from the daughter cells and carry out the resorption of a volume of bone on one of the surfaces. In human adult bone, this phase lasts one month on the average. It then ceases and after a short time is followed by the *formative* phase. New osteoblasts appear and begin forming new bone at the sites of previous resorption. When skeletal balance is maintained, the same mass of bone that was removed in approximately one month is replaced in about three. However, it is usually oriented differently from the previous bone and is a distinct functional unit of bone. This is most clearly illustrated by the fact that the interface between the site of previous resorption and subsequent formation is identifiable by a cement line when an undecalcified bone section is viewed histologically.

Within the unit of new bone, the osteocytes communicate with one another by means of canaliculi within the bone structure, and with the cells of the bone envelope overlying the unit. However, there are no canaliculi that cross the cement lines and no direct communication between osteocytes in one unit with those in another. This shows that bone is organized in distinct functional or metabolic units. In cortical bone, these units are synonymous with haversian systems or osteons. It is possible to subdivide the bone metabolic units, in terms of skeletal remodeling, into those that are active and those that are inactive. In the normal adult, inactive units, as defined in this manner, account for over 95 per cent of all bone metabolic units. However, it must be emphasized that these units, which are inactive in the remodeling sense, are active in maintaining mineral homeostasis (see p. 680).

Active bone metabolic units of skeletal remodeling are characterized by evidence of surface cell activity, either resorption or formation. The total number of these active surfaces is a measure of the overall rate of skeletal remodeling. The ratio between formation and resorption sites is one measure of the balance between formation and resorption within the skeleton.

The cellular events underlying the various phases of the life cycle of a bone metabolic unit are not completely understood. It is clear that mitoses are seen only in the mesenchymal, or osteoprogenitor, cells. These are followed by the appearance of a group of daughter cells (Fig. 11–10). It has been a generally held belief that these daughter cells could give rise to either osteoclasts or osteoblasts under appropriate stimuli. This ignores a cardinal feature of bone remodeling, however. The sequence of events is always activation $\longrightarrow$ resorption $\longrightarrow$ formation. An osteoclastic

phase always precedes but never follows an osteoblastic phase.

A logical alternative to the general view is that the progression of cells is osteoprogenitor cells $\longrightarrow$ preosteoclasts $\longrightarrow$ osteoclasts $\longrightarrow$ preosteoblasts $\longrightarrow$ osteoblasts $\longrightarrow$ osteocytes (Fig. 11–10). Such a model of cellular events would account for nearly all the observations concerning bone and bone cell turnover. An alternative to this model is one in which products of osteoclastic bone cell activity regulate and are necessary for the flow of daughter cells into osteoblasts (Fig. 11–10).

Bone Cells: Internal Remodeling

During the process of bone formation, after osteoblasts have elaborated an extracellular matrix, they become incorporated into the matrix as successive osteoblastic cell layers begin to produce matrix. They cease matrix synthesis and assume the role of *osteoid osteocytes*, in which they are responsible for the elaboration of the *matrix calcification granules or vesicles*. Upon initiation of matrix calcification, this function stops, and they

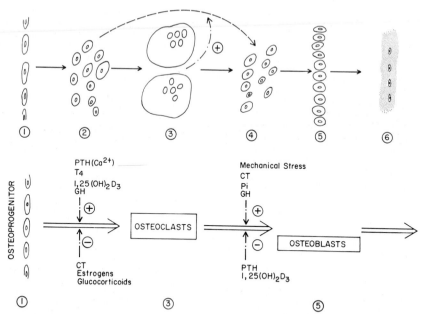

Figure 11–10. The sequence of cellular events in an active bone metabolic unit. *Top,* the five cellular pools involved in the life cycle of such a unit: ① osteoprogenitor cells; ② preosteoclasts; ③ osteoclasts; ④ postosteoclasts or preosteoblasts; ⑤ osteoblasts; and ⑥ osteocytes. The proposed sequence is a direct progression of cells from ① to ⑥. Others have proposed, however, that the daughter cells of the osteoprogenitor cells can proceed directly to either osteoclasts or osteoblasts. If this is the case, all the present data argue that the activity of the osteoclasts regulates this flow; however, the weight of evidence favors the direct progress. *Bottom,* the three bone cell pools which can be measured: ① osteoprogenitor cells; ② osteoclasts; and ③ osteoblasts. The width of the block is an attempt to represent the number of cells in the pool, and the height an attempt to represent their activity (see also Fig. 11–17). When skeletal homeostasis or the balance between resorption and formation is maintained, the total area of the two blocks should be equal. Also shown are the factors that control the activation of osteoprogenitor cells into osteoclasts and the modulation of osteoclasts to osteoblasts. The model provides a cellular basis for the sequence of events in bone remodeling discussed by Frost (1964): (1) activation, (2) resorption, and (3) formation (A $\longrightarrow$ R $\longrightarrow$ F). The broken arrow from cell pool ② to ④ indicates an alternate possibility in which the daughter cells ② give rise to preosteoblasts ④ directly, with no obligatory osteoclastic phase, but in which some metabolic product of osteoclastic activity regulates ($-\cdot\rightarrow$) the flow of daughter cells ② to preosteoblasts ④. Operationally, this relationship would be similar to the direct pathway inasmuch as a coupling between the osteoclastic and osteoblastic phases of bone remodeling would exist. (Modified from Rasmussen, H., and Bordier, P.: *The Physiological and Cellular Basis of Metabolic Bone Disease.* Baltimore, Williams and Wilkins Co., 1973.)

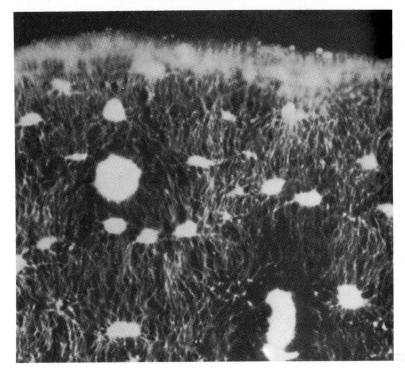

Figure 11–11. Photomicrograph of a section of rat bone in which the lacunar-canalicular system, the mini-circulation of bone, has been injected with a fluorescent dye. The picture dramatically illustrates the extensive canalicular system that interconnects the osteocytes within the bone and also connects them to the cells in the surface envelope of bone. (Figure kindly supplied by Dr. David Baylink.)

are then incorporated into the mineralized bone as mature osteocytes. The most important structural feature of all osteocytes is their numerous protoplasmic extensions, which pass through numerous small canaliculi within the bone tissue and join with similar extensions from adjacent osteocytes (Fig. 11–11). The entire osteocyte population, within a functional bone unit, forms a syncytium of cells that are joined one with another and to the mesenchymal cells (or surface osteocytes) on the bone surface. Within this unit there is a flow of liquid, the *minicirculation* of bone. Although no direct measurement of its ionic composition has been made, indirect estimates of its composition indicate it is high in K^+ and Cl^- and low in calcium (0.5 mM versus 1.3 mM in plasma). The mechanism by which this liquid circulates is not known. It has been shown that, after intravenous injection of the protein, horseradish peroxidase, this protein is found along the surface of osteocytes in their *lacunae* and along their canalicular extensions. This indicates that the mesenchymal cell envelopes of bone do not represent tight membranes, in that proteins of 40,000 M.W. readily pass through them. It seems likely that eventually it will be found that some type of countercurrent fluid circulation takes place in this minicirculation, and that the entry and egress of hormones, nutrients, and cell catabolites is entirely by an extracellular flow rather than, as has been proposed, by a system of extracellular entry and intracellular exit.

From the functional point of view, the importance of this minicirculation is that osteocytes are exposed to, and respond to, changes in the concentration of circulating ions and hormones. There is unequivocal evidence that osteocytes are capable at different points in their life cycle of making new

bone and of resorbing old bone. There is a small amount of woven bone normally seen immediately next to osteocytes and forming the internal wall of their lacunae and canaliculi. There is some evidence to suggest that this bone can be resorbed and re-formed more rapidly than the overlying dense lamellar bone. It thus constitutes a mobile reservoir of bone mineral functioning in mineral homeostasis in a manner similar to that of glycogen in blood sugar homeostasis. The amount of this bone in each lacuna or canaliculus is small, but the total lacunar-canalicular surface is 5 to 10 orders of magnitude greater than the total external surfaces of bone, so that in the aggregate this mobile reserve may represent as much as 5 g. of calcium. Since the total calcium content of the extracellular fluids is normally 1.0 to 1.5 g., this mobile bone reservoir is of potential significance in mineral homeostasis.

A crude index of the rate of calcium removal from this bone pool over a long period of time may be the extent of osteocytic osteolysis, assessed from the percentage of the total osteocytes seen to be enlarged in undecalcified bone sections. This percentage is increased in hyperparathyroidism and decreased in states characterized by excess CT secretion, e.g., medullary carcinoma. The percentage is also increased in hyperthyroidism and decreased in hypothyroidism.

HORMONAL CONTROL OF MINERAL HOMEOSTASIS AND SKELETAL REMODELING

There are three hormones of primary importance in the regulation of mineral homeostasis: PTH, CT, and $1,25(OH)_2D_3$. In addition, all three influence skeletal remodeling, but this process is also controlled by thyroxine, the adrenal glucocorticoids, the gonadal hormones, and growth hormone. Because of these differences, it is worthwhile discussing separately the hormonal control of mineral homeostasis and that of skeletal remodeling. In doing so, however, it is necessary to bear in mind that the two processes and their controlling factors do overlap.

Control of Skeletal Remodeling

The major determinants of skeletal remodeling are: (1) the rate at which new bone metabolic units are activated; and (2) the balance between resorption and formation within the units. More precisely, these events are determined by: (1) the rates of flow of bone mesenchymal cells into osteoclasts; (2) the activity of these osteoclasts; (3) the rate of conversion of osteoclasts to osteoblasts; and (4) the activity of these osteoblasts. The situation can be represented diagrammatically in terms of six cell pools (Fig. 11–10). The first, which is essentially of infinite size, is the mesenchymal, or osteoprogenitor, pool. The second is the pool of daughter cells, or preosteoclasts, which arise by mitotic division from the osteoprogenitor cells when a new bone metabolic unit is activated. The third is the pool of active osteoclasts. The rate of bone resorption will depend upon the total size of this cellular pool and the activity of the individual cells within it. The size of the pool is determined by the rate of entry of cells into this phase and the length of their stay. The fourth pool is that of preosteoblasts. As drawn in Figure 11–10, this pool is derived from the osteoclasts. There is some uncertainty about this hypothesis, however. An alternative possibility is that the preosteoblast can be derived directly from the pool of daughter cells (pool 2). If this is the case, the rate of flow of cells from pools 2 to 4 is controlled in some manner by the activity of the cells (osteoclasts) in pool 3. Hence, from an operational point of view, the two alternatives are equivalent in that resorption precedes formation and determines the flow of cells into pools 4 and 5. The fifth pool contains the active osteoblasts. Its size depends upon the rate of flow of cells from pool 4 (preosteoblasts) into pool 5 and the length of time each cell remains in this pool before becoming an osteocyte (pool 6). The osteocyte pool is extremely large compared with pools 2 through 5. The rate of bone formation depends upon both the size of the osteoblast pool and the activity of the individual cells within this pool.

Unfortunately, it is not possible to determine the size of all these different cellular pools. It is possible, however, to determine by quantitative histologic examination of bone biopsy material the size of the pool of active osteoclasts or the extent of active bone resorption surfaces and the size of the pool of active osteoblasts or bone formation surfaces. Thus the situation can be simplified to a consideration of three pools: progenitor cells, osteoclasts, and osteoblasts (Fig. 11–10). Two parameters of each of the two pools of active bone surface remodeling cells can be depicted: the size of the cell pool (the width of the box) and the relative activity of the cells (the height of the box). The size of these cellular pools and the activity of the respective pools are regulated by a complex set of hormonal and ionic factors, which are summarized in Figure 11–10.

Because the flow of cells is always from progenitor cells to osteoclasts and then to osteoblasts, it becomes immediately obvious that the overall size of the combined pools of active bone cells (osteoblasts plus osteoclasts) is determined by the rate of flow of cells from the osteoprogenitor cells to osteoclasts, i.e., the rate at which new active bone metabolic units are formed. Regardless of the total size of the combined pool of active bone cells, however, it is the relative distributions and activities of cells between osteoclasts and osteoblasts which determine skeletal balance. An imbalance in skeletal remodeling in favor of resorption can be seen with normal (osteoporosis), low (glucocorticoid-induced osteoporosis), or high (hyperparathyroidism and hyperthyroidism) rates of osteoprogenitor cell activation. Likewise, an imbalance in favor of formation can be seen with normal (osteopetrosis), low (hypothyroidism and hypoparathyroidism), or high (certain renal osteodystrophies and acromegaly) rates of osteoprogenitor cell activation. These various disease states will be discussed more fully in succeeding sections of this chapter. Finally, it is possible to maintain skeletal balance even with very high rates of formation of metabolic units of new active bone, as may be seen in Paget's disease of bone (see p. 767).

There are two nonhormonal factors of considerable importance in the control of skeletal remodeling, particularly in determining the balance between formation and resorption. These are the mechanical stresses placed upon the skeleton and the concentration of inorganic phosphate in plasma and extracellular fluids. The major effect of both appears to be that of increasing the flow of cells from osteoclasts to osteoblasts. In both cases, the result is to increase formation and decrease resorption, resulting in a new balance of skeletal remodeling in favor of formation.

Control of Mineral Homeostasis

The importance of the three primary hormones to calcium and phosphate homeostasis is illustrated by the changes in calcium and phosphate metabolism that are noted in their absence (Figs. 11–3 and 11–12).

The effect of complete removal of both thyroid and parathyroid glands upon calcium homeostasis is illustrated in Figure 11–3 by the responses of normal and thyroidectomized dogs to standard intravenous infusions of calcium and ethylenediaminetetraacetic acid (EDTA). In the normal animal, the rapid infusion of calcium leads to a rise in plasma calcium, and the infusion of EDTA to a fall. In both instances, the plasma calcium returns to the control level within 3 to 4 hours. Similar in-

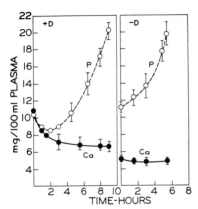

Figure 11–12. The changes in plasma calcium (○-----○) and plasma phosphate (●———●) as a function of the time after parathyroidectomy in vitamin D–fed (+D, left) and vitamin D–deficient rats (−D, right).

fusions into thyroparathyroidectomized animals lead to a greater initial deviation in plasma calcium, and the concentration does not return to the control value, even 24 hours after infusion has been terminated. Clearly the thyroparathyroidectomized animal is less able to adjust to either calcium excess or deprivation.

The importance of vitamin D and parathyroid hormone to calcium and phosphate homeostasis is illustrated in Figure 11–12. Deficiency of vitamin D leads to hypocalcemia in rats on normal mineral intakes. Removal of the parathyroid glands in the vitamin D–fed (+D) animals leads to a fall in plasma calcium, accompanied by an initial fall in plasma phosphate, followed by a dramatic rise. Parathyroidectomy in the vitamin D–deficient (−D) animal leads to no change in plasma calcium but to an immediate and dramatic rise in plasma phosphate. Thus, in normal animals, continuing parathyroid function is necessary to maintain normal levels of both plasma calcium and plasma phosphate, and in the −D animal, the hormone appears unable to alter the deranged calcium metabolism but continues to exert its characteristic effect upon phosphate metabolism.

Parathyroid Hormone

Parathyroid hormone, a polypeptide, is the only known secretory product of the parathyroid glands. These glands first appear as recognizable structures in the Amphibia, and they are present in all higher forms. There are some data showing that bony fish respond to bovine parathyroid extracts, but there is no conclusive evidence that they possess parathyroid glands.

Anatomy and Histology of Parathyroid Glands

Description of Parathyroid Glands

In man, there are usually two parts of parathyroid glands situated close to the posterior surface of the thyroid gland (one at each of the upper and lower poles); however, their number and location may vary considerably. About one of every ten glands is found in an aberrant location (usually in the mediastinum, occasionally within the thyroid, and rarely behind the esophagus). The mean size of a single human gland is approximately $5 \times 5 \times 3$ mm.; the combined weight of the four glands is about 120 mg. Children's parathyroids weigh approximately half this amount. The parathyroid glands are derived from the third and fourth branchial pouches. The superior glands develop from the fourth, and the inferior from the third. The latter migrate caudally during development.

The glands are reddish or yellowish brown and have distinct stalks (containing the blood vessels and the nerves) which enter each gland independently and serve as identifying features. In addition, each gland is surrounded by an ill-defined fibrous capsule and has a rich capillary plexus stemming from its blood vessels, a few nonmedullated nerve fibers along these vessels, a few indefinite bands of fibrous tissue and lymphatics (but no lymphoid follicles), and (after puberty) islands of fat cells between the cords of parenchymal cells. The normal epithelial cells (Fig. 11–13, A) are of two types: the chief cells, and the oxyphil cells. In hyperplasia, however, a third cell type, the water clear cell, is also seen (Fig. 11–13, C).

Chief Cells

The chief cells have been classified into two types, the light and the dark. The light cells are rich in glycogen, have a small Golgi apparatus and scant endoplasmic reticulum, and contain few secretory granules. They are considered to be inactive cells not secreting hormone and are seen characteristically in the rim of normal cells surrounding an adenoma. The dark chief cells are poor in glycogen and rich in secretory granules and have prominent Golgi and endoplasmic reticulum. They are considered to be actively engaged in synthesizing hormone and to be the main source of PTH. Both the water clear and oxyphil cells are derived from chief cells, and both cell types are apparently capable of secreting hormone. The secretory polarity of the chief cells is indicated by the fact that the nuclei are situated basally, and the Golgi apparatus appears apically. This orientation is very pronounced in hyperfunctioning glands. Studies of the fine structure of the parathyroid glands, using the electron microscope, have shown that the secretory cells contain cytoplasmic inclusions intimately associated with the Golgi complex. These inclusions are small dark vesicles (40 to 50 mμ) and are similar to those seen in other glandular tissues. The inclusions are considered to represent an initial stage in the formation of the secretory droplets; these droplets also are seen as larger bodies (60 mμ) in the cytoplasm not necessarily associated with the Golgi apparatus. In the hyperactive gland, there is an increase in the ribonucleoprotein particles and an increase in the number of small inclusions associated with the

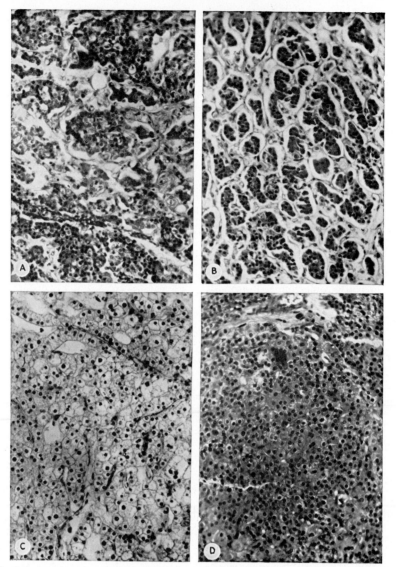

Figure 11–13.   Photomicrographs of parathyroid tissue from a normal gland (*A*), from an adenoma (*B*), from a gland with hyperplasia of the water clear cells (*C*), and from a gland with secondary hyperplasia of the chief cells (*D*). All four photomicrographs were taken at about the same magnification (× 360). In *D* there are many more cells than in *A* but they are equal in size, while in *C* the cells are much larger than in either *A* or *D*. In *C* there also is an increase in the total number of cells. Note the solid masses of cells in *B*. (The author is indebted to Dr. Benjamin Castleman for these histologic sections.)

Golgi complex, which suggests that these inclusions are the intracellular form of PTH. This is supported further by the observation that the number of these droplets varies directly with the functional activity of the gland, and by the further observation that the hormone is associated with a particulate cellular fraction that sediments with the mitochondrial fraction.

Oxyphil Cells

The distinguishing features of the oxyphil cells are these: (1) they contain no glycogen; (2) they appear after puberty; and (3) they vary in size, but usually range from 11 to 14 μ in diameter (a little larger than the usual type of chief cell). They have not been identified with any special function.

Water Clear Cells

These cells appear in small numbers in normal parathyroid tissue but are particularly prominent in certain hyperplastic glands. They are large polygonal cells, usually 10 to 15 μ in diameter, but they may have a diameter of 40 μ; there is a conspicuous lack of cytoplasm (Fig. 11–13, *C*).

Chemistry

The parathyroid hormone isolated from bovine parathyroid tissue is a single polypeptide chain of

PARATHYROID HORMONE

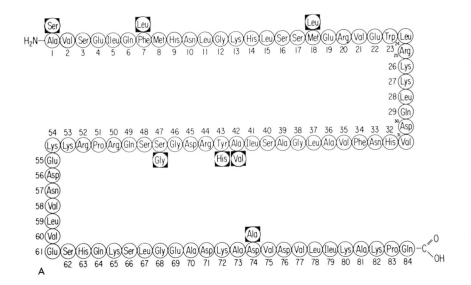

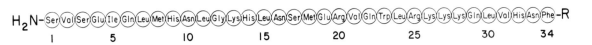

HUMAN PARATHYROID HORMONE

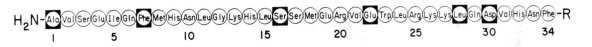

BOVINE PARATHYROID HORMONE

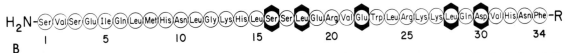

PORCINE PARATHYROID HORMONE

Figure 11–14. *A,* The structure of bovine parathyroid hormone (circles). The porcine hormone differs from the bovine by the substitution of the seven amino acids represented in the blocks. The biologic activity resides in the first 29 to 32 residues on the N-terminal region of the molecule. (Figure kindly supplied by Dr. Bryan Brewer.) *B,* A comparison of the structure of the N-terminal (1 to 34) portions of human, bovine, and porcine PTH. The boxed residues indicate the loci at which the bovine and porcine sequences differ from the human hormone. The sequence of the human hormone was determined by Brewer et al. (74). (This figure was kindly supplied by these authors before publication.)

84 amino acid residues (Fig. 11–14). However, a fragment of this hormone, consisting of the 33 or 34 amino acids at the N-terminal region of the molecule, is sufficient for the peptide to exert its characteristic biologic effects. The porcine hormone is of similar size but differs in amino acid composition (Fig. 11–14, *A*). The human hormone has been shown to be of a comparable size, and the N-terminal portion (34 amino acid residues) has been shown to differ from both the bovine and the porcine hormones (Fig. 11–14, *B*).

Until recently, it had been assumed that the "native" hormone extracted from the parathyroid glands was the molecular species circulating in the peripheral blood. However, this now appears not to be the case. Two, and possibly three, forms of PTH have been identified.

A possible larger precursor to bovine parathyroid hormone has been found in slices of parathyroid tissue. It contains 15 to 20 more amino acids than does the "native" hormone and has a molecular weight of approximately 11,500 compared with 9500 for the "native" hormone. This *proparathyroid hormone* combines with antibodies against PTH, and it contains the tryptic peptides usually found in bovine PTH plus two additional ones. When parathyroid tissue is incubated *in vitro* with [C^{14}] amino acids, radioactivity is detected first in proparathyroid hormone and then in the hormone. All of these data are consistent with the concept that the initial biosynthetic product in parathyroid tissue is a proPTH with a molecular weight of 11,500, which is normally converted to a molecule of 9500 molecular weight for storage and secretion.

The introduction of radioimmunoassay as a method for the detection of circulating PTH led to the discovery of several distinct immunologic forms of PTH in human peripheral blood. Similarly, when human parathyroid adenoma tissue is cultured *in vitro*, it continues to secrete biologically active, but immunoheterogeneous, parathyroid hormone. Three predominant species have been identified in human plasma. The first appears identical to the predominant form of the hormone isolated from parathyroid tissue, having a molecular weight of approximately 9500. It reacts best with antibovine antibodies. The second is a smaller species with a molecular weight of approximately 7000 which reacts best with antiporcine antibodies. The third is the smallest species, having a molecular weight in the range of 4500. The conversion of the larger to the smaller species has been demonstrated *in vitro*. A partially purified, calcium-regulated peptidase which catalyzes this conversion has been demonstrated in parathyroid tissue and liver. The activity of this enzyme is inhibited by Ca^{2+}. The product of this conversion, the 7000-molecular-weight species, is able to induce the biologic effects of bovine PTH (M.W. 9500) when administered to thyroparathyroidectomized rats. Moreover, the third species, purified from human plasma, has been found to activate renal adenyl cyclase.

The proPTH is normally found in small amounts within parathyroid tissue. Its conversion to the 9500-M.W. species normally takes place within the parathyroid cells. In some patients with parathyroid adenomas, however, some of this proPTH is probably released into the blood stream and is detected there as a larger immunoreactive species. The 9500-M.W. hormone is the predominant form in the normal gland. It is secreted as such, and, in part, may be hydrolyzed within the parathyroid tissue at the time of its secretion. Peripheral conversion to the 7000 and 4500 M.W. species also takes place and may be of greater importance, because the PTH found in the venous effluent from human parathyroid tissue is predominantly the 9500-M.W. species. In contrast, this species may represent 50 per cent or less of the total circulating PTH in peripheral blood, the remainder being the 7000 and 4500-M.W. species. The half-lives of the two species in the peripheral

circulation also differ. The 9500-M.W. species has a half-life of approximately 30 minutes; the 7000-M.W. species, of 2 to 4 hours.

When acute hypocalcemia is induced in man or experimental animals, the initial change (within the first ten minutes) in PTH concentration takes place almost entirely in the 9500-M.W. pool. Only later does the concentration of the smaller species increase.

There are conflicting views of the importance of the three peripheral forms of circulating PTH. One view is that only the 9500-M.W. material is biologically active, and the smaller species represent a degradation product. This view is based on the tenuous concept that antibodies against the N-terminal, biologically active portion of bovine PTH do not detect, or react poorly with, the 7000-M.W. species of human PTH. However, the N-terminal portions of bovine and human PTH are dissimilar in structure, so such an interpretation is uncertain. The other view is that the smaller species are the major biologically active forms of the hormone. This view is supported by the facts that: (1) these species, when purified from human plasma or from the culture media of human adenomatous tissue, are biologically active; (2) measurement of the amounts of these hormones in the peripheral circulation is a better means of discriminating between normal and hyperparathyroid human subjects than is measurement of the amount of the 9500-M.W. species; (3) the degree of osteocytic osteolysis and the number of osteoclasts per unit of bone surface in bone biopsies obtained from patients with primary hyperparathyroidism both have correlated closely with the concentration of the 7000-M.W. species in peripheral blood but not with the 9500-M.W. species; and (4) at least one patient with presumed idiopathic hypoparathyroidism has been found to have hypocalcemia associated with high circulating concentrations of the 9500-M.W. PTH species but normal or low concentrations of the 7000-M.W. species, suggesting a deficiency of the enzyme that catalyzes this conversion. Alternatively, the hormone found in this patient's plasma may be structurally abnormal, so that both the biologic activity and immunologic determinants in its N-terminal portion are altered.

Assay of Parathyroid Hormone Activity

Three different types of assay have been employed for the detection of parathyroid hormone: (1) biologic assay *in vivo* based upon either the calcium mobilizing or the phosphaturic actions of the hormone; (2) biologic assay *in vitro* using either isolated mitochondria or bones grown in tissue cultures; and (3) radioimmunoassay *in vitro*.

Biologic Assay

The most widely used biologic assay is based upon the calcium-mobilizing activity of PTH. A commonly used procedure (Munson) is to inject rats with PTH immediately after parathyroidectomy and bleed them six hours later. In the control group, plasma calcium concentration usually falls to 6 mg. per 100 ml., and in the experimental group, the plasma calcium does or does not fall, depending upon hormone concentration.

Another method is to place rats weighing 120 g. on a low-calcium diet, 0.02 per cent calcium for four days, then surgically parathyroidectomize them under light ether anesthesia. Immediately thereafter, they are injected with the hormone or vehicle without hormone and bled six hours later by cardiac puncture. The hormone is given subcutaneously as a suspension in sterile sesame oil. Six animals are employed in each group, and each assay contains a control group not receiving hormone and two groups each receiving a different amount of the standard. The assay is capable of detecting as little as 10 μg. of purified bovine parathyroid hormone and is useful in the range from 10 to 80 μg. Potency can be estimated with an error of $\pm$20 per cent. The assay is not capable of detecting hormone in biologic fluids. Its major use has been in the purification and characterization of parathyroid polypeptides.

A number of methods have been described for assaying parathyroid hormone *in vivo*, in which phosphaturia is used as an index of activity. None has gained wide acceptance because the methods are less precise and less specific. Nevertheless, in suitably prepared rats, the infusion of as little as 1 to 3 μg. of hormone per hour leads to a significant phosphaturia, indicating that this response is a more sensitive index of hormonal activity than is the standard calcium assay.

The biologic activity of PTH can be measured in rat embryonic bone *in vitro*. The bone is labeled by injecting 300 to 500 μC. of Ca^{45} into pregnant rats on the seventeenth day of pregnancy and by sacrificing them two days later. The embryos are taken from the mothers, and their forelimbs are removed and cultured on watch glasses in a medium of serum and Eagle's medium containing varying amounts of parathyroid hormone. After 72 hours of culture, the medium is analyzed for Ca^{40} and Ca^{45}, and the results are expressed as the ratio of counts in the treated to those in the control. This method is capable of measuring hormone concentrations in the range of 0.3 to 1.0 μg. per ml. The bioassay is not sufficiently sensitive, however, to detect PTH activity in small quantities of human blood plasma.

Radioimmunoassay

The most sensitive method for detecting parathyroid hormone in biologic fluids is a radioimmunoassay similar to that used for insulin (Ch. 9) and growth hormone (Ch. 2). Antibodies prepared against either bovine or porcine PTH are used because purified human PTH is not available as an antigen. Most success has been achieved with the antiporcine antibody. A few studies using both an-

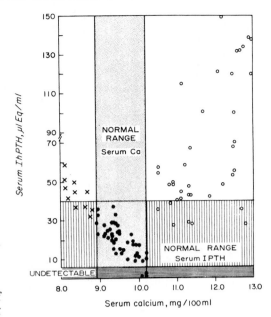

o   Surgically proved parathyroid adenomata

•   Normal

x   Hypocalcemia, no renal disease; not hypothyroid

Figure 11–15. Serum immunoreactive PTH plotted against serum calcium concentration in normal human subjects, patients with primary hyperparathyroidism, and patients with hypocalcemia of various etiologies other than hypoparathyroidism. (From Arnaud, C. D., Tsao, H. S., et al.: *J. Clin. Invest.* 50:21, 1971.)

tiporcine and antibovine hormone have shown that there are at least two species of circulating PTH. As noted above, the best correlation between various indices of disease and circulating PTH is obtained by measuring the amount of 7000-M.W. PTH using an antiporcine antibody. This method can be used routinely to detect the hormone in the blood plasma from normal human subjects, and also, when the hormone is measured in conjunction with the plasma calcium concentration, to discriminate between normal individuals and normocalcemic subjects with primary hyperparathyroidism (Fig. 11–15).

This discrimination depends upon the fact that, as the plasma calcium concentration rises in a normal person, PTH concentrations fall. Hence, normal subjects with plasma calcium concentration in the high normal range have the lowest PTH values, but patients with primary hyperparathyroidism have inappropriately high PTH values for the plasma calcium concentration.

The use of the radioimmunoassay to measure the concentration of PTH in human plasma has shown that patients with hypocalcemia from chronic renal disease and various forms of vitamin D deficiencies all have elevated concentrations of the two smaller species of PTH but may or may not have increased concentrations of the 9500-M.W. species. In these patients, there is an inverse correlation between the amount of PTH and the serum calcium concentration (Fig. 11–15), as would be expected if the plasma ionized calcium concentration were a prime regulator of PTH secretion.

Regulation of Secretion

Much older indirect evidence had indicated that the major factor controlling parathyroid hormone secretion is the plasma level of calcium. First, an inverse relationship was noted between the size of the glands and the calcium content of the diet; second, perfusion of the thyroparathyroid glands of the dog with blood containing low concentrations of calcium led to the appearance in the venous blood of a hypercalcemic principle; and third, hyperplasia of the parathyroid glands was noted in a variety of clinical states associated with hypocalcemia. More recently, it has been noted that a lowering of the plasma calcium level leads to an increased uptake of amino isobutyric acid (AIB) by the parathyroid gland but not by other tissues.

More direct evidence has come from studies of the effects of various ions upon amino acid uptake, hormone synthesis, and hormone release in parathyroid glands grown *in vitro*. The following changes have been noted when the glands are cultured in a low-calcium rather than a high-calcium medium: (1) an increased release of bone-mobilizing activity, presumably parathyroid hormone; (2) an increased rate of amino acid or AIB uptake; (3) an increased rate of incorporation of orotic acid into RNA and of amino acid into protein; and (4) a marked morphologic change of the plasma membranes of the cells. The effects upon RNA and protein synthesis are blocked by actinomycin, but those upon amino acid transport are not. Changes in magnesium concentration do not influence the various parameters in this system.

The results of tissue culture studies have been confirmed *in vivo* by more refined methods. Direct measurements of hormone secretion rates have been made in cows and pigs by radioimmunoassay. These studies show that PTH concentrations increase in plasma when hypocalcemia is induced by the infusion of the chelating agent, EDTA, and decrease when hypercalcemia is induced by the infusion of calcium. The converse pattern is observed with CT secretion. When antibodies prepared against porcine PTH and porcine CT are used, the effect of changes in serum calcium concentration upon the concentrations of these two hormones shows that there is direct correlation between serum calcium concentration and CT concentration in the range of serum calcium from 9.5 to 15 mg. per 100 ml. (Fig. 11–16). Conversely, there is an inverse correlation between serum calcium concentration and PTH concentration in the range of 4 to 10 mg. calcium per 100 ml. (Fig. 11–16). These data illustrate that the fullest control of serum calcium concentration is achieved in the range of 9 to 10.5 mg. per 100 ml., the normal physiologic range of concentration. Over this range, there is dual hormonal control.

The one situation in which hypocalcemia is not

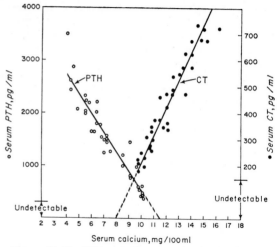

Figure 11–16. PTH and CT concentrations in pig serum plotted against serum calcium concentration. The serum calcium concentration was changed radically by the infusion of calcium or EGTA, an agent that chelates calcium (From Arnaud, C. D., Tsao, H. S., et al.: *J. Clin. Invest.* 50:21, 1971.)

associated with an increase in plasma PTH concentration, even though functioning parathyroid tissue is present, is severe hypomagnesemia. In patients with very low plasma magnesium concentrations, hypocalcemia develops, but PTH concentrations do not rise. When these subjects receive an infusion of Mg^{2+}, however, plasma PTH increases and is followed by an increase in the plasma calcium concentration. These data show that Mg^{2+} is required for the secretion of PTH in hypocalcemic humans.

There are two other factors of physiologic importance which may play a role in regulating PTH secretion. These are CT and vitamin D metabolites. In the case of CT, addition of this hormone to parathyroid tissue grown in organ culture leads to a release of PTH. The concentration of CT necessary to evoke such a response, however, is well above the normal circulating concentration of CT, and this may represent a pharmacologic rather than physiologic action of CT.

The other factor, vitamin D or its metabolites, does seem to have a physiologic role. When vitamin D is administered to vitamin D–deficient humans, the concentration of PTH in peripheral blood falls within the first 24 to 36 hours, despite the fact that the plasma calcium concentration has not changed or has even fallen. A logical interpretation of these results is that vitamin D increases the uptake of calcium into parathyroid cells, which is interpreted by these cells as an increase in plasma calcium concentration, i.e., vitamin D changes the set point around which plasma calcium concentration regulates PTH secretion.

Another feature of PTH secretion worthy of comment is the biphasic nature of this process after an acute stimulus to secretion. For example, in a human subject with Paget's disease with high rates of skeletal remodeling, the injection of CT will induce a rapid fall in plasma calcium concentration and a biphasic increase in PTH secretion. An initially very sharp rise in PTH concentration is followed by a more prolonged rise. Only the latter phase is closely correlated to changes in plasma calcium concentration. These data suggest that there is a small initial secretory pool of PTH within the glands, which is released immediately by any hypocalcemic stimulus, and a larger pool (possibly reflecting new hormone synthesis), which maintains secretory rate as an inverse function of plasma calcium concentration.

Function of PTH

In considering the function of a hormonal agent, one applies teleological reasoning. That is why interpretation of the function of a hormone depends to a considerable extent upon the point of view of the investigator. Nevertheless, in order to gain perspective, it is useful to consider, in general terms, the function or functions a particular hormone serves in bodily homeostasis. In the case of PTH, its major functions appear to be the regulation of the rate of activation of bone metabolic units and the maintenance of plasma calcium concentration at a level sufficient to ensure the optimal functioning of a wide variety of cells, such as the beta cells of the pancreas, other endocrine cells, and nerve and muscle cells in general. It also functions as a tropic hormone, regulating the renal synthesis of $1,25(OH)_2D_3$ from $25(OH)D_3$.

Effects of PTH: General

The major target organs for PTH action are kidney and bone. It also acts upon the intestine, but its effect may be indirect, being achieved by controlling the renal synthesis of $1,25(OH)_2D_3$.

The most important effects of PTH are to: (1) increase the plasma calcium concentration and decrease the plasma phosphate concentration; (2) increase the urinary excretion of phosphate and hydroxyproline-containing peptides but decrease the urinary excretion of calcium; (3) increase the rate of skeletal remodeling and the net rate of bone resorption; (4) increase the extent of osteocytic osteolysis in bone and increase the number of both osteoclasts and osteoblasts upon bone surfaces; (5) increase the rate of conversion of $25(OH)D_3$ to $1,25(OH)_2D_3$ in renal tissue; (6) activate adenyl cyclase in the cells of its target tissues; (7) cause an initial increase in calcium entry into cells of its target tissues; (8) alter the acid-base balance of the body; and (9) increase the gastrointestinal absorption of calcium.

Effects of PTH: Intestine

There is little doubt that parathyroid hormone promotes the absorption of calcium from the gastrointestinal tract in experimental animals and man. This has been demonstrated by (1) metabolic balance studies in man and experimental animals; (2) isotopic studies of calcium absorption in intact experimental animals and man (Fig. 11–39); (3) the loss of Ca^{45} from ligated loops of small intestine *in situ*; (4) the transport of calcium in isolated everted sacs of small intestine; and (5) uptake and release of calcium by isolated intestinal villi from normal and parathyroidectomized rats.

Three additional features of this PTH-mediated effect are that (1) it is not observed immediately after PTH administration but several hours later; (2) it has not been demonstrated *in vitro* after direct addition of PTH to intestinal sacs from parathyroidectomized animals; and (3) it is not observed in vitamin D–deficient animals.

Notwithstanding, the belief has persisted that PTH has a direct effect upon intestinal function, that of promoting the intestinal absorption of calcium. However, with the discovery that $1,25(OH)_2D_3$ is the biologically active metabolite of vitamin D_3 in the intestine (p. 703) and that PTH stimulates the renal synthesis of this metabolite (p. 703), it seems more likely that the effect of PTH upon intestinal calcium transport is mediated indirectly via its effects upon calciferol metabolism.

Effects of PTH: Bone

Classically, PTH has been considered the principal hormonal agent that controls bone resorption. However, the effects of this hormone are considerably more complex than originally supposed and are most easily considered in terms of the model of cellular events depicted in Figures 11–10 and 11–17.

The response of bone to PTH is biphasic (Table 11–4): the first, or immediate, phase depends upon the effect of PTH on bone cell activity; the second depends upon the effect of PTH on the size of active bone cell pools.

When PTH is administered to a parathyroidectomized animal, it has the immediate effects of increasing osteocytic and osteoclastic osteolysis by increasing the activity of both types of cells and by decreasing bone matrix synthesis through decreasing the activity of osteoblasts. These effects are seen within a few minutes following hormone administration; they are most easily observed by observing the effects that the hormone has upon the urinary excretion of calcium and hydroxyproline as well as upon plasma calcium concentration. PTH increases the concentrations of all three. These immediate effects are not blocked by the prior administration of inhibitors of RNA or protein synthesis.

In addition to this immediate effect upon bone cell activity, PTH also increases the size of the osteoclast pool by two actions: an inhibition of the flow of cells from osteoclasts to osteoblasts, and, most importantly, an activation of new groups of osteoprogenitor cells in the endosteal bone cell envelope (Figs. 11–10 and 11–17). This activation leads to waves of mitotic cell divisions and to the formation of preosteoclasts and, eventually, of new

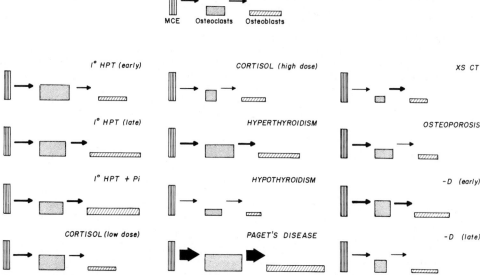

Figure 11-17. A model of the cellular events in the endosteal bone surface in adult human beings with a variety of metabolic bone diseases (see also Fig. 11-10). In the normal human being, the osteoprogenitor cells of the mesenchymal cell envelope (MCE) are activated first to osteoclasts which resorb bone, and these, in turn, then undergo modulation to osteoblasts which form bone. Each such bone remodeling unit has a lifetime of a few months. The number of such units present at any time is determined by the rate of activation of cells in the MCE. Within each unit, the sequence of resorption followed by formation may result either in net resorption, net formation, or skeletal balance, depending upon nutritional and hormonal factors. The sum of the activities of all such units can be depicted in terms of the size and activity of two cellular pools: osteoclasts (resorption) and osteoblasts (formation). These pools are represented schematically as blocks. The width of the block represents the size of the cell pool, and the height, the activity of these cells. For example, primary hyperparathyroidism leads first to (1) an increase in both size and activity of the osteoclast pool, and (2) a decrease in the size and activity of the osteoblast pool [1° HPT (early)]. However, as the disease progresses, the size of the osteoblast pool becomes greater than normal, although these cells appear less active than normal.

osteoclasts. The more important of these two effects is the latter, and if PTH administration is sustained, the enlarged osteoclast pool leads to a secondary increase in the flow of cells into the osteoblast pool, with a resultant increase in bone formation as well as bone resorption. Resorption is usually greater than formation, however, so that a net negative skeletal balance is observed in hyperparathyroidism.

The effects of PTH upon bone cell populations develop slowly over a matter of hours, differing from species to species, but requiring 12 to 24 hours in man. These effects are accompanied by an early increase in DNA synthesis, followed by increases in RNA and protein synthesis. As resorption increases, there is an increase in the release of lysosomal enzymes; as the secondary osteoblastic proliferation occurs, there is an increase in the rate

TABLE 11-4. CHARACTERISTICS OF THE TWO OSTEOLYTIC PHASES SEEN IN BONE FOLLOWING AN INCREASE IN PTH CONCENTRATION

Characteristic	Phase	
	Early Response	Late Response
Time of onset	Minutes to hours	Hours to days
Cells affected	Osteocytes and osteoclasts already present	Preosteoclasts and endosteal mesenchymal cells; periosteal mesenchymal cells
Result of effect	Increase in resorptive activity of individual cells and increase in flow of Ca^{2+} from deep bone to bone surface	Increase in number of osteoclasts and, secondarily, increase in osteoblast number
Magnitude of response	Limited or small	Potentially unlimited or large
Effect of vitamin D deficiency	Reduced response to PTH	Greatly reduced response to PTH
Sensitivity to PTH	Relatively sensitive	Relatively insensitive
Constant presence of PTH	Necessary	Unnecessary

of collagen biosynthesis. These slowly developing effects upon cell proliferation and modulation are blocked by inhibitors of RNA and protein synthesis.

The characteristic features of adult human bone in primary hyperparathyroidism are an increase in the number of active bone metabolic units, an increase in osteoclasts per unit surface of bone, and an increase in osteoblasts per unit surface of bone. These osteoblasts appear less active than normal, so that the major reason for the increase in bone formation is an increase in the number, but not the activity, of the osteoblasts.

In physiologic circumstances, the major effect of parathyroid hormone is exerted upon cells in the endosteal and haversian cell envelopes. In hyperparathyroidism, however, activation of osteoprogenitor cells occurs in the periosteal bone cell envelope as well, leading to the formation of active bone metabolic units on the periosteal surface, which in turn leads to the characteristic subperiosteal bone erosion seen radiographically in primary hyperparathyroidism (Fig. 11–53).

Effects of PTH: Kidney

Direct infusion of parathyroid hormone into a renal artery leads to unilateral phosphaturia. The effect is rapid (within 5 to 10 minutes) and is brought about by a change in tubular rather than glomerular function. This dramatic phosphaturia was one of the earliest known effects of parathyroid hormone. It so dominated the attention of most investigators that it obscured the fact that hormonal action upon the renal tubule leads not only to increased excretion of potassium, bicarbonate, sodium, and amino acids but also to decreased excretion of calcium, magnesium, ammonia, and titratable acidity. Urinary pH and the urinary excretion of C-AMP also increase. In acidotic animals, the hormone does not increase urinary pH but continues to promote Na^+ and K^+ loss, whereas in sodium-depleted animals, it increases urinary pH and the excretion of K^+.

The changes in renal electrolyte excretion are associated with a mild hyperchloremic systemic acidosis and a decrease in the total buffering capacity of the blood; and it has been argued that the primary effect of PTH is upon acid-base balance, leading to changes in bone mineral metabolism. The experimental support for this point of view is limited, however.

A site of action of PTH in the kidney has been localized to the proximal tubule. By micropuncture methods, it has been shown that PTH blocks the proximal tubular reabsorption of Na^+, Ca^{2+}, and HPO_4^{2-}. It appears to do so either by blocking $Na^+ \rightleftarrows H^+$ exchange in this portion of the nephron or by inhibiting the nonelectrogenic reabsorption of Na^+ and Cl^-. If this were the only effect of the hormone, it could probably also account for the hormone-induced increase in K^+ excretion by an increase in distal tubular $Na^+ \rightleftarrows K^+$ exchange. However, it is difficult to account for one of the

other major effects of PTH by this single proximal tubular action. PTH decreases the proximal tubular reabsorption of calcium. If the sodium load to the kidney is increased, the excretion of both Na^+ and Ca^{2+} increases. Nevertheless, when PTH is given, even though Na^+ excretion increases, *that of calcium decreases*. This effect of PTH upon the tubular reabsorption of calcium appears to be due to an action of the hormone directly upon the distal nephron. It remains possible that the change in K^+ excretion is also a reflection of this distal tubular effect. The decrease in H^+ excretion may also reflect, in part, a blockage of proximal tubular HCO_3^- reabsorption.

Although the effect of PTH on the tubular reabsorption of phosphate has been considered of major importance, more and more evidence indicates that the ability of PTH to enhance the renal tubular reabsorption of calcium is of prime importance in maintaining plasma calcium homeostasis.

The importance of this effect of PTH can be most easily demonstrated if the rate of calcium excretion is plotted against the serum calcium concentration in normal subjects given calcium infusions and in patients with hypo- and hyperparathyroidism (Fig. 11–18). What these data illustrate is that patients with hyperparathyroidism, although they may have hypercalciuria when compared with normal controls, have very low rates of calcium excretion for their serum calcium (or more correctly, their filtered load). If a normal subject had a serum calcium concentration of 12 mg. per 100 ml., for example, his rate of calcium excretion would be approximately 0.8 mg. per 100 ml. of his glomerular filtrate. Yet the patients with primary hyperparathyroidism have rates in the range of 0.2 mg. per 100 ml. Conversely, patients with hypoparathyroidism may have normal rates of excretion if their serum calcium concentrations are 7

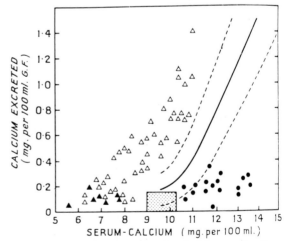

Figure 11–18. The urinary excretion of calcium as a function of serum [Ca^{2+}] in normal subjects [solid line ± 2 (SD) – dotted lines] and in patients with hypoparathyroidism ($\triangle$) and hyperparathyroidism ($\bullet$). The shaded area represents the normal physiologic situation. (From Nordin, B. E. C., and Peacock, M.: *Lancet* 2:1280, 1969.)

mg. per 100 ml. or below but extremely high rates if their serum calcium concentrations are 9 to 10 mg. per 100 ml.

The other important action of PTH upon the kidney is that of regulating the conversion of $25(OH)D_3$ to $1,25(OH)_2D_3$ and $24,25(OH)_2D_3$ (24,25-dihydroxycholecalciferol). PTH acts as a tropic hormone. When its concentration rises in blood, the conversion of $25(OH)D_3$ to $1,25(OH)_2D_3$ is increased and its conversion to $24,25(OH)_2D_3$ decreased. These effects are discussed more fully in later sections of this chapter.

Effects of PTH: Other Cells and Tissues

There is still doubt about the effects of PTH upon soft tissues. Its administration *in vivo* leads to an increase of hepatic calcium exchange without activation of hepatic adenyl cyclase. The problem is that of determining whether these changes in cellular calcium flux represent a direct effect of PTH or are a reflection of PTH-induced changes in vitamin D metabolism.

The one other tissue in which there is considerable evidence of a direct effect of PTH is the thymus. When thymocytes are isolated from the thymus gland of a young animal, there are two predominant cell types. The more numerous, representing 85 to 90 per cent of the cells, are small, mature lymphocytes which do not undergo further mitotic division. The remainder are larger lymphoblasts, which are either in mitosis or capable of being stimulated to enter into mitosis. It is only the larger lymphoblasts that respond to PTH and CT.

When a culture of immature thymus cells is incubated in the presence of colchicine, cells undergoing mitosis become arrested in metaphase, in which case they are easily recognized microscopically and counted. The percentage of cells (total population) arrested in metaphase is altered by PTH, Ca^{2+}, C-AMP, and CT. When no calcium is added to the medium, approximately 4.5 per cent of the cells are found to be in metaphase after a standard time of incubation (Fig. 11–19). If the calcium concentration is increased to 2.4 mM, 6.5 per cent of the cells are in metaphase. If PTH is added in the absence of calcium, it has little effect, but if the calcium concentration is 0.6 mM, then the addition of PTH leads to nearly a doubling of the number of cells in metaphase (Fig. 11–19). The addition of C-AMP causes a similar change, and CT blocks both the PTH- and C-AMP-induced increase. These cellular responses are similar to those of the osteoprogenitor cells *in vivo* in that PTH stimulates and CT inhibits mitotic division.

Modifiers of PTH Effects

In the ensuing discussion of the action of other hormones upon bone and mineral metabolism, their effects will be related to the actions of PTH, primarily because PTH action can serve as a useful

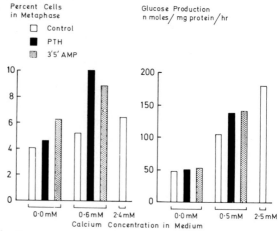

Figure 11–19. *Left*, the relationship between per cent of cells in metaphase and the presence of PTH, C-AMP, or calcium ion in the incubation medium of isolated thymocytes *in vitro*. *Right*, rate of glucose production as a function of PTH, 3',5'-AMP, and calcium concentration in isolated renal tubules. (From Rasmussen, H.: *Amer. J. Med. 50*:567, 1971.)

focus around which to center such a discussion. It is also useful to discuss several other factors that modify the effects of PTH upon bone, in particular, the concentrations of phosphate, pyrophosphate, and calcitonin (Table 11–5). Moreover, it is worth contrasting the effects of PTH with those of exogenous C-AMP because of the role of C-AMP in PTH action.

When PTH is administered, one of its first effects in both bone and kidney is to cause an increase in C-AMP concentration, which leads to an increase in the urinary excretion of this nucleotide. The infusion of C-AMP or its dibutyryl analogue into a thyroparathyroidectomized animal will lead to an increase in urinary phosphate excretion and an increase in the excretion of both calcium and hydroxyproline-containing peptides, with an associated rise in plasma calcium and a fall in phosphate concentration. These changes indicate that the infusion of C-AMP will mimic in a qualitative sense the gross physiologic effects of PTH, even though there are significant quantitative differences in their effects. For example, if the relative amounts of PTH and C-AMP are adjusted so

TABLE 11–5. COMPARISON OF EFFECTS OF PHOSPHATE, CALCITONIN, AND PYROPHOSPHATE ON THE RESPONSE OF THE TPX ANIMAL TO PTH INFUSION

Parameter	Pi	CT	PPi
Urinary calcium	Decrease	Decrease	Decrease
Plasma calcium	Decrease	Decrease	Decrease
Urinary HOP	No change	Decrease	Decrease
Urinary 3',5'-AMP	Small increase	No change	Decrease
Plasma phosphate	Small increase	Decrease	Decrease
Osteocytic osteolysis	No change	Decrease	Decrease
Osteoblastic activity	Increase	No change	?

that they cause comparable changes in plasma calcium concentration, it is found that the fall in plasma phosphate after C-AMP administration is much greater and the increase in hydroxyproline-containing peptides much less than those seen after PTH administration. Likewise, there are very significant differences in their effects when they are added to bone grown in tissue culture, with PTH being a more effective agent in inducing the activation of new osteoclasts from progenitor cells.

Another similarity between PTH and C-AMP is that CT infusion blocks the increase in calcium and hydroxyproline peptide excretion seen after either PTH or C-AMP infusion. Likewise, phosphate infusion will induce a decrease in the plasma calcium concentration in thyroparathyroidectomized (TPX) animals maintained on either PTH or C-AMP infusions. On the other hand, pyrophosphate blocks the bone-mobilizing effects of PTH but not those of C-AMP.

Of greatest interest are the agents that inhibit the effects of PTH upon bone (Table 11–5). These include CT, pyrophosphate, and phosphate. As shown in Table 11–5, even though all three cause a decrease in the plasma calcium concentration and the urinary excretion of calcium in TPX animals maintained on a constant infusion of PTH, their effects are not comparable. Neither CT nor phosphate inhibits the PTH-induced increase in C-AMP excretion, but pyrophosphate does. Both CT and pyrophosphate decrease urinary hydroxyproline excretion, but phosphate does not. The effect of pyrophosphate appears to be mediated, in part at least, by an inhibition of adenyl cyclase, but clearly the other two agents do not inhibit the activity of this enzyme. Their effects are more complex. Those of CT are considered in more detail later. However, those of phosphate are of special interest and will be dealt with here.

In terms of the model of cellular events in bone depicted in Figure 11–17, phosphate has several important effects. It increases the activity of osteoblasts and increases the flow of cells from osteoclasts to osteoblasts. This means that its most immediate effect is that of increasing the synthesis of collagen by osteoblasts, both directly by its effect upon their activity and indirectly by increasing the size of the osteoblast pool. If the phosphate concentration is raised sufficiently, the size of the osteoclast pool falls, and the rate of bone resorption falls. This is due, however, to the regulation of the flow of cells from osteoclasts to osteoblasts. There is no evidence to suggest that phosphate alters the rate of activation of osteoprogenitor cells, but there are theoretical grounds for thinking it might inhibit the process of activation.

The effect of phosphate upon the balance bebween bone resorption and formation is of great importance. Phosphate is the one known agent that, when given to a patient with primary hyperparathyroidism, will restore skeletal remodeling to a state of balance. In patients with renal osteodystrophy and secondary hyperparathyroidism, the plasma phosphate concentration can be suffi-

ciently high to induce a net positive balance in favor of bone formation. This is the basis for the osteosclerosis that is often seen in this disease.

Under some circumstances, particularly in parturient paresis in cattle and in vitamin D deficiency, calcium ions are capable of modifying PTH action.

Mode of Action of PTH: Bone

The two most immediate effects of PTH upon bone cells are (1) an increase in C-AMP concentration, and (2) an increase in the uptake of calcium into the cell (Fig. 11–20). These effects appear to be independent effects of the hormone, because even though exogenous C-AMP will induce an increase in bone resorption, it will not stimulate calcium uptake by bone cells. On the basis of these facts and data from a variety of other systems, it has been possible to develop a hypothesis as to the mode of action of PTH upon bone cells. A schematic representation of this model is shown in Figure 11–21. The central features of the model are that PTH has at least two primary effects upon bone cells: it activates adenyl cyclase, and it stimulates the entry of calcium into the cell. The activation of adenyl cyclase leads to an increase in C-AMP concentration within the cell cytosol, which in turn stimulates the activity of one or more of the protein kinases and enhances the efflux of calcium from the mitochondrial calcium pool. This effect may be mediated by regulating the activity of a membrane-bound protein kinase in the mitochondrial membrane, but this point remains to be established.

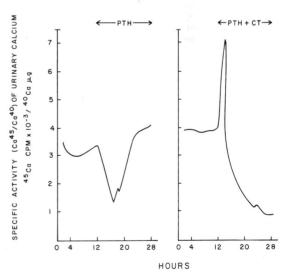

Figure 11–20. The change in urinary specific activity (Ca^{45}/Ca^{40}) in TPX −D rats given Ca^{45} three weeks prior to TPX, then given an infusion of PTH or PTH + CT. Note that PTH caused an initial fall in specific activity and CT a rise. Similar responses are seen in +D animals. These changes are thought to indicate an immediate effect of PTH upon calcium uptake into bone cells, and of CT upon calcium efflux from bone cells. (From Rasmussen, H., and Feinblatt, J.: *Calcif. Tissue Res.* 6:265, 1971.)

CALCIUM HOMEOSTASIS

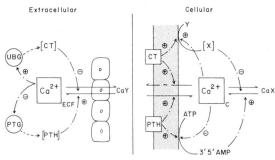

Figure 11–21. A schematic representation of the dual feedback control of extracellular and cellular calcium homeostasis. UBG: ultimobranchial gland or C cells of thyroid; PTG: parathyroid gland; CaY: bone calcium; CaX: mitochondrial calcium; $\boxed{Ca^{2+}}$: calcium concentration in cytosol; Y and X: postulated precursor and product of a CT-controlled intracellular process that leads to the synthesis of X, an intracellular regulator of mitochondrial calcium transport.

The combined action of PTH upon calcium entry into the cell and of C-AMP upon efflux of calcium from the mitochondria leads to an increase in cytosolic calcium. Thus both cytosolic Ca^{2+} and C-AMP concentrations increase, and both agents serve as second messengers within the cell. In addition, their concentrations are mutually regulated because $[Ca^{2+}]$ in the cytosol acts as a negative feedback regulator of adenyl cyclase activity.

These two second messengers have several important actions within bone cells. One of the most important, in terms of the ability of PTH to activate osteoprogenitor cells to divide and produce preosteoclasts and osteoclasts, is the effect of Ca^{2+} upon DNA synthesis and mitosis. The physiologic implication of this effect will be discussed subsequently (p. 693). Another effect which may be related to the ability of PTH to inhibit collagen synthesis in osteoblasts is that it alters carbohydrate metabolism, causing a fall in α-ketoglutarate concentration. This dicarboxylic acid has been shown to be an obligatory substrate in the protocollagen hydroxylase reaction which is responsible for the hydroxylation of the proline residues in this macromolecule.

It is not yet known in detail how the changes in cytosolic calcium and C-AMP lead to an increase in the activity of osteocytes and osteoclasts, causing thereby an increase in bone resorption. The problem is that the biochemical basis of the process of bone resorption remains to be established. It is a complex process which normally involves the simultaneous destruction of matrix and mineral. Matrix destruction requires some type of collagenase activity. Such enzymatic activity has been detected in bone, but it has not been well characterized.

One theory that has been advanced to account for resorption is that the major factor involved is the release of lysosomal enzymes, mainly because when PTH is added to bone grown in tissue culture, there is an increase in the release of lysosomal enzymes associated with the increase in bone resorption. Two findings which raise doubts about the validity of this theory are that (1) lysosomes do not contain collagenase, yet this is an enzyme of key importance in the destruction of bone matrix; and (2) there is, in addition to an increase in bone resorption after PTH, an increase in the turnover of bone cells which undergo a successive sequence of modulatory events involving considerable changes in cell structure. It remains possible that the increase in lysosomal enzyme activities is more a reflection of this change rather than a reflection of the resorptive activities of the osteolytic cells.

Another aspect of the biochemical effects of PTH upon bone that has attracted considerable interest is the increase in citrate and lactate production the hormone induces. Under some circumstances, there is a good correlation between resorption and citrate production, but under others this is not so. It now seems clear that, although citrate production is a part of the normal response to PTH, it is not an indispensable part of this response. The situation with lactate is less clear. The production of acids at the site of resorption would aid greatly in the dissolution of bone mineral, and the changes in citrate and lactate production may be secondary consequences of an increase in the H^+ gradient across the cell membrane of bone cells after PTH action.

Physiologic Implications

One of the most interesting features of the model depicted in Figure 11–21 is the possible way in which phosphate alters the cellular response to PTH. As discussed previously, there is an intimate relationship between calcium and phosphate within the cell cytosol and the pool of insoluble calcium phosphate within the mitochondria (Fig. 11–1). The latter serves as a buffer system for Ca^{2+}, HPO_4^{2-}, and H^+. It is this relationship which helps to determine the cellular response to changes in phosphate concentration. If isolated cells are treated with a standard dose of PTH and then exposed to increasing amounts of phosphate in the medium, the total cellular uptake of calcium increases, but the amount of C-AMP also increases. The major part of the additional calcium, however, can be shown by isotopic studies to be taken up into the mitochondrial calcium pool. A logical interpretation of the cellular effects of phosphate is as follows: an increase in extracellular phosphate leads to an increase in the amount of phosphate entering the cell cytosol. As cytosolic phosphate concentration increases, it stimulates the uptake of calcium by the mitochondria, and cytosolic calcium concentration falls. This leads, in turn, to (1) a relief of the inhibition of adenyl cyclase, with a resultant rise in C-AMP concentration; and (2) an increase in the amount of calcium entering the cell. The latter effect, plus the fact that the increase in cytosolic C-AMP causes an increase in mitochondrial calcium efflux, means that a new steady state is attained in which cytosolic C-AMP concentration is higher and cytosolic calcium concentration lower than in cells maintained in a low-phosphate environment.

An additional aspect of phosphate metabolism in bone concerns the effect of phosphate deficiency upon bone turnover. A deficiency of phosphate has two important consequences: it blocks mineralization and enhances resorption. Hence, severe phosphate deprivation leads to rickets or osteomalacia. In contrast, calcium deficiency leads to osteoporosis.

A feature seen in the model shown in Figure 11–21 is that, in order for PTH to enhance the process of bone resorption, it must first increase the uptake of calcium into bone cells. On the basis that the initial effect of PTH is that of inducing a fall in plasma calcium concentration, it seems likely that the calcium taken up by the bone cells must come from the bulk extracellular fluids and not from bone mineral. This can be represented schematically as in Figure 11–22. There is a "feed-forward" loop, so that an initial increase in cellular calcium uptake is required to initiate bone resorption.

Such a relationship must also be of importance

in the acute cellular responses to PTH, because when $CaCl_2$ was infused into chicks together with PTH, the plasma calcium concentration was significantly higher one hour later in the animals receiving both $CaCl_2$ and PTH than in those receiving PTH alone. The amount of calcium administered with the PTH, however, was insufficient to account for the elevation of plasma calcium concentration, clearly implying that the calcium acted as an amplifying modifier of the action of PTH.

If a change in cytosolic calcium ion concentration is an important signal for the activation of osteoprogenitor cells and their conversion to osteoclasts, then the model shown in Figure 11–22 predicts that, in conditions of extreme hypocalcemia, PTH would be ineffective in enhancing bone resorption. This situation is comparable to that encountered in parturient paresis in cattle.

Parturient paresis occurs in large milk producers at the time of calving. The sequence of events follows a rather typical pattern. During the last months of pregnancy, if the cattle are on a good diet, there is a marked increase in the absorption of calcium from the gut, much of which is retained by the fetal skeleton. At this time, the rate of remodeling of the maternal skeleton is usually low, so that relatively few active bone metabolic units are present. Shortly before, during, and for several days after parturition, the cow fails to eat, and simultaneously milk production begins. The consequence is a dramatic and rapid fall in plasma calcium concentration, which may reach a value as low as 2 mg. per 100 ml. This profound hypocalcemia is accompanied by a flaccid paralysis and by derangements of energy metabolism, including hyperglycemia. Plasma PTH concentration is *elevated,* however, and the administration of this hormone does not correct the hypocalcemia. Successful therapy requires the administration of calcium. This is successful even though plasma PTH concentrations fall. The administration of one or two large doses of calcium leads to the return of the plasma calcium concentration to near normal, even though milk production continues and calcium is removed from the body. A logical interpretation of these events can be made by reference to the model depicted in Figure 11–22. Prepartum, the rate of skeletal remodeling is low. There are very few osteoclasts upon bone surfaces. Hence, when PTH increases because of the hypocalcemia, the increase in activity of the few osteoclasts and of the osteocytes is insufficient to restore the plasma calcium concentration to normal. This normally leads to the activation of new osteoprogenitor cells by PTH and then an increase in the size of the osteoclast pool (Fig. 11–17). However, the effect of PTH upon osteoprogenitor cell activation requires time. In the cow, it may take as long as 48 to 72 hours for a new population of osteoclasts to appear. The activation also requires a change in the concentration of cytosolic calcium (Fig. 11–22), which in turn is partially dependent upon the calcium concentration in the extracellular fluids, because one of the primary effects of PTH is that of stimulating calcium uptake by these cells (Fig. 11–22). If

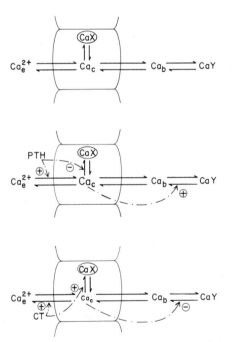

Figure 11–22. A schematic representation of the relationship between the concentration of calcium in the extracellular fluids ($Ca_e{}^{2+}$), the cell cytosol (Ca_c), mitochondria (CaX), the bone extracellular fluid (Ca_b), and the bone mineral (CaY). When PTH acts, it stimulates the uptake of calcium from $Ca_e{}^{2+}$ to Ca_c, and via C-AMP, it inhibits the uptake of calcium into CaX. This leads to an increase in the concentration of Ca_c, which acts as a feed-forward signal to stimulate bone resorption and increase the flow of calcium from CaY to Ca_b and, eventually, to $Ca_e{}^{2+}$. CT acts in the opposite sense. The most important feature of this model is that if $Ca_e{}^{2+}$ and CaX are too low PTH will be ineffective in raising Ca_c and, therefore, of increasing bone resorption.

the extracellular calcium concentration falls below some critical level, however, then PTH is ineffective in causing an increase in cytosolic calcium concentration and thus in the activation of new cells.

The reason that this situation is not normally seen is that only in the special circumstance that a profound hypocalcemia develops very rapidly will the response of the system fail. Once the hypocalcemia is profound, then merely increasing PTH concentration will not restore the response, but increasing the extracellular calcium concentration will restore it.

There is no exact counterpart to this parturient paresis in humans. However, the model depicted in Figure 11–22 accounts for the response of the bone cells to calcium infusion or ingestion in patients with osteomalacia and hypocalcemia. These patients have a relatively low osteoclast count upon the surface of their bones, particularly when compared with patients with primary hyperparathyroidism. In the latter patients, there is a direct correlation between osteoclast count and plasma PTH concentration. The correlation is inverse in patients with osteomalacia, however. This means that in patients with vitamin D deficiency, there is a significant reduction in the size of the osteoclast pool relative to that predicted by the concentration of circulating PTH. The administration of PTH leads to little change in these patients, but the administration of vitamin D leads to a marked increase in osteoclast number, even though plasma PTH concentration falls (p. 705). Moreover, if patients with osteomalacia are given sufficient calcium to cause a sustained increase in the plasma calcium concentration, the *osteoclast count* upon the endosteal bone surface *increases,* even though the *plasma PTH concentration falls.* The model depicted in Figure 11–22 accounts for these results in a logical fashion, particularly if once assumes that the bone cells of the vitamin D–deficient animal are unable to take up and retain calcium to the same extent as normal cells.

Mode of Action of PTH: Kidney

Extensive studies of the effects of PTH upon kidney tubules and isolated kidney tubule cells grown in tissue culture have established the following facts: (1) PTH activates adenyl cyclase; (2) PTH stimulates the uptake of calcium into these cells, but exogenous C-AMP does not; (3) both PTH and exogenous C-AMP enhance the efflux of radioactive calcium from prelabeled cells; (4) both PTH and C-AMP enhance the rate of gluconeogenesis from a variety of substrates, including pyruvate, malate, and α-ketoglutarate; (5) the stimulation of gluconeogenesis by either agent is dependent upon the extracellular calcium concentration; (6) increasing the phosphate concentration in the medium induces an increase in calcium uptake and a reduction in calcium efflux, an increase in C-AMP concentration in PTH-treated cells, but a fall in PTH-mediated gluconeogenesis; and (7) an in-

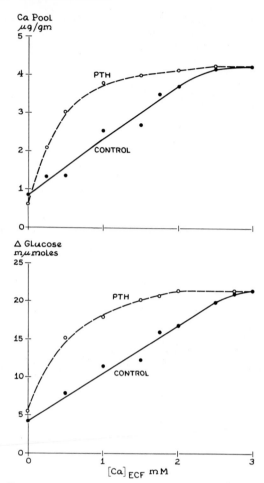

Figure 11–23. The effect of changing extracellular fluid calcium concentration, in the absence and presence of PTH, upon the uptake of calcium by isolated kidney cells (upper) and upon gluconeogenesis in isolated renal tubules (lower). [From the work of Borle (70) and Rasmussen et al. (37).]

crease in the extracellular calcium ion concentration in the absence of PTH will also enhance the rate of gluconeogenesis.

When the effects of PTH and changes in extracellular calcium ion concentration upon the size of the intracellular calcium pool and upon the rates of glucose formation from pyruvate are compared (Fig. 11–23), there is a striking similarity. In the absence of extracellular calcium, PTH is obviously ineffective in increasing the size of the intracellular calcium pool, but it is also ineffective in increasing the rate of gluconeogenesis. In the absence of PTH, an increase in the external calcium concentration from 0.05 to 2.5 mM leads to a nearly linear increase in the size of the intracellular pool and in the rate of glucose formation. As the extracellular calcium ion concentration rises above 2.5 mM, there is no further increase in the size of the intracellular pool nor in the rate of gluconeogenesis. When the external Ca^{2+} concentration is between 0.05 and 2.5 mM, the addition of PTH causes an increase in both the size of the pool and the rate of glucose formation. At very low or very high external Ca^{2+} concentrations, however, the effect of PTH is less marked. Thus, in the renal cell, just as in the bone cell, the response to PTH is dependent upon the extracellular calcium ion concentration.

In contrast, if the concentration of C-AMP is measured in renal tubule cells treated with a maximal dose of PTH, an inverse relationship is found between C-AMP concentration and extracellular Ca^{2+} concentration.

The effects of PTH and exogenous C-AMP upon calcium exchange in renal tubule cells can be interpreted in terms of the model depicted in Figure 11–21. PTH has two primary effects upon the cell surface: (1) it stimulates adenyl cyclase, and (2) it enhances the uptake of calcium into the cell. The activation of adenyl cyclase leads to an increase in C-AMP concentration within the cell, which causes an increase in the rate of calcium efflux from the mitochondria. This model is similar to that developed to account for the action of PTH upon bone cells. It argues that a second messenger of great importance in PTH action is the concentration of Ca^{2+} in the cell cytosol. The inverse relationship between C-AMP concentration and extracellular Ca^{2+} concentration in PTH-treated renal cells can be explained if it is assumed that an increase in cytosolic $[Ca^{2+}]$ acts as an inhibitor of adenyl cyclase.

These results indicate that PTH acts upon bone and renal cells through a basically similar mechanism. In the case of kidney cells, it has not yet been possible to define the relationship between this model of the action of PTH, which is based upon metabolic studies *in vitro*, with the major physiologic effects of PTH upon the tubular reabsorption of electrolytes.

Mode of Action of PTH: Isolated Thymocytes

Another cell type that responds to PTH is the isolated thymocyte. In this cell type, PTH increases the rate of mitotic division and DNA synthesis. Similar changes have been reported in bone marrow cells. Superficially, the responses of thymocytes to PTH resemble the responses of kidney (Fig. 11–19) and bone cells. PTH stimulates C-AMP accumulation, and the effect of PTH and exogenous C-AMP requires calcium. It has been proposed, however, that the primary effect of PTH is to stimulate calcium entry, which in turn blocks phosphodiesterase and leads thereby to an increase in C-AMP within the cell.

Calcitonin

Calcitonin (CT) is a small polypeptide hormone secreted by the ultimobranchial body in fish, amphibians, reptiles, and birds. In mammals, calcitonin is secreted by specialized cells of ultimobranchial origin, found primarily in the thyroid but, in some cases, in the parathyroid and thymus tissue as well.

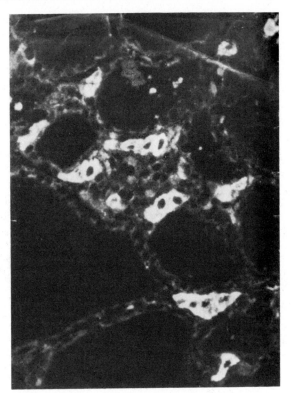

Figure 11–24. The thyroid C cells labeled by an immunofluorescent technique specific for calcitonin. Note the unstained acinar cells in the background. (Figure kindly supplied by Dr. A. G. E. Pearese.)

Source

This hormone originates in specialized "C" cells, which in the mammalian thyroid are derived embryologically from the ultimobranchial organs. They exist as small groups of interstitial or parafollicular cells in thyroid tissue. They are rich in mitochondria and secretory vesicles and contain high concentrations of α-glycerophosphate dehydrogenase activity. They have been identified as the source of calcitonin by immunofluorescent techniques (Fig. 11–24).

The C cell of the mammalian thyroid and the ultimobranchial cells of lower forms all arise embryologically from the neural crest. Cells of the adrenal medulla have a similar neuroectodermal origin, which explains why medullary carcinoma of the thyroid and pheochromocytoma both contain catecholamines and may occur in the same individual.

Chemistry

The structure of the porcine, bovine, salmon, and human hormones has been determined, and synthetic human hormone has been prepared and shown to be biologically active. The amino acid sequences of these four hormones are shown in Figure 11–25. The amino-terminal end of all four is identical, consisting of a seven-membered ring enclosed by an intrachain disulfide bridge. All four molecules consist of a single sequence of 32 amino

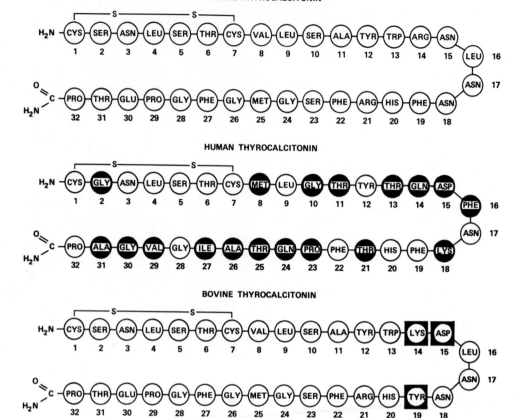

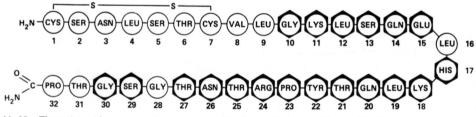

Figure 11–25. The amino acid sequences of porcine, human, bovine, and salmon calcitonin. The blackened symbols represent residues in the other hormones which differ from those found in the porcine hormone.

acid residues (3000 M.W.), and the C-terminal amino acid, proline, is identical in all four. Moreover, the residues in positions 9 and 28 are identical, but differences exist in all other positions. At the present time, it appears as though the entire molecule is essential for biologic activity.

One of the most surprising features of the salmon hormone is that, on a weight basis, it is a more potent hypocalcemic agent than any of the mammalian hormones when administered to mammals, including man.

Assay

Calcitonin can be assayed *in vivo* by a method that depends upon the ability of CT to lower serum calcium concentration in suitably prepared rats.

The best results have been obtained from young rats weighing 75 to 150 g. The animals are maintained on a low-calcium diet for four days. Then, under light ether anesthesia, 0.5 ml. of the control or hormone solution is injected into the external jugular vein, and a sample (1.0 ml.) of blood is obtained either by cardiac puncture or phlebotomy one hour later. The index of precision using this method is approximately 0.20, when two doses of standard and unknown are compared under suitable circumstances.

If the rats are more uniformly selected (100 ± 3 g.), the response is slightly more sensitive, and the index of precision is 0.15 to 0.20. The method is capable of detecting 0.05 µg. of porcine calcitonin.

Radioimmunoassays were originally developed for the porcine hormone. These have been used successfully in the study of mineral homeostasis in the pig but have been found unsuitable for the assay of calcitonin concentrations in normal human plasma. More recent work with the synthetic human hormone, however, has led to the development of assays suitable for clinical use. In normal adult human subjects, the circulating concentration of calcitonin in plasma ranges from 0.02 to 0.40 ng. per ml., with the majority of individuals having values below 0.10 ng. per ml. This value rises 1.5- to 3-fold in most normal human beings after a standard calcium infusion of 15 mg. of calcium per kilogram of body weight over a 4-hour period.

The hormone (at least the immunoreactive component) is stable and can be detected in urine at a concentration of less than 1 ng. per ml.

The most thoroughly studied examples of excess secretion of CT are patients with medullary carcinoma of the thyroid. In such patients, the circulating CT concentration may range from high normal to nearly 540 ng. per ml. Interestingly, CT concentrations are not usually increased in the plasma of patients with primary hyperparathyroidism, and the amount of hormone in their thyroid tissue is less than normal.

Regulation of Secretion: CT

The only known, physiologically important regulator of the rate of CT secretion is the concentration of calcium ion in the plasma and extracellular fluids. The rate of CT secretion is a direct function of the plasma calcium concentration when the total calcium concentration is above 9 mg. per 100 ml. (Fig. 11–16). Below this level, CT is undetectable in normal human plasma, because present-day radioimmunoassays are not sufficiently sensitive to measure very low (<0.05 ng. per ml.) concentration of CT.

The only other ionic factor that has been shown to stimulate CT secretion is an increase in Mg^{2+} concentration. Only high and nonphysiologic concentrations of Mg^{2+}, however, will induce secretion, and at present there is no evidence that a change in plasma Mg^{2+} concentration is normally an important regulator of CT secretion *in vivo*.

One of the most interesting aspects of the control of CT secretion is that related to calcium ingestion. In experiments on young animals, calcitonin secretion increases after a high calcium meal, but the increase takes place before a significant rise in plasma calcium concentration is observed. It is possible that secretion is due to a small, undetectable rise in plasma ionized calcium concentration. It has also been shown, however, that the injection of either gastrin or pancreozymin will induce an increase in the circulating concentration of calcitonin, while the injection of pentagastrin into normal adult human beings gives variable results, with the majority of individuals showing no rise in CT secretion but a few showing a significant increase.

Function of CT

There are at least three functions attributed to CT. In terms of plasma calcium homeostasis, the first proposed function is that of protecting the young organism against postprandial hypercalcemia. In this function, the stimulation of calcitonin secretion by gastrin is considered part of an endocrine reflex arc which anticipates, in a sense, the potentially dangerous rise in plasma calcium concentration. It has proved difficult to establish a similar function for CT in the normal human adult.

The second proposed function is related to both plasma calcium homeostasis and bone remodeling. One of the most impressive features of the physiology of calcitonin is its age-related effectiveness (Fig. 11–26). When administered on the basis of a unit of weight or of surface area, CT is a much more effective hypocalcemic agent in the young than in the old animal. Thus a 2-week-old animal may be 50 to 100 times more sensitive to CT administration than a fully grown one. In contrast, the effectiveness of PTH is, at most, two times greater in young than in mature animals (Fig. 11–26). The effectiveness of CT shows a direct correlation with the rate of bone remodeling, or osteoclast count, on endosteal bone surfaces. As the remodeling rate falls with skeletal maturation, CT effectiveness declines. If the remodeling rate is increased by disease (e.g., Paget's disease) or by the administration of PTH, then CT becomes more effective. As can be seen from these observations, a major function of CT is that of regulating the rate of skeletal remodeling.

The third function of CT is that of controlling fluid and electrolyte homeostasis in lower animals. For example, salmon calcitonin, which is a very potent hypocalcemic agent in man, has little or no hypocalcemic activity in fish, including salmon. On the other hand, CT in man, in addition to its effects upon calcium metabolism, produces a natriuresis

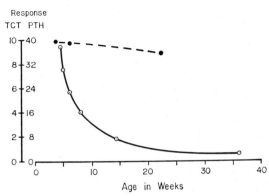

Figure 11–26. The effect of the age of rats upon relative response to PTH (●-----●) and CT (○———○). Note particularly the marked decrease in responsiveness to CT with age. This decreased responsiveness is directly related to the decrease in rate of skeletal remodeling with age. (From Copp, D. H.: *Ann. Rev. Pharmacol.* 9:327, 1969.)

and a decrease in body fluid volume. A similar effect has been described in the eel. Its function in lower forms may be to permit fish to adjust to changes in osmotic environment.

Effects of CT: General

The most readily observable effects of CT in young animals or older animals with elevated rates of skeletal remodeling are upon plasma calcium and phosphate concentrations. CT administration causes a fall in the concentration of both. If the early time course of CT action is observed, however, it is found that CT causes an initial short increase in the release of calcium from the skeleton before inducing a profound inhibition of this release (Fig. 11–20). This initial release may be of sufficient magnitude, under the proper experimental conditions, to cause a transient increase in plasma calcium concentration. It is noteworthy that these changes are the opposite of those induced by PTH administration.

Effects of CT: Bone

The most important effects of CT upon bone are three in number: (1) to decrease the resorptive activity of osteoclasts and osteocytes, (2) to decrease the rate of activation of osteoprogenitor cells to preosteoclasts and osteoclasts, and (3) to increase the modulation of osteoclasts to osteoblasts (Fig. 11–10).

Serial biopsies of the bones of young rabbits given CT reveal a very striking decrease in osteoclast count, starting within 15 minutes after hormone administration. The osteoclasts withdraw from the bone surface, round up, and then undergo transformation to mononucleated cells. These changes, along with histologic evidence that CT blocks the osteocytic osteolysis induced by PTH administration, are clearly related to the initial hypocalcemic effects of CT. If CT administration is continued, however, the rate of activation of osteoprogenitor cells to osteoclasts decreases, i.e., there is a decrease in the rate of formation of new active bone metabolic units. As a consequence, both bone resorption and bone formation fall following long-term CT administration because of the coupling between these two bone surface cell pools. Thus the effect of CT upon bone formation is biphasic. Initially, by inducing a modulation of osteoclasts to osteoblasts, CT induces an increase in the rate of bone formation and a decrease in bone resorption, with a net positive skeletal balance. This phase in man may last from weeks to one or two months. As the rate of activation of the osteoprogenitor cells declines, however, the size of the osteoclast pool decreases, and, as a consequence, the rate of modulation of osteoclasts to osteoblasts also declines, and the extent of bone forming surface falls.

The implications of these facts, in terms of the therapeutic use of CT, are clear. CT is *not* an agent that will induce a long-term increase in bone formation.

When CT is given before PTH to thyroparathyroidectomized (TPX) animals, it blocks the effects of PTH upon hydroxyproline excretion (Table 11–5), osteocytic osteolysis, and activation of new bone metabolic units. Both *in vivo* and *in vitro,* however, continued administration of CT with PTH often leads to an escape phenomenon, in that the effects of PTH become manifest even though CT administration has continued. The physiologic importance of this phenomenon is not clear, because in patients with medullary carcinoma of the thyroid and excessive CT secretion, bone biopsies reveal extremely low rates of skeletal remodeling in spite of secondary hyperparathyroidism. These observations imply that in man long-term excessive secretion of CT has a continuous and long-term effect upon skeletal remodeling.

The other feature of CT action upon bone relating to PTH action is that CT blocks neither of the initial effects of PTH upon bone cells. If CT is given to a TPX animal at the same time as or before PTH, it does not block the PTH-induced increase in calcium uptake or the PTH-induced activation of adenyl cyclase. On the contrary, CT given with PTH leads to a greater rise in C-AMP concentration than PTH given alone, and PTH given with CT does not block the initial CT-induced mobilization of calcium from bone. These facts demonstrate that CT does not act at the cellular level as an antiparathyroid hormone. This conclusion is supported by the fact that CT blocks the bone resorption induced by the infusion of exogenous C-AMP or its dibutyryl derivative just as effectively as it blocks PTH-induced resorption.

Finally, it is of interest that the two hormones, CT and PTH, have opposite effects upon the membrane potential of osteoclasts. PTH treatment leads to a fall, and CT to a rise, in membrane potential.

Effects of CT: Intestine

There is considerable uncertainty concerning the effects of CT upon gastrointestinal function. CT is just as effective a hypocalcemic agent in a young animal whose gastrointestinal tract has been removed as in a normal control. Likewise, in most studies of absorption of calcium from isolated gut loops *in vivo,* CT has not been found to increase calcium absorption. On the other hand, the perfusion of high concentrations of CT into an isolated loop of small intestine (principally duodenum) has led to a decrease in calcium absorption.

The present evidence speaks against an important direct effect of this hormone upon intestinal calcium absorption. A physiologically important effect of CT upon calcium absorption, however, may be mediated by an inhibition of the renal conversion of $25(OH)D_3$ to $1,25(OH)_2D_3$ (p. 703).

Effects of CT: Kidney

Careful studies of the effects of CT and PTH upon renal electrolyte excretion in hypoparathy-

TABLE 11-6. COMPARISON OF THE EFFECTS OF CT AND PTH UPON URINARY ELECTROLYTE EXCRETION IN MAN

Electrolyte Excreted	CT	PTH
Phosphate	Increase	Increase
Calcium	Increase	Decrease
Hydrogen	No change	Decrease
Chloride	Increase	Little or no change
Potassium	Very slight increase	Significant increase
Magnesium	Increase	Decrease
Sodium	Increase	Increase
Other Parameters		
Body weight	Decrease	No change
Systemic acidosis	None	Present

roid and normal human beings have shown that, even though both hormones induce a decrease in tubular phosphate reabsorption, they do so by different mechanisms. The contrasting effects of the two hormones upon renal electrolyte excretion in man are summarized in Table 11-6. The most striking differences are that CT infusion leads to a Na^+, Cl^-, and Ca^{2+} diuresis, with little change in H^+ excretion, while PTH infusion leads to a Na^+ and K^+ diuresis associated with H^+ and Ca^{2+} retention, and no change in Cl^- excretion. The CT-induced NaCl diuresis leads to a loss of body weight, i.e., a decrease in extracellular fluid volume, which results in a secondary rise in plasma renin and aldosterone secretion. The injection of CT leads to no significant alteration in body acid-base balance, but PTH injection leads to a mild systemic hyperchloremic metabolic acidosis.

CT does not stimulate renal adenyl cyclase or alter the urinary excretion of C-AMP, and it does not block the PTH-induced rise in urinary C-AMP excretion. In patients with medullary carcinoma, urinary calcium excretion is not elevated, bone resorption and turnover are greatly diminished, and both plasma calcium and phosphate are usually normal.

The physiologic significance of the effects of CT upon renal electrolyte excretion remains to be elucidated. There is some evidence that CT affects electrolyte transport in other tissues, e.g., it apparently causes a decrease in gastric acid and fluid secretion and may be an important regulator of osmotic balance in fish.

The other known effect of CT upon renal function is that of inhibiting the renal conversion of $25(OH)D_3$ to $1,25(OH)_2D_3$.

Mode of Action of CT

On the basis of the following facts, a model of CT action in bone has been developed (Fig. 11-21). CT causes (1) an immediate release of calcium from bone (presumably from bone cells); (2) a later profound inhibition of this release; (3) a retention of calcium by isolated cells; (4) no change, or often an increase, in C-AMP concentration in bone tissue; and (5) an inhibition of bone citrate production. The major effects of CT in this model are an initial stimulation of calcium efflux from cells and the generation of a second messenger, as yet unidentified, which stimulates the retention of calcium by mitochondria. As a consequence of these actions, the concentration of cytosolic calcium falls. This leads, in turn, to the relief of inhibition of adenyl cyclase and a rise in C-AMP. The nature of this proposed second messenger remains to be established.

Alternatively, it has been suggested that CT activates bone cell adenyl cyclase directly, and that the distinction between CT and PTH is that they act upon different cell types within bone.

The model depicted in Figure 11-21 emphasizes that, at both the cellular and physiologic levels, PTH and CT do not act as complete antagonists, so that both the cellular and physiologic consequences of CT action are not exactly opposite to those of PTH. Nevertheless, in terms of their most important physiologic actions, CT does inhibit, and PTH stimulate, osteoprogenitor cell activation; and CT stimulates, and PTH inhibits, the modulation of osteoclasts to osteoblasts (Fig. 11-10). At the cellular level, although both hormones increase the concentration of C-AMP, they do so by different mechanisms, and these mechanisms are related to the differences in their effect upon cell calcium metabolism.

Although, in a general way, the model depicted in Figure 11-21 accounts for the known effects of CT upon bone, it is less satisfactory when the renal effects of CT are considered. There is no evidence that CT alters renal intracellular C-AMP concentration or the renal excretion of C-AMP. The difficulties in defining the cellular mode of action of CT in the kidney are threefold. The first is that, at present, data from micropuncture studies of the portion of the nephron affected by CT are lacking. The second is that species differences exist in the renal response to CT. The third is that it has become apparent only in recent years that there are two modes of renal tubular sodium reabsorption. When the cellular basis of each mode is more clearly defined, it may become possible to define more clearly the mode of CT action.

Comparison of Cellular and Extracellular Calcium Homeostasis

There is a striking similarity, in the operational sense, in the way in which the concentrations of plasma calcium in the organism and cytosolic calcium in the cell are regulated (Fig. 11-21). In each instance, there is a reservoir of un-ionized calcium, bone mineral calcium, and mitochondrial calcium, respectively, in rapid exchange with an ionic pool. In both systems, there appear to be dual feedback control loops which respond to a change of calcium ion concentration in either direction and which in turn regulate the synthesis or secretion or both of the respective controlling elements.

Cholecalciferols

The third major hormone involved in regulating mammalian calcium metabolism and skeletal remodeling is vitamin D_3, or cholecalciferol. This agent, which can either be ingested in the diet or manufactured in the skin, has long been considered a vitamin. It can equally well be considered a hormone, however, and this latter point of view will be adopted herein.

The hormonal nature of this substance is most clearly established by a consideration of its historical role in human nutrition. As long as man was primarily an outdoor hunter, his needs for vitamin D were largely supplied by the synthesis of this compound in his skin. With the rise of urban life in temperate regions, this source of vitamin D was lessened. The real turning point, however, came with the industrial revolution. Rickets and osteomalacia developed in epidemic proportions in factory workers. With this transition in human activity, cholecalciferol became an essential dietary constituent for northern, urban man but not for rural, tropical man.

A most interesting feature of cholecalciferol physiology is its evolution. Cholecalciferol is produced in the stratum granulosum of human skin. Its synthesis is catalyzed by the ultraviolet (UV) rays of the sun of the wavelength 290 to 320 millimicrons. The rate of synthesis in Caucasian skin can be quite high, but in both Negroes and Orientals, the rates are considerably lower. In the Negro, this is due to a constitutive melanization of a more superficial layer of the skin, and in the Oriental, a constitutive keratinization. Both these processes protect these individuals from excessive production of cholecalciferol by largely excluding UV light below 430 millimicrons. In Caucasians, the reversible tanning induced by continued exposure to sunlight serves to reduce the penetration of UV light and thus the rate of cholecalciferol synthesis. It can be considered an induced rather than a constitutive protective device.

On the basis of present paleontologic evidence, it seems clear that human beings first evolved in tropical regions, and that they, in common with their primate ancestors had dark, hairy skins.

Both features appeared necessary for the protection of the organism from excessive production of cholecalciferol, even though both increased the heat retention of the organism. As human migrations took place into subtropical and temperate regions of the earth, a major adaptation was that of a lighter skin. Without this adaptation, severe rickets would have resulted. Hence light skin gave these migrants a very marked adaptive advantage.

From the medical point of view, individual and societal mobility has altered population distributions. One of the consequences is that the American Negro, for example, has a higher dietary requirement for vitamin D than does the American Caucasian. This is particularly true in the winter months when the natural vitamin D content of the diet falls markedly. This seasonal change in the vitamin D content of food is, of course, less marked in tropical than in temperate climates.

Chemistry

The single most important fact about cholecalciferol, in the hormonal sense, is that it must undergo further metabolic transformations before exerting its biologic effects. To date, four metabolites of cholecalciferol that possess biologic activity have been identified (Fig. 11–27):

1. 25-hydroxycholecalciferol [25(OH)D_3]
2. 1,25-dihydroxycholecalciferol [1,25(OH)$_2D_3$]
3. 25,26-dihydroxycholecalciferol [25,26(OH)$_2D_3$]
4. 24,25-dihydroxycholecalciferol [24,25(OH)$_2D_3$]

Other less well characterized biologically inactive metabolites have been noted. Previous reports of the identification of 21,25(OH)$_2D_3$ were incorrect, and it has been shown that the correct structure of this metabolite is 24,25(OH)$_2D_3$.

In addition to these natural metabolites, there are a number of other closely related sterols with similar biologic properties. These include calciferol

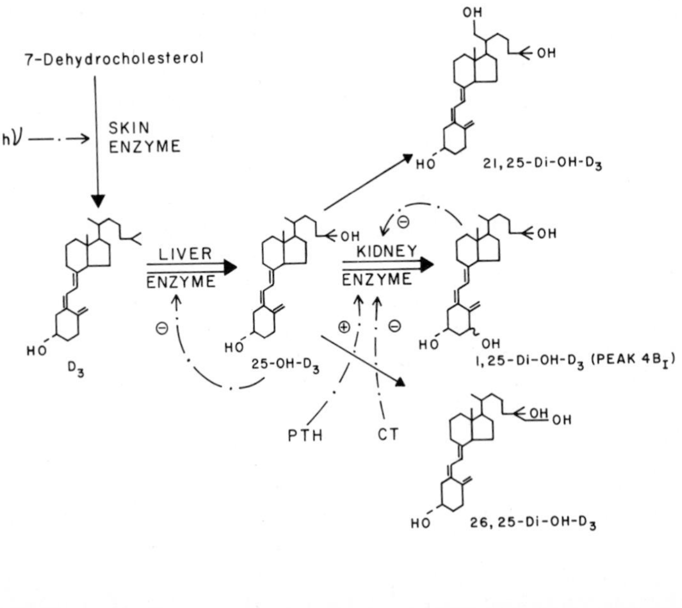

Figure 11–27. The metabolism of vitamin D. The symbol hν denotes ultraviolet light, which acts with an enzyme in the skin to stimulate the conversion of 7-dehydrocholesterol to vitamin D_3, which then undergoes further metabolism in the liver and kidney. The metabolic product of major physiologic importance is 1,25(OH)$_2$ D_3.

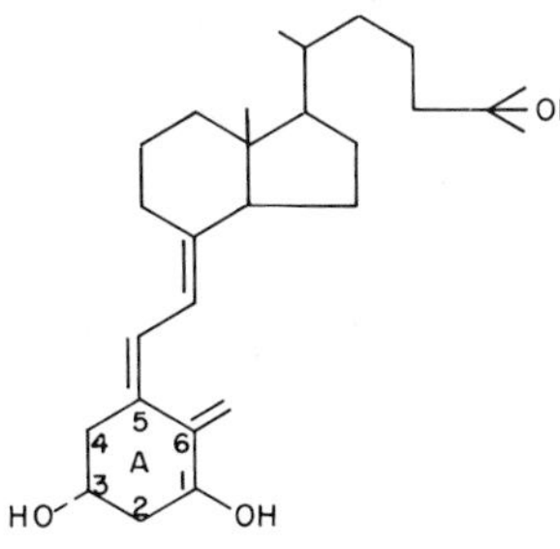

1, 25 (OH)$_2$ D$_3$

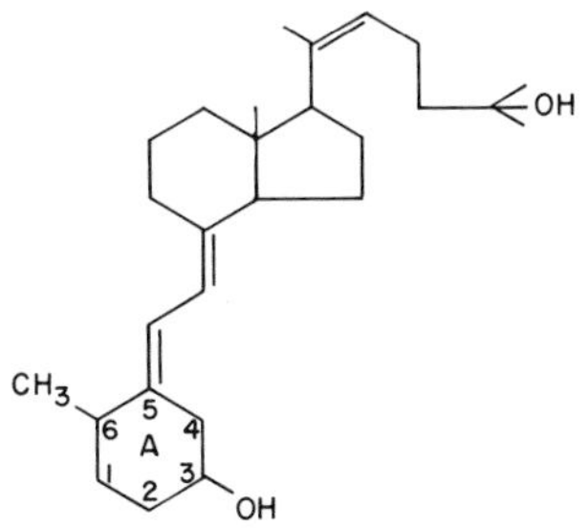

25 (OH) DHT

Figure 11–28. The structure of 25-dihydrotachysterol and 1,25-dihydroxycholecalciferol.

(vitamin D$_2$), which is made by the irradiation of the plant sterol, ergosterol, and which, when administered to mammals, undergoes transformation to types of metabolites [25(OH)D$_2$ and 1,25(OH)$_2$D$_2$] similar to those derived from cholecalciferol.

A sterol of considerable interest is dihydrotachysterol, because it has enjoyed widespread therapeutic use in human disease. In this compound, ring A is rotated 180 degrees, so that, in an extended configuration, the hydroxyl in position 3 occupies a position sterically equivalent to the hydroxyl in position 1 in 1,25(OH)$_2$D$_3$ (Fig. 11–28). All present evidence shows that, when DHT is administered to a mammal, it undergoes transformation to 25-DHT, just as do vitamins D$_2$ and D$_3$, but that hydroxylation of position 1 of DHT does not take place. This means that the major active metabolite of DHT is apparently 25-DHT, in contrast to vitamin D$_3$, whose major active metabolite, under physiologic circumstances, at least, is 1,25(OH)$_2$D$_3$.

Another class of synthetic analogues of considerable interest comprises the 5,6-trans-isomers of vitamin D$_3$ and 25(OH)D$_3$. In these two compounds, just as in dihydrotachysterol, the A ring of the molecule is rotated 180 degrees from the natural configuration, so that the hydroxyl in position 3 of these synthetic compounds occupies a position sterically equivalent to the 1-hydroxyl in 1,25(OH)$_2$D$_3$. Both 5,6-trans-D$_3$ and 5,6-trans-25(OH)D$_3$ are biologically active when administered to anephric rats, which is taken to mean that neither agent must undergo further transformation in order to exert its biologic effects.

The most interesting feature of their actions is

that 5,6-trans-D$_3$ stimulates both intestinal calcium absorption and the mobilization of calcium from bone when given to vitamin D–deficient animals, while 5,6-trans-25(OH)D$_3$ acts only upon the intestinal absorption of calcium and does not induce the mobilization of bone mineral. Although these observations have been taken as evidence that the receptor site in bone is able to combine with 5,6-trans-D$_3$ but not with 5,6-trans-25(OH)D$_3$, an alternative possibility is that the 5,6-trans-D$_3$, but not the 5,6-trans-25(OH)D$_3$, is capable of undergoing further metabolic transformation.

In any case, if biologically active analogues of vitamin D$_3$ can be found that are relatively specific in terms of the end organ upon which they act, such analogues should eventually prove therapeutically significant.

Assay

The assay for vitamin D activity in biologic materials still depends primarily upon a biologic assay: either the ability to induce the healing of rickets or at least to induce the deposition of bone mineral in rachitic bone, or the ability to induce an increase in the intestinal transport of calcium. Both kinds of assays require administration of the vitamin or its metabolite *in vivo* and the subsequent determination of either an increase in bone mineral deposition or in calcium absorption. The latter is the more useful. It can be carried out in one of two ways.

In the standard assay for vitamin D$_3$, vitamin D–deficient chicks, weighing 170 to 190 g., are given the vitamin, either by intracardiac injection or by stomach tube. A standard dose of Ca^{45} is then administered by stomach tube 24 to 40 hours after the vitamin D has been given. The animal is killed one hour later, bled, and the radioactivity in the plasma measured. Alternatively, the chick can be anesthetized 24 to 50 hours after vitamin D administration and a loop of duodenum tied off, which is then washed and filled with a standard amount of Ca^{45}. The loop is then replaced in the abdomen and excised 30 minutes later. It is ashed, and the Ca^{45} remaining in the excised loop is measured.

The two methods give similar results. They are capable of measuring 25(OH)D$_3$ in the range of 20 to 200 ng.

The difficulty with standardizing either assay lies in the fact that the time course of action of vitamin D$_3$, 25(OH)D$_3$, and 1,25(OH)$_2$D$_3$ differs significantly. The peak response in the chick to vitamin D$_3$ administration is reached at 40 hours, that to 25(OH)D$_3$, 2 to 4 hours sooner, but that to 1,25(OH)$_2$D$_3$, at only about 8 hours. In the case of 1,25(OH)$_2$D$_3$, the effects of a single small dose upon calcium absorption is over in 24 hours. A time lapse of 24 to 40 hours between administration of vitamin or metabolite and Ca^{45} administration is suitable for the assay of either D$_3$ or 25(OH)D$_3$ but is clearly unsuitable for the assay of 1,25(OH)$_2$D$_3$. In order to assay this metabolite, a time lapse of 6

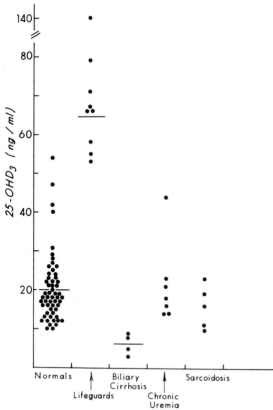

Figure 11–29. The concentration of 25(OH)D₃ in human plasma as measured by a protein-binding assay in normal individuals, lifeguards, and patients with biliary cirrhosis, uremia, and sarcoidosis. (Figure kindly supplied by Dr. John Haddad.)

the measurement of vitamin D activity in human blood.

When vitamin D_3 undergoes conversion to $25(OH)D_3$, this metabolite binds to a specific plasma protein. Also, a $25(OH)D_3$-binding protein has been identified and partially purified from the renal tissue of rachitic rats. With this purified protein, a competitive binding assay using H^3-$25(OH)D_3$ has been developed capable of detecting 1 to 5 ng. of $25(OH)D_3$. This assay will detect $25(OH)D_3$ in normal human plasma. The normal values are in the range of 20 ng. per ml. (Fig. 11–29), and these values increase upon exposure to sunlight, as seen in lifeguards in whom the value may be three to four times the normal (Fig. 11–29).

One disease in which an increased sensitivity to vitamin D_3 has been postulated is sarcoidosis. It is of interest that the $25(OH)D_3$ concentration in the plasma of such patients is normal (Fig. 11–29).

The concentration of $25(OH)D_3$ in human plasma also increases as a function of the vitamin D intake. This is most clearly seen in patients with the X-linked vitamin D–resistant rickets (Fig. 11–30). but normal individuals respond in a similar fashion. In patients on very high doses of vitamin D, the concentration of $25(OH)D_3$ in plasma may reach values as high as 350 ng. per ml. — a value 15 times the normal (Fig. 11–30).

Metabolism

Vitamin D_3 is the natural form of vitamin D in man. It is synthesized in the skin from 7-dehydrocholecalciferol by a photochemical reaction. This pathway can, under natural conditions, supply the bodily needs of man. Because of social and cultural factors, however, the extent of exposure of the skin of the typical urban man is insufficient to meet the body's needs. Dietary supplementation in the form of either vitamin D_3 or vitamin D_2 is then necessary in order to meet physiologic needs.

Regardless of whether it is made naturally in the skin or taken as a dietary constituent, vitamin D_3 (and vitamin D_2) must undergo metabolic conversion before exerting its biologic effects (Fig. 11–27). The first step is the conversion of D_3 to $25(OH)D_3$

to 10 hours is optimal, but this is unsuitable for the assay of D_3.

A feature of these assays is their insensitivity. The normal concentration of $25(OH)D_3$ in human plasma is in the range of 20 ng. per ml., whereas the range of sensitivity of the calcium absorption assays is 50 to 200 ng. per ml. Moreover, these assays will not differentiate between $25(OH)D_3$ and D_3. Hence they have not been widely applied to

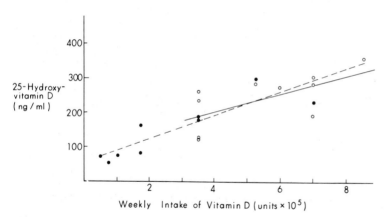

Figure 11–30. The concentration of 25(OH)D₃ in plasma of patients (●) with vitamin D-resistant rickets and in control subjects (○) as a function of the weekly intake of vitamin D₃. (From Haddad, J. G., Jr., Chyu, K., et al.: *J. Lab. Clin. Med.* 81:22, 1973.)

(Fig. 11–27). This hydroxylation is unusual in that most steroid hydroxylation reactions involve a secondary hydrogen, whereas D_3 to $25(OH)D_3$ involves a tertiary hydrogen. The enzyme responsible for controlling this hydroxylation is mitochondrial in location and requires a cytoplasmic factor (? protein) for its activity:

$$D_3 + H^+ + TPNH + \frac{1}{2}O_2 \rightleftharpoons TPN^- + 25(OH)D_3$$

The reaction exhibits product inhibition, so that, as $25(OH)D_3$ concentration increases, the rate of conversion of D_3 to $25(OH)D_3$ decreases. This means that, as the amount of vitamin D_3 ingested or made in the skin increases, the percentage converted immediately decreases, and the remainder is stored, primarily as vitamin D_3. However, the end-product control of this hydroxylation is not complete, so that, as the amount of vitamin D ingested or the amount made in the skin increases, the concentration of $25(OH)D_3$ in plasma also increases (Fig. 11–30). Thus both D_3 and $25(OH)D_3$ represent storage forms of vitamin D.

Early studies pointed to the liver as the site of the 25-hydroxylation reaction, but more recent data suggest that other organs, e.g., kidney and intestine, also can catalyze the conversion of D_3 to $25(OH)D_3$. The relative importance of these different organs in the overall metabolism of D_3 under physiologic circumstances is not known, nor has it yet been established whether bone also possesses this enzymatic activity.

When very large amounts of vitamin D_3 are administered for therapeutic reasons, the amount of $25(OH)D_3$ may increase tenfold or more (Fig. 11–30). Under these circumstances, $25(OH)D_3$ may begin to exert biologic effects directly rather than serving as a precursor for further metabolites. Normally, however, $25(OH)D_3$ is converted to at least three other metabolites (Fig. 11–27): $1,25(OH)_2D_3$, $24,25(OH)_2D_3$, and $25,26(OH)_2D_3$. Most attention has been directed toward $1,25(OH)_2D_3$. This is the major metabolite of $25(OH)D_3$ detected in intestine, kidney, and bone, but $25,26(OH)_2D_3$ is more prevalent in the plasma.

The site of synthesis of $25,26(OH)_2D_3$ is not established, but both $24,25(OH)_2D_3$ and $1,25(OH)_2D_3$ are synthesized from $25(OH)D_3$ in the kidney. The rates of synthesis of these two metabolites are reciprocally related and controlled by the same factors. These reactions appear to take place in the mitochondria and, like the hepatic 25-hydroxylation reaction, appear to require a cytoplasmic factor.

A major reason for the delay between vitamin D administration and the expression of its biologic effects is the slowness with which $25(OH)D_3$ is converted to $1,25(OH)D_3$. When the latter metabolite is administered to a D–deficient chick, it begins to exert an effect within two hours and exerts its maximal effect in approximately eight hours. In contrast, when $25(OH)D_3$ is given, 6 to 8 hours elapse before any effect is detectable, and maximal expression of its biologic effects is not seen before 36 to 40 hours. Clearly, then, the conversion of

$25(OH)D_3$ to $1,25(OH)_2D_3$ is the rate-limiting step in vitamin D metabolism. The rate of this reaction is also controlled by the plasma calcium concentration. It was originally supposed that this effect was direct, but it is now evident that changes in plasma calcium concentration exert their effects indirectly by altering the rates of secretion of PTH and CT. These two hormones have opposite effects. In physiologic concentrations, PTH stimulates and CT inhibits the conversion of $25(OH)D_3$ to $1,25(OH)_2D_3$. The physiologic implications of this hormonal control of calciferol metabolism are considered later (p. 708).

A second feature of the hormonal control of renal calciferol metabolism relates to the synthesis of $24,25(OH)_2D_3$. At least *in vivo*, when $1,25(OH)_2D_3$ synthesis increases, the synthesis of $24,25(OH)_2D_3$ declines and vice versa. The importance of this reciprocal control is not established, primarily because little is known about the physiologic role of $24,25(OH)_2D_3$. Very little of this metabolite is found in either intestine or bone; hence, it seems most unlikely that it is of importance in the metabolism of either of these organs. It is possible that $24,25(OH)_2D_3$ acts primarily on the kidney. It has been shown, for example, that $25(OH)D_3$ is more effective than $1,25(OH)_2D_3$ in stimulating the renal tubular reabsorption of phosphate, but that the effect of $25(OH)D_3$ is not immediate, requiring 30 minutes or more before being expressed. These results suggest that $25(OH)D_3$ may have to undergo conversion to another metabolite before acting upon renal electrolyte transport. One possible metabolite which might both be made in and act upon the kidney is $24,25(OH)_2D_3$.

Less is known about the pathways by which vitamin D and its metabolites undergo inactivation, degradation, and excretion. The present evidence suggests that the liver is the major site of these transformations, and the bile the major excretory route. It is presumed that this group of compounds is handled biochemically in a manner similar to that by which steroids are handled, including esterifications and possibly other hydroxylations. Of great practical importance is the fact that at least part of the degradative or inactivating pathways involves the hepatic microsomal oxidases of mixed function, which play such an important role in the metabolism of many drugs. The practical consequence of this is that, in humans receiving large doses of anticonvulsant drugs, such as Dilantin or phenobarbital, there is a marked hypertrophy of the smooth endoplasmic reticulum and an associated increase in the amount of the microsomal oxidases. This leads to an increase in the rate of catabolism of vitamin D or its metabolites or both, which may be sufficient to induce a relative deficiency of vitamin D, leading to rickets or osteomalacia.

Function of Vitamin D

The major physiologic functions of vitamin D and its metabolites are (1) to increase the retention of calcium and phosphate by the organism, and (2) to control the mineralization of bone matrix. Another function, related to the first two, is that of allowing PTH to exert its normal effects upon bone.

In a functional sense, vitamin D can be thought to act in such a way as to cause the retention of sufficient mineral ions to ensure the proper calcification of bone, and PTH to maintain the proper ratio of calcium to phosphate in the extracellular fluids.

Effects of Vitamin D and Metabolites: General

In discussing the effect of vitamin D or its metabolites, it is important to distinguish between physiologic and pharmacologic effects.

The physiologic effects of vitamin D depend upon the parathyroid status of the organism. In discussing these effects, it is most convenient to begin with a resumé of the effects of the administration of vitamin D (or its metabolites) on a vitamin D–deficient organism. In such an organism on an otherwise normal diet, hypocalcemia, hypophosphatemia, and secondary hyperparathyroidism exist.

The changes in electrolyte balance, plasma electrolyte concentrations, and bone structure seen in vitamin D deficiency in man depend upon the stage of the disease. The signs and symptoms are most marked in growing children, and three stages of the disease can be recognized (Table 11–7). Stage I is characterized by hypocalcemia, normal plasma phosphate, slightly elevated plasma PTH concentrations, and radiologic evidence of bone demineralization. These patients respond to exogenous PTH with an increase in plasma calcium concentration and renal phosphate excretion. Stage II cases are normocalcemic, with low plasma phosphate, aminoaciduria, and frank rickets and osteomalacia. These patients also have elevated concentrations of circulating PTH but still respond to large doses of exogenous PTH with a rise in plasma calcium concentration. In stage III, hypocalcemia and hypophosphatemia both exist along with aminoaciduria, even higher circulating PTH concentrations, and florid rickets. They do not respond to exogenous PTH. The progression from one stage to another

may take place relatively rapidly, from a few days to weeks.

It seems that compensatory parathyroid hyperplasia takes time to develop, and early in the D-deficient state, the circulating PTH is insufficient to maintain a normal plasma calcium concentration. As the parathyroids hypertrophy a normal plasma calcium level is reestablished at the expense of phosphate homeostasis. When phosphate depletion occurs, bone mineralization fails, and rickets develops. As this progresses, less and less calcified bone surface is available for resorption, and less and less bone mineral is mobilized, in spite of a continuing increase in PTH concentration, until the point is reached at which PTH is no longer effective in mobilizing bone mineral.

When vitamin D is given to a vitamin D–deficient human, there is often, in the next 16 to 48 hours, a transient further fall in the plasma calcium and plasma phosphate concentrations and a fall in plasma PTH concentration. This is followed by a progressive increase in plasma calcium and phosphate and a further fall in plasma PTH concentration. Urinary phosphate concentration falls, and urinary calcium excretion usually rises. The most marked metabolic change is the increase in calcium and phosphate absorption from the intestine. In the D-deficient man, the absorption of both calcium and phosphate is greatly reduced, but within 48 hours after vitamin D treatment, calcium absorption increases markedly.

The excretion of hydroxyproline-containing peptides may be normal or slightly increased in the D-deficient animal, but after administration of vitamin D, there is always a significant increase in the excretion of these peptides. Likewise, plasma alkaline phosphatase is usually elevated in the untreated patient and increases significantly after the institution of therapy. Eventually, after weeks or months of therapy, these indices return to normal values.

Effects of Vitamin D: Bone

The two most striking changes in bone in advanced vitamin D deficiency are a failure of the normal mineralization of bone matrix, leading to the accumulation of unmineralized osteoid, and a decrease in osteoclast count and bone resorption surface in relation to the concentration of circulating parathyroid hormone. For example, if the osteoclast count is plotted against the plasma PTH concentration in patients with primary hyperparathyroidism, there is a direct, nearly linear correlation between the two. In contrast, in osteomalacia with secondary hyperparathyroidism, the correlation is an inverse one. The more advanced the disease, the higher the circulating PTH concentration, but the fewer the osteoclasts per unit of *calcified* bone surface. The other striking change in bone, in addition to the increase in osteoid, is a lack of a normal calcification front in this osteoid.

When either vitamin D_3, 25(OH)D_3, or 1,25(OH)$_2$$D_3$ is administered to a D-deficient

TABLE 11–7. STAGES OF VITAMIN D DEFICIENCY IN MAN

Biochemical or Morphologic Index	Stage		
	I	*II*	*III*
Plasma calcium	↓	N	↓
Plasma phosphate	N	↓	↓
Alkaline P-tase	↑	↑ ↑	↑ ↑
Aminoaciduria	N	↑	↑
Radiographic evidence of disease	Demineralization	Rickets	Rickets
Phosphaturia	↑	↑ ↑	↑ ↑
Responsiveness to exogenous PTH	++	+	−

human or animal, one of the earliest changes seen in bone is the reestablishment of a normal calcification front in the osteoid surfaces. This change may *precede* an increase in plasma *calcium or phosphate concentration* or both and is probably responsible for the fall in plasma calcium and phosphate concentrations seen after the initiation of vitamin D therapy. The fact that vitamin D treatment leads to a reestablishment of the normal calcification front in osteoid surface before there is any positive change in the mineral ion product of the extracellular fluids is unequivocal evidence that vitamin D (via its metabolites) *acts directly upon bone.* An extremely important feature of this physiologic action of vitamin D_3 upon bone is that it requires the presence of parathyroid hormone.

The other change in bone, following vitamin D administration, is an increase in osteoclast count on the endosteal bone surfaces. This change may also precede the increase in the concentration of calcium and phosphate in the extracellular fluids, and it is another indication that vitamin D has a direct action upon bone. This action also requires the presence of PTH.

One of the reasons that there has been continued debate as to whether or not vitamin D has a direct action upon bone, particularly on bone mineralization, has been the evidence that one can induce bone mineralization *in vivo* in patients with vitamin D deficiency osteomalacia (stage I) simply by feeding sufficient phosphate to increase the extracellular phosphate concentration. When the bone is examined after such therapy, however, an important distinction is evident. Vitamin D administration leads to the reestablishment of a normal calcification front and the orderly mineralization of the bone from the old mineralized bone to the surface osteoblast layer. In contrast, phosphate therapy leads to a patchy remineralization which begins at the osteoblast surface, does not reestablish a calcification front, and may leave behind islands of uncalcified or poorly calcified matrix.

A lack of vitamin D interferes with events in the epiphyseal growth plate. In the normal sequence of events, the cells in the hypertrophic zone of the epiphyseal plate accumulate mineral ions as electron-dense deposits in their mitochondria. This mineral is then transported out of the cells as membrane-bound matrix calcification granules, which initiate the mineralization of the cartilaginous matrix. There are two views as to this sequence. In one, the mitochondria themselves migrate to the cell periphery and transfer the mineral to endocytotic vesicles of the cell membrane. In the other, the mineral is transferred intracellularly from mitochondria to the Golgi region, where it is incorporated into vesicles that are eventually secreted.

In either case, once mineralization is initiated, the primary cartilaginous matrix becomes calcified. This primary calcified cartilage is a very transient stage, because it normally undergoes rapid resorption by chondroclasts, after which woven bone is laid down on the very thin spicules of surviving calcified cartilage. The woven bone itself then undergoes resorption to be replaced, in turn, by lamellar bone.

In the absence of vitamin D, intracellular mineral accumulation does not take place, calcification of the cartilaginous matrix does not occur, and this, in turn, blocks the cycles of woven bone and lamellar bone remodeling. As a consequence, the epiphyseal plate thickens as more primordial cartilaginous matrix is formed.

The striking cellular change in the area of the cartilaginous matrix is the virtual absence of chondroclasts. Thus a major effect of D deficiency on all bone surfaces is the failure for surface resorption cells, chondro- and osteoclasts to develop normally in spite of secondary hyperparathyroidism. In both cartilage and bone, the administration of either vitamin D or calcium will lead to an increase in osteoclast or chondroclast number. Thus three factors are of importance in regulating the activation of mesenchymal cells into preosteoclasts and osteoclasts: PTH, vitamin D, and the calcium ion concentration.

Mode of Action: Bone

The present evidence favors the view that, in bone as in the intestine, the physiologically important metabolite of vitamin D is $1,25(OH)_2D_3$. In physiologic amounts, this compound in some manner changes the responsiveness of bone cells to PTH. When either $1,25(OH)_2D_3$ or $25(OH)D_3$ is added to bone grown in organ culture in the absence of PTH, it will stimulate osteoclastic proliferation and the resorption of bone. The difference is that $1,25(OH)_2D_3$ is 50 to 100 times more effective than $25(OH)D_3$. These data predict that, in pharmacologic amounts, both $1,25(OH)_2D_3$ and $25(OH)D_3$ should induce bone resorption *in vivo* in parathyroidectomized animals. This is the case, but the amount of $1,25(OH)_2D_3$ needed to induce bone mobilization in a parathyroidectomized animal is 30 to 100 times that needed to permit PTH to induce its normal physiologic effects in bone.

A point of key importance in developing a model of $1,25(OH)_2D_3$ action upon bone is that vitamin D deficiency does not change the initial effects of PTH and CT upon bone cells. Thus PTH causes an initial uptake of calcium into bone, and CT an initial release of calcium from bone (Fig. 11–20) in the vitamin D–deficient (−D) animal, just as they do in the vitamin D–fed (+D) animal. In addition, PTH activates adenyl cyclase in −D bone cells, and the steady-state concentration of C-AMP may actually be higher in such cells than in normal cells exposed to the same concentration of PTH. These data, in conjunction with the data relating to bone cells, mean that, even though the −D bone cells exhibit a normal biochemical response to PTH initially, these initial biochemical changes do not lead to the normal changes in bone cell populations. In particular, the size of the osteoclast pool does not increase, and therefore there is no sustained increase in bone resorption.

The other facts of importance in relation to the

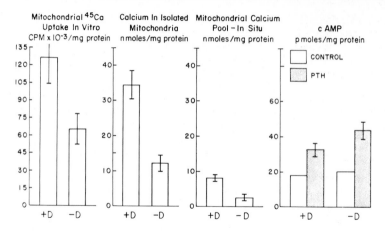

Figure 11–31. A summary of the effects of vitamin D deficiency (−D) upon (1) the ability of isolated kidney mitochondria to accumulate radiocalcium *in vitro;* (2) the total calcium content of isolated kidney mitochondria; (3) the size of the mitochondrial calcium pool *in situ* in isolated intestinal cells; and (4) the renal content of C-AMP in TPX rats given a standard dose of PTH.

cellular effects of vitamin D are summarized in Fig. 11–31. These data also show that the mitochondria isolated from −D kidney cells contain less calcium than do those from +D cells and are less able to accumulate calcium from a standard medium *in vitro*. In addition, if the size of cellular calcium pools is estimated in the intact intestinal cells by kinetic means, the intramitochondrial pool of calcium in the −D cells is considerably smaller than in the +D cells.

The final point relates to the effect of calcium administration upon osteoclast count on the bone surfaces of −D humans. When calcium is administered to patients with nutritional osteomalacia and hypocalcemia, the plasma calcium concentration increases, *PTH concentrations decrease* but still remain higher than normal, and *the osteoclast count increases*.

All these data can be incorporated into a model of vitamin D action on bone cells (Fig. 11–32), which is directly related to the previous model of PTH action (Fig. 11–21). In the model represented in Figure 11–32, PTH exerts two simultaneous effects: an increase in calcium entry into the cell and an activation of adenyl cyclase. The resulting increase in C-AMP leads to a shift of calcium from the mitochondrial to the cytosolic pool. This effect, plus the primary effect of PTH upon calcium entry, leads to an increase in cytosolic calcium ion concentration, which is one of the key second messengers responsible for activating the osteoprogenitor cells and thereby increasing the size of the osteoclast pool. Because of a decreased rate of entry of calcium into cells or mitochondria or both in −D animals, the mitochondrial calcium pool and the extracellular calcium pool are both reduced in size. As a consequence, when PTH acts, even though calcium entry increases and adenyl cyclase is activated, the resulting changes in intracellular calcium distribution are less marked than normal. In particular, the cytosolic calcium concentration, which was less than normal to begin with, does not increase to the same extent as in the cells of +D animals. If one now increases the extracellular cal-

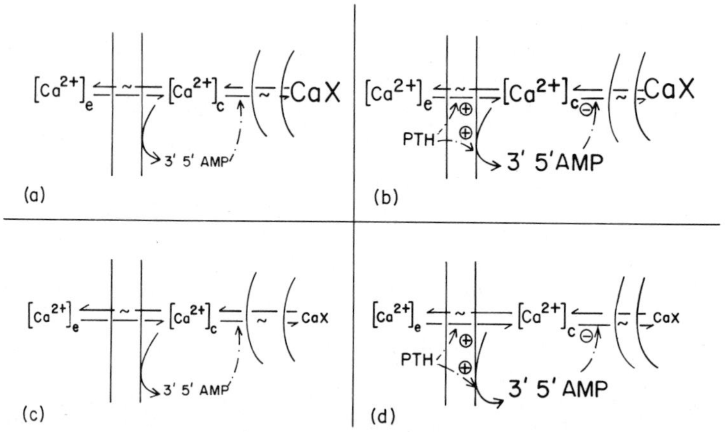

$$[Ca^{2+}]_e \rightleftarrows \sim \rightleftarrows [Ca^{2+}]_c \rightleftarrows (\sim (\sim CaX$$

(a)

$$[Ca^{2+}]_e \rightleftarrows \sim \rightleftarrows [Ca^{2+}]_c \rightleftarrows (\sim (\sim CaX$$

(b)

$$[Ca^{2+}]_e \rightleftarrows \sim \rightleftarrows [Ca^{2+}]_c \rightleftarrows (\sim (\sim CaX$$

(c)

$$[Ca^{2+}]_e \rightleftarrows \sim \rightleftarrows [Ca^{2+}]_c \rightleftarrows (\sim (\sim CaX$$

(d)

Figure 11–32. A schematic representation of how vitamin D deficiency influences the cellular response to PTH. *A*, Normal control bone cell. *B*, Normal cell treated with PTH. PTH increases calcium entry into the cell and blocks calcium uptake into mitochondria via an increase in 3′,5′-AMP. The net result is an increase in cytosolic calcium [Ca²⁺]ₒ. The combined increase in 3′,5′-AMP and cytosolic calcium concentrations is the signal for increase in osteoclastic activity and osteoclast number (see Fig. 11–17). *C*, Vitamin D–deficient cell in which mitochondrial calcium pool (CaX) is depleted and extracellular calcium concentration is reduced. *D*, Response of −D cell to PTH. Because of a decrease in both [Ca²⁺]ₑ and CaX, PTH does not increase [Ca²⁺]ₒ to the same extent as it does in normal cells, in spite of a normal or supernormal increase in 3′,5′-AMP concentration.

cium ion concentration, however, the cytosolic calcium ion concentration increases, activation of osteoprogenitor cells takes place, and the size of the osteoclast pool increases.

As outlined, the hypothesis emphasizes the important second messenger function of cytosolic calcium. It seems most likely, however, that both C-AMP and cytosolic calcium play a role in the activation of osteoprogenitor cells. It is not yet clear whether the control of mitosis in thymocytes by calcium, PTH, and C-AMP is a valid model of the control of these events in bone cells, but it is clear that an increase in PTH stimulates mitosis in thymocytes by a calcium-dependent process that involves C-AMP.

The precise mechanism by which $1,25(OH)_2D_3$ acts to alter cell calcium metabolism is yet to be established. It could have a primary action on the calcium permeability of the cell membrane or the mitochondrial membrane or both. The nature of this membrane action remains to be elucidated.

Effects and Mode of Action of Vitamin D: Intestine

A major target tissue for $1,25(OH)_2D_3$ action is the intestinal mucosa. In this tissue, the sterol increases the active transcellular transport of calcium and the calcium-dependent transport of phosphate. The sterol also increases the growth and maturation of the intestinal mucosal cells.

Under physiologic circumstances, the major vitamin D metabolite found in the intestine is $1,25(OH)_2D_3$. Moreover, $1,25(OH)_2D_3$ acts more rapidly than either D_3 or $25(OH)D_3$ in stimulating the intestinal transport of calcium when administered to $-D$ animals. Finally, $1,25(OH)_2D_3$ is 10 to 100 times more potent than $25(OH)D_3$ in stimulating calcium absorption in isolated perfused intestinal loops from $-D$ animals.

The mode of action of $1,25(OH)_2D_3$ upon the intestine is not yet known. There are several possibilities (Fig. 11–33). The sterol may act by stimulating gene expression, with the resultant gene product being a calcium-binding protein. In this hypothesis, the proposed sequence is as follows: (1)

binding of $1,25(OH)_2D_3$ to a cytoplasmic receptor; (2) uptake of the sterol-receptor complex by the nucleus; (3) activation of a specific gene locus responsible for coding the mRNA for calcium-binding protein synthesis; (4) increase in the synthesis of this mRNA; (5) a resulting increase in calcium-binding protein (CaBP) synthesis; and (6) an increase in transcellular calcium transport as a consequence of the increase in CaBP.

The experimental evidence in support of this hypothesis is as follows: (1) the amount of calcium-binding protein increases after vitamin D administration; (2) both DNA and RNA synthesis increase; (3) labeled $1,25(OH)_2D_3$ is located in the nuclear fraction of the cell when the animal is treated with labeled $25(OH)D_3$ and the mucosal tissue is then removed from the animal, homogenized, and fractionated; and (4) this nuclear binding precedes the change in transcellular calcium transport.

Against this hypothesis is the following evidence: (1) $1,25(OH)_2D_3$ will produce an increase in intestinal calcium absorption even in animals treated with sufficient actinomycin D to markedly inhibit RNA synthesis in intestinal cells; (2) even though, under some circumstances, the change in calcium transport and change in CaBP content are correlated, there are other conditions in which this is not the case; (3) by immunofluorescent antibody techniques, the major part of the CaBP is localized in the goblet cells, even though these secretory cells are not thought to be involved in the transepithelial transport of calcium; and (4) the CaBP is not localized in the mucosal brush border, even though physiologic evidence supports the concept that at least one of the important changes produced in this tissue by $1,25(OH)_2D_3$ is a change in function of the brush border.

An alternative hypothesis argues that the major site of action of $1,25(OH)_2D_3$ in the intestine is at the brush border or the inner mitochondrial membrane or both. In this hypothesis, the rate-limiting steps in transcellular calcium transport are either the active or passive movement of calcium from the intestinal contents across the mucosal brush border into the cell or its uptake into mitochondria (Fig. 11–33). This hypothesis is supported by considerable physiologic evidence. Moreoover, if a

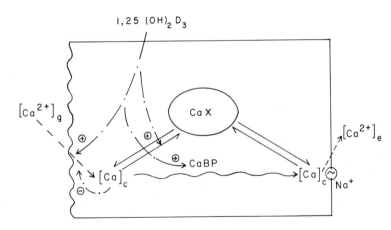

Figure 11–33. Possible sites of action of $1,25(OH)_2D_3$ upon intestinal mucosal cells. These include (1) a stimulation of calcium entry into the cell across the brush border, (2) a stimulation of calcium uptake by mitochondria, and (3) a stimulation of the synthesis of a calcium-binding protein (CaBP).

series of electron micrographs are prepared of mucosal cells from −D animals as a function of time after the treatment of such animals, a characteristic sequence of events can be observed. If the animals are fed calcium, the major tissue site of calcium localization is along the membrane surfaces of the microvilli of the brush border. After vitamin D therapy, however, large numbers of electron-dense granules appear in the mitochondria of the intestinal cells, and fewer calcium granules are seen along the membrane surface of the microvilli. The appearance of the mitochondrial granules corresponds in time to the increase in transcellular calcium transport.

Two interpretations of these observations are possible. On the one hand, vitamin D may alter the calcium permeability of the mucosal surface membrane and allow calcium to enter the cell. On the other, vitamin D may alter the calcium-accumulating properties of the intestinal cell mitochondria, and mitochondrial calcium exchange may be an obligatory aspect of transcellular calcium transport. In all likelihood, $1,25(OH)_2D_3$ exerts its effects upon both membranes (cell and mitochondrial). The problem is to define the physiologic significance of a change in mitochondrial calcium exchange in relation to a change in transcellular calcium transport. Two possible roles for this mitochondrial activity have been proposed: (1) the mitochondrial calcium exchange and accumulation act as a buffer system controlling the $[Ca^{2+}]$ of the cell cytosol and thus act in parallel with the transcellular transport system; or (2) the accumulation of calcium within the mitochondria is an obligatory step in the process of transcellular transport and thus acts in series with the other elements involved in transcellular transport. Present data are insufficient to allow a choice to be made between these two alternatives.

Effects of Vitamin D: Kidney

Until recently there has been considerable controversy regarding a direct effect of vitamin D upon renal function. With the availability of the various active metabolites of vitamin D, this controversy has been resolved. The infusion of either $25(OH)D_3$ or $1,25(OH)_2D_3$ will produce an increased proximal tubular reabsorption of both calcium and phosphate within 30 to 60 minutes. The $25(OH)D_3$ is more active than $1,25(OH)_2D_3$ and is probably the physiologically important metabolite in vivo, although it remains possible that $24,25(OH)_2D_3$, or some other metabolite of $25(OH)D_3$, is the physiologically important renal hormone. The effect of $25(OH)D_3$ is blocked by PTH, CT, or calcium infusion.

Nothing is known of the cellular basis for this effect of $25(OH)D_3$, but it is of considerable interest that it develops more rapidly than do the effects of $1,25(OH)_2D_3$ in intestine or bone.

Integrated Control of Extracellular Calcium Homeostasis

The discussion of the separate hormones in the preceding sections has emphasized that, in the adult, the two hormones of major importance in the maintenance of extracellular calcium homeostasis are parathyroid hormone and vitamin D or its active metabolites and that the three organs of major importance are kidney, intestine, and bone. In considering how the activities of the two hormones and the responses of the three organs are integrated so as to achieve extracellular mineral homeostasis, it is possible to discuss the situation in two ways. In the first, it is useful to consider the manner in which the responses of the three organs to PTH are integrated in maintaining plasma calcium homeostasis. In the second, one can discuss the interrelated nature of PTH and vitamin D metabolites in this homeostatic system.

From data obtained from both man and experimental animals, it is possible to define in a semiquantitative fashion the contribution of the different organs in the time course of response to PTH. This can be most graphically illustrated by plotting the retention of calcium in the extracellular fluids against time in a hypoparathyroid human who is receiving an infusion of PTH sufficient to maintain his plasma calcium concentration at 9 mg. per 100 ml., and in whom, at time zero, the rate of PTH infusion is increased sufficiently so that, when a new steady state is achieved, the plasma calcium is 10.8 mg. per 100 ml. (Fig. 11–34).

Immediately after the increase in PTH infusion rate, the plasma and urinary calcium concentrations fall because of the uptake of calcium by bone and kidney cells. Within one hour, the plasma calcium concentration begins to rise because of two effects: (1) an increased renal tubular reabsorption of calcium, and (2) the stimulation of osteocytic osteolysis and osteoclastic bone resorption by preformed osteoclasts (Fig. 11–34). In addition, a small contribution to net retention of calcium in the extracellular fluids will be made by the inhibition of calcium uptake at bone-forming surfaces (not shown in Fig. 11–34). These renal and early osseous effects predominate during the first 8 to 16 hours. With time, however, the labile bone mineral pool around the osteocytes becomes depleted, and the contribution of this pool declines. Moreover, as plasma calcium concentration rises, the urinary excretion of calcium increases, so that, after 12 hours, the kidney is no longer responsible for any further retention of calcium. Plasma calcium continues to rise, however, because after a delay of 8 to 10 hours, PTH, through its control of $1,25(OH)_2D_3$ production, stimulates the intestinal absorption of calcium. Moreover, after this period of time, the hormone has induced an increase in the size of the osteoclast pool, with a progressive increase in the contribution of osteoclastic bone resorption to the mobilization of calcium from bone. As the plasma calcium concentration continues to increase, even

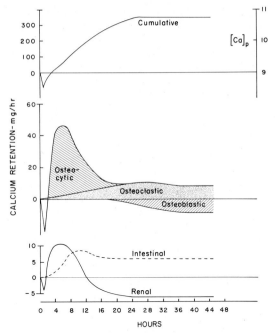

Figure 11-34. A hypothetical re-creation of the sequence of events when the rate of PTH infusion to a PTX human is increased at time zero so that, at the new steady state, the plasma calcium concentration rises from 9.0 to 10.8 mg. per 100 ml. Retention of calcium in the extracellular fluids is plotted as a function of time. The upper panel represents total retention; the middle, the retention due to the activities of the different bone cells; and the lower, the retention due to changes in renal or intestinal calcium transport. Note that, after 40 hours, the increased retention due to increased intestinal absorption and increased osteoclastic bone resorption is balanced by increased renal excretion (decreased retention) and increased bone mineralization.

though PTH continues to exert its effect upon the tubular reabsorption of calcium, the filtered load of calcium increases to such an extent that the urinary loss of calcium exceeds the rate at time zero, and the kidney is now responsible for a continuing loss of calcium from the extracellular pool. This loss is more or less compensated for by an increase in the intestinal absorption of calcium, however. In addition, the secondary osteoblastic response to PTH has begun in bone, and, with time, the rate of new bone formation and mineralization balances the rate of increased osteoclastic resorption. A new steady state is achieved in which the plasma calcium concentration has stabilized and the rate of skeletal remodeling has increased (Fig. 11-34).

This hypothetical reconstruction is based upon an ideal situation in which the vitamin D status of the animal is normal and the dietary intake of calcium and phosphate is optimal.

In an operational sense, the organization of this system is similar to that involved in controlling plasma glucose homeostasis, with the early renal and osteocytic responses being analogous to the mobilization of glucose from glycogen, and the later intestinal and osteoclastic responses being analogous to gluconeogenesis.

Of key importance in integrating these organ responses are the interrelated effects of PTH and vitamin D metabolites. Their activities are coordinated in a very complex but elegant fashion (Fig. 11-35). The primary feedback relationship is between PTH secretion rate and plasma calcium concentration. When plasma calcium concentration falls, PTH secretion rises. The increased plasma PTH acts primarily on two organs, kidney and bone, causing in both a shift of calcium into the extracellular fluids. The hormone also stimulates the renal synthesis of $1,25(OH)_2D_3$ from $25(OH)D_3$. The resulting increase in plasma $1,25(OH)_2D_3$ leads to an increase in the intestinal absorption of calcium and an enhancement of the effect of PTH upon bone. Both these effects of $1,25(OH)_2D_3$ also cause a net increase of extracellular fluid calcium (Fig. 11-35). They constitute, in the operational sense, positive feed-forward loops in this control system, serving to amplify the initial calcium-mobilizing effects of PTH.

Other Hormones

Although PTH, CT, and $1,25(OH)_2D_3$ are the hormones most directly involved in regulating both mineral homeostasis and skeletal remodeling, a number of other hormones do act on one or the other of these physiologic systems. Of particular importance in clinical medicine are the effects of thyroxine, growth hormone, the adrenal corticoids,

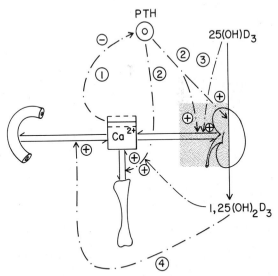

Figure 11-35. The relationships between PTH, $25(OH)D_3$, and $1,25(OH)_2D_3$ in mammalian plasma calcium homeostasis. When plasma calcium concentration falls, it acts as a signal ① for an increase in PTH secretion. The increase in PTH acts directly upon kidney ② and bone ② to increase the movement of calcium into the ECF. The effect on the kidney supplements that of $25(OH)D_3$ upon calcium reabsorption ③. In addition, PTH stimulates the renal conversion of $25(OH)D_3$ to $1,25(OH)_2D_3$. The latter metabolite acts as a feed-forward signal to enhance the effect of PTH upon net bone resorption, and also acts, with a time delay, to enhance the intestinal absorption of calcium ④. The shaded area signifies the importance of the renal effects in terms of integrating the responses of the three major organs—kidney, intestine, and bone.

and estrogens upon skeletal remodeling. Most aspects of the chemistry, biochemistry, and physiology of these agents are discussed in detail in other chapters of this volume; hence, only the most relevant features of their actions upon bone will be discussed here.

Thyroxine

The thyroid hormones, thyroxine and triiodothyronine, influence mineral metabolism and bone turnover. In patients with hyperthyroidism, there are (1) a marked increase in cellular Ca^{2+} and Mg^{2+} turnover; (2) a marked increase in bone mineral exchange; (3) a significant increase in bone remodeling (Figs. 11–17 and 11–45), with histologic evidence of increased bone resorption and formation, but with a balance in favor of resorption, so that osteoporosis may developed with increased urinary calcium excretion; (4) a decrease in the gastrointestinal absorption of calcium; (5) an increase in plasma phosphate; and (6) histologic evidence of subperiosteal bone resorption. In addition, patients with hyperthyroidism may have hypercalcemia, which may or may not be due to an associated hyperparathyroidism.

In patients without hyperparathyroidism, the hypercalcemia may be due to one of several factors: (1) accelerated bone turnover, with decreased renal clearance of calcium; (2) potentiation of PTH action; or (3) potentiation of $1,25(OH)_2D_3$ action.

In patients with hypothyroidism, skeletal remodeling is very low (Figs. 11–17 and 11–45), with often a more profound inhibition of resorption than formation, associated with an increase in the intestinal absorption of calcium.

Normally in patients with either hyper- or hypothyroidism, the plasma calcium concentration is normal in spite of the marked changes in skeletal remodeling, emphasizing again the dissociation between skeletal remodeling and plasma mineral homeostasis.

Present evidence, admittedly incomplete, suggests that plasma PTH concentrations are normal or high in hypothyroid patients, and normal or low in hyperthyroid patients. The fact that normal PTH concentrations are found in patients with hypothyroidism and extremely low rates of skeletal remodeling indicates that the presence of thyroxine is necessary for PTH action upon bone cell activation. This may also be true for the action of $1,25(OH)_2D_3$. In addition, it is possible that $1,25(OH)_2D_3$ synthesis is impaired in hypothyroidism, because vitamin D therapy is relatively ineffective in inducing a rise in plasma calcium concentration in hypoparathyroid patients with associated hypothyroidism. Conversely, however, in states of excess thyroxine production or administration, PTH is not necessary in order for this hormone to stimulate bone remodeling.

Estrogens

The effects of estrogens upon bone metabolism have been of great interest for the past 30 years because of the therapeutic use of estrogens in the treatment of osteoporosis. Unfortunately, in spite of 30 years' experience, there is no clear-cut evidence that these therapeutic agents are of lasting value in the treatment of this disease, because their short-term and long-term effects differ.

The short-term administration of estrogens leads to a shift in the balance of bone surface activities in favor of formation. This is apparently due to an inhibition by estrogens of PTH-induced bone resorption.

It is important to bear in mind that, in the normal life of a bone metabolic unit (activation⟶ resorption⟶formation), the activation phase usually lasts a few days, the resorption phase a few weeks, but the formation phase several months. Because of this, when estrogen shifts the balance of surface activities in favor of formation, a positive calcium balance will ensue, and this balance may remain positive for several months. Unfortunately, it does not persist. The long-term administration of estrogen leads to an inhibition of osteoprogenitor cell activation (Fig. 11–10), which means that the rate of both resorption and formation falls. This leads to a tendency toward hypocalcemia and secondary hyperparathyroidism; skeletal remodeling falls, and net bone formation is not maintained.

Adrenal Cortical Steroids

The relation of adrenal steroids to bone metabolism is also important in osteoporosis. Osteoporosis is a prominent sign of Cushing's disease or overproduction of adrenal glucocorticoids. It is also a common and often serious complication of prolonged adrenal corticoid therapy in collagen diseases (e.g., rheumatoid arthritis).

Administration of cortisol or other adrenal corticoids causes a decrease in the intestinal absorption of, and the renal tubular reabsorption of, calcium. If given to parathyroidectomized animals maintained on a constant dose of PTH, cortisol will induce hypocalcemia. If given to animals with intact parathyroid glands, it will induce a rise in plasma PTH concentration.

The effect of cortisol upon skeletal remodeling in bone depends upon the dose of steroid given. In low doses (0.5 to 2.5 mg. per kg. per day), cortisol leads to an inhibition of bone formation but an increase in resorption (Fig. 11–17). This is due to an inhibition of the modulation of osteoclasts to osteoblasts. In addition, the rate of osteoprogenitor cell activation, as measured by mitotic rate of a standard bone cell population, increases. None of these changes, except for a slight decline in bone formation, is seen in parathyroidectomized animals. These results argue that the major changes in skeletal remodeling after the administration of low doses of cortisol are due to (1) a direct inhibition of the modulation of osteoclasts to osteoblasts (Fig. 11–17), and (2) the secondary hyperparathyroidism resulting from the cortisol-induced inhibition of intestinal and renal tubular calcium absorption.

In higher doses of cortisol (>5 mg. per kg. per day), the rate of osteoprogenitor cell activation falls (Fig. 11-17), so that, in spite of secondary hyperparathyroidism, there is a decrease in the rate of formation of new osteoclasts; hence, the skeletal remodeling rate declines, but an imbalance in favor of resorption persists.

In addition to these effects of cortisol upon the size of active bone cell pools, cortisol in low or high doses directly inhibits the activity of osteoblasts, i.e., it inhibits bone collagen synthesis.

The mode of action of cortisol, either in bone or intestine, remains to be elucidated. There is some evidence that cortisol has an anti-vitamin D-like activity. Careful analysis shows, however, that vitamin D will still act in rachitic animals treated with adrenal steroids and will still induce the synthesis of the intestinal calcium-binding protein. On the other hand, cortisol therapy decreases, and vitamin D therapy increases, the ability of isolated mitochondria to take up and retain calcium *in vivo* or *in vitro*.

Thus the mitochondria reflect in some way the opposing effects of vitamin D and adrenal glucocorticoids upon intestinal calcium transport. The problem is to define the role of the mitochondria in transcellular calcium transport. This has yet to be accomplished.

Growth Hormone

One of the major target organs for the action of growth hormone in the growing organism is the skeleton. Without this hormone, skeletal growth slows, and dwarfism results. It now appears likely that the effects of this hormone are mediated not directly but indirectly via somatomedin (see Ch. 2). A discussion of this aspect of growth hormone is out of place here. Growth hormone does have effects upon the skeleton and upon mineral metabolism in the adult, however.

It is not yet known whether, in the adult human, growth hormone is necessary for skeletal homeostasis, but it is clear that mineral homeostasis can be maintained in adults without growth hormone. On the other hand, acromegaly, the syndrome of excessive growth hormone secretion in the adult, leads to changes in the skeleton. The most striking effect is an increase in skeletal remodeling in both the periosteal and endosteal bone cell envelopes. In the periosteal envelope, the balance greatly favors bone formation, so that periosteal new bone growth occurs, particularly in the flat bone and vertebral bodies. This increase in the cortical thickness of bones is the most striking skeletal effect of growth hormone. It is associated with an increase in endosteal remodeling, which leads to an imbalance in favor of resorption, so that cancellous bone, in particular, decreases in volume.

The cellular basis for the growth hormone–induced changes in skeletal remodeling is not known.

In addition to its effects upon the skeleton, growth hormone induces an increase in calcium and phosphate absorption in the intestinal tract and an increased tubular reabsorption of calcium and phosphate. As a consequence, plasma phosphate concentrations are high in acromegaly.

Because growth hormone induces a positive balance in regard to skeletal mass, it has been proposed as a therapeutic agent in the treatment of osteoporosis.

SKELETAL AND MINERAL HOMEOSTASIS

The endoskeleton subserves two important functions: supporting and protecting the organism, and regulating mineral metabolism. In order to subserve the first function, an amount of calcified bone sufficient to ensure sufficient strength and rigidity to withstand the ordinary mechanical forces to which the organism is normally subjected is required. The maintenance of a sufficiently strong endoskeleton, *skeletal homeostasis,* is achieved by the regulation of the rates of bone formation and bone resorption. The regulation of mineral balance, *mineral homeostasis,* is also achieved by regulating the rates of these two processes, as well as that of mineral accretion. In a normal organism in mineral balance, the two operate effectively as a single mechanism and are obviously interrelated. In various disorders, however, skeletal homeostasis is compromised in order to maintain mineral homeostasis. Conversely, in a few primary disorders of bone, mineral homeostasis becomes deranged.

Skeletal Homeostasis

The mature skeleton is a dynamic organ undergoing constant destruction and renewal. At any given time, some 3 to 5 per cent of the total organ is being actively remodeled. The remodeling serves the important function of molding the structure of bone to best resist the mechanical stresses to which it is subjected. In the young adult, resorption and formation are balanced, so that there is little net change in total skeletal mass. The mechanisms whereby this balance is maintained are not completely understood, although an important facet of this control is mechanical stress or pressure in regulating bone formation. The most dramatic confirmation of the importance of this factor is the *osteoporosis*—decreased bone density—that occurs in young adults suddenly immobilized by paralytic poliomyelitis. Bone formation rate as assessed by microradiography falls dramatically, and bone resorption rate either remains normal or increases. The result is a dramatic loss in total bone mass, the rate being sufficient under some circumstances to exceed the ability of the kidney to excrete calcium (400 to 500 mg. per day), with consequent hypercalcemia.

Experiments carried out with dead or living bone have shown that bone can serve as a transducer, converting mechanical energy to electrical energy. When a bone segment is subjected to deforming pressure, i.e., bending stress rather than compression, an electric potential and a direct electric current are generated. The current is characterized by an initial surge, dropping in a few seconds to a steady current output and persisting as long as the stress is maintained. When the mechanical force is relieved, the flow of current is momentarily reversed, and then it ceases. The amplitude of the potential generated is dependent upon the rate and magnitude of the deformation, and its polarity is determined by the direction of deformation. Areas under compression develop negative potentials. When living bones are subjected to deformation *in vivo*, the areas under compression are the surfaces on which increased osteoblastic activity is observed. The mechanism whereby this pressure electricity, or *piezoelectricity*, is generated is not known, but organized bone containing both collagen and hydroxyapatite is required. One suggestion is that the functional unit formed between the apatite-collagen complex operates as a stress-sensitive series of positive-negative (PN) junctions similar to those seen in certain semiconductors. Several other characteristics of bone under pressure are similar to those of a semiconductor.

The possible importance of these stress-induced direct currents in bone is twofold: (1) they may be important in directing the pattern of aggregation of the macromolecules forming the bone matrix; and (2) they may influence the activity of the osseous cells, leading thereby to a change in rate of macromolecular synthesis. There is experimental evidence to indicate that both effects can be brought about by changes in current flow. Particularly striking are the changes seen when electrodes are placed in bone and a current is passed across them. When current in the range of 10 μamp. is passed, increased osteoblastic activity is noted at the negative electrode and either no change or slight resorption at the positive. This current is of the same order of magnitude as that generated by bone deformation *in vitro*.

These facts can be incorporated into a scheme compiled from present knowledge of *skeletal homeostasis*. Basically, the system is a negative feedback loop, as illustrated in Figure 11–36 (see also

Fig. 11–10). An increase in the deforming pressure upon a given bone segment leads to the generation of an electric current, the collagen-apatite complex serving as a transducer of mechanical to electrical energy. The increased current acts upon bone cells, the second transducer, converting an electrical signal to a chemical one, and resulting in a conversion of osteoclasts to osteoblasts and, eventually, an increase in matrix synthesis. The maturation and calcification of this increased matrix lead to increased bone mass, which in turn leads to a more rigid bone; that is, the degree of deformation produced by a given mechanical pressure will be less; hence, the system exhibits negative feedback, with bone cell activity being the dependent variable and mechanical force the independent one. A second independent variable is *osteolysis*. Increased osteolysis leads to decreased bone mass and hence has the effect of increasing the piezoelectric output from a given mechanical stress. Thus both the activity and number of bone-forming cells are altered in response to these piezoelectric effects.

The mechanisms by which piezoelectric effects regulate bone cell function are not established, but in the light of the recent evidence showing the great importance of ions as regulators of the functions of bone cells, it is logical to suppose that electrical impulses cause changes in membrane characteristics and therefore in ionic fluxes. The latter in turn alter cell function.

Mineral Homeostasis

The value of continual bone remodeling, aside from serving as a means whereby the skeleton can most effectively fulfill its supportive role, is that it makes available metabolically active surfaces which can serve as sites for regulating mineral balance. Mineral homeostasis means calcium and phosphate homeostasis primarily, although bone may also play a role in magnesium homeostasis and is a reservoir of body sodium.

Because of its importance in the regulation of membrane function and other physiologic activities, the concentration of calcium in the plasma and extracellular fluids is maintained constant in the face of even extreme calcium deprivation. Bone is a major reservoir of calcium in the organism; hence, calcium homeostasis in times of calcium deprivation is achieved by a net shift of calcium from bone to extracellular fluids. The agent of prime importance in this regard is the parathyroid hormone. Increased PTH is released by a fall in plasma calcium and acts upon bone to increase osteolytic activity and decrease osteoblastic. Thus, in spite of diminished bone mass and a presumed increase in piezoelectric stimulus, bone biosynthesis does not keep pace with bone resorption; that is, skeletal mass decreases. From the point of view of calcium homeostasis, this alteration in both parameters of bone metabolism makes sense, because if bone biosynthesis did not diminish or actually increased to keep pace with osteolysis, and if plasma phosphate were maintained at a suffi-

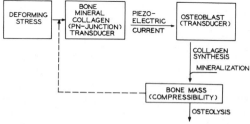

Figure 11–36. A schematic representation of the feedback relationships between stress, bone mass, bone formation and bone resorption (osteolysis). The bone mineral collagen complex acts as a mechanical transducer, converting mechanical (deforming) stress into electrical energy. The amount of current generated is a function of the magnitude of the deforming pressure and the thickness of the bone. The current acts upon osteoblasts to transduce an electrical into a chemical signal, which leads to increased collagen biosynthesis. This, when calcified, leads to increased bone mass, which in turn leads to a decreased current output because it minimizes the effect of a given mechanical force. Osteolysis, by decreasing bone mass, has the opposite effect. (Modified from the concept of R. Becker.)

cient level to ensure nucleation of bone mineral, then the calcium mobilized by osteolysis would be returned to the skeleton and no net gain in extracellular calcium would result.

The skeleton is also involved in phosphate homeostasis, although in a strikingly different fashion. Phosphate deficiency leads to minimal parathyroid gland activity, because of the associated hypercalcemia, and to osteomalacia. Stated another way, when phosphate deficiency lowers phosphate levels, its deposition on bone collagen ceases; hence, no mineralization of bone collagen ensues, and phosphate is conserved for critical metabolic functions. In this instance, however, bone collagen biosynthesis is not inhibited. Nevertheless, skeletal homeostasis, i.e., the maintenance of a constant mass of calcified supporting tissue, is again subservient to mineral homeostasis.

The most interesting aspect of phosphate deficiency is that, if severe, it leads to an increase in the rate of bone resorption, even though plasma PTH concentration is low. Because of the low PTH level, the kidney does not retain the calcium mobilized from bone, and the individual, or organism, goes into negative calcium balance. Thus there is a net loss of bone and a net loss of bodily calcium in an attempt to maintain plasma phosphate concentration. Conversely, in calcium deficiency with a secondary rise in plasma PTH concentration, urinary phosphate excretion is markedly enhanced in an effort to maintain calcium concentration.

It is clear that, as long as a relative balance between bone formation and bone resorption is maintained, the absolute rates of skeletal remodeling can change dramatically without altering plasma calcium or phosphate homeostasis. The most striking examples of this are Paget's disease and thyrotoxicosis, in which high rates of skeletal remodeling are observed but in which plasma electrolyte concentrations are normal, and hypothyroidism and osteopetrosis, in which plasma electrolyte concentrations are normal in spite of extremely low rates of skeletal remodeling.

These disease states in man illustrate the importance of organs other than bone in mineral homeostasis. For example, the rates of skeletal remodeling are often as high in patients with thyrotoxicosis as in those with primary hyperparathyroidism, although hypercalcemia and hypophosphatemia are rarely seen in the former but are the rule in the latter. Likewise, the rates of skeletal remodeling are just as low in hypothyroidism as in hypoparathyroidism, although hypocalcemia and hyperphosphatemia are rarely seen in the former but are the rule in the latter. In all these situations, the determining factors are to be found in the renal tubule and gastrointestinal tract. In particular, the regulation of the renal tubular reabsorption of calcium is of key importance (Fig. 11-35).

METABOLIC BONE DISEASE

As originally defined by Albright, metabolic bone disease is a generalized disorder of bone arising as a consequence of disturbance in general body metabolism. All the bones are involved, but it is not uncommon for some to exhibit a more pronounced alteration than others. In fact, nearly all metabolic bone diseases show characteristic and distinct patterns of skeletal involvement. In contrast, localized bone disorders are restricted in distribution, always being clearly delineated from areas of normal bone. As with most classifications, however, certain disorders are difficult to categorize. For example, Paget's disease has been considered a localized condition of bone, even though 90 per cent or more of the skeleton may be involved. In any case, as our knowledge advances, disorders grouped into one category will undoubtedly be reclassified.

The usual classification of the major metabolic bone diseases, based upon combined histologic (Fig. 11-37) and radiographic criteria, is this: (1) osteoporosis—a decrease in radiographic density and less total bone which is histologically normal in terms of cellular appearance, degree of mineralization, and organization (Fig. 11-37); (2) osteomalacia (and rickets)—characterized radiographically by typical changes in the epiphyses (rickets) and pseudofractures and histologically by decreased mineralization, i.e., presence of excess osteoid (Fig. 11-37); (3) osteopetrosis—radiologically dense bone, which is immature histologically and has not undergone normal remodeling; and (4) *osteitis fibrosa cystica*—radiographic evidence of cysts, localized erosion, and absence of lamina dura and histologic evidence of marked osteoclastic activity and secondary fibrosis (Fig. 11-37).

The introduction of several new tools has permitted a more accurate assessment of bone formation and bone resorption rates and has led to a reclassification based upon more dynamic criteria. Before this classification is considered, a brief discussion of the tools used in studying bone is presented.

Methods of Study

There have been two general approaches to the assessment of bone formation and resorption rates. One has been the use of radiographic or isotopic methods *in vivo,* and the other, the assessment of these parameters by an analysis of bone biopsies *in vitro.* The latter methods have included labeling the bones *in vivo* with tracer or bone-seeking substances, such as tetracycline, prior to removal of the bone specimen; the assessment of these rates by a detailed quantitative analysis of microradiographs of standard sections of undecalcified bone obtained in as standard a fashion as possible; and quantitative histology of bone, in which the various types of bone surfaces are identified in standard sections of cancellous and cortical bone and their extent quantified.

In some respects, quantitative histologic and microradiologic evaluation of bone parameters give similar results, but there are important differences between the results obtained by the two methods, particularly in regard to the measurement and interpretation of extent of resorption

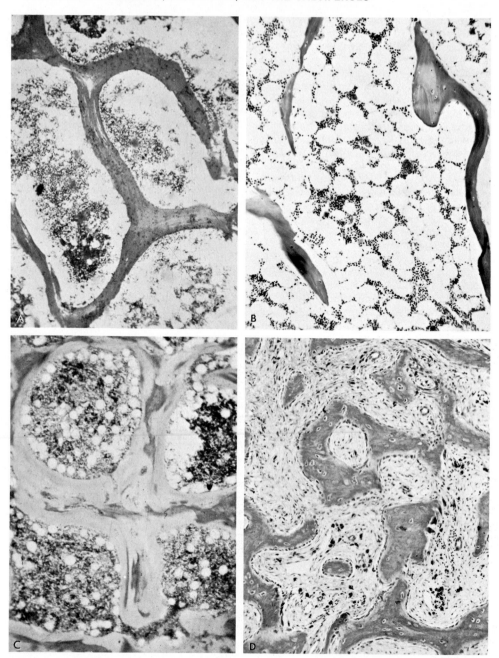

Figure 11–37. The histologic appearance of human bone in various disease states: *A,* normal, *B,* osteoporosis, *C,* osteomalacia, and *D,* osteitis fibrosa. The only change in osteoporosis is a decrease in total mass of mineralized tissue. In osteomalacia, large amounts of osteoid are present; in osteitis, the marrow is replaced by fibrous tissue, large numbers of resorptive cells with osteoclasts are apparent, and the osteocytic lacunae are enlarged. (Hematoxylin and eosin stain, × 120.) (Kindly supplied by Dr. Benjamin Castleman.)

surfaces. These differences are of a fundamental significance because they lead to quite different conclusions as to the pathogenesis of certain metabolic bone diseases, particularly osteoporosis.

Methods In Vivo

Radiography

The radiologic study of bone density and bone changes is an important diagnostic tool in the evaluation of patients with metabolic bone disease. By standard methods, it is possible to discern characteristic changes in bone shadows which are pathognomonic of osteitis fibrosa cystica, osteoporosis, rickets, osteomalacia, Paget's disease, and related conditions. These changes are described in the discussion of the particular disorder. It is important to emphasize that the three most common disorders are osteoporosis, osteomalacia, and osteitis fibrosa cystica, and that each may be caused by one of several etiologic agents. For example, osteitis fibrosa cystica and hyperparathyroidism are often considered synonymous, but osteitis can be seen in conditions other than hyperparathyroidism, and primary or secondary hyperparathyroidism can lead to osteoporosis and possibly even to osteomalacia rather than to osteitis. Thus it is important to distinguish between specific diseases and the more limited number of skeletal derangements with which they may be associated.

Photon Absorption

Although radiography is an important means of detecting qualitative changes in bone structure, it has not proved particularly useful for measuring bone mineral content. Bone mineral content can be measured very accurately *in vivo* by the use of photon absorption techniques. In the standard method, a monochromatic beam of low-energy photons from a radioactive source as I^{125} or Am^{241} is allowed to pass through a specific portion of a long bone (midshaft of the radius), and the intensity of the emergent beam is measured with a collimated scintillation detector.

In the adult, if the measurement is made at a point 3 cm. from the distal end of the radius, then primarily cancellous bone is measured, and if it is made at a point 8 cm. from the distal end of the radius, then cortical bone is measured. Total mass at these sites usually varies in the same direction in various disease states. For example, bone mineral content at either site is reduced in osteoporosis, hyperparathyroidism, osteomalacia, and often in hyperthyroidism. In acromegaly, however, cancellous bone mass may decrease at the same time that cortical mass increases.

The method is quite reproducible, having a coefficient of variation of 2.5 per cent. By this technique, it has been possible to show that Caucasians have a lower bone mass, or bone mineral content, than do Negroes, confirming earlier autopsy evidence. In addition, the technique has established unequivocally that normal women after the age of 45 to 50 have a progressive decrease in bone mass. A similar less-marked change is observed after the age of 60.

This direct method *in vivo* is highly reliable, is easy to use, and is enjoying increased application. It has reaffirmed the important role of physical exercise in controlling bone mass. Even in older subjects, a program of physical activity and physical therapy has been shown to lead to a significant increase in bone mass.

At present, this method is clearly the most useful technique for the *in vivo* assessment of skeletal homeostasis. It is particularly useful in the study of the response of osteoporotic subjects to therapy.

Balance Studies

The metabolic balance study has an important place in the diagnosis of, and evaluation of therapeutic efficacy in, metabolic bone disease. The principle of this technique is to place the patient on a standard and constant intake, then to measure the total intake and output of the various minerals of interest, e.g., calcium, magnesium, sodium, potassium, phosphate, and nitrogen. The procedure is costly and time-consuming, but does yield valuable information that is unobtainable by other means. For example, some disorders of mineral or bone metabolism are associated with normal concentrations of calcium, phosphate, magnesium, and phosphatase in the plasma, despite which there may be a considerable negative or positive balance or a shift in the ratio of fecal to urinary excretion of one or more minerals. Although net shifts of mineral into and out of bone can be assessed by this means, it is not possible to evaluate bone formation and resorption separately.

Tracer Techniques

The most widely employed technique for assessing *in vivo* the rates of bone turnover has been the use of either radioactive (Ca^{45}, Ca^{47}) or stable (Sr) tracers as a means of measuring skeletal dynamics. The greatest experience has been gained with radiocalcium, and the results with other methods are in general agreement with those obtained with this method.

Following the injection of a tracer dose of radiocalcium into an experimental animal or a human, the change of plasma specific activity (Ca^{45}/Ca^{40}) with time follows a series of exponential decay curves which vary somewhat in different conditions. By one of several mathematical devices, it is possible to calculate an accretion rate, A. This is defined by the equation,

$$qR = ES + A \int_0^t Sdt$$

where q is activity of tracer injected (microcuries)

R = fractional retention as a function of time, t
S = specific activity of blood as a function of time
E = a rapidly exchangeable calcium pool.

The last is necessary to correct for the rapid disappearance of isotope during the early time intervals. Formerly, it was considered to represent an exchangeable compartment in bone, but recent evidence indicates that it may represent soft-tissue calcium as well.

The formulation omits any influence of resorption, which is considered to be negligible during the early part of the study.

Several methods have been employed for solving this equation. One of the most useful calculates A from the values and slopes of S and R at a single time point

$$A = \frac{qR(\lambda - \lambda_r)}{S + \lambda_s I}$$

where $\lambda_s = \frac{1}{s} \left(\frac{ds}{dt} \right)$ the rate constant of the

curve s at time t
λ_r = the rate constant for R
and I = the time integral of S from time zero to t.

By this means, A is calculated. A typical value of 500 mg. of calcium per day is considered normal for a 70-kg. man. This is a value two to five times larger than values obtained *in vitro* (see below).

Often some 4 to 10 days after the injection of isotope, a break in the specific activity curve is observed, indicating a return of isotope from bone to blood. The difference in slope observed after the break compared with that expected of an exponential function has been used as an index of bone resorption. There is considerable question, however, whether such a calculation is valid. The fundamental assumption is that the skeleton traps calcium in only two ways. Studies in experimental animals indicate, however, that a significant percentage of the calcium, particularly in adult animals, labels the total bone mineral in a diffuse fashion which is clearly unrelated to accretion, and which exchanges with a time constant considerably greater than that estimated for the rapidly exchangeable pool. In fact, it would appear that 50 per cent or more of the isotope taken up by bone resides in this diffuse component. Hence it is possible, although not established, that the break in the plasma specific-activity curve represents an exchange of isotope out of this compartment and does not represent resorption. This, coupled with the fact that part of the exchangeable compartment is probably soft-tissue calcium, indicates that the true situation is considerably more complex than usually assumed. Hence estimates of alterations in accretion rates in disease states may err considerably, depending upon the relative importance of true accretion versus long-term exchange in the particular disorder. This is particularly striking in kinetic studies carried out in patients with defective mineralization and osteomalacia. Most have shown high accretion rates which contrast in a striking fashion to those estimated by other means. In all likelihood, the relatively poorly mineralized bone seen in these disorders has a relatively higher component of long-term exchangeable calcium.

Another feature of the results obtained by kinetic analysis is the relationship between the rates of bone mineral accretion and resorption in humans with a variety of metabolic bone diseases. In nearly all cases (Fig. 11–38), an increase in resorption is associated with an increase in formation, emphasizing again the link between resorption and formation in the adult skeleton.

A particularly useful application of isotopic methods in man has been the use of Ca^{47} in the measurement of intestinal absorption of calcium in a variety of disease states. In this technique, the appearance of Ca^{47} in bone or in an entire limb is measured as a function of time after the administration of Ca^{47} by mouth and compared with the time course of change after the intravenous administration of a similar dose of isotope. The results are analyzed by a suitable mathematical protocol and plotted as the fraction of the total dose absorbed per unit time (Fig. 11–39).

In the normal human subject, there is a delay of 5 to 10 minutes before absorption begins; peak ab-

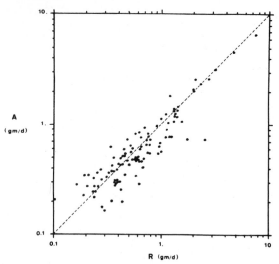

Figure 11–38. The relationship between the rate of mineral accretion (A) and mineral resorption (R) in patients with a variety of metabolic bone diseases. The dotted line represents the state in which R balances A. (From Harris, W. H., and Heaney, R. P.: *New Eng. J. Med. 280*:193, 1969.)

sorption rate is reached in 30 to 60 minutes, depending upon the amount of nonradioactive calcium given, and is essentially complete in three hours (Fig. 11–39). The rate is extremely low in nontropical sprue and vitamin D deficiency. It is somewhat reduced in hypoparathyroidism and hyperthyroidism and increased in idiopathic hypercalciuria, hypothyroidism, and hyperparathyroidism.

Neutron Activation Analysis

Another technique which has not yet received widespread application, but which may become quite useful in the assessment of skeletal balance and long-term response to therapy, is the estimation of total body calcium by the technique of neutron activation. In this procedure, the subject is exposed to whole-body neutron irradiation, which gives rise to the short-lived calcium isotope Ca^{49} ($T_{1/2} = 8.9$ min.) from the small amount of the stable and naturally occurring calcium isotope Ca^{48}. After exposure, the subject is placed in a whole-body counter and the amount of total body calcium estimated from the radioactive decay of Ca^{49}. The technique is highly reproducible and has a coefficient of variation of less than 2 per cent.

The potential usefulness of this technique is similar to that of estimation of skeletal mass by photon absorption. The advantage of neutron activation is that it estimates total body calcium and not the mass of a single, small cross section of one bone. Its disadvantage is that it requires considerably more elaborate equipment. In addition, the biologic effects of repeated exposures to neutron irradiation are still a matter of dispute. It seems unlikely that short and infrequent exposures represent a risk, but clearly the risk from the photon

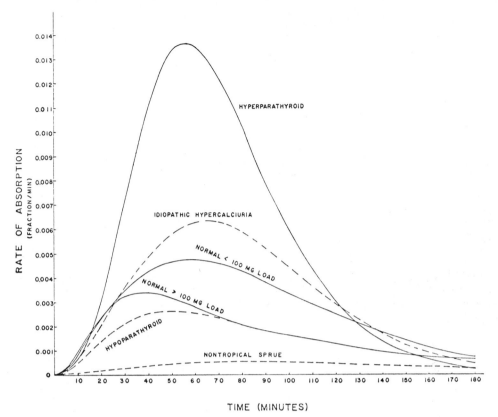

Figure 11–39. The rate of intestinal absorption of a standard dose of oral calcium in normal patients with high and low calcium intakes and in patients with sprue, hypoparathyroidism, idiopathic hypercalciuria, and hyperparathyroidism. (From Birge, S. J., Peck, W. A., et al.: *J. Clin. Invest.* 48:1705, 1969.)

absorption technique is less. Both procedures should turn out to be most useful in long-term studies in which estimation of changes in skeletal mass are an important parameter either in following the natural course of a particular disease or in the estimation of the therapeutic efficacy of a particular drug.

Hydroxyproline Excretion

When collagen is destroyed, it is first degraded into soluble peptides containing hydroxyproline (HOP). These are further degraded, for the most part, to carbon dioxide and urea, but a small percentage circulates in the plasma and is excreted in the urine. The excretion of hydroxyproline has come to be regarded as an independent index of bone resorption in various clinical disorders. As discussed elsewhere in this chapter (p. 670), the interpretation of changes in hydroxyproline excretion is not as simple as is generally supposed. A point of particular importance in establishing standard basal conditions is that some 8 to 10 per cent of the hydroxyproline in dietary gelatin and collagen appears in the urine, and this can cause significant increases in urinary HOP under normal dietary conditions. In addition, a small but variable, and often significant, portion of the urinary

hydroxyproline is derived from recently synthesized collagen. This portion is an indicator of the rate of collagen synthesis rather than of the rate of destruction.

The excretion of HOP varies with age and decreases considerably after puberty. Typical values of urinary HOP as a function of age are shown in Table 11–8, and changes of HOP in various clinical disorders are summarized in Table 11–9. A wide variety of disorders leads to increased excretion, and it is clear that no simple relationship exists between urinary hydroxyproline excretion and rate of bone resorption.

Considerably more information is needed concerning the intimate details of collagen metabolism in these various states before it is possible to

TABLE 11–8. URINARY HYDROXYPROLINE EXCRETION IN HUMANS AS A FUNCTION OF AGE

Age	*HOP mg./24 hr./m.²
0–1 yr.	50–190
1–10 yr.	40–90
11–14 yr.	40–110
Adults	10–30

*Hydroxyproline excretion per day per square meter of body surface.

TABLE 11–9. URINARY HYDROXYPROLINE EXCRETION IN VARIOUS DISEASE STATES

State	Change
Hypopituitarism	↓ in children, n in adults
Acromegaly	↑
Hypothyroidism	↓
Hyperthyroidism	↑
Hypoparathyroidism	↓
Hyperparathyroidism	↑ or n
Paget's disease	↑
Rickets and osteomalacia	↑
Extensive fractures	↑
Neoplasia in bone	↑
Osteoporosis	↑ or n
Marfan's syndrome	↑ or n
Malnutrition	↓
Cushing's syndrome	n

↑ = Increase; ↓ = decrease; n = normal.

correlate the changes in hydroxyproline excretion with the metabolism of bone measured by a variety of other techniques. Changes in hydroxyproline excretion have proved useful as guides to therapy in certain states, particularly acromegaly and hypo- and hyperthyroidism.

Methods In Vitro

Tetracycline Labeling

The first localization of a dye in bones was observed nearly 200 years ago, but only recently has this knowledge been used as the basis for estimating the rates of bone formation and bone remodeling. The principle of this technique is that bone is examined after one or more injections of a marker compound into the organism. The important assumption is that the marker localizes solely in areas of bone formation. Several different compounds have been employed, but the one most fully evaluated is the antibiotic tetracycline. This substance localizes at the sites of initiation of calcification in newly forming bone and then remains in the bone until the bone undergoes resorption. The tetracycline is detected by fluorescence microscopy. If two doses of the antibiotic are given at least 10 days apart, they will outline, in active haversian systems or at bone surfaces, a thin layer of bone. The distance between the two lines is a measure of the *rate of appositional growth* at the particular site. From this and the total surface labeled, it is possible to determine the fraction of the volume of bone tissue added within a given volume of bone, per unit time, in a particular part of the skeleton. If one is able to estimate the total volume of bone and to assume that the sample gives a representative figure of appositional rate, then the *bone formation rate* (BFR) can be calculated. It is important to point out that this measure (BFR) is in reality a measure of the rate of mineral accretion. Under normal conditions, it measures the rate of new matrix formation as well, because there is a constant relationship between matrix formation

and subsequent mineralization. However, when applied to conditions in which defective mineralization is involved, such as rickets and the osteomalacias, formation rates measured by tetracycline labeling are usually decreased. The presence of a considerable amount of uncalcified osteoid indicates that true bone formation, i.e., rate of bone collagen synthesis, is certainly more rapid than rate of mineral accretion. Hence, in these situations, estimations of bone formation rates appear invalid, and the true value will be obtainable only when a method for measuring the rate of collagen formation independently of mineralization is available.

Some studies have been done in experimental animals contrasting values of "bone formation rate" obtained by tetracycline labeling with accretion rates obtained with radioisotopes of calcium. Invariably the latter technique gives higher values than does the former, for instance, a factor of two to five times, and these differences become more marked with age. The values for bone formation rate obtained by tetracycline labeling are similar to those obtained by microradiography. They indicate that the rate of new bone formation represents approximately 2 to 5 per cent of the total skeleton per year in the adult. Stated another way, this represents 50 to 100 mg. of calcium per day. Thus, if bone formation ceased entirely and resorption continued at a normal rate, approximately 50 per cent of the skeleton would disappear in ten years.

The BFR becomes minimal at age 35 and then increases to age 65. These figures are similar to the data obtained with microradiography. Formation and resorption are balanced in young adults aged 20 to 35. Before this age, bone formation is greater (skeletal growth), and after this age resorption is normally greater (1.3 to 1.8 times) than formation. The BFR is reduced in postmenopausal osteoporosis, hypoparathyroidism, vitamin D–resistant rickets, and hypercorticism and is increased in osteogenesis imperfecta.

No direct measure of bone resorption rate is possible with the technique of tetracycline labeling, but an assessment of the rate has been made by measuring, on routine micrographs, the total surface showing the scalloped appearance, which is characteristic of osteoclastic activity (Howship's lacunae). The rate of the resorptive activity at any given surface has been estimated indirectly from the fact that in young adults bone resorption and formation are presumably balanced. Also, the total surface involved in resorptive activity in a given bone sample is less than the total surface involved in bone formation (tetracycline labeling), and the rate of appositional growth can be measured by the tetracycline method. From these data, it has been estimated that the rate of linear appositional resorption is equal to that of appositional accretion, i.e., 1 μ per day.

The application of the technique to abnormal situations depends upon the following assumptions: (1) osteoclastic resorption is the sole means of bone destruction — an obviously incorrect deduction; (2)

the rate of linear resorption at a given surface is always the same, regardless of age and metabolic state—a most unlikely assumption; and (3) each Howship's lacuna indicates an active resorption site—a most unlikely assumption.

Microradiography

The principle of this technique is the production of a microradiograph of a standard section (100 μ) of bone, employing soft x-rays. The degree of grayness in the microradiograph is related to the mineral density. Typical radiographs are shown in Figure 11–40. When viewed with a microscope, the bone surfaces can be identified by their characteristic appearance as inactive surfaces, bone-forming surfaces, and bone-resorbing surfaces. The inactive surfaces have a high density with a sclerotic edge. Bone-forming surfaces appear of low density and smooth, and bone-resorbing surfaces are of high density and uneven appearance. Sites of active bone formation identified by microradiography are the sites where tetracycline localizes. The percentage of the total surface involved in each process is assessed by quantitative means, as is the fraction of the total area occupied by bone. From the total surface involved in each type of activity and the amount of surface per unit volume, it is possible to calculate bone formation and resorption rates,

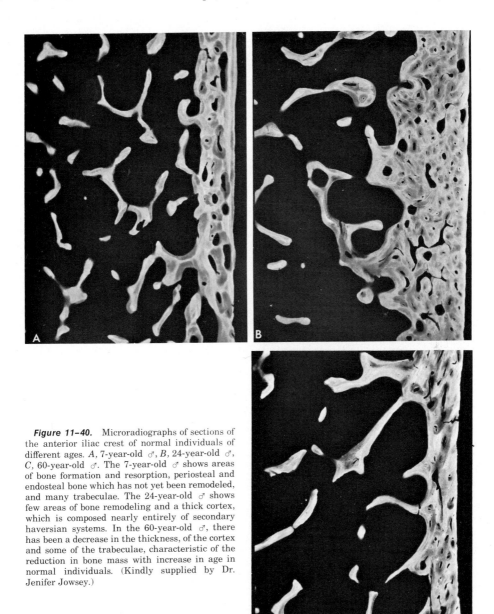

Figure 11–40. Microradiographs of sections of the anterior iliac crest of normal individuals of different ages. *A*, 7-year-old ♂, *B*, 24-year-old ♂, *C*, 60-year-old ♂. The 7-year-old ♂ shows areas of bone formation and resorption, periosteal and endosteal bone which has not yet been remodeled, and many trabeculae. The 24-year-old ♂ shows few areas of bone remodeling and a thick cortex, which is composed nearly entirely of secondary haversian systems. In the 60-year-old ♂, there has been a decrease in the thickness, of the cortex and some of the trabeculae, characteristic of the reduction in bone mass with increase in age in normal individuals. (Kindly supplied by Dr. Jenifer Jowsey.)

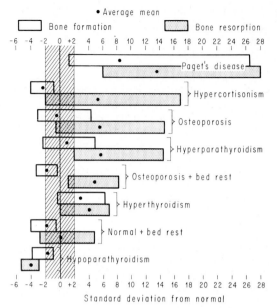

Figure 11–41. The extent of bone formation and bone resorption surfaces measured by quantitative microradiography in patients with a variety of metabolic bone diseases. (Kindly supplied by Dr. Jenifer Jowsey.)

using the assumption that an appositional rate of growth of 1 μ per day occurs at each surface of formation, and a rate of destruction of 1 μ per day occurs at each resorptive surface. These values are taken from tetracycline-labeling measurements made in normal young adults. This application to bones from patients with altered bone metabolism may not always be valid. Nevertheless, bone formation calculated by this means is similar to calculations obtained with tetracycline. Typical microradiographs of human bone from individuals of different ages are shown in Figure 11–40. When the length of surface involved in formation or resorption in a certain area is plotted as a percentage of the inactive surface in the same area, the values indicate the same general trend with age as those obtained with a tetracycline marker.

In Figure 11–41 are shown the deviations from normal of these two parameters in bone obtained from patients with a variety of metabolic bone diseases, and in Figure 11–42 are illustrated typical microradiographs obtained of bone from a patient with hyperparathyroidism, Paget's disease, and vitamin D–resistant rickets. Of particular importance is the fact that bone resorption rates as measured by this method change much more dramatically under most circumstances than do bone formation rates. These findings will be considered in more detail in relation to similar measurements made by histologic methods.

The major assumptions underlying this technique which remain to be validated are (1) that the linear rates of mineral apposition or of bone resorption remain the same regardless of the physiologic condition of the bone; (2) that all so-called resorptive surfaces are active at the time of measurement; and (3) that all so-called bone-forming surfaces are active.

Quantitative Histologic Examination of Bone

An alternate means of assessing the metabolic events in bone is the quantitative histologic evaluation of stained, undecalcified sections of bone from standard biopsy sites, either the iliac crest or a full-thickness biopsy of the ilium. In this type of analysis (Fig. 11–43), six or more other parameters are evaluated: (1) the total extent of bone surface; (2) the total resorption surface (TRS); (3) the active resorption surface (ARS); (4) the active formation surface (AFS); (5) the total osteoid surface; and (6) the percentage of the osteoid surface covered by a calcification front. In addition, the total volume of cancellous bone, the number of osteoclasts, and the percentage of enlarged osteocytic lacunae (representative of osteocytic osteolysis) may also be measured.

The relative values of these parameters as a function of age in the normal human are shown in Figure 11–44. The most striking difference between these results and those obtained with microradiography is that, by quantitative bone histology, the percentage of the total surface of calcified bone covered by *active resorption surface does not change with age*, but the *total resorption surface decreases*. The same qualitative changes are observed in patients with senile or postmenopausal osteoporosis, except that, in these, the decrease in extent of bone formation surface is more marked than in age-matched controls.

The major difference between the results of quantitative histologic analysis and those by microradiography involves the change in resorption surface. It seems clear that quantitative microradiography cannot distinguish between active and inactive resorption surfaces, but quantitative histology can. Thus, in osteoporosis, both techniques measure an increase in total resorption surface, but quantitative histology detects no increase in active resorption surface or osteoclast count. In contrast, in most metabolic bone diseases other than osteoporosis, there is a simultaneous increase or decrease in both active and total bone resorption surface (TRS) (Fig. 11–45).

The changes in ARS, TRS, and AFS in a variety of metabolic bone diseases are shown in Figure 11–45. In thyrotoxicosis, Paget's disease, and hyperparathyroidism, all three increase dramatically, and in hypothyroidism, medullary carcinoma, and hypoparathyroidism, all three decrease dramatically. These data emphasize two points: (1) in most metabolic bone diseases, when the extent of active resorption surface increases or decreases, there is a proportional increase or decrease in the extent of total resorption surface; and (2) in nearly all metabolic bone diseases, when active resorption increases, active formation increases.

On the basis of the model of cellular events in

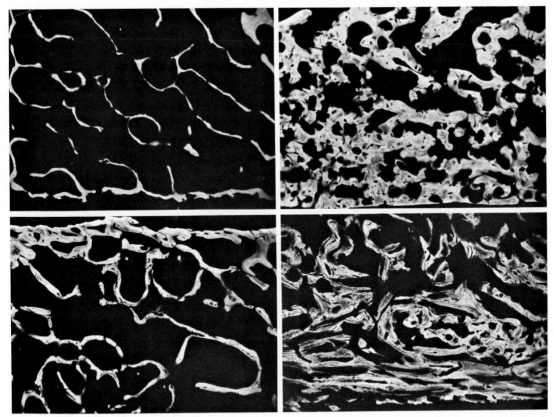

Figure 11–42. Microradiograph (upper left) of iliac crest from a 50-year-old ♂ with osteoporosis. There has been complete loss of cortex, and the remaining trabeculae are thin. Both are characteristic changes of osteoporosis. Cortical bone (upper right) of an individual with Paget's disease of bone. The microradiograph demonstrates the high levels of resorption and formation that are taking place. Microradiograph (lower left) of iliac crest of an adult man with primary hyperparathyroidism. There are enlarged osteocyte lacunae present in the trabeculae, an appearance which has been experimentally associated with increased levels of parathyroid hormone. Microradiograph (lower right) of iliac crest of a growing child with vitamin D–resistant rickets. There are areas of decreased mineral density surrounding the osteocyte lacunae, an appearance characteristic of excessive mineral deficiency and especially evident in this particular disorder. (Kindly supplied by Dr. Jenifer Jowsey.)

Figure 11–43. A schematic representation of the various bone surfaces which are measured by quantitative histologic methods. (From Rasmussen, H., and Bordier, P.: *The Physiological and Cellular Basis of Metabolic Bone Disease.* Baltimore, Williams and Wilkins Co., 1973.)

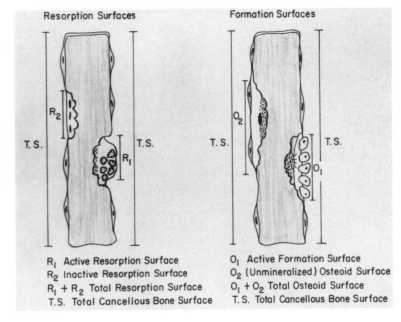

Resorption Surfaces   Formation Surfaces

R_1 Active Resorption Surface
R_2 Inactive Resorption Surface
$R_1 + R_2$ Total Resorption Surface
T.S. Total Cancellous Bone Surface

O_1 Active Formation Surface
O_2 (Unmineralized) Osteoid Surface
$O_1 + O_2$ Total Osteoid Surface
T.S. Total Cancellous Bone Surface

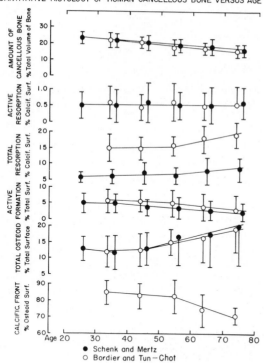

QUANTITATIVE HISTOLOGY OF HUMAN CANCELLOUS BONE VERSUS AGE

● Schenk and Mertz
○ Bordier and Tun–Chot

Figure 11–44. A plot of various parameters of bone remodeling in humans as a function of age, as determined by Schenk and Mertz and by Bordier and Tun-Chot. The only difference between the two sets of data is in the estimation of total resorption surface. This difference is due to a difference in the criteria selected to assesss this parameter. (From Rasmussen, H., and Bordier, P.: *The Physiological and Cellular Basis of Metabolic Bone Disease.* Baltimore, Williams and Wilkins Co., 1973.)

bone remodeling, it is possible to categorize the various metabolic bone diseases and, particularly, to redefine the nature of Paget's disease and osteoporosis (Fig. 11–17).

In these models of metabolic bone diseases, it is necessary to reiterate the basic features of the normal cellular events (Fig. 11–10). The sequence of steps is (1) *activation* of a new group of osteoprogenitor cells, with the resultant production of a new group of daughter cells which give rise to osteoclasts; (2) *resorption* by osteoclasts of old bone; (3) conversion of osteoclasts to preosteoblasts; (4) *formation* of new bone by osteoblasts at the site of previous resorption; and (5) cessation of new bone growth. The size of the two active cell pools, osteoclast and osteoblast, can be estimated by quantitative histologic methods. It is less easy to gauge the activity of the individual cells within the pool, although in many instances there is indirect evidence of changes in activity, e.g., long-continued parathyroid administration leads to an increase in the size of the pool of osteoblasts, but the individual cells within this pool are less active than normal.

There are three major determinants of cell pool size: (1) the rate of activation of osteoprogenitor cells into osteoclasts; (2) the rate of modulation of

osteoclasts to osteoblasts; and (3) the rate of modulation of osteoblasts to osteocytes, i.e., the rate of their bone-forming activity. Over long periods of time, the most important of these is the rate of osteoprogenitor cell activation. If the rate of osteoprogenitor cell activation falls to very low values as in hypothyroidism, excess calcitonin secretion (medullary carcinoma of the thyroid) or hypoparathyroidism, then the size of both active bone cell pools decreases dramatically (Figs. 11–17 and 11–45). As a consequence, the rate of skeletal remodeling declines markedly. It is of importance to note that, even though the rate of skeletal remodeling declines to the same extent in all three diseases, it is only in hypoparathyroidism that this decline is normally associated with hypocalcemia, emphasizing again the importance of the function of other organs, particularly the kidney, in plasma mineral homeostasis.

In contrast, in both hyperthyroidism and hyperparathyroidism, there is a significant increase in the size of both active bone cell pools (Figs. 11–17 and 11–45) and thus in skeletal remodeling. In these circumstances, the balance of remodeling activity favors resorption, so that the volume of cancellous bone declines.

These results indicate that, at the level of bone cell activation and modulation, PTH and thyroxine have similar effects. They both increase the rate of osteoprogenitor cell activation and thus the total size of the active bone cell pool, but both lead to a decrease in rate of flow of osteoclasts to osteoblasts or a decrease in activity of the osteoblasts or both. This leads to a decrease in formation relative to resorption, even though the absolute rates of both activities have increased.

In the case of hyperparathyroidism, at least, the administration of large amounts of phosphate will

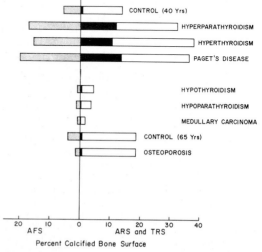

Figure 11–45. A summary of quantitative histologic measurement of active formation surface (stippled), total resorption surface (white plus black), and active resorption surface (black) in human metabolic bone diseases. [Based on the data of Bordier reported in Rasmussen and Bordier (12).]

correct this imbalance (Fig. 11–17). Phosphate acts to increase the flow of osteoclasts to osteoblasts and to increase the activity of these osteoblasts, so that the relative balance between resorption and formation is shifted in favor of the latter. The extreme example of this shift is seen in some cases of renal osteodystrophy, in which phosphate retention and secondary hyperparathyroidism coexist, and in which excessive new bone formation may lead to osteosclerosis.

Paget's disease is also characterized by a marked increase in the rate of osteoprogenitor cell activation and in the size of the pools of both types of active bone cells (Figs. 11–17 and 11–45). The distinctive feature of the cells in this disease is their heterogeneity. For example, in hyperparathyroidism, even though the number of both osteoclasts and osteoblasts may increase markedly, both types of cells are uniform in appearance. The osteoblasts are relatively the same size and have the same staining characteristics, and the osteoclasts usually contain 8 to 12 nuclei. In contrast, in Paget's disease, osteoclasts with 100 or more nuclei are observed next to those with 3 to 5 nuclei, and there is a marked variability in the size and staining characteristics of the osteoblasts. Another feature of Paget's disease is the correlation between resorption and formation. Patients with the highest rates of resorption also have the highest rates of formation (Fig. 11–38). From all these facts, it is most logical to conclude that *Paget's disease in bone represents a benign neoplasia or hyperplasia.* The normally tightly controlled activation of osteoprogenitor cells has become deranged, but the normal coupling sequence of activation ———→ resorption ———→ formation remains.

Senile osteoporosis represents the converse – normal activation but a decoupling between resorption and subsequent formation (Figs. 11–17 and 11–45). Much of the morphologic data can be explained if one assumes that osteoprogenitor cell activation is fairly normal, and that the resorption phase that follows is also normal. There is a delay, however, between the end of this phase and the initiation of formation. This will lead to an increase in total resorption surface with time, but a decrease in active formation surface will be seen histologically (Figs. 11–17, 11–44, and 11–45).

This interpretation of events is quite different from that made on the basis of microradiographic analysis (Fig. 11–41), in which an absolute increase in resorption rate was postulated as the underlying defect in skeletal remodeling in osteoporosis. Far from being a question of purely academic interest, this difference in interpretation has immediate practical import because it determines, in large part, the possible therapeutic strategies to be employed in the treatment of this condition.

It is readily apparent that quantitative histologic analysis of bone, as recently refined by Bordier and by Schenk, has become an extremely important tool in the study and analysis of metabolic bone disease in man.

Classification of Metabolic Bone Diseases

In classifying metabolic bone disease, four terms should be considered: (1) bone remodeling rate, (2) bone formation rate, (3) bone accretion rate, and (4) bone resorption rate. The second and fourth indicate respectively the rates of formation and destruction of bone, and the first, the overall rate of the combined processes. Hence, if (2) and (4) are both increased or decreased to a similar extent, bone remodeling will be respectively increased or decreased without any net change in skeletal mass.

Four general groups of metabolic bone diseases can be distinguished as having: (1) a normal amount of calcified bone and increased or decreased bone remodeling; (2) an increased amount of calcified bone, because of an imbalance between resorption and formation; (3) a decreased amount of calcified bone, because of imbalance; and (4) disorders of mineral accretion.

The various disorders in each category are summarized in Table 11–10. In some instances, the bone disease may be a mixture; for example, osteoporosis of some degree is commonly seen in patients with many forms of osteomalacia. Equally important, the same general metabolic disorder, e.g., hyperparathyroidism, may lead to several different types of bone disease, such as osteoporosis, osteitis fibrosa, normal amounts of calcified bone with increased remodeling, and even osteomalacia.

In this classification (Table 11–10), osteitis fibrosa cystica and osteoporosis are both considered states of skeletal imbalance characterized by an excess of resorption over formation. Both conditions can be produced by the same derangement in mineral metabolism, and it would appear that osteitis is only an aggravated or more severe form of osteoporosis, although this may be an oversimplification. Osteoporosis is associated with a negative calcium balance. Plasma calcium is usually normal, with the exception of those rare cases associated with primary hyperparathyroidism, and there should be little or no stimulus to increase thyrocalcitonin production. On the other hand, the most common cause of osteitis fibrosa cystica is primary hyperparathyroidism, in which plasma calcium is characteristically elevated. This in turn may alter thyrocalcitonin production. Thus the bones may well be exposed to a different hormonal environment in the two states, and this difference may be of considerable importance in determining the nature of the bone response.

Symptomatology

There is a wide range of symptoms associated with various metabolic bone diseases and disruption of calcium homeostasis. Most of these will be considered in the discussion of the individual diseases. However, two particular manifestations deserve special consideration: bone pain and muscu-

TABLE 11–10. CLASSIFICATION OF
METABOLIC BONE DISORDERS

1. Normal amount of calcified bone with altered remodeling rates
   A. Increased bone destruction balanced by increased bone formation
      1. Hyperthyroidism
      2. Mild hyperparathyroidism
      3. Paget's disease
      4. Fluorosis
   B. Decreased bone formation balanced by decreased bone destruction
      1. Hypothyroidism
      2. Hypoparathyroidism
      3. Medullary carcinoma of the thyroid
2. Increased amount of calcified bone — osteosclerosis
   A. Increased formation with normal resorption
      1. Metastatic tumors
      2. Adrenal virilizing tumor
      3. Acromegaly
      4. Some cases of renal osteodystrophy
   B. Normal formation with decreased resorption
      1. Osteopetrosis
      2. Lead poisoning
      3. Phosphorus poisoning
3. Decreased amount of calcified bone — osteoporosis and osteitis fibrosa cystica
   A. Normal or increased formation — increased resorption
      1. Idiopathic osteoporosis
      2. Hyperparathyroidism
      3. Osteogenesis imperfecta
      4. Hyperthyroidism
      5. Hypogonadism
      6. Neoplasia without bone metastases
      7. Adrenal hypercorticism, mild
   B. Decreased formation with normal or increased resorption
      1. Immobilization
      2. Adrenal hypersecretion
4. Disorders of mineral accretion
   A. Disturbances with normal plasma calcium and phosphate
      1. Healing scurvy
      2. Conditions with rapid rates of bone formation
      3. Hypophosphatasia
   B. Disturbances with decreased levels of plasma calcium or phosphate or both
      1. Vitamin D deficiency
      2. Familial osteomalacia and rickets (see Table 11–11 for more complete classification)

the bath, and climbing stairs. The patients with severe weakness exhibit a characteristic waddling gait. They are usually incapable of standing on one leg. Symptoms related to the upper extremities are less dramatic but may be elicited. The weakness can be objectively demonstrated by asking the patient to perform suitable tasks, e.g., climbing stairs.

The pathogenesis of this weakness is not known. One characteristic feature of all these cases, however, is some degree of hyperparathyroidism, and the most severe weakness is seen when this coexists with vitamin D deficiency (relative or absolute). Parathyroid hormone has been found to alter the rates of passage of magnesium and calcium into and out of cells, as well as the distribution of these cations across the membrane of isolated mitochondria *in vitro*. There is also good evidence that the hormone leads to a depletion of phosphate from soft tissues. Thus it is possible that the muscular weakness is brought about by change in intracellular electrolyte concentrations. This may be a direct effect upon the coupling between excitation and contraction or upon the energy-producing systems in the cell or both.

PATHOLOGIC CONSIDERATIONS: PRIMARY DISORDERS OF PARATHYROID GLAND FUNCTION

The common disorders of the parathyroid glands fall into two main categories: those associated with hypofunction (hypoparathyroidism) and those associated with hyperfunction (hyperparathyroidism).

Idiopathic or Postoperative Hypoparathyroidism

Etiology

The most common cause of hypoparathyroidism is damage to or removal of the parathyroid glands in the course of an operation on the thyroid gland. When the glands or their blood vessels have merely been damaged and not removed, the tissue often regenerates, so that the clinical manifestations disappear in a few months. Damage to the parathyroid glands following hemorrhage, infection, or thyroid gland irradiation (x-ray or radioiodine) is very rare.

A much less common cause of hypoparathyroidism is idiopathic lack of function. Most cases are children, and approximately twice as many females as males are affected. It is not known why all four glands cease functioning. Hypoparathyroidism does not occur as a consequence of panhypopituitarism, which is good evidence that the cessation of parathyroid gland function is not the result of a deficiency in a tropic hormone of the anterior pituitary. Some cases of idiopathic hypoparathyroidism appear to be familial. A rare syndrome

lar weakness. The two are often associated in the same patient. Diffuse, poorly localized pain in the lower extremities, pelvis, and lower back is common in osteomalacia and either primary or secondary hyperparathyroidism, as well as in conditions involving various forms of renal tubular failure. The pain is described as constant, nagging, and difficult to relieve. It is usually bilateral and is often associated with bone tenderness, especially of ribs and shins. Local stress or weight bearing increases the pain. This may lead to difficulty in walking, which complaint may also arise in part because of the muscular weakness.

Muscular weakness ranging from a generalized feeling of weakness to profound and incapacitating loss of muscle strength is commonly seen in primary vitamin D deficiency and in both primary and secondary hyperparathyroidism. The weakness involves particularly the trunk and limb girdle. It leads to a sense of heaviness in the legs and to difficulty in standing, getting in and out of

(DiGeorge syndrome) has been described in which hypoparathyroidism occurs along with abnormal cellular immunity. Convulsions in infancy may be the result of a transitory deficiency of parathyroid hormone appearing shortly after birth. Hypoparathyroidism in the newborn infant may be a prenatal compensation for hyperparathyroidism in the mother.

The possibility also exists that hypoparathyroidism may arise because of the secretion of an immunologically detectable but biologically inactive parathyroid peptide or because of a disorder of parathyroid hormone metabolism.

Incidence

The incidence of postoperative hypoparathyroidism is about 1 to 10 cases in each 100 operations involving the thyroid gland; it is more common when a total resection is attempted. Idiopathic hypoparathyroidism is very rare, and only about 150 cases have been reported in the world literature. Unrecognized cases probably exist, however, and if these go untreated and unrecognized, the patients may be classified as mentally retarded or epileptic and eventually become institutionalized. For example, a survey of hypoparathyroid subjects shows that a lag of from 2 to 6 years may exist between the first visit to a physician and the establishment of the correct diagnosis.

Pathology of the Parathyroid Glands

In postoperative hypoparathyroidism, any glandular tissue that is present is found to have degenerated. In idiopathic hypoparathyroidism, the epithelial cells are either diminished in number or absent. They are partially or completely replaced by fat cells. Apart from that, however, the glands appear grossly normal.

Pathologic Physiology

Cessation of parathyroid function leads to a fall in plasma calcium level, and an initial fall followed by a rise in plasma phosphate level. Urinary calcium excretion rises acutely, then falls to low levels as plasma calcium falls. Urinary phosphate excretion falls. All of these changes can be accounted for by the effects of PTH upon (1) the mobilization of calcium and phosphate from bone, (2) the retention of calcium and enhanced excretion of phosphate by the kidney, and (3) the decreased absorption of calcium and phosphate from the intestine. Changes in magnesium metabolism are less well characterized, but an initial magnesium diuresis without significant change in plasma magnesium has been observed.

In spite of a dramatic change in the concentrations of plasma calcium and phosphate, bone mineralization is normal, bone resorption falls, and bone formation is normal initially and then declines (Fig. 11–17). Hence the bones are often slightly more dense than normal, and in longstanding cases rather striking osteosclerosis may be seen.

The major signs and symptoms are directly attributable to the decreased level of plasma ionized calcium. This leads to increased neuromuscular excitability. The basis of this change is due to the fact that calcium plays an important but incompletely defined role in membrane function, particularly in controlling sodium and potassium transport. It is also involved in the coupling of excitation to contraction in skeletal muscle. In this regard, there is some evidence indicating that intracellular calcium actually increases, at least in some tissues, following parathyroidectomy. This may be the basis for the abnormal, metastatic calcification seen in the basal ganglia. The pathogenesis of the abnormalities in dentition and in the epidermis is not known, although the abnormalities are presumed to be directly related to the changes in mineral metabolism.

Symptomatology

The most prominent feature is tetany or its equivalent; about 70 per cent of patients with hypoparathyroidism have this initial complaint. Tetany, in an overt form, is ushered in by numbness and tingling of the extremities; a feeling of stiffness in the hands, feet, and lips; cramps of the extremities; and carpopedal spasm. These symptoms are in rare instances followed by laryngeal stridor and generalized convulsions. The characteristic position of carpal spasm is one of flexion at the elbow, wrist, and metacarpophalangeal joints; extension at the interphalangeal joints; and adduction of the thumb—"accoucheur's hand." Asphyxia as a result of laryngeal spasm may be fatal, although it is uncommon. The laryngeal stridor may be mistaken for bronchial asthma, and the generalized convulsions, for epilepsy. Manifestations of tetany may be mistaken for intrinsic disease in the structures involved. Psychiatric symptoms include emotional lability, irritability, anxiety, depression, delirium, delusions, and other features of psychoses. Patients with chronic hypoparathyroidism, unless continuously and adequately treated, usually show mental retardation.

In latent tetany, patients may complain for several decades of muscular weakness, fatigue, palpitation, and numbness or tingling of the extremities before the diagnosis is suspected and established. The condition should be considered in all patients with mild, variable, recurrent, or vague symptoms of this nature.

Signs

Tetany

Two signs can be elicited which will reveal latent tetany. *Chvostek's sign* is a twitch of the facial muscles, notably those of the upper lip, when a sharp tap is given over the facial nerve in front of the ear. The test is *usually* positive in untreated hypoparathyroidism but also may be positive in approximately 10 per cent of normal adults. *Trousseau's sign* is the induction of carpopedal spasm by reducing the circulation in the arm with a blood pressure cuff. The constriction should be maintained at a sufficient pressure to stop the blood flow for 3 minutes before the test is considered to be negative. This test is rarely positive in normal adults.

Other Signs

Epidermal lesions are commonly found in patients with long-standing hypoparathyroidism. Coarse scaliness of the skin; cutaneous pigmentation; thin patchy hair on the head, axillae, pubis, eyelids, and eyebrows; atrophic, brittle, or deformed fingernails and toenails (with horizontal ridges); and exfoliative dermatitis have been reported. Skin infections, especially moniliasis, are not infrequent. Lenticular cataracts are very common; early calcium deposits in the lens may be detected with the slit lamp. Later changes include zonular opacities, nuclear degeneration, vacuoles, fissures, or diffuse opacities. Aplasia or hypoplasia occurs in teeth that develop after onset of the disease. In a child stricken at about 10 years of age, this may result in blunting of the roots of the molar teeth, a diagnostic sign of some importance (Fig. 11–46). The crowns of hypoplastic teeth show defects in the enamel, yellow spots, horizontal grooves, and punctate holes. Radiographically, bones often appear unusually dense. Symmetrical, bilateral, punctate calcifications of the basal ganglia are sometimes found, and bilateral cerebellar calcification is also common. The Q-T interval in the electrocardiogram is prolonged, primarily as a result of a lengthening of the Q_0-T_c interval, and often is associated with an abnormal T wave. The electroencephalogram may be abnormal. Bilateral choked discs have been seen in a few cases. The reason for this is obscure. This change is most common, however, in very young patients, 1 to 3 years old, and is often associated with grand mal seizures. In this group of patients, a primary diagnosis of epilepsy is often made. This then leads to anticonvulsant therapy with diphenylhydantoin or phenobarbital or both. Both drugs alter the metabolism of vitamin D (p. 757) and are likely to exacerbate the hypocalcemia and thus create the need for increasing anticonvulsant medication. Once the nature of the basic disease is recognized and hypocalcemia is corrected therapeutically, the need for anticonvulsant medication disappears. It is not yet clear, however, whether the high intracranial pressure can be prevented by early therapy. In the usual case, when therapy is instituted, a long period of time ensues before all evidence of increased intracranial pressure subsides.

Laboratory Findings

In young patients with a total absence of parathyroid gland function, the plasma total calcium level may fall as low as 4 mg. per 100 ml., the diffusible calcium level as low as 3 mg. per 100 ml., and the plasma inorganic phosphate level may range from 6 to 16 mg. per 100 ml. In all cases, the plasma total protein level should be determined to eliminate the possibility that the hypocalcemia is the result of a reduced protein-bound calcium fraction. The plasma alkaline phosphatase level usually is normal or slightly low. Plasma citrate is reduced, but plasma magnesium is usually normal. Blood urea nitrogen is normal. Hydroxyproline excretion in the urine is reduced, and there is histologic and microradiographic evidence of decreased bone turnover, with both formation and resorption reduced, but with a tendency for the latter to be more severely restricted (Figs. 11–41 and 11–45). When plasma calcium falls below 7 to 8 mg. per 100 ml., the urinary calcium excretion is diminished, but the renal threshold for calcium is often low, pre-

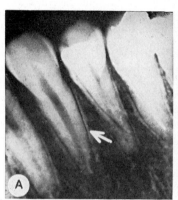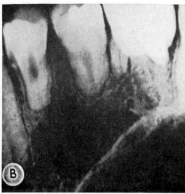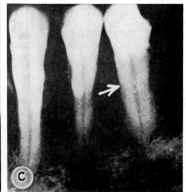

Figure 11–46. X-ray films of the teeth of a normal individual (*A*), of a patient with hypoparathyroidism (*B*), and of a patient with hyperparathyroidism and overt bone disease (*C*). Note that the lamina dura is present in *A* (arrow) and *B* and absent in *C* (arrow). Note the hypoplasia (blunted ends) of the teeth in *B*. (Modified from Albright, F., and Reifenstein, E. C.: *The Parathyroid Glands and Metabolic Bone Disease.* Baltimore, Williams and Wilkins Co., 1948.)

sumably because there is no direct effect of parathyroid hormone upon renal tubular retention of calcium. Because of this, urinary calcium excretion at normal levels of plasma calcium is marked when these patients are treated with vitamin D.

Direct measurement of plasma PTH by radioimmunoassay is now possible and has confirmed the fact that, in nearly all these patients, immunoreactive PTH is low or undetectable in their blood plasma (see p. 684). Moreover, with the discovery that PTH activates renal adenyl cyclase, it was shown that PTH stimulates the excretion of C-AMP in the urine of normal subjects. In patients with idiopathic or postsurgical hypoparathyroidism, the urinary excretion of C-AMP is somewhat reduced (3.2 ± 0.3 nmoles per mg. creatinine, compared with the normal of 3.9 ± 0.3). When such patients are given PTH, however, they usually exhibit a very striking rise in the urinary excretion of C-AMP, in contrast to patients with pseudohypoparathyroidism, in whom PTH infusion causes a very small increase in C-AMP excretion. These differences in C-AMP excretion are a useful diagnostic aid in differentiating idiopathic hypoparathyroidism from pseudohypoparathyroidism and appear to be a more reliable means of making this differentiation than the classical Ellsworth-Howard test, in which phosphate excretion is measured.

Diagnosis

Acute hypoparathyroidism usually can be diagnosed with ease if the condition is suspected. Numbness of the phalanges, laryngeal stridor, "epileptic" seizures, and psychologic changes in young patients are the most common symptoms. In older individuals, a history of recent thyroid surgery followed by any of the symptoms mentioned should suggest the possibility of this disorder. When hypoparathyroidism has become chronic, the symptoms may be vague and the diagnosis may be overlooked. The disease should be suspected in any patient with a past history of neck surgery who presents vague symptoms of cramps, cataracts,

lethargy, or any of a large variety of manifestations usually attributed to psychoneurosis or psychosis. The diagnosis can be established readily by the characteristic chemical findings of a low plasma calcium level combined with a high plasma phosphate level.

Differential Diagnosis

Hypoparathyroidism must be differentiated from two other syndromes: other states which cause tetany, and pseudohypoparathyroidism. The latter disorder is discussed below.

Tetany is brought about by a change in muscle-membrane stability (Table 11–11). It can be induced either by an alkalosis, which increases the binding of calcium to protein and organic anions, without causing a change in the total calcium concentration, or by a change in the total calcium concentration, which leads to a proportional decrease in the ionized calcium. The absolute level of ionized calcium at which tetany will become manifest depends upon the rate of change in the calcium concentration. If the calcium-ion concentration falls rapidly in acute hypoparathyroidism, severe tetany will develop at a calcium-ion concentration high enough to prevent obvious tetany in chronic hypocalcemia.

The tetany of alkalosis can be diagnosed readily from these findings: (1) a history of alkali ingestion, hyperventilation, or vomiting; (2) normal total plasma calcium and inorganic phosphate concentrations; (3) a normal level of urinary calcium; and (4) an alkaline plasma and urine. The cause of tetany in this condition is probably an effect of the change in pH upon membrane excitability and not a major change in calcium ion concentration. Hyperventilation from an emotional disturbance is the most common cause of tetany associated with an alkalosis. There usually is a history of similar attacks under stress, and during an attack, the respirations are rapid. Rebreathing into a paper bag usually results in prompt alleviation of the symptoms.

TABLE 11–11. CHEMICAL FINDINGS IN TETANY

Type of Tetany	Plasma Alkaline Phosphatase	Urinary Calcium	Plasma Carbon Dioxide Combining Power	Plasma Chloride
Low calcium				
Low phosphate				
Rickets and osteomalacia	H	0	N	N
Osteitis fibrosa after operation				
High phosphate				
Hypoparathyroidism	N	0	N	N
Normal calcium and phosphate (alkalosis)				
Hyperventilation	N	N	L	N or H
Vomiting	N	N or H	H	L
Excess alkali	N	N	H	N
Primary hyperaldosteronism	N	N	H	L

H = high; N = normal; L = low; 0 = absent.

TABLE 11–12. SUMMARY OF THE IMPORTANT CHANGES IN RENAL (AZOTEMIC) OSTEITIS, PRIMARY HYPERPARATHYROIDISM, SIMPLE RICKETS, RENAL (AZOTEMIC) RICKETS, AND PHOSPHATE DIABETES

	Renal Osteitis	Primary HPT	Simple† Rickets	Renal Rickets	Phosphate Diabetes
Plasma Ca	n or ↑	↑	↓ or n	↓	n
Plasma P*	↑	n or ↓	↓	↑	↓
Plasma citrate	↑	↑	↓	n or ↓	n or ↓
Ca × P	↑	n	↓	n	↓
BUN*	↑↑	n	n	↑	n
Alk P-tase	↑↑	↑	↑↑	↑	↑ or n
Fecal Ca	↑	n or ↓	↑	↑	↓
Urine Ca	↓	↓	↓	↓	↓
Bone mass	↓	↓	↓	↑	n or ↑
Parathyroid glands	Grossly enlarged	Adenoma, enlarged	Slightly enlarged	Slightly enlarged	
Response to exogenous PTH	↓	↓	↓	↓	n or ↓
Metastatic calcification	Present	Rare	Absent	Rare	Absent
Skeletal turnover		↑		n or ↓	↓
Muscular weakness	Conspicuous	Conspicuous in patients with bone disease	Conspicuous	Conspicuous	Conspicuous

*BUN and plasma phosphate show highly positive correlation in both renal rickets and renal osteitis.
†Vitamin D–deficiency rickets or osteomalacia.

Hypokalemic alkalosis is found occasionally in patients with primary hyperaldosteronism. Frank tetany is rare in this condition; when it does occur, it usually can be differentiated from that of hypoparathyroidism by the chemical findings in the plasma. The pathogenesis of the latent tetany in primary hyperaldosteronism is not clear. The alkalosis probably is an important factor, but alterations in the intracellular and extracellular potassium levels also may play a role. Further investigation of the calcium and phosphate metabolism is needed in patients with primary hyperaldosteronism.

Hypocalcemia (with or without tetany) occurs very commonly in rickets or osteomalacia; the various conditions which result in this osseous disorder are outlined in Tables 11–12 and 11–13. The hypocalcemia of osteomalacia usually can be differentiated from that of hypoparathyroidism by the chemical findings in the plasma (Table 11–14) and by the characteristic radiographic appearance of the bones.

An additional cause of hypocalcemia is hypomagnesemia. In such cases, both plasma calcium and magnesium concentrations are low and plasma phosphate high.

Occasionally in the osteomalacia resulting from renal insufficiency, there is plasma phosphate retention coupled with a low plasma calcium level. The chemistry then may be confused with that of hypoparathyroidism. However, azotemia and a disturbance in the acid-base equilibrium with acidosis are present in renal insufficiency and are absent in hypoparathyroidism. Tetany is rare in the osteomalacia resulting from renal insufficiency, because the associated acidosis inhibits this manifestation. However, tetany may develop if the acidosis is eliminated by therapy with alkali before the hypocalcemia has been corrected. The chemical findings of value in the differential diagnosis of hypoparathyroidism and certain bone disorders are given in Table 11–14.

Certain manifestations of hypoparathyroidism suggest epilepsy, brain tumor, bronchial asthma,

TABLE 11–13. CHANGES IN PLASMA, URINE, AND TISSUES OF PATIENTS WITH SIMPLE RICKETS AND WITH VARIOUS RENAL TUBULAR DISORDERS

	Plasma						Urine					Tissue
	Ca	P	pH	Alk P-tase	BUN	Citrate	P	Ca	Glucose	A.A.	Prot.	Cystine
Vitamin D deficiency	n or ↓	↓	n	↑	n	↓	↑	↓	n	↑	n	O
Tubular disorders Pi alone	n	↓	n	↑ or n	n	n or ↓	↑	↓	n	n	n	O
Fanconi	n or ↓	↓	n	↑	n	n or ↓	↑	↓	↑	↑	n	O
Faconi with acidosis	n or ↓	↓	↓	↑	n or ↑	↓	↑	↑	↑	↑	n or ↑	O
Fanconi with cystine storage (Lignac)	n or ↓	↓	↓	↑	n or ↑	↓	↑	↑	↑	↑	n or ↑	+
Renal tubular acidosis	n or ↓	↓	↓	↑	n	—	↑	↑	n	n	n	O
Azotemic osteodystrophy	↓ or n	↑ or n	↓	↑	↑	↓	↓	↓	n	n	↑	O
Hypophosphatasia	n or ↑	n	n	↓↓	n	—	n	n	PE*	n	n	O

*Increased excretion of phosphoethanolamine.

TABLE 11–14. CHEMICAL FINDINGS IN DISEASES OF CALCIUM AND SKELETAL HOMEOSTASIS

Disease	Plasma							Urine					
	Ca	Mg	P	P-tase	TP	BUN	Cl	Ca	TRP	HOP	AA	CA	AcA
Hyperparathyroidism	↑	N↓	↓N	N↑	N	N↓	↑	↑N	↓N	↑N	↑N	↓	↓
Hypoparathyroidism	↓	N	↑	N	N	N	N↓	↓	↑	↓N	N	N	N
Vitamin D intoxication	↑	↑	N⇅	N↑	N	N↑	N↑	↑	N↓	N↓	N	N↓	N↓
Sarcoidosis	↑	—	↓N	N	↑	N	N↓	↑	↓N	N	—	↓	—
Milk alkali syndrome	↑	N	N↑	N	N	↑	↓	N	N↓	N	—	↓	—
Multiple myeloma	N↑	N	N↑	N↑	↑	↑	N↓	↑	↓	N	—	—	—
Acute bone atrophy	↑	N	↑N	N	N	N	N	↑	N	↑	—	N	N
Paget's disease	N↑	N	N	↑↑	N	N	N	↑	N	↑	—	N	N
Osteoporosis	N	N	N	N	N	N	N	N↑	N	N↑	N	N	N
Osteomalacia	↓	↑N↓	↓	↑	N	N	N↑	↓	↓N	↓↑	↑	N	↓N
Malignant neoplasm with osseous metastasis	↑	N	N	N	N	N	N↓	↑	N	↑	N	N	N
Malignant neoplasm without osseous metastasis	↑	N	↓N	N↑	N	N	↑	N↑	↓N	↑	—	↓	↓
Hyperthyroidism	↑N	N	N↓	N↑	N	N	N↓	↑	N	↑	N	↓	N
Osteopetrosis	N	N	N	N	N	N	N	↓	N	↓↑	N	N	N
Idiopathic hypercalciuria	N	N	↓	N	N	N	N	↑	↓N	N	N	N	N

TRP = tubular reabsorption of phosphate; HOP = hydroxyproline excretion; AA = amino acid excretion; CA = renal concentrating ability; AcA = renal acidifying ability; TP = total protein.

arthritis (because of the muscle spasm), or a psychiatric disturbance. Therefore, in all patients suspected of having these conditions, hypoparathyroidism should be carefully excluded. Abnormal brain wave patterns in the electroencephalogram can result from hypocalcemia. These will disappear if 10 ml. of a 10 per cent calcium gluconate solution is given intravenously. However, chronic hypocalcemia leads to organic deterioration in the brain; therefore, hypoparathyroidism cannot be excluded if no change in the brain waves is produced by the injection of the calcium.

Tetany has been described as a manifestation of magnesium deficiency. However, the disordered neuromuscular function of magnesium deficiency differs from hypocalcemic tetany and is characterized by absence of cramps, negative Trousseau's sign, convulsive seizures with or without a positive Chvostek's sign, extreme irritability, muscle weakness, and gross tremors. The signs are often nonspecific, and diagnosis is difficult. The picture is further complicated by the report of hypocalcemia as a result of primary hypomagnesemia. Treatment of hypomagnesemia with oral or intravenous calcium does not stop the tremors or convulsions.

Treatment

The major objective in the treatment of hypoparathyroidism is to elevate the plasma calcium concentration to approximately 9 mg. per 100 ml. The most natural form of therapy would be replacement therapy employing parathyroid hormone. Unfortunately, purified or synthetic parathyroid hormone is not yet commercially available, so that vitamin D or dihydrotachysterol (DHT) combined with oral calcium supplements is the major therapeutic agent employed. In addition, because many patients with surgical hypoparathyroidism may have some degree of thyroid deficiency, thyroid function must be assessed and replacement therapy initiated when indicated. This is particularly important because the effectiveness of vitamin D therapy is greater in euthyroid than in hypothyroid patients.

Acute hypocalcemic episodes following thyroid or parathyroid surgery can usually be effectively managed by intravenous administration of calcium gluconate. This should be infused slowly and in doses of 10 ml. of a 10 per cent solution. Oral calcium therapy should be instituted as soon as feasible. If the hypocalcemia and tetany occur after removal of a parathyroid adenoma, conservative measures, i.e., calcium therapy, should be given a trial of several weeks, because the remaining atrophic parathyroid tissue may respond and regain sufficient function to maintain plasma calcium concentration. On the other hand, severe hypocalcemia and tetany after total thyroidectomy are usually indications of permanent hypoparathyroidism. A few of these patients may recover parathyroid function, however, in the first few postoperative weeks.

Therapy in chronic hypoparathyroidism consists of either vitamin D (25,000 to 100,000 units daily) or dihydrotachysterol (0.1 to 5.0 mg. daily) supplemented with oral calcium (2 to 3 g. daily). The calcium can be given as the lactate, gluconate, or chloride. In most instances, any of the three is effective. In a few patients, however, the administration of calcium chloride is more effective than the others. This may be related to improved intestinal absorption of this acid salt or the fact that, because it is acidic, it helps counteract the metabolic alkalosis of hypoparathyroidism. In a rare patient who has become resistant to therapy, the administration of oral magnesium (1 to 2 g. daily) has led to improvement. The underlying mechanism by which magnesium acts is not known.

There are several theoretical reasons why DHT

is a better therapeutic agent than vitamin D, but in practice it has not yet been established that this is the case. Because of this and the fact that vitamin D is less expensive than DHT, vitamin D is recommended. The use of thiazides as an adjunct to vitamin D therapy has been recommended on the basis of the observation that this class of drugs increases the renal tubular reabsorption of calcium. More data are needed before it is possible to evaluate its effectiveness.

The major difficulty with the treatment of hypoparathyroidism is that recurrent episodes of hyper- and hypocalcemia are common even in conscientious patients. The therapeutically effective and the toxic doses of vitamin D are often close to each other. In addition, because vitamin D acts slowly, it is difficult to anticipate therapeutic effectiveness. Likewise, because of the prolonged storage of vitamin D in the body, once hypercalcemia develops, it may persist for months, even if no further sterol is given.

Hypercalcemia is a serious complication that requires prompt treatment. Patients should be taught to recognize the symptoms of hypercalcemia and seek medical advice when they occur. Hypercalcemia can usually be effectively controlled by elimination of vitamin D and calcium therapy, hydration, and the administration of furosemide. If necessary, a short course of CT can be given. It might also be possible to increase the catabolism of vitamin D by the administration of barbiturates.

A major difference between the actions of vitamin D and PTH upon the kidney is their respective effects upon distal tubular reabsorption of calcium: PTH increases this process, but vitamin D does not. Thus, when the plasma calcium concentration is raised to 9 mg. per 100 ml. by vitamin D, there is a considerably greater urinary excretion of calcium than if a similar elevation of plasma calcium concentration had been induced by PTH administration. As a consequence, the therapeutic objective when employing vitamin D is to maintain the plasma calcium concentration in the vicinity of 9 mg. per 100 ml.

The only reliable procedure for following the therapeutic response is to measure the concentration of calcium in the plasma at frequent intervals. During the initial period of sterol therapy, the plasma calcium level should be determined every week to two weeks. After the dosage of calciferol has been stabilized, the determination should be carried out three to four times per year or at any time that the patient or his family observes changes in his mental functioning or his behavior. Hypervitaminosis D is a constant threat and requires prompt attention if renal damage is to be avoided.

The treatment of young, growing patients with idiopathic hypoparathyroidism is often a more difficult problem than the treatment of patients with the postsurgical disease. There is a very marked variability in the need for vitamin D_3 or dihydrotachysterol. The latter is still in general use in the treatment of children with this disease. From recent knowledge of DHT and vitamin D_3 metabolism, it seems that there may be good reason to use

DHT (p. 702). In any case, the amount of vitamin D_3 or DHT needed to obtain a therapeutic response may vary from 0.1 mg. to more than 5 mg. per day. Of particular note, the need for vitamin D treatment may vary considerably as a function of the time of year, with a significant increase in dose requirement during the winter months and a reduction during the summer.

One of the unanswered questions in the use of vitamin D as a pharmacologic agent to treat hypoparathyroidism is the form of the vitamin which exerts the beneficial effects. It may well be that $25(OH)D_3$ rather than $1,25(OH)_2D_3$ is the effective metabolite, but more data are necessary to establish this point.

One aspect of the effect of vitamin D in the treatment of this disease concerns the changes in renal phosphate excretion. The physiologic effect of vitamin D is to increase the proximal tubular reabsorption of phosphate. When used in large doses in the treatment of hypoparathyroidism, however, it has the opposite effect, that of decreasing tubular phosphate reabsorption. It is not yet clear whether this is a direct effect of the vitamin D metabolites or is due to the increase in plasma calcium. In favor of the latter is the finding that the constant infusion of calcium into a hypoparathyroid subject at a rate sufficient to elevate the plasma calcium concentration into the normal range will cause an increase in urinary phosphate excretion and a fall in plasma phosphate.

Pseudohypoparathyroidism

Pseudohypoparathyroidism is a rare genetic disorder involving bone and mineral metabolism. It is probably inherited as an X-linked dominant trait with variable penetrance and is characterized by signs and symptoms similar to those of hypoparathyroidism. Failure to respond to parathyroid hormone, a round face, short stature, strabismus, possibly mental retardation, brachydactylia—especially of the metacarpal and metatarsal bones as a result of early epiphyseal closure (Fig. 11–47)—and ectopic subcutaneous calcifications are also seen. Hypometabolism and abnormal glucose tolerance, similar to what is seen in diabetes, have been described in some patients. The disease may coexist with Turner's syndrome.

Several patients have been described who lack the skeletal manifestations of the disease but have the biochemical abnormalities. Others have been described in whom plasma calcium and phosphate are normal, but in whom the skeletal abnormalities and ectopic bone are present—so-called pseudo-pseudohypoparathyroidism. Several of these patients have developed hypocalcemia in the later course of their disease, indicating the existence of a continuous spectrum rather than two distinct entities.

In the typical patient, the diagnosis is first made at the age of 5 to 10 years. The initial complaint may be related to either the skeleton or the neuromuscular system. Tetany, convulsions, and muscular weakness are common. The tetany is usually

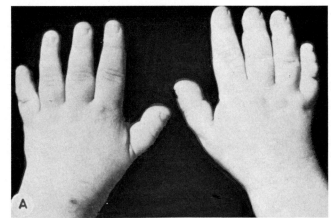

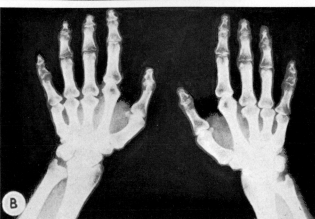

Figure 11–47. Photograph and x-ray film of hands of a patient with pseudohypoparathyroidism. Note that all digits except the thumbs and index fingers are shorter than normal. The shortness results mainly from short metacarpals. (Modified from Albright, F., and Reifenstein, E. C.: *The Parathyroid Glands and Metabolic Bone Disease.* Baltimore, Williams and Wilkins Co., 1948.)

less severe than in idiopathic hypoparathyroidism. On the other hand, metastatic subcutaneous calcification is considerably more common. Plasma calcium is low and plasma phosphate high, but plasma PTH concentration is elevated. The infusion of a large dose of purified bovine parathyroid hormone has been noted to cause a transient but definitely subnormal phosphaturia and a subnormal excretion of C-AMP.

In some cases, this lack of responsiveness to parathyroid hormone is limited to one end-organ (the kidney), because another end-organ (bone) often shows evidence of osteitis fibrosa cystica by both radiologic and histologic examinations. The changes are associated with an increased plasma alkaline phosphatase activity. These observations are consistent with the finding of parathyroid hyperplasia in untreated cases of pseudohypoparathyroidism. Hence the sequence of events in some cases of pseudohypoparathyroidism may be the following: (1) a genetically determined inability of the renal tubules to respond to parathyroid hormone; (2) phosphate retention with a rise in the plasma phosphate level; (3) hypocalcemia; (4) stimulation of parathyroid hormone secretion and parathyroid gland hyperplasia; and (5) increased bone resorption secondary to the increase in the circulating parathyroid hormone, with a tendency to ectopic calcification. If this is the true situation,

however, an unanswered question is why, in these patients with renal phosphate retention and secondary hyperparathyroidism, plasma calcium does not increase to the same extent as that seen in patients with renal rickets (Table 11–12). Part of the answer may lie in what happens to calcium in the renal tubule, which has not been adequately investigated in these patients, and the possibility that high plasma phosphate inhibits bone resorption and enhances bone formation.

There are two other measurements of great value in distinguishing true from pseudohypoparathyroidism. The plasma PTH concentration, which is normally high in untreated patients with pseudohypoparathyroidism and can be suppressed by calcium infusion, is low or undetectable in patients with hypoparathyroidism. There is also a striking difference in the response to PTH infusion. The infusion of PTH into patients with hypoparathyroidism results in a very marked increase in both C-AMP and phosphate excretion and an initial decrease in calcium excretion. In contrast, patients with pseudohypoparathyroidism have very little response to PTH in terms of either C-AMP or phosphate excretion. The infusion of dibutyryl C-AMP into such patients, however, produces changes in C-AMP and renal electrolyte excretion similar to those seen when it is infused into patients with hypoparathyroidism.

These data argue that the principal defect is a defective renal receptor site for PTH or an altered adenyl cyclase. Two confusing findings, however, which are yet to be explained are that: (1) in some of these patients, vitamin D therapy leads to the restoration of a normal renal response to PTH; and (2) at autopsy, normal amounts of PTH-sensitive adenyl cyclase have been found in renal homogenates from these patients. More information is needed in regard to both of these points before their significance is clear.

The usual therapy is similar to that discussed for idiopathic hypoparathyroidism. Upon treatment with vitamin D, the abnormalities in plasma electrolytes are corrected, and there is rapid healing of the osteitis. The short stature and other changes persist. Usually, the dose of vitamin D required to maintain plasma calcium in these patients is smaller than needed in idiopathic hypoparathyroidism.

Secondary Hypoparathyroidism: Phosphorus Depletion

There is as yet no unequivocal evidence of a syndrome of secondary hypoparathyroidism in man. The presumption is that hypoparathyroidism exists in patients with hypercalcemia due to causes other than primary hyperparathyroidism, but direct confirmation of this presumption is lacking. Likewise, the changes observed in the syndrome of phosphorus depletion in man may involve a reactive hypoparathyroidism.

This presumed syndrome is of both practical and theoretical interest. It has been induced in man by the prolonged administration of nonabsorbable antacids, such as magnesium-aluminum hydroxide. It is characterized by hypophosphatemia, hypophosphaturia, hypercalciuria with increased bone resorption, and increased intestinal calcium absorption. These signs are associated with anorexia, debility, muscle weakness, bone pain, and malaise. It is of practical importance because, although it does not occur spontaneously, it may occur as a consequence of medical therapy.

Hyperfunction of the Parathyroid Glands: Primary Hyperparathyroidism

Primary hyperparathyroidism is a disorder of mineral metabolism characterized by a defect in the normal feedback control of PTH secretion by the plasma calcium concentration. Secondary hyperparathyroidism is a disorder characterized by a primary disruption of mineral homeostasis, leading to a compensatory increase in parathyroid gland function and size.

Etiology

The etiology of primary hyperparathyroidism is unknown. Most patients have a simple adenoma, which functions autonomously, so that hormone secretion continues even when plasma calcium is high. There has been considerable speculation that the development of the adenoma is due to long-continued overactivity of the gland as a consequence of hypocalcemia of unknown cause. The support for this is indirect and consists of the following: (1) the disease is rare before puberty; (2) the disease is two to three times more common in females than in males; and (3) experimental hyperparathyroidism can be produced by long-continued calcium deprivation. There is usually no clear-cut history indicating calcium deprivation, however, or other information indicative of abnormalities in calcium metabolism. Moreover, in some patients, a genetic factor is clearly operative, particularly in the group with chief-cell hyperplasia.

Incidence

Hyperparathyroidism is the most common disorder involving the parathyroid glands. The exact incidence of this disorder is difficult to determine, but in recent years there has been a progressive increase in the frequency of the diagnosis in all the large series of reported cases. This increase is the result primarily of a growing awareness of the possibility of the diagnosis and a wider application of the various diagnostic procedures. For example, at the Mayo Clinic, 15 cases were diagnosed during the 15 years preceding 1945, and 370 cases during the 15 years after 1945 (a 25-fold increase). One of every 700 to 800 patients seeking medical attention may have the disease.

Pathology

Primary hyperparathyroidism is associated with five pathologic disorders: single adenoma, multiple adenomas, carcinoma, primary water-clear-cell hyperplasia, and chief-cell hyperplasia or multiple adenomatosis. The relative incidence of these pathologic states in 751 cases of hyperparathyroidism is shown in Table 11–15.

TABLE 11–15. PATHOLOGIC CLASSIFICATION OF PRIMARY HYPERPARATHYROIDISM*

	Per Cent
Neoplasia	
Benign	
Single adenoma	83.0
Multiple adenoma	4.3
Carcinoma	1.7
Hyperplasia	
Water-clear cell	7.6
Chief-cell†	3.6

*Based upon 751 cases.
†Associated with polyendocrine disorders. The reported incidence may be too low, because some authors classify this disorder as multiple adenoma.

Single Parathyroid Adenoma

By far the largest number of cases are associated with a single adenoma. This is usually an encapsulated, lobulated, brownish tumor, 2 to 200 times larger than the normal gland. The tumor is usually larger in patients with skeletal involvement than in those with purely renal manifestations of the disease; a rough correlation exists between tumor size and plasma calcium concentration. The tumors appear more commonly in the inferior parathyroids, usually within 3 cm. of the lower poles of the thyroid gland. Some 10 per cent are situated within the mediastinum.

The chief-cell adenoma, consisting of solid masses of small chief cells similar to those seen in the normal gland, is the most common, but the adenoma may contain predominantly water-clear or oxyphil cells or a heterogeneous mixture of several cell types. In most cases, it is possible to distinguish a rim of normal tissue. A small number of apparently nonfunctioning oxyphil adenomas have been described.

Multiple Adenomas

These are similar to single adenomas in size, histologic picture, and location, except that two or even three glands may be involved. A familial incidence of multiple adenomas has been reported.

Primary Clear-Cell Hyperplasia

This is a condition characterized by enlargement of all four glands. The glands are usually 30 to 100 times normal size and are composed entirely of large water-clear cells. The cytoplasm of the cells is absolutely clear upon routine histologic examination, and the cells often tend to arrange themselves in alveolae (Fig. 11–16). There are at present no clues to the pathogenesis of these striking changes, nor is it possible to distinguish on clinical grounds this form of hyperparathyroidism from that associated with adenomas.

Primary Chief-Cell Hyperplasia

The classification of this condition is in dispute. Some pathologists consider that the condition is hyperplasia of all four glands, whereas others contend that there are adenomas of all four glands. Histologically, the glands are composed of irregular masses of chief cells, with nets of water-clear or oxyphil cells, indistinguishable from the pattern seen in secondary parathyroid hyperplasia of the type seen in renal rickets. There may be a considerable difference in the size of the four glands, and usually the superior glands are larger than the inferior. On occasion, a normal-sized gland has been reported.

This pathologic state is important because it is a genetic disorder, characterized as an autosomal dominant trait with high penetrance and variable expressivity, and is associated with one or more of the following: peptic ulcer, pancreatitis, functioning adenomas of the pancreatic islets, functioning or nonfunctioning adenomas of the pituitary, functioning adenomas of the thyroid or adrenal or both, tumors of the adipose tissue, and diffuse gastric polyposis.

Parathyroid Carcinoma

Carcinoma of a parathyroid gland associated with hyperparathyroidism is very rare. About 45 unquestionable cases have been reported. The functioning malignant tumors generally are larger than the adenomas and are clinically palpable. They tend to grow slowly; to recur locally after excision; and to metastasize to the regional lymph nodes, the lungs, and the liver. These tumors usually are associated with severe hyperparathyroidism, including bone involvement, and are very resistant to x-ray therapy.

Nonfunctioning Parathyroid Tumors

Primary nonfunctioning carcinomas of the parathyroid glands have been reported but are not accepted generally because of the difficulty in establishing the origin of the tumor. Oxyphil adenomas and metastatic carcinomatous lesions occur but are very rare. Gross and microscopic cysts are commonly found in normal glands and in hyperplastic or adenomatous parathyroid tissue. Most of these nonfunctioning tumors arise, as do the adenomas, in the lower two parathyroid glands. These tumors usually do not produce symptoms. When they do, the manifestations are pressure on local structures, including the recurrent laryngeal nerve.

In addition to the forms of primary hyperparathyroidism listed in Table 11–15, all of which involve pathologic alterations of the glands themselves, there is a form of hyperparathyroidism caused by secretion of this hormone (or at least a peptide with biologic effects of PTH) by nonparathyroid tumors. This syndrome of ectopic or pseudohyperparathyroidism produces the signs and symptoms of primary hyperparathyroidism, but the hormone circulating in the plasma of many of these patients differs immunologically from that in the plasma of patients with primary hyperparathyroidism.

Pathologic Physiology

An increase in the rate of PTH secretion leads first to changes in osteocytic osteolysis and in renal electrolyte excretion, including an increase in phosphate and a decrease in Ca^{2+} and H^+ excretion. These changes lead to a rise in plasma calcium, a fall in plasma phosphate, and a slight systemic hypercholoremic acidosis. In addition, the hormone stimulates the renal synthesis of

$1,25(OH)_2D_3$ (Fig. 11–27), which, in turn, stimulates the intestinal absorption of calcium and, in concert with PTH, acts upon bone to enhance bone resorption by stimulating the activation of osteoprogenitor cells and by inhibiting the modulation of osteoclasts to osteoblasts (Figs. 11–10 and 11–17). The latter effect leads to an initial decrease in osteoblast number. In addition, PTH acts to inhibit collagen synthesis by preformed osteoblasts. After this phase, however, if hypersecretion of PTH continues, there is a secondary increase in osteoblast pool size, so that the rate of bone formation increases (Fig. 11–17). This is usually insufficient to reestablish skeletal balance, i.e., resorption continues to exceed formation, but if sufficient phosphate is ingested, skeletal balance will be reestablished (Figs. 11–10 and 11–17).

The problem of defining the reason why some patients with primary hyperparathyroidism appear to have minimal bone disease whereas others have marked changes in bone is yet to be completely solved. There are several possible explanations. One is the possibility of more than one form of PTH with each form having somewhat organ-specific actions. In spite of the fact that multiple circulating forms of PTH have been discovered, there is no evidence that the different forms act specifically on different target organs, so at present there is no convincing evidence in support of different forms of PTH being responsible for different clinical disorders.

A second possibility is that, in patients without bone disease, there is a compensatory increase in CT secretion, which is sustained and which blocks the osseous effects of PTH without blocking its renal effects. As yet, there is no direct evidence in support of this alternative. In patients with evident bone disease and hypercalcemia, plasma CT concentrations have been found to be normal or low and the CT content of the thyroid gland low. This suggests that CT secretion cannot be sustained over long periods of time, even if a hypercalcemic stimulus is sustained over the same time period.

A third possibility is that the phosphate content of the diet, or the other factors regulating phosphate metabolism, are sufficient to maintain plasma phosphate concentration high enough so that skeletal homeostasis is maintained even though skeletal remodeling is slightly increased.

Finally, present evidence shows that, in general, patients with overt bone disease have higher concentrations of circulating PTH in their plasma and at operation have larger adenomas. This suggests that it may be a matter of quantitative rather than qualitative difference. With small adenomas, only the function of the more sensitive organ, the kidney, is significantly altered, but with large adenomas and higher rates of hormone secretion, significant changes in skeletal remodeling ensue.

Another aspect of the pathophysiology of the bone disease in primary hyperparathyroidism relates to the effect of this hormone upon vitamin D metabolism. There are two features of this relationship that are of interest. On the one hand, the

administration of $25(OH)D_3$ or vitamin D_3 may be of practical value in the diagnosis of primary hyperparathyroidism (p. 742). On the other, it is evident that the physiologic changes seen in mineral metabolism in patients with hyperparathyroidism are the result of not only the direct effects of PTH upon organ function but also the changes in the concentrations and actions of vitamin D metabolites (Fig. 11–27). It is even possible to suggest that the relative vitamin D deficiency of hyperparathyroidism is a protective adaptation in limiting the hypercalcemia.

As noted previously (Fig. 11–16), a major factor regulating the rate of PTH secretion is the plasma calcium concentration. When the plasma calcium concentration falls below approximately 10 mg. per 100 ml., the rate of PTH secretion increases. The secreted hormone, by acting upon kidney and bone, causes an increase in plasma calcium concentration, which, in turn, acts as a negative feedback signal, shutting off further hormone secretion. The system operates as though there were a calciostat in the parathyroid cells that normally operates around a set point of 10 mg. per 100 ml. plasma calcium concentration (Fig. 11–48). In terms of this model, it is possible to envision two alternative ways in which inappropriate secretion of PTH could take place: (1) the set point around which secretion is controlled is altered; or (2) secretion is autonomous, i.e., there is no longer effective feedback control (Fig. 11–48). From the experimental point of view, these two possibilities are readily distinguishable by examining the effect of calcium infusion upon PTH secretion. In the normal individual, calcium infusion leads to a suppression of PTH secretion. In an individual with an altered set point, calcium infusion should also cause suppression, only the plasma calcium concentration would have to be higher than normal. In an individual in whom autonomous secretion were occurring, calcium infusion should not cause suppression.

In the past, the general assumption was that most patients with primary hyperparathyroidism fell into the class of autonomous secretors. The use of the radioimmunoassay for PTH has revealed, however, that, contrary to expectation, nearly all patients with primary hyperparathyroidism show a suppression of plasma PTH concentration (particularly the 9000-M.W. species) during, and immediately following, calcium infusion. Parenthetically, it is of interest that patients with medullary carcinoma and CT hypersecretion exhibit increased plasma CT concentrations after calcium infusion. Hence both types of endocrine tumor usually respond to the natural control variable with a change in secretion rate. Aside from their theoretical interest, these findings are of practical import, because suppression of PTH secretion by calcium infusion cannot be used to distinguish patients with primary hyperparathyroidism from normals.

The most common presenting complaints in patients with primary hyperparathyroidism are related to the genitourinary tract (Table 11–15). Of particular importance is the occurrence of renal

PTG

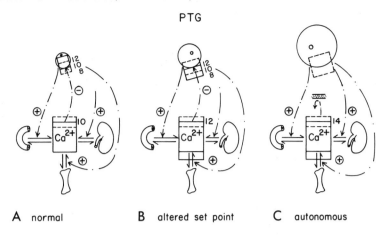

Figure 11–48. The nature of the possible alteration in feedback relationship in primary hyperparathyroidism. *A,* Normal. Calciostat in the parathyroid gland (PTG) operates around a set point of 10 mg. per 100 ml. *B,* Set point altered. The gland still responds to changes in plasma calcium concentration with changes in secretion rate, but the set point is now 12 mg. per 100 ml. *C,* Autonomous secretion. Calciostat no longer responds to changes in plasma calcium concentration.

A normal   **B** altered set point   **C** autonomous

calculi. The formation of these calculi is usually attributed to calcium and phosphate precipitation in the urine, i.e., the product of the concentrations of these two ions exceeds their solubility product. In this view, the formation of calculi is principally, if not entirely, determined by extracellular events. There are a number of observations, however, which speak against this view. Firstly, there is no simple relationship between stone formation and $Ca^{2+} \times HPO_4^{2-}$ product. Secondly, hypercalciuria and hyperphosphaturia may often be greater in hypoparathyroid patients treated with enough vitamin D to increase their plasma calcium concentration to normal than in patients with primary hyperparathyroidism, yet stone formation is not seen in the former but is observed in the latter. Thirdly, in patients with idiopathic hypercalciuria, phosphate therapy is highly effective in preventing stone formation, but even though urinary calcium excretion declines, the calcium × phosphate product does not change (Figs. 11–49 and 11–50). Fourthly, studies of the development of renal stones in hyperparathyroid experimental animals have shown that the earliest renal changes occur within the cells of the distal portion of the proximal nephron. In these cells, the mitochondria swelled, following which calcium deposits within the apical portion of the cells were observed. Many of these deposits were within mitochondria, but the cells also contained vacuoles within which needle-like mineral crystals were evident. The cells became progressively more densely calcified, and eventually the luminal portion sloughed off into the tubular lumen, leaving behind only a thin portion of cytoplasm, the nucleus and some other cell organelles along the basement membrane, which eventually regenerated to form a normal tubular cell.

These events argue that the initial calcific deposits in the kidney form within cells and not in the tubular fluid, and that when they have been extruded into the tubular lumen they act as sites for the progressive growth of calculi. In this view, the effects of PTH on cellular mineral exchange and cellular calcium accumulation are major determinants of the eventual formation of renal calculi.

Symptomatology

Hyperparathyroidism is a chronic disease of variable symptomatology which exhibits exacerbations and remissions. The history and symptoms can be so characteristic as to lead readily to the diagnosis, or the picture can be so perplexing as to suggest disorders ranging from psychoneurosis and psychosis to arthritis. As measured by radioisotope or microradiographic techniques, 60 to 65 per cent of patients with primary hyperparathyroidism have osseous involvement, but bone involvement that is detectable by x-ray film or bone biopsy is present in only about 30 per cent of the cases. Recognizable renal signs or symptoms are present in about 80 per cent. The two occur together in 48 per cent of the cases. Between 2 and

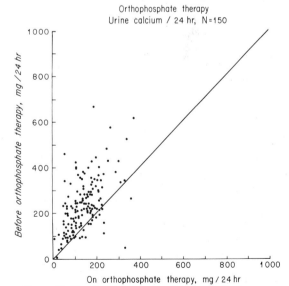

Figure 11–49. A plot of urinary calcium excretion in a group of patients with idiopathic hypercalciuria before and after oral phosphate therapy. The solid line represents the idealized situation in which phosphate therapy would have no effect upon calcium excretion. The appearance of nearly all the dots above the line indicates that phosphate therapy reduced calcium excretion in most subjects. [From Smith, L. H., Thomas, W. C., Jr., et al., In *Calcium Urolithiasis,* A Symposium, 1973 (in press). Kindly supplied by Dr. L. H. Smith.]

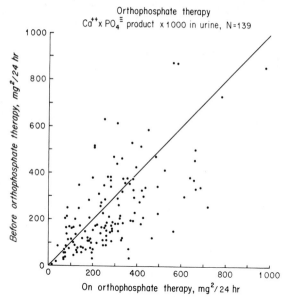

Orthophosphate therapy
$Ca^{++} \times PO_4^{\equiv}$ product $\times 1000$ in urine, N=139

Figure 11–50. A plot of the calcium × phosphate ion concentration product in the urine of a group of patients with idiopathic hypercalciuria, illustrating that this product did not change with oral phosphate therapy. Compare with Figure 11–49. [From Smith, L. H., Thomas, W. C., Jr., et al., In *Calcium Urolithiasis,* A Symposium, 1973 (in press). Kindly supplied by Dr. L. H. Smith.]

10 per cent of the cases of primary hyperparathyroidism show no apparent renal damage and no bone involvement that can be detected by x-ray film or bone biopsy (Table 11–16).

Symptoms Associated with Renal Disease

The most characteristic symptoms are renal colic and hematuria from the renal calculi, the passing of "sand" or small renal calculi, and dull back pain. Urinary tract infection may occur with its train of symptoms.

Symptoms Associated with Bone Disease

There may be a long history of vague skeletal pains, often considered to be manifestations of some form of rheumatism. At times the pain may be severe and may be mistaken for arthritis or neu-

TABLE 11–16. PRESENTING SYMPTOMS IN PATIENTS WITH HYPERPARATHYROIDISM

	Percentage
Skeletal symptoms	8.0
Fracture	1.0
Local bone tumor	0.5
Urinary symptoms	60.0
Hypertension	1.0
Gastrointestinal symptoms	10.0
Muscular weakness or generalized fatigue	6.0
Psychiatric complaints	4.0
Discovered on routine chemical screening	3.0–8.0

ritis. Rarely, the bones of the jaw become so soft that the teeth fall out, or there is a history of repeated fractures from slight trauma. When bone deformities are present, they are accompanied by appropriate symptoms.

Symptoms Associated with Gastrointestinal Tract

The gastrointestinal manifestations of hypercalcemia are anorexia, nausea, vomiting, constipation, and vague abdominal pains. These symptoms may be a major feature in the history of the disease. The symptoms may be characteristic of a duodenal ulcer; in fact, in some series, as many as 24 per cent of patients with hyperparathyroidism have been found to have an ulcer. Conversely, in a recent survey of patients with a duodenal ulcer, 1.3 per cent were found to have hyperparathyroidism. Repeated episodes of acute upper abdominal pain radiating to the back, with nausea and vomiting, may be indicative of recurrent episodes of pancreatitis.

Symptoms Associated with Central Nervous System

Marked aberrations of mental function may be present, particularly in patients with acute and severe disease. Mental retardation and spells of unconsciousness, confusion, delusions, and hallucinations have been reported. More often, the patient complains of a number of typically psychoneurotic symptoms, with or without other signs of the illness. In general, the personality structure and adjustment of the patient determine the psychologic manifestations associated with hyperparathyroidism.

Symptoms Associated with Hypercalcemia

If the hypercalcemia is marked, the patient may complain of generalized muscular weakness, anorexia, lethargy, dryness of the nose, difficulty in swallowing, nausea, thirst, constipation, weight loss, fatigability, cardiac irregularities, insomnia, apathy, and severe occipital headaches. Polyuria and polydipsia are very common and may be of such magnitude as to suggest diabetes insipidus or diabetes mellitus. In the absence of more specific symptoms, the disease may be extremely difficult to diagnose.

Signs

The signs of hyperparathyroidism can be divided into those that result from the renal disease, those that result from the bone disease, and those that are associated with hypercalcemia.

Signs Associated with Renal Disease

The signs relating to the urinary tract consist of those that result from hypercalciuria and hyperphosphaturia, the formation of kidney stones and of calcium deposits in the kidney tubules. The presence of kidney stones in hyperparathyroidism can be detected by x-ray, since the stones are largely either calcium oxalate or calcium phosphate, both of which produce an opaque shadow. The chemical composition of renal calculi often can be determined from the x-ray appearance of the stones *in vivo*. Calcium phosphate stones may form "staghorns," while those of calcium oxalate do not. Calcium oxalate stones have a crystalline structure, with radiations from a central point; calcium phosphate stones grow in concentric layers.

The deposition of calcium in the collecting tubules of the kidney produces nephrocalcinosis, which is a serious complication. Patients who have nephrocalcinosis usually have nephrolithiasis as well. Nephrocalcinosis may lead to serious impairment of renal function, manifested by copious excretion of dilute urine and, in the later stages, by uremia, edema, and hypertension. Anemia may be present in patients with hyperparathyroidism complicated by marked renal damage. A most serious aftermath of the renal involvement is hypertension, which may persist after correction of the underlying disorder, even in those patients with little apparent permanent renal damage.

Signs Associated with Bone Disease

The bone disease that occurs as a manifestation of hyperparathyroidism has three main features: generalized decalcification, bone cysts, and the so-called "brown tumors."

Radiographic evidence of generalized decalcification includes a loss of density in all bones, the absence of the lamina dura surrounding the teeth (Fig. 11–46, C), the resorption of subperiosteal bone in the metacarpals and phalanges of the fingers (Fig. 11–51), and the characteristic, even, groundglass or moth-eaten appearance of the skull (Fig. 11–52). The most characteristic and helpful sign is subperiosteal bone resorption (Fig. 11–53), which often appears first on the radial side of the middle phalanges. In some cases, the only finding is generalized decalcification, i.e., osteoporosis. On histologic examination, osteitis fibrosa generalisata resulting from either primary or secondary hyperparathyroidism shows increased formation and increased resorption and many osteoclasts (Figs. 11–37 and 11–45). There is also an increase in the amount of osteoid, with a normal percentage of calcification front; an increased number of osteoblasts which, from their staining characteristics, appear less active than normal; and a loss of normal trabecular architecture with replacement of lamellar by woven bone, giving the ground-glass appearance often seen by radiography of the bones in the skull and maxilla. Microradiographic examination usually shows increased bone formation and increased resorption (Figs. 11–41 and 11–42), with the balance in favor of resorption.

The bone disease results in many types of deformities — bending of the long bones and deformities of the pelvis, similar to those seen in osteomalacia (which may lead to a waddling gait or to inability to walk), and of the vertebrae. The vertebral deformities are not characteristic of the bone disease in hyperparathyroidism but are found in all conditions in which there is a decreased amount of calcified bone (Table 11–9). There may be a decrease in stature or the pigeon-breast deformity, in which the neck seems to disappear into the thorax. The bones in this disease are more brittle than in osteomalacia, so that fracture rather than bending is the rule. Since bone cysts and brown tumors give the same appearance on radiography, it is not possible to distinguish between them. After removal of the hyperfunctioning parathyroid tissue, the bone tumors disappear and are replaced by bone, but the cysts remain as radiolucent areas.

Signs Associated with Hypercalcemia

The decreased excitability of the neuromuscular apparatus can be demonstrated by electrical reactions, since about twice as much galvanic current is required to excite a peripheral nerve in hyperparathyroidism as in the normal state. In many patients, muscular weakness of a profound degree can be detected by objective means. The increased hypotonicity of the muscles leads to unusual flexibility of the limbs. Hypercalcemia from any cause leads to a shortening of the Q-T interval on the electrocardiogram.

Hyperparathyroid patients seem to have a decrease in auditory acuity and sometimes difficulty in focusing the eyes. Calcium phosphate crystals may be deposited in the conjunctiva of the palpebral fissure; this apparently is a manifestation of hypercalcemia. Band keratitis is associated with hypercalcemia, particularly in hyperparathyroidism. Metastatic calcification rarely occurs, in contrast to the situation in hypervitaminosis D, in which it is quite common.

Laboratory Findings

The most important changes in blood chemistry are those in plasma calcium, phosphate, chloride, and immunoreactive PTH (Table 11–14). In addition, plasma alkaline phosphatase activity is elevated in patients with bone disease. Persistent hypercalcemia, either detected because of signs and symptoms of the disease or found upon routine blood analysis, is the most common reason for evaluating the patient. These patients usually have an increase in total plasma calcium, but patients with hyperparathyroidism have been described in whom total plasma calcium concentration is normal but the ionized calcium concentration is high. The determination of the ionized calcium, however, employing commercially

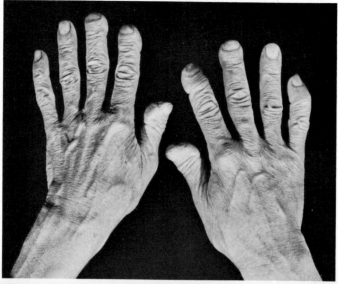

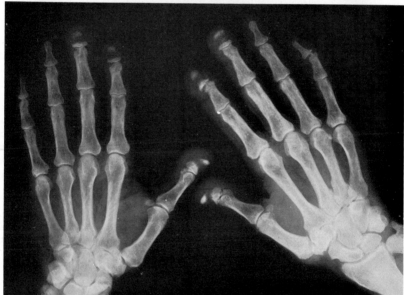

Figure 11–51. Marked periosteal bone erosion in the terminal phalanges of a patient with primary hyperparathyroidism. The erosion has been so extensive that clubbing has resulted.

available calcium ion–sensitive electrodes, remains primarily a research procedure and has not been widely employed in routine analysis. The accurate measurement of the total plasma calcium concentration and the total protein remains the most important of the procedures for the initial evaluation of patients suspected of having this disease. With the increasing availability of radioimmunoassays and other tests, however, a small but significant number of patients with normocalcemic hyperparathyroidism have been diagnosed. Measurement of the other plasma electrolytes is of less value but, in selected cases, can be most helpful. Plasma phosphate is low or in the low normal range, and plasma citrate is high or in the high normal range. The alkaline phosphatase activity is high only in patients with overt bone disease.

Plasma [Mg^{++}] is normal or low but has not been measured in a large number of these patients. The plasma chloride is usually above 102 mEq. per liter in patients with hyperparathyroidism and below this value in other forms of hypercalcemia. The plasma bicarbonate follows the converse pattern. This finding may be a useful diagnostic aid. All the findings may be altered if significant renal damage develops, accompanied by a rise in BUN.

Bone turnover is nearly always increased if studied by means of isotope (Ca^{47} or Ca^{45}) kinetics, and bone resorption rates are increased if measured by microradiography (Fig. 11–41) or by quantitative histology (Fig. 11–45).

The urinary excretion of calcium is normal in 20 to 30 per cent of cases and high in the remainder, but it is inappropriately low for the concentration

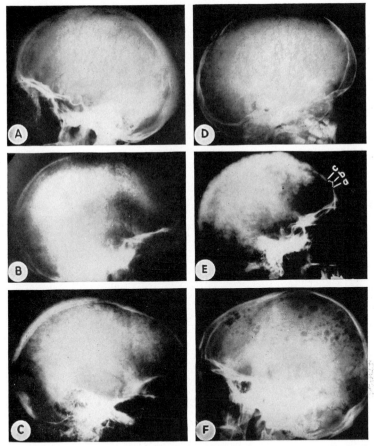

Figure 11–52. X-ray films to contrast the appearance of different types of skulls. Normal skull (*A*); thin, moth-eaten skull of osteitis fibrosa generalisata (*B*); thick, moth-eaten skull of osteitis fibrosa generalisata (*C*); thin, well-calcified skull of osteogenesis imperfecta (*D*); overgrown, fuzzy skull of Paget's disease (*E*); and skull of multiple myeloma peppered with sharply punched-out areas (*F*). Note in the skull of Paget's disease (*E*) the transition from normal bone to Paget's disease: *a,* end of normal bone; *b,* zone of increased bone destruction; and *c,* beginning of overgrowth of bone. (From Albright, F., and Reifenstein, E. C.: *The Parathyroid Glands and Metabolic Bone Disease.* Baltimore, Williams & Wilkins, 1948.)

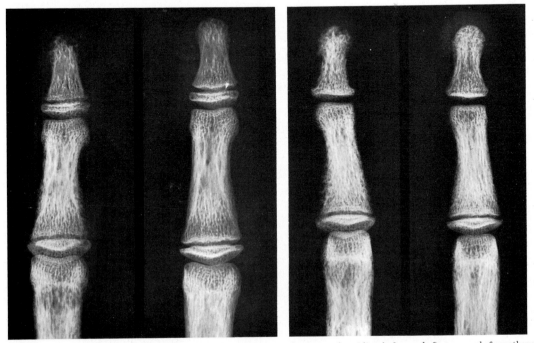

Figure 11–53. Radiographs of distal phalanges of boys with primary hyperparathyroidism before and after removal of parathyroid adenoma (left) and with hyperparathyroidism secondary to azotemic osteodystrophy (right) compared before and during treatment with vitamin D. Note similarity of lesions before treatment in both instances and similarity in healing after treatment. Healing is not complete in either case. (Figure produced by the Department of Medical Illustration, Manchester Royal Infirmary, and kindly supplied by Dr. S. W. Stanbury.)

of plasma calcium (Fig. 11–18). The hypercalciuria may fall when the patient is placed upon a low-calcium diet. The percentage of the filtered phosphate which is reabsorbed (TRP) is usually less than normal but is quite variable. The excretion of hydroxyproline is increased in patients with overt bone disease, and increased urinary hydroxyproline has been reported in patients "without bone disease." Potassium excretion may also be increased. The ability to both concentrate and acidify the urine is usually impaired in patients with hyperparathyroidism. The loss of concentrating ability is commonly seen in patients with any form of hypercalcemia, but the decreased ability to form an acid urine is more likely a direct effect of the multiple actions of the hormone upon the kidney tubule. Aminoaciduria is quite common and is also seen in vitamin D deficiency, in which it may also be due to the associated secondary hyperparathyroidism.

Restriction of dietary phosphate has been proposed as a diagnostic test on the grounds that a high phosphate intake can reverse the classical chemical abnormalities of hypercalcemia and hypophosphatemia (Fig. 11–54). Dietary phosphate restriction, however, has not led to an increase in plasma calcium in most patients with proven hyperparathyroidism, but in some instances there is a definite rise in plasma calcium which may be most helpful. The test is particularly useful in patients with some degree of renal failure.

The response to intravenous calcium infusion was proposed as a diagnostic aid on the basis that the infusion of calcium should lead to a fall in hormone secretion rate and thence to a decrease in urinary phosphate excretion, which can be most accurately measured by changes in net renal tubular reabsorption of phosphate. Further evidence indicates, however, that calcium mobilizes phosphate from cells and leads to renal phosphate retention independent of effects upon PTH secretion. The test will not distinguish patients with hyperparathyroidism from patients with other forms of hypercalcemia. Both false-negative and false-positive responses are observed. The test is not widely used.

The study of the kinetics of calcium turnover with the tracers Ca^{47}, Ca^{45}, or Sr indicates that nearly all patients with hyperparathyroidism have high turnover values. This is not always so, however, and the interpretation of these kinetic studies, which are time consuming and have not proved of great diagnostic value, is open to some uncertainty (p. 715).

The hypercalcemia of vitamin D excess, sarcoidosis, and hypercalcemia associated with invasive malignant lesions usually responds to adrenal corticoid therapy with a relatively prompt fall in plasma calcium. In contrast, the administration of corticoids to patients with hyperparathyroidism usually does not alter plasma calcium levels, although this is not invariably the case. This test (p. 742) has proved a useful diagnostic aid; however, its use is attended by some danger, unless the patient is allowed several weeks to recover from the suppression of adrenal function before being subjected to parathyroid exploration. If the operation is to be carried out shortly after this test, the patient should be given adrenal steroids before, during, and after surgery in order to avoid the risk of adrenocortical insufficiency.

Hyperparathyroidism may be distinguished from other forms of hypercalcemia by means of the parathyroid hormone infusion test. This test is based upon the fact that parathyroid hormone leads to a significant increase in urinary phosphate excretion in most patients, but hormone infusion in patients with hyperparathyroidism leads to no change. The test is reliable only when creatinine and phosphate clearances are measured before and during hormone infusion. The test has proved to be the most specific of all those designed to assess renal phosphate handling and is particularly useful in distinguishing cases of minimal hyperparathyroidism with predominantly renal signs and symptoms from other causes of renal calculi and hypercalciuria. The test should be even more reliable if purified hormone rather than crude extract were to become available, thereby minimizing the renal hemodynamic effects of the extract. The infusion of hormone into hyperparathyroid subjects leads to only a minimal change in TRP (2 to 6 per cent) but to a significant decrease (10 to 30 per cent) in patients with other forms of hypercalcemia.

Special Laboratory Tests

Radioimmunoassay

The use of radioimmunoassay has proved of immense value in the diagnosis of this disease (Fig. 11-15). Antibodies prepared against the porcine hormone appear to discriminate better between normals and patients with hyperparathyroidism than do antibodies against the bovine hormone. There is as yet no radioimmunoassay that employs the human hormone as standard. If the plasma PTH concentration is related to the plasma calcium concentration, however, then the assay gives, with the appropriate antibody, nearly complete discrimination between normals and patients with primary hyperparathyroidism (Fig. 11-15).

The value of immunoreactive PTH (IPTH) is a function of age, being highest in the year-old infant, declining between 4 and 14 years, and then increasing to adult values (Fig. 11-55). Over this same time, plasma phosphate falls dramatically in the first 6 years of life, remains relatively constant for the next 4 to 5 years, then falls again over the next 6 to 8 years to its adult value (Fig. 11-55). Plasma total calcium concentration follows a similar pattern, but the changes are less marked than those of phosphate concentration. There is no correlation between age-related changes in plasma total calcium concentration and PTH concentration (Fig. 11–55), but if ionized concentration is measured, there is a negative correlation with

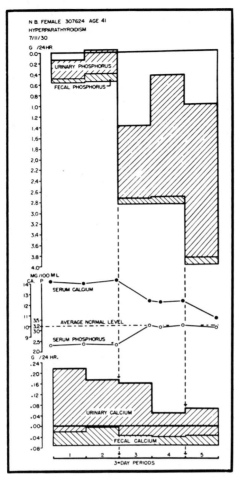

Figure 11–54. The effect of a high intake of phosphate on the metabolic manifestations of hyperparathyroidism. The phosphate balance data are given at the top, the serum calcium and inorganic phosphate values in the middle, and the calcium balance data at the bottom of the chart. The study is charted in three-day periods. During periods 1 and 2, the phosphate intake was 0.55 g. per 24 hours; during periods 3 and 4, it was 2.84 g. per 24 hours; and during period 5, it was 3.97 g. per 24 hours. Throughout the study, the calcium intake was 0.073 g. per 24 hours. The metabolic balance data are charted according to the method described by Reifenstein, Albright, and Wells: intake is represented by the distance from the zero or baseline to the bottom line, the fecal values are plotted from the bottom line upward, and the urinary values are plotted from the top of the fecal values upward. When the sum of the urinary and fecal excretions rises above the baseline, the patient is in a positive balance (white area below the baseline).

Note that during the first 6 days of the study (periods 1 and 2), the patient on the low-phosphate and low-calcium intake showed the characteristic metabolic features of hyperparathyroidism: hyperphosphaturia, hypophosphatemia, hypercalcemia, and hypercalciuria. During the last 9 days of the study (periods 3, 4, and 5), when the phosphate intake was increased to high levels while the calcium intake remained low, the urinary phosphate excretion increased tremendously, but a positive phosphate balance was achieved, the serum inorganic phosphate level rose to normal, the serum total calcium level fell to normal, and the urinary calcium excretion fell to normal. The fecal calcium excretion also fell during the high phosphate intake. At the end of the experiment, the only metabolic abnormality that remained to indicate the underlying parathyroid hyperfunction was hyperphosphaturia. A reciprocal relationship between the calcium ion activity and the phosphate ion activity in the plasma at a high level of parathyroid hormone activity is clearly demonstrated. The hyperparathyroidism was proved subsequent to the study, by the removal of a parathyroid adenoma. The parathyroid hyperfunction in this patient was associated with extensive bone involvement. Attention is called to the fact that a high phosphate intake is not recommended as therapy in hyperparathyroidism because of two dangers, the induction of metastatic calcification and the production of calcium phosphate renal calculi. (Modified from Albright, F., and Reifenstein, E. C.: *The Parathyroid Glands and Metabolic Bone Disease.* Baltimore, Williams and Wilkins Co., 1948.)

PTH concentraion; i.e., when PTH is highest, ionized calcium is lowest. In contrast to the situation in children, there is a highly significant correlation between total calcium concentration and PTH in the adult (Fig. 11–15).

Most of these changes occur during the growth period, during which the incidence of primary hyperparathyroidism is very low. Less than 1 per cent of all cases of primary hyperparathyroidism

occur in patients under the age of 18 years. As emphasized in Figure 11-15, in adults it is necessary to record the PTH value in relation to the plasma calcium concentration in order to discriminate between normal individuals and patients with primary hyperparathyroidism.

Radioimmunoassay may also assist in the preoperative location of the site of the suspected parathyroid adenoma and perhaps even in the

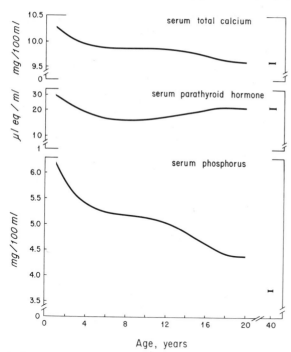

Figure 11–55. The change in total serum calcium, phosphate, and PTH with age in normal human subjects (From Arnaud, S., Goldsmith, R. S., et al.: *Pediat. Res.* 7:485, 1973.)

marily research techniques and have not proved simple and reliable enough for routine use.

The best present technique employs a calcium-sensitive electrode (Orion Corporation). By this technique, plasma is collected anaerobically under vacuum in a heparinized tube and the cells separated from the plasma by centrifugation. Aliquots of the plasma are passed through a flow-through cell in which the electrode resides. The normal values are 4.3 ± 0.4 mg. per 100 ml. Unfortunately, the electrode is sensitive to changes in magnesium concentration and is difficult to standardize. Nonetheless, under optimal conditions, it has been successfully employed to demonstrate an increase in plasma ionized calcium in some patients with so-called normocalcemic hyperparathyroidism, i.e., patients with primary hyperparathyroidism but normal total plasma calcium concentrations.

Therapeutic Response to Vitamin D_3 or 25(OH)D_3

Although not yet standardized as a test, one of the simplest and potentially most useful presumptive tests for hyperparathyroidism may be the response of patients to the administration of vitamin D_3 or 25(OH)D_3. When patients with primary hyperparathyroidism are given a single 5 mg. dose of vitamin D_3 (Fig. 11-56), the plasma calcium concentration increases over the next several days. In contrast, there is no such rise in normal controls (Fig. 11-56). A similar response is observed when 25(OH)D_3 is given to patients with primary hyperparathyroidism. Unfortunately, this response cannot be considered of diagnostic value until more data become available, except in the rare instance of a patient with primary hyperparathyroidism manifesting the signs and symptoms of osteomalacia with a normal plasma calcium concentration.

The Corticosteroid Therapeutic Test

The corticosteroid therapeutic test is a simple procedure based upon the observation that the

preoperative differentiation of hyperplasia from adenoma. A venous catheter is inserted into the femoral vein and then passed, under fluoroscopic observation, into the innominate and jugular veins, where blood samples are taken at various levels on both sides of the neck. These samples are then subjected to radioimmunoassay for PTH. The values in the venous effluent from the parathyroid glands are generally 10 to 15 times higher than in the peripheral circulation. If there is a significant difference between the concentration of PTH in the venous samples collected from the two sides of the neck, this difference has been found to indicate the size of the adenoma with a high degree of reliability. This technique may be particularly helpful in cases of earlier unsuccessful surgery.

Unfortunately, the radioimmunoassay for PTH is not easy to set up. Because of this, it is not yet generally available, and other less direct methods for assessing the possibility of PTH hypersecretion still find an important place in the differential diagnosis of primary hyperparathyroidism.

Plasma Ionized Calcium

Although in most cases of primary hyperparathyroidism the total plasma calcium concentration is the only parameter of plasma calcium distribution measured, there are techniques for measuring the ionized fraction. Theoretically, the measurement of the plasma ionized calcium concentration should be the more meaningful and informative measurement in all cases; practically, however, the techniques for its measurement are still pri-

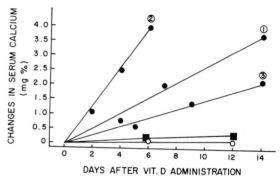

Figure 11–56. The effect of vitamin D administration upon the serum calcium concentration in three subjects with primary hyperparathyroidism (●————●), in normal subjects (○————○), and in patients with osteoporosis (■————■). (Figure supplied by Dr. Philippe Bordier.)

hypercalcemia of sarcoidosis is eliminated by therapy with adrenal cortical hormones. The test consists of oral administration of 100 to 200 mg. per day of cortisone for 5 or 6 days. The plasma calcium level is determined daily. The suppression of hypercalcemia with the restoration of the plasma calcium concentration to the normal range by the administration of this steroid is good evidence against hyperparathyroidism. However, a lack of response does not necessarily establish the diagnosis of parathyroid hyperfunction, because the steroid therapy may fail to suppress hypercalcemia in conditions other than hyperparathyroidism. Also, there are several reports which suggest that, in some patients with hyperparathyroidism, the plasma calcium level falls during the steroid therapy. Nevertheless, the corticosteroid therapeutic test has proved to be of some assistance in evaluating hypercalcemia.

The Phosphate Deprivation Test

The phosphate deprivation test is based on the observation that, in persons on a normal calcium intake, a marked restriction of the phosphate intake results in a fall in plasma phosphate level and as a consequence a rise in the plasma calcium level. Theoretically, the plasma phosphate level of patients with parathyroid hyperfunction should fall lower and the plasma calcium level should rise higher during the phosphate restriction because of the increased amount of parathyroid hormone. The individual under study eats the same diet for three days. The diet must be *low* in phosphate (under 350 mg. per day), it must be *normal* in calcium, and it must be *adequate* in calories. The effectiveness of the low-phosphate aspect of the diet can be increased by simultaneously administering aluminum salts (aluminum hydroxide gel or basic aluminum carbonate) to decrease the absorption of phosphate from the gastrointestinal tract. Blood samples for determining the fasting plasma concentrations of the total calcium, the inorganic phosphate, and the total protein are taken on the morning that the three-day diet is started and daily thereafter for four consecutive mornings.

On this regimen, a few patients with normocalcemic hyperparathyroidism will exhibit a significant increase in the concentration of calcium in their plasma. If, however, in addition to phosphate deprivation, the patients are given chlorothiazide, 1 g. twice daily for three days, the number of patients exhibiting such a rise increases. Thus this simple test is particularly useful in patients with normocalcemia and hypercalciuria but some normal subjects may have an increase in plasma calcium concentration after combined phosphate deprivation and chlorothiazide therapy.

Parathyroid Hormone Infusion Test

A procedure for evaluating parathyroid function is based upon the measurement of the tubular reabsorption of phosphate (TRP) in patients before and after the administration of parathyroid extract. The test is valid only if the BUN is below 50 mg. per 100 ml. of plasma and the plasma creatinine is less than 1.6 mg. per 100 ml. The patient is told to drink three to four glasses of milk a day for three days before the test is begun. The patient is then hospitalized, placed upon NPO after the evening meal, and told to void at 8 P.M. An infusion of 5 per cent dextrose in water is given over the next 11 hours at a rate of 90 ml. per hr. A blood sample is taken at the midpoint of the infusion; urine is collected for 13 hours from the start of the infusion and analyzed for phosphate and creatinine. TRP is calculated as follows:

$$TRP = \left[1 - \left(\frac{UP \times SC}{UC \times SP} \right) \right]$$

where UP = phosphate in 12-hour urine; UC = creatinine in 12-hour urine; SC = plasma creatine; and SP = plasma phosphate. The procedure is repeated on the second day, with the addition of 200 units of parathyroid extract in the infusate. The difference in TRP between day 1 and day 2 is an index of tubular responsiveness to parathyroid hormone. In patients with hyperparathyroidism, a difference of only 2 to 7 per cent is found, whereas in patients with hypercalcemia from other causes, the difference is 12 to 30 per cent, with a decrease on the second day.

Diagnosis

The diagnosis of the typical case of hyperparathyroidism with hypercalcemia and osteitis fibrosa cystica is relatively easy once it has been considered. Nor is it difficult to distinguish this form of bone disease from other metabolic bone diseases. The difficulty in diagnosis lies in two general areas: consideration of the diagnosis, and differentiation of mild cases from other causes of renal calculi or hypercalcemia. Occasionally, it is also difficult to distinguish primary hyperparathyroidism with renal failure from secondary hyperparathyroidism with primary renal disease.

Consideration of the Diagnosis

The manifestations of hyperparathyroidism are so protean that the disorder should be considered in any differential diagnosis of conditions involving a number of systems. The presenting symptoms in 751 proven cases are shown in Table 11-16. By far the largest group have symptoms referable to either the skeleton or the kidneys or, very commonly, to both. A significant percentage of patients manifest gastrointestinal symptoms of either ulcer or recurrent pancreatitis. Hyperparathyroidism has been recognized in an increasing number of patients because they complained of muscular weakness, fatigue, or vague psychiatric disorders or simply by chance estimation of their plasma calcium concentration. This emphasizes the probability of the existence of many unrecognized cases of the disease. The data in Table 11-16 give a historical view of our present experience, but they do not emphasize the fact that many more mild cases are being recognized now than was formerly the case.

Laboratory Investigation of Suspected Case

The more care and precision with which serum calcium determinations are done, the higher the number of mild cases of this disease that will be discovered. In addition to methodology, the time of collection and the handling of the blood sample are important. The following sources of error have been recognized: (1) an elevation due to venous stasis at the time of collection, which can be corrected by simultaneous measurement of blood specific gravity (for every increase of 1 unit in the third decimal place of the plasma specific gravity determined by the copper sulfate method, 0.25 g. per 100 ml. of calcium should be subtracted from the observed value); (2) exposure of the blood sample to cork stoppers; (3) prolonged storage of blood without separation of plasma from cells, leading to a low value; and (4) a lowering produced by high-phosphate diet. The plasma protein concentration should also be measured and the plasma calcium concentration corrected for any change. A change of 1.0 g. per 100 ml. of protein (albumin) corresponds to a parallel change in total calcium concentration of 0.8 mg. per 100 ml.

Plasma calcium determinations should be done routinely upon all patients with calcium-containing renal calculi, nephrocalcinosis, pancreatitis, and duodenal and gastric ulcers and upon any patients with generalized weakness or vague bone pains. The detection of a small but increasing number of unsuspected cases by means of a routine calcium determination at the time of hospital admission or office visit raises the important philosophic problem of when and how often routine chemical determinations are warranted. Recent developments in the automation of routine chemical procedures and in data processing should shortly allow for the routine determination of plasma calcium and other chemical elements in the blood of all patients seeking medical advice.

In a suspected case of hyperparathyroidism, at least three consecutive plasma calcium values should be obtained. At the same time, plasma protein should be determined to rule out the possibility that the rise in plasma calcium is due to increased protein. Paper electrophoresis of the plasma proteins is most helpful in differentiating cases of multiple myeloma and sarcoidosis from hyperparathyroidism. Alkaline phosphatase, plasma pH, bicarbonate, Cl^-, BUN, and pCO_2 should be done routinely. Routine x-ray examination should be made of kidneys, ureter, and bladder, as well as hands, teeth, and skull. Further radiograms are indicated for patients with elevated alkaline phosphatase, any patients suspected of having malignant lesions, or those with

skeletal symptoms. A 24-hour urine calcium test, with the patient on an 850-mg. calcium diet, is useful because urinary calcium is usually elevated in hyperparathyroidism. Measurements of urinary hydroxyproline may be particularly helpful in differentiating hyperparathyroidism from idiopathic hypercalciuria, particularly if the level does not change upon calcium infusion. However, urinary hydroxyproline is not always increased in hyperparathyroidism and may be elevated in other disorders associated with hypercalcemia, e.g., thyrotoxicosis.

The use of the more specialized tests depends upon the particular diagnostic problem and will be discussed more fully later. These problems fall into four categories: the differential diagnosis of osteitis fibrosa cystica; the differential diagnosis of hypercalcemia; the differential diagnosis of cases with renal calculi, hypophosphatemia, hypercalciuria, and minimal deviations of plasma calcium level; and the problem of a coexistent disease also leading to hypercalcemia. Because of the importance of laboratory investigations in distinguishing these conditions, the chemical findings in the various disorders are summarized in Table 11-14.

Differential Diagnosis of Osteitis Fibrosa Cystica

The four causes of osteitis fibrosa cystica are primary or secondary hyperparathyroidism, severe acidosis, neoplasms producing a parathyroid-like polypeptide, and thyrotoxicosis. There is considerable doubt that acidosis per se ever causes clinically detectable osteitis, and both neoplasms producing parathyroid-like polypeptides and thyrotoxicosis lead to hypercalcemia with or without osteitis. These conditions are discussed later.

The causes and manifestations of secondary hyperparathyroidism are discussed on page 753. When primary hyperparathyroidism has led to renal failure, distinction from secondary hyperparathyroidism with primary renal disease may be difficult. The history may be of considerable help, particularly if there have been repeated episodes of renal calculi, or, conversely, a clear-cut history of chronic renal disease or acute renal disease in the past. The plasma calcium concentration is usually normal or elevated in patients with primary hyperparathyroidism, even when the BUN is moderately elevated, whereas in those with chronic renal disease, it is usually low. The situation is made more difficult because some patients with long-standing renal disease and secondary hyperparathyroidism develop parathyroid adenomas.

A number of localized bone diseases may be mistaken for osteitis fibrosa cystica but can usually be distinguished radiographically or by the lack of characteristic chemical findings.

Polyostotic Fibrous Dysplasia

A disorder which may be mistaken for hyperparathyroidism with bone disease is polyostotic fibrous dysplasia (sometimes called Albright's syndrome). This peculiar disease shows a disseminated osteitis fibrosa of both hyperostotic and hypoöstotic types, with a segmental distribution that suggests a neurologic or embryologic relationship; areas of brown cutaneous pigmentation, with a distribution suggesting some connection between them and the bone lesions; and sexual and somatic precocity in females but not in males. It can be differentiated from hyperparathyroidism because the bone lesions are not generalized. Furthermore, the bone lesions are hyperostotic as well as hypoöstotic, which is most unusual in hyperparathyroidism. The blood chemistry is normal in polyostotic fibrous dysplasia, although there may be some elevation of the plasma alkaline phosphatase level if there are extensive bone lesions. Precocity in females and areas of pigmentation, when present, aid further in the differentiation of the two syndromes. There is some evidence suggesting that the sexual precocity is caused by lesions in the walls of the third ventricle.

Neurofibromatosis

In neurofibromatosis there may be radiolucent defects at the ends of the long bones, in the skull, in the vertebrae, or at other points where nerves penetrate bone. There are areas of brownish skin pigmentation resembling those of polyostotic fibrous dysplasia in color but more regular in outline. In addition, there are neurocutaneous lesions, often in a segmental distribution. Neurofibromatosis can be differentiated from hyperparathyroidism with overt bone disease because the plasma calcium and phosphate levels are normal.

Osteitis Deformans (Paget's Disease)

Osteitis deformans is a localized disease of bone remodeling (Figs. 11-17, 11-41, and 11-45). The diagnosis is made (1) by the characteristic appearance of the lesions on x-ray film, particularly when the condition is found in the skull (see Fig. 11-52, E); (2) by the coarse trabeculation with a marked increase in density, when it is found in the long bones; and (3) by a marked tendency to overgrowth of bone. The plasma calcium level is usually normal, and alkaline phosphatase very high. The latter may increase considerably when sarcomatous transformation of the osteitis deformans has occurred. These findings are very different from those of bone disease with hyperparathyroidism. Hypercalcemia occurs only when patients with osteitis deformans are immobilized and acute osteoporosis of disuse is superimposed on the underlying bone condition. These immobilized patients also have hyperphosphatemia, and there is no difficulty in distinguishing the condition from hyperparathyroidism. The plasma calcium level or the urinary calcium excretion or both of patients with Paget's disease who are immobilized should be determined at frequent intervals in order to detect any ten-dency toward the development of hypercalcemia or any marked increase in urinary calcium excretion, because the risk of developing renal lithiasis or nephrocalcinosis is high in these patients. The chemical findings of value in the differential diagnosis of osteitis deformans and certain bone and related disorders are given in Table 11-14.

Solitary Cystic Bone Lesions

Solitary cystic bone lesions occur which, upon biopsy, are indistinguishable from those of osteitis fibrosa generalisata. These lesions are found particularly at the ends of the long bones, where not infrequently they lead to pathologic fractures. The fact that the plasma calcium, phosphate, and alkaline phosphatase levels are normal serves to indicate that such cysts are not manifestations of an underlying metabolic bone disease.

Epulis

Epulis, a lesion of the alveolar process of the jaw, usually is a fibroma or a giant-cell sarcoma. A tumor of similar appearance may occur in the jaw in hyperparathyroidism with bone disease. This latter condition always should be ruled out when an epulis is found. The lesion is differentiated from that of hyperparathyroidism by the normal plasma levels for calcium, phosphate, and alkaline phosphatase activity and by the absence of hypercalciuria.

Neoplasms with Osseous Metastasis

Radiologically, the bone lesions of metastatic malignant disorders usually can be differentiated from those of hyperparathyroidism because of the sharply demarcated areas of involvement. Plasma calcium levels may be high, with hypercalciuria and kidney stones. The plasma phosphate level usually is normal, occasionally is elevated, and infrequently is decreased. The plasma alkaline phosphatase level may be elevated. A demonstration of a primary focus in the breast, prostate, kidney (hypernephroma), bronchus, or thyroid is helpful in establishing the diagnosis. The hypercalcemia, which is the finding in metastatic malignant lesions most likely to lead to the suspicion of hyperparathyroidism, is discussed elsewhere (p. 748). The chemical findings of value in the differential diagnosis of neoplasia with osseous metastasis and certain bone and related disorders are given in Table 11–14.

Other Bone Diseases

There is another large group of conditions manifesting bone lesions which might occasionally be mistaken for primary hyperparathyroidism with bone disease. These include lymphoma, benign metastasizing hemangioma, Gaucher's disease, xanthomatosis, and chronic radium poisoning.

Differential Diagnosis of Hypercalcemia

The largest group of patients who must be distinguished from patients with hyperparathyroidism are those with hypercalcemia from causes other than osteitis fibrosa cystica. In patients with unequivocal hypercalcemia, the symptoms and signs may closely mimic those of hyperparathyroidism. Hypercalcemia may occur in all of these: hypervitaminosis D (vitamin D intoxication); idiopathic hypercalcemia of infancy; hypophosphatasia; acute adrenal insufficiency (Addison's disease); hyperthyroidism; sarcoidosis; milk-alkali syndrome; neoplasia (lung, kidney, or bladder) without osseous metastases; acute osteoporosis of disuse (following immobilization in patients with fractures, poliomyelitis, Paget's disease, or acidosis); multiple myeloma; and neoplasia with osseous metastases (spontaneously or during gonadal steroid therapy). In all of these disorders, the hypercalcemia may be associated with hypophosphatemia, so that the determination of the plasma phosphate concentration may be of no assistance in the differential diagnosis (Table 11–14). The measurement of the total protein concentration and the albumin/globulin (A/G) ratio in the plasma is useful, because hyperglobulinemia is rare in hyperparathyroidism. When it is present, it usually indicates multiple myeloma or sarcoidosis. The carbon dioxide combining power of the plasma is normal or slightly low in hyperparathyroidism but often is high in hypercalcemia from other causes.

The most useful test is the measurement of plasma immunoreactive PTH. It is high in patients with primary hyperparathyroidism but low in patients with the other conditions except the syndrome of ectopic hyperparathyroidism related to neoplasia in organs other than the parathyroids.

Hypercalciuria is the rule in all patients with hypercalcemia except for those with the milk-alkali syndrome. Radiologic investigation may aid in the differential diagnosis of the hypercalcemia in patients with malignant disease (particularly of the lung, kidney, or bladder) with or without osseous metastases; otherwise these conditions may be difficult to differentiate from hyperparathyroidism.

Hypervitaminosis D (Vitamin D Intoxication)

Patients receiving excessive amounts of vitamin D (50,000 units per day or more) may develop the syndrome of vitamin D poisoning. This is manifested by' hypercalcemia with hyperphosphatemia or even, in some cases, hypophosphatemia; impaired renal function; hyposthenuria; albuminu-

ria; polyuria and polydipsia; anorexia; lethargy; and constipation. These result from enhanced bone resorption, increased urinary phosphate excretion, and enhanced calcium and phosphate absorption from the intestine. If the intoxication with vitamin D is severe, dehydration and acute failure of renal function may occur, leading to a rapidly rising plasma phosphate, [K^+], and BUN and finally to death from the electrolyte imbalance. The chemical findings of value in the differential diagnosis of hypervitaminosis D and certain bone and related disorders are given in Table 11–14.

Vitamin D is potent and potentially harmful; it should be used with caution. It is contraindicated for conditions such as arthritis, in which no physiologic need exists.

When intoxication has been recognized, prompt therapy is indicated. These measures should include cessation of vitamin D therapy, adequate hydration, restriction of calcium and phosphate intake, and treatment with adrenal steroids to suppress hypercalcemia. Patients may require 50 to 100 mg. per day of hydrocortisol 1 to 2 weeks in order to control acute hypercalcemia.

Idiopathic hypercalcemia has been described in infants. It resembles hypervitaminosis D in many respects. This disorder is considered to result from either an excessive intake of vitamin D or a defect in the enzymatic inactivation of this vitamin. A few patients with this disorder, however, have been found to have primary hyperparathyroidism. For this reason, the measurement of immunoreactive PTH is mandatory in all patients with this syndrome.

Adrenal Cortical Insufficiency (Addison's Disease)

Adrenal cortical insufficiency may be accompanied by hypercalcemia and hypophosphatemia and thus superficially be confused with hyperparathyroidism. Such patients, however, usually have the other more characteristic symptoms and signs of adrenal cortical insufficiency. Furthermore, the hypercalcemia of patients with adrenal cortical hypofunction responds dramatically to the administration of *small* doses of adrenal cortical hormones. The chemical findings of value in the differential diagnosis of adrenal cortical insufficiency and certain bone and related disorders are given in Table 11–14.

Hyperthyroidism

Patients with hyperthyroidism frequently have hypercalciuria and hyperphosphaturia, usually associated with normocalcemia. In acute or severe cases, however, there may be an increased rate of bone turnover and hypercalcemia, manifestations which suggest the diagnosis of hyperparathyroidism. The sequence of events in hyperthyroidism may be as follows: (1) an increased resorption of bone from the action of the excessive amount of thyroid hormone; (2) hypercalcemia from the accelerated bone resorption; (3) a decreased production of PTH as a result of the hypercalcemia; (4) a compensatory decrease in bone resorption because of the decreased amount of parathyroid hormone; (5) a compensatory decrease in the tubular reabsorption of calcium because of the decreased amount of parathyroid hormone; and (6) hypercalciuria from the decreased tubular reabsorption of calcium. These compensatory alterations usually are adequate to maintain the plasma calcium concentration in the physiologic range. In severe hyperthyroidism, however, the excessive bone resorption may lead to hypercalcemia in spite of the compensatory underproduction of PTH.

Recognizable osteitis fibrosa generalisata rarely occurs in patients with hyperthyroidism. Other patients with a marked degree of thyroid hyperfunction have disturbances in protein metabolism, a negative nitrogen balance, and osteoporosis. Some patients also have disorders of magnesium metabolism, but the relationship of these to the bone disease is not known. The presence of the other more characteristic manifestations of hyperthyroidism usually aids in differentiating this condition from hyperparathyroidism. The chemical findings of value in the differential diagnosis of hyperthyroidism and certain bone and related disorders are given in Table 11–14.

Sarcoidosis

In sarcoidosis one may find bone changes, hypercalcemia, hypercalciuria, a high plasma alkaline phosphatase level, and kidney stones. The plasma phosphate concentration may be normal or low. The presence of hyperproteinemia and hyperglobulinemia as well as the characteristic dermal and pulmonary changes aids in establishing the diagnosis. The bone lesions of sarcoidosis are found primarily in the hands and feet, and usually there is no generalized decalcification. The corticosteroid therapeutic test (p. 742) may be helpful, because the administration of adrenal cortical steroids eliminates the hypercalcemia of sarcoidosis but usually does not affect that of hyperparathyroidism. The chemical findings of value in the differential diagnosis of sarcoidosis and certain bone and related disorders are given in Table 11–14.

Milk-Alkali Syndrome

Another interesting syndrome results from prolonged and excessive intake of milk and alkali. Patients with this syndrome exhibit the following: hypercalcemia without hypercalciuria; a normal or high plasma phosphate level; impaired renal function with azotemia, decreased excretion of phenolsulfonphthalein, and a fixed specific gravity of the urine; conjunctival calcium deposits and band keratitis; mild alkalosis; and a lowering of the plasma calcium level with clinical improvement when the patient is placed on a low-calcium diet.

These patients can be distinguished from those with hyperparathyroidism by the lack of hypercalciuria and by the response, usually rapid, to a low-calcium diet. Furthermore, the rate of bone turnover is normal in contrast to the increased rate in patients with hyperparathyroidism. The chemical findings of value in the differential diagnosis of the milk-alkali syndrome and certain bone and related disorders are given in Table 11–14. Excessive intake of milk and alkali may be seen in patients with primary hyperparathyroidism because of the incidence of peptic ulcer in this latter disease. As a consequence, hyperparathyroidism and this syndrome may coexist.

Neoplasia without Osseous Metastasis (Pseudohyperparathyroidism)

In recent years there has developed an increasing awareness of a condition which closely mimics the chemical abnormalities of hyperparathyroidism. This condition is the development of hypercalcemia in patients with malignant tumors of various organs (particularly the kidney, bladder, and lung) in the absence of obvious osseous metastases.

The syndrome may result from the secretion of a PTH-like peptide from the malignant tumor. This peptide appears to be structurally larger than the normal circulating peptides and can be distinguished from them by its different reaction to appropriate antisera. In general, for any degree of hypercalcemia found in the plasma of patients with pseudohyperparathyroidism, the measured IPTH is lower than that in patients having the same degree of hypercalcemia but suffering from primary hyperparathyroidism.

A similar syndrome may appear in patients in whom no detectable circulating immunoreactive PTH is present, In these patients, the evidence seems quite clear that the tumor is producing a substance other than PTH. A prime candidate is prostaglandin E_2. This compound has been shown to stimulate bone resorption and bone adenyl cyclase, and to be produced in large quantities by mouse fibrosarcomas. In addition, animals with these tumors suffer from hypercalcemia, and evidence an increase in bone resorption.

It is particularly important to recognize the syndrome of pseudohyperparathyroidism, because its chemical manifestations (other than plasma IPTH) are identical to those of the primary disease. In general, this disease is more common in elderly patients. Careful clinical and radiologic studies are necessary in all older patients with suspected hyperparathyroidism to rule out the presence of tumors in other sites. The use of the radioimmunoassay is of particular value.

Acute Osteoporosis of Disuse

The one important exception to the lack of change in the plasma calcium and phosphate levels in osteoporosis (see p. 768) occurs in the rapidly induced osteoporosis of disuse. When rapid bone formation has been going on and it is suddenly stopped by immobilization, the plasma calcium level may become elevated. This situation is found in rapidly growing children and active adults who experience sudden paralysis (as with poliomyelitis), and in individuals with excessive bone repair compensatory to increased bone destruction from a localized condition such as Paget's disease. Thus immobilization may aggravate the condition of patients with hypercalcemia or systemic osseous disease. Since hyperphosphatemia also occurs in acute osteoporosis of disuse, usually there is no difficulty in distinguishing this condition from hyperparathyroidism. The calcium intake should be restricted in immobilized patients, and the plasma calcium level or the urinary calcium excretion should be determined at frequent intervals in order to detect any tendency toward the development of hypercalcemia. Evidence that bone formation is decreased in acute osteoporosis of disuse is obtained from microradiography (Fig. 11–41) and from the fact that there is a fall in the elevated plasma alkaline phosphatase activity of adults who have had excessive bone formation compensatory to bone resorption prior to the immobilization. The hypercalcemia of acute osteoporosis of disuse responds rapidly to treatment with fluids (intravenously), a low-calcium high-phosphate diet, and mobilization. It is aggravated by the administration of calcium and vitamin D. The chemical findings of value in the differential diagnosis of acute osteoporosis of disuse and certain bone and related disorders are given in Table 11–14.

Osteoporosis as well as osteitis fibrosa cystica can occur in patients with hyperparathyroidism. Usually, this can be readily differentiated from other causes of osteoporosis by the chemical findings. However, idiopathic osteoporosis may coexist with other conditions causing hypercalcemia. In patients with hyperparathyroidism who sustain a fracture and are immobilized, the hypercalcemia may be mistaken for that arising from acute osteoporosis of disuse.

Multiple Myeloma

Although hypercalcemia and hypercalciuria are present in about 40 per cent of the cases of multiple myeloma, the phosphate concentration in the plasma usually is normal or high. Nephrolithiasis occurs in about 10 per cent of the patients. A very small number of patients, however, have been reported with plasma phosphate levels as low as those found in hyperparathyroidism. The plasma alkaline phosphatase level is rarely elevated in multiple myeloma, which is an important point in differentiating this disorder from hyperparathyroidism (Table 11–14). Although in most cases of multiple myeloma the osseous involvement is visible radiographically as sharply demarcated lytic lesions (Fig. 11–52, F), in a few cases it appears as a diffuse infiltration (particularly of the spine) that is difficult to distinguish from the decreased density observed in osteitis fibrosa generalisata. The presence of an increased amount of circulating globulin with a characteristic M spike, the presence of Bence Jones protein in the urine, and the finding of plasma cells in the bone marrow are of considerable aid in the diagnosis of multiple myeloma and in the differentiation of this condition from hyperparathyroidism. The chemical findings of value in the differential diagnosis of multiple myeloma and certain bone and related disorders are given in Table 11–14.

Neoplasia with Osseous Metastasis

The characteristic chemical findings in patients with osseous metastases from a primary neoplasm in the breast, prostate, kidney, bronchus, or thyroid are these: hypercalciuria; kidney stones; a plasma phosphate level that is usually normal but occasionally elevated and very infrequently decreased; a plasma alkaline phosphatase level that may be elevated; and a plasma calcium level that is usually normal. In certain patients with these tumors, a rapidly developing hypercalcemia occurs. In some patients with malignant mammary or prostatic lesions, a similar rapidly progressing hypercalcemia occurs, a complication of gonadal hormone therapy during the first weeks of treatment, about as frequently as spontaneous hypercalcemia (with or without steroid medication) takes place in the untreated cases. Hypercalcemia should be suspected in such a case when the patient suddenly develops anorexia, nausea, vomiting, dryness of the nose and throat, or all these symptoms. In the later stages, renal damage results from the prolonged hypercalcemia and hypercalciuria, and there may be an associated impairment of the calcium excretory mechanism with further aggravation of the hypercalcemia. When hypercalcemia is present, the radiologic appearance of the metastatic bone lesions usually helps in differentiating this condition from hyperparathyroidism (Table 11–14).

Differential Diagnosis of Renal Calculi and Nephrocalcinosis

The most common presenting symptoms in cases of hyperparathyroidism are related to the urinary tract. Conversely, in large series of patients with renal calculi, 5 to 10 per cent have been found to have hyperparathyroidism; and in those with nephrocalcinosis, the lesion has been associated with hyperparathyroidism in 30 to 40 per cent of cases.

Diffuse nephrocalcinosis is found in a variety of conditions. Besides hyperparathyroidism, the most common causes are renal tubular acidosis (p. 760) and pyelonephritis. Nephrocalcinosis due to these causes is associated with normal values of plasma calcium and usually low plasma phosphate values. Once it has been established that the stones contain calcium (either phosphate or oxalate), hyperparathyroidism must be excluded. The factors involved in the formation of such stones include hypercalciuria; anatomic defects in the urinary tract favoring stasis; dehydration; the presence in the urine of mucoprotein, polysaccharide constituents, or protein; and conditions which lead to an alkaline urine (such as urinary tract pathogens that split urea to form ammonia, and alkalosis resulting from diet, drugs, or acid depletion by vomiting). In patients with calcium calculi and no overt bone disease, hypercalciuria points toward primary hyperparathyroidism, and the finding of hypercalcemia and hypophosphatemia establishes the diagnosis.

Normocalcemic Hyperparathyroidism

Even though the use of the proper radioimmunoassay for PTH (Fig. 11–15) and of an automated technique for the measurement of plasma calcium are of major importance in distinguishing subjects with hyperparathyroidism from normal subjects, there is a group of patients in whom the plasma calcium concentration is normal upon repeated examination, yet who have signs or symptoms which raise the possibility that they do have primary hyperparathyroidism. These patients fall into two classes: those with and those without evidence of vitamin D deficiency.

In the group of subjects with normocalcemia and osteomalacia, the problem is that of defining whether the patient has a primary deficiency of vitamin D and a secondary hyperparathyroidism, or whether he or she suffers from primary hyperparathyroidism and a secondary relative deficiency of vitamin D. The distinction between the two is most easily made by the response of the patient to vitamin D therapy. In patients with primary hyperparathyroidism, the administration of therapeutic amounts of vitamin D leads to a significant increase in the plasma calcium concentration. Conversely, in subjects with primary vitamin D deficiency, vitamin D administration usually results in an initial fall in plasma calcium concentration during the first several days of therapy which is followed by a return to normal values but never to frank hypercalcemia.

The other group of normocalcemic hyperparathyroid patients usually has the signs and symptoms of recurrent renal calculi and must be distinguished from a group of patients with so-called idiopathic hypercalciuria. With the increasing sophistication of diagnostic methods, the distinction between these two groups of patients has become more difficult rather than easier, strongly suggesting that changes in parathyroid physiology are important factors in the etiology of renal calculi in all these patients.

Idiopathic Hypercalciuria and Normocalcemic Hyperparathyroidism

One of the most difficult diagnostic problems is that of differentiating between primary hyperparathyroidism and idiopathic hypercalciuria. The presenting complaints in nearly all these patients are related to the passage of calcium-containing stones. The major chemical abnormality is hypercalciuria. This term is rather imprecise, however, and means different things to different people. Nordin has suggested classifying hypercalciuria into absolute or relative. Absolute hypercalciuria is defined as a 24-hour urine calcium of 400 mg. in men or 300 mg. in women on a normal calcium intake of 1 g. It may be due to a high rate of intestinal absorption or a high rate of net bone resorption. Clearly, only in the case of resorptive hypercalciuria will the urinary calcium excretion remain high when the subject is placed on a restricted dietary intake of calcium.

A more meaningful definition is that for relative hypercalciuria, i.e., a greater than normal excretion of calcium in the urine for a given intake of dietary calcium. This type of hypercalciuria is seen in patients with hypoparathyroidism in whom the plasma calcium is elevated either by calcium infusion or vitamin D therapy. It is also observed in patients with so-called idiopathic hypercalciuria. In over 50 per cent of these patients, the intestinal absorption of both calcium and phosphate but not that of xylose is increased (Fig. 11–39), which is very suggestive of an increase in vitamin D–like or $1,25\ (OH)_2D_3$ activity in these patients.

From these observations it has been suggested that the primary defect in these patients is the hyperabsorption of calcium in the intestinal tract. If this is the case, the therapeutic objective is to reduce the dietary intake of calcium to low values and thereby decrease the urinary excretion of calcium. This form of therapy has not proved uniformly successful, however.

Perhaps the reason for this lack of success relates, in part, to the evidence that a significant number of these patients have hyperparathyroidism. For example, in one series of 19 patients with idiopathic hypercalciuria, 8 developed hypercalcemia when put on combined phosphate deprivation and chlorothiazide (Fig. 11–57). Four out of five of these patients who underwent operation were found to have parathyroid adenomas. In another study, approximately 10 per cent of 285 patients

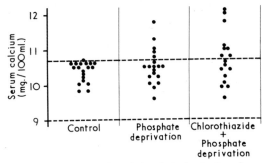

Figure 11–57. The effect of phosphate deprivation alone or with chlorothiazide therapy upon serum calcium concentration in subjects with idiopathic hypercalciuria. (From Adams, P., Chalmers, T. M., et al.: *Brit. Med. J.* 4:582, 1970.)

were found to have increased values of plasma IPTH.

These data all raise the possibility that the disease is of primary renal origin, with defective tubular reabsorption of calcium leading to a urinary calcium leak, an increase in PTH secretion, and, in turn, an increase in the renal synthesis of $1,25(OH)_2D_3$ and thereby to an increase in the intestinal absorption of calcium. If this is the sequence of events, it is then quite possible that hyperfunctioning parathyroid tissue will be found in many such patients.

Of particular note has been the success of oral phosphate therapy in the treatment of this disease. When neutral phosphate is given in daily divided doses of 1.5 to 2.5 g. per day, over 90 per cent of patients with recurrent stone formation respond successfully with cessation of stone formation; even a loss of stone mass is often seen. The major effect of phosphate therapy is to cause a decrease in urinary calcium excretion (Fig. 11–49) without changing plasma calcium concentration. The urinary excretion of phosphate increases so that the calcium × phosphate product does not change (Fig. 11–50). Plasma phosphate falls slightly, and plasma IPTH does not change consistently.

The mechanism by which phosphate acts is not known. It is known, however, that the tubular reabsorption of calcium and that of phosphate are interrelated, and it seems likely that phosphate has a direct effect upon renal cell function that is related to the increased tubular reabsorption of calcium. In this regard, it is of considerable interest that patients with the syndrome of phosphorus depletion have a hypophosphaturia and hypophosphatemia associated with hypercalciuria, clearly indicating that phosphate level affects renal calcium reabsorption, although in these cases it is possible that the hypercalciuria is associated with a physiologic hypoparathyroidism.

Associated Diseases

In a few patients, hyperparathyroidism has been found to coexist with other conditions which lead to hypercalcemia: sarcoidosis, malignant disorders, and hyperthyroidism. The parathyroid hyperfunction has usually been uncovered when the usual therapeutic measures in these diseases have failed to relieve the hypercalcemia.

Polyendocrine Adenomatosis.   Some patients with hyperparathyroidism have pre-existing manifestations of hyperactivity of some other endocrine organ. Particularly common is the so-called Zollinger-Ellison syndrome, with islet-cell tumors of the pancreas and intractable duodenal ulcers. These patients may have one or more of the following: hyperparathyroidism due to primary chief-cell hyperplasia (or multiple adenomatosis); rarely, Cushing's syndrome due to adenomas of the adrenal cortex; functioning or nonfunctioning tumors of the anterior pituitary, particularly those leading to acromegaly; gastric polyposis; and lipomas. The disease is inherited as an autosomal dominant

with a high degree of penetrance. The expression of the disease in different members of the same kindred varies considerably. Every patient with the Zollinger-Ellison syndrome or with intractable duodenal ulcer should be thoroughly investigated for possible parathyroid hyperfunction. The pathogenesis of the ulcer in these cases is strongly correlated with the presence of α cell tumor of the pancreatic islets which produces gastrin. The ulcer may be due to hyperparathyroidism, islet-cell tumor producing a gastrin-like substance, an independent expression of the underlying genetic abnormality, and adrenal cortical hyperfunction. The recognition of this small group of patients with hyperparathyroidism is of practical importance in their operative management, and every patient with hyperparathyroidism should be considered to have this condition until proven otherwise.

Hyperparathyroidism in Children

Primary hyperparathyroidism before puberty is extremely rare, but 25 cases in children below the age of 10 years have been reported. In one patient, the disease had the radiologic appearance of rickets. Moreover, at least 3 patients with idiopathic hypercalcemia of infancy have been reported, in whom high plasma IPTH was measured and in whom hyperplastic parathyroid tissue was found at operation.

Hyperparathyroidism and Pregnancy

Maternal hyperparathyroidism occurs in a small percentage of pregnancies. It has been discovered in the mother by finding hypocalcemia in the newborn. The degree of hypercalcemia is usually slight to moderate. Bone disease may be present but usually is not. The concentration of calcium in the amniotic fluid and in the fetal plasma is higher than normal, but the latter falls shortly after birth, resulting in many instances in tetany. The plasma alkaline phosphatase activity of the newborn is elevated, but there is no evidence of bone disease. The mother's milk contains less calcium than normal. The incidence of stillbirth and neonatal death appears to be increased. The evidence suggests that the maternal hormone does not cross the placental barrier, but that maternal hypercalcemia and hypophosphatemia lead to hypoplasia of the fetal parathyroid glands.

Calcium Intoxication

A few patients with severe hyperparathyroidism have acute and rapidly progressive symptoms, including weakness, anorexia, nausea, vomiting, thirst, polyuria, and disturbances in mentation and behavior. The plasma calcium is usually 16 mg. per 100 ml. or above, the BUN is elevated, ectopic calcifications may be apparent on radiography, and hypochloremic alkalosis (from vomiting) is frequent. The alkalosis may be due to K^+ depletion, which often accompanies prolonged or severe hypercalcemia. A short Q-T interval on the electrocardiogram with some degree of heart block may be most helpful in suggesting the diagnosis. Similar symptoms and signs are noted in other cases of severe hypercalcemia, e.g., malignant neoplasm with osseous metastases, milk-alkali syndrome, and vitamin D intoxication.

The diagnosis of this state is not easy and should be considered in any patient in whom vomiting, altered mental or behavioral state, and hypertension are seen. Once the diagnosis of calcium intoxication has been made, the differential diagnosis may also prove difficult. In most instances, however, the history, radiologic appearance of the bone, and the other guides enumerated earlier should help. Patients with malignant neoplasms without osseous metastases may be extremely difficult to distinguish from those with hyperparathyroidism. Any patient with a plasma calcium level above 16 mg. per 100 ml. should be regarded as in critical condition and should receive intensive care.

The three major therapeutic means by which plasma calcium concentration can be lowered are (1) inducing a saline diuresis; (2) administering neutral phosphate; and (3) administering calcitonin. If the plasma calcium concentration is above 15 mg. per 100 ml., the initial treatment of choice is intravenous phosphate, which should be given as a neutral salt. A dose of 50 mmoles can be safely administered over a period of 6 to 8 hours. At the same time intravenous infusion of saline should be initiated and maintained so that the dehydration is corrected. With correction of dehydration and administration of saline, the plasma K^+ may fall and supplemental I.V. K^+ may be required. Hence it is important to monitor urine output and plasma Na^+, K^+, and Ca^{2+} during the course of therapy. If phosphate is given too rapidly, severe hypocalcemia and even death may occur, but if it is given at the recommended rate, it is usually effective in lowering plasma $[Ca^{2+}]$. If it is not effective, the intravenous administration of CT at a rate of 0.2 mg. per hr. can be employed. When the plasma $[Ca^{2+}]$ is below 15 mg. per 100 ml., then intravenous saline plus furosemide in a dose of 40 to 80 mg. will usually induce a calcium diuresis and cause a fall in plasma calcium concentration. Once the patient has been well hydrated, if hypercalcemia persists, then phosphate should be administered as well.

Surgical Treatment

The only well-established and effective treatment of hyperparathyroidism is surgical removal of the malfunctioning parathyroid tissue. Any patient capable of undergoing the operative procedure should be so treated. In a few instances, however, operation cannot be done for these reasons: (1) repeated failure to find the abnormal parathyroid tissue at previous operations; (2) other medical conditions for which surgery is contraindicated; (3) refusal of the patient to submit to surgery; and (4) unoperable but functioning metastases. Several alternative methods of therapy have been tried with some success in this group of patients.

Even though, in general, surgical intervention remains the treatment of choice, there is an increasing number of mildly hyperparathyroid patients who exhibit minimal elevation of plasma calcium and IPTH and who show either no progression or regression of symptoms and signs of the disease. The natural course of the disease is not known in these patients. At least one prospective five-year study is now under way, however, in an attempt to establish this natural history and the possible criteria that can be safely employed in deciding on a policy of watchful waiting.

Preoperative Management

The patient should be placed on an ordinary diet while awaiting operation. Plasma magnesium should be measured, and if it is low, the patient should be given supplemental magnesium by mouth. If the cortisone-suppression test has been employed in preoperative studies, at least two weeks should elapse before surgery. If the plasma calcium concentration is above 11.5 mg. per 100 ml., supplemental oral phosphate can be given preoperatively.

Surgical Considerations

Surgery of the parathyroid glands in hyperparathyroidism involves two considerations: the location of the glands, and the amount of tissue to be removed. The operation should be performed by a surgeon who has made a special study of the appearance and location of the parathyroid glands and who can distinguish them from small lymph nodes and collections of fat. He should be aware that about 10 per cent of parathyroid tumors have been found in the anterior or posterior mediastinum, and that patients may have anywhere from three to six glands rather than the usual four.

Once the pathologic parathyroid tissue has been located, the surgeon must decide how much tissue to remove. An attempt should be made to identify all the parathyroid glands before any tissue is excised. Single or multiple adenomas usually are removed *in toto*. However, multiple adenomas do occur, and the removal of one adenoma is no guarantee that another is not present. A surgeon with experience can tell whether the size of the pathologic lesion is commensurate with the clinical degree of hyperparathyroidism. If all four glands are found to be enlarged, a frozen section should be made in order to learn whether the condition is secondary hyperplasia or primary chief-cell hyperplasia. If primary chief-cell hyperplasia is present, the surgeon should remove three of the glands *in toto* and leave behind 50 mg. of the fourth gland with a good blood supply.

Postoperative Course and Management

Patients without Overt Bone Disease. If the patient has had no radiologically recognizable signs of osteitis fibrosa generalisata, the postoperative course is not particularly remarkable. The plasma calcium level falls to the normal range within 1 day, but the plasma phosphate level may not return to normal for 6 to 10 days. Urinary phosphate falls promptly to undetectable levels and remains thus for 2 to 3 days. This is associated with striking oliguria. The onset of oliguria usually provides the earliest clinical evidence of a successful operation. Urinary calcium declines as plasma calcium falls.

Patients with Overt Bone Disease. In hyperparathyroidism associated with osteitis fibrosa generalisata, the removal of the entire quantity of pathologic tissue at one operation will usually result in a fall in the plasma calcium. The maximal fall usually occurs 4 to 10 days after operation. The plasma phosphate level may fall even farther. Calcium and phosphate practically disappear from the urine. Several factors contribute to these changes. There is usually an increase in osteoid volume, and, following surgery, this osteoid undergoes rapid mineralization. There is an abrupt fall in rate of bone resorption and a rise in bone formation as the bone cell population shifts from osteoclastic to osteoblastic activity. Furthermore, during the development of the osteitis fibrosa generalisata, the reduction in the skeletal mass has decreased the weight-bearing capacity of the bones, so that they have become more sensitive to and more responsive to mechanical stress. This results in a compensatory increase in osteoblastic activity, with increased formation of bone matrix. The surgical removal of the hyperfunctioning parathyroid tissue does not immediately bring about an increase in the skeletal mass to normal. Thus the increased activity of the osteoblasts continues until the mass of the calcified bone has reached a weight-bearing capacity that no longer provides a stimulus for increased osteoblastic activity; in other words, skeletal homeostasis is reestablished. During the period when these adjustments are taking place, the osteoblasts continue to produce an increased amount of bone matrix. The process of calcifying this matrix draws the available mineral from the plasma into the "hungry bones." The result is an intractable form of tetany, with a low calcium level and a low phosphate level in the plasma.

Therapy consists of placing the patient on a high milk and calcium intake. More severe symptoms can usually be treated with infusions of calcium gluconate given twice daily. When the bone disease is particularly severe, or is associated with renal failure, supplemental vitamin D_3 is indicated, starting with a dose of 6 to 8 mg. per day for 2 days, and continuing with 4 mg. per day for 2 days, and 2 mg. per day until significant changes in symptomatology and plasma electrolytes are evident. The vitamin D can usually be stopped within 1 to 4 months after surgery. A particularly useful guide to therapy is the plasma alkaline phosphatase level. When this falls to normal, it is indicative of healing of the bone disease. Plasma magnesium should also be measured postoperatively, and if hypomagnesemia is found, it should be treated.

The repair processes in bone usually continue beyond the point at which a normal amount of calcified bone tissue has been laid down. As a result, the end-state of healed osteitis fibrosa generalisata is often over-dense bone. The true bone cysts, which contain fluid, remain as bone cysts, but the pseudocysts (those that contain fibrous tissues, such as the brown tumors [osteoblastomas or osteoclastomas]) become reorganized and are eventually filled with bone. The radiolucent areas often become more radiodense than normal with healing, giving a radiographic pattern unique to healed osteitis fibrosa cystica.

Patients with Renal Manifestations. If the hyperparathyroidism has been complicated by renal manifestations, the postoperative course is usually not remarkable, but the long-term prognosis is poor. When the renal damage has progressed to acidosis and phosphate retention, secondary hyperparathyroidism may be superimposed on the primary disorder; under these circumstances, it usually is advisable to remove less parathyroid tissue at the operation. When renal involvement is early or mild, there is usually some improvement in function after the hypercalciuria is eliminated. In cases that respond favorably, the improvement in renal function may take place very gradually over a period lasting from months to more than a year. In some cases, the renal damage is permanent or progressive.

Patients with Persistent or Recurrent Manifestations. If the hypercalcemia of hyperparathyroidism (with or without overt bone or renal disease or both) persists for 7 or more days after the operation or recurs after an apparently satisfactory improvement has taken place, the presence of a second adenoma or a metastasis from a carcinoma of the parathyroid glands should be suspected. Radiation and repeated excision have been recommended as therapeutic measures for malignant parathyroid tumors. Some patients with solitary adenomas, who respond to surgery with a fall in calcium, oliguria, and symptomatic improvement, have a recurrence of hypercalcemia within 2 to 4 weeks. Reoperation reveals a second adenoma in another gland previously assumed to be normal.

Long-Term Follow-Up

Once a patient has had the diagnosis of primary hyperparathyroidism established and has been successfully treated, it is important that he understand the possibility that, even if a single adenoma was the cause of his disease, his disease may recur. For this reason, yearly determination of plasma calcium should be carried out along with clinical examination and evaluation.

Medical Treatment

There is, at present, no well-established alternative to the surgical removal of hyperfunctioning parathyroid tissue. As noted above, however, a prospective study of the need for surgical intervention is being carried out at the Mayo Clinic in the hope of establishing the natural progression of this disease in its mild form. Until this study is complete, surgical intervention should be the recommended therapy. There are, however, instances in which this is not possible, either because of concurrent disease, unwillingness on the part of the patient, or repeated unsuccessful attempts to locate the hyperfunctioning tissue. In these cases, two therapeutic alternatives exist, neither of which has been used long enough or in a sufficient number of patients to assess its effectiveness.

The first is the long-term use of daily, or twice-weekly, injections of human CT at a dose of 0.5 to 1.0 mg. The administration of this hormone will induce a sustained fall in plasma calcium concentration in hyperparathyroid patients, particularly in those with overt bone disease. Theoretically, CT administration, by increasing the renal excretion of calcium and phosphate, might lead to an increased incidence of renal calculi, but practically the opposite has usually been observed. The other potential failure of this type of treatment is an escape phenomenon observed in CT-treated hyperparathyroid animals in whom, after several days or weeks of therapy, the plasma calcium concentration returns to normal values. This phenomenon has been observed less often in man, however, and the concentration will respond to the addition of oral phosphate to the therapeutic regimen. There has not been, to date, any careful evaluation of this form of treatment. The most important reason for its not being widely used is the likelihood that the underlying hypersecretion of PTH will increase in intensity, and it will be a stimulus for a further hyperplasia of the hyperfunctioning tissue.

The second form of medical management is the use of oral phosphate in the amount of 1.5 to 2.5 g. per day. When phosphate is given to a patient with overt bone disease, hypercalcemia, and hypercalciuria, its administration leads to a fall in plasma calcium concentration and a decrease in urinary calcium excretion (Fig. 11–54). Moreover, it will lead to an increase in osteoblastic activity and an increase in the rate of modulation of osteoclasts to osteoblasts (Fig. 11–17), which may be sufficient to reestablish a balance in skeletal remodeling. The original concept that this form of therapy is attended by the danger of ectopic and renal calcification has been proved incorrect. In addition, in patients with idiopathic hypercalciuria, some of whom may have mild hyperparathyroidism, the administration of phosphate leads to a very striking decrease in stone formation. To date, there have been few careful studies of the use of long-term phosphate therapy in the treatment of the mild form of the disease characterized by renal stone formation, slight hypophosphatemia, and a plasma calcium concentration below 11 mg. per 100 ml. There are theoretical reasons to think that such therapy might be successful, however, particularly since the use of phosphate therapy in patients with osteoporosis or idiopathic hypercalciuria (Figs. 11–49 and 11–50) has led to a decrease in calcium excretion without a significant change in plasma calcium concentration and *with no increase in the concentration of plasma IPTH.* Thus phosphate therapy may well lead to a fundamental change in cellular calcium metabolism and in transcellular calcium transport, minimizing the derangement of mineral metabolism in this group of patients. A prospective study of this form of medical management appears to be warranted on the basis of our present evidence.

An alternative approach to the medical treatment of hyperparathyroidism is the use of pituitary growth hormone (GH) or sex hormones or both. GH administered to hyperparathyroid patients leads to significant retention of calcium, phosphate, and nitrogen. Long-term testosterone therapy leads to similar changes and to a return of plasma calcium concentration toward normal. Estradiol has similar effects in afflicted females. The effects of GH and the sex hormones appear additive in most patients. The experience with these measures is very limited, but the results are of considerable theoretical interest and do suggest that hyperparathyroid patients with unoperable disease can be managed by medical means. Nevertheless, it is important to reemphasize that, at present, the treatment of choice is surgical removal of the malfunctioning tissue.

SECONDARY DISORDERS OF PARATHYROID GLAND FUNCTION

In a large number of conditions, a change in PTH activity is thought to play a role in the pathogenesis of the chemical or pathologic abnormalities. The most common of these primarily involve the kidney, bone, gastrointestinal tract, or other endocrine organs. Many involve possible alterations in the activity and metabolism of, or sensitivity to, vitamin D.

Secondary Hypoparathyroidism

Only when animals are fed a diet abnormally low in phosphate is parathyroidectomy followed by no change in the plasma calcium concentration. Rarely, if ever, does one encounter such a situation in clinical practice. Hence it is most unlikely that there are many instances in which prolonged underproduction of this hormone plays a significant role in the pathogenesis of disease in man. There are types of vitamin D–resistant rickets in which this may occur, however (see below).

There are several conditions in which a decreased end-organ responsiveness to PTH has been considered an important aspect of the disease. The situation in pseudohypoparathyroidism has already been discussed, and the relationship in various forms of rickets will be discussed later. One other such disease is osteopetrosis.

Osteopetrosis (Marble Bone Disease; Albers-Schönberg Disease)

Osteopetrosis is a rare disease which appears in either a severe form at birth or a milder form in adolescence. The severe form is inherited as an autosomal recessive trait and is characterized primarily by a lack of bone remodeling. The bones become increasingly dense, with characteristic club-shaped metaphyses and with nearly complete obliteration of the marrow cavity. The latter leads to anemia, hepatosplenomegaly, abnormal bleeding tendencies, and an immature blood cell pattern. The cranial bones fail to enlarge, with consequent disorders of cranial nerve function, blindness, increased intracranial pressure, and eventually death. The disease is nearly always fatal.

Histologic examination of the bone indicates that osteoclasts are virtually absent; the structure is highly immature, with many areas of endochondrial bone. Evaluation by more modern techniques indicates that the rate of bone formation is normal but that of bone resorption markedly decreased. A curious feature of nearly all cases is that x-ray films show signs of fluctuating activity of the osteosclerotic process, as indicated by alternating transverse bands of greater and less density.

In spite of this bone pattern, affected individuals characteristically absorb greater than normal amounts of calcium from the diet, excrete very little calcium in the urine, and are in marked positive calcium balance.

The chronic or benign form of the disease is characterized by survival to adulthood without involvement of the blood-forming tissue. The bones are characteristically dense and also show evidence of fluctuating activity and a histologic picture indistinguishable from that of the severe form.

Clinically, the patients usually show skeletal deformities, often short stature, and a propensity to fracture. Peculiarly, the rate of fracture healing is normal, but remodeling of the callus is delayed.

Plasma calcium, phosphate, and alkaline phosphatase are normal (Table 11–14), in spite of a markedly positive calcium balance. An elevation of the acid phosphatase has been reported. Few long-term studies have been carried out, but the scant evidence available indicates that these individuals are less responsive than are normal persons to exogenous PTH, and none of the measures which lead to increased bone resorption in experimental animals leads to significant calcium mobilization in individuals with this disease. These data indicate a decreased responsiveness of bone to PTH.

Etiology

The etiology is unknown. The disease is presumed to represent an inborn error of metabolism.

In all likelihood, it is primarily a defect in bone remodeling. There may be decreased responsiveness to PTH. This alone would be insufficient to account for the continued osteoblastic activity. The reason for the disturbance of skeletal homeostasis is not known. A peculiar aspect of the disease is the continued high rate of calcium absorption and retention. This has led some authors to propose that the primary defect lies in the gastrointestinal tract. If this were the case, the tendency to hypercalcemia might well lead to an increased production of thyrocalcitonin and an enhanced production of bone, with a concomitant suppression of PTH release and of PTH action upon bone. Against this interpretation is the fact that the disease has been diagnosed *in utero*.

Osteopetrosis also occurs sporadically in adults as a consequence of intoxication by fluoride, phosphorus, or strontium and is sometimes a consequence of primary blood dyscrasias.

Similar disorders of bone are seen as genetic diseases in mice (gray-lethal) and rats (ia). The etiology of these diseases is unknown, but one suggestion is that they represent primary overproduction of calcitonin. The more likely explanation, however, is that there is a primary defect in bone resorption.

Treatment

There is no satisfactory therapy for osteopetrosis. A severe restriction of calcium intake combined with phytate or cellulose phosphate has been reported to be beneficial, but considerably more experience is needed to evaluate this approach. All cases deserve more thorough genetic and biochemical characterization.

Secondary Hyperparathyroidism

There are a number of disorders of mineral and bony metabolism in which secondary hyperparathyroidism is thought to exist. The reasons for believing this are as follows: (1) similarities between the clinical disorder and those induced in experimental animals; (2) enlarged and presumably hyperfunctioning parathyroid glands at autopsy; (3) evidence of hyperfunction by one of several indirect means; (4) the presence of osteitis fibrosa cystica or of osteoporosis; (5) dramatic changes in calcium or phosphate metabolism following parathyroidectomy; and (6) an increase in plasma PTH concentration as measured by radioimmunoassay.

The most important groups of patients with secondary hyperparathyroidism are those suffering either from simple vitamin D deficiency or from vitamin D deficiency secondary to gastrointestinal or renal disease (Table 11–12). In present-day practice in the United States and western Europe, the latter group are by far the more important. They are also most significant from the theoretical point of view, because the pathogenesis of these disorders is not well understood.

Simple Rickets and Osteomalacia

Rickets and osteomalacia are diseases of infancy and adulthood, respectively, characterized by a lack of normal mineralization of bone and disordered calcium, magnesium, and phosphate metabolism associated with abnormalities of growth and neuromuscular function. The diseases are caused by a lack of exposure to sunlight or, more often, a dietary lack of vitamin D. This can be either an absolute lack of the vitamin; an alteration in the metabolism of vitamin D, leading to an increase in the individual's need for vitamin D; or the result of an inability to absorb a normal amount of this vitamin from the intestine. The last of these is encountered in the malabsorption syndromes seen in pancreatic disease, biliary disease, celiac disease, and sprue and following gastrectomy.

Incidence

Simple rickets is an uncommon disease in the United States because of the addition of vitamin D to milk. It is still seen, however, in certain rural areas and among infants living in the slums of large metropolitan areas. Negro infants are particularly susceptible. Osteomalacia, the adult counterpart of simple rickets, is extremely rare, except in association with the various causes of malabsorption already noted.

Pathologic Physiology

A lack of vitamin D leads to a diminished retention of both dietary calcium and phosphate and alters the sensitivity of bone cells to the osteolytic actions of PTH. As a result, plasma calcium and phosphate both fall. The fall in plasma calcium leads to a stimulation of PTH secretion, which in turn leads to restoration of a nearly normal plasma calcium concentration because of increased bone mobilization, and a further fall in plasma phosphate because of increased phosphaturia. Eventually the plasma phosphate falls enough that normal mineralization of bone ceases. However, bone (collagen) formation continues, with the eventual production of a large mass of uncalcified matrix—*osteoid* (Fig. 11–37). When this osteoid begins to form a significant amount of the bone mass, the bone bends or develops classic pseudofractures (Fig. 11–58). When the degree of vitamin D deficiency becomes severe, bone resorption decreases in spite of increased levels of PTH, and hypocalcemia and tetany ensue. For reasons not at all clear, the patients develop muscular weakness, bone pain and tenderness, and a waddling gait. These manifestations may be due to phosphate deficiency. In addition to phosphaturia, aminoaciduria and reduced urinary calcium excretion are common.

Signs and Symptoms

Rickets. The earliest symptoms usually are apathy and muscular weakness. These are followed by abdominal distention, irritability, frontal bossing, delayed closure of the anterior fontanelle, deformities of the limbs, and beading of the ribs. Tetany is a rare and late manifestation. Vitamin D deficiency may produce minimal signs in starved or malnourished infants.

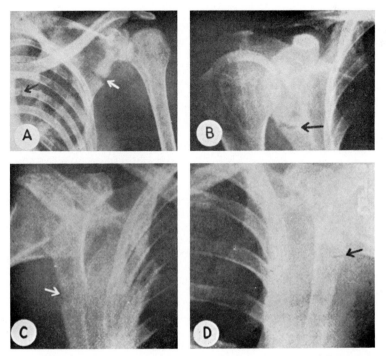

Figure 11–58. X-ray films of bone lesions in four patients with osteomalacia. Note the pseudofractures (arrows) in the scapulae. Osteomalacia with pseudofracture is called Milkman's syndrome. Note the decrease in bone density in case *C*. (Modified from Albright, F., and Reifenstein, E. C.: *The Parathyroid Glands and Metabolic Bone Disease.* Baltimore, Williams and Wilkins Co., 1948.)

Osteomalacia. An early symptom and often the only one is muscular weakness, which is particularly noticeable as a difficulty in mounting stairs. This is followed by poorly localized skeletal pains, which are often considered to be rheumatic. As the disease progresses, the pains become severe, and the patient develops a waddling gait and eventually marked bone tenderness and skeletal deformities. These manifestations are associated with a variety of intestinal complaints when the osteomalacia is due to malabsorption, e.g., steatorrhea; a past history of gastric surgery; and biliary, pancreatic, or liver disease.

Radiologic examination in rickets may reveal little change in the early stage of the disease. The first abnormalities appear in the epiphyses, where widening and irregularity of the epiphyseal lines are seen. This often leads to cupping of the metaphyses, and eventually fractures, bowing, and pseudofractures appear.

The radiologic hallmarks of osteomalacia are the pseudofractures (Fig. 11–58). These are straight bands of rarefaction, perpendicular or oblique to the bone surface. On either side of these radiolucent zones are denser shadows. The pseudofractures are often bilateral and symmetrical, and their sites often correspond to the position of the circumflex arteries crossing the particular bone. At other sites they appear as a result of stress. The vertebrae characteristically have a ground-glass appearance.

The histologic finding characteristic of osteomalacia is an excess of osteoid tissue (Fig. 11–37). Early in the course of the disease, increased osteoclastic activity may be observed, but this usually is not seen in the more advanced disease. Similarly, microradiography reveals a normal extent of bone resorption.

Laboratory Findings

The laboratory findings in simple rickets and osteomalacia are shown in Tables 11–12 and 11–13, in which they are contrasted with those seen in primary and secondary hyperparathyroidism with osteitis fibrosa cystica and other common forms of osteomalacia. The important changes are a marked decrease in calcium and phosphate absorption from the intestine, low plasma phosphate and citrate, normal or low plasma calcium, and an elevated plasma alkaline phosphatase. These changes are associated with aminoaciduria and decreased urinary calcium.

If the basis of the osteomalacia is malabsorption, the gastric acidity is often low, steatorrhea is present, and macrocytic anemia is common. The plasma magnesium may also be low. A flat oral glucose tolerance test is frequently present, and in some patients evidence of vitamin A deficiency or vitamin K deficiency or both may be seen.

Diagnosis

Once considered, the diagnosis is not difficult, particularly when the classic biochemical and ra-diographic changes are found (Tables 11–12 and 11–14). The difficulty lies in defining the etiology. In rare instances, the cause is a dietary lack which the history will usually reveal. More often it is malabsorption, and a thorough investigation of gastrointestinal function should be carried out.

Osteomalacia and rickets due to vitamin D deficiency of whatever cause must be differentiated from a variety of other conditions considered jointly as "vitamin D–resistant rickets." These conditions are classified and discussed in the succeeding pages (Table 11–12).

Treatment

Therapy consists of supplying adequate amounts of vitamin D and providing sufficient calcium and phosphate in the diet to induce healing of the bones. In uncomplicated vitamin D deficiency, a dose of 2000 I.U./day is usually sufficient to produce a cure. If the patient with apparently uncomplicated osteomalacia or rickets does not respond promptly to this management, further investigation into this "resistance" is necessary. In patients with steatorrhea, up to 50,000 I.U. per day may be necessary, presumably because the vitamin is poorly absorbed. If medical treatment improves the steatorrhea, this dose may be too large and may produce vitamin D intoxication. Usually, it is wise to supplement the diet with calcium, e.g., calcium lactate 10 to 15 g. per day.

The one form of osteomalacia or rickets which may respond better to treatment with $25(OH)D_3$ than with the parent vitamin is that associated with liver disease. Presumably, in severe liver disease, the conversion of D_3 to $25(OH)D_3$ is impaired; and under these circumstances, the $25(OH)D_3$ metabolite would be expected to bypass this block in metabolism.

Patients with deficiency rickets also respond to treatment with 25-hydroxycholecalciferol. Treatment with 2,000 U. per day (50 μg.) has been shown to be as effective in curing the disease as is vitamin D_3 therapy. At present, there appears to be no advantage to this form of treatment in patients with deficiency rickets.

Whether one employs vitamin D_3 or its metabolite, $25(OH)D_3$, for the treatment of deficiency rickets, an immediate worsening of hypocalcemia and tetany is commonly seen after the initiation of sterol therapy. Supplemental intravenous calcium may be necessary during this period, which may last several days. This very characteristic response to vitamin D therapy is one of the lines of evidence which support the concept that vitamin D or, more correctly, its active metabolite has a direct action on bone, leading to an increase in bone mineralization.

Vitamin D–Dependent or Pseudo-Deficiency Rickets

In addition to the classical cases of simple dietary deficiency rickets, it has been recognized that an increasing number of children develop rickets on a normal intake of vitamin D but are cured by treatment with doses of vitamin D 3 to 10 times that required in ordinary deficiency.

These children display all the signs and symptoms of classical rickets, but careful dietary history often fails to reveal a deficiency of vitamin D in their diets. Furthermore, upon the usual therapeutic dose of vitamin D_3 or $25(OH)D_3$, the rickets is not healed. Nevertheless, when 3 to 10 times more vitamin D_3 is given, they respond with complete healing and a period of increased growth in which they catch up in size to their peer group, and they then maintain normal growth rates. As long as they are maintained upon an increased intake of vitamin D, they will attain normal size and apparently be normal in every other respect.

The basis of this disease is not yet clear, but there appears to be either an increase in the catabolism of vitamin D_3 or a decreased sensitivity of target tissues to the action of $1,25(OH)_2D_3$. An iatrogenic pseudodeficiency due to increased catabolism is seen in patients on long-term anticonvulsant therapy.

Iatrogenic Pseudodeficiency Rickets

An increased incidence of rickets and osteomalacia has been observed in patients with epilepsy. In most of these studies, an inverse correlation has been noted between the degree of hypocalcemia and the total dose of anticonvulsant therapy. In addition, the plasma concentration of $25(OH)D_3$ has been found low in a third of such patients so tested and inversely correlated with the total drug dosage. In this one third, the serum $25(OH)D_3$ concentration was positively correlated with vitamin D intake (Fig. 11–59), but at any given level of vitamin D intake, the mean $25(OH)D_3$ concentration was lower in the patients than in normal controls (Fig. 11–59).

Studies in both human beings and experimental animals have shown that treatment with either phenobarbital, diphenylhydantoin, or a combination of the two leads to an increased rate of conversion of labeled vitamin D_3 to $25(OH)D_3$ and an

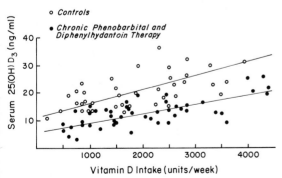

Figure 11–59. The plasma $25(OH)D_3$ concentration as a function of vitamin D intake in a group of normal subjects and in a group on long-term anticonvulsant therapy. (From Hahn, T. J., Hendin, B. A., et al.: *New Eng. J. Med., 287:*900, 1972.)

increase in the rate of turnover of this metabolite, with an increased rate of appearance of polar-inactive metabolites of both. Moreover, hepatic microsomes from treated animals have been shown to catalyze the more rapid conversion of both labeled vitamin D_3 and $25(OH)D_3$ to these inactive metabolites *in vitro*.

These studies have led to the conclusion that osteomalacia and hypocalcemia in epileptics treated with chronic anticonvulsant therapy is due to an accelerated conversion of vitamin D_3 and $25(OH)D_3$ to inactive metabolites by drug-induced hepatic microsomal enzymes.

The relative importance of the conversion of vitamin D_3 directly to inactive metabolites, instead of its initial conversion to $25(OH)D_3$ followed by catabolism to an inactive metabolite, is not yet clear. Preliminary studies of the therapeutic efficacy of $25(OH)D_3$ in this condition, however, suggest that it may be more effective than vitamin D_3. This possibility remains to be validated.

The importance of recognizing the effect of anticonvulsant therapy upon vitamin D metabolism is twofold: (1) the complication of hypocalcemia and rickets or osteomalacia can be prevented by the institution of prophylactic vitamin D therapy; and (2) the treatment of epileptic seizures in patients with hypoparathyroidism must be recognized as constituting an extremely complicated therapeutic situation.

Prophylaxis consists of the administration of additional vitamin D to all patients on long-term anticonvulsant therapy. The addition of 4000 to 8000 I.U. of dietary vitamin D_3 per week should be sufficient in the majority of cases. Although not yet in widespread use, the measurement of plasma $25(OH)D_3$ in all these patients may prove to be the simplest and most direct means of assessing the need for and efficacy of vitamin D therapy.

The combination of hypoparathyroidism and epilepsy requires careful consideration. In several instances, children with epilepsy who later proved to have hypoparathyroidism have been started upon anticonvulsant therapy without adequate evaluation of their parathyroid status. The need for anticonvulsant medication has been progressive, with larger and larger doses becoming necessary to control symptoms. When hypocalcemia, usually of a severe degree, i.e., 4 to 5 mg. per 100 ml., has been recognized, large doses of vitamin D_3 or dihydrotachysterol have been required initially to correct the hypocalcemia. As the plasma calcium has risen, the need for anticonvulsant medication has declined and often has been eliminated entirely. If in such cases seizures did continue, however, the reinstatement of anticonvulsant therapy led to a rapid fall in plasma calcium concentration and an increased need for vitamin D. Because of these relationships, this therapeutic situation is difficult to manage. In most instances, calcium and vitamin D should be given without other medication to hypocalcemic patients in an effort to control symptoms. Anticonvulsant therapy should be employed only if seizures occur when the patient is normocalcemic. In this regard, it is worth noting that the plasma calcium concentratiom may fall in the night, leading to convulsions in the early morning hours.

Perhaps the most important lesson from these patients is the need to evaluate carefully all children with epilepsy to make certain they do not have hypoparathyroidism before instituting therapy, and to reevaluate the parathyroid and calcium status of all patients exhibiting a progressive need for anticonvulsant medication.

Rickets and Osteomalacia Associated with Renal Diseases

Altered bone structure and metabolism are common complications of many types of renal disease (Table 11–12), but the exact incidence of upset calcium balance is not known. Significant changes in one or more parameters of bone or mineral metabolism are a common feature of acute renal disease. Chronicity of the renal disease leads to one form or another of renal osteodystrophy in a significant percentage of patients. A particularly frequent accompaniment of renal disease is an increase in fecal calcium excretion. Osteomalacia or rickets, osteitis fibrosa, or a mixture of the two is often seen. Osteosclerosis may also be present. Osteodystrophy is most commonly associated with chronic renal failure and azotemia, i.e., a combined glomerular and tubular dysfunction. Less commonly, it is associated with various renal tubular disorders (Tables 11–12 and 11–14).

Osteodystrophy of Renal Failure — Azotemic Osteodystrophy

Incidence

Various pathologic studies of patients dying of renal failure indicate that between 55 and 80 per cent have demonstrable pathologic changes in their bones. This may take the form of rickets or osteomalacia, osteitis fibrosa, or a combination thereof.

Pathophysiology

Stanbury in his careful studies of these conditions has recognized two general types: those with predominantly osteitis fibrosa, and those with primarily osteomalacia or rickets. A summary of the salient features of these two types is given in Tables 11–12 and 11–13, and a comparison is made with the findings in primary hyperparathyroidism, simple rickets, and renal tubular rickets or phosphate diabetes.

Azotemic Osteomalacia. The patients with rickets or osteomalacia have hypocalcemia, and their phosphate levels are lower than those seen in patients with predominantly osteitis. Plasma phosphate may be normal in spite of an elevated BUN. These abnormalities are associated with muscular weakness, bone pain and tenderness, and other signs typical of simple vitamin D deficiency. Slight parathyroid gland hyperplasia and a lack of response to the usual doses of parathyroid extract are characteristically observed. Metastatic calcification in soft tissue is rarely present. Calcium balance shows high fecal and low renal excretion of calcium — the pattern of vitamin D deficiency. The rickets or osteomalacia may be indistinguishable radiographically and histologically from that seen in classic vitamin D deficiency rickets, although with renal disease, some degree of associated osteitis fibrosa is more common.

Azotemic Osteitis. Patients with renal osteodystrophy associated with osteitis fibrosa usually have a higher BUN and presumably a more advanced degree of renal failure. Commonly, they have metastatic calcification and grossly enlarged parathyroid glands. Calcium balance shows high fecal calcium. The radiologic and histologic changes may be indistinguishable from those seen in primary hyperparathyroidism (Fig. 11–53), although evidence of associated osteomalacia is the rule. Because long-continued overactivity of the parathyroid glands may lead to renal impairment, it is possible that an occasional patient has primary hyperparathyroidism leading to renal failure and subsequent secondary hyperparathyroidism, but this sequence of events is rare. There is every indication that patients with osteitis fibrosa represent a later stage in renal failure; patients may progress from predominantly azotemic rickets to predominantly osteitis, with a concomitant rise in both plasma calcium and plasma phosphate.

The most logical explanation of these changes is that the development of chronic renal disease leads to a relative (rather than absolute) vitamin D deficiency. This in turn leads to a state in which the bones become unresponsive to normal or somewhat increased amounts of circulating PTH, and both plasma calcium and plasma phosphate fall. The fall in plasma calcium leads to increased PTH secretion, but this increase is insufficient to mobilize significant calcium and phosphate from bone because of the unresponsiveness of this organ. A complicating factor, however, may be the appearance of osteoid which acts as a trap for any calcium that is mobilized. In any case, the long-continued stimulus to glandular hyperactivity leads eventually to a greatly enhanced rate of PTH secretion, sufficient to cause significant bone mobilization. The elevation of plasma calcium and phosphate leads to the consequent healing of the rickets or osteomalacia and the appearance of osteitis fibrosa cystica. In some instances, the hyperactive glands become autonomous.

The hypothetical interpretation of events is supported by experimental evidence in the rat, as well as by the fact that treatment with moderate to large doses of vitamin D of patients with defective mineralization leads to healing of the rickets, a decrease in fecal calcium, a rise in plasma and urinary calcium, and a rise in plasma phosphate and citrate. These changes are similar to those seen in patients with simple rickets.

The nature of the relative vitamin D deficiency

which apparently underlies these conditions is not clear. The plasma levels of vitamin D are usually normal; hence, a lack of absorption appears not to be involved. There is some evidence that the conversion of vitamin D_3 to $25(OH)D_3$ is also normal (Fig. 11-29), but that the renal synthesis of $1,25(OH)_2D_3$ from $25(OH)D_3$ is impaired. It is possible that hepatic microsomal hydroxylase activity is increased in this state and may contribute to the altered metabolism of vitamin D.

A striking aspect of the therapeutic response to vitamin D in some patients is a marked improvement in the bone and a significant decrease in fecal calcium without a striking change in either plasma calcium or plasma phosphate. These observations have been interpreted as evidence that vitamin D has a direct effect upon mineral accretion (see p. 703). It is not yet clear whether the therapeutic response is mediated by an increase in plasma $25(OH)D_3$ or $1,25(OH)_2D_3$.

The other feature of the bone changes in many patients with renal osteodystrophy is an increase in bone mass. The bones, particularly the vertebrae, become denser than normal, particularly in patients with signs primarily of hyperparathyroidism. This hyperostosis is rare in adults with primary hyperparathyroidism. The difference in skeletal balance can be attributed to the differences in plasma phosphate concentration. In patients with renal osteodystrophy, the hyperparathyroidism is associated with a high plasma phosphate concentration. Phosphate is a major stimulus for the modulation of osteoclasts to osteoblasts (Figs. 11-10 and 11-17). As a consequence, the overall rate of skeletal remodeling is increased, but the balance of remodeling activities is in favor of formation.

A similar type of hyperostotic hyperparathyroidism can be produced experimentally in the horse simply by feeding a high-phosphate diet. Moreover, in very young rats, the administration of small daily doses of PTH will induce a net increase in bone mass. Here, as well, the key factor in determining the hyperostosis is the high plasma phosphate concentration.

The single most important factor in the pathogenesis of the bone disease in renal osteodystrophy is the retention of phosphate. When patients are ingesting a 1200-mg. phosphate diet and the glomerular filtration rate (GFR) falls below 70 ml. per min., the tubular reabsorption of phosphate falls. As the GFR falls lower, phosphate retention increases, and secondary hyperparathyroidism ensues. If phosphate intake is severely restricted, however, TRP remains high even in patients with a GFR of 20 ml. per min. Under these conditions, no phosphate retention is seen, and, as a consequence, there is no increase in plasma PTH concentration.

Phosphate stimulates PTH secretion indirectly. It lowers the plasma calcium concentration, which, in turn, stimulates PTH secretion. The mechanism by which hypocalcemia is sustained, in spite of hyperparathyroidism, is complex. Several factors that contribute to the hypocalcemia are (1) the

phosphate-induced net balance in favor of bone formation; (2) a disturbance in vitamin D metabolism, with a decrease in $1,25(OH)_2D_3$ concentrations in the blood; and (3) an intrinsic defect in the intestinal absorption of calcium in uremic patients unrelated to the synthesis or amount of $1,25(OH)_2D_3$.

Diagnosis

A diagnosis of azotemic osteitis should be considered in all patients with chronic renal disease and particularly in those in whom muscular weakness, bone tenderness, knock-knees, and/or bone pains are prominent complaints. Once it is suspected, a combination of laboratory and x-ray examinations (Table 11-12) will verify its presence or absence.

Treatment

The most important therapeutic agents are the D vitamins. Vitamins D_2, D_3, and crystalline dihydrotachysterol (DHT) have all been used with comparable therapeutic results. The dose needed in a given patient is unpredictable, although it is invariably large compared with the normal daily requirement. A safe procedure is to initiate therapy with 1.25 to 1.50 mg. of vitamin D (50,000 to 60,000 I.U.) and continue for at least 3 weeks before increasing the dose. A dose of 10 mg. or more may be required eventually in some patients, whereas others will respond adequately to 1.0 mg. Acidosis if present should be corrected by the administration of sodium bicarbonate. Therapeutic response can be assessed by measuring plasma calcium, phosphate, and phosphatase; by serial roentgenograms; and by noting symptomatic improvement. The end-point of therapy is to obtain healing of the bone lesions, if possible. Once this is achieved, the patients should be maintained on vitamin D and bicarbonate. The dose of vitamin should be reduced from that needed to induce healing. In some patients, vitamin D therapy has allowed the resumption of nearly normal activity and survival for years in a productive capacity. The addition of phosphate precipitants (aluminum hydroxide) to the diet may also be of value.

The administration of vitamin D to patients with predominant osteitis usually results in healing of their bone lesions. However, in certain patients there is no change in the bone lesions, although there is a rise in plasma calcium. This may point to autonomous parathyroid gland overactivity, either hyperplasia or adenoma, and is an indication for subtotal parathyroidectomy. In the group of patients with normal or high plasma calcium before therapy, this possibility should be considered.

The fact that 25-hydroxy-dihydrotachysterol [25(OH)DHT] does not undergo renal conversion to a 1-hydroxy derivative before exerting its biologic effects (p. 702) suggests that DHT may be most useful in treating patients with advanced renal disease in whom the synthesis of $1,25(OH)_2D_3$ is impaired. It also has the advantage that 25-DHT does not act as a feedback inhibitor of its own synthesis. Therapeutic use of DHT has not been widespread, but in studies to date administration of 0.125 to 0.25 mg. per day has been found effective in curing the osteomalacia in patients with renal disease, whereas in similar patients, 1.25 to 2.5 mg. per day of vitamin D_3 was ineffective in curing the bone disease. Thus DHT may have an important place in the treatment of this particular bone disease. Alternatively, $25(OH)D_3$ may prove useful, but experience with this compound is at present limited. Therapeutic responses in a few patients have shown it to be less effective than DHT.

The appearance of normo- or hypercalcemia in patients with the most advanced azotemic osteitis and with low GFR is a fairly frequent phenomenon. It suggests autonomous functioning of the previous hyperplastic parathyroid tissue. If they are examined carefully, however, it is found that, in most patients, the secretion of PTH is suppressible by calcium infusion. Nonetheless, the mass of parathyroid tissue is large, and even in the "suppressed" state, the rate of secretion may be significant. In addition, even though total plasma calcium is high in these patients, the ionized calcium is usually low or normal.

These changes in parathyroid function are important considerations in the therapeutic management, either with dialysis or a renal transplant, of patients with chronic renal diseases. Clearly, the most important consideration is the stage of the disease at which either form of therapy is instigated.

In patients with hyperphosphatemia, hypocalcemia, and osteitis, the first step is to control the plasma calcium and phosphate concentrations during an initial period of dialysis before transplant or during prolonged dialysis. The plasma calcium concentration is maintained at near-normal values by a combination of 6 to 8 mg. per 100 ml. calcium in the dialysate of patients dialyzed for 18 hours a week and dietary aluminum hydroxide sufficient to lower the plasma phosphate to 3 to 4 mg. per 100 ml. It is recommended that the aluminum hydroxide therapy be instituted before the patient is dialyzed against this high-calcium solution. On this regimen, the high plasma PTH values fall slowly over a period of several months and eventually may reach the normal range. Also on this regimen, the osteomalacic component of the disease heals; patients can be maintained for long periods of time without bone disease. Renal transplantation in these patients is usually not complicated by postoperative hypercalcemia.

The most difficult therapeutic problems are those in patients with hypercalcemia, either before or shortly after the start of therapy. Most of these patients can be managed medically by the control of dialysate calcium concentration and oral aluminum hydroxide therapy. It is important to understand that the hypersecretion of parathyroid hormone may persist for several months, even on a good regimen. In those patients whose plasma PTH concentration has been followed by serial radioimmunoassays, however, no patient has shown persistent autonomous secretion of PTH, i.e., there is a progressive fall in PTH concentration with time. Also, with time, changes in the calcium concentration in the dialysate may be necessary for proper therapy.

These procedures are contingent upon the extent of dialysis. If a particular center has, on the average, patients undergoing dialysis for 30 rather than 18 hrs. a week, a regimen employing a calcium concentration of 8 mg. per 100 ml. in the dialysate could lead to hypercalcemia and its attendant complications. Regardless of the particular regimen, by careful measurement of plasma calcium, phosphate, and IPTH, it should be possible to adjust the therapeutic program so as to optimize these values and to prevent bone disease secondary to long-term dialysis.

Rickets and Renal Tubular Dysfunction

Rickets or osteomalacia is a common occurrence in a large number of distinct but rare disorders of renal tubular function, in which, in most instances, there is no loss of glomerular function. In some patients, particularly those with cystine storage disease, glomerular filtration is often impaired, leading eventually to azotemic osteodystrophy.

The rickets is radiographically indistinguishable from that seen in simple vitamin D deficiency, but it is distinguishable by its appearance in microradiographs of the affected bone (Fig. 11–42) and by the fact that large doses of vitamin D are necessary to induce a cure. At least six distinct types of renal tubular or presumed renal tubular disorders are associated with rickets or osteomalacia. The abnormal findings in plasma, urine, and tissue are recorded in Table 11–13 and compared with those seen in simple rickets and renal osteodystrophy. The four nearly universal findings are hypophosphaturia, hypophosphatemia, increased fecal calcium excretion, and elevated plasma alkaline phosphatase. Plasma calcium is usually normal or slightly low.

Simple Vitamin D–Resistant Rickets; Phosphate Diabetes

This is, in many instances, a familial sex-linked disorder transmitted as a dominant with full penetrance. The one universal finding is low plasma phosphate, with a high clearance of phosphate by the kidney without other evidence of abnormal renal function. This may be associated with rickets or osteomalacia. Short stature is the rule. In patients with rickets, the disease usually manifests itself between 6 months and 2 years of age. In some instances, it may appear in early adult life. Particularly common is relative shortening of the long bones. In nearly one third of the cases, there is no positive family history, and the condition is believed to be an X-linked recessive trait. A few affected adults have an associated increase in urinary glycine excretion.

The cause of the disease is unknown. Three general theories as to its pathogenesis have been advanced: (1) the primary disorder is an inability to absorb calcium normally, and this in turn leads to secondary hyperparathyroidism, followed by increased excretion of phosphate, lowering of plasma phosphate, and rickets; (2) the primary defect is altered phosphate transport in the renal tubule; and (3) the metabolism of vitamin D is abnormal.

The following facts support the first hypothesis: (1) infusion of calcium intravenously leads to increased retention of phosphate and to a rise in plasma phosphate, which is interpreted as suppression of parathyroid gland activity; (2) hyperplastic parathyroid glands are sometimes found post mortem; (3) some evidence of a fibrotic reaction in bone, the appearance of mineralization defects around osteocytic lacunae, and microradiographic evidence of increased rates of bone turnover have been described.

On the basis of present evidence, however, it is most likely that the second hypothesis is correct, i.e., that the renal defect is primary, because (1) there is a decrease in the tubular transport maximum for phosphate (TmP) in these patients but not in those with primary hyperparathyroidism; (2) calcium deficiency in experimental animals is associated with osteoporosis, not osteomalacia, and is presumed to represent a situation in which secondary hyperparathyroidism exists; (3) patients, when untreated, have normal or low concentrations of circulating PTH; (4) exogenous PTH does not increase phosphate excretion in these patients, even when the concentration of endogenous plasma PTH is normal; (5) plasma phosphate concentration rarely returns to normal, even with adequate vitamin D therapy and restoration of normal calcium absorption; (6) intravenous infusion of phosphate initiates bone healing, and when this occurs, there is a prompt increase in calcium absorption from the gut; (7) parathyroidectomy does not bring plasma phosphate back to normal, even though plasma calcium falls; (8) the parathyroid glands generally appear normal at autopsy; (9) oral phosphate loads in these subjects lead to increased urinary phosphate excretion without a change in plasma phosphate, whereas similar phosphate loads in hyperparathyroid patients lead to a rise in plasma phosphate; (10) the urinary excretion of phosphate may exceed the filtered load when these patients are given oral phosphate loads (this is not seen in patients with primary hyperparathyroidism); and (11) there is a defect in the intestinal mucosal absorption of phosphate in these patients.

The most direct evidence for a primary renal tubular defect in this disease is the fact that plasma PTH concentrations are normal, but these patients exhibit no increase in phosphate excretion when given PTH. When they are infused with calcium, however, there is an increase in the tubular reabsorption of phosphate, even though PTH concentration falls, indicating that (1) the PTH-dependent phosphate transport system in the kidney is

lost, but a calcium-dependent phosphate transport system continues to operate; or (2) the kidney is responding to a decrease in circulating PTH, i.e., the kidney is unusually sensitive to low concentrations of endogenous PTH.

In spite of this impressive evidence of a primary renal lesion, it is not yet clear what factors are involved in the pathogenesis of the osteomalacia. At least two important factors may be involved: (1) an alteration in vitamin D metabolism; and (2) a direct effect of phosphate deficiency upon bone formation and bone mineralization.

As discussed previously (p. 667), experimental phosphate deficiency in animals and iatrogenic phosphate deficiency in man may both lead to osteomalacia, presumably because the lack of phosphate impairs mineralization of bone matrix. Moreover, experimental phosphate deficiency, even in hypoparathyroid animals, leads to an increase in bone resorption and a decrease in bone formation. A delay in bone mineralization more profound than the decrease in rate of bone formation is also observed. A combination of osteomalacia and osteoporosis is seen. It is possible that similar changes in these patients are directly related to the hypophosphatemia. It also remains possible that the bone cells have a disorder of phosphate metabolism similar to that in the kidney cells, but there is, at present, no direct evidence in support of this hypothesis.

In terms of vitamin D metabolism, it is clear that these patients have normal concentrations of $25(OH)D_3$ in their plasma, but it is not yet known whether the renal synthesis of $1,25(OH)_2D_3$ is normal. It is possible that phosphate deficiency may, by altering cellular calcium metabolism and C-AMP concentrations, alter the rate of $1,25(OH)_2D_3$ synthesis and contribute, thereby, to the pathogenesis of this disease.

Diagnosis is made on the basis of the characteristic signs and symptoms of rickets. Tetany is rarely observed. Muscular weakness is uncommon. The laboratory and radiographic evidence (Tables 11-12 and 11-13), the family history, plasma phosphate determinations upon as many members of the family as possible, and the response to vitamin D are all helpful in establishing the diagnosis. The conditions from which it must be distinguished are the other forms of rickets associated with renal tubular lesions. The important evidence in making this choice is derived from various laboratory determinations (Table 11-12). In addition to the changes noted in Table 11-12, low plasma magnesium has been reported in some patients.

There is continuing controversy concerning treatment of this condition. Some experts argue for a therapy based primarily on vitamin D, and others for one on phosphate. In most instances, the treatment with phosphate, particularly if it is given in divided doses over the entire day, will induce at least partial healing and growth. Additional phosphate in a dosage of 2.0 to 5.0 g. per day is usually possible, although when phosphate therapy is initiated, diarrhea may result.

The combined use of vitamin D (50,000 to 250,000 I.U. per day) and neutral phosphate (2.5 to

4.0 g. per day) has given the most impressive therapeutic results. Plasma phosphate concentrations usually rise after each ingestion of phosphate and then fall to control levels over the next several hours. For this reason, it appears necessary to give the phosphate in five or six divided doses at regularly spaced intervals throughout the day. On this regimen some patients, in addition to having their rickets cured, undergo a growth spurt. It has been suggested that the decreased growth in these patients is related to the altered oxygen affinity of their red cells, resulting from the hypophosphatemia (p. 668). It seems more likely, however, that the phosphate deficiency inhibits skeletal growth and remodeling. Combined phosphate and vitamin D therapy reestablishes higher plasma phosphate concentrations and responsiveness to PTH. As a consequence, the activation of bone metabolic units is increased and the modulation of osteoclasts to osteoblasts enhanced. It is also possible that epiphyseal growth and mineral turnover is increased, leading to the growth spurt.

Treatment with $25(OH)D_3$ rather than vitamin D_3 has been tried, but there is no evidence of its therapeutic superiority.

Hypophosphatemic Osteomalacia Associated with Tumors

A small number of patients with a sporadic form of vitamin D–resistant rickets or osteomalacia have been described in whom the osteomalacia has been associated with skin or bone tumors. These patients have appeared with the usual signs and symptoms of the X-linked disease and have responded poorly to phosphate or vitamin D therapy or both. Each has had a complete remission of symptoms following excision of a tumor, however. The size and nature of the tumor have varied from sclerosing hemangiomas and giant-cell granulomas to malignant neurinomas.

This evidence, admittedly incomplete, raises the possibility that the tumors in these patients have been secreting a phosphaturic agent which leads to the development of a syndrome similar clinically to that produced by an X-linked renal defect in tubular phosphate reabsorption. This in turn reemphasizes the likelihood that phosphate deficiency in the X-linked disease is the primary determinant of the osseous manifestations of the disease.

The most important practical lesson is that, in all patients with acquired hypophosphatemic osteomalacia, a very careful search for cutaneous and osseous tumors should be made, and if any are found, regardless of their size, they should be excised in hopes of "curing" this disease.

Vitamin D Intoxication

Overdosage with vitamin D is a serious medical problem because of the danger of irreversible renal damage. It is characterized by anorexia, irritability, lassitude, weight loss, and an increase in plasma calcium, phosphate, and BUN. All patients on large doses of this vitamin should be instructed to report any such symptoms promptly and should be followed at regular and frequent intervals in order to minimize the danger.

Fanconi's Syndrome

In 1936 Fanconi recognized several cases of vitamin D–resistant rickets with low plasma phosphate, hyperphosphaturia, systemic acidosis, glycosuria, and excess excretion of organic acids in the urine. Since that time, a variety of patients have been described with acidosis, rickets, or osteomalacia, and hyperphosphaturia with one or all of these manifestations, including in some cases cystinosis, or cystine deposits in the tissues. In Table 11–13 these cases have been classified into two groups: those with and those without cystinosis. Other authors have included numerous subclasses: those characterized by increased phosphate and glucose excretion with minimal acidosis, those with phosphaturia and aminoaciduria without glucosuria, and those with all three. It is obvious that more than one condition is included under the term *Fanconi's syndrome*. Characteristically the disease occurring in early life is associated with cystine storage, whereas the disease appearing in adult life usually is not. In all instances, renal calcification and renal calculi are rare, in contrast to the situation in renal tubular acidosis (see below).

The disease associated with cystinosis is transmitted as a simple recessive trait. It usually appears during the first few months of life and is characterized by vomiting, retarded development, polyuria, polydipsia, and muscle weakness with or without the other signs of rickets. Several cases have been detected in which the renal lesions have been present without the signs of bone disease. The evolution of the disease has been followed by careful observation from birth of the siblings of known patients. There is no detectable abnormality for 4 to 6 months; then growth slows, and anorexia and vomiting develop. This state is followed by the appearance of cystine crystals in the cornea and lymph nodes and of increased excretion of amino acids and glucose in the urine. The serum phosphate then falls, and urinary phosphate excretion rises. Several months later, rickets appears. The renal lesions are progressive in spite of therapy, and glomerular insufficiency eventually develops, followed by uremia and death. Thus the bones in the early stage of the disease resemble those seen in simple rickets, unless growth is severely retarded, in which case pseudofractures may be observed without significant changes in the epiphyses. As renal failure develops, the bone lesions resemble those seen in azotemic osteodystrophy.

The important pathologic findings are (1) cystine deposits throughout the reticuloendothelial system and the cornea of the eye; and (2) abnormal thinning of segments of the proximal renal tubules, which are shortened, often accompanied by flattening and atrophy of the epithelium lining the distal tubules.

The pathogenesis of the bone disease and the disordered calcium and phosphate metabolism is complex. The excretion of phosphate in the urine is high, and the excretion of both calcium and phosphate by the gut is high. This leads to low plasma phosphate, which may be responsible in large part for the development of the rickets or osteomalacia. Under these conditions, one would expect the parathyroids to be normal or hypoactive. Normal glands have been noted in many patients, but hypertrophy has been noted in others. The latter case is common when the uremic phase of the disease develops. There is no evidence upon which to decide whether the lack of calcium and phosphate absorption by the gut represents a primary defect or is related in some way to the renal disorder. The picture is complicated by acidosis and often by potassium deficiency as well, both of which can alter the renal disposition of calcium and phosphate.

Although the classic disease in children has a genetic basis, a number of acquired diseases can be associated with similar metabolic derangements. These include multiple myeloma; uranium, lead, and cadmium poisoning; ingestion of outdated tetracyclines; and Wilson's disease. The latter is of particular interest because of the suggestion that Fanconi's syndrome may result from the accumulation of some abnormal metabolic product, possibly cystine, in various tissues. In this regard, it is possible and even likely that the high levels of tissue cystine lead to inactivation of numerous SH-containing enzymes.

A point of considerable interest is that vitamin D administration or the infusion of calcium intravenously can temporarily nullify the resorptive defects in the kidneys of patients in the early stage of the disease. The basis for this is unknown. Treatment is aimed at correcting the rickets, acidosis, and K^+ deficiency. Large doses of vitamin D are required, and the same considerations apply as discussed in the treatment of other vitamin D–resistant states. Supplemental oral phosphate may also be of value.

Renal Tubular Acidosis

The clearest example of a primary renal tubular lesion leading to osteomalacia or rickets is renal tubular acidosis. This is a rare genetic disorder transmitted as a dominant trait with variable penetrance. The disease is characterized by acidosis with high plasma chloride and low bicarbonate, associated with an inability to excrete an acid urine, i.e., below pH 6.0. This inability is associated with an increased excretion of fixed base, Na, K, Ca, and Mg, which may lead to sodium depletion with possible dehydration, potassium depletion with associated weakness and paralysis, increased excretion of both calcium and phosphate, and lowered excretion of citrate. Osteomalacia, urinary calculi, and nephrocalcinosis are commonly seen, and ability to form a concentrated urine is impaired because of hypokalemia, nephrocalcinosis or both. The plasma calcium is usually normal, the plasma phosphate low, and the alkaline phosphatase elevated (Table 11–13). Tetany is rarely seen.

An incomplete form of the disease has been described with these features: an inability to excrete an acid urine, associated with an increased excretion of ammonia and in some instances of calcium; a decreased excretion of citrate without systemic acidosis; no alterations in plasma calcium or phosphate; and no osteomalacia. The transition from the incomplete to the complete form has been observed.

The primary defect appears to be an inability of the distal renal tubule to maintain a steep hydrogen ion gradient between blood and tubular urine. This inability is presumed to be the result of an increased permeability of these cells to H^+.

The presumed course of events leading to the osteomalacia is as follows: (1) hypercalciuria with a tendency to hypocalcemia; (2) stimulation of parathyroid gland activity; (3) increased mobilization of calcium and phosphate from bone; (4) increased excretion of phosphate in the urine with a fall in plasma phosphate; (5) increased urinary phosphate excretion as a direct consequence of the metabolic acidosis; (6) the combination of (3), (4), and (5), leading to a striking decrease in plasma phosphate and a normal or slightly depressed plasma calcium. These changes lead in turn to osteomalacia. The basis of the nephrocalcinosis appears to be multifactorial, including increased calcium and phosphate in the urine, decreased citrate in the urine, inability to form an acid urine, and altered intracellular electrolytes with possibly a decreased intracellular pH.

An additional possibility is that the disorder in renal function and renal cell electrolyte distribution alters the renal synthesis of $1,25(OH)_2D_3$ and contributes to the development of the osteomalacia.

The signs and symptoms of the rickets or osteomalacia are in general indistinguishable from those seen in vitamin D deficiency states, except that normocalcemia is the rule, tetany is very rare, and acidosis is present (Table 11–13) along with hypokalemia. Moreover, nephrocalcinosis and renal calculi do not occur in simple rickets. The laminae durae are usually well preserved, and the bone disease is an osteomalacia with pseudofractures both radiologically and histologically.

When renal tubular acidosis was discovered, the major factor in the pathogenesis of the bone disease was considered to be the hypercalciuria with resultant hyperparathyroidism. This appears unlikely for the following reasons: idiopathic hypercalciuria without acidosis does not lead to osteomalacia; urinary calcium excretion is not always high in these patients; plasma phosphate may be in the same range as that seen in primary hyperparathyroidism and may be accompanied by significant acidosis. The combination of hyperparathyroidism and metabolic acidosis leads characteristically to osteitis fibrosa cystica, not osteomalacia. Thus some other factor must be operative in these patients with renal tubular acidosis. One is a direct renal loss of phosphate, which may lead to a phosphate deficiency that is known to produce osteomalacia, and the second is the possibility that a relative lack of $1,25(OH)_2D_3$ may exist. Few balance studies have been done in these patients, but in the few reported instances in which patients have been treated initially with relatively small doses of vitamin D, a marked increase in calcium retention and a decrease in fecal calcium excretion was observed.

The disease is readily controlled by treatment with an alkali, either sodium bicarbonate or Shohl's solution (a mixture of citric acid and sodium citrate, 140 g. and 90 g., respectively, in 1 liter of water) administered in doses of 50 to 100 ml. three times a day. Potassium can be given as the citrate salt when needed. The major danger in alklai therapy is precipitating tetany in a patient with severe osteomalacia. If rickets or osteomalacia is present, supplemental vitamin D is recommended. A dose of 2000 to 5000 I.U. per day is usually sufficient and should be discontinued when healing has occurred, because relapse does not usually occur if the acidosis is controlled. Supplemental calcium may be needed initially, particularly in patients with hypocalcemia and in those in whom tetany is induced by alkali therapy.

The prognosis depends upon the degree of permanent renal damage present before initiation of adequate therapy. Nephrocalcinosis predisposes to pyelonephritis, which may further injure the kidney. If adequate and sustained treatment is instituted early in the course of the disease, the prognosis is good.

Hypophosphatasia

Hypophosphatasia is a rare genetic disease of bone which has several of the radiographic features of rickets. The disease is probably inherited as an autosomal recessive trait and is characterized biochemically by a lack of alkaline phosphatase in bone, plasma, and leukocytes and by the excretion of phosphoethanolamine in the urine. Normal or increased concentrations of calcium and phosphate are seen in the plasma. Urinary hydroxyproline excretion is decreased and that of pyrophosphate increased (Table 11–13). The major clinical abnormalities are related to the bones. Upon x-ray examination, they resemble those in simple rickets, except that the widened epiphyses are notched and irregular rather than smooth and cupped. Often there is evidence of subperiosteal bone formation. Patients surviving into adult life usually give a history of rickets followed by an asymptomatic period, and as adults x-ray examination may reveal pseudofractures. These changes lead to genu valgum, short stature, and premature synostosis of the skull, recognized radiographically by absence of demonstrable bone over large areas of the skull. This radiolucent area is uncalcified osteoid, which may lead to increased cranial pressure and exophthalmos. Histologically the bones appear similar to those seen in rickets, with evidence of poorly arranged collagen and decreased osteoclastic activity.

The finding of normal amounts of collagen in the absence of normal levels of alkaline phosphatase seems to indicate that the defect is not in collagen biosynthesis but rather in the extracellular maturation of the collagen or in the calcification of mature collagen.

In view of the recent evidence implicating alkaline phosphatase in the function of the matrix calcification granules, the most likely explanation is that, in the absence of this enzyme, these granules do not form, or they form but fail to accumulate mineral; hence, defective mineralization follows. Just as in patients with vitamin D deficiency treated with phosphate, however, if the plasma electrolyte concentrations are maintained at a high level, then a patchy mineralization of the matrix will take place.

In this view, the only useful therapy would be to increase the ion product in the extracellular fluids by the administration of phosphate. This form of therapy has been used with some success, and its success contrasts with the failure of vitamin D therapy to alter the course of the disease.

The most striking fact about this disease is that the concentrations of plasma calcium are normal or high, and those of phosphate are normal in spite of a clearly deranged metabolism of bone mineral, which emphasizes again the distinction between mineral and skeletal homeostasis.

PRIMARY DISORDERS OF C-CELL FUNCTION

The only recognized disorder of C-cell function is medullary carcinoma of the thyroid with hypersecretion of calcitonin.

Primary Hypercalcitoninemia: Medullary Carcinoma

Etiology and Incidence

The only known cause of continued hypersecretion of calcitonin is medullary carcinoma of the thyroid. The etiology of this condition is unknown. Over 50 per cent of the cases exhibit a familial incidence, and the pattern of inheritance indicates an autosomal dominant mode of transmission. The disease is rare, occurring in one of every several thousand patients seeking medical attention. It represents approximately 6 per cent of all patients with thyroid carcinoma.

Pathology

The disease represents a carcinoma developing in the parafollicular area, or C cells, of the thyroid gland. It seems clear that the carcinoma can arise in multiple foci within a single gland. It is characterized histologically by a marked degree of aneuploidy and an amyloid stroma. In spite of its malignant appearance histologically, the tumor usually grows slowly and spreads to the local lymph nodes. Hematogenous dissemination occurs in the late stages of the disease. Before the advent of assays for plasma CT, the tumors usually grew to a considerable size before the patient sought medical attention. Nearly all these tumors, however, even the most undifferentiated, secrete excessive amounts of CT, and it is now possible with radioimmunoassay to detect very small tumors (see p. 696).

Another feature of this disease is the very common association with pheochromocytomas, parathyroid adenomas, and rarely with ACTH-secreting tumors. Both the pheochromocytomas and ACTH-secreting tumors arise from chromaffin tissue, which has the same histologic and histochemical characteristics as the thyroid C cells. It has been suggested that these all represent primary chromaffin neoplasms with differing endocrine expression. In support of this thesis are kindred in which nearly all afflicted members have both medullary carcinoma and pheochromocytoma with a high incidence of ACTH-secreting tumors, and other kindred in which only medullary carcinoma or pheochromocytoma occurs. In individuals of the first group, either one of the tumors may become manifest years before the other.

There are at least five separate forms of this disease which have been recognized: (1) a sporadic nonfamilial type; (2) a familial type; (3) a familial type with associated pheochromocytoma; (4) a familial type with pheochromocytoma and hyperparathyroidism; and (5) a neuroma phenotype.

In contrast, the appearance of parathyroid adenomas often seems to follow the development of medullary carcinoma. Because of this, it has been argued that the parathyroid dysfunction represents a reactive response to the long-continued hypersecretion of CT. It remains distinctly possible, however, that the high incidence of parathyroid hyperplasia and adenomas is an additional manifestation of the primary disease, particularly in view of the fact that patients from families with a high incidence of medullary carcinoma may have

elevated PTH concentrations at a time when their CT values are normal (Fig. 11–60).

The syndrome of parathyroid adenoma, medullary carcinoma, and pheochromocytoma is distinct from the syndrome of multiple endocrine adenomatosis which usually includes the association of parathyroid hyperplasia with functioning islet-cell tumors of the pancreas, and with adenomas of the pituitary adrenals and thyroid. Intractable peptic ulcer may also coexist with gastrin-secreting islet-cell tumors.

In addition to functioning endocrine tumors, patients with medullary carcinoma often have multiple neuromas. The patients are frequently described as having an appearance similar to that of patients with Marfan's syndrome without, however, either the ocular or osseous lesions seen in this condition.

Pathophysiology

The principal effect of hypersecretion of CT of long duration is upon skeletal remodeling. Quantitative histologic examination of the bones of patients with this disease reveals a very marked reduction in the rate of both bone formation and bone resorption (Fig. 11–45). These changes are consistent with the model of cellular events depicted in Figure 11–10. The major actions of CT upon the bone cell population are two in number: (1) to increase the rate of modulation of osteoclasts to osteoblasts; and (2) to decrease the rate of activation of osteoprogenitor cells. When hypersecretion is of long duration, the second effect becomes of predominant importance, leading to a striking decrease in skeletal remodeling. The implication of these skeletal effects of CT is obvious. *Long-term CT administration in the adult will not increase bone formation.* On the contrary, it will decrease it (Fig. 11–17).

Perhaps the most surprising aspect of the med-

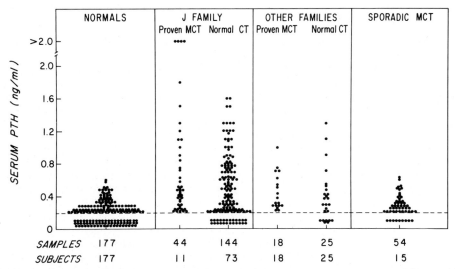

Figure 11–60. The serum PTH concentration in normal human subjects, in patients with proven medullary carcinoma of the thyroid and elevated serum CT concentrations, and in members of the same kindred without medullary carcinoma or elevated serum CT concentrations. The major point is that many of the kindred without increased concentrations of CT in serum did, nevertheless, have elevated concentrations of parathyroid hormone. (From Melvin, K. E. W., Miller, H. H., et al.: *New Eng. J. Med.* 285:1115, 1971.)

ullary carcinoma is that, in most of these patients, the plasma calcium concentration is normal or only slightly decreased, and the plasma phosphate is normal. The latter is surprising in view of the well-established acute effects of CT upon plasma phosphate concentration.

On the one hand, these observations reemphasize the fact, made repeatedly throughout this chapter, that mineral homeostasis can be maintained in conditions in which skeletal remodeling is either very rapid or very slow. There is no simple relation between the two. Of critical importance is the balance between bone formation and resorption rather than the overall rate of skeletal remodeling.

The other feature of these observations which is of considerable theoretical interest is the apparent lack of any long-term renal effect of CT in terms of phosphaturia and hypophosphatemia. Nonetheless, in patients with medullary carcinoma, nephrocalcinosis and renal calculi sometimes occur. These develop even though the rate of urinary excretion of calcium and phosphate is not high. This observation increases the likelihood that renal calcification develops because of changes in intracellular electrolyte metabolism and not because of extracellular events in the tubular lumens. Unfortunately, detailed studies of renal function in terms of acid and ammonia production, concentrating ability, response to exogenous PTH or C-AMP, and C-AMP excretion have not yet been reported. These data are needed in order to assess the association of hyperparathyroidism and normal plasma phosphate excretion. It would be of considerable interest if prolonged excessive plasma CT were found to block the phosphaturic effect of PTH.

Nothing is yet known about the gastrointestinal absorption of calcium in this condition or about possible alterations in vitamin D metabolism, but both represent important areas for further investigation.

Signs and Symptoms

If a medullary carcinoma is present without either pheochromocytoma or ACTH-secreting tumors, there may be few symptoms. The most common reason for seeking medical advice is the appearance of a thyroid nodule or goiter. Presentation because of a metastatic nodule is also common. In spite of the high incidence of pheochromocytoma, only a few patients present with the signs and symptoms of this disease. The signs and symptoms of hyperparathyroidism are not usually seen, except that nephrocalcinosis and urinary calculi are commonly observed.

Diagnosis

The single most important laboratory test is the radioimmunoassay for CT (p. 696). Of particular value is the measurement of CT concentration before and after a standard calcium infusion. In normal control subjects, the basal concentration is usually less than 0.10 ng. per ml. and never exceeds 0.38 ng. per ml. After the infusion of calcium gluconate for 4 hours at a rate of 15 mg. calcium per kg. body weight, the calcitonin concentration rises an average of two- to threefold but never exceeds 0.55 ng. per ml. In patients with medullary carcinoma, the basal values range from 0.30 to 1.8 ng. per ml., and after calcium infusion they rise severalfold to values from 2.9 to 29.0 ng. per ml. In those few patients with normal resting CT values, calcium infusion leads to a much greater than normal increase in CT secretion.

Using this assay, it is possible to show a rough correlation between plasma CT concentration after calcium infusion and the size of the tumor.

Treatment

The usefulness of the CT assay is that the disease can be detected at an early stage in affected siblings and in children in a particular kindred. Once the diagnosis is established, even without any detectable neck mass or other signs of the disease, total thyroidectomy with removal of the lymph nodes in the central zone of the neck is the only treatment. Even with small tumors the disease nearly always affects both lobes of the thyroid and often has already extended to the central cervical lymph nodes.

Dissection requires removal of the inferior parathyroids, which are almost always found hyperplastic. Because of this, transient postsurgical hypocalcemia is often seen, which may be a consequence of both the removal of hyperplastic parathyroid tissue and the release of CT from the manipulated thyroid gland.

Because of the high incidence of tumor recurrence, once patients have undergone thyroid surgery, they should be reevaluated at yearly intervals. This follow-up should include the assay of plasma CT after calcium infusion, since this is the only known diagnostic procedure which will detect the reappearance of functioning neoplastic tissue.

Secondary Hypercalcitoninemia

There is no known clinical syndrome in which a secondary increase in calcitonin secretion plays a role in its pathogenesis. It has been thought that patients with primary hyperparathyroidism without overt bone disease may be examples of a condition in which a secondary increase in CT secretion is sufficient to inhibit the osseous effects of the PTH without blocking its renal effects. To date, however, in those patients with primary hyperparathyroidism and definite hypercalcemia in whom CT assays have been performed, the values are usually normal. In such patients, measurement of the content of CT in their thyroid glands at the time of parathyroid surgery usually shows a significant decrease in CT content. These facts suggest that, in most patients with primary hyperparathyroidism, CT secretion may be high initially in response to the hypercalcemic stimulus, but if long-sustained, the hypercalcemia leads to a depletion of CT within the thyroid gland, after which the rate of CT synthesis is not rapid enough to maintain elevated plasma CT concentrations.

Hypocalcitoninemia

One of the unsettled problems in calcitonin physiology is that of determining its physiologic function in adult man. After total thyroidectomy, hypercalcemia is rarely, if ever, a problem. If patients without thyroids who are maintained on thyroxine, however, are subjected to a standard calcium infusion, they do exhibit an abnormally slow rate of disappearance of calcium from their plasma similar to the phenomenon observed in thyroparathyroidectomized dogs (Fig. 11–3). Under normal circumstances of dietary calcium intake, these same patients exhibit no postprandial hypercalcemia. Furthermore, examination of bone from such patients shows no evidence of increased skeletal remodeling or imbalance between formation and resorption.

Hence it must be concluded that, in adult man, deficiency or undersecretion of calcitonin does not lead to a recognizable clinical syndrome, and its roles in mineral homeostasis and skeletal remodeling are relatively unimportant.

THERAPEUTIC USES OF CALCITONIN IN THE TREATMENT OF DISORDERS OF SKELETAL HOMEOSTASIS

In spite of the fact that CT plays a minor physiologic role in the adult human, it has been recommended as a therapeutic agent in the treatment of certain diseases of the skeleton. In particular, it has been employed in the treatment of Paget's disease and postmenopausal osteoporosis. In order to discuss these uses of calcitonin, it is first necessary to consider the cellular basis of these two diseases. Both Paget's disease and osteoporosis represent disorders of skeletal, as opposed to mineral, homeostasis.

Paget's Disease

Paget's disease of bone is characterized by localized areas of increased skeletal remodeling. It was originally considered an inflammatory disease; on the basis of the model of cellular events depicted in Figure 11–10, however, it is best characterized as a benign hyperplasia or neoplasia of bone which leads to an increase in the activation of osteoprogenitor cells or bone metabolic units (Fig. 11–17). The most striking features of the disease are that (1) in general, the rates of increase in bone formation and resorption parallel each other (Figs. 11–38, 11–41, and 11–45), as is predicted by the model of cellular events (Fig. 11–10); (2) the new bone laid down is largely of the woven variety; (3) because of the rapid bone turnover and production of woven bone, the bone develops a characteristic mosaic pattern (Fig. 11–42); (4) the osteoclasts

vary greatly in size and in number of nuclei; (5) the osteoblasts vary greatly in size and staining characteristics; (6) plasma calcium concentration is usually normal, plasma phosphate is usually normal but may be high, and plasma alkaline phosphate and urinary calcium and hydroxyproline are elevated; (7) late in the course of the disease, osteosarcoma may develop; and (8) the disease is a primary disorder of skeletal remodeling, as shown by the fact that localized areas of intense remodeling exist next to areas of normal bone, i.e., it is not a generalized metabolic disease of bone.

Incidence

The disease is quite common, being diagnosed at autopsy in approximately 3 per cent of persons over 40. It is rarely seen in patients under 40, and it is seen with increasing frequency with advancing age. Probably less than 30 per cent of all patients, however, have symptomatic disease that is recognized before death. Even when recognized, the disease is only slowly progressive but may eventually lead to marked disability.

Signs and Symptoms

The cardinal features of the disease are (1) skeletal deformity; (2) bone pain; (3) symptoms, including deafness, related to compression of cranial or spinal nerves from bone overgrowth; (4) an increase in blood flow through the affected regions of bone, which may lead to a significant increase in skin temperature over the affected area, and, of greater seriousness, if the bone involvement is extensive, to high-output congestive heart failure; (5) normocalcemia in general (Table 11–14), but hypercalcemia may develop if a patient is immobilized; and (6) hypercalciuria and increased urinary hydroxyproline excretion (Table 11–14).

Diagnosis

The diagnosis can usually be made on clinical grounds and by x-ray (Fig. 11–52). Histologic examination of the affected bone is also useful. The only diagnostic difficulty comes in making certain that, in cases with hypercalcemia, coexistent hyperparathyroidism is not present. Likewise, it is important to be aware of the fact that osteosarcoma eventually occurs in a small percentage of these patients. It is usually a rapidly progressing tumor.

Treatment

The most successful form of therapy at present is the prolonged administration of human calcitonin. Other forms of therapy that have been recommended are mithramycin, diphosphonates, and fluoride. These will not be discussed here. Three aspects of CT therapy will be considered: (1) indications for its use; (2) the dosage and course of therapy; and (3) the results of therapy, and the implications in terms of the pathogenesis of the disease and the cellular basis of skeletal remodeling.

Indications

Not all patients with Paget's disease require treatment. At present the major indications for CT use are (1) bone pain; (2) prevention of further deformity; and (3) congestive heart failure.

Bone pain is probably the most common symptom, but its cause is not known. Nevertheless, it can be severe and persistent. Congestive heart failure is a rare feature of the disease and indicates extensive involvement of the skeleton. Deformity of some degree is quite common, and it may be difficult to decide in an individual case whether therapy is warranted. Hypercalciuria occurs in 10 to 20 per cent of patients and is usually also indicative of very active disease. It is not clear whether increased hydroxyproline excretion or plasma alkaline phosphatase should be used as indications for therapy, but they have proved of great value in following the course of CT therapy.

The other unknown factor is whether long-term CT therapy will decrease the incidence of the development of sarcoma. Insufficient data are available upon which to make this decision.

Dose and Course of Treatment

When patients with Paget's disease are given CT either intravenously or intramuscularly, there is a very rapid decrease in the urinary excretion of hydroxyproline and calcium. Bone biopsies reveal a striking decrease in osteoclast count. Long-term daily administration of 0.5 to 1.0 mg. of CT leads to a progressive fall in hydroxyproline excretion, until nearly normal rates of excretion are observed after several months of therapy. Plasma alkaline phosphatase also declines, but at a slower rate, and after 4 months or more of therapy, it will often fall into the normal range. In patients with the most severe form of the disease, these values may not return to normal even after 6 to 12 months of treatment.

Long-term treatment relieves bone pain. Bone biopsies reveal a decrease in both bone formation surfaces and bone resorption surfaces. Moreover, the new bone has a normal lamellar structure.

The dose of CT needed to induce these changes varies in different patients. There is as yet insufficient experience to determine an optimal dosage schedule. Some patients have responded to a dose as small as 0.5 mg. once a week, whereas others have shown an incomplete response on this dose schedule.

The disadvantages of this therapy are that (1) CT can only be given by injection; and (2) CT administration may lead to flushing, tingling, nausea, and a sense of uneasiness for 30 or more minutes after its administration. Some patients complain of not feeling well while on the hormone.

Salmon and porcine CT have also been used successfully in the treatment of this disease, but patients treated with these peptides have developed neutralizing antibodies against them, so their use is not to be recommended.

Implications

All our present evidence supports the view that Paget's disease represents a hormone-sensitive benign neoplasia of bone in which the neoplastic cells carry out their normal remodeling function, albeit in a disordered manner. The most compelling fact about CT therapy is that it leads to a decrease first in bone resorption and then in formation. This sequence is exactly what would be predicted on the basis of the model of cellular events in Figure 11–10, and it emphasizes the fact that the two processes in skeletal remodeling are coupled and sequential in nature. This explains why both are increased in this disease and why both decrease following CT therapy.

Osteoporosis

Osteoporosis is the most common generalized disorder of bone. It is characterized as a state of insufficient calcified bone (Table 11–14 and Figs. 11–37, 11–41, 11–42, and 11–45) and is the end result of a number of disease states that affect the skeleton.

Etiology and Pathogenesis

A few causes of osteoporosis are recognized: adrenal cortical hyperfunction, hyperparathyroidism, hyperthyroidism, acromegaly, prolonged calcium deficiency, and prolonged immobilization. In some young individuals it appears without cause, however, and in many older people, particularly postmenopausal women, no single etiologic agent has been identified.

The development of postmenopausal osteoporosis ultimately depends upon a long-sustained imbalance between rates of bone formation and bone resorption in favor of resorptive activity (Figs. 11–17, 11–41, 11–42, and 11–45). Two general theories have been advanced to account for the development of this disease: (1) the major defect is a decreased rate of new bone formation; and (2) the major defect is enhanced bone resorption.

In order to discuss these alternatives, it is necessary first to reconsider the normal sequence of age-related events in the human skeleton (Figs. 11–9, 11–41, 11–44, and 11–45). From the age of 35 to 40 onward, there is normally a progressive loss of skeletal mass. This loss is predominantly due to a sustained imbalance between resorption and formation upon the endosteal and haversian bone surfaces. In fact, there is a slight positive balance of formation upon the periosteal surface (Fig. 11–9). In view of this normal age-related loss of skeletal mass, it is difficult to decide whether senile osteoporosis represents a distinct disease entity or an exaggeration of this normal physiologic change. On the one hand, it has been proposed that the mass of the skeleton at age 40 is the prime determinant of whether or not a given individual will develop the disease. In this view, persons with a more massive skeleton at age 40 and those with a smaller skeletal mass lose bone mass at the same rate with age, with the consequence that the person with the smaller skeleton develops a skeleton so thin as to lead to a high incidence of fractures in later life. In support of this are the facts that men, having greater skeletal mass than women, are less prone to senile osteoporosis; and that Negroes, having a greater skeletal mass than whites, also have a lesser incidence of senile osteoporosis. On the other hand, the incidence of osteoporosis is low in Orientals, in spite of the fact that their average skeletal mass at age 40 is less than that of Caucasians. This observation has raised a question as to the possible importance of genetic and cultural factors.

Among the latter, one of the most important may be physical activity. Older women in Oriental countries continue to perform heavy manual labor, whereas this is not the rule in western society. In Europeans with osteoporosis, there is a very good correlation between the ash weight of the lumbar vertebrae and the weight of the psoas muscle. The inference from this correlation is that one of the major determinants of muscle mass is physical activity, and in turn, the greater the physical activity and muscle mass, the greater the deforming stress placed upon bone, with a greater stimulus to the modulation of osteoclasts to osteoblasts resulting in net bone formation (Figs. 11–10 and 11–36). This shift in bone remodeling activity in favor of bone formation leads to an increase in skeletal mass.

Direct support for this hypothesis is the fact that, using photon absorption techniques to assess skeletal mass *in vivo* (p. 713), it has been shown that a program of increasing physical activity in a group of women over 50 years old led to a significant increase in skeletal mass.

A second cultural factor of possible importance is nutrition. A number of studies have suggested that deficiencies of calcium or vitamin D intake or both may contribute to the pathogenesis of the disease by leading to a relative calcium deficiency, secondary hyperparathyroidism, and negative skeletal balance. The evidence in support of this viewpoint is not decisive, however.

When the bones of patients with crush fractures of the vertebral spine (an objective criterion of osteoporosis) are compared with those of age-matched controls, the only difference found by quantitative histologic analysis is a more profound reduction in active bone formation surface (Fig. 11–45). Both groups exhibit a significant increase in total resorption surface. These findings, although indicating a difference in degree, emphasize only the similarity of skeletal changes in aging to those in osteoporosis and leave unresolved the question of whether or not there is a clear distinction between the disease and the physiologic state.

There have been two general theories as to the pathogenesis of this disease. Albright's original thesis was that the disease represented a failure of bone formation. Examination of bone biopsy material by microradiography, however, showed that there was a marked increase in extent of total resorption surface but little change in extent of formation surface (Fig. 11–41), hence the proposal that the primary change in skeletal homeostasis was an increase in active bone resorption. On the basis of this and the known inhibitory effects of CT upon bone resorption, CT was recommended as a therapeutic agent in this disease.

There was one unexplained observation, however – a discrepancy between microradiographic and ordinary histologic analysis of osteoporotic bone. The discrepancy was that, in spite of the fact that the extent of resorption measured microradiographically in osteoporosis was as high as in primary hyperparathyroidism (Fig. 11–41), there were few osteoclasts present upon the endosteal surfaces in osteoporotic bone but numerous osteoclasts in the bone of hyperparathyroid subjects.

Quantitative histologic analysis has been instrumental in explaining this discrepancy and in defining the likely pathogenesis of skeletal loss. When undecalcified stained bone sections from osteoporotic subjects are examined by quantitative histologic means, it is clear that the total resorption surface is increased (Fig. 11–45), but the active resorption surface decreases, as does the active formation surface. Likewise, the osteoclast count is normal or low, and the osteoclasts contain less than the normal number of nuclei. In addition, there is an increase in the number of terminal seams, i.e., areas in which active bone formation has ceased but the remaining osteoid has not yet become mineralized. These data clearly imply that total resorption surface can be measured by microradiography, but the distinction between active and inactive resorption surfaces cannot be made by this method. Likewise, microradiographic estimation of formation surfaces includes both active and inactive osteoid seams, so that by using this method, the extent of active formation surface is overestimated, as is active resorption surface.

From the model of cellular events in Figure 11–10, a logical sequence of events during the development of osteoporosis would be the following: (1) the activation of osteoprogenitor cells continues at a normal or slightly reduced rate; (2) these cells progress to osteoclasts which contain fewer nuclei and which may be less active than normal; and (3) the major defect is in the modulation of osteoclasts to osteoblasts (Figs. 11–10 and 11–17) and in the subsequent function of these osteoblasts. As a consequence, there is a delay between the cessation of active resorption and the initiation of subsequent formation. With time, this leads to an increase in total resorption surface, of which an increasing percentage is inactive rather than active surface. Moreover, there appears to be a delay between matrix formation and its ultimate mineralization, leading to an increase in the number of terminal osteoid seams.

In this view, the primary defect is in the process of bone cell modulation and in osteoblast function. This view is supported by the fact that the plasma

PTH concentrations are normal and not high in most osteoporotic subjects.

A question of major importance is whether or not this defect in bone cell modulation is an irreversible consequence of the aging process, or whether, by appropriate means, it can be reversed. The answer appears to be that it is not an irreversible indicator of senility. Two observations, in particular, point to this conclusion. The first is that a well-controlled program of physical activity in a group of elderly subjects has been shown to induce a definite increase in skeletal mass. The second is that treatment of osteoporotic subjects with fluoride leads to a definite and often striking increase in bone mass. Unfortunately, much of the bone is poorly organized structurally and fails to mineralize, so that it is structurally poor bone. Examination of bone from osteoporotic subjects treated with fluoride shows an increase in active resorption surface and total resorption surface, but a much more marked increase in active bone formation surface, i.e., osteoblastic proliferation. It also reveals a marked increase in the extent of osteoid. Thus fluoride stimulates the activation of osteoprogenitor cells and the modulation of osteoclasts to osteoblasts, with a resulting increase in bone matrix synthesis, but simultaneously blocks the subsequent mineralization of this new matrix.

These data show that the bone cells in osteoporotic subjects can be stimulated to restore the balance or reverse the negative skeletal balance characteristic of this disease. Clearly, however, fluoride, because it inhibits mineralization, is not totally satisfactory as an agent with which to treat this disease. A proper therapeutic balance of fluoride and vitamin D therapy, however, has been reported to result in a net increase in the amount of calcified bone in osteoporotic subjects, but vitamin D therapy has not been universally successful in inducing mineralization of the osteoid that appears during fluoride therapy.

From a combination of the above reasoning and the previous discussion of the action of CT upon bone cell turnover (Fig. 11-10) and the appearance of bone in patients with medullary carcinoma (Fig. 11-45), it is clear that CT should not be an effective therapeutic agent in osteoporosis. This has proved to be the case. CT treatment has not produced a sustained positive calcium or skeletal balance in osteoporotic patients. It remains possible that, if used with another agent capable of inducing the activation of osteoprogenitor cells, CT might then help to shift the active bone cell population to osteoblasts (Fig. 11-10).

Therapeutic Implications

At present, there is no satisfactory form of treatment for this disease. It is obvious that in most instances it develops slowly over a period of years, and that the ideal medical management should be concerned with prevention rather than cure. In terms of events in the skeleton (Fig. 11-10), it becomes clear that in order to rebuild bone mass or prevent its loss, two processes need to be influenced.

One process is the activation of osteoprogenitor cells to form new metabolic units in bone. The most effective agent to bring this about is PTH. Unfortunately, PTH also blocks the modulation of osteoclasts to osteoblasts (Fig. 11-10). It also seems clear that GH will activate these cells, particularly those in the periosteal bone cell envelope. It is possible that $1,25(OH)_2D_3$ or some synthetic metabolite of vitamin D_3 will also prove effective as an activator of osteoprogenitor cells.

The other process is that of the modulation of osteoclasts to osteoblasts (Fig. 11-10). Unfortunately, PTH inhibits this process also. The three recognized factors that stimulate this conversion are CT, phosphate, and the mechanical stresses related to physical activity. In addition, it seems likely that fluoride, by stabilizing the mineral crystal structure, inhibits the resorptive action of osteoclasts and thereby increases the flow of osteoclasts to osteoblasts.

It seems possible that an effective therapy may be developed by the proper combination of these various therapeutic agents: vitamin D metabolites, PTH, phosphate, fluoride, physical activity, and GH.

REFERENCES

Conference Proceedings and Monographs

Albright, F., and Reifenstein, E. C.: *The Parathyroid Glands and Metabolic Bone Disease.* Baltimore, Williams and Wilkins Co., 1948.

Barzel, U. S. (ed.), *Osteoporosis.* New York, Grune and Stratton, 1970.

Cuthbert, A. (ed.), *Calcium and Cellular Function.* London, Macmillan and Co., Ltd., 1970.

Frost, H. M. (ed.), *Bone Biodynamics.* Boston, Little, Brown and Co., 1964.

Frost, H. M.: *Mathematical Elements of Lamellar Bone Remodeling.* Springfield, Ill., Charles C Thomas, 1964.

Frost, H. M.: *The Bone Dynamics in Osteoporosis and Osteomalacia.* Springfield, Ill., Charles C Thomas, 1966.

Garn, S. M.: *The Earlier Gain and the Later Loss of Cortical Bone.* Springfield, Ill., Charles C Thomas, 1970.

Hioco, D. J. (ed.), *Phosphate et Métabolisme Phosphacalcique.* Paris, Laboratoires Sandoz, 1971.

MacIntyre, I. (ed.), Calcium metabolism and bone disease, In *Clinics in Endocrinology and Metabolism.* Vol. 1. London, W. B. Saunders, Ltd., 1972.

Neuman, W. F., and Neuman, M. W.: *The Chemical Dynamics of Bone Mineral.* Chicago, University of Chicago Press, 1958.

Nichols, G., Jr., and Wasserman, R. H. (eds.), *Cellular Mechanisms for Calcium Transfer and Homeostasis.* New York, Academic Press, 1971.

Rasmussen, H., and Bordier, P.: *Bone Cells, Mineral Homeostasis and Skeletal Remodeling.* Baltimore, Williams and Wilkins Co., 1973.

Shelling, D. H.: *The Parathyroids in Health and Disease.* St. Louis, C. V. Mosby Co., 1935.

Talmage, R. V., and Belanger, L. F. (eds.), *Parathyroid Hormone and Thyrocalcitonin (Calcitonin).* Amsterdam, Excerpta Medica, 1968.

Talmage, R. V., and Munson, P. L. (eds.), *Calcium, Parathyroid Hormone and the Calcitonins.* Amsterdam, Excerpta Medica, 1972.

Vaughan, J. M.: *The Physiology of Bone.* Oxford, Clarendon Press, 1970.

Reviews

Aurbach, G. D., Kentmann, H. T., et al.: Structure, synthesis, and mechanism of action of parathyroid hormone. *Recent Progr. Hormone Res.* 28:353, 1972.

Borle, A. B.: Membrane transfer of calcium. *Clin. Orthop.* 52:267, 1967.

Copp, D. H.: Calcitonin and parathyroid hormone. *Ann. Rev. Pharmacol.* 9:327, 1969.

Copp, D. H.: Endocrine regulation of calcium metabolism. *Ann. Rev. Physiol.* 32:61, 1970.

DeLuca, H. F.: The role of vitamin D and its relationship to parathyroid hormone and calcitonin. *Recent Progr. Hormone Res.* 27:479, 1971.

Glimcher, M. J., and Krane, S. M.: The organization and structure of bone, and the mechanism of calcification, In *A Treatise On Collagen.* Vol. II. London, Academic Press, 1968.

Grant, M. E., and Prockop, D. J.: Biosynthesis of collagen. *New Eng. J. Med.* 286:194, 1972.

Harris, W. H., and Heaney, R. P.: Skeletal renewal and metabolic bone disease. *New Eng. J. Med.* 280:193, 1969.

Hirsch, P. F., and Munson, P. L.: Thyrocalcitonin. *Physiol. Rev.* 49:548, 1969.

Irving, J. T., and Wuthier, R. E.: Histochemistry and biochemistry of calcification with special reference to the role of lipids. *Clin. Orthop.* 56:237, 1968.

Kimberg, D. V.: Effects of vitamin D and steroid hormones on the active transport of calcium by the intestine. *New Eng. J. Med.* 280:1396, 1969.

Lehninger, A. L.: Mitochondria and calcium transport. *Biochem. J.* 119:129, 1970.

Melvin, K. E. W., Tashjian, A. H., Jr., et al.: Studies in familial (medullary) thyroid carcinoma. *Recent Progr. Hormone Res.* 28:399, 1972.

Posner, A. S.: Crystal chemistry of bone mineral. *Physiol. Rev.* 49:760, 1969.

Prockop, D. J., and Kivirikko, K. J.: Relationship of hydroxyproline excretion in urine to collagen metabolism. *Ann. Intern. Med.* 66:1243, 1967.

Raisz, L. G., and Bingham, P. J.: Effect of hormones on bone development. *Ann. Rev. Pharmacol.* 12:337, 1972.

Rasmussen, H.: Parathyroid hormone: Nature and mechanism of action. *Amer. J. Med.* 30:112, 1961.

Rasmussen, H.: Mitochondrial ion transport mechanism and physiological significance. *Fed. Proc.* 25:903, 1966.

Rasmussen, H.: Cell communication, calcium ion, and cyclic adenosine monophosphate. *Science* 170:404, 1970.

Rasmussen, H.: Ionic and hormonal control of calcium homeostasis. *Amer. J. Med.* 50:567, 1971.

Rasmussen, H., Feinblatt, J., et al.: Effect of ions upon bone cell function. *Fed. Proc.* 29:1190, 1970.

Rasmussen, H., Goodman, D. B. P., et al.: The role of cyclic AMP and calcium in cell activation. *CRC Crit. Rev. Biochem.* 1:95, 1972.

Steendijk, R.: Metabolic bone disease in children. *Clin. Orthop.* 77:247, 1971.

Talmage, R. V.: Morphological and physiological considerations in a new concept of calcium transport in bone. *Amer. J. Anat.* 129:467, 1970.

Urist, M. R., and Craven, P. L.: Bone cell differentiation in avian species: With comments on multinucleation and morphogenesis. *Fed. Proc.* 29:1680, 1970.

Wallach, S., Chausmer, A. B., et al.: Hormonal effects on calcium transport in liver. *Clin. Orthop.* 78:40, 1971.

Weidmann, S. M.: Calcification of skeletal tissues. *Int. Rev. Connect. Tissue Res.* 1:339, 1963.

Literature

Adams, P., Chalmers, T. M., et al.: Idiopathic hypercalciuria and hyperparathyroidism. *Brit. Med. J.* 4:582, 1970.

Adams, P. H., Jowsey, J., et al.: Effects of hyperthyroidism on bone and mineral metabolism in man. *Quart J. Med.* 36:1, 1967.

Adams, T. H., Wong, R. G., et al.: Studies on the mechanism of action of calciferol. II. Effects of the polyene antibiotic, filipin, on vitamin D–mediated calcium transport. *J. Biol. Chem.* 245:4432, 1970.

Agus, Z. S., Puschett, J. B., et al.: Mode of action of parathyroid hormone and cyclic adenosine-3′-5′-monophosphate on renal tubular phosphate reabsorption in the dog. *J. Clin. Invest.* 50:617, 1971.

Albright, F.: A page out of the history of hyperparathyroidism. *J. Clin. Endocr.* 8:637, 1948.

Anast, C., Mohs, J. M., et al.: Evidence for parathyroid failure in magnesium deficiency. *Science* 177:606, 1972.

Anderson, H. C., Matsuzawa, T., et al.: Membranous particles in calcifying cartilage matrix. *Trans. N.Y. Acad. Sci.* 32:619, 1970.

Arnaud, S., Goldsmith, R. S., et al.: Serum parathyroid hormone, blood minerals, and growth: Interrelationships in normal children, 1972 (in press).

Arnaud, C. D., Sizemore, G. W., et al.: Human parathyroid hormone: Glandular and secreted molecular species. *Amer. J. Med.* 50:630, 1971.

Arnaud, C. D., Tsao, H. S., et al.: Radioimmunoassay of human parathyroid hormone in serum. *J. Clin. Invest.* 50:21, 1971.

Aurbach, G. D., and Chase, L. R.: Cyclic-3′,5′-adenylic acid in bone and the mechanism of parathyroid hormone. *Fed. Proc.* 29:1179, 1970.

Balsan, S., and Garabedian, M.: 25-hydroxycholecalciferol: A comparative study in deficiency rickets and different types of resistant rickets. *J. Clin. Invest.* 51:749, 1972.

Bassett, C. A. L.: Biologic significance of piezoelectricity. *Calcif. Tissue Res.* 1:252, 1968.

Baud, C. A.: Submicroscopic structure and functional aspects of the osteocyte. *Clin. Orthop.* 56:227, 1968.

Baylink, D., Stauffer, M., et al.: Formation mineralization and resorption of bone in vitamin D–deficient rats. *J. Clin. Invest.* 49:1122, 1970.

Baylink, D., Wergedal, J., et al.: Formation, mineralization, and resorption of bone in hypophosphatemic rats. *J. Clin. Invest.* 50:2519, 1971.

Bell, N. H., Avery, S., et al.: Effects of dibutyryl cyclic adenosine-3′,5′-monophosphate and parathyroid extract on calcium and phosphorus metabolism in hypoparathyroidism and pseudohypoparathyroidism. *J. Clin. Invest.* 51:816, 1972.

Bernard, G. W.: An electron microscopic study of initial intramembranous ossification. *Amer. J. Anat.* 125:271, 1969.

Bijvoet, O. L. M.: Relation of plasma phosphate concentration to renal tubular reabsorption of phosphate. *Clin. Sci.* 37:23, 1969.

Bijvoet, O. L. M., van der Sluys Veer, J., et al.: Effects of calcitonin on patients with Paget's disease, thyrotoxicosis or hypercalcemia. *Lancet* 1:876, 1968.

Bijvoet, O. L. M., van der Sluys Veer, J., et al.: Natriuretic effect of calcitonin in man. *New Eng. J. Med.* 284:681, 1971.

Bingham, P. J., Brazell, I. A., et al.: The effect of parathyroid extract on cellular activity and plasma calcium levels *in vivo. J. Endocr.* 45:387, 1969.

Birge, S. J., Peck, W. A., et al.: Study of calcium absorption in man: A kinetic analysis and physiologic model. *J. Clin. Invest.* 48:1705, 1969.

Bonnucci, E.: The locus of initial calcification in cartilage and bone. *Clin. Orthop.* 78:108, 1971.

Bordier, P., Miravet, L., et al.: Bone changes in adult patients with abnormal thyroid function (with special reference to ^{45}Ca kinetic and quantitative histology). *Proc. Roy. Soc. Med. 60(II)*:1132, 1967.

Bordier, P., Tun-Chot, S., et al.: Histological measurement of bone formation and resorption in Paget's disease: Effects of human calcitonin therapy. *Europ. J. Clin. Invest.*, 1973 (in press).

Borle, A. B.: Le turn-over du calcium dans l'organisme et les principaux points d'impact hormonaux. *Extrait de Problèmes Actuels d'Endocrinologie et de Nutrition. (Série No. 15)*:5, 1972.

Boyle, I. T., Gray, R. W., et al.: Regulation by calcium of *in vivo* synthesis of 1,25-dihydroxycholecalciferol and 21,25-dihydroxycholecalciferol. *Proc. Nat. Acad. Sci.* (USA) 68:2131, 1971.

Brewer, H. B., Jr., and Ronan, R.: Bovine parathyroid hormone: Amino acid sequence. *Proc. Nat. Acad. Sci.* (USA) 67:1862, 1970.

Brewer, H. B., Jr., Schlueter, R. J., et al.: Isolation and characterization of bovine thyrocalcitonin. *J. Biol. Chem.* 245:4232, 1970.

Brewer, H. B., Jr., Fairwell, T., et al.: Human parathyroid hormone: Amino acid sequence of the amino terminal residues, 1–34. *Proc. Nat. Acad. Sci.* (USA) 69:3585, 1972.

Bricker, N. S.: On the pathogenesis of the uremic state. *New Eng. J. Med.* 286:1093, 1972.

Cameron, J. R., Mazess, R. B., et al.: Precision and accuracy of bone mineral determination by direct photon absorptiometry. *Invest. Radiol. 3*:41, 1968.

Cannigia, A., Gennari, C., et al.: Initial increase of plasma radioactive calcium after intravenous injection of calcitonin in man. *Clin. Sci. 43*:171, 1972.

Carlsson, A.: The cause of hypophosphatemia and hypocalcemia in vitamin D deficiency. *Acta Physiol. Scand. 31*:308, 1954.

Chance, B.: The energy-linked reaction of calcium with mitochondria. *J. Biol. Chem. 240*:2729, 1965.

Chase, L. R., and Aurbach, G. D.: The effect of parathyroid hormone on the concentration of adenosine-3',5'-monophosphate in skeletal tissue *in vitro. J. Biol. Chem. 245*:1520, 1970.

Chase, L. R., Melson, G. L., et al.: Pseudohypoparathyroidism: Defective excretion of 3',5'-AMP in response to parathyroid hormone. *J. Clin. Invest. 48*:1832, 1969.

Cooper, C. W., Schwesinger, W. H., et al.: Thyrocalcitonin: Stimulation of secretion by pentagastrin. *Science 172*:1238, 1971.

DeLong, A., Feinblatt, J., et al.: The effect of pyrophosphate infusion on the response of the thyro-parathyroidectomized rat to parathyroid hormone and adenosine-3',5'-cyclic monophosphate. *Calcif. Tissue Res. 8*:87, 1971.

Dent, C. E.: Rickets and osteomalacia from renal tubule defects. *J. Bone Joint Surg. 34B*:266, 1952.

Donaldson, C. L., Hulley, S. B., et al.: Effect of prolonged bed rest on bone mineral. *Metabolism 19*:1017, 1970.

Doyle, F. H.: Radiology of the skeleton in endocrine disease. *Proc. Roy. Soc. Med. 60*:1131, 1967.

Doyle, F. H.: Age-related bone changes in women. *J. Physiol. 202*:25P, 1969.

Fleisch, H., Russell, R. G. G., et al.: Diphosphonates inhibit hydroxyapatite dissolution *in vitro* and bone resorption in tissue culture and *in vivo. Science 165*:1262, 1969.

Fleisch, H., Russell, R. G. G., et al.: Prevention by a diphosphonate of immobilization osteoporosis in rats. *Nature* (London) *223*:211, 1969.

Fleisch, H., Russell, R. G. G., et al.: Effect of pyrophosphate on hydroxyapatite and its implications in calcium homeostasis. *Nature* (London) *212*:901, 1966.

Fournier, A. E., Arnaud, C. D., et al.: Etiology of hyperparathyroidism and bone disease during chronic hemodialysis II. *J. Clin. Invest. 50*:599, 1971.

Fournier, A. E., Johnson, W. J., et al.: Etiology of hyperparathyroidism and bone disease during chronic hemodialysis I. *J. Clin. Invest. 50*:592, 1971.

Fraser, D. R., and Kodicek, E.: Unique biosynthesis by kidney of a biologically active vitamin D metabolite. *Nature* (London) *228*:764, 1970.

Fraser, D., Kooh, S. W., et al.: Hyperparathyroidism as the cause of hyperaminoaciduria and phosphaturia in human vitamin D deficiency. *Pediat. Res. 1*:425, 1967.

Gaillard, P. J.: Parathyroid gland and bone *in vivo. Schweiz. Med. Wschr. 87*(Suppl. 14):447, 1957.

Gaillard, P. J.: Bone culture studies with thyrocalcitonin. *Proc. Kon. Nederl. Akad. Wet.* (Biol. Med.) *70*:309, 1967.

Garn, S. M., Rohmann, C. G., et al.: Bone loss as a general phenomenon in man. *Fed. Proc. 26*:1729, 1967.

Glimcher, M., and Katz, E. P.: The organization of collagen in bone: The role of noncovalent bonds in the relative insolubility of bone collagen. *J. Ultrastruct. Res. 12*:705, 1965.

Glorieux, F., and Scriver, C. R.: Loss of a parathyroid hormone-sensitive component of phosphate transport in X-linked hypophosphatemia. *Science 175*:997, 1972.

Glorieux, F. H., Scriver, C. R., et al.: Prevention of dwarfism and rickets in X-linked hypophosphatemia. *New Eng. J. Med. 287*:481, 1972.

Goldsmith, R. S., Furszyler, J., et al.: Control of secondary hyperparathyroidism during long-term hemodialysis. *Amer. J. Med. 50*:692, 1971.

Goldsmith, R. S., and Ingbar, S. H.: Inorganic phosphate treatment of hypercalcemia of diverse etiologies. *New Eng. J. Med. 274*:1, 1966.

Greenberg, B. G., Winters, R. W., et al.: The normal range of serum inorganic phosphorous and its utility as a discriminant in the diagnosis of congenital hypophosphatemia. *J. Clin. Endocr. 20*:364, 1960.

Giedmondsson, T. V., MacIntyre, I., et al.: The isolation of thyrocalcitonin and a study of its effect in the rat. *Proc. Roy. Soc. Med. 164B*:460, 1965.

Haas, H. G., Dambacher, M. A., et al.: Renal effects of calcitonin and parathyroid extract in man. *J. Clin. Invest. 50*:2689, 1971.

Haddad, J. G., Jr., Chyu, K., et al.: Serum concentration of 25-hydroxyvitamin D_3 in sex-linked hypophosphatemic vitamin D–resistant rickets. *J. Lab. Clin. Med. 81*:22, 1973.

Hahn, T. J., Hendin, B. A., et al.: Effect of anticonvulsant therapy on serum 25-hydroxycalciferol. *New Eng. J. Med. 287*:900, 1972.

Haussler, M. R., Boyce, D. W., et al.: A rapidly acting metabolite of vitamin D. *Proc. Nat. Acad. Sci* (USA) *68*:177, 1971.

Hellman, D. E., Au, W. Y. W., et al.: Evidence for a direct effect of parathyroid hormone on urinary acidification. *Amer. J. Physiol. 209*:643, 1965.

Isaksson, B., Lindholm, B., et al.: A critical evaluation of the calcium balance technic. II. Dermal calcium losses. *Metabolism 16*:303, 1967.

Jee, W. S. S., Roberts, W. E., et al.: Interrelated effects of glucocorticoid and parathyroid hormone upon bone remodelling, In *Calcium, Parathyroid Hormone, and The Calcitonins.* Talmage, R. V., and Munson, P. L. (eds), Amsterdam, Excerpta Medica Foundation, 1972, p. 430.

Johnston, C. C., Smith, D. M., et al.: *In vivo* measurement of bone mass in the radius. *Metabolism 17*:1140, 1968.

Jowsey, J., and Detenbeck, L. C.: Importance of thyroid hormones in bone metabolism and calcium homeostasis. *Endocrinology 85*:87, 1969.

Jowsey, J., Riggs, B. L., et al.: Effects of prolonged administration or porcine calcitonin in postmenopausal osteoporosis. *J. Clin. Endocr. 33*:752, 1971.

Jowsey, J., Riggs, B. L., et al.: Effect of combined therapy with sodium fluoride, vitamin D and calcium in osteoporosis. *Amer. J. Med. 53*:43, 1972.

Jubiz, W., Canterbury, J. M., et al.: Circadian rhythm in serum parathyroid hormone concentration in human subjects: Correlation with serum calcium, phosphate, albumin, and growth hormone levels. *J. Clin. Invest. 51*:2040, 1972.

Kalu, D. N., Pennock, J., et al.: Parathyroid hormone and experimental osteosclerosis. *Lancet 1*:1363, 1970.

Kaye, M., Chatterjee, M. B., et al.: Arrest of hyperparathyroid bone disease with dihydrotachysterol in patients undergoing chronic hemodialysis. *Ann. Intern. Med. 73*:225, 1970.

Kimberg, D. V., Baerg, R. D., et al.: Effect of cortisone treatment on the active transport of calcium by the small intestine. *J. Clin. Invest. 50*:1309, 1971.

Krane, S. M., Muñoz, A. J., et al.: Urinary polypeptides related to collagen synthesis. *J. Clin. Invest. 49*:716, 1970.

Lafferty, F. W.: Pseudohyperparathyroidism. *Medicine 45*:247, 1966.

Lawson, D. E. M., Fraser, D. R., et al.: Identification of 1,25-dihydroxycholecalciferol, a new kidney hormone controlling calcium metabolism. *Nature* (London) *230*:228, 1971.

Lee, W. R., Marshall, J. H., et al.: Calcium accretion and bone formation in dogs: An experimental comparison between the results of Ca^{45} kinetic analysis and tetracycline labelling. *J. Bone Joint Surg. 47B*:157, 1965.

Lichtman, M. A., Miller, D. R., et al.: Reduced red cell glycolysis, 2,3-diphosphoglycerate, and adenosine triphosphate concentration, and increased hemoglobin-oxygen affinity caused by hypophosphatemia. *Ann. Intern. Med. 74*:562, 1971.

Loomis, W. F.: Skin pigment regulation of vitamin D biosynthesis in man. *Science 157*:501, 1967.

Lotz, M., Zisman, E., et al.: Evidence for a phosphorus-depletion syndrome in man. *New Eng. J. Med. 278*:409, 1968.

Martin, J. H., and Matthews, J. L.: Mitochondrial granules in chondrocytes, osteoblasts and osteocytes: An ultrastructural and microincineration study. *Clin. Orthop. 68*:273, 1970.

Matthews, J. L., and Martin, J. H.: Intracellular transport of calcium and its relationship to homeostasis and mineralization. *Amer. J. Med. 50*:589, 1971.

Mawer, E. B., Backhouse, J., et al.: Evidence for formation of 1,25-dihydroxycholecalciferol during metabolism of vitamin D in man. *Nature (New Biol.) 232*:188, 1971.

Mears, D. C.: Effects of parathyroid hormone and thyrocalcitonin on the membrane potential of osteoclasts. *Endocrinology* 88:1021, 1971.

Melvin, K. E. W., Miller, H. H., et al.: Early diagnosis of medullary carcinoma of the thyroid gland by means of calcitonin assay. *New Eng. J. Med.* 285:1115, 1971.

Merz, W. A., and Schenk, R. K.: Quantitative structural analysis of human cancellous bone. *Acta Anat.* (Basel) 74:140, 1969.

Merz, W. A., and Schenk, R. K.: A quantitative histological study on bone formation in human cancellous bone. *Acta Anat.* (Basel) 76:1, 1970.

Merz, W. A., Schenk, R. K., et al.: Paradoxical effects of vitamin D in fluoride-treated senile osteoporosis. *Calcif. Tissue Res.* 4(Suppl.):49, 1970.

Meunier, P., Bernard, J., et al.: The measurement of periosteocytic enlargement in primary and secondary hyperparathyroidism. *Israel J. Med. Sci.* 7:483, 1971.

Murad, F., Brewer, H. B., Jr., et al.: Effect of thyrocalcitonin on adenosine 3'-,5'-cyclic phosphate formation by rat kidney and bone. *Proc. Nat. Acad. Sci.* (USA) 65:446, 1970.

Nordin, B. E. C., and Peacock, M.: Role of kidney in regulation of plasma-calcium. *Lancet* 2:1280, 1969.

Owen, M.: Cell population kinetics of an osteogenic tissue I. *J. Cell Biol.* 19:33, 1963.

Pautard, F. G. E.: A molecular survey of calcification, In *Calcified Tissues, 1965* (Davos, 1965). Proc. Third European Symposium. Fleisch, H., Blackwood, H. J. J., and Owen, M. (eds.), New York, Springer Verlag, 1966, p. 108.

Pechet, M. M., Bobadilla, E., et al.: Regulation of bone resorption and formation. Influences of thyrocalcitonin, parathyroid hormone, neutral phosphate and vitamin D_3. *Amer. J. Med.* 43:696, 1967.

Peck, W. A., Brandt, J., et al.: Hydrocorticose-induced inhibition of protein synthesis and uridine incorporation in isolated bone cells *in vitro*. *Proc. Nat. Acad. Sci.* (USA) 57:1599, 1967.

Perris, A. D., MacManus, J. P., et al.: The parathyroid glands and mitotic stimulation in rat bone marrow after hemorrhage. *Amer. J. Physiol.* 220:773, 1971.

Petruska, J. A., and Hodge, A. J.: A subunit model for the tropocollagen macromolecule. *Proc. Nat. Acad. Sci.* (USA) 51:871, 1964.

Purnell, D. C., Smith, L. H., et al.: Primary hyperparathyroidism: A prospective clinical study. *Amer. J. Med.* 50:670, 1971.

Puschett, J. B., Moranz, J., et al.: Evidence for a direct action of cholecalciferol and 25-hydroxycholecalciferol on the renal transport of phosphate, sodium, and calcium. *J. Clin. Invest.* 51:373, 1972.

Pyrah, L. N., Hodgkinson, A., et al.: Primary hyperparathyroidism. *Brit. J. Surg.* 53:16, 1966.

Raisz, L. G.: Bone resorption in tissue culture: Factors influencing the response to parathyroid hormone. *J. Clin. Invest.* 44:103, 1965.

Raisz, L. G., Au, W. Y. W., et al.: Thyrocalcitonin and bone resorption studies employing a tissue culture bioassay. *Amer. J. Med.* 43:684, 1967.

Raisz, L. G., Trummel, C. L., et al.: 1,25-dihydroxycholecalciferol: A potent stimulator of bone resorption in tissue culture. *Science* 175:768, 1972.

Ramp, W. K., and Neuman, W. F.: Some factors affecting mineralization of bone in tissue culture. *Amer. J. Physiol.* 220:270, 1971.

Rasmussen, H., and Feinblatt, J.: The relationship between the actions of vitamin D, parathyroid hormone, and calcitonin. *Calcif. Tissue Res.* 6:265, 1971.

Rasmussen, H., and Tenenhouse, A.: Thyrocalcitonin, osteoporosis and osteolysis. *Amer. J. Med.* 43:711, 1967.

Rasmussen, H., Wong, M., et al.: Hormonal control of the renal conversion of 25-hydroxycholecalciferol to 1,25-dihydroxycholecalciferol. *J. Clin. Invest.* 51:2502, 1972.

Richens, A., and Rowe, D. J. F.: Disturbance of calcium metabolism by anticonvulsant drugs. *Brit. Med. J.* 4:73, 1970.

Riggs, B. L., Arnaud, C. D., et al.: Parathyroid function in primary osteoporosis. *J. Clin. Invest.* 52:181, 1973.

Riggs, B. L., Arnaud, C. D., et al.: Immunologic differentiation of primary hyperparathyroidism from hyper-

parathyroidism due to non-parathyroid cancer. *J. Clin. Invest.* 50:2079, 1971.

Riggs, B. L., Randall, R. V., et al.: The nature of metabolic bone disorder in acromegaly. *J. Clin. Endocr.* 34:911, 1972.

Robinson, C. J., Rafferty, B., et al.: Calcium shift into bone: A calcitonin-resistant primary action of parathyroid hormone, studied in rats. *Clin. Sci.* 42:235, 1972.

Sampson, H. W., Matthews, J. L., et al.: An electron microscopic localization of calcium in the small intestine of normal, rachitic, and vitamin D–tested rats. *Calcif. Tissue Res.* 5:305, 1970.

Sanderson, P. H., Marshall, F., et al.: Calcium and phosphorus homeostasis in the parathyroidectomized dog; evaluation by means of ethylene diamine tetraacetate and calcium tolerance tests. *J. Clin. Invest.* 39:661, 1960.

Saville, P. D., and Smith, R.: Bone density, breaking force and leg muscle mass as functions of weight in bipedal rats. *Amer. J. Phys. Anthrop.* 25:35, 1966.

Smith, J. W.: Molecular pattern in native collagen. *Nature* (London) 219:157, 1968.

Smith, L. H., Thomas, W. C., Jr., et al.: Orthophosphate therapy in calcium renal lithiasis, 1972 (in press).

Suh, S. M., Csima, A., et al.: Pathogenesis of hypocalcemia in magnesium depletion. *J. Clin. Invest.* 50:2668, 1971.

Talmage, R. V., Anderson, J. J. B., et al.: The influence of calcitonins on the disappearance of radiocalcium and radiophosphorus from plasma. *Endocrinology* 90:1185, 1972.

Tashjian, A. H., Howland, B. G., et al.: Immunoassay of human calcitonin. *New Eng. J. Med.* 283:890, 1970.

Taylor, A. N., and Wasserman, R. H.: Vitamin D_3–induced calcium-binding protein, partial purification, electrophoretic visualization, and tissue distribution. *Arch. Biochem.* 119:536, 1967.

Triffitt, J. T., Terepka, A. R., et al.: A comparative study of the exchange *in vivo* of major constituents of bone mineral. *Calcif. Tissue Res.* 2:165, 1968.

Vaes, G.: Excretion of acid and of lysosomal hydrolytic enzymes during bone resorption induced in tissue culture of parathyroid extract. *Exp. Cell Res.* 39:470, 1965.

Walker, D. G.: The induction of osteopetrotic changes in hypophysectomized, thyroparathyroidectomized, and intact rats of various ages. *Endocrinology* 89:1389, 1971.

Wallach, S., Bellavia, J. V., et al.: Thyroxine-induced stimulation of hepatic cell transport of calcium and magnesium. *J. Clin. Invest.* 51:1572, 1972.

Walser, M.: Protein-binding of inorganic phosphate in plasma of normal subjects and patients with renal disease. *J. Clin. Invest.* 39:501, 1960.

Walser, M.: The separate effects of hyperparathyroidism, hypercalcemia of malignancy, renal failure, and acidosis on the state of calcium phosphate and other ions in plasma. *J. Clin. Invest.* 41:1454, 1962.

Wasserman, R. H., Corradino, R. A., et al.: Vitamin D–dependent calcium-binding protein: Purification and some properties. *J. Biol. Chem.* 243:3978, 1968.

Wasserman, F., and Yaeger, J. A.: Fine structure of the osteocyte capsule and of the wall of the lacunae in bone. *Z. Zellforsch.* 67:636, 1965.

Whitfield, J. F., MacManus, J. P., et al.: The possible mediation by cyclic AMP of parathyroid hormone-induced stimulation of mitotic activity and deoxyribonucleic acid synthesis in rat thymic lymphocytes. *J. Cell. Physiol.* 75:213, 1970.

Woodhouse, N. J. Y., Bordier, P., et al.: Human calcitonin in the treatment of Paget's bone disease. *Lancet* 1:1139, 1971.

Woodhouse, N. J. Y., Doyle, F. H., et al.: Vitamin-D deficiency and primary hyperparathyroidism. *Lancet* 2:283, 1971.

Wu, K., Jett, S., et al.: Bone resorption rates in physiological, senile, and postmenopausal osteoporosis. *J. Lab. Clin. Med.* 69:810, 1967.

Young, R. W.: Cell proliferation and specialization during endochondral osteogenesis in young rats. *J. Cell Biol.* 14:357, 1962.

CHAPTER 12

Neuroendocrinology

By Seymour Reichlin

INTRODUCTION: NEUROENDOCRINOLOGY AND NEUROSECRETION

Neuroendocrinology concerns the interactions of the nervous system with the endocrine glands. Through the integrated function of these structures animals respond metabolically and behaviorally to alterations in both the internal and external environments. Neuroendocrine reactions also play a major role in the regulation of reproduction. Dominant themes in neuroendocrine physiology are those of control, regulation, communication, integration, and homeostasis, all functions in which the nervous system and blood-borne chemical secretions are of paramount importance.

A sharp distinction has generally been made between the mechanism of neural control of the endocrine as contrasted with the control of the exocrine glands. Exocrine glands such as sebaceous and salivary glands are innervated by secretomotor nerve fibers derived from the autonomic nervous system. Control of these structures is mediated by neurotransmitters such as norepinephrine and acetylcholine released from nerve endings which abut on the glandular cells. Analogous secretomotor innervation of anterior pituitary, thyroid, adrenocortical, and gonadal secretory cells has not been convincingly demonstrated, although sympathetic fibers do innervate the vascular supply to these organs and may alter function to some degree by modulating regional blood flow. Vasomotor regulation of endocrine glands is not considered to be of physiologic importance.

The sharp distinction between the role of the autonomic nervous system in the control of exocrine as compared with endocrine function, taught as a general principle of endocrinology for many years, has recently been modified by the demonstration that the secretions of the pineal gland and of the renal juxtaglomerular apparatus (JG apparatus) are both controlled by postganglionic sympathetic nerve fibers. Although the secretion of insulin and glucagon is regulated directly by regional concentrations of glucose, presumably sensed by intrinsic "glucoreceptors" in islet cells, there is also evidence for an interaction of the glucose stimulus with controls exerted by both adrenergic and cholinergic neurotransmitters mediated by local autonomic nerve fibers.

Neural control of the anterior and posterior lobes of the pituitary gland is exerted by neurosecretory neurons of the hypothalamus. The phenomenon of neurosecretion is central to the development of current ideas about neuroendocrine control of the pituitary gland. As first delineated by Ernst Scharrer, neurosecretion was viewed as a specific secretory product of a neuron possessing the characteristic feature of a hormone in being borne in the blood to the target organ. Vasopressin and its associated carrier substance (both secretory products of the supraoptico-hypophysial neurons) is the prototype of neurosecretion. Working as he did with histochemical stains, Scharrer initially restricted the use of the term *neurosecretion* to specifically stainable secretory granules in neurons. Extensive ultrastructural studies of neurons by electron microscopy have now broadened the concept of neurosecretion to include all secretory products of neurons which enter the bloodstream and act as hormones.

In higher animals, the major neurosecretory systems are the supraoptico- and paraventriculohypophysial neurons which constitute the neurohypophysis, and the neurons of the base of the hypothalamus which secrete hypophysiotropic hormones into the blood supplying the anterior pituitary gland.

Neurosecretory neurons of this type are of ancient lineage from a phylogenetic point of view and are of major importance in determining many behavioral, developmental, and metabolic functions even in primitive forms. For example, molting in the silkworm is induced by the coordinated secretion of ecdysone and juvenile hormone under the control of neurosecretory neurons of the protocerebrum, and in crustaceans water balance and reproduction are under the control of neurosecretory neurons.

Neurosecretory cells retain the characteristic functional and structural properties of neurons in addition to possessing secretory capacity. These cells propagate electrical action potentials, have dendrites and Nissl substance, are acted upon by other neurons through synapses, and react to neural transmitter substance such as acetylcholine and norepinephrine. In a general sense, indeed, all neurons have a secretory function because the transmission of the nerve impulse across the synaptic space depends upon the release at nerve terminals of excitatory chemicals such as acetylcholine or norepinephrine which are synthesized within the nerve itself. Escape of these substances into the general circulation occurs but is unimportant from a functional point of view. On the other hand, the secretions of neurosecretory neurons are not released into synaptic spaces but instead enter the circulation and, in true hormone fashion, affect organs at remote sites. It is now recognized that there is an active cell body–to–axon terminal axoplasmic flow in neurons of all types. Neuroendocrine cells are specialized in that the secretory product synthesized for export into the general circulation is a hormone.

Although not neurosecretory in the narrow sense, several other glands derived embryologically from neural tissue secrete neurohormones into the blood. The best known of these is the adrenal medulla, which is a functional analogue of a postsynaptic sympathetic ganglion cell of neural crest origin. The adrenal medulla is innervated by preganglionic sympathetic nerve fibers. Several neural structures derived from ependymal cell lining of the cerebral ventricles have endocrine functions. One is the pineal gland, innervated by postganglionic nerve fibers. Others, of unknown function, are the subcommissural organ and certain other specialized ependymal derivatives.

Taken together, the specialized neural structures which possess endocrine function serve as the major controlling links between the brain and the endocrine system. Wurtman has applied the term "neuroendocrine transducer" to cells of this type because they are capable of translating neural activity to a hormonal output. Neurons affecting glandular function are in turn governed by other neurons and by their metabolic and hormonal environment. Specialized neuronal receptors sensitive to changes in both the internal and the external environments can thus modulate endocrine function. These receptors also serve to generate adaptive and sexual behavior. At the highest level, the central nervous system integrates the varied neural and hormonal mechanisms to maintain the integrity of the individual organism and the perpetuation of the species.

For convenience of presentation, the neural structures which serve an endocrine function have been listed in Table 12–1 under the designation of

TABLE 12-1. THE NEUROHORMONAL GLANDS

Gland	Secretion
Adrenal medulla	Epinephrine Norepinephrine
Neurohypophysis	Vasopressin Oxytocin

Median eminence of
hypothalamus
	Hypophysiotropic hormones*
	   Corticotropin releasing factor (CRF)
	   Thyrotropin releasing
	      hormone (TRH)
	   Somatotropin releasing factor (SRF)
	   Somatotropin inhibiting factor (SIF)
	      (Somatostatin)
	   Gonadotropin releasing hormone
	      (GNRH, LRH)
	   Prolactin inhibiting factor (PIF)
	   Prolactin releasing factor
	      (PRF, TRH)
	   Melanocyte stimulating hormone
	      inhibiting factor (MIF)
	   Melanocyte stimulating hormone
	      releasing factor (MRF)

Pineal gland	Melatonin
Subcommissural organ	Reissner's fiber

*The current terminology of the hypothalamic releasing factors refers to substances of established identity as releasing *hormones*. Biologic activities as yet unsupported by chemical identification are termed releasing *factors*. A single substance, gonadotropin releasing hormone, appears to have both luteinizing hormone releasing activity (LRF) and follicle stimulating hormone releasing activity (FRF). TRH is also listed under prolactin releasing factor because in some species TRH acts like a PRF.

"neurohormonal glands." This chapter deals with the functions and diseases of the neurohormonal glands and their neuroendocrine interactions. More consideration is given to the neurohypophysis in Chapter 3, the pineal in Chapter 13, the JG apparatus in Chapter 20, and the adrenal medulla in Chapter 5.

ANATOMY AND PHYSIOLOGY OF THE NEUROHORMONAL GLANDS

Hypothalamic-Pituitary Unit
(Figs. 12-1 and 12-2)

The pituitary gland and the hypothalamus are so closely related that an understanding of the structure and function of this region requires their description as a unit. The pituitary gland is divided into a glandular portion (adenohypophysis, anterior lobe), an intermediate lobe (pars intermedia), and a neural lobe which is a direct downgrowth of tissue from the base of the hypothalamus. The neurohypophysis consists of specialized tissue at the base of the hypothalamus, together with the neural stalk and the neural lobe. The neurohypophysial portion of the hypothalamus which forms the base of the third ventricle is funnel-shaped, a resemblance which gave rise to the term *infundibulum* and to the charming hypothesis of Vesalius that animal spirits (cerebrospinal fluid) drained mucus ("pituita") from the

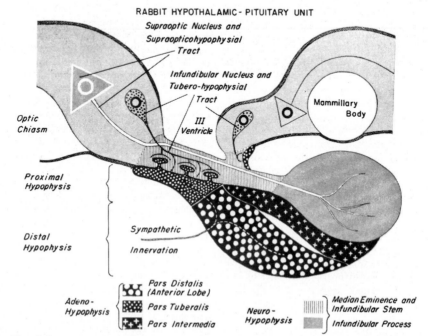

Figure 12-1. Hypothalamic-pituitary unit. Semidiagrammatic sagittal section of the rabbit brain demonstrating the anatomic relation between the base of the hypothalamus and the pituitary gland. Unlike conventional diagrams, this figure (adapted from Spatz) emphasizes two distinct neurovascular transmission systems. One system, best known, is the supraoptico-hypophysial tract, which arises in the supraoptic nuclei and terminates in relation to blood vessels of the neural lobe. The other system, whose neurons arise in the tuberal region of the hypothalamus, terminates in relation to the blood vessels of the median eminence. In view of its role in neurohumoral regulation of anterior lobe function, this region of the brain may be considered the "median eminence gland." (Reproduced from Reichlin. S.: *New Eng. J. Med.* 269:1182, 1963, with permission.)

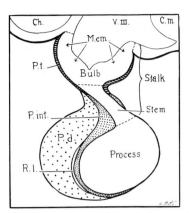

Figure 12–2. The structure and standard nomenclature of the hypothalamic-pituitary unit are outlined in this diagram of the hypophysis of a macaque monkey *(Macaca mulatta)*. Bulb, infundibular "bulb" of "infundibulum"; Ch., optic chiasma; C.m., mamillary body; M.em., median eminence; P.d., pars distalis; P.t., pars tuberalis; P. int., pars intermedia; Process, infundibular process (neural lobe); R.l., residual lumen; Stem, infundibular stem; V.III., third ventricle. (Reproduced from Rioch, D. M., Wislocki, G. B., et al.: *Res. Publ. Ass. Nerv. Ment. Dis. 20*:3, 1940, with permission.)

the base of the hypothalamus which is termed the *median eminence* of the *tuber cinereum*. Although the median eminence is anatomically classified as part of the neurohypophysis, and is traversed by fibers of the supraoptic and paraventricular neurons, this structure is primarily related to control of the anterior pituitary. In the median eminence transfer of neurosecretions of hypophysiotropic neurons of the hypothalamus to the pituitary blood supply takes place.

By gross examination the hypothalamus is readily outlined by several landmarks. Anteriorly it is bounded by the optic chiasm, posteriorly by the mamillary bodies, and laterally by the sulci formed with the temporal lobes. The smooth, rounded base of the hypothalamus is termed the *tuber cinereum,* and its central region, the *median eminence,* from which descends the *pituitary stalk.* In fresh specimens (with blood-filled vessels) or India ink-perfused specimens, the extent of the median eminence can be easily determined because it is coextensive with the distribution of the primary plexus of the hypophysial-portal circulation (Fig. 12–3). Dorsally, the hypothalamus is delineated from the thalamus by the hypothalamic sulcus.

The Neurohypophysis

As part of the integrated neural response to water deficiency, which includes induction of the

brain into the nose via this structure. The central portion of the infundibulum is enveloped from below by the pars tuberalis portion of the anterior pituitary gland and is penetrated by numerous capillary loops of the primary portal plexus of the hypophysial-portal circulation. This neurovascular complex forms a small but conspicuous structure at

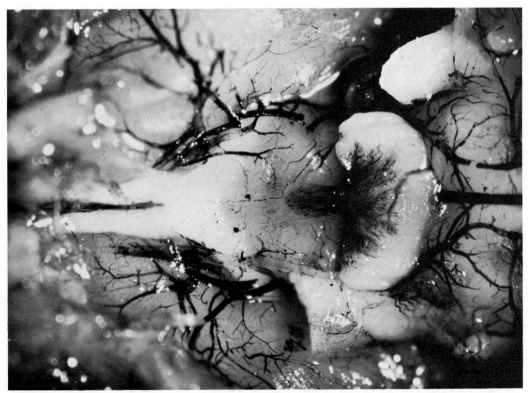

Figure 12–3. Vascular structure of the hypophysial-portal circulation of the rat. The brain has been perfused with India ink solution. The dense tuft at the base corresponds to the distribution of the primary portal plexus and pars tuberalis, forming a mantle surrounding the median eminence.

sensation of thirst and of drinking behavior, the neurohypophysis acts to conserve water through the release of vasopressin. This pattern of integrated behavioral and neuroendocrine response is typical of many homeostatic regulations in which the hypothalamus is involved. Oxytocin, the other hormone of the neurohypophysis, is released as part of a nervous reflex response to stimulation of the nipples.

The neural lobe develops embryologically as a downgrowth from the ventral diencephalon and retains its neural connections and its neural character in adult life. The dominating features of the neurohypophysis are the supraoptico-hypophysial and paraventriculo-hypophysial nerve tracts (Figs. 12-1 and 12-4). These unmyelinated nerve tracts arise from the supraoptic and paraventricular nuclei respectively within the hypothalamus itself; they descend through the infundibulum and the neural stalk to terminate in the neural lobe.

Hormone Synthesis, Transport, and Secretion

Vasopressin and oxytocin are synthesized mainly in the cell bodies of the supraoptic and paraventricular neurons. There is evidence, largely adduced by Sachs and collaborators, that the neurohypophysial hormones are synthesized together with the carrier proteins, neurophysin I and neurophysin II, by ribosomes, the complex serving as a prohormone for vasopressin and oxytocin. Like all neurosecretions, these hormones are transported in small vesicles, enclosed by a membrane. Secretory vesicles with the hormones flow down the axons by axoplasmic streaming to the neural lobe where they are stored (Fig. 12-4).

This view of neurohypophysial hormone production and transport is based on several lines of evidence. Vasopressin and oxytocin can be extracted from both the hypothalamus and the neural lobe. If the passage from brain to neural lobe is interrupted experimentally, either by section or by ligation of the neural stalk, stainable neurosecretory material accumulates above the block and disap-

pears below it. Radioactive precursors of the neurohypophysial hormones appear first in the supraoptic and paraventricular nuclei, which suggests that the hypothalamus is the initial site of hormone synthesis. However, measurement of specific activity of labeled vasopressin isolated from various parts of the dog hypothalamus and neural lobe indicates that a modest amount of the hormone is synthesized in the neural lobe as well. Isolated guinea pig hypothalami form vasopressin, oxytocin, and neurophysin in incubation media; isolated neural lobe does not.

Two kinds of vesicles are found in the terminals of the supraoptic-hypophysial neurons: the neurosecretory vesicle, related to hormone synthesis and transport; and a second kind, termed the *synaptic vesicles,* which are found characteristically in presynaptic nerve terminals in other parts of the nervous system. The latter are considered by neurologists to be storage vesicles for acetylcholine, which is released in "quantal" packets in response to a nerve action potential. These vesicles may contain other neurohormones or transmitters as well.

In the neural lobe, the neurosecretory vesicles accumulate in palisade formation in dilated nerve endings (Fig. 12-5). Fibers of the supraoptic and paraventricular tracts terminate on delicate basement membranes separated from the basement membranes of capillaries by a narrow perivascular space (Fig. 12-6). This anatomic relation of nerve ending to capillary wall is characteristic of endocrine cells in general. The posterior lobe neurons thus present the peculiar morphology of a nerve cell modified to act as an endocrine organ.

In the process of secretion, nerve action potentials are propagated along the axon, resulting in the disappearance of neurosecretory material from nerve endings in the neural lobe. There is general agreement that the neurosecretory vesicles, like glandular secretions of the anterior pituitary and the pancreatic islets, are released from nerve endings by the process of reverse pinocytosis. The neurohypophysial hormones leave the cell together with neurophysin in fixed ratio. This has been shown in incubation systems. In whole animals, including the human, plasma neurophysin can be shown to rise under conditions of increased neurohypophysial activity.

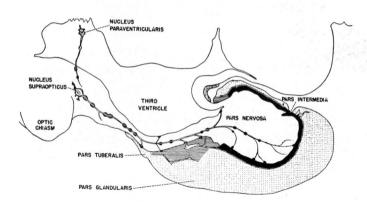

Figure 12–4. Course of the neurosecretory substance from hypothalamic cell body, along neural stalk, to neurohypophysis. This diagram illustrates the concept of cell body formation of oxytocin-vasopressin and passage of the material down the stalk to a storage site in the neural lobe. The dilated areas on the axons have been thought in the past to represent extraneuronal accumulation of neurosecretory material (NSM). Electron microscopy now shows that all of the NSM is within the axon itself. Most of the fibers are unmyelinated. (Reproduced from Bargmann, W., and Scharrer, E.: Amer. Sci. *39*:225, 1951, with permission.)

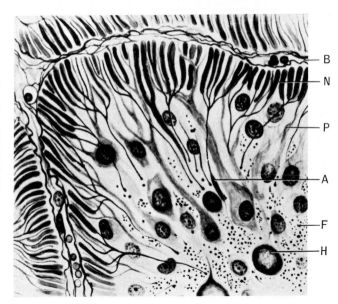

Figure 12–5. Pattern of nerve endings in the neurohypophysis of the opossum *(Didelphis virginiana)*. Simple form of opossum neurohypophysis allows easy demonstration of enlarged, clublike dilations of supraoptico-hypophysial nerve endings in relation to blood vessels of the neural lobe. B, Blood vessel-collagenous septal layer; N, palisade zone, formed by nerve fiber terminals coated with a rocklike formation of neurosecretory substance; P, pituicyte fibers; A, axons with neurosecretion; F, nerve fibers from the supraoptico-hypophysial tract; H, Herring bodies. (Reproduced from Bodian, D.: *Bull. Johns Hopkins Hosp. 89:*354, 1951, with permission.)

Recently it has been suggested that the pituicyte, a glial cell erroneously considered in the past to secrete vasopressin and oxytocin, may serve as a phagocytic cell to degrade neurosecretory vesicles and neurophysin, the carrier substance of oxytocin and vasopressin. The secretions of the neurohypophysis stimulate both the metabolic and protein synthetic activity of the glial cells.

Douglas and colleagues have demonstrated convincingly that the process of secretion is coupled to the entry of Ca^{++} into the secretory cell. In the "stimulus-secretion coupling" process, nerve cell depolarization apparently leads to inward flux of Ca^{++}. The intimate details of how Ca^{++} entry then activates the release process are not known. It has been proposed that the entrant Ca^{++} in the presence of ATP causes contraction of microtubular elements analogous to the actomyosin response in skeletal muscle (thus pulling the secretory granule towards the plasma membrane) or alters the adherence of the secretory granule to the plasma membrane.

The function of the "peptidergic" neurosecretory neurons is in turn affected by neural influences mediated by cholinergic and adrenergic fibers. That the supraoptic neuron is "cholinergic" is supported by considerable evidence. For example, acetylcholine injected directly into the supraoptic nucleus of the dog induces an antidiuresis; the anticholinesterase, di-isopropyl fluorophosphate (DFP), injected into the supraoptic nucleus, induces first an antidiuresis and later prolonged diabetes insipidus. DFP injected into the supraoptic nucleus can induce the release of oxytocin as well. The cell bodies of the supraoptic and paraventricular nuclei stain specifically for true cholinesterase (further evidence for the role of acetylcholine as a neurotransmitter substance). The clinical finding that nicotine injection or inhalation produces an antidiuresis is also an illustration of its cholinergic function. Cholinergic influences are also capable of inhibitory effects. In addition, catecholaminergic neurons exert an inhibitory influence on neuronal function, and sympathetic amines have been identified by histochemical methods in nerve fibers that end on cell bodies in the supraoptic and paraventricular nuclei.

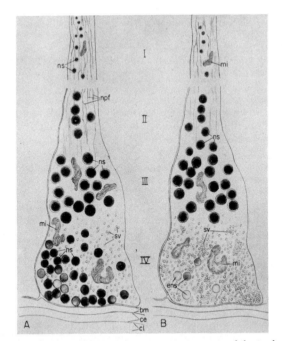

Figure 12–6. Diagram of a neurosecretory axon of the toad, from a control animal *(A)* and from a chronically dehydrated one *(B)*. When these electron microscopic observations were made, they were initially interpreted to indicate that the neurosecretory substances were dissociated in situ and the neurohypophysial hormone released by diffusion. Most recent work indicates that secretion takes place by reverse pinocytosis. The roman numerals refer to different portions of axon from stalk to terminus; ns, neurosecretory granules; npf, neuroprotofibrils; mi, mitochondria; bm, basement membrane; ce, capillary endothelium; cl, capillary lumen. (Reproduced from Gerschenfeld, H. M., Tramezzani, J. H., et al.: *Endocrinology 66:*741, 1960, with permission)

Regulation of Hormone Release

The most important stimulus to the release of vasopressin is hypertonicity of the blood perfusing the head. It has been shown by neurophysiologic methods that when hypertonic saline is introduced into the carotid artery, the activity of certain neurons in the supraoptic nucleus (but not the paraventricular nucleus) becomes accelerated. This neuronal activation — and accompanying release of vasopressin — is functional proof that some type of "osmoreceptor" exists within the perfusion area of the internal carotid artery. Whether the osmoreceptor neuron is different from the vasopressin neurosecretory neuron has not been established. For a time, attention was given to vesicular structures in the hypothalamus believed to respond to changes in blood tonicity by alterations in size. These structures were postulated by Jewell and Verney to be sensory organs which altered vasopressin release reflexly. These anatomic findings are artifacts. Changes in osmolarity more likely alter the electrical properties of the membranes of the osmoreceptor cell, thereby changing its firing rate.

Closely related to regulation of vasopressin secretion by osmoreceptors (and thus to the mechanisms for conservation of water) is their function in regulating thirst. Neurophysiologic studies have shown that the sensation of thirst (as contrasted with the sensation of dry mouth) results from an internally perceived signal arising from the hypothalamus in response to local hyperosmolarity or to peripheral volume receptors which sense a decrease in the effective intravascular blood volume. Thirst sensation may be mediated by cholinergic neurons (as is supraoptico-hypophysial function) since it has been shown that local intrahypothalamic injections of cholinergic drugs stimulate drinking behavior as well as antidiuresis. Recently, angiotensin II has been proposed as a regulator of thirst sensation and antidiuresis, which may be of importance in modulating the central nervous system effects of NaCl concentration. The intrahypothalamic injection of this polypeptide hormone (derived from enzymatic breakdown of a circulating plasma prohormone) leads to increased fluid intake in animals and to antidiuresis. In situations in which angiotensin II circulates in increased amount, as for example in hypovolemic shock, fluid intake is markedly enhanced.

The neurohypophysial neurons also are affected by blood volume receptors believed to be located in the left atrium and in other vascular areas. In addition, the secretion of vasopressin is affected by various parts of the "visceral brain" and the reticular activating system — regions involved in the maintenance of consciousness and in emotional expression.

The influence of "higher" neural centers on vasopressin secretion is evidenced by stress-induced antidiuresis in both man and animals, and by the experimental induction of diuresis or antidiuresis by hypnotic suggestion or by psychological conditioning. Drugs such as morphine also stimulate ADH release. When the supraoptico-hypophysial system is deprived of neural input from other parts of the brain (as by the production of a hypothalamic "island"), neurons in this region are electrically more active than normal. This denervation hyperfunction of the neurohypophysis may provide the explanation for the syndrome of "inappropriate ADH secretion" (Chapters 3 and 30) which occurs in certain kinds and locations of brain damage, but the validity of this hypothesis has not been established. It has also been proposed that "inappropriate ADH secretion" in comatose patients is due to prolonged and immobile recumbancy which leads to persistent activation of volume receptors.

The phenomenon of milk "let down" is another example of neural control of neurohypophysial function first recognized in animal husbandry. Suckling in dairy animals is followed by the appearance of the milk at the teat after some delay. The young animal does not begin to obtain milk until after 30 seconds or more. A neurogenic reflex is responsible for this effect. The stimulus of suckling, transmitted from afferent nerve endings in the nipple, is conducted through the spinal cord, midbrain, and finally to the hypothalamus, where it triggers the release of oxytocin from the neurohypophysis. The oxytocin released causes contraction of the myoepithelial cells which encircle mammary acini and expel the milk into the nipple. In the absence of this reflex contraction, milk cannot be obtained from even a full breast: for example, nursing rats cannot obtain milk from their posterior-hypophysectomized mothers until injections of oxytocin are given.

This reflex is accompanied by changes in hypothalamic neuronal function and can be blocked by specific neural lesions and also by certain types of neural stimuli. In cows, "let down" can be abolished by a strange or threatening environment, and similar blockade has been noted in painfully stressed rabbits. Pain or fright inhibits milk "let down" in the rabbit by central nervous system action or by epinephrine causing central inhibition of oxytocin release.

Milk "letdown" occurs in women in response to suckling and in some women to a conditioned stimulus such as the hungry crying of their baby. Milk "let down" may be inhibited by emotional stress and triggered by sexual excitement.

Secretion of vasopressin and of oxytocin are independent. For example, in lactating women, antidiuretic hormone secretion can be achieved by hypertonic saline infusion without producing "let down," and the suckling stimulus induces "let down" without accompanying antidiuresis. On the basis of ablative studies in rats, it has been postulated that oxytocin is secreted by the paraventricular nuclei and vasopressin by the supraoptico-hypophysial system, a differentiation supported by electrophysiologic studies of neuron populations.

Damage to the neurohypophysis or to its central controlling input leads to diabetes insipidus. Excessive secretion by the neurohypophysis can also occur due to an abnormality of the neural regulating system. The syndromes of excessive or deficient

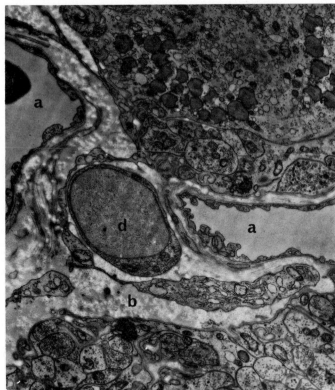

Figure 12–7. Electron micrograph of hamster median eminence. The median eminence is made up of densely packed nerve endings distributed in relation to the perivascular space of the primary portal capillaries in a schema resembling in principle the distribution of nerve endings in the neurohypophysis. The nerve endings shown here in cross-section profiles contain a variety of vesicles, both large and small, of differing electron density which are thought to contain neurosecretions. Mitochondria are also found. Note that nerves end in close relation to a basement membrane. The path of secretion is from nerve endings, through axon basement membrane, perivascular connective tissue space, capillary basement membrane, and finally endothelium. This is the characteristic arrangement of glandular cells throughout the endocrine system. Symbols: a, capillary lumen; b, perivascular space; c, nerve endings; d, nucleus of supporting (connective tissue) cell. (Courtesy of Karl M. Knigge, unpublished, 1966.)

vasopressin secretion, the chemistry and mechanisms of action of the neurohypophysial hormones, and the overall problem of water balance are presented in Chapter 3.

The Median Eminence Gland

Harris and Green were the first to recognize fully the functional significance of the fact that nearly all of the blood which reaches the anterior pituitary has first traversed capillary plexuses located in the median eminence and adjoining neural stalk. Their postulate, now termed the *portal vessel–chemotransmitter hypothesis,* was that these vessels formed part of a neurovascular link by which the hypothalamus, through the mediation of neurohumoral substances, regulated the secretion of the anterior pituitary tropic hormones. Anatomic and physiologic evidence for this view is outlined in the following sections.

Anatomy
(Figs. 12–1, 12–3, 12–7, and 12–8)

The median eminence consists of a neural component (the infundibulum of the hypothalamus), a vascular component (the hypophysial-portal capillaries and veins), and an epithelial component (the pars tuberalis of the adenohypophysis). Electron microscopic studies show that the infundibulum is

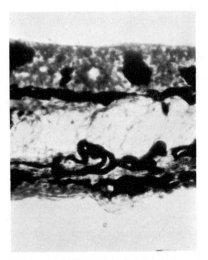

Figure 12–8. Capillary loops of the neural stalk of the rat. A photomicrograph of the neural stalk of a rat perfused with India ink demonstrates the peculiar hairpin loops of the primary hypophysial-portal plexus which penetrate and ramify in the neural portion of the stalk. Similar structures are found in the median eminence. On this vascular structure are postulated to end nerve endings secreting anterior pituitary tropic hormone releasers. Upper part, tuberalis portion; lower part, beginning of anterior lobe at stalk-gland junction.

composed mainly of densely packed nerve endings, capillaries with conspicuous perivascular spaces, supporting cells resembling neurohypophysial pituicytes, and specialized ependymal cells (the tanycyte) which traverse the median eminence from the lumen of the third ventricle to the outer mantle plexus. The nerve endings are the terminals of axons which arise chiefly in the ventral hypothalamus: the capillaries form the primary plexus of the portal circulation.

Relationships of nerve ending, basement membrane, interstitial space, and capillary wall are identical in plan to those in the neural lobe, and thus the process of secretion at median eminence terminals is probably analogous to the stimulus-secretion mechanism of the neurohypophysis. The large perivascular space contact area and the peculiar vessels in this region, which have fenestrations typical of those seen in ordinary endocrine glands, account for the observation that the neurohypophysis including the median eminence, unlike most of the brain, is particularly permeable to molecules such as thyroxine, trypan blue, and growth hormone.

Although axons of the supraoptic and paraventricular-hypophysial tract pass through the median eminence on their way from cells of origin in the hypothalamus to termination in the neural lobe, experimental studies have shown that median eminence function is distinct from neural lobe function. For example, dehydration in birds leads to a discharge of neurosecretory material from the neural lobe without change in median eminence neurosecretory substance. In contrast, ovulation depletes the stainable material from the median eminence without altering the appearance of the neural lobe.

The form of the blood vessels in the primary plexus varies somewhat from species to species. In man, capillaries form loops which are part of spiral structures termed *gomitoli*. These penetrate the infundibulum and stalk. Arterioles of the stalk and median eminence of man have highly muscular walls, suggesting that hemodynamic changes in these vessels might affect pituitary function, but evidence to support this point of view is lacking. Reflex constriction of these vessels following postpartum hemorrhage has been suggested as a factor in the genesis of pituitary infarction. More recently, the finding of disturbed hypothalamic regulatory function in some cases of Sheehan's syndrome (postpartum hemorrhage) has made it appear likely that the stalk region may also be infarcted as a major manifestation of this syndrome.

Detailed studies of the arterial supply to the primary portal plexus and pituitary have explained the characteristic pattern of infarction observed after surgical or traumatic interruption of the pituitary stalk. Blood reaches the plexus of the median eminence and upper stalk by way of the superior hypophysial artery, a branch of the internal carotid. This plexus is drained by the long portal veins which run along the stalk and finally reach the pituitary sinusoids. The capillary plexus in the lower portion of the stalk is supplied by the inferior hypophysial artery and is drained by short portal veins which enter the pituitary almost directly. Section of the pituitary stalk generally interrupts the long portal veins and causes infarction of the vascular territory supplied by these vessels; a

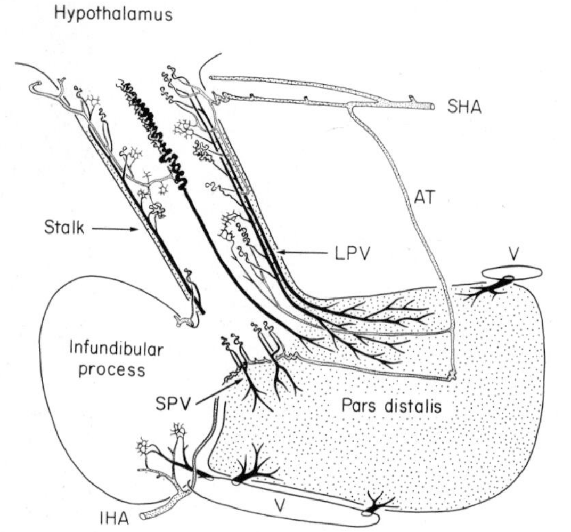

Figure 12–9. Diagram of blood supply of human pituitary gland (in sagittal section) to explain the distribution of the infarcted and surviving areas in the anterior lobe after transection of the pituitary stalk. Section of the stalk severs the long portal vessels (LPV) and thus deprives the greater part of the anterior lobe or pars distalis of its blood supply, causing a massive infarct. The circulation through the short portal vessels (SPV) is not interrupted, and consequently a small area of the anterior lobe adjacent to the neural lobe survives. Hypophysiotropic hormone deficiency can also occur as a consequence of infarct of the stalk-median eminence region. SHA, superior hypophysial artery; IHA, inferior hypophysial artery; V, venous sinus draining anterior lobe. (Reproduced from Adams, J. H., Daniel, P. M., et al., *Brit. Med. J.* 1:193, 1965/66, with permission.)

small zone in the region of the intermediate lobe escapes infarction because it is supplied by the intact short portal veins (Fig. 12–9).

The third component of the median eminence, the pars tuberalis, is in the form of a thin glandular sheath around the infundibulum and pituitary stalk. In some animals the epithelial component may make up as much as 10 per cent of the total glandular tissue of the pituitary, and several pituitary tropic hormones have been extracted from this region. Moreover, nerve fibers can be traced to the pars tuberalis. These findings to the contrary, the bulk of studies indicate that the pars tuberalis does not have an important physiologic function but serves merely as the region through which arteries and veins of the hypophysial-portal circulation are conducted.

The Portal Vessel–Chemotransmitter Hypothesis

The hypophysial portal-chemotransmitter hypothesis of pituitary control was introduced as an explanation of how the anterior pituitary gland, which is devoid of secretomotor nerve fibers, could be influenced by the nervous system. According to this hypothesis, neurohumoral substances released from nerve endings in the median eminence enter capillaries of the primary plexus of the hypophysial-portal circulation and are carried by the portal veins of the hypophysial stalk into the sinusoids of the anterior lobe. Releasing factors may also be transported from the third ventricle to the median eminence by ependymal tanycytes. Various lines of indirect evidence provided the initial basis for the portal vessel–chemotransmitter concept, including the inability to demonstrate nerve endings on the glandular cells of the adenohypophysis, the existence of the hypophysial portal circulation throughout the vertebrates, and the fact that the direction of blood flow in the portal vessels is from the hypothalamus to the pituitary gland.

Further indirect support of the portal chemotransmitter hypothesis came from the study of pituitary stalk section and of pituitary transplantation. If regeneration of the portal vessels is prevented, pituitary stalk section in various species, including man, is followed by gonadal failure, thyroid inactivity, adrenal involution, and growth failure, all to a degree intermediate between that of normal and hypophysectomized animals. The ablative studies (stalk section and hypothalamic lesions) on which the conclusion that the function of the pituitary was largely but not completely dependent upon the hypothalamus was based probably did not produce complete hypophysiotropic hormone deficiency. With the recognition of syndromes of hypophysiotropic failure in the human (see below), it now appears that at least certain functions of the anterior pituitary, such as growth hormone and TSH secretion, are virtually completely dependent upon hypothalamic stimulation. The neural component of the pituitary stalk does not regenerate, but the portal vessels do. Following experimental section of the stalk, restitution of anterior lobe function is correlated with regeneration of these vessels.

Transplantation experiments indicate that the median eminence blood supply is of special significance for the control of anterior pituitary secretion. If displaced to the kidney capsule, to the anterior chamber of the eye, or in a subcutaneous pocket, the pituitary gland does not support normal growth or normal thyroid, adrenal, or gonadal function. Greep was the first to show that the median eminence was a privileged site for pituitary transplants: only in this site is the transplant capable of supporting cyclic sexual function, pregnancy, and other pituitary tropic activities.

Although such experiments suggest that the portal vessel connection to the pituitary gland has special functional significance, disturbed blood supply and inadequate nutrition are alternate explanations for the poor glandular performance of displaced tissue. This criticism is answered in part by the fact that even small remnants of pituitary tissue situated within the sella can maintain normal growth and normal thyroid, adrenal, and gonadotropic function, and that the isolated pituitary gland (as by stalk section or transplantation) can secrete supernormal quantities of prolactin (see below).

Direct effects of the hypothalamus on the pituitary have been further studied by transplanting pituitary fragments into the hypothalamus itself, using stereotaxic methods. Work of this type has permitted the delineation within the ventral hypothalamus of "fields" where the hypophysiotropic hormones are found. Transplants in this region show normal differentiation of cellular detail and granulation, support normal testicular function, and restore other tropic functions toward normal. Thus, in considering the hypothalamic basis of neural control of the anterior pituitary, one may speak of the median eminence "gland," in which are located nerve terminals which secrete the hypophysiotropic hormones in relation to the primary plexus, and a somewhat more extensive area in the basal hypothalamus, in which the hypophysiotropic substances are found which correspond to the axons and cell bodies of the tubero-hypophysial tract (Fig. 12–10).

The most direct proof of the portal vessel–chemotransmitter hypothesis has been the isolation of the biologic activity of growth hormone releasing factor (SRF), thyrotropic releasing factor (TRH), prolactin inhibitory factor (PIF), and luteinizing hormone releasing factor (LRH) from portal vessel blood by Porter and colleagues; the isolation of hypothalamic releasing factors from stalk median eminence tissue; and the chemical identification

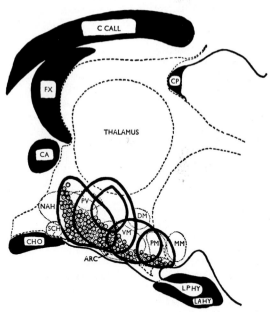

Figure 12–10. Diagrammed here is the "hypophysiotropic area" of the hypothalamus. Pituitaries transplanted into various regions of the brain show morphologic differentiation and some tropic function. This observation indicates that there is a "field" of hypophysiotropic neurons within the hypothalamus. These probably correspond to the cell bodies of the tracts to the median eminence.

(---), Outline of third ventricle; (. . .), midsagittal projection of main hypothalamic nuclei; (−), borders of five relatively midline pituitary grafts; (✿), PAS-positive basophils; ARC; arcuate nucleus; CA, anterior commissure; C CALL, corpus callosum; CHO, optic chiasma; CP, posterior commissure; DM, dorsomedial nucleus; FX, fornix; LAHY, anterior lobe of hypophysis; LPHY, posterior lobe of hypophysis; MM, medial mammillary nucleus; NAH, anterior hypothalamic nucleus; PM, premammillary nucleus; PV, paraventricular nucleus; SCH, suprachiasmic nucleus; VM, ventromedial nucleus. (Reproduced from Halasz, B., Pupp, L., et al.: *J. Endocr.* 25:147, 1962, with permission.)

and synthesis of two of these substances, TRH and LRH (see below). The hypophysiotropic area and median eminence have also been shown to synthesize TRH and LRH from precursor amino acids by a nonribosomal mechanism.

Secretions of the Median Eminence: Hypophysiotropic Hormones

In his review of the history of the portal vessel–chemotransmitter hypothesis, Harris gives priority for the notion of a neurohumoral control of anterior lobe function to Hinsey and Markee (1933) and to Friedgood (1936). Although acetylcholine and epinephrine were the subject of the earliest direct studies of neurohumoral control of anterior lobe function, evidence now available indicates that these well established "classic" synaptic transmitters are not direct regulators of anterior lobe function, although they exert effects at the hypothalamic level.

The search for hypothalamic neurohumors with anterior pituitary regulating properties focused upon extracts of stalk median eminence (SME) and hypothalamus. Such hypophysiotropic materials have been called releasing *factors* (Table 12–1) after the first description of corticotropin releasing factor (CRF). This term was introduced by Saffran and his colleagues to describe a substance extracted from hypothalamic tissues which stimulated the release of ACTH from pituitary fragments maintained in organ culture. At the present time, the term releasing *factor* is still applied to substances of unknown chemical nature, while substances with established chemical identity, such as TRH and LRH (thyrotropin releasing hormone, luteinizing hormone releasing hormone), have been called releasing *hormone.*

Since the first disclosures of hypophysiotropic actions of hypothalamic extracts, intense efforts have been made in many laboratories to identify the hypothalamic factors regulating each of the tropic hormones of the anterior pituitary gland, to describe their chemical properties, and to determine the factors controlling their secretion. Although these materials have been named releasing factors, they also have stimulatory effects on other secretory functions, such as differentiation and hormone synthesis.

Three exceptions to the rule that hypothalamic factors stimulate the pituitary gland are the factors concerned with regulation of prolactin, growth hormone, and MSH secretion. For each of these hormones, both inhibitory and stimulatory hypothalamic factors have been identified by bioassay. For the other pituitary functions (FSH, LH, TSH, and ACTH), only excitatory hypophysiotropic hormones have been identified. These releasing factors have peculiar and somewhat unexpected effects on specific pituitary cell types. For example, TRH does not alter ACTH secretion but has minor and variable effects on the secretion of GH and the gonadotropins, is a very potent releaser of prolactin both in the human and certain animals, and

releases GH in acromegaly. LRH stimulates both LH and FSH release but has no effect on the other anterior pituitary secretions. The median eminence gland thus assumes a hormonal virtuosity which rivals the anterior pituitary itself. Analysis of the mechanism of action of the releasing factors is reviewed in the chapter on the anterior pituitary. Current chemical knowledge of each of these factors and its physiologic effects is discussed in the following sections.

Thyrotropin Releasing Hormone (TRF, TRH)

The most dramatic neuroendocrine discovery made during the period between the present and previous editions of this text was the elucidation of the structure of TRH, accomplished virtually simultaneously by teams of investigators associated with the laboratories of Guillemin and of Schally. Identification was soon followed by synthesis and clinical testing. It has also been shown that TRH is biosynthesized enzymatically by nonribosomal systems limited to the hypophysiotropic area of the hypothalamus. The discovery of TRH has, in a sense, established the portal vessel–chemotransmitter hypothesis and permitted the proof of many of the earlier experimental formulations. Moreover, knowledge gained from TRH chemistry made it possible to elucidate the structure of LRH (luteinizing hormone releasing hormone) and will aid immeasurably in identifying the other substances, especially difficult because of their presence in extremely minute amounts in hypothalamic tissue.

TRH proves to be an extremely simple substance, a tripeptide amide (pyro) Glu-His-Pro-NH$_2$ (Fig. 12–11). Although some substituent forms are potent, an intact amide group and the cyclized glutamic acid terminus are essential for activity. TRH is relatively stable under most circumstances, it can be absorbed by mouth but is degraded in plasma. Following injection in the human or in the rat, plasma TSH levels rise rapidly and dramatically, a change being detected within 3 minutes, which is maximal 10 to 20 minutes after injection (Fig. 12–12). The material is extremely potent; as little as 15 mcg. are detectable, and near maximal effects are exerted by a dose of 400 mcg. Except for mild nausea and urinary urgency, no serious side effects have been detected. The effect of the brief pulse of TSH released from the anterior pituitary by a single injection of TRH is apparently not sufficient to give reliably significant changes in plasma thyroxine levels, but plasma triiodothyronine levels are raised predictably by this material. Prolonged infusion raises both T$_3$ and T$_4$ levels. TRH has proven useful in evaluating pituitary TSH reserve. Patients with hypopituitarism due to pituitary destruction do not respond to this agent, whereas patients with hypothalamic disease do respond; although the initial response is usually delayed, it may exceed that of the normal response. Use of this agent has made it possible to differen-

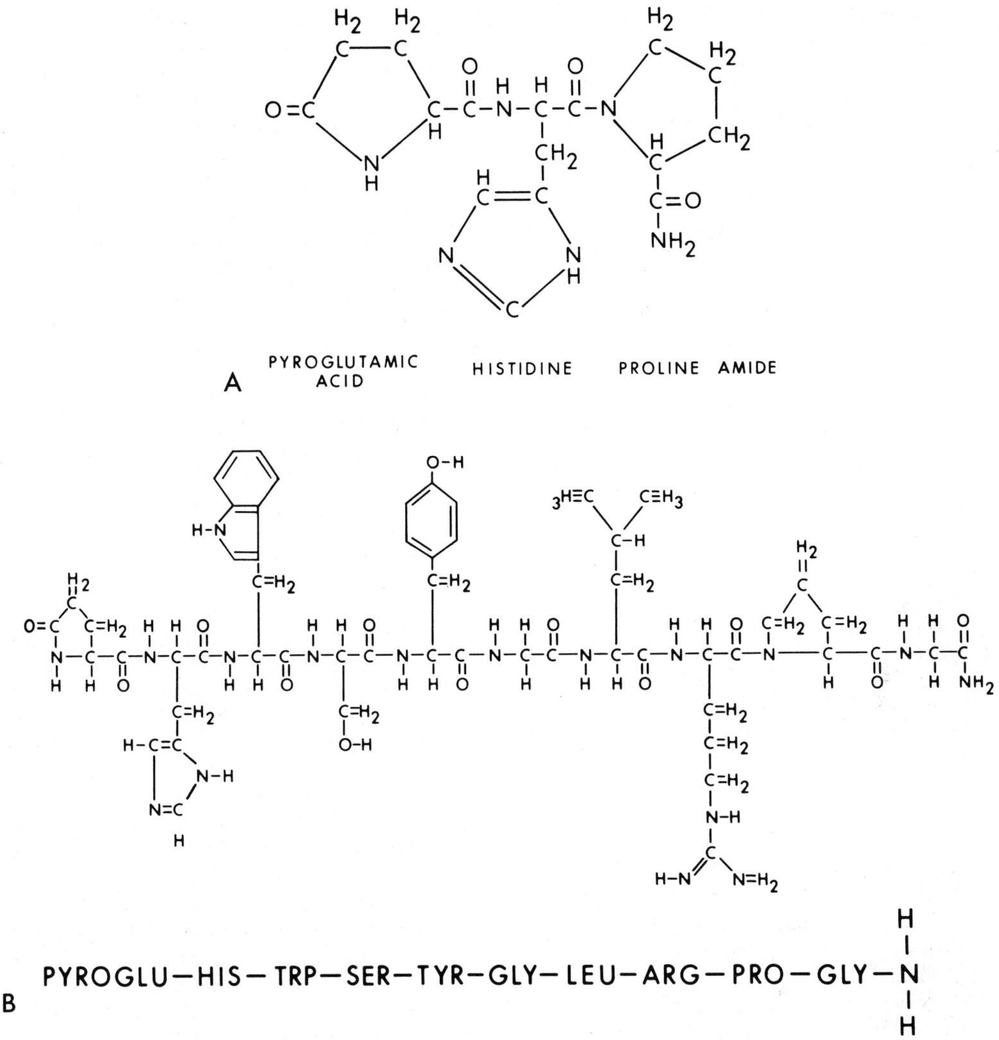

PYROGLUTAMIC ACID   HISTIDINE   PROLINE AMIDE

A

PYROGLU — HIS — TRP — SER — TYR — GLY — LEU — ARG — PRO — GLY — N

B

Figure 12–11. *A,* Formula of thyrotropin releasing hormone (TRH); *B,* formula of luteinizing hormone releasing hormone (LH-RH). Since LH-RH has intrinsic FSH-RH activity, it is possible that only one molecule, which could then be called gonadotropin releasing hormone (Gn-RH), is the gonadotropic regulatory hormone.

tiate between pituitary and hypothalamic causes of isolated TSH deficiency, to identify a syndrome of isolated TRH deficiency, and to demonstrate that a large proportion of children with idiopathic growth failure (with associated panhypopituitarism) are TRH responsive and, therefore, must be suffering from hypophysiotropic failure.

Advantage has also been taken of the fact that the pituitary TSH secretory response to TRH injection is modulated by the thyroid status of the individual. Thyroid hormone excess inhibits response to TRH, and deficiency sensitizes the pituitary to the effects of TRH. These interactions (as discussed below) are operative over the physiologic range of plasma thyroid hormone levels; TRH reserve proves to be a good guide to effective tissue thyroid hormone level in the anterior pituitary gland.

The effects of TRH were believed to be relatively specific, with only occasional changes in growth hormone and LH levels being observed in clinical testing. However, the recent introduction of sensi-

tive techniques for measuring prolactin in human plasma made it possible to show that TRH was an extremely potent prolactin releasing hormone, that threshold effects for prolactin release were of the same order of magnitude as those for TSH release, and, as in the case of TSH secretion, that prolactin secretory response to TRH was modulated by thyroid hormone levels (Fig. 12–12).

The physiologic significance of TRH effects on prolactin release has not as yet been determined. Since the threshold for effects on prolactin secretion is close to the threshold for effects on TSH secretion, it is likely that TRH may play a role in the tonic stimulation of prolactin secretion. However, the many instances in which the secretion of TSH and prolactin are dissociated indicate different hypothalamic mechanisms of control. Also, much work indicates that the major component of hypothalamic control of prolactin secretion is tonic inhibitory, not stimulatory.

Finally, there may be species differences or sev-

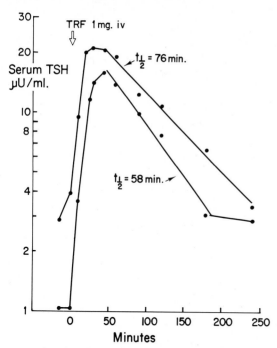

Figure 12–12. Effect of intravenous injection of TRF on plasma TSH in the human. (Reproduced from Hershman, J. M., and Pittman, J. A., Jr.: *New Eng. J. Med.* 285:997–1006, 1971, with permission.)

eral types of PRF since in the rat even relatively large amounts of TRH do not release prolactin, whereas crude hypothalamic extracts are quite active in this regard. TRH does release prolactin from pituitary tumor cell cultures derived from rat lines.

Some information has been gained about the metabolic fate of TRH. The material is degraded in plasma quite rapidly, and there is some excretion in the urine. Specific pituitary cell membrane receptors for TRH have been identified, and a pituitary deamidase has been reported which inactivates this material.

Gonadotropic Hormone Releasing Factors (LRH)

With sensitive assay techniques capable of detecting release of luteinizing hormone from the anterior pituitary into the blood, systemic injections of hypothalamic extracts from various species including man have been shown to have LH releasing effects in laboratory animals and in the human (Fig. 12–13). Similar extracts injected directly into the adenohypophysis induce ovulation in rats, rabbits, and hamsters and, when added to incubated pituitary tissue, increase the release of LH into the medium.

That LRF plays a physiologic role in the release of LH is suggested by the fact that cyclic changes in the hypothalamic concentration of LRF appear to correlate with estrus in the rat, a decrease in stored LRF occurring during proestrus when

plasma LH levels are rising. The blood of hypophysectomized rats contains measurable quantities of LRF which disappear after the destruction of the ventral hypothalamus. Bioassayable LRF is detectable in the peripheral blood of normal women at midcycle at a time when the ovulatory LH surge is occurring. As is discussed below, LH secretion and the ovulatory surge of LH is abolished by lesions of the basal-ventral hypothalamus; electrical stimulation of the median eminence of the hypothalamus causes a release of LH; and transplantation of pituitary fragments into the "hypophysiotropic area" of the hypothalamus restores the normal basophilic granules of the gonadotropic cells and stimulates enough gonadotropin release to permit the development of normal testicular function. These observations taken together have made the existence of an LRF substance a virtual certainty.

In a series of brilliant experiments culminating with the isolation of a purified peptide from pig hypothalamic tissue with LRF activity, Schally and collaborators succeeded in determining from a total of only 200 nanomoles of material the structure of LRF. This material proves to be a decapeptide (Fig. 12–11). Like TRH, the amino terminal is a pyroglutamic acid residue, and the carboxy terminal has a substituted amide group, a property shared not only with TRH, but with vasopressin, oxytocin, and a number of other small peptide hormones, including calcitonin, gastrin, and glucagon. A synthetic peptide of this structure proves to have high LRF potency in animals and in the human (Fig. 12–13), as shown by effects on plasma levels of LH determined by radioimmunoassay. The synthetic compound (in common with the natural compound) induces ovulation in experimental animals and in the human (when given by slow intravenous injection). Both natural and synthetic LRF materials are receiving wide evaluations and have already been shown to be of value in identifying pituitary failure and in differentiating between various causes of anovulation in the human.

LRH, unlike TRH, is quite stable in whole blood and is not excreted in the urine in appreciable amounts; like TRH, however, it disappears rapidly from the circulation after injection. It is likely that LRH interacts with pituitary cell membranes, but this has not as yet been demonstrated.

FSH Releasing Factor

The biologic data which provided the basis for postulating the existence of a follicle stimulating hormone releasing factor are generally similar to those which supported the existence of LRF. They include demonstration of potency of crude extracts, both in whole animals (including the human) and in isolated incubation systems, and of the effects of hypothalamic ablation and stimulation. As the purification of LRF became more and more precise, it became apparent that the most pure preparations of native LRF possessed intrinsic FSH stimulating properties (Fig. 12–13). It was proposed by White, and later by Schally and by Guillemin and their

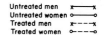

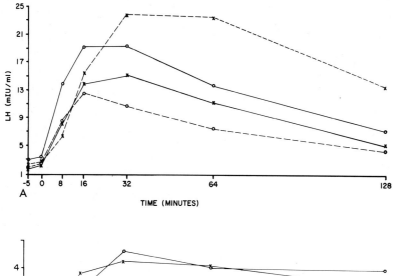

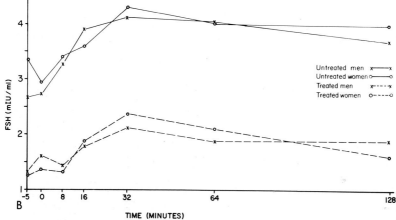

Figure 12–13.   Mean plasmá LH *(A)* and FSH *(B)* levels after administration (I.V.) of synthetic LH-RH to four groups of subjects. The treated group received ethinyl estradiol or Lyndiol. (Reproduced from Kastin, A. J., Schally, A. V., et al.: *J. Clin. Endocr. 34:* 753, 1972, with permission.)

collaborators, that LRF and FSH-RF were one and the same compound. With the synthesis of LRF, this suspicion was confirmed. The synthetic has both LRF and FSH activities, a property which has led to the proposal that the material be called gonadotropin releasing hormone (GnRH). It is possible, however, to demonstrate under experimental and spontaneously occurring conditions, that the secretion of LH does not parallel the secretion of FSH. This is well shown in the human where, during the follicular phase of development, FSH levels are relatively high as compared with the postovulatory period, a difference which contrasts with that for LH secretion. At midcycle, however, both LH and FSH rise in an identical pattern. If there is but one gonadotropic hormone, it would appear reasonable to postulate that the pituitary response to the GnRH is conditioned by prior steroid treatment which alters both pituitary hormone content and pituitary sensitivity to the effects of the releasing factor. On the other hand, two types of LRH with different FRF potency may also exist.

Growth Hormone Releasing and Inhibiting Factors (SRF, SIF)

Extracts of stalk median eminence tissue stimulate the release of growth hormone from pituitary gland incubates and raise plasma levels of growth hormone as determined by immunoassay in a number of species including the rat, monkey, and man (Fig. 12–14). A material potent in releasing pituitary GH from incubated glands has been isolated from hypophysial-portal blood, providing the final proof of the relevant hormonal nature of the material. The injection of hypothalamic extracts directly into the portal circulation of rats has also been shown to bring about the release of GH.

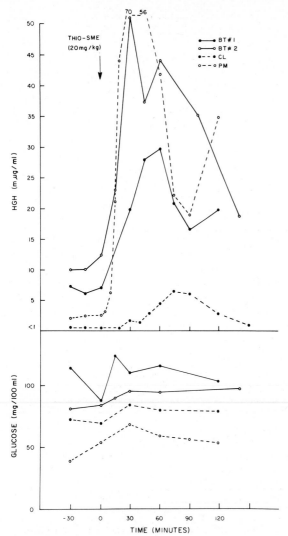

Figure 12–14. Effect of a partially purified hypothalamic extract on plasma GH in the human. Thio-SME refers to thioglycolate-treated hypothalamic extract. This chemical procedure inactivates the vasopressin contaminant, itself capable of producing a nonspecific release of GH. (Reproduced from Root, A. W.: *Human Pituitary Growth Hormone.* Springfield, Illinois, Charles C Thomas, 1972, p. 146, with permission.)

hypothalamic extracts and propose a dual form of control analogous to that which appears to regulate prolactin secretion (see below). A GH release-inhibiting polypeptide consisting of fourteen amino acids has been isolated from sheep hypothalamic extract by Guillemin and collaborators. The synthetic material, christened "somatostatin," is effective in animals and man.

Corticotropin Releasing Factor (CRF)

Although CRF was the first of the releasing factors to be recognized, its chemical nature is still unknown. A substance acting to release ACTH has been isolated from blood draining the primary portal plexus. Evidence has also been presented that CRF enters the general circulation and the cerebrospinal fluid. This material disappears after destruction of the "adrenotropic" region of the hypothalamus. Stress also has been shown to deplete the median eminence of CRF activity, and a few patients treated with purified hypothalamic fractions have responded with a rise in plasma corticoid levels, an effect thought to be due to induced ACTH release (Fig. 12–15).

Vasopressin was initially thought to be CRF because it is secreted during stress and releases ACTH both *in vivo* and *in vitro,* and because hypothalamic lesions which cause diabetes insipidus also block reflex ACTH discharge. However, several lines of evidence indicate that although vasopressin may under certain circumstances serve as *a* CRF, it is not *the* CRF. The secretion of ACTH and of vasopressin, though usually occurring under similar circumstances, is independent under certain conditions such as hypoglycemic stress or intracarotid hypertonic saline injection. The most convincing evidence that vasopressin is not essen-

Despite this unequivocal biologic evidence, the chemical nature of SRF has not been established with certainty. One of the main problems in this field has been that of assay methodology, there being disagreement as to the critical means needed to demonstrate the existence of an SRF substance. A pure compound capable of causing a decrease in the pituitary content of GH in the rat and a release of GH from pituitary incubates was reported by Schally and collaborators, but this material does not release GH into the blood as measured by radioimmunoassay, whereas crude materials are capable of doing so. The precise nature of SRF and of the GH depletor are still unknown, but most evidence suggests that SRF is a peptide substance.

Several major groups of workers report the presence of a growth hormone inhibitory substance in

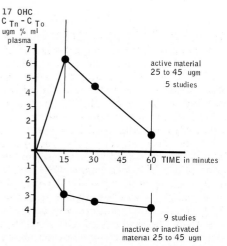

Figure 12–15. Variations of the plasma 17-OH corticoid concentration in normal individuals receiving a single intravenous injection of purified corticotropin releasing factor (electrophoretic fraction DΔ). Bottom of diagram, control studies. (Reproduced from Guillemin, R.: *Diabetes* 8:352, 1959, with permission.)

tial for ACTH discharge comes from studies of rats with hereditary diabetes insipidus. Such animals are incapable of synthesizing vasopressin yet have nearly normal adrenocortical responses to stress. Similar studies have been made in humans with idiopathic diabetes insipidus. Microinjections of vasopressin in threshold amounts trigger ACTH release when introduced into the median eminence but not into the anterior pituitary, providing further evidence that vasopressin is *not* CRF.

Prolactin Regulating Factors (PIF, PRF)

In keeping with the observation that the hypothalamus exerts an *inhibitory* effect on prolactin secretion (see below) is the observation that hypothalamic extracts contain a substance inhibitory to prolactin release, particularly evident in incubation systems. This material was termed "PIF" by Meites and collaborators. PIF has been identified in portal vessel blood by Kamberi, Porter, and their collaborators, again satisfying the critical requirement of evidence for physiologic significance of a hypophysiotropic hormone.

The view that PIF is the principal prolactin regulator in the mammal seems to be well founded, but a number of authors have reported that mammalian hypothalamic tissue contains a substance stimulatory to prolactin release. In the human, TRH is a highly potent prolactin releaser (Fig. 12–16); the dose response characteristics of TRH are such as to suggest that TRH may play a role in maintaining basal stimulation of prolactin secretion. In the rat, TRH does not appear to be a prolac-

tin releasing factor, crude extracts of hypothalamus being highly potent in this regard, far out of proportion to their TRH content. It seems most reasonable to suppose, on the basis of current evidence, that there is a dual inhibitory and excitatory control system for prolactin regulation.

The precise structures of PIF and PRF are unknown, but on the basis of their behavior in solvent systems and on Sephadex columns, it is believed that they are small peptides.

Melanocyte Stimulating Hormone Regulatory Factors (MIF, MSF)

Much physiologic evidence suggests that intermediate lobe function, like that of prolactin secretion, is tonically inhibited by the hypothalamus. For example, the intermediate lobe becomes larger than normal in rats with lesions of the hypothalamus. Transplantation of the pituitary gland in the frog leads to increased MSH secretion as reflected in changes in skin coloration. In harmony with these physiologic observations is the claim that extracts of rat hypothalamus inhibit the release of MSH from rat pituitary glands *in vitro*. This material has been called MIF by Kastin and collaborators. The nature of MIF has been proposed by both Celis, Walter, and collaborators, and by Kastin and his collaborators to be a tripeptide, proline leucine glycinamide (Pro-Leu-Gly-NH$_2$), which has the special attribute of being the side chain of oxytocin. According to Celis and collaborators, the side chain is split from the remainder of the oxytocin molecule (which thus serves as a prohormone) by a specific hypothalamic peptidase, in turn controlled by the gonadal hormonal status of the animal. However, this claim is not accepted by all workers, and there may, in fact, be more than one inhibitor of MSH release. A hypothalamic fraction which stimulates MSH release has also been reported.

Neurotransmitter Control of Secretion of Hypophysiotropic Hormones

In the foregoing section, emphasis has been placed on the neurosecretory neurons responsible for the synthesis and release of the peptide hypophysiotropic hormones which serve as the functional link between the nervous system and the anterior pituitary. This "neurotransducer" peptidergic neuron is in turn brought under the control of the remainder of the brain through the mediation of neurotransmitter synapses of a more conventional type (Fig. 12–17). In keeping with the special properties of the peptidergic hypophysiotropic neurons, however, nerve fibers impinging upon them belong to a special class of neurotransmitters which have very limited distribution in the brain. The principal transmitters involved in the control of the hypophysiotropic neurons are dopamine, norepinephrine, and serotonin (Fig. 12–18).

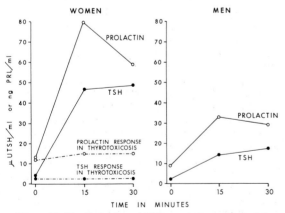

RESPONSE TO I.V. TRH 800 μg IN HUMANS (BOWERS et al, 1971)

Figure 12–16. Prolactin and TSH secretory response to injection of TRH in humans. This figure shows that TRH induces discharge of both prolactin and of TSH, that the effect in females is greater than in males (presumably due to estrogen sensitization of the pituitary), and that thyrotoxicosis inhibits the response of both prolactin and TSH to TRH. The inhibitory effect on TRH response is noted at the upper limit of the normal range of thyroid hormone levels and is a very sensitive test of minor degrees of thyroid hormone excess. Although TRH is a potent PRF, there is evidence that there is another PRF material physiologically connected to prolactin regulation. (Replotted from data of Bower, S., Friesen, H. G., et al.: *Biochem. Biophys. Res. Comm.* 45:1033, 1972.)

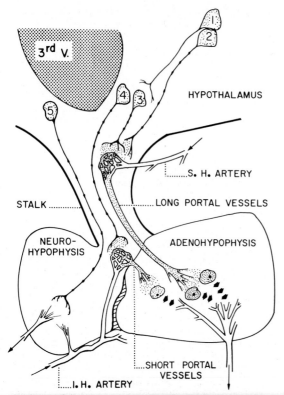

Figure 12–17. Neural control of pituitary gland. This figure summarizes the types of neural inputs into pituitary regulation. Neuron five represents the peptidergic neurons of the supraoptico-hypophysial and paraventriculo-hypophysial tracts, with hormone-producing cell bodies in the hypothalamus and nerve terminals in the neural lobe. Neurons four and three are the peptidergic neurons of the tubero-hypophysial tract, which secrete the hypophysiotropic hormones into the substance of the median eminence in anatomical relationship to the primary plexus. Neuron three ends in the median eminence. Neuron four ends low in the stalk. Neuron one represents a monoaminergic neuron ending in relation to the cell body of the peptidergic neuron. Neuron two represents a monoaminergic neuron ending on terminals of the peptidergic neuron to give axo-axonic transmission as proposed by Schneider and McCann. Neurons one and two are the functional links between the remainder of the brain and the peptidergic neuron. (Reproduced from Gay, V. L.: *Fertility and Sterility* 23:50, 1972, by permission of the Williams and Wilkins Company.)

The three transmitters are collectively referred to as monoamines. Dopamine and norepinephrine are referred to as catecholamines because they possess the characteristic dihydroxy substituents in the benzene ring. Monoaminergic pathways have been identified by a histochemical technique which reveals characteristic fluorescence after formaldehyde vapor treatment, and by the use of radioac-

tive neurotransmitters which characteristically are taken up by specific binding structures in nerve endings. Schematic distribution of monoaminergic neurons in the central nervous system is shown in Fig. 12–19.

From the results of electrical stimulation and lesion studies, it is apparent that various regions of the limbic system (that portion of the brain often referred to as the "visceral brain") can alter the neural inputs into the hypothalamus. These include the hippocampus, the amygdaloid nucleus, and interacting neurons. How these structures specifically influence neuroendocrine control of the anterior pituitary will be dealt with in the sections on individual hormone regulation.

It should be recognized that the function of monoaminergic neurotransmitters in altering peptidergic neuron function (including the neurohypophysial neurons) is analogous to certain other important neuroendocrine control systems located outside of the brain proper. These include the noradrenergic innervation of the pineal gland (derived from the superior cervical ganglion of the sympathetic chain) which ends in relation to the pinealocyte, of the noradrenergic neurons which end on renal juxtaglomerular cells where they control the secretion of the enzyme, renin, and of the pancreatic beta cell which is capable of both stimulation and inhibition of insulin release (see Chapters 9, 13, and 20).

Norepinephrine appears to be the major central monoamine transmitter stimulating secretion of LRH and TRH. Dopamine is stimulatory to release of PIF and GH-RF. Serotonin appears to stimulate prolactin release and growth hormone release. The secretion of ACTH is tonically *inhibited* by a catecholaminergic link in CRF control.

The clinical neuropharmacologist has available a number of drugs which interfere with one or more aspects of the synthesis, storage, uptake, and degradation of the biogenic amines (Table 12–2) [see Chapter 13 (pineal) and Chapter 5 (adrenal medulla)]. In general, drugs of this type may interfere with enzymes which are rate limiting in the formation of the transmitter and may interfere with the storage phase, the release phase, the receptor reaction, and the intrasynaptic degradation of the transmitter. Some agents act through the formation of false transmitters. By this is meant the incorporation of a precursor analogue into a neurotransmitter analogue of low potency. Some examples of the clinical effectiveness of certain drugs in altering anterior pituitary function in the human are the effects of reserpine in causing anovulation (through inhibition of cyclic LH re-

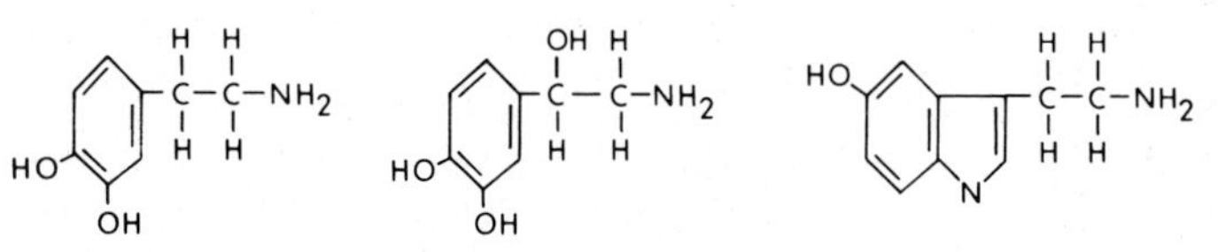

DOPAMINE   NOREPINEPHRINE   SEROTONIN

Figure 12–18. Structures of the three monoaminergic neurotransmitters involved in regulation of the hypophysiotropic (peptidergic) neurons. For descriptions of pathways of synthesis and degradation of the catecholamines, dopamine and norepinephrine, see Chapter 5, Part II; for the indolamines, such as serotonin, see Chapter 13.

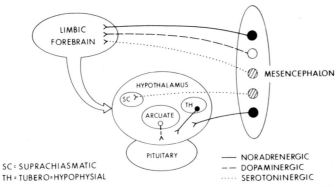

Figure 12–19. Major monoaminergic pathways involved in regulation of hypophysiotropic function. The peptidergic neurons of the hypothalamus are, in turn controlled by monoaminergic fibers. Dopaminergic pathways arise in the arcuate nucleus of the hypothalamus and noradrenergic pathways from the tubero-hypophysial nucleus (TH). Noradrenergic fibers from the mesencephalon also reach the hypothalamus and may interact with hypophysiotropic neurons. Within the mesencephalon, all three types of monoaminergic fibers arise; these are distributed to the limbic forebrain, which exerts effects on the hypothalamus through more conventional neural routes. In addition, the mesencephalon contributes a serotoninergic pathway to the suprachiasmatic nucleus of the hypothalamus (SC).

lease), the effects of chlorpromazine, which blunts the growth hormone secretory response to hypoglycemic stress and has been used to treat acromegaly, and imipramine, a tricyclic antidepressant which proves to be efficacious in inhibiting the nocturnal surge of GH secretion characteristic of the first hour or two of sleep. Imipramine is believed to act by blocking the uptake of norepinephrine and serotonin at nerve endings. Other drugs which block or blunt reflex GH release are alpha adrenergic blockers such as Dibenzyline. Amphetamines bring about the release of both growth hormone and ACTH in man. This class of drugs is believed to act by stimulating the release of norepinephrine from the endings of sympathetic nerve fibers in the brain and possibly by blocking reuptake of norepinephrine. The list of clinically effective drugs is quite large, and the search for drugs of this type which might affect individual pituitary functions is clearly quite important from a therapeutic point of view and is now being subject to intense research activity.

In order to understand the signficance of experiments in which monoamines or analogues are administered or to understand how various drugs can alter the function of the monoaminergic synapses (and thus alter hypophysiotropic function), it is necessary to review the enzymatic pathways of monoamine biosynthesis and the nature of the release, reuptake, and destructive mechanisms at the syn-

TABLE 12–2. CLINICALLY USEFUL PSYCHOPHARMACEUTICAL DRUGS INFLUENCING HYPOTHALAMIC MONOAMINE SYNTHESIS AND ACTION

Name	Mode of Action*
Reserpine	Blocks uptake and storage of norepinephrine, dopamine, and serotonin in preganglionic nerve endings. Interferes with monoamine transmitter control.
Chlorpromazine (Thorazine)	Interferes with uptake of norepinephrine at receptor and increases norepinephrine turnover.
L-Dopa	Increases monoamine activity by increasing substrate pool of dopamine and norepinephrine.
Iproniazid, imipramine, pargyline	Increase effectiveness of monoamines by inactivating metabolic destruction by the enzyme monoamine oxidase of norepinephrine, dopamine, and serotonin.
Tranylcypromine (Elavil), Cocaine	Increase noradrenergic effects by inhibiting norepinephrine uptake at presynaptic nerve terminals. This makes more norepinephrine available at receptors.
Amphetamines	Increase norepinephrine effects by discharging norepinephrine at terminals. Partially mimic norepinephrine and eventually may block postganglionic receptor.
Dibenzyline (Dibenamine)	Peripheral alpha-adrenergic blocker. Interferes with some central noradrenergic effects, but mechanism is not fully known.
Promethazine (Propranolol)	Peripheral beta-adrenergic blocker. Interferes with some central noradrenergic effects, but mechanism is not fully known.
Alpha-methyldopa (Aldomet)	Overall effect is to interfere with noradrenergic effects, but precise mode of action is unknown.

*Mode of action is the principal one. Several drugs have overlapping effects with other types of action.

apse. These have been worked out in elegant fashion by Axelrod and collaborators and are described in more detail in Chapters 5 and 13.

The best recognized neurotransmitter system of control of hypophysiotropic function is that for prolactin regulation, derived largely from the work of Kamberi, Porter, and their colleagues. Dopamine (infused into the third ventricle of the rat) inhibits the release of prolactin, presumably by stimulating the release of the prolactin inhibiting factor, PIF. In contrast, serotonin stimulates the release of prolactin, which may be due to inhibition of the secretion of PIF or the release of a prolactin releasing substance. Clinical expression of these effects comes from the finding that L-dopa, a precursor of dopamine, inhibits prolactin release in the human and has been used successfully in the management of nonpuerperal galactorrhea.

This agent, unlike dopamine, is capable of penetrating the blood-brain barrier. The amino acid precursor of serotonin, L-tryptophan, when given to humans, is unique among amino acids in causing release of prolactin. Dopamine injected into the rat third ventricle or L-dopa in the human brings about the release of growth hormone. Intraventricular dopamine also brings about the release of FSH and LH in the rat, but the dopamine precursor, L-dopa, when administered to the human in doses which release GH, does not alter gonadotropic function in the monkey. Intraventricular norepinephrine releases GH.

Neuroendocrine Aspects of Control of Specific Pituitary Tropic Hormones

Anatomical aspects of hypophysiotropic control are summarized in Figure 12–20.

General Considerations: Servo-Engineering Concepts in Neuroendocrinology

For each of the pituitary control systems, one can identify a hormonal feedback control exerted on the pituitary or hypothalamus or both and important interactions with relevant visceral, behavioral, and environmental functions. These are summarized in Figs. 12–21, 12–23, 12–24, 12–26, and 12–30.

In the neuroendocrine literature, servo-engineering concepts and formulations have been liberally applied to describe endocrine control systems. To clarify these terms, a brief account of feedback control is presented in this section together with a review of specific controls for hormonal systems described in following sections.

Most hormonal systems form part of a homeostatic feedback loop in which the controlled variable (generally the plasma hormone level or some function of it) determines the rate of secretion of the hormone. Most hormonal systems are, in fact, neg-

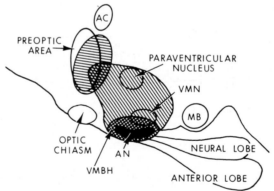

Figure 12–20. Anatomic localization of hypothalamic hypophysiotropic functions. This is a highly schematized diagram of the rat hypothalamus. Hypophysiotropic neuron cell bodies are generally distributed throughout the hypophysiotropic area. Stimulation at sites anywhere in this region is capable of eliciting release of TSH, FSH, LH, and prolactin. The medial-basal hypothalamus is the site of the "final common pathway" of neurons destined to end in the median eminence. This includes both peptidergic neurons and the terminals of the monoaminergic neurons (largely arcuate nucleus in origin) which end here. Stimulation here is capable of eliciting release of TSH, FSH, LH, prolactin, ACTH, and GH. Destruction of this region produces panhypophysiotropic hormone deficiency. All pituitary secretions are reduced except for prolactin and MSH, both of which are elevated. The ventromedial nucleus (together with the medial-basal hypothalamus) are the only hypothalamic sites electrically excitable for GH release. Lesions of the ventromedial nucleus produce GH deficit, hyperinsulinemia and hypophagia. The preoptic region is a site of input into the more basal hypothalamic regions for TSH regulation and gonadotropic regulation. Thermoreceptor neurons here are capable of stimulating TSH release, as well as stimulating autonomic body temperature regulation. In roughly the same region, the areas responsible for cyclic LH release in the female are located, in addition to the areas responsible for timing the onset of puberty. Stimulation here triggers TSH release and LH release. Lesions block cold-induced TSH discharge and produce an ovulation with constant anestrus.

The paraventricular nucleus is electrically excitable for oxytocin release and TSH release. The mammillary body is endocrinologically silent.

Receptor sites generating sexual behavior in response to estrogens and androgens are somewhat variable in different species. In rats they are localized chiefly in the medial-basal hypothalamic and preoptic area. The principal site of feedback for control of prolactin, growth hormone, ACTH, and gonadotropins is the medial-basal hypothalamus

Abbreviations: AC, anterior commissure; VMN, ventromedial nucleus; AN, arcuate nucleus; MB, mammillary body; VMBH, ventromedial-basal hypothalamus.

ative feedback systems (see below), but examples of positive feedback control can be cited. All the negative and positive feedback systems in which the pituitary is involved have nervous system inputs which either alter the "set point" of the feedback control system or introduce an "open loop" element of control.

Some definitions used in feedback control models should be clarified: these are largely borrowed from servo-engineering, and the mathematical modeling of these systems provides an important tool for the analysis and investigation of endocrine function. The mathematical basis of feedback systems is useful, particularly for research; the concepts are relatively simple and can be grasped at an intuitive level.

A *system* is a set of components related in such a way as to act as a unit.

A *control system* is a system so arranged as to regulate itself or another system.

An *input* is the stimulus applied to a control system from a source outside of the system so as to produce a specified response from the control system.

An *output* is the actual response of a control system.

An *open loop* control system is one with the control action independent of output.

A *closed loop* control system is one where control action depends upon (is a function of) output.

A *negative feedback* system is one in which the control action is a function of output in such a way that the output *inhibits* the control action.

A *positive feedback* system is a closed loop control system in which the output *accelerates* the control action.

All negative feedback systems have a "controlled variable" which is the factor (in the case of homeostatic functions) which the system is designed to maintain. For example, thyroid hormone levels are the controlled variable of the pituitary-thyroid axis, blood calcium is the controlled variable of the parathyroid-calcitonin-skeleton axis, blood glucose is the controlled variable in the pancreas-liver axis.

All feedback systems, negative or positive, have a "sensor element" capable of detecting the concentration of the controlled variable. Information gained by the sensor is used to determine the output of the controlling system. In *engineering* formulations of feedback, there are three elements of executive control of the controlled variable. There is a "sensing" element, which detects the concentration of the controlled variable; there is a "reference input," which may be defined as an absolute measure of what the controlled variable should be; and there is an "error signal," which is a function of the difference between what the sensor senses the controlled variable to be and what the reference input determines it *should* be. The magnitude of the error signal and the direction of its deviation (negative or positive) determines the output of the system. The reference input can be considered the "set point" of the system. An ex-

ample of these terms can be found in the common household thermostat. The reference input is the preferred temperature on the thermostat. There is a thermometer which detects the actual room temperature (the sensor). When the temperature sensed by the detector is different from the reference input, the furnace is either turned off or turned on until the error signal is minimized. In common furnace applications, the error signal is either off or on, but in more complex systems it is apparent that the error signal might determine output in a more sophisticated way; that is, a large error signal might call for a large burst of heat, and a small error signal might call for a small burst of heat.

Hormonal feedback control systems resemble their engineering analogues in that the concentration of the hormone in the blood (or some function of the hormone) regulates the output of the controlling gland. Hormonal feedback control systems differ from the engineering formulation system in that the sensor element and the reference input element are not readily distinguishable. Rather than having a reference input signal with which the controlled variable is compared, thus providing an error signal to determine gland output, the controlled variable has a more or less direct regulatory influence on the secretory process. This becomes more clear when specific systems are discussed.

The following types of neuroendocrine feedback control can be identified:

1. Simple closed loop negative feedback systems.

2. Closed loop negative feedback system with open loop transient controls.

3. Closed loop negative feedback system with positive feedback elements and open loop neural transients.

4. Open loop control with negative feedback elements.

Examples are given of each of these systems in the following section.

TSH Secretion

As outlined in Chapter 2, secretion of TSH is related to secretion of thyroid hormone through a classic feedback control system. Most early students of the pituitary-thyroid axis tacitly assumed that feedback control was exerted directly on the pituitary gland (Fig. 12–21). However, the possibility that thyroxine might exert its inhibitory effects through a primary action on the hypothalamus (see below) made it necessary to reexamine the assumption that thyrotroph cells are intrinsically sensitive to thyroxine concentration. The validity of this assumption has been verified by studying thyrotropin regulation in animals with pituitary stalk section, hypothalamic lesions, or pituitary transplants, all of which remove the pituitary gland from the influence of the brain. From these experiments and others in which minute amounts of thyroxine or triiodothyronine were in-

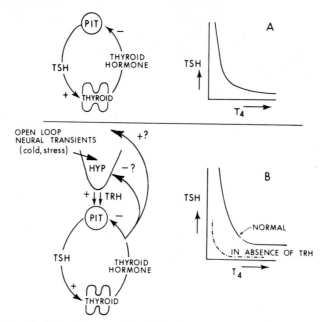

Figure 12–21. Pituitary-thyroid axis: closed loop negative feedback system with positive feedback elements and open loop neural transients.

At the simplest level of conceptualization (*A*), the pituitary and thyroid glands are functionally related in a closed loop negative feedback manner. When thyroid hormone is administered, TSH release is inhibited; when thyroid hormone levels fall, TSH secretion is stimulated. The function of this negative feedback can be illustrated in humans and in animals by fractional replacement of T_4 to thyroidectomized individuals. Plasma TSH is a curvilinear function of plasma thyroid hormone. In man, this relationship has been determined: plasma TSH is a function of the *log* of the plasma thyroid hormone level. The pituitary is the principal target of thyroid hormone in negative feedback.

If one examines the system more closely, it is apparent that there is a regulatory input into the system from the hypothalamus through the mediation of the hypophysiotropic hormone, TRH (*B*). The level at which the controlled variable is maintained, in this case the circulating thyroid hormone, is set by the hypothalamus. There is now some suggestion that thyroid hormone may act on the hypothalamus to stimulate the secretion of TRH (in which case it is acting as a positive feedback stimulus), and also some evidence that thyroid hormones may inhibit the activity of the hypothalamus under conditions as yet not well understood. This would be regarded as an example of negative feedback. In addition, the secretion of TSH is altered by neural open loop transients related to cold exposure (in which case TRH secretion "breaks through" the feedback control) and by conditions of stress (in which case the secretion of TSH is inhibited, presumably by a reduction in the hypothalamic input).

If one neglects for the moment the possibility of a negative feedback at the hypothalamic level, it appears that the interaction of a positive and a negative feedback loop provides a hypothetical mechanism by which the controlled variable (in this case thyroid hormone) can be programmed genetically. Thus thyroid hormones stimulate the output of TRH and inhibit the pituitary; the precise controlled T_4 blood level will be the resultant of the characteristic biochemical responses of these two interacting systems. Since both excitatory effects of T_4 at the pituitary and hypothalamic level are probably mediated by protein synthetic responses, this mechanism provides a means by which the mechanisms for maintenance of the controlled variable can be inherited. This generalization has not as yet been proved but may apply to other feedback systems for pituitary control.

jected directly into the gland, it has been concluded that the pituitary gland is autonomously sensitive to thyroid hormone concentration.

Although feedback effects are qualitatively normal in animals with the pituitary gland deprived of neural influences from the hypothalamus (Fig. 12–21), baseline thyroid function is markedly reduced. This finding has been taken to mean that the hypothalamus determines the "set point" of blood thyroid hormone. Tonic control of baseline TSH secretion is believed to be accomplished through the secretion of TRH into the hypophysial-portal vessels. Thus the function of the thyrotroph cell is stimulated by TRH and inhibited by thyroid hormone acting locally on the pituitary gland.

Thyroxine (or triiodothyronine) blocks the pituitary response to TRF. This reaction takes almost an hour to develop and appears to be mediated by a suppressor protein induced by the thyroactive material. Pretreatment with antibiotic inhibitors of protein synthesis blocks the inhibitory ac-

tion of thyronine on the response to TRH without interfering with TRH action directly. The interaction of thyroxine with TRH effects occurs over the physiologic range of plasma thyroid hormone levels (in both animals and man), permitting the conclusion that the TRH-thyroxine interaction is of major importance in negative feedback control of TSH secretion.

The occurrence of thyroid hormone feedback effects directed at the hypothalamic level has been controversial. The bulk of experiments have utilized direct microinjection studies; these suffer from the defect that injected T_4 or T_3 may be taken up in the median eminence and directly enter the pituitary by way of the portal vessels. There are several experiments in which T_4 implants into the preoptic hypothalamus appear to have inhibited TSH secretion under experimental conditions in which diffusion was not likely to have occurred. On the other hand, studies of control of the activity of TRH synthetase, the enzyme which forms TRH in the hypothalamus, indicate that thyroxine excess stimulates, and thyroxine deficiency inhibits, formation of this enzyme. If the concentration of enzyme is an indication of the rate of TRH synthesis and release, it would mean that thyroid hormone exerts a *positive* feedback effect on the hypothalamic component of TSH regulation. By this formulation, the plasma thyroid hormone level, which is the controlled variable in the pituitary-thyroid axis, is determined by the characteristics of the inhibitory effects of thyroid hormone on the pituitary and the excitatory effects on TRH secretion. Since both the inhibitory effects on the pituitary and the stimulatory effects at the hypothalamic level involve the formation of new protein, it would then be concluded that the fundamental action of thyroid hormone in determining its set point of control is based on stimulation of protein synthesis, an effect which appears to underlie its actions in all other thyroid-sensitive structures. This hypothesis provides an explanation of the mechanism of genetic control of the "set point" of thyroid hormone level in the blood. It should be emphasized that this proposed hypothesis has not been established (Fig. 12–21).

The region of the anterior hypothalamus between the paraventricular nucleus and the anterior lip of the median eminence appears to be responsible for TSH regulation (Fig. 12–20). Lesions in this region reduce thyroid function and block the usual thyroid activation which ordinarily follows exposure to the cold. Electrical stimulation of this region activates TSH release (Fig. 12–22), as does stimulation of the preoptic region.

The hypothalamic component of TSH control integrates thyroid activity with mechanisms for regulation of body temperature. Body temperature is controlled by a region in the anterior hypothalamus which contains neurons sensitive to even slight blood temperature changes in the brain ("core temperature"). This region is anatomically adjacent to the "thyrotropic area." If the anterior

hypothalamus is cooled, heat production and conservation mechanisms are activated and body temperature rises. If this region is heated, heat dissipation mechanisms are activated. Local cooling of the anterior hypothalamus and adjacent regions not only causes fever but activates the thyroid gland as well. Fever induced by usual measures inhibits thyroid function in animals.

One can bring about central cooling in rats by use of sympatholytic drugs which inactivate peripheral vasoconstriction. TSH release is induced. The existence of peripheral cold receptors mediating TSH regulation can be demonstrated in animals exposed to cold which manifest a slight rise in intrahypothalamic temperature. Newborn babies also act like rats in their thyroid response to external cooling. The characteristic postpartum rise in plasma TSH and PBI can be duplicated by placing newborns into room temperature after a period of time in an incubator. External cooling is much less effective in stimulating pituitary-thyroid function in adults. In rats, the increased thyroid function in chronic cold adaptation involves both increased thyroxine clearance from the gut due to increased food intake, increased hypothalamic drive, and a disproportionate elevation of triiodothyronine relative to thyronine.

Hypothalamic mechanisms for body temperature control and thyroid regulation are also related to control of food intake. As is outlined in Chapter 18 food seeking is governed by hypothalamic drive, a function which can be activated by central cooling of the hypothalamus. These observations indicate that within the small compass of the hypothalamus is an organized neural network (possibly noradrenergic) which controls body heat production and dissipation through a variety of autonomic, endocrine, and behavioral means.

The pituitary-thyroid axis is also affected by other hormones, particularly estrogens and adrenal corticoids, and by physical stress, which usually inhibits thyroid function. Estrogen admin-

Figure 12–22. Plasma thyroid stimulating hormone (TSH) response in individual rats following electrical and sham stimulation. The gray bar represents the period of stimulation. A prompt rise in plasma TSH is observed while the anesthetized controls show a gradual fall over the period of observation. (Reproduced from Martin J., and Reichlin, S.: *Science 168*:1366, 1970, with permission.)

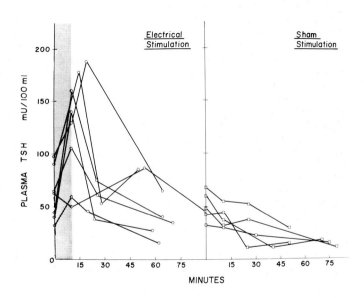

istration brings about a transient increase in TSH secretion and sensitizes the pituitary to the effects of TRH. Cortisol apparently acts on the hypothalamus to inhibit the release (or synthesis) of TRH.

Much has been written about the thyroid response to emotional stress, a traditional view derived initially from clinical experience with thyrotoxicosis. The first published report of the disease by Parry in 1825 included a case which was apparently precipitated in an invalid girl by a frightening episode with a runaway wheel chair. Subsequent authors emphasize acute and chronic emotional stress in the history of patients with thyrotoxicosis; a personality constellation typical of the disease has been described, and a large literature on thyroid function in mental disorder has accumulated (see below). Evidence that the nervous system affects the pituitary-thyroid axis has added to the speculation that emotional stress can increase TSH secretion and that Graves' disease may be a psychosomatic syndrome produced by disordered hypothalamic-pituitary-thyroid function.

Despite masses of information relating neural function to TSH regulation, convincing evidence that emotional stress can increase thyroid function in man has not been presented. In fact, most studies with animals, with few exceptions, indicate that emotional stress *inhibits* the pituitary-thyroid axis, and well-controlled experiments in man have failed to show any effect on thyroid function from a variety of emotionally stressful conditions. The psychosomatic theory of Graves' disease as a *hypothalamic-thyrotropic* hormone disorder has been disproven by the disclosure that TSH levels are not elevated in this disorder (see Chapter 4). Recent psychological studies have shown that the disordered brain function of individuals with Graves' disease is partly secondary to thyroid overactivity and is restored toward normal by appropriate therapy of the thyroid gland. That psychological factors may be important in the pathogenesis of Graves' disease has not been ruled out, but current data indicate that psychological stress does not produce its effect on the thyroid through the hypothalamic-pituitary system.

ACTH Secretion

Secretion of ACTH is regulated both by feedback from adrenocortical hormones and by a neuroendocrine mechanism (Fig. 12–23). Feedback regulation is readily demonstrated by treatment with exogenous steroids which cause adrenal atrophy or by adrenalectomy which causes plasma ACTH concentration to rise (see Chapter 5 for discussion of the pituitary-adrenal axis in man). Neural control is demonstrated by the wide variety of stimuli which increase ACTH secretion and plasma corticoid levels. A partial list of these includes acute trauma and burns, surgical operations, electroshock therapy, exercise, hypoglycemia, pyrogen administration, and emotional stress.

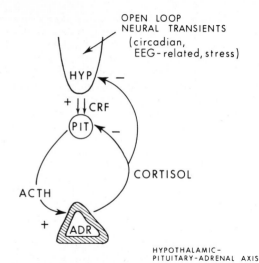

Figure 12–23. The pituitary-adrenal axis: closed loop negative feedback system with open loop transient controls.

The secretion of ACTH by the pituitary stimulates the release of cortisol, the principal glucocorticoid secretion of the adrenal gland. Glucocorticoid levels in turn regulate the output of ACTH. High cortisol levels inhibit, and low glucocorticoid levels stimulate, ACTH secretion. There is evidence that the feedback limb of cortisol effect is directed largely at the pituitary gland [here designated as a negative (−) function] and probably also at the neural control system. In addition to the negative feedback elements, the hypothalamus drives ACTH secretion through the release of the hypothalamic hormone, corticotropin-releasing hormone, CRF. The neural component of control is influenced by various nonfeedback neural transients. Some of these neural transients are themselves subject to feedback control by circulating cortisol levels, and others are unaffected by circulating cortisol. Neural factors include the circadian rhythm generated by intrinsic brain rhythms and linked to light-dark changes, sleep stage-related transients, and emotional and physical stress. Some workers have formulated this control system to signify that the central nervous system can determine the "set point" for plasma cortisol level; in addition, some neurogenic effects "break through" even maximum steroid treatment.

The ACTH-releasing substance that appears in the blood of stressed hypophysectomized rats (CRF) is no longer found after production of large ventral hypothalamic lesions, and, as indicated above, abundant evidence indicates ACTH-releasing factors in extracts of this region. Thus the ventral hypothalamus–median eminence is regarded as essential in the neural regulation of ACTH release, acting by the release of CRF into the hypophysial-portal circulation.

Considerable evidence also exists for a suprahypothalamic regulatory system which is both excitatory and inhibitory and involves portions of the "visceral brain," notably the amygdaloid nuclei and the reticular activating system. The inhibitory component of this system is probably adrenergic. These structures are probably involved in the psychic stimulation of ACTH release and the circadian rhythm of ACTH output. Although the ventral hypothalamus and median eminence appear from most studies to be essential for ACTH regulation in the normal animal, certain experiments indicate an extrahypothalamic source of CRF.

A plausible model of control of pituitary-adrenal function can be developed along lines analogous to the pituitary-thyroid axis (Fig. 12–23). It is proposed that the secretion of the adrenotropic cell is controlled by two interacting influences, a stimulatory component from the hypothalamus (CRF) and an inhibitory component responsive to the direct effects of cortisol at the pituitary level. The latter effect is dependent upon corticoid-induced new protein synthesis. Stress, circadian rhythms, and other stimuli release CRF which "breaks through" the steroid-inhibited pituitary. Higher doses of steroid are then required to suppress the CRF effect. The brain thus provides a variable "set point" of steroid control of the pituitary adrenostat. Some stimuli, such as severe nerve stimulation will break through even supramaximal corticoid levels. Still unresolved is the question of whether glucocorticoids influence CRF secretion. Corticoids are selectively taken up by cells in the hippocampus and septum; direct application of cortisol to nerve cells in the brain reduces single electrical activity of single units, and changes in hypothalamic CRF content are induced by cortisol treatment. The latter observations indicate that corticoids influence CRF secretion in some way but have not definitely clarified the role of feedback effects of glucocorticoids on the brain in the regulation of the pituitary-adrenal axis.

Neuroendocrine Aspects of the Regulation of Sexual Function

Every component of the patterned reproductive activity of the higher vertebrates depends upon a close interplay between neural and endocrine events. Perpetuation of the species obviously requires the accurate correlation of overt mating behavior with the internal events of gametogenesis in ovary and testis. This correlation of behavior and readiness for insemination is achieved by complex neuroendocrine mechanisms involving the brain, the pituitary, and the sex steroid hormones. But the role of the nervous system in regulating pituitary-gonadal function extends beyond the integration of reproductive behavior and the production of reproductive cycles. Neural influences also determine the timing of onset of puberty. Neuroendocrine factors are also involved in initiating and maintaining lactation and, in most vertebrates, with parental behavior.

Most information about neural control of pituitary-gonadal interactions has been obtained from animals, from which only general extrapolations to humans can be made. However, that neural control is involved in pituitary-gonadal function in man is clear from other avenues of investigation, e.g., alterations in human gonadal function following hypothalamic lesions, emotional disturbance, psychopharmacologic drugs, or electroshock therapy (see below).

The hypothalamus operates at several levels of control in reproductive regulation (Fig. 12–20). The median eminence and the tubero-hypophysial neurons maintain the basal secretion of FSH and LH by releasing gonadotropic releasing hormones into the hypophysial-portal vessels. When these regions are destroyed in animals or man as indicated above, gonadotropic hormone secretion is abolished and gonadal atrophy results.

Control of the Midcycle Ovulatory LH Surge: the "Female" Brain

The hypothalamus, exerting a second level of control of hypophysiotropic hormone secretion, triggers the surge of luteinizing hormone release which brings about ovulation. The factors which determine when this ovulatory LH surge occurs are complex and vary among different species of animals. In certain species, such as rabbit and cat, ovulation occurs only when the female has been successfully mounted by the male. This ovulatory reflex (which can also be induced by electrical or mechanical stimulation of the uterine cervix) involves the hypothalamus and the release of LRH into the hypophysial-portal circulation. In other species, such as the human and rat, ovulation occurs as part of the regular cycle of recurrent LH secretion. The precise mechanism underlying the regularly recurring ovulatory LH "surge" has not been fully established. Until fairly recently, it was believed that the release of ovulatory hormone was determined in turn by an endogenous *hypothalamic* rhythm. This view was supported by the findings that the rhythm of LH release in the rat is linked to the timing of light and darkness to which the animal is exposed, and that recurring ovulation can be blocked by the use of centrally acting drugs at critical stages of the cycle. In the human this endogenous rhythm is not altered by light but can be distorted by "psychic stress," psychopharmacologic drugs (see below), and certain diseases.

More recently it has become apparent that cyclic LH release in the rat, the human, and the monkey is due to the effect of preovulatory estrogen secretion by the ovary and not by a brain-determined rhythm (Fig. 12–24) (see Chapter 7). Rising plasma estrogen levels could provoke release of LH either by increasing the secretion of LRH or by enhancing the sensitivity of the pituitary to a constant level of LRH. Work in this area is controversial. The primate pituitary is not sensitized to LRH by estrogens, and it has been shown that bioassayable LRH appears in the blood of women at midcycle, findings which support the interpretation that estrogens exert a *positive* feedback effect on LRH secretion. If this interpretation proves to be correct, it would mean that a short "pulse" of estrogen at a critical stage in the cycle can stimulate the hypothalamus (Fig. 12–24). Other examples of estrogen stimulation of the hypothalamus are the hastening of onset of puberty in rats, presumably by stimulating brain maturation, and the stimulation of psychic changes in sexual receptivity.

Positive stimulatory effects of estrogen on gona-

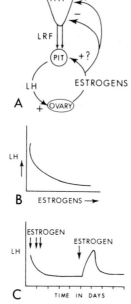

Figure 12–24. Pituitary-gonad axis: closed loop negative feedback system with positive feedback elements and open loop neural transients.

Hormone secretion by the ovary is regulated by two gonadotropic hormones, FSH (follicle stimulating hormone) and LH (luteinizing hormone). The secretion of the gonadotropic hormones is regulated by hypothalamic hormones, current evidence indicating that only one releasing factor, designated LH-RF or GnRF, is responsible for control of both hormones.

At the simplest level of formulation (as with the pituitary-thyroid axis), the level of estrogen in plasma is observed to control LH secretion (A). When plasma estrogens are elevated, LH secretion is inhibited. When plasma estrogen levels are low, the secretion of LH is enhanced. Thus plasma LH can be shown to be a negative function of plasma estrogen concentration (B). The precise target for estrogen in bringing out this negative inhibition is still not firmly established, but most work indicates that the effect is mediated at the hypothalamic level [here designated as a (−), presumably through inhibition of the secretion of LRF. The situation is not that simple, however, for it has also been shown that estrogen transients (such as occur after administration of estrogens in animals or humans and in the spontaneous phases of the estrus cycle) are capable of stimulating the release of LH (C). The site of action of the positive hormone transient has not been fully established. There is evidence that the positive feedback element may be exerted at the level of the pituitary (by sensitizing the LH-releasing mechanism to estrogens) or at some hypothalamic level which leads to the release of LRF. In humans, the latter explanation is most probable. In addition, the secretion of LRF by the hypothalamus is subject to open loop neural transients, such as sexual stimulation, which in some species may trigger LH secretion, and emotional stress, which in many species, including the human, can inhibit LH secretion.

the hypothalamus duplicates the results of systemic administration.

To explain how both positive and negative stimulatory effects can follow estrogen administration, one may speculate that there are two populations of estrogen-sensitive LRH secreting neurons whose response to the sex steroid are different. Brief, intense estrogen stimulation (as at the midcycle preovulatory period) excites the stimulatory neurons; chronic estrogen administration inhibits a population of neurons.

Characteristically, normal adult *male* rodents lack an intrinsic neural mechanism for producing the ovulatory surge of LH secretion in response to estrogen administration. Studies of rats and mice have shown that the "female" pattern of hypothalamic function, *i.e.,* the capacity to release LH in response to androgens, is present at birth in males as well as in females. The "female" pattern of hypothalamic function is suppressed in the male rat when the developing brain is exposed to androgens at a critical developmental period (between birth and 5 days of age). This reaction is analogous to the effects of androgen on the differentiation of the internal and external genitalia. Unlike the rat, however, the castrated male monkey maintained on estrogens shows a surge of LH and FSH secretion following injection of estrogen. If this is shown to be true for the human, it would indicate that there is not a critical period of androgenization of the gonadotropic regulatory mechanism in primates. Nevertheless, there may be some kind of androgen-induced brain change even in humans, because prenatally masculinized genetic female humans show a predominance of tomboyish behavior prepubertally and, as adults, display behavioral patterns and interests more commonly associated with male predominance. It is emphasized (see below also) that the direction of sexual interest of prenatally masculinized females is determined by the psychological rearing pattern and not by the hormonal environment. In recent years it has been proposed that subtle psychological changes may be produced in higher mammals by alterations in endocrine environment *in utero.* Such disorders as transsexualism and homosexuality have been theorized as possibly being related in some cases to altered prenatal brain differentiation analogous to the finding that the neonatally androgenized female rat permanently loses characteristic female sexual behavior (even when given estrogens), and the neonatally castrate male rat never attains typical mounting behavior as an adult, even with full replacement androgen therapy.

Timing of Puberty

A third level of hypothalamic control, imposed upon the other two, is the determination of time of onset of puberty. Long before puberty begins, the gonads and secondary sexual structures are capable of being stimulated by exogenous hormones,

dotropin are generally looked upon as being paradoxical because under most circumstances estrogens inhibit gonadotropic secretion. The castrate man or woman or castrate animal has high LH and FSH plasma levels, and these are suppressed by administering exogenous steroids. Compensatory hyperfunction of the gonads after partial removal is also prevented by estrogen administration. These more obvious effects of sex steroids have usually been considered to be due to suppression of LRH secretion, because localized deposition of estrogen in various critical parts of and the pituitary gland is capable of releasing gonadotropins when stimulated by LRF. In the human, a negative feedback system of pituitary-gonad secretion occurs before puberty; the positive component appears at puberty. It is characteristic of the prepubertal state that the adult pattern of pituitary and gonadal secretion does not appear, even though these glands are capable of normal function.

Clinical analysis of hypothalamic disease and destruction of various parts of the brain in experimental animals have shown that certain regions of the hypothalamus tonically inhibit gonadotropin secretion before puberty. Donovan and Van der Werfften Bosch have argued that since feedback control of gonadotropin secretion from estrogens appears to involve hypothalamic and not pituitary receptors, the fundamental change in the advance toward sexual maturity is a reduction in hypothalamic sensitivity to feedback effects of gonadal hormone. According to this interpretation, the infantile hypothalamus is more sensitive to estrogens and androgens and therefore maintains the low gonadotropin levels characteristic of the prepubertal state. As the brain matures, this sensitivity to the inhibitory actions of gonadal steroids decreases, allowing the secretion of gonadotropin to increase. This maturation toward decreasing sensitivity to hormone feedback is analogous to other maturational changes in the developing brain, which include changes in behavior, intelligence, and personality. McCann suggests that hypothalamic lesions, both clinical and experimental, bring on precocious puberty by reducing the size of the area from which pituitary-inhibiting stimuli arise. Such an interpretation agrees well with clinical data on destructive lesions of the hypothalamus (see below).

Pubertal development in the human is accompanied by the capacity to respond to estrogen with *increased* LH secretion. Both components are probably responsible for onset of puberty. The time of onset of pubertal brain function depends upon genetic and environmental factors. In humans, the secular trend for decreasing age of onset of puberty demonstrable by study of records over the past century and comparisons of different population groups indicates that the trigger for puberty is a critical factor related to body size. This is the probable explanation of why improved nutrition and freedom from disease have been followed by decreasing age of onset of menarche. Moderately obese girls have earlier puberties than do normally weighted girls, and individuals (or rats) with malnutrition fail to develop normal pituitary-ovarian function.

Effect of Sex Steroids on the Brain

Not only does feedback action of sex steroids on the central nervous system play an important role in regulating gonadotropin secretion, but also the direct effects of sex steroids on the brain markedly alter sexual behavior. After castration, female cats refuse to mate and the genital tract becomes atrophic, both responses resulting from estrogen lack and both readily reversed by systemic replacement treatment. Minute implants of estrogens in certain hypothalamic regions restore normal sexual behavior with amounts of sex hormone which do not reverse atrophic genital changes. These observations indicate that the cat's brain is sensitive to estrogens and capable of inducing the full range of sexual behavior. Estrogen chemoreceptor function of the hypothalamus can also be demonstrated by radioautographic localization of labeled estrogenic hormones after systemic administration. The estrogen concentrates in areas corresponding to those from which physiologic effects are obtained after local implantations. Specific cytoplasmic and nuclear estrogen-binding proteins analogous to those found in the uterus have been identified in this region. It is apparent that sex drive is generated by a neural signal from an estrogen receptor located within the hypothalamus. This generation of a basic drive is analogous to hunger drive in hypoglycemia, to thirst following hyperosmolarity, and to temperature-safeguarding behavior following central cooling or heating.

Progesterone blocks the ovulatory surge of LH release but, by itself, does not inhibit either FSH or the tonic component of LH secretion. The effect on ovulation is the basis for the use of the oral contraceptive progestational agents. Adding small, otherwise ineffective, amounts of estrogen to progesterone leads to complete inhibition of LH secretion. Recent neurophysiologic studies indicate that progesterone acts on certain hypothalamic neurons to decrease their rate of spontaneous firing and to elevate their threshold of excitability to reflex stimulation from the uterine cervix. In this regard, it should be recalled that progesterone in the human acts on the hypothalamus to raise body temperature. This mechanism is responsible for the postovulatory rise in basal body temperature commonly used as an index of ovulation. The hypothalamus is not the only structure in which excitability is decreased by progesterone. Spontaneous and electrically or pharmacologically stimulated contractions of the uterus are also inhibited by progesterone.

Although it has appeared reasonable to believe that the suppressive effects of progesterone are exerted on the hypothalamic component of control, a number of recent studies have indicated that progesterone and synthetic gestagens of the type used in contraceptive (i.e., chlormadinone) block the effect of LRF at the pituitary level rather than in the hypothalamus. Progesterone action is thus analogous to thyroid hormone and cortisol feedback. As in the case of estrogens in which negative feedback effects also predominante, progesterone under certain conditions can also elicit gonadotropic stimulatory responses. For example, progesterone can hasten the onset of puberty and induce an ovulatory LH surge if given to an estrogen-primed woman. Factors determining the nature and direction of the gonadotropic response to progesterone and the site of its action in each of these activities remain to be clarified.

The hypothalamus is capable of maintaining gonadal function, estrus cycling, and patterned mating behavior, but it is important to recognize that nerve pathways exist which bring the hypothalamus under the influence of the "visceral brain," now recognized to be the anatomic substrate of emotion. Through these pathways, emotional states in both humans and animals can alter gonadotropic function. Functional relations of hypothalamus, pituitary, and ovary gonadotropic control are schematically outlined in Fig. 12–24.

This brief description of the hypothalamus emphasizes its pivotal role in integrating the behavioral response to sex hormones with the regulatory action of the hypothalamus on gonadal secretion. The relevance of hypothalamic function to human sexual function is discussed below.

Lactation

The sequence of hormonal events responsible for growth of the breast and for lactation are fully as complicated as those of the ovarian cycle, a not unexpected circumstance in view of the mammal's late phylogenetic development (see Chapter 7). This system has been worked out most completely in the rat, where duct growth appears to require the combined action of corticoids, growth hormone, and estrogen; in addition, progesterone and prolactin are needed for growth of the alveolar lobules. Milk secretion is initiated when progesterone and estrogen are withdrawn simultaneously but only in the continued presence of prolactin, insulin, and the adrenal corticoids. During pregnancy, placental lactogen and pituitary prolactin are secreted in increased amounts. Delivery of the child initiates lactation mainly because of the sudden withdrawal of estrogen and progesterone when the placenta is lost. Once lactation has developed, its maintenance depends on continued secretion of prolactin. As Selye showed many years ago, the continued secretion of milk after delivery depends upon prolactin released after mechanical stimulation of the nipples by suckling. Reflex discharge of prolactin from the pituitary gland is abolished by denervation of the nipples or by lesions in the spinal cord and brainstem. Impulses carried over these pathways ultimately impinge upon the hypothalamus where they bring about the release of prolactin (Fig. 12–25). Release of prolactin has usually been attributed to an inhibition of the secretion of the hypophysiotropic hormone PIF (prolactin inhibiting factor), which led to an "unleashing" of prolactin secretion. This may in fact be the case, but, in addition, evidence has accumulated indicating that the hypothalamus contains a prolactin releasing factor, and it is possible that PRF is released in response to suckling. The short time course of suckling-induced prolactin release and the finding

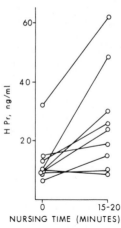

PLASMA PROLACTIN RISE AFTER NURSING IN WOMEN

Figure 12–25. Illustrated here is the change in plasma prolactin level which follows nursing in the human. (Data of Valverde, R. C., Friesen, H. G., and Reichlin, S., 1972, unpublished.)

that prolactin secretion (like GH secretion) is extremely labile further support the existence of PRF.

Suckling brings about two additional neurogenic responses: milk "let down" and gonadotropic hormone inhibition. Milk "let down" refers to the appearance of milk in the nipple ducts a few seconds after institution of nipple stimulation. Contraction of the myoepithelial cells of the breast parenchymal acinus is responsible for the appearance of milk in the larger ducts, a response due to the direct effect of oxytocin, in turn released by neural stimuli reaching the paraventricular nuclei. Inhibition of the release of the FSH- and LH-releasing factors by a suckling-induced reflex results in the inhibition of ovarian function and of ovulation responsible for amenorrhea and infertility of the nursing mother. It is probable that suckling-induced gonadotropin inhibition is due to suckling-induced prolactin secretion acting through short-loop feedback effects on the hypothalamus. The inhibitory effects of suckling on gonadotropin secretion decline with time; therefore menstrual periods and conception may still occur during lactation. Prolactin release also declines with passage of time after delivery.

In addition to stimulation of the breast, prolactin has in certain species an important supporting role in maintaining the corpus luteum. Thus it is also termed luteotropic hormone (LTH). Under the influence of LTH, the rat corpus luteum persists and secretes progesterone. In a normal rat ovarian cycle, LTH is not secreted and corpus luteum does not persist. However, after various neural stimuli, including mechanical or electrical stimulation of the uterine cervix, electroshock to the head, severe stress, certain psychopharmacologic drugs, and copulation with sterile males, LTH is released and the corpus luteum persists and secretes progesterone. This condition, termed *pseudopregnancy,* is mentioned here because of certain similarities it has to the human syndrome termed *persistent corpus luteum* (PCL) and also to pseudocyesis (see below). Recent evidence also suggests (contrary to prior belief) that, in the primate as well as the rat, prolactin is luteotropic.

Used as a test of prolactin (LTH) release, persistent functioning of the corpus luteum has revealed that LTH secretion increases when the pituitary gland is transplanted from the median eminence or if the basal portions of the hypothalamus are destroyed. These observations have been important links in the chain of evidence proving that the hypothalamus exerts tonic inhibitory control over prolactin secretion.

Neural elements regulating prolactin secretion are also identifiable in humans. Galactorrhea not infrequently follows section of the pituitary stalk in women operated upon for metastatic breast carcinoma whose pituitary glands are otherwise free from disease. Less commonly, irritation of the thoracic-spinal nerve segments, as by thoracotomy or herpes zoster, initiates persistent lactation. Certain psychopharmacologic drugs also initiate lactation in women, an effect readily produced in the laboratory animal. This effect is due to excessive stimulation of the breast by prolactin, as shown in both animals and the human, by elevations in radioimmunoassayable prolactin. Various human tumors and inflammatory lesions of the hypothalamic-pituitary region on occasion result in galactorrhea, and, in at least one of these syndromes, psychiatric disorders are common (see below, non-puerperal galactorrhea). Plasma prolactin levels are reduced by L-dopa in normal and abnormal states of prolactin secretion in women.

From these studies on neural control of prolactin secretion, it appears reasonable to hypothesize that all the stimuli reported to induce a release of prolactin, including psychopharmacologic drugs and the human galactorrhea syndrome, ultimately produce their major effect by altering secretions of prolactin regulating hormones, PIF and probably PRF. Current views of prolactin regulation are summarized in Figure 12–26.

GH Regulation

Neural Pathways

The major early observations from which neural control of GH secretion was inferred were the demonstration that spontaneous disease of the hypothalamus in man, or induced hypothalamic damage or pituitary stalk section in animals, induced a degree of growth retardation which could not be restored by treatment with substitution therapy (omitting GH); that growth was abolished in animals by transplantation of the pituitary away from the hypothalamus; that lesions of the hypothalamus led to a decrease in pituitary GH concentration; and that a growth hormone stimulating sub-

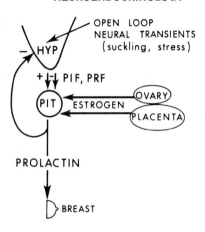

HYPOTHALAMIC REGULATION
OF PROLACTIN SECRETION

Figure 12–26. Prolactin secretion: open loop control with negative feedback elements.

As in the case of GH (see Fig. 12–30), the predominant regulatory influence of prolactin secretion is by open loop neural transients which cause the release of prolactin-releasing factor or the inhibition of prolactin-inhibiting factor, shown as a dual hypothalamic control. Suckling, emotional stress, and endogenous sleep rhythms are the most important neural transients involved. As in the case of GH, there is negative feedback loop control of the secretion of the hypothalamic hormones which regulate prolactin secretion. This negative feedback control is probably more important in the case of prolactin secretion. As with GH regulation, the estrogen secretion of the ovary (and placenta) sensitizes the pituitary to the effects of PRF, despite the fact that these glands are not a functional part of a feedback loop.

stance (effective in organ incubates) could be demonstrated in hypothalamic extracts. These observations arose at a time when GH was primarily linked to growth stimulation and therefore made little teleologic sense in relating a role of the brain to the regulation of growth. With the newer understanding that GH secretion is episodic and influenced by many stimuli [see Chapter 2 (Pituitary)], including psychic factors, endogenous sleep rhythms, and exercise, neural control has emerged as the centrally important mechanism of GH regulation, although the teleologic significance of this fact is still not fully understood.

The first clear-cut evidence, using modern immunoassay techniques, that GH secretion was under control of the nervous system was the study by Roth, Glick, Berson, and Yalow, who demonstrated that pituitary stalk section in the human blocked hypoglycemia-induced GH discharge. This observation has been supported by a number of more complete studies in humans which indicate that either stalk section or a variety of spontaneously occurring hypothalamic diseases block reflex GH discharge. In some series of patients subjected to stalk section, a few may still manifest reflex GH discharge. Such cases may represent incomplete operations, regrowth of the hypophysial-portal vessels (as demonstrated by Harris in his classic studies of regulation of estrus in the rat), or the release into the general blood stream of growth hormone releasing substance from the hypothal-

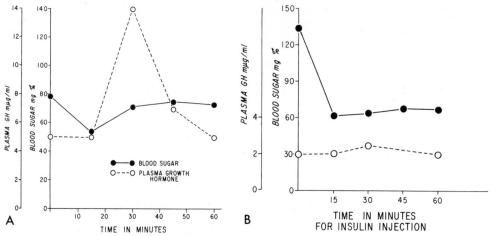

Figure 12--27. *A*, Blood glucose and plasma GH response to hypoglycemia in the squirrel monkey. As in man, insulin (0.15 U. per kg.) lowered the blood glucose level and stimulated the release of growth hormone. *B*, Blood glucose and plasma GH response to hypoglycemia in a squirrel monkey with an electrolytic lesion in the anterior median eminence. In this animal, GH levels failed to rise despite the fact that blood glucose concentrations fell as much as in the normal animal. Animals of this type have been described as manifesting "growth hormone blockade." (Reproduced from Abrams, R., Parker, M., et al.: *Endocrinology* 78:605, 1966, with permission.)

amus which reaches the pituitary through the general circulation. With time, hypoglycemic responses gradually decline. In the human, reflex growth hormone discharge has been found to be one of the most sensitive indicators of hypothalamic-pituitary disease. These include tumors of many kinds, granulomatous disease, and several forms of metabolic disturbance. The anatomic localization of hypothalamic areas subserving GH regulation in the human have not as yet been established, but it has been shown that electrical stimulation of posterior hypothalamus in man does indeed result in an increase in plasma radioimmunoassayable GH.

Studies in humans, though specific in the sense that reliable signs of GH secretion are available, have not permitted precise identification of neural pathways underlying growth hormone secretion. This has depended upon animal studies, utilizing either ablation or stimulation techniques. Electrolytic lesions of the stalk of the squirrel monkey will inhibit reflex GH responses to induced hypoglycemia (Fig. 12–27) or emotional stress. Damage to as little as one third of the stalk is sufficient to block GH responses. The hypothalamic areas responsible for these effects are the median eminence and perhaps the inferior portion of the mammillary bodies.

Using electrical stimulation methods, neural control pathways have been worked out most clearly in the rat. Electrical stimulation of the ventromedial nucleus and medial-basal hypothalamus provoke a prompt rise in plasma GH, hormone levels thereafter gradually falling with the same decay constants as GH (Fig. 12–28). Stimulations elsewhere in the hypothalamus, such as in the preoptic area and the paraventricular nuclei, although they lead to release of TSH, have no effect on plasma GH, thus confirming the specificity of GH controlling areas.

Extrahypothalamic sites of GH regulation must exist in view of the marked lability of GH secretion and its response to a wide variety of neural inputs including spontaneous variations with sleep cycle. A tonic neural *inhibitory* influence on GH secretion

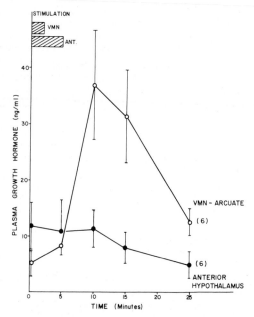

Figure 12–28. Effect on plasma GH of electrical stimulation of the ventromedial hypothalamic nucleus of the rat. This figure shows the marked increase in plasma GH levels which follows electrical stimulation of the ventromedial nucleus of the rat. The ventromedial nucleus and ventral-basal hypothalamus are the only hypothalamic regions capable of this response, although certain extrahypothalamic sites may also cause this change (see Fig. 12–29). Note the very short latent period of the response. The ventromedial nucleus is also important in that it has an effect on insulin secretion and satiety sensation and is the site of glucoreceptors. (Reproduced from Martin, J.: *Endocrinology* 91:107–115, 1972, with permission.)

MAJOR AFFERENT PATHWAYS TO THE VENTROMEDIAL–ARCUATE COMPLEX IN THE RAT

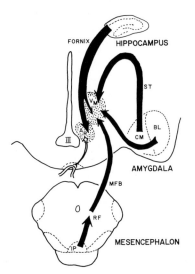

Figure 12–29. Neural pathways involved in GH regulation. This diagram illustrates the varied pathways by which impulses from the limbic system (visceral brain) ultimately impinge upon the ventromedial nucleus, which in turn is capable of stimulating GH release through the mediation of GH-RF. Pharmacologic blocking studies show that the pathways between the extrahypothalamic regions and the ventromedial nucleus are catecholaminergic, whereas those between the ventromedial nucleus and the stalk-median eminence region are not catecholaminergic. (Reproduced from Martin, J.: *Endocrinology 91*:107–115, 1972, with permission.)

is revealed by experiments in which the hypothalamus is isolated from anterior neural connections by the Halasz technique. Such animals have high plasma growth hormone levels and grow at a more rapid rate than do sham-operated controls. Extrahypothalamic pathways capable of stimulating GH secretion have been demonstrated to include a number of areas in the "visceral brain" (Fig. 12–29). Since both GH release and slow wave sleep changes in the EEG are produced by hippocampal stimulation, it has been postulated that this region is responsible for the generation of slow wave sleep–related GH discharge.

Glucoreceptors and Hypothalamic Control of GH Secretion

A number of established physiologic facts have made it appear almost certain that GH responses to hypoglycemia and hyperglycemia are mediated by glucose-sensitive neural structures. The existence of hypothalamic neurons electrically responsive to shifts in blood glucose has been demonstrated in the region of the ventromedial nucleus (VMN), and this region appears to be glucoreceptive for appetite regulation as well. Moreover, the VMN is one of the primary areas mediating GH secretion. Small amounts of glucose infused into the median eminence of the hypothalamus of the

squirrel monkey during the course of an insulin tolerance test in which peripheral glucopenia had been produced blocked the expected GH discharge. Critical to the evaluation of the site of the glucose receptive neurons is the distribution of glucose after infusion. Unfortunately, the site of the "glucoreceptor" cannot be identified precisely because tracer glucose diffuses throughout the ventricular system, as shown by studies of radioactivity after intrahypothalamic injection of C^{14} glucose. These results nevertheless support the existence of central nervous system glucose-sensitive structures capable of altering GH secretion. When small amounts of 2-deoxyglucose were injected into various regions of the hypothalamus of the rhesus monkey (a procedure causing local blockade of glucose effect), GH hypersecretion was produced in those animals in which the infusion had been into the lateral hypothalamus, an observation which suggests the existence of a highly localized neuronal system sensitive to tissue glucose deficit and linked to the regulation of GH secretion. Similar studies of deoxyglucose effects on gastric secretion in the rat also indicate a lateral hypothalamic localization of hypoglycemia-sensitive neurons.

Contrary to expectations, GH release is not elicited from the VMN area by local injection of 2-deoxyglucose. This observation may be interpreted to mean that the lateral hypothalamus is sensitive to *falling* levels of plasma glucose, and that the VMN is sensitive to *rising* levels of glucose. Such a formulation is compatible with current views about reciprocal medial and lateral hypothalamic control of food intake, in which food drive is controlled by the lateral hypothalamus and satiety by the VMN. It has been reasonably well established that *changing* glucose level is a stimulus for the alteration of GH secretion, not any fixed homeostatically maintained glucose level. Glucoreceptor regulation is probably involved in the inhibition of exercise-induced GH discharge by glucose administration, and "adaptation" of glucoreceptors may be responsible for the abnormalities in GH regulation seen in poorly regulated diabetes (see Chapter 9).

Short Loop Feedback Control

Several of the anterior pituitary hormones appear to be capable of influencing their own secretions through effects of the tropic hormone on a regulatory area of either hypothalamus or pituitary (independent of the target glands). The lack of a classic feedback mechanism for the control of GH has made it reasonable to consider that a short loop feedback might play a relatively important role in regulation of this hormone (Fig. 12–30).

The earliest clue that GH might regulate its own secretion directly was the observation that the characteristic regranulation of pituitary acidophils, observed when thyroid hormone is administered to a thyroxine-deficient animal, is delayed and reduced by simultaneous administration of

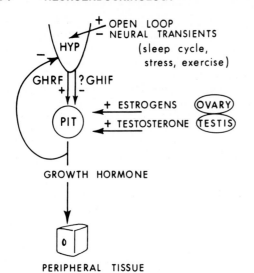

Figure 12–30. Hypothalamic-pituitary axis for regulation of growth hormone secretion: open loop control with negative feedback elements.

In two particular systems for anterior pituitary regulation, those for growth hormone and for prolactin, the predominant control is from neural transients. Neither of these hormones exerts effects on target glands (as for example, the thyroid or adrenal), but each of these hormones is capable of exerting a negative influence on its own secretion through effects at the hypothalamic level. The relative importance of these negative feedback components is unknown. Feedback loops of this type have been called "short loop feedback" to contrast with loops involving target organs.

The secretion of GH is regulated by the secretion of the hypothalamic hormone, GH-RF. The secretion of the GH-RF is affected by neural transients correlated with the sleep cycle and by falling blood sugar levels; moreover, it is triggered by emotional stress and by exercise. GH may exert a negative feedback effect at the hypothalamus. Sensitivity of the pituitary to the effects of GH-RF is modulated by the sex steroids, so that the ovary and the testis can influence GH secretion even though these glands are *not a functional part of the GH feedback loop*. GHIF (growth hormone inhibiting factor) or "somatostatin" may play a role also.

growth hormone. Other more substantial evidence is the demonstration that rats bearing mammotropic-somatotropic tumors have reduced pituitary GH levels and that the pituitaries of such animals synthesize GH *in vitro* at a reduced rate.

In the human, the infusion of GH has been shown to interfere with subsequent hypoglycemia-induced GH discharge, and in the Laron type of dwarf, believed to have a deficiency of tissue responsiveness to GH (and presumably of the GH-sensitive receptor), plasma GH levels are exceedingly high.

Perhaps the most convincing evidence for a role of GH in regulating GH secretion is the demonstration that an infusion of GH administered two hours prior to either hypoglycemic or vasopressin-induced stress blocks the expected GH discharge in the rhesus monkey.

None of these studies satisfactorily demonstrates that GH is acting directly on a specific regulatory area in hypothalamus or pituitary or indirectly through stimulation of a metabolic product. In fact, since GH effects on bone are mediated through a plasma factor termed somatomedin (a

factor believed to be deficient in the Laron dwarf who manifests high GH levels), it is possible that somatomedin is the intermediate step in control; however, if such be the case its site of action in GH regulation is unknown. Several studies suggest that GH may interfere both with GH-RF release and with pituitary responsiveness to GH-RF. The physiologic importance of short loop feedback control awaits further study.

Pherhormones

Every owner of a female dog in heat becomes unpleasantly aware of the fact that the dog emits a scent infinitely attractive to male dogs in the neighborhood. This phenomenon is an example of a response mediated by a pherhormone, the term applied to chemical substances secreted by one animal which arouse either behavioral or hormonal changes in another individual of the same species. In nonvertebrate forms such as moths, pherhormones are of great importance in regulating many aspects of activity and behavior. In sheep and goats, the onset of estrus behavior and ovulation is accelerated if males are placed with the flock. In the female mouse, gonadotropic function is very strikingly altered by the presence of a male. In the absence of a male, estrus cycles tend to be irregular and may become prolonged. In the presence of the male, sexual cycles become synchronized, and on the third night after contact with the male, estrus behavior and mating occur. This response, termed the Whitten effect, can be induced merely by exposing the females to the urine-contaminated bedding of the male. In the Bruce effect, female mice successfully mated with familiar males will fail to carry pregnancy to term if permitted to come in contact with the urine of a strange male or a male from a different strain of mice. Female rats deprived of their olfactory bulbs will not build nests for their young or retrieve them. In monkeys, fatty acids formed in the vagina at estrus, presumably as a consequence of hormonally altered bacterial flora, arouse grooming behavior in the male.

Little is known about the role of pherhormones in human sexual activity. Perfumes have been used since antiquity for purposes of enhancing the sexual attractiveness of women. Interestingly, certain of the ingredients forming the base of perfume (musk and civet) are derived from the glands of animals who use these secretions as sexual attractants. The ability to detect certain kinds of smells is hormone-dependent in women and is heightened at midcycle. There is a statistically significant correlation between the timing of the menstrual cycle in women living together as roommates compared to those who are separated. The basis of this synchronization of cycles is unknown, but the role of pherhormones in this response is strongly suggested. It should be emphasized that a pherhormone may act without the necessary conscious awareness of the stimulus being perceived. The role of pherhormones in human function is largely unknown, but may prove to be more important than is generally recognized.

Sleep-related Endocrine Rhythms

Sensitive immunoassay methods capable of detecting minute-by-minute changes in plasma hormone level have revealed unexpected periodic phenomena in pituitary secretion, some of which are related to phases of the sleep cycle and which may become disordered as a consequence of abnormal brain function. The secretion of growth hormone occurs in periodic bursts, reaching a maximum within an hour of falling asleep, and is chiefly related to slow wave sleep. Nocturnal growth hormone secretion is of major importance for total GH secretion since more than two thirds of total GH secretion occurs during the night. Children have much greater nocturnal GH secretion than do adults, and there are functional consequences (such as impaired glucose tolerance) occurring as a response to the nocturnal GH secretion. Glucose administration does not block nocturnal GH secretion nor do alpha receptor blockers. On the other hand, fatty acids are inhibitory of nocturnal secretion. Prolactin secretion also occurs in bursts at night.

The release of ACTH is largely, but not exclusively, related to rapid eye movement (REM) sleep; as in the case of GH, the highest values for plasma ACTH and cortisol are achieved at night. Unlike GH secretion, which is *sleep*-related, the diurnal rhythm of ACTH secretion is related to day–night cycle. In children, the appearance of puberty is heralded by the onset of bursts of REM sleep-related gonadotropic hormone release which disappear with full sexual maturity.

Changes in endocrine function at night are probably related to the intrinsic electrical activity of the limbic system. Loss of circadian rhythms of ACTH secretion are the earliest signs of abnormality in hypothalamic disease. In Cushing's disease, the loss of episodic ACTH and GH secretion (even after therapy) has been taken to mean that there is an intrinsic hypothalamic abnormality in this disease. Children with impaired growth may show normal stress-responsive GH discharge but abnormal nocturnal GH secretion; severe growth deficiency may result from loss of nocturnal sleep-related GH secretion.

An important practical consequence of sleep-related endocrine rhythms is the recognition that adequate evaluation of endocrine function requires study over the full twenty-four hours of one day. An important theoretical consequence of this new information is that the bulk of anterior pituitary secretion is under open loop nonhomeostatic control.

Ependymal Cell Secretory Structures (Fig. 12–31)

Lining the ventricles of the brain and the central canal of the spinal cord are ependymal cells which in most places form cuboidal, usually ciliated, epithelium. In several areas of the third ventricle, cells have been modified into structures which are of actual or presumptive neuroendocrine interest. Most important of these is the pineal gland, derived embryologically from the ependymal cells of the roof of the third ventricle (See Chapter 13). Others are the subcommissural organ, the subfornical organ, and the specialized ependyma of the floor of the third ventricle at the site of the median eminence and the infundibular recess. The choroid plexus, also an ependymal derivative, forms a

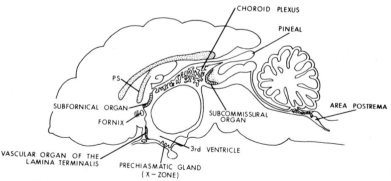

Figure 12–31. Topographical overview of the major periventricular organs of the rabbit on a semischematic sagittal section. The choroid plexus may also have endocrine function. All four periventricular organs are derived from ependyma and apparently have a secretory function as inferred from ultramicroscopic and histochemical demonstration of structures resembling secretory granules. The subfornical organ lies under and behind the fornix as the limbs separate to descend into the hypothalamus. The subcommissural organ lies in the roof of the cerebral aqueduct connecting the third and fourth ventricles. The prechiasmatic organ, also called the X-zone, refers to the specialized ependyma of the floor of the fourth ventricle, which may have a transport function in translocating materials from the third ventricle to the portal vessels of the primary portal plexus of the hypothalamus. The area postrema may play a role in the transport of substances from the ventricular system to the extraventricular cerebrospinal fluid. All these structures are unusual in that they do not have the usual blood-brain barrier. Most ependyma are joined by "tight junctions" which prevent entry of particulate cerebrospinal fluid materials into the underlying brain. (PS = psalterium) [Redrawn from Weindl, A.: *Z. Zellforsch.* 67:740–775, 1965, with modifications from Knowles, F.: *J. Neurovisc. Relat.* (Suppl. IX), pp. 97–110, 1969, with permission.]

lipolytic compound identical with one formed by the pineal.

The Subcommissural Organ

The subcommissural organ (SCO) is a poorly understood structure which has persisted through evolutionary development from fish to man. It is considered here because of experiments and clinical studies in which the organ was claimed to have a function in regulating water and salt balance. The SCO is a collection of columnar cells lining the roof of the caudal end of the third ventricle, where it enters the aqueduct connecting the third and fourth ventricles. This region is beneath the habenular commissure and is adjacent to the pineal recess (to the apex of which is attached the pineal gland). Cells of the SCO differ from the usual ependymal cell in being much taller and in containing secretory granules which stain selectively with various histochemical reagents. An outstanding peculiarity of the SCO in animals studied so far (except for the human) is that the cells secrete into the lumen of the aqueduct a substance which is relatively insoluble in cerebrospinal fluid. This secretion forms a cordlike structure (Reissner's fiber) which is extruded through the aqueduct and through the fourth ventricle and spinal cord lumen to terminate in the caudal spinal canal.

Reissner's fiber contains mucopolysaccharides and apparently breaks down at its termination in the sacral spinal cord, but in some species, such as the rat, the tip of the fiber forms a coil much as a rope would under similar mechanical circumstances. In man, intracellular secretory granules are identifiable in the SCO, but Reissner's fiber is absent. The SCO secretion in man is therefore presumed to be relatively more soluble than in other animals and is absorbed directly from the cerebrospinal fluid. In addition to drainage into the cerebrospinal fluid (which is characteristic of ependyma in general, there may be drainage into regional capillaries as well. The subcommissural organ has no direct nerve supply, and its anatomic localization adjacent to the pineal gland does not appear to be functionally significant.

Among the clues suggesting that SCO secretion might be involved in water regulation is the observation of Wislocki and Leduc, that the secretory granules stain somewhat like the granules of the neurohypophysis, which are known to be involved in ADH secretion. The hypothesis that the SCO is involved in water balance has been tested by studying the effects of hydration and dehydration on the histologic appearance of the SCO, the effect of lesions of the SCO on water intake and on sodium balance, and the effects of SCO extracts on water excretion and aldosterone secretion. Work with lesions in experimental animals has not been decisive because of the difficulty in producing complete but selective ablation in a region of complex neural connections, and studies of histologic changes in the organ in relation to dehydration have been conflicting. It has been claimed that SCO extracts control thirst, as indicated by a decline in water intake when rats are injected with such extracts. Perhaps the most important question about the subcommissural organ concerns its role in aldosterone regulation. The earlier experiments of Farrell and co-workers on epithalamic control of aldosterone regulation did not adequately differentiate between pineal and SCO effects, and it has been claimed that extracts of this region both inhibit and excite aldosterone secretion.

No firm conclusion can be drawn at this time about the function of the SCO, but a peculiar syndrome has been described in the human with tumors in this region of the brain. Unlike the normal individual, in whom sodium restriction increases aldosterone secretion, several patients with "pretectal" disease have been described who do not respond in the usual way to low-salt diets. These cases are believed to be the clinical counterpart of animals with epithalamic destruction, but since the validity of the animal model is itself in question, further extrapolation to the human is not possible.

The Subfornical Organ

The subfornical organ (SFO) is another peculiar glomuslike ependymal structure of suspected neuroendocrine function. It consists of both neurosecretory neurons and modified ependymal cells found at the junction between the lamina terminalis and the tela choroidea of the third ventricle. Its name is derived from its location under the fornices. The neurons of the SFO receive cholinergic innervation which has been traced to cells in the midbrain, and the electron microscopic appearance of the SFO suggests a neurosecretory gland capable of secretion into the lumen of the ventricle. The intensity of staining of the neurosecretory material is modified by anesthesia, stress, hyperosmotic challenge, alcohol injection, and estrogen administration. The histologic changes are of unknown significance and have been related by some workers to the control of salt and water balance by the central nervous system.

Unusual ependymal cells are also found in the lining of the floor of the third ventricle. These cells are specialized so that the ventricular face shows large clublike villi projecting into the ventricular space and long processes upon capillaries of the primary portal plexus. The presence of vesicles and granules within these cells and the fact that a number of substances introduced into the third ventricle are found rapidly in the anterior pituitary gland (despite the presence of "tight junctions" between the ependymal lining cells) have led to the suggestion that these cells are involved in the transport of releasing factors and other brain secretory products from the ventricular fluid to the pituitary circulation. The terms "prechiasmatic gland" and X-zone have been applied to this region.

HUMAN NEUROENDOCRINE DISEASE

General Considerations

Almost all endocrine disorders in organic brain disease arise from direct hypothalamic damage (Table 12–3). The notable exception to this generalization is the syndrome of inappropriate antidiuretic hormone (ADH) secretion (see Chapter 3), which occurs in various cerebral disorders including stroke, encephalopathy, and head injury. A variety of neural factors may be responsible for the

TABLE 12–3. ETIOLOGY OF DISEASES OF THE HYPOTHALAMUS

Neoplasms	Pituitary tumor
	Chromophobe adenoma
	Eosinophilic adenoma
	Basophil adenoma
	Hamartoma
	Craniopharyngioma
	Astrocytoma
	Hyperplasia (congenital malformation)
	Infundibuloma
	Pinealoma (Germinoma)
	Ependymoma
	Ganglioneuroma
	Plasmacytoma
	Neurofibroma
	Medulloblastoma
	Microgliomatosis
	Perithelial sarcoma
	Angioma
	Malignant hemangioendothelioma
	Cyst of choroid plexus
	Cyst of third ventricle
	Lipoma
	Metastatic carcinoma
	Leukemia
	Meningioma
Inflammatory lesions	Viral encephalitis
	Epidemic encephalitis
	Smallpox
	Measles
	Varicella
	Rabies inoculation
	Granulomatous lesions
	Tuberculosis
	Boeck's sarcoid
	Reticuloendotheliosis
	Hand-Schüller-Christian disease
	Eosinophilic granuloma
	Histiocytosis X
Degenerative lesions	Tuberous sclerosis
	Encephalomalacia
	Gliosis of unknown cause
	Tay-Sachs disease
	Atrophy of unknown cause
Physical agents	Stalk section (surgical)
	Rupture of stalk due to head injury
	Foreign body in the hypothalamus
	Radiation necrosis
Vascular lesions	Arteriosclerosis and encephalomalacia
	Aneurysm of circle of Willis
	Rupture of aneurysm of circle of Willis
	Periventricular anoxia of newborn
Miscellaneous forms of encephalopathy	Systemic lupus erythematosus
	Acute intermittent porphyria
	CO_2 narcosis

inappropriate ADH syndrome. These include direct irritative lesions of the supraoptic nuclei (as has been reported in lupus encephalitis, persistent stimulation of pain pathways, and continued stimulation of ADH by stretch receptors in the right side of the heart in patients who lie supine due to coma or severe paralysis. In experimental animals, severing the input into the supraoptic nuclei leads to persistent increase in electrical activity of the supraoptico-hypophysial neurons, but hypersecretion of ADH has not been demonstrated in this experimental model as yet. Another nonhypothalamic endocrine disorder of brain origin is impaired aldosterone secretory response in patients with disease of the pretectal area, but this is exceedingly uncommon and unassociated with specific clinical manifestations of endocrine disturbance. Diffuse brain disease may also cause a loss of the normal diurnal variation in adrenal steroid and GH secretory pattern. Apart from these disorders, most neuroendocrine disease syndromes in man are due to either functional or organic disturbances of the hypothalamus. Deficit syndromes are most common, but paroxysmal hypothalamic disorders may occur, including hypothalamic epilepsy with periodic elevation of 17-hydroxycorticoid excretion to extremely high levels.

Psychic abnormalities are common in hypothalamic disease, including manifestations such as violent rage, attacks of laughing or crying, disturbed sleep pattern, excessive sexuality, and serious behavior disturbance. Somnolence or pathologic wakefulness have been observed, as have bulimia and malignant anorexia. These are analogous to the situation in the experimental animal caused by ventromedial nuclear damage or lateral hypothalamic damage respectively. Patients with hypothalamic damage may show hyper- or hypothermia or unexplained variations in body temperature and, in fact, may appear clinically as cases of pyrexia of unknown etiology. Pathologic disturbances in sweating or acrocyanosis are observed, and sphincter control may be disturbed. On rare occasions, these individuals have "diencephalic epilepsy."

Patients with hypothalamic disease are seldom seen with precisely localized lesions which have led to precisely defined deficits of anterior lobe function. Pituitary stalk section gives rise to one of the most clear-cut of the hypothalamic endocrine syndromes.

Pituitary Stalk Section in Man

Pituitary stalk sectioning in animals has been studied extensively to determine the effect of the hypothalamus on pituitary function. In recent years, this procedure has been used in humans as an alternative to the technically more difficult hypophysectomy for treating metastatic carcinoma of the breast and diabetic microangiopathy. Destructive lesions of this region, such as tumors or granulomas, or traumatic rupture of the stalk result in similar effects. From study of such patients, much is now known about the relative autonomy of pituitary control in humans.

The results of stalk section are due to damage to the neural stalk, loss of hypophysiotropic hormones, and interference with blood supply to the gland. Diabetes insipidus (DI) develops in approximately 80 per cent of these patients, depending somewhat upon the level of stalk section. If section is close to the hypothalamus, diabetes insipidus is almost a constant finding, whereas, if the section is close to the diaphragma sella, the incidence is much lower. These differences depend upon damage to neurohypophysial neurons within the stalk and infundibulum. The classic three phases of diabetes insipidus, i.e., transient polyuria followed by normal water control and then by total ADH deficiency, are observed in about half the cases.

Menses cease following both stalk section and hypophysectomy, but gonadotropic failure is less severe in the former than in the latter. Secondary sex characteristics are better maintained and urinary gonadotropins though reduced are still detectable, whereas hypophysectomy results in complete loss of detectable gonadotropins. Urinary excretion of 17-hydroxy- and 17-ketosteroids and plasma hydroxycorticoids falls after either procedure, but the change after stalk section may take much longer to develop and 17-hydroxy-steroid excretion may be transiently elevated after stalk section. ACTH reserve as estimated by the metyrapone test is abolished by hypophysectomy or stalk section, but response to vasopressin injection or to pyrogens may be preserved in the stalk-sectioned individual. Persistence of response despite successful section of the stalk has been attributed to the release into the systemic blood of the releasing factor, which thus bypasses the hypophysial-portal circulation. A similar mechanism has been invoked to explain persistent GH response after stalk section. This explanation is at least theoretically reasonable: in experimental animals, a number of releasing factors have been demonstrated in peripheral blood, and in humans, both LRF and GH-RF activity have been similarly shown.

The most striking differences between patients with section of the pituitary stalk and those with hypophysectomy relate to the secretion of growth hormone and prolactin. The basal GH level is normal in stalk-sectioned patients, but in most cases GH response to hypoglycemic stimulation is blocked or reduced. Where it persists, it may gradually decrease with time. In the hypophysectomized individual, both the response to hypoglycemia and baseline GH function are depressed. Stalk-sectioned patients develop increased prolactin levels, and in a few, the increased prolactin level leads to galactorrhea. Of course this does not occur in hypophysectomized individuals.

Hypophysiotropic Hormone Deficiency

With the recent introduction of clinical testing of pituitary function with native or synthetic TRH and LRH, it has been possible to identify syndromes of hypothalamic hypophysiotropic hormone deficiency. By analogy with earlier methods of examining adrenal reserve with ACTH or thyroid reserve with TSH, isolated TRH deficiency has been identified in several cases as a cause of isolated pituitary-thyroid failure and isolated LRH deficiency as a cause of hypogonadotropic hypogonadism and of functional amenorrhea. In a large series of children with idiopathic hypopituitarism with varying patterns and degrees of pituitary insufficiency, the majority of those with TSH deficiency were shown to be responsive to the TSH stimulating effects of TRH. This means that such cases have TRH failure. Since other pituitary tropic hormones are also deficient, it appears almost certain that analogous hypophysiotropic hormonal deficiencies are the fundamental defect in control. If this is the case, it suggests that occult brain damage, either infectious, traumatic, or due to other unknown factors, may underlie most cases of idiopathic hypopituitarism. Many of these cases deserve the more accurate designation of "panhypophysiotropic failure."

Isolated prolactin deficiency unresponsive to drugs such as chlorpromazine (which raise prolactin levels in the normal person) has also been reported; it has not as yet been established whether this is a pituitary or hypothalamic disorder. It is likely that when all the releasing hormones become available it will be possible to identify accurately isolated or combined failure of each of the anterior pituitary secretions and the relevant hypophysiotropic hormones.

Diseases of Gonadotropin Regulation

Precocious Puberty

Race, geography, nutrition, and genetic endowment all influence the time of onset of puberty. The work of Frisch and Revelle indicates that the crucial factor for initiation of puberty is the achievement of a critical body weight. This observation may explain the secular trend in earlier age of menarche which has been noted in successive generations for more than a hundred years. In a large group of normal women in the United States studied in 1964 and 1965, mean age at menarche was 12.6 years ±1.1 year (SD). Testicular growth begins at a mean age of 11.8 years with a standard deviation of 1 year.

Despite these variations in timing of puberty, it is generally agreed that the diagnosis of precocious puberty is warranted when sexual maturation begins before the age of 8 in girls or 10 in boys. The term *precocious puberty*, when applied without qualification, refers to "true" precocious puberty, a condition in which normal pituitary-gonadal function is activated at an abnormally early age. *Pseudoprecocious puberty* applies to those disorders in which secondary sexual characteristics develop without maturation of the gonads because secretion of androgenic or estrogenic hormones is abnormal. Rarely, disease of the gonads or adrenal glands or teratoma causes feminization of prepubertal boys or masculinization of prepubertal girls, but such conditions are not properly classified under the heading of precocious puberty.

In girls, several incomplete forms of "true" precocious puberty have been recognized: "precocious thelarche," defined by Wilkins as the premature development of breasts in young girls without other sexual manifestations, and precocious "adrenarche" or "pubarche," referring to the premature development of pubic or axillary hair or both. The pathophysiology of these forms of fractional maturation has not been fully elucidated. They are important to recognize because they are benign and must be differentiated from disorders of excessive androgen or estrogen secretion.

True precocious puberty arises in all cases from disturbed function of the brain (which may or may not be associated with demonstrable structural abnormalities), whereas pseudoprecocious puberty is due to disease of the gonads or adrenal glands or, rarely, other hormone-producing tissues. Of exquisite rarity is the intracranial chorioepithelioma of pineal origin, which causes pseudoprecocious puberty by the secretion of excessive amounts of testosterone rather than through a neurogenic mechanism. True precocious puberty is characterized by an adult pattern of sexual function (in girls menstrual cycles, in boys testicular development and spermatogenesis). Pseudoprecocity in girls is manifested by hyperestrogenism and in boys by androgenization without testicular maturation. This chapter is concerned mainly with the etiology and manifestations of true (or neurogenic) precocious puberty.

Incidence and Causes

From a compilation of 770 cases, Wilkins concluded that precocious puberty of all types was twice as common in girls as in boys and in girls is far less indicative of serious disease. Most prematurely developed girls (80 per cent) have no demonstrable structural abnormality of brain, pituitary gland, or ovary, whereas more than 60 per cent of sexually precocious boys have serious organic disease. In girls, ovarian tumors account for 15 per cent of the cases of precocious development and intracranial lesions for only 4 per cent. In boys, 20 per cent of the cases of precocious development are due to intracranial disease, 25 per cent to adrenal disease, and less than 10 per cent to lesions of the testicle. Certain peculiar and inexplicable sex differences have been observed in the incidence of true sexual precocity. "Idiopathic" precocious puberty is 4 to 10 times as common in girls than boys; polyostotic fibrous dysplasia of Albright (a cause of precocious puberty) rarely occurs in boys; and hypothyroidism as a cause of precocious puberty has been recognized almost exclusively in girls. In contrast, precocious puberty due to pineal tumors occurs but with the rarest exceptions in boys.

Idiopathic Sexual Precocity

This category encompasses the largest proportion of cases of premature but otherwise normal sexual development. This disorder is diagnosed by exclusion of organic disease of the central nervous system and other known causes of the syndrome. A few pedigrees have been described in which true precocious puberty appeared as a genetically determined disorder, including one family in which four generations were involved. With a few exceptions, almost all such cases have been reported in males. Familial incidence has been estimated to account for less than 10 per cent of the idiopathic disorder. The familial variety of this condition is presumed due to a genetically determined early maturation of the hypothalamic gonadotropin regulatory areas. When carefully studied, most children with "idiopathic" precocious puberty reveal diffuse electroencephalographic abnormalities. These include abnormal slowing with paroxysmal activity or paroxysmal activity alone. The paroxysmal activity includes spikes, sharp waves, and spike wave patterns. Girls with premature pubarche (premature appearance of pubic and axillary hair) also have a high incidence of EEG abnormality. Thus, so-called idiopathic precocious puberty appears in many cases to be due to unrecognized brain disorder without other neurologic manifestations. A continuum of clinical disease probably embraces those precociously developed children who have normal EEG tracings, abnormal tracings without convulsive disorder, and those manifesting precocious puberty plus convulsive disorder. The identification of hypophysiotropic failure as a cause of idiopathic hypopituitarism in children (see above) permits the inclusion of this disorder as a part of the idiopathic hypothalamic deficiency spectrum. In some instances, hypophysiotropic loss is progressive with time. At the extreme of this continuum are children with unmistakable evidence of severe brain damage, including behavior disturbance and mental retardation.

Neurogenic Precocious Puberty with Demonstrable Structural Changes

Hypothalamic regions affecting timing of puberty have not been well localized in humans. Most individuals who come to autopsy due to hypothalamic disease have widespread damage to the hypothalamus. Furthermore, localization of lesions is rendered more difficult by the diffuse neurologic organization of the hypothalamus; compensatory functions may develop if the damage progresses slowly enough. Nevertheless, approximately two thirds of cases of precocious puberty caused by destructive lesions in humans is due to damage behind the median eminence, a finding which is in contrast to experimentally produduced sexual precocity in the rat, which involves lesions of the anterior hypothalamus.

Hamartoma of the Hypothalamus. A possible exception to the rule that neurologic lesions induce precocious puberty by damaging structures that normally inhibit gonadotropin secretion is the hypothalamic hamartoma. As used in neuropathology, the term *hamartoma* refers to a tumorlike collection of normal tissue lodged in an abnormal location. The hypothalamic hamartoma consists of a sharply encapsulated nodule of nerve tissue which is attached to the posterior hypothalamus at a point between the anterior portion of the mamillary body and the posterior region of the tuber cinereum. These tumors must be clearly differentiated (and have not always been so differentiated) from low-grade malignant gliomas, such as the astrocytoma, which may also induce precocious puberty by invading the hypothalamus.

The hypothalamic hamartoma grows into the cisternal space between the cerebral peduncles, often adapting itself to the pyramidal shape of the space, and may produce signs of early puberty before any hypothalamic pressure or local damage has resulted to surrounding nerve tissue. Reported tumors of this type number less than 50, but a careful search showed miniature "hamartomatous" nodular formations of the tuber cinereum in 21 per cent of 121 normal brains. Patients with significant disease may be those in whom these normal minute formations continue to grow. Hypothalamic hamartomas do not cause precocious puberty in every case. Some evidence suggests that the critical factor for the development of precocious puberty may be the presence of neuronal connections between the hamartoma and the hypothalamus. The hypothalamic hamartoma is made up of neurons resembling those of the hypothalamus, particularly the tuber cinereum, and has been likened by Richter (93) to an "accessory hypothalamus." In a few well-studied cases, neurons have been described ending in the region of the tuber cinereum, and some have been noted to contain neurosecretory substance analogous to that found in the supraoptico-hypophysial nerve system.

No special clinical features sharply distinguish these patients from those with other types of brain tumor-induced precocious puberty. Distribution by sex is not characteristic; symptoms reportedly have occurred as early as 3 months of age. Although abnormal neurologic findings are rare at the time precocious puberty is first noted, the majority of these patients have progressive manifestations of hypothalamic involvement, such as internal hydrocephalus with headache, visual disturbance, papilledema, obesity, convulsive disorder, and behavioral changes. Almost always the lesion is fatal before the age of 20 years, but one case surviving to age 62 has been reported (Wolman). These lesions have proved to be virtually untreatable so far because of their inaccessibility and their resistance to radiation therapy.

Neurons from this structure may increase the excitability of the gonadotropin controlling center and overcome normal inhibitory impulses. Alternatively, precocious puberty might be caused by gonadotropin releasing factors synthesized by cells of the hypothalamic hamartoma, many of which

resemble those of the tuberal-hypophysial tract. Although neurosecretory material has been demonstrated by histochemical stains, no physiologic studies of tumor tissue have been made.

Brain Tumors.   Brain tumors can cause sexual precocity if the hypothalamus is involved directly. Craniopharyngiomas usually induce hypopituitarism by destroying the pituitary stalk and ventral hypothalamus, but this lesion occasionally induces premature puberty with or without associated deficiency of other pituitary tropic hormones. Gliomas and astrocytomas in the region of the brainstem and third ventricle, optic nerve, tuber cinereum, and temporal lobe have all been reported to cause this syndrome. As with gliomas located elsewhere in the brain, these disorders have been noted in association with neurofibromatosis (von Recklinghausen's disease). Internal hydrocephalus due to any cause may produce precocious puberty provided the pituitary stalk has not been stretched or damaged. When the latter occurs, gonadal atrophy and hypogonadism may be the result.

Tumors of the Pineal Gland and the "Ectopic Pinealomas."   As discussed in Chapter 13, interest in the pineal gland as a regulator of sexual function was first aroused by clinical reports of precocious puberty in boys in association with pineal tumors. When the hypothalamus came to be recognized as regulating the timing of puberty, analysis of clinical material indicated that pineal tumors caused difficulty by their effects on hypothalamic function (in which case they act as any other destructive brain lesion in the region of the diencephalon). More recently, studies in experimental animals have again suggested that pineal tumors may have endocrine function and have reawakened speculation about the gonadotropin regulating function of the pineal gland.

Neuropathologists do not fully agree about the classification of neoplasms of the pineal gland. The dominant view is that of Dorothy Russel, who points out that most lesions in the region of the pineal gland are not true neoplasms of the pineal parenchymal cells but are in fact atypical teratomas.

The term *pinealoma* should be used to refer to tumors of the pineal parenchymal cell; these have also been called *pineoblastomas* or *pineocytomas* according to their maturity. The more common teratoma of this region only superficially resembles the pineal cell and, like teratomas in other sites, may be composed of a mixture of well-differentiated tissues of adult type and may show an organoid pattern. Sometimes derivatives of all three germ layers are identified. They may appear as dermoid cysts, some with teeth, bones, and cartilage. Many of these tumors contain elements similar to or identical with the seminoma of the testis and thus are termed *seminomatous pinealomas* or, by preference, *germinomas*.

Although the pineal gland and region is the most common site of these tumors, they also occur relatively frequently around the infundibulum, where they result in a striking association of diabetes insipidus, visual disturbance, and precocious puberty. These lesions as well as those occurring in other brain sites (cerebellum or quadrigeminal plate) have been called *ectopic pinealomas* — a misnomer because they are teratomas similar to those occurring in the pineal region and not neoplasms of pineal cell origin. To make matters more confusing, at least one of these so-called ectopic pinealomas has been found to contain enzymes unique to the normal pineal gland. The teratoma may metastasize outside the brain. In one series of teratomas of the pineal gland and hypothalamus, 10 per cent metastasized to the spinal cord causing spinal cord compression. These lesions are markedly sensitive to radiation therapy, which should be considered following surgical decompression in emergency situations. Almost all of the teratomatous lesions occur in males. When they occur in girls, precocious puberty only rarely has been noted. The true pinealoma, unlike the more common teratoma of the pineal gland, resembles the cerebellar medulloblastoma or (even more rarely) the pineal parenchymal cell. Other rare lesions in this region are astrocytomas, spongioblastomas, ependymomas, choroid-plexus papillomas, and glioblastomas.

The relationship of pineal tumors to the occurrence of precocious puberty has been much studied in efforts to determine whether the pineal is truly involved in the regulation of puberty in the human by a humoral mechanism as it appears to be in animals. Precocious puberty proves not to be a uniform or even a common finding in pineal disease. In 65 pineal tumors studied by Ringertz and co-workers, not a single case of sexual precocity was noted; only seven of these patients were younger than 11 years of age. Thus these disorders are not common before puberty and, when they do occur before puberty, do not commonly hasten sexual maturation. In a study of 177 subjects by Bing and co-workers, 56 were less than 15 years of age and of these only one third had sexual precocity. Whenever precocious puberty was caused by pineal tumor, neuroanatomic evidence indicated extension beyond the pineal region, such as internal hydrocephalus or invasion of the third ventricle or of the hypothalamus. Clinical evidence of hypothalamic involvement, such as diabetes insipidus, polyphagia, somnolence, obesity, or behavioral disturbance, was noted in 71 per cent of cases. These neuroanatomic studies strongly support the view that neoplasms of the pineal gland produce damage by secondary structural neuroendocrine effects on the hypothalamus.

In light of these data, the studies of Kitay bear careful review. This author found that nonparenchymal tumors were three times more likely to produce precocity than were parenchymal tumors. He postulated that the high incidence was due to pineal destruction with the loss of a pineal secretion believed to inhibit development of sexual maturity. Though an interesting speculation, and compatible with extensive work in animals, Kitay's conclusion that "precocious puberty in patients with pineal tumor is not caused by pressure on the hypothalamus" cannot be based on histologic type, unless one makes a correlation with the extent of neurologic damage. When this has been done, as by Bing and colleagues, the close correlation with hypothalamic damage is convincing. In a few cases, precocity or infantilism may be due to altered pineal secretion (see above), but if such exist, they are exceedingly rare.

Hypothyroidism. The association of true precocious puberty with juvenile hypothyroidism is well known but rare, only 12 cases having been reported by 1965. Hypothyroidism induces the disorder since it is readily shown that replacement treatment with thyroid hormone restores prepubertal gonadotropic function. This syndrome has occasionally been associated with galactorrhea, ovarian cysts, enlargement of the sella turcica, and hyperpigmentation. Although it is primarily a disease of girls, at least two boys have also been described with hypothyroidism-induced sexual precocity. Various etiologic theories have been proposed, but the one suggested by Van Wyk and Grumbach has been most widely quoted. These authors suggest that cross specificity exists in feedback control of the pituitary gonadotropins by the thyroid hormone so that gonadotropic cells respond to thyroid deficiency as do thyrotrophs.

Consideration of two facts leads to an alternate hypothesis. In any case in which the cause of precocious puberty is known specifically, the defect has been found to lie in the brain without exception. Secondly, hypothyroidism is known to impair neural function (see below). It seems more reasonable to suppose that this disorder is due to depression of hypothalamic gonadotropin regulating areas by hypothyroid encephalopathy. The association with galactorrhea is rationalized (as it is in the cases caused by tranquilizer drug therapy or pituitary stalk secretion) as being due to a loss of normal prolactin inhibiting factor (PIF), also a possible manifestation of hypothyroidism-induced brain depression. The possible role of TRH hypersecretion in causing galactorrhea in hypothyroidism will be discussed below. The occasional cases in which hyperpigmentation occurs may be explained by the fact that intermediate lobe secretion, like that of prolactin, appears from studies in experimental animals to be under tonic inhibitory control by the hypothalamus.

Fibrous Dysplasia (Albright's Syndrome). Precocious sexual development is a common manifestation of Albright's syndrome of fibrous dysplasia of bone, occurring in 10 of 37 carefully studied cases in the Massachusetts General Hospital series. The pathogenesis of this aspect of the disorder has not been well clarified and perhaps should not be included as a form of true precocity, because no female and only one male have developed prepubertal gonadal maturation. The manifestations of the syndrome resemble those of isosexual pseudoprecocity, the vaginal bleeding being of the estrogen breakthrough type. Unlike true precocious puberty, the normal order of sexual development—breast growth, pubic hair growth, and finally menstruation—is often not followed; some subjects have vaginal bleeding before the age of 8 years and only later develop other signs of maturation at the normal age for puberty. Furthermore, in three persons in whom ovarian histology was studied, no evidence of ovulation or luteinization was obtained, a finding which is not typical of true precocity. These patients ultimately develop normal menstrual periods and may conceive. At one time, sexual precocity was thought to be due to bony abnormalities of the base of the skull which distorted the hypothalamus. This view has not been supported by study of subsequent cases. One patient reportedly had a hamartomatous abnormality of the hypothalamus. In the few individuals in whom autopsy has been done, this abnormality was not again found, so it must be concluded that no consistent neurologic abnormality has been observed. Rarely male children with sexual precocity and the Albright syndrome have been described. Hypothyroidism also occurs in an unusually high proportion of patients with Albright's syndrome (seven of 34 in the MGH series).

Manifestations of Neurogenic Precocious Puberty.   The most striking manifestations of precocious puberty are due to the effects of the gonadal steroids on secondary sexual characteristics and skeletal growth and maturation. Precocity usually occurs after 3 years of age, but medical curiosities have been described in which breast development and pubic hair were present in girls at birth, with menses as early as 6 weeks of age, while in boys, penile growth has been noted as early as the fifth month of life. These precocious children are capable of precocious procreation as well. The famous Peruvian child, Lina Medina, menstruated at 8 months of age and gave birth at 5 years 8 months to a 6½ pound child. In the literature of the nineteenth century is mention of a boy who fathered a child before the age of 7.

Due to the stimulation of skeletal and muscular growth, precociously pubertal children grow more rapidly, show an advanced skeletal age and muscular development, but ultimately suffer from short adult stature because of premature maturation with closure of the epiphyses. In girls, obesity is commonly associated with precocity, and there may be some degree of mental dullness. Surprisingly, dental development does not parallel skeletal development but is appropriate to the chronological age. Precociously developed girls rarely become precociously interested in boys. For example, in Jolly's series, only one child in 50 was noted to have precocious sexual interests.

Among the special psychological characteristics of sexually precocious boys (regardless of etiology), as pointed out by Money and Alexander, are: "a tendency to high IQ . . .; increased energy expenditure, especially in infancy; a possible increased incidence (by no means universal) of behavior tantrums and impulsive anger; early occurrence of the capacity for frankly sexual imagery in dreams and daydreams, its content, however, determined by cognitional experience; and early establishment of the capacity for erotic and sexual arousal in relation to visual imagery and visual perception as well as tactile sensation. . . .

The psychological maturation of males with physical sexual precocity otherwise keeps in step with that of boys of the same chronological and/or social age."

Not uncommonly girls with precocious puberty have ovarian enlargement, sometimes with follicular cyst formation. This has been recognized in association with hypothyroidism and also with idiopathic precocity. This manifestation is emphasized because granulosa cell tumors of the ovary may also appear with precocious estrogenization and palpable ovarian mass, and because these follicular cysts, when diagnosed by laparotomy, should not be removed. When due to hypothyroidism, ovarian cysts may regress after thyroid hormone therapy, and, for this reason, a therapeutic test is indicated.

Differential Diagnosis of Precocious Puberty

The differential diagnosis of the cause of true precocious puberty is somewhat different in boys and girls. In girls, the main differential diagnosis lies between the "idiopathic" disorder, Albright's syndrome, and central nervous system disease. The idiopathic form is diagnosed for the most part by exclusion, but it should be recognized that the majority of these children have obesity, some mental retardation, and abnormal EEG patterns either singly or in combination. Albright's syndrome is recognized by the occurrence of areas of skin pigmentation or the appearance of the characteristic bone lesion with disseminated rarefaction or both (see Chapter 11). The most common ovarian tumor causing sexual development (pseudoprecocious puberty) is the granulosa cell tumor. Wilkins pointed out that in every reported case, a palpable abdominal tumor existed by the time that sexual precocity was apparent. Rarely, chorioepitheliomas and luteomas cause precocity. Neither of these lesions may be associated with palpable ovarian masses, in which case their recognition is exceedingly difficult.

Neurogenic precocity is diagnosed more readily if other evidence indicates neurologic disease. If neurologic examination and routine skull films are normal, more extensive neurodiagnostic studies such as pneumoencephalography are usually not warranted in view of the low incidence of hypothalamic tumor as a cause of this syndrome in girls. Associated manifestations of hypothalamic disease warrant full neurologic diagnostic evaluation. In female precocity, plasma gonadotropin (FSH and LH) is usually appropriate to the stage of sexual development, not the chronological age, but a low gonadotropin measurement does not exclude this diagnosis. Reports of plasma gonadotropins in pubarche and thelarche have been conflicting, some indicating levels appropriate for age and others indicating slight elevations.

In boys, true precocious puberty can be distinguished from pseudoprecocity by physical examination of the testes and by measurement of urinary 17-ketosteroid excretion. Since true precocity is due to precocious but *normal* gonadal stimulation, the testes will be enlarged toward those of the normal male, and, in time, spermatogenesis can be demonstrated by testicular biopsy. In contrast, precocity due to abnormal androgen production will be manifested by inhibited testicular growth and function. Certain rare exceptions have been due to testicular tumors (of testicular or aberrant adrenocortical origin), but these would not show spermatozoal maturation.

In true neurogenic precocity, 17-ketosteroid excretion, though detectably higher than normal for children of comparable age, does not reach the normal values of adolescent males. Although neurogenic precocity is due to precocious gonadotropin secretion, determining gonadotropins by urinary excretion studies is not useful in differential diagnosis unless elevation can be demonstrated. Insufficient data have accumulated using plasma gonadotropin assay to provide criteria to differentiate neurogenic precocity in males from pseudoprecocity. The use of Clomid and of LRF in differential diagnosis has not been evaluated adequately as yet. When physical examination and 17-ketosteroid determinations fail to clarify the diagnosis, testicular biopsy will settle the question. Because of the high frequency of serious neurologic disease as a cause of sexual precocity in males, careful neurologic evaluation is mandatory. Associated findings of hypothalamic or pineal disorder should be carefully assessed, and neurosurgical evaluation is often required. Albright's syndrome, considered to be a disease occurring only in girls, has now been recognized in boys and should be considered as a rare cause of the syndrome in males.

Management. The only cases of true precocious puberty which are treatable specifically are due to hypothyroidism and brain tumor. For the remainder, management is chiefly psychological for both the parents and the child. Hormonal management with long-acting progesterone derivatives such as medroxyprogesterone acetate (MPA, Provera), 100 to 150 mg. IM every two weeks, is worth a trial since in most girls precocious menses and breast growth regress, although ultimate height is unchanged by therapy. For unexplained reasons, some girls do not improve, and in at least one third of patients, including those in whom menses cease, tests of gonadotropin secretion may not change significantly.

Boys appear, in most instances, to respond well to MPA, and limited experience suggests that the ultimate stature (otherwise low) may be restored to normal. The effect of gestagens in reversing androgen-induced precocious puberty is well supported by experimental data in rats. No other form of gonadotropin suppressive therapy, such as estrogen or androgen administration, is rational, nor is direct treatment of the pituitary with x-irradiation or surgery.

Case management for the most part involves psychological handling. The Johns Hopkins group, notably Money and Hampson, have studied this problem and have formulated many helpful suggestions on the rearing and management of sexually precocious children. Their original articles should be read in detail.

Psychogenic Amenorrhea

Cessation of normal menstrual cycles in young, nonpregnant women who have no demonstrable structural abnormality of brain, pituitary, or ovary occurs in several clinical syndromes. These are pseudocyesis (false pregnancy), anorexia nervosa, and a large group of poorly defined conditions, loosely called "psychogenic" or "hypothalamic" amenorrhea. This entire group of disorders is often associated with gross psychopathology or with psychic stress and is usually temporary. Depending upon the degree and type of gonadotropin deficiency present, the ovarian abnormality in these cases ranges from failure of ovulation to severe degrees of estrogen loss. Abnormalities in the timing of ovulation represent the mildest form of this disorder. All of these disorders probably arise from functional abnormalities in the hypothalamic gonadotropin regulating areas. Certain tranquilizer drugs, such as reserpine and chlorpromazine, may block ovulation and delay menses.

Pseudocyesis

Pseudocyesis is one form of neurogenic amenorrhea. In this condition, a woman firmly believes herself to be pregnant and develops many of the signs and symptoms of pregnancy. These include amenorrhea, abdominal enlargement, sensation of fetal movements, breast changes, gastrointestinal symptoms, and even labor pains. Although amenorrhea is the rule, normal or regular menses were reported in 52 of 444 women diagnosed as having pseudocyesis. About half of the subjects have amenorrhea for 9 months, but in a few individuals it persists longer.

Abdominal distention, which superficially resembles the pregnant state, is extremely common and has misled even competent obstetricians. This manifestation may be due to obesity, tympanites, urinary and fecal retention, or marked contraction of the diaphragms forcing the abdominal contents down and outward, and it resembles the hysterical bloating and lordosis described by Alvarez. The sensation of fetal movements in the fourth and fifth months may be misinterpreted sensations from the bowel or contractions of abdominal muscles. The breast changes consist of swelling and tenderness and may include secretion of milk and colostrum and an increase in the size of papillae. In some respects, breast changes are similar to those described under nonpuerperal galactorrhea (see below). Even experienced physicians occasionally report the uterus to be enlarged and compatible with early pregnancy. In a study carried out in a university hospital, one in 250 maternity clinic admissions was due to pseudocyesis, and every patient in the study had been diagnosed by at least one physician as having been pregnant. In the author's experience, pseudocyesis has become a rare disease.

The specific hormonal disturbance in these cases has not been precisely established. Physical examination suggests that estrogen secretion is normal or increased, and biopsies indicate secretory changes in the endometrium. Prolactin was demonstrable in the urine of each of five studied cases. One may presume that the endocrine manifestations are attributable to a reasonably normal rate of FSH secretion, tonic high LH release without the ovulatory surge, and increased prolactin secretion, a syndrome loosely attributed to "persistent corpus luteum." Experience using modern assay methods for prolactin and gonadotropins is too meager to allow proof of these assertions.

That PCL (persistent corpus luteum) may account for the manifestations of pseudocyesis is suggested by the finding of persistent progesterone effects, including secretory endometrium and softening of the cervix. In a few cases in which laparotomy was performed, corpora lutea beyond the normal 14-day life of this structure were observed. Lactation (which may occur even in nulliparous virgins suffering from pseudocyesis) is probably due to excessive prolactin secretion through a mechanism analogous to that of nonpuerperal galactorrhea (see below).

How pseudocyesis or the PCL syndrome comes about following psychological disturbance is not established. Much is known about pseudopregnancy in rats, for, in this species, sterile mating or certain physical and psychic stresses can prolong the life of the corpus luteum long beyond the normal span. In the rat, this condition is due to neurogenic inhibition of the hypothalamic structures which normally inhibit prolactin secretion. Thus an inhibitory area is inhibited, the pituitary gland is "unleashed," and the increased prolactin (which is luteotropic in the rat) stimulates and maintains the growth and function of the corpus luteum. In humans, good evidence that prolactin is luteotropic has not been advanced, and only limited studies of prolactin secretion in pseudocyesis have been made. Therefore, pseudocyesis in the human cannot be related with certainty to pseudopregnancy in the rat. Galactorrhea when it occurs may be due to associated prolactin excess.

Although this syndrome has been recognized from the time of Hippocrates, psychological aspects of pseudocyesis have not been adequately studied. Pseudocyesis arises in some women who desperately wish, or feel the need, to *be* pregnant and in others who fear that they *are* pregnant. Hysteria has been diagnosed in some cases and is probably present in the majority of women with pseudocyesis. Treatment of pseudocyesis (or of hysteria, for that matter) is not easy. In one series of 27 patients, the patients were simply told that they were not pregnant. Only 13 "accepted" the diagnosis, and of these most again developed pseudocyesis within a few months. Fried and his co-workers strongly advise against bluntly telling the patient that she is not pregnant: it does not cure the disease, it causes confusion and hostility, and it may lead to suicide. Psychotherapy, which may be quite superficial, is recommended. Some physicians produce menstrual flow with progesterone or testosterone or perform a curettage to confirm to the patient that she is not pregnant.

Anorexia Nervosa

Amenorrhea is an almost constant accompaniment of anorexia nervosa. Although starvation and inanition themselves can produce amenorrhea, many patients with anorexia nervosa develop amenorrhea *before* the onset of weight loss, indicating that the changes in gonadotropic hormone secretion can be a direct effect of the disease itself. As starvation proceeds, however, both neural and nutritional factors influence pituitary-ovarian function.

Psychiatrists are not in general agreement as to the classification of anorexia nervosa. Bliss and Branch diagnose this disorder in any patient who has lost 25 pounds or more for psychologic reasons, but this definition does not adequately indicate that there are different types of psychic anorexia. As outlined by King, two kinds of anorexia nervosa syndromes exist, a secondary variety which is a symptom of another psychiatric illness, such as schizophrenia, depressive illness, and phobic anxiety states, and a primary variety in which the psychopathologic manifestations are centered around food and the eating process.

By tradition, the endocrinologist sees cases of anorexia nervosa because of the occurrence of amenorrhea and because of the fallacious legacy left by Simmonds in his description of "pituitary cachexia."

Usually, the differential diagnosis between hypopituitarism and anorexia nervosa is easy to make by clinical means. In anorexia nervosa, the clinical picture is dominated by the disturbance in food intake and other psychological abnormalities. The patient may have been obese at one time and may alternate between obesity and emaciation. The patient may induce vomiting or deny being hungry or craving food. In hypopituitarism, anorexia which is usually but not always present is rarely as severe as in anorexia nervosa, and other manifestations of hypopituitarism are more prominent. Delirium, psychosis, and other behavioral disturbance can, of course, be a manifestation of hypopituitarism. In anorexia nervosa, except for amenorrhea and genital tract atrophy, endocrine functions remain normal, so that such persons retain pubic and axillary hair, which are dependent upon adrenal androgens. Primary anorexia nervosa seldom occurs in men.

Differential diagnosis by means of laboratory tests provides an interesting teaching exercise. In anorexia nervosa and in hypopituitarism, urinary gonadotropic hormones fall. In both of these disorders, urinary excretion of adrenal cortical steroid metabolites is low, but in anorexia nervosa, as constrasted with hypopituitarism, blood levels of corticoids are normal or above normal; such patients are usually hyper-reactors to the metyrapone test of ACTH reserve. Functional inhibition of gonadotropin secretion is shown by refractoriness to clomiphene therapy (in three of three patients), in contrast to cases of functional amenorrhea of other causes, 80 per cent of which respond to clomiphene. Thyroid function, as determined by PBI and thyroidal I^{131} uptake, is almost always normal or borderline low normal in anorexia nervosa. A further difference between anorexia nervosa and hypopituitarism is the plasma growth hormone level; the starved individual often manifests abnormally high levels of this hormone and almost always has hypoglycemia-induced GH discharge, whereas the hypopituitary patient has low GH levels and is unresponsive to hypoglycemia. Patients with anorexia nervosa show an LH secretory response to injections of LRH.

Severe anorexia nervosa is sometimes manifested by severe hypokalemia and mild hyponatremia which on occasion may prove fatal. This syndrome of sodium and potassium deficiency is associated with secondary hyperaldosteronism (see Chs. 5 and 20). In some individuals, self-induced vomiting or cathartic abuse may be the cause of the severe electrolyte depletion. In others, fluid loss is not adequately documented. Hypokalemia is not observed in hypopituitarism.

Curiously, despite the traditional interpretation that these patients have serious psychosexual conflicts, it has been reported that three women who became pregnant after hormone-induced ovulation successfully carried pregnancy to term, and two of the three resumed normal cycling after delivery. Women with anorexia nervosa may also improve if given estrogen replacement, but this therapy has not been studied systematically.

"Psychogenic" Amenorrhea of Other Types

Disturbed menstrual function is well recognized as a consequence of emotional upset both in normal women and in patients suffering from severe mental disease. Anorexia nervosa and pseudocyesis described earlier are the most clearly defined psychiatric syndromes in which these disturbances occur. Besides these disorders, amenorrhea may occur as a response to relatively trivial events, such as going away to college, or to serious stress, such as electroshock therapy. Concentration camp internees gave dramatic evidence that psychic factors affect menstrual rhythm. In the concentration camp of Theresienstadt, 800 interned women were studied by Bass. Fully 54 per cent of the women exposed to extreme conditions of crowding and threat of danger stopped menstruating. Poor food and physical damage were shown not to be the cause of this difficulty because 60 per cent of the affected cases became manifest within the first month of imprisonment, and in 94 per cent, the periods had returned within 18 months despite continued privation and danger. The literature is replete with anecdotes of menstrual disturbance following dramatic stressful events of many types, and the claim has been made based on interpretation of endometrial biopsy in four cases that normal endocrine cycling was arrested "precisely" at the time of shock.

A chronic form of the disease (and the most common cause of secondary amenorrhea in nonpregnant women) occurs without obvious or superficially apparent psychic disorder, although psychiatric observations have been interpreted to indicate that these individuals display significantly higher incidence of psychosexual immaturity, "oral conflicts," and schizoid traits than control groups. Manifestations and hormonal excretion pattern in the chronic disorder are like those seen in the more clearly evident neurogenic amenorrhea, but whether these represent "functional" disorder of hypothalamic mechanisms for regulating FSH and LH secretion is not known. Simple irregularity of periods or infrequency (oligomenorrhea) may be a mild manifestation of neurogenic disorder of gonadotropic regulation.

Hormone Function in Psychogenic Amenorrhea

Various patterns of hormonal defect displayed in psychogenic amenorrhea are not fully understood. As a rule, cyclical LH release is abolished, as manifested by absence of ovulation, presence of a monophasic body temperature curve, absence of secretory changes in endometrial biopsy, and virtual lack of pregnanetriol in the urine. This pattern resembles the syndrome produced experimentally in the rat by preoptic hypothalamic lesions and is probably a functional disturbance of the LH regulating region. Varying degrees of estrogen deficiency are found in some women, and the deficiency may approach that of the typical menopause in severity. This disturbance must be due to more severe LH deficiency with variable degrees of FSH deficiency, a syndrome comparable to that produced by lesions of the anterior median eminence in experimental animals. In one study of functional amenorrhea, four of sixteen patients resumed normal cycling within the first month of medical supervision. In the others, no consistent secretory pattern of plasma gonadotropins emerged. Three types were recognized by Boon and collaborators. Type I had sustained low levels of LH and FSH; type II had normal LH and FSH values, with occasional rises into the ovulatory range but without evidence of ovulation; and type III had sustained elevated LH or FSH levels or both without evidence of ovulation.

A curious and unexplained finding in certain cases of psychogenic amenorrhea is that the endometrium may become relatively refractory to stimulation by endogenous estrogen and progesterone. This observation has been interpreted to indicate that the brain may affect uterine function by mechanisms other than those involving the pituitary-ovarian axis. Recent studies indicate that a significant proportion of women with oligomenorrhea and secondary amenorrhea (20 and 13 per cent respectively) have hyposmia (normal incidence 0.4 per cent). This group may be analogous to the hypogonadotropic hypogonadal men (see next section) who also display hyposmia. The occurrence of this manifestation, helpful in clinical differential diagnosis, is likely a reflection of abnormality in function of the hypothalamic gonadotropic regulatory area. Unfortunately, gonadotropin secretion patterns have not been correlated with hyposmic patterns. It is likely that such patients have a distinct form of psychogenic amenorrhea, because in the usual case, menses are readily provoked by hormone administration and often with Clomid.

Management

Many case reports have been published claiming success from treatment by psychotherapy or by parasympathomimetic drugs. Menstrual cycles can be restored in some individuals by cyclical use of progesterone, and when this is unsuccessful, by cyclical estrogen-progesterone therapy (see Chapter 7). Ovulation is produced in a high proportion (up to 80 per cent) of patients of this type by means of Clomid therapy. Human menopausal gonadotropin plus human chorionic gonadotropins can be used if Clomid fails (see Chapter 7). The choice of therapy depends upon the severity of emotional disturbance and its influence on other spheres of body function and behavior and the therapeutic goals in the individual case, which may be the psychological reassurance of normal femininity and of the potential capacity to conceive, restoration of periodic vaginal bleeding, or repair of tissue estrogen deficiency.

Massive obesity is commonly associated with amenorrhea, and normal cycles may be restored when weight reduction is accomplished. Although these reactions probably involve the hypothalamus, the precise mechanism of the response is unknown.

Failure to develop gonadotropic function at the normal time is seen in disease of the pituitary and hypothalamus and as a variation within the normal range. Very rarely gonadotropic function may never develop in an otherwise normal girl: the fundamental cause of this difficulty has not been established.

Neurogenic Hypogonadism in the Male

Since gonadotropin secretion in the male as well as in the female is regulated by the hypothalamus,

hypogonadotropic hypogonadism might be expected to arise sometimes from neurogenic causes. Indeed, organic disorders of the hypothalamus such as tumor, encephalitis, microcephaly, Friedreich's ataxia, and demyelinating disorders can cause gonadal failure, but the largest proportion of men with hypogonadotropic hypogonadism do not have clinically detectable structural disease of the pituitary gland and have otherwise normal pituitary function (see Chapter 2). Experimental work in animals fosters the speculation that such cases may be due not only to intrinsic defects in pituitary gonadotrope cells but also to failure of proper maturation of hypothalamic gonadotropin regulating areas.

This speculative view cannot be confirmed in most cases until additional experience with LRH stimulation tests has been accumulated, but in one category of gonadotropin deficiency, reasonable evidence exists for a primary neurogenic disorder. In this disease, called Kallman's syndrome or "olfactory-genital dysplasia," hypogonadism is associated with anosmia or hyposmia and often with other neurologic defects, such as color blindness and nerve deafness. Dystrophic bone changes also occur. Pathologic examination of the brains of such individuals reveals that the olfactory defect is due, in some instances, to agenesis or maldevelopment of the olfactory lobes. In view of the close anatomic and physiologic connections between the rhinencephalon and sex-regulating areas of the hypothalamus (described earlier), failure to develop gonadotropic function is very probably due to maldevelopment of the hypothalamus. Kallman's syndrome is a genetic disorder thought to be inherited as an X-chromosomal dominant gene with incomplete penetrance. In such pedigrees, one may find males with hyposmia but with normal male sexual development, and females with hyposmia who as a rule have normal gonadotropic function. In other more usual forms of pituitary hypogonadism, sensitivity of the sense of smell is enhanced. This clinical difference between gonadotropin failure due to pituitary disease and that associated with Kallman's syndrome has been stated to be of value in differential diagnosis. Sporadic cases without family history also occur. An unexplained accompaniment of hypogonadotropism is the relative nonresponsiveness of the testes to exogenous gonadotropins (as compared with usual gonadotropin deficiency.) Bardin and colleagues have noted that "both ends of the pituitary-gonad axis are abnormal." Pituitary responses to LRF injection may also be much below normal in some but not all cases.

Psychogenic impairment of testicular function has received little study. Acute battle stress leads to decreased urinary secretion of testosterone in most men, as does the stress of officer training school. Decreased beard growth is apparently noted during long periods of sexual abstinence; the relation to testosterone secretion is unknown. Orgasm is not associated with increased LH secretion, and the viewing of a sexually arousing movie is similarly without effect on plasma LH levels.

A well-established neurogenic cause of hypogonadism is that observed following inflammatory or traumatic lesions of the spinal cord, occasionally in association with gynecomastia. Such cases are associated with loss of sensation in the genital area. Since LH secretion can be triggered in certain animals by stimulating the uterine cervix, and since the secretion of prolactin in the human can be induced by irritative lesions of the thoracic spinal nerves, maintenance of gonadotropic function may reasonably be expected to depend somewhat upon neural stimuli from the genital region. Convincing data in the human on this point have not been published.

In any discussion of hypogonadotropic hypogonadism, mention must be made of Fröhlich's syndrome (adiposogenital dystrophy). As first reported in 1901, the affected patient, a boy, had hypogonadism and obesity due to a pituitary tumor. A similar syndrome can readily be produced in experimental animals by damaging the median eminence and the ventromedial nuclei of the hypothalamus, clearly the result of disturbed FSH and LH release together with loss of sense of satiety. In humans, tumors and various inflammatory or degenerative lesions can produce the same disorder.

On the other hand, the overwhelming majority of obese children with delayed sexual development brought to endocrinologists do not have any structural damage to the hypothalamus. In some, the seeming failure of penile growth may be due merely to the presence of a large pubic fat pad. In most, the problem is constitutional delayed puberty in association with obesity of the usual type. Whether there is a functional disorder of the hypothalamus in these cases is not known. Many endocrinologists suspect that obesity in some way can delay onset of puberty. It is important to reassure the patient and his parents about the benign nature of this condition. The use of testosterone or chorionic gonadotropin injections is sometimes but not usually indicated for psychological reasons, but the administration of these hormones without a strict weight reduction regimen does not ameliorate the obesity (see Chapter 6).

Disorders of Prolactin Regulation

Nonpuerperal Galactorrhea

Lactation occurs abnormally in various clinical disorders unrelated to the puerperium. The basic pathophysiologic mechanism in all of these cases is probably excessive prolactin secretion occurring in patients whose breasts have been developed by insulin, growth hormone, adrenal corticoids, estrogens, and progesterone. In normal pregnancy, lactation is initiated when progesterone and estrogen levels fall, but whether a similar sequence—ovarian steroid secretion followed by ovarian steroid withdrawal—is required for development of nonpuerperal galactorrhea is not known

with certainty. In many of these cases, estrogen insufficiency is not clinically evident, but in others, as in pituitary stalk section or hypothalamic tumor, gonadotropin deficiency may be marked. The first recognized subjects with nonpuerperal galactorrhea, now termed the *Chiari-Frommel syndrome*, manifested persistent lactation, amenorrhea, and gonadal atrophy after pregnancy; mental disorders, including schizophrenia-like manifestations, are common. These manifestations seem due most likely to hypothalamic disorder, but the etiology of the disease is not known.

A second group of nonpuerperal galactorrheics is now recognized in whom the disease occurs spontaneously, with or without menstrual disturbance, and often with no antecedent pregnancy. These persons are often designated as suffering from the Forbes-Albright syndrome; about half have clinical evidence of pituitary tumor, which in a few instances appeared to be chromophobe adenomas (see Chapter 2). The other patients with the Forbes-Albright syndrome have no evidence of pituitary tumor, and in this type the etiology is unknown.

Galactorrhea may occur in patients with craniopharyngioma, sarcoidosis, and other inflammatory or neoplastic disease of the infundibulum or stalk. A similar syndrome is produced by administration of alpha-methyldopa or large doses of phenothiazine or reserpine, all of which are pharmacologic depressants of hypothalamic function. Hypothyroidism may also bring about lactation; in this circumstance, unlike in the usual hypothyroid patient, plasma prolactin levels are consistently elevated. One interpretation of this phenomenon is that hypothyroid encephalopathy (like other forms of brain impairment) can inhibit PIF secretion. Based on the recent demonstration that TRH is a potent prolactin releasing factor in the human (Fig. 12–16), an alternative explanation is that hypothyroidism-induced TRH secretion stimulates prolactin release. However, studies reported from the author's laboratory indicate that hypothyroidism is associated with a marked decrease in hypothalamic TRH synthetase activity, thus suggesting that TRH secretion is not enhanced in hypothyroidism. It is also possible (as suggested by Turkington) that hypothyroidism acts by increasing the sensitivity of the anterior pituitary to endogenous prolactin releasing factor (PRF or TRH). In addition to disturbances of the hypothalamic-pituitary unit, galactorrhea may result from prolonged irritative lesions of the anterior chest wall, notably post-thoracotomy or after herpes zoster of the thoracic segments. Even prolonged mechanical stimulation of the nipples as by suckling has been known to initiate lactation in nonpregnant or even virgin women. A foster mother may thus be enabled to suckle her adopted child.

The treatment of nonpuerperal galactorrhea is directed at the cause when possible. The idiopathic variety may respond to administration of estrogen or oral contraceptive agents, even though estrogen stimulates prolactin secretion by its action on both the hypothalamus and the pituitary gland. In this case it is effective by a direct action on the breast to inhibit the action of prolactin. Nipple stimulation should also be avoided as this may be a factor which prolongs lactation. Turkington has shown that L-dopa effectively reduces prolactin secretion in patients suffering from idiopathic galactorrhea and even in those with tumors. These observations confirm the role of dopamine as a stimulator of PIF secretion (already shown in the rat) and also indicate that the tumor is not fully autonomous (i.e., free of hypothalamic influence). One can speculate that the tumor might arise from sustained deficiency of PIF. In many cases no treatment is effective, and slight lactation may persist for many years. Local anesthesia of thoracic spinal segments has been reported to stop lactation in thoracotomy-induced disease, but has not been reported on in other forms of galactorrhea.

Neurogenic Disturbances in Growth Hormone Secretion and Growth

Lesions of the Central Nervous System

Growth disturbance is now recognized to follow a number of central nervous system disorders. Of course, direct pituitary damage or gross lesions of the pituitary stalk or hypothalamus will bring about growth hormone deficiency and growth insufficiency. As noted above, the majority of children with idiopathic hypopituitarism associated with low TSH secretion, in addition to growth hormone deficiency, have elevated plasma prolactin levels and relatively normal plasma TSH secretion in response to exogenous TRH injection, findings which suggest that the disorder is one of hypophysiotropic failure. A group of idiopathic dwarfs with GH failure have malformations of the prosencephalon, as shown by malformations of the hypothalamus, optic nerve dysplasia (with coloboma), and, frequently, absence of the septum pellucidum.

Maternal Deprivation Syndrome

Growth failure is also observed as a functional and potentially reversible disorder in children subject to severe psychological trauma. In most instances, growth retardation in severely disturbed children is due to caloric deficit, but a well defined group of these patients suffering from the syndrome of maternal deprivation prove to have growth failure despite adequate caloric intake. Such children have functional growth hormone deficiency, documented by persistently low plasma GH values, and failure to respond to the usual stimuli, such as hypoglycemia and arginine. A smaller group have deficiencies of ACTH-adrenal secretion. Because the provision of close personal attention and psychological treatment restores

growth and the secretion of growth hormone, it is reasonable to conclude that the entire syndrome is due to psychologically determined inhibition of GH secretion. Gardner has suggested that associated sleep disorder may be the cause of the GH deficiency.

Acromegaly

The suggestion that the excess growth hormone secretion observed in acromegaly may, in certain instances, be due to an increased release of the growth hormone releasing factor (GH-RF) has come from the demonstration that the secretion of growth hormone in certain acromegalics is to some degree subject to physiologic controls (i.e., suppressed to some extent by hyperglycemia, increased by hypoglycemia, inhibited by the drug chlorpromazine), and from the fact that GH-RF-like material has been demonstrated in the plasma of some individuals with this disease. Further evidence for a neural abnormality of GH regulation in acromegaly is the demonstration that a proportion of such patients have paradoxical increases in GH levels after glucose ingestion and paradoxical decreases in plasma GH following the ingestion of L-dopa which in normal individuals *stimulates* GH release.

Cerebral Gigantism

As summarized by Milunsky and colleagues, cerebral gigantism is a distinct and characteristic entity, the major features of which include gigantism with macrocrania and prognathism, mental retardation, dolichocephaly, high arched palate, characteristic facies with frontal bossing, hypertelorism, antimongoloid obliquity of the palpebral fissures, and some form of neuromuscular disturbance, such as clumsiness, awkward gait, or ataxia. Growth rates are extremely rapid during the first four to five years of life and gradually become normal thereafter. In almost all cases, the cerebral ventricles are dilated (mainly lateral and third ventricular), convulsions occur, and nonspecific abnormal electroencephalograms are seen. Chromosomes have been normal in all cases reported, but the disease was apparently associated with Klinefelter's syndrome in one individual who continued to grow abnormally after puberty (Reardon, personal communication). The growth disturbance in a few cases begins *in utero,* the macrocrania presenting difficulties at childbirth, and the permanent teeth erupt about two years earlier than normal.

Although a superficial consideration would make it seem reasonable to propose that there is an excess of growth hormone secretion in these patients, repeated studies have now confirmed without doubt that cerebral gigantism is *not* associated with elevated radioimmunoassayable growth hormone. In fact, insulin-induced hypoglycemia may provoke only sluggish GH discharge, and in at least one case, a paradoxical elevation was observed after glucose administration.

The nature of this disorder is still obscure. Possibilities include an intrinsic disturbance in tissues throughout the body (including brain) which makes them unusually susceptible to the effects of normal amounts of growth hormone. Another possibility is that the brain is capable of stimulating growth through hormonal effects exerted by as yet unrecognized secretory products (of the brain itself) or stimulated by the pituitary. In this regard, it is important to recall that normal growth has, on occasion, been observed in the absence of detectable growth hormone. This has been observed in otherwise normal individuals and as a special feature of the "catch-up" growth phase observed in a proportion of children after removal of craniopharyngiomas. In such children, growth far in excess of normal occurs for a few months in the absence of detectable plasma GH.

Diencephalic Syndrome

Tumors in the region of the hypothalamus and third ventricle may occasionally produce the diencephalic syndrome in children. The cardinal features of this disease are striking and complete absence of subcutaneous fat despite normal or increased appetite, cachexia and impaired growth after an initial period of accelerated growth, overalertness and euphoria, and increased locomotor activity. Such children prove to have persistently high growth hormone levels suppressible with glucose. GH levels have been reported to return to normal after radiotherapy. Pimstone and collaborators suggest that the marked wasting of fat is due to GH excess, but this seems unlikely since a similar finding is not observed in acromegaly.

Diseases of Thyrotropin Regulation

Hypothalamic Hypothyroidism

The occurrence of TRH failure in association with other pituitary hormone deficiencies has been alluded to above in reference to idiopathic hypopituitarism. In addition to this complex of hypophysiotropic hormone deficiencies, several patients have now been recognized who have thyroid gland failure due to isolated TRH deficiency (hypothalamic hypothyroidism, tertiary hypothyroidism). This disorder is recognized by the fact that such individuals have low thyroid function, which can be stimulated by TSH injection, and low plasma TSH levels, which can be stimulated by injections of TRH. It is possible that many cases previously considered as having monotropic TSH deficiency with myxedema may prove to fall largely into this cate-

gory. Even in Sheehan's syndrome, a disorder attributed to pituitary infarction, TSH deficiency may arise from infarction of the pituitary stalk or median eminence since some of such cases respond to TRH.

Familial Thyroid Hormone Unresponsiveness

Theoretically, it is possible that patients with hyperthyroidism due to an excess of TRH secretion can ultimately be identified. Such patients would truly have neurogenic thyrotoxicosis. One such patient may have been identified, but proof of TRH excess has not been established. Several patients have been observed who do manifest inappropriately high TSH levels in association with increased thyroid function, as shown by goiter, high I^{131} uptake, and high plasma thyroid hormone levels. Rather than suffering from TRH excess, as might be superficially presumed, these individuals prove to be suffering from defective thyroid hormone tissue responsiveness; they are not hypermetabolic, and the abnormal thyroid function is secondary to loss or blunting of the negative feedback loop component of the pituitary-thyroid axis (see discussion above). In normal humans, adrenal corticoids inhibit TSH secretion, presumably due to effects on hypothalamic TRH production or on pituitary responsiveness to TRH. In patients with thyroid hormone resistance, adrenal corticoids are as effective as in normals in suppressing TSH; thus this defect is truly an isolated one of thyroid hormone response in regulation of TSH secretion.

Diseases of Adrenocorticotropin Regulation

Cushing's Disease

Of all pituitary hypersecretory disorders, Cushing's disease comes closest to fitting the theoretical prediction of what a disease caused by primary excess of hypophysiotropic hormone secretion ought to be. In this disorder, there is an elevated "set point" for plasma cortisol levels, manifested by an excessively high threshold for feedback inhibition, and high plasma ACTH. Patients with Cushing's disease may show spontaneous remissions or recurring bouts of hypercortisolism, and such individuals lose their normal sleep-related ACTH and GH secretory discharge patterns, which do not return to normal even when adrenal overactivity has been rectified. Histologic abnormalities in the hypothalamus were described by Heinbecker. Hypothalamic tumors may cause Cushing's Syndrome, and the syndrome "paroxysmal ACTH discharge" has been recognized as a nervous system disease. In the case reported by Wolf and collaborators, paroxysms of cortisol hypersecretion were associated with paroxysmal EEG disturbance, and the patient responded well to treatment with chlorpromazine. In patients with depressive illness, impaired suppression of adrenal cortical function by standard doses of cortisol has been noted.

Despite these suggestive clinical observations, direct proof of a neurogenic etiology of the usual case of Cushing's disease still awaits proof of CRF hypersecretion.

Neurogenic Deficiency of ACTH Secretion

ACTH failure occurs in idiopathic hypopituitarism of childhood. Since most of these cases appear to be due to hypophysiotropic failure (see above), it is reasonable to assume that the associated adrenal cortical deficiency is due to failure of CRF secretion. Functional inhibition of CRF secretion is probably the basis of the impaired responsiveness of the adrenal cortex to stressful stimuli and to metyrapone in children suffering from maternal deprivation syndrome. Although failure of GH secretion is the most common of the endocrine manifestations of this disorder, adrenal cortical unresponsiveness also occurs in a small proportion of individuals. Changes in adrenal cortical function in the emotionally deprived child may well be the manifestation in the human of the well-established finding in experimental animals that the responsiveness of the pituitary-adrenal system is profoundly affected by the early postnatal psychological environment.

EFFECTS OF HORMONES ON THE BRAIN

Psychological disturbances may occur in virtually every disease of the endocrine organs. In some, e.g., hypothyroidism, behavioral changes may overshadow in severity and significance all other manifestations. The purpose of this section is to summarize the behavioral and psychologic aspects of endocrine disease and to outline the knowledge (surprisingly meager) of the mechanisms of their production. The excellent reviews by Michael and Gibbons, Smith and collaborators, McEwen and collaborators, and Levine give important details and a full bibliography.

Brain Function in Adrenocortical Disease

Cushing's Syndrome

The majority of patients with spontaneously occurring Cushing's disease have some mental change. Disorder severe enough to be termed psychotic occurs in 5 to 20 per cent of cases. Depression is the most common manifestation, and (in contrast to drug-induced Cushing's disease) elevation of mood or frank euphoria is very uncommon. Some individuals develop irritability, difficulty in concentrating, insomnia, paranoid delusions, and hallucinations; a wide range of other disturbances occur but all less commonly. These include excitement, anxiety, apathy verging on stupor, and typical delirium manifested by impaired consciousness, disorientation, and loss of recent memory. The acute organic brain syndrome of Cushing's disease is not readily differentiated from the acute brain syndrome of other causes. Schizophrenia-like illness is also recognized. Many patients with Cushing's disease have been treated unwittingly for functional psychosis; when the condition has been recognized and appropriately treated, dramatic improvement in mental state has been described.

Patients treated with pharmacologically large doses of glucocorticoids often show significant alterations in mood. Euphoria and cheerfulness are observed in three fourths and are accompanied often by increased appetite and occasionally by increased libido. Depression occurs less often but may be severe, and patients occasionally become depressed enough to attempt suicide. This finding is true of spontaneous Cushing's syndrome as well. Acute toxic psychosis with "organic" features also occurs. Some question exists as to whether these effects are dose related. In certain patients, dose dependency can be demonstrated so that effective therapeutic dosage with anti-inflammatory steroids may require adjustment to the smallest amount that does not produce cerebral manifestations. Other patients may have psychosis on one occasion and not on another despite the fact that they are receiving the same dose of medication. Most evidence indicates that occurrence of this illness is not related to the patient's premorbid personality. Prior mental disease is not a contraindication to steroid therapy; such patients do not run a greater than normal risk of steroid-induced psychosis.

Addison's Disease

From the earliest description of adrenocortical deficiency, significant change in personality and behavior has been regarded as an almost universal manifestation of this disorder. "Addisonian encephalopathy" in its severe form is recognizable as a typical organic psychosis or delirium, manifested by memory deficit, clouding of consciousness, and even stupor and unconsciousness. In milder cases apathy, depression, fatigue, poverty of thought, and lack of initiative are common. The patients are seclusive, irritable, and negativistic.

Associated evidence of organic brain disturbance is given by the EEG, which shows diffuse, high amplitude, slow activity. Detailed testing by Henkin and associates reveals the patient with adrenal insufficiency to have a lowered threshold of sensitivity to taste, smell, and hearing. Although detection threshold is low, judgment and discrimination of sensory input is impaired. The addisonian patient is notoriously hypersensitive to narcotic agents, particularly the barbiturates. These changes in brain function are due principally to glucocorticoid and not to mineralocorticoid deficits. This is known from the fact that administration of salt and DOCA neither repairs the abnormal EEG nor raises sensory thresholds to normal and only partially rectifies the personality disorder. Use of cortisone and other glucocorticoids, on the other hand, completely heals the behavioral, perceptual, and EEG disturbances.

Mechanism of Corticoid Effects on the Brain

In recent years, the physiologic basis for these neural defects has been better defined but is still not fully understood. Sophisticated electrophysiologic studies have shown that the conduction rate of nerve impulses along neurons is not altered by glucocorticoid deficiency, but the latency of transmission at central synapses is notably prolonged. This is particularly marked in multisynaptic systems such as the reticular-activating system, the tonic activity of which is responsible for maintaining alertness and other functions. High dosages of glucocorticoids decrease the latency of synaptic delay. Much progress has been made in elucidating the molecular basis of glucocorticoid action on nerve cells. In common with the other steroid hormones, the major site of action is on the nucleus, in a manner analogous to steroid-induced responses in peripheral tissues. Labeled corticoids localize to specific binding proteins in the septum and hippocampus by a saturable process and to the remainder of the brain by a nonsaturable mechanism. In all sites, corticoids are principally localized to cell nuclei, and this is especially so in the hypothalamus. Corticoids appear to stimulate RNA synthesis in these cells and to regulate important enzymes, certain of which may be rate limiting for synthesis of neurotransmitters. Aldosterone probably regulates Na^+ and K^+ flux in brain cells as it does in toad bladder and renal tubule. Local effects of the corticoids probably are responsible for certain negative feedback effects (as shown by inhibition of single neuron unit activity) and their biochemical and behavioral effects.

Brain Function in Thyroid Disease

Hypothyroidism

The oft-quoted Myxedema Commission of 1888 set up by the Clinical Society of London found in a population of severely ill patients that fully a third had frank and unmistakable psychosis with delusions, dementia, or mania. Dr. R. Asher, who applied A. J. Cronin's term, "myxedema madness,"

observed 14 cases over a 3-year period in London. The extreme form of hypothyroid encephalopathy is myxedema coma, which may have a fatal outcome (see Chapter 4).

These dramatic cases aside, close study of hypothyroid individuals reveals a high proportion with mental disturbance. The slowness and marked latency of response is readily noted, but in addition mood and affect are altered, and psychologic tests indicate mild delirium which, unless searched for, is not readily detectable. A peculiar facetiousness is common, resembling the *Witzelsucht* of patients with frontal lobe tumors. The jocularity of an anemic old woman with croaking voice is one of the most characteristic clinical clues to the endocrinologist. Often patients are depressed and retarded, but illness resembling schizophrenia is observed including paranoid delusions or hallucinations. Mania and excitement may occur. Laboratory evidence of organic brain disorder in hypothyroidism is not hard to find. The EEG in severe cases shows slowing of the dominant frequency, which is roughly proportional to metabolic rate and depressed voltage as well. Cerebral blood flow and cerebral oxygen utilization are decreased in proportion to the severity of the clinical manifestations. Surprisingly, seizures may occur in hypothyroid encephalopathy; seizures are not more common than normal in thyrotoxicosis.

Although most patients improve after thyroxine treatment, a certain proportion do not. Some of these probably have coincidental psychosis of the usual types rather than myxedema psychosis, but in other cases, organic brain deficit apparently related to long-standing thyroid deficiency does not clear following replacement therapy. Such individuals probably have suffered permanent brain damage from hypothyroidism. Further clinical evidence of the organic brain disturbance in myxedema is abnormal sensitivity to the depressant action of drugs such as morphine and phenothiazines which act on the central nervous system. Reduction in fractional turnover of drugs with a resultant elevation in blood level contributes to the depressant effect in myxedema. The effect of thyroid hormone deficit in the developing brain is well known in the patient with cretinism. Prolonged hypothyroidism may also affect peripheral nerves, giving rise to the clinical picture of "myxedema peripheral neuritis" (see Chapter 4).

Hyperthyroidism

Emotional lability, anxiety, "tension," over-reactiveness, poor ability to concentrate, restlessness, tremor, sleep disturbance, and even frank psychosis are extremely common in thyrotoxicosis (see Chapter 4). A minority of patients, particularly the elderly, become depressed, withdrawn, and apathetic and lose their appetites. In extremely "toxic" patients, delirium and coma may supervene; indeed, the occurrence of organic delirium in thyrotoxicosis is one of the hallmarks of thyroid storm. Detailed psychological testing has revealed an "organic brain damage" pattern in many. In some of these patients, even after treatment, the organic deficit persists although much reduced, suggesting that severe hyperthyroidism may cause irreversible brain damage. Thyroid encephalopathy is probably not due to a simple increase in cellular metabolism.

The role of premorbid personality disturbance in the pathogenesis of Graves' disease is still the subject of debate, some authors reporting a high incidence of psychological abnormality or stressful life situations or both prior to onset of the disease, and others claiming that such abnormalities are due to the disease itself. Based on the demonstration of *low* TSH levels in Graves' disease, it can be confidently concluded that this disorder is not due to an excessive TSH secretion secondary to hypothalamic abnormality.

Mechanism of Thyroid Hormone Effects on the Brain

In past years, it appeared reasonable to attribute the changes in brain function in hypothyroidism simply to a lowering of oxygen consumption of neurons. More recently, the role of thyroid hormone in regulating protein metabolism in general has been emphasized (see Chapter 4). The possibility must be considered, therefore, that the cerebral disturbance in hypothyroidism is also due to impaired nucleoprotein and protein synthesis in neurons and synapses. Clear-cut data support this contention for the developing brain, but such has not been demonstrated in mature brains. In the thyroidectomized newborn rat, nerve cells fail to reach their normal size, branching of neuronal dendrites is much less extensive, synaptic endings are fewer and smaller, and development of enzyme systems is impaired as is RNA synthesis. These changes appear to be responsible for the delay in maturation of electrical activity and behavior patterns and to account for decreased intelligence. Protein synthetic defect plays an unmistakable role in cretinism. As outlined by Sokoloff, the effects of thyroxine in stimulating brain metabolic rate and brain protein synthesis depend upon the responsiveness of the mitochondria; those from immature brain respond, while those from adult brain do not. The function of thyroxine in regulating all aspects of protein turnover and neurotransmitter synthesis in the adult brain has not been defined.

The neurophysiologic basis of thyrotoxic encephalopathy has not been established and, in fact, is enigmatic at this time. Surprisingly, cerebral oxygen consumption is not increased in the human with Graves' disease; brain tissue oxygen consumption (measured in laboratory animals), unlike that of liver and skeletal muscle, is unaltered by thyroid administration, and isolated brain mitochondria (unlike those from muscle, kidney, or liver) fail to swell or "uncouple" when exposed to excess thyroxine. These results indicate that hypothyroid encephalopathy is probably not due to a simple increase in cellular metabolism.

Pituitary Disease

As might be expected from the fact that hypothyroidism, adrenocortical failure, and hypogonadism individually may give rise to mental disturbance, pituitary disease with its secondary changes in all three of these functions is almost invariably accompanied by personality disorder. For example, in one review of 78 case reports of hypopituitarism, only six patients were free of psychological disturbances. At least a third of hypopituitary patients become profoundly dependent and develop psychological invalidism. Apathy, depression, drowsiness, loss of initiative and drive, and fatigue are the most common manifestations. As pointed out by Michael and Gibbons, "apathy, indifference and inactivity may become so profound that patients rarely leave their living quarters, they lie in bed for much of the day and they neglect even their personal hygiene." Severe contractures may occur. A striking feature of hypopituitarism is the dramatic loss of libido in both men and women which occurs almost uniformly. A chronic brain syndrome with typical organic features of disorientation and loss of memory is common, and its extreme form is recognizable as hypopituitary coma (see Chapter 2).

The test of therapy reveals that adrenal corticoid deficiency is the major factor contributing to the mental disturbance of patients with hypopituitarism, and few observations in clinical medicine are more gratifying than that of the confused or stuporous patient who may within an hour become alert and mentally clear following intravenous therapy with hydrocortisone. After corticoid replacement, thyroxine is further restorative, but return of libido requires for most individuals of either sex replacement doses of androgenic hormones. In women, increased sense of well-being follows the administration of estrogen.

After all of these known replacements have been supplied, and in presumably physiologic amounts, certain patients with panhypopituitarism still show some apathy, lack of drive, and chronic fatigue.

The basis for this residual deficiency is unknown, but possibly it is due to growth hormone deficiency. In view of the profound effects of this hormone on various metabolic functions, it would be surprising if this were not the case, but data to prove this point are lacking. Beyond the report by Raben that growth hormone increased libido, virtually nothing is known about its effects on psychologic function. The effects of prolactin in this regard are also unknown. Prolactin has a wide range of behavioral effects in lower forms, including the induction of maternal behavior and migratory drive, but no behavioral changes in the human have been definitely established.

Gonadal Steroids and Human Sexual Function

Androgens and Male Sexual Function

Androgenic hormone is required during adolescent development to bring about normal libidinal drive and potency; after these have been fully established, acquired androgenic deficiency may be quite severe before normal male sexual function is seriously impaired, and the onset of impotence and loss of libido may be gradual as compared with the loss of androgenic function. It is frequently stated in the literature that sex drive and potency in normally androgenized men is relatively independent of testosterone level, but there are differences from individual to individual. Most men with androgen deficiency who are receiving replacement therapy note a rather close correlation between treatment and psychologic effects, even over a few days. Estrogen therapy in males dramatically inhibits potency and sex drive.

Although androgen effects on libido and sex drive are much emphasized, its effects on personality are not limited specifically to the sexual sphere. Aggressiveness, drive, and the rambunctious behavior of the teenager are well-recognized effects of androgen stimulation. Among the psychological side effects of androgen treatment, if the hormone is given in excess, are insomnia, increased pressure of thought, and irritability. Hypogonadal men characteristically show marked passivity, poverty of ideation, and a lack of drive and general vigor, and have a higher than normal incidence of psychoneurotic symptoms. Patients suffering from Klinefelter's syndrome (who, in addition, have a chromosome abnormality) have a higher than normal incidence of psychosis, criminal psychopathy, disorders of sex identification, and transsexualism.

The personality deficits of the adult eunuch arise in part from the interaction of the physically and sexually inadequate individual with his environment, but an additional important organic component may be androgen deficiency during brain development. This conclusion is suggested by the fact that testosterone treatment, if delayed until adulthood, rarely restores psychosexual maturity, drive, and assertiveness to normal; therefore, treatment with androgen replacement should not be delayed too long in the hypogonad boy, a point emphasized by many clinicians (see Chapter 6). In experimental animals, a smaller dose of androgen replacement is required to prevent loss of sex drive than is required to restore it when once lost.

In men under the age of 50, loss of libido is almost always due to factors such as neurotic conflict, depression, poor health, fatigue, and fear of erectile failure. Testosterone deficiency is not demonstrable in such cases, and testosterone treatment does not benefit the patient beyond its use as a placebo.

The question of testosterone deficiency as a cause of impotence in healthy older men is the subject of the most notorious chapter in the history of endocrinology. Definitive studies by Kinsey and collaborators now indicate that male sexual drive and potency reach peak levels in the second decade of life and decline progressively thereafter. This decline cannot be attributed to androgen deficiency because testosterone secretion is maintained at approximately the same level in almost all men until the sixth decade. More likely, the normal decline in male sexual vigor with age represents maturation and then aging of neural structures involved in sexual behavior. These changes may be analogous to the well-recognized changes in other mental functions which accompany the aging of man and are a continuation of the neural changes in sexual function that begin with the determination of onset of puberty.

We are on less certain ground when the question of the male climacteric is raised. Approximately 15 per cent of older men show evidence of testicular aging by biopsy and by hormonal studies of testosterone and gonadotropin secretion. A proportion of such men are said to lose libido and to manifest the autonomic and nervous changes which are characteristic of the menopause, and to have a restoration of these functions after testosterone administration. As emphasized by Heller and Myers, this syndrome is not a normal part of the aging process, it is uncommon, and it may occur even in young men. Other workers dispute the existence of the male climacteric and dismiss the syndrome as being a manifestation of psychoneurosis. In view of the uncertain status of this question and the availability of modern diagnostic tests for gonadal function, it appears reasonable to evaluate testicular deficiency as a cause of loss of libido or potency in men suspected of having the syndrome of the male climacteric and to judge each case on its merits.

Female Sexual Function

Hormonal regulation of psychosexual function in women is more complex than in men, involving adrenal androgens as well as cyclic changes in estrogen and progesterone secretion. The most clear-cut fact about hormones and female sexuality concerns the importance of adrenal androgens. As demonstrated by Sutherland and collaborators, adrenalectomy or hypophysectomy leads to almost complete loss of libido and sex drive, and this loss can be reversed by treatment with testosterone. Analogous findings are observed in spontaneously occurring pituitary-adrenal disease and are helpful in both diagnosis and management. High dosage androgen therapy leads in some cases to enhanced, even pathologic, sexual drive. Whether these pathologic changes are due only to clitoral enlargement and hypersensitivity (which has been well demonstrated) or to an additional central component as well has not been clearly established.

The major importance of the psychic component in female sexuality as compared to the male makes it difficult to evaluate the effects of estrogen and progesterone. It is often stated that spontaneous or induced menopause with its loss of ovarian function has little effect on sex drive or the capacity for orgasm, and that the loss of fear of pregnancy may, in fact, increase sexual interest and the frequency of sexual intercourse. Many estrogen-deficient women, on the other hand, note a loss of sexual interest which is restored by replacement therapy. Moreover, the regressive changes in the female genitalia induced by estrogen deficiency – thinning and friability of the vulva and vagina and decrease in sexual secretions – may lead to dyspareunia. Loss of a sense of well-being also contributes to the loss of sexual feeling in the post-menopausal woman. Masters and Johnson state that the single most important factor in maintenance of sexual function in older women is continued sexual activity, but they also emphasize the importance of adequate replacement therapy to prevent vulvar and vaginal involution. Most physicians are relatively conservative in their use of endocrine replacement in menopausal women and fail to take account of the sexual functioning of the patient, as well as the presence of unpleasant vasomotor menopausal symptoms.

Even more complex are the changes in female sexuality which accompany the normal menstrual cycle. These are deeply intertwined with conscious and unconscious conflicts over the significance of the menses themselves. Studies with animals in which sex drive and behavioral "heat" are closely associated with high estrogen levels would lead one to suggest that women should show heightened sexual receptivity at midcycle. Viewed teleologically, the timing of gonadal readiness might be expected to coincide with behavioral acceptance.

This supposition based on work in lower animals does not appear to hold true uniformly in the human. Although sexual feeling varies throughout the menstrual cycle and, on the average, is maximum on the fourteenth day of the cycle (Moos and collaborators) not all women have a peak of sexual interest around the time of ovulation, and some demonstrate increased sexual desire just before and just after the menses. Most women have a decline in sexual feeling during the luteal (postovulatory) phase of the cycle, considered by most workers to coincide with the effects of progesterone on the brain.

The syndrome of "premenstrual tension" begins as estradiol and progesterone secretion begins to fall rapidly from its postovulatory peak, and is maximum when sex steroid levels are approaching their nadir. The mechanism of this syndrome has not been fully established. Normally, menstruating women show maximum "negative" affect immediately after, and immediately before, their menses. This is true for both anxiety and hostile feelings. As pointed out by Moos, a "large proportion of women who commit suicide or engage in criminal acts of violence and who as pilots have serious and fatal airplane accidents do so during the menstrual or premenstrual phases of the

cycle." About half of the occurrences of industrial sickness, acute psychiatric admissions, and acute medical and surgical admissions coincide with the four premenstrual and four menstrual days. Half of the children attending clinic with minor respiratory complaints did so during these same menstrual days of the mother.

The normal pattern of anxiety and hostile feelings is observed in women taking sequential contraceptives but not in those taking combined therapy with estrogens and gestagens. It appears that gestagens prevent the occurrence of the usual midcyclic peak of estrogen-induced well-being. Oral contraceptives of the combined type are said to be particularly, but not uniformly, likely to inhibit libido.

Another good example of the relation of estrogens to human brain function is seen in the menopause. Emotional instability and the "hot flash" which occur in 80 per cent of women are relieved by estrogen treatment. Fuller Albright believed that gonadotropin excess was the cause of hot flashes, but this does not seem to be true since they occur occasionally in hypopituitarism, are not induced by treatment with FSH or LH, and do not occur in girls who have congenital ovarian failure, even though they have high gonadotropin levels. The observation that clomiphene, an antiestrogen, causes hot flashes *before* gonadotropins rise and not after withdrawal of the drug (during the time of major ovulatory gonadotropin rise) further indicates that the hot flash and associated mental symptoms probably represent an estrogen deficiency syndrome. This may be analogous to the withdrawal syndromes of morphine or barbiturate addiction.

Mechanism of Female Sex Steroid Action on the Brain

Actions of progesterone on the brain have been well established. This steroid, in common with certain others, acts directly upon the hypothalamic temperature regulating area to raise the "set point" for body temperature control. This reaction is the basis for the postovulatory temperature rise in the basal body temperature curve of normal women. The hypothalamic locus of action of progesterone has been demonstrated by its feedback effects in regulation of gonadotropins in animals and in recent electrophysiologic studies in rats, which show that progesterone depresses the excitability threshold of hypothalamic neurons to reflex stimuli from the genital area and to direct electrical stimulation. In this respect, the effect of progesterone on hypothalamic neurons is similar to the effect exerted on the neuromuscular excitability of the estrogen-treated uterus. The molecular basis of sex steroid action on the brain has received much study following principles of steroid hormone action developed from experiments on estrogen and progesterone action on reproductive organs. In fact, sexual behavior should be looked upon as a sex hormone-dependent secondary sexual characteristic. Estradiol is localized to the preoptic area, hypothalamus, and amygdaloid region (areas previously shown to be involved in gonadotropin and behavioral regulation). Most of the steroid is localized in nuclei, where it may produce both increases and decreases in RNA synthesis (according to specific functions affected). Local estrogen effects probably account for increased hypothalamic monoamine oxidase at proestrus, altered turnover of H^3-norepinephrine, and altered histochemical staining of hypothalamic neurons. It appears that the behavioral effects and negative feedback effects of estrogens involve RNA formation since both estrogen-induced estrus and estrogen-induced gonadotropin inhibition are blocked by treatment with actinomycin D, an antibiotic inhibitor of RNA transcription.

Endocrine Changes in Homosexuality and Transsexualism

The bulk of clinical data supports the view that gonadal function is normal and appropriate to the genetic sex of patients with homosexuality, and that the orientation of sexual interest is not influenced by male or female sex steroids. Very recently, new data have appeared suggesting that there may be disturbances of sex steroid secretion in homosexuals after all. It has been reported that the more extremely feminine groups of male homosexuals have significantly lower than normal testosterone levels, whereas the more masculine groups of lesbians have higher than normal female levels of testosterone and a high incidence of menstrual irregularities. It has not been established whether these changes are due to the homosexual state, are dependent upon the behavior of these particular groups of homosexuals (since sex steroid secretion is affected by emotional state), or are independently caused by the same basic pathologic process that causes the abnormal psychological orientation. This area of research merits close study because of the large number of homosexual individuals in the general population.

In patients with transsexualism (defined as a disorder in which the patient feels himself to be the opposite of, and has a sexual orientation opposite to, his genetic sex), gonadal function is also appropriate to genotype. The endocrinologist is called upon to prescribe appropriate treatment to reverse secondary sexual characteristics and often to advise patients and others in positions of authority as to the management and advisability of the sex reversal process. This complex and rapidly developing area is discussed in detail by Money and collaborators.

Effects of Peptide Hormones on Brain Function

Little attention has been paid in the past to the direct effects of the peptide hormones on brain function, most emphasis having been given to the more obvious disturbances and changes induced by altered thyroid and steroid status. More recently, a number of important manifestations of peptide hormone action on the brain have been recognized. Because they probably will prove to be important as more work is carried out, they will be summarized in brief as a miscellaneous group of possibly related phenomena.

Certain of the pituitary peptide hormones appear capable of regulating their own secretion through operation of a short loop feedback control at the hypothalamic level. Thus prolactin implants in the hypothalamus inhibit prolactin release, growth hormone implants inhibit GH release, LH implants inhibit LH release, and ACTH implants inhibit ACTH release. An apparent exception to this phenomenon is TSH, which does not inhibit TSH secretion (in most but not all studies).

The reflex release of FSH during copulation in the rabbit appears to be responsible for mediating the sleeplike EEG state of postcoital female rabbits, and FSH is reported to alter catecholamine metabolism in the hypothalamus. The hypophysectomized rat is psychologically conditioned with great difficulty, if at all. This deficit is not restored by adrenal steroid replacement but by ACTH, which has a direct effect on the brain. The specific amino acid sequence responsible for the behavioral effect of ACTH has been studied; it proves to be a small polypeptide. Whether this peptide is involved in other forms of learning is unknown. As mentioned earlier, prolactin exerts marked effects on maternal behavior in lower animals; its effects in the human are unknown. Many women who nurse their children describe this experience and the period of nursing as one of special tranquillity, but it is not known at present whether this is a response to the mother-baby psychological interaction or to the *persistent* high levels of prolactin in the nursing mother.

Changes in learned behavior and EEG results have been reported to follow injections of α and β MSH both in animals and in humans. An interaction in potentiating dopamine effects has been reported as a possible basis for the observation that MSH ameliorates parkinsonism in some cases. TRH has been reported to alleviate depression through direct effects on the brain.

Perhaps the most interesting peptide hormone effects may prove to be those of angiotensin II. When given systemically to man or animals or by cerebral-ventricular injection to animals, this drug stimulates drinking behavior and the release of ADH. The effects of hypertonic salt injection into the third ventricle are potentiated by angiotensin II, which has led to the suggestion that this hormone enhances the uptake of salt by osmoreceptors, as it enhances the uptake of salt by vascular structures elsewhere. The human in shock develops severe thirst, a manifestation which may be related to the increased circulating levels of angiotensin II. Anephric humans have blunted thirst responses. The thirst following hypovolemia may be a behavioral response to altered renal function.

The actions of peptide hormones on brain have not been elucidated; conceivably they could act through the cyclic AMP mechanism (as peptide hormones do in the rest of the body), since the brain is rich in adenyl cyclase and cyclic AMP, and striking functional and behavioral changes can be induced by localized intracerebral injections of cyclic AMP derivatives. What should come as a sobering and provocative thought is that many of these peptide hormone-induced changes in brain function have been recognized only recently, and there may be other circulating peptide hormones as yet unrecognized which exert profound effects on many aspects of mind and behavior.

Mental Disturbances in Hyperinsulinism and Parathyroid Disorder

Abnormal brain function is among the most important manifestations of patients with hypoglycemia, hypocalcemia, and hypercalcemia. The extensive literature on this subject is reviewed in Chapter 10 (hyperinsulinism) and Chapter 11 (parathyroid disorder).

Benign Intracranial Hypertension (BIH)

General Considerations

This disorder, sometimes termed *pseudotumor cerebri* or *otitic hydrocephalus,* presents a characteristic clinical syndrome which includes headache, nausea, vomiting, papilledema, blurred vision, and increased intracranial pressure. As pointed out by Joynt and Sahs (194), neurologic disturbance is remarkably slight despite the degree of intracranial pressure; sixth nerve weakness is the chief localized neurologic deficit. The disturbance is transient, lasting weeks or months, and the prognosis is excellent. In most cases, the basic pathologic process appears to be chronic cerebral edema as indicated by biopsy and by the pneumoencephalographic demonstration of small ventricles. The etiology of this disorder is quite varied and includes sagittal or lateral sinus thrombosis, otitis media (so-called otitic hydrocephalus), head injury, vitamin A intoxication, and chlortetracycline administration. Instances of iron deficiency anemia, pernicious anemia, sarcoidosis, and a number of other rare diseases have been reported as causes of this condition.

Endocrine Causes

Several endocrine disorders have also been associated with benign intracranial hypertension. Absolute or relative adrenocortical deficiency is an important cause of this disease. It is observed in Addison's disease or following a sudden reduction in the dosage of corticoids being used as anti-inflammatory agents, particularly in children. Although the detailed pathologic physiology of this condition has not been established, it is probable that corticoids affect the permeability of cerebral capillaries (as they affect capillaries elsewhere), and that corticoid deficiency leads to increased capillary permeability and to altered fluid balance in the supportive oligodendroglia cells. Oligodendroglia make up a significant fraction of the non-neuronal space of the brain and play a trophic function in support of nerve cells. The symptoms of cerebral edema due to established brain disease such as brain tumor respond dramatically to high-dosage treatment with glucocorticoids, a clinical finding which further indicates an effect of this hormone on fluid balance in the brain. High dosage of glucocorticoids also inhibits the formation of cerebrospinal fluid, an additive factor in therapeutic response in hydrocephalus.

Hypoparathyroidism is another well-established endocrine cause of idiopathic brain edema which should be considered in differential diagnosis of any patient with unexplained papilledema and headache. The precise pathogenesis of this disease is unknown, but the condition is probably related to the effect of calcium deficiency on cerebral blood vessels or oligodendroglia fluid transport (not parathyroid hormone per se), since it is alleviated by treatment with calcium and vitamin D.

Other endocrinopathies associated with idiopathic cerebral edema are much less clear-cut. In 102 patients studied by Greer, 8 were pregnant, 10 were pubertal girls who had begun to menstruate from 10 months before to 2 months after the onset of cerebral edema, and 4 were mature women who had suffered from amenorrhea for 3 to 5 months before the onset of signs and symptoms of benign intracranial hypertension. Nonpuerperal galactorrhea also is observed in association with this disorder, but it is not known whether the cerebral edema causes both the lactation and the amenorrhea or is an associated manifestation of the same underlying disorder. Obesity, oral contraceptives, and diabetes mellitus have also been reported in association with BIH. This disorder is usually benign and self-limited and has been successfully treated by ventriculography, subtemporal decompression, and therapy with adrenocortical steroids or acetazolamide (Diamox). Fine judgment is necessary to determine which case should be managed by endocrine means and which requires full neurosurgical evaluation, particularly since high-dosage steroids – a logical form of therapy – may also produce striking amelioration of neurologic signs and symptoms, even in patients with well-established mass lesions of the brain.

REFERENCES

General Reviews and Anatomy

Harris, G. W.: *Neural Control of the Pituitary Gland.* Baltimore, Williams & Wilkins, 1955.

Reichlin, S.: Medical Progress, Neuroendocrinology. *New Eng. J. Med. 269*:1182–1191, 1246–1250, 1296–1303, 1963.

Harris, G. W., and Donovan, B. T. (eds.), *The Pituitary Gland.* Vol. 2. London, Butterworth & Co., Ltd., 1966.

Szentogothai, J., Flerko, B., et al.: *Hypothalamic Control of the Anterior Pituitary.* Budapest, Academiai Kiado, 1968.

Martini, L., and Ganong, W. F. (eds.), *Neuroendocrinology.* New York, Academic Press, Vol. 1, 1966, Vol. 2, 1967.

Brown-Grant, K., and Cross, B. A. (eds.), Recent studies on the hypothalamus. *Brit. Med. Bull. 22,* No. 3, 1966.

Reichlin, S.: Function of the hypothalamus. Amer. J. Med. *43*:477–485, 1967.

Martini, L., and Ganong, W. F. (eds.), *Frontiers in Neuroendocrinology.* Vol. 1, 1969. Vol. 2, 1971. Vol. 3, 1973. New York, Oxford University Press, (in press).

Martini, L., and Motta, M. (eds.), *The Hypothalamus.* New York, Academic Press, 1970.

Donovan, B. D.: *Mammalian Endocrinology.* London, Mc-Graw-Hill, 1970.

Knigge, K. M., Scott, D. E., et al. (eds.), *Brain-Endocrine Interaction. Median Eminence: Structure and Function.* Basel, S. Karger, 1972.

Harris, G. W.: Humours and hormones: The Sir Henry Dale Lecture for 1971. *J. Endocr. 53*:i–xxiii, 1972.

Bibliographic Reviews in Neuroendocrinology. Published periodically by U.C.L.A. Brain Information Service.

Weitzman, M., (ed.), *Bibliographica Neuroendocrinologica.* Albert Einstein School of Medicine, Department of Anatomy. Published periodically.

Brown, G. M., and Martin, J. B.: Neuroendocrine relationships, In *Progress in Neurology and Psychiatry.* Spiegel, E. (ed.), 1973 (in press).

Hypophysiotropic Hormones of the Hypothalamus

McCann, S. M., and Porter, J. C.: Hypothalamic pituitary stimulating and inhibiting hormones. *Physiol. Rev. 49*:240–284, 1969.

Meites, J. (ed.), *Hypophysiotropic Hormones of the Hypothalamus: Assay and Chemistry.* Baltimore, Williams & Wilkins, 1970.

Geschwind, I. I.: Mechanism of action of hypothalamic adenohypophysiotropic factors, In *Hypophysiotropic Hormones of The Hypothalamus: Assay and Chemistry* Meites, J. (ed.), Baltimore, Williams & Wilkins, 1970, pp. 218–319.

McCann, S. M.: Mechanism of action of hypothalamic-hypophyseal stimulating and inhibiting hormones, In *Frontiers in Neuroendocrinology.* Vol. 2. Martini, L. and Ganong, W. F. (eds.), New York, Oxford University Press, 1971, pp. 209–235.

Gay, V. L.: The Hypothalamus: Physiology and clinical use of releasing factors. *Fertility and Sterility 23*:50–63, 1972.

Burgus, R., Dunn, T. F., et al.: Structure moleculaire du facteur hypothalamique hypophysiotrope TRF d'origine ovine: evidence par spectrometrie de masse de la sequence PCA-His-Pro-NH₂. *C. R. Acad. Sci.* (Paris) *269*:1870–1873, 1969.

Bowers, C. Y., Schally, A. V., et al.: Porcine thyrotropin releasing factor is (pyro)glu-his-pro (NH₂). *Endocrinology 86*:1143–1153, 1970.

Schally, A. V., Nair, R. M. G., et al.: Isolation of the luteinizing hormone and follicle-stimulating hormone-releasing hormone from porcine hypothalami. *J. Biol. Chem. 246*:7230–7236, 1971.

Schally, A. V., Kastin, A. J., et al.: Hypothalamic follicle-stimulating hormone (FSH) and luteinizing hormone (LH)-regulating hormone: Structure, physiology and clinical studies. *Fertility and Sterility 22*:703–721, 1971.

Guillemen, R., Burgus, R.: The hormones of the hypothalamus. Sci. Amer. *227*(5):24–33, 1972.

Reichlin, S., and Mitnick, M. A.: Biosynthesis of hypophysiotropic hormones, In *Frontiers in Neuroendocrinology.* Vol. 3. Martini, L., and Ganong, W. F. (eds.), New York, Oxford Press, 1973, pp. 61–88.

Fleischer, N., and Guillemin, R.: Clinical applications of hypothalamic-releasing factors, In *Advances in Internal Medicine.* Vol. 18. Stollerman, G. H., (ed.),

Chicago, Year Book Medical Publishers, 1972, pp. 303–323.

Brazeau, P., Vale, W., et al.: Hypothalamic polypeptide that inhibits the secretion of immunoreactive pituitary growth hormone. *Science 179*:77–79, 1973.

Bowers, C. Y., Friesen, H. G., et al.: Prolactin and thyrotropin release in man by synthetic pyroglutamyl-histidyl-prolinamide. *Biochem. Biophys. Res. Comm. 45*:1033, 1972.

Neurotransmitter Control of Secretion of Hypophysiotropic Function

Wurtman, R. J.: Brain monoamines and endocrine function. Neurosciences Research Program Bulletin. Vol. 9. 1970, pp. 172–297.

Porter, C. C.: *Chemical Mechanisms of Drug Action.* Springfield, Ill., Charles C Thomas, 1970, pp. 83–102.

Cooper, J. R., Bloom, F. E., et al.: *The Biochemical Basis of Neuropharmacology.* New York, Oxford University Press, 1970.

Boyd, A. E., 3rd, Lebovitz, H. E., et al.: Stimulation of human-growth-hormone secretion by L-dopa. *New Eng. J. Med. 283*:1425–1429, 1970.

Frohman, L. A.: Clinical neuropharmacology of hypothalamic releasing factors. *New Eng. J. Med. 286*:1391–1397, 1972.

Fuxe, K., and Hokfelt, T.: Participation of central monoamine neurons in the regulation of anterior pituitary function with special regard to the neuro-endocrine role of tubero-infundibular dopamine neurons, In Bargmann, W., and Scharrer, B. (eds.), *Aspects of Neuroendocrinology,* New York, Springer-Verlag, 1970.

Hillarp, N. A., Fuxe, K., et al.: Demonstration and mapping of central neurons containing dopamine, noradrenaline, and 5-hydroxytryptamine and their reactions to psychopharmaca. *Pharmacol. Rev. 18,* Part 1:727–741, 1969.

Neuroendocrine Control of Specific Pituitary Tropic Hormones

TSH

Reichlin, S.: Control of TSH secretion, In Werner, S. C., and Ingbar, S. (eds.), *The Thyroid,* New York, Harper and Row, 1971.

Reichlin, S., Martin, J. B., et al.: The hypothalamus in pituitary-thyroid regulation. *Recent Progr. Hormone Res. 28*:229–286, 1972.

Hershman, J. M., and Pittman, J. A., Jr.: Control of thyrotropin secretion in man. *New Eng. J. Med. 285*:997–1006, 1971.

Martin, J. B.: Neural control of thyrotropic hormone secretion. *New Eng. J. Med.,* 1973 (in press).

ACTH

Ganong, W. F.: The central nervous system and the synthesis and release of adrenocorticotropic hormone. In *Advances in Neuroendocrinology.* Nalbandov, A. V. (ed.), Urbana, University of Illinois Press, 1963, pp. 92–149.

Kreiger, D. T., and Kreiger, H. P.: Aldosterone excretion in pretectal disease. *J. Clin. Endocr. 24*:1055–1066, 1964.

Liddle, G. W., Island, D., et al.: Normal and abnormal regulation of corticotropin secretion in man. *Recent Progr. Hormone Res. 18*:125–153, 1962.

Mulrow, P. J.: Neural and other mechanisms regulating aldosterone secretion, In *Neuroendocrinology.* Martini, L., and Ganong, W. F., (eds.), New York, Academic Press, 1966.

Yates, F. E., and Urquhart, J.: Control of plasma concentration of adrenocortical hormones. *Physiol. Rev. 42*:359–443, 1962.

Kendall, J. W.: Feedback control of adrenocorticotrophic hormone secretion, In *Neuroendocrinology.* Vol. 2. Martini, L., and Ganong, W. F. (eds.), New York, Oxford University Press, 1971, pp. 177–208.

Gonadotropins

Everett, J. W.: Central neural control of reproductive functions of the adenohypophysis. *Physiol. Rev. 44*:373–431, 1964.

McCann, S. M., and Ramirez, V. D.: The neuroendocrine

regulation of hypophyseal luteinizing hormone secretion. *Recent Progr. Hormone Res.* 20:131–170, 1964.

Schwartz, N.: A model for the regulation of ovulation in the rat. *Recent Progr. Hormone Research* 25:1–43, 1969.

Odell, W. D., and Moyer, D. L.: *Physiology of Reproduction.* St. Louis, C. V. Mosby, 1971.

Vande Wiele, R. L., Bogumil, I., et al.: Mechanisms regulating the menstrual cycle in women. *Recent Progr. Hormone Res.* 26:63–103, 1970.

Ross, G. T., Cargille, C. M., et al.: Pituitary and gonadal hormones in women during spontaneous and induced ovulatory cycles. *Recent Progr. Hormone Res.* 26:1–48, 1970.

The Neuroendocrinology of Human Reproduction, Mack, H. C., and Sherman, A. I. (eds.), Springfield, Charles C Thomas, 1971.

Malacara, J. M., Seyler, L. E., Jr., et al.: Luteinizing hormone releasing factor activity in peripheral blood from women during the midcycle luteinizing hormone ovulatory surge. *J. Clin. Endocr.* 34:271–278, 1972.

Gorski, R. A.: Gonadal hormones and the perinatal development of neuroendocrine function, In *Frontiers in Neuroendocrinology.* Martini, L., and Ganong, W. F. (eds.), New York, Oxford University Press, 1970, pp. 237–290.

PROLACTIN

Meites, J.: Control of mammary growth and lactation, In *Neuroendocrinology.* Martini, L., and Ganong, W. F. (eds.), New York, Academic Press, 1966, pp. 669–707.

Nicoll, C. S.: Aspects of the neural control of prolactin secretion, In *Frontiers in Neuroendocrinology.* Martini, L., and Ganong, W. F. (eds.), New York, Oxford University Press, 1970, pp. 291–330.

Frantz, A. G., Kleinberg, D. K., et al.: Studies on prolactin in man. *Recent Progr. Hormone Res.* 28:527–590, 1972.

Meites, J., Lu, K. H., et al.: Recent studies on functions and control of prolactin secretion in rats. *Recent Progr. Hormone Res.* 28:471–526, 1972.

GROWTH HORMONE

Glick, S. M., Roth, J., et al.: The regulation of growth hormone secretion. *Recent Progr. Hormone Res.* 21:241–283, 1965.

Knobil, E.: The pituitary growth hormone: an adventure in physiology. *The Physiologist* 9:25–44, 1966.

Brown, G. M., and Reichlin, S.: Psychological and neural regulation of growth hormone secretion. *Psychosom. Med.* 34:45–61, 1972.

Reichlin, S.: Regulation of somatotrophic hormone secretion, In *American Physiological Society Handbook of Physiology* (in press).

Martin, J. B.: Neural control of growth hormone secretion. *New Eng. J. Med.,* 1973 (in press).

Pherhormones

Michael, R. A.: Neuroendocrine factors regulating primate behavior, In *Frontiers in Neuroendocrinology.* Martini, L., and Ganong, W. F. (eds.), New York, Oxford University Press, 1970, pp. 359–398.

McClintock, M. K.: Menstrual synchrony and suppression. *Nature* (London) 229:244–245, 1971.

Periventricular Organs

Knigge, K. M., Scott, D. E., et al. (eds.), *Brain-Endocrine Interaction. Median Eminence: Structure and Function.* Basel, S. Karger, 1972, pp. 1–368.

Weindl, A.: Auf Morphologie und Histochemie von Subfornicalorgan Organum Vasculosum Laminae Terminalis und Area Postrema bei Kaninchen und Ratte. *Z. Zellforsch.* 67:740–775, 1965.

Akert, K.: The mammalian subfornical organ. *J. Neurovisc. Relat.* (Suppl. IX), 1969, pp. 78–93.

Knowles, F.: Ependymal secretion, especially in the hypothalamic region. *J. Neurovisc. Relat.* (Suppl. IX), 1969, pp. 97–110.

Oksche, A.: The subcommissural organ. *J. Neurovisc. Relat.* (Suppl. IX), 1969, pp. 111–139.

Gilbert, G. J.: The subcommissural organ and water-electrolyte metabolism, In *Thirst.* Proceedings 1st International Symposium on Thirst in the Regulation of Body Water. Wayne, M. J. (ed.), New York, The Macmillan Co., 1964, pp. 457–471.

Upton, P. D., Dunihue, F. W., et al.: Subcommissural organ and water metabolism. *Amer. J. Physiol.* 201:711–713, 1961.

Wislocki, G. B., and Leduc, E. H.: The cytology of the subcommissural organ, Reisner's fiber, periventricular glial cells and posterior collicular recess of the rat's brain. *J. Comp. Neurol.* 101:283–299, 1954.

Rudman, D., Del Rio, A. E., et al.: Comparison of lipolytic and melanotropic factors in bovine pineal gland. *Endocrinology* 90:1139–1146, 1972.

Human Neuroendocrine Disease

Bauer, H. G.: Endocrine and other clinical manifestations of hypothalamic disease. *J. Clin. Endocr.* 14:13–31, 1954.

Oppenheimer, J. H.: Abnormalities of neuroendocrine functions in man, In *Neuroendocrinology.* Vol. 2. Martini, L., and Ganong, W. F. (eds.), New York, Academic Press, 1967.

Rothballer, A.: Some endocrine manifestations of central nervous system disease: an approach to clinical neuroendocrinology. *Bull. N. Y. Acad. Med.* 42:257–283, 1966.

Kahana, L., Kahana, S., et al.: Endocrine manifestations of intracranial extrasellar lesions, In *An Introduction to Clinical Neuroendocrinology.* Bajusz, E. (ed.), Baltimore, Williams & Wilkins, 1967, pp. 254–272.

Peake, G. T., and Daughaday, W. H.: Disturbances of pituitary function in central nervous system disease. *Med. Clin. N. Amer.* 52:357–369, 1968.

Krieger, D. T., Ross, F. R., et al.: Response to dexamethasone suppression in central nervous system disease. *J. Clin. Endocr.* 26:227–230, 1966.

Krieger, D. T., Glick, S., et al.: A comparative study of endocrine tests in hypothalamic disease. Circadian periodicity of plasma 11-OHCS levels, plasma 11-OHCS and growth hormone response to insulin hypoglycemia and metyrapone responsiveness. *J. Clin. Endocr.* 28:1589–1598, 1968.

Reeves, A. G., and Plum, F.: Hypophagia, rage and dementia accompanying a ventromedial hypothalamic neoplasm. *Arch. Neurol.* (Chicago) 20:616–624, 1969.

Killeffer, F. A., and Stern, W. E.: Chronic effects of hypothalamic injury (report of a case of near total hypothalamic destruction resulting from removal of a craniopharyngioma). *Arch. Neurol.* (Chicago) 22:419–429, 1970.

Heuser, G., Batzdorf, U., et al.: Advances in human neuroendocrinology. *Ann. Intern. Med.* 73:783–807, 1970.

Pituitary Stalk Section

Adams, J. H., Daniel, P. M., et al.: Some effects of transection of the pituitary stalk. *Brit. Med. J.* 2:1619–1625, 1964.

Dugger, G. S., VanWyk, J. J., et al.: The effects of pituitary-stalk section on thyroid function and gonadotropic hormone secretion in women with mammary carcinoma. *J. Neurosurg.* 19:589–593, 1962.

Ehni, G., and Eckles, N. E.: Interruption of the pituitary stalk in the patient with mammary cancer. *J. Neurosurg.* 16:628–651, 1959.

Li, M. C., Rall, J. E., et al.: Thyroid function following hypophysectomy in man. *J. Clin. Endocr.* 15:1228–1238, 1955.

Lipsett, M. B., West, C. D., et al.: Adrenal function after hypophysectomy in man. *J. Clin. Endocr.* 17:356–363, 1957.

VanWyk, J. J., Dugger, G. S., et al.: The effect of pituitary stalk section on the adrenal function of women with cancer of the breast. *J. Clin. Endocr.* 20:157–172, 1960.

Antony, G. J., Van Wyk, J. J., et al.: Influence of pituitary stalk section on growth hormone, insulin, and TSH secretion in women with metastatic breast cancer. *J. Clin. Endocr.* 29:1238–1250, 1969.

Turkington, R. W., Underwood, L. E., et al.: Elevated serum prolactin levels after pituitary-stalk section in man. *New Eng. J. Med.* 285:707–710, 1971.

Hypophysiotropic Failure

Costom, B. H., Grumbach, M. M., et al.: Effect of thyrotropin-releasing factor on serum thyroid-stimulating hormone (an approach to distinguishing hypothalamic from pituitary forms of idiopathic hypopituitary dwarfism). *J. Clin. Invest. 50*:2219–2225, 1971.

Pittman, J. A., Jr., Haigler, E. D., et al.: Hypothalamic hypothyroidism. *New Eng. J. Med. 285*:844–845, 1971.

Disease of Gonadotropin Regulation

PRECOCIOUS PUBERTY

Donovan, B. T., and Van der Werff ten Bosch: *Physiology of Puberty.* Baltimore, Williams & Wilkins, 1965.

Jolly, H.: *Sexual Precocity.* Springfield, Ill., Charles C Thomas, 1955.

Wilkins, L.: *The Diagnosis and Treatment of Endocrine Disorders in Childhood and Adolescence.* Springfield, Ill., Charles C Thomas, 1965.

Liu, N., Grumbach, M. M., et al.: Prevalence of electroencephalographic abnormalities in idiopathic precocious puberty and premature pubarche: bearing on pathogenesis and neuroendocrine regulation of puberty. *J. Clin. Endocr. 25*:1296–1308, 1965.

Richter, R. B.: True hamartoma of the hypothalamus associated with pubertas praecox. *J. Neuropath. 10*:368–383, 1951.

Stotijn, C. P. J., and Nauta, W. J. H.: Precocious puberty and tumor of the hypothalamus. *J. Nerv. Ment. Dis. 111*:207–224, 1950.

Bing, J. F., Globus, J. H., et al.: Pubertas praecox: a survey of the reported cases and verified anatomical findings. *J. Mount Sinai. Hosp. N. Y. 4*:935–965, 1938.

Cohen, R. A., Wurtman, R. J., et al.: Combined Clinical Staff Conference at the National Institutes of Health. Some clinical, biochemical and physiological actions of the pineal gland. *Ann. Intern. Med. 61*:1144–1161, 1964.

Kitay, J. I.: Pineal lesions and precocious puberty, a review. *J. Clin. Endocr. 14*:622–625, 1957.

Ringertz, N., Nordestam, H., et al.: Tumors of the pineal region. *J. Neuropath. 13*:540–561, 1954.

Russell, D. S., Rubinstein, L. J., et al.: Pineal neoplasm, In *Pathology of Tumours of the Nervous System.* London, Edward Arnold, 1963, pp. 173–183.

Weinberger, L. M., and Grant, F. C.: Precocious puberty and tumors of the hypothalamus. *Arch. Intern. Med. 67*:762–792, 1941.

Wurtman, R. J., and Kammer, H.: Melatonin synthesis by ectopic pinealoma. *New Eng. J. Med. 244*:1233–1237, 1966.

Jenner, M. R., Kelch, R. P., et al.: Hormonal changes in puberty. IV. Plasma estradiol, LH and FSH in prepubertal children, pubertal females and in precocious puberty, premature thelarche, hypogonadism and in a child with a feminizing ovarian tumor. *J. Clin. Endocr., 34*:521–530, 1972.

Husband, P., and Snodgrass, J. A. I.: McCune-Albright syndrome with endocrinological investigations. *Amer. J. Dis. Child 119*:164–167, 1970.

Rifkind, A. B., Julin, H. E., et al.: Suppression of urinary excretion of luteinizing hormone (LH) and follicle stimulating hormone (FSH) by medroxygesterone acetate. *J. Clin. Endocr. 29*:506–513, 1969.

Teller, W. M., Murset, G., et al.: Urinary C_{19} and C_{21} steroid patterns in isosexual precocious puberty during long-term treatment with gestagons. *Acta Paediat. Scand. 58*:385–392, 1969.

Castleman, B., and McNeely, B. U.: Case 25–1971 (germinoma). Case Records of the Massachusetts General Hospital. *New Eng. J. Med. 284*:1427–1434, 1971.

Wood, L. C., Olichney, M., et al.: Syndrome of juvenile hypothyroidism associated with advanced sexual development: report of two new cases and comment on the management of an associated ovarian mass. *J. Clin. Endocr. 25*:1289–1295, 1965.

Futterweit, W., and Goodsell, C. H.: Galactorrhea in primary hypothyroidism: Report of two cases and review of the literature. *Mount Sinai J. Med. N. Y. 37*:584–589, 1970.

Hampson, J. G., and Money, J.: Idiopathic sexual precocity in the female. Report of 3 cases. *Psychosom. Med. 17*:16–35, 1955.

Money, J., and Hampson, J. G.: Idiopathic sexual precocity in the male: management: report of a case. *Psychosom. Med. 17*:1–15, 1955.

Money, J., and Alexander, D.: Psychosexual development and absence of homosexuality in males with precocious puberty. *J. Nerv. Ment. Dis. 148*:111–123, 1969.

PSYCHOGENIC AMENORRHEA

Björo, K.: Secondary oligo-amenorrhea. *Acta Obstet. Gynec. Scand.* (Suppl. 6) *41*:5–47, 1962.

Kelley, K., Daniels, G. E., et al.: Psychological correlations with secondary amenorrhea. *Psychosom. Med. 16*:129–147, 1954.

Sturgis, S. H.: *The Gynecologic Patient.* New York, Grune & Stratton, 1962.

Reifenstein, E. C.: Psychogenic or "hypothalamic" amenorrhea. *Med. Clin. N. Amer. 30*:1103–1114, 1946.

Backer, M. H., Jr., and Cavanagh, D.: Psychogenic amenorrhea. *Med. Clin. N. Amer. 52*:339–355, 1968.

Boon, R. C., Schalch, D. S., et al.: Plasma gonadotropin secretory patterns in patients with functional menstrual disorders and Stein-Leventhal syndrome: Response to clomiphene treatment. *Amer. J. Obstet. Gynec. 112*:736–748, 1972.

PSEUDOCYESIS

Bivin, G. D., and Klinger, M. P.: *Pseudocyesis.* Bloomington, Principia Press, Inc., 1937.

Fried, P. H., Rakoff, A. E., et al.: Pseudocyesis: a psychosomatic study in gynecology. *J.A.M.A. 145*:1329–1335, 1951.

Moulton, R.: The psychosomatic implications of pseudocyesis. *Psychosom. Med. 4*:376–389, 1942.

Schopbach, R. R., Fried, P. H., et al.: Pseudocyesis: a psychosomatic disorder. *Psychosom. Med. 14*:129–134, 1952.

ANOREXIA NERVOSA

Bliss, E. L., and Branch, C. H. H.: *Anorexia Nervosa, Its History, Psychology and Biology.* New York, Hoeber, 1960.

King, A.: Primary and secondary anorexia nervosa syndromes. *Brit. J. Psychiat. 109*:470–479, 1963.

Landon, J., Greenwood, F. C., et al.: The plasma sugar, free fatty acid, cortisol, and growth hormone response to insulin and the comparison of this procedure with other tests of pituitary and adrenal function. II. In patients with hypothalamic or pituitary dysfunction or anorexia nervosa. *J. Clin. Invest. 45*:437–449, 1966.

Nemiah, J. C.: Anorexia nervosa: a clinical psychiatric study. *Medicine 29*:225–267, 1950.

Russell, G. F.: Metabolic, endocrine and psychiatric aspects of anorexia nervosa. *Sci. Basis Med. Ann. Rev.* pp. 236–255, 1969.

NEUROGENIC HYPOGONADISM

Bors, E., Engle, E. T., et al.: Fertility in paraplegic males. *J. Clin. Endocr. 10*:381–398, 1950.

Nowakowski, H., and Lenz, W.: Genetic aspects in male hypogonadism. *Recent Progr. Hormone Res. 17*:53–89, 1961.

Rose, R. M., Bourne, P. G., et al.: Androgen responses to stress. II. Excretion of testosterone, epitestosterone, androsterone and etiocholanolone during basic combat training and under threat of attack. *Psychosomatic Med. 31*:418–436, 1969.

Bardin, C. W., Ross, G. T., et al.: Studies of the pituitary-Leydig cell axis in young men with hypogonadotropic hypogonadism and hyposomia: Comparison with normal men, prepuberal boys, and hypopituitary patients. *J. Clin. Invest. 48*:2046–2056, 1969.

Boström, K., and Brun, A.: Testicular changes in association with malformation of the central nervous system and mental retardation. *Acta Path. Microbiol. Scand. 79*:249–256, 1971.

Marshall, J. R., and Henkin, R. I.: Olfactory acuity, menstrual abnormalities and oocyte status. *Ann. Intern. Med. 75*:207–211, 1971.

Naftolin, F., Harris, G. W., et al.: Effect of purified luteinizing hormone releasing factor on normal and hypogonadotrophic anosmic men. *Nature* (London) *232*:496–497, 1971.

Disease of Growth Hormone Regulation

Kaplan, S., Grumbach, M., et al.: A syndrome of hypopituitary dwarfism, hypoplasia of optic nerve and malformation of prosencephalon: Report of 6 patients (abstract). *Pediat. Res. 4*:480, 1970.

Costom, B. H., Grumbach, M. M., et al.: Effect of thyrotropin-releasing factor on serum thyroid-stimulating hormone (An approach to distinguishing hypothalamic from pituitary forms of idiopathic hypopituitary dwarfism). *J. Clin. Invest. 50*:2219–2225, 1971.

Powell, G. F., Brasel, J. A., et al.: Emotional deprivation and growth retardation simulating idiopathic hypopituitarism. *New Eng. J. Med. 276*:1279–1283, 1967.

Krieger, I., and Mellinger, R. C.: Pituitary function in the deprivation syndrome. *J. Pediat. 79*:216–225, 1971.

Sherman, L., and Kolodny, H. D.: The hypothalamus, brain catecholamines and drug therapy for gigantism and acromegaly. *Lancet i*:682–685, 1971.

Kenny, F. M., Iturzaeta, N. F., et al.: Iatrogenic hypopituitarism in craniopharyngioma: Unexplained catch-up growth in three children. *J. Pediat. 72*:766–775, 1968.

Hagen, T. C., Lawrence, A. M., et al.: *In vitro* release of monkey pituitary growth hormone by acromegalic plasma. *J. Clin. Endocr. 33*:448–451, 1971.

Lawrence, A. M., Goldfine, I. D., et al.: Growth hormone dynamics in acromegaly. *J. Endocr. 31*:239–247, 1970.

Goodman, H. G., Grumbach, M. M., et al.: Growth and growth hormone. *New Eng. J. Med. 278*:57–68, 1968.

Cerebral gigantism

Bejar, R. L., Smith, G. F., et al.: Cerebral gigantism: Concentrations of amino acids in plasma and muscle. *J. Pediat. 76*:105–111, 1967.

Milunsky, A., Cowie, V. A., et al.: Cerebral gigantism in childhood. A report of 2 cases and a review of the literature. *Pediatrics 40*:395–402, 1967.

Diencephalic syndrome

Pimstone, B. L., Sobel, J., et al.: Secretion of growth hormone in the diencephalic syndrome of childhood. *J. Pediat. 76*:886–889, 1970.

Disease of Thyrotropin Regulation

Pittman, J. A., Jr., Haigler, E. D., et al.: Hypothalamic hypothyroidism. *New Eng. J. Med. 285*:844–845, 1971.

Refetoff, S., DeWind, L. T., et al.: Familial syndrome combining deaf-mutism, stippled epiphyses, goiter and abnormally high PBI: Possible target organ refractoriness to thyroid hormone. *J. Clin. Endocr. 27*:279–294, 1967.

Cushing's disease

Krieger, D. T., and Glick, S. M.: Growth hormone and cortisol responsiveness in Cushing's syndrome. Relation to a possible central nervous system etiology. *Amer. J. Med. 52*:25–40, 1972.

Disease of prolactin regulation

Brown, D. M., Jenness, R., et al.: A study of the composition of milk from a patient with hypothyroidism and galactorrhea. *J. Clin. Endocr. 25*:1225–1230, 1965.

Dowling, T. J., Richards, J. B., et al.: Nonpuerperal galactorrhea. *Arch. Intern. Med.* (Chicago) *107*:151–159, 1961.

Rabinowitz, P., and Friedman, I. S.: Drug-induced lactation in uremia. *J. Clin. Endocr. 21*:1489–1493, 1961.

Clinical Pathological Conference. Recant, L., and Lacy, P. (eds.), Non-puerperal galactorrhea, amenorrhea and visual loss. *Amer. J. Med. 33*:591–602, 1962.

Turkington, R. W.: Phenothiazine stimulation test for prolactin reserve. The syndrome of isolated prolactin deficiency. *J. Clin. Endocr. 34*:247–249, 1972.

Turkington, R. W.: Secretion of prolactin by patients with pituitary and hypothalamic tumors. *J. Clin. Endocr. 34*:159–164, 1972.

Friesen, H., Webster, B. R., et al.: Prolactin synthesis and secretion in a patient with the Forbes-Albright syndrome. *J. Clin. Endocr. 34*:192–199, 1972.

Effects of Steroid and Thyroid Hormones on the Brain

Michael, R. P., and Gibbons, J. L.: Interrelationships between the endocrine system and neuropsychiatry. *Int. Rev. Neurobiol. 5*:243–302, 1963.

Michael, R. A. (ed.), *Endocrinology and Human Behavior.* New York, Oxford University Press, 1968.

Ford, D. H. (ed.), *Influence of Hormones on the Nervous System.* Basel, S. Karger, 1971.

Smith, C. K., Barish, J., et al.: Psychiatric disturbance in endocrinologic disease. *Psychosom. Med. 34*:69–86, 1972.

Henkin, R. I., McGlone, R. E., et al.: Studies in auditory thresholds in normal man and in patients with adrenal cortical insufficiency: the role of adrenal cortical steroids. *J. Clin. Invest. 46*:429, 1967.

Woodbury, D. M., and Vernadakis, A.: Influence of hormones on brain activity, In *Neuroendocrinology.* Vol. 2. Martini, L., and Ganong, W. F. (eds.), New York, Academic Press, 1967.

Chambers, W. F., Freedman, S. L., and Sawyer, C. H.: The effects of adrenal steroids on evoked reticular responses. *Exp. Neurol. 8*:458–469, 1963.

Cameron, M. P., and O'Connor, M. (eds.), *Brain-Thyroid Relationships.* Ciba Foundation Study Group No. 18. London, J. & A. Churchill, 1964.

McEwen, B. S., Zigmond, R. E., et al.: *Biochemistry of Brain and Behavior.* Bowman, R. E., and Datta, S. P. (eds.), New York, Plenum Press, 1970, pp. 123–167.

Relkin, R.: Effect of endocrine on central nervous system, In *Recent Advances in Medicine and Surgery. New York J. Med. 69*:2133–2265, 1969.

Henkin, R. I.: The neuroendocrine control of perception, In *Perception and its Disorders.* Vol. 48. Hamburg, D. (ed.), Baltimore, Williams and Wilkins, 1970, pp. 54–107.

Levine, S.: *Hormones and Behavior.* New York, Academic Press, 1972.

Effect of Peptide Hormones on the Brain

Fitzsimons, J. T.: The hormonal control of water and sodium intake, In *Frontiers in Neuroendocrinology.* Vol. II. Martini, L., and Ganong, W. F. (eds.), New York, Oxford University Press, 1971, pp. 103–128.

Andersson, B.: Thirst and brain control of water balance. *American Scientist 59*:408–415, 1971.

Butterfield, W. J. H., Abrams, M. E., et al.: Insulin sensitivity of the human brain. *Lancet i*:557–560, 1966.

DeWied, D.: Pituitary control of avoidance behavior, In *The Hypothalamus.* Martini, L., and Fraschini, F. (eds.), New York, Academic Press, 1970, pp. 1–8.

Kastin, A. J., Miller, L. H., et al.: Psycho-physiologic correlates of MSH activity in man. *Physiol. Behav. 7*:893, 1971.

Lande, S., Witter, A., et al.: Pituitary peptides – an octapeptide that stimulates conditioned avoidance acquisition in hypophysectomized rats. *J. Biol. Chem. 246*:2058–2062, 1971.

Gonadal Steroids and Sexual Function

Gorski, R. A.: Gonadal hormones and the perinatal development of neuroendocrine function, In *Frontiers in Neuroendocrinology.* Martini, L., and Ganong, W. F. (eds.), New York, Oxford University Press, 1971.

Barraclough, C. A.: Modifications in reproductive function after exposure to hormones during the prenatal and early postnatal period, In *Neuroendocrinology.* Martini, L., and Ganong, W. F. (eds.), New York, Academic Press, 1966.

Gorski, R. A., and Whalen, R. E. (eds.), *Brain and Behavior.* Proceedings of the Third Conference on the Brain and Gonadal Function. Berkeley and Los Angeles, University of California Press, 1966.

Levine, S., and Mullins, R. F., Jr.: Hormonal influences on brain organization in infant rats. *Science 152*:1585–1592, 1966.

Huffer, V., Scott, W. H., et al.: Psychological studies of adult male patients with sexual infantilism before and after androgen therapy. *Ann. Intern. Med. 61*:255–268, 1964.

Salmon, U. J., and Geist, S. H.: Effect of androgens upon libido in women. *J. Clin. Endocr. 3*:235–238, 1943.

Schon, M., and Sutherland, A. M.: The role of hormones in

human behavior. III. Changes in female sexuality after hypophysectomy. *J. Clin. Endocr. 20*:833–841, 1960.

Waxenberg, S. H., Drellich, M. G., et al.: The role of hormones in human behavior. I. Changes in female sexuality after adrenalectomy. *J. Clin. Endocr. 19*:193–202, 1959.

Winokur, G.: *Determinants of Human Sexual Behavior.* Springfield, Ill., Charles C Thomas, 1963.

Green, R., and Money, J.: *Transsexualism and Sex Reassignment.* Baltimore, Johns Hopkins University Press, 1969.

Masters, W. H., and Johnson, V. E.: *Human Sexual Inadequacy.* Boston, Little, Brown & Co., 1970.

Masters, W. H., and Johnson, V. E.: *Human Sexual Response.* Boston, Little, Brown and Co., 1966.

Kinsey, A. C., Pomeroy, W. B., et al.: *Sexual Behavior in the Human Male.* Philadelphia, W. B. Saunders Co., 1948, pp. 226–238.

Heller, C. G., and Myers, G. B.: The male climacteric, its symptomatology, diagnosis and treatment. *J.A.M.A. 126*:472, 1944.

Money, J., and Alexander, D.: Psychosexual development and absence of homosexuality in males with precocious puberty. *J. Nerv. Ment. Dis. 148*:111–123, 1969.

Moos, R. H., Kopell, B. S., et al.: Fluctuations in symptoms and moods during the menstrual cycle. *J. Psychosom. Res. 13*:37–44, 1969.

Paige, K. E.: Effects of oral contraceptives on affective fluctuations associated with the menstrual cycle. *Psychosom. Med. 33*:515–537, 1971.

Loraine, J. A., Adamopoulos, D. A., et al.: Patterns of hormone excretion in male and female homosexuals. *Nature* (London) *234*:552–554, 1971.

Goy, R. W., and Resko, J. A.: Gonadal hormones and behaviour of normal and pseudohermaphroditic nonhuman female primates. *Recent Progr. Hormone Res. 28*:707–733, 1972.

Michael, R. P., Zump, D., et al.: Neuroendocrine factors in the control of primate behavior. *Recent Progr. Hormone Res. 28*:665–706, 1972.

Benign Intracranial Hypertension

Dees, S. C., and McKay, H. W., Jr.: Occurrence of pseudotumor cerebri (benign intracranial hypertension) during treatment of children with asthma by steroids. *Pediatrics 23*:1143–1151, 1959.

Joynt, R. J., and Sahs, A. L.: Endocrine studies in pseudotumor cerebri. *Trans. Amer. Neurol. Ass. 87*:110–113, 1962.

Paterson, R., Di Pasquale, N., et al.: Pseudotumor cerebri. *Medicine 40*:85–97, 1961.

Feldman, M. H., and Schleziner, N. S.: Benign intracranial hypertension associated with hypervitaminosis A. *Arch. Neurol.* (Chicago) *22*:1–7, 1970.

CHAPTER 13

The Pineal Organ

By Richard J. Wurtman and
Daniel P. Cardinali*

INTRODUCTION

Fourteen years have elapsed since the discovery of the pineal hormone, melatonin (41); since then, interest in the physiology of the pineal organ has grown steadily, as has knowledge of the pineal's contribution to the economy of the body (71, 66). The "melatonin hypothesis" of pineal function, put forth in 1965 (70), is now well supported. This hypothesis, which we will discuss in detail, holds that the mammalian pineal organ synthesizes and secretes melatonin at a rate inversely dependent on environmental lighting, and that the pineal receives signals about the lighting milieu via a complex pathway involving the retinae, the brain, and the sympathetic neurons to and from the superior cervical ganglia.

Knowing what the pineal or any other organ *does* is a major first step towards understanding its physiologic function in the body, or what it is *for*. We characterize what a hormone-secreting organ does by defining its *input-output relations*. We identify its primary input and output signals (i.e., what it secretes and in response to what) and determine the general shape of their quantitative relationship. Characterization of what the organ is for is intrinsically more difficult; the investigation must demonstrate in intact organisms that the hormone's concentration in plasma or another biologic fluid actually does change under physiologic circumstances, and that such a change causes parallel changes in the functional activity of another distant "target organ." For the pineal this means demonstrating that when the pineal secretes sufficient melatonin to cause its plasma or cerebrospinal fluid (CSF) levels to rise, another important change results in the brain or some other organ. We will describe in this chapter our current understanding of what the pineal does and how it is modified in some pathologic situations; we will also speculate as to what the pineal might be for.

NEURAL AND ENDOCRINE COMMUNICATIONS

Three types of cells mediate communications between organs: neurons, neuroendocrine transducers, and endocrine cells (68, 69); the mammalian pineal is a member of the second group. Like other neuroendocrine transducers, it converts a neuronal input (i.e., a neurotransmitter released at a synapse) to an endocrine output; the secretion of melatonin. Other examples of neuroendocrine transducer cells include adrenomedullary chromaffin cells, which secrete epinephrine in response to acetylcholine released from the medulla's preganglionic neurons; renin-secreting juxtaglomerular cells of the kidney; the "releasing-factor" cells of the median eminence; the vasopressin-secreting cells of the supraoptic hypothalamic nuclei; and the beta cells of the pancreatic islets. These cells all respond to humoral as well as to neuronal inputs; however, their uniqueness derives from their ability to translate "nerve language" into "gland language." We will briefly discuss the major differences between these two languages.

The transmission of a neuronal signal across a synapse to neurons and neuroendocrine transducers is mediated by a specific neurotransmitter substance (e.g., acetylcholine, norepinephrine, or sero-

*These studies were supported in part by grants from the U. S. National Institutes of Health (AM–11709) and the U. S. National Institute of Environmental Sciences (ES–00616).

tonin) which is released into the synaptic cleft from the presynaptic cell. The neurotransmitter then diffuses across a short distance to reach a specialized receptor zone on the postsynaptic cell, where it alters the flux of specific ions and the activity of adenyl cyclase or other membrane enzymes triggering specific biochemical processes within the cell. Nearly all the compounds thought to function as neurotransmitters are chemically similar. They are low-molecular-weight water-soluble amines or possibly amino acids, and they are rapidly deactivated by enzymes or by physical processes such as reuptake into their neurons of origin. Hence their concentrations in blood tend to be very low. Hormonal signals are transmitted via the blood stream; the array of chemicals used by the body for this purpose is far broader than the current list of probable neurotransmitters. Hormones are not chemically similar; for example, insulin is water-soluble, while testosterone is highly nonpolar. Thyroxine is a low-molecular-weight amino acid, while TSH is a large glycoprotein, and so forth.

Perhaps the most characteristic difference between the transmission of signals by neurotransmitters and that by hormones is the technique used to achieve "privacy." Nervous systems obtain privacy by anatomic means: a given neuron transmits signals only to the small number of cells with which it makes direct synaptic contact or which lie within a few hundred angstroms of its terminal endings. When the acetylcholine is emitted after a specific neuron fires, it can theoretically carry information to billions of neurons within the brain. However, only a much smaller number of cells actually receives sufficient information from the cholinergic nerve terminals to become activated. In contrast, hormones attain privacy biochemically. A given signal may be distributed via the circulatory system to every cell in the body; because the signal is chemically coded, only a relatively small number of cells (i.e., those able to decode the signal) can understand the information.

To demonstrate that the pinealocyte or any other cell functions as a neuroendocrine transducer, one must show that the cell receives a direct innervation (i.e., by electron microscopic evaluation), and that the cell's ability to secrete appropriate amounts of its hormone under various physiologic conditions is impaired when this innervation is interrupted. Terminals of postganglionic sympathetic neurons (whose cell bodies lie outside the cranial cavity in the superior cervical ganglia) have been identified in the vicinity of pineal parenchymal cells, sometimes forming true synapses. Furthermore, indirect evidence has been obtained that the parenchymal cells receive and respond to impulses (i.e., norepinephrine quanta) from these neurons. The functional activity of the pineal, identified by its ability to produce more or less melatonin in response to lighting conditions and time of day, is severely disturbed if its sympathetic input is removed.

The pineal's identity as a neuroendocrine trans-

ducer, as opposed to an endocrine gland, allows one to understand its apparent failure to function after transplantation. In contrast to the thyroid or the adrenal cortex, the pineal cannot function simply by reestablishing an adequate circulation. A generation of scientists failed to recognize the pineal's similarity to the adrenal medulla and its differences from true glands. This failure was partly responsible for delayed entry of the pineal into twentieth century experimental science.

EMBRYOLOGIC DEVELOPMENT AND ANATOMY OF THE PINEAL ORGAN

In all vertebrates the pineal originates as a neuroepithelial evagination protruding from the roof of the diencephalon; in man, this pineal anlage is first observed at the start of the second fetal month. The pineal of the adult human is a conical organ that lies within the posterior border of the corpus callosum and between the superior colliculi. It weighs about 120 mg. and is mostly enveloped by pia mater from which blood vessels, unmyelinated nerve fibers, and stroma of connective tissue penetrate the organ. The pinealocyte, the characteristic parenchymal cell of the mammalian pineal, derives from the neuroepithelial matrix layer and is no longer overtly similar to the pineal photoreceptor cells of most lower vertebrates. [Photoreceptor cells contain characteristic subcellular organelles (i.e., "outer segments" and lamellar bodies) which mediate cellular response to light.] In addition to pinealocytes, the pineal also contains modified glial cells. The pineal organ is richly irrigated by a well-developed vascular system; the proportion of the cardiac output received by each gram of pineal is among the highest in the body (27). This extremely rich vascular supply constitutes evidence against the hypothesis that the pineal is merely vestigial in mammals. Numerous cytoplasmic processes from the pinealocytes terminate within the perivascular spaces that surround its capillaries. The pineal itself is surrounded by CSF; whether the pineal secretes hormones into the blood, the CSF, or both has not been determined.

The mammalian pineal is innervated almost solely by autonomic postganglionic fibers originating in the superior cervical ganglia (34), a remarkable peculiarity for an organ which is at least embryologically part of the brain. Postganglionic sympathetic fibers reach the pineal along its blood vessels or by coalescing into two unmyelinated nerves, the nervi conarii, which penetrates the distal pole of the organ. The sympathetic fibers terminate near the pineal parenchymal cells, and some actually form synapses. These nerve terminals generally exhibit the 400 Å. granular vesicles characteristic of sympathetic neurons elsewhere in the body. Chemical and fluorescence microscopy studies have demonstrated the presence of norepinephrine and serotonin in the pineal; the norepinephrine is confined to the nerve endings, while serotonin is present both in the pinealocytes and in the sympathetic nerve terminals.

Another peculiarity of the human pineal is its tendency to calcify (71). Soon after birth, human pinealocytes begin to produce and secrete a "ground substance" of unknown chemical composition which serves as the matrix for subsequent calcification. The composition of the calcium salts deposited (mostly calcium hydroxyapatite) does not differ from those found in bone and tooth. Most studies based on x-ray evidence have concluded that the calcification of the human pineal is absent at birth and appears in most humans only after puberty (18). This has been taken to indicate that the pineal degenerates at puberty. Two lines of evidence argue against this hypothesis (71). First, activity of the pineal enzymes related to melatonin biosynthesis does not decrease significantly with age, even among highly calcified organs taken at autopsy from the very old (51, 71). Second, many pineals taken at autopsy from children who died before the age of 10 years have been significantly calcified. The functional significance of pineal calcification remains entirely unexplained, but radiologically observable pineal calcification is so uncommon during the first decade of life that its presence should lead the physician to suspect the possibility of a pineal tumor.

PINEAL INDOLES

Isolation, Biosynthesis, and Metabolism

The isolation of melatonin, a specific pineal constituent that reproduces many of the effects of pineal extracts and reverses the endocrine sequelae of pinealectomy, was a landmark in the history of pineal research. Since 1917 we have known that the skin of frogs and tadpoles blanches rapidly when the animals are fed extracts of bovine pineals; forty years later, the skin-lightening principle in these extracts was shown to be melatonin (5-methoxy,N-acetyltryptamine) by Aaron Lerner and his associates at Yale University (41). As little as 10^{-13} g. per ml. of melatonin visibly changes the amphibian skin; this effect was used by Lerner to trace the skin-lightening compound through the various extraction and purification steps required for its identification and is now widely used to bioassay the melatonin in pineal extracts. Melatonin apparently has no obvious effects on the melanocytes responsible for the pigmentation of the human skin (45). In place of dermatologic actions, melatonin has come to exert effects on another neuroectodermal derivative, the brain.

When isolated, melatonin differed from all indoles previously identified in mammals in that it contained a methoxy side chain; this suggested to Axelrod and Weissbach that melatonin was synthesized by the O-methylation of a 5-hydroxy compound, perhaps derived from serotonin. Soon these investigators identified the hypothesized O-methylating enzyme, hydroxyindole-O-methyl transferase (HIOMT), in pineals of various mammals (5). HIOMT catalyzes the transfer of a methyl group from S-adenosylmethionine to N-acetylserotonin, which causes the formation of 5-methoxy, N-acetyltryptamine, or melatonin (Fig. 13–1). HIOMT activity is highly concentrated within the pineal; however, it has also been detected in other mammalian organs, e.g., the retina (12) and the harderian gland (64), a relatively small orbital structure in humans. The high degree of HIOMT localization in the pineal allows the enzyme to be used as a "marker," for example, in differentiating true pinealomas from pineal tumors of glial or other origin (73).

Melatonin has a unique distribution: most of the indole present in a mammal at any time is located within the pineal; the amount of melatonin present in human pineal obtained at autopsy varies from 0.05 to 0.4 μg. per g. (43). There is only indirect evidence that melatonin is actually secreted from the

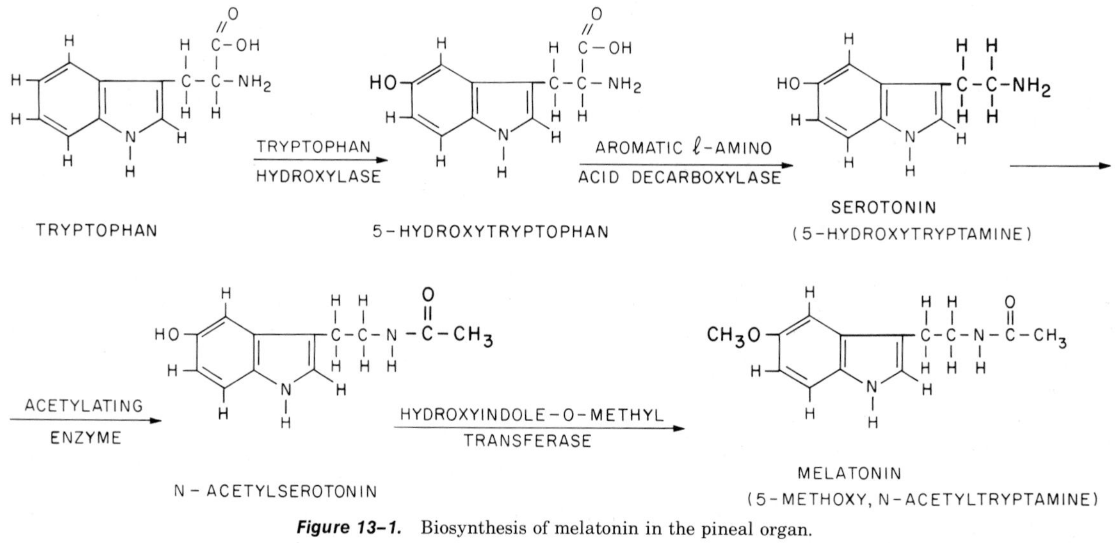

Figure 13–1.   Biosynthesis of melatonin in the pineal organ.

human pineal; it is found in human plasma and urine and in certain tissues (e.g., peripheral nerves) which lack the HIOMT activity necessary for its synthesis.

The metabolic pathway for melatonin biosynthesis is shown in Figure 13–1. Pinealocytes take up the amino acid, tryptophan, from the circulation, and an enzyme, tryptophan hydroxylase, catalyzes its hydroxylation to 5-hydroxytryptophan. The amino acid is subsequently decarboxylated to 5-hydroxytryptamine, or serotonin, through the action of the enzyme, aromatic-L-amino acid decarboxylase. Serotonin is present in high concentrations in the pineals of most mammals (71); a portion of this amine, like the serotonin in other organs, is deaminated by monoamine oxidase (MAO), then oxidized to 5-hydroxyindoleacetic acid. More significant is the conversion of another portion of serotonin to melatonin: it is first acetylated by serotonin-N-acetyltransferase, an acetylating enzyme probably found in many tissues, to form N-acetylserotonin and is then converted to melatonin through the action of HIOMT. Both of the potentially charged groups in serotonin (i.e., the 5-hydroxy and the amine) are thus blocked, and the resulting melatonin is highly nonpolar. HIOMT also catalyzes the synthesis of other methoxyindoles in the pineal; these include methoxytryptophol and methoxyindoleacetic acid. Melatonin ultimately enters the general circulation, either by direct secretion from the pinealocytes or indirectly via the CSF.

The concentration of melatonin in human blood displays a characteristic 24-hour rhythm, with maximal values during darkness (44). Melatonin's lipid solubility is compatible with the observation that much of the indole in human plasma is bound to serum albumin (11). This complex is readily dissociable, however, and the presence of the binding protein apparently does not modify the biologic activity of the melatonin (11). Circulating melatonin is taken up and concentrated within several organs, especially in the gonads (71). The methoxyindole passes easily across the blood-brain barrier, thus differing from serotonin, for example, which is polar at physiologic pH. Isotopically labeled melatonin injected into the CSF is taken up unevenly within the brain; it becomes concentrated within the hypothalamus and the midbrain (3, 9). The labeled melatonin disappears rapidly from both the bloodstream and the brain. Although the central nervous system actively metabolizes melatonin (through yet undefined pathways), the liver appears to be the major site of melatonin inactivation in the body; the methoxyindole is first hydroxylated to 6-hydroxymelatonin by a microsomal NADPH-requiring enzyme (40), and this hydroxylated product is then conjugated with glucuronic or sulfuric acid and excreted into the urine.

Control of Melatonin Synthesis in the Pineal

By using a light microscope, Holmgren, a Swedish anatomist, observed in 1918 that the pineal region of the frog and dogfish contained cells that resembled retinal photoreceptors; he thus suggested that the pineals of these species functioned as a "third eye." Although mammalian pinealocytes lack these organelles and do not give rise to axons to the brain, their biochemical activity continues to be influenced by environmental lighting. Operating via an indirect neuronal pathway described below, light exposure determines HIOMT activity as well as the activities of several other pineal enzymes involved in melatonin biosynthesis (e.g., aromatic-L-amino acid decarboxylase, serotonin-N-acetyltransferase) (71). At least three major structural changes have occurred in the phylogenetic development of the mammalian pineal, all of which are involved in pineal responses to light.

1. A new cell type, the pineal parenchymal cell or pinealocyte, developed, lacking subcellular organelles specialized for photoreception, but containing other organelles (i.e., an abundant endoplasmic reticulum) characteristic of secretory cells.

2. A new and unique pattern of pineal innervation, first described by Kappers in 1960 (34), appeared: the abundant postganglionic sympathetic nerves to the pineal, which originated in the superior cervical ganglia, terminate not, as expected, on blood vessels, but on or near the pineal parenchymal cells. These nerves mediate the brain's control of the pineal.

3. A portion of the optic tract containing fibers whose cell bodies lie in the retina became diverted to form a special nerve bundle, the inferior accessory optic tract, which transmits the portion of the photic input that ultimately reaches the pineal (49).

Biochemical and pharmacologic studies using organ cultures of individual rat pineals have clarified somewhat the mechanisms involved in the sympathetic control of mammalian pineal function. Thus the addition of norepinephrine, the postganglionic sympathetic neurotransmitter, or of dibutyryl cyclic AMP stimulates C^{14}-melatonin synthesis from C^{14}-tryptophan (4, 30); norepinephrine also increases the adenyl cyclase activity and cyclic AMP content of the rat pineal (62, 65). Norepinephrine stimulation of melatonin biosynthesis is mediated by beta adrenergic receptors, inasmuch as this effect is blocked by propranolol but not by phenoxybenzamine (74). The probable sequence of events linking environmental lighting with the production of melatonin appears to be that the lack of photic input (i.e., darkness) increases the activity of the postganglionic sympathetic neurons to the pineal, releasing norepinephrine from the nerve terminals. The norepinephrine, via a beta receptor, activates the adenyl cyclase in the pineal parenchymal cells, thereby enhancing the activity of several of the enzymes in the melatonin biosynthetic pathway (tryptophan hydroxylase, serotonin-N-acetyltransferase, and HIOMT). In support of this theoretical model, light acting via the eyes has been demonstrated to decrease the electrical impulses reaching the pineal via its sympathetic nerves (63) and to lower pineal norepinephrine levels as well (72). The exposure of rats to continuous illumination also reduces the activity of pineal HIOMT (71) and serotonin-N-acetyltransferase (39) and the melatonin content of the pineal (54).

The characteristic decrease in pineal HIOMT activity caused by placing rats in an environment of continuous illumination has been useful for defining the pathways through which retinal responses to light influence the pineal and perhaps other neuroendocrine organs (49). The extent of this decrease appears to depend on the spectral composition of the light source. The action spectrum for photic inhibition of pineal HIOMT resembles the absorption spectrum for retinal rhodopsin (10) (i.e., yellow-green light is very effective, while red and ultraviolet are ineffective), which suggests that the same photopigment mediates both the visual and the neuroendocrine effects of light in mammals. The retinal projection that mediates the photic control of the pineal uses one of the two sets of accessory optic tracts generally found in mammals, the inferior accessory optic tract. This nerve bundle leaves the main optic tract just caudal to the optic chiasm; it then runs within the medial forebrain bundle in the lateral hypothalamus to terminate near the junction of the hypothalamus and the mesencephalon in the nucleus of the inferior accessory optic tract (Fig. 13–2). If the inferior accessory optic tracts are transected within the medial forebrain bundle (or if one bundle is cut and the ipsilateral eye removed), the pineal is effec-

tively "blinded," even though vision is preserved (49). It has not yet been possible to trace the path taken by photic input to the pineal between the nucleus of the inferior accessory optic tract and the preganglionic fibers to the superior cervical ganglia. Most likely, the transmission of this information through the midbrain, pons, medulla, and spinal cord involves multisynaptic systems.

Environmental lighting is not the only factor affecting the sympathetic tone to the pineal and the rate of melatonin synthesis; for example, testosterone acts postnatally on the brain to cause long-term modifications in pineal HIOMT activity (31). The stress of immobilization or of insulin-induced hypoglycemia causes major increases in the serotonin-N-acetyltransferase activity and in the melatonin contents of the rat pineal. These changes are manifest within two hours of the onset of the stress, and they appear in spite of the fact that the test animals continue to be exposed to environmental lighting (42a).

Biologic Effects

The most thoroughly investigated physiologic actions of melatonin in mammals are those involving the neuroendocrine apparatus (Table 13–1) (55, 71). Melatonin injections inhibit various aspects of gonadal, thyroid, and adrenal function and, in particular, decrease ovarian weight, inhibit pregnant mares' serum gonadotropin induced by ovulation (42), and delay pubescence in immature rats; melatonin also reduces the frequency of vaginal estrus in mature rats.

The absence of the pineal seems to cause some stimulation of the hypophysiogonadal axis (Table 13–1). Usually pinealectomy produces gonadal hypertrophy (71), the degree of which is related to both the interval between pinealectomy and autopsy and the age at pineal ablation. Prepubertal pinealectomy in female rats results in premature sexual development, manifested by earlier vaginal opening and increased ovarian weight. In males, pinealectomy at 20 to 30 days of age causes enlargement of the accessory sexual organs (71), including the seminal vesicles and ventral prostate; it also enhances the secretion of testosterone (36). Pinealectomy in adult female rats increases the frequency of estrous vaginal smears, and in adult males increases the weight of the testes and accessory sexual organs. Pineal ablation is associated with increases in the LH and FSH contents of the rat hypophysis, whereas implants of melatonin within the hypothalamus or brainstem exert an opposite effect, decreasing the LH content of the rat pituitary gland (25). These results have been confirmed by observations that perfusion with melatonin of the third ventricle lowers plasma LH (32) and FSH (33) and blocks ovulation in mature rats, while it delays the opening of the vagina in immature animals (25). The direct perfusion of the hypophysis with melatonin does not modify plasma gonadotropin concentrations; hence melatonin appears to act on the brain to suppress the secretion

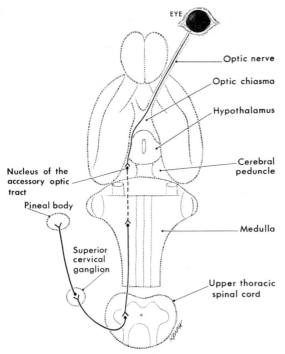

EYE

Optic nerve

Optic chiasma

Hypothalamus

Cerebral peduncle

Nucleus of the accessory optic tract

Pineal body

Medulla

Superior cervical ganglion

Upper thoracic spinal cord

Figure 13–2. Schematic diagram of pathway taken by light impulses between the retina and the pineal of the rat (Reproduced from Wurtman, R. J., Axelrod, J., et al.: *The Pineal.* New York, Academic Press, 1968, with permission.)

TABLE 13–1. ENDOCRINE EFFECTS OF PINEALECTOMY IN MAMMALS

Gonadal Function

Rat   Increased ovarian and uterine weight* (71)
       Earlier vaginal opening* (57)
       Increased proportion of vaginal smears showing estrous phases* (71)
       Increased weight of testes, seminal vesicles, and prostate* (71)
       Reversion of the inhibitory effects of darkness (with or without anosmia) on gonadal function in normal and androgenized rats* (55)
       Increased LH and FSH levels in pituitary* (25)
       Increased prolactin levels in pituitary; decreased levels in plasma†† (58)
       Earlier ovulation following PMS treatment* (22)
       Induction of ovulation in anovulatory rats with pre-optic lesions* (47)

Hamster   Blocked decreases in gonadal activity which follow blinding or maintenance under 23 hours of darkness† (55)

Ferret   Blocked gonadal activation by increases in the length of the photoperiod† (28)

Pituitary

Rat   Increased pituitary weight* (71)
       Increased number of mitoses†† (7)
       Decreased neurosecretory activity of the supraoptic hypothalamic nucleus†† (21)
       Counteracted inhibition of growth hormone secretion in blinded rats† (61)
       Increased pituitary MSH* (35)

Thyroid

Rat   Increased thyroid weight* (71)
       Increased I^{131} uptake* (17)
       Increased thyroid hormone secretion rate* (60)

Adrenal Cortex

Rat   Increased adrenal weight* (71)
       Increased aldosterone secretion†† (37)
       Increased corticosterone secretion* (37)

Parathyroid

Rat   Hypertrophy of parathyroid cells† (48)
       Muscular spasms and death in thyroparathyroidectomized rats† (56)

---

*Effect reversed by the administration of melatonin.
†Effect not reversed by the administration of melatonin.
††Melatonin effects not investigated.

---

of LH-releasing factor. The position of the hypothalamus and brainstem as melatonin target organs is also suggested by the finding that intraperitoneal injections of the hormone rapidly elevate the serotonin contents of these brain regions (1). The antigonadal effects of exogenous melatonin may also result from direct actions on the gonads themselves or on the accessory organs, inasmuch as melatonin is a potent inhibitor of testicular androgen production (13, 24) and of the androgenic effects of testosterone on the prostate and seminal vesicles (19).

Another methoxyindole produced in the pineal through the action of HIOMT, 5-methoxytryptophol, also suppresses gonadal growth when administered systemically (46) and modifies pituitary gonadotropin levels when implanted in the brain (25). In contrast to melatonin, this compound appears to exert its primary action on FSH secretion. Thus the possibility should be considered that the mammalian pineal produces a family of chemically related hormones that influences different aspects

of gonadal function. A nonindolic presumably peptide substance (or substances) which suppresses compensatory ovarian hypertrophy has been isolated from the mammalian pineal (6, 23); however, its identity and physiologic control remain unknown.

Pinealectomy is followed by hypertrophy of the thyroid gland in a number of mammalian species (30, 71) (Table 13–1). This effect does not seem to involve pituitary TSH since it also occurs in hypophysectomized rats (30). Pineal removal increases the uptake of I^{131} by the rat thyroid (17), as well as the rate at which the thyroid loses I^{131} (presumably an index of thyroid hormone secretion). Conversely, subcutaneous administration of melatonin inhibits the thyroid enlargement that follows pinealectomy and depresses I^{131} uptake (20, 60). The increase in plasma TSH observed after melatonin administration (52) suggests that the antithyroidal effects of the pineal indole are exerted at the level of the thyroid cells rather than via the brain or pituitary. It is not clear that the effects of pineal compounds on thyroid function are of sufficient magnitude to be physiologically significant.

The pineal also appears to inhibit certain aspects of adrenocortical function (Table 13–1). Pinealectomy reportedly causes a threefold increase in the concentrations of aldosterone in rat adrenal venous blood and of corticosteroids in rat plasma (37). Melatonin, 5-methoxytryptophol, and 5-hydroxytryptophol significantly decrease plasma corticosterone levels after acute injections into the lateral ventricles of rats (50). The intravenous administration of melatonin causes a rapid depletion of rat pituitary MSH (35). High MSH levels are observed in pinealectomized animals or in rats kept in continuous light; this suggests that the effect of injected melatonin simulates an action of the endogenous hormone. Removal of the pineal produces muscular spasms and death in thyroparathyroidectomized rats without significantly modifying the plasma calcium level (which is already low because of parathyroidectomy) (56); the effects of melatonin on this phenomenon have not yet been described. In summary, exogenous melatonin reverses many of the endocrine changes that occur after pinealectomy (Table 13–1). Thus exogenous melatonin probably acts in pinealectomized animals as the endogenous hormone does in intact rats.

Melatonin also exerts other pharmacologic effects on the central nervous system. Its administration produces distinct effects on EEG activity, sleep, and behavior in various experimental animals (26, 29) and suppresses the adventitious movements induced by L-dopa in mice (16). Melatonin administration to normal human subjects is followed by a general electrophysiologic pattern of deactivation (i.e., slowing of the major EEG rhythm, sleep, and rise of the convulsive threshold) without major changes in behavior (2). The pineal hormone has also been reported to ameliorate the EEG alterations characteristic of temporal epilepsy and some of the motor disorders seen in Parkinson's disease (2).

SIGNIFICANCE OF THE CONTROL OF PINEAL FUNCTION BY ENVIRONMENTAL LIGHTING

The capacity of pineal enzymes to respond rapidly to changes in environmental lighting has an obvious corollary: the normal daily cycle of light and darkness to which most animals and humans are exposed generates a parallel rhythm in melatonin production; this provides the rest of the body with a circulating "time signal." Thus the question, "What do pineal hormones do?" can now be rephrased as, "What other organs in the body respond to changes in methoxyindole secretion?" Many pineal functions undergo 24-hour rhythmic variations (14). These include enzyme activities (e.g., HIOMT, serotonin-N-acetyltransferase, adenyl cyclase, catechol-O-methyltransferase); contents of monoamines (e.g., norepinephrine, serotonin); levels of cyclic AMP, RNA, and proteins; incorporation of P^{32} into macromolecules; and, of course, melatonin concentration itself. The amount of melatonin in human plasma, measured by bioassay, also undergoes a 24-hour rhythm, attaining peak values during the night. Little information is thus far available on the possible role of the pineal in producing 24-hour rhythms that have been observed in such other mammalian functions as body temperature, adrenocortical secretion, sleep, and eating behavior. The pineal could provide the rhythmic signals that generate these rhythms; alternatively, it might serve to modify the phasing of an intrinsic oscillatory mechanism. In the sparrow, pinealectomy abolishes the body temperature rhythm as well as the rhythm of locomotor activity observed in animals kept in darkness (8). In rats, pinealectomy modifies the rate at which the activity rhythm becomes entrained to a new lighting schedule (53).

An area in which the pineal has a relatively well-characterized function is the control of the gonadal responses to environmental light. When most birds or mammals are exposed to continuous light or darkness or are blinded, marked changes occur in the timing of gonadal maturation and in the subsequent ovulatory cycles (15, 67). Blind humans exhibit a significant acceleration of menarche; blinded rats show the opposite response. Hamsters kept in continuous darkness develop a pronounced atrophy of the gonads; this effect is blocked by pinealectomy. The particular gonadal response of each mammalian species to light seems to depend on whether the species is monoestrous or polyestrous (that is, whether it normally ovulates once a year, in the spring or the fall, or at regular intervals throughout the year). Examples of polyestrous species are rats (every 4 or 5 days), guinea pigs (every 12 to 14 days), and human beings (every 29 days). The gonadal response of each species also seems to depend on whether its members are spontaneously active during the daylight hours or during the nighttime. Gonadal maturation is accelerated in most avian species by exposure to artificial "long days" (i.e., days in which light is present for nearly 14 hours). The stimula-tory effect of light is inhibited by removing the pineal, suggesting that this organ may mediate the photic stimulation of gonadal maturation in birds. The avian pineal appears to be directly sensitive to light; hence its physiologic function probably differs significantly from that of the mammalian organ in that the former may directly transform photic energy to a hormonal output [i.e., the avian pineal may function as a photoendocrine transducer (14)].

The neural and neuroendocrine pathways connecting the retinae and the mammalian gonads are not yet completely defined. One such pathway involves the pineal organ as described above; another may utilize direct retinohypothalamic connections which could modify the secretion of gonadotropin.

PINEAL PATHOLOGY

Two pineal lesions have been of some interest for clinical medicine: (1) pineal calcification, which, as described above, is a ubiquitous autopsy finding, and (2) pineal tumors, which often are associated with endocrine sequelae. Pineal tumors may be divided into several distinct categories by their microscopic appearance (38, 71). Somewhat more than half may be classified as true pinealomas; these contain clusters of two distinct cell types, i.e., large, spheroidal epithelial cells and small, dark-staining cells that have an ultrastructure indistinguishable from that of the lymphocytes. About 10 to 15 per cent of all reported pineal tumors have been teratomas; these may contain mucus-secreting columnar epithelial cells, adenocarcinoma tissue, and other areas resembling thyroid, muscle, cartilage, bone, or nerve. Like other midline teratomas, these pineal tumors are often malignant. The origin of the remaining pineal tumors has usually been vascular or glial. Several explanations have been offered for the existence of two distinct cell types within classic parenchymal pinealomas. The tumors might arise from embryonic rests; hence their appearance is similar to that of the normal gland during one phase of its prenatal development (late in prenatal life the human pineal contains two types of cells arranged in a mosaic pattern which is not dissimilar from the pattern in true pinealomas). In support of this theory, pineal embryonic rests without evidence of neoplastic degeneration have been observed in normal brains. Alternatively, the two apparent cell types might actually reflect a single clone of cells. It has also been proposed that the presence of cells resembling lymphocytes in pinealoma results from an immune reaction to the tumor on the part of the host. That the large cells in true pinealomas are of pineal origin is suggested by the presence of measurable HIOMT activity in tumor specimens (73).

The natural history of a pineal tumor is related to its size and histologic appearance. Tumors that originate within the pineal gland usually become clinically manifest because of symptoms that arise from their location (e.g., internal hydrocephalus, elevated CSF pressure, and oculomotor signs such as Parinaud's syndrome); less frequently, medical attention is initially sought because of the appearance of precocious puberty. About one third of all boys below the normal age of sexual maturation who are afflicted with pineal tumors develop precocious puberty. This neoplasm may account for as much as 10 to 15 per cent of all cases of precocious sexual development seen in males. For unexplained reasons, pineal tumors are rare among girls and have not been associated with precocious menarche. It has been suggested that the precocious sexual development that appears in male pinealoma patients is a nonspecific consequence of the pressure that these tumors exert on surrounding brain tissue. There is growing evidence, however, against the "pressure hypothesis" (38, 71). Thus the endocrine effects of a tumor do not appear to be related to its size, its effect on CSF pressure, or the extent to which it has invaded local brain tissues. The endocrine effects are, however, related to histologic appearance; most often precocious puberty develops in patients with nonparenchymal tumors, while most cases of delayed pubescence or of secondary gonadal failure are associated with parenchymal pinealomas. Finally, the demonstration that a pineal hormone, melatonin, influences normal sexual maturation in experimental animals supports the hypothesis that precocious puberty develops in certain pinealoma patients because the damaged pineal fails to release an inhibitory hormone.

Parenchymal pinealomas frequently show a good, if temporary, clinical remission following irradiation. Patients generally receive 3,000 to 5,000 rads; radiation is administered over a wide portal because pinealomas not infrequently metastasize throughout the ventricles and the subdural space. Japanese surgeons have reported encouraging results following the surgical extirpation of pinealomas; however, this method is complicated by the relative inaccessibility of the pineal. A small number of tumors with the histologic aspect of pinealomas originate elsewhere in the brain at some distance from the normal pineal organ. These "ectopic pinealomas" usually arise in the hypothalamus, in the region of the infundibulum. Hence, patients generally present a picture similar to that seen with craniopharyngioma, with a clinical triad of bitemporal hemianopsia, hypopituitarism, and diabetes insipidus. Many ectopic pinealomas show a good clinical response to irradiation.

SUMMARY

The pineal has undergone marked changes as vertebrates have evolved from amphibians to mammals. The amphibian pineal is a photoreceptor which sends information to the brain; the mammalian pineal is an endocrine organ which has no direct connection to the central nervous system and whose metabolism is controlled by environ-

mental lighting via an indirect pathway involving its peripheral sympathetic nerves.

The mammalian pinealocytes are *neuroendocrine transducers:* they respond to a neurotransmitter (i.e., norepinephrine) released from their sympathetic neurons by synthesizing and secreting a family of biologically active compounds, the methoxyindoles, of which melatonin is the prototype. Melatonin acts via the brain and, perhaps, directly to depress the rate of gonadal maturation and to interfere with subsequent gonadal function and cyclicity; it also may modify thyroid and adrenal cortex function. In rats, and presumably in human beings, exposure to darkness stimulates melatonin synthesis, while light suppresses it. Melatonin is secreted into the blood or CSF and apparently acts on the brain to influence several physiologic processes that share a tendency towards time dependency (i.e., that vary cyclically or with age); these include the onset of puberty, ovulation, and sleep. Considerable information is available about the factors that control pineal function; much less is known about the uses to which the body puts melatonin and other possible pineal secretions. Tumors that destroy the pineal organ often cause precocious puberty in young boys, and tumors that are able to synthesize melatonin may inhibit gonadal function.

REFERENCES*

1. Anton-Tay, F., Chou, C., et al.: *Science 162*:277, 1968.
2. Anton-Tay, F., Diaz, J. L., et al.: *Life Sci. 10*:841, 1971.
3. Anton-Tay, F., and Wurtman, R. J.: *Nature* (London) *221*:474, 1969.
4. Axelrod, J., Shein, H. M., et al.: *Proc. Nat. Acad. Sci. USA 62*:544, 1969.
5. Axelrod, J., and Weissbach, H.: *J. Biol. Chem. 236*:211, 1961.
6. Benson, B., Matthews, M. J., et al.: *Acta. Endocr. 69*:257, 1972.
7. Bindoni, M., and Raffaele, R.: *J. Endocr. 41*:451, 1968.
8. Binkley, S., Kluth, E., et al.: *Science 174*:311, 1971.
9. Cardinali, D. P., Hyyppä, M. T., et al.: *Neuroendocrinology* 1973 (in press).
10. Cardinali, D. P., Larin, F., et al.: *Proc. Nat. Acad. Sci. USA. 69*:2003, 1972.
11. Cardinali, D. P., Lynch, H. J., et al.: *Endocrinology 91*:1213, 1972.
12. Cardinali, D. P., and Rosner, J. M.: *Endocrinology 89*:301, 1971.
13. Cardinali, D. P., and Rosner, J. M.: *Steroids 18*:25, 1971.
14. Cardinali, D. P., and Wurtman, R. J., In *Pineal Physiology.* Altschule, M. D. (ed.), Cambridge, Harvard University Press, 1973 (in press).
15. Cardinali, D. P., and Wurtman, R. J., In *Physiological Anthropology.* Damon, A. (ed.), Cambridge, Harvard University Press, 1973 (in press).
16. Cotzia, G. C., Tang, L. C.. et al.: *Science 173*:450, 1971.
17. Csaba, G., Kiss, J.. et al.: *Acta. Biol. Acad. Sci. Hung. 19*:35, 1968.
18. Daramola, G. F., and Olowu, A. O.: *Neuroendocrinology 9*:41, 1972.
19. Debeljuk, L., Feder, V. M., et al.: *Endocrinology 87*:1358, 1970.
20. DeProspo, N. D., Safinski, R. J., et al.: *Life Sci. 8*:837, 1969.
21. DeVries, R. A. C., and Kappers, J. A.: *Neuroendocrinology 8*:359, 1971.

*For complete bibliography up to 1968, see Wurtman et al. (71).

22. Dunaway, J. E.: *Neuroendocrinology 5*:281, 1969.
23. Ebels, I., Moszkowska, A., et al.: *J. Neurovisc. Relat. 32*:1, 1970.
24. Ellis, L. G.: *Endocrinology 90*:17, 1972.
25. Fraschini, F., Collu, R., et al.: In *The Pineal Gland*. Wolstenholme, G. E. W., and Knight, J. (eds.), Ciba Foundation Symposium. London, Churchill, Livingstone, 1971, p. 259.
26. Geller, I.: *Science 173*:456, 1971.
27. Goldman, J., and Wurtman, R. J.: *Nature* (London) *203*:87, 1964.
28. Herbert, J., In *The Pineal Gland*. Wolstenholme, G. E. W., and Knight, J. (eds.), Ciba Foundation Symposium. London, Churchill, Livingstone, 1971, p. 303.
29. Hishikawa, Y., Cramer, H., et al.: *Exp. Brain Res. 7*:84, 1969.
30. Houssay, A. B., and Pazo, J. H.: *Experientia 24*:813, 1968.
31. Hyyppä, Cardinali, D. P., et al.: *Neuroendocrinology* 1973 (in press).
32. Kamberi, I. A., Mical, R. S., et al.: *Endocrinology 87*:1, 1970.
33. Kamberi, I. A., Mical, R. S., et al.: *Endocrinology 88*:1288, 1971.
34. Kappers, J. A.: *Anat. Rec. 136*:220, 1960.
35. Kastin, A. J., and Schally, A. V.: *Nature* (London) *213*:1238, 1967.
36. Kinson, G. A., and Peat, F.: *Life Sci. 10*:259, 1971.
37. Kinson, G. A., Wahid, A. K., et al.: *Gen. Comp. Endocr. 8*:445, 1967.
38. Kitay, J. I., and Altschule, M. D.: *The Pineal Gland*. Cambridge, Harvard University Press, 1954.
39. Klein, D. C., and Weller, J. L.: *Science 169*:1093, 1970.
40. Kopin, I. J., Pare, C. M. B., et al.: *Biochim. Biophys. Acta 40*:377, 1960.
41. Lerner, A. B., Case, J. D., et al.: *J. Amer. Chem. Soc. 81*:6084, 1959.
42. Longenecker, D. E., and Gallo, D. G.: *Proc. Soc. Exp. Biol. Med. 137*:623, 1971.
42a. Lynch, H. J., Eng, J. P., et al.: *Proc. Nat. Acad. Sci.* (USA) 1973 (in press).
43. Lynch, H. J., Ralph, C. L., et al.: Unpublished results.
44. Lynch, H. J., and Wurtman, R. J.: Unpublished results.
45. MacGuire, J., and Möller, H.: *Nature* (London) *208*:495, 1965.
46. McIsaac, W. M., Taborski, R. G., et al.: *Science 145*:63, 1968.
47. Mess, B., Heizer, A., et al.: In *The Pineal Gland*. Wolstenholme, G. E. W., and Knight, J. (eds.), Ciba Foundation Symposium. London, Churchill, Livingstone, 1971, p. 229.
48. Miline, R., and Krstíc, R.: *Ann. Endocr.* (Paris) *24*:233, 1966.
49. Moore, R. Y., Heller, A., et al.: *Arch. Neurol.* (Chicago) *18*:208, 1968.
50. Motta, M., Schiaffini, O., et al.: In *The Pineal Gland*. Wolstenholme, G. E. W., and Knight, J. (eds.), Ciba Foundation Symposium. London, Churchill, Livingstone, 1971, p. 279.
51. Otani, T., Gyorkey, F., et al.: *J. Clin. Endocr. 28*:349, 1968.
52. Panda, J. N., and Turner, C. W.: *Acta Endocr. 57*:363, 1968.
53. Quay, W. B.: *Physiol. Behav. 5*:353, 1970.
54. Ralph, C. L., Mull, D., et al.: *Endocrinology 89*:1361, 1971.
55. Reiter, R. J., and Fraschini, F.: *Neuroendocrinology 5*:219, 1969.
56. Reiter, R. J., Sorrentino, S., et al.: *Life Sci. 11*:123, 1972.
57. Relkin, R.: *Endocrinology 88*:415, 1971.
58. Relkin, R.: *J. Endocr. 53*:179, 1972.
59. Shein, H. M., and Wurtman, R. J.: *Science 166*:519, 1969.
60. Singh, D. V., and Turner, C. W.: *Acta Endocr. 69*:35, 1972.
61. Sorrentino, S., Reiter, R. J., et al.: *Neuroendocrinology 7*:105, 1971.
62. Strada, S. J., Klein, D. C., et al.: *Endocrinology 90*:1470, 1972.
63. Taylor, A. N., and Wilson, R. W.: *Experientia 26*:267, 1970.
64. Vlahakes, G., and Wurtman, R. J.: *Biochim. Biophys. Acta 261*:194, 1972.
65. Weiss, B.: *Ann. N. Y. Acad. Sci. 185*:507, 1971.
66. Wolstenholme, G. E. W., and Knight, J. (eds.), *The Pineal Gland*. Ciba Foundation Symposium. London, Churchill, Livingstone, 1971.
67. Wurtman, R. J., In *Neuroendocrinology*. Vol. 2. Martini, L., and Ganong, W. F. (eds.), New York, Academic Press, 1967, p. 19.
68. Wurtman, R. J., In *The Neurosciences*. Second Study Program. Schmitt, F. O. (ed.), New York, The Rockefeller University Press, 1970, p. 350.
69. Wurtman, R. J.: *Fed. Proc.* 1973 (in press).
70. Wurtman, R. J., and Axelrod, J.: *Scientific American 213*:50, 1965.
71. Wurtman, R. J., Axelrod, J., et al.: *The Pineal*. New York, Academic Press, 1968.
72. Wurtman, R. J., Axelrod, J., et al.: *J. Pharmacol. Exp. Ther. 157*:487, 1967.
73. Wurtman, R. J., and Kammer, H.: *New Eng. J. Med. 274*:1233, 1966.
74. Wurtman, R. J., Shein, H. M., et al.: *J. Neurochem. 18*:1683, 1971.

CHAPTER 14

The Gastrointestinal Hormones

By James E. McGuigan

The gastrointestinal hormones are polypeptides which are produced in the mucosal endocrine cells of the stomach and small intestine. Gastrointestinal hormones participate in the stimulation, inhibition, and regulation of the motor and secretory activities of a variety of organs, including the stomach, small intestine, liver, biliary tract, and pancreas. There are three major gastrointestinal hormones about which information has been accumulated concerning their structures, physiologic activities, mechanisms of release, neurohumoral relationships, and, in some instances, their partici-

pation in disease. These hormones include gastrin, secretin, and cholecystokinin-pancreozymin.

The discovery and description of secretin, the first hormone ever to be recognized, by Bayliss and Starling (1) in 1902 introduced the discipline of endocrinology and initiated the functional concept of hormones and chemical messengers. The second substance identified as a hormone was gastrin; its activity in stimulating gastric acid secretion was described by John Edkins (2) in 1905. The polypeptide hormone cholecystokinin-pancreozymin was originally thought to be two distinct substances. The term "cholecystokinin" was applied to material which could be extracted from small intestinal mucosa and which stimulated gallbladder contraction (3). The term "pancreozymin" was applied to a substance also derived from small intestinal mucosa which stimulated pancreatic enzyme secretion (4). It has now been proved that both of these stimulated functions are produced by a single polypeptide hormone which has been termed cholecystokinin-pancreozymin (5). (Some prefer the term cholecystokinin alone, acknowledging the earlier discovery of cholecystokinin activity.) In this chapter the three well-substantiated gastrointestinal hormones will be discussed in detail. Available information on other, possibly hormonal, substances and activities within the gastrointestinal tract will also be mentioned.

The gastrointestinal hormones were identified during the search for physiologic agents that stimulated and regulated exocrine secretion and activity of the gut. The well-characterized members of the gastrointestinal hormone group were recognized as stimulating such activities, and they could be demonstrated in extracts from the gastrointestinal mucosa. Until relatively recently, advances in the understanding of the gastrointestinal hormones were impaired by the lack of pure preparations for study. Advances in protein chemistry techniques have now led to the isolation of pure materials, and the development of radioimmunoassay has provided methods for sensitive and specific measurement of some of these hormones.

In general, as will become apparent from examination of the activities of the gastrointestinal hormones, there are extensive areas of overlapping and much functional interplay among the gastrointestinal hormones. Although the nervous system may modify both the release and the effects of the gastrointestinal hormones, the hormones can act independently of the nervous system inasmuch as they evoke their anticipated responses even in denervated target glands.

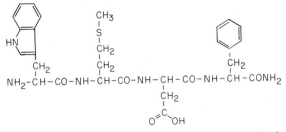

Figure 14–2. The physiologically active carboxyl-terminal tetrapeptide amide region of gastrin (Try. Met. Asp. Phe.-NH$_2$).

GASTRIN

In 1964 Gregory and Tracy (6) reported the isolation and characterization of gastrins I and II from hog gastric antral mucosa; they identified them as each containing 17 amino acids (heptadecapeptides) in a single, linear polypeptide chain. Gastrins I and II, which were isolated separately during purification, differ only in that gastrin II contains a sulfated tyrosine in position 12, while gastrin I contains a nonsulfated tyrosine in position 12. Subsequently, gastrin heptadecapeptides have been isolated and their amino acid sequences documented from several other species, including man (7), dog, cat, cow, and sheep (Fig. 14–1). These molecules differ from one another only by one or two amino acid residues contained in the midportion of the molecule. The spectrum of activities of the intact gastrin heptadecapeptides is shown by the carboxyl-terminal tetrapeptide amide (8). Therefore, part or all of this segment of the molecule contains the activity of gastrin (Fig. 14–2). On an equimolar basis, the tetrapeptide amide is approximately one-sixth to one-tenth as potent as is intact heptadecapeptide gastrin. For most activities, gastrins I and II are equally potent. Pentagastrin, a synthetic pentapeptide (which contains the active site tetrapeptide amide region of the gastrin molecule) has been used widely in pharmacologic and clinical studies and is under evaluation as an agent to test gastric acid secretory responsiveness. Although gastrin has been proved to play an important role in the regulation of gastric acid secretion in man and other mammals, the physiologic importance of many of the other activities of gastrin, often demonstrable in apparently pharmacologic doses, has not yet been clarified.

Substitutions in the tetrapeptide amide portion of the gastrin molecule, particularly in the car-

boxyl-terminal region, greatly reduce or abolish activity. Deamidization of the gastrin tetrapeptide or the heptadecapeptide eliminates physiologic activity. Both terminal groups of the gastrin heptadecapeptide are blocked, the amino by pyroglutamyl condensation and the carboxyl by amidization. The gastrin heptadecapeptides possess a strong net negative charge, conferred by the abundance of dicarboxylic acids, which results in strong electrophoretic migration to the anode and absorption by anion exchange resins. Recently, Yalow and Berson (9, 10) demonstrated that the major fraction of gastrin circulating in the blood is more basic and larger than the heptadecapeptide, having a molecular weight of approximately 7,000 (contrasted to approximately 2,100 for the heptadecapeptide). It has been suggested that the larger and more basic form ("big gastrin") is composed of the heptadecapeptide plus a peptide of approximately 5,000 molecular weight, perhaps attached to its amino terminus. Radioimmunoassay and bioassay of physiologic activity suggest that the larger form of gastrin and the heptadecapeptide are approximately equally potent in stimulating gastric acid secretion. The precise relationship between basic gastrin and the heptadecapeptide has not yet been clarified. Incubation of basic gastrin with trypsin has been shown to yield a fragment with size and charge characteristics indistinguishable from heptadecapeptide gastrin; basic gastrin is not altered by 8 M urea, 0.2 M hydrochloric acid, or neuraminidase. There is some evidence that basic gastrin may be somewhat slower than heptadecapeptide gastrin in its onset and disappearance of activity. More recent studies indicate an even larger form of immunoreactive gastrin ("big, big gastrin") in plasma and extracts from jejunal mucosa.

Activities

Gastrin is the most powerful known stimulant of gastric acid secretion (Table 14–1). On a molar basis, it is approximately 1,500 times as potent as its nearest rival, histamine. In addition to stimulating gastric acid secretion, gastrin also stimulates the gastric mucosa to secrete pepsin (6) and "intrinsic factor" (11). Although substantially less potent than secretin in this respect, gastrin stimu-

STRUCTURES OF GASTRIN MOLECULES FROM VARIOUS SPECIES

	1	2	3	4	5	6	7	8	9	10	11	12	13	14	15	16	17
HUMAN	⌐Glu.*	Gly.	Pro.	Try.	Leu.	Glu.	Glu.	Glu.	Glu.	Glu.	Ala.	Tyr.**	Gly.	Try.	Met.	Asp.	Phe.-NH$_2$
HOG								Met.									
COW and SHEEP						Val.				Ala.							
DOG								Met.		Ala.							
CAT											Ala.						

 •⌐Glu is pyroglutamyl.
 •• Tyr-HSO$_3$ in gastrin II.

Figure 14–1. Primary structure of gastrin heptadecapeptides from several mammalian species.

TABLE 14–1. PRIMARY ACTIONS OF THE MAJOR GASTROINTESTINAL HORMONES

Hormone	Gastric Acid Secretion	Pancreatic Bicarbonate Secretion	Pancreatic Enzyme Secretion	Gallbladder Contraction
Secretin	Strong inhibitor	Strong stimulant	Weak stimulant	*
Gastrin	Strong stimulant	Weak stimulant	Strong stimulant	Weak stimulant
Cholecystokinin-pancreozymin	Weak stimulant†	Weak stimulant	Strong stimulant	Strong stimulant

*Weak stimulant when given with cholecystokinin-pancreozymin.
†Inhibitor of gastrin-mediated gastric acid secretion.

lates water and bicarbonate secretion by the pancreas, liver, and Brunner's glands (Table 14–2). Gastrin is almost as potent as cholecystokinin-pancreozymin in stimulating pancreatic enzyme secretion (12). Gastrin stimulates the release of secretin by the small intestinal mucosa, both by a direct hormonal effect and by stimulating acid secretion, which in turn evokes secretin release. In high doses, gastrin is capable of promoting insulin release by pancreatic islet beta cells and can inhibit absorption of sodium by the ileum (13). Pentagastrin, which contains the carboxyl-terminal tetrapeptide amide active portion of the gastrin molecule, has been shown to stimulate volume secretion by both jejunum and ileum in dogs; this has been achieved at concentrations which are submaximal for acid secretion, thereby suggesting the possibility that gastrin may, under normal (physiologic) conditions, stimulate intestinal fluid secretion. Gastrin causes contraction and increases tone of the lower esophageal sphincter (14) and causes smooth muscle contractions of the stomach, small and large intestine, gallbladder, and uterus and relaxes the sphincter of Oddi (15) (Table 14–2). Gastrin pentapeptide, in causing weak antral contractions, appears to be an inhibitor of the rate of gastric emptying; if such an effect is physiologic, gastrin, while stimulating acid and pepsin secretion, would appear to delay the delivery of gastric contents into the duodenum by reducing the rate of gastric emptying. Gastrin would also appear to reduce regurgitation of gastric juice in the esophagus by its effect on the distal esophageal sphincter mechanism. These actions may be viewed as protective in respect to the exposure of acid to the duodenum and the esophagus. Gastrin also stimulates the growth of the gastric mucosa, resulting in increases in the parietal cell mass and the associated capacity to secrete hydrochloric acid. Gastrin administration increases gastric, pancreatic, and small intestinal blood flow. Rapid intravenous injection of supramaximal doses of gastrin inhibits gastric acid secretion in the dog but not in man (16).

Hormonal stimulation of gastric acid secretion by gastrin and vagal stimulation are intimately interrelated (17–23); gastrin stimulates acid secretion directly and augments the acid secretory response of the gastric mucosa to vagal stimulation, and, in turn, vagal stimulation lowers the threshold for the acid secretory response of the gastric mucosa to gastrin. Following antrectomy, acid secretion in response to vagal stimulation is decreased, and following vagal transection, acid secretory responses to administered gastrin are greatly reduced.

TABLE 14–2. DEMONSTRABLE ACTIONS OF THE MAJOR GASTROINTESTINAL HORMONES

Activity	Gastrin	CCK-PZ	Secretin
Water-electrolyte secretion			
Stomach	↑	↑*	↓
Pancreas	↑	↑	↓
Liver	↑	↑	↑
Brunner's glands	↑	↑	↑
Water-electrolyte absorption			
Ileum	↓	↓ ↑†	↓ ↑†
Gallbladder	0	0	↓
Enzyme secretion			
Stomach and pancreas	↑	↑	↑
Pancreatic islet secretion			
Insulin	↑	↑	↑
Glucagon	0	↑	↓
Smooth muscle			
Lower esophageal sphincter	↑	↓	↓
Stomach	↑	↑	↓
Pyloric sphincter	↓	↑	↓
Intestine	↑	↑	↓
Ileocecal sphincter	↓	NT	NT
Gallbladder	↑	↑	↑
Sphincter of Oddi	↓	↓	NT
Growth and amino acid uptake			
Gastric mucosa	↑	NT	↓
Pancreas	↑	↑	0
Metabolic			
Lipolysis	0	0	↑
Glycogenolysis	0	0	0
Glucose absorption			
Jejunum	↓	↑	NT

*Inhibition of gastrin-mediated water and electrolyte secretion.
†Conflicting results.
NT = Not tested; ↑ = increase; ↓ = decrease; 0 = no effect.

Distribution

The major location of gastrin is the mucosa of the gastric antrum (the pyloric gland area) and most proximal duodenum; there is progressively less gastrin as one proceeds distally along the upper small intestine (24). Extracts of the antral mucosa reveal that antral gastrin is mainly heptadecapeptide gastrin. Extracts of proximal duodenal mucosa of man contain approximately as much gastrin as does antral mucosa, in about equal proportions of basic gastrin and heptadecapeptide gastrin. Smaller amounts of gastrin are also found in the mucosa of the upper jejunum. The relative abundance of basic gastrin increases distally so that, in the proximal jejunal mucosa, only basic gastrin and "big, big gastrin" are found. Using immunofluorescence (25) and immunoelectronmicroscopic (26) techniques, gastrin has been identified in cytoplasmic granules of endocrine cells interspersed along the course of the antral pyloric glands. These cells are in contact with, and form a portion of, the glandular luminal surfaces. Gastrin cells are most numerous in the midportion of the antral glands, and the granules are most frequent in the portion of cytoplasm adjacent to the basement membrane and least numerous in the cytoplasmic region adjacent to the luminal surface of these endocrine cells. The granules average 180 nm. in diameter. The gastrin-containing cells have been designated "gastrin cells" or "G cells." Gastrin has also been shown to be present in granules in the cytoplasm of the delta cells of pancreatic islets (27, 28). Infrequent, scattered endocrine cells in small intrapancreatic ducts have also been shown to possess cytoplasmic gastrin-containing granules.

Release

The release of gastrin from the antral mucosa into the circulation is promoted by vagal stimulation or by acetylcholine in contact with the antral mucosa (29). Insulin-induced hypoglycemia, with resulting vagal stimulation, evokes gastrin release (30). Gastrin release is also stimulated after eating (31), particularly after a protein-containing meal. The importance of cholinergic reflexes in stimulating gastrin release after eating has been challenged because it appears that gastrin release after eating is enhanced rather than reduced by prior atropine administration (32). Antral distention stimulates gastrin release by cholinergic reflexes, principally the short or local reflexes within the wall of the stomach. The increase in serum gastrin levels following calcium ingestion and intravenous infusion suggests that calcium may also play a role in stimulating gastrin release (33 to 35). Gastrin release is effectively stimulated by the presence of amino acids in the stomach; amino acids vary greatly in their capacity to stimulate gastrin release, glycine being the most potent. Acid in the gastric antrum strongly inhibits gastrin release to all stimuli, thereby indicating the presence of a strong negative feedback control mechanism, with gastrin and hydrochloric acid functioning as a closed loop in the regulation of gastrin-mediated acid secretion. It is believed that the acid acts on the gastrin cell in inhibiting gastrin release, inasmuch as, even after local anesthetic application to the gastric mucosa, the acid prohibits acetylcholine-stimulated gastrin release.

Interactions with Other Gastrointestinal Hormones

The gastrointestinal hormones share many physiologic properties. For example, both gastrin and cholecystokinin-pancreozymin (CCK-PZ) are capable of stimulating gastric acid secretion. However, gastrin is a potent stimulant to acid secretion, while CCK-PZ is relatively weak. Secretin, on the other hand, is an inhibitor of gastric acid secretion. CCK-PZ inhibits gastrin-stimulated acid secretion in species such as man and the dog in which the efficacy of gastrin exceeds that of CCK-PZ. In species such as the rat and cat, in which CCK-PZ has equal efficacy to gastrin, inhibition of gastrin-mediated gastric acid secretion by CCK-PZ is not seen. It is believed that CCK-PZ and gastrin act on the same receptor site (36). Gastrin and CCK-PZ are structurally similar, sharing an identical carboxy-terminal pentapeptide amide sequence (37). The competitive kinetics of inhibition of gastrin-mediated secretion by CCK-PZ are comparable to those of two agents acting on the same receptor site. It is believed that the receptor sites for gastrin and secretin, although separate, interact (36). Secretin inhibition of gastrin-mediated acid secretion appears not to be competitive.

Serum Gastrin Concentrations in Man

Because of the development of radioimmunoassay techniques (38 to 41), it is now possible to measure gastrin in human serum and plasma. A variety of techniques have been evolved, usually by means of antibodies produced in rabbits (38 to 40) or guinea pigs (41). With most antibodies used for radioimmunoassay of gastrin, there is detectable cross-reactivity with CCK-PZ. With antibodies against human gastrin I or crude tissue gastrin, immunologic cross-reactivity with CCK-PZ is minimal and does not interfere with radioimmunoassay measurement of gastrin. Normal fasting serum gastrin concentrations are less than 200 pg. per ml., with average values in most laboratories approximating 70 pg. per ml.

Serum gastrin concentrations, both for normal individuals and for patients with peptic ulcer disease, have been found to be lowest during early morning hours (3 A.M. to 7 A.M.), highest during the day, and beginning to fall about 10 P.M. (42). These observations may represent circadian rhythm effects or be the result of specific physiologic stimulation, including eating, or both.

In some studies, increases in mean serum gastrin concentrations have been noted with increasing age. This is thought to reflect the decrease in gastric acid secretion accompanying chronic gastritis and gastric atrophy, the incidence of which increases progressively with age (43). In general, there is an inverse relationship between fasting serum gastrin concentrations and rates of acid secretion (44). When patients with impaired acid secretion are excluded, it is doubtful that fasting serum gastrin levels increase with age. As previously indicated, a low pH of gastric contents constitutes a potent mechanism for inhibition of gastrin release. The absence of secreted gastric acid would create an environment permitting greater than normal gastrin release. Mean serum gastrin concentrations have been shown to be increased in patients with pernicious anemia (43). The elevated levels are believed, in major part, to be due to the absence in these patients of gastric acid within the stomach. The result is a marked increase in serum gastrin concentration. Fasting serum gastrin concentrations in patients with pernicious anemia are usually elevated, averaging approximately 1,000 pg. per ml.; they may be as high as 10,000 pg. per ml. Placement of 0.1 N hydrochloric acid in the stomachs of hypergastrinemic patients with pernicious anemia results in marked reductions towards, but not completely to, normal serum gastrin levels (41). Hyperplasia of gastrin cells in the gastric mucosa of patients with pernicious anemia (45) may also contribute to the hypergastrinemia of pernicious anemia.

Although increases in portal venous gastrin have been demonstrated with insulin-induced hypoglycemia, these increases are small, and peripheral serum gastrin concentrations in response to insulin-induced hypoglycemia are variable and small in magnitude.

The Zollinger-Ellison Syndrome

The Zollinger-Ellison syndrome (ulcerogenic islet cell tumor) (46) is characterized by severe ulcer disease of the upper gastrointestinal tract, markedly elevated rates of gastric acid secretion, and the presence of non-beta islet cell tumors usually, but not invariably, located in the pancreas. It has now been well established that the Zollinger-Ellison syndrome results from the release of large amounts of gastrin from the tumors, which are rich in gastrin (47, 48) and thereby merit the term "gastrinomas" (49). Up to 50 per cent of the gastrin in pancreatic Zollinger-Ellison tumors has been identified as basic gastrin. Fasting serum gastrin concentrations in patients with the Zollinger-Ellison syndrome are increased, ranging from 300 pg. per ml. to 350,000 pg. per ml. Intravenous calcium infusion (15 to 20 mg./3 hr.) in patients with Zollinger-Ellison tumors results in marked increases in both serum gastrin concentrations and rates of acid secretion (33, 50). The increases in both acid secretory rates and gastrin levels exceed those observed with calcium infusion in normal patients or in patients with common duodenal ulcer disease. In normal individuals and in patients with common peptic ulcer disease (non-Zollinger-Ellison), feeding a test meal results in increases in serum gastrin concentrations, whereas in patients with Zollinger-Ellison tumors, there is no rise in serum gastrin after eating (51). The absence of evidence of significant postprandial gastrin release in Zollinger-Ellison patients is consistent with the thesis that persistent gastric hyperchlorhydria has suppressed secretion in the gastrin cells of the antral and duodenal mucosa, that the test meal probably exerts little neutralizing effect on the acid in the stomach, and that the tumor itself is not stimulated to release gastrin in response to food. Thus the serum gastrin profile in a patient with the Zollinger-Ellison syndrome is that of fasting hypergastrinemia which does not increase after eating but is associated with marked increases after intravenous infusion of calcium.

In normal man, secretin administration appears to inhibit gastrin-mediated gastric acid secretion and also results in lowering of serum gastrin concentrations (52). In some patients with the Zollinger-Ellison syndrome, secretin administration has been followed by increases rather than decreases in serum gastrin levels (53), which have also been associated with increases in serum calcium concentrations. The mechanism of this effect is not known.

Diarrhea, which is found in approximately one third of patients with the Zollinger-Ellison syndrome, probably results from both effects of hypersecreted acid on the small intestinal mucosa and direct hormonal effects of gastrin on intestinal transport of fluid and electrolytes. Steatorrhea in patients with Zollinger-Ellison tumors is due to the irreversible denaturation of pancreatic lipase at low pH that results from the voluminous gastric secretion of hydrochloric acid into the upper small intestine.

Gastrin and Common Duodenal Ulcer Disease

Important questions remain concerning hypergastrinemia in duodenal ulcer disease, which is commonly, although not invariably, associated with increased rates of gastric acid secretion. In some patients with duodenal ulcer disease, acid secretory rates both in the basal state and in response to stimulation with histamine may be as high as those found in patients with the Zollinger-Ellison gastrinomas. In view of the increased rates of acid secretion in these patients and the capacity of acid to inhibit gastrin release, it might be expected that serum gastrin levels would be lower than normal in patients with duodenal ulcer disease; this prediction has not been borne out (54). Although results are not uniform, fasting serum gastrin concentrations in duodenal ulcer patients have been reported by most investigators to be either normal or slightly increased (not increased to the levels of patients with gastrinomas). Our own studies, as well as those of several other groups of investigators, have shown neither increased nor decreased fasting serum gastrin levels in duodenal ulcer patients. In response to eating, however, serum gastrin levels are higher in patients with duodenal ulcer disease than in control subjects (55). Results in duodenal ulcer patients suggest that secretion of gastrin is not normally responsive to feedback inhibition of gastrin release by acid within the stomach. Patients with duodenal ulcer also are more sensitive to administered pentagastrin and secrete more gastric acid in response to intravenous pentagastrin than do patients without ulcer (56). In spite of the failure to demonstrate striking fasting hypergastrinemia, the findings that serum gastrin levels are not appropriately reduced (in response to increased acid in the stomach) and that they are higher than normal in response to food suggest the importance of gastrin in the acid hypersecretory state which frequently characterizes duodenal ulcer disease.

Gastrin and Gastric Ulcer Disease

Since there is an inverse relationship between gastric acid secretion and serum gastrin concentrations, and since gastric acid secretory rates tend to decrease in gastric ulcer patients, we expect, and in some instances find, moderate elevations of serum gastrin (57). However, apart from this relationship, there is no general trend of serum gastrin elevation in gastric ulcer patients. These findings have failed to support the suggestion that gastric stasis, with resulting excessive production and release of gastrin, is the cause for gastric ulcer.

Gastrin and the Lower Esophageal Sphincter

Gastrin may play a major role in the regulation of the lower esophageal sphincter, the mechanism of which is exquisitely sensitive to gastrin, with contractions induced *in vitro* by concentrations as low as 10 pg. per ml. Patients with achalasia have normal fasting serum gastrin concentrations; however, their lower esophageal sphincters exhibit hypersensitivity to injected gastrin (58). It has been suggested that the persistent increase in tone of the distal esophageal sphincter in achalasia may result from enhanced sensitivity of the sphincter to gastrin. In experimental animals, injection of antibodies to gastrin, which neutralize the effects of gastrin *in vivo*, lowers the distal esophageal sphincter pressure. This observation provides additional support for the role of gastrin in maintaining lower esophageal sphincter pressure. The role of gastrin in maintaining the competency of the distal esophageal sphincter in normal man and the extent to which alterations in its activity account for sphincter incompetence remain to be clarified (59).

SECRETIN

Secretin, the first hormone ever recognized, was described by Bayliss and Starling in 1902 (1). Secretin is the most powerful known stimulant of pancreatic water and bicarbonate secretion (Table 14–1). Secretin has been isolated from both duodenal and jejunal mucosa (60). Porcine secretin has been purified, its chemical structure determined (61), and it has been synthesized (62). Secretin contains 27 amino acids in a single chain. It is of interest to note that, in 14 of the 27 loci, the amino acid residues are identical to those of pancreatic glucagon (Fig. 14–3). Unlike gastrin and CCK-PZ, it appears that the entire polypeptide is required for biologic activity; no minimum fragment with activity has been identified. Secretin bears no structural similarity to the other major gastrointestinal hormones, gastrin and CCK-PZ.

Activities

Secretin is approximately five times as potent as CCK-PZ or gastrin in stimulating pancreatic bicarbonate secretion in dogs. In cats, stimulants other than secretin evoke virtually no response in bicarbonate secretion; however, they do strikingly augment the activities of secretin. Maximum pancreatic bicarbonate and enzyme secretion in response to administration of both secretin and CCK-PZ exceeds that for either agent alone (63).

The only known stimulant to release secretin from the mucosa of the upper small intestine is acid. Eating is followed by brisk increases in pancreatic flow rates. Inasmuch as extremely limited acidification of the duodenal mucosa occurs after eating, it is reasonable to conclude that CCK-PZ participates with secretin in effecting the increase in volume of the pancreatic secretions that follow ingestion of a meal. Secretin stimulates bicarbonate and water secretion in the intra- and extrahepatic biliary ducts and by Brunner's glands (Table 14–2), but it does not stimulate secretion of bile salts or bile pigments (64). Although a potent stimulant of pepsin secretion by the stomach, secretin alone among the major gastrointestinal hormones inhibits gastric acid secretion (Table 14–1). Secretin inhibits smooth muscle contraction in the stomach, small and large intestines, and in the lower esophageal sphincter. Secretin has inhibitory effects on the motor activity of the upper small intestine, and, since the dose producing such responses is small, it is possible that this hormone may act physiologically as an inhibitor of intestinal motor activities. In addition, secretin relaxes the sphincter of Oddi. It increases the strength of contractions induced by CCK-PZ and gastrin but, when administered alone, does not cause gallbladder contractions. Secretin reduces absorption of water and sodium by the ileum and gallbladder, inhibits the release of gastrin, and stimulates insulin release.

In view of the major structural similarities between secretin and glucagon, it comes as no surprise that secretin shares many of the physiologic properties of glucagon (65). Secretin increases cardiac output by increasing both stroke volume and heart rate. It increases blood flow to the pancreas and the small intestine and decreases hepatic arterial blood flow. Secretin is more powerful than glucagon in promoting lipolysis by activation of

STRUCTURES OF SECRETIN AND GLUCAGON

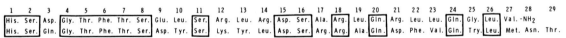

Figure 14–3. Amino acid sequence of porcine secretin (*above*) and glucagon (*below*). The boxes enclose areas of identical amino acids in both peptides.

adenyl cyclase. Secretin stimulation of exocrine pancreatic secretion may be inhibited by glucagon, perhaps reflecting an inhibition related to the structural similarities between the molecules of secretin and glucagon.

Distribution and Release

With the use of immunofluorescent methods, human secretin has been located in the cytoplasm of endocrine cells in the mucosa of the duodenum and the first portion of the jejunum (66). The secretin-containing cells have been designated S cells. Secretin-containing cells could not be demonstrated in mucosa from the stomach or ileum. The cells that contained secretin were in contact with the luminal surface of the duodenum and the jejunum. Secretin-containing cells have small cytoplasmic granules (averaging 100 to 150 nm.) of varying electron density. The secretin-containing cells were shown to be distinct from cells exhibiting immunoreactivity with antibodies to glucagon (presumed to contain enteroglucagon).

The only known stimulant to the release of secretin is hydrogen ion in contact with the mucosa of the upper small intestine. The threshold for secretin release is pH 4.5; with reduction of pH 4.5 toward 3.0, increasing amounts of secretin are released, and below pH 3.0 there is no further increase. The rate of secretin release is related to the length of small intestinal mucosa in which the pH is reduced. This in turn reflects the rate of acid entrance into the duodenum. After eating, only the first 10 centimeters of small intestine achieve pH levels below the threshold for secretin release.

Clinical Applications

In man, maximum pancreatic bicarbonate secretion is reached with administration of one to two clinical units of secretin (GIH Research Units, Karolinska Institute, Stockholm) administered as a single intravenous injection. Secretin administration is used widely to assess pancreatic exocrine function. In patients with pancreatic exocrine insufficiency resulting from such diseases as chronic destructive pancreatitis, increases in bicarbonate secretion in response to secretin administration usually fail to occur, and the maximum bicarbonate concentration fails to exceed 90 mEq. per liter. Patients with carcinoma of the pancreas often do not exhibit expected increases in the volume of pancreatic secretion following secretin administration.

Secretin administration results in neutralization of the contents of the duodenal bulb, possibly chiefly because it stimulates secretion of pancreatic bicarbonate (although gastrin effects on acid secretion are also reduced). A potential role for secretin administration in the treatment of duodenal ulcer patients (67) is currently under investigation.

Radioimmunoassay of Secretin

It is expected that the role of secretin in normal physiology and in disease will be further clarified by the development of sensitive and specific radioimmunoassay techniques for measurement of secretin in serum and body tissues. Absolute values of serum secretin are not known. The following results of secretin measurements by radioimmunoassay were obtained from a single laboratory and may be in great part due to success in radiolabeling secretin, which, by virtue of the absence of a tyrosine residue, constitutes a formidable task (68). Increases in serum secretin have been reported, as would be anticipated, following continuous intraduodenal infusion of hydrochloric acid (69). It has also been reported that eating a meal increases serum secretin concentrations. Oral and intraduodenal glucose administration has been followed by a brief sharp increase in serum secretin levels, reaching a peak value at 5 to 10 minutes and returning to near basal concentrations at 30 to 40 minutes (68 to 70). Intravenous glucose administration had no effect on serum secretin levels (70). Confirmation and extension of these observations by other groups of investigators are awaited.

CHOLECYSTOKININ-PANCREOZYMIN

Cholecystokinin-pancreozymin (CCK-PZ) is a single hormone with two major properties. It was originally described as stimulating gallbladder contraction (3) and pancreatic enzyme secretion (4) (Table 14–1). Porcine CCK-PZ has been isolated from duodenal and jejunal mucosa; it is a single-chain polypeptide consisting of 33 amino acid residues (71). The carboxyl-terminal pentapeptide of CCK-PZ is identical to that of gastrin, and the tyrosyl residue is esterified with sulfate as in gastrin II (71). The carboxyl-terminal octapeptide portion of CCK-PZ is more potent than the intact molecule.

Activities

CCK-PZ, like the other gastrointestinal hormones, performs a wide variety of activities (Table 14–2). In many respects, its functions are similar to those of gastrin; however, it has the capacity to inhibit gastrin activity. Other activities of CCK-PZ are similar to those of secretin, to which it bears no structural relationship. CCK-PZ, alone among the major gastrointestinal hormones, is a powerful stimulant to gallbladder contraction (gastrin is much less potent). CCK-PZ is a powerful stimulant to pancreatic enzyme synthesis and secretion and augments the water-bicarbonate response of the pancreas to secretin. Neither pancreatic enzyme secretion nor gallbladder contraction in response to CCK-PZ administration is reduced by vagotomy or atropine (72). In man CCK-PZ stimulates gastric acid secretion; however it inhibits gastrin-mediated acid secretion by the stomach. CCK-PZ stimulates Brunner's glands and hepatic bile secretion. It shares the properties of other major gastrointestinal hormones in promoting pepsin secretion by the gastric mucosa. CCK-PZ stimulates release of both glucagon and insulin from pancreatic islets (73) and may serve important functions in preventing hypoglycemia after ingestion of a high-protein meal. CCK-PZ relaxes the sphincter of Oddi and inhibits gastric motility and the distal esophageal sphincter mechanism. Small and large intestinal motor activity are stimulated by CCK-PZ. CCK-PZ stimulates both growth of the pancreas and amino acid uptake by pancreatic tissue. Blood flow to the small bowel and pancreas are markedly increased in response to cholecystokinin-pancreozymin administration.

Distribution and Release

CCK-PZ is contained in the mucosa of the duodenum and jejunum in man. It is released into the circulation from the mucosa of the upper small intestine in response to intraluminal acid, amino acids, and fatty acids. Impaired secretion of CCK-PZ has been identified in patients with celiac sprue, a disorder associated with damage to the mucosa of the small intestine, particularly of the duodenum and jejunum (74). In patients with celiac sprue, gallbladder and pancreatic functions are normal following intravenous administration of CCK-PZ; however, pancreatic enzyme secretion and expulsion of gallbladder contents are reduced in response to intraluminal administration of amino acids. The failure to absorb nutrients in patients with celiac sprue may be in part due to impaired release of CCK-PZ, resulting in incomplete digestion of the luminal contents and malabsorption due to the destructive mucosal lesion.

It is probable that only L-amino acids are effective in stimulating CCK-PZ release (75). The length of intestine exposed to the stimulant is the primary determinant for the amount of CCK-PZ released. CCK-PZ release is not stimulated by intact proteins. In contrast to amino acids, hydrogen ion is a weak stimulant to CCK-PZ release. Release of CCK-PZ, but not its effects on the pancreas, is believed to be dependent upon cholinergic influences (76).

Caerulein — A Structurally Related Peptide

Caerulein (77), a naturally occurring polypeptide (isolated from the skin of the Australian frog, *Hyla caerulea*), bears structural and functional relationships to both gastrin and CCK-PZ. This agent, which possesses a carboxyl-terminal penta-peptide region identical to that of CCK-PZ and gastrin molecules and has an adjacent sulfated tyrosyl, exhibits powerful CCK-PZ activity. Caerulein stimulates gastric acid secretion in the fasting state but can act as a competitive inhibitor of gastrin-mediated acid secretion (78), observations

which have stimulated the search for synthetic competitors of acid secretion with negligible gastrinlike activity which may be useful in the management of clinical states associated with hypersecretion of gastric hydrochloric acid.

OTHER GASTROINTESTINAL HORMONES

A state of advanced, albeit imperfect, knowledge of the aforementioned major gastrointestinal hormones — gastrin, secretin, and CCK-PZ — has been reached in terms of their structures, sites of origin, and target organs and in terms of the multiple factors controlling their release and physiologic activity. An assortment of substances that may act upon the gastrointestinal tract or be extracted from portions of the gut have been suggested; one or more of these may reach "hormone status" as further investigation into their nature proceeds. Some available information about these candidate hormones is provided below.

Urogastrone

Urogastrone (79) is a polypeptide which has been isolated in pure form from urine and is a well-recognized inhibitor of gastric hydrochloric secretion. Its site of origin, molecular size, and amino acid sequence have not been reported.

Enterogastrone

Enterogastrone is a term for a compound originating in the small intestine with the capacity to inhibit gastric acid secretion and emptying. Several hormones, including secretin and CCK-PZ, also have enterogastrone-like activity. Whether enterogastrone exists as a hormonal substance separate from the established and evolving gastrointestinal hormones remains to be established.

Bulbogastrone

The term bulbogastrone (80) has been applied to a material which has been extracted from the mucosa of the initial portion of the duodenum and which has the capacity to inhibit gastrin-mediated gastric acid secretion. Its failure to stimulate pancreatic secretion establishes that this material is neither secretin nor cholecystokinin-pancreozymin. Its chemical structure is not yet known.

Gastric Inhibitory Polypeptide

Another polypeptide with substantial structural homology to secretin and glucagon has been isolated from the small intestine. This material (81), which has been designated gastric inhibitory polypeptide (GIP), is released from the mucosa of the small intestine in response to lipid in the lumen; it inhibits both gastric motility and gastric acid secretion, as well as small intestinal secretions. (GIP may be considered an enterogastrone.)

Intestinal Glucagon-like Material

In response to glucose ingestion, a material is released from the mucosa of the small intestine which demonstrates immunologic cross-reactivity with antibodies to pancreatic alpha cell glucagon; this material (82 to 84) has been variously described as "enteroglucagon," "gut glucagon," or as having "glucagon-like immunoreactivity" (GLI). The physiologic importance of GLI has not been established. It consists of at least two components, both of which are immunologically distinguishable from pancreatic glucagon. While it appears that a component of GLI can stimulate insulin secretion, the amounts released in response to glucose ingestion are probably unable to produce such an effect. One component is similar to pancreatic glucagon both in its molecular size and in its glycogenolytic and hyperglycemic activities. The second GLI fraction has a molecular size larger than that of glucagon and similar hyperglycemic and glycogenolytic activities, but it binds much less to glucagon antibodies.

Vaso-inhibitory Peptide

An additional polypeptide designated vaso-inhibitory peptide (VIP) has been isolated from the small intestine of the hog (85). This peptide has potent and diverse biologic actions producing systemic vasodilatation, hypotension, increased cardiac output, respiratory stimulation, and hyperglycemia. The peptide, which has 28 amino acid residues, is structurally distinct from the kinins, "substance P," glucagon, and secretin. The role of VIP in normal physiology has not been identified; however, several potential physiologic activities are suggested for it, including the possibility that it may participate in the control of blood sugar and intestinal blood flow. The hyperglycemic properties of VIP suggest that it may be related to one of the glucagon-like factors demonstrable in extracts of small intestinal mucosa. VIP appears to be inactivated principally in the liver, so that it is doubtful that its physiologic activities extend beyond the splanchnic circulation. With hepatic insufficiency and possible impaired VIP inactivation, it is conceivable that VIP could express some systemic symptoms. VIP activities are similar to those exhibited by some patients with cirrhosis, including increased cardiac output, peripheral vasodilatation, relative impairment of renal blood flow, and abnormal glucose tolerance.

PANCREATIC CHOLERA

The term "pancreatic cholera" has been applied to a clinical syndrome characterized by severe hypokalemia and profuse diarrhea, frequently accompanied by shock, reduced intravascular volume, and salt and water depletion in association with pancreatic islet cell tumors (86 to 89). (Synonyms include Verner-Morrison syndrome and WDHA syndrome.) Many but not all of these patients exhibit histamine-fast achlorhydria. In others, reduced or normal rates of acid secretion are observed. The diarrhea is voluminous, with stool volumes approximating 6 liters per day with exacerbated symptoms and sometimes amounting to 10 liters. Electrolyte depletion results from the losses of huge amounts of potassium and sodium in the diarrheal fluid. During treatment, replacement of fluid and electrolytes must be vigorous in order to keep up with and correct losses. Unlike the Zollinger-Ellison syndrome, neither gastric acid hypersecretion nor ulcerations of the upper gastrointestinal tract are components of the syndrome. Although these patients exhibit no chemical evidence of increased circulating serotonin or serotonin metabolites, several have exhibited facial and trunk flushing similar to that observed in the carcinoid syndrome (90).

Clinical and Laboratory Abnormalities

With clinical exacerbation, the serum potassium is markedly reduced; it is always less than 3 mEq. per liter and in some instances less than 2 mEq. per liter. Hypokalemia is accompanied by reduced serum bicarbonate levels, reflecting excess bicarbonate losses via the gastrointestinal tract. Fluid depletion may be profound and may be reflected in prerenal azotemia with elevated serum creatinine levels. Serum chloride and sodium may be normal or somewhat, but not profoundly, depressed. Severe and sustained hypokalemia may lead to the development of hypokalemic nephropathy. Daily fecal potassium losses may average 200 to 400 mEq. per day (89). In about 50 per cent of patients with pancreatic cholera, hypercalcemia is found (89); usually this is in the absence of parathyroid adenomas, which have, however, been found in several of these patients. Following resection of the pancreatic tumors, there is a disappearance of the diarrheal abnormalities; gastric acid secretion returns to normal; often plasma calcium levels return to normal; and glucose intolerance, which is also found in approximately half of these patients, becomes normal. It is possible that the tumors liberate parathyroid hormone or a parathyroid hormone-like substance, or that they may stimulate the parathyroids to release parathyroid hormone. It is presently believed that these pancreatic tumors release one or more hormones which provoke water and electrolyte losses from the gut and inhibit gastric acid secretion. The development of hypokalemic nephropathy may be reflected in the loss of ability to concentrate urine, as well as in an increased incidence of urinary tract infections.

The diagnosis is established in these patients by demonstration of an islet cell tumor in the absence of other explanations for profound diarrhea. Certain proof of the diagnosis is provided by correction of the metabolic abnormalities following resection of the tumor.

The nature of the endocrine agent responsible for the abnormalities observed in the pancreatic cholera syndrome has not been identified. Secretin has been proposed as a possible candidate (91); however, this has not been proven. Evidence against secretin includes the observation that relatively little diarrhea in man follows secretin administration. Additional evidence is supplied by normal pancreatic function tests with normal responses to exogenous secretin (87, 92) and inconclusive or negative results from testing most pancreatic cholera tumor extracts for secretin activity. Extracts of tumor tissue have been shown to inhibit water, chloride, and sodium transport by the hamster ileum (93). They have also inhibited histamine- and pentagastrin-stimulated gastric acid secretion (94). Glucagon, gastrin, prostaglandins, and kallikrein activities have not been found in these tumors (94, 95). GIP has also been suggested as a possible cause.

The tumors are approximately equally divided between adenomas and malignant tumors. A small portion of patients have been found to have islet hyperplasia in the absence of recognizable tumors. The tumors are indistinguishable by standard light microscopy from Zollinger-Ellison tumors. The treatment of choice is resection of the pancreatic tumors, after which metabolic sequelae usually disappear if tumor resection is complete. Steroid therapy (20 mg. prednisone or greater per day) has been effective in the treatment of most patients in whom complete resection of the tumor has not been possible (96).

HISTAMINE IN GASTRIC ACID SECRETION

Except for gastrin, histamine is the most potent agent thus far identified in stimulating gastric acid secretion. Histamine, which is nearly ubiquitous in the body, has been shown to abound in many tissues including the gastric mucosa. Histamine has been suggested by many as a final chemoactive agent in stimulating the parietal cell to produce hydrochloric acid; however, when the evidence is examined, certain proof is lacking that histamine plays such a role (97). The most persuasive evidence in favor of a role for histamine in stimulating the parietal cell has been obtained in rats and not in man, where the bulk of evidence is against such a role (98). The peak concentration of histamine in the gastric mucosa resides in the same area as do the parietal cells. Gastrin and other gastric acid secretory stimulants cause histamine to be released in the gastric mucosa of rats; however, this is not proven in man. Although histamine is found in the enterochromaffin-like cells of the rat (99, 100), in man and in other species it is located in granules of mast cells (101). In patients with duodenal ulcer disease, a disorder associated with increased rates of acid secretion, increases in the concentration of gastric mucosal histamine are not found (102). Unlike classic histamine-releasing substances, gastrin does not cause the release of histamine from isolated gastric mucosal tissues *in vitro*. There is no evidence that plasma histamine concentrations increase during gastrin stimulation of gastric acid secretion. Experiments indicate that gastrin is not a general histamine releaser; however, they do not exclude the possibility that histamine may be released and exert its effect locally. Free urinary histamine increases after ingestion of protein, but there is no evidence that this histamine originates in the stomach or has a relationship to gastrin secretion. Histidine decarboxylase, which may be found in the gastric mucosa of rats, has not been conclusively demonstrated in the gastric mucosa of man.

If histamine remains unproven as a physiologic chemostimulator of gastric acid secretion, is there another physiologic role for it? It is conceivable that histamine in the gastrointestinal tract, as well as in other sites, has some important effect on the microcirculation (98). It is also conceivable that gastrin causes histamine to be released from granules of storage cells in the vicinity of the parietal cells, where it causes local vasodilation. This might explain the well-recognized vasodilator effects of gastrin. Furthermore, it is possible that blood vessels in the immediate vicinity of the parietal cells have special, heightened sensitivity to histamine, thereby increasing blood flow and hence increasing sources of fluid for secretion.

In spite of its recognized effects on smooth muscle, there is no evidence for a role for histamine in gastrointestinal motility.

EFFECTS OF OTHER HORMONES ON THE GASTROINTESTINAL TRACT

Hormones other than those viewed as primarily gastrointestinal have been shown to produce a variety of effects on components of the gastrointestinal tract.

Glucagon produces multiple effects on the gastrointestinal tract. It inhibits secretion of acid and pepsinogen by the stomach but stimulates hepatic bile flow. Glucagon inhibits sodium and water absorption by both jejunum and ileum and reduces pancreatic enzyme and bicarbonate secretion. It decreases smooth muscle activity of the stomach, small intestine, gallbladder, and the sphincter of Oddi.

In man, reduction of blood glucose to a concentration of 45 mg. per 100 ml. or less by *insulin* administration stimulates both acid and pepsinogen secretion by the stomach. Insulin-induced hypoglycemia also stimulates chief cells of the neck region of the gastric glands to secrete a mucoprotein or soluble mucus which is chemically and physically distinct from the secretion of the surface cells. Although injected insulin produces augmentation of gastric contraction in dogs and rats, it does not do so in man. Hypoglycemia induced by insulin results in increased motility of the empty stomach in normal man. These insulin effects are inhibited if blood glucose concentration is maintained. The hypoglycemic effect following insulin administration does not result in stimulation of acid secretion when the vagus nerves have been divided.

Glucocorticoids have been shown to reduce basal pancreatic volume and bicarbonate and amylase secretion but to have no effect on the pancreatic response to secretin administration. In lower animals, glucocorticoids induce more rapid cellular differentiation of small intestinal mucosal epithelial cells. *Hydrocortisone* increases alkaline phosphatase and sucrase activities in embryonic intestinal mucosal cells of lower species. Slight reductions in sodium and reciprocal increases in potassium concentrations of ileal fluid are produced by 9α-fluorohydrocortisone in man. *Aldosterone* in normal humans has been shown to increase the rate of mean net sodium absorption by the colon.

Parathyroid hormone appears to play an important role in stimulating the absorption of calcium by the small intestine. Malabsorption of calcium occurs in hypoparathyroidism and is presumed due to insufficient parathyroid hormone to promote adequate calcium absorption.

Serotonin (5-hydroxytryptamine) is capable of stimulating small and large intestinal motility. Serotonin may serve as a neural transmitter between sensory and motor neurons in the peristaltic reflex. During peristalsis, serotonin is released into intestinal venous blood. Serotonin has been shown to induce ileal spasm in patients who have ileostomies but to inhibit gastric and colonic motility in man. Serotonin relaxes isolated samples of teniae coli in humans. Serotonin, which decreases distally in the small intestine, is contained in mucosal enterochromaffin cells. It is believed that these intestinal cells are the source of serotonin contained in platelets, inasmuch as removal of the gastrointestinal tract lowers blood concentrations of serotonin. Reserpine causes serotonin release from intestinal enterochromaffin cells. It is believed that this release of serotonin from enterochromaffin cells on distention plays an important role in the initiation and maintenance of peristalsis, possibly by sensitizing intestinal mechanoreceptors to deformation. In man, the stomach, lower small intestine, and large intestine are not stimulated by intravenous serotonin.

Administration of *thyroid hormone* and hyperthyroidism in man are associated with increases in bile acid production. In hypothyroid patients, there is a preponderance of bile acids conjugated with glycine. However, with correction of hypothyroidism, the ratio of glycine-conjugated to taurine-conjugated bile acids decreases to normal values. In experimental animals, thyroid hormone decreases cholesterol absorption by the small intestine.

REFERENCES

1. Bayliss, W. M., and Starling, E. H.: Mechanism of pancreatic secretion. *J. Physiol.* (London) 28:325, 1902.
2. Edkins, J. S.: Chemical mechanism of gastric secretion. *Proc. Roy. Soc. Med.* 76:376, 1905.
3. Ivy, A. C., and Oldberg, E.: Observations on the cause of gall-bladder contraction and evacuation. *Proc. Soc. Exp. Biol. Med.* 25:251, 1928.
4. Harper, A. A., and Raper, H. S.: Pancreozymin, stimulant of secretion of pancreatic enzymes in extracts of small intestine. *J. Physiol.* (London) 102:115, 1943.
5. Jorpes, E., and Mutt, V.: Cholecystokinin and pancreozymin; one single hormone? *Acta Physiol. Scand.* 66:1966.
6. Gregory, R. A., and Tracy, H. J.: The constitution and properties of two gastrins extracted from hog antral mucosa. *Gut* 5:103, 1964.
7. Beacham, J., Bentley, P. H., et al.: Synthesis of human gastrin I. *Nature* (London) 209:585, 1966.
8. Morley, J. S., Tracy, H. J., et al.: Structure-function relationships in the active C-terminal tetrapeptide sequence of gastrin. *Nature* (London) 207:1356, 1965.
9. Yalow, R. S., and Berson, S. A.: Size and charge distinctions between endogenous human plasma gastrin in peripheral blood and heptadecapeptide gastrins. *Gastroenterology* 58:609, 1970.
10. Yalow, R. S., and Berson, S. A.: Further studies on the nature of immunoreactive gastrin in human plasma. *Gastroenterology* 60:203, 1971.
11. Irvine, W. J.: Effect of gastrin I and II on secretion of intrinsic factor. *Lancet* 1:736, 1965.
12. Preshaw, R. M., Cooke, A. R., et al.: Stimulation of pancreatic secretion by a humoral agent from the pyloric gland area of the stomach. *Gastroenterology* 49:617, 1965.
13. Gingell, J. C., Davies, M. W., et al.: Effect of a synthetic gastrin-like pentapeptide upon the intestinal transport of sodium, potassium and water. *Gut* 9:111, 1968.
14. Castell, D. O., and Harris, L. D.: Hormonal control of gastroesophageal-sphincter strength. *New Eng. J. Med.* 282:886, 1970.
15. Lin, T. M., and Spray, G. F.: Effect of pentagastrin, cholecystokinin, caerulein and glucagon on the choledochal resistance and bile flow of conscious dogs. *Gastroenterology* 56:1178, 1969.
16. Emas, S., and Grossman, M. I.: Differences in response between dogs and cats to large doses of gastrin on gastric secretion. *Gut* 8:267, 1967.
17. Thein, M. P., and Schofield, B.: Release of gastrin from the pyloric antrum following vagal stimulation by sham feeding in dogs. *J. Physiol.* (London) 148:291, 1959.
18. Andersson, S., and Grossman, M. I.: Effect of vagal denervation of pouches on gastric secretion in dogs with intact or resected antrums. *Gastroenterology* 48:449, 1965.
19. Cooke, A. R., Nahrwold, D. L., et al.: Comparison of endogenous and exogenous gastrin in stimulation of acid and pepsin secretion. *Amer. J. Physiol.* 213:432, 1967.
20. Olbe, L., Ridley, P. T., et al.: Effects of gastrin and histamine on vagally induced acid and pepsin secretion in antrectomized dogs. *Acta Physiol. Scand.* 72:492, 1968.
21. Payne, R. A., Cox, A. G., et al.: Effect of vagotomy on gastric acid secretion stimulated by pentagastrin and histamine. *Brit. Med. J.* 4:456, 1967.
22. Konturek, S. J., Wysocki, A., et al.: Effect of medical and surgical vagotomy on gastric response to graded doses of pentagastrin and histamine. *Gastroenterology* 54:392, 1968.
23. Emas, S., and Grossman, M. I.: Effect of truncal vagotomy on acid and pepsin responses to histamine and gastrin in dogs. *Amer. J. Physiol.* 212:1007, 1967.
24. Berson, S. A., and Yalow, R. S.: Nature of immunoreactive gastrin extracted from tissues of the gastrointestinal tract. *Gastroenterology* 60:215, 1971.
25. McGuigan, J. E.: Gastric mucosal intracellular localization of gastrin by immunofluorescence. *Gastroenterology* 55:315, 1968.
26. Greider, M. H., Steinberg, V., et al.: Electron microscopic identification of the gastrin cell of the human antral mucosa by means of immunocytochemistry. *Gastroenterology* 63:572, 1972.
27. Lomsky, R., Langr, F., et al.: Immunohistochemical demonstration of gastrin in mammalian islets of Langerhans. *Nature* (London) 223:618, 1969.
28. Greider, M. H., and McGuigan, J. E.: Cellular localization of gastrin in the human pancreas. *Diabetes* 20:389, 1971.
29. Cooke, A. R., and Grossman, M. I.: Comparison of stimulants of antral release of gastrin. *Amer. J. Physiol.* 215:314, 1968.
30. McGuigan, J. E., Jaffe, B. M., et al.: Immunochemical mea-

surements of endogenous gastrin release. *Gastroenterology* 59:499, 1970.

31. McGuigan, J. E., and Trudeau, W. L.: Studies with antibodies to gastrin: radioimmunoassay in human serum and physiological studies. *Gastroenterology* 58:139, 1970.

32. Walsh, J. H., Yalow, R. S., et al.: The effect of atropine on plasma gastrin response to feeding. *Gastroenterology* 60:16, 1971.

33. Trudeau, W. L., and McGuigan, J. E.: Effects of calcium on serum gastrin levels in the Zollinger-Ellison syndrome. *New Eng. J. Med.* 281:862, 1969.

34. Reeder, D. D., Jackson, B. H., et al.: Influence of hypercalcemia on gastric secretion and serum gastrin concentration in man. *Ann. Surg.* 172:540, 1970.

35. Reeder, D. D., Conlee, J. L., et al.: Calcium carbonate antacid and serum gastrin concentration in duodenal ulcer. *Surg. Forum* 22:308, 1971.

36. Grossman, M. I.: Gastrin, cholecystokinin, and secretin act on one receptor. *Lancet* 1:1088, 1970.

37. Mutt, V., and Jorpes, J. E.: Isolation of aspartylphenylalanine amide from cholecystokinin-pancreozymin. *Biochem. Biophys. Res. Commun.* 26:392, 1967.

38. McGuigan, J. E.: Immunochemical studies with synthetic human gastrin. *Gastroenterology* 54:1005, 1968.

39. McGuigan, J. E.: Studies of the immunochemical specificity of some antibodies to human gastrin. *Gastroenterology* 56:429, 1969.

40. Hansky, J., and Cain, M. D.: Radioimmunoassay of gastrin in human serum. *Lancet* 2:1388, 1969.

41. Yalow, R. S., and Berson, S. A.: Radioimmunoassay of gastrin. *Gastroenterology* 58:1, 1970.

42. Feurle, G., Ketterer, H., et al.: Circadian serum gastrin concentrations in control persons and in patients with ulcer disease. *Scand. J. Gastroent.* 7:177, 1972.

43. McGuigan, J. E., and Trudeau, W. L.: Serum gastrin concentrations in pernicious anemia. *New Eng. J. Med.* 282:358, 1970.

44. Trudeau, W. L., and McGuigan, J. E.: Relations between serum gastrin levels and rates of gastric hydrochloric acid secretion. *New Eng. J. Med.* 284:408, 1971.

45. Creutzfeldt, W., Arnold, R., et al.: Gastrin and G-cells in the antral mucosa of patients with pernicious anemia, acromegaly, and hyperparathyroidism, and in a Zollinger-Ellison tumor of the pancreas. *Europ. J. Clin. Invest.* 1:461, 1971.

46. Zollinger, R. M., and Ellison, E. H.: Primary peptic ulcerations of the jejunum associated with islet cell tumors of the pancreas. *Ann. Surg.* 142:709, 1955.

47. Gregory, R. A., Grossman, M. I., et al.: Nature of the gastric secretagogue in Zollinger-Ellison tumours. *Lancet* 2:543, 1967.

48. McGuigan, J. E., and Trudeau, W. L.: Immunochemical measurement of elevated levels of gastrin in serum of patients with pancreatic tumors of the Zollinger-Ellison variety. *New Eng. J. Med.* 278:1308, 1968.

49. Grossman, M. I.: Gastrointestinal hormones: Some thoughts about clinical applications. *Scand. J. Gastroent.* 7:9, 1972.

50. Basso, N., and Passaro, E.: Calcium-stimulated gastric secretion in the Zollinger-Ellison syndrome. *Arch. Surg.* 101:399, 1970.

51. Berson, S. A., and Yalow, R. S.: Radioimmunoassay in gastroenterology. *Gastroenterology* 62:1061, 1972.

52. Hansky, J., Soveny, C., et al.: Effect of secretin on serum gastrin as measured by radioimmunoassay. *Gastroenterology* 61:62, 1971.

53. Isenberg, J. I., Walsh, J. H., et al.: Unusual effect of secretin on serum gastrin, serum calcium and gastric acid secretion in a patient with suspected Zollinger-Ellison syndrome. *Gastroenterology* 62:626, 1972.

54. Trudeau, W. L., and McGuigan, J. E.: Serum gastrin levels in patients with peptic ulcer disease. *Gastroenterology* 59:6, 1970.

55. McGuigan, J. E., and Trudeau, W. L.: Differences in rates of gastrin release in normal individuals and patients with duodenal ulcer disease. *New Eng. J. Med.* 288:64, 1973.

56. Isenberg, J., Walsh, J. H., et al.: Effect of graded doses of pentagastrin on gastric acid secretion in duodenal and non-duodenal ulcer subjects. *Gastroenterology* 62:764, 1972.

57. Trudeau, W. L., and McGuigan, J. E.: Relations between serum gastrin levels and rates of gastric hydrochloric acid secretion. *New Eng. J. Med.* 284:408, 1971.

58. Cohen, S., Lipshutz, W., et al.: Role of gastrin supersensitivity in the pathogenesis of lower esophageal sphincter hypertension in achalasia. *J. Clin. Invest.* 50:1241, 1971.

59. Cohen, S., and Harris, L.: Does hiatus hernia affect competence of the gastroesophageal sphincter? *New Eng. J. Med.* 284:1053, 1971.

60. Jorpes, J. E., and Mutt, V.: Biological activity and amino acid composition of secretin. *Acta Chem. Scand.* 15:790, 1961.

61. Mutt, V., and Jorpes, J. E.: Proceedings of the 4th International Symposium on Chemistry of Natural Products, Stockholm, 1966. *Pure Appl. Chem.* 14:1, 1966.

62. Bodansky, M., Ondetti, M. A., et al.: Synthesis of heptacosapeptide amide with the hormonal activity of secretin. *Chem. Industr.* 42:1757, 1966.

63. Henriksen, F.: The maximum pancreatic secretion in dogs. *Scand. J. Gastroent.* 3:140, 1968.

64. Wheeler, H. O., and Mancusi-Ungaro, P. L.: Role of bile ducts during secretin choleresis in dogs. *Amer. J. Physiol.* 210:1153, 1966.

65. Ross, G.: Cardiovascular effects of secretin. *Amer. J. Physiol.* 218:1166, 1970.

66. Polak, J., Coulling, I., et al.: Immunofluorescent localization of secretin and enteroglucagon in human intestinal mucosa. *Scand. J. Gastroent.* 6:739, 1971.

67. Grossman, M. I.: Treatment of duodenal ulcer with secretin: A speculative proposal. *Gastroenterology* 50:912, 1966.

68. Young, J. D., Lazarus, L., et al.: Radioimmunoassay of secretin in human serum. *J. Nucl. Med.* 9:641, 1968.

69. Chisholm, D. J., Young, J. D., et al.: The gastrointestinal stimulus to insulin release. I. Secretin. *J. Clin. Invest.* 48:1453, 1969.

70. Chisholm, D. J., Kraegen, E. W., et al.: Comparsion of secretin response to oral, intraduodenal, or intravenous glucose administration. *Horm. Metab. Res.* 3:180, 1971.

71. Mutt, V., and Jorpes, J. E.: Isolation and primary structure of porcine cholecystokinin-pancreozymin. Paper presented at Nobel Symposium XVI, Frontiers in Gastroenterology, Stockholm, July, 1970.

72. Henriksen, F. W.: Effect of vagotomy or atropine on the canine pancreatic response to secretin and pancreozymin. *Scand. J. Gastroent.* 4:137, 1969.

73. Dupre, J., Curtis, J. D., et al.: Effects of secretin, pancreozymin or gastrin on the response of the endocrine pancreas to administration of glucose or arginine in man. *J. Clin. Invest.* 48:745, 1969.

74. DiMagno, E. P., Go, V. L. W., et al.: Impaired cholecystokinin-pancreozymin secretion, intraluminal dilution, and maldigestion of fat in sprue. *Gastroenterology* 63:25, 1972.

75. Meyer, J., and Grossman, M. I.: Comparison of D- and L-phenylalanine as pancreatic stimulants. *Gastroenterology* 58:1046, 1970.

76. Crider, J. O., and Thomas, J. E.: Secretion of pancreatic juice after cutting the extrinsic nerves. *Amer. J. Physiol.* 141:730, 1944.

77. Erspamer, V., and Asero, B.: Identification of enteramine specific hormone of enterochromaffin cell system, or 5-hydroxytryptamine. *Nature* (London) 169:800, 1952.

78. Agosti, A., Biasioli, S., et al.: Action of caerulein on gastric secretion in man. *Gastroenterology* 59:727, 1970.

79. Gregory, H.: Some polypeptides influencing gastric-acid secretion. *Amer. J. Dig. Dis.* 15:141, 1970.

80. Uvnäs, B.: Role of duodenum in inhibition of gastric acid secretion. *Scand. J. Gastroent.* 6:113, 1971.

81. Brown, J. C., and Dryburgh, J. R.: A gastric inhibitory polypeptide. II. The complete amino acid sequence. *Canad. J. Biochem.* 49:867, 1971.

82. Samols, E., Tyler, J., et al.: Immunochemical glucagon in human pancreas, gut and plasma. *Lancet* 2:727, 1966.

83. Unger, R. H., Ketterer, H., et al.: Distribution of immunoassayable glucagon in gastrointestinal tissues. *Metabolism* 15:865, 1966.

84. Valverde, I., Rigopoulon, E. J., et al.: Demonstration and

characterization of a second portion of glucagon-like immunoreactivity in jejunal extracts. *Amer. J. Med. Sci. 255*:415, 1968.

85. Said, S. I., and Mutt, V.: Polypeptide with broad biological activity: isolation from small intestine. *Science 169*:1217, 1970.

86. Verner, J. V., and Morrison, A. B.: Islet cell tumor and a syndrome of refractory watery diarrhea and hypokalemia. *Amer. J. Med. 25*:374, 1958.

87. Marks, I. N., Bank, S., et al.: Islet cell tumor of the pancreas with reversible watery diarrhea and achlorhydria. *Gastroenterology 52*:695, 1967.

88. Matsumoto, K. K., Peter, J. B., et al.: Watery diarrhea and hypokalemia associated with pancreatic islet cell adenoma. *Gastroenterology 50*:231, 1966.

89. Kraft, A. R., Tomkins, R. K., et al.: Recognition and management of the diarrheal syndrome caused by non-beta islet cell tumors of the pancreas. *Amer. J. Surg. 119*:163, 1970.

90. Shafer, W. H., McCormack, L. J., et al.: Non-beta islet cell carcinoma of the pancreas, with flushing attacks and diarrhea. *Cleveland Clin. Quart. 32*:13, 1965.

91. Zollinger, R. M., Tomkins, R. K., et al.: Identification of the diarrheogenic hormone associated with non-beta islet cell tumors of the pancreas. *Ann. Surg. 168*:502, 1968.

92. Gjone, E., Fretheim, B., et al.: Intractable watery diarrhoea, hypokalaemia, and achlorhydria associated with pancreatic tumour containing gastric secretory inhibitor. *Scand. J. Gastroent. 5*:401, 1970.

93. Gardner, J. D., and Cerda, J. J.: *In vitro* inhibition of intestinal fluid and electrolyte transfer by a non-beta islet cell tumor. *Proc. Soc. Exp. Biol. Med. 123*:361, 1966.

94. Semb, L. S., Gjone, E., et al.: Bioassay for gastric secretory inhibitor in extract of pancreatic tumor from patient with WDHA syndrome. *Scand. J. Gastroent. 5*:409, 1970.

95. Andersson, H., Dotevall, G., et al.: Pancreatic tumor with diarrhoea, hypokalemia and hypochlorhydria. *Acta Clin. Scand. 138*:102, 1972.

96. Verner, J. V.: Clinical syndromes associated with non-insulin producing tumors of the pancreatic islets, In *Non-Insulin Producing Tumors of the Pancreas.* Demling, L., and Ottenjann, R. (eds.), Stuttgart, Georg Thieme Verlag, 1968, p. 125.

97. Grossman, M. I.: Some aspects of gastric secretion. *Gastroenterology 52*:882, 1967.

98. Watson, N. G.: Histamine and the parietal cell. *Amer. J. Dig. Dis. 16*:921, 1971.

99. Hakanson, R., Lilja, B., et al.: Properties of a new amine-storing cell system in the gastric mucosa of the rat. *Europ. J. Pharmacol. 1*:188, 1967.

100. Thunberg, R.: Localization of cells containing and forming histamine in the gastric mucosa of the rat. *Exp. Cell Res. 47*:108, 1967.

101. Hakanson, R., Owman, C., et al.: Amine mechanisms in enterochromaffin and enterochromaffin-like cells of the gastric mucosa in various mammals. *Histochemie 21*:189, 1970.

102. Smith, A. N.: The distribution and release of histamine in human gastric tissues. *Clin. Sci. 18*:533, 1959.

CHAPTER 15

The Prostaglandins

By James B. Lee

HISTORICAL ASPECTS

The prostaglandins (PG's) are a unique group of cyclic fatty acids with vast and potent biologic ef-

fects involving almost every organ system in a variety of species including the human. Biologic activity ascribable to these compounds was first discovered in the early 1930's independently by Kurzrok and Lieb (27), Goldblatt (18), and von Euler (49), who observed that extracts of seminal vesicles or human semen caused contraction of the isolated uterus and lowering of blood pressure. Von Euler further characterized the responsible compounds as fatty acids and named them prostaglandins. Some twenty five years later in 1960 Bergström and his co-workers isolated and identified in sheep seminal vesicles two classes of prostaglandins, prostaglandin E (PGE) (10) and prostaglandin F (PGF) (11). Biologic activity ultimately ascribable to a third class, prostaglandin A (PGA), was discovered in rabbit kidney medulla in 1963 (32). This third class of prostaglandins, originally called medullin, was first isolated in 1965 from rabbit kidney medulla (30) and subsequently identified as PGA_2 by Lee and his co-workers (28, 31).

Since the isolation and identification of the prostaglandins, there has been an explosive and exponential increase in the prostaglandin literature to the extent that well over 600 articles dealing with these compounds appeared in the literature in 1972 in contrast to a single article appearing in 1961. This has occurred in large part because of the diversity of potent biochemical and physiologic effects that these compounds exert, as well as because of their ubiquitous distribution in mammalian tissues.

Since the prostaglandin literature is so voluminous, no attempt will be made to cite all the sources of the information in this chapter. The interested reader is referred to several reviews and symposia for a more detailed presentation and bibliography (9, 21, 29, 39, 40).

STRUCTURAL-FUNCTIONAL RELATIONSHIPS

The structures of the most common naturally occurring prostaglandins are shown in Figure 15–1. It is evident that these compounds are all com-

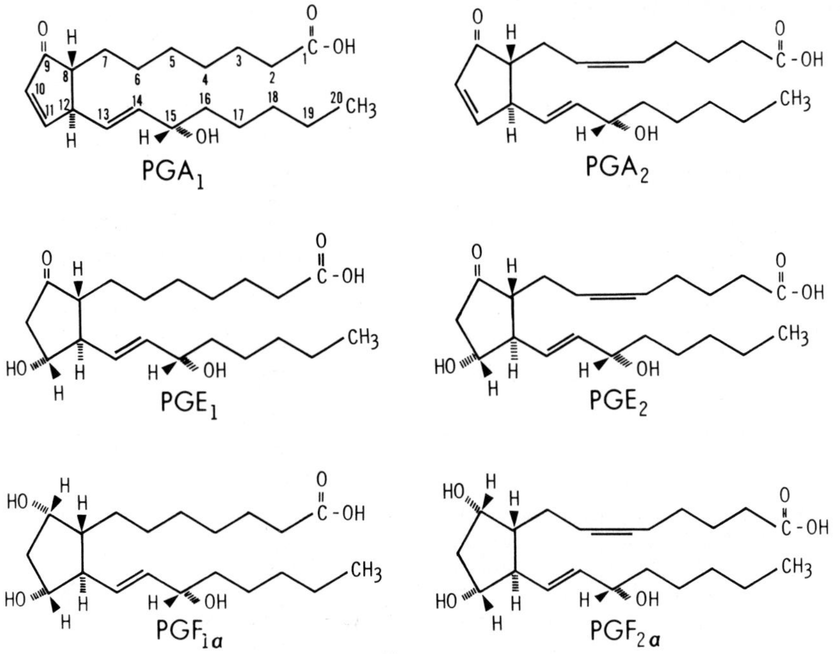

Figure 15–1. Structures of the most commonly occurring biologically active prostaglandins.

posed of a 20-carbon carboxylic acid containing a cyclopentane ring, a hypothetical structure referred to as prostanoic acid. However, they contain various degrees of substitution and unsaturation in the ring as well as in the aliphatic side chains. Depending on the class of prostaglandin, they may either relax vascular smooth muscle with consequent lowering of blood pressure or contract nonvascular smooth muscle, such as intestines and uterus, or both.

PGA$_1$, which has only blood pressure effects with no nonvascular smooth muscle stimulatory activity, contains a ketone at C-9 and a double bond at C-10 in the five-membered ring. PGA$_1$ is so named because it has one double bond at C-13 in the side chain. PGA$_2$, which has almost the same biologic effects as PGA$_1$, differs only in that it has two double bonds in the side chain, the additional bond being at C-5.

PGE$_1$, which has both blood pressure-lowering and nonvascular smooth muscle-stimulating activity, differs from PGA$_1$ in that a water molecule is introduced at ring position C-10, 11, and the double bond is eliminated. Again, PGE$_2$ resembles PGE$_1$ except that it has an additional double blond in the side chain at C-5.

PGF$_{1\alpha}$ and PGF$_{2\alpha}$, which have no blood pressure-lowering properties, retain their nonvascular smooth muscle-stimulating activity and differ from PGE$_1$ and PGE$_2$ in that the ketone in the ring at C-9 is reduced to a hydroxyl group. This reduction results in two possible stereochemical compounds, of which only PGF$_{1\alpha}$ and PGF$_{2\alpha}$ are naturally occurring. The structural-functional properties of the prostaglandins are summarized in Figure 15–2.

PGE$_3$ and PGF$_{3\alpha}$ have been described but occur in smaller concentrations and in far fewer tissues. PGB$_1$ and PGB$_2$ are also normally occurring but in relatively minute amounts. The latter compounds are formed by isomerization of the double bond of the PGA's from the Δ^{10} position to the Δ^{8-12} position, a change which results in a loss of all biologic activity. The widespread occurrence of the prostaglandins is evidenced by their isolation and full structural elucidation from such tissues as seminal vesicles, seminal fluid, renal medulla, lung, iris, brain, thymus, and menstrual fluid. In this regard, it is noteworthy that PG-2's predominate over PG-1's and PG-3's.

STRUCTURE	COMPOUND	EFFECT ON BLOOD PRESSURE	NON-VASCULAR SMOOTH MUSCLE STIMULATING ACTIVITY
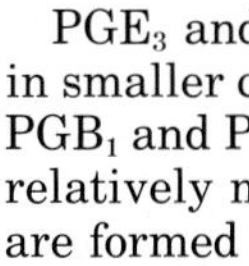	PGA	DECREASE	INACTIVE
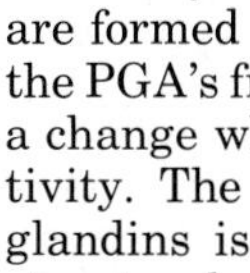	PGE	DECREASE	VERY ACTIVE
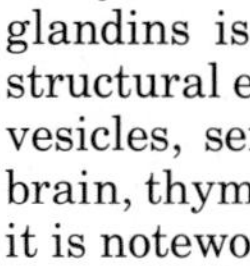	PGF	TRANSIENT INCREASE	VERY ACTIVE

Figure 15–2. Structural-functional relationships among the principal prostaglandin classes.

BIOSYNTHESIS AND METABOLISM

Prostaglandin Formation

The immediate precursors of prostaglandin synthesis are essential unsaturated fatty acids. It is now believed that they are needed in the diet because they play a pivotal role in being converted to prostaglandins (6, 8). The precursor for PGE_1 and $PGF_{1\alpha}$ is 8, 11, 14-eicosatrienoic acid (dihomo-γ-linolenic acid), and that for PGE_2 and $PGF_{2\alpha}$ is 5, 8, 11, 14-eicosatetraenoic acid (arachidonic acid). It has also been shown that PGE_3 and $PGF_{3\alpha}$ can be formed from 5, 8, 11, 14, 17-eicosapentaenoic acid. The transformation of unsaturated fatty acids to prostaglandins is catalyzed by PG synthetase, an enzyme specifically inhibited by essential fatty acid analogues and a number of anti-inflammatory agents, including indomethacin and aspirin. Figure 15–3 shows that, in the case of PGE_1 and $PGF_{1\alpha}$, the mechanism of biosynthesis involves (1) reduction of two of the double bonds in the fatty acid, (2) isomerization of the Δ^{12} double bond with introduction of a molecular oxygen at C-9, 11, and 15, and (3) subsequent cyclization to the cyclic endoperoxide. The endoperoxide is then converted to either PGE_1 or $PGF_{1\alpha}$. The latter two compounds are not generally interconvertible, both being formed from the same endoperoxide

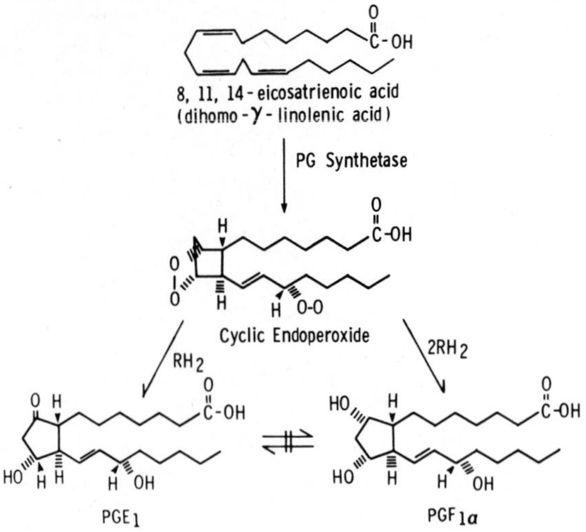

Figure 15–3.   Mechanisms of biosynthesis of PGE_1 and $PGF_{1\alpha}$.

precursor. A similar mechanism exists for the synthesis of PGE_2 and $PGF_{2\alpha}$ from arachidonic acid. The exact mechanism of PGA formation has not been studied intensively, but it is believed to be the result of chemical dehydration at C-10, 11 with introduction of a double bond at this site (Fig. 15–4). There is little free unsaturated fatty acid inside

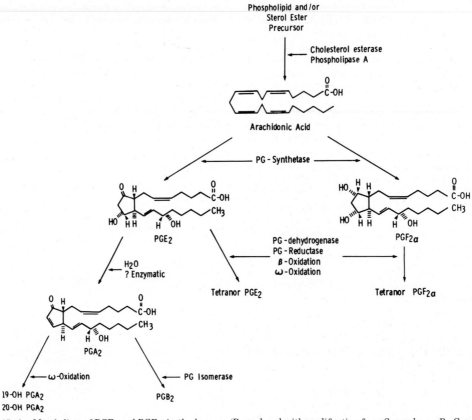

Figure 15–4.   Metabolism of PGE_2 and $PGF_{2\alpha}$ in the human. (Reproduced with modification from Samuelsson, B., Granström, E., et al.: *Ann. N. Y. Acad. Sci. 180*:139, 1971, with permission.)

cells, and it is believed that these precursors are stored as membrane phospholipids or as membrane sterol esters or both. There is evidence that the major rate-limiting enzymes in prostaglandin synthesis are not only PG synthetase but also cholesterol esterase and phospholipase A, which catalyze the hydrolysis of the unsaturated fatty acids from cholesterol and phospholipids respectively.

Prostaglandin Degradation

Figure 15–4 summarizes the overall synthesis and metabolism of PGA_2, PGE_2, and $PGF_{2\alpha}$. After production of PGA_2, there are at least two mechanisms of inactivation. The first is ω-oxidation in the liver to yield the inactive metabolites 19-hydroxy PGA_2 and 20-hydroxy PGA_2. The second is formation of the metabolite PGB_2, catalyzed by blood prostaglandin isomerase activity, which results in isomerization of the Δ^{10} double bond to Δ^{8-12}.

Newly synthesized PGE_2 is converted to its inactive tetranor metabolite by (1) oxidation at C-15 by PG dehydrogenase, (2) reduction of the Δ^{13} double bond by PG reductase, (3) β-oxidation, and (4) ω-oxidation. Three tetranor metabolites of $PGF_{2\alpha}$ are formed. The metabolism of PGE_1 and $PGF_{1\alpha}$ yields the same metabolites as that of PGE_2 and $PGF_{2\alpha}$ respectively. Although PG synthetase and the inactivating enzymes are ubiquitously distributed in virtually every tissue, PG synthetase has its highest activity in renal medulla and seminal vesicles, while the PG-inactivating enzymes have their highest activity in renal cortex, lung, and liver, apparently in that order.

Prostaglandin Release

Table 15–1 illustrates that a variety of physiologic stimuli will evoke release of prostaglandins. The significance of PGE or PGF release remains unclear since these two groups of prostaglandins are extensively metabolized by the lung and thus cannot qualify as true circulating hormones. It appears likely that prostaglandins are released into the venous circulation by many heterogeneous stimuli, but as Horton has noted (21), "prostaglandin" release has been estimated in most studies by relatively nonspecific bioassay procedures. Until more sensitive and specific methods are available, conclusions about the release of prostaglandin-like compounds should be made with caution. It appears that release into the venous circulation reflects an increase in prostaglandin synthesis within a particular tissue or organ, leading to a functional change in that system, followed by a secondary "overflow" release of PGE and PGF into the blood for eventual metabolism in the lung.

BIOLOGIC ACTIONS

The biologic actions of the prostaglandins are the most varied of any naturally occurring com-

TABLE 15–1.   RELEASE OF PROSTAGLANDINS FROM TISSUES*

Site	Stimulus
Cat superfused somatosensory cortex	Spontaneous
	Sensory nerve stimulation
	Contralateral cortical stimulation
Cat superfused cerebellar cortex	Spontaneous
Cat perfused cerebral ventricles	Spontaneous
Dog perfused cerebral ventricles	Spontaneous
	5-Hydroxytryptamine
Frog superfused spinal cord	Spontaneous
	Sensory nerve stimulation
Rat phrenic nerve–diaphragm in vitro	Electrical stimulation
	Norepinephrine
Rat epididymal fat pad in vitro	Nerve stimulation
	Norepinephrine
Rat gastrointestinal tract	Pentagastrin
	Histamine
	Vagal stimulation
	Carbachol
	5-Hydroxytryptamine
Dog blood-perfused spleen	Nerve stimulation
	Epinephrine
	Colloidal particles
Cat Ringer-perfused adrenals	Acetylcholine
Guinea pig Ringer-perfused lungs	Phospholipase A
Dog Ringer-perfused lungs	Stretch
Rabbit eye	Mechanical stimulation
Frog intestine in vitro	Spontaneous
Human medullary carcinoma of the thyroid in vivo	Spontaneous
Rat carrageenin pouch	Inflammatory response
Dog kidney	Ischemia
Guinea pig uterus	Distention, estrogen

*From Horton, E. W.: *Prostaglandins. Monographs on Endocrinology*, Vol. 7. Berlin-Heidelberg-New York, Springer-Verlag, 1972, p. 36, with permission.

pound. The nonvascular actions of the prostaglandins are closely linked to changes in $3',5'$-cyclic AMP (C-AMP). In this regard, it is important to note that unlike other hormones affecting C-AMP, the same prostaglandin can in some tissues increase and in others decrease adenyl cyclase and C-AMP. A role for prostaglandin interaction with C-AMP in the cardiovascular system has yet to be established.

Cardiovascular-Renal System

Antihypertensive Renal Function

A growing body of evidence suggests that the kidney, in addition to secreting the well-known renal pressor hormones, such as those of the renal renin-angiotensin system, also has an antihypertensive endocrine function. It is thought that the state of hypertension may be the result of a deficiency of renal vasodepressor substances which allow pressor mechanisms to act unopposed in bringing about peripheral arteriolar constriction and an ensuing rise in blood pressure (Fig. 15–5). The isolation from the rabbit renal medulla of the vasodilating prostaglandin, medullin (sub-

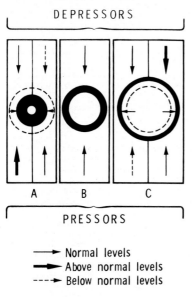

DEPRESSORS

A   B   C

PRESSORS

—→ Normal levels
━▶ Above normal levels
---→ Below normal levels

A. HYPERTENSION (vasoconstriction)
B. NORMOTENSION
C. HYPOTENSION (vasodilatation)

Figure 15–5. Schematic illustration of a possible interaction between vasodepressor and vasoconstrictor influences on blood pressure regulation. According to this hypothesis, normotension (*B*) will result when pressor mechanisms are equally offset by depressor mechanisms. The stage of hypertension (*A*) is expected to occur when there is a relative or absolute deficiency of depressor mechanisms, while hypotension (*C*) is expected when there is an absolute or relative deficiency of pressor systems. (Reproduced from Lee, J. B.: *Physiologist 13*:379, 1970, with permission.)

TABLE 15–2. DIFFERENCES BETWEEN PGA AND PGE

	PGA	PGE
Mechanism of hypotensive effect	Indirect peripheral arteriolar dilation	Direct peripheral arteriolar dilation
Metabolism by lung	Minor degree	Major degree
Renal oxidative metabolism and Na-K ATPase	Marked decrease	No effect
Effect on nonvascular smooth muscle	None	Contraction

sequently renamed PGA_2), provided the first demonstration that the kidney possessed a specific antihypertensive compound (28, 30). The vasodepressor prostaglandin, PGE_2, was also located and identified in rabbit renal medulla (31). However, its effects on nonvascular smooth muscle, its rapid metabolism by the lung, and its different metabolic and hypotensive mechanisms seem to exclude PGE_2 as a circulating antihypertensive hormone (Table 15–2).

Blood Pressure-Lowering Effects in Normotensive Animals

A sustained intravenous infusion of PGA_1 or PGA_2 results in an initial fall in blood pressure (the result of peripheral arteriolar dilatation), leading to a fall in total peripheral resistance and a reflex baroreceptor-mediated acceleration in heart rate. Evidence has accumulated that the splanchnic vascular bed largely mediates the hypotensive action of PGA. Thus intra-arterial administration of PGA or PGE compounds to normotensive animals results in an increase in regional blood flow in the carotid, coronary, cutaneous, splanchnic, femoral, brachial, and renal systems. However, only intra-arterial administration into the splanchnic bed results in a concomitant fall in blood pressure. This suggests that hypotension induced by PGA or PGE is largely the result of

splanchnic arteriolar dilatation. Support for this hypothesis is provided by the observation that, upon intravenous administration of PGA to dogs, the fall in blood pressure is accompanied by a simultaneous rise in splanchnic blood flow and an unchanged or decreased flow to most other vascular beds. Within 10 to 15 minutes, blood pressure returns to the preinjection level despite continued PGA administration. This is a reflection of adaptive pressor mechanisms being elicited to offset the unphysiologically low blood pressure fall induced by prostaglandin. Similar observations have been made in normotensive humans after intravenous PGA_1 administration. PGA has little positive or negative chronotropic or inotropic effect on the isolated perfused heart, indicating that its hypotensive effects are peripherally mediated. During PGA_1 or PGA_2 administration, there is a redistribution of renal blood flow from medulla to cortex, with an associated rise in total blood flow, natriuresis, kaliuresis, and diuresis, leading to a reduction in plasma volume. However, the natriuresis with PGA's may be due not only to changes in blood flow but also to metabolic inhibition of NA-K ATPase (Table 15–2), which results in a decrease in active sodium reabsorption.

The biochemical mechanism of arteriolar dilation by prostaglandin is unknown but does not appear to involve histaminergic, cholinergic, or adrenergic mechanisms. It is likely that PGA or PGE compounds act on postsynaptic vascular smooth muscle, leading to vasodilatation that is probably mediated in part by a decrease in NA-K ATPase. There is little evidence implicating C-AMP in the vascular mechanism of PGA action. PGE causes an immediate fall in blood pressure when injected into the aorta, whereas with PGA, a delayed blood pressure fall occurs, suggesting that PGA is acting through an indirect mechanism. These prostaglandins are also physiologic, but not pharmacologic, inhibitors of norepinephrine- and angiotensin-mediated arteriolar constriction. The cardiovascular effects of PGA and PGE are summarized in Table 15–3.

Antihypertensive Effects in Hypertensive Humans

The first prostaglandin administered to a hypertensive human being was PGA_2 isolated from the

TABLE 15–3. INTRAVENOUS CARDIOVASCULAR EFFECTS OF PGA AND PGE IN THE NORMOTENSIVE DOG

	PGA and PGE*
Blood pressure	Lowered
Peripheral arterioles	Dilated
Total peripheral resistance	Lowered
Heart rate	Reflex increase
Myocardial contractility	Unchanged
Regional blood flow given IA	Increased†
Regional blood flow given IV	
Splanchnic	Increased
Coronary	Decreased
Carotid	Unchanged or decreased
Femoral	Unchanged or decreased
Renal cortical	Increased
Renal medullary	Decreased
Sodium and potassium excretion	Increased
Urine flow	Increased
Plasma volume	Decreased

*Given IV in large amounts, allowing part to escape degradation by lung and act systemically. When given in equimolar amounts at which PGA has an intravenous effect (10^{-6} M), PGE has no systemic circulating action because of its metabolism by the lung.

†Except in the nasal vascular beds where flow is decreased.

kidney as medullin (28). Blood pressure fell from hypertensive to normotensive levels as a result of peripheral arteriolar dilatation, and there was a reflex increase in heart rate and cardiac output. In a series of 20 hypertensive patients, PGA_1 produced similar effects (33, 34). Its administration to the human being differed most notably from its administration to normotensive animals in that the lowering of blood pressure from hypertensive to normotensive levels in the human being is not transitory but lasts as long as the compound is infused.

The initial effect of PGA_1 is an increase in renal cortical blood flow (Fig. 15–6), which is associated with a marked natriuresis, kaliuresis, and diuresis, leading to a 10 per cent fall in blood volume. The effects are probably in large part the result of hemodynamic changes in the peritubular capillaries. At the end of this period (stage I) when blood pressure remains elevated, there is extrarenal arteriolar dilation and a fall in blood pressure to normotensive levels (stage II). This leads to a decrease in renal perfusion pressure in stage II offsetting the renovasodilatory effects so that renal blood flow, sodium and potassium excretion, and urine flow return to control preinjection levels when pressure normalized (Fig. 15–6). Therefore, normotension produced by PGA_1 does not lead to a compromise in renal blood flow but is associated with normal salt and water excretion. PGA_1 and PGA_2 appear to act as "ideal" antihypertensive compounds in that they reverse many of the abnormalities observed in the state of essential hypertension. Thus they favorably affect total peripheral resistance, renal resistance, cardiac output, baroreceptor activity, plasma volume, and sodium and water balance, all factors intimately involved in the genesis of human essential hypertension.

Reproductive System

Prostaglandins of the E and F (but not A) classes have marked effects on the reproductive system of nonprimates and primates, including the human. Their main actions are (1) to stimulate gravid uterine muscle to contract, (2) to produce luteolysis and decreased progesterone secretion, and (3) to act at the pituitary-hypothalamic level as mediators of luteinizing hormone releasing factor (LRF) on luteinizing hormone (LH) secretion. Most of these actions involve stimulation of adenyl cyclase activity, leading to a rise in intracellular C-AMP.

The Estrous Cycle

Ovulation is followed by the development of the corpus luteum and increased progesterone secretion. According to Caldwell et al. (13) summarizing recent studies (Fig. 15–7), the most likely series of events leading to luteolysis in the sheep is as follows: during the secretory phase the maturing follicle secretes increased quantities of estradiol

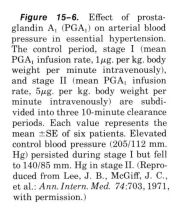

Figure 15–6. Effect of prostaglandin A_1 (PGA_1) on arterial blood pressure in essential hypertension. The control period, stage I (mean PGA_1 infusion rate, 1 µg. per kg. body weight per minute intravenously), and stage II (mean PGA_1 infusion rate, 5 µg. per kg. body weight per minute intravenously) are subdivided into three 10-minute clearance periods. Each value represents the mean ±SE of six patients. Elevated control blood pressure (205/112 mm. Hg) persisted during stage I but fell to 140/85 mm. Hg in stage II. (Reproduced from Lee, J. B., McGiff, J. C., et al.: *Ann. Intern. Med.* 74:703, 1971, with permission.)

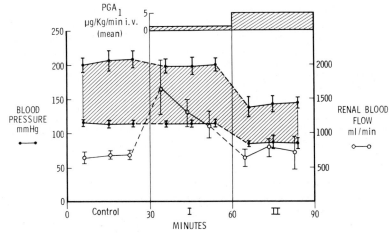

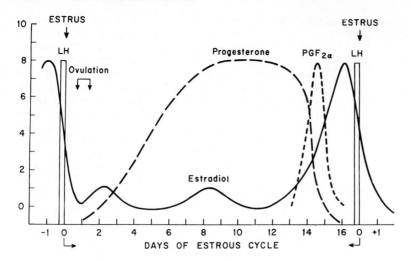

Figure 15–7. A model of the sheep estrous cycle, indicating the key role played by $PGF_{2\alpha}$ in producing the demise of the corpus luteum. (Reproduced from Caldwell, B. V., Tillson, S. A., et al.: *Prostaglandins* 1:217, 1972, with permission.)

which cause a rise in $PGF_{2\alpha}$ (previously called "uterine luteolysin"). This in turn results in luteolysis and a diminution in progesterone production. The subsequent continuing increase in estradiol then stimulates pituitary LH secretion, which, in a critical concentration relative to FSH, initiates ovulation and repetition of the cycle. The mechanism by which $PGF_{2\alpha}$ acts as a luteolysin is unknown, but its action may be the result of either a reduction in luteal blood flow or a direct inhibition of progesterone synthesis. Although early studies *in vitro* revealed a paradoxical increment in progesterone synthesis and in C-AMP, recent investigations reveal a decrease in progesterone synthesis (7, 37). This is most likely the result of inhibition by $PGF_{2\alpha}$ of luteal cholesterol synthetase, allowing greater esterification of cholesterol esters with concomitant decrease of progesterone precursor and hence of progesterone synthesis (7). The route by which uterine $PGF_{2\alpha}$ reaches the ovary in the sheep is by a countercurrent mechanism, whereby $PGF_{2\alpha}$ in the uterine vein is transferred to the ovarian artery which is anatomically closely interwoven with the vein (36). Since hysterectomy does not alter the normal ovarian estrous cycle in the human, a uterine-ovarian countercurrent system of this type is unlikely. However, human fallopian tube $PGF_{2\alpha}$ may have a luteolytic role, since fallopian tube fluid contains $PGF_{2\alpha}$. The occurrence of a normal estrous cycle after hysterectomy in the human may be explained by the fact that distal fallopian tubes are generally not removed during this procedure. Evidence of an LH ovulatory surge conditioned by $PGF_{2\alpha}$-mediated luteolysis is supported by the observation that ovulation is inhibited by indomethacin (5) and aspirin, potent inhibitors of prostaglandin synthesis. Furthermore, PGF levels rise sharply during the preovulatory phase in normal ewes and ewes treated with progesterone plus estrogen but not with progesterone alone (13). Lastly, hysterectomized ovariectomized ewes have negligible PGF plasma levels.

Evidence that the luteolytic action of $PGF_{2\alpha}$ may also, at times, be mediated via the pituitary-hypothalamus axis is twofold: (1) hypothalamic extracts increase pituitary adenyl cyclase and LH release, and $PGF_{2\alpha}$ increases pituitary C-AMP; and (2) prostaglandin antagonists block stimulation of LH release by LRF.

Abortion

Karim and Filshei (24) and Roth-Brandel et al. (41) first observed the induction of therapeutic abortion in women with high success rates in mid trimester by intravenous injection. However, subsequent investigation revealed many side effects, particularly nausea and vomiting. The most successful route appears to be a single injection of $PGF_{2\alpha}$ into the amniotic cavity. Success rates of close to 100 per cent have been reported with a mean duration of labor of 22 hours (2). Side effects were few, and the number of incomplete abortions was relatively low (25 per cent). The most immediate clinical application of prostaglandins appears to be in mid-trimester abortion by intra-amniotic injection. Suction curettage still remains preferable to prostaglandin administration during the first trimester. Although prostaglandins have been suggested as effective "hindsight" oral contraceptive agents, little confirmational evidence has yet been forthcoming.

Induction of Labor

$PGF_{2\alpha}$ and PGE_2 are potent oxytocics whether given orally, parenterally, or instilled locally in the gravid uterus (25). The intravenous infusion rate necessary to induce labor is 0.5 to 2.0 μg per minute for PGE_2 and 5.0 to 10.0 μg. per minute for $PGF_{2\alpha}$, and there are relatively few side effects. The delivery duration ranges from 30 minutes to almost 20 hours, depending on the state of inducibility. Similar degrees of inducibility with $PGF_{2\alpha}$ and oxytocin have been noted in difficult and easily inducible patients (3). Although extremely effective oxytocics, PGE and PGF seem to offer little immediate clinical advantage over oxytocin since they are equally effective and act by similar mechanisms. Of immediate physiologic interest is the fact that $PGF_{2\alpha}$ is present in amniotic fluid, and its concentration rises in the blood of women in labor, suggesting that endogenous $PGF_{2\alpha}$ may be an important factor in the normal induction of labor. In addition, its presence in menstrual fluid, together with its activity in constricting gastrointestinal smooth muscle, suggests a role for $PGF_{2\alpha}$ in the production of the pain of dysmenorrhea by causing gastrointestinal or uterine contractions or both. The future clinical use of $PGF_{2\alpha}$ in labor induction is uncertain, but its highly desirable mechanism of action and its natural occurrence in the female reproductive system may ultimately make it a more attractive agent than oxytocin.

Hematopoietic System

Platelets

When endothelium is damaged, platelets are known to adhere to subendothelial connective tissue, leading to a release reaction involving secretion of such agents as catecholamines, serotonin, and ADP, which leads in turn to further platelet aggregation, a phenomenon intricately involved in the intrinsic clotting process. In 1966 Kloeze found that PGE_1 markedly inhibits the aggregation reaction, while PGE_2 is a potent stimulator (26). Subsequent studies revealed that platelets normally contain PGE_2 and $PGF_{2\alpha}$, that they are released during the clotting process, and that their synthesis and release are inhibited by aspirin, a potent PG synthetase inhibitor (45). The effect of PGE_2 on platelet aggregation induced by adenosine diphosphate (ADP) is biphasic; it has little effect during the initial phases of aggregation but produces a prolonged secondary aggregation after exposure to ADP (44).

The mechanism by which PGE_1 and PGE_2 inhibit or stimulate platelet aggregation appears to involve C-AMP (Table 15–4), which in itself is an inhibitor of platelet aggregation. The inhibitor PGE_1 induces a rise in C-AMP by a combination of adenyl cyclase activation and phosphodiesterase

inhibition, whereas the stimulator PGE_2 decreases C-AMP primarily by inactivation of adenyl cyclase and has little effect on phosphodiesterase. Aspirin, which inhibits the secondary phase of platelet aggregation, has no effect on C-AMP levels but does inactivate phosphodiesterase. PGA and PGF compounds which have little action on platelet aggregation are also devoid of C-AMP effects, strongly suggesting that the inhibition and stimulation of platelet aggregation by PGE_1 and PGE_2, respectively, are mediated by C-AMP.

Erythrocytes

Red cells normally undergo "deformity" as they pass through the capillary system. The degree of deformity may be an important determinant of red cell survival and control of the microcirculation. Furthermore, such deformability is highly dynamic, changing in response to sex, time of day, and a variety of hormones, including prostaglandins. The effect of PGE_1 is to increase deformability, whereas PGE_2 decreases it (1). $PGF_{2\alpha}$ is without effect except during certain periods of the menstrual cycle. In turkey erythrocytes, unlike in other cells, PGE_1 does not affect epinephrine-stimulated C-AMP accumulation (43). The significance of these effects, particularly with regard to red cell survival and the state of the microcirculation, remains to be clarified.

The Inflammatory Response

Local Inflammation

The inflammatory response is characterized by increased vascular permeability and vasodilatation with a subsequent migration of leukocytes leading to the classical signs of redness, heat, pain, and swelling. The induction of the response is multifold and includes burns, trauma, carrageenin administration, infection, and inflammatory diseases of unknown etiology such as rheumatoid arthritis. Bradykinin, serotonin, and histamine released into inflammatory areas by leukocytes have all been proposed as mediators of the response, but the specific agents involved and their interrelationships and mechanisms remain obscure.

Recent evidence has accumulated that prostaglandins may be important mediators of inflammation. In the first place, PGE and PGA but not PGF compounds markedly increase histamine-mediated vascular permeability and elicit all the classic signs of inflammation with the notable exception of skin pain. Secondly, prostaglandins have been shown to prolong the delayed phase of the acute inflammatory response when invasion of leukocytes occurs. PGE_1 is leukotactic in this regard; it has been shown to be released into local areas of inflammation. The separation of the inflammatory effects of PGE and PGA from the effects of simulta-

TABLE 15–4. EFFECT OF PROSTAGLANDINS ON PLATELET FUNCTION

	Platelet Aggregation*	C-AMP	Adenyl Cyclase	Phospho-diesterase
PGE_1	↓ ↓ ↓	↑ ↑ ↑	↑ ↑ ↑	↓ ↓
PGE_2	↑ ↑	↓ ↓	↓ ↓	0

*Induced by ADP.

↑ = Augmentation; ↓ = inhibition, PGA_1, $PGF_{1\alpha}$; and $PGF_{2\alpha}$ either do not affect or only minimally inhibit platelet aggregation, with slight increases in C-AMP.

neously released histamine and serotonin has been achieved in histamine- and serotonin-blocked rats, in which the delayed phase of acute inflammation mediated by PGE_2 persists. Lastly, Änggård and Jonsson (4) have demonstrated all the necessary precursors and enzymes for prostaglandin synthesis in human skin. In addition, they identified PGE_2 in the skin following burns and have suggested that it is an important capillary vasodilator mediator in the delayed phase of the acute inflammatory response.

Systemic Inflammation

Common systemic manifestations of inflammation are headache and fever, which are classically alleviated by such anti-inflammatory analgesic, antipyretic agents as aspirin, indomethacin, phenylbutazone, and aminopyrine, all compounds which markedly inhibit prostaglandin synthesis by inhibiting prostaglandin synthetase. There is strong evidence that the headache and fever are prostaglandin-mediated. There is a strong negative correlation between a variety of the effects of aspirin and PGE (Table 15–5). Firstly, pyrogen-induced fever is accompanied by a rise in hypothalamic prostaglandin content, and injections of PGE_1 into the third ventricle of cats produce a striking hyperthermia. Secondly, the classical analgesic, headache-relieving properties of aspirin may be the result of inhibition of PGE synthesis, since PGE_1 produces severe headaches when infused into man. Lastly, the anti-inflammatory action of aspirin has been shown to be most likely the result of inhibition of PGE synthesis, since the concentration of the latter is dramatically reduced in inflammatory exudates of aspirin- and indomethacin-treated animals. The anti-inflammatory action of corticosteroids is not believed to involve prostaglandin release, synthesis, or action. Although the evidence is circumstantial, it is likely that most, if not all, of the antiphlogistic actions of the nonsteroidal, anti-inflammatory agents are mediated, at least in part, by inhibition of PGE synthesis (48).

The Immune Response

Bronchial Asthma

Although the cause and mechanisms of human bronchial asthma are unknown, certain important facts are well established. In general, beta adrenergic stimulating agents such as isoproterenol result in bronchodilatation associated with a rise in intracellular C-AMP, whereas beta blocking agents or cholinergic stimulation leads to bronchoconstriction associated with a fall in intracellular C-AMP. There is increased evidence that asthma is a systemic disorder associated with partial beta adrenergic blockade since (1) asthmatic patients exhibit a reduced generalized metabolic response to epinephrine, (2) the peripheral lymphocytes show a decreased antigenic inactivation by cate-

TABLE 15–5. ASPIRIN AND PROSTAGLANDINS

	Aspirin	PGE
Fever	↓	↑
Headache	↓	↑
Local inflammation	↓	↑
Gastric HCl production	↑	↓
Experimental peptic ulceration	↑	↓
Cutaneous pain	0	0
Muscle pain	↓	?

↑ = Augmentation; ↓ = inhibition; 0 = no effect.

cholamines, and (3) there is a reduction in the rise of lymphocytic C-AMP in response to isoproterenol in blood from asthmatics as compared with controls (46).

The possibility of involvement of prostaglandins in asthma stems from the observation that PGE_1 and PGE_2 relax human bronchiolar smooth muscle *in vitro*, while $PGF_{2\alpha}$ contracts these muscles and inhibits the bronchodilating effect of isoproterenol (Table 15–6). Of great clinical interest is the fact that patients with bronchial asthma respond to cold temperatures with profuse nasal congestion and bronchiolar constriction, and that PGE_1 administration results in nasal vasoconstriction and bronchiolar dilation in such patients (15). There is one group of asthmatic patients whose disease is aggravated by aspirin, suggesting that in this group the bronchiolar constriction may be the result of aspirin inhibition of PGE_2 synthesis. Since both PGE_2 and $PGF_{2\alpha}$ have been demonstrated in human lung, it has been suggested that this disorder may arise in part from a decreased $PGE_2/PGF_{2\alpha}$ ratio.

Arthritis

Intradermal injection of complete Freund's adjuvant produces a severe polyarthritis which is prevented or inhibited by subcutaneous administration of PGE_1 and PGE_2, but not by PGA or PGF, compounds (53) (Table 15–6). It has been suggested that one mechanism by which PGE_2 might alleviate experimental arthritis is immunologic, involving inhibition of sensitized lymphocytic migration into the affected joints by increasing lymphocytic C-AMP. Drugs that increase the latter compound have been shown to decrease lymphocyte-mediated cytolysis of target cells (19). Paradoxically PGE_1 and PGE_2 in smaller doses appear to produce experimental arthritis and are capable of evoking such signs of inflammation as pain, swelling, heat, and redness. At present, the role of PGE's in inflammation in both experimental and human rheumatoid arthritis is unknown.

Immediate Hypersensitivity

One model of immediate hypersensitivity is antigen-induced histamine release from IgE antibody-sensitized basophils and from the lung, a reaction which is inhibited by catecholamines and

TABLE 15–6. EFFECT OF PROSTAGLANDINS ON THE IMMUNE RESPONSE

	C-AMP Intact Lymphocytes	Immediate Hyper-sensitivity	Leukocyte C-AMP*	Delayed Hyper-sensitivity	Lymphocyte Transformation†	Lymphocyte C-AMP	Adjuvant Arthritis	Bronchial Smooth Muscle
PGE_1	↑↑↑	↓↓↓	↑↑↑	↓↓↓‡	↓↓↓	↑↑↑	↓↓↓	↓↓↓
PGE_2	↑↑	↓↓↓	↑↑↑	↓↓↓	↓↓	↑↑↑	↓↓↓	↓↓↓
$PGF_{1\alpha}$	↑	0	0	0	↓	↑	N.T.	N.T.
$PGF_{2\alpha}$	N.T.	N.T.	↑	N.T.	N.T.	N.T.	0	↑↑↑
PGA_1	↑↑↑	N.T.	↑↑	N.T.	↓↓↓	↑↑↑	N.T.	N.T.
PGA_2	↑↑↑	N.T.	N.T.	N.T.	↓↓	↑↑	0	N.T.

*Values pertain to the immediate hypersensitivity reaction.
†As measured by DNA, RNA, and protein synthesis in phytohemagglutinin-stimulated lymphocyte proliferation.
‡Lymphocyte C-AMP levels elevated.
↑ = Augmentation; ↓ = inhibition; 0 = no effect; N.T. = not tested.

C-AMP, PGE_1, and PGE_2 but not by $PGF_{1\alpha}$. The effect of catecholamines is on beta adrenergic receptors, since their inhibition of histamine release can be blocked by propranolol, whereas no such inhibition occurs with PGE_1. In addition, catecholamine inhibition of histamine release is associated with a rise in leukocyte C-AMP which is blocked by propranolol, whereas the rise in C-AMP with prostaglandins is not so inhibited. PGE_1 and PGE_2 are the most potent of all the prostaglandins, while the PGA and PGF classes are almost inactive (Table 15–6). The evidence at present suggests that PGE compounds increase C-AMP, leading to decreased histamine release using a receptor other than that used by catecholamines.

Delayed Hypersensitivity

C-AMP and catecholamines inhibit the delayed hypersensitivity reaction. The most potent inhibitors, however, are prostaglandins PGE_1 and PGE_2, while $PGF_{1\alpha}$ (35) is inactive (Table 15–6). Again, as in acute hypersensitivity, the effect of the catecholamines but not of the PGE's is blocked by propranolol. Furthermore, PGE_1 inhibition is associated with a C-AMP increase in mononuclear cells. The possible therapeutic implication for such sensitivity reactions as bronchial asthma is noteworthy in that prostaglandins are able to bypass beta adrenergic stimulation of adenyl cyclase and lead to an independent rise in C-AMP which, at least theoretically, could act as a second messenger in inhibiting the hypersensitivity reaction.

Lymphocyte Transformation

Catecholamines stimulate adenyl cyclase in human lymphocytes, leading to a rise in C-AMP. A similar rise in C-AMP can be elicited by PGE and PGA compounds but to a much lesser degree by the PGF class (Table 15–6). The rise in C-AMP is not blocked by propranolol as is that of isoproterenol-induced C-AMP, suggesting a non-beta adrenergic mechanism for the prostaglandins. Phytohemagglutinin-induced lymphocyte transformation (measured by protein DNA and RNA synthesis) is inhibited by C-AMP as well as by PGA and PGE

(38) (Table 15–6); in fact, cell morphology concomitantly returns toward normal under the influence of C-AMP. Prostaglandins have been found in high concentrations in human colonic carcinomas (23), where they may act to promote regional vascularization or possibly in a compensatory fashion to retard cell division.

Gastrointestinal System

Intestinal Secretion

Intravenous administration of PGE_1, PGE_2, and PGA_1 to animals or humans or both inhibits the stimulation of gastric hydrochloric acid (HCl) secretion by histamine, pentagastrin, and food ingestion (51). Furthermore, in the rat, PGE_1 reduces the incidence of experimental ulcer formation resulting from pyloric ligation, a finding which has led to speculation that hypersecretion of gastric HCl causing Zollinger-Ellison syndrome and peptic ulcer may be due to a deficiency of prostaglandins normally located in and released from the stomach. Since C-AMP reduces gastric HCl secretion, it has been postulated that the mechanism of prostaglandin inhibition may be through activation of adenyl cyclase. Alternatively, a reduction in gastric mucosal blood flow could be the underlying mechanism.

PGE_1, PGA_1, and $PGF_{2\alpha}$ inhibit the absorption of sodium and water by the small intestine to such a degree that, with PGE and PGF, profuse watery diarrhea similar to that observed with cholera toxin occurs. In fact, both cholera toxin and PGE_1 produce a rise in mucosal adenyl cyclase and C-AMP, which itself inhibits intestinal sodium and water transport. From these observations the hypothesis has arisen that cholera toxin induces diarrhea by increasing intestinal prostaglandin release, leading to an elevation of C-AMP.

Intestinal Motility

PGE and PGF compounds which are normally present in the gastrointestinal tract are released by various stimuli and produce rhythmic contraction of longitudinal smooth muscle *in vitro* and, in the human being, *in vivo*. They appear to inhibit intestinal motility in the dog *in vivo*. It is believed that prostaglandins act directly on smooth muscle since the effects are only partially blocked by atropine. The role of prostaglandins in normal peristalsis remains to be clarified.

Metabolic and Endocrine Systems

Adipose Tissue

The lipolytic effect of glucagon, ACTH, and epinephrine is inhibited by PGE$_1$ *in vitro* (47). The lipolytic agents act by increasing fat-cell adenyl cyclase activity with a subsequent enhanced conversion of ATP to C-AMP (12). Theophylline, by inhibiting phosphodiesterase activity, also increases C-AMP and lipolysis. PGE$_1$ is antilipolytic; however, it does not inhibit the lipolytic activity of C-AMP, suggesting that the mechanism of antilipolytic activity of PGE$_1$ is through adenyl cyclase inhibition. The effects of experiments *in vivo* are conflicting, with reports of both lipolytic and antilipolytic effects of PGE$_1$ in dogs and in humans.

Thyroid

In contrast to the inhibiting effects on adipose-tissue adenyl cyclase, PGE$_1$ stimulates adenyl cyclase in slices of dog thyroid, resulting in an increase in C-AMP. Many of the effects of PGE$_1$ mimic those of TSH (enhanced glucose oxidation, conversion of H^3-adenine to H^3-C-AMP, P^{32} incorporation into phospholipids, and increased colloid droplet formation), suggesting that TSH may act by elevating PGE$_1$ concentration (Table 15–7). Field has presented evidence, however, which dissociates the C-AMP effects of other prostaglandins from thyroid hormone production (16), a phenomenon which is largely dose-dependent. This suggests a far more complicated mechanism of action than simple adenyl cyclase activation. However, support for TSH stimulation of thyroid prostaglandin production is derived from the fact that it is known

the thyroid contains large amounts of prostaglandin-like compounds (probably PGE$_1$, PGE$_2$, and PGF$_{2\alpha}$), and that TSH stimulates both thyroid prostaglandin production and hormonogenesis. Both hormonogenesis and the accompanying adenyl cyclase rise are inhibited by prostaglandin antagonists.

The only clinical prostaglandin syndromes so far described are associated with malignant amine-peptide-secreting tumors, notably medullary carcinoma of the thyroid. The clinical picture is characterized by profuse watery diarrhea and abdominal cramps, which may be the result of excessive PGE$_2$ or PGF$_{2\alpha}$ secretion or both by the tumor. The syndrome is associated with an increased incidence of pheochromocytoma.

Adrenals

PGE$_2$ accelerates corticosterone production as does ACTH (17). Since C-AMP also activates steroidogenesis, it has been suggested that PGE$_2$ activates adenyl cyclase in the adrenals, a situation analogous to that in the thyroid.

Central Nervous System

In the unanesthetized chick and mouse, PGE$_1$ has sedative, tranquilizing, and anticonvulsive effects. In the mouse, ptosis and ataxia result from the PGE$_1$ administration (20). In the cat, intraventricular administration of PGE$_1$ produces a loss of spontaneous movements and a catatonic-like state lasting up to 24 to 48 hours.

Although PGF$_{2\alpha}$ is without effect on intraventricular administration, intravenous administration of PGF$_{2\alpha}$ in the chick causes extension of the limbs and dorsiflexion of the neck. Horton and Main (22) showed that limb extension is the result of an increased gastrocnemius muscle tension secondary to an action of PGF in augmenting central but not peripheral spinal reflexes. Presumably, PGE$_1$ may have (1) a high inhibitory action of spinal reflexes and (2) a spinal excitatory action. From these considerations as well as the demonstration that PGE (but not PGF) antagonizes norepinephrine inhibition of Purkinje cell discharge (14), it has been suggested that certain prostaglandins may serve as central nervous system neurotransmitters.

TABLE 15–7. COMPARATIVE EFFECTS OF PGE$_1$ (μg. per ml.) AND TSH ON VARIOUS PARAMETERS OF THYROID METABOLISM *IN VITRO**

Parameter	PGE$_1$		TSH
Adenyl cyclase	↑	.02	↑
^{3}H-Cyclic AMP	↑	1	↑
Cyclic AMP	↑	1	↑
^{14}CO$_2$	↑	1	↑
^{32}Phospholipid	↑	100	↑
Colloid droplets	↑	1	↑

*Adapted from Field, J., Dekker, A., et al.: *Ann. N.Y. Acad. Sci.* 180:278, 1971, with permission. While PGA$_1$, PGF$_{2\alpha}$, and PGB$_1$ produce similar effects, the concentrations necessary to elicit a response are generally 100 times greater.

Ocular Effects

PGE$_2$ and PGF$_{2\alpha}$ are normal constituents of the eye synthesized and released by the iris. Administration of PGE$_1$, PGE$_2$, or PGF$_{2\alpha}$ produces a marked miosis in all species studied, which is antagonized by norepinephrine. In the rabbit but not in most other species, PGE$_1$ and PGE$_2$ cause an increased intraocular pressure believed to be the result of intraocular vasodilatation (50). As with miosis, the effect is inhibited by norepinephrine. PGE$_1$-like material has been extracted from human aqueous humor and found to be significantly higher in patients with open-angle glaucoma than in patients with cataract, suggesting an etiologic role for PGE_1 in the production of glaucoma (52). Lastly, PGE's have also been implicated in the etiology of uveitis.

MECHANISMS OF ACTION

Metabolic

3',5'-Cyclic AMP

It is obvious from the data presented in this chapter that a major action of prostaglandins is activation of adenyl cyclase in a wide variety of tissues and cell systems. Where prostaglandins give rise to an increase in C-AMP, target-cell function is almost inevitably enhanced (Table 15–8). Conversely, where cell function is depressed by prostaglandins, there is a decrease in C-AMP (Table 15–9).

Figure 15–8 illustrates a suggested mechanism by which prostaglandins exert a role in the transmission of the message of such tropic hormones as LH, TSH, and ACTH. The tropic hormone interacts with a membrane receptor, which leads to an increase in prostaglandin synthetase and prostaglandin production. The prostaglandins in turn activate membrane adenyl cyclase, possibly through a specific prostaglandin receptor. The resultant increase in C-AMP generated from ATP then produces its action on cell function. Prostaglandins

TABLE 15–9. TISSUES IN WHICH PROSTAGLANDINS* INHIBIT HORMONALLY INDUCED RESPONSES†

Tissue	Hormone	Response
Toad bladder	Vasopressin	Water transport
Rabbit kidney tubules	Vasopressin	Water transport
Rat adipocytes‡	Epinephrine	Lipolysis
	ACTH	
	TSH	
	Glucagon	
	Growth hormone	
Cerebellar Purkinje cells	Norepinephrine	Inhibition of discharge frequency

*PGE_1 most effective at <0.28 μM.
†From Shaw, J. E., Gibson, W., et al.: *Ann. N.Y. Acad. Sci.* 180:241, 1971, with permission.
‡Inhibition associated with decreased cyclic AMP accumulation.

would act as a second messenger and C-AMP as a third messenger. The most puzzling aspect, however, is the remarkable nonspecificity of prostaglandin action, augmenting C-AMP accumulation in some systems and inhibiting it in others. Unlike other stimulators of adenyl cyclase, whose action is restricted to a particular target cell (parathyroid hormone increases C-AMP in kidney and bone but not in other tissues), prostaglandins have effects on almost every cell line with the notable exception of vascular smooth muscle. Specificity, therefore, must reside and be inherent in each cell line in a manner yet to be demonstrated. Furthermore, as Horton has suggested (21), the fact that prostaglandins interact with C-AMP does not identify their biochemical mechanisms of action, which still remain to be defined. It is highly likely that, with the possible exception of PGA's, the prosta-

TABLE 15–8. TISSUES WHERE PROSTAGLANDINS INCREASE ACCUMULATION OF CYCLIC 3', 5'-AMP*

Tissue	Species	Prostaglandin (μM) most active	
Lung	Rat	PGE_1	2.8
Spleen	Rat	PGE_1	2.8
Diaphragm	Rat	PGE_1	2.8
Adipose	Rat	PGE_1	2.8
Leucocytes	Human	PGE_1	–
Platelets†	Human	PGE_1	0.28
Platelets	Human	PGE_1	0.01
Platelets	Human	PGE_1	0.1
Platelets	Rabbit	PGE_1	0.1
Platelets	Rabbit	PGE_1	0.15
Liver	Rat	PGE_1	–
Anterior pituitary†	Rat	PGE_1	2.8
Aorta	Rat	PGE_1	2.8
Bone	Rat	PGE_1	–
Gastric mucosa†	Guinea pig	PGE_1	–
Kidney	Dog, rat	PGE_1	–
Heart	Guinea pig	PGE_1	0.01
		$PGF_{1\alpha}$	0.01
Corpus luteum†	Cow	PGE_2	28
Thyroid†	Dog	PGE_2	
Erythrocytes†	Rat	PGE_2	0.03

*From Shaw, J. E., Gibson, W., et al.: *Ann. N.Y. Acad. Sci.* 180:241, 1971, with permission.
†Indicates those tissues in which prostaglandins increase adenyl cyclase activity.

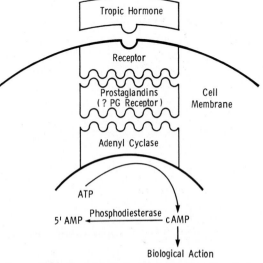

Figure 15–8. Postulated role of the interaction of prostaglandins and C-AMP in the transmission of the trophic hormone message. [Reproduced with modification from Speroff, L., et al.: Prostaglandins and reproduction, In *Prostaglandins.* Lee, J. B. (ed.), New York, Medcom (in press, 1973), with permission.]

glandins will be found to function as local intracellular mediators responding to regional stimuli specific to the tissues involved.

Na-K ATPase

The demonstration that PGA (but not PGE) inhibits Na-K ATPase in renal cortex and medulla *in vitro* (Table 15–2) has raised speculation that this enzyme may also be an important prostaglandin target. The inhibition is associated with a reduction in oxygen consumption and glucose oxidation. Since energy production in the kidney is largely confined to active sodium transport, it is likely that the natriuresis mediated by PGA may be the result of a decrease in ATP available for sodium reabsorption secondary to an inhibition of Na-K ATPase-linked active transport. That such a mechanism might also underlie the vasodilatory effects of PGA_1 is suggested by the fact that inhibition of vascular smooth muscle contraction by PGA_1 is abolished by ouabain, a relatively specific inhibitor of Na-K ATPase.

Vascular

The Microcirculation

The mechanism by which PGE and PGA compounds dilate peripheral arterioles is unclear, but it is probably by postsynaptic myogenic relaxation of vascular smooth muscle without involvement of adrenergic, histaminergic, or cholinergic nerve endings. A second mechanism involves interaction with well-established pressor systems, since the pressor responses to angiotensin, vasopressin, and norepinephrine are blunted or abolished by PGA's and PGE's. There is no current evidence that C-AMP is involved in the vascular response to prostaglandins. As mentioned previously, inhibition of Na-K ATPase may be included.

Blood Pressure Regulation

Figure 15–9 illustrates a schema of a proposed mechanism by which either renomedullary PGA_2 or PGE_2 might function as an intrarenal antihypertensive hormone. Behavioral hypertensive stimuli, such as intellectual activity, fright, and anxiety, cause elevation in blood pressure associated with intrarenal cortical vasoconstriction so that renocortical blood flow remains unchanged (the so-called autoregulation of the kidney). However, blood flow to the renal medulla is not believed to be autoregulated to this degree. With each elevation in arterial blood pressure, there is a corresponding rise in medullary blood flow, which might signal the release of PGA_2 or PGE_2 or both by the renomedullary interstitial cells. This might lead to intrarenal circulation of PGA_2 or PGE_2 or both from renal medulla to cortex and subsequently produce cortical vasodilatation. In this fashion,

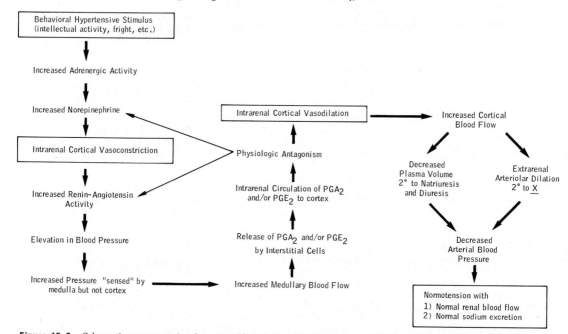

Schema of a Proposed Mechanism by Which Either Renomedullary
PGA_2 or PGE_2 May Function as an Intrarenal Antihypertensive "Hormone"

Figure 15–9. Schematic representation for a possible intrarenal role of the renomedullary prostaglandins in the regulation of systemic blood pressure and maintenance of normotension. [Reproduced from Lee, J. B., In *Prostaglandins in Cellular Biology.* Ramwell, P. W., and Pharriss, B. B. (eds.), New York, Plenum Publishing Corp., 1972, p. 399, with permission.]

relief of the intrarenal cortical vasoconstriction occasioned by the original hypertensive stimulus would take place. The enhanced cortical blood flow would lead to (1) natriuresis and decreased plasma volume, and (2) extrarenal arteriolar dilatation due either to prostaglandin or to unknown vasoactive compounds (designated $\underline{X}$). These effects would all result in a decrease in arterial blood pressure, with subsequent reduction in renal arteriolar perfusion pressure and sodium excretion. The resulting normotension would be associated with normal renal blood flow and normal sodium and water excretion. Alternatively, PGA_2 (but not PGE_2, since it is metabolized by the lung) could be released into the systemic circulation and exert generalized peripheral arteriolar dilatation.

Since PGA_2 and PGE_2 decrease outer medullary flow and increase cortical flow, a deficiency of such prostaglandins would be expected to result in decreased renal cortical flow, an observation repeatedly demonstrated in patients with essential hypertension. Thus systemic hypertension resulting from activation of renal pressor systems might result from cortical ischemia induced by such reduction in cortical blood flow. It can be hypothesized that hypertension could result from intrarenal vasoconstriction associated with a deficiency of renomedullary prostaglandins whose normal function might be to regulate cortical medullary blood flow distribution. According to this hypothesis, blood pressure control would reside within the kidney itself, and renal prostaglandins would not necessarily have to be secreted into the systemic circulation in order to regulate blood pressure.

THERAPEUTIC IMPLICATIONS

Although only preliminary human trials with prostaglandins have been undertaken, they hold promise as one of the most revolutionary therapeutic substances ever discovered. The most immediate applications are summarized in Table 15–10. It is unlikely that the PGE and PGF classes can ultimately be given intravenously because of their side effects, particularly with regard to their gastrointestinal effects. If, as it is postulated, they normally act as local regulators (hormones by definition circulate), new delivery routes will have to be devised to produce a specific therapeutic response in one organ (such as a PGE aerosol for bronchial asthma) which would not result in an undesirable effect in a different organ (such as the effect of PGE in stimulating contraction of the uterus). The synthesis of a number of prostaglandin analogues with more specific actions offers an alternative in obviating their nonspecific effects.

In contrast to PGE's and PGF's, PGA's can be given intravenously to produce antihypertensive effects since they do not stimulate nonvascular smooth muscle contraction. It is also possible that they may be effective orally and that their action is prolonged by production of analogues that are metabolized at a slower rate. The difference between prostaglandins and most pharmaceuticals is that the former are naturally occurring, and their administration may constitute specific replacement therapy (such as the use of oral or parenteral PGA_2 in human beings with essential hypertension, whose disorder may be a genetic or acquired deficiency of PGA_2).

The investigation of prostaglandin action holds great promise for revealing as yet undiscovered cellular events. Although there has probably been excessive exuberance for the therapeutic potential of prostaglandins in some areas, it remains likely that further study of these compounds will markedly increase the understanding of many basic biologic processes and provide innovative and possibly revolutionary avenues of medical therapy.

TABLE 15–10. POTENTIAL THERAPEUTIC APPLICATIONS OF THE PROSTAGLANDINS

Hypertension
Bronchial asthma
Anaphylactic shock
Edema
Induction of labor
Induction of abortion
Gastric hyperacidity and peptic ulceration
Coronary and deep venous thrombosis
Nasal congestion
Infertility
Glaucoma (prostaglandin antagonist)
Cholera and Zollinger-Ellison syndrome
    (prostaglandin antagonist)
Burns (prostaglandin antagonist)

REFERENCES

1. Allen, J. E., and Rasmussen, H.: Some effects of vasoactive hormones on the mammalian red blood cell, In *Prostaglandins in Cellular Biology*. Ramwell, P. W., and Pharriss, B. B. (eds.), New York, Plenum Press, 1972, p. 27.
2. Anderson, G. G., Hobbins, J. C., et al.: Midtrimester abortion using intra-amniotic prostaglandin $F_{2\alpha}$. *Prostaglandins* 1:147, 1972.
3. Anderson, G. G., Hobbins, J. C., et al.: Intravenous prostaglandins E_2 and $F_{2\alpha}$ for the induction of term labor. *Amer. J. Obstet. Gynec.* 112:382, 1972.
4. Änggård, E., and Jonsson, C. E.: Formation of prostaglandins in the skin following a burn injury, In *Prostaglandins in Cellular Biology*. Ramwell, P. W., and Pharriss, B. B. (eds.), New York, Plenum Press, 1972, p. 269.
5. Armstrong, D. T., and Grinwick, D. L.: Blockade of spontaneous and LH-induced ovulation in rats by indomethacin, an inhibitor of prostaglandin biosynthesis. *Prostaglandins* 1:21, 1972.
6. Beerthuis, R. K., Nugteren, D. H., et al.: The biosynthesis of prostaglandins. *Biochim. Biophys. Acta* 90:204, 1964.
7. Behrman, H. R., MacDonald, G. J., et al.: Regulation of ovarian cholesterol esters: Evidence for the enzymatic sites of prostaglandin-induced loss of corpora luteum function. *Lipids* 6:791, 1971.
8. Bergström, S., Danielsson, H., et al.: The enzymatic formation of prostaglandin E_2 from arachidonic acid. *Biochim. Biophys. Acta* 90:207, 1964.
9. Bergström, S., and Samuelsson, B. (eds.), *Nobel Symposium II, Prostaglandins*. Stockholm, Almqvist and Wiksell, 1967.
10. Bergström, S., and Sjövall, J.: The isolation of prostaglandin E from sheep prostate glands. *Acta Chem. Scand.* 14:1701, 1960.

11. Bergström, S., and Sjövall, J.: The isolation of prostaglandin F from sheep prostate glands. *Acta Chem. Scand.* 14:1693, 1960.

12. Butcher, R. W., Pike, J. E., et al.: The effect of prostaglandin E_1 on adenosine 3′,5′-monophosphate levels in adipose tissue, In *Nobel Symposium II, Prostaglandins.* Bergström, S., and Samuelsson, B. (eds.), Stockholm, Almqvist and Wiksell, 1967, p. 133.

13. Caldwell, B. V., Tillson, S. A., et al.: The effects of exogenous progesterone and estradiol on prostaglandin F levels in ovariectomized ewes. *Prostaglandins* 1:217, 1972.

14. Coceani, F., Puglisi, L., et al.: Prostaglandins and synaptic activity in spinal cord and cuneate nucleus. *Ann. N. Y. Acad. Sci.* 80:289, 1971.

15. Cuthbert, M. F.: Effect on airways resistance to prostaglandin E_1 given by aerosol to healthy and asthmatic volunteers. *Brit. Med. J.* 4:723, 1969.

16. Field, J., Dekker, A., et al.: *In vitro* effects of prostaglandins on thyroid gland metabolism. *Ann. N. Y. Acad. Sci.* 180:278, 1971.

17. Flack, J. D., Jessup, R., et al.: Prostaglandin stimulation of rat corticosteroidogenesis. *Science* (New York) 163:691, 1969.

18. Goldblatt, M. W.: Depressor substance in seminal fluid. *Chem. Industr.* 52:1056, 1953.

19. Henney, C. S., and Lichtenstein, L. M.: The role of cyclic AMP in the cytolytic activity of lymphocytes. *J. Immun.* 107:610, 1971.

20. Horton, E. W.: Action of prostaglandins E_1, E_2 and E_3 on the central nervous system. *Brit. J. Pharmacol.* 22:189, 1964.

21. Horton, E. W.: *Prostaglandins.* Berlin, Springer-Verlag, 1972.

22. Horton, E. W., and Main, I. H. M.: Further observations on the central nervous actions of prostaglandins $F_{2\alpha}$ and E_1. *Brit. J. Pharmacol.* 30:568, 1967.

23. Jaffe, B. M., Parker, C. W., et al.: Prostaglandin release by human cells *in vitro*, In *Prostaglandins in Cellular Biology.* Ramwell, P. W., and Pharriss, B. B. (eds.), New York, Plenum Press, 1972, p. 207.

24. Karim, S. M. M., and Filshei, G. M.: Therapeutic abortion using prostaglandin $F_{2\alpha}$. *Lancet* 1:157, 1970.

25. Karim, S. M. M., Twissell, R. R., et al.: Induction of labor with prostaglandin $F_{2\alpha}$. *Brit. Med. J.* 4:621, 1968.

26. Kloeze, J.: Influence of prostaglandins on platelet adhesiveness and platelet aggregation, In *Nobel Symposium II, Prostaglandins.* Bergström, S., and Samuelsson, B. (eds.). Almqvist and Wiksell, Stockholm, 1967, p. 241.

27. Kurzrock, R., and Lieb, C. C.: Biochemical studies of human semen II. *Proc. Soc. Exp. Biol. Med.* 26:268, 1930.

28. Lee, J. B.: Chemical and physiological properties of renal prostaglandins with emphasis on the cardiovascular effects of medullin in essential human hypertension, In *Nobel Symposium II, Prostaglandins.* Bergström, S., and Samuelsson, B. (eds.), Almqvist and Wiksell, Stockholm, 1967, p. 197.

29. Lee, J. B.: Prostaglandins. *Physiologist* 13:379, 1970.

30. Lee, J. B., Covino, B. G., et al.: Renomedullary vasodepressor substance, medullin: Isolation, chemical characterization and physiological properties. *Circ. Res.* 7:57, 1965.

31. Lee, J. B., Crowshaw, K., et al.: The identification of prostaglandin E_2, $F_{2\alpha}$ and A_2 from rabbit kidney medulla. *Biochem. J.* 105:1251, 1967.

32. Lee, J. B., Hickler, R. B., et al.: Sustained depressor effects of renal medullary extract in the normotensive rat. *Circ. Res.* 13:369, 1963.

33. Lee, J. B., Kannegiesser, H., et al.: Hypertension and the renomedullary prostaglandins: A human study of the antihypertensive effects of PGA_1. *Ann. N. Y. Acad. Sci.* 180:218, 1971.

34. Lee, J. B., McGiff, J. C., et al.: Antihypertensive renal effects of prostaglandin A_1 in patients with essential hypertension. *Ann. Intern. Med.* 74:703, 1971.

35. Lichtenstein, L. M., and Henney, C. S.: Prostaglandin inhibition of immediate and delayed hypersensitivity *in vitro*, In *Prostaglandins in Cellular Biology.* Ramwell, P. W., and Pharriss, B. B. (eds.), New York, Plenum Press, 1972, p. 293.

36. McCracken, J. A., Baird, D. T., et al.: Factors affecting the secretion of steroids from the transplanted ovary in the sheep. *Recent Progr. Hormone Res.* 27:537, 1971.

37. O'Grady, J. P., Kohorn, E. I., et al.: Inhibition of progesterone synthesis *in vitro* by prostaglandin $F_{2\alpha}$. *J. Reprod. Fertil.* 30:153, 1972.

38. Parker, C. W.: The role of prostaglandins in the immune response, In *Prostaglandins in Cellular Biology.* Ramwell, P. W., and Pharriss, B. B. (eds.), New York, Plenum Press, 1972, p. 173.

39. Ramwell, P. W., and Pharriss, B. B. (eds.), *Prostaglandins in Cellular Biology.* New York, Plenum Press, 1972.

40. Ramwell, P. W., and Shaw, J. E. (eds.), *Prostaglandin Symposium of the Worcester Foundation for Experimental Biology.* New York, John Wiley and Sons, 1968.

41. Roth-Brandel, U., Bygdeman, M., et al.: Prostaglandins for induction of therapeutic abortion. *Lancet* 1:191, 1970.

42. Samuelsson, B., Granström, E., et al.: Metabolism of prostaglandins. *Ann. N. Y. Acad. Sci.* 180:139, 1971.

43. Shaw, J. E., Gibson, W., et al.: The effect of PGE_1 on cyclic AMP and ion movements in turkey erythrocytes. *Ann. N. Y. Acad. Sci.* 180:241, 1971.

44. Shio, H., and Ramwell, P. W.: Prostaglandin E_1 and E_2: Qualitative difference in platelet aggregation, In *Prostaglandins in Cellular Biology.* Ramwell, P. W., and Pharriss, B. B. (eds.), Plenum Press, New York, 1972, p. 77.

45. Smith, J. B., and Willis, A. L.: Aspirin selectively inhibits prostaglandin production in platelets. *Nature New Biol.* 231:235, 1971.

46. Smith, J. W., and Parker, C. W.: The responsiveness of leukocyte cyclic AMP to adrenergic agents in patients with asthma. *Proc. Cent. Soc. Clin. Res.* 43:76, 1970.

47. Steinberg, D., Baughan, M., et al.: Effects of prostaglandin E opposing those of catecholamines on blood pressure and on triglyceride breakdown in adipose tissue. *Biochem. Pharmacol.* 12:764, 1963.

48. Vane, J. R.: Inhibition of prostaglandin synthesis as a mechanism of action for aspirin-like drugs. *Nature New Biol.* 231:232, 1971.

49. von Euler, U. S.: Zur Kenntnis der pharmakologischen Wirkungen von nativsekreten und extrakten männlicher accessorischer Geschlectsdrüsen. *Arch. Exp. Path. Pharmakol.* 175:78, 1934.

50. Waitzman, M. B., and King, C. D.: Prostaglandin influences on intraocular pressure and pupil size. *Amer. J. Physiol.* 212:329, 1967.

51. Wilson, D. E., Cosmos, P., et al.: Inhibition of gastric secretion in man by prostaglandin A_1. *Gastroenterology* 61:201, 1971.

52. Wyllie, A. M., and Wyllie, J. H.: Prostaglandins and glaucoma. *Brit. Med. J.* 3:615, 1971.

53. Zurier, R. B., and Weissmann, G.: Effect of prostaglandins upon enzyme release from lysosomes and experimental arthritis, In *Prostaglandins in Cellular Biology.* Ramwell, P. W., and Pharriss, B. B. (eds.), New York, Plenum Press, 1972, p. 151.

CHAPTER 16

Cyclic Nucleotides and Hormone Action

By Joel G. Hardman

Historical Background
(2, 12, 13, 16, 17, 36, 39, 44, 45, 46, 48)

The elucidation by E. W. Sutherland, T. W. Rall, and their colleagues of the hepatic glycogenolytic action of glucagon and epinephrine was a signal development in biomedical research. Not only did the work of these investigators provide an understanding of how some hormones control blood glucose levels, but also, more importantly, it revealed a mechanism by which many hormones bring about at least some of their actions in a variety of cell types.

By 1951 it was known from the work of Sutherland and Cori that epinephrine and glucagon accelerated the rate of hepatic glycogen breakdown by increasing the amount of active glycogen phosphorylase in the liver. Attempts to show effects of the hormones on the activity of phosphorylase in cell-free systems were unsuccessful, however.

Realizing that a knowledge of the fundamental properties of liver phosphorylase would be essential to an understanding of how hormones regulated the enzyme, Sutherland and his colleagues in the early 1950's set about to purify the enzyme and to find out what happened to it when it became ac-

tivated. Liver phosphorylase was found to exist in interconvertible active and inactive forms. Inactivation of the active form of the enzyme was shown to be accompanied by the release of inorganic phosphate from the protein, a reaction catalyzed by another enzyme, phosphorylase phosphatase. Reactivation of the inactive form of enzyme was found to result from the incorporation into the protein of the terminal phosphate group from ATP in a reaction catalyzed by a third enzyme, phosphorylase kinase.

With this information in hand, Rall, Sutherland, and Berthet were able to perform a landmark experiment in 1956 demonstrating that epinephrine and glucagon could bring about the activation of phosphorylase in a cell-free system, a homogenate of cat liver. The key to the success of this experiment was the fortification of the homogenate with Mg^{++} and ATP, which were required for the kinase reaction. The hormones seemed to work by increasing the activity of the kinase.

The next logical step—attempting to demonstrate the hormone effects in the soluble fraction of the homogenate—yielded surprising results. In spite of the presence of inactive phosphorylase, the phosphatase, and the kinase in the soluble fraction, epinephrine and glucagon were devoid of action on phosphorylase activity when the insoluble fraction of the homogenate was removed by low-speed centrifugation.

Thus the hormones were shown to act not directly on the phosphorylase system but indirectly by way of a process that required the presence of a particulate fraction of the liver. In short order, this process was shown to involve the formation of a heat-stable, small molecule by the particulate fraction. Epinephrine and glucagon stimulated the formation of this substance, which was able to bring about the activation of phosphorylase when added to the soluble fraction of the liver. The substance was shown to be a nucleotide formed from ATP, and it could be produced by particulate fractions of several different tissues.

At about the same time, Dr. David Lipkin and

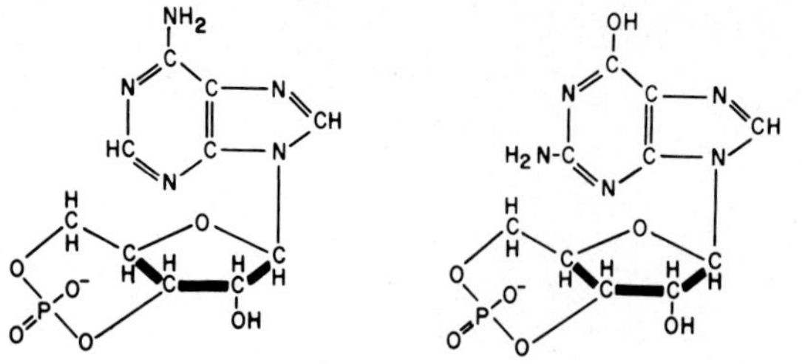

CYCLIC AMP   **CYCLIC GMP**

Figure 16–1. Structural formulas for cAMP and cGMP.

his colleagues were attempting to identify a product formed nonenzymatically from ATP when it was heated with Ba(OH)$_2$. The Sutherland group in Cleveland and the Lipkin group in St. Louis were put in touch with each other after they both wrote to Dr. Leon Heppel in Bethesda, asking him for an enzyme to help in the characterization of what seemed to Dr. Heppel to be similar substances. The two groups soon found that they were indeed studying the same compound, and its identity was established as adenosine 3′,5′-monophosphate, or cyclic AMP (cAMP) (Fig. 16–1).

By 1959, R. C. Haynes and his associates had demonstrated that ACTH could stimulate the accumulation of cAMP in the adrenal cortex, and that cAMP could mimic the actions of ACTH to activate phosphorylase and to stimulate steroidogenesis in that tissue. During the next decade, further work from Sutherland's laboratory and from several other laboratories indicated that cAMP was a mediator of diverse effects of a number of hormones in a variety of cell types.

In 1963, Ashman and his associates reported the presence in rat urine of another cyclic nucleotide, guanosine 3′,5′-monophosphate, or cyclic GMP (cGMP) (Fig. 16–1). These investigators were searching for organic phosphate compounds in urine, and, following the injection of inorganic ^{32}P into rats, they could identify two radioactive organic compounds in urine. One of these was cAMP, and the other was cGMP. Three years later the excretion of cGMP in rats was shown to vary with altered hormonal states and to vary independently of that of cAMP, suggesting that the metabolic pathways of the two cyclic nucleotides were under separate hormonal control. The existence of separate biosynthetic systems for cGMP and cAMP and the presence of cGMP in tissues was reported in 1969.

Beginning with the observation by George and co-workers that acetylcholine raised cGMP in the perfused rat heart, a growing list of agents has been shown to raise concentrations of this nucleotide in many cell types. Often agents that raise cGMP have effects that appear to be functionally opposite to effects of agents that raise cAMP, an example being the myocardial effects of acetylcholine, which raises cGMP, and of beta adrenergic agents, which raise cAMP. Such situations have led to the suggestion by Goldberg and associates

that cGMP and cAMP in general play antagonistic regulatory roles. Although cGMP has not been unequivocally shown to mediate the action of any hormone, there is substantial evidence to suggest its involvement in cellular regulatory mechanisms.

The "Second Messenger" Concept (39, 45, 47, 48)

Sutherland and his associates conceived a role for cAMP in the actions of some hormones as that of a "second messenger." A hormone released from an endocrine gland (or a neurotransmitter substance released from a nerve ending), the "first messenger," interacts with its receptor on the plasma membrane of its target cell (Fig. 16–2). As a result of the hormone-receptor interaction, there is an increase (or perhaps in some cases a decrease) in the activity of the enzyme, adenylate cyclase, which is associated with the plasma membrane and apparently closely associated morphologically with the hormone receptor. An increase in the activity of adenylate cyclase leads to an increase in the rate of formation of cAMP, which in turn alters certain enzyme activities or other cell processes and thereby elicits responses that are characteristic for the cell and the hormone involved.

Because individual cell types have functional receptors for only certain hormones, hormones that raise the cAMP content in some cell types do not raise it in all cell types. Because different cAMP-sensitive processes survive or arise during cell differentiation, an increase in cAMP content does not cause the same response in all cell types. Thus glucagon does not stimulate steroid hormone formation by the adrenal cortex, because it does not raise the cAMP content there, and it does not stimulate steroid hormone formation by the liver, even though it raises the cAMP content there, because biosynthetic pathways for steroid hormones are absent.

Sutherland and his associates suggested three criteria that should be satisfied to implicate cAMP

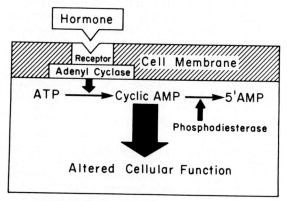

Figure 16–2. Schematic representation of the role of cAMP as a "second messenger" in hormone action, as suggested by Sutherland and associates. (From Liddle, G. W., and Hardman, J. G.: *New Eng. J. Med. 285*:560, 1971.)

as the primary mediator of a hormone action in a certain tissue. The hormone should stimulate adenylate cyclase activity in a cell-free system of the tissue in point; the hormone should increase the content of cAMP in an intact cell system of the tissue in a manner that is appropriate with respect to the time course and dose-response relation of the familiar effect of the hormone; finally, cAMP itself should reproduce the effect of the hormone when the nucleotide is added to an intact cell system. All three of these criteria have been met for several hormones, but only one or two have been met for others. Extending the criteria to include cGMP and its possible role in hormone action, in no case have all three criteria been fulfilled as yet.

The concept of cAMP as a "second messenger" does *not* imply (a) that cAMP is unique in playing such a role, (b) that cAMP is responsible for *all* the actions of hormones that work through cAMP to produce some of their effects, or (c) that all hormones use a "second messenger" system.

Cyclic Nucleotide Functions not Involving Hormones (4, 5, 13, 18, 20, 30, 33, 34, 35, 39, 52)

This chapter deals with aspects of the roles or possible roles of cyclic nucleotides only in hormone actions. In so limiting a discussion of cyclic nucleotides, it is probable that some of their most fundamental biologic functions will be ignored. Recent findings from many laboratories indicate that cyclic nucleotides are involved in regulatory processes that were important to primitive life forms before the evolution of endocrine systems or hormones as they are commonly thought of.

Cyclic AMP levels in bacteria rise when certain foodstuffs in the medium become exhausted, and the elevated levels of the nucleotide then participate in the synthesis of enzymes that the bacteria need to metabolize other foodstuffs. In the complex life cycle of cellular slime molds, cAMP seems to function extracellularly, in a sense as a hormone itself, to promote the aggregation of free swimming amoebae and the differentiation of some of the aggregated cells to function as specialized parts of a primitive multicellular organism. An abundance of evidence points to possible roles for cAMP and cGMP in cell division, and abnormalities in the metabolism of one or both of these compounds have been suggested to be of great importance in cell transformation. Physiologic stimuli other than hormones may act on cells in higher organisms via changes in cyclic nucleotide metabolism; a possible role for cAMP in visual excitation is suggested by the presence in outer rod segments from vertebrate retina of a large amount of an adenylate cyclase that is reported to be inactivated by light.

In all probability, the role of cyclic nucleotides in hormone action is only one of many regulatory functions served by these substances. As systems of cell to cell communication arose during evolution of multicellular organisms, messages sent from one cell to another in the form of some hormones were probably translated through cyclic nucleotide–regulated systems that were already established and important in adaptive processes in single-celled organisms.

Effects of Cyclic Nucleotides in Hormone-Sensitive Tissues (4, 13, 16, 18, 19, 22, 23, 29, 39, 45)

Cyclic AMP can produce many diverse effects when added to various intact and broken cell systems (Table 16-1). In most if not all of the examples shown in the table, the effect of cAMP is at least qualitatively similar to that produced by a hormone. For example, the effects of exogenous cAMP on the liver in general mimic effects of glucagon and epinephrine, and the effects of cAMP on steroidogenesis in the adrenal and corpus luteum mimic effects of ACTH and LH, respectively. The probable role of protein kinase in mediating many effects of cAMP will be discussed in a later section.

Cyclic AMP, a highly polar compound at physiologic pH, is often ineffective when applied to intact cells or is effective only in such high concentrations that its effects are difficult to evaluate. A series of acylated derivatives of cAMP, the most commonly used ones being the N^6-butyryl and the $N^6,O^{2'}$-dibutyryl derivatives, often have been much more effective than the parent compound in producing effects on intact cells. The effects of these derivatives are assumed, although not always established, to be like those produced by native, endogenous cAMP. The greater effectiveness of the derivatives, compared with exogenous cAMP itself, may result from their reduced polarity and presumed greater ability to enter cells (and then perhaps be converted to cAMP), or from their ability to inhibit phosphodiesterase, which thereby elevates the level of endogenous cAMP.

Effects of exogenous cGMP in hormone-sensitive tissues have been less extensively studied than have those of cAMP. Often exogenous cGMP is ineffective when cAMP or one of its derivatives is effective in reproducing the effect of a certain hormone. In other cases, cGMP elicits responses from intact cells that are qualitatively similar to those elicited by exogenous cAMP. In a few cases, derivatives of cGMP have been reported to produce effects that appear to be functionally antagonistic to those produced by cAMP or a derivative of it. For example, dibutyryl cGMP is said to reproduce acetylcholine effects in reducing the rate of contraction of cultured myocardial cells and in producing depolarization of the postganglionic membrane of the superior cervical ganglion. The antigen-stimulated release of histamine and slow-reacting substance A from human lung fragments is reported to be enhanced by acetylcholine and by 8-bromo-cGMP. In all three of these cases, dibutyryl cAMP is said to produce effects that are functionally opposite to those produced by the derivatives of cGMP. Whether or not these derivatives of cGMP are suitable models for the parent compound in biologic systems is unknown.

TABLE 16–1. A PARTIAL LIST OF EFFECTS OF CYCLIC AMP IN VARIOUS CELL-FREE AND INTACT CELL SYSTEMS*

Enzyme or Process Affected	Tissues	Change in Activity or Rate
Protein kinase	Several	Increased
Phosphorylase	Several	Increased
Glycogen synthetase	Several	Decreased
Phosphofructokinase	Liver fluke	Increased
Lipolysis	Adipose	Increased
Clearing factor lipase	Adipose	Decreased
Amino acid uptake	Adipose	Decreased
Amino acid uptake	Liver and uterus	Increased
Synthesis of several enzymes	Liver	Increased
Net protein synthesis	Liver	Decreased
Gluconeogenesis	Liver	Increased
Ketogenesis	Liver	Increased
Steroidogenesis	Several	Increased
Water permeability	Epithelial	Increased
Ion permeability	Epithelial	Increased
Calcium resorption	Bone	Increased
Renin production	Kidney	Increased
Discharge frequency	Cerebellar Purkinje	Decreased
Membrane potential	Smooth muscle, superior cervical ganglion	Increased
Tension	Smooth muscle	Decreased
Contractility	Cardiac muscle	Increased
HCl secretion	Gastric mucosa	Increased
Fluid secretion	Insect salivary glands	Increased
Amylase release	Parotid gland	Increased
Insulin release	Pancreas	Increased
Thyroid hormone release	Thyroid	Increased
Calcitonin release	Thyroid	Increased
Release of other hormones	Anterior pituitary	Increased
Histamine release	Mast cells	Decreased
Melanin granule dispersion	Melanocytes	Increased
Aggregation	Platelets	Decreased
Proliferation	Thymocytes	Increased
Cell growth	Tumor cells	Decreased

*Compiled by Sutherland, E. W.: Studies on the mechanism of hormone action. *Science* 177:401-408, August, 1972. Copyright 1972 by the American Association for the Advancement of Science.

Cyclic Nucleotide Concentrations in Tissues (11, 13, 39, 42)

The concentrations of cAMP and cGMP in tissues represent only a very small fraction of the total adenine or guanine nucleotide content. The total adenine nucleotide concentration of most tissues of the rat is between 2 and 5 mmoles/kg. wet weight; about 90% of this is ATP. Cyclic AMP concentrations generally fall between 0.1 and 1.0 μmole/kg. wet weight, about 0.01% of the ATP concentrations. Cyclic GMP makes up a similarly small percentage of the total guanine nucleotide content. Concentrations of cGMP are usually between 0.01 and 0.1 μmole/kg. wet weight, about 10% or less of cyclic AMP concentrations. Relative concentrations of cAMP and cGMP vary considerably, however; the concentration of cAMP in the rat liver under basal conditions is nearly 100 times that of cGMP, whereas the two cyclic nucleotides are present in the cerebellum in almost equal concentrations.

In all likelihood, neither the cyclic nucleotides nor their triphosphate precursors are uniformly distributed throughout the intracellular space. There is some indication, from experiments in which the adenine nucleotides of intact cells have been labeled with radioactive adenine or adenosine, that more than one pool of ATP exists. Other types of data suggest that at least a substantial fraction of the cAMP that exists in the basal state is in a sequestered or metabolically inert pool. For example, the basal concentration of cAMP, if uniformly distributed throughout the cell, would be high enough to produce maximum activation of cAMP-dependent protein kinase as discussed later, based on the enzyme's behavior in cell-free systems, yet the protein kinase in intact cells is known to be in a predominantly inactive state under basal conditions. Furthermore, low but effective glycogenolytic concentrations of glucagon or epinephrine can produce a marked increase in the amount of cAMP extruded from the perfused rat liver, while causing only barely detectable changes in the tissue concentration of cAMP, suggesting that the newly synthesized and presumably metabolically active cAMP may be in a pool that at times represents only a small fraction of the total cell content of the nucleotide.

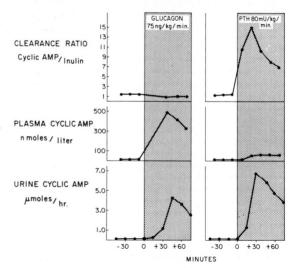

Figure 16–3. Effects of glucagon and parathyroid hormone on urine and plasma cAMP, and on the ratio of cAMP clearance/inulin clearance in a human subject. (From Kaminsky, N. I., Broadus, A. E., et al.: *J. Clin. Invest.* 49:2387, 1970.)

Cyclic Nucleotides in Extracellular Fluids (7, 9, 13, 31, 39)

Cyclic AMP and cGMP are found in plasma, urine, seminal plasma, milk, and cerebrospinal fluid. The cyclic nucleotides are the only nucleotides normally excreted in urine. Virtually all of the cGMP in human urine is derived from plasma by glomerular filtration. Only part of the cAMP in urine is derived from plasma; normally one-third to one-half the cAMP in urine is derived from renal tissue.

Cyclic AMP levels in extracellular fluids often reflect actions of hormones to raise concentrations of the nucleotide in certain organs. Glucagon raises the concentration of cAMP in the liver, and some of the nucleotide exits from the hepatocytes and appears in plasma and then in urine (Fig. 16–3). Parathyroid hormone raises the concentration of cAMP in the kidney, and the cAMP that exits from tubular cells appears largely in the urine and only minimally in plasma (Fig. 16–3). Plasma and urine levels of cAMP also can be increased by beta adrenergic agents, and levels of cGMP can be increased by alpha adrenergic agents.

The finding that some hormones can increase the concentration of cyclic nucleotides in extracellular fluids has raised the possibility that altered levels might be detectable in certain endocrinopathies

and perhaps be of some diagnostic value. Although it is too early to say how valuable such determinations will be, studies by Broadus, Chase, Murad, and their associates and by others suggest a cause for optimism.

Cyclic AMP concentrations in plasma are normally between 1 and 3×10^{-8} M; cGMP concentrations in plasma are lower than those of cAMP, but only by two- to threefold, not by ten- to a hundredfold as in most tissues. The plasma levels of both nucleotides appear to be far too low to produce any effects on intact cells, since concentrations of 10^{-5} to 10^{-2} M are usually required to produce effects on various intact cells *in vitro*. Very high local concentrations of cyclic nucleotides in extracellular fluids and possible effects of these on some cell types cannot be ruled out, however. Indeed, concentrations of cAMP in milk and seminal plasma have been observed in the 10^{-5} M range.

Cyclic Nucleotide Biosynthesis (4, 13, 15, 16, 18, 39, 48)

Cyclic AMP is formed from ATP by a reaction catalyzed by the Mg^{++}- or Mn^{++}-requiring enzyme, adenylate cyclase; the other product of this reaction is inorganic pyrophosphate (Fig. 16–4). In mammalian cells, adenylate cyclase is largely if

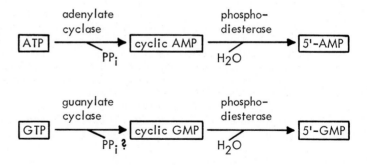

Figure 16–4. Established pathways of the biosynthesis and degradation of cyclic nucleotides. Formation of pyrophosphate in the guanylate cyclase reaction has not been established. Separate phosphodiesterases may or may not be involved in the hydrolysis of the cyclic nucleotides.

not entirely associated with plasma membranes. There have been suggestions that some of the enzyme may be associated with other structures, for example, sarcoplasmic reticulum in skeletal muscle and heart. The insolubility and relative instability of mammalian adenylate cyclase have precluded a high degree of purification. Adenylate cyclase from some bacteria is a soluble protein, and extensive purification of this material has been achieved.

Cyclic GMP is formed from GTP by a reaction catalyzed by the enzyme, guanylate cyclase (Fig. 16–4). Unlike adenylate cyclase, guanylate cyclase is usually found in both soluble and particulate fractions of most mammalian tissues, although it may be predominantly associated with either the soluble or the particulate fraction in a given tissue. The subcellular distribution of the particulate form of guanylate cyclase has not been extensively studied. Whether or not there are important differences in the properties of the particulate and soluble forms of the enzyme is not known.

Guanylate cyclase requires Mn^{++} for maximum activity, differing generally in this regard from adenylate cyclase, which usually uses either Mn^{++} or Mg^{++}, but which in a few cases also has an absolute or near absolute requirement for Mn^{++} (this appears to be true of adenylate cyclase from sperm and from some lower organisms). Although adenylate and guanylate cyclases are distinct and separable enzymes in most if not all tissues thus far examined, it has not been possible to rule out absolutely the possibility that a single enzyme may in some cases have both adenylate and guanylate cyclase activity.

Cyclic Nucleotide Degradation (10, 13, 15, 18, 32, 39, 49)

The only established pathway for the biochemical degradation of cAMP and cGMP is hydrolysis of the $3'$ bond, yielding the corresponding $5'$-nucleoside monophosphate (Fig. 16–4). This reaction is catalyzed by one or more cyclic nucleotide phosphodiesterases, which occur in both soluble and particulate fractions of most if not all cells.

Cyclic nucleotide phosphodiesterases can be found in two or more soluble forms in homogenates of most cell types. Different forms of the enzyme have been separated by ion-exchange chromatography, gel filtration, and other means. These forms seem to differ in their apparent molecular weights, relative and perhaps absolute substrate specificity, kinetic behavior, and in some cases sensitivity to cations or to synthetic inhibitors. Thompson and Appleman have demonstrated in a variety of tissues the presence of one form of phosphodiesterase that has a much higher apparent affinity for cGMP than for cAMP, and another form that has a higher apparent affinity for cAMP than for cGMP. Phosphodiesterase activity associated with particulate fractions of at least some tissues seems to have a higher affinity for cAMP than for cGMP. Whether the different forms of phosphodiesterase represent distinct molecular species or different configurational or oligomeric forms of a single enzyme has not been made clear. While the physiologic significance of the apparent multiplicity of form is uncertain, the implication is that there is a preferential degradative pathway for each of the cyclic nucleotides.

The possibility of a pathway for the degradation of cyclic nucleotides not involving phosphodiesterase has not been ruled out. Murad and coworkers have reported formation in cell-free systems of an unidentified substance that seems to inhibit the ability of cAMP to activate liver phosphorylase. There is some indication that this substance is formed from cAMP. If so, this would mean that a second pathway for cAMP degradation exists, since $5'$-AMP, the product of the phosphodiesterase reaction, does not interfere with cAMP effects on phosphorylase activity.

In addition to enzyme-catalyzed degradation, cyclic nucleotide "inactivation" could be brought about by a translocation of the nucleotide from one cell compartment to another or by extrusion of the nucleotide from the cell. Makman and Sutherland observed that cAMP was extruded rapidly from *Escherichia coli* in the presence of a high glucose concentration, which caused a lowering of the intracellular concentration of cAMP. Other studies by Davoren and Sutherland indicated that avian erythrocytes could extrude cAMP against a concentration gradient. Such observations indicate that in at least some cell types there is a process for cyclic nucleotide extrusion that is more complicated than simple passive diffusion. This process may be useful to the cell in controlling its cyclic nucleotide concentrations. Whether or not such a system is important in mammalian cells is unknown, but this possibility is suggested by the fact that several mammalian organs can rapidly extrude cAMP when its formation is stimulated by hormones.

Effects of Hormones and other Agents on Cyclic Nucleotide Metabolism (4, 6, 11, 12, 13, 18, 26, 27, 28, 38, 39, 40, 41, 43, 48, 50)

Cyclic AMP

The concentration of a cyclic nucleotide in a cell can be raised either by accelerating its synthesis or by inhibiting its degradation. Hormones that can increase cAMP levels in intact cells in all cases studied seem to do so by increasing the rate of conversion of ATP to cAMP. There is no established case of a hormone raising cAMP by inhibiting its degradation, although some drugs are inhibitors of cyclic nucleotide phosphodiesterase in cell-free systems, and some of these agents, notably the methyl xanthines, caffeine and theophylline, can increase the concentrations of both cAMP and cGMP in intact cells.

TABLE 16–2. SOME HORMONES AND OTHER AGENTS THAT HAVE BEEN SHOWN TO INCREASE CYCLIC AMP CONCENTRATIONS IN INTACT CELLS OR TO STIMULATE ADENYLATE CYCLASE ACTIVITY IN CELL-FREE SYSTEMS

Agent	Tissue
Catecholamines* (beta-component)	Many
Dopamine*	Superior cervical ganglion
Glucagon*	Liver, fat, heart, pancreatic islets
Secretin	Fat, liver
ACTH*	Adrenal cortex, fat
Angiotensin II	Adrenal cortex
Vasopressin*	Toad bladder, kidney, pituitary gland
Oxytocin	Kidney, toad bladder
Luteinizing hormone* (ICSH)	Corpus luteum, ovary, testis
Follicle stimulating hormone	Testis
Melanocyte stimulating hormone	Frog skin (dorsal)
Parathyroid hormone*	Kidney, bone
Calcitonin	Kidney, bone
Histamine*	Mast cells, brain, gastric mucosa
Hypothalamic extract	Pituitary gland
Thyrotropin releasing factor	Pituitary gland
Prostaglandins*	Many

*Hormones for which all three criteria discussed in the text for mediation by cAMP have been met in one or more tissues.

Hormones that can rapidly increase cAMP levels in intact cells or that can increase adenylate cyclase activity in cell-free systems include the catecholamines and many, but not all, peptide hormones (Table 16–2). Although not fitting the classical definition of hormones, agents such as histamine, dopamine, serotonin, prostaglandin E_1, and angiotensin II also increase cAMP levels in some cell types.

Studies, initially from Sutherland's laboratory and subsequently from the laboratories of Rodbell and other investigators, have shown that some hormones are capable of increasing adenylate cyclase in cell-free homogenates, rigorously washed particulate material, or purified plasma membranes from heart, liver, adipose tissue, and other hormone-sensitive tissues. Studies by Rodbell and associates and by others indicate a close relationship between the amount of a hormone that binds to plasma membranes and the degree of activation of adenylate cyclase in the membranes produced by the hormone. Such observations suggest a close functional and anatomical relationship between hormone receptors and the catalytic moiety of adenylate cyclase.

A number of lines of evidence suggest that hormonal activation of adenylate cyclase involves a more complicated process than simple binding of a hormone to the enzyme. Adenylate cyclase from at least some hormone-sensitive tissues can be dispersed with detergents, but the enzyme usually loses its sensitivity to hormones in the process. According to Levey, specific phospholipids can restore responsiveness of detergent-dispersed adenylate cyclase from the myocardium to specific hormones. The restoration of responsiveness does not appear to be a result of any effect of the phospholipid on hormone binding. Rodbell and associates have shown that very low concentrations of GTP can enhance the responsiveness of membrane-bound adenylate cyclase to hormones while, in at least some instances, reducing the amount of hormone bound. From the work of Lefkowitz and associates, it appears that calcium is required for the activation of adrenal adenylate cyclase by ACTH but not for the binding of ACTH to its receptor.

Robison and associates have suggested that hormone receptors might be analogous to allosteric regulatory subunits of adenylate cyclase, being oriented so that the site of hormone attachment is on the external surface of the cell. Others have suggested the existence of a functional if not morphologic coupling system between the hormone receptor and adenylate cyclase. At present such conjecture cannot be confirmed experimentally, because the inability to achieve extensive purification of adenylate cyclase from hormone-sensitive cells makes it difficult if not impossible to define precisely the relationship between a hormone receptor and the catalytic function of adenylate cyclase. Thus a clear understanding of the molecular basis of hormonal activation of adenylate cyclase must await new techniques or experimental approaches.

Several hormones and other agents can lead to a reduced concentration of cAMP in various cell types under some conditions. These substances include specific hormone antagonists, such as beta adrenergic receptor blocking agents, which can prevent catecholamine effects to increase cAMP in intact tissues or to increase the activity of adenylate cyclase in cell-free systems.

In addition to receptor blocking agents, another group of chemically heterogeneous substances prevents hormone-induced elevations in cAMP in several cell types without any apparent selectivity as to the type of hormone involved. These substances seem to work not by interfering with hormone-receptor interactions but by interfering with the expression of these interactions. Agents that fall in this category are insulin, prostaglandin E₁, alpha adrenergic agents, melatonin, nicotinic acid, and perhaps other agents. The reader should not infer that these agents work by a common mechanism to reduce cAMP concentrations, for this is not known. On the other hand, the possibility cannot be ruled out.

How these agents prevent hormone-induced elevations in cAMP concentrations is not clear. Insulin has been claimed by some investigators to inhibit adenylate cyclase in cell-free systems, but other investigators have been unable to confirm such an effect. Still other investigators have observed small increases in phosphodiesterase activity when the enzyme is prepared from intact cells exposed to insulin but not when insulin is added to the enzyme in a cell-free system. It is not clear whether or not small effects on phosphodiesterase

can account for the ability of insulin to lower cAMP levels in some cells, and it does not appear that the effect of insulin on phosphodiesterase is a direct one. Similarly, the ability of alpha adrenergic agents and other substances to lower cAMP cannot clearly be linked to a direct effect on either adenylate cyclase or phosphodiesterase.

It is important to keep in mind that these substances do not appear to be able to reduce cAMP levels in all cell types on which they have effects. For example, the well-known effects of insulin on heart and skeletal muscle appear not to be accompanied by a detectable reduction in cAMP concentration, and the effects of alpha adrenergic agents to cause contraction of smooth muscle, at least in general, are not accompanied by a detectable reduction in cAMP concentration. Therefore the reduction in cAMP following exposure of tissues to insulin and some other agents may be a secondary phenomenon occurring in some but not all types of target cells and probably participating in, but not primarily causing, the overall response to the agent.

Cyclic GMP

Agents that have been shown to increase the level of cGMP in intact cells (Table 16–3) usually do not elevate and may even reduce the level of

TABLE 16–3. SOME AGENTS THAT HAVE BEEN SHOWN TO INCREASE CYCLIC GMP CONCENTRATIONS IN INTACT CELLS*

Tissue	Source	Agents
Heart ventricle	Rat	Acetylcholine
Heart ventricle	Calf	Acetylcholine
Cerebellum	Mouse	Maaloxone, oxotremorine, D-amphetamine, electroconvulsive shock (postictal depression)
Cerebellum	Rabbit	Acetylcholine, histamine
Cerebral cortex	Mouse	Oxotremorine, atropine
Cerebral cortex	Rabbit	Acetylcholine
Forebrain	Mouse	Electroconvulsive shock (postictal depression)
Lung	Rabbit	Methacholine
Uterus	Rat	Oxytocin, serotonin, methacholine, prostaglandin F₂
Ductus deferens	Rat	Carbachol, acetylcholine, K⁺, norepinephrine
Intestinal smooth muscle	Guinea pig	Acetylcholine, histamine, serotonin, K⁺
Submaxillary gland	Rat	Methacholine
Anterior pituitary	Rat	Hypothalamic extract
Ova	Sea urchin	Sperm
Platelets	Human	Epinephrine, collagen
Lymphocytes	Human	Phytohemagglutinin, concanavalin A, acetylcholine, insulin†
Plasma	Human	Norepinephrine, epinephrine
Urine	Human	Norepinephrine epinephrine Parathyroid hormone, Ca⁺⁺
Urine	Rat	Calcitonin, parathyroid hormone
Urine	Dog	Methacholine
Bacteria	Escherichia coli	Glucose

*This list was compiled by Goldberg, N. D., O'Dea, R. F., et al. Cyclic GMP, In *Advances in Cyclic Nucleotide Research,* Vol. III. Greengard, P., and Robison, G. A. (eds.), New York, Raven Press, © 1973; references may be found in their article.
†The effect of insulin on cyclic GMP in lymphocytes was observed by Goldberg and associates (personal communication) after the list was compiled.

cAMP in the same cell type. At least some of these agents, however, can increase cAMP levels in other cell types and occasionally even in the same cell type. Different receptors are probably involved when an agent raises both cyclic nucleotides. This seems clear for catecholamines, which interact with beta receptors, at least in most cases, to raise cAMP and which seem to work through alpha receptors when they raise cGMP.

Agents that can raise cGMP in intact cells, as tested thus far, have been incapable of affecting the activity of guanylate cyclase in cell-free systems. As of this writing, only one hormone, secretin, has been reported to stimulate the activity of guanylate cyclase in cell-free systems (Thompson et al., 1973). It is not known whether or not secretin can elevate cGMP concentrations in any intact cells.

At least some of the agents that increase cGMP concentrations in cells require the presence of extracellular Ca^{++} to do so, and alterations in extracellular Ca^{++} concentrations lead to alterations in cGMP levels in some tissues. Thus Ca^{++} can be shown to increase the activity of guanylate cyclase in cell-free systems under some conditions. For these reasons, Schultz and co-workers have suggested that alterations in guanylate cyclase activity can occur secondary to hormone-induced alterations in cytoplasmic Ca^{++} concentrations. Secondary effects of hormones on adenylate cyclase activity via alterations in local concentrations of Ca^{++} or other ions also is a possibility. In cell-free systems Ca^{++} is usually inhibitory to adenylate cyclase activity, but it also is usually inhibitory to cyclic nucleotide phosphodiesterase. There is some evidence, however, that small amounts of Ca^{++} may be required for activities of some adenylate cyclases and phosphodiesterases. Thus alterations in cytoplasmic Ca^{++} could conceivably alter cyclic nucleotide levels in intact cells in either a positive or a negative direction by potential effects on either cyclase or phosphodiesterase systems.

Although there is little reason to believe that steroid hormones bring about their familiar effects by directly and rapidly altering cyclic nucleotide levels (the same can be said for thyroid hormone and some peptide hormones), these substances may have actions that involve in other ways cyclic nucleotides or cyclic nucleotide–sensitive processes. For example, the presence of glucocorticoids seems to be required for normal expression of the effects of cAMP on carbohydrate and lipid metabolism in some tissues. It is possible that such substances have effects on protein synthesis or electrolyte distribution that alter the synthesis or sensitivity of enzymes that participate in cyclic nucleotide action or metabolism.

for all effects of some hormones, perhaps even in cells where those hormones raise cAMP. Several agents that are known to raise cAMP in some cell types can produce effects in other cell types that are not related to a rise in cAMP but may in some instances even be related to a fall in cAMP. These agents include catecholamines and their alpha and beta effects, prostaglandin E_1, histamine, antidiuretic hormone, oxytocin, and angiotensin II. Indeed, even insulin, which can lower cAMP in fat and liver, can be shown to elevate cAMP in fat and muscle under some conditions; moreover, acetylcholine, which usually has no effect on or reduces cAMP levels, is reported to raise cAMP in intestinal smooth muscle under some conditions.

Thus one is led to consider the possibility that many hormones are capable of bringing about effects by at least two distinct mechanisms, one of which is an elevation of cAMP and another of which either is independent of a change in cAMP or is associated with a reduction in cAMP. Rasmussen has offered evidence that hormones that can raise cAMP also can stimulate the uptake of calcium into the cell independently of their effect on cAMP. Batzri and co-workers have obtained evidence that, in parotids, a beta adrenergic effect (cAMP elevation and stimulated amylase secretion) and an alpha adrenergic effect (potassium release) occur simultaneously in the same cell. Whether or not all hormones that can raise cAMP have the ability to elicit effects by another mechanism, perhaps involving elevated cytoplasmic calcium or, in other words, having the functional equivalents of adrenergic beta and alpha activities, remains to be firmly established. It is possible that the full expression of many familiar hormone effects may depend on the simultaneous occurrence of "beta- and alpha-equivalent" effects.

Whether or not cGMP plays a role in "alpha-equivalent" effects, perhaps analogous to the role of cAMP in "beta-equivalent" effects, remains to be established. As discussed above, elevated tissue concentrations of cGMP have been shown to occur in response to alpha adrenergic compounds, histamine, acetylcholine, and insulin under conditions in which cAMP levels are not elevated or are reduced, and elevated levels of cGMP seem to occur secondarily to an increased cytoplasmic calcium concentration in at least some cases. With a few exceptions, and perhaps very important exceptions, cGMP has not yet been shown to be able to reproduce effects of agents that increase its concentration in tissues. It is probably premature, therefore, to conclude that cGMP mediates (or co-mediates with calcium) effects of agents that increase its levels in cells, at least in all cases.

Possible Multiple Mechanisms of Hormone Action (1, 3, 13, 21, 26, 37, 43)

Although cAMP appears to mediate a number of hormone effects in many tissues, an increase in the concentration of this nucleotide does not account

Mechanisms of Action of Cyclic Nucleotides (8, 13, 14, 18, 23, 24, 25, 26, 33, 34, 35, 39, 51)

The only well-documented mechanism of cAMP action in mammalian cells is that elucidated by E. G. Krebs and his colleagues—the activation of one or more enzymes that catalyze the transfer of the terminal phosphate of ATP to a protein. Such enzymes, which are widely distributed in nature, are usually referred to as *cAMP-dependent protein kinases*. These enzymes are quite insensitive to cGMP, but protein kinases selectively stimulated by cGMP have been shown to exist in arthropods and in mammalian cerebellum. Other protein kinases in various cell types are insensitive to both cyclic nucleotides. Although cAMP-dependent protein kinase is very insensitive to cGMP, extremely high concentrations of this nucleotide can activate the enzyme. This is of no physiologic importance, but it may explain cAMP-like effects of high concentrations of cGMP applied to intact cells.

The activation by cAMP of protein kinase results from the binding of cAMP to a regulatory subunit which, without cAMP bound to it, restrains the activity of the catalytic subunit of the enzyme. When cAMP binds to the regulatory subunit, the two subunits dissociate, and the catalytic subunit is then freely active. This interaction was expressed by Brostrom and co-workers as follows:

$$RC + cAMP \rightleftharpoons R\text{-}cAMP + C$$

in which R is the regulatory subunit and C is the catalytic subunit of protein kinase. This process appears to be a dynamic equilibrium and can be reversed by removing or reducing the concentration of cAMP.

The substrate proteins for the cAMP-activated protein kinases may either gain or lose certain properties as a result of the incorporation of phosphate. For example, muscle phosphorylase kinase is activated through a protein kinase–catalyzed phosphorylation, whereas muscle glycogen synthetase is inactivated by the same process. This reciprocal effect of protein kinase on the activities of these two enzymes provides for more efficient glycogenolysis.

Many other proteins can be phosphorylated by cAMP-dependent protein kinases *in vitro*. Whether or not all of these phosphorylations occur *in vivo* and result in alterations of cell function is not known. Several criteria have been proposed by Krebs and associates for the mediation of cAMP effects by protein phosphorylation. These criteria, along with several proteins that are substrates for cAMP-dependent protein kinases *in vitro*, are given in Table 16–4.

With phosphorylase kinase, glycogen synthetase, and triglyceride lipase, the altered enzyme activity clearly is associated with alteration of important biochemical processes (glycogenolysis, glycogenesis, and lipolysis, respectively). Since casein is an effective substrate for cAMP-dependent protein kinases from most tissues, the ability of a protein to serve as a substrate for a protein kinase *in vitro* does not necessarily mean that an important physiologic process is altered as a result of its phosphorylation *in vivo*. It is possible that phosphorylation of histones or of ribosomal protein could be involved in effects of cAMP on protein synthesis, that phosphorylation of microtubular pro-

TABLE 16–4. CRITERIA FOR MEDIATION OF cAMP EFFECT BY PROTEIN PHOSPHORYLATION*

Substrate	1	2	3	4	5	6
Phosphorylase kinase	+	+	+	+	−	+
Glycogen synthetase	+	+	+	+	−	+
Triglyceride lipase	+	+	+	+	−	±
Histone F$_1$	+	+	±	−	+	−
Other	+	+	−	−	−	−
Protamine	+	−	−	−	+	±
Ribosomal proteins	+	+	±	−	+	−
Membrane proteins	+	+	−	−	+	−
Casein	+	+	−	−	−	−
Phosvitin	+	+	−	−	−	−
RNA polymerase	+	+	+	−	−	−
Polynucleotide phosphorylase	+	−	+	−	−	−
Microtubular protein	+	+	−	−	−	−
Troponin	+	+	−	−	−	−

*From Krebs, E. G. (24) and Walsh, D. A., and Ashby, C. D.: *Recent Progr. Hormone Res. 29:*329, 1973.

+ = Criterion satisfied; − = criterion not yet satisfied.
The number at the top of each column indicates the criterion from the list.

(1) Cell type involved contains a cAMP-dependent protein kinase.
(2) Protein which bears a functional relationship to cAMP-mediated process is phosphorylated *in vitro*.
(3) *In vitro* phosphorylation of protein leads to modified function.
(4) Stoichiometric correlation exists between *in vitro* phosphorylation and modified function.
(5) Demonstration of phosphorylation *in vivo* in response to cAMP.
(6) Demonstration of modified function *in vivo* in response to cAMP.

tein could be involved in effects on secretory processes, or that phosphorylation of troponin could be involved in an effect on muscle contraction. As can be seen in Table 16–4, however, evidence is lacking in varying degrees to firmly document the physiologic significance of the phosphorylation of these and several other potentially important substrates for cAMP-dependent protein kinases. At least some tissues contain what appear to be multiple forms of cAMP-dependent protein kinases. These forms, separable by ion exchange chromatography or other techniques, in some cases appear to have quite similar, and in other cases clearly different, physical properties. The possibility exists that the ability of cAMP to alter a variety of processes in one tissue, e.g., glycogenolysis, gluconeogenesis, ketogenesis, and ureogenesis in liver, involves activation of different protein kinases for the different processes. A single protein kinase, however, could also bring about multiple effects by using several substrates.

Kuo and Greengard have suggested that all effects of cAMP are brought about through the activation of protein kinases. This could be the case in mammalian cells, but Pastan and his associates have shown that the capacity of cAMP to promote the synthesis of messenger RNA in *Escherichia coli* seems to be independent of a protein kinase. These effects of cAMP require a receptor protein for cAMP, but this receptor protein does not appear to be associated with a protein kinase. The cAMP–receptor protein complex appears to stimulate the synthesis of specific messenger RNA in cell-free extracts of bacteria by binding to DNA in such a way that the binding of RNA polymerase is facilitated. Whether or not analogous mechanisms exist in higher organisms has not yet been documented.

REFERENCES

1. Andersson, R., Lundholm, L., et al.: Role of cyclic AMP and Ca^{++} in metabolic and mechanical events in smooth muscle, In *Advances in Cyclic Nucleotide Research*. Vol. 1. Greengard, P., Paoletti, R., et al. (eds.), New York, Raven Press, 1973.
2. Ashman, D. F., Lipton, R., et al.: Isolation of adenosine 3′,5′-monophosphate and guanosine 3′,5′-monophosphate from rat urine. *Biochem. Biophys. Res. Commun.* 11:330, 1963.
3. Batzri, S., Selinger, Z., et al.: Potassium ion release and enzyme secretion: Adrenergic regulation by α and β-receptors. *Science* 174:1029, 1971.
4. Bitensky, M. W., and Gorman, R. E.: Cellular responses to cyclic AMP, In *Progress in Biophysics and Molecular Biology*. Butler, J. A. V., and Noble, D. (eds.), Oxford, Pergamon Press, 1973.
5. Bonner, J. T.: Cyclic AMP in the cellular slime molds, In *The Role of Adenyl Cyclase and Cyclic 3′,5′-AMP in Biological Systems. Fogarty International Center Proceedings No. 4*. Rall, T. W., Rodbell, M., et al. (eds.), Washington, U.S. Govt. Printing Office, 1971.
6. Breckenridge, B. M.: Cyclic AMP and drug action. *Ann. Rev. Pharmacol.* 10:19, 1970.
7. Broadus, A. E., Hardman, J. G., et al.: Extracellular cyclic nucleotides. *Ann. N.Y. Acad. Sci.* 185:50, 1971.
8. Brostrom, C. O., Corbin, J. D., et al.: Interaction of the subunits of adenosine 3′,5′-cyclic monophosphate–dependent protein kinase of muscle. *Proc. Nat. Acad. Sci. USA* 68:2444, 1971.
9. Chase, L. R., Melson, G., et al.: Pseudohypoparathyroidism: Defective excretion of 3′,5′-AMP in response to parathyroid hormone. *J. Clin. Invest.* 48:1832, 1969.
10. Davoren, P. R., and Sutherland, E. W.: The effect of L-epinephrine and other agents on the synthesis and release of adenosine 3′,5′-phosphate by whole pigeon erythrocytes. *J. Biol. Chem.* 238:3009, 1963.
11. Exton, J. H., Lewis, S. B., et al.: The role of cyclic AMP in the interaction of glucagon and insulin in the control of liver metabolism. *Ann. N.Y. Acad. Sci.* 185:85, 1971.
12. George, W. J., Polson, J. B., et al.: Elevation of guanosine 3′,5′-cyclic phosphate in rat heart after perfusion with acetylcholine. *Proc. Nat. Acad. Sci. USA* 66:398, 1970.
13. Goldberg, N. D., O'Dea, R. F., et al.: Cyclic GMP, In *Advances in Cyclic Nucleotide Research*. Vol. II. Greengard, P., and Robison, G. A. (eds.), New York, Raven Press, 1973.
14. Greengard, P., and Kuo, J. F.: On the mechanism of action of cyclic AMP, In *Role of Cyclic AMP in Cell Function. Advances in Biochemical Psychopharmacology*. Vol. 3. Greengard, P., and Costa, E. (eds.), New York, Raven Press, 1970.
15. Hardman, J. G., Beavo, J. A., et al.: The formation and metabolism of cyclic GMP. *Ann. N.Y. Acad. Sci.* 185:27, 1971.
16. Hardman, J. G., Robison, G. A., et al.: Cyclic nucleotides. *Ann. Rev. Physiol.* 33:311, 1971.
17. Haynes, R. C., Koritz, S. B., et al.: Influence of adenosine 3′,5′-monophosphate on corticoid production by rat adrenal glands. *J. Biol. Chem.* 234:1421, 1959.
18. Jost, J. P., and Rickenberg, H. V.: Cyclic AMP. *Ann. Rev. Biochem.* 40:741, 1971.
19. Kaliner, M., Orange, R. P., et al.: Immunological release of histamine and slow reacting substance of anaphylaxis from human lung. IV. Enhancement by cholinergic and alpha adrenergic stimulation. *J. Exp. Med.* 136:556, 1972.
20. Konijn, T. M.: Cyclic AMP as a first messenger, In *Advances in Cyclic Nucleotide Research*. Vol. 1. Greengard, P., Paoletti, R., et al. (eds.), New York, Raven Press, 1972.
21. Kono, T., and Barham, F. W.: Effects of insulin on the levels of cAMP and lipolysis in fat cells (abstract). *Fed. Proc.* 32:535, 1973.
22. Krause, E. G., Halle, W., et al.: Effect of dibutyryl cyclic GMP on cultured beating rat heart cells, In *Advances in Cyclic Nucleotide Research*. Vol. 1. Greengard, P., Paoletti, R., et al. (eds.), New York, Raven Press, 1972.
23. Krebs, E. G.: Protein kinases, In *Current Topics in Cellular Regulation*. Horecker, B. L., and Stadtman, E. R. (eds.), New York, Academic Press, 1972.
24. Krebs, E. G.: The mechanism of hormonal regulation by cyclic AMP. *Proceedings of the Fourth International Congress of Endocrinology* (June, 1972, Washington, D.C.). Amsterdam, Excerpta Medica Foundation, 1973 (in press).
25. Kuo, J. F., and Greengard, P.: An adenosine 3′,5′-monophosphate dependent protein kinase from *Escherichia coli. J. Biol. Chem.* 244:3417, 1969.
26. Larner, J.: Insulin and glycogen synthase. *Diabetes 21* (Suppl. 2):428, 1972.
27. Lefkowitz, R. S., Roth, J., et al.: Effects of calcium on ACTH stimulation of the adrenal: Separation of hormone binding from adenyl cyclase activation. *Nature* (London) 228:864, 1970.
28. Levey, G. S.: Restoration of norepinephrine responsiveness of solubilized myocardial adenylate cyclase by phosphatidylinositol. *J. Biol. Chem.* 246:7405, 1971.
29. Makman, R. S., and Sutherland, E. W.: Adenosine 3′,5′-phosphate in *Escherichia coli. J. Biol. Chem.* 240:1309, 1965.
30. McAfee, D. A., and Greengard, P.: Adenosine 3′,5′-monophosphate: Electrophysiological evidence for a role in synaptic transmission. *Science* 178:310, 1972.
31. Murad, F., and Pak, C. Y. C.: Urinary excretion of adenosine 3′,5′-monophosphate and guanosine 3′,5′-monophosphate. *New Eng. J. Med.* 286:1382, 1972.
32. Murad, F., Rall, T. W., et al.: Conditions for the formation, partial purification and assay of an inhibitor of adenosine 3′,5′-monophosphate. *Biochim. Biophys. Acta* 192:430, 1969.
33. Pastan, I.: Cyclic AMP. *Sci. Amer.* 227:97, 1972.
34. Pastan, I., and Perlman, R.: Cyclic AMP in bacteria. *Science* 169:339, 1970.
35. Pastan, I., Perlman, R. L., et al.: Regulation of gene expression in *Escherichia coli* by cyclic AMP. *Recent Progr. Hormone Res.* 27:421, 1971.
36. Rall, T. W., Sutherland, E. W., et al.: The relationship of epinephrine and glucagon to liver phosphorylase. III. Reactivation of liver phosphorylase in slices and in extracts. *J. Biol. Chem.* 218:483, 1956.
37. Rasmussen, H.: Cell communication, calcium ion, and cyclic adenosine monophosphate. *Science* 170:404, 1970.
38. Robison, G. A., Butcher, R. W., et al.: Adenyl cyclase as an adrenergic receptor. *Ann. N.Y. Acad. Sci.* 139:703, 1967.
39. Robison, G. A., Butcher, R. W., et al.: *Cyclic AMP*. New York, Academic Press, 1971.
40. Rodbell, M., Birnbaumer, L., et al.: The glucagon-sensitive adenyl cyclase system in plasma membranes of rat liver. V. An obligatory role of guanyl nucleotides in glucagon action. *J. Biol. Chem.* 246:1877, 1971.
41. Rodbell, M., Krans, H. M. J., et al.: The glucagon-sensitive adenyl cyclase system in plasma membranes of rat liver. III. Binding of glucagon: Method of assay and specificity. *J. Biol. Chem.* 246:1861, 1971.
42. Sattin, A., and Rall, T. W.: The effect of adenosine and adenine nucleotides on the cyclic adenosine 3′,5′-phosphate content of guinea pig cerebral cortex slices. *Molec. Pharmacol.* 6:13, 1970.
43. Schultz, G., Hardman, J. G., et al.: Cyclic nucleotides and smooth muscle function, In *Asthma: Physiology, Immunopharmacology and Treatment*. Austen, F., and Lichtenstein, L. (eds.), New York, Academic Press, 1974.

44. Sutherland, E. W.: Hormonal regulatory mechanisms, In Liebecq, C. (ed.), *Proceedings of the Third International Congress of Biochemistry,* Brussels, 1955. New York, Academic Press, 1956.

45. Sutherland, E. W.: Studies on the mechanism of hormone action. *Science 177:*401, 1972.

46. Sutherland, E. W., and Cori, C. F.: Effect of hyperglycemic-glycogenolytic factor and epinephrine on liver phosphorylase. *J. Biol. Chem. 188:*531, 1951.

47. Sutherland, E. W., Øye, I., et al.: The action of epinephrine and the role of the adenyl cyclase system in hormone action. *Recent Progr. Hormone Res. 21:*623, 1965.

48. Sutherland, E. W., and Rall, T. W.: The relation of adenosine 3′,5′-phosphate and phosphorylase to the actions of cat-echolamines and other hormones. *Pharmacol. Rev. 12:*265, 1960.

49. Thompson, W. J., and Appleman, M. M.: Characterization of cyclic nucleotide phosphodiesterases of rat tissues. *J. Biol. Chem. 246:*3145, 1971.

50. Thompson, W. J., Williams, R. H., et al.: Activation of guanyl cyclase and adenyl cyclase by secretin. *Biochim. Biophys. Acta 302:*329, 1973.

51. Walsh, D. A., and Ashby, C. D.: Protein kinases: Aspects of their regulation and diversity. *Recent Progr. Hormone Res. 29:*329, 1973.

52. Whitfield, J. F., Rixon, R. H., et al.: Calcium, cyclic adenosine 3′,5′-monophosphate, and the control of cell proliferation. A review. *In Vitro 8:*257, 1973.

CHAPTER 17

Protein Metabolism and Hormones

By Keith L. Manchester

Many hormones influence the rate of growth and the size attained of a variety of individual organs in the body or of the body as a whole (Table 17–1). The protein content of cells is in a constant state of dynamic turnover. Growth is therefore achieved when the rate of protein formation is in excess of the rate of catabolism, while in the adult the two processes are in overall balance. In seeking to understand how the various hormones control growth, it is logical to look at their influence on the sequential steps of protein synthesis and also on those of catabolism, though very little is known about the mechanism of protein breakdown. Concentrating attention on protein metabolism alone, however, is a gross oversimplification, since growth and development often include cell division and differentiation. These are very complex processes, also subject to hormonal regulation, whose mechanisms, let alone control, are as yet little understood.

REACTIONS OF PROTEIN SYNTHESIS

The main steps in the formation of a protein molecule are shown in Figure 17–1 (3, 12). In building up such a molecule, a precise number of amino

TABLE 17–1. HORMONES CONTROLLING GROWTH

Hormone	Organ(s) Stimulated	Hormone Deficiency State
Thyroxine	Many	Myxedema
Growth hormone	Many, including liver, fat tissue, and muscle	Dwarfism
Insulin	Many, including liver, fat tissue, and muscle	Diabetes
Estrogen	Uterus, mammary gland, hen oviduct	
Androgen	Prostate, seminal vesicles, muscle, kidney	Eunuchoidism
ACTH	Adrenal gland	Hypoadrenocorticism
TSH	Thyroid	Hypothyroidism
FSH and LH	Testes, ovaries	Hypogonadism
Prolactin	Mammary gland	Hypolactation
Glucosteroid	Many, but inhibits protein synthesis in all but liver	Addison's disease

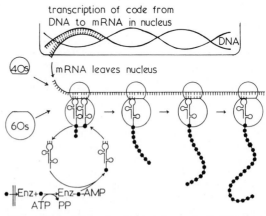

Figure 17–1. Mechanism of protein synthesis. Messenger RNA is formed in the nucleus. In the cytoplasm 40S and 60S ribosomal subunits attach to the messenger and, in the presence of appropriate aminoacyl-tRNA's and other factors, translation of the messenger proceeds. Puromycin inhibits protein synthesis because it structurally resembles aminoacyl-tRNA and causes premature chain termination when it is inserted in the growing peptide chain in place of the appropriate amino acid. Actinomycin binds strongly to DNA, particularly to deoxyguanosine residues. It therefore prevents transcription.

881

TABLE 17–2. THE GENETIC CODE*

First Letter		Second Letter				Third Letter
		U	C	A	G	
U		UUU $\}$ Phe UUC UUA $\}$ Leu UUG	UCU UCC $\}$ Ser UCA UCG	UAU $\}$ Tyr UAC UAA UAG	UGU $\}$ Cys UGC UGA UGG Trp	U C A G
C		CUU CUC $\}$ Leu CUA CUG	CCU CCC $\}$ Pro CCA CCG	CAU $\}$ His CAC CAA $\}$ Gln CAG	CGU CGC $\}$ Arg CGA CGG	U C A G
A		AUU AUC $\}$ Ile AUA AUG Met	ACU ACC $\}$ Thr ACA ACG	AAU $\}$ Asn AAC AAA $\}$ Lys AAG	AGU $\}$ Ser AGC AGA $\}$ Arg AGG	U C A G
G		GUU GUC $\}$ Val GUA GUG	CGU GCC $\}$ Ala GCA GGG	GAU $\}$ Asp GAC GAA $\}$ Glu GAG	GGU GGC $\}$ Gly GGA GGG	U C A G

*Each amino acid is coded by a triplet of three bases, of which the first two seem to be more precisely defined than the third. Note that there are, for example, up to six possible codes for leucine, serine, and arginine, the different tRNA molecules for the same amino acid being known as isoaccepting species. AUG, which codes for methionine, is believed to signal the beginning of the translation of a section of mRNA. GUG can also code for methionine when present in other than the initiation position. UAA, UAG, and UGA indicate chain termination, but they also seem capable of recognizing lysyl, arginyl, and seryl-tRNA's.

acids of a precise kind [there are normally 20 varieties to choose from (Table 17–2)] have to be joined together by peptide linkage in a defined order. To do this, a template molecule is required which contains the information of which amino acids, how many, and in what order they are to be linked. A form of ribonucleic acid (RNA) called *messenger RNA* (mRNA) serves this function. It is a single-stranded polynucleotide whose sequence of bases determines which amino acids are to be linked. This is possible by virtue of the *genetic code* in which triplets of bases in the polynucleotide chain, or *codons*, correspond to individual amino acids (Table 17–2). Thus, if one starts at one end or one point of the mRNA strand and reads off the bases in threes, it is possible to *translate* the information coded in it into a sequence of amino acids.

The main store of information in the cell is in the *chromosomes,* in particular, in the DNA located in the nucleus. Messenger RNA is formed by *transcription* of appropriate lengths of the DNA chains, a process in which, by the action of the enzyme *RNA polymerase,* nucleotide units from ATP, GTP, CTP, and UTP are linked together in a sequence determined by the order of bases in the DNA according to the principle of base pairing. Although DNA is relatively stable, the mRNA's of the animal cell are short-lived and are turning over with half-lives estimated to range from 2 to 80 hours. Thus continuing synthesis of protein, which occurs even in nongrowing cells, requires continuous synthesis of mRNA, which, since it is formed in the nucleus, must move to the cytoplasm for translation.

There are two other types of RNA in the cell involved in protein synthesis, *ribosomal* and *transfer* RNA (formerly called "soluble" RNA to distinguish it from ribosomal RNA, which is par-

ticulate). Ribosomal RNA, together with a number of proteins, comprises the ribosomes, structures which in higher organisms are quite large, with a molecular weight of about 4×10^6 daltons. The unit ribosome (called 80S from its sedimentation coefficient, 80 Svedberg units) is readily dissociated in solutions low in bivalent cations or of high ionic strength into two subunits. The smaller one (40S) with a molecular weight of 1.6×10^6, consists of a single strand of RNA (M.W. 0.8×10^6, 18S) and about 30 separate protein species, and the larger unit (60S) consists of two strands of RNA (M.W. 1.7×10^6, 28S, and 4×10^4, 5S) and about 40 different protein species.

The ribosomes, together with transfer RNA (tRNA) and various soluble proteins, constitute the machinery by which the information of mRNA is translated and a protein synthesized. Some of the ribosomes in the cell normally exist as separated subunits. In the presence of a number of as yet incompletely identified proteins (initiation factors), initiation of the synthesis of the polypeptide chain takes place. First the 40S subunit and a tRNA molecule (usually methionyl-tRNA) attach to a specific point on the mRNA molecule, followed by the 60S subunit. The resulting ribosome is now ready to move along the messenger molecule (or the messenger through the ribosome), during which process the triplet codons are "read" and a polypeptide chain built up, provided that the necessary amino acids are available.

Amino acids cannot be used directly by ribosomes but must first be activated and attached to the appropriate tRNA molecule. With the aid of ATP, the activating enzymes of which there must be at least 20 varieties, one for each amino acid, select the individual amino acids. The activating enzyme-amino acid-complex reacts with the appropriate tRNA molecule to form an aminoacyl transfer RNA complex, in which the amino acid is linked through its carboxyl group to the 3-position of the ribose of the terminal adenosine of the nucleotide sequence. Transfer RNA has a molecular weight of about 25,000 and is believed to fold itself up into a cloverleaf shape. It has a triplet of bases at the end of the molecule opposite to the site of attachment of the amino acid that "recognizes" by base pairing triplets of bases in the mRNA. This is the point at which translation of the RNA base code into an amino acid sequence takes place. Because for many of the amino acids there are several possible triplets, there are also several different tRNA species accepting certain amino acids (Table 17–2). In the presence of the ribosome and other proteins called *elongation factors,* the appropriate tRNA molecule attaches to the next three bases adjacent to the three used by the previous tRNA molecule. Catalyzed by the ribosomal proteins, the amino acid (or, as translation proceeds, *the peptide chain*) attached to one tRNA molecule is transferred to the amino group of the amino acid of the incoming aminoacyl-tRNA molecule. So the peptide chain grows. At the end of the mRNA sequence undergoing translation, there is a *termination* codon, which is not used to code for any amino acid, and at this point the peptide chain detaches as the completed polypeptide. These steps are all summarized in Figure 17–1. When protein synthesis takes place in a cell, the supply of amino acids to the cell needs to be maintained.

POSSIBLE POINTS OF REGULATION

In a process as complex as protein formation, there are obviously many points at which regulation could occur. They can be briefly listed as follows:

1. Both amino acid activation and synthesis of the peptide bond consume ATP and other nucleoside triphosphates, as does RNA synthesis. Lack of energy is thus likely to slow down growth processes. This, however, is a rather crude and unspecific form of control.

2. Lack of availability of amino acids is also a potential limitation. This may apply either to amino acids in general or to one particular amino acid, since protein synthesis cannot proceed in the absence of any amino acid, unless the protein being synthesized should happen not to contain it. The quantities of the different amino acids in cells in free form cover a wide range. Alanine, glycine, and the dicarboxylic acids and their amides are usually present in large amounts. Leucine, isoleucine, valine, phenylalanine, tyrosine, tryptophan, methionine, and cysteine are present in much smaller quantities and would be obvious candidates as the species limiting the rate of protein synthesis. To date there is no clear evidence that in normal or endocrine-induced conditions the availability of any particular amino acid or of amino acids in general is the critical factor controlling the rate of protein formation. A characteristic feature of the action of many hormones is, however, that they stimulate uptake of amino acids by responsive tissues, and fast-growing tissues in general have a greater capacity for accumulation of amino acids than they do when their growth rate slows down.

3. Since protein synthesis is dependent on RNA, the rate of RNA production is important. The quantity of RNA in tissues with a high rate of protein synthesis (e.g., liver) is much greater than in others (e.g., muscle). The RNA content of tissues declines with age as the growth rate falls; conversely, during regeneration or hypertrophy, there is a marked rise. Cellular RNA is mainly ribosomal (ca. 70 per cent), with tRNA and nuclear RNA making up the rest (15 per cent each). The quantity of mRNA is too small to measure directly. An increase in the RNA content of cells means primarily an increase in the quantity of all the entities involved in protein formation and, as such, will be expected to increase the capacity for protein synthesis. In appropriate organs, marked stimulation in the level of RNA is seen following treatment with most of the hormones listed in Table 17–1.

An increase in the content of RNA can arise from a decrease in its rate of catabolism (both ribosomal and transfer RNA have half-lives of 50 to 100 hours) or from enhanced rates of synthesis. This rise would result from enhancement of the activity of RNA polymerase, as well as from an increasing availability of DNA for transcription (10). Control at this point appears to be of considerable importance, and many hormones can influence transcription, as will be discussed in more detail later. Regulation of the availability of DNA for transcription may influence not only the amount of RNA synthesized but also, particularly where messenger RNA is concerned, which messenger RNA molecules are transcribed and, therefore, which proteins are made. This becomes important in regard to the changes in enzyme activities in response to the hormones listed in Table 17–3.

Synthesis of rRNA takes place in the nucleolus; it involves a form of RNA polymerase different from that involved in the synthesis of mRNA and tRNA, which occurs in the nucleoplasm. The nucleolar polymerase appears to turn over much more rapidly than the polymerases of the nucleus as a whole, and this fact may explain why the nucleolar polymerase and rRNA synthesis show early and large responses to hormones.

4. A ribosome is not able to synthesize protein unless attached to mRNA. The rate of synthesis of protein able to be catalyzed by a given amount of RNA will therefore be proportional to the number of ribosomes attached to mRNA (constituting polysomes), as opposed to those that are free and hence inactive. In general, it is believed that the majority of ribosomes in tissues are contained in polysomes, but the proportion may decline in endocrine deficiency states (e.g., in diabetes or in the hypophysectomized animal), presumably because of a diminished rate of initiation for reasons yet to be determined.

TABLE 17–3.   HEPATIC ENZYME ACTIVITIES ENHANCED OR SUPPRESSED IN RESPONSE TO VARIOUS HORMONES

	Enhanced	Suppressed
Insulin	Glucokinase	Glucose-6-phosphatase
	Glycogen synthetase	Phosphoenolpyruvate carboxykinase
	Phosphofructokinase	Pyruvate carboxylase
	Pentose pathway dehydrogenases	Hydroxyglutaryl-CoA saturase
	Pyruvate kinase	Urea cycle enzymes
	Glycerol kinase	Transaminases
	Malic enzyme	
	Citrate cleavage enzyme	
	Microsomal fatty acid desaturase	
Growth Hormone	Ornithine decarboxylase	Amino acid–degrading enzymes
Thyroxine	α-Glycerophosphate dehydrogenase	
	Cytochrome oxidase	
	Cytochrome c	
	NAD-isocitric dehydrogenase	
	Mitochondrial membrane formation	
Glucocorticoids	Glucose-6-phosphatase	
	Phosphoenolpyruvate carboxykinase	
	Pyruvate carboxylase	
	Tyrosine transaminase	
	Tryptophan pyrrolase	
	Amino acid–degrading enzymes	
Prolactin	Lactose synthetase	

5. Once initiation has taken place, it is possible that the rate of translation of the messenger may vary. Thus availability of the appropriate aminoacyl-tRNA molecules will limit how fast the ribosome may read out the codons of the messenger. How fully and how rapidly tRNA takes up amino acids depend among other things on the activity of the amino acid-activating enzymes; these decline in diabetes and estrogen deficiency and have been observed to rise in activity with muscle hypertrophy and insulin administration.

It is clear from the foregoing that there are many points in the overall process of protein formation at which regulation can take place and where hormones can interact. This is summarized in Table 17–4. In fact, a moment's thought will show that if protein synthesis is to proceed effectively there has to be a degree of coordination between the various steps. The logical consequence of this is that endocrine stimulation of the overall process of protein synthesis must involve enhancement of activity all along the line—at the stage of increasing the availability of amino acids, of mRNA to translate, and of ribosomes with which to translate it and at the stage of amino acid activation, initiation, and peptide elongation together with the appropriate enzymes and other protein factors. Thus it is not surprising to find effects of hormones on all these stages, a coordinated response for which parallels exist in the switching on or off of growth of bacteria and for which a term "pleiotypic response" has been coined. While a lot has been learned about the effects of individual hormones over the years, we still await the cardinal discovery of how the coordinated response is initiated or restrained.

To reach our present understanding of how the

TABLE 17–4.   INFLUENCE OF HORMONES ON THE DIFFERENT STAGES OF PROTEIN AND RNA METABOLISM*

	Insulin	Growth Hormone	Thyroxine	Estrogen	Androgen
Enhanced amino acid transport	+	+		+	
Enhanced activity of cytosol fractions in support of amino acid incorporation by ribosomes	+	+			
Enhanced activity of isolated ribosomes in protein synthesis	+	+	+	+	+
Enhanced rate of polysome formation (initiation)	+	+	+	+	+
Enhanced ability of isolated ribosomes to respond to poly(U)	−	+	+	−	−
Enhanced rate of ribosome formation	+	+	+	+	+
Enhanced activity of RNA polymerase	+	+	+	+	+

*The table condenses an enormous number of observations in a rather arbitrary manner. Fuller details are to be found in the bibliography (See 5, 6, 7, and 14 for reviews).
Lack of a sign indicates lack of available data.

overall process of protein formation is controlled, it has obviously been necessary to study separately the various steps and the influence of hormones on them. This is possible in several ways. The various stages may lend themselves to individual investigation, e.g., charging of tRNA can be studied without the involvement of ribosomes, the activity of ribosomes can be investigated in cell-free systems without nuclear influence, and synthesis of RNA by isolated nuclei or polymerases can be followed. Alternatively, it is sometimes possible to inhibit one stage in the overall process in order to isolate other steps. The drugs puromycin and cycloheximide (11) inhibit protein synthesis and thus allow dissociation of the effects of hormones on protein synthesis from those on amino acid uptake by cells. Actinomycin inhibits RNA synthesis and thus allows dissociation of the effects of hormones regulating stages in translation from those involved in transcription. An additional technique designed to study the activity of ribosomes uncomplicated by that of their associated mRNA is to supply ("to prime") them with synthetic messenger, a chemically synthesized sequence of nucleotides, the most popular of which has been poly (U) coding for (poly) phenylalanine (Table 17–2). Initiation of the translation of poly (U) is probably different from that with a natural messenger. This is an advantage in that initiation occurs more easily, but it is a disadvantage in that the system is "unnatural."

INDIVIDUAL HORMONES

Since control of the growth rates of particular organs is likely to involve some or all of the steps described in the previous section, it is not surprising that there are many points of similarity in the action of the different hormones. This is illustrated in the extensive overlap of points of action listed in Table 17–4. To take but one example, testosterone, growth hormone, and thyroxine all enhance the activity of RNA polymerase in liver and muscle, but the result of the stimulation is not the same in metabolic terms, i.e., the end result is different for each hormone.

There are, on the other hand, significant differences in the mode of action of several hormones; for example, the influence of insulin can be detected very shortly after its administration or application to responsive tissues and is not prevented by actinomycin, which blocks synthesis of RNA. The effects of thyroxine or triiodothyronine on protein synthesis, however, are not seen for many hours after injection and are prevented by actinomycin. The effects of sex steroids are similarly sensitive to the drug, whereas many of those of growth hormone are not. It is therefore possible to separate the various hormones and their responses by this criterion into two groups: (1) those whose action appears to be primarily outside the nucleus (e.g., insulin and growth hormone operating primarily through translational control), and (2) those whose primary site of action appears to be in the nucleus (e.g., thyroxine and steroid hormones) and which stimulate transcription.

Insulin

The ability of insulin to lower the level of blood amino acids as well as of glucose has been known for many years, as has the negative nitrogen balance associated with insulin deficiency. Interest in the possibility that insulin has an important influence on protein metabolism unrelated to or independent of its effect on carbohydrate metabolism arose from observations that the hormone stimulates the incorporation of labeled amino acids into the protein of isolated muscle preparations (5, 6). Thus, for example, when insulin is added to medium containing labeled amino acids in which isolated rat diaphragm is being incubated, the presence of the hormone enhances the rate of incorporation of the amino acids into the protein of the tissue, and this effect is independent of whether or not glucose is added to the medium. Since one of the major actions of insulin on carbohydrate metabolism in muscle is to enhance glucose transport, when insulin stimulates amino acid incorporation in the absence of added glucose, glucose metabolism is presumably not involved. Moreover, as indicated above, this effect of insulin on protein synthesis is virtually immediate.

Since the labeled amino acids that are incorporated into protein in these experiments have to enter the tissue before encountering the ribosomes, it is possible that the stimulation of incorporation into protein results from enhancement of their transport from the medium into the cell. It is clear that insulin does enhance the rate of entry of certain amino acids but probably not of all. The interpretation of the incorporation experiments is complicated by the difficulty in knowing the specific activity of the intracellular amino acid pool and, in particular, of amino acids in use by the ribosomes, but recent work with heart muscle suggests that the stimulation of incorporation results from a real enhancement of the rate of protein anabolism. How these effects are brought about is not yet known. The actions of insulin are not dependent on synthesis of RNA, since they are seen in the presence of actinomycin.

The decrease in the blood amino acid level is likely to result not only from an increased uptake of amino acids by tissues, principally muscle, but also from a diminished rate of release. It seems likely that in the muscle of diabetic animals there is a smaller proportion of ribosomes contained in polysomes because there is a slowing down or defect in the rate of initiation. This appears to be speedily corrected by insulin, leading to increase towards normal of the proportion of ribosomes attached to mRNA. It has been suggested in the past that ribosomes from diabetic tissues may have some defect, in particular a lack of some specific protein possibly associated with the larger (60S) subunit, but it seems likely at present that such observations have technical explanations (7).

The action of insulin on nitrogen metabolism is thus multifactorial, and the hormone is a good example of a "pleiotypic effector." It is believed that the first action of the hormone is to combine with a receptor on the surface of or in the membrane of responsive cells. This interaction results in effects on carbohydrate and fat metabolism, and, independently, stimulation of amino-acid transport, of polysome assembly, of the activity of amino acid-activating enzymes, as well as suppression of protein catabolism. Over a longer period, there is an increase of RNA concentrations and, in the liver, an increase of polymerase activity and a change in the level of a variety of specific enzymes involved in glucose and fat metabolism (Tables 17–3 and 17–4). How all these actions follow from the initial interaction of the hormone with its membrane receptor is not known. That many of them are not directly related to membrane phenomena suggests the involvement of an intracellular effector ("second messenger"), but the identity of this messenger, if indeed it exists, remains to be discovered. At least as far as muscle and adipose tissue are concerned, it is unlikely to be cyclic AMP, though effects of insulin on synthesis and degradation of this nucleotide may be important in the liver. In this respect, insulin antagonizes the enhancement of hepatic protein degradation induced by glucagon, the action of the latter hormone facilitating mobilization of amino acids for gluconeogenesis.

What still remains complicated about the action of insulin on protein metabolism is, first, that insulin deficiency does not slow down protein synthesis in all tissues or even in all types of muscle; heart, for example, shows relatively little change in diabetes. Second, while it is clear that insulin is required for proper growth to occur and for the adult to retain nitrogen equilibrium, it has never been possible to show growth-promoting effects of the hormone in normal animals as is, for example, possible with growth hormone.

Growth Hormone

The stunting of growth following ablation of the anterior pituitary and the gigantism that can result from excessive administration of growth hormone are well known (13). Until recently, the actions of growth hormone have been less well characterized than those of insulin, and, as befits a large molecule, the origin of its effects has proved difficult to pin down. Like insulin, growth hormone, when added to incubated diaphragm muscle, stimulates uptake of glucose and amino acids and promotes incorporation of the latter into protein. However, while insulin will stimulate these processes in muscle from normal animals, growth hormone stimulates them in muscle only after hypophysectomy. The significance of this has not been sufficiently established.

Ribosomal preparations from hypophysectomized animals show a subnormal rate of incorporation of amino acids, but the rate is enhanced after growth hormone is administered to the tissue donors. It is likely that growth hormone raises the proportion of ribosomes in polysomes, i.e., enhances the rate of initiation of protein synthesis, and there is some evidence that the functional capacity of the ribosomes themselves is changed.

Also, activity of the smaller (40S) subunit appears deficient in the hypophysectomized animal. The capacity of growth hormone to enhance incorporation can be seen when it is added to a liver perfusate, provided that the level of amino acids is raised appreciably above the normal plasma value. Indeed, a similar effect is also seen with liver slices, and under these conditions addition of growth hormone enhances precursor incorporation into RNA, an effect abolished by cycloheximide.

Growth hormone treatment promotes the activity of RNA polymerase and the synthesis of RNA, which is reflected in a change in the RNA content of a number of tissues. Its administration to immature hypophysectomized animals enhances nuclear replication, the effect being delayed some 12 to 48 hours. Growth hormone administration also raises the level in serum of a sulfation factor capable (as growth hormone itself is not) of enhancing incorporation of chondroitin sulfate into cartilage, an important feature of skeletal growth, and this same factor is also potent in promoting incorporation of thymidine into nuclei. Skeletal growth is also facilitated by the hormone's promotion of collagen synthesis in skin and bone. So far, relatively few enzymes or specific proteins have been shown to change their activity or content in response to the hormone. Nothing, moreover, is yet known of the existence or nature of a binding site for the hormone, but presumably for so large a molecule this will be on the cell membrane. It is interesting to note that when, after acute denervation, diaphragm muscle loses sensitivity to insulin, it likewise loses its capacity to respond to growth hormone added in vitro.

The other hormones of the anterior pituitary stimulate release of hormones by target glands. Over longer periods they also have tropic effects on these organs. Little is known of the mechanisms involved in the tropic effects, but they are likely to exhibit many of the features seen in the action of testosterone and estradiol.

Thyroxine

Thyroxine and related derivatives are best known for their influence on the maintenance of the oxygen consumption of tissues and the basal metabolic rate (BMR). Stunting of growth and cretinism are characteristics of thyroid deficiency, and in amphibia, thyroxine plays an important role in inducing metamorphosis and developmental processes. As stated above, thyroxine stands in contrast to insulin and growth hormone in vitro in the slowness of onset of its effects; as many as 48 hours elapse between injection of a low dose of thyroxine to a thyroidectomized animal and the subsequent rise in BMR, though other changes, such as enhanced heart rate, decreased cardiac glycogen, and raised sensitivity to lipolytic effects of epinephrine, precede this increased oxygen consumption. The slow pace of change provides the opportunity to plot the time course and sequence of events (14).

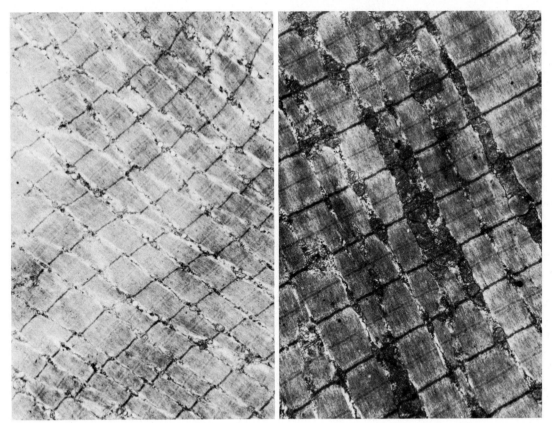

Figure 17-2. Longitudinal section through the central portion of contracted rat gastrocnemius muscle ($\times$ 18,000). On the left is that of a normal animal, on the right that of a thyroidectomized rat three weeks after treatment with thyroxine (18 μg. per 100 g. body weight every fourth day). (By kind permission of Dr. J. R. Tata.)

The rise in oxygen consumption (particularly noticeable in the heart) results from an increase in the number of mitochondria, which, in muscle, increase in size and in their relative proportion of cristae to matrix (Fig. 17-2). Synthesis of mitochondrial proteins (membrane proteins) occurs partly in the mitochondria; however, the cytochromes (except cytochrome a + a_3), respiratory chain components, and citric acid cycle enzymes are synthesized outside on cytoplasmic ribosomes. The eventual rise in BMR after thyroxine administration appears to be preceded by an increase in the capacity of isolated hepatic ribosomes and mitochondria to incorporate amino acids into protein. This alteration results from some increase in intrinsic ribosomal functional ability, as indicated by an increase in response to poly (U). These changes are observed within 30 hours of thyroxine injection, and by this time there is a substantial increase in the number of ribosomes. There is also a measurable increase in the quantity of cytochromes and of mitochondrial glycerol phosphate dehydrogenase.

Within 3 to 4 hours after hormone injection, increased incorporation of precursors into nuclear RNA is observable. This represents one of the earliest effects of the hormone. RNA synthesis is inhibited in the presence of actinomycin, and it is therefore not surprising that the presence of actinomycin at this point prevents response to the hormone. What form of receptor exists for thyroxine and what steps are involved after this in leading to changing rates of RNA synthesis remain to be learned. If an important aspect of response to the hormone is the synthesis of additional ribosomes and, as a result of this, the building up of new mitochondria, it is not of special significance that the effects of the hormone take time to become manifest. With our present understanding of how ribosomes function, their synthesis alone could not be expected to determine selective synthesis of specific proteins. It must be concluded, therefore, that the enhancement of RNA synthesis includes mRNA synthesis, and that the rise in polymerase activity of both the nucleolus and the nucleoplasm must be selective in regard to the areas of DNA transcribed. In the hypothyroid state, the rate of turnover of mitochondrial protein and DNA appears to be slow and to rise in response to thyroid treatment. As with insulin, an increase in protein content may result from a diminished rate of catabolism.

Estrogen

Growth changes in the uterus during the menstrual cycle are controlled by estradiol (2, 9). Its administration to immature or to mature ovariectomized female animals leads to rapid growth of the uterus. A lot of the early increase in weight is due to uptake of water, but between 6 and 24 hours after the hormone administration, there is an increase in the RNA content of the tissue, together with a rise in protein. These changes are prevented by simultaneous administration of puromycin or actinomycin. A measurable increase in RNA implies increased formation of ribosomes, and, indeed, the proliferation and enlargement of nucleoli, the source of rRNA, can be seen. After ovariectomy, the activity of ribosomes isolated from the uterus declines transiently, while their response to poly (U) increases. Treatment with estrogen increases their endogenous incorporating capacity but decreases their response to poly (U). This suggests that a greater proportion of the new ribosomes are to be found in functional polysomes.

Unlike insulin and growth hormone, there is good evidence that steroid hormones penetrate their target tissues (8). From both nucleus and cytoplasm, proteins capable of binding specifically to the appropriate steroid can be isolated. There is, therefore, good evidence that estrogens have a nuclear site of action. Within two minutes of injection, molecules of estradiol become bound to specific non-histone chromatin proteins, and a substantially increased incorporation of precursors into RNA can be seen shortly after, although enhancement of their uptake into the cell may partly explain this rise. As might be expected, the activity of RNA polymerase increases; there is an increase in the rate of synthesis of RNA chains rather than, as might be thought, an increase in the number of chains initiated. There is also an enhanced rate of uptake of certain amino acids.

It has been suggested that the action of estradiol involves two phases. In the first, after binding to nuclear elements, there is stimulation of transcription of specific regions of the genome, with the formation of new RNA species, which results in rapid synthesis of a few specific, probably acidic, proteins. This occurs within a few minutes and during the first few hours of estrogen action. In the second phase, these new proteins enhance synthesis of RNA in bulk, thus leading to increased protein formation. This is an amplification step seen from four or so hours onwards. It is not readily possible in this later stage to identify individual proteins whose synthesis is increased out of proportion to others.

Androgen

The story for androgen is very similar to that for estrogen when seminal vesicles and prostate gland are substituted for uterus (1, 16, 17), except that an important function of the male sexual tissues as opposed to the uterus is to secrete proteinaceous materials. After castration the glands shrink to a small proportion of their normal size. There is some decrease in DNA, as well as marked loss of RNA. Androgen reverses these changes, and the increase in RNA it brings about results in the appearance of many new ribosomes. As they do in the uterus, these ribosomes have a greater intrinsic capacity for amino acid incorporation and a lower response to poly (U) than is seen with ribosomes from the untreated organs. There is a rise in RNA polymerase activity, and the effects of the hormone are inhibited by actinomycin. A large proportion of the ribosomes of the prostate appear to be membrane-bound, as might be expected for a secretory tissue, and androgen administration to castrated males promotes membrane formation. Marked increase in the rate of respiration and in the density of mitochondria in epithelial cells is seen.

A significant feature of the mode of testosterone action is its reduction to dihydrotestosterone in the nucleus. Like estradiol it becomes protein-bound on entry into the cell; autoradiographic evidence indicates its localization within chromosomes, where it is bound to acidic proteins from which it is only slowly released.

Testosterone and other androgens affect the musculature. They promote amino acid incorporation in the muscle of castrate animals and elevate polymerase activity (4). Moreover, anabolic steroids can counteract the inhibitory influence of glucocorticoids on protein synthesis in muscle. Testosterone also has an anabolic influence on the kidney. With these tissues, increase in mass results from cell hypertrophy, whereas prostate and seminal vesicles undergo hyperplasia as well.

Glucocorticoids

The glucocorticoids are not generally considered anabolic. When large doses are given to experimental animals, a rapid loss of weight occurs, and the rates of amino acid incorporation into protein are decreased in muscle, spleen, lymphocytes, reticulocytes, and bone cells. The mechanism by which the steroids act is not known, but the various steps seem to be mainly the reverse of what is found with other hormones; there is decreased amino acid uptake, decreased RNA polymerase, and decreased incorporating activity by isolated ribosomes.

The liver stands apart from other tissues in that corticoid treatment can lead to variable changes depending on dose. At moderate levels, the liver increases in relative mass. Precursor incorporation into RNA is markedly increased, as is synthesis of specific enzymes, particularly those concerned with gluconeogenesis and amino acid degradation (Table 17–3). The glucocorticoids, therefore, have a directive influence on the form of proteins being synthesized by the liver, which they achieve through influence both on transcription and on post-transcriptional events (15).

Studies of the adrenalectomized rat show an early increased rate of amino acid incorporation into protein by ribosomes of isolated muscle and by hepatic ribosomes that, at least in the latter case, wears off with time. Loss of adrenal cortical function does not enhance growth rates.

Prolactin

Development of the mammary gland during pregnancy to enable it to synthesize and secrete lactose and specific milk proteins is under the control of prolactin. However, mammary gland development is an excellent example of the coordinated (synergistic) activity of several hormones, since prolactin is effective only in conjunction with steroid hormones and other protein hormones. Differentiation of the mammary epithelial cells into secretory alveolar cells involves cell division and proliferation for which insulin, estrogen, and progesterone are necessary, together with cortisone if the other steroids are to exert their maximum effect. The presence of prolactin then induces a rapid rise in RNA synthesis, followed by increased formation of protein. As is to be expected, inhibitors of protein and RNA synthesis prevent the action of prolactin. Ovine prolactin has many growth hormone-like effects in man, including induction of nitrogen retention.

SUMMARY

It is not possible yet to provide any unified picture of how hormones act, if indeed there will ever be such a picture to present; but in general terms, the mechanisms seem to result either from an action of the hormone at the cell membrane (e.g., insulin), with no nuclear involvement, or from the probable binding of the hormone to a specific protein (e.g., steroid hormones), which brings about transfer of the hormone to the nucleus, where the hormone or a derivative in some way stimulates transcription and the production of new RNA. Elucidation of the means by which binding of hormone to the cell membrane can influence intracellular events and of the detailed action of hormones in the nucleus are likely to be two extremely important areas for future investigation.

REFERENCES

1. Frieden, E. H.: Sex hormones and metabolism of amino acids and proteins, In *Actions of Hormones on Molecular Processes.* Litwack, G., and Kritchevsky, D. (eds.), New York, Academic Press, 1964, p. 509.
2. Hamilton, T. H.: Control by estrogen of genetic transcription and translation. *Science 161*:649, 1968.
3. Lucas-Lenard, J., and Lipmann, F.: Protein biosynthesis. *Ann. Rev. Biochem. 40*:409, 1971.
4. Kochakian, C. D.: Mechanism of anabolic action of androgens, In *Mechanism of Hormone Action.* Karlson, P. (ed.), New York, Academic Press, 1965, p. 192.
5. Manchester, K. L.: Sites of hormonal regulation of protein metabolism, In *Mammalian Protein Metabolism.* Vol. IV. Munro, H. N. (ed.), New York, Academic Press, 1970, p. 229.
6. Manchester, K. L.: Insulin and protein synthesis, In *Biochemical Actions of Hormones.* Vol. I. Litwack, G. (ed.), New York, Academic Press, 1970, p. 267.
7. Manchester, K. L.: Effect of insulin on protein synthesis. *Diabetes 21*:447, 1972.
8. McKerns, K. V. (ed.), *The Sex Steroids: Molecular Mechanisms.* New York, Appleton-Century-Crofts, 1971.
9. Means, A. R., and O'Malley, B. W.: Mechanism of estrogen action: Early transcriptional and translational events. *Metabolism 21*:357, 1972.
10. Paul, J.: General theory of chromosome structure and gene activation in eukaryotes. *Nature* (London) *238*:444, 1972.
11. Pestka, S.: Inhibitors of ribosome functions. *Ann. Rev. Biochem. 40*:697, 1971.
12. Schreiber, G.: Translation of genetic information on the ribosome. *Angew. Chem.* (Eng.) *10*:638, 1971.
13. Tanner, J. M.: Human growth hormone. *Nature* (London) *237*:433, 1972.
14. Tata, J. R.: Regulation of protein synthesis by growth and developmental hormones, In *Biochemical Actions of Hormones.* Vol. I, Litwack, G. (ed.), New York, Academic Press, 1970, p. 89.
15. Tomkins, G. M., Gelehrter, T. D., et al.: Control of specific gene expression in higher organisms. *Science 166*:1474, 1969.
16. Williams-Ashman, H. G.: Ribonucleic acid and protein synthesis in male accessory reproductive glands and its control by testosterone, In *Mechanisms of Hormone Action.* Karlson, P. (ed.), New York, Academic Press, 1965, p. 214.
17. Williams-Ashman, H. G., and Reddi, A. H.: Androgenic regulation of tissue growth and function, In *Biochemical Actions of Hormones.* Vol. II. Litwack, G. (ed.), New York, Academic Press, 1972, p. 257.

CHAPTER 18

Disorders of Lipid Metabolism

By Edwin L. Bierman and
    John A. Glomset

INTRODUCTION

Four interrelated disorders of lipid metabolism, all affected by hormones and diet, account for much of the morbidity and mortality in clinical medicine. These are obesity, hyperlipidemia, atherosclerosis, and cholelithiasis. Although the last two in particular are usually associated with specialties other than endocrinology, i.e., cardiology and surgery, it is likely that physicians interested in endocrinology and metabolism will be increasingly involved in their management. Emphasis in the future will certainly be on prevention, and there is reason to believe that this will require long-term control of triglyceride and cholesterol metabolism, with attention to all four disorders. Although current understanding of lipid metabolism and hormone-lipid interrelationships is far from complete and rational preventive care is not yet possible, enough is known to formulate a tentative framework of pathophysiologic concepts as an aid to following the rapid developments in this area. Furthermore, an understanding of the numerous hormone-lipid interrelationships as discussed in other chapters has become crucial to the student of endocrinology. Particular lipids, especially phospholipids, comprise important structural components of all membranes, and those in plasma membranes are likely to play a central role in the mechanism of action of a variety of hormones. Many hormones are intimately linked to the transport of fat as fuel, and disordered lipid metabolism is often an early sign of an altered endocrine state. Conversely, altered lipid metabolism can profoundly influence hormone production, distribution, and action.

The aim of this chapter is to provide such a pathophysiologic framework of lipid metabolism and hormone-lipid relationships, then a discussion of present knowledge concerning obesity, hyperlipidemia, atherosclerosis, and cholelithiasis in relation to it. Emphasis has been given to triglyceride, fatty acids, and cholesterol, because of the very close relationship between disordered triglyceride and cholesterol metabolism and these major diseases. The metabolism of phospholipids and specific lipid-binding proteins and peptides is undoubtedly important in this context as well, but a more detailed discussion is beyond the scope of this chapter.

TRIGLYCERIDE METABOLISM: FAT AS A FUEL

Aside from its role in insulating the body against heat loss, the major function of triglyceride is to provide an efficient storage form for energy. The importance of triglyceride as a fuel can be appreciated from the fact that enough is usually stored to support many weeks of fasting, whereas carbohydrate is stored in amounts sufficient to last only a few hours (Cahill). The advantages of triglyceride are that it yields more than twice as many calories per gram as either carbohydrate or protein and that it requires less than half the amount of intracellular water for storage. Both advantages depend upon the long-chain fatty acid components of triglyceride, which yield large amounts of energy when oxidized and which are only slightly soluble in water. The same properties, however, necessitate the special mechanisms of transport and metabolic control discussed below.

Digestion and Absorption

Human diets contain highly variable amounts of triglyceride (fat) provided by both plant and animal foods. Typical "western" diets provide as much as 40 per cent of the total calories in the form of triglyceride, but on a world-wide scale, this type of diet is geographically as well as historically unusual. The less affluent most often consume much less triglyceride and much more carbohydrate.

Most dietary triglyceride is absorbed in the duodenum and proximal jejunum after undergoing

TABLE 18–1. MAJOR ORGANIC COMPONENTS OF HUMAN GALLBLADDER BILE*

	mg. per ml. Bile
Dihydroxycholanic acids	48.9
Cholic acid	32.2
Phospholipid†	27.3
Protein	5.0
Cholesterol	3.0
Bilirubin	2.8

*From Nakayma and Miyake: *J. Lab. Clin. Med. 67*:78, 1966.
†>95% lecithin (Phillips).

partial hydrolysis. The water-insoluble triglycerides of food spontaneously aggregate into large oil droplets when mechanically mixed with the aqueous secretions of the gastrointestinal tract. Transfer of triglyceride from these oil droplets across mucosal cell membranes is extremely inefficient, but upon partial hydrolysis, smaller aggregates (micelles) can be formed, greatly increasing the total surface area and facilitating transfer. The events that occur during hydrolysis are schematically illustrated in Figure 18–1. Conjugated cholic and dihydroxycholanic acids from bile (Table 18–1), secreted into the intestinal lumen in response to dietary fat, act as detergents to disrupt and disperse the oil droplets (Hofmann and Small). They are able to do this because of their unique configuration. The polar hydroxyl groups all project from the same side of the relatively flat ring structure (Fig. 18–2), creating a hydrophilic side, which spontaneously aligns towards the aqueous phase, and a hydrophobic side which associates with the surface of the oil droplets. This association causes the oil droplets to become negatively charged, because of the acidic groups of the bile acids, and promotes their dispersion. Bile acids also promote the action of the triglyceride hydrolase secreted in pancreatic juice. This enzyme attacks the triglyceride of the oil droplets, mainly

Figure 18–1. Schematic representation of events during the hydrolysis and absorption of triglyceride. ✶— , conjugated bile salt; ← , free fatty acid; ✶— , monoglyceride. (From Senior, J. R.: *J. Lipid Res. 5*:495, 1964.)

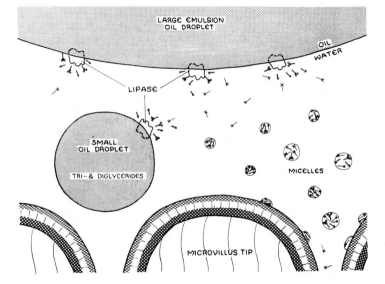

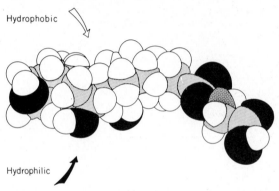

Hydrophobic

Hydrophilic

Figure 18–2. Model of taurocholic acid. Black areas are oxygen atoms, gray areas carbon atoms, white areas hydrogen atoms.

forming monoglycerides and free fatty acids. This causes a large increase in the area of the oil-water interface, because bile acids combine with the monoglycerides and free fatty acids to form micelles, i.e., aggregates which are so small (about 50 Å. in diameter) that they yield a clear solution in aqueous media.

The surface area of the intestinal mucosa also is enlarged. Finger-like villi project into the lumen and are covered by epithelial cells which themselves have an enlarged surface because of the presence of microvilli (Fig. 18–3). Since the micelles formed by digestion are small enough to enter the spaces between the microvilli, they can come into direct contact with a large part of the mucosal surface, and rapid transfer of monoglyceride and free fatty acids into the cells can occur. Within the cells, the monoglyceride, free fatty acids, and the small amount of free glycerol formed during digestion are reconverted into triglyceride (Fig. 18–4), packaged into lipoproteins, and secreted into the lymph. These processes occur rapidly, as can be demonstrated by sequential electron microscopy. Within 20–30 minutes after the introduction of fat into the intestinal lumen, the Golgi region is crowded with lipid, and within one hour, the lipid can be observed in the extracellular space at the base of the cell, ready for entrance into the lymphatic system (Fig. 18–3).

The enzymic reactions within the mucosal cells include not only reformation of triglyceride but also formation of phospholipid, unesterified cholesterol, cholesteryl ester, and specific proteins (lipoprotein apoproteins), which have a high capacity to bind lipids. Apparently the phospholipid, unesterified cholesterol, and apoproteins form a hydrophilic surface "coat" surrounding the more hydrophobic triglycerides and cholesteryl esters. The finished products of this activity, observed within the Golgi region, are lipid-rich particles of dimensions comparable to those of the chylomicrons and very-low-density lipoproteins (VLDL) of thoracic-duct lymph (750–6,000 Å). The composition of the particles probably differs somewhat from that of lymph particles, however, because rapid changes occur upon mixing chylomicrons with plasma (Bierman and Strandness; Minari and Zilversmit),

and similar changes probably begin to occur as soon as the particles are secreted from the mucosal cells into the lymph.

Chylomicrons isolated from human thoracic duct lymph contain more than 95 per cent triglyceride and less than 1 per cent protein (Table 18–2), but the highly specific components of the protein appear to be major determinants of the stability and ultimate fate of the particles. These apoproteins are being studied so intensively at present that even the nomenclature is in a state of flux. In the following we shall use the terminology of Alaupovic, who distinguishes three major classes of apoproteins, apo-A, apo-B, and apo-C, which contain a variety of polypeptides and which are present in human chylomicrons (Kostner and Holasek). Little is known about the function of apo-A in chylomicrons, but apo-B apparently plays an important structural role, since patients who lack this protein are unable to release absorbed lipid into the lymph (Isselbacher et al.; Ways et al.). Apo-C, the major peptide class of chylomicrons, consists of several peptides and affects the subsequent metabolism of chylomicrons. Several authors (Scanu and Wisdom) have reported activation of the enzyme, lipoprotein lipase (LPL), by one or more of the apo-C peptides, and Brown and Baginski have recently found that another of the apo-C peptides inhibits the enzyme. These functional effects are likely to be of great physiologic importance, since the LPL reaction appears to be the first step in the removal of chylomicrons from plasma.

Lipoprotein Lipase (LPL)

Normally chylomicrons begin to appear in plasma soon after a fatty meal and reach a maximum concentration within 4–5 hours. Because chylomicrons are so large that they scatter light, they frequently cause turbidity of the plasma (post-alimentary lipemia). Studies using chylomicrons labeled with radioactive triglyceride have demonstrated their rapid removal from the plasma and have shown that the fate of the triglyceride depends on nutritional and hormonal factors. Partial hydrolysis of the chylomicron triglyceride by LPL is believed to occur at the lumenal surface of capillary cells, where tight complexes with infused chylomicrons can be demonstrated by electron microscopy (Fig. 18–5). Evidence from several sources suggests that LPL absorbed on the cell surface initiates the hydrolysis (Robinson). This enzyme, also referred to as "post-heparin lipolytic activity" (PHLA) or "clearing factor" lipase because it is partially released into plasma upon injection of heparin and can sometimes "clear" lipemic plasma, appears initially to form free fatty acids and partial glycerides. Subsequently, the partial glycerides may be further hydrolyzed within pinocytotic vacuoles of the capillary cells (Blanchette-Mackie and Scow). Finally, free fatty acids are presumably released into the extravascular space, where they become available for uptake by tissue cells or for recirculation into the plasma.

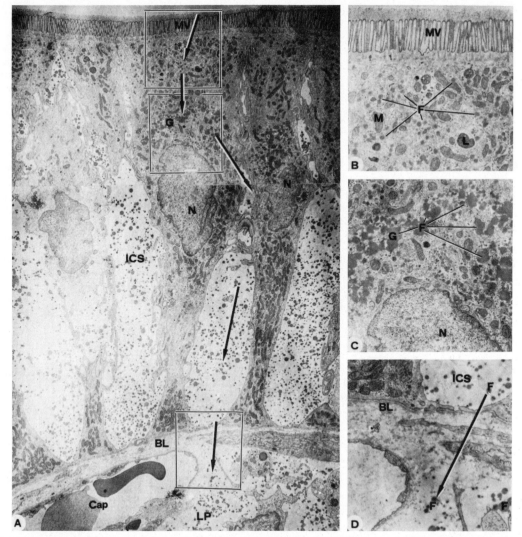

Figure 18–3. Fat absorption in the jejunum of man. The large picture on the left (*A*) is a montage of electron micrographs of absorptive cells at the tip of a villus fixed with osmic acid and embedded in epon. (× 5,000). The three outlined areas (*B, C, D*) are shown to the right at a greater magnification (× 12,000). This biopsy was obtained with a peroral biopsy tube 60 minutes after a fat meal had been given intragastrically. The large arrows delineate the sequential movement of fat, F, seen as dark grayish globules, from the lumen to the apical area of the cell, then to the Golgi area, G, the intercellular space, ICS, and, finally to the lamina propria, LP, where they will enter lacteals. MV, microvilli; M, mitochondrion; N, nucleus; BL, basal lamina; L, lysosome; Cap, capillary. (Courtesy of Dr. Stanley S. Shimoda, Division of Gastroenterology, University of Washington.)

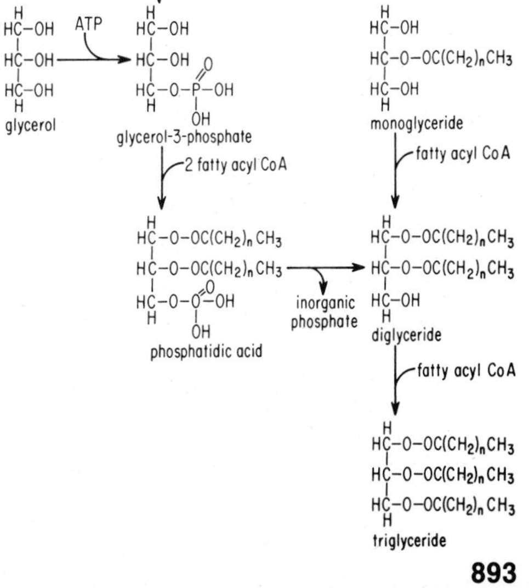

Figure 18–4. Synthesis of triglyceride within the mucosal cell. Note that the major pathway utilizes the monoglyceride formed during digestion. ATP, adenosine triphosphate; CoA, coenzyme A.

TABLE 18–2. LYMPH CHYLOMICRONS (Obtained by thoracic duct cannulation from human subject fed corn oil.)*

	Protein†	Triglyceride‡	Phospholipid	Cholesterol‡
Chylomicron	0.58%	96.5%	2.9%	0.6%
"Membrane"	11.5%	43.0%	52.8%	4.8%

*From Zilversmit, D. B.: *J. Clin. Invest.* 44:1610, 1965.
†Per cent total weight.
‡Per cent total lipid.

The liberated glycerol reenters the bloodstream and is mainly metabolized by the liver and kidney.

Because LPL appears to be a rate-limiting factor in chylomicron removal and appears to direct the flow of chylomicron fatty acid into tissues, and because it has been implicated in diseases asso-ciated with hypertriglyceridemia (see section on hyperlipidemia), the factors that influence the distribution and activity of the enzyme are of special interest. LPL activity has been demonstrated in several tissues (Robinson), but adipose tissue, heart, and the mammary gland have received the most attention. The activity in adipose tissue decreases during fasting and in diabetes, is higher in the fed state, and is highest in animals that have been fasted and subsequently refed (Bezman et al.). In contrast, the activity of heart muscle increases during prolonged fasting (Hollenberg). In mammary tissues, enzyme activity is relatively low until parturition, when it increases as much as tenfold (McBride and Korn). The factors responsible for these changes are best understood for adipose tissue. Evidence exists that the LPL of this tissue is synthesized by the fat cells, though only a

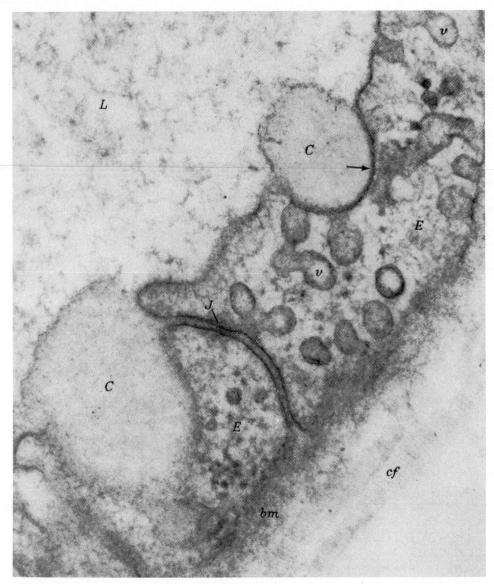

Figure 18–5. Detail of the capillary endothelium of a rat mammary gland 10 minutes after the intravenous injection of chyle. L, capillary lumen; C, chylomicron; E, endothelium; J, cell junction; v, vesicle; bm, basement membrane; cf, collagen fiber. Lead citrate stain (× 140,000). [From Schoefl, G. I., and French, J. E.: *Proc. Royal Soc.* (Biol.) *169*:153, 1968.]

relatively small proportion of the total tissue activity can be demonstrated within the cells themselves (Cunningham and Robinson). The fat cells synthesize LPL in the presence of glucose and insulin but not in the presence of agents that increase intracellular free fatty acid levels (Patten). They also release the enzyme in the presence of glucose and insulin (Stewart and Schotz). Although subsequent events remain to be clarified, the released enzyme presumably becomes associated with the vasculature, possibly after being activated by heparin released from adipose tissue mast cells. The bound enzyme appears to have a short half-life, and this causes the total activity of the tissue to be highly dependent on glucose and insulin. Studies *in vivo* show multiphasic release into the circulation after heparin administration (Brunzell et al., 1972a) consistent with this scheme. Note that glucose and insulin not only increase adipose tissue LPL activity, thereby directing the flow of chylomicron fatty acids into the extracellular space surrounding the adipocyte, but also stimulate intracellular reesterification of this fatty acid by promoting the formation of glycerol phosphate within the cell.

Production of Triglyceride from Carbohydrate

When dietary fat is replaced by carbohydrate, endogenous synthesis of fatty acid increases in both adipose tissue and the liver. This biosynthesis also is dependent upon glucose and insulin. Fatty acids synthesized within fat cells are esterified to glycerol phosphate formed from glucose and converted to triglyceride for storage. Those synthesized in the liver also are converted mainly to triglyceride, but most of the newly formed triglyceride is packaged into very-low-density lipoproteins, secreted into the plasma, and removed within minutes to hours by mechanisms probably similar to those involved in removal of chylomicron triglyceride.

The pathways of fatty acid biosynthesis and the mechanisms that control them appear to be similar in adipose tissue and liver. Fatty acids are synthesized from two-carbon units and hydrogen, both of which are mainly derived from glucose. Activated two-carbon units (acetyl CoA) are formed from pyruvate within the mitochondria by the pyruvate dehydrogenase reaction (see Ch. 9). Since fatty acid biosynthesis occurs outside the mitochondria, the two-carbon units must be transferred across the relatively impermeable mitochondrial membrane. The principal pathway of transfer appears to involve condensation of acetyl CoA with oxalacetate to form citrate. The citrate is transferred across the membrane by a membrane carrier protein or permease and reconverted to acetyl CoA and oxalacetate outside the mitochondria by cleavage in the presence of ATP and CoA (Srere; Spencer and Lowenstein) (Fig. 18–6). Eight acetyl CoA molecules are required for synthesis of one molecule of palmitic acid (16 carbon atoms). One acetyl group appears to be transferred directly to a carrier protein-enzyme complex (fatty acid synthetase). The remaining seven are first carboxylated by a key enzyme, acetyl CoA carboxylase, to form malonyl CoA (Fig. 18–7). Subsequently, the malonyl groups are successively transferred to fatty acid synthetase and condensed to form a long hydrocarbon chain. With each transfer of a malonyl group, one molecule of CoA and one of CO_2 are released. At each step, four atoms of hydrogen, transferred from two molecules of NADPH, are required to convert the elongated chain into a saturated hydrocarbon. The NADPH appears to be derived from two separate pathways, the "pentose shunt" (Ch. 9), which produces two molecules of NADPH during the oxidation of glucose-6-phosphate and 6-phosphogluconate, and the "malic enzyme" pathway. In the latter, the oxalacetate produced by the citrate cleavage reaction (Fig. 18–

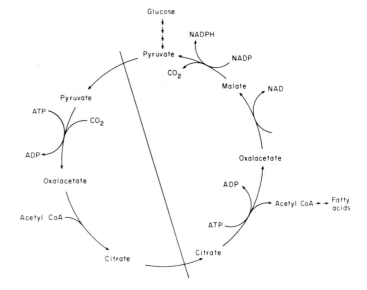

Figure 18–6. Schematic drawing showing reactions by which intramitochondrial citrate is converted to extramitochondrial acetyl CoA and NADPH.

1. Acetyl Co A carboxylase

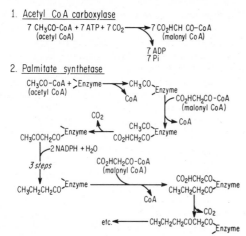

2. Palmitate synthetase

Figure 18-7. Schematic representation of the formation of palmitic acid in the extramitochondrial fluid. ATP, adenosine triphosphate; ADP, adenosine diphosphate; CoA, coenzyme A; Pi, inorganic phosphate.

6) is first reduced by NADH to form malate. Then the malate is reoxidized by NADP in the presence of "malic enzyme" (malic dehydrogenase) (Lardy et al.) to form NADPH, pyruvate, and CO_2. Palmitic acid synthesized by this sequence of condensation and reduction steps can be activated to form palmityl CoA and directly esterified to form triglycerides and other lipids or it can be elongated or dehydrogenated or both to form other fatty acids. Elongation occurs within the mitochondria or in association with the endoplasmic reticulum (microsomes). Dehydrogenation occurs in the endoplasmic reticulum closely coupled to chain elongation.

The rate of fatty acid biosynthesis is highest on hypercaloric, high carbohydrate diets, low on fat-rich diets, and lowest during prolonged starvation or diabetes. The factors that cause these differences are not completely understood, but some potential mechanisms of fine and coarse control have been identified. For example, acetyl CoA carboxylase may be subject to allosteric regulation, since high concentrations of citrate cause the enzyme to form an active aggregate, whereas increased concentrations of long-chain fatty acyl CoA rapidly promote disaggregation to a smaller inactive form (Lane and Moss). Pyruvate dehydrogenase is an example of a different and probably more important type of control (Jungas). In the presence of substances that increase tissue concentrations of cyclic AMP (see Ch. 10), this enzyme is phosphorylated and thereby inactivated, whereas, in the presence of glucose and insulin, the enzyme is rapidly dephosphorylated to its active form. The activation or inactivation of pyruvate dehydrogenase appears at least partly to explain the rapid changes in fatty acid biosynthesis noted in various physiologic conditions, but slower changes in the concentrations of other enzymes also occur, and these appear to explain more long-term physiologic effects. Thus the rates of biosynthesis of glucokin-

ase, the citrate cleavage enzyme, acetyl CoA carboxylase, fatty acid synthetase, glucose-6-phosphate dehydrogenase, 6-phosphogluconate dehydrogenase, and malic enzyme all are coordinately affected by diet, producing a coarse control of fatty acid biosynthesis.

Whether fatty acids are synthesized slowly or rapidly by liver cells, very-low-density lipoproteins (VLDL) are still formed and secreted into the plasma. They can be recognized in the Golgi region of the cell prior to secretion. Like chylomicrons, they contain large amounts of triglyceride, probably surrounded by a "coat" of protein, phospholipid, and unesterified cholesterol. Although the apoproteins of freshly secreted human or primate VLDL have not yet been studied, human VLDL have been isolated from plasma and contain mainly apoprotein B and C (Brown et al.). Again, the B apoproteins probably are of structural importance, whereas the C apoproteins facilitate the hydrolysis of VLDL triglyceride by lipoprotein lipase.

Release of Fatty Acids from Adipose Tissue Stores

Net release of free fatty acids and glycerol from adipose tissue triglyceride occurs during several physiologic conditions, including exercise, stress, and fasting, as well as in uncontrolled diabetes. Hormones play an important part in this release. Some hormones, and perhaps autonomic nervous stimulation (Table 18-3), increase lipolysis within minutes by promoting formation of cyclic AMP, which stimulates a protein kinase that activates a rate-limiting triglyceride hydrolase, "hormone-sensitive lipase" (Fig. 18-8). Thyroid hormone appears to increase the sensitivity of adipose tissue to these hormones, whereas insulin and prostaglandin PGE_1 inhibit their action, apparently by blocking formation of cyclic AMP (Butcher). Growth hormone stimulates lipolysis in a different way. *In vitro*, in the presence of dexamethasone, it increases release of free fatty acids from adipose tissue but only after a time lag of about two hours (Fain et al.). This effect can be inhibited by ac-

TABLE 18-3. HORMONES THAT AFFECT LIPOLYSIS IN VITRO

Rapid Stimulation
Epinephrine
Norepinephrine
ACTH
Glucagon
Secretin
α MSH
β MSH
Arginine vasopressin

Slow Stimulation
Growth hormone
Cortisone

Suppression
Insulin
Prostaglandin (PGE_1)

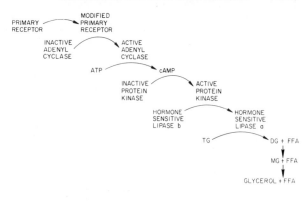

Figure 18-8. Cascade of reactions involved in the activation of hormone-sensitive lipase. (From Steinberg, D., and Huttunen, J. K., In *Advances in Cyclic Nucleo-tide Research.* Vol. 1. Greengard, P., Paoletti, R., et al. (eds.), New York, Raven Press, 1972, pp. 47–62.)

tinomycin and puromycin, which suggests that the biosynthesis of new protein is involved. Once the effect has developed, however, it is insensitive to agents that block protein synthesis but is sensitive to inhibition by insulin. This suggests that the new protein synthesized is the hormone-sensitive triglyceride hydrolase. The synergism between growth hormone and corticosteroids and the relatively long time lag are of interest because both features characterize the action of growth hormone *in vivo.* Why so many hormones activate free fatty acid release is not known; however, the hormones involved in the rapid mobilization of free fatty acids seem to be different from those involved in the slower release of free fatty acids during growth, fasting, or diabetes. Fain et al. have suggested that the hormones may not be equally sensitive to inhibition by insulin, and that this differential sensitivity may permit a fine control of free fatty acid release during different physiologic conditions.

Fate of Plasma Free Fatty Acids

When glycerol and free fatty acids are released from adipose tissue, they circulate briefly in the plasma. If lipolysis is brisk, the plasma concentrations of these metabolites rise. The rise only partially reflects the rate of lipolysis, however, since uptake by the tissues is proportional to the concentration in the plasma. The glycerol is mainly metabolized in the kidney and the liver, where it is phosphorylated by glycerophosphokinase and either reutilized for triglyceride formation or used for gluconeogenesis (Wagle et al.). The fatty acids circulate as albumin complexes. Their disposal is greatly dependent upon blood flow. During intense exercise, when the flow of blood through the splanchnic bed is reduced, they are largely oxidized in muscle. Those taken up by the liver are either reconverted to triglyceride or other lipids and secreted as VLDL, oxidized to CO_2, or converted into ketone bodies, depending on nutritional and hormonal conditions. In the presence of glucose or fructose and insulin, conversion to VLDL triglyceride predominates, possibly because of the reactions shown in Figure 18–9. During fasting or in diabetes, when glucose or insulin or both are diminished, most of the fatty acids are oxidized or converted into ketone bodies.

Fatty Acid Oxidation and Ketogenesis

Both oxidation and ketogenesis occur within the mitochondria. Neither free fatty acids nor their CoA derivatives formed outside the mitochondria readily penetrate mitochondrial membranes, but the soluble fluid of the cell (cytosol) contains an enzyme which reversibly transfers fatty acyl groups from CoA to carnitine, and acylcarnitine derivatives can enter the mitochondria. Once inside, a second enzyme (Kopec and Fritz) causes essentially irreversible transfer of the acyl groups back to CoA, thus effectively preventing the fatty acids from returning to the cytosol. The fatty acyl CoA derivatives then enter the β-oxidation pathway and contribute to the formation of reduced coenzymes (NADH and FADH) and acetyl CoA.

When small amounts of fatty acids are oxidized, the reduced coenzymes largely enter the electron transport pathway within the mitochondria and yield ATP and H_2O. The acetyl CoA condenses with oxalacetate to form citrate and is either transported across the mitochondrial membrane by the permease system and reconverted to fatty acid, or oxidized to CO_2 by the enzymes of the citric acid cycle. During fasting and in uncontrolled diabetes, however, the flow of free fatty acids into the liver is greatly increased. Moreover, degradation of hepatic triglycerides also is increased. Under these conditions, production of VLDL triglyceride from these fatty acids is limited, and reduced coenzymes and acetyl CoA within the mitochondria accumulate. The acetyl CoA molecules then condense successively to form acetoacetyl CoA and hydroxymethylglutaryl CoA, whereupon the latter is cleaved to yield acetoacetate and acetyl CoA. This causes the release of CoA, which can then be used in the metabolism of additional fatty acids by the β-oxidation pathway. In addition, the free acetoacetate formed can be reduced by the excess mitochondrial NADH to form β-hydroxybutyrate, thus liberating NAD for use in β-oxidation. Alternatively, it can decompose spontaneously to yield acetone, which accounts for the increased concentrations of all three metabolites in the plasma during ketogenesis.

The fate of the blood ketones, like that of the blood fatty acids, depends on nutritional and hormonal conditions. After a short period of fasting, acetoacetate and β-hydroxybutyrate are mainly

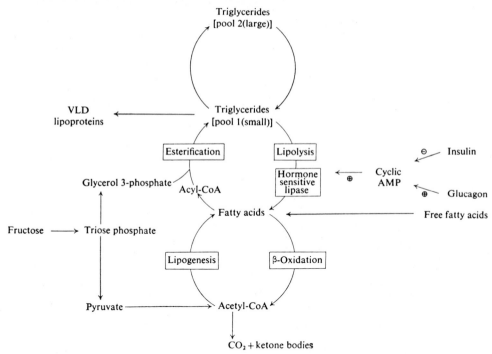

Figure 18-9. Scheme showing role of hormones in hepatic metabolism of fatty acids. Note that glucose as well as fructose contributes to the formation of triose phosphate. (From Topping, D. L., and Mayes, P. A.: *Biochem. J. 126*:295, 1972.)

metabolized by peripheral tissues such as muscle, but after longer periods, the brain apparently develops the capacity to metabolize these substrates (Cahill). In muscle, the acetoacetate and β-hydroxybutyrate must be converted into derivatives of mitochondrial CoA before being cleaved to acetyl CoA and oxidized via the citric acid cycle. Since fatty acids taken up from the blood by muscle also must be converted into derivatives of mitochondrial CoA before they can be metabolized, the two substrate types compete with each other. Moreover, both compete for the CoA ordinarily utilized by the pyruvate dehydrogenase reaction in converting pyruvate derived from glucose to acetyl CoA. This competition, along with the conversion of pyruvate dehydrogenase to its less active phosphorylated form in the presence of increased concentrations of free fatty acids (Wieland et al.) may partially account for the decreased utilization of glucose by muscle noted during fasting and diabetes (Randle et al.).

Summary: Hormonal Effects

Adipocyte triglyceride is formed from fatty acids provided either by dietary fat or biosynthesis. Fatty acids from dietary fat are largely transported to adipose tissue as chylomicrons. Those formed by biosynthesis either arise within fat cells or are formed in the liver and transported to adipose tissue as VLDL triglycerides. Formation of triglyceride within adipocytes and liver is dependent upon the availability of glucose and insulin.

Both increase adipose tissue lipoprotein lipase, both are required for the formation of triglyceride glycerol, and both are required for fatty acid biosynthesis. Glucose and insulin also diminish release of free fatty acids from adipocytes in two ways. Insulin blocks activation of a cyclic AMP–dependent, intracellular, hormone-sensitive triglyceride hydrolase by epinephrine, ACTH, and other hormones and by promoting reesterification of hydrolyzed fatty acid. Control of these processes within adipose tissue affects the concentration of circulating plasma triglyceride in two ways. Under some conditions, increased free fatty acid release from adipose tissue causes increased formation and release of VLDL triglyceride by the liver. Under other conditions, i.e., fasting and diabetes, adipose tissue LPL is diminished, and this increases the concentration of VLDL and especially chylomicron triglyceride in plasma by slowing the rate of their removal.

The availability of glucose and insulin also appears to determine the fate of free fatty acids taken up by the liver. In the absence of one or both, only a small proportion of the free fatty acids is converted to triglyceride and secreted as VLDL (Basso and Havel). This reduced capacity to form and secrete VLDL triglyceride, coupled with the limited ability of the liver to oxidize the large amounts of fatty acid to CO_2 (McGarry and Foster), accounts at least partially for the greatly increased formation of ketone bodies observed in diabetes. Finally, lack of insulin apparently contributes to the ketosis of diabetes in still another way, by decreasing the utilization of acetoacetate by peripheral tissues

(Balasse and Havel). This effect probably depends on the role of insulin in controlling plasma free fatty acid levels, since fatty acids compete with acetoacetate for mitochondrial CoA.

CHOLESTEROL METABOLISM

Form and Function

Cholesterol is important as a precursor of bile acids and steroid hormones, but particularly as a component (with phospholipids) of plasma membranes and plasma lipoproteins. Its wedge-like shape (Fig. 18–10) and single hydrophilic hydroxyl group apparently adapt it uniquely for intercalation between molecules of phospholipid (Demel et al.). "Mosaics" formed by this intercalation appear to contribute importantly to the structure of outer cell membranes (plasma membranes) and plasma lipoproteins. Apparently, the presence of cholesterol in these mosaics markedly decreases the permeability of membranes to water soluble compounds (deKruyff et al.). The water insolubility of cholesterol and the inability of most tissues to degrade it presumably contribute to its value as a cell membrane constituent, but, as in the case of triglyceride, its hydrophobic properties complicate the processes of transport and metabolism.

Transport of Cholesterol

No dietary requirement for cholesterol exists, since most mammalian cells, particularly in the liver and intestine, can synthesize cholesterol

TABLE 18–4. CHOLESTEROL CONTENT OF SOME COMMON FOODS*

Food	Cholesterol (mg./100 g. wet weight)
Eggs	470–650
Butter	280
Lobster, shrimp, oysters, roe	>200
Liver, kidney, brain, tripe, sweetbreads, heart, lung	>150
Cheese	130–160
Cream (35% fat)	124
Meat	70–140
Fish	60–90
Fowl	60–90
Milk (skim)	3
Cottage cheese	1

*From Kritchevsky, D.: *Cholesterol.* New York, John Wiley & Sons, 1958.

(Dietschy and Wilson). "Western" diets, however, rich in eggs, dairy products, and meat (Table 18–4) generally provide 0.5 to 1.0 g. of exogenous cholesterol per day, and this cholesterol contributes significantly to body pools. A considerable proportion of the cholesterol of food is esterified, and the esters are probably not directly absorbed. Pancreatic juice contains a cholesteryl ester hydrolase, however, which in the presence of trihydroxy bile acids catalyzes the hydrolysis of cholesteryl esters in the intestinal lumen to form free fatty acids and unesterified cholesterol. The latter mixes with the unesterified cholesterol of food, bile, and possibly desquamated mucosal cells, and considerable amounts can be absorbed. The process of absorption is not well understood, but it seems to be passive rather than active, and the following events probably occur. Unesterified cholesterol in the intestinal lumen is taken up by mixed micelles of bile acid and free fatty acid, monoglyceride, or lysolecithin. As a component of these micelles, cholesterol then enters the spaces between the microvilli of the mucosal cells and, during collisions with the microvillar membranes, becomes available for net transfer into the cell. When net transfer occurs, it is probably to replace mucosal unesterified cholesterol that has been incorporated onto the surfaces of newly formed chylomicrons or intestinal VLDL or that has been esterified within the cell and incorporated into the triglyceride-rich "cores" of these lipoproteins (Fig. 18–11). If net transfer does not occur, but free fatty acids, monoglycerides, or lysolecithin molecules are taken up, the micelles are disrupted and cholesterol precipitates, no longer capable of being absorbed (Simmonds et al.).

The intracellular mechanism by which cholesterol is transferred from the microvillar membrane to the site of lipoprotein synthesis has not been delineated. It is not even certain that chylomicrons secreted into the intestinal lymph contain enough unesterified cholesterol to form a fully stable surface "coat" since Minari and Zilversmit have shown that dog lymph chylomicrons rapidly take up additional unesterified cholesterol immediately

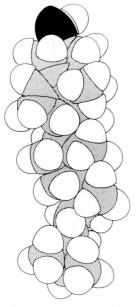

Figure 18–10. Schematic representation of the molecular size and shape of unesterified cholesterol.

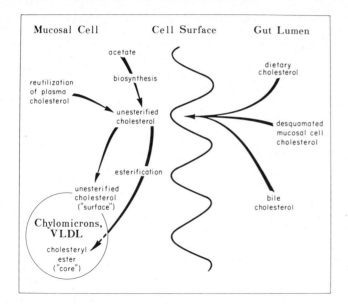

Figure 18–11. Alternate sources of the cholesterol of chylomicrons and VLDL formed by cells of the intestinal mucosa. (From Glomset, J. A., and Norum, K. R.: *Advances Lipid Res., 11*:1, 1973.)

upon being mixed with dog plasma. Nevertheless, the amount of chylomicron cholesterol secreted into the intestinal lymph can be estimated by assuming that approximately 100 g. of chylomicron triglyceride is secreted each day and that the content of chylomicron unesterified and esterified cholesterol is 1.6 per cent and 1.4 per cent, respectively (Kostner and Holasek). If these assumptions are valid, then the amounts of cholesterol secreted as chylomicron unesterified cholesterol and cholesteryl ester are about 2 g./day and 1 g./day, respectively (Glomset and Norum).

Within minutes after chylomicrons and intestinal VLDL enter the plasma, the triglyceride of these lipoproteins begins to be removed by lipoprotein lipase (LPL) (see page 892). Removal of the cholesterol of these lipoproteins, however, does not occur by the same mechanism or at the same time. Instead, cholesterol continues to circulate in the plasma, associated with one or more chylomicron remnants (Redgrave). Experiments in rats have shown that the cholesteryl esters of these remnants are removed relatively rapidly and then hydrolyzed by a liver cholesteryl ester hydrolase (Stein et al.). The fate of the unesterified cholesterol, phospholipid, and apoproteins remains to be fully clarified (see below).

Cholesterol enters the plasma not only as a component of chylomicrons and intestinal VLDL, but also as a component of hepatic VLDL. The liver is able to synthesize all of the cholesterol required from acetyl CoA by a multistage series of condensation reactions (Fig. 18–12) similar to that present in most cells. The reaction sequence is at least partially inhibited in most subjects, however, because of feedback inhibition by dietary cholesterol (Siperstein). Cholesterol biosynthesis in the liver appears to be particularly sensitive to dietary cholesterol, perhaps because of the liver's special role in metabolizing the cholesterol of chylomicrons. Studies have shown that cholesterol accumulates in the smooth and rough endoplasmic reticulum of liver cells when rats are fed high-

cholesterol diets (Pronczuk and Fillios) and that this is associated with decreased activity of an enzyme that acts as an important regulator of cholesterol biosynthesis (Shapiro and Rodwell).

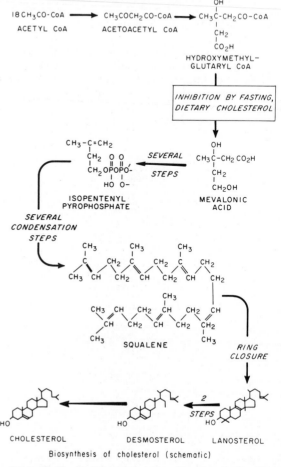

Figure 18–12. Partial representation of reactions involved in cholesterol biosynthesis.

FLOTATION RATE (DENSITY)	DESIGNATION (ELECTROPHORETIC MOBILITY)	SOURCE	MAJOR APOPROTEINS	MAJOR LIPIDS "CORE"/"SURFACE"	DIRECT ENZYMIC ATTACK BY
$S_f > 400$	CHYLOMICRONS	GUT	APO C,B,A	TG/UC,PC	LPL
$S_f\ 20 - 400$	VLDL (PRE β)	LIVER, GUT	APO C,B	TG/UC,PC	LPL
(1.006 g/ml) − −					
$S_f\ 0 - 20$	LDL (β)	PLASMA CHYLOMICRONS, VLDL, OTHER ?	APO B	CE/UC,PC,S	LCAT (?)
(1.063 g/ml) − −					
$F_{1.20}\ 0 - 9$	HDL (α_1)	PLASMA CHYLOMICRONS ? LIVER, OTHER ?	APO A,C	PC/UC,PC	LCAT
(1.21 g/ml) − −					
	ALBUMIN APOPROTEINS	LIVER, ?	APO A	FFA, LYSO PC	

Figure 18–13. Schematic representation of the classes of lipoproteins in human plasma. Apo A-C = apoprotein A-C; TG = triglyceride; UC = unesterified cholesterol; CE = cholesteryl ester; PC = phosphatidylcholine (lecithin); LYSO PC = lysolecithin; S = sphingomyelin; FFA = free fatty acid; LPL = lipoprotein lipase; LCAT = lecithin: cholesterol acyltransferase.

This enzyme, hydroxymethylglutaryl CoA reductase, catalyzes the essentially irreversible formation of mevalonic acid, the first committed metabolite in the biosynthesis of cholesterol. Decreased activity of this enzyme diminishes formation of hepatic cholesterol and somewhat limits the effect of diet on hepatic cholesterol levels.

In some species, hepatic VLDL contain both unesterified cholesterol and cholesteryl ester. Human liver, however, appears to lack the acyl CoA:cholesterol acyltransferase that forms these esters (Stokke) and presumably secretes VLDL that only contain surface unesterified cholesterol. The amount of this cholesterol that enters the plasma each day is difficult to evaluate, but it is probably of the order of 1 to 3 g. (Glomset and Norum). As mentioned earlier, the triglyceride of hepatic VLDL is hydrolyzed by peripheral LPL, just as in the case of the triglyceride of chylomicrons. Thus the unesterified cholesterol of the hepatic VLDL can be presumed to become associated with "remnants" not unlike those formed from chylomicrons and intestinal VLDL. Indeed, one of the most interesting possibilities now being investigated is that these remnants are eventually converted to the low-density lipoproteins (LDL) and high-density lipoproteins (HDL) classically recognized in the plasma of fasting subjects.

Before considering this possibility, the physical and chemical properties of the four lipoprotein classes usually identified in plasma (Fig. 18–13) should be recalled. These four are chylomicrons, VLDL, LDL, and HDL—or chylomicrons, pre-β lipoproteins, β lipoproteins, and α_1 lipoproteins—depending on whether one uses a nomenclature based on ultracentrifugation or electrophoresis. As mentioned earlier, chylomicrons and VLDL mainly contain triglyceride and smaller quantities of cholesteryl ester, surrounded by a surface "coat" of unesterified cholesterol, phospholipid, and apoprotein. Apoproteins A, B, and C all are present, but apoproteins B and C predominate, and the relative amount of apoprotein B is inversely proportional to lipoprotein size (Eisenberg et al.). In contrast to chylomicrons and VLDL, LDL and HDL contain relatively little triglyceride. Instead, the predominant "core" lipid is cholesteryl ester, and once again the "surface" lipids are lecithin and unesterified cholesterol. Moreover, very little apo-C is present. LDL mainly contain apo-B, and HDL mainly contain apo-A. The arbitrary divisions and the static picture conveyed by this classification scheme have been useful for some purposes but have failed to convey the functional relationships among the four lipoprotein classes. Indeed, these relationships are only now beginning to emerge.

A major interrelationship among lipoprotein classes is dependent on LPL. There is evidence (Bilheimer et al.) that attack by this enzyme on chylomicrons and large VLDL produces not only smaller VLDL but also LDL and some HDL. A schematic representation of the formation of small VLDL, LDL, and HDL "remnants," consistent with the lipoprotein "families" whose existence in plasma has long been emphasized by Alaupovic, is shown in Figure 18–14.

Another functional relationship is dependent on lecithin:cholesterol acyltransferase (LCAT). This enzyme circulates in plasma as an HDL complex

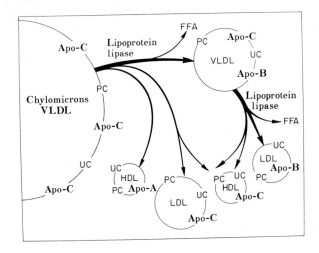

Figure 18–14. Possible formation of lipoprotein "remnants" by the action of lipoprotein lipase on chylomicrons and large VLDL. Apo-A, Apo-B, and Apo-C = apoprotein A-C; UC = unesterified cholesterol; PC = phosphatidylcholine; FFA = free fatty acids. (From Glomset, J. A., and Norum, K. R.: *Advances Lipid Res.*, *11*:1, 1973.)

(Glomset), and forms cholesteryl esters by catalyzing the transfer of fatty acids from HDL lecithin to HDL unesterified cholesterol (Fig. 18–15). This indirectly affects the lipids of other lipoproteins in two important ways. First, because unesterified cholesterol and lecithin readily equilibrate among lipoproteins, these lipids undergo non-enzymic net transfer from lipoproteins like VLDL to HDL (Fig. 18–16). Second, the LCAT reaction, for reasons that are not clearly understood, promotes non-enzymic exchange of HDL cholesteryl ester for the triglyceride of other lipoproteins (Nichols and Smith). Thus the net effect of the reaction is to diminish the unesterified cholesterol and lecithin and increase the cholesteryl ester of all plasma lipoproteins, not just HDL. Calculations of the rate of the reaction suggest that the amount of unesterified cholesterol converted into cholesteryl ester each day is of the order of that which enters plasma on the surfaces of chylomicrons and VLDL (Glomset and Norum). Moreover, patients who have familial LCAT deficiency (Norum et al.) have abnormal, unesterified cholesterol- and lecithin-rich particles in the plasma, and these are presumably derived from the surfaces of chylomicrons since

they markedly diminish in concentration when the patients are fed fat-free diets (Glomset et al.). This suggests that the role of the LCAT reaction is to dispose of the surface unesterified cholesterol and lecithin once the triglyceride of chylomicrons has been hydrolyzed by LPL (Schumaker and Adams). The effects of the pathologic accumulation of unesterified cholesterol and lecithin in plasma are not completely clear, but the patients who lack LCAT develop hemolytic anemia and ultimately renal failure, and this is associated with increased erythrocyte cholesterol and probably also increased glomerular cholesterol (Glomset and Norum).

Whether other enzyme reactions alter plasma lipoproteins as they circulate is not known. Furthermore, neither the reactions involved in the ultimate uptake of the various lipoprotein "products" of the LPL and LCAT reactions nor the ultimate sites of lipoprotein removal have been fully identified. Therefore, the best that can be done at present is to assume that the liver is important in the removal of lipoprotein cholesterol on the basis of its extremely important role in *cholesterol* catabolism and excretion.

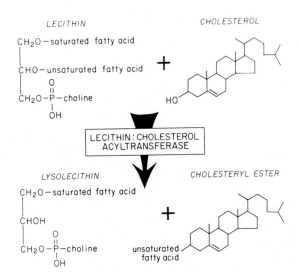

Figure 18–15. Principal reaction catalyzed by lecithin: cholesterol acyltransferase. (From Glomset, J. A.: *J. Lipid Res.* *9*:155, 1968.)

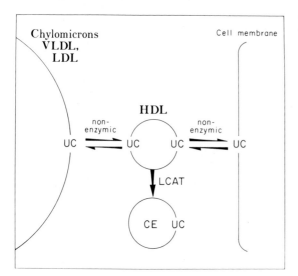

Figure 18–16. Non-enzymic exchange of unesterified cholesterol among plasma lipoproteins and plasma membranes coupled with the essentially irreversible esterification of HDL cholesterol by the LCAT reaction results in net transfer to HDL. (From Glomset, J. A., and Norum, K. R.: *Advances Lipid Res.*, *11*:1, 1973.)

Hepatic Metabolism of Cholesterol

Although the mechanisms by which lipoproteins are removed from the plasma are unknown, it is likely that cholesteryl ester hydrolases are involved (Goodman; Stokke), and since one of these is a lysosomal enzyme (Stokke), lysosomes are apparently involved. In any event, the unesterified cholesterol released by the cholesteryl ester hydrolases presumably mixes with that provided directly by incoming plasma lipoproteins as well as that provided by biosynthesis. This "pool" of unesterified cholesterol can either be used for the formation of lipoproteins (VLDL and probably some HDL) or for the formation of bile. The unesterified cholesterol used for bile formation is either converted into bile acids and secreted or it is secreted directly.

Conversion into bile acids occurs by a series of reactions located in the endoplasmic reticulum, cytosol, and mitochondria (Fig. 18–17). In dogs and

rats, this conversion increases severalfold when the animals are fed cholesterol. In man, however, the response appears to be much more limited, and increased amounts of cholesterol are secreted instead (Quintao et al.). This important species difference may predispose humans to the formation of cholesterol gallstones. Why humans are unable to increase bile acid formation in response to dietary cholesterol is not understood, but it may depend on the 7 α-hydroxylase that catalyzes the first step in bile acid formation. It is generally agreed that this step is an important control point in bile acid biosynthesis (Boyd and Percy-Robb), and its negative feedback control by bile acids has already been demonstrated.

The mechanisms that promote the direct secretion of cholesterol in bile are not understood, but it has been established that bile acids promote the secretion of biliary lecithin (Entenmann et al.) and that bile acids and lecithin together form micelles which can solubilize cholesterol. Bile containing these micelles is stored in the gallbladder and released into the intestine in response to fatty meals. Within the intestinal lumen, the micelles are presumably disrupted as the bile salts participate in the hydrolysis and transport of dietary fat. The lecithin is partially hydrolyzed by a pancreatic lecithinase, and the cholesterol mixes with that of the diet. A substantial recirculation (enterohepatic circulation) of each of these bile components occurs, however, since the bile salts are very efficiently absorbed by an active mechanism in the distal ileum (Dietschy and Wilson) and return to the liver complexed to the albumin of the portal blood; the lecithin (resynthesized in the mucosa) and cholesterol return to the liver as components of chylomicrons and VLDL. Nevertheless, a small proportion of the bile acids and a considerably larger proportion of the bile cholesterol escape reabsorption during each recirculation of the bile, and since the number of recirculations per day has been estimated to be as great as ten, a substantial amount of cholesterol and bile acid is lost in the feces.

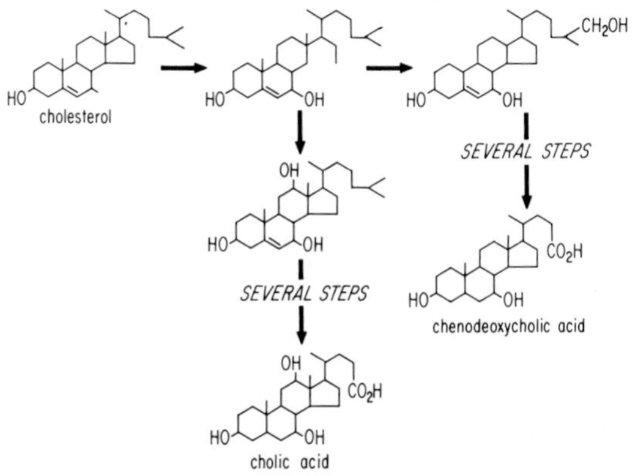

Summary: Hormonal Effects

Adequate amounts of cholesterol for the body's needs are provided by biosynthesis, so that dietary cholesterol is superfluous and increases body pools, particularly in the plasma and bile. There is no evidence that absorption of dietary cholesterol is regulated by hormones. Instead, absorption seems to be a passive process, dependent on the amount of unesterified cholesterol required for "packaging" the triglyceride of chylomicrons and intestinal VLDL and on the amount of cholesterol esterified within mucosal cells and included in the "cores" of these lipoproteins. The amount of dietary cholesterol absorbed probably depends also on the amount of endogenous cholesterol provided by the bile and desquamated mucosal cells and on local biosynthesis within the mucosal cells.

Much of the body's cholesterol, and particularly that of the plasma pool, is formed within the liver,

Figure 18–17. Principal steps in the conversion of cholesterol to bile acids.

where a variety of controls are operative. Both dietary cholesterol and fasting decrease cholesterol synthesis by the liver, and hypoinsulinism has a similar effect (Lehner et al.). Furthermore, hepatic cholesterol biosynthesis is under circadian control, even in fasted or adrenalectomized animals. Finally, cholesterol biosynthesis is decreased in hypothyroidism and increased in hyperthyroidism.

The concentration of cholesterol in blood plasma depends not only on the amount of cholesterol absorbed and biosynthesized but also on the rates at which chylomicrons, VLDL, LDL, and HDL enter and leave the plasma. These rates appear to be affected by several hormones, including estrogens, androgens, adrenal steroids, glucagon, insulin, and thyroid hormone (Margolis and Capuzzi). The latter is of particular interest because of its effect on the concentration of LDL, the major carrier of cholesterol in the plasma. In hypothyroidism, both the rate of LDL formation and the rate of LDL clearance from the plasma are slowed, and a new steady state concentration of LDL is reached which is considerably higher than that in euthyroid or hyperthyroid individuals.

The mechanisms involved in lipoprotein removal from the plasma are unknown, but they are likely to be influenced by the mechanisms of secretion of cholesterol and bile acids in bile, and here, too, hormones appear to be important. Thyroid hormones are known to increase bile steroid secretion in both man (Miettinen) and experimental animals, and the effects of estrogens on bile acid formation (Kritchevsky et al.) and bile flow have been demonstrated in rats and mice. Biliary secretion of cholesterol and bile acids plays a major role in regulating body cholesterol pools, because significant amounts of these components escape reabsorption during repeated daily enterohepatic circulations and are excreted in the feces. This is the main means by which cholesterol input through ingestion and biosynthesis is balanced by cholesterol output.

OBESITY

Obesity is the most common disorder of triglyceride metabolism in man and is closely linked to the other disorders discussed in this chapter (hyperlipidemia, atherosclerosis, and gallstones). It is also one of the oldest documented metabolic disturbances in recorded history. A limestone statuette dating from the stone age has been unearthed (Venus of Willendorf, Fig. 18–18) which appears to be the most ancient example of obesity, antedating the development of agriculture by about 10,000 years. Although almost prehistoric, the ancient Venus has the body build of the present-day, middle-aged, fat woman (Fig. 18–19). Similar historical evidence for obesity is found in Egyptian mummies and Greek sculpture. Despite the prevalence of this abnormality throughout centuries characterized by markedly different environmental stresses and dietary habits, the disorder

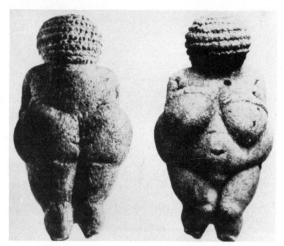

Figure 18–18. Venus of Willendorf. Limestone statuette, circa early Stone Age, 22,000 B.C.

persists, and we are not much closer to elucidation of its pathogenesis or elaboration of long-term successful measures for therapy.

Definition and Measurement

It is not clear whether obesity represents a "disease" or a common clinical manifestation of a group of disorders. The definition is necessarily arbitrary, since body weight (more accurately, quantity of body fat) is continuously distributed in populations with no clear break between individuals who are obese and individuals who are thin. A definition of obesity could be made easier if there were a distinct point at which a clear influence of obesity on morbidity and mortality begins. This is not the case, however, since there is a continually progressive excess mortality for increasing degrees of overweight based on insurance company actuarial standards (Fig. 18–20). Moreover, the metabolic, physiologic, and pathophysiologic consequences (see below) appear to increase continuously with the degree of deviation above average weight.

Body weight, although the simplest index of obesity, is not always the best reflection of the relative proportion of adipose tissue in the body or of total adipose mass. The latter needs to be determined or estimated if knowledge of the degree of excess adiposity is desirable. Weight adjusted to body size gives a better indication. For clinical purposes, per cent ideal body weight (relative weight) based on insurance company tables (Table 18–5) usually gives a rough approximation of the degree of adiposity. For common usage, obesity can be defined as that body weight over 20 per cent above this ideal body weight for a given population.

A variety of methods for assessment of total body fat, such as body density, x-ray, distribution of fat-soluble gases, total body water, and total body potassium-40, have been used for research purposes. In addition, a variety of anthropometric measurements (limb and trunk diameters, circumfer-

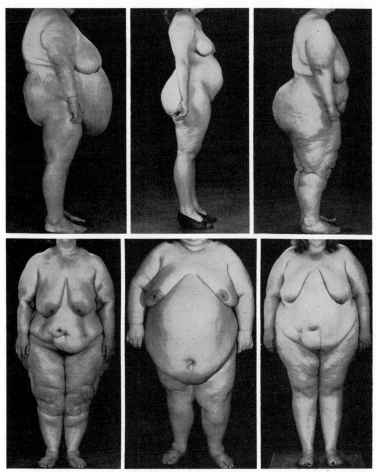

Figure 18–19. Note marked variations in distribution of fat. *Top center,* This patient consulted the Obstetrics Clinic many times for question of pregnancy, which she never had. *Lower left,* This patient preserved sufficient pride to place the mammae beneath a girdle and to substitute pseudomammae, but not enough pride to reduce her 325 pounds. *Lower center,* Chronic hospitalization was necessary because of incapacitation from obesity. *Lower right,* This patient's hyperphagia began exactly 1 day after she fell from a ladder and injured her head, at age 11. The correlation indicating hypothalamic injury seemed excellent in this patient, but such occurrences are rare.

ences, and skin-fold thicknesses) have been used to derive regression equations which correlate closely with per cent body fat determined by independent means (Steinkamp et al.). The weight/height^2 index is the most useful anthropometric measurement and the simplest to obtain; it deemphasizes the effect of stature on body weight and also correlates closely with adiposity (Edwards and Whyte; Grace and Goldrick). Tables for the distribution of subscapular and triceps skin-fold thickness measurements in large populations have been published (Mayer, 1966; Montoye et al.), which also provide an accurate guide. Mayer (1966) suggests that triceps skin-fold thickness greater than 23 mm. in men and 30 mm. in women should be defined as obesity.

Clinical Types

Although it has been clear for some time that there are two clinical types of obesity, little metabolic or physiologic evidence has been available until recently to support such a clinical concept. In one type (lifelong obesity), patients give a characteristic history. Although generally of normal birth weight, they tend to have been heavier as children since early grade school, to have a large spurt in weight gain during puberty, and (in females) to give a history of irreversibly gaining weight with each successive pregnancy. These individuals usually have tried all available methods and fads promoted for caloric restriction and weight reduction to no permanent avail. After successful weight loss regardless of the program, they usually return gradually to approximately their prereduction level of overweight. These individuals tend to be grossly obese (more than 150 per cent of ideal body weight) adults.

The other clinical type (adult-onset obesity) is much more common and essentially represents "middle-age spread." These individuals give a history of being thin or of average weight until age 20 to 40, when weight gain associated with a more sedentary existence and other environmental factors begins. This type of weight gain in adult life is

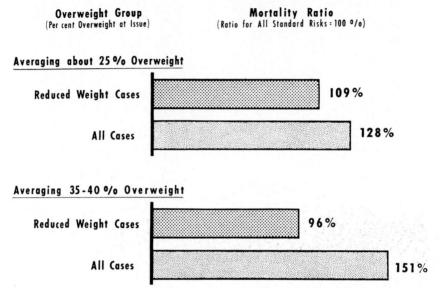

MORTALITY OF OVERWEIGHT MEN SUBSEQUENT TO WEIGHT REDUCTION AND OF ALL OVERWEIGHT MEN

Cases Accepted for Ordinary Insurance in 1935-53, Traced to Policy Anniversary in 1954

Overweight Group
(Per cent Overweight at Issue)

Mortality Ratio
(Ratio for All Standard Risks = 100 %)

Averaging about 25 % Overweight

Reduced Weight Cases — **109%**

All Cases — **128%**

Averaging 35-40 % Overweight

Reduced Weight Cases — **96%**

All Cases — **151%**

Figure 18-20. The high mortality rate associated with marked obesity falls to a normal level with loss of obesity. (Build and Blood Pressure Study, 1959, published by the Society of Actuaries.)

extremely common as evidenced by a cross-sectional analysis of a total, free-living community — Tecumseh, Michigan (Fig. 18–21). It appears that there is a gradual increase in relative body weight (compared with ideal) until the middle years, after which there is some decline. Since this is not a longitudinal study of the same individuals throughout life, it is possible that the reason for this decline in relative weight in later years reflects the increased morbidity and mortality associated with overweight. It is rare to find markedly obese individuals in retirement or old age homes.

A possible explanation for weight gain during adult life that does not appear to be tenable is a decrease in basal energy utilization with aging (Table 18–6). If one examines changes in basal oxygen consumption with age, one observes a slight decline during adult life (Fig. 18–22). Body composition is changing, however, even at constant body weight. There is a larger proportion of body

TABLE 18–5.   DESIRABLE WEIGHTS FOR MEN AND WOMEN*
(According to height and frame; ages 25 and over)

Height (in Shoes)†	Weight in Pounds (in Indoor Clothing)			Height (in Shoes)†			
	Small Frame	Medium Frame	Large Frame		Small Frame	Medium Frame	Large Frame
	Men				Women		
5′ 2″	112–120	118–129	126–141	4′10″	92– 98	96–107	104–119
3″	115–123	121–133	129–144	11″	94–101	98–110	106–122
4″	118–126	124–136	132–148	5′ 0″	96–104	101–113	109–125
5″	121–129	127–139	135–152	1″	99–107	104–116	112–128
6″	124–133	130–143	138–156	2″	102–110	107–119	115–131
7″	128–137	134–147	142–161	3″	105–113	110–122	118–134
8″	132–141	138–152	147–166	4″	108–116	113–126	121–138
9″	136–145	142–156	151–170	5″	111–119	116–130	125–142
10″	140–150	146–160	155–174	6″	114–123	120–135	129–146
11″	144–154	150–165	159–179	7″	118–127	124–139	133–150
6′ 0″	148–158	154–170	164–184	8″	122–131	128–143	137–154
1″	152–162	158–175	168–189	9″	126–135	132–147	141–158
2″	156–167	162–180	173–194	10″	130–140	136–151	145–163
3″	160–171	167–185	178–199	11″	134–144	140–155	149–168
4″	164–175	172–190	182–204	6′ 0″	138–148	144–159	153–173

*Prepared by the Metropolitan Life Insurance Company. Derived primarily from data of the Build and Blood Pressure Study, 1959, Society of Actuaries.
†1-inch heels for men and 2-inch heels for women.
Body build is often difficult to place in these categories. Other indices are therefore advantageous, as discussed in the text.

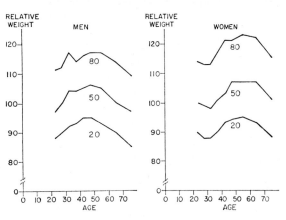

Figure 18-21. Relative weight index for males and females (29th, 50th, and 80th percentiles) throughout adulthood from a cross-sectional study of a total community–Tecumseh, Michigan. (From Montoye, H. J., Epstein, F. H., et al.: *Amer. J. Clin. Nutr. 16*:417, 1965.)

fat and a smaller proportion of lean body mass with age, so that basal oxygen consumption in terms of lean body mass, predominantly muscle and bone, may actually be virtually constant with age. Therefore, adult-onset obesity simply may reflect an imbalance between caloric intake and utilization, based on the fact that such individuals do not reduce their caloric intake with age appropriately for their change in body composition. Ahrens has calculated that the daily caloric requirement for weight maintenance of adults decreases 43 calories per decade for males and 27 calories per decade for females.

These two broad clinical types of obesity were recognized by Albrink and Meigs, who proposed that adult-onset obesity is mainly central in location (the "middle-age spread"), while lifelong obesity might be peripheral as well as central. For peripheral localization of adiposity, skin-fold thickness of the forearm or the triceps is measured and compared with skin-fold thickness over the tip of the scapula. Weight gain during adult life is significantly correlated with costal, scapular, and, to a lesser extent, triceps skin-fold thickness but not with ulnar skin-fold thickness. Thus forearm fat is minimally influenced by adult-onset obesity, while adipose tissue of the trunk is most influenced by weight gain during adult life.

Pathophysiology

A possible pathophysiologic basis for these clinical observations was first proposed by Bjurulf, who suggested that some forms of obesity might be due to increased numbers of cells. Proof of this hypothesis was provided by the elegant experiments of Hirsch and his co-workers. They demonstrated that grossly obese humans (lifelong) characteristically have an increase in adipose cell number as well as adipose cell size. After weight reduction, adipose cell size shrinks, but hypercellularity remains fixed (Fig. 18-23).

Adult-onset obesity (after age 20) appears to be characterized predominantly by adipose cell hypertrophy, with only minimal increase in cell number. Adipose cell number appears to be fixed very early in life. In studies with rats, animals subjected to overnutrition before weaning maintained larger numbers of adipose cells throughout life than did litter mates subjected to undernutrition prior to weaning (Knittle and Hirsch). Weight changes during adult life did not influence the cell number of these animals. Preliminary studies in man (Hirsch and Knittle) also have shown that adipose

TABLE 18-6. POSSIBLE FACTORS IN THE PATHOGENESIS OF OBESITY
(Adipocyte Hypertrophy)

Excessive Lipid Deposition
  Increased food intake
  Hypothalamic lesions
  Adipose cell hyperplasia
  Hyperlipogenesis

Diminished Lipid Mobilization
  Decrease in lipolytic hormones
  Defective adipose cell lipolysis
  Abnormality of autonomic innervation

Diminished Lipid Utilization
  Aging
  Defective lipid oxidation
  Defective thermogenesis
  Inactivity

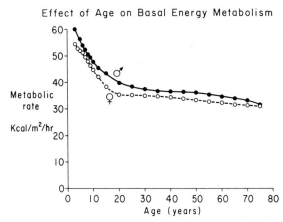

Effect of Age on Basal Energy Metabolism

Figure 18-22. Values for basal metabolic rate (kilocalories per square meter per hour) for normal males and females. (From *Handbook of Biological Data*, National Academy of Sciences, National Research Council. Spector, W. S. (ed.), Philadelphia, W. B. Saunders, 1961.)

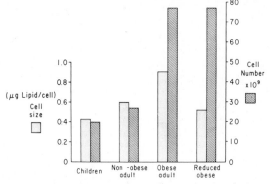

Figure 18-23. A comparison of adipose cell size and adipose cell number in non-obese children and adults and in obese adults before and after weight reduction. (Adapted from the data of Hirsch, J., Knittle, J., et al.: *J. Clin. Invest. 45*:1023, 1966.)

cell number is determined early in life, which has profound implications with regard to the effect of feeding patterns during infancy and early childhood on the subsequent development of lifelong obesity. It has been shown that excessive weight gain within the first six months of life is correlated with overweight at the age of 6–8 years, and thus it appears that the rapidity of weight gain in infancy is a better guide to the risk of obesity in later years than is the weight of the parents (Eid). Although less than a third of obese adults were overweight children, most overweight children become obese adults (Knittle). The familial aggregation of obesity (from Mayer, 1965: fewer than 10 per cent of children are overweight when both parents are thin; 50 per cent are overweight when one parent is obese; 80 per cent are overweight when both parents are obese), then, could be explained in part by a familial aggregation of eating patterns, particularly as applied to nutrition in early life. There also appears to be some genetic influence, since body weights of identical twins are correlated more closely than are those of fraternal twins (Newman et al.).

Experimental Obesity

Support for this concept has been derived from studies of experimental obesity in man by Sims and co-workers (1968, 1971). They force-fed volunteers to produce 20–30 per cent increments in weight (Fig. 18–24) associated with centripetal distribution of excess fat, which was predominantly due to an increase in adipose cell size without a change in adipose cell number. Prompt, spontaneous reversal of adipose increment and cell size was achieved at the termination of the experimental forced feeding.

Studies of experimental obesity in animals also lend some support to these concepts. Genetically transmitted obesity in rodents is characterized by adipose cell hyperplasia as well as hypertrophy, while experimentally induced obesity, such as that which can be obtained by destruction of the ventromedial nucleus of the hypothalamus, is associated with hypertrophy alone (Johnson and

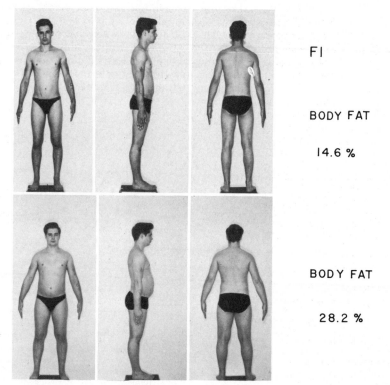

Figure 18-24. Experimental obesity in a human volunteer before (top) and after (bottom) overfeeding. (Courtesy of E. A. Sims.)

TABLE 18–7. TYPES OF OBESITY

	Hyperplastic	Hypertrophic
History	Lifelong	Adult-onset
Fat distribution	Peripheral and central	Central ("middle-age spread")
Adipose cellularity	↑ cell number and ↑ cell size	↑ cell size only
Insulin resistance	Related to cell size	Related to cell size
Metabolic consequences	Related to cell size	Related to cell size
Long-term response to R_x	Poor	Fair

Hirsch). The only experimental manipulation thus far made which produces a significant change in adipose cell number in adults is a change in very early infantile nutrition. A summary of these two broad general categories of obesity is given in Table 18–7.

Etiology

Little is known of the etiologic basis for adipose cell hyperplasia. Only in rare instances of hypothalamic obesity in man, in which damage to the ventromedial hypothalamic nucleus occurs as a result of tumor or trauma, can an etiology be defined and, with surgical removal of the tumor, obesity cured. This hypothalamic center appears to regulate the deposition of adipose tissue triglyceride. Formerly its role as an appetite or satiety center was emphasized (ventrolateral nucleus = feeding center; ventromedial nucleus = inhibitory or satiety center). Thus this center has been thought by many to be related to obesity in man via inappropriate hyperphagia derived at the hypothalamic level. Recent studies (Frohman et al.; Hustvedt and Løvø), however, have shown that experimentally induced hypothalamic lesions alter insulin levels and lipogenesis independent of changes in food intake. Anomalous insulin secretion after hypothalamic injury in man has also been observed (Bray et al.), and it is possibly linked to the development of obesity in these individuals. In any event, the relevance to the common types of human obesity of experimental animal models in which obesity is produced by injury to the hypothalamus is open to question. For a thorough description of the various genetic experimental animal models of obesity, the reader is referred to a recent review by Bray.

Cerebral and emotional influences on eating patterns surely play a role in obesity, but, aside from overt psychiatric disturbances, the general role of altered behavioral patterns in the etiology of obesity has been difficult to define, and a specific type of personality associated with obesity has yet to be distinguished. Cultural influences and socioeconomic status have a strong influence on the prevalence of obesity. As Stunkard has pointed out, every social factor studied has been strongly correlated with obesity and thus must be considered a determinant. No less important, habit and environment appear to influence appetite regulation. The experiments of Schacter have clearly indicated that external cues differentially affect behavior of obese and normal subjects. It appears that obese individuals are stimulated by environmental influences such as ready availability of food, flavor, time of day, and the like. In contrast, thin individuals appear to be stimulated to eat by internal cues presumably related to physiologic appetite regulation. In simplest terms, a non-obese individual eats when hungry, an obese person eats because it's time to eat and the food is appetizing. If food is not readily available or is not appetizing, as shown by the ingenious "black box" feeding experiments of Campbell et al., in which subjects fed themselves through an automatic liquid formula dispensing device without being able to monitor the amount of intake, an obese individual will actually consume far fewer calories than will his thin control counterpart. In addition to eating behavior influencing the degree of adiposity, the reverse is also true. Profound adiposity, particularly of the lifelong type, leads to numerous psychological and psychiatric disturbances which may not be reversible with weight reduction (in fact in some instances may be exacerbated) (Bruch).

Metabolic Features

Regardless of the cause or type of obesity, the metabolic consequences are predictable. They appear to relate only to fat cell size, and virtually all metabolic disturbances tested are inducible with weight gain (Sims et al., 1971) and reversible with weight reduction. Thus, although numerous hormonal imbalances have been described in obesity, they are likely to be consequences of rather than causes of the obese state.

The metabolic alteration with the most profound influence on metabolism is the acquired resistance to the action of insulin on glucose translocation in fat and muscle cells that appears to be a direct function of increased fat cell size. Insulin resistance associated with adiposity has been demonstrated both *in vivo*, by the observation that peripheral glucose uptake across the forearm in response to either exogenous or endogenous insulin is less in obesity (Rabinowitz and Zierler; Butterfield et al.), and *in vitro*, by studies of the metabolism of glucose in isolated fat cells (Salans et al.). Since Bjorntorp's studies showed that physical training decreased hyperinsulinemia in obesity without diminishing adiposity, muscle metabolism presumably plays an important but as yet unknown role in the insulin resistance of obesity. One of the consequences of this resistance to the action of insulin appears to be a feedback compensatory hyperinsulinism. The beta cells of the pancreatic islets are stimulated by an unknown mechanism to produce more insulin, and beta-cell hypertrophy eventually results. The signal is as yet unknown but may be neuronal, hormonal, or may involve small changes in glucose, fatty acids, or specific amino acids (Felig et al.). In any case, the result is an increase in circulating insulin levels (both basal and in response to a variety of stimuli), which is directly related to the degree of adiposity (Fig. 18–

25) and is reversible with weight reduction (Bagdade, 1968; Bierman et al., 1968; Kalkhoff et al.). It is not simply a matter of body weight or fat-free body size that is associated with hyperinsulinemia, since very muscular individuals who are heavy do not appear to have hyperinsulinism. Compensatory hyperinsulinism appears to be a common pathway for a multitude of other factors which produce resistance peripherally to the action of insulin (Fig. 18–26).

The emergence of adult-onset diabetes mellitus in the population may well be profoundly influenced by the degree and duration of obesity (Ogilvie). One concept is that prolonged hyperinsulinism might lead to beta-cell "exhaustion" in those individuals who are genetically susceptible. As is well known, when the pressure is off after successful weight reduction, glucose intolerance is reversed (Newburgh and Conn). Thus glucose intolerance in the obese adult may represent "high-output failure," in which the beta cell has failed to compensate fully for the degree of peripheral insulin resistance associated with adiposity. Abnormal growth hormone regulation has been associated with obesity (lack of a normal rise with starvation, hypoglycemia, or arginine stimulation), but the significance of this finding and its relation to the glucose intolerance of obesity is not understood. These changes in insulin and growth hormone regulation in obesity can be found even in early childhood (Parra et al.).

Fatty acid mobilization appears to be less affected by the insulin resistance associated with adiposity. Impairment of the insulin effect on lipolysis would be expected to lead to enhancement of fat mobilization. In simple obesity (uncomplicated by glucose intolerance), however, lipolysis does not appear to be increased, as reflected by normal to low plasma free fatty acid and glycerol levels (Bagdade et al., 1969), unimpaired braking of lipolysis after oral glucose, and apparently normal stimulation after administration of fat-mobilizing hormones. Furthermore, studies *in vivo* of human forearm metabolism (Rabinowitz and Zierler) have

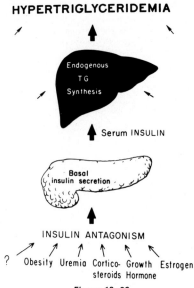

HYPERTRIGLYCERIDEMIA

Figure 18–26

shown no increase in arteriovenous free fatty acid output by subcutaneous tissue in simple obesity. Björntorp and Ostman) have shown that plasma glycerol levels appear to be correlated with fat cell number but not fat cell size. Thus it appears likely that, in other studies in which elevated free fatty acid and glycerol plasma levels and turnover rates have been reported in obese subjects, enhanced lipolysis was a function of the presence of adipose tissue hyperplasia or concomitant glucose intolerance. Furthermore, it is doubtful that enhanced lipolysis, when present, plays a major regulatory role in the hyperinsulinism of obesity. Alternatively, there is little evidence that decreased lipolysis, or resistance to normal fat mobilizing stimuli (hormonal, neuronal), plays an etiologic role in adipose cell hypertrophy (Table 18–6).

The peculiar "resistance to ketosis" attributed to obese patients refers to the prolonged interval of fasting (usually more than 2–3 days), in comparison to thin individuals, before ketonuria is observed. This parallels the prolonged decline in elevated insulin levels in obesity observed during total fasting (Bagdade et al., 1972), which suggests that the liver remains well insulinized during fasting in obesity for a longer period of time, resulting in a diversion of fatty acids to nonketogenic pathways (McGarry and Foster). (There is no evidence that the insulin resistance of adipose tissue and muscle associated with adiposity extends to the liver.) Higher insulin levels would also explain the often observed delay and blunted, increased mobilization of fatty acids when obese patients begin fasting. In addition, the "resistance" of obese individuals to the hypoglycemia induced by ethanol after fasting (Arky and Freinkel) may reflect expanded hepatic glycogen reserves consequent to hyperinsulinemia.

Although lipoprotein lipase [the enzyme in adipose tissue responsible for assimilation of triglyc-

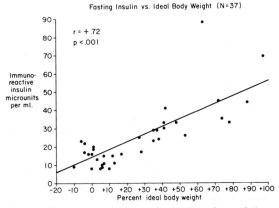

Fasting Insulin vs. Ideal Body Weight (N=37)

r = +.72
p <.001

Figure 18–25. Basal serum insulin levels in thin and obese men plotted as a function of per cent ideal body weight (an index of adiposity). (Adapted from Bagdade, J. D., Bierman, E. L., et al.: *J. Clin. Invest.* 46:1549, 1967.)

eride fatty acids into the fat cell from circulating triglyceride-rich lipoproteins (see p. 892)] appears to be sensitive to the availability of insulin, no abnormalities in obesity have yet been described.

Other alterations in adipose cell metabolism in obesity have been sought, particularly those involving lipogenesis. Bray has demonstrated a deficiency of intramitochondrial glycerophosphate dehydrogenase in human obesity which theoretically could have effects on lipogenesis; however, "hyperlipogenesis" has not been demonstrable in man. The recent demonstration by Miller et al. that increased thermogenesis can be induced in man as well as animals by increased caloric intake raises the intriguing possibility that defects in adaptive thermogenesis might be associated with obesity.

Another metabolic consequence of obesity is hypertriglyceridemia, which may result in part from the associated hyperinsulinism. Triglyceride levels in populations are correlated with relative body weight, skin-fold thickness, and particularly with weight gain in adult life (Albrink et al.). In a variety of studies recently reviewed by Bierman, Porte, et al., circulating insulin levels are significantly associated with triglyceride levels, and, since insulin is one of the factors involved in endogenous triglyceride-rich lipoprotein secretion by the liver (see page 898), a hypothetical pathway can be devised to explain these results (Fig. 18–26). In hypertriglyceridemic individuals, it is of interest that the hyperinsulinemia is correlated with both relative body weight and fat cell size (Bagdade et al., 1971; Bjorntorp et al., 1971). In such individuals, both hyperinsulinemia and hypertriglyceridemia are reversible with weight reduction (Bierman and Porte). Both hyperinsulinemia and increased endogenous triglyceride production rates have been produced with overfeeding in an experimental animal model for obesity, the desert sand rat (Robertson et al.). The role of obesity in determining the serum lipid levels in populations as a whole is suggested by the superimposibility of age-related curves of relative body weight, plasma triglycerides, and plasma cholesterol in males and females (Fig. 18–27).

Serum cholesterol levels are less closely linked with obesity, but nevertheless a significant relationship exists (Montoye et al., 1966). This could be explained in part by the observation that cholesterol turnover (production rate) appears to be related to the degree of adiposity (Nestel et al.; Miettinen). This relationship may be linked to the increased propensity of obese individuals to develop gallstones (see section on gallstones).

The influence of obesity on glucose and lipid levels also may be related to the increased tendency for obese individuals to develop all the complications of atherosclerosis (see p. 929). Possible mechanisms linking obesity, altered carbohydrate and fat metabolism, and atherosclerosis are indicated in Figure 18–28. The metabolic and endocrine alterations produced as a consequence of human obesity are summarized in Table 18–8. For further discussion of the metabolic aspects of obesity, the reader is referred to recent reviews by Gordon; Bjorntorp and Ostman; Bortz; and Salans and Wise. From metabolic considerations alone, it would appear appropriate to define obesity in terms of adipose tissue fat cell size.

Physiologic Features

The physiologic consequences of obesity lead to a variety of clinical manifestations and diseases (Table 18–9). Every organ system appears to be involved. In the respiratory system, alveolar hypoventilation eventually leads to carbon dioxide retention and somnolence (the Pickwickian

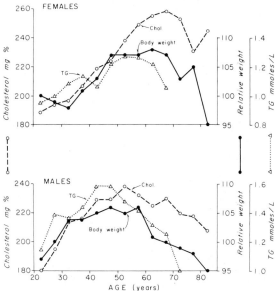

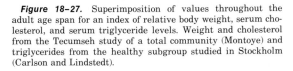

Figure 18–27. Superimposition of values throughout the adult age span for an index of relative body weight, serum cholesterol, and serum triglyceride levels. Weight and cholesterol from the Tecumseh study of a total community (Montoye) and triglycerides from the healthy subgroup studied in Stockholm (Carlson and Lindstedt).

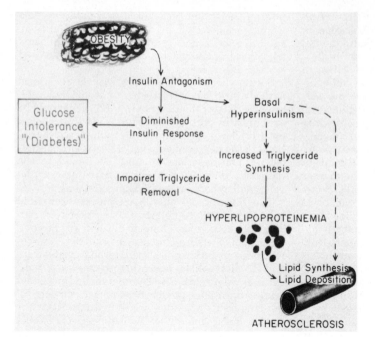

Figure 18-28

syndrome). In the cardiovascular system, cor pulmonale is common, and nonspecific myocardial lesions have been described. Obese individuals appear particularly prone to sudden death, and they often develop angina pectoris (Kannel et al., 1967). Nonspecific gastrointestinal symptoms (bloating, dyspepsia) are frequent. A fatty liver is common, with abnormalities in bromsulfophthalein excretion reaching an incidence as high as 85 per cent among obese individuals. In addition to the arterial lesions of atherosclerosis, varicose veins are common. Flabby and redundant skin produces moist folds, resulting in a propensity to fungal and yeast skin lesions (particularly in the axillae, perineal region, and under the breasts). Gallstones and cholecystitis are more common in obese individuals (see p. 931). Osteoarthritis is more common and severe. Amenorrhea and oligomenorrhea are common. The incidence of toxemia of pregnancy is increased.

Endocrine Features and Differential Diagnosis

Endocrine lesions as specific primary causes of adiposity are relatively uncommon. It is clear, however, that hormones influence the regulation of fat deposition. This may involve a general effect on adipocyte metabolism throughout the body (e.g., insulin; thyroid hormone) or characteristic regional effects (e.g., glucocorticoids; estrogen). Hyperinsulinism can lead to adiposity, as well as vice versa, as exemplified by patients with insulinoma. Individuals with this tumor are only rarely markedly obese, however.

Although much attention has been paid to hypothyroidism and milder degrees of "hypometabolism" as a cause of obesity, and vast quantities of thyroid extract have been administered for treatment, there is little evidence for deficiency of thyroid hormone secretion as a primary cause in most cases. Most of the weight gain associated with the development of myxedema is due to the accumulation of fluid (Ch. 4) rather than to adipose mass. Furthermore, the administration of thyroid hormone to obese patients may result in a loss of lean body mass exceeding the loss of fat (Kyle et al.) and in increased appetite. Circulating thyroid

TABLE 18-8. METABOLIC AND ENDOCRINE CONSEQUENCES OF OBESITY

↓ Sensitivity to insulin (muscle, adipose tissue)
Hyperinsulinemia
↓ Glucose tolerance; hyperglycemia
Hyperaminoacidemia
Hypertriglyceridemia
Hypercholesterolemia
↓ Growth hormone responses
"Resistance" to ketosis
↑ 17-Hydroxycorticoid excretion

TABLE 18-9. PATHOPHYSIOLOGIC CONSEQUENCES OF OBESITY

System	Condition
Respiratory	Alveolar hypoventilation (Pickwickian syndrome)
Cardiovascular	Hypertension
	Cor pulmonale
	Varicose veins
Gastrointestinal	Fatty liver
	Gallstones
Musculoskeletal	Osteoarthritis

hormone levels (Glennon), thyroidal I[131] uptake, and Achilles reflex times are usually normal.

The fat deposition associated with hyperadrenocorticism (Cushing's syndrome) is characteristic (Ch. 5). Helpful diagnostic clinical features, in addition to fat distribution, that distinguish the much more common obese individual with mild hypertension and glucose intolerance from obesity secondary to adrenal hypersecretion include thick rather than thin skin, pale rather than purplish striae, absence of plethora, preservation of muscle strength, and absence of osteoporosis. Laboratory tests are also helpful. Polycythemia in obesity (in contrast to Cushing's syndrome) is found rarely and appears to be associated with cor pulmonale when present. Higher than normal urinary excretion rates of hydroxycorticoids and an increase in cortisol turnover may be present (Simkin), but these changes correlate with the increase in lean body mass associated with obesity. Blood cortisol levels tend to be normal in obesity and are suppressible, and the diurnal rhythm in adrenal steroid secretion appears to be maintained (Schteingart and Conn).

Gonadal deficiency certainly is not a common cause of obesity. Although in animals it has been shown that castration is often followed by obesity, this association has been much less prominent in man. Nevertheless, it has been observed to occur, particularly when the castration is performed after puberty. Moreover, some eunuchoid males are found to be somewhat obese and tend to lose some of the obesity after the administration of testosterone. Women with the Stein-Leventhal syndrome tend to be obese (Ch. 7). Presumably the obesity results from the secretion by the ovary of steroids with actions similar to those of some of the adrenal steroids. Gonadal hormones do not constitute a satisfactory therapeutic measure for obesity unless there is definite evidence of their deficiency.

With classic hypersomatotropinism (acromegaly), obesity is not a characteristic feature. Furthermore, there is no increase in plasma levels of growth hormone in randomly selected obese patients. In fact, with fasting, hypoglycemia, exercise, and arginine stimulation, the expected rise in circulating growth hormone is much more sluggish in obesity (Roth et al.; Beck et al.; Rabinowitz). Therefore, treatment of obesity with various pituitary hormones has little rational basis. Although daily subcutaneous injections of human chorionic gonadotropin have been advocated by some to promote weight loss, controlled studies indicate no beneficial effect from this form of therapy.

Hypothalamic syndromes resulting from lesions affecting the ventromedial nucleus are extremely rare causes of obesity in man. In the case of gross lesions found in the vicinity of the hypothalamus, e.g., craniopharyngioma (Fig. 18–29) or lesions due to trauma, obesity associated with hypogonadotropic hypogonadism and in some instances with diabetes insipidus is part of the syndrome. It is not clear to what extent impairment of the secretion of hypothalamic pituitary releasing factors might contribute to the obesity.

Obesity also rarely may be present in early child-

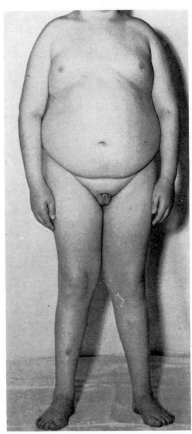

Figure 18–29. Boy aged 19 with craniopharyngioma which was associated with hypogonadotropic hypogonadism and excess fat in hip, abdominal, and pectoral regions. Genu valgum is apparent.

hood as part of a variety of congenital syndromes such as adiposogenital dystrophy (Fröhlich's syndrome), Prader-Labhart-Willi syndrome, Laurence-Moon-Biedl syndrome, Bongiovanni-Eisenmenger syndrome, and pseudohypoparathyroidism. The cause of the obesity in these syndromes remains unknown, although structural or functional hypothalamic defects have been postulated (Dunn).

Unusual distributions of adiposity can occur. Partial lipodystrophy is an unusual variation of congenital lipodystrophy (lipoatrophy), in which subcutaneous fat is totally absent from a portion of the body and hypertrophied in the remainder (Steinberg and Gwinup). In multiple lipomatosis, a frequently familial disorder characterized by localized, discrete, subcutaneous fat deposits throughout the body (Fig. 18–30), stored triglyceride in lipoma cells appears to be unavailable for mobilization even during starvation, despite the morphologic and biochemical resemblance of these cells to the more usual adipose tissue cells (Gelhorn and Benjamin).

Treatment

The prognosis for treatment of obesity appears to vary with the clinical type. Lifelong obesity is frus-

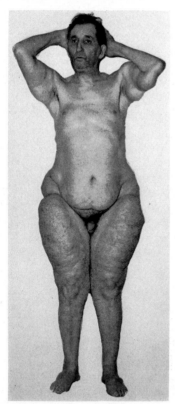

Figure 18–30. Unusual variety of lipomatosis.

TABLE 18–10. RATIO OF DEATH RATE OF OBESE TO STANDARD RISK INDIVIDUALS ANALYZED AS TO CAUSE OF DEATH (BARR)

Condition	Men	Women
Diabetes	3.83	3.72
Cirrhosis of liver	2.49	1.47
Appendicitis	2.23	1.95
Biliary calculi	2.06	2.84
Chronic nephritis	1.91	2.12
Cerebral hemorrhage	1.59	1.62
Coronary disease	1.42	1.75
Auto accidents	1.31	1.20
Suicides	0.78	0.73
Tuberculosis	0.21	0.35

Although there have been many suggestions that the macronutrient composition of the calorically restricted diet is important for successful weight reduction, there is no firm evidence that a calorie is anything more or less than a calorie, regardless of the food source from which it is derived. Bortz et al. (1967), Kinsell et al., and others have clearly shown that the rate of weight loss on low-calorie diets high in protein is the same as the rate on diets high in fat or high in carbohydrate. Previous observations which indicated less rapid weight loss with high-carbohydrate, low-calorie diets have been attributed to short-term treatment in which changes in salt and water balance obscure changes in weight. It is apparent that an obese individual has a marked propensity to retain sodium during weight reduction and that this tendency is transiently exaggerated by carbohydrate in the diet (Elsbach and Schwartz; Bortz et al., 1967; Bloom and Azar). Meal frequency may play a role in the degree of success; frequent feedings may be more likely to promote weight loss than less frequent consumption of larger loads, which may lead to abnormal eating patterns, such as the night-eating syndrome described by Stunkard et al. Fabry and his associates report that obesity is more common in individuals who eat less frequently; however, Bortz et al. (1966) could find no evidence of an effect of feeding frequency on the rate of weight loss in obese subjects studied in a metabolic ward. Appetite suppressants (usually amphetamine derivatives) are of limited utility, since their effect is transient and rarely leads to more than a 10 per cent weight reduction (London and Schreiber; Mayer, 1966). Total starvation has been promoted as a rapid route to achieve or start weight loss (Drenick et al., 1964, 1970). However, the additional metabolic and other consequences of prolonged total starvation, such as unexplained anemia, body potassium depletion, hyperuricemia, gout, ketosis, lactic acidosis, liver function abnormalities, arrhythmias, hypotension, and, rarely, sudden death (Lawlor and Wells; Cubberley et al.), have limited the utility of this form of treatment. Furthermore, it has been shown that the additional weight loss achieved by total starvation over that achieved by a 600–800 calorie diet is achieved by a selective loss in lean body mass rather than by additional loss of fat mass (Benoit et al.; Ball et

trating to treat and leads to much grief on the part of both physician and patient. In view of the poor results after long-term follow-up of a variety of weight reduction schemes (which may be very successful over the short term), this form of obesity may be virtually irreversible. It is a common experience in obesity clinics that less than 5 per cent of the markedly (presumably lifelong) obese patients ever attain normal weight, and few can maintain a short-term weight loss in excess of 40 pounds (Stunkard; Glennon; Bray et al., 1972). On the other hand, adult-onset obesity should be amenable to treatment, so that most of the metabolic and pathophysiologic consequences of enlarged adipose cell mass should be avoidable. Furthermore, excess mortality associated with obesity (Table 18–10) appears to be preventable (Fig. 18–20).

In general, obesity can be treated by reduction of caloric intake or increase of caloric expenditure or both. In special circumstances, particularly as applied to lifelong obesity, surgical techniques to decrease gastrointestinal adsorption of food and to decrease fat storage capacity by resection of large amounts of tissues have been used. Weight loss can be achieved by caloric restriction, regardless of the nature of the diet. The amount of weight loss depends largely on the degree of negative energy balance that is attained. Unfortunately, oxygen consumption declines in parallel with weight loss (Dole; Bray), making it more difficult to maintain a steady degree of weight loss over the long term.

al.). Thus a minimal quantity of protein and carbohydrate in weight reduction diets appears necessary, although the body has an unusual capacity to conserve nitrogen. In principle, it is clear that the aim of a weight reduction diet should be to keep normal body composition as well as to attain normal weight. There is no evidence to support the superiority of any form of low-calorie diet over that of any other. Thus a practical dietary recommendation for long-term management of obesity would be 15–20 cal./kg. ideal body weight, containing 20 per cent protein, 45 per cent carbohydrate, and 35 per cent fat calories. Substitution of one or more meals each day by fixed composition liquid formulas appears to have contributed to successful initiation of weight loss in many individuals. Where psychological problems appear prominent, emotional support may be necessary. The success of weight reduction groups for many individuals indicates that support of the "group therapy" type may be a useful adjunct.

The most common method for promoting caloric expenditure in obese individuals is increased exercise. Obese patients, particularly adolescent females, are consistently less active than are thin individuals (Stunkard). In practice, obese individuals on weight reduction diets tend spontaneously to decrease their activity further, perhaps to compensate for decreased caloric intake in an attempt to preserve their fat mass. Exercising animals appear to gain less weight than do free-eating sedentary controls as a result of both an increase in caloric expenditure and a decrease in food intake (Oscai and Holloszy). Exercise results in a significant decrease in the percentage of body fat, with a proportional increase in lean body mass. Sedentary calorie-restricted animals have a higher fat content than do exercising animals of the same weight. Thus exercise does appear to influence both body composition and food intake and should be part of reducing regimens. Exercise alone, however, does not appear to be an effective means of weight reduction, since the caloric equivalent of most activities is easily nullified by small amounts of food intake (Table 18–11).

Thyroid extract has been widely used to increase the oxygen consumption of obese patients regardless of whether or not they suffer from hypothyroidism or "hypometabolism." Studies of body composition have shown that the accelerated weight loss from superimposition of thyroid extract on a low-calorie diet is due to a differential loss of lean body mass rather than to loss of fat tissue. Numerous other medications have been promoted for their ability to help achieve weight loss in obese individuals. Evaluation of these becomes a problem, since the routine of frequent physician visits, weight measurement, emotional support, medication, and diet itself promotes weight loss, and it is difficult to ascribe success to a particular medication. Furthermore, weight loss may result predominantly from loss of fluid, as with the widely dispensed diuretics, rather than from loss of adipose mass.

An ileal bypass operation has been proposed for the treatment of severe and refractory obesity in an attempt to prevent early morbidity and mortality in such individuals. This surgical procedure has been devised to eliminate functionally a sufficient length of jejunum and ileum to produce weight loss and to reduce serum lipids without producing clinical steatorrhea. The distal ileum is essentially completely by-passed. Unfortunately, as reviewed by Drenick et al. (1970) and Juhl et al., by-pass surgery has been followed in several instances by massive fatty changes in the liver, cholestasis, fibrosis, interstitial inflammation, and fatal hepatic necrosis. At the present time, caution in the use of this experimental procedure is warranted. There is increasing rationale for adipectomy in the management of lifelong obesity, since the disorder is characterized by adipose cell hyperplasia. Experimental studies in animals, however, lead to little optimism, since adipectomy of large adipose deposits has been followed by compensatory hypertrophy of remaining fat cell mass (Liebelt et al.).

TABLE 18–11. ENERGY EQUIVALENTS OF TYPICAL FOODS EXPRESSED IN TERMS OF VARIOUS ACTIVITIES*

| Food | Calories | Minutes of Activity | | | | |
		Reclining	Walking	Bicycling	Swimming	Running
Apple (large)	100	78	19	12	9	5
Beer (1 glass)	114	88	22	14	10	6
Bread and butter	78	60	15	10	7	4
Carrot	42	32	8	5	4	2
Cookie (1 plain)	15	12	3	2	1	1
Chicken (½ fried)	232	178	45	28	21	12
Egg (boiled)	77	59	15	9	7	4
Ham (2 slices)	167	128	32	20	15	9
Hamburger	350	269	67	43	31	18
Milk (1 glass)	166	128	32	20	15	9
Orange (medium)	68	52	13	8	6	4
Pie, apple (⅙)	377	290	73	46	34	19
Pork chop (loin)	314	242	60	38	28	16
Spaghetti (1 serving)	400	310	77	49	36	21

*Adapted from Mayer, J.: *Overweight. Causes, Cost and Control.* New Jersey, Prentice-Hall, 1968, pp. 80–81.

Thus it can no longer be assumed that obesity is simply the result of overeating and that every fat person is simply an overfed normal one. Certainly, most slightly overweight middle-aged individuals are fundamentally normal but have eaten a little too much and exercised much too little. The grossly overweight patient who has had his problem throughout life suffers from a disorder that we do not yet understand and have been unable to cure.

HYPERLIPIDEMIA

Definition and Classification

Hyperlipidemia consists of an excessive accumulation of one or more of the major lipids transported in plasma and is usually a manifestation of an underlying disorder in lipid metabolism. For clinical purposes, hyperlipidemia may manifest as hypercholesterolemia or hypertriglyceridemia, or both. Thus levels of the lipid-carrying molecular aggregates—the lipoproteins (p. 901)—are elevated (hyperlipoproteinemia). The older term "lipemia" or "hyperlipemia" refers to the turbid or lactescent plasma visible when the large, triglyceride-rich particles accumulate (p. 892).

Aside from producing overt signs and symptoms such as xanthoma, lipemia retinalis, and acute abdominal crises, elevated plasma concentrations of certain lipids and lipoproteins are associated with an increased risk of atherosclerotic disease. It is this risk which is generally used as the guideline for arbitrarily deciding which lipid levels are abnormally high. Although there is a continuous gradient of risk throughout the population (see p. 928), individuals whose triglyceride or cholesterol levels are in the upper 5 per cent for their age and sex are most likely to develop atherosclerotic complications. Consequently, such persons have been arbitrarily defined as hyperlipidemic (Table 18–12). Thus, as with obesity, the definition of "disease" is somewhat arbitrary, since there are continuous distributions of both plasma levels and morbidity risk in the population. Also, since populations vary widely, it is meaningless to select arbitrary limits for normality that can be usefully applied to all populations. Ultimately the level at which preventive treatment can be successfully applied will influence our definition of abnormality.

Excessive lipid accumulation in plasma can result from either defective removal from plasma or excessive endogenous production or both. These abnormalities may be primary or may occur as a result of other diseases, such as endocrine disorders (diabetes or hypothyroidism, for example), or as a result of therapy with certain drugs.

The primary forms of hyperlipidemia are generally divided into familial, in which clear evidence of a genetic predisposition ("monogenic" or "polygenic") is based on the presence of the disorder in closely related family members, and sporadic, in which neither genetic nor known secondary factors

TABLE 18–12. MEAN AND UPPER 95th PERCENTILE VALUES FOR PLASMA CHOLESTEROL AND TRIGLYCERIDE IN ADULTS*

Age (Years)	Cholesterol (mg./100 ml. plasma)		Triglyceride (mg./100 ml. plasma)	
	Mean	95th Percentile	Mean	95th Percentile
Males				
20–29	190	255	75	155
30–39	210	275	80	160
40–49	220	285	85	165
50–59	230	295	95	175
60+	220	300	100	180
Females				
20–29	190	255	65	145
30–39	205	270	75	155
40–49	220	285	85	165
50–59	235	300	100	180
60+	250	315	110	190

*Data derived by regression analysis from 950 spouse controls from the Seattle myocardial infarction study (Goldstein et al.). Values in the 95th percentile approximate +2 standard deviations above the mean for cholesterol. Since triglyceride levels are not normally distributed, mean and percentiles were derived from logarithmic transformation of raw values. Normal childhood and adolescent values are considerably lower.

appear to play a role. The primary and secondary hyperlipidemias are generally characterized, however, by similar symptoms and laboratory abnormalities, and the metabolic sequelae appear to be identical.

Differentiation between primary and secondary hyperlipidemia, which is sometimes extremely difficult, is the cornerstone of successful therapy, since the secondary hyperlipidemias may be corrected simply by treatment of the causative disease, when possible, or by withdrawal of the offending medication.

Hyperlipidemia has been classified into five types, based on the specific electrophoretic patterns of the various lipoproteins (Fredrickson and Levy). Thus excess chylomicrons have been designated as Type I hyperlipoproteinemia, excess beta lipoproteins as Type II, excess broad-beta lipoproteins (mobility between very-low- and low-density lipoproteins) as Type III, excess pre-beta lipoproteins as Type IV, and an excess of both chylomicrons and pre-beta lipoproteins as Type V.

Classification solely by this morphologic method, however, does not reflect the pathophysiologic or genetic mechanisms responsible for the disorders. A single mechanism may lead to several different lipoprotein patterns, and conversely, a single pattern may reflect a variety of diseases or mechanisms. Table 18–13 presents a classification of hyperlipoproteinemias based both on lipoprotein pattern and pathophysiologic characteristics. The common secondary causes of lipid disorders and the types of associated hyperlipoproteinemia are depicted in Table 18–14. Discrete familial hyperlipidemic disorders that have been defined are summarized in Table 18–15. These more comprehensive classifications clearly elucidate the dis-

TABLE 18–13. CLASSIFICATIONS OF HYPERLIPOPROTEINEMIA MORPHOLOGIC VS. PATHOPHYSIOLOGIC CHANGES

	I Chylomicrons	V Chylomicrons + Pre-β	IV Pre-β	III Broad-β	IIA β	IIB β + Pre-β
↓ *Removal*						
LPL deficiency	+	+				
LPL depletion		+	+			+
Remnant accumulation				+		
?↓ LDL removal					+	+
Production ↑		+	+			+
Plasma TG/CHOL ratio						

Plasma TG/CHOL ratio

TABLE 18–14. SECONDARY HYPERLIPIDEMIA

Cause of Hyperlipidemia	Lipoprotein Pattern					
	I Chylomicrons	V Chylomicrons + Pre-β	IV Pre-β	III Broad-β	IIA β	IIB β + Pre-β
Endocrine						
Diabetes						
Severe	+	+				
Moderate		+	+	+		+
Mild		+	+	+		
Corticosteroid R$_x$						
High dose	+	+				
Low dose or						
Cushing's syndrome			+		+	+
Hypothyroidism		+	+	+	+	+
Hypopituitarism		+	+			
Estrogen or						
oral contraceptive R$_x$		+	+			
Nonendocrine						
Renal disease						
Nephrotic syndrome		+	+		+	+
Uremia		+	+			
Alcohol		+	+			
Dysglobulinemia	+	+		+	+	
Glycogen storage disease	+	+				
Congenital lipodystrophy		+	+			

TABLE 18–15. GENETIC HYPERLIPIDEMIAS

Disorder	Plasma Lipoprotein Pattern	Genetic Mechanism	Estimated Gene Frequency
Familial hypercholesterolemia (monogenic)	IIA, IIB	Autosomal dominant	1–2/1,000
Familial hypercholesterolemia (polygenic)	IIA, IIB	Polygenic	—
Familial hypertriglyceridemia	IV, V	Autosomal dominant	2/1,000
Familial combined hyperlipidemia	IIA, IIB, IV, V	Autosomal dominant	3–5/1,000
Broad-beta disease	III, IV, V	?Autosomal dominant	1/5,000
Lipoprotein lipase deficiency	I, V	Autosomal recessive	Rare

orders for purposes of diagnosis; they also yield a better understanding of the rationale for different approaches to therapy.

Triglyceride Removal Defects

Lipoprotein Lipase Deficiency

Since impaired LPL activity leads to defective removal of all triglyceride-rich lipoproteins, it produces either a predominance of chylomicrons derived from dietary fat (Type I lipoprotein pattern) or a combined predominance of chylomicrons and VLDL derived from the liver (Type V). This accumulation may vary in type with age (children have less VLDL) and diet (fat ingestion increases the concentration of chylomicrons).

Although LPL deficiency may occasionally be seen in its congenital form, it is more frequently acquired, as in severe insulin-dependent diabetes, hypothyroidism, prolonged, high-dose corticosteroid therapy, dysgammaglobulinemia, and acute pancreatitis (Bagdade, Porte, et al., 1967, 1970; Glueck et al., 1969).

The Type I pattern is more likely to occur in the familial disorder, manifesting itself in childhood with typical episodes of eruptive xanthoma and with the acute abdominal pain of pancreatitis. On the other hand, the Type V pattern is more frequent in adults, largely because they accumulate more endogenous lipoproteins of the pre-beta variety than do children.

Regardless of underlying cause or age of onset, hyperchylomicronemia can be associated with the following physical findings: lipemia retinalis, acute pancreatitis, and eruptive xanthoma due to deposits of chylomicrons in the skin (Parker et al.). The xanthomas are usually located over extensor surfaces of the arms, lower extremities, buttocks, or back and often wax and wane with dietary fat content and the degree or duration of the disorder.

In the laboratory, hyperchylomicronemia may easily be recognized by a characteristic creamlike layer atop fresh plasma after centrifugation or brief refrigeration. Diagnosis of lipoprotein lipase deficiency is suggested by findings of a markedly elevated plasma triglyceride level accompanied by normal or only slightly increased cholesterol measurements, and it is confirmed by subnormal lipoprotein lipase activity in post-heparin plasma (post-heparin lipolytic activity, or PHLA) (Fredrickson et al.).

Impaired Lipoprotein Lipase Function

This disorder, which usually manifests itself in a Type V (or, less frequently, Type IV) lipoprotein pattern, appears to be related to a defect in the function of LPL, despite the fact that the usual assay for this enzyme (post-heparin lipolytic activity measurement) is normal. Studies of triglyceride transport have shown that, in some individuals, LPL can be depleted by prolonged infusions of

heparin (Brunzell et al., 1972a). In these individuals, as yet an unknown proportion of individuals with hypertriglyceridemia, the synthesis of LPL appears to be unable to compensate for the reactions that deplete the enzyme.

The fact that approximately 90 per cent of these lipemic patients are also moderately severe diabetics and that the severity of the lipoprotein abnormality seems to be directly related to the height of the fasting blood glucose (Brunzell et al., 1972a) suggests that insulin deficiency is responsible for the impaired lipoprotein lipase activity. (This is described further in the section on hypertriglyceridemia and impaired glucose tolerance.)

Excessive Triglyceride Production

"Endogenous" Lipemia

Although a specific defect has not been demonstrated, this disorder appears to result from accelerated hepatic production of pre-beta lipoproteins (VLDL) (Reaven et al.; Nikkilä). In its mildest, most frequent form, endogenous lipemia has a Type IV lipoprotein pattern (increased pre-beta). When increased lipogenesis is more marked, however, removal mechanisms are unable to assimilate all the lipids additionally derived from the diet. In these situations, chylomicrons derived from exogenous fat may build up as well, leading to a Type V lipoprotein pattern.

Endogenous lipemia is not associated with xanthomas unless hyperchylomicronemia supervenes. The familial form, however, which occurs quite frequently, is associated with an increased prevalence of premature coronary atherosclerosis (Goldstein et al.), especially when combined with increased beta lipoproteins (see combined hyperlipidemia). Basal triglyceride levels are characteristically elevated, and since the VLDL which accumulate also contain significant amounts of cholesterol, total serum or plasma cholesterol may also show an increase.

Increased production of pre-beta migrating, triglyceride-rich VLDL often occurs during weight gain, during the last trimester of pregnancy, or during therapy with corticosteroids or estrogenic agents. Estrogen-containing oral contraceptive steroid agents have been shown to produce uniformly a 50–100 per cent increase in plasma triglyceride levels (Hazzard et al., 1969); in some individuals, gross hypertriglyceridemia has been unmasked (Zorilla et al.). Hypertriglyceridemia also has been observed as a consequence of nonnephrotic chronic renal failure (Bagdade et al., 1968b). In the primary form of the disorder, however, no such stimuli may be demonstrable.

Because of the markedly elevated triglyceride levels observed in these patients following high-carbohydrate, fat-free diets, it was once believed that their metabolic defect was related specifically to carbohydrate, and the disorder was termed "carbohydrate-induced lipemia." It is now clear, however, that "carbohydrate induction" is a normal

TABLE 18–16. PROBLEM-ORIENTED FLOW SHEET FOR HYPERTRIGLYCERIDEMIA

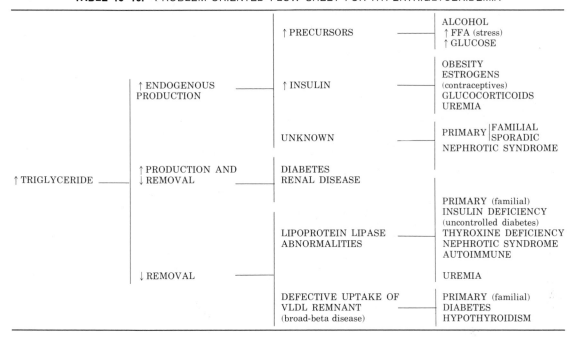

phenomenon, since healthy subjects have been found to double basal triglyceride levels in response to fat-free diets (Bierman and Porte; Glueck, Levy, et al.). The distinguishing feature in patients with "endogenous" lipemia is abnormal triglyceride regulation in the basal state after ingestion of normal amounts of carbohydrate and fat. Increasing the proportion of carbohydrate in the diet accentuates the hypertriglyceridemia but does not cause it.

Most patients with primary endogenous lipemia share characteristics other than their lipoprotein accumulation, namely obesity, mild glucose intolerance without clinical diabetes, and hyperinsulinism—factors which may contribute to excessive production of triglyceride. (This phenomenon is described in the section, Hypertriglyceridemia and Impaired Glucose Tolerance.)

"Mixed lipemia" occurs when removal defects are associated with factors promoting triglyceride synthesis, such as excess alcohol intake; it also occurs in certain diabetics (Havel; Bierman, Porte, et al., 1970). Thus hypertriglyceridemia as a clinical "problem" can be conveniently dissected in terms of some currently held views regarding pathophysiology (Table 18–16).

By-Product Accumulation

"Broad-Beta" Disease

Whether lipoprotein lipase function is completely normal in this disorder is not yet known. It is characterized, however, by accumulation of an apparent by-product of lipoprotein lipase action—a cholesterol-rich "remnant" produced by the enzyme's degradation of triglyceride-containing lipoproteins (see p. 901). This cholesterol-rich lipoprotein separates by density with VLDL but has the electrophoretic β mobility of LDL. Although it may occasionally be acquired (Hazzard and Bierman, 1971), Broad-beta disease is predominantly familial, inherited either with an autosomal dominant or recessive pattern (Fredrickson and Levy). As with most other inherited lipoprotein disorders, the patients are extremely prone to develop both coronary and peripheral vascular atherosclerosis at an early age.

Diagnosis of the disease is strongly suggested by findings of (1) tuberous and planar xanthomas which are almost pathognomonic when they are present (Fig. 18–31), (2) both plasma triglycerides and cholesterol levels elevated in approximately a 1:1 ratio, and (3) a Type III lipoprotein pattern on paper or agarose electrophoresis (since these "remnants" have a mobility intermediate between prebeta and beta lipoproteins, the pattern presents as a broad smear between those two lipoprotein zones). For a definitive diagnosis, however, preparative ultracentrifugation and VLDL compositional analysis are usually required, particularly in asymptomatic patients (Hazzard et al., 1972).

Defective Low-Density Lipoprotein Removal

Hyperbetalipoproteinemia; Hypercholesterolemia

This widespread disorder, whose primary form was recognized early as "essential hypercholes-

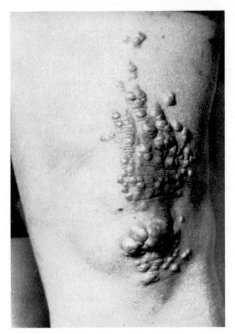

Figure 18–31.   Xanthoma tuberosum of knee.

terolemia," is characterized by an accumulation of the cholesterol-rich beta lipoproteins (Type II), apparently because of a delay in their catabolism (Langer et al.).

Both familial (monogenic and polygenic) and sporadic varieties of hyperbetalipoproteinemia are prevalent and may be associated with obesity (see p. 911). Beta lipoprotein elevation also occurs secondary to hypothyroidism, in which the removal rate appears to be decreased (Walton et al.), and to the nephrotic syndrome, in which production may be increased (Scott et al.). Occasionally it occurs in patients with acute intermittent porphyria (Lees et al.) or with myeloma (Cohen et al.), in which an abnormal globulin is believed to bind to beta lipoprotein and diminish its clearance rate (Savin). Hypercholesterolemia is also frequently seen in patients with obstructive liver disease in whom an abnormal cholesterol-rich lipoprotein accumulates (LP-X) (Seidel et al.), and it may occur in those who have ingested excessive amounts of dietary cholesterol or saturated fats (Fredrickson and Levy).

Regardless of the cause of accumulation of these cholesterol-rich lipoproteins, the risk of coronary atherosclerosis is high, and cardiovascular complications are frequent. Familial hypercholesterolemia expresses early in life (Schrott et al.) and has been documented in cord blood samples (Glueck et al., 1971).

Severe hypercholesterolemia is associated with a specific kind of xanthoma, the tendinous xanthoma, which may be nodular or diffuse but which usually appears on the extensor forearm tendons, Achilles tendons, or tendons of the hand. These typically appear during the first decade of life in individuals with the homozygous form of this autosomal dominant disorder.

Combined Hypertriglyceridemia and Hypercholesterolemia

Frequently associated with coronary atherosclerosis, this disorder was only recently recognized as a distinct entity (Goldstein et al.; Rose et al.); the precise pathophysiologic mechanisms have not yet been established. Although the pattern of increased beta and pre-beta lipoproteins has been tentatively classified by the World Health Organization as Type II-B hyperlipoproteinemia (Beaumont et al.), this familial disease may present with a variety of lipoprotein types (II-B, II, or IV) in affected individuals in the same family.

In a recent study by Goldstein and colleagues of 500 consecutive three-month survivors of myocardial infarction in Seattle, in which more than 2,600 relatives were tested, this disorder was the most frequent genetic type (Fig. 18–32). It was associated with 30 per cent of the cases of myocardial infarction in patients who had hyperlipidemia (one-third of all cases), while familial hypertriglyceridemia accounted for 14 per cent, and familial hypercholesterolemia (hyperbetalipoproteinemia) only 10 per cent. At present, diagnosis can be established only by family studies; both plasma cholesterol and triglycerides are elevated, and electrophoretic analysis shows a combined pattern of elevated beta and pre-beta lipoproteins in the majority of family members.

Hypertriglyceridemia and Impaired Glucose Tolerance

Alterations in fat transport often resulting in hypertriglyceridemia are well-recognized concomitants of both mild glucose intolerance and clinical diabetes. In large groups of diabetics, elevated

GENETIC ANALYSIS OF HYPERLIPIDEMIA IN 164 M.I. SURVIVORS

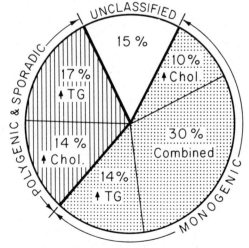

Figure 18–32

plasma triglyceride levels coexist in about one third of patients (Bierman and Porte) and appear to be related to the critical role of insulin in both the removal of triglyceride-rich lipoproteins from plasma ("diabetic lipemia") and their production ("endogenous lipemia"). These more distinct abnormalities appear to be extremes of a spectrum, since mixed anomalies appear to merge between them.

Severe Glucose Intolerance:
Diabetic Lipemia

Insulin availability appears to be necessary for normal function of lipoprotein lipase (see page 895); thus the extreme insulin deficiency associated with severe, uncontrolled diabetes mellitus leads to diabetic lipemia, an acquired form of lipoprotein lipase deficiency.

LPL activity, indirectly assessed as plasma postheparin lipolytic activity (PHLA), is low in patients with the diabetic lipemia syndrome (Bagdade, Porte, et al., 1967). Although this disorder was recognized in 5 per cent of diabetics before the insulin era, it is now relatively rare. When it occurs, the underlying enzyme deficiency is reversed with appropriate insulin repletion; it promptly restores normal PHLA, improves triglyceride removal, and reduces plasma triglyceride levels.

Diabetic lipemia can be mimicked by brief withdrawal of insulin from insulin-dependent juvenile diabetics; the enzyme activity decreases and triglyceride levels rise within 48 hours (Bagdade et al., 1968a). The diabetic lipemia syndrome has also been observed as a complication of acute pancreatitis and during prolonged treatment with high doses of corticosteroids (Bagdade, 1969, 1970).

Moderate Glucose Intolerance:
Lipoprotein Lipase Depletion

More subtle insulin deficiency occurs in patients with less severe diabetes, those with mild, fasting hyperglycemia in the range of 130–160 mg./100 ml. Recent studies by Brunzell and co-workers have demonstrated PHLA abnormalities in these individuals despite normal levels by standard assay. In contrast to normally sustained levels of PHLA during a five-hour infusion of a large dose of heparin, the PHLA levels of these subjects consistently drop significantly after the second hour, and this seems to reflect impaired synthesis of enzyme. The severity of this "PHLA depletion" appears to be related to the degree of insulin deficiency, judged by fasting glucose levels, but contrasts with the gross PHLA deficiency which is immediately evident after intravenous heparin in the diabetic lipemia syndrome. A comparable phenomenon has been observed in alloxan diabetic rats (Atkin and Meng).

Most clinical diabetics with hypertriglyceridemia fall into this category, which really represents

another acquired form of "removal" lipemia, in which either chylomicrons (Type I), pre-beta lipoproteins (Type IV), or both (Type V) accumulate in plasma. As with severe insulin-deficient diabetics, these persons will respond to replacement therapy. Either oral antidiabetic agents or insulin corrects the removal defect and subsequently lowers triglyceride levels. When this syndrome occurs in a diabetic under management,' it usually indicates that therapy is suboptimal and that treatment requires reevaluation.

Mixed lipemia (defective removal plus overproduction) occurs in this group; treatment of hyperglycemia may correct the triglyceride removal defect, thereby unmasking endogenous lipemia.

Mild Glucose Intolerance:
"Endogenous" Lipemia

By a completely different mechanism, excess insulin associated with the obese patient who frequently has mild glucose intolerance leads to another lipid defect, an acquired form of overproduction hypertriglyceridemia. This form may also be seen in well-treated diabetics (see above). Aside from its effect on lipoprotein lipase activity, insulin (among other substances) appears to act on the liver to promote VLDL production (Topping and Mayes), presumably by enhancing lipogenesis and lipoprotein packaging and by preventing hepatic triglyceride breakdown (see Figs. 18–9 and 18–26). A variety of patient studies recently reviewed (Bierman, Porte, et al., 1970) have shown that elevated serum-immunoreactive insulin levels (IRI), both in the basal state and after glucose stimulation, are directly related to plasma triglyceride levels in normal subjects as well as in those with endogenous lipemia.

The fact that most patients with endogenous lipemia are also mildly glucose-intolerant (fasting glucose levels are frequently normal, however) led to the idea that the glucose intolerance was causing the hypertriglyceridemia. It is now apparent that early insulin responses to glucose are similar in patients with hypertriglyceridemia and in subjects with normal triglyceride levels who have comparable degrees of mild glucose intolerance (Bagdade et al., 1971), and correction of glucose intolerance during oral sulfonylurea therapy does not lower triglyceride levels (Belknap et al.). This suggests that glucose intolerance, with its associated abnormality of early insulin release, is not etiologically related to hypertriglyceridemia. Conversely, hypertriglyceridemia does not appear to cause the glucose intolerance (see below).

Obesity is the most prevalent of several secondary factors (Fig. 18–26) that induce endogenous hypertriglyceridemia by invoking mechanisms which impair the action of insulin on glucose translocation in peripheral tissue. This reduced responsiveness (insulin "resistance" or "antagonism") by some unknown process is "sensed" by the pancreas, which secretes additional insulin. The hyperinsulinemia associated with adiposity is well documented (see p. 909). The basal hyperinsulinemia often observed in persons with endogenous lipemia is fully accounted for by the degree of coexisting adiposity (Bagdade et al., 1971). Moreover, correlations between adiposity and plasma triglyceride levels have been observed in both sexes, at all ages, using such indices of adiposity as relative weight, skin-fold thickness, and actual measurements of per cent body fat (recent review by Bierman, Porte, et al., 1970).

Most patients with endogenous lipemia and mild glucose intolerance have a long history of obesity. As might be expected, obesity-related hypertriglyceridemia responds dramatically to weight reduction, which reverses basal hyperinsulinemia, hypertriglyceridemia, and glucose intolerance. On the other hand, correction of mild glucose intolerance does not decrease triglyceride levels, nor does lowering of triglyceride levels with pharmacologic agents affect either glucose or insulin levels in these individuals.

The other forms of hypertriglyceridemia associated with hyperinsulinemia respond to reduction or removal of the offending hormone or drug or to correction of a causative disorder.

Hyperlipidemia and Hypothyroidism

In addition to the elevated, cholesterol-rich, beta lipoprotein levels (p. 901) frequently observed in hypothyroidism, deficiency of thyroid hormone exerts profound effects on triglyceride transport, often leading to hypertriglyceridemia. The severity of the effect is in large part related to the degree of hormone deficiency, whether primary or secondary to pituitary disorders, and thus the presence or absence of hypertriglyceridemia or hypercholesterolemia offers little diagnostic aid in the differentiation between primary and secondary hypothyroidism.

Availability of adequate thyroid hormone is essential for normal activity of lipoprotein lipase. In hypothyroidism, low LPL appears to be reciprocally related to hypertriglyceridemia, and the abnormalities are reversible with thyroid replacement (Porte et al.). As with insulin deficiency, the degree and type of triglyceride-rich lipoprotein accumulation may vary in severity and type with diet and age. Reversible hypertriglyceridemia associated with low LPL has recently been reported in a 14-month-old cretin (Baum et al.).

The normal removal of chylomicron and VLDL remnants (p. 901) also appears to be affected by hypothyroidism, since a Type III lipoprotein pattern and all the features of "broad-beta" disease can become clinically manifest with thyroid insufficiency and reversible with treatment (Hazzard and Bierman, 1973).

Although fatty acid mobilization from adipose tissue may be decreased in hypothyroidism, thereby reducing fatty acid flux to the liver, diminished hepatic production of triglyceride-rich lipoproteins is presumably insufficient to fully counterbalance impairment of removal.

Thus a wide variety of patterns of hyperlipoproteinemia can be produced by hypothyroidism (Table 18–14). In a large series of patients with primary myxedema reported by Koppers and Palumbo, the majority of patients (53 per cent) were hyperlipidemic, with increased pre-beta or beta lipoprotein levels or both. In addition, the broad-beta pattern and fasting chylomicronemia were not unusual. Although individuals with hypothyroidism appear to be excessively predisposed to atherosclerosis, the role of these varieties of secondary hyperlipidemia in that regard is unknown.

Laboratory Tests in Differential Diagnosis

The first step in the diagnosis of hyperlipidemia is routine quantitative measurement of both cholesterol and triglyceride levels in fasting serum or plasma. When values are above normal (exceed the 95th percentile matched for age and sex, Table 18–12) and verified at least once more, a combination of personal, dietary, and family histories, a thorough examination, and laboratory tests are necessary to define the specific lipid disorder accurately.

Further studies of plasma obtained after an overnight fast may yield additional information regarding the underlying abnormality. The formation of a cream layer in the cold always indicates the presence of chylomicrons, which often points to a deficiency in triglyceride removal. When a high concentration of triglyceride-rich VLDL is present, the plasma also appears turbid. For practical purposes, completely clear plasma or serum suggests a normal triglyceride level and rules out disorders of chylomicron and VLDL transport.

Because lipoproteins carry varying amounts of triglyceride and cholesterol, the relative degree of elevation of these two lipids in whole plasma is often helpful. In hyperchylomicronemia, the triglyceride-cholesterol ratio is high, 10:1 or higher. In hyperbetalipoproteinemia, the triglyceride-cholesterol ratio may be as low as 0:5 or less, and in broad-beta disease the ratio is about 1:1. On the other hand, in the common combined disorder, since both beta and pre-beta may be increased in varying proportions, ratios of lipids in plasma can be misleading.

Electrophoretic studies, which are used to define semiquantitatively an abnormal lipoprotein pattern, may provide additional aid in selected circumstances. Electrophoresis is usually not necessary, however, when serum measurements show only an elevated cholesterol level. In such instances, there is a very close correlation between serum cholesterol and beta lipoprotein cholesterol levels. Occasionally, in certain individuals (usually younger females), a mildly increased serum cholesterol may be due to elevated alpha (high-density) lipoprotein levels. These can be distinguished by precipitation methods. In situations with marked degrees of hypertriglyceridemia, on the other hand, electrophoretic studies are often insufficient for definitive diagnosis. Not infrequently, high levels of triglycerides will produce a smearing effect, so that some of the patterns merge. For example, it is often difficult to distinguish between Types III, IV, and V by paper or agarose electrophoresis alone. While determination of plasma lipoprotein patterns by this method may be confirmatory or provide clues for further work-up, the analysis alone does not define disease or distinguish discrete genetic disorders, such as familial hypercholesterolemia, from the newly discovered combined hypercholesterolemia and hypertriglyceridemia. In some situations, only ultracentrifugation of plasma will provide an answer (will define broad-beta disease); in others, more detailed family studies are most helpful.

Guidelines for Therapy

Before a therapeutic program for hyperlipidemia is undertaken, the possible secondary causes should be thoroughly investigated since these are very frequent. In general, a thorough history plus laboratory tests for thyroid and liver function, serum glucose, and plasma and urine protein levels will elucidate the secondary disorders. These may be simpler to treat, since it is usually only a matter of withdrawal of inciting pharmacologic agents or treatment of the underlying illness.

When secondary causes cannot be elucidated, it must be assumed that the disorder is either familial or sporadic. Although diet and drugs are the treatment mainstays of hyperlipidemia, therapy must be aimed at the pathophysiology associated with the disorder rather than at a particular lipoprotein pattern, which often is nonspecific.

Diet

Provided the patient will cooperate, dietary restriction alone is often very effective in lowering blood lipids in most hyperlipidemias. The exception is hypercholesterolemia, where optimal diet alone rarely achieves more than a 20 per cent reduction in cholesterol levels (Lees and Wilson; Evans et al.). In all primary or sporadic disorders, however, dietary therapy should always be attempted initially. Only when the patient proves refractory should pharmacologic agents be considered.

Lipoprotein lipase deficiency, in which hypertriglyceridemia is aggravated by dietary fat, is best handled simply by restriction of fat intake and optionally substituting short- or medium-chain triglycerides. None of the available medications is very effective in this disorder. When severe insulin deficiency is causing the enzyme deficiency, the patient should be vigorously treated with insulin. In lipemia associated with impaired lipoprotein lipase activity in conjunction with hyperglycemia, either insulin or oral antidiabetic agents are effective in correcting the disorder.

Most other types of hyperlipidemia respond to a basic diet that is low in cholesterol and saturated fat. Since obesity aggravates the lipid disorders, this diet should be hypocaloric until the patient achieves ideal body weight. Such a diet most likely will contain a higher proportion of carbohydrate, but in most instances this is of little concern, even in patients with endogenous lipemia. Although triglyceride levels are reportedly highest on high carbohydrate diets, this only occurs in the postabsorptive state following an overnight fast. Studies of twenty-four hour patterns of triglyceride levels have shown them to be actually lower on high carbohydrate diets compared with diets higher in fat than carbohydrate (Schlierf and Stossberg).

Thus a disproportionate restriction of carbohydrates in the diet of these patients is not usually justified. If hypertriglyceridemia persists after ideal weight is achieved, however, avoidance of excessive intake is indicated. Alcohol, which may increase triglyceride production by altering the caloric balance and directly stimulating hepatic syntheses (Kudzma and Schonfeld), should be discouraged in patients with any disorder in the transport of VLDL. In patients with hypercholesterolemia, particular emphasis must be placed on lowering the intake of cholesterol-containing foods. Decreasing the dietary intake from the average American consumption of 750–1,000 mg./day to less than 250 mg. is an essential step in therapy, since dietary cholesterol will accumulate beyond the ability of the body to reduce the amount synthesized and increase the amount excreted (see p. 903) (Fig. 18–33). Saturated fat intake should also be curtailed, since these fatty acids also appear to raise serum cholesterol levels. Cholesterol and saturated fat usually occur in the same foods, however, so that the dietary regimen would probably be identical. Dietary management has been shown to reduce cholesterol levels during the first year of life in infants with familial hypercholesterolemia (Glueck et al., 1971).

The value of substituting unsaturated for saturated fat in diets for patients with hypercholesterolemia is debatable. It is not known whether a

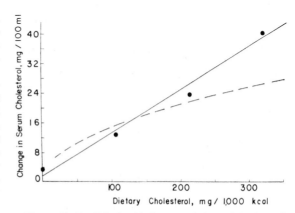

Figure 18–33. Relationship between cholesterol intake and the change in serum cholesterol following 21 days on a cholesterol-free formula diet of constant fatty acid composition. The broken line shows predicted values based on the equation of Keys et al. (1965) (From Mattson, F. H., Erickson, B. A., et al.: *Amer. J. Clin. Nutr.* 25:589, 1972.)

diet high in unsaturated fats will be more efficient in lowering cholesterol levels than restriction of cholesterol and saturated fats without the substitution. Furthermore, the long-term effects of highly unsaturated fat diets remain unknown, and the mechanism by which unsaturated fat appears to lower cholesterol levels may not necessarily be by increasing cholesterol excretion but could include redistribution of the sterol between plasma and tissues.

Pharmacologic Agents

When dietary restrictions or weight reduction or both are ineffective, or the patient fails to cooperate, a number of agents may be added to the therapeutic regimen. Drugs which act by reducing hepatic triglyceride production—clofibrate, nicotinic acid, phenformin—all are effective (Bierman, Brunzell, et al., 1970; Carlson, Gustafson et al.; Stout and Bierman; Strisower et al.; Berkowitz) in disorders involving this mechanism: endogenous lipemia, mixed lipemia, and broad-beta disease. Patients with the last disorder have been found to respond particularly well to combined weight reduction and clofibrate (Fredrickson and Levy).

Certain anabolic and progestational agents, such as oxandrolone and norethindrone, have been found by Glueck et al. (1969) to be effective in some patients with primary removal disorders, perhaps by enhancement of the effect of lipoprotein lipase.

By directly diverting cholesterol and bile acids from the intestines to the feces, bile acid binding agents, such as cholestyramine and the experimental drug colestipol, enhance cholesterol excretion and interfere with enterohepatic recycling. Consequently, these agents are useful in lowering plasma cholesterol levels in patients with hypercholesterolemia. Although dextrothyroxine has been shown to reduce both plasma cholesterol and triglyceride levels by 10–15 per cent, presumably by stimulating removal processes more than synthetic, this drug has been withdrawn from a large, secondary, drug prevention trial because of a higher mortality and morbidity among patients with coronary heart disease treated with the drug (Stamler). It is quite likely that the lipid-lowering action of thyroid hormone and its analogues is not separable from the stimulating effect on tissue oxygen consumption.

Combinations of drugs are seldom indicated except in the severe familial monogenic form of hypercholesterolemia—when cholesterol levels move above 700 mg./100 ml. In these highly resistant patients, a combination of nicotinic acid and a bile acid binding agent may help improve the picture. Perhaps in the future, combined therapy—for example, cholestyramine (or its analogue, colestipol) coupled with clofibrate—may prove useful in the newly recognized genetic disorder of combined hypertriglyceridemia and hypercholesterolemia. The value of drug therapy has not yet been established, however.

Surgery

A number of medical centers are currently performing ileal by-pass operations on patients with severe, resistant familial hypercholesterolemia (Scott). The procedure results in increased excretion of cholesterol degradation products in the stool. At present, however, the surgical approach should be regarded as experimental, for little is known about the long-term effects of the surgery itself.

Comment

The association between hypertriglyceridemia, hypercholesterolemia, and atherosclerotic disease in persons with and without hyperglycemia has been amply confirmed in a variety of population studies (Ostrander; Carlson and Böttiger). Although various factors have thus far been implicated, the mechanisms that account for this relationship are yet to be clearly elucidated; they are discussed in more detail in the section on atherosclerosis.

The rationale for treating symptomatic hyperlipidemia is obvious. Treatment of asymptomatic disorders is based on the yet unproved "lipid hypothesis"—that lowering lipid levels will decrease morbidity and mortality from associated atherosclerosis. The decision who should be treated and when is not yet on a rational footing and must await controlled intervention trials aimed at this question.

ATHEROSCLEROSIS

Atherosclerosis has been defined as "a variable combination of changes of the intima of arteries . . . consisting of the focal accumulation of lipids, complex carbohydrates, blood and blood products, fibrous tissue and calcium deposits, and associated with medial changes" (WHO Study Group). Because of its connection with coronary heart disease, cerebrovascular disease, and peripheral vascular disease, atherosclerosis is associated with higher morbidity and mortality than is any other disorder in the western world. Progress toward clarification of its etiology has been slow for several reasons, however. First, it tends to develop insidiously for many years in ostensibly healthy individuals, and no satisfactory method is available for directly studying this important phase of the disease. Second, when clinical symptoms finally develop, atherosclerosis is usually advanced and is only one of a complex group of precipitating factors. This makes evaluation of the course of the primary disease process even more difficult. Finally, because of the difficulty of making satisfactory studies of man *in vivo*, conclusions with respect to pathogenesis and therapy have had to depend on statistical correlations between the incidence or prevalence of overt vascular disease and plasma lipid concentrations, hypertension, obesity, diabetes, etc.; the study of specimens obtained at autopsy; and investigations of experimental atherosclerosis in animals. Despite these difficulties, there is strong evidence that lipids play an important role in atherosclerosis, and they have repeatedly been implicated in connection with the pathogenesis, prophylaxis, and treatment of the disease. Consequently, it is important that those involved in the management of diseases of lipid metabolism be acquainted with present knowledge in this area.

Pathogenesis

Structural Factors and Definitions

Normal arteries vary not only in size and degree of branching but also in histologic and chemical composition. This also is true of the arteries most prone to develop atherosclerosis, including the aorta and the coronary and cerebral arteries. Nevertheless, all arteries are composed of three more or less distinguishable layers: the intima, the media, and the adventitia. The *intima* is the primary focus of the developing atherosclerotic process. It is composed of several elements. First, a single layer of endothelial cells borders on the arterial lumen. Next to this are variable numbers of smooth muscle cells and variable amounts of collagen and other extracellular connective tissue components. Finally, the intima is limited by a layer of elastic tissue, the *internal elastic lamina*. The overall thickness of the intima increases with age because of proliferation of smooth muscle cells and is particularly pronounced at sites of arterial branching. This thickening appears to be corre-

lated with the susceptibility of arteries to atherosclerotic change. The *media* of arteries like the coronaries is mainly composed of smooth muscle cells surrounded by an extracellular matrix of collagen, elastic fibers, and proteoglycans. In the larger arteries, layers of elastic tissue are particularly prominent. The *adventitia* is mainly composed of loose connective tissue.

Fatty Streaks. The earliest macroscopically detectable fatty change in arteries is the so-called fatty streak, regarded by many pathologists as an early stage of atherosclerosis. This is a small, yellow-gray area that is characteristically flat and does not compromise the arterial lumen. The yellow-gray color is largely caused by lipid within smooth muscle cells, macrophages, and "foam" cells (Figs. 18–34 and 18–35). The lipid is mainly cholesterol (Table 18–17), most of which is esterified to oleic and palmitic acid. Little phospholipid or triglyceride appears to be present, since the relative content of these lipids in fatty streaks is less than that in lesion-free intima. Despite the presumed relation between fatty streaks and fibrous atherosclerotic plaques, the prevalence and location of fatty streaks are not generally correlated with the prevalence and location of fibrous lesions. Fatty streaks occur in all populations studied, irrespective of the propensity of these populations to develop clinical vascular disease. They begin in childhood (in the aorta) and in late adolescence (in the coronary and cerebral arteries), increase with age, and do not necessarily "progress" into fibrous lesions. Even in populations susceptible to atherosclerosis, the location of fatty streaks in the aorta and the extent of intimal involvement do not parallel the location and extent of fibrous lesions. Only

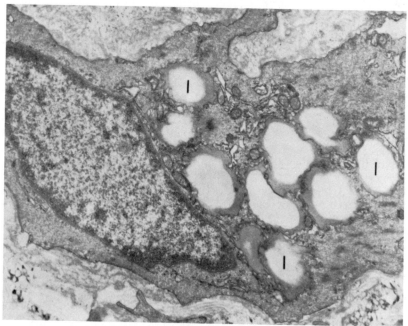

Figure 18–34. Electron micrograph ($\times$ 15,000) of smooth muscle cell in fatty streaks in human intima. Lipid inclusions are labeled *1*. They are irregular in contour and lined by a single membrane. The lipid is moderately electron-dense; the central portion of the inclusions is electron-lucent, probably because of extraction of a portion of the lipid during tissue processing. (From Greer, J.: *Lab. Invest. 14*:1764, 1965.)

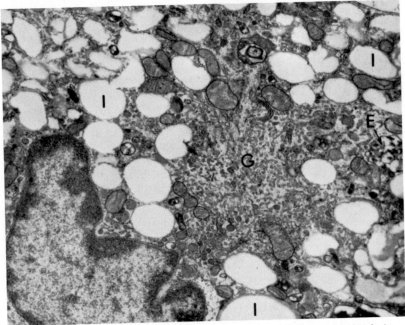

Figure 18–35. Electron micrograph (× 15,250) of foam cell in fatty streak in human intima. Lipid inclusions are labeled *I*, as in Figure 18–34. Vesicles and membranes of a large Golgi zone (G) are present. (From Greer, J.: *Lab. Invest.* 14:1764, 1965.)

in the coronary arteries have better correlations been observed (Geer et al.).

Fibrous Plaques. Fibrous plaques differ from fatty streaks not only in prevalence and location but also in appearance, composition, and effects. They are pearly white, considerably larger than fatty streaks, and cause the intimal surface to bulge outward into the lumen. A major part of the lipid is extracellular, often mixed with what appears to be cell debris to form "gruel." Although this lipid, like that of fatty streaks, is mainly cholesteryl ester (Table 18–17), linoleic rather than oleic acid is the principal esterified fatty acid. Consequently, the composition of the cholesteryl ester resembles that of plasma lipoprotein cholesteryl ester rather than fatty streak cholesteryl ester. Another distinctive feature of fibrous plaques is the presence of large numbers of smooth

muscle cells and large amounts of collagen (Table 18–18). These usually form a cap between the lumen and the extracellular lipid, and, in older individuals, the collagen is the cap's dominant component. The presumption is that many of the smooth muscle cells have disintegrated and contributed to the lipid-rich extracellular gruel. In older individuals, too, fibrous plaques contain increasing amounts of calcium. These *complicated lesions* are the ones that frequently are associated with clinical symptoms. With increasing cell degeneration and accumulation of gruel, the wall of the artery becomes progressively weaker, and rupture of the intima can occur, causing aneurysm and death by hemorrhage. Alternatively, arterial emboli can form when fragments of diseased intima dislodge into the arterial lumen, or stenosis and impaired organ function can occur as smaller arteries gradually become occluded by widespread atherosclerotic thickening (Fig. 18–36). Stenosis of

TABLE 18–17. LIPID DISTRIBUTION IN DIFFERENT TYPES OF PLAQUE

	Normal Intima†	Fatty Streaks*	Fatty Nodules*	Fibrous Plaques*	Calcified Fibrous Plaques*
Total Lipid (mg./100 mg. dry tissue)	11	28	61	47	50
Percentage Distribution					
Cholesteryl ester	42	60	65	54	56
Unesterified cholesterol	13	12	14	18	22
Triglyceride	15	10	9	11	7
Phospholipid	29	18	14	16	15

†Age group 40–59. (Data from Smith, E. B., Evans, P. H., et al.: *J. Atherosclerosis Res.* 7:177, 1967.)
*Without amorphous lipid. (Reproduced from Smith, E. B.: *J. Atherosclerosis Res.* 5:231, 1965.)

TABLE 18–18. CONNECTIVE TISSUE COMPONENTS AND LIPIDS OF DIFFERENT TYPES OF LESION

	Collagen (Calculated) (mg./100 mg. protein)	Mucopolysaccharide (Calculated) (mg./100 mg. protein)	Total Lipid (mg./100 mg. protein)
Fatty streaks and nodules	26 (24)*	3.0 (2.6)	31 (9)
Fibrous plaques	41 (25)	2.5 (2.6)	47 (11)
Calcified plaques	61 (24)	1.2 (3.0)	109 (9)

*Controls given in parentheses. (From Smith, E. B.: *J. Atherosclerosis Res.* 5:241, 1965.)

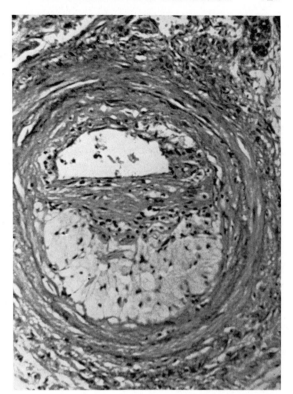

Figure 18–36. A cross section of a small artery with a large, eccentric aggregation of intimal smooth muscle cells loaded with lipid. (Courtesy of S. L. Robbins).

the coronaries can cause sudden death from ischemic heart disease following what would otherwise be trivial alterations in coronary blood supply and demand. In those who survive an acute ischemic episode, thrombosis can subsequently lead to complete occlusion. This has been documented in about 50 per cent of the patients who die of acute ischemic heart disease (Crawford; Roberts and Buja). A scheme that generally summarizes these concepts is shown in Figure 18–37.

Etiologic Factors

Injury to the Arterial Wall. Since atherosclerosis tends to be focal rather than generalized, its pathogenesis ultimately will have to be explained in terms of local factors that affect the biology of the arterial wall. Thus hemodynamic and structural factors probably influence the biochemistry of arterial cells and predispose specific regions of selected arteries to atherosclerosis. One suggested possibility is that turbulent blood flow or shear associated with bending and branching of arteries locally "injures" the arterial wall and induces platelet aggregation and the formation of organized microthrombi (French, 1970). Another is that increased intimal permeability to blood proteins occurs either because of turbulence or because of disruption of tissue architecture at arterial sites close to branch points that are more firmly anchored and less able to evenly dissipate stresses caused by pulse waves (French, 1966).

One reason why intimal permeability is thought to be so critical is that it presumably influences the ingress of blood proteins like LDL and fibrinogen, which have been identified in arteries and may play an important role in atherosclerosis. A second reason is that the proliferation of smooth muscle

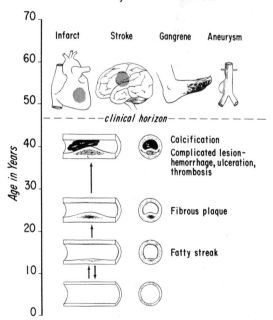

Figure 18–37. Diagrammatic concept of the pathogenesis of atherosclerosis. (From McGill, H., et al., In *Atherosclerosis and Its Origin*. Sandler, M., and Bourne, J. (eds.), New York, Academic Press, 1963.)

cells associated with the formation of fibrous plaques may depend on increased intimal permeability. Experimental removal of the arterial endothelium immediately promotes proliferation of smooth muscle cells and causes the formation of a raised lesion (Stemerman and Ross). This proliferation may occur because removal of the endothelium greatly increases intimal permeability and thereby the availability of specific blood proteins required for smooth muscle cell growth (Ross and Glomset). A third reason why intimal permeability is important is that it plays a major role in the nutrition of the arterial wall. Neither the intima nor the inner media of arteries is supplied by vasa vasorum, so the cells of these regions must obtain nutrients solely by diffusion from the lumen. Thus increased endothelial permeability might first promote smooth muscle cell proliferation and the formation of connective tissue proteins and by so doing paradoxically compromise the nutrition of more deeply situated cells.

Lipids. Many factors probably interact to produce fibrous and complicated lesions, but lipids are clearly of special importance. As shown in Tables 18–17 and 18–18, one-third to one-half of the calcium-free dry weight of atherosclerotic plaques is lipid, more than 70 per cent of which is cholesterol. In addition, the risk of developing atherosclerotic heart disease is directly correlated with plasma cholesterol concentrations both within (Fig. 18–38) and among populations. Finally, atherosclerosis can be induced not only in rabbits but also in animals as similar to man as the nonhuman pri-

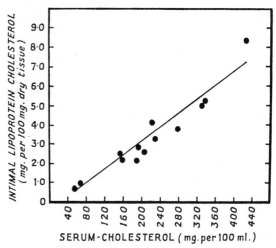

Figure 18–39. Immunologically detectable low-density lipoprotein in the intima of arteries as a function of low-density lipoprotein concentration in plasma. (From Smith, E. B., and Slater, R. S.: *Lancet* 1:463, 1972.)

mate by dietary measures that increase the concentration of cholesterol in plasma.

The mechanism by which cholesterol and other lipids accumulate in plaques is not yet understood, but three possible sources of the lipid have been proposed: local biosynthesis within the arterial wall, the platelets of encrusted mural thrombi, and plasma lipoproteins that have filtered into the intima. Probably all three are involved to some extent. Nevertheless, most of the extracellular cholesterol is probably derived from the plasma. One reason for believing this has already been mentioned, i.e., the similarity in fatty acid composition between the cholesteryl esters of plaques and of plasma lipoproteins. A second reason is that isotopic studies of the plaque cholesterol of humans and experimental animals have indicated that biosynthesis by the cells of the arterial wall is too limited to account for more than a small proportion of the total cholesterol present. A third reason is that LDL have been demonstrated in the intima of arteries (Smith and Slater), and that the concentration of these lipoproteins is directly related to their concentration in plasma (Fig. 18–39), which in turn is directly related to the risk of developing atherosclerotic heart disease (Fig. 18–38).

If most of the lipid of plaques is derived from plasma lipoproteins, why does it accumulate in arteries, and how does the accumulated lipid affect the biology of the arterial wall? These unanswered questions appear to be of central importance to our understanding of the pathogenesis of atherosclerosis. Smith and her colleagues have already shown that fine droplets of extracellular lipid are present even in arteries that have a normal macroscopic appearance, and that this lipid is rich in cholesteryl ester and increases with age (Fig. 18–40). Since the percentage of linoleic acid present also increases with age and approaches that of the cholesteryl esters of plasma lipoproteins, it is

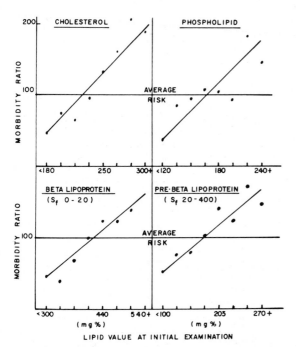

Figure 18–38. Risk of developing overt coronary heart disease (morbidity ratio) as a function of plasma lipid and lipoprotein concentrations. (From Kannel, W. B., Garcia, M. J., et al.: *Hum. Path.* 2:129, 1971.)

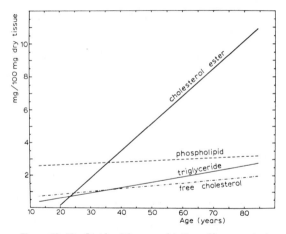

Figure 18–40. Lipids of the normal intima of human arteries as a function of age. (From Smith, E. B., Evans, P. H., et al.: *J. Atheroscler. Res.* 7:171, 1967.)

highly likely that this "perifibrous" lipid is derived from plasma lipoproteins. Presumably, all that is required for this lipid to accumulate is some non-enzymic or enzymic mechanism that would alter the lipoproteins in such a way as to render them insoluble and thus incapable of diffusing out of the intima. One possibility is that lipoproteins absorb to the intimal connective tissue matrix. Since both LDL and VLDL readily form complexes with sulfated polysaccharides of the type found in the arterial wall, absorption of this type might explain the association between plasma VLDL or triglyceride concentrations (Fig. 18–38; Carlson and Böttiger; Goldstein et al.) and coronary heart disease. Another possibility is that LDL or VLDL, trapped within extracellular connective tissue matrices, undergo slow, spontaneous denaturation or precipitate after being attacked by extracellular enzymes. Should this be so, the biologic disposal mechanisms of the organism, very poorly understood in the case of the artery, might be inadequate to cope with the problem.

Intracellular lipid probably accumulates primarily through direct uptake of extracellular lipoprotein. Uptake of medium lipoproteins by arterial cells grown in culture has been demonstrated by several investigators, and uptake probably also occurs *in vivo*, since Smith and Slater found that the concentration of soluble LDL immediately surrounding fatty streaks is considerably lower than that in normal intima. Once taken up by arterial cells, the lipoproteins are presumably degraded by lysosomal esterases and proteases and the cholesterol reesterified within the cell. The effect of the accumulated cholesteryl ester on the subsequent fate of the cells has not yet been clarified, although the presumption is that cell damage and ultimately cell death occur, and that this contributes to the formation of fibrous plaques.

Another question that arises in connection with the "atherogenicity" of plasma lipoproteins is whether or not a risk-free concentration of plasma lipoprotein cholesterol exists. Studies of the comparative geography of atherosclerosis suggest that plasma cholesterol concentrations below approximately 140–150 mg./100 ml. tend to be correlated with relative freedom from atherosclerotic heart disease, but prospective studies in western countries have not yet provided information with regard to this point because of the relatively small proportion of individuals older than 40 who have plasma cholesterol concentrations below 175 mg./100 ml. They have indicated, however, that individuals who have plasma cholesterol concentrations below 175 mg./100 ml. are at lower risk than are individuals who have plasma cholesterol concentrations of 200 mg./100 ml. Thus most individuals who have "normal" plasma cholesterol concentrations by commonly used standards do not have *optimal* concentrations. Below the arbitrary upper concentration limits used to define "hyperlipidemia" (Table 18–12), a 75 mg./100 ml. increment in the concentration of plasma cholesterol is still associated with an increased risk of developing atherosclerotic heart disease equivalent to that of aging ten years (Westlund and Nicolaysen).

Other Risk Factors. In western populations, several other risk factors, including hypertension, obesity, diabetes, male sex, and age, have been correlated with the incidence of atherosclerotic heart disease. These factors appear to exacerbate the effects of high plasma lipid concentrations but apparently do not cause extensive atherosclerosis by themselves, since populations that exhibit a high prevalence of hypertension, obesity and diabetes, but low plasma lipid concentrations, do not seem to be at high risk of developing coronary heart disease.

Like that of plasma lipids, the effect of hypertension on atherosclerotic heart disease is almost linear. Presumably, intimal permeability increases progressively with increasing blood pressure and influences the metabolism of arterial cells. Although the response of these cells is only now being studied, evidence is already available that experimental hypertension increases the content of sulfated mucopolysaccharide in the aorta (Hollander et al.).

It is largely because obese individuals tend to be hypertensive and have higher plasma lipid concentrations that they are at increased risk of developing coronary heart disease. If they are compared to thin individuals who have similar degrees of hypertension and similar plasma lipid concentrations, the effect of obesity largely disappears (Keys et al., 1972). Only when sudden death is considered separately from myocardial infarction that occurs at rest (Kannel et al., 1967) does a distinct, independent effect of obesity emerge, presumably because obesity increases the cardiac work load and thereby the burden of physical activity on an already compromised coronary circulation. However, regardless of whether or not obesity is considered an independent risk factor, its frequent association with hypertension, hyperlipidemia and hyperglycemia (see below), all potentially reversible with weight reduction should focus particular attention on this problem.

That diabetics are particularly susceptible to atherosclerotic vascular disease as well as microangiopathy has long been appreciated. Definitive proof that hyperglycemia is a risk factor for coronary heart disease independent of hypercholesterolemia or hypertension, however, was only recently obtained in prospective studies (Ostrander). It is still not clear that hyperglycemia is a risk factor independent of hypertriglyceridemia, since the two are closely correlated (see the section, Hyperlipidemia). Studies in animals have not yet clarified this question. Indeed, the effect of diabetes has been found to differ in different species. Diabetic rats and monkeys (Lehner et al.) are more susceptible to atherosclerosis. However, alloxan diabetes actually protects against the atherosclerosis induced in rabbits by feeding them cholesterol (Duff and McMillan).

Sex is another factor that influences the incidence of atherosclerosis, at least in Caucasians. Particularly in the coronary arteries but also in the aorta, the prevalence of atherosclerotic plaques is greater in males than in females. In addition, prospective studies such as that done in Framingham (Kannel et al., 1967) have shown that the incidence of coronary heart disease in males is about twice that in females, and that an even greater differential exists among males and females below the age of fifty. The basis for this sex differential remains to be explained. There is no direct evidence that it is caused by estrogens, since the incidence of coronary heart disease rises almost linearly with age in females and does not appear to be affected by menopause. Furthermore, the sex differential is not universal, since very little if any difference in the incidence of atherosclerosis can be demonstrated among male and female Negroes (Tejada et al.), and even the sex differential in Caucasians is obliterated in diabetics. Nevertheless, sex hormones do affect risk factors associated with coronary heart disease, and this has led some investigators to fear that the sex differential may be reversed in normal females taking oral contraceptives. Thus estrogen-containing oral contraceptives tend to increase plasma lipid levels, impair carbohydrate tolerance, promote hypertension, and alter blood coagulation (Hazzard et al., 1969; Ygge et al.; Chidell).

Other risk factors that have been identified include smoking, physical activity, and psychological behavior pattern. For a discussion of these and other risk factors, the reader is referred to a recent review by Epstein and Ostrander.

Prevention and Treatment

Obviously a great need exists for a rational therapeutic approach to atherosclerosis, but such an approach is unfortunately not yet at hand. One problem has been that treatment has seldom been attempted until after the onset of clinical symptoms, i.e., after the primary disease process has progressed to the point where little hope of regression seems justified. Consequently, it is not surprising that attempts at therapy have met with relatively little success. A second problem is that, while most investigators would agree that prevention of atherosclerosis is the only rational approach, this might have to be begun in childhood and would certainly have to be carried out for decades. The paradox is that ultimate proof of the efficacy of a given therapeutic regimen probably will demand this type of long-term approach in a large population, whereas many physicians not unreasonably feel that before such long-term therapy is begun proof of efficacy should already be at hand. Fortunately, a means of circumventing this dilemma may be provided by the series of Lipid Clinics recently established throughout the United States by the National Institute of Heart and Lung Diseases. These clinics will conduct carefully designed attempts to reduce plasma lipid concentrations in individuals defined as having hyperlipidemia and who are thus at high risk of developing atherosclerotic disease. Although these individuals may not necessarily respond in the same way as individuals who have lower concentrations of plasma lipids, the evidence obtained may provide the necessary impetus for large-scale therapeutic trials in the general population.

In the meantime, what can be done? Apart from surgery to improve the coronary circulation (Baue), the approach usually advocated is to treat where possible the recognized risk factors. For a general review of the problem, the reader is referred to a recent review by Dawber and Thomas, and for detailed discussions of obesity and hyperlipidemia to earlier sections of the present chapter. The dietary measures recommended to mitigate hyperlipidemia can be applied generally to reduce serum lipid levels in anyone concerned about the risk of developing atherosclerotic vascular disease. Furthermore, more rigorous dietary approaches can be justified for offspring of families with known forms of primary hyperlipidemia (see p. 916). The long-term use of pharmacologic agents is more controversial. As for the therapeutic use of hormones, both thyroid hormones and estrogens have been tried but were later discontinued because of side effects. Justification for hormone therapy exists only when deficiency is to be corrected, as in the case of diabetes and hypothyroidism.

CHOLESTEROL GALLSTONES

Gallstones occur frequently in Western countries and appear to be increasing in prevalence in newly "westernized" countries like Japan (Miyake and Johnston). Some gallstones are mainly composed of bile pigments or insoluble calcium salts but most contain at least 70–80 per cent cholesterol and at times as much as 98 per cent cholesterol. These cholesterol-rich stones are of particular interest because of increasing evidence that they are formed when hepatic cholesterol excretion exceeds the normal solubilizing capacity of the bile. In other words, "cholesterol cholelithiasis" can be considered a "disease" of cholesterol metabolism. In the following presentation, the prevalence of gallstones in various population groups, the factors believed to solubilize cholesterol in bile, and recent studies that directly pertain to gallstone formation in man will be briefly discussed.

For additional details, the reader should consult recent reviews by Small and by Bouchier, and for discussion of other factors related to cholelithiasis (infection, stasis, hemolytic anemia, etc.), the reader is referred to a review by Bockus.

Many studies have demonstrated that the prevalence of gallstones increases with age. For example, in a recent review of a large necropsy series, the overall incidence of gallstones in females was 27.1 per cent whereas the incidence in females between the ages of 80 and 89 was 38.0 per cent, and a qualitatively similar relation was found in males (Torvik and Hoivik). The cause of the apparent increase with age is not understood. The tendency to form gallstones may be a simple function of age in all individuals. On the other hand, a process of selection may be operative, i.e., the mechanisms that promote gallstone formation may favor longevity by protecting individuals from premature vascular disease. Studies of Indians from the southwestern United States seem to support this concept (see below). Most authors agree that cholesterol gallstones occur more frequently in females than in males. For example, in the study by Torvik and Hoivik, the overall incidence of gallstones in males (12.7 per cent) was less than half that found in females, and a similar sex-related difference was found by Friedman et al. and by Horn (Fig. 18-41). The study by Horn and a recent study by Hove and Geill are of interest, since they suggest that the sex differential tends to diminish in aged individuals. The effect of parity may explain part of the sex differential. In Horn's study, the incidence of gallstones in women below the age of 50 increased in proportion to the number of children they had borne, although women with no children still had a higher incidence of gallstones than had men. Another factor that affects the relative incidence of gallstones is body weight. In Horn's study, women below the age of 50 who had gallstones were 25 pounds heavier on the average than were women without gallstones. Furthermore, Van der Linden found a small but probably significant correlation between subscapular and lateral skin-fold thickness and the incidence of surgically verified cholelithiasis in women. He found the correlation less obvious, however, than is

suggested by the catch phrase "fat, fertile female" found in some textbooks.

It has been suggested from time to time that the incidence of cholelithiasis may be affected by various endocrine abnormalities, such as hypothyroidism and diabetes. Both thyroid hormone and insulin are known to affect sterol metabolism, and untreated hypothyroidism and diabetes are characterized by high serum lipid levels (see the section, Hyperlipidemia). So far no evidence is available, however, that cholelithiasis occurs more frequently in myxedema, and in fact several cases of coincident cholelithiasis and hyperthyroidism are known (Bockus). In the case of diabetes, evidence is conflicting, possibly because of the relation between diabetes and obesity (see p. 909). In two large autopsy series, the incidence of gallstones was found to be almost twice as high in diabetics as in nondiabetics (Robertson and Dochat; Lieber). Nevertheless, Feldman and Feldman reviewed the findings of 1,319 autopsies and found that gallstones were no more prevalent in diabetics than in nondiabetics.

Solubilization of Cholesterol in Bile

Although cholesterol is essentially insoluble in water, significant amounts are solubilized in bile (Table 18-1), because of the combined presence of bile acids and lecithin (Isaksson, Small). Physical studies of bile acid-lecithin-water mixtures (Small et al.) suggest the presence of mixed micelles of the general composition and shape indicated in Figure 18-42. Studies in model systems (Admirand and Small) have shown that mixed micelles of bile and lecithin can solubilize up to three times as much cholesterol as can solutions of bile acids alone. Nevertheless, the ability of these mixed micelles to solubilize cholesterol is limited, as is readily seen when the conditions for optimal solubilization of cholesterol are expressed in terms of triangular coordinates (Fig. 18-43). Moreover, the composition of normal bile can be shown to be compatible with complete solubilization, whereas that of bile containing gallstones is supersaturated with cholesterol (Fig. 18-44). Thus it is apparent that understanding of the pathology of cholesterol stone formation and ultimate treatment or prevention of the disease must be sought in terms of the factors that regulate the proportions of cholesterol, bile salts, and lecithin in the bile.

Bile Secretion

The hepatic mechanisms of bile secretion are not yet understood, although bile acids, secretin, and polyunsaturated fatty acids (Campbell et al., 1972) are recognized choleretics. Furthermore, it is clear that the relative proportions of bile acids, lecithin, cholesterol, and water are not rigidly fixed. Thus, in some American Indian tribes, the prevalence of cholesterol gallstones is unusually high. (It approaches 80 per cent in women.) These Indians consume a diet similar in lipid content to that of white Americans but have higher concentrations of bil-

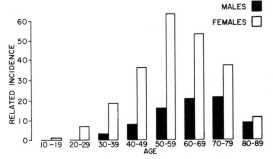

Figure 18-41. Incidence of cholelithiasis in Birmingham males and females as a function of age. "Related incidence" is the ratio of the number of cases in each group to the population (of Great Britain) in the corresponding group (number of cases per million population). (From Horn, G.: *Brit. Med. J.* 2:732, 1956.)

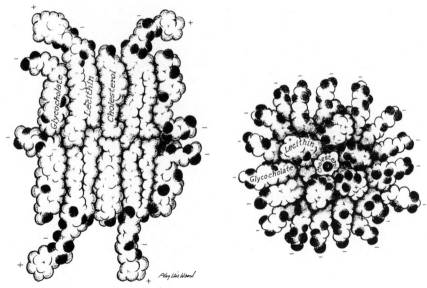

Figure 18–42. Schematic drawing of a bile micelle based on molecular models of unesterified cholesterol, glycocholic acid, and lecithin. Left side = sagittal section through micelle; right side = micelle seen from top; dark areas = oxygen atoms.

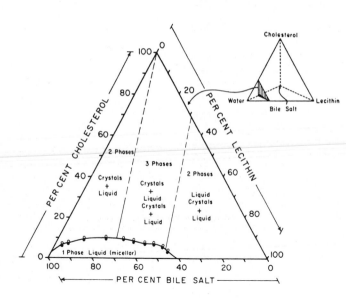

Figure 18–43. Triangular phase diagram showing the physical state of all possible combinations of bile salts, lecithin, and cholesterol in aqueous solutions containing 10% solids and 90% water. Line separating open and closed circles indicates maximum amount of cholesterol solubilized by any mixture of lecithin and bile salt. (From Admirand, W. H., and Small, D. M.: *J. Clin. Invest. 47*:1048, 1968.)

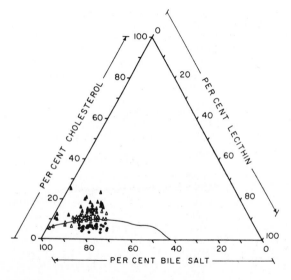

Figure 18–44. Triangular phase diagram showing composition of gallbladder bile from normal subjects (closed circles), patients with cholesterol or mixed gallstones but no microcrystals (open triangles), and patients with gallstones and microcrystals (closed triangles). (From Admirand, W. H., and Small, D. M.: *J. Clin. Invest. 47*:1046, 1968.)

iary cholesterol and lower concentrations of plasma cholesterol (Grundy et al., 1973). Furthermore, their bile acid pools are unusually small (Vlahcevic et al.). Apparently, the increased concentrations of biliary cholesterol relative to bile acid lead to gallstone formation, while the low concentrations of plasma cholesterol are associated with relative freedom from cardiovascular disease. Even in the same individual, however, the relative concentrations of biliary components vary. Both increased cholesterol intake (Quintao et al.) and increased cholesterol production in obese individuals (Miettinen, 1971; Grundy et al., 1972) cause increased excretion of biliary cholesterol without markedly affecting bile acid excretion. Moreover, the secretion of water by bile duct canaliculi, affected by bile acids, secretin, and estrogens (Gumucio and Valdiviesco), appears to undergo cyclic daily (McSherry et al.) as well as monthly variations. All of these factors may well promote gallstone formation in obese Western women.

Treatment and Prevention

Cholesterol crystals form and grow to clinically manifest size in the gallbladder, but rational prevention will have to be directed toward the super-saturated bile. A basis for this type of preventive management is likely to be provided within the not too distant future, since techniques are now available for determining the effects of diet and drugs on bile secretion in man (Grundy and Metzger). Already it seems likely that restriction of calories and cholesterol will be important, especially since gallstones can be produced experimentally in monkeys simply by feeding butter and cholesterol (Osuga and Portman). This should be considered particularly in patients being treated with polyunsaturated fats or clofibrate to reduce plasma cholesterol concentrations, since both forms of treatment can increase cholesterol excretion (Connor et al.; Grundy et al., 1972). Another approach recently introduced by Thistle and Schoenfield is to dissolve preexisting gallstones by increasing bile acid concentrations through oral administration of chenodeoxycholic acid. When 0.75–4.5 g. of this acid were given daily to seven women with gallstones, the gallstones diminished in four of the women over a period of 6–22 months, while liver function and morphology remained normal (Danzinger et al., 1972). Plans are being made to test this promising result in a large field study.

REFERENCES

Admirand, W. H., and Small, D. M.: The physiochemical basis of cholesterol gallstone formation in man. *J. Clin. Invest.* 47:1043, 1968.

Ahrens, E. J., Jr.: The use of liquid formula diets in metabolic studies: 15 years' experience, In *Advances in Metabolic Disorders.* Vol. 4. Levine, R., and Luft, R. (eds.), New York, Academic Press, 1970.

Alaupovic, P.: Apolipoproteins and lipoproteins. *Atherosclerosis* 13:141, 1971.

Albrink, M. J., and Meigs, J. W.: Interrelationship between skinfold thickness, serum lipids and blood sugar in normal men. *Amer. J. Clin. Nutr.* 15:225, 1964.

Albrink, M. J., Meigs, J. W., et al.: Weight gain and serum triglycerides in normal men. *New Eng. J. Med.* 266:484, 1962.

Arky, R. A., and Freinkel, N.: Alcohol hypoglycemia. V. Alcohol infusion to test gluconeogenesis in starvation with special reference to obesity. *New Eng. J. Med.* 274:426, 1967.

Atkin, E., and Meng, H. C.: Release of clearing factor lipase (lipoprotein lipase) in vivo and from isolated perfused hearts of alloxan diabetic rats. *Diabetes* 21:149, 1972.

Bagdade, J. D.: Basal insulin and obesity. *Lancet* 2:630, 1968.

Bagdade, J. D.: Diabetic lipaemia complicating acute pancreatitis. *Lancet* 2:1041, 1969.

Bagdade, J. D., Bierman, E. L., et al.: Significance of basal insulin levels in the evaluation of the insulin response to glucose in diabetic and nondiabetic subjects. *J. Clin. Invest.* 46:1549, 1967.

Bagdade, J. D., Bierman, E. L., et al.: The influence of obesity on the relationship between insulin and triglyceride levels in endogenous hypertriglyceridemia. *Diabetes* 20:664, 1971.

Bagdade, J. D., Bierman, E. L., et al.: Counter-regulation of basal insulin secretion during alcohol hypoglycemia in diabetic and normal subjects. *Diabetes* 21:65, 1972.

Bagdade, J. D., Porte, D., Jr., et al.: Diabetic lipemia: a form of acquired fat-induced lipemia. *New Eng. J. Med.,* 276:427, 1967.

Bagdade, J. D., Porte, D., Jr., et al.: Acute insulin withdrawal and the regulation of plasma triglyceride removal in diabetic subjects. *Diabetes* 17:127, 1968a.

Bagdade, J. D., Porte, D., Jr., et al.: Hypertriglyceridemia: a metabolic consequence of chronic renal failure. *New Eng. J. Med.* 279:181, 1968b.

Bagdade, J. D., Porte, D., Jr., et al.: The interaction of diabetes and obesity on the regulation of fat mobilization in man. *Diabetes* 18:759, 1969.

Bagdade, J. D., Porte, D., Jr., et al.: Steroid-induced lipemia. *Arch. Intern. Med.* 125:129, 1970.

Balasse, E. O., and Havel, R. J.: Evidence for an effect of insulin on the peripheral utilization of ketone bodies in dogs. *J. Clin. Invest.* 50:801, 1971.

Ball, M. F., Kyle, L. H., et al.: Comparative effects of caloric restriction and metabolic acceleration on body composition in obesity. *J. Clin. Endocr.* 27:273, 1967.

Basso, L. V., and Havel, R. J.: Hepatic metabolism of free fatty acids in normal and diabetic dogs. *J. Clin. Invest.* 48:537, 1970.

Baue, A.: Survey for coronary artery disease. *J.A.M.A.* 208:849, 1969.

Baum, D., Guthrie, R., et al.: An abnormality of triglyceride metabolism in infantile hypothyroidism. *Amer. J. Dis. Child.* 125:612, 1973.

Beaumont, J. L., Carlson, L. A., et al.: Classification of hyperlipidaemias and hyperlipoproteinaemias. *Bull. WHO* 43:891, 1970.

Beck, P., Koumans, J. H. T., et al.: Studies of insulin and growth hormone secretion in human obesity. *J. Lab. Clin. Med.* 64:654, 1964.

Belknap, B. H., Bagdade, J. D., et al.: In *Tolbutamide After Ten Years.* Butterfield, W. J. H., and Van Westering, W. (eds.), Amsterdam, Excerpta Medica, No. 149, 1967.

Benoit, F. L., Martin, R. L., et al.: Changes in body composition during weight reduction in obesity. *Ann. Intern. Med.* 63:604, 1965.

Berkowitz, D.: Long-term treatment of hyperlipidemic patients with clofibrate. *J.A.M.A.* 218:1002, 1971.

Bezman, A., Felts, J. M., et al.: Relation between the incorporation of triglyceride fatty acids and heparin-released lipoprotein lipase from adipose tissue slices. *J. Lipid Res.* 3:427, 1962.

Bierman, E. L., and Porte, D., Jr.: Carbohydrate intolerance and lipemia. *Ann. Intern. Med.* 68:926, 1968.

Bierman, E. L., and Strandness, D. E.: Formation of secondary fat particles from lymph chylomicrons in the dog. *Amer. J. Physiol.* 210:13, 1966.

Bierman, E. L., Bagdade, J. D., et al.: A concept of the pathogenesis of diabetic lipemia. *Trans. Ass. Amer. Physicians* 79:348, 1966.

Bierman, E. L., Bagdade, J. D., et al.: Obesity and diabetes: the odd couple. *Amer. J. Clin Nutr.* 21:1434, 1968.

Bierman, E. L., Brunzell, J. D., et al.: On the mechanisms of action of Atromid-S on triglyceride transport in man. *Trans. Ass. Amer Physicians* 83:211, 1970.

Bierman, E. L., Porte, D., Jr., et al.: Hypertriglyceridemia and glucose intolerance in man, In *Adipose Tissue, Regulation and Metabolic Functions*. Jeanrenaud, B., and Hepp, D. (eds.), New York, Academic Press, 1970.

Bilheimer, D., Eisenberg, S., et al.: The metabolism of very low density lipoproteins. I. Preliminary in vitro and in vivo observations. *Biochim. Biophys. Acta* 260:212, 1972.

Björntorp, P., and Ostman, J.: Human adipose tissue dynamics and regulation, In *Advances in Metabolic Disorders*. Vol. 5. Levine, R., and Luft, R. (eds.), New York, Academic Press, 1971.

Björntorp, P., DeJounge, K., et al.: The effect of physical training on insulin production in obesity. *Metabolism* 19:631, 1970.

Björntorp, P., Gustafson, A., et al.: Relationships between adipose tissue cellularity and carbohydrate and lipid metabolism in a randomly selected population, In *Atherosclerosis: Proceedings of the Second International Symposium*. Jones, R. J. (ed.), New York, Springer-Verlag, 1970.

Björntorp, P., Gustafson, A., et al.: Adipose tissue fat cell size and number in relation to metabolism in endogenous hypertriglyceridemia. *Acta Med. Scand.* 190:363, 1971.

Bjurulf, P.: Atherosclerosis and body-build with special reference to size and number of subcutaneous fat cells. *Acta Med. Scand.* 166 (Suppl. 349):1, 1959.

Blanchette-Mackie, E. J., and Scow, R. O.: Sites of lipoprotein lipase activity in adipose tissue perfused with chylomicrons. Electron microscope and chemical study. *J. Cell Biol.* 51:1, 1971.

Bloom, W. L., and Azar, G. J.: Similarities of carbohydrate deficiency and fasting. *Arch. Intern. Med.* 112:333, 1963.

Bockus, H.: Cholelithiasis, In *Gastroenterology*. Vol. 3. Bockus, H. (ed.), Philadelphia, W. B. Saunders Co., 1965.

Bortz, W. M.: Metabolic consequences of obesity. *Ann. Intern. Med.* 71:833, 1969.

Bortz, W. M., Wroldsen, A., et al.: Weight loss and frequency of feeding. *New Eng. J. Med.* 274:376, 1966.

Bortz, W. M., Wroldsen, A., et al.: Fat, carbohydrate, salt and weight loss. *J. Clin. Nutr.* 20:1104, 1967.

Bouchier, I. A. D.: Gallstone formation. *Lancet* 1:711, 1971.

Boyd, G. S., and Percy-Robb, I. W.: Enzymatic regulation of bile acid synthesis. *Amer. J. Med.* 51:580, 1971.

Bray, G. A.: Effect of caloric restriction on energy expenditure in obese patients. *Lancet* 2:397, 1969.

Bray, G. A., and York, D. A.: Genetically transmitted obesity in rodents. *Physiol. Rev.* 51:598, 1971.

Bray, G. A., Davidson, M. D., et al.: Obesity: A serious symptom. *Ann. Intern. Med.* 77:797, 1972.

Brown, W. V., Levy, R. I., et al.: Studies of the proteins in human plasma very low density lipoproteins. *J. Biol. Chem.* 244:5687, 1969.

Brown, W. V., and Baginsky, M. L.: Inhibition of lipoprotein lipase by an apoprotein of human very low density lipoprotein. *Biochim. Biophys. Res. Commun.* 46:375, 1972.

Bruch, H.: *The Importance of Overweight*. New York, W. W. Norton, 1957.

Brunzell, J. D., Porte, D., Jr., et al.: PHLA depletion: a defect in plasma triglyceride removal related to hyperglycemia. *Diabetes* 21 (Suppl. 1):342, 1972a.

Brunzell, J. D., Smith, N. D., et al.: Evidence for multiphasic release of postheparin lipolytic activity. *J. Clin. Invest.* 51:16a, 1972b.

Butcher, R. A.: The role of cyclic AMP in the actions of some lipolytic and anti-lipolytic agents, In *Adipose Tissue, Regulation and Metabolic Functions*. Jeanrenaud, B., and Hepp, D. (eds.), New York, Academic Press, 1970.

Butterfield, W. J. H., Hanley, T., et al.: Peripheral metabolism of glucose and free fatty acids during oral glucose tolerance tests. *Metabolism* 14:851, 1965.

Cahill, G. F., Jr.: Starvation in man. *New Eng. J. Med.* 282:668, 1970.

Campbell, C. B., Cowley, D. J., et al.: Dietary factors affecting biliary lipid secretion in the rhesus monkey. A mechanism for the hypocholesterolaemic action of polyunsaturated fat. *Europ. J. Clin. Invest.* 2:332, 1972.

Campbell, R. G., Hashim, S. A., et al.: Studies of food-intake regulation in man. Responses to variations in nutritive density in lean and obese subjects. *New Eng. J. Med.* 285:1402, 1971.

Carlson, L. A.: The effect of nicotinic acid treatment on the chemical composition of plasma lipoprotein classes in man, In

Advances in Experimental Medicine and Biology. Vol. 4. Holmes, W. L., Carlson, L. A., et al. (eds.), New York, Plenum Press, 1969.

Carlson, L. A., and Böttiger, L. E.: Ischaemic heart disease in relation to fasting values of plasma triglycerides and cholesterol. *Lancet* 1:865, 1972.

Carlson, L. A., and Lindstedt, S.: The Stockholm prospective study. 1. The initial values for plasma lipids. *Acta Med. Scand.* Suppl. 493:1, 1968.

Chidell, M. P.: Oral contraceptives and blood pressure. *Practitioner* 205:58, 1970.

Chirico, A., and Stunkard, A. J.: Physical activity and human obesity. *New Eng. J. Med.* 263:935, 1960.

Cohen, L., Blaisdell, R. K., et al.: Familial xanthomatosis and hyperlipidemia, and myelomatosis. *Amer. J. Med.* 40:299, 1966.

Connor, W. E., Witiak, D. T., et al.: Cholesterol balance and feral neutral steroid and bile acid excretion in normal men fed dietary fats of different fatty acid composition. *J. Clin. Invest.* 48:1363, 1969.

Crawford, T.: Morphological aspects in the pathogenesis of atherosclerosis. *J. Atherosclerosis Res.* 1:3, 1961.

Cubberley, P. T., Polster, S. A., et al.: Lactic acidosis and death after the treatment of obesity by fasting. *New Eng. J. Med.* 272:628, 1965.

Cunningham, V. J., and Robinson, D. S.: Clearing factor lipase in adipose tissue. Distinction of different states of the enzyme and the possible role of the fat cell in the maintenance of tissue activity. *Biochem. J.* 112:203, 1969.

Danzinger, R. G., Hofmann, A. F., et al.: Dissolution of cholesterol gallstones by chenodeoxycholic acid. *New Eng. J. Med.* 286:1, 1972.

Dawber, T. R., and Thomas, H. E., Jr.: Prevention of myocardial infarction. *Progr. Cardiovasc. Dis.* 13:343, 1971.

deKruyff, B., Demel, R. A., et al.: The effect of cholesterol and epicholesterol incorporation on the permeability and on the phase transition of intact Acholeplasma laidlawii cell membranes and derived liposomes. *Biochim. Biophys Acta* 255:331, 1972.

Demel, R. A., Bruckdorter, K. R., et al.: Structural requirements of sterols for the interaction with lecithin at the air-water interfall. *Biochim. Biophys. Acta* 255:304, 1972.

Dietschy, J. M., and Wilson, J. D.: Regulation of cholesterol metabolism. *New Eng. J. Med.* 282:1128, 1179, 1241, 1970.

Dole, V. P.: Body fat. *Sci. Amer.* 201:71, 1959.

Drenick, E. J., Simmons, F., et al.: Effect on hepatic morphology of treatment of obesity by fasting, reducing diets and small-bowel bypass. *New Eng. J. Med.* 282:829, 1970.

Drenick, E. J., Swendseid, M. E., et al.: Prolonged starvation as treatment for severe obesity. *J.A.M.A.* 187:100, 1964.

Duff, G. L., and McMillan, G. C.: Effect of alloxan diabetes on experimental cholesterol atherosclerosis in the rabbit. *J. Exp. Med.* 89:611, 1949.

Dunn, H. G.: The Prader-Labhart-Willi syndrome: Review of the literature and report of nine cases. *Acta Pediat. Scand.* (Suppl.) 186:1, 1968.

Edwards, K. D. G., and Whyte, H. M.: The simple measurement of obesity. *Clin. Sci.* 22:347, 1962.

Eid, E. E.: Follow-up study of physical growth of children who had excessive weight gain in first six months of life. *Brit. Med. J.* 2:74, 1970.

Eisenberg, S., Bilheimer, D. W., et al.: On the apoprotein composition of human plasma very low density lipoprotein subfractions. *Biochim. Biophys. Acta* 260:329, 1972.

Elsbach, P., and Schwartz, I. L.: Salt and water metabolism during weight reduction. *Metabolism* 10:595, 1961.

Entenmann, C., Holloway, J., et al.: Bile acids and lipid metabolism. I. Stimulation of bile lipid excretion by various bile acids. *Proc. Soc. Exp. Biol. Med.* 127:1008, 1968.

Epstein, F. H., and Ostrander, L. D., Jr.: Detection of individual susceptibility toward coronary disease. *Progr. Cardiovasc. Dis.* 13:324, 1971.

Evans, D. W., Turner, S. M., et al.: Feasibility of long-term plasma-cholesterol reduction by diet. *Lancet* 1:172, 1972.

Fabry, P., Hejl, Z., et al.: The frequency of meals: its relation to overweight, hypercholesterolemia, and decreased glucose-tolerance. *Lancet* 2:614, 1964.

Fain, J., Koraceu, U., et al.: Effect of growth hormone and dexamethasone on lipolysis and metabolism in isolated fat cells of the rat. *J. Biol. Chem.* 240:3522, 1965.

Feldman, M., and Feldman, M., Jr.: The incidence of cholelithiasis, cholesterosis, and liver disease in diabetes mellitus. *Diabetes* 3:305, 1954.

Felig, P., Marliss, E., et al.: Plasma amino acid levels and insulin secretion in obesity. *New Eng. J. Med.* 271:811, 1969.

Fredrickson, D. S., Ono, K., et al.: Lipolytic activity of postheparin plasma in hyperglyceridemia. *J. Lipid Res.* 4:24, 1963.

Fredrickson, D. S., and Levy, R. I.: Familial hyperlipoproteinemia, In *The Metabolic Basis of Inherited Disease.* 3rd ed. Stanbury, J. B., Wyngaarden, J. B., et al. (eds.), New York, McGraw-Hill, 1972.

French, J. E.: Atherosclerosis in relation to the structure and function of the arterial intima, with special reference to the endothelium. *Int. Rev. Exp. Path.* 5:253, 1966.

French, J. E.: Formation and fate of a thrombus, In *Atherosclerosis. Proceedings of the Second International Symposium on Atherosclerosis.* Jones, R. J. (ed.), New York, Springer-Verlag, 1970.

Friedman, G. D., Kannel, W. B., et al.: The epidemiology of gallbladder disease: observations in the Framingham study. *J. Chronic Dis.* 19:273, 1966.

Frohman, L. A., Bernardis, L. L., et al.: Plasma insulin and triglyceride levels after hypothalamic lesions in weanling rats. *Amer. J. Physiol.* 216:1496, 1969.

Galton, D. J., and Bray, G. A.: Metabolism of α-glycerol phosphate in human adipose tissue in obesity. *J. Clin. Endocr.* 27:1573, 1967.

Geer, J. C., McGill, H. C., et al.: Histologic characteristics of coronary artery fatty streaks. *Lab. Invest.* 18:565, 1968.

Gellhorn, A., and Benjamin, W.: Effect of aging on the composition and metabolism of adipose tissue in the rat, In *Adipose Tissue.* Renold, A. E., and Cahill, G. F., Jr. (eds.), Baltimore, Williams and Wilkins, 1965.

Glennon, J. A.: Weight reduction — an enigma. *Arch. Intern. Med.* 118:1, 1966.

Glennon, J. A., and Brech, W. J.: Serum protein-bound iodine in obesity. *J. Clin. Endocr.* 25:1673, 1965.

Glomset, J. A.: The plasma lecithin: cholesterol acyltransferase reaction. *J. Lipid Res.* 9:155, 1968.

Glomset, J. A.: Plasma lecithin:cholesterol acyltransferase, In *Blood Lipids and Lipoproteins: Quantitation, Composition and Metabolism.* Nelson, G. J. (ed.), New York, John Wiley & Sons, 1972.

Glomset, J. A., and Norum, K. R.: The metabolic role of lecithin: cholesterol acyltransferase. Perspectives from pathology. *Advances Lipid Res.* 11:1, 1973.

Glomset, J. A., Norum, K. R., et al.: Evidence for abnormal disposal of chylomicrons in familial lecithin:cholesterol acyltransferase deficiency. *European J. Clin. Invest.,* 3:231, 1973.

Glueck, C. J., and Tsang, R. C.: Pediatric familial type II hyperlipoproteinemia: effects of diet on plasma cholesterol in the first year of life. *Amer. J. Clin. Nutr.* 25:224, 1972.

Glueck, C. J., Brown, W. V., et al.: Amelioration of hypertriglyceridemia by progestational drugs in familial type-V hyperlipoproteinemia. *Lancet* 1:1290, 1969.

Glueck, C. J., Heckman, F., et al.: Neonatal familial Type II hyperlipoproteinemia: cord blood cholesterol in 1800 births. *Metabolism* 20:597, 1971.

Glueck, C. J., Kaplan, A. P., et al.: A new mechanism of exogenous hyperglyceridemia. *Ann. Intern. Med.* 71:1051, 1969.

Glueck, C. J., Levy, R. I., et al.: Immunoreactive insulin, glucose tolerance, and carbohydrate inducibility in types II, III, IV, and V hyperlipoproteinemia. *Diabetes* 18:739, 1969.

Goldstein, J. L., Hazzard, W. R., et al.: Genetics of hyperlipidemia in coronary heart disease. *Trans. Ass. Amer. Phys.,* Vol. LXXXV, 1972.

Goodman, D. S.: Cholesterol ester metabolism. *Physiol. Rev.* 45:747, 1965.

Gordon, E. S.: Metabolic aspects of obesity, In *Advances in Metabolic Disorders.* Vol. 4. Levine, R., and Luft, R. (eds.), New York, Academic Press, 1970.

Grace, C. S., and Goldrick, R. B.: Fibrinolysis and body build. *J. Atherosclerosis Res.* 8:705, 1968.

Grundy, S. M., and Metzger, A. L.: A physiological method for estimation of hepatic secretion of biliary lipids in man. *Gastroenterology* 62:1200, 1972.

Grundy, S. M., Ahrens, E. H., Jr., et al.: Mechanisms of action of clofibrate on cholesterol metabolism in patients with hyperlipidemia. *J. Lipid Res.* 13:531, 1972.

Grundy, S. M., Metzger, A. L., et al.: Mechanisms of lithogenic bile formation in American Indian women with cholesterol gallstones. *J. Clin. Invest.* 51:3026, 1972.

Gumucio, J. J., and Valdiviesco, V. D.: Studies on the mechanism

of the ethynylestradiol impairment of bile flow and bile salt excretion in the rat. *Gastroenterology* 61:339, 1971.

Gustafson, A., Bjorntorp, P., et al.: Metformin administration in hyperlipidemic states. *Acta Med. Scand.* 190:491, 1971.

Havel, R. J.: Pathogenesis, differentiation and management of hypertriglyceridemia, In *Advances in Internal Medicine.* Vol. 15. Stollerman, G. H. (ed.), Year Book Medical Publishers, 1969.

Hazzard, W. R., and Bierman, E. L.: Impaired removal of very low density lipoprotein (VLDL) "remnants" in the pathogenesis of broad-β disease (Type III hyperlipoproteinemia). *Clin. Res.* 19:476, 1971.

Hazzard, W. R., and Bierman, E. L.: Aggravation of broad-β disease (Type III hyperlipoproteinemia) by hypothyroidism. *Arch. Intern. Med.* 130:22, 1972.

Hazzard, W. R., Lingren, F. R., et al.: Very low density lipoprotein subfractions in a subject with broad-β disease (Type III hyperlipoproteinemia) and a subject with endogenous lipemia (Type IV). Chemical composition and electrophoretic mobility. *Biochim. Biophys. Acta* 202:517, 1970.

Hazzard, W. R., Porte, D., Jr., et al.: Heterogeneity of very low density lipoproteins in man: evidence for a functional role of a β migrating fraction in triglyceride transport and its relation to broad-β disease (Type III hyperlipoproteinemia). *J. Clin. Invest.* 49:40a, 1970.

Hazzard, W. R., Porte, D., Jr., et al.: Abnormal lipid composition of very low density lipoproteins in the diagnosis of broad-beta disease (Type III hyperlipoproteinemia). *Metabolism* 21:1009, 1972.

Hazzard, W. R., Spiger, M. J., et al.: Studies on the mechanisms of increased plasma triglyceride levels induced by oral contraceptives. *New Eng. J. Med.* 280:471, 1969.

Hirsch, J., and Knittle, J. L.: Cellularity of obese and nonobese human adipose tissue. *Fed. Proc.* 29:1516, 1970.

Hirsch, J., Knittle, J., et al.: Cell lipid content and cell number in obese and nonobese human adipose tissue. *J. Clin. Invest.* 45:1023, 1966.

Hofmann, A. F., and Small, D. M.: Detergent properties of bile salts: Correlation with physiological function. *Ann. Rev. Med.* 18:333, 1967.

Hollander, W., Kramsch, D. M., et al.: Arterial wall metabolism in experimental hypertension of coarctation of the aorta of short duration. *J. Clin. Invest.* 47:1221, 1968.

Hollenberg, C. H.: The effect of fasting on the lipoprotein lipase activity of rat heart and diaphragm. *J. Clin. Invest.* 39:1282, 1960.

Horn, G.: Observations on the aetiology of cholelithiasis. *Brit. Med. J.* 2:732, 1956.

Hove, E., and Geill, T.: Serum cholesterol and incidence of gallstones. *Geriatrics* 23:114, 1968.

Hustvedt, B. E., and Løvø, A.: Correlation between hyperinsulinemia and hyperphagia in rats with ventromedial hypothalamic lesions. *Acta Physiol. Scand.* 84:29, 1972.

Isaksson, V.: Dissolving power of LBS for cholesterol. *Acta Soc. Med. Ups.* 59:298, 1953.

Isselbacher, K. J., Scheig, R., et al.: Congenital β-lipoprotein deficiency: An hereditary disorder involving a defect in the absorption and transport of lipids. *Medicine* 43:347, 1964.

Johnson, P. R., and Hirsch, J.: Cellularity of adipose depots in six strains of genetically obese mice. *J. Lipid Res.* 13:2, 1972.

Juhl, E., Christoffersen, P., et al.: Liver morphology and biochemistry in 8 obese patients treated with jejunoileal anastomosis. *New Eng. J. Med.* 285:543, 1971.

Jungas, R. L.: Hormonal regulation of pyruvate dehydrogenase. *Metabolism* 20:43, 1971.

Kalkhoff, R. K., Kim, H. J., et al.: Metabolic effects of weight loss in obese subjects. Changes in plasma substrate levels, insulin and growth hormone responses. *Diabetes* 20:83, 1971.

Kannel, W. B., Garcia, M. J., et al.: Serum lipid precursors of coronary heart disease. *Hum. Path.* 2:129, 1971.

Kannel, W. B., LeBauer, E. J., et al.: Relation of body weight to development of coronary heart disease. The Framingham Study. *Circulation* 35:734, 1967.

Keys, A., Anderson, J. T., et al.: Serum cholesterol response to changes in the diet. II. The effect of cholesterol in the diet. *Metabolism* 14:759, 1965.

Keys, A., Aravanis, C., et al.: Coronary heart disease: overweight and obesity as risk factors. *Ann. Intern. Med.* 77:15, 1972.

Kinsell, L. W., Gunning, B., et al.: Calories do count. *Metabolism* 13:195, 1964.

Knittle, J. L.: Obesity in childhood. A problem in adipose tissue cellular development. *J. Pediat.* 81:1048, 1972.

Knittle, J. L., and Hirsch, J.: Effect of early nutrition on the development of rat epididymal fat pads: cellularity and metabolism. *J. Clin. Invest.* 47:2091, 1968.

Kopec, B., and Fritz, I. B.: Properties of a purified carnitine palmitoyltransferase, and evidence for the existence of other carnitine acyltransferases. *Canad. J. Biochem.* 49:941, 1971.

Koppers, L. E., and Palumbo, P. J.: Lipid disturbances in endocrine disorders. *Med. Clin. N. Amer.* 56:1013, 1972.

Kostner, G., and Holasek, A.: Characterization and quantitation of the apolipoproteins from human chylomicrons. *Biochemistry* 11:1217, 1972.

Kritchevsky, D., Tepper, S., et al.: Influence of sex and sex hormones on the oxidation of cholester-26-C14 by rat liver mitochondria. *J. Lipid Res.* 4:188, 1963.

Kudzma, D. J., and Schonfeld, G.: Alcoholic hyperlipidaemia: induction by alcohol but not by carbohydrate. *J. Lab. Clin. Med.* 77:384, 1971.

Kyle, L. H., Ball, M. F., et al.: Effect of thyroid hormone on body composition in myxedema and obesity. *New Eng. J. Med.* 275:12, 1966.

Lane, M. D., and Moss, J.: Regulation of fatty acid synthesis in animal tissues, In *Metabolic Pathways.* 3rd ed. Vol. V. Vogel, H. J. (ed.), New York, Academic Press, 1971.

Langer, T., Strober, W., et al.: The metabolism of low density lipoprotein in familial type II hyperlipoproteinemia. *J. Clin. Invest.* 51:1528, 1972.

Lardy, H. A., Foster, D. O., et al.: Hormonal control of enzymes participating in glucogenesis and lipogenesis. *J. Cell. Comp. Physiol.* 66:39, 1965.

Lawlor, T., and Wells, D. G.: Metabolic hazards of fasting. *Amer. J. Clin. Nutr.* 22:1142, 1969.

Lees, R. S., and Wilson, D.E.: The treatment of hyperlipidemia. *New Eng. J. Med.* 284:186, 1971.

Lees, R. S., Song, C. S., et al.: Hyperbeta-lipoproteinemia in acute intermittent porphyria. *New Eng. J. Med.* 282:432, 1970.

Lehner, N. D. M., Clarkson, T. B., et al.: The effect of insulin deficiency, hypothyroidism, and hypertension on atherosclerosis in the squirrel monkey. *Exp. Molec. Pathol.* 15:230, 1971.

Lesser, G. T., Kumar, I., et al.: Changes in body composition with age. *Ann. N. Y. Acad. Sci.* 110:578, 1963.

Liebelt, R. A., Ichinoe, S., et al.: Regulatory influences of adipose tissue on food intake and body weight. *Ann. N. Y. Acad. Sci.* 131:559, 1965.

Lieber, M.: Incidence of gallstones and their correlation with other diseases. *Ann. Surg.* 135:394, 1952.

London, A. M., and Schreiber, E. D.: A controlled study of the effects of group discussions and an anorexiant in outpatient treatment of obesity. *Ann. Intern. Med.* 65:80, 1966.

Margolis, S., and Capuzzi, D.: Serum-lipoprotein synthesis and metabolism, In *Blood Lipids and Lipoproteins: Quantitation, Composition and Metabolism.* Nelson, G. J. (ed.), New York, John Wiley & Sons, 1972.

Mattson, F. H., Erickson, B. A., et al.: Effect of dietary cholesterol on serum cholesterol in man. *Amer. J. Clin. Nutr.* 25:589, 1972.

Mayer, J.: Genetic factors in human obesity. *Ann. N. Y. Acad. Sci.* 131:412, 1965.

Mayer, J.: Some aspects of the problem of regulation of food intake and obesity. *New Eng. J. Med.* 274:610, 622, 722, 1966.

Mayer, J.: *Overweight: Causes, Cost and Control.* Englewood Cliffs, New Jersey, Prentice-Hall, 1968.

McBride, O. W., and Korn, E. D.: The lipoprotein lipase of mammary gland and the correlation of its activity to lactation. *J. Lipid Res.* 4:17, 1963.

McGarry, J. D., and Foster, D.W.: Regulation of ketogenesis and clinical aspects of the ketotic state. *Metabolism* 21:471, 1972.

McSherry, C. K., Glenn, F., et al.: Composition of basal and stimulated hepatic bile in baboons, and the formation of cholesterol gallstones. *Proc. Nat. Acad. Sci. USA* 68:1564, 1971.

Miettinen, T. A.: Mechanism of serum cholesterol reduction by thyroid hormones in hypothyroidism. *J. Lab. Clin. Med.* 71:537, 1968.

Miettinen, T. A.: Cholesterol production in obesity. *Circulation* 44:842, 1971.

Miller, D. S., Mumford, P., et al.: Gluttony. 2. Thermogenesis in overeating man. *Amer. J. Clin. Nutr.* 20:1223, 1967.

Minari, O., and Zilversmit, D. B.: Behavior of dog lymph chylomicron lipid constituents during incubation with serum. *J. Lipid Res.* 4:424, 1963.

Miyake, H., and Johnston, C. G.: Gallstones: Ethnological studies. *Digestion* 1:219, 1968.

Montoye, H. J., Epstein, F. H., et al.: The measurement of body fatness. A study in a total community. *Amer. J. Clin. Nutr.* 16:417, 1965.

Montoye, H. J., Epstein, F. H., et al.: Relationship between serum cholesterol and body fatness, an epidemiologic study. *Amer. J. Clin. Nutr.* 18:397, 1966.

Nestel, P. J., Whyte, H. M., et al.: Distribution and turnover of cholesterol in humans. *J. Clin. Invest.* 48:982, 1969.

Newburgh, L. H., and Conn, J. W.: A new interpretation of hyperglycemia in obese middle-aged persons. *J.A.M.A. 112*:7, 1939.

Newman, J., Freeman, F., et al.: *Twins, a Study of Heredity and Environment.* Chicago, University of Chicago Press, 1937.

Nichols, A. V., and Smith, L.: Effect of very low density lipoproteins on lipid transfer in incubated serum. *J. Lipid Res.* 6:206, 1972.

Nikkilä, E. A.: Control of plasma and liver triglyceride kinetics by carbohydrate metabolism and insulin, In *Advances in Lipid Research.* Vol. 7. Paoletti, R., and Kritchevsky, D. (eds.), New York, Academic Press, 1969.

Norum, K. R., Glomset, J. A., et al.: Familial lecithin:cholesterol acyltransferase deficiency, In *The Metabolic Basis of Inherited Disease.* 3rd ed. Stanbury, J. B., Wyngaarden, J. B., et al. (eds.), New York, McGraw-Hill, 1972.

Ogilvie, R. F.: Sugar tolerance in obese subjects. A review of sixty-five cases. *Quart. J. Med.* 4:345, 1935.

Oscai, L. B., and Holloszy, J. O.: Effects of weight changes produced by exercise, food restriction, or overeating on body composition. *J. Clin. Invest.* 48:2124, 1969.

Osuga, T., and Portman, O. W.: Relationship between bile composition and gallstone formation in squirrel monkeys. *Gastroenterology* 63:122, 1972.

Ostrander, L. D., Jr.: Hyperglycemia and vascular disease in Tecumseh, Michigan, In *Early Diabetes.* Camerini-Davalos, D., and Cole, H. S. (eds.), New York, Academic Press, 1970.

Ostrander, L. D., Jr., Neff, B. J., et al.: Hyperglycemia and hypertriglyceridemia among persons with coronary heart disease. *Ann. Intern. Med.* 67:34, 1967.

Parker, G., Bagdade, J. D., et al.: Evidence for the plasma chylomicron origin of lipids accumulating in diabetic eruptive xanthomas: a correlative lipid biochemical, histochemical and electron microscopic study. *J. Clin. Invest.* 49:2172, 1970.

Parra, A., Schultz, R. B., et al.: Correlative studies in obese children and adolescents concerning body composition and plasma insulin and growth hormone levels. *Pediat. Res.* 5:605, 1971.

Patten, R. L.: The reciprocal regulation of lipoprotein lipase activity and hormone-sensitive lipase activity in rat adipocytes. *J. Biol. Chem.* 245:557, 1970.

Phillips, G.: The lipid composition of human bile. *Biochim. Biophys. Acta* 41:361, 1960.

Porte, D., Jr., O'Hara, D. D., et al.: The relation between postheparin lipolytic activity and plasma triglyceride in myxedema. *Metabolism* 15:107, 1966.

Pronczuk, A., and Fillios, L. C.: Changes in cholesterol concentrations in rough and smooth endoplasmic reticulum and polysomal profiles in rats fed cholesterol. *J. Nutr.* 96:46, 1968.

Quarfordt, S. H., Levy, R. I., et al.: On the lipoprotein abnormality in Type III hyperlipoproteinemia. *J. Clin. Invest.* 50:754, 1971.

Quintao, E., Grundy, S. M., et al.: Effects of dietary cholesterol on the regulation of total body cholesterol in man. *J. Lipid Res.* 12:233, 1971.

Rabinowitz, D.: Hormonal profile and forearm metabolism in human obesity. *Amer. J. Clin. Nutr.* 21:1438, 1968.

Rabinowitz, D., and Zierler, K.: Forearm metabolism in obesity and its response to intra-arterial insulin. Characterization of insulin resistance endurance for adaptive hyperinsulinism. *J. Clin. Invest.* 41:2173, 1962.

Randle, P., Garland, P., et al.: The glucose fatty acid cycle. Its role in insulin sensitivity and the metabolic disturbance of diabetes mellitus. *Lancet 1*:785, 1963.

Reaven, G. M., Hill, D. B., et al.: Kinetics of triglyceride turnover of very low density lipoproteins of human plasma. *J. Clin. Invest.* 44:1826, 1965.

Redgrave, T. G.: Formation of cholesteryl ester-rich particulate lipid during metabolism of chylomicrons. *J. Clin. Invest.* 49:465, 1970.

Roberts, W. C., and Buja, L. M.: The frequency and significance of coronary arterial thrombi and other observations in fatal acute myocardial infarction. *Amer. J. Med.* 52:425, 1972.

Robertson, H., and Dochat, G.: Pregnancy and gallstones: collective review. *Surg. Gynec. Obstet.* 78:193, 1944.

Robertson, P., Gavareski, D. J., et al.: Accelerated triglyceride secretion: A metabolic consequence of obesity. *J. Clin. Invest.*, 52:620, 1973.

Robinson, D. S.: The function of the plasma triglycerides in fatty acid transport. *Compr. Biochem.* 18:51, 1970.

Rose, H. G., Kranz, P. D., et al.: Characteristics of combined hyperlipoproteinemia. *Circulation* 44 (Suppl. II):11, 1971.

Ross, R., and Glomset, J. A.: Atherosclerosis: a problem in the biology of the arterial smooth muscle cell. *Science, 180*:1332, 1973.

Roth, J., Glick, S. M., et al.: Secretion of human growth hormone: physiologic and experimental modification. *Metabolism* 12:577, 1963.

Salans, L. B., and Dougherty, J. W.: Effect of insulin upon glucose metabolism by adipose cells of different size. Influence of cell lipid and protein content, age and nutritional state. *J. Clin. Invest.* 50:1399, 1971.

Salans, L. B., Knittle, J. L., et al.: The role of adipose cell size and adipose tissue insulin sensitivity in the carbohydrate intolerance of human obesity. *J. Clin. Invest.* 47:153, 1968.

Salans, L. B., and Wise, J. K.: Metabolic studies of human obesity. *Med. Clin. N. Amer.* 54:1533, 1970.

Savin, R. C.: Hyperglobulinemic purpura terminating in myeloma, hyperlipemia and xanthomatoses. *Arch. Derm.* 96:679, 1965.

Scanu, A., and Wisdom, C.: Serum lipoproteins. Structure and function. *Ann. Rev. Biochem.* 41:703, 1972.

Schacter, S.: Obesity and eating. *Science* 161:751, 1968.

Schlierf, G., and Stossberg, V.: Diurnal patterns of plasma triglyceride, free fatty acid, blood sugar and insulin levels on high-fat and high-carbohydrate diets in normals and in patients with primary endogenous hyperglyceridemia, In *Atherosclerosis: Proceedings of the Second International Symposium.* Jones, R. J. (ed.), New York, Springer-Verlag, 1970.

Schteingart, D. E., and Conn, J. W.: Characteristics of the increased adrenocortical function observed in many obese patients. *Ann. N.Y. Acad. Sci.* 131:388, 1965.

Schrott, H. G., Goldstein, J. L., et al.: Familial hypercholesterolemia in a large kindred. *Ann. Intern. Med.* 76:711, 1972.

Schumaker, V. N., and Adams, G. H.: Circulating lipoproteins. *Ann. Rev. Biochem.* 38:113, 1969.

Scott, H. W., Jr.: Metabolic surgery for hyperlipidemia and atherosclerosis. *Amer. J. Surg.* 123:3, 1972.

Scott, P. J., White, B. M., et al.: Low-density lipoprotein peptide metabolism in nephrotic syndrome: a comparison with patterns observed in other syndromes characterized by hyperlipoproteinaemia. *Australas. Ann. Med.* 1:1, 1970.

Seidel, D., Alaupovic, P., et al.: A lipoprotein characterizing obstructive jaundice. I. Method for quantitative separation and identification of lipoproteins in jaundiced subjects. *J. Clin. Invest.* 48:1211, 1969.

Shapiro, D. J., and Rodwell, V. W.: Regulation of hepatic 3-hydroxy-3-methylglutaryl coenzyme A reductase and cholesterol synthesis. *J. Biol. Chem.* 246:3210, 1971.

Simkin, B.: Urinary 17-ketosteroid and 17-ketogenic steroid excretion in obese patients. *New Eng. J. Med.* 264:974, 1961.

Simmonds, W. J., Hofman, A. F., et al.: Absorption of cholesterol from a micellar solution: intestinal perfusion studies in man. *J. Clin. Invest.* 46:874, 1967.

Sims, E. A. H., Goldman, R. F., et al.: Experimental obesity in man. *Trans. Ass. Amer. Phys.* 81:153, 1968.

Sims, E. A. H., Horton, E. S., et al.: Inducible metabolic abnormalities during development of obesity. *Ann. Rev. Med.* 22:235, 1971.

Siperstein, M. D.: Regulation of cholesterol biosynthesis in normal and malignant tissues, In *Current Topics in Cellular Regulation.* Horecker, B. L., and Stadtman, E. R. (eds.), New York, Academic Press, 1970.

Small, D. M.: The formation of gallstones. *Advances Intern. Med.* 16:243, 1970.

Small, D. M., Penkett, S. A., et al.: Studies on simple and mixed bile salt micelles by nuclear magnetic resonance spectroscopy. *Biochim. Biophys. Acta* 176:178, 1969.

Smith, E. B.: The influence of age and atherosclerosis on the chemistry of aortic intima. *J. Atherosclerosis Res.* 5:224, 1965.

Smith, E. B., and Slater, R. S.: Relationship between low-density lipoprotein in aortic intima and serum-lipid levels. *Lancet* 1:463, 1972.

Smith, E. B., Evans, P. H., et al.: Lipid in the aortic intima: the correlations of morphological and chemical characteristics. *J. Atheroscler. Res.* 7:171, 1967.

Spencer, A. F., and Lowenstein, J. M.: Citrate content of liver and kidney of rat in various metabolic states and in fluoracete poisoning. *Biochem. J.* 103:342, 1967.

Spencer, F. C., and Glassman, E.: Surgical procedures for coronary artery disease. *Ann. Rev. Med.* 23:229, 1972.

Srere, P. A.: The citrate cleavage enzyme. I. Distribution and purification. *J. Biol. Chem.* 234:2544, 1959.

Stamler, J.: The Coronary Drug Project: Findings leading to further modifications of its protocol with respect to dextrothyroxine. *J.A.M.A.* 220:996, 1972.

Stein, O., Stein, Y., et al.: The metabolism of chylomicron cholesteryl ester in rat liver. *J. Cell Biol.* 43:410, 1969.

Steinberg, D., and Huttunen, J. K.: The role of cyclic AMP in activation of hormone-sensitive lipase of adipose tissue. *Fed. Proc.* 1:47, 1972.

Steinberg, T., and Gwinup, G.: Lipodystrophy: A variant of lipoatrophic diabetes. *Diabetes* 16:715, 1967.

Steinkamp, R. C., Cohen, N. L., et al.: Measures of body fat and related factors in normal adults. II. A simple clinical method to estimate body fat and lean body mass. *J. Chronic Dis.* 18:1291, 1965.

Stemerman, M. B., and Ross, R.: Experimental atherosclerosis. I. Fibrous plaque formation in primates. An electron microscopic study. *J. Exp. Med.* 136:769, 1972.

Stewart, J. E., and Schotz, M. D.: Studies on release of lipoprotein lipase activity from fat cells. *J. Biol. Chem.* 246:5749, 1971.

Stokke, K. T.: The existence of an acid cholesterol esterase in human liver. *Biochim. Biophys. Acta* 270:156, 1972.

Stout, R. W., and Bierman, E. L.: The lipid-lowering effect of phenformin in hypertriglyceridemia: the role of insulin and free fatty acids. *Diabetes* 21:380, 1972.

Strisower, E. H., Adamson, G., et al.: Treatment of hyperlipidemias. *Amer. J. Med.* 45:488, 1968.

Stunkard, A. J.: Environment and obesity: recent advances in our understanding of regulation of food intake in man. *Fed. Proc.* 27:1367, 1968.

Stunkard, A. J., and McLaren-Hume, M.: The results of treatment for obesity. *Arch. Intern. Med.* 103:79, 1959.

Stunkard, A. J., Grace, W. J., et al.: The night-eating syndrome: a pattern of food intake among certain obese patients. *Amer. J. Med.* 19:78, 1955.

Tejada, C., Strong, J. P., et al.: Distribution of coronary and aortic atherosclerosis by geographic location, race, and sex. *Lab. Invest.* 18:509, 1968.

Thistle, J. L., and Schoenfield, L. J.: Lithogenic bile among young Indian women. *New Eng. J. Med.* 284:177, 1971.

Topping, D. L., and Mayes, P. A.: The immediate effects of insulin and fructose on the metabolism of the perfused liver: changes in lipoprotein secretion, fatty acid oxidation and esterification, lipogenesis and carbohydrate metabolism. *Biochem. J.* 126:295, 1972.

Torvik, A., and Hoivik, B.: Gallstones in an autopsy series. *Acta Chir. Scand.* 120:168, 1960.

Van der Linden, W.: Some biological traits in female gallstone disease patients. *Acta Chir. Scand.* Suppl. 269, 1961.

Vlahcevic, Z. R., Bell, C. C., Jr., et al.: Relationship of bile acid pool size to the formation of lithogenic bile in female Indians of the Southwest. *Gastroenterology* 62:73, 1972.

Wagle, S., Gaskins, R., et al.: Studies on glucose synthesis by rat liver and kidney cortex slices. *Life Sci.* 5:655, 1966.

Walton, K. W., Scott, P. J., et al.: Alterations of metabolism and turnover of I^{131} low density lipoprotein in myxedema and thyrotoxicosis. *Clin. Sci.* 29:217, 1965.

Ways, P. O., Permentier, C. M., et al.: Studies on the absorptive defect for triglyceride in abetalipoproteinemia. *J. Clin. Invest.* 46:35, 1967.

Westlund, K., and Nicolaysen, R.: Serum cholesterol and risk of mortality and morbidity. A 3-year follow-up of 6,886 men. *Scand. J. Clin. Lab. Invest.* 18 (Suppl. 87): 1, 1966.

Wieland, O., VonFuncke, H., et al.: Interconversion of pyruvate dehydrogenase in rat heart muscle upon perfusion with fatty acids or ketone bodies. *FEBS Letters* 12:295, 1971.

World Health Organization Study Group: Classification of atherosclerotic lesions. Tech. Rep. Ser. No. 143, 1958.

Ygge, J., Brody, S., et al.: Changes in blood coagulation and fibrinolysis in women receiving oral contraceptives. Comparison between treated and untreated women in a longitudinal study. *Amer. J. Obstet. Gynec.* 104:87, 1969.

Zorilla, E., Hulse, M., et al.: Severe endogenous hypertriglyceridemia during treatment with estrogen and oral contraceptives. *J. Clin. Endocr.* 28:1793, 1968.

CHAPTER 19

Summarization of the Effects of Hormones on Water and Electrolyte Metabolism

By Alexander Leaf and
Grant W. Liddle

The hormones that are of greatest importance in regulating water and electrolyte metabolism exert their principal effects on renal function. By far the most important of these hormones are the antidiuretic hormone (ADH) of the posterior pituitary and aldosterone, the sodium-retaining hormone of the adrenal cortex. These two hormones are of major significance in the homeostatic regulation of water and electrolyte balance under ordinary physiologic conditions. Other hormones have relatively minor significance under ordinary conditions but may assume importance under pathologic conditions.

SEQUENCE OF EVENTS IN RENAL METABOLISM OF WATER AND ELECTROLYTES

1. *Glomerular filtration* is the initial event in the formation of urine. In a normal man, the daily glomerular filtrate includes more than 150 liters of water, 20,000 mEq. of sodium, and 14,000 mEq. of chloride. The fact that approximately 99 per cent of the filtered water, sodium, and chloride is reabsorbed by the renal tubules indicates the existence of a very delicate balance between the processes of filtration and reabsorption. This balance is influenced by hemodynamic, metabolic, pharmacologic, and hormonal factors. Although the regulation of glomerular filtration rate (GFR) is primarily nonhormonal, increases in GFR result from increases in the levels of thyroid hormones, growth hormone, and glucocorticoids. Sodium-retaining steroids and ADH may indirectly increase GFR by promoting expansion of body fluid compartments. Other things being equal, an increase in GFR leads to an increase in excretion of water and electrolytes.

2. The *proximal convoluted tubule* reabsorbs two thirds or more of the filtered sodium, chloride, and water and usually virtually all the bicarbonate. Parathyroid hormone acts on this portion of the renal tubule to inhibit sodium, bicarbonate, and phosphate reabsorption. Since the sodium is subsequently largely reabsorbed at some more distal site, a marked phosphaturia and a mild hyperchloremic acidosis result. Calcitonin administered in pharmacologic amounts to humans also causes a modest initial sodium diuresis with an accompanying weight loss of approximately one kilogram. Since the sodium diuresis occurs with an aminoaciduria and phosphaturia, the site of action of calcitonin is thought to be in the proximal tubule. The much sought after "natriuretic hormone" (or "third factor") is also thought to inhibit sodium chloride reabsorption in this segment of the nephron. The increased salt and water excretion by the hypothyroid rat is associated with a decreased reabsorption of sodium in the proximal tubule, as well as in the distal nephron, and may be caused by a generalized decrease in sodium-potassium adenosine triphosphatase in the absence of thyroid hormone.

3. The *ascending limb of the loop of Henle* actively reabsorbs sodium and chloride against a concentration gradient but is relatively impermeable to water. Consequently, the fluid leaving this seg-

ment is hypotonic, and the interstitial fluid adjacent to the loop is very hypertonic. It is not known whether hormones influence this process.

4. The *distal convoluted tubule* reabsorbs sodium, chloride, and water and "secretes" hydrogen and potassium ions into the urine. Ammonia synthesized by the tubular epithelium diffuses into the tubular lumen where, in the presence of hydrogen ion, it is converted into the ammonium ion. All these processes are stimulated by aldosterone-like steroids and inhibited by aldosterone antagonists (spironolactones).

In the primate, it seems that the hypotonic fluid emerging from the loop of Henle undergoes little change in tonicity during either diuresis or antidiuresis as it passes through the distal convoluted tubule. ADH has little or no effect in reducing the relative impermeability to water of the epithelium lining the distal convoluted tubule.

5. The *collecting duct* passively reabsorbs water and certain other small molecules such as urea. In the absence of ADH, the collecting duct is relatively impermeable to water, and the large volume of hypotonic fluid entering it from the distal con-

voluted tubule passes through producing a copious dilute urine. In the presence of ADH, the permeability of the collecting duct epithelium to water and urea increases, allowing them to diffuse along their concentration gradients into the very hypertonic interstitial fluid of the renal medulla. (This hypertonicity is created and maintained by reabsorption of large quantities of sodium and chloride by the ascending limbs of the loops of Henle.) Thus, in the presence of ADH, a small volume of concentrated urine is finally excreted.

HORMONAL REGULATION OF WATER AND ELECTROLYTE METABOLISM

The principal effects of hormones are listed in Table 19–1. More detailed consideration is given in the following paragraphs.

Pituitary Hormones

The *antidiuretic hormone (ADH) of the human posterior pituitary* has been identified as arginine

TABLE 19–1.   EFFECTS OF HORMONES ON FLUID AND ELECTROLYTES

Hormone	Mechanism	Effect
Antidiuretic hormone	Increases permeability of tubule cells of collecting duct to water and to urea, permitting their reabsorption from urine.	Decreases volume and increases concentration of urine with resultant conservation of body water. In excess, it can cause water retention, overexpansion of body water, dilution of intracellular and extracellular fluids, increased GFR, decreased secretion of aldosterone, and increased sodium excretion.
Aldosterone	Increases sodium reabsorption in distal portions of nephron.	Decreases sodium and chloride excretion with resultant conservation of extracellular fluid volume. Also increases urinary potassium, titratable acid, and ammonium. In excess, it may overexpand extracellular fluid compartment, causing either edema or hypertension with potassium depletion and alkalosis.
Cortisol	1. Increases distal sodium reabsorption (similar to aldosterone).	1. Decreases sodium excretion and increases excretion of potassium, ammonium, and titratable acids (similar to aldosterone).
	2. Increases GFR.	2. Increases excretion of water.
	3. Correction of pathologic stimulus to secondary aldosterone hypersecretion.	3. Natriuresis.
Estrogens	Similar to aldosterone.	Inconstant sodium retention.
Progesterone	Aldosterone antagonist.	Increases sodium excretion and decreases potassium excretion.
Growth hormone	General tissue anabolism.	Retention of intracellular and extracellular water and electrolytes in quantities appropriate for growth.
Androgens	Similar to growth hormone plus aldosterone?	Retention of intracellular and extracellular water and electrolytes.
Thyroid hormones	1. Increase cardiac output, renal blood flow, and tubular reabsorption of sodium.	Variable increased or decreased excretion of water and electrolytes.
	2. Dissolution of myxedema.	
Parathyroid hormone	1. Reduces proximal tubular reabsorption of phosphate, sodium, and bicarbonate; increases reabsorption of calcium.	1. Increases phosphate, bicarbonate, sodium, and potassium in urine.
	2. Dissolution of bone.	2. Increases calcium excretion with hypercalcemia.
Calcitonin	Reduces proximal tubular reabsorption of phosphate, sodium, calcium, and magnesium.	Increases sodium, phosphate, potassium, calcium, and magnesium excretion with pharmacologic doses.
Catecholamines	1. Circulatory effects.	Water diuresis with alpha adrenergic stimuli.
	2. Alpha adrenergic blockade of renal effects of vasopressin.	Antidiuresis from beta adrenergic stimuli.
	3. Beta adrenergic simulation of ADH action on renal tubule, or by release of ADH.	
Prostaglandins	Modify action of ADH on renal tubule.	Increase water and sodium excretion.

vasopressin. This hormone promotes the conservation of water by increasing the water-permeability of the cells lining the distal portions of the nephron. The studies of Orloff and Handler have shown an increase in adenosine 3',5'-monophosphate concentrations in cells that respond to ADH, and it is established that this intracellular intermediary in some manner increases the permeability of such cells primarily to water but also to urea.

ADH is secreted in response to dehydration, and its ultimate effect is to overcome dehydration. The supraoptico-hypophysial system is so sensitive to small changes in the concentration of extracellular fluid that even a slight increase in extracellular osmolality stimulates the secretion of ADH. The hormone acts on the cells of the distal nephron to increase their permeability to water and urea but not to larger molecules generally. The collecting ducts are surrounded by the extremely hypertonic interstitial fluid of the renal medulla. Therefore, in the presence of ADH, water reaching the collecting duct can be drawn by osmotic forces across the cells lining the duct into the hypertonic interstitial space of the renal medulla and thus regain access to the circulation. In this way, urinary solutes are concentrated and water is conserved. The water that is reabsorbed serves to dilute extracellular fluids and thereby tends to correct the hyperosmolality that initially stimulated the secretion of ADH.

A decrease in the osmolality of extracellular fluid below approximately 280 mOsm. per kg. of water normally leads to cessation of ADH secretion. In the absence of ADH, the kidneys excrete "free" water (water in excess of the quantity required to make urine iso-osmotic with plasma). The loss of free water from the body increases the concentration of extracellular solutes, which ultimately results in the resumption of ADH secretion.

Clinical disorders of ADH physiology include pathologic deficiencies and pathologic excesses of the hormone, as well as renal disorders characterized by limited responsiveness to the hormone.

Diabetes insipidus is characterized by limited capacity of the supraoptico-hypophysial system to secrete ADH because of a variety of disorders affecting the hypothalamus.

In addition to extracellular hypertonicity, there are numerous physiologic and pharmacologic stimuli to ADH secretion. These include such factors as hypovolemia, pain, nicotine, and cholinergic agents. It should not be surprising, therefore, that patients might sometimes be encountered who seem to be secreting ADH "inappropriately" when considered from the narrow viewpoint that ADH should be regulated only by the osmolality of extracellular fluids. One form of "inappropriate ADH excess" is the production of ectopic ADH by certain tumors of the lung. Tumors of other organs, as well as a diversity of other conditions in the lung, have been associated with the syndrome of inappropriate ADH secretion. Such patients may continue to elaborate hypertonic urine even though serum osmolality is distinctly subnormal. This causes excessive water retention, overexpansion of body fluid compartments, increased GFR, and decreased aldosterone secretion with increased urinary sodium despite hyponatremia. This sequence of events may produce marked dilution of the body fluids and clinical water intoxication. Curtailment of water intake is an important part of the therapeutic management of such patients in order to avoid the development of central nervous system dysfunction from water intoxication.

Certain renal disorders are characterized by limited responsiveness to ADH. One of these is a familial disorder referred to as "nephrogenic diabetes insipidus." In addition, in patients with hypokalemia or hypercalcemia, the kidney may lose its ability to generate a normal degree of hypertonicity of the medullary interstitial fluid. Such kidneys, therefore, lack the osmotic gradient that is necessary to draw water from the collecting duct into the interstitium. The defect does not represent a disturbance in ADH physiology per se, and normal urinary concentrating capacity cannot be restored in such patients by treatment with ADH.

Growth hormone promotes retention of both the constituents of protoplasm and extracellular fluid. In so doing it promotes a positive sodium, chloride, and water balance, as well as a positive potassium, phosphorus, and nitrogen balance. Over prolonged periods, growth hormone induces renal hypertrophy which is accompanied by increased renal blood flow and GFR. The precise mechanism through which growth hormone diminishes urinary excretion of various electrolytes is unknown. The effects of growth hormone upon electrolyte excretion can be demonstrated in either the presence or absence of the adrenal glands. Injections of growth hormone frequently induce increased calcium excretion.

Thyroid-stimulating hormone, prolactin, gonadotropic hormones, and adrenocorticotropic hormone (ACTH) have not been shown to exert any major direct effect upon electrolyte or fluid metabolism. Indirect effects are more properly attributable to the hormones of the thyroid, gonads, and adrenal cortex, which will be considered in subsequent paragraphs.

The important role of hormones in the control of lactation falls beyond the scope of this chapter.

Adrenocortical Hormones and Related Steroids: Physiologic Considerations

Mechanisms through which corticosteroids influence fluid and electrolyte metabolism are as follows:

1. Increased renal tubular ion transport (aldosterone-like action).

2. Aldosterone antagonism (spironolactone-like action).

3. Increased GFR (property of glucocorticoids).

4. Correction of pathologic stimulus to hypersecretion of aldosterone.

5. Tissue catabolism.

Aldosterone: Physiologic Effects. Of the naturally occurring steroids, aldosterone is by far the most potent regulator of electrolyte excretion. The hormone binds to specific protein receptors in the responsive renal cells, where, it is postulated, it induces the DNA-directed synthesis of RNA with subsequent formation of new protein. The role of this protein remains controversial but is thought either to facilitate entry of sodium into the transporting cells or to provide these cells with an increased energy supply for active sodium transport. In either case, its net effect is to enhance sodium transport (reabsorption).

In the distal nephron, the action of aldosterone is manifested by increased reabsorption of sodium and chloride from tubular lumen and increased secretion of potassium and hydrogen ions into the tubular lumen. The reabsorption of sodium and chloride tends to increase the osmolality of extracellular fluid. An increase in extracellular osmolality stimulates the secretion of ADH, and ADH facilitates the renal conservation of water. Thus sodium, chloride, and water are commonly retained or excreted together, and aldosterone can be said to promote, indirectly, the renal tubular reabsorption of water.

Factors Controlling the Secretion of Aldosterone. The mechanism regulating the secretion of aldosterone is separate from that controlling the secretion of the other major adrenal steroids, and it is appropriately responsive to changes in body hydration. The important studies of Davis and others have established the fact that the renin-angiotensin system is the principal mediator of the adrenocortical response to changes in body hydration. The question of what regulates the secretion of aldosterone has thus become transformed into the question of what regulates the secretion of renin. As summarized in Figure 19–1, conditions that reduce extracellular fluid volume, and conditions that result in sequestration of venous blood all tend to stimulate the production of renin, thereby increasing the formation of angiotensin. Angiotensin not only acts directly on the vascular system as a pressor agent but also stimulates adrenocortical production of aldosterone. Teleologically, this sequence of events makes good sense, for all the aforementioned stimuli to renin, angiotensin, and aldosterone production are conditions that tend to decrease the "effective" blood volume. Since aldosterone promotes sodium retention,

it helps to expand the extracellular fluid compartment and thus, indirectly, supports the circulation.

Renin production and, therefore, aldosterone secretion are also increased in some patients with renal artery stenosis and in some with diffuse renovascular disease associated with malignant hypertension.

In normal subjects in whom postural and dietary influences on renin production are held constant at all times, there is a diurnal rhythm in plasma renin activity, with lowest levels occurring in the afternoon. The diurnal rhythm in plasma renin activity is probably the major factor leading to a diurnal rhythm in aldosterone secretion; the latter too is characterized by a decrease in the afternoon.

Although angiotensin appears under many circumstances to be the principal regulator of aldosterone secretion, it is not the only one. ACTH has at least a transient stimulatory effect on the secretion of aldosterone. If the administration of ACTH is continued for more than a few days, however, its effect on aldosterone secretion disappears even though its stimulatory effect on the secretion of other adrenal steroids persists.

Aldosterone secretion is also influenced by the concentration of potassium in body fluids. Potassium depletion diminishes the secretion of aldosterone. Again, this is a biologically useful relationship: an excess of potassium stimulates the production of a potassium-wasting hormone, and a deficiency of potassium has the opposite effect.

Other Corticosteroids Having Aldosterone-like Activity. A very large number of corticosteroids, including most compounds with "glucocorticoid activity," share to varying degrees the electrolyte-regulating activity of aldosterone.

11-Desoxycorticosterone (DOC) is an aldosterone-like compound which is of historical importance because it was for many years the principal corticosteroid used in the treatment of Addison's disease. Although DOC is an important intermediate in adrenal biosynthesis of corticosterone and aldosterone, it is not itself released into the blood in biologically significant quantities except under abnormal circumstances. Faulty conversion of DOC to corticosterone is observed in patients with the "hypertensive" variety of congenital adrenal hyperplasia and in individuals treated with a chemical inhibitor of 11-beta-hydroxylase such as 2-methyl-1,2-bis(3-pyridyl)-1-propanone (metyrapone). Under such conditions, DOC is secreted in appreciable quantities and causes (acutely) sodium retention and potassium loss and (over a sufficient period) hypertension.

Corticosterone has electrolyte-regulating activity which is qualitatively similar to that of aldosterone, but it has less than 1 per cent of the potency of aldosterone. In certain animals, including the rat, corticosterone is the principal glucocorticoid. In man, corticosterone is secreted in quantities of the order of 5 mg. per day. Compared with cortisol (hydrocortisone), it is of little importance as a glucocorticoid, and compared with aldosterone, it is of little importance normally as a regulator of electrolyte metabolism.

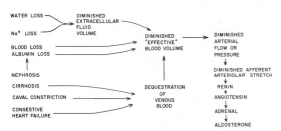

Figure 19–1. A common mechanism through which various physiologic factors might stimulate aldosterone secretion.

Aldosterone Antagonists. Aldosterone antagonists are steroids which reverse the effects of aldosterone-like steroids on electrolyte and water excretion. The clearest examples of aldosterone antagonists are the synthetic steroids known as "spironolactones." These compounds have little or no effect upon fluid or electrolyte metabolism when administered in the absence of aldosterone-like steroids, but in the presence of aldosterone-like steroids, the spironolactones cause an increase in excretion of sodium, chloride, and water while diminishing the excretion of potassium, ammonium, and titratable acid. It has been demonstrated that the spironolactones are competitive inhibitors of aldosterone and that they block the attachment of aldosterone-like steroids to a specific receptor substance within cells of the renal tubules. Landau has shown that progesterone is an aldosterone antagonist. It, and possibly other naturally occurring steroids, also acts by competitively blocking the binding of aldosterone-like steroids to specific receptor proteins within the cytosol and nuclei of responsive cells.

Steroids Which Modify GFR. Glucocorticoids commonly cause transient increases in glomerular filtration rate. With increased glomerular filtration rate, there tends to be an increase in excretion of water and electrolytes.

Steroids Which Modify "Secondary Aldosteronism." Anti-inflammatory steroids may affect fluid and electrolyte metabolism indirectly by correcting a pathologic stimulus to excessive aldosterone secretion. For example, by promoting healing of the renal lesion leading to the nephrotic syndrome, anti-inflammatory steroids might indirectly correct the hypoalbuminemia, thus increasing "effective" blood volume, thereby bringing about a decrease in the production of renin, angiotensin, and aldosterone and facilitating the excretion of excess sodium, chloride, and water.

Catabolic Steroids. One of the characteristic properties of glucocorticoids is that of shifting the balance between protein anabolism and catabolism in favor of the latter. One aspect of the protein-wasting process is the wasting of potassium. Therefore, a catabolic steroid may promote an increase in potassium excretion.

Multiple Actions of Steroids. Certain steroids, such as cortisol, may exert multiple actions influencing fluid and electrolyte metabolism. Cortisol mimics aldosterone in its effect upon renal tubular cation transport, thus causing sodium retention and potassium loss. However, cortisol may also be effective in increasing glomerular filtration rate and in correcting certain pathologic conditions leading to the hypersecretion of aldosterone; through these mechanisms, cortisol sometimes promotes sodium loss. Since it is a catabolic steroid, cortisol may also promote potassium wasting as part of a tissue-wasting process. In addition, cortisol tends to promote the excretion of "free-water," an action which is most easily observed when the steroid is administered to patients with adrenal insufficiency. This free-water diuresis is not due to antagonism of the action of ADH on the renal tubule but has been attributed to antagonism of the release of ADH, to an increase in GFR, or to a reduction in permeability to water of renal tubule cells in the absence of ADH. However, it appears that maintaining a normal sodium balance in the adrenalectomized dog in the absence of glucocorticoid hormones may correct the defect in water diuresis.

Adrenocortical Hormones: Clinical Disorders

Effects of Combined Deficiency of Aldosterone and Cortisol. The effects of steroids upon water and electrolyte metabolism can be deduced from observations of patients with deficiencies or pathologic excess of these hormones. In Addison's disease, a combined deficiency of cortisol and aldosterone results in impairment of ion transport in a number of organs. There is an increased tendency to lose sodium and a diminished tendency to lose potassium in gastrointestinal secretions, sweat, and urine. The consequences of adrenal insufficiency with respect to renal function are especially important. There is impairment of renal tubular capacity to reabsorb sodium and to secrete potassium, hydrogen, and ammonium. Consequently, the patient withstands sodium deprivation, acid loading, and potassium loading very poorly. Loss of sodium is accompanied by loss of chloride and water and, consequently, by depletion of extracellular fluid. Blood volume decreases. Blood pressure falls, in part because of reduced blood volume and in part because, in the absence of corticosteroids, the responsiveness of arterioles to norepinephrine is diminished. Cardiac size decreases. Cardiac output diminishes. Renal blood flow and glomerular filtration rate decrease, resulting in prerenal azotemia. There is impaired ability to excrete a water load. Hyperkalemia and mild acidosis result from impaired renal tubular secretion of potassium, hydrogen, and ammonium ions in the distal nephron. Sodium depletion may be accelerated by poor food intake and by diarrhea. This set of circumstances culminates in vasomotor collapse and is referred to clinically as addisonian crisis.

In some cases of virilizing congenital adrenal hyperplasia, there is a deficiency of both cortisol and aldosterone, leading to a "salt-losing" disorder similar to that observed in Addison's disease.

Isolated Deficiency of Cortisol. This disorder is observed in patients with Addison's disease who are treated only with aldosterone or DOC. The latter steroids tend to reverse all the aforementioned abnormalities of electrolyte and fluid metabolism. GFR usually remains subnormal, however, and the ability to excrete a water load remains impaired. Appetite, vigor, and normal "organic" metabolism are not restored by aldosterone or DOC alone. A similar derangement of adrenal steroid pattern is observed in patients with ACTH deficiency; they lack the capacity to secrete normal quantities of cortisol but retain the capacity to secrete fairly adequate quantities of aldosterone. The hyponatremia of such patients is usually due not to aldosterone deficiency but to cortisol deficiency and its consequent impairment of free-water excretion. Cortisol is uniquely valuable in bringing about rapid correction of the lethargy, hypotension, nausea, and vomiting of the patient in addisonian crisis. Cortisol is especially effective in raising the glomerular filtration rate and in restoring the ability of the addisonian patient to excrete free water.

Isolated Deficiency of Aldosterone. This disorder is observed in patients with Addison's disease who are treated only with cortisol. The administration of cortisol to the patient with Addison's disease helps to reverse all the aforementioned abnormalities in fluid and electrolyte metabolism. However, cortisol is not a very potent sodium-retaining agent. If one were to treat all addisonian patients with cortisol alone, it would be necessary in many cases to give doses large enough to produce mild Cushing's syndrome in order to obtain optimal sodium conservation. In order to prevent hypotension, acidosis, azotemia, weakness, and anorexia in patients with Addison's disease, it is usually desirable to give an aldosterone substitute, such as DOC or fludrocortisone, as well as adequate quantities of sodium chloride.

Aldosterone Excess. The effects of a chronic excess of aldosterone are observed clinically in the syndrome of *primary aldosteronism.* Primary actions of aldosterone are on electrolyte transport with increased reabsorption of sodium and chloride and increased excretion of potassium, hydrogen ion, and ammonium. In time, a secondary shift in electrolyte metabolism occurs. After retaining a few hundred milliequivalents of sodium, a patient with a normal circulatory system establishes a new steady state with his sodium output equal to his intake. Sodium is not retained to the point of producing overt edema. The patient with primary aldosteronism is often able to excrete an acute sodium load more readily than the normal individual. This adaptation depends upon the integrity of the circulatory system and is possibly related to a slightly expanded "effective blood volume," decreased responsiveness of the sympathetic nervous system, decreased production of renin and angiotensin, and increased GFR. The ultimate development of hypertension is probably due, at least in part, to occult sodium retention.

Excessive loss of potassium in the urine results in hypokalemia, depletion of intracellular potassium, elevation of serum bicarbonate, and elevation of serum pH. Increased myocardial irritability may occur, together with electrocardiographic changes such as T-wave depression and appearance of U waves. Muscular weakness is common, and paresthesias and tetany are sometimes encountered. Potassium depletion frequently causes a nephropathy characterized by degenerative changes in cells of the proximal convoluted tubules and collecting ducts. There may be diminished ability to elaborate concentrated urine. This difficulty may result in polyuria and polydipsia; nocturia is especially common. Some patents with primary aldosteronism develop hypernatremia. The precise mechanism is not clear.

A distinguishing feature of the patient with steroid-dependent potassium wasting is that he continues to excrete large amounts of potassium (for example, more than 25 mEq. per day) despite the fact that his serum potassium concentration is distinctly subnormal (e.g., 3.0 mEq. per liter or less). A high potassium clearance with low serum potassium is characteristic of patients with primary aldosteronism. In contrast, patients with potassium depletion due to gastrointestinal losses or patients who are recovering from potassium depletion due to diuretic agents usually excrete very small amounts of potassium in the urine as long as the serum potassium remains low.

The need for a reliable set of diagnostic tests for primary aldosteronism has long been felt. Hypertension is a nonspecific manifestation. Hypokalemia is neither limited to primary aldosteronism nor is it invariably present in this disease. Even the demonstration of an elevated aldosterone secretory rate does not prove that a patient has primary aldosteronism; alternatively, he might have secondary aldosteronism. A useful adjunct in diagnosis is the measurement of plasma renin activity. In primary aldosteronism, the autonomous secretion of aldosterone by an adrenal adenoma leads to sodium retention, expansion of extracellular fluid volume, and suppression of renin production by the kidneys. In contrast, in secondary aldosteronism the production of abnormally large quantities of aldosterone is "secondary" to increased renin production. The combination of high aldosterone secretory rate and low plasma renin activity, therefore, might be considered pathognomonic of primary aldosteronism.

Secondary aldosteronism is the term given to a group of disorders in which extraordinary quantities of aldosterone are secreted as a physiologic response to some extra-adrenal disorder. Conditions which cause a decrease in effective blood volume (simple dehydration, sodium depletion, hypoalbuminemia, exsanguination, or venous sequestration of blood such as occurs in hepatic cirrhosis and congestive heart failure) lead to increased production of renin and angiotensin and, secondarily, to increased aldosterone secretion. Circulatory insufficiency not only stimulates secretion of aldosterone but also tends to compromise glomerular filtration rate. The two processes act synergistically in causing sodium retention. Hypersecretion of aldosterone alone does not lead to overt edema formation in the absence of renal failure or some circulatory disorder. On the other hand, unless renal function is severely impaired (because of intrinsic renal disease or severe circulatory failure), aldosterone-like steroids must be present in order to reduce sodium excretion to less than about 20 mEq. per day. Thus, two factors, one circulatory and one hormonal, ordinarily coexist in the pathogenesis of edema.

Although secondary aldosteronism is usually not characterized by potassium depletion, deficiency of this cation is often seen as a complication of therapy. Diuretic therapy tends to diminish extracellular fluid volume and, therefore, often leads to further increases in renin, angiotensin, and aldosterone production. The more aldosterone, the greater the tendency of the kidneys to respond to conventional diuretics by excreting potassium rather than sodium. The spironolactones, by acting as aldosterone antagonists, work synergistically with conventional diuretics in promoting sodium excretion while diminishing the potassium-excreting effect of the conventional agents.

Aldosterone Secretion in Response to ADH Excess and Deficiency. Although ADH has no direct effect upon aldosterone secretion, it may have an indirect effect mediated by changes in total body hydration. Thus, if water loading is carried out in the presence of large quantities of ADH, whether exogenous or endogenous, expansion of all fluid compartments will occur, suppressing the secretion of aldosterone. As a consequence of decreased aldosterone secretion, sodium excretion rises and potassium excretion falls. As a further consequence of extracellular and intravascular fluid compartment expansion, GFR increases, and this too leads to an increase in sodium excretion. Overhydration is also reflected in dilution of serum electrolytes. The overall picture of ADH excess may, then, comprise "water intoxication," hyponatremia, and excretion of large quantities of sodium in the urine. The syndrome of ADH excess is sometimes confused with adrenal insufficiency; however, the former is associated physiologically with overexpansion of all body fluid compartments and a normal or supernormal circulatory system, whereas the latter is associated with reduced extracellular fluid volume and insufficiency of circulation. Furthermore the latter must be corrected by steroids, but the former responds to curtailment of water intake.

Deficiency of ADH (diabetes insipidus) permits the loss of excessive quantities of free water in the urine. The consequent dehydration stimulates the secretion of aldosterone, which promotes sodium retention and potassium excretion by the kidneys. A further effect of dehydration is a fall in GFR, and this too results in a decrease in sodium excretion.

Cortisol Excess. The effect of a chronic excess of cortisol is observed in patients with Cushing's syndrome, either spontaneous or iatrogenic. The most severe excesses of cortisol are often encountered in patients with Cushing's syndrome due to ACTH produced by tumors of "nonendocrine" tissues. The disturbances of fluid and electrolyte metabolism are similar to those observed in primary aldosteronism. The mechanisms are probably the same, involving primarily increased potassium excretion and increased sodium reabsorption by the renal tubules.

Other Hormones

Parathyroid hormone has as its major physiologic role the regulation of calcium and phosphorus metabolism. It promotes the renal excretion of phosphate and enhances renal tubular reabsorption of calcium. At the same time, it promotes resorption of calcium salts from bone, with resultant hypercalcemia and hypercalciuria, the latter in spite of the direct, but weak, effect to increase tubular reabsorption of calcium. The hypercalcemia and hypercalciuria may indirectly cause a renal tubular disorder characterized by loss of concentrating ability, hyposthenuria, polyuria, dehydration, and polydipsia. Depending in part upon the degree of nephrocalcinosis or renal stone formation resulting from the hypercalciuria, there is often other evidence of renal malfunction as well.

Parathyroid hormone reduces reabsorption of sodium and bicarbonate, as well as phosphate, in the proximal tubule. Most of the sodium is subsequently reabsorbed at more distal sites, and this may cause some increased potassium secretion. Thus the net effect will be phosphate and bicarbonate loss with a modest increase in sodium and potassium in the urine. The bicarbonate loss results in systemic acidosis, and it has been shown that a mild hyperchloremic acidosis may be associated with hyperparathyroidism, and slight metabolic alkalosis may be seen in hypoparathyroidism in man.

Calcitonin also has as its major physiologic role the regulation of calcium and phosphate metabolism. Injections of calcitonin peptides into hypoparathyroid patients promptly increase the renal clearance of inorganic phosphate, sodium, potassium, calcium, and magnesium. These changes in excretion are similar to those following parathyroid hormone injection, except that the initial effect, as mentioned, of parathyroid hormone is to reduce urinary calcium and magnesium clearance. The natriuresis in the first two days of continuous infusion of calcitonin in man may cause a weight loss of some 0.5 to 1.5 kilograms until a new steady state is achieved by an enhanced secretion of renin and aldosterone in response to the shrinkage of extracellular fluid volume. Since the effects of sodium excretion are accompanied by phosphaturia and aminoaciduria, it is presumed that calcitonin reduces proximal tubular reabsorption of these substances by an action on membrane bound adenyl cyclase which is, however, distinct from the adenyl cyclase that mediates the renal effects of either parathyroid hormone or vasopressin.

Insulin has no significant direct effect upon water and electrolyte metabolism. Hyperglycemia resulting from insulin deficiency may, however, result in a sufficient increase in solute load presented to the renal tubules to cause "osmotic diuresis," with loss of water and electrolytes in the urine. The polyuria results in systemic dehydration and polydipsia. An increase in ketone body formation resulting from insulin deficiency leads to acidosis. The increase in anion load which is presented to the kidney results in increased hydrogen ion and ammonium ion excretion, as well as increased excretion of "fixed" cations such as sodium and potassium. Increased phosphate excretion also occurs as a consequence of acidosis. The diuresis of uncontrolled diabetes mellitus may result in severe dehydration with loss of extracellular fluid volume, loss of blood volume, hypotension, and peripheral vascular collapse. Diminished renal blood flow leads to prerenal azotemia. The acidosis worsens as renal excretion of acid diminishes. The renal insufficiency may lead to a deceptive increase in serum potassium and phosphate and obscure the existence of total body deficits of these "intracellular" ions.

Insulin induces a transient decrease in serum potassium and inorganic phosphate concentrations, attributable to the increased hepatic and muscular uptake of these substances during glycogen synthesis. With glycogen storage there also is water storage

Glucagon has not been shown to influence electrolytes or water in any important direct manner.

Catecholamines have little, if any, direct effect on water and electrolyte metabolism. However, interestingly they do modulate the effects of another hormone, namely ADH. Thus both epinephrine and norepinephrine inhibit the water permeability response of the toad bladder to low concentrations of vasopressin, and this effect is reversed by alpha adrenergic blocking agents (phenoxybenzamine or phentolamine) but not by beta adrenergic blocking agents (propranolol). Furthermore, beta adrenergic stimulation in the dog with intravenous isoproterenol significantly increases urinary osmolality and decreases free water clearance. However, at present it is uncertain whether this antidiuretic action results from a release of ADH from the hypothalamus or from a direct effect of isoproterenol on the water permeability of the renal tubular epithelium. The physiologic importance of these effects is not clear, but the diuresis associated with the tension of an important interview or examination may be explained by the anti-ADH effect of catecholamines on the renal tubule.

Gonadal hormones, such as estradiol and testosterone, have slight sodium-retaining activity, presumably through promoting sodium reabsorption by the renal tubules. This effect is slight and inconstant.

Progesterone administered in large doses (50 to 100 mg. per day) in a setting of high mineralocorticoid activity will increase sodium excretion and decrease urinary potassium consistent with its action as an aldosterone antagonist. However, in such high doses its protoplasmic catabolic action with release of potassium may actually enhance potassium loss.

Thyroid hormones (thyroxine and triiodothyronine) have no major direct effect on renal excretion of water and electrolytes, although some increased salt and water excretion in the hypothyroid rat is associated with decreased reabsorption of sodium, which may be associated with the generalized decrease in sodium-potassium-dependent adenosine triphosphatase in the absence of thyroid hormone. As metabolic stimulants, however, thyroid hormones exert an important influence on the circulatory system, causing increased cardiac output, increased renal blood flow, and increased GFR. Chronic lack of thyroid hormone permits accumulation of myxedema fluid. Treatment of the myxedematous patient with thyroid hormones results in mobilization of myxedema fluid with increased urinary excretion of water, sodium, and chloride. Congestive heart failure, resulting either from myxedema heart disease or thyrotoxic heart disease, may be associated with accumulation of edema fluid. Correction of the thyroidal abnormality may permit recovery from congestive heart failure with increased renal excretion of sodium, chloride, and water. Water turnover may be increased by thyroid hormone; in patients with diabetes insipidus, this may aggravate the symptoms of polyuria and polydipsia. The mechanisms resulting in increased urinary volume include (1) increased solute "load" (especially nitrogenous products, sodium, and chloride) resulting from a general increase in metabolic activity and increased food intake, and (2) increased glomerular filtration rate.

Angiotensin.   The importance of angiotensin in regulating electrolyte excretion has only recently been appreciated. Through its effect on aldosterone secretion, angiotensin promotes sodium conservation. In addition, however, angiotensin has direct effects on renal function that are not mediated by the adrenal cortex. When administered in small doses to normal subjects or to patients with Addison's disease, angiotensin causes decreases in glomerular filtration rate, sodium excretion, and urinary volume. When it is administered in much larger doses to patients with cirrhosis and ascites or to certain patients with essential hypertension, angiotensin can cause an increase in sodium and water excretion, presumably by inhibiting tubular reabsorption of these substances.

Prostaglandins.   Both prostaglandins A and E have been isolated from renal medulla (see Ch. 15) When infused into human beings, they promote salt and water excretion and a lowering of blood pressure in some hypertensive subjects. Urinary volume, sodium excretion, free water clearance, and renal plasma flow are increased by infusion of prostaglandin E_1 directly into one renal artery of anesthetized dogs. The increase in free water clearance is not prevented by concomitant administration of vasopressin. This finding is consistent with the effect of prostaglandin E_1 in blocking the osmotic water flow response to low concentration of vasopressin in the isolated collecting tubule and in toad bladder. The actions of prostaglandin on sodium and water transport are associated with changes in adenyl cyclase activity and cyclic AMP content of responsive tissues.

Vitamin D.   This vitamin, which shows increasingly the attributes of a hormone, also has been found to have modest direct effects on the renal tubular reabsorptive processes. Both cholecalciferol and 25-hydroxycholecalciferol depressed sodium excretion as well as that of calcium and phosphate. The effects on phosphate were antagonized by parathyroid hormone.

HOMEOSTASIS IN FLUID AND ELECTROLYTE METABOLISM

Since the water and electrolyte composition of the body remains relatively constant in the face of extreme variations in external circumstances, it is obvious that mechanisms must exist for conservation of these materials when in deficit and their rapid excretion when in excess.

Expansion of the extracellular fluid compartment as a result of high sodium intake or the action of sodium-retaining steroids leads to suppression of renin, angiotensin, and aldosterone production and increased glomerular filtration. These processes facilitate sodium excretion. Depletion of extracellular fluid resulting from restricted sodium intake and renal or extrarenal losses of sodium leads to increased renin, angiotensin, and aldosterone production and decreased glomerular filtration. These processes tend to prevent further loss of sodium in the urine.

If water loss exceeds water intake, the resulting increase in osmolality of body fluids stimulates secretion of antidiuretic hormone. At the same time, a decrease in fluid volume leads to a decrease in glomerular filtration. Increased antidiuretic hormone and pronounced decreases in glomerular filtration both result in conservation of free water. On the other hand, a "positive water balance" results in decreased osmolality, which suppresses the secretion of antidiuretic hormone. Concurrently, expansion of fluid compartments leads to an increase in glomerular filtration. Diminution of ADH and increased GFR both facilitate excretion of free water.

Extreme abnormalities of potassium concentration in body fluids are potentially life threatening, and it is not surprising, therefore, that compensatory mechanisms exist which adjust the body content of this ion with considerable precision. High serum potassium levels tend to stimulate aldosterone secretion, and aldosterone accelerates the excretion of potassium by the kidneys. Depletion of body potassium tends to suppress aldosterone secretion, thus facilitating renal conservation of potassium. Other nonhormonal mechanisms are also of importance in regulating potassium excretion.

REFERENCES

Agus, Z. S., Puschett, J. B., et al.: Mode of action of parathyroid hormone and cyclic adenosine 3',5'-monophosphate on renal tubular phosphate reabsorption in the dog. *J. Clin. Invest.* 50:617, 1971.

Bartter, F. C.: The role of aldosterone in normal homeostasis and in certain disease states. *Metabolism* 5:369, 1956.

Baulieu, E. E., and Robel, P.: *Aldosterone. A Symposium.* Oxford, Blackwell Scientific Publications, 1964.

Baumann, E. J., and Kurland, S.: Changes in the inorganic constituents of blood in suprarenalectomized cats and rabbits. *J. Biol. Chem.* 71:281, 1926.

Berliner, R. W., Levinsky, N. G., et al.: Dilution and concentration of the urine and the action of antidiuretic hormone. *Amer. J. Med.* 24:730, 1958.

Bijvoet, O. L. M., Veer, J., et al.: Natriuretic effect of calcitonin in man. *New Eng. J. Med.* 284:681, 1971.

Blizzard, R. M., Liddle, G. W., et al.: Aldosterone excretion in virilizing adrenal hyperplasia. *J. Clin. Invest.* 38:1442, 1959.

Brown, J. J., Davies, D. L., et al.: Influence of sodium deprivation and loading on the plasma-renin in man. *J. Physiol.* (London) 173:408, 1964.

Conn, J. W., Fajans, S. S., et al.: Metabolic and clinical effects of corticosterone (compound B) in man, In *Proceedings of the Second ACTH Clinical Conference.* Vol. 1. Mote, J. R. (ed.), New York, Blakiston Co., 1951, p. 221.

Conn, J. W.: Primary aldosteronism, a new clinical syndrome. *J. Lab. Clin. Med.* 45:3, 1955.

Coppage, W. S., Island, D., et al.: Inhibition of aldosterone secretion and modification of electrolyte excretion in man by a chemical inhibitor of 11β-hydroxylation. *J. Clin. Invest.* 38:2101, 1959.

Davis, J. O.: Mechanisms of salt and water retention in congestive heart failure; the importance of aldosterone. *Amer. J. Med.* 29:486, 1960.

Davis, J. O., et al.: The role of the renin-angiotensin system in the control of aldosterone secretion. *J. Clin. Invest.* 41:378, 1962.

Duncan, L. E., Liddle, G. W., et al.: The effect of changes in body sodium on extracellular fluid volume and aldosterone and sodium excretion by normal edematous men. *J. Clin. Invest.* 35:1299, 1956.

Genest, J.: Angiotensin, aldosterone and human arterial hypertension. *Canad. Med. Ass. J.* 84:403, 1961.

Grantham, J. J., and Orloff, J.: Effect of prostaglandin E₁ on the permeability response of the isolated collecting tubule to vasopressin, adenosine 3',5'-monophosphate and theophylline. *J. Clin. Invest.* 47:1154, 1968.

Gross, F., Brunner, H., et al.: Renin-angiotensin system, aldosterone, and sodium balance. *Recent Progr. Hormone Res.* 21:119, 1965.

Haas, H. G., Dambacher, J. G., et al.: Renal effects of calcitonin and parathyroid extract in man. *J. Clin. Invest.* 50:2689, 1971.

Handler, J. S., Bensinger, R., et al.: Effect of adrenergic agents on toad bladder response to ADH, 3',5'-AMP, and theophylline. *Amer. J. Physiol.* 215:1024, 1968.

Henneman, P. H., et al.: Effects of human growth hormone in man. *J. Clin. Invest.* 39:1223, 1960.

Kagawa, C. M., Sturtevant, F. M., et al.: Pharmacology of a new steroid that blocks salt activity of aldosterone and desoxycorticosterone. *J. Pharmacol. Exp. Ther.* 126:123, 1959.

Kleeman, C. R., Czaczkes, J. W., et al.: Mechanisms of impaired water excretion in adrenal and pituitary insufficiency. IV. Antidiuretic hormone in primary and secondary adrenal insufficiency. *J. Clin. Invest.* 43:1641, 1964.

Klein, L. A., Liberman, B., et al.: Interrelated effects of antidiuretic hormone and adrenergic drugs on water metabolism. *Amer. J. Physiol.* 221:1657, 1971.

Landau, R. L., and Lugibihl, K.: Inhibition of the sodium-retaining influence of aldosterone by progesterone. *J. Clin. Endocr.* 18:1237, 1958.

Langford, H. G.: Tubular action of angiotensin. *Canad. Med. Ass. J.* 90:332, 1964.

Liddle, G. W.: Effects of anti-inflammatory steroids on electrolyte metabolism. *Ann. N. Y. Acad. Sci.* 82:854, 1959.

Liddle, G. W.: Aldosterone antagonists. *Arch. Intern. Med.* (Chicago) 102:998, 1958.

Liddle, G. W., Duncan, L. E., et al.: Dual mechanism regulating adrenocortical function in man. *Amer. J. Med.* 21:380, 1956.

Lieberman, A. H., and Luetscher, J. A.: Some effects of abnormalities of pituitary, adrenal, or thyroid function on excretion of aldosterone and the response to corticotropin or sodium deprivation. *J. Clin. Endocr.* 20:1004, 1960.

Luetscher, J. A.: Studies of aldosterone in relation to water and electrolyte balance in man. *Recent Progr. Hormone Res.* 12:175, 1956.

Manitius, A., Levitin, H., et al.: On the mechanism of impairment of renal concentrating ability in potassium deficiency. *J. Clin. Invest.* 39:684, 1960.

Manitius, A., Levitin, H., et al.: On the mechanism of impairment of renal concentrating ability in hypercalcemia. *J. Clin. Invest.* 39:693, 1960.

Michael, U. F., Barenberg, R. L., et al.: Renal handling of sodium and water in the hypothyroid rat. *J. Clin. Invest.* 51:1405, 1972.

Muldowney, E. P., Carroll, D. V., et al.: Correction of renal bicarbonate wastage by parathyroidectomy. *Quart. J. Med.* 40:487, 1971.

Oliver, J., et al.: The renal lesions of electrolyte imbalance. I. The structural alterations in potassium-depleted rats. *J. Exp. Med.* 106:563, 1957.

Orloff, J., and Handler, J. S.: The cellular mode of action of antidiuretic hormone. *Amer. J. Med.* 36:686, 1964.

Porter, G. A., Bogoroch, R., et al.: On the mechanism of action of aldosterone on sodium transport: the role of RNA synthesis. *Proc. Nat. Acad. Sci.* USA *52*:1326, 1964.

Porter, G. A., and Edelman, I. S.: The action of aldosterone and related corticosteroids on sodium transport across the toad bladder. *J. Clin. Invest. 43*:611, 1964.

Puschett, J. B., Moranz, J., et al.: Evidence for a direct action of cholecalciferol and 25-hydroxycholecalciferol on the renal transport of phosphate, sodium and calcium. *J. Clin. Invest. 51*:373, 1972.

Relman, A. S., and Schwartz, W. B.: The kidney in potassium depletion. *Amer. J. Med. 24*:764, 1958.

Sartorius, O. W., Calhoon, D., and Pitts, R. F.: The capacity of the adrenalectomized rat to secrete hydrogen and ammonium ions. *Endocrinology 51*:444, 1952.

Sawyer, W. H., Munsick, R. A., et al.: Antidiuretic hormones. *Circulation 21*:1027, 1960.

Schrier, R. W., Lieberman, R., et al.: Mechanism of antidiuretic effect of beta adrenergic stimulation. *J. Clin. Invest. 51*:97, 1972.

Sharp, G. W. G., and Leaf, A.: Biological action of aldosterone *in vitro. Nature* (London) *202*:1185, 1964.

Sharp, G. W. G., and Leaf, A.: The mechanism of action of aldosterone. *Physiol. Rev. 46*:593, 1966.

Thorn, G. W., et al.: Clinical and metabolic changes in Addison's disease following the administration of compound E acetate (11-dehydro, 17-hydroxycorticosterone acetate). *Trans. Ass. Amer. Physicians 62*:233, 1949.

Ufferman, R. C., and Schrier, R. W.: Importance of sodium intake and mineralocorticoid hormone in the impaired water excretion in adrenal insufficiency. *J. Clin. Invest. 51*:1639, 1972.

Weston, R. E., et al.: Homeostatic regulation of body fluid volume in nonedematous subjects. *Metabolism 9*:157, 1960.

Wolff, H. P., Koczorek, K. R., et al.: Endocrine factors. *J. Chronic Dis. 9*:554, 1959.

CHAPTER 20

The Renin-Aldosterone Axis and Blood Pressure and Electrolyte Homeostasis

By John H. Laragh

The interrelationships of a group of hormones, now recognized as the renin-angiotensin-aldosterone system, have only recently been exposed. Angiotensin and aldosterone were studied separately until 1960, when a direct relationship between the activity of these renal and adrenal hormones was established with the discovery by Laragh and associates that angiotensin infusion selectively stimulates aldosterone secretion in normal man. Since then the role of this interaction in electrolyte and blood pressure homeostasis has been increasingly appreciated.

The renin-angiotensin-aldosterone system seems to have been organized primarily for the simultaneous regulation of the interrelated functions of sodium and potassium balance and blood pressure-volume homeostasis. This humoral system is a major, but certainly not the sole, regulator of these vital homeostatic functions, and its activity is coordinated with those of other neurovascular, humoral, and local cellular mechanisms.

THE SYSTEM DESCRIBED

The renin-angiotensin-aldosterone system regulates sodium balance, fluid volume, and blood pressure as follows (Fig. 20–1): when, as the result of such events as hemorrhage, sodium depletion, fluid transudation, or alimentary loss, effective blood volume contracts and arterial pressure falls, the kidney's perfusion is reduced, and it secretes renin into the blood stream. Renin, acting enzymatically, hydrolyzes a plasma globulin to release angiotensin I, which is then rapidly hydrolyzed to angiotensin II by pulmonary and plasma-converting enzymes. Angiotensin II, in addition to its pressor action, stimulates aldosterone secretion. Aldosterone acts on the kidney distal tubules to cause sodium retention. This positive sodium balance leads to a secondary retention of water and expansion of the extracellular fluids. Thus angiotensin and aldosterone together act to raise the blood pressure and restore renal perfusion, thereby compensating the system and shutting off the initial signal to renal renin release.

Arterial blood pressure is additionally supported by a coordinated interaction between plasma angiotensin levels and available sodium ions. Since induced sodium retention enhances and sodium depletion diminishes the pressor activity of angiotensin, the product of these two factors determines vascular tone.

Simultaneously, the renin-angiotensin system regulates potassium homeostasis. This activity tends to stabilize plasma potassium levels and avoids dangerous hyperkalemia which may develop in patients with adrenal insufficiency after a meal of high potassium content. Increases in plasma potassium levels act directly on the adrenal cortex to stimulate aldosterone release. Aldosterone acts to promote K^+ loss, at the same time

B.P. = VASOCONSTRICTION X VOLUME
(angio)   (aldo)(Na)

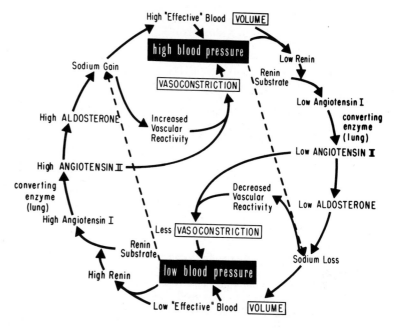

Figure 20–1. The renin-angiotensin-aldosterone system and sodium-volume-blood pressure homeostasis.

stimulating Na^+ reabsorption by the Na^+–K^+ ion exchange transport system. As the plasma potassium level falls, aldosterone secretion is accordingly reduced. At the same time, increases in plasma potassium act directly on the kidney to inhibit renin release, whereas hypokalemia is a potent stimulus for renin secretion. Thus renal conservation or elimination of potassium ions is closely related to opposite changes in both renin and aldosterone secretion.

The ultimate signal(s) inducing renin release has not yet been identified, but it appears to involve (1) a pressure- or stretch-sensitive receptor in the renal afferent arterioles, (2) a distal tubular macula densa receptor responsive to changes in sodium supply, (3) changes in autonomic nerve activity, and (4) changes in potassium balance. Additionally, increases in plasma angiotensin levels may "feed back" to retard further renin secretion, and humoral agents may be involved in the mediation (Table 20–1).

TABLE 20–1.   MECHANISMS FOR RENIN SECRETION

Renal Receptors
   Afferent arteriolar barostat
   Macula densa natriastat
Other Mediators
   Nervous system and catecholamines
   Plasma potassium level
   Plasma angiotensin II feedback suppression
   Other humoral agents:
     Vasopressin
     Cyclic AMP
     Prostaglandin
     Renin-stimulating hormone?

The renin-angiotensin-aldosterone system has two effector hormones: angiotensin II and aldosterone.

Angiotensin II is an octapeptide with three striking physiologic actions: (1) in constricting the arterioles, it is by weight the most potent pressor substance known; (2) it acts directly on the kidney to cause sodium retention with lower dosages and natriuresis with larger amounts; and (3) it acts on the adrenal cortex to evoke a prompt and sustained increase in aldosterone secretion. The concentration of angiotensin II in human venous plasma normally ranges from 1 to 10 ng. per 100 ml.

Aldosterone, the second effector hormone of the system, is an adrenal corticosteroid, unique because of its 18-aldehyde configuration. It acts primarily on the renal tubules to increase the reabsorption of sodium chloride and to promote the elimination of potassium ions. Like angiotensin II, aldosterone is present in relatively minute amounts. In blood, its level is approximately .0001 of that of cortisol. In man, it ranges from 1 to 10 pg. per ml. in venous plasma.

In this system, both the renin substrate and the converting enzymes are ordinarily present in sufficient amounts so that their concentrations are not physiologically rate-limiting for the formation of angiotensin II. Therefore, a relatively small change in the concentration of renin in plasma is usually the major determinant of the final concentration of circulating angiotensin II. By changing the plasma concentrations of the effector components, angiotensin II and aldosterone, this hormonal interaction simultaneously regulates (1) body sodium and water content and thus hydrostatic pressures, (2) arterial blood pressure, and (3) potassium balance.

ABNORMALITIES OF ALDOSTERONE AND RENIN SECRETION IN MAN

Major Categories of Disease Involving Oversecretion of Aldosterone

In man, increased secretion of aldosterone may participate in the pathogenesis of (1) disorders characterized chiefly by potassium wastage, (2) conditions in which there is progressive sodium retention and edema formation, and (3) states characterized mainly by arterial hypertension. The major naturally occurring disorders that involve pathologic oversecretion of aldosterone are summarized in Table 20–2. They are divided into two main groups, primary and secondary aldosteronism.

Primary Aldosteronism

The term "primary" means that the oversecretion arises from an autonomous aldosterone-secreting adrenal cortical adenoma. The resulting disease is the expression of increased aldosterone secretion in an otherwise healthy patient. The characteristic abnormalities—potassium wastage, polyuria, muscle weakness, hypokalemic alkalosis, and mild arterial hypertension—are entirely corrected by the removal of the offending adenoma.

Pseudoprimary Aldosteronism

A significant fraction of patients with the clinical syndrome of primary aldosteronism are found at laparotomy to exhibit bilateral adrenal hyperplasia instead of an isolated adenoma. Patients with such hyperplasia appear to have a different pathophysiologic basis for adrenal overactivity, one perhaps involving an extra-adrenal humoral stimulus to both glands. Unlike patients with primary aldosteronism, they are usually not cured of hypertension by adrenal surgery. The condition has therefore been tentatively called pseudoprimary aldosteronism.

Secondary Aldosteronism

Secondary aldosteronism may be defined as increased aldosterone secretion due to stimulation of the adrenal glands from sources extraneous to them. Discrete adrenal tumors are absent, and the oversecretion is the result of bilateral adrenal cortical hyperfunction. In secondary aldosteronism, the oversecretion is usually associated with and seems to be a consequence of other major disturbances, such as nephrosis, cirrhosis, or heart failure. Increased aldosterone secretion also occurs in various forms of hypertensive vascular disease, and for reasons presented below, this too may be considered a form of secondary aldosteronism.

Oversecretion of Aldosterone in Edematous States. Since the report of Deming and Leutscher, it has become generally recognized that patients with nephrosis, cirrhosis, or heart failure excrete increased amounts of urinary aldosterone while becoming edematous.

We have observed marked adrenal cortical hypersecretion of aldosterone in these edematous states, especially in nephrosis and cirrhosis. In general, the values observed in heart failure were considerably lower than those observed in cirrhosis or nephrosis, and in the case of advanced right-sided heart failure, the aldosterone secretion rates were sometimes not significantly increased at all. Furthermore, there was a paradoxical response pattern in heart failure. Sodium administration, which may further embarrass the circulation, induces more, not less, aldosterone secretion; diuretic therapy, which consistently increases aldosterone secretion in normal subjects, may lower it in heart failure, presumably because the sodium diuresis allows cardiac performance to improve. In contrast, hypersecretion of aldosterone in nephrosis and cirrhosis is usually unaffected by changes in dietary salt.

These observations suggest that hemodynamic factors per se may be more important than hormonal factors in the edema of congestive heart failure, whereas hormonal factors appear to predominate in the pathogenesis of the edema of nephrosis and cirrhosis. Furthermore, these findings perhaps suggest a fundamental difference in the nature of the stimulus for aldosterone secretion under these conditions. All of these disorders are characterized by a tendency for fluid to transude out from the vascular bed, but there are differences in distribution. In heart failure, total blood volume is increased, and there is a generalized increase in venous back pressure. However, in cirrhosis and nephrosis, the effective blood volume and the oncotic pressure may be greatly reduced. Furthermore, central venous pressure is not elevated in cirrhosis or nephrosis. With more study, it may be possible to show how certain of these altered circulatory dynamics are critically involved in eliciting increased aldosterone secretion as part of a homeostatic response.

Aldosterone Secretion in Malignant Hypertension. The physiologic derangements observed in the syndrome of malignant hypertension are of

TABLE 20–2.　OVERSECRETION OF ALDOSTERONE

I. Adrenal in origin
  (a) Primary aldosteronism due to adenoma
  (b) Pseudoprimary aldosteronism (bilateral adrenal hyperplasia)
II. Secondary aldosteronism (from extra-adrenal stimulation)
  (a) Edematous states:
    1. Cirrhosis
    2. Nephrosis
    3. Heart failure
  (b) Hypertensive states:
    1. Malignant hypertension
    2. Malignant or severe hypertension due to unilateral renal disease
  (c) Alkalotic normotensive states:
    1. Juxtaglomerular cell hyperplasia with potassium wastage and retarded growth

special interest to this discussion because an analysis of this problem led to an understanding of the renin-angiotensin-aldosterone system and its involvement in other disorders.

An early study revealed that, unlike in other forms of hypertension, aldosterone secretion was consistently and strikingly elevated in malignant hypertension. This syndrome is expressed clinically by neuroretinopathy, severe accelerating hypertension, and evidence of advancing renal disease, and pathologically by necrotizing arteriolitis. The hyperaldosteronism of malignant hypertension is usually accompanied by hypokalemic alkalosis, probably the result of aldosterone excess acting on the kidney. This pattern is still apparent even when renal failure has developed.

The hyperaldosteronism that accompanies malignant hypertension, unlike primary aldosteronism, is in most cases not related to the presence of an adrenal tumor. Therefore, it seemed important to establish the extra-adrenal stimulus that might elevate aldosterone secretion in malignant hypertension. Since patients with malignant nephrosclerosis have a tendency to hypokalemic alkalosis, aldosterone stimulation cannot be attributed to increased plasma potassium. In fact, it has been possible to effect further increases in aldosterone secretion by rectifying plasma potassium values. None of the hemodynamic faults, such as those observed in edematous states that might elevate aldosterone, is associated with this disorder. All of these considerations led our group to suspect that in these patients there was another stimulus to the adrenals, probably arising in the kidneys, which are the major site of pathologic change. The studies that defined this renal-adrenal relationship are discussed below.

Renal Juxtaglomerular Cell Hyperplasia (Bartter's Syndrome). Renal juxtaglomerular cell hyperplasia is a very rare disorder described by Bartter and his associates in 1962. It is characterized clinically by chronic renal potassium wastage, hypokalemic alkalosis, and retarded growth and development. Hyperplasia of the renal juxtaglomerular cells occurs but is associated with normotension and the absence of edema. Marked oversecretion of aldosterone occurs in this disorder and is accompanied by marked hypersecretion of renin.

The pathophysiology has been the subject of some debate. Bartter himself proposed that the primary defect might be an unresponsiveness of the arterioles to angiotensin, leading to hypersecretion of renin and aldosterone and chronic kaliuresis. We have suggested as an alternative that the syndrome can be an expression of renal injury or disease, with a sodium-losing tubular lesion inducing the hyper-reninemia, hyperaldosteronism, and K+ wastage. It is possible that either one or the other of these mechanisms applies in patients with the syndrome. It is certainly true too that other forms of sodium-losing renal diseases can be associated with compensatory increases in renin and aldosterone secretion without elevating the blood pressure.

Physiologic Relationships Leading to Definition of the Renal-Adrenal Axis

Angiotensin as a Potent Stimulus to Aldosterone Secretion in Man

The elevated blood pressure and renal involvement that characterize malignant nephrosclerosis led us to suspect a renal pressor substance as the appropriate stimulus for the observed marked increases in aldosterone secretion. Our opinion was reinforced by the fact that both the malignant hypertensive state and the aldosteronism of unilateral renal disease could be rectified by removal of the offending kidney. Therefore, we investigated the effects of intravenous infusions of the renal pressor peptide angiotensin and were able to demonstrate that this peptide consistently increases aldosterone secretion in normal subjects. These studies further demonstrated that the stimulation is a specific process that cannot be duplicated by other pressor agents. Furthermore, stimulation occurs without an accompanying increase in adrenal cortisol secretion, and it persists for as long as the angiotensin infusion is applied. Maximum stimulation occurs using doses of angiotensin which are only mildly pressor. Because this stimulation is persistent and selective, angiotensin fulfills the requirements of a tropic hormone for the secretion of aldosterone.

The Renal-Adrenal Hormonal System: Its Relation to Malignant Hypertension and to Other Forms of Primary and Secondary Aldosteronism

Our results permitted proposal of a renal-adrenal interaction for normal control of sodium balance, a derangement of which appears to be involved in the pathogenesis of malignant hypertension. Thus, in malignant hypertension, the kidney appears to have developed a critical degree of damage. When this critical renal damage develops, a sequence is set in motion: renin, secreted into the blood stream in excessive amounts, interacts with the circulating renin substrate to release more angiotensin II; angiotensin II, in addition to raising blood pressure inappropriately by constricting arterioles, also stimulates excessive secretion of aldosterone by the adrenal cortex.

In normal subjects, a feedback loop is closed as aldosterone induces sodium retention and volume expansion and the increased renin secretion ceases. However, in malignant hypertension, because of kidney damage, a vicious cycle develops. The induced aldosteronism cannot turn off the renin secretion, perhaps partly because it cannot induce appropriate sodium retention in the damaged target organ, kidney. A situation results in which there is too much angiotensin and too much aldosterone in the blood at the same time, leading to more renal and vascular damage. We believe that this vicious cycle is crucial to the pathogenesis of the malignant hypertension syndrome.

Indeed, experiments have shown that the simultaneous administration of large doses of angiotensin and aldosterone produces the necrotizing vasculitis so characteristic of malignant hypertension. Neither agent alone has had this effect. Moreover, in man, total nephrectomy can reverse malignant vasculitis.

Conversely, the benign nature of primary aldosteronism may be attributed to the absence of renin and angiotensin. Thus aldosterone, secreted autonomously in the absence of renal damage, would suppress renal release of renin and prevent the initiation of the vicious cycle that seems to occur in malignant hypertension.

If this is the sequence of events in malignant hypertension, it would seem that oversecretion of aldosterone in this disorder, although not necessarily related to its initiation, is an appropriate consequence of renal damage and contributes to its pathogenesis.

Other studies indicate that the normotensive forms of secondary aldosteronism, in which renin and angiotensin are also presumably increased, are not necessarily accompanied by vascular damage. The secondary aldosteronism in cirrhosis of the liver is a case in point. This disorder is accompanied by the overall abnormal ion distribution usual in edema. Despite the avid renal retention of sodium, cirrhosis is not accompanied by high blood pressure. Patients with cirrhosis also have extremely reduced pressor responses to infusions of angiotensin and, in fact, may rapidly develop tachyphylaxis to pressor effects of drugs. The notable tendency for displacement of sodium and water out of the vascular tree in edematous states may account for the absence of hypertension and of vascular damage in the presence of excess aldosterone and angiotensin.

Human Disorders of Renin Secretion: A Physiologic Classification of Hyperaldosteronism

The studies cited above, indicating that renin, via the generation of angiotensin II, is a potent stimulus for eliciting increased aldosterone secretion, make possible reclassification of most of the naturally occurring disorders or physiologic derangements involving increased aldosterone secretion (see Tables 20–3 and 20–4). That practically all of these disorders can be classified by relating them to associated abnormalities in plasma renin activity provides strong additional, albeit circumstantial, evidence in support of the idea that renin and angiotensin do, in fact, constitute the major hormonal control system involved in regulating the secretion of aldosterone. Indeed, there are to date very few naturally occurring examples of either physiologic or pathologic hypersecretion of aldosterone that cannot be explained and analyzed

TABLE 20–3. DISORDERS WITH SUPPRESSED PLASMA RENIN ACTIVITY

With Adrenal Cortical Disease
(a) Hypertensive states:
    1. Primary aldosteronism (discrete, usually single, adrenal adenoma)
    2. Pseudoprimary or idiopathic aldosteronism (usually bilateral adrenal cortical hyperplasia)
    3. Glucocorticoid-suppressible aldosteronism
    4. Adrenal carcinoma with mineralocorticoid excess
    5. Adrenal enzyme defects with oversecretion of other mineralocorticoids

Without Adrenal Cortical Disease
(a) Hypertensive states:
    1. Low-renin essential hypertension
    2. Certain patients with renal parenchymal diseases
    3. Liddle's syndrome
    4. Licorice or mineralocorticoid ingestion
(b) Normotensive states:
    1. Renal parenchymal diseases
    2. Autonomic disorders with postural hypotension
    3. Uninephrectomized subjects
    4. Drug-induced adrenergic blockers

in terms of theoretically appropriate abnormalities in plasma renin activity.

This relationship is particularly useful in distinguishing primary from secondary forms of aldosteronism because, characteristically, primary aldosteronism due to an oversecreting autonomous adenoma or pseudoprimary aldosteronism due to diffuse and adrenal cortical hyperplasia are both associated with suppression of renal renin secretion to subnormal levels. Except for these two conditions and some other even more unusual adrenal gland disorders, all other instances of hyperaldosteronism that have been identified in man can be associated with a prior increase in renal renin secretion, with hyperangiotensinemia appearing

TABLE 20–4. DISORDERS WITH INCREASED PLASMA RENIN ACTIVITY

With Consequent Secondary Aldosteronism
(a) Hypertensive states:
    1. Malignant or severe hypertension
    2. Unilateral renal disease with malignant or severe hypertension
    3. High-renin forms of essential hypertension
    4. Renal parenchymal diseases
    5. Renin-secreting tumors
    6. Oral contraceptive–induced hypertension
(b) Edematous normotensive states:
    1. Cirrhosis
    2. Nephrosis
    3. Congestive heart failure
(c) Hypokalemic normotensive states:
    1. Juxtaglomerular cell hyperplasia (Bartter's syndrome)
    2. Other nephropathies with sodium or potassium wastage
    3. Alimentary disorders with electrolyte loss
(d) Physiologic:
    1. Dietary sodium depletion
    2. Diuretic usage, laxative abuse
    3. Reduced effective blood volume states (hemorrhage, dehydration, upright posture)

Without Consequent Secondary Aldosteronism
(a) Adrenal cortical insufficiency
(b) Potassium depletion states (alimentary)

to be the direct stimulus to the adrenal for aldosterone oversecretion.

Perhaps surprisingly, practically all observed instances of abnormally suppressed plasma renin activity in man have been associated with some degree of high blood pressure. The only exceptions to this are certain normotensive patients with renal disease. Moreover, such suppression of plasma renin levels is not necessarily associated with any demonstrable adrenal cortical dysfunction, as evidenced by the fact that many, perhaps 30 per cent, of all patients with common essential hypertension exhibit suppressed plasma renin levels.

According to the proposed renin-adrenal hormonal interaction, the lowest plasma renin levels of all would be expected in response to primary excessive adrenal secretion of mineralocorticoid hormones. Similarly, the highest levels of plasma renin might be expected to occur with failure of adrenal cortical function, as in Addison's disease or after total adrenalectomy. In these cases, the feedback loop cannot be closed by an adrenal cortical response, and the initial signal for renin release persists and escalates. The same picture, a high renin and low aldosterone pattern, may result from potassium depletion. Potassium is as effective as angiotensin itself in stimulating aldosterone secretion. Its deficit has been shown to retard normal adrenal cortical capacity for aldosterone production, and it also affects the kidney in such a way as to stimulate renin secretion.

Table 20–3 shows that, among naturally occurring situations associated with increased plasma renin levels, there are two main types of disorders. The first seems to have as a common mechanism either some compromise of, or deficit in, the so-called "effective" blood volume (total extracellular fluid volume or sodium space), or else this type of disorder is associated with a fall in arterial blood pressure or filling capacity. The second type of stimulus for renin secretion involves certain intrinsic diseases of the kidney. In both mechanisms, the high plasma renin levels can be envisaged as the result of a physiologic response to volume depletion, which can be induced by internal sequestration of blood, hemorrhage, vomiting, diarrhea, diuretics, or various nephropathies. Following the first line of reasoning, the high plasma renin levels found in cirrhosis with ascites or nephrosis result from the sequestration or transudation of fluid out of the circulation, thereby compromising venous return and the normal filling of the renal arterial bed. In congestive heart failure, poor forward pumping of blood and reduced effective blood volume may signal renin release.

As indicated previously, the increased renin secretion of advanced or malignant hypertensive disease can be related to a critical degree of renal damage. Other renal diseases in which tubular dysfunction is reflected in faulty sodium conservation and volume depletion (e.g., renal tubular acidosis, Bartter's syndrome) may also be associated with hyper-reninemia and hyperaldosteronism.

Renin and Aldosterone Secretion in Essential Hypertension

Let us next consider the large problem of patients with benign essential hypertension. In this category, the role of the renal-adrenal axis remains to be fully clarified. A connection between salt metabolism, adrenal cortical activity, and high blood pressure has long been suspected. It has been known, for example, that experimental Goldblatt hypertension can be prevented or corrected by adrenalectomy and that the feeding of salt alone or accompanied by a sodium-retaining steroid can cause hypertension in various species of animal.

The analysis of the relationship of aldosterone and renin secretions to human hypertensive disease poses a particularly difficult problem because patients with essential hypertension may not represent a homogenous etiologic group. Furthermore, the disorder has an insidious onset, and it is often accompanied by occult renal and cardiac complications that, by themselves, might influence the renal-adrenal axis.

Conceptually, it is of fundamental importance to establish whether or not the renal-adrenal axis is abnormal in uncomplicated essential hypertension. Our own earlier measurements indicated that aldosterone secretion and its response to fluctuations in electrolyte balance are most often normal in benign essential hypertension. Other investigators have reported similar findings. In support of these results, it should be noted that these patients are not potassium depleted, a circumstance that may be taken as strong evidence against hyperaldosteronism, because aldosterone excess almost invariably brings about a potassium deficit.

More recently, with the availability of reliable methods for measuring renin and angiotensin, we have investigated the question of whether or not subtle abnormalities in the renin-angiotensin system might be involved in the initiation or pathogenesis of essential hypertension. In a study of 219 patients, simultaneous measurements of plasma renin activity and of aldosterone excretion were related to concurrent daily rates of sodium excretion. The designation of low, normal, or high values for each hormone was made against an index drawn from normal volunteers studied over the same wide and continuous range of sodium balance.

Three major categories of patients with essential hypertension can be identified with respect to plasma renin. Plasma renin activity was subnormal in 27 per cent, normal in 57 per cent, and abnormally increased in 16 per cent of patients. These groups were then further classified with respect to aldosterone excretion to develop a total of eight different categories representing eight different patterns of renin and aldosterone secretion. Thus, with the development of more precise methodology, subtle abnormalities in aldosterone and more flagrant variations in renin have been identified in the population with essential hypertension.

This biochemical "profiling" of hormonal patterns appears to have physiologic relevance. When the observed hormonal patterns were related to the natural history of the disease, it was found that the rate of renin secretion, and also perhaps of aldosterone secretion, was closely related to the risk of heart attack and stroke. Thus none of the 59 patients with low plasma renin suffered a heart attack or stroke, while those with normal or high renin values had significantly greater incidences of these complications. The higher mean age but similar deviation of hypertension of the low-renin group added further weight to the postulate of a protective role for the low-renin condition.

These observations are in keeping with earlier observations on the relationship of excessive renin and aldosterone secretion to the severe vascular disease of malignant hypertension. They suggest that renin and aldosterone secretion may also be involved in a more subtle way in the vascular injury that so often complicates hypertensive disease. Further analysis of these hormonal patterns in essential hypertension promises to define further the nonhomogeneity of this group of patients and may well be useful in understanding causations, forecasting prognosis, and applying specific therapy.

Renin and Aldosterone Secretion in the Hypertension of Renal Disease

Despite many clinical and experimental studies following the description of Goldblatt hypertension in 1934, it is still difficult to assign a causal role to increased renin secretion in this condition, because many reports have described normal or even low circulating plasma renin levels in significant fractions from experimental animals or patients with this disorder, as well as in hypertensive patients with a whole variety of bilateral parenchymal renal diseases.

This dilemma perhaps may be explained by the existence of two different mechanisms for experimental or clinical renal hypertension, only one of which involves an increased renin secretion. A recent study by Brunner and associates supports this idea, which perhaps provides a rational explanation for the clinical problem posed by patients who appear to have renal hypertension but who, nonetheless, fail to exhibit increases in their plasma renin levels.

In this experimental study, two types of renal hypertension were examined in rats. In each type there was partial occlusion of one renal artery by a clamp, but in one type the opposite kidney was removed, and in the second type the opposite kidney was left in place. In the first type, no beneficial effects were observed from administration of either angiotensin antibody or of a specific peptide inhibitor of angiotensin. However, in the second type, hypertension was completely corrected by either of these procedures. The findings, therefore, describe both renin and non-renin–dependent types of experimental renal hypertension.

The reason for these two different types of renal hypertension, which exhibit different contributions of renin, may be related to differences in their states of sodium balance. Other studies have shown that, with unilateral renal artery constriction, the untouched contralateral kidney appeared to become a sodium-wasting kidney, perhaps from exposure to the systemic arterial hypertension.

Taken altogether, these results suggest that, in experimental renal hypertension, as in other situations, blood pressure is determined by the product of plasma renin activity and the state of sodium balance. Accordingly, in the one-kidney model, hypertension results largely from excessive body sodium content, whereas in the two-kidney model, increased plasma renin activity plays a more predominant role. This concept gains considerable support from reports relating the pressor activity of angiotensin to the state of sodium balance in man and from experimental studies demonstrating that the activity of angiotensin receptors is directly related to the state of sodium balance.

It seems likely that there are clinical counterparts of these two pressor mechanisms. Indeed, clinical renal hypertension may present the whole spectrum of possible variation between the two extremes illustrated by the experimental models. Accordingly, in chronic bilateral renal disease with hypertension, both volume-dependent and renin-dependent types are well recognized. In the former, reduction of body sodium by diuretics or by ultrafiltration can restore the blood pressure to normal. In the latter group, total nephrectomy, by reducing inappropriately high renin, will correct the hypertension. Undoubtedly, between these two extremes there are patients with renal hypertension in whom more subtle but inappropriate increases in either body sodium relative to renin or in renin relative to body sodium are operating to cause high blood pressure.

Cybernetics of the Hormonal System in Sodium, Potassium, and Blood Pressure Homeostasis

In the light of information from clinical and experimental studies, the renin-angiotensin-aldosterone mechanism appears to play a major role in the normal regulation of electrolyte balance and arterial blood pressure.

It is perhaps appropriate now to consider in more detail just how the proposed hormonal system might operate to accomplish simultaneously the coordinated control of body sodium and water content, to which is linked potassium balance and arterial blood pressure. In dealing with this question, it is also appropriate to consider to what extent various disorders of electrolyte and fluid balance and of arterial pressure might be explained in terms of disturbance of the hormonal interaction.

In this analysis, it will be assumed for reasons discussed already that (1) angiotensin II is the major tropic hormone for stimulating aldosterone secretion, (2) plasma levels of angiotensin II ordinarily are largely determined by commensurate changes in plasma renin levels, so that, in analyzing the system, changes in plasma renin are a reliable index of changes in angiotensin II, and (3) aldosterone secretion, however, is not solely dependent on angiotensin II and also responds to a similar degree to changes in potassium balance.

There appear to be two loci where perturbations in electrolyte and blood pressure homeostasis are detected and transduced. The adrenal cortex perceives changes in potassium balance, and the kidney is responsive to changes in sodium balance or fluid pressure. Signals so received then induce appropriate changes in the two effector hormones of the system, *angiotensin II* and *aldosterone.* Normally these effectors, in restoring homeostasis, turn off the initial signal.

Sodium-Linked Potassium Homeostasis

The defense of plasma potassium levels within a relatively narrow range, despite wide variations in intake, is one of the most closely guarded homeostatic functions. In this defense, the direct effect of plasma potassium levels on aldosterone secretion can be viewed as part of a system which protects the organism from dangerous hyperkalemia via an aldosterone-induced kaliuresis. Thus, adrenalectomized animals or patients with adrenal insufficiency are prone to hyperkalemia and cardiac arrest after a potassium meal. Conversely, in various states of potassium depletion, the retarding effect of hypokalemia on aldosterone secretion operates to promote renal K$^+$ conservation. Potassium depletion also simultaneously stimulates renal renin secretion and vice versa. However, there is as yet little information about the role of angiotensin II in potassium homeostasis. Perhaps worthy of further study in this regard are the observations that angiotensin natriuresis in normal subjects only occurs when potassium is given concurrently. The maintenance of potassium balance also invokes coordinated changes in renal sodium transport, as will be discussed.

Double-Cycle Feedback for Sodium and Potassium Homeostasis

The data discussed in this chapter provide the basis for a cybernetic scheme for coordinated regulation of sodium and potassium homeostasis. Figure 20–2 in the upper panel describes the "double-cycle feedback" cybernetic system, involving renin (angiotensin) and aldosterone, which simultaneously controls sodium and potassium homeostasis.

The Sodium Cycle. The outer cycle in the figure describes the system for regulation of sodium balance via changes in renin and aldosterone secretion. In this cycle, any stimulus producing sodium or volume depletion activates renal renin

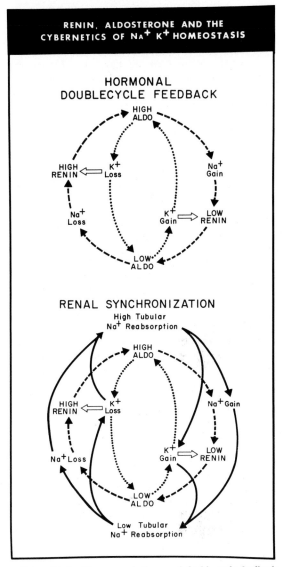

Figure 20–2. *Upper panel,* Hormonal double-cycle feedback system for simultaneous sodium and potassium homeostasis. *Lower panel,* Complementary intrarenal physical factors in renal tubular sodium transport coordinated with dynamic changes in the hormonal system. (From Laragh, J. H., Sealey, J. E., et al.: *Amer. J. Med. 53*:649, 1972.)

secretion, and this, in turn, stimulates aldosterone secretion. Aldosterone then causes sodium retention with attendant hydremia. This effect, by restoring renal perfusion, operates to turn off the original signal for renin secretion and bring the aldosterone secretory rate back to the null point.

The Potassium Cycle. The inner cycle in the figure describes the system which maintains potassium balance. Ingested potassium ions, by raising plasma potassium, stimulate aldosterone secretion. Aldosterone, in turn, by acting on the renal tubules, restores plasma potassium to normal by promoting renal potassium excretion. As potassium levels in the blood fall, aldosterone secretion is again retarded and restored to the null point. Simultaneously, changes in plasma K^+ also produce direct effects on renal renin secretion, so that a rising plasma potassium suppresses renin secretion and vice versa. It should be noted that the concurrently induced changes in plasma renin activity tend to modulate the effects of potassium on the aldosterone secretory mechanism, so that while potassium stimulates aldosterone secretion, this action is dampened by a concurrently induced fall in plasma renin activity. Accordingly, potassium would exert a much greater stimulatory effect on aldosterone secretion if plasma renin levels remained constant.

Intrarenal hemodynamic adjustments support and amplify the activity of these hormones in maintaining both sodium and potassium homeostasis. The effect of these changes in intrarenal physical factors on sodium and potassium balance are illustrated in the lower panel of Figure 20–2. Accordingly, a high sodium intake produces volume expansion, a rise in glomerular filtration rate and in renal blood flow, and changes in intrarenal physical factors, all of which operate to promote renal sodium excretion. These changes also facilitate potassium excretion, because more sodium is delivered to the potassium secretory site in the distal tubule, thereby amplifying the effect of aldosterone and thus increasing potassium excretion. However, potassium wastage is prevented by the high sodium diet–induced fall in aldosterone excretion which concurrently promotes potassium retention and sodium elimination. Completely opposite renal physical effects occur under circumstances of salt and water depletion. This compensatory system is not perfect, since sodium depletion does lead to some potassium retention and very high salt diets might induce K^+ depletion, suggesting that the changes in intrarenal physical factors overcompensate for the hormonal changes.

Deviations in potassium balance can affect renal tubular transport mechanisms either by a direct action or by modifying renal hemodynamic and physical factors. Thus potassium depletion causes increased sodium reabsorption from proximal tubules and resultant decreased sodium delivery to the distal tubule. Clinically, this may cause sodium retention and gross edema even though aldosterone secretion is sharply reduced. Conversely, potassium gain, as can be illustrated by infusing potassium into the renal artery or the peritubular capillaries, can lead to depressed proximal tubular sodium reabsorption, and this may account for the renin-inhibitory action of K^+ consequent to diverting more Na^+ distally to a macula densa natriastat receptor.

Sodium-Linked Blood Pressure Homeostasis

As indicated already, the maintenance of sodium balance, body fluid volumes, and blood pressure constitutes a closely coordinated homeostatic function. Perturbations of this homeostasis from a whole variety of stimuli are initially perceived by the kidney as a fall in arterial pressure or as a reduction in tubular sodium supply, either of which induces renal secretion of renin. This leads to angiotensin II formation and thus to increased aldosterone secretion. The pressor and sodium-retaining effects of these two hormones together operate to restore body fluid volume and renal perfusion, thereby shutting off the initial signal for renin release.

The two effector hormones, angiotensin II and aldosterone, are admirably equipped for these purposes. Thus *angiotensin II* (Fig. 20–1) has three major physiologic actions: (1) it constricts the arterioles to raise arterial pressure, (2) it stimulates adrenal aldosterone secretion, and (3) it acts on the kidney to produce renal sodium retention (not shown in Fig. 20–1). Teleologically, it appears that angiotensin is designed to protect the organism from arterial hypotension or sodium loss or volume contraction. That is to say, it seems to act to maintain tissue perfusion. *Aldosterone* works in concert with angiotensin. It acts primarily on the kidney to increase sodium reabsorption, but it has the additional role of maintaining potassium balance by acting on the kidney to promote potassium secretion. Notwithstanding, before accepting this control system as presented, it is appropriate to consider certain seeming paradoxes in its behavior as they occur in physiologic and pathologic situations.

Participation in Physiologic or Secondary Aldosteronism

In view of the fact that angiotensin II is the most potent pressor substance known, the consistent absence of arterial hypertension in many typical examples of secondary aldosteronism (e.g., sodium depletion, cirrhosis, and nephrosis) requires an explanation. If angiotensinemia does in fact occur in sodium depletion of normal subjects as well as in the edematous states, why is there no accompanying increase in arterial pressure? The answer might possibly reveal a role for angiotensin in essential hypertension and in other hypertensive disorders. Therefore, let us now consider the proposed renin-angiotensin-aldosterone hormonal mechanism in relation to this question.

Dependence of the Vasoactivity of Angiotensin on the State of Sodium Balance

An explanation for the lack of arterial hypertension in states of secondary aldosteronism with presumed angiotensinemia may have been provided by studies of patients with a typical form of secondary hyperaldosteronism, i.e., patients with cirrhosis and ascites, in whom a reduced pressor responsiveness to angiotensin was demonstrated. Such reduced sensitivity was apparent both in acute studies and during infusions lasting several days. The finding seems important because it indicates that increased amounts of angiotensin could circulate and account for hyperaldosteronism without also causing arterial hypertension. This effect could be nonspecific because sodium-depleted subjects (and patients forming edema) are less responsive in general to pressor agents. Indeed, a reduced sensitivity to norepinephrine was actually observed in these patients.

However, other studies have been able to offer a reasonable explanation for clinical examples of both the *increased* and *decreased* sensitivity to angiotensin. These studies involved the prolonged infusion of angiotensin or of norepinephrine into normal subjects, patients with cirrhosis and ascites, and patients with arterial hypertension. Changing pressor sensitivity to angiotensin could be directly related to concurrently induced changes in the state of sodium balance. In normal subjects, as prolonged angiotensin infusion produced progressive sodium retention, pressor sensitivity increased, so that less and less angiotensin was required to maintain the pressor response. In contrast, sodium-depleted normal subjects and cirrhotic subjects exhibited a much reduced sensitivity. Furthermore, in the cirrhotic subjects, in whom it was possible to give even larger doses of angiotensin because of their pressor unresponsiveness, a paradoxical and striking natriuresis occurred, and with this, negative sodium balance pressor sensitivity declined even more. Angiotensin infusions in patients with arterial hypertension also produced natriuresis, and again this negative sodium balance was followed by a declining pressor reactivity to the drug. These studies indicate that angiotensin-induced changes in sodium balance can determine vascular reactivity to the peptide. The experiments further suggest that it was an intravascular accumulation of sodium ions that accounted for the increased sensitivity, because patients with the sodium retention of edema did not exhibit increased sensitivity.

These observations perhaps explain the slowly developing hypertension described in rabbits maintained on initially subpressor infusions of angiotensin, the slowly developing pressor response of rats given renin, the increased pressor response to renin of deoxycorticosterone-treated animals, and the greatly reduced pressor response to angiotensin reported in patients with Addison's disease.

The relationship between angiotensin and available sodium ions may be summarized as follows: (1) in normal subjects, angiotensin causes renal sodium retention and a concomitant *increasing* pressor sensitivity; (2) angiotensin stimulates aldosterone secretion and thus amplifies vascular reactivity by increasing renal sodium retention; (3) however, this sodium-retaining activity of angiotensin appears to have a specific renal feedback component, because with inordinate pressure rises or with larger amounts of exogenous angiotensin, natriuresis (or "escape" from sodium retention) occurs. This natriuresis is greater than that produced by other pressor substances (e.g., norepinephrine), suggesting, in addition, a specific natriuretic action of angiotensin. Taken as a whole,

these results suggest an internally controlled system for the regulation of arterial pressure determined by both the blood level of angiotensin and the available sodium ions. The results suggest that, during angiotensin-induced sodium retention, diminishingly small blood levels of angiotensin can act to induce and maintain arterial hypertension, without at the same time being sufficient to increase aldosterone secretion. On the other hand, in normal subjects completely deprived of sodium and in patients forming edema (i.e., transuding), relatively large amounts of angiotensin are unable to raise the blood pressure.

Altered Vascular Receptor Affinity as a Determinant of the Vasoactivity of Angiotensin

A recent study provides more direct evidence for the existence of specific angiotensin II vascular receptors, changes in the activity of which appear to be a determinant of changes in the vasoactivity of angiotensin, with the resultant changes in sodium balance described above. Receptor affinity, as evaluated by determining the amount of angiotensin antibody required to block the blood pressure response to exogenous angiotensin II, was determined in normotensive rats and in various types of hypertensive rats with low, normal, or high salt intakes. Using the immunologic approach, Brunner and his associates found that the binding affinity of angiotensin receptors for exogenous angiotensin was greatly increased by a high-salt diet in normal animals and that it was also greatly increased in animals with various forms of experimental hypertension. These results provide further evidence that there is an important interrelationship between angiotensin pressor responsiveness and sodium balance. They indicate again that angiotensin could, by induction of this mechanism, participate in the pathogenesis of various types of experimental hypertension, even when circulating levels of the hormone itself are not elevated.

Participation of the Renal-Adrenal System in Hypertensive Diseases

Quite unlike the states of physiologic and secondary aldosteronism, where hypertension is not ordinarily observed, it is clear that, in the appropriate settings, high blood pressure can be a cardinal expression of derangements in the renal-adrenal hormonal system. High blood pressure only seems to result when the circulation remains intact, so that any excess fluid retention due to aldosterone excess is reflected in vascular expansion relative to vascular capacity; a steady state results which is characterized by "escape" or a tendency to rapidly excrete any added fluid. This tendency may be viewed as a pressure natriuresis, in which the central circulation is intolerant of any further distention. In the edematous states, on the other hand, fluid increments "leak" rapidly from the central circulation, so that similar vascular-bed filling relative to its capacity does not occur, and the blood pressure remains normal or low. Accordingly, in the edematous states, decompression of the circulation occurs via transudation which precludes a blood-pressure rise, whereas in hypertensive states, the kidney is the run-off site, resisting further increased arterial pressure by natriuresis.

It is apparent from these considerations that hypertension can result either (1) when the vascular bed is overfilled from a fluid surfeit, or (2) when the vascular bed is inappropriately vasoconstricted relative to the available fluid volume. If this reasoning, invoking two interrelated factors, is correct, one might predict that, in extreme situations, there could occur two forms of chronic hypertension, one which would be entirely due to volume excess, and the other almost entirely related to excessive vasoconstriction (i.e., to excessive pressor activity).

Thus: BP = volume × vasoconstriction

or   BP = (aldosterone) (Na$^+$) × (angiotensin II)

Using this hypothesis, blood pressure is determined by the product of a volume factor and a vasotonic or pressor factor (both of which can be determined by the renal-adrenal hormone axis). In this relationship, the vasoconstrictor component is amplified or dampened by concurrent changes in sodium balance, as described above.

For simplicity, in this analysis we shall assume normal cardiac performance, so that the heart has not yet "failed" from any volume or resistance overload. Admittedly, changes in cardiac performance could modify the blood pressure level determined by the other two components. Notwithstanding, let us now consider to what extent various forms of hypertensive disease might be explained in terms of volume and vasoconstrictor factors.

"Volume" Hypertension. This term describes that extreme in which hypertension seems to be largely due to, or associated with, a maintained excess of sodium and water. In terms of the equation given above, vasoconstrictor activity (i.e., angiotensin II) is minimal or absent in this state. Thus plasma renin activity measurements approach zero. The "volume" factor is maximally excessive because of either (a) excess dietary salt (experimental salt hypertension); (b) excess mineralocorticoid with adequate dietary salt, as in experimental mineralocorticoid hypertension and in primary aldosteronism in man; or (c) inability to excrete dietary salt, as in certain forms of chronic renal disease and in nephrectomized man. Physiologically, this type of hypertension would be characterized by minimal vasoconstrictor activity (low plasma renin), dilated and distended arterioles, high plasma and extracellular fluid volumes, and a low blood viscosity and hematocrit. In patients with mineralocorticoid excess, hypokalemia and alkalosis would also be apparent. In all these patients, hypernatriuresis of administered saline would be a prominent feature unless masked by renal dysfunction.

This form of hypertension can be controlled by volume depletion with measures such as a low-salt diet, diuretic therapy, or vigorous ultrafiltration using a hemodialyzer. In patients with mineralocorticoid excess, appropriate adrenal surgery or pharmacologic blockade provides an additional specific corrective measure.

"Vasoconstrictor" Hypertension. This term refers to hypertensive disorders in which arteriolar vasoconstriction is the predominant factor. In terms of the present discussion, it is defined simply as a physiologic excess of renin and angiotensin II. (Theoretically, increased autonomic nervous activity or excess norepinephrine should produce an extremely similar picture. In fact, norepinephrine and angiotensin II may synergize or amplify each other, and they may act, at least in part, at similar sites.)

This form of hypertension in its fullest expression is exemplified by human malignant hypertension due to either bilateral or unilateral renal disease and by its experimental counterpart, malignant Goldblatt hypertension. In these states, plasma angiotensin II remains markedly elevated. Typically, this is accompanied by secondary aldosteronism and hypokalemia.

Physiologically, this hypertension is characterized by maximal arteriolar vasoconstriction. While one would expect plasma and extracellular fluid volume to be increased because of the aldosteronism, this volume influence is countered by the vasoconstriction and resultant pressure natriuresis of the severe hypertension, so that the "volume" component in this hypertension may be reduced, especially in the extreme forms. Thus the hematocrit and blood viscosity may be high and the plasma volume reduced. However, as in volume hypertension, hypernatriuresis of administered saline is a prominent feature.

This form of hypertension is controlled by measures that neutralize or eliminate the excessive renin secretion. Thus appropriate unilateral or bilateral nephrectomy can produce dramatic reversal of the hypertension. Short of this, drugs which control renin secretion, such as propranolol or alpha-methyldopa, can also be of striking benefit. As one might expect, diuretics are of little value here, and they may even produce adverse effects by further stimulating renin secretion. For the same reason, adrenalectomy may not help. Actually, saline infusion may benefit some of these patients by restoring plasma volume, which would suppress renin and the blood pressure.

Vasoconstrictor and Volume Factors in Renal Hypertension

Let us then consider to what extent blood pressure elevations in renal hypertension might be explained by the product of renin activity and the state of sodium balance, with the latter also acting secondarily to amplify or dampen the activity of angiotensin II, as already described.

In dealing with this problem, it should be appreciated that there are two models of experimental renal hypertension which appear to express the two different mechanisms. Two-kidney hypertension (one renal artery maintained partially constricted and the other untouched) is characterized by a high plasma renin level, volume contraction with sodium wastage from the untouched kidney, and a striking drop in blood pressure with administration of either an angiotensin antibody or antagonist. Thus this form seems to fit the requirements of a vasoconstrictor form of hypertension. On the other hand, one-kidney renal hypertension (one renal artery partially constricted, the other kidney removed) in its established form seems to be largely a "volume" hypertension. Accordingly, the latter is characterized by low or normal plasma renin and no effect on blood pressure of angiotensin antibody administration. Here, because of reduced nephron mass, the volume expansion is probably related to a relative inability to excrete sodium.

In clinical renal hypertension may be found the whole spectrum of possible variation between the two extremes illustrated by the experimental models. Accordingly, in chronic bilateral renal diseases with hypertension, both volume-dependent and renin-dependent types are well recognized. In the former, reduction of body sodium by diuretics or by ultrafiltration can restore the blood pressure to normal. In the latter group, total nephrectomy, by reducing inappropriately high renin, will correct the hypertension. Undoubtedly, between these two extremes there are patients with renal hypertension in whom more subtle but inappropriate increases either in volume relative to renin or in renin relative to volume are operating to cause high blood pressure.

The Renal-Adrenal Vasoconstrictor and Volume Factors in the Rubric of Essential Hypertension

As indicated already, a variety of abnormal patterns in renin and aldosterone secretion have been described among patients classified as so-called essential hypertension. It is worth considering here how these abnormal patterns might emerge, assuming that the hypertension in its established form is (1) largely vasoconstrictor-initiated, (2) largely hypervolemic-initiated, or (3) an abnormal interaction of the two factors.

Vasoconstrictor-Initiated Essential Hypertension

For this sequence let us assume that the process begins as a primary renal disturbance with a subtle increase in renin secretion, angiotensin formation, and then aldosterone secretion. A sequence similar to that observed in the infusion studies of normal subjects would ensue. Sodium retention (due to increased aldosterone) and the increased angiotensin would together raise arterial pressure. Increased sodium retention would progressively tend to suppress the excess renin secretion. Thus the amount of angiotensin required to maintain an elevated blood pressure would fall to normal or nearly normal levels because of the increased sodium balance. A point could be reached where angiotensin blood levels would no longer suffice to cause excess aldosterone secretion. This chain of events could produce sustained high blood pressure with no other apparent residual abnormality except for a subtle change in amount or distribution of body sodium ions.

This hypothesis of a mechanism leading to elevated blood pressure in the absence of discernible physiologic fault is in keeping with numerous theories that essential hypertension is a disorder of a regulatory system in which the hypertension has compensated for the system. That is, the initial defect has been masked by a series of readjustments involving feedback mechanisms and changes in the autoregulatory activity by the kidney.

Physiologically, in its established state, this hypertension would exhibit normal or slightly high renin and aldosterone secretion. These patterns actually occur in a large number of patients with essential hypertension.

Volume-Initiated Essential Hypertension

Several mechanisms might produce hypertension associated with chronic, albeit subtle, volume expansion. Thus, as in animal models, the chronic ingestion of a very-high-sodium diet theoretically might be a cause. In fact, the amounts required on a weight basis may exceed those usually ingested by man. Such hypertension would be expected to exhibit a subnormal renin-secretory and a subnormal aldosterone-secretory pattern. Actually, this hormonal pattern occurs in about 30% of hypertensive patients who have low plasma renin activity.

A second possible mechanism for chronic volume-expansion hypertension could involve an impaired renal capacity to excrete the amounts of sodium occurring in average diets. Since most hypertensive patients excrete sodium abnormally rapidly, this seems an unlikely causal mechanism unless the hypertension has actually overcompensated for the initial renal defect. Both renin and aldosterone also might be expected to be low in this situation. However, since a renal disturbance is postulated, abnormal renin secretion could be an attendant part.

Another possible mechanism for volume-induced hypertension could result from a primary renal inability to excrete ingested potassium ions. This would lead to elevated plasma potassium levels and thus to increased aldosterone secretion, volume expansion, increased vascular sensitivity, and suppressed plasma renin activity. In the compensated state, potassium balance would be restored to normal, and the established hypertension would be sustained by aldosterone-induced sodium retention with increased vascular sensitivity to angiotensin. This thesis has the attraction of an experimental basis, since potassium gain is known both to stimulate aldosterone and to suppress renin. Moreover, low renin secretion with an inappropriately high aldosterone secretion is a rather common pattern among patients with essential hypertension.

A fourth mechanism for volume-induced essential hypertension involves a primary adrenal disturbance with increased secretion of aldosterone or of another mineralocorticoid. As indicated elsewhere, this leads to volume expansion and suppressed plasma renin levels, but in this situation, unlike the first three, potassium depletion with hypokalemia is almost invariably observed.

Pathophysiologic Implications of "Vasoconstrictor" Hypertension as Contrasted with "Volume" Hypertension

This functional classification of hypertensive states appears to have pathophysiologic correlations in both experimental models and naturally-occurring situations. Thus vasoconstrictor forms of hypertension appear to have more devastating consequences than do volume-expansion forms. In this context, renin-induced forms of hypertension, such as malignant hypertension, are associated with severe vascular injury, and the injection of renin into experimental animals also produces severe vascular injury. Conversely, primary aldosteronism with suppressed renin and a large volume component is usually a benign form of hypertensive disease exhibiting little evidence of vascular injury or target organ damage in the brain, kidneys, and heart. The benign nature of this form of hypertension relative to the vasoconstrictor form may be explained by the more adequate delivery of oxygen and nutrition to the tissues associated with the increased blood volume and relatively dilated arterioles.

While more documentation is required, it now appears that these relationships may also obtain in a more subtle way in various types of essential hypertension. Thus it has been found that patients with low-renin forms of essential hypertension are significantly less prone to the development of heart attacks or strokes than are patients with either normal or high levels of plasma renin activity. If these relationships continue to be observed, they could have important implications for classifying, determining prognosis, and planning treatment.

Meanwhile, from a physiologic standpoint, the data suggest that, given an equal degree of hypertension, arterial-tree distention with hemodilution and low viscosity constitutes, from a biophysical standpoint, a less deleterious situation than does the vasoconstrictor state characterized by a high-resistance arterial tree and a constricted vasculature perfused by a high-viscosity blood.

Pharmacologic Corroboration of the Thesis

The effects of various types of antihypertensive drugs on blood pressure and on the renin system provide both theoretical and practical corroboration for this functional characterization of hypertensive disorders in terms of either predominantly vasoconstrictor or volume factors. Moreover, the interactions of these various antihypertensive drugs with the renin system now provide a rational basis for their well-known variations in effectiveness in different patients.

Accordingly, antihypertensive drugs which produce volume depletion — thiazide diuretics and aldosterone antagonists — are especially effective not only in primary aldosteronism but also in a wide spectrum of patients with low-renin forms of essential hypertension. Conversely, preliminary data indicate that these drugs are often ineffective in high-renin forms of hypertensive disease. Moreover, in certain of these latter patients, the induced volume depletion may worsen the situation significantly by exciting more renin secretion, vasoconstriction, and hemoconcentration.

The converse also appears to hold: antiadrenergic drugs such as reserpine, methyldopa, and propranolol often produce strikingly antihypertensive effects in patients with essential, renal, or malignant hypertension whether the renin levels are high or normal. Also, preliminary data indicate that these agents are ineffective, often produce unpleasant side effects, and may even be contraindicated in the low-renin forms of hypertension. The latter contraindication results from their effects of impairing cardiac performance without, at the same time, acting to reduce the cardiac work imposed by the chronic volume overload.

In a third category of antihypertensive drugs (those which reduce arteriolar tonus, such as hydralazine and nitroprusside), more study is required. However, these agents usually induce reflex sympathetic discharge with increased renin secretion. More work is also needed on the net effects of combination therapy on the renal-adrenal hormone-controlled vasoconstrictor-volume equation.

Meanwhile, the potential for better characterization and understanding of hypertensive disorders by evaluating individual pharmacologic responses seems particularly bright. Moreover, such an approach enables more specific and individually tailored long-term therapy.

The ongoing elucidation of the cybernetics of the renin-angiotensin-aldosterone system has led to a working hypothesis for hormonal control of blood pressure, blood volume, and electrolyte homeostasis. From an analysis of possible sequences leading to various forms of chronic hypertension, it appears that changes in fluid volume and arterial vasoconstriction work together to maintain blood pressure. Derangement in the renin-angiotensin-aldosterone system leads to changes in the balance of these two components which can lead to sustained hypertension. Specific pharmacologic correction of the initial derangement in the hormonal system can result in lowering of the blood pressure.

SUMMARY

A large constellation of clinical and experimental evidence has accumulated which characterizes the renin-angiotensin-aldosterone hormonal concatenation. By changing the plasma concentrations of its two effector components, angiotensin II and aldosterone, the system works to regulate simultaneously (1) body sodium and water content and thus hydrostatic pressures, (2) potassium balance, and (3) arterial blood pressure.

In this system, the kidney, responding to various stimuli perceived as a fall in arterial pressure or in tubular sodium supply, releases renin. Renin liberates angiotensin from a specific circulating plasma globulin. Angiotensin, in turn, stimulates the secretion of aldosterone by the adrenal cortex. Angiotensin and aldosterone together act to restore sodium balance and arterial pressure, thus shutting off the initial signal for renin release.

More specifically, angiotensin II acts directly to restore blood pressure by causing arteriolar vasoconstriction. The pressor effect is amplified by the sodium-retaining actions of angiotensin which, acting directly on the kidneys and via stimulation of aldosterone secretion, induces renal sodium retention. The increased sodium helps to maintain blood pressure not only by increasing the vasoconstrictor action of angiotensin but also by volume expansion with an increased filling of the vascular bed. Thus the renin-angiotensin-aldosterone system maintains blood pressure both by reducing the capacity of the system (vasoconstriction) and by increasing the volume of the vascular tree through increased sodium and thus water retention.

At the same time as this sodium-linked blood-pressure homeostasis is maintained, sodium-linked potassium homeostasis is accomplished by two direct but opposing effects of changes in plasma potassium levels on aldosterone and on renin secretion.

Specific derangements of the renal-adrenal cybernetic system are involved in the pathogenesis of the edematous states of heart failure, cirrhosis, and nephrosis and in certain hypertensive disorders, notably malignant hypertension, primary (adenoma) and pseudoprimary (hyperplasia) adrenal cortical aldosteronism, renovascular hypertension, and oral contraceptive-induced hypertension.

Abnormalities in the renal-adrenal system also occur in the large population of patients with other forms of hypertensive disease, including essential hypertension. In this problem, a cybernetic analysis can be applied in which the chronic hypertension is considered to be the product of two influences, a vasoconstrictor factor and a volume component, each of which may be largely determined by the activity of the renal-adrenal system. This analysis appears to have meaningful pathophysiologic and pharmacologic coordinates.

Accordingly, predominantly vasoconstrictor hypertension is largely renin-induced, and it is associated with arteriolar vasoconstriction, hemoconcentration, and, with time, evidences of vascular injury. It can be corrected by drugs that reduce renin secretion. This group includes patients with malignant hypertension, more severe forms of renal hypertension, and high-renin and some normal-renin essential hypertension.

On the other hand, predominantly volume-factor hypertension is characterized by undue sodium and water retention, a relatively distended or open arterial tree, hemodilation and low blood viscosity, and, with time, less evidence of target organ vascular damage. It can be corrected by volume-depleting natriuretic drugs. This group of patients includes those with primary and pseudoprimary aldosteronism, syndromes of aberrant mineralocorticoid excess, and a large subfraction of patients with essential hypertension in whom aldosterone is normal or nearly normal.

Areas of uncertainty still exist and should be given special attention. Elucidation of these may finally offer a complete explanation for the genesis of a host of common diseases characterized by hypertension or abnormal sodium or potassium metabolism.

REFERENCES

Ames, R. P., Borkowski, A. J., et al.: Prolonged infusions of angiotensin II and norepinephrine and blood pressure, electrolyte balance, aldosterone and cortisol secretion in normal man and in cirrhosis with ascites. J. Clin. Invest. 44:1171, 1965.

Biglieri, E. G., Stockigt, J. R., et al.: Adrenal mineralocorticoids causing hypertension. Amer. J. Med. 52:623, 1972.

Brunner, H. R., Baer, J., et al.: The influence of potassium administration and potassium deprivation on plasma renin in normal and hypertensive subjects. J. Clin. Invest. 49:2128, 1970.

Bartter, F. C., Provone, P., et al.: Hyperplasia of the juxtaglomerular complex with hyperaldosteronism and hypokalemic alkalosis. Amer. J. Med. 33:811, 1962.

Brunner, H. R., Chang, P., et al.: Angiotensin II vascular receptors: their avidity in relationship to sodium balance, the autonomic nervous system, and hypertension. J. Clin. Invest. 51:58, 1972.

Brunner, H. R., Kirshman, J. D., et al.: Hypertension of renal origin: evidence for two different mechanisms. Science 174:1344, 1971.

Brunner, H. R., Laragh, J. H., et al.: Essential hypertension: renin and aldosterone, heart attack and stroke. New Eng. J. Med. 286:441, 1972.

Bühler, F. R., Laragh, J. H., et al.: Propranolol inhibition of renin secretion: a specific approach to diagnosis and treatment of renin-dependent hypertensive diseases. New Eng. J. Med. 287:1209, 1972.

Cannon, P. J., Leeming, J. M., et al.: Juxtaglomerular cell hyperplasia and secondary hyperaldosteronism (Bartter's syndrome): a reevaluation of the pathophysiology. Medicine 47:107, 1968.

Deming, Q. B., and Leutscher, J. A., Jr.: Bioassay of desoxycorticosterone-like material in urine. Proc. Soc. Exp. Biol. Med. 73:171, 1950.

Dustan, H. P., Tarazi, R. C., et al.: Physiologic characteristics of hypertension. Amer. J. Med. 52:610, 1972.

Gross, F.: The renin-angiotensin system and hypertension. Ann. Intern. Med. 75:777, 1971.

Guyton, A. C., Coleman, T. G., et al.: Arterial pressure regulation. Overriding dominance of the kidneys in long-term regulation and in hypertension. *Amer. J. Med.* 52:584, 1972.

Laragh, J. H.: The role of aldosterone in man: evidence for regulation of electrolyte balance and arterial pressure by renal-adrenal system which may be involved in malignant hypertension. *J.A.M.A.* 174:293, 1960.

Laragh, J. H.: Hormones and pathogenesis of congestive heart failure: Vasopressin, aldosterone and angiotensin II. Further evidence for renal-adrenal interaction from studies in hypertension and cirrhosis. *Circulation* 25:1015, 1962.

Laragh, J. H.: Evaluation and care of the hypertensive patient. *Amer. J. Med.* 52:565, 1972.

Laragh, J. H., Baer, L., et al.: Renin, angiotensin and aldosterone system in pathogenesis and management of hypertensive vascular disease. *Amer. J. Med.* 52:633, 1972.

Laragh, J. H., Sealey, J. E., et al.: Patterns of adrenal secretion and urinary excretion of aldosterone and plasma renin activity in normal and hypertensive subjects. *Circ. Res.* (Suppl. 1) 18 & 19:158, 1966.

Laragh, J. H., Sealey, J. E., et al.: The control of aldosterone secretion in normal and hypertensive man: abnormal renin-aldosterone patterns in low renin hypertension. *Amer. J. Med.* 53:649, 1972.

Laragh, J. H., and Stoerk, H. C.: A study of the mechanism of secretion of the sodium-retaining hormone (aldosterone). *J. Clin. Invest.* 36:383, 1957.

Sealey, J. E., Bühler, F. R., et al.: Aldosterone excretion: physiologic variations in man measured by radioimmunoassay or double isotope dilution. *Circ. Res.* 31:367, 1972.

Sealey, J. E., Clark, I., et al.: Potassium balance and the control of renin secretion. *J. Clin. Invest.* 49:2119, 1970.

Sealey, J. E., Gerten-Banes, J., et al.: The renin system: variations in man measured by radioimmunoassay or bioassay. *Kidney International* 1:240, 1972.

Tobian, L.: Interrelationship of electrolytes, juxtaglomerular cells and hypertension. *Physiol. Rev.* 40:280, 1960.

Tobian, L.: A viewpoint concerning the enigma of hypertension. *Amer. J. Med.* 52:595, 1972.

Vander, A. J.: Control of renin release. *Physiol. Rev.* 47:359, 1967.

CHAPTER 21

Hormones and the Formed Elements of the Blood

By John W. Adamson and
Clement A. Finch*

Cellular proliferation in all tissues is normally under precise regulation, and the formed elements of the blood are no exception. The production of erythrocytes, granulocytes, and platelets is believed to be under the control of specific humoral regulators. In addition, the number and function of the formed elements are influenced by the levels of various hormones. While the latter changes are of little consequence in themselves, they are useful in reflecting abnormalities of hormonal function and in explaining deviations from normal of the formed elements.

THE ERYTHRON

Primary Hormonal Regulation by Erythropoietin

Erythropoietin is the primary hormone which regulates erythropoiesis (38). This glycoprotein has been substantially purified (9,200 units per

mg.) from anemic sheep plasma by Goldwasser and Kung (21). While this preparation is electrophoretically homogeneous, it has not yet been demonstrated to be pure, and its exact chemical composition is unknown. The molecular weight of erythropoietin is believed to be about 45,800, and it contains 70 per cent protein and 30 per cent carbohydrate, of which 10.8 per cent is sialic acid. The presence of sialic acid prevents the rapid hepatic degradation of the molecule and is therefore critical for hormonal activity *in vivo*.

The kidney is responsible for the major part of erythropoietin production. Within the kidney an enzymelike factor, erythrogenin, acts on a plasma substrate presumably synthesized in the liver to generate the active hormone, erythropoietin (22). The activating substance is found in the light mitochondrial fraction of centrifuged kidney homogenates.

The regulation of erythropoietin production is determined in a general sense by the relationship between the oxygen supply to the kidney and the metabolic needs of that organ. When the hemoglobin concentration of blood or its arterial saturation falls, there is a logarithmic increase in erythropoietin production as monitored by urinary excretion of the hormone (1). Conversely, erythropoietin excretion falls with red cell transfusion. Erythropoietin production is also affected by changes in the availability of oxygen in the blood. An increase in hemoglobin affinity for oxygen (a left shift of the oxygen-hemoglobin dissociation curve) which decreases tissue oxygen tension increases erythropoietin and hemoglobin production; the opposite occurs with a decreased hemoglobin affinity for oxygen.

The most important action of erythropoietin is to increase the number of developing erythroid precursors within the marrow by inducing differentiation of erythropoietin-responsive stem cells (38). The underlying mechanism involves a sequential

*This work was supported by research grant HL–06242 from the National Institutes of Health. Dr. Adamson is the recipient of Research Career Development Award AM–70222–01 of the National Institute of Arthritis, Metabolic and Digestive Diseases.

production of messenger, ribosomal precursor, and transfer RNA (28, 29, 37). In addition to the increased number of maturing erythroid forms, erythropoietin has other recognizable effects on erythropoiesis. With increased hormonal stimulation, mitotic intervals of marrow normoblasts are moderately shortened; the amount of hemoglobin synthesized per cell is increased; and the reticulocyte, which normally spends up to three days in the human marrow, is released prematurely (33, 50).

More detailed knowledge of erythropoietin metabolism and of the biochemical aspects of its action has been seriously limited by difficulties in hormone measurement. Presently, the most widely used and best standardized quantitative technique is a bioassay employing the polycythemic mouse. In this assay animal, endogenous erythropoiesis is reduced markedly, and the erythropoietic stimulating activity of sera or other biologic materials is more apparent. Activity is usually quantitated by comparing the amount of injected radioiron appearing in newly formed red cells in mice receiving test material with that in groups of animals receiving known doses of an International Reference Preparation.* Serum assays are useful for determining significant increases in erythropoietin, but urinary concentrates must be employed to detect normal or subnormal levels (2). Unfortunately, these bioassay methods are difficult to standardize and are of limited availability. Assays *in vitro*, using freshly harvested marrow cells or immunologic techniques (40), are being evaluated but at the present time cannot be considered satisfactory substitutes.

In the clinical setting, increased erythropoietin production may be recognized by its effect on reticulocyte release from the marrow, and this can be assessed in two ways. First, the marrow radioiron transit time, which reflects primarily the period of reticulocyte maturation in the marrow, will shorten predictably with increased erythropoietin stimulation (16). Second, the prematurely released reticulocytes, or "shift cells," may be recognized in the peripheral blood film by their larger size and basophilic appearance (52).

While erythropoietin regulates red cell production through its effect on proliferation, the availability of iron also determines the amount of hemoglobin synthesized. In man, where iron supply is particularly limited, the effect of increased erythropoietin on marrow proliferation and hemoglobin synthesis is usually limited by the plasma iron level. Because of this, changes in reticulocyte delivery, which are independent of iron supply, are more useful in evaluating erythropoietin stimulation than is the amount of red cell production.

The hemoglobin concentration of the blood may be increased or decreased by appropriate changes in erythropoietin production (Table 21–1). Increased erythropoietin production most frequently occurs in response to a limitation in oxygen avail-

---

*Available from the World Health Organization, International Laboratory for Biological Standards, National Institute of Medical Research, Mill Hill, London, N.W. 7, England.

TABLE 21–1.

Erythropoietin production is increased through:
  I. Physiologic regulation
      A. Changes in renal oxygen supply
          Decreased oxygen content (anemia or dilutional)
          Increased hemoglobin affinity for O_2
      B. Hormonal changes
          Testosterone
  II. Pathologic states
      A. Unilateral ischemic renal disease
      B. Autonomous production
          Neoplasm
          Familial disorder

---

ability, as seen with inadequate oxygen loading of arterial blood (high altitude hypoxia, pulmonary disease, vascular shunting), and is also seen in conditions which modify hemoglobin affinity for oxygen (Table 21–1). The latter effects are best illustrated by certain mutant hemoglobins. A number of these mutants have increased oxygen affinity and an associated increase in hemoglobin concentration, while others have reduced oxygen affinity which favors oxygen unloading to tissue and results in a decreased hemoglobin concentration.

Impaired production of erythropoietin is most frequently seen with renal disease (3). While some erythropoietin production may persist, it is less than that expected for the degree of anemia present. In such patients, the blood creatinine and urea nitrogen usually exceed 5 mg. per 100 ml. and 50 mg. per 100 ml., respectively. Reflecting the decreased erythropoietin production, there is neither the expected shortening of marrow transit time nor an appearance of "shift cells" in circulation. Discrepancies do occur between impairment in excretory function of the kidney and in erythropoietin production: with uremia associated with arteriolar damage (hemolytic-uremic syndrome), there may be renal excretory failure but increased erythropoietin production; with radiation damage to the kidney, the opposite may occur (19).

Reduced erythropoietin production may occur in chronic inflammation but is complicated by an associated reduction in iron supply to the marrow and a moderate shortening of red cell life span. Thus it is difficult to define the relative importance of erythropoietin suppression in this setting. Evidence for reduced hormone production includes direct measurements of erythropoietin levels (73) and measurements of marrow transit time (16).

It is in the polycythemic states that the measurement of erythropoietin production has been shown to be of the greatest clinical value. Hypoxic stimulation, autonomous erythropoietin production, and autonomous erythropoiesis (polycythemia vera) all have distinct patterns of erythropoietin response with changes in the hemoglobin concentration (Fig. 21–1). Excessive erythropoietin output is seen with a variety of neoplasms that produce erythropoietin or erythropoietin-like material. The tumors most frequently associated are the hyper-

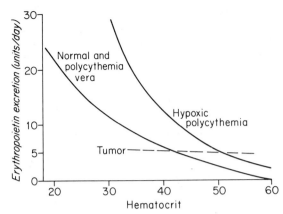

Figure 21–1. Patterns of erythropoietin excretion by polycythemic patients whose hematocrits were lowered by phlebotomy. (From Finch, C. A.: *The Red Cell Manual,* University of Washington, Seattle, 1970.)

nephroma, hepatoma, cerebellar hemangioblastoma, uterine leiomyoma, and pheochromocytoma (42). It has been suggested on the basis of preliminary evidence that hypernephromas produce increased quantities of erythrogenin (53), while hepatomas produce increased quantities of plasma substrate material (26). The active material produced by these tumors resembles erythropoietin from normal sources (60).

General Effects of Hormones on the Erythron

Oxygen transport by the red cell may be affected in several ways by hormones (Table 21–2). *Testosterone* and its derivatives are some of the most potent hormones in increasing hemoglobin synthesis and are primarily responsible for the 1 to 2 g. higher hemoglobin concentration in the male compared with the female (Table 21–1). In large doses, androgens will increase hemoglobin synthesis and hemoglobin concentration in both sexes. This stimulating effect of androgens has prompted their use in the treatment of patients with aplastic anemia and chronic renal disease, conditions in which beneficial responses have been well documented (62, 65). The effect is not well understood but apparently depends upon the presence of a significant degree of pre-existing erythroid proliferation (more than one-fifth normal) (5). Since erythropoietin excretion may increase as much as tenfold with androgen administration (4), and since the

TABLE 21–2. POSSIBLE EFFECTS OF HORMONES ON THE ERYTHRON

1. Direct effect on the production of erythropoietin or its precursors
2. Direct effect on bone marrow
3. Indirect effect on metabolic (oxygen) requirements
4. Effect on hemoglobin function (oxygen hemoglobin dissociation characteristics)
5. Alteration of blood volume

erythropoietic action of androgens is blocked by procedures that interfere with the production or circulation of erythropoietin (20, 63), at least part of the action of this hormone is thought to be mediated by erythropoietin. At the same time it is difficult to ascribe the effectiveness of androgens in marrow aplasia solely to increased erythropoietin production, since markedly elevated levels of the hormone already exist. Recent studies *in vitro* and in small animals suggest a direct action, particularly of the 5β-OH steroid derivatives, on cellular proliferation and hemoglobin synthesis (27, 48). An entirely unrelated action of testosterone—that of decreasing hemoglobin oxygen affinity—has been demonstrated in patients with renal anemia (51).

Adrenal glucocorticoids also affect hemoglobin concentration, but the mechanism of action is unclear. Male subjects with adrenal insufficiency whose plasma volume was maintained by deoxycorticosterone had an average hemoglobin concentration of 13.3 g. per 100 ml. (8), whereas with Cushing's disease, the hemoglobin concentration is often increased to 1 to 2 g. above normal (56). Experience with the use of glucocorticoids in man suggests that they have little effect on erythropoiesis except indirectly as changes in the plasma volume occur. On the other hand, glucocorticoids have been found effective in treating two forms of red cell aplasia: the congenital anemia of infancy (Diamond-Blackfan syndrome) (6) and erythroid aplasia in certain adults (18). In the latter instance, the effectiveness of glucocorticoids used in conjunction with other immunosuppressive agents such as 6-mercaptopurine suggests that the anemia may be mediated by immune mechanisms directed against the developing normoblast or against erythropoietin itself (39).

The effect of *thyroxine* on red cell production is illustrated by the normocytic normochromic anemia which follows extirpation of the thyroid in animals and which is corrected by thyroxine administration (24). However, reports in man of the hematologic effects of hypothyroidism are inconsistent. Thus Larsson (41) reported normochromic anemia (hemoglobin < 11.5 g. per 100 ml.) in 23 of 48 patients, while Tudhope and Wilson (68) found only 4 instances of normochromic normocytic anemia (hemoglobin < 12 g. per 100 ml. in females and < 13.9 g. per 100 ml. in males) among 116 patients with hypothyroidism. To complicate this further, iron deficiency occurs with the menorrhagia seen with hypothyroidism, and megaloblastic changes may occur as a result of either folate or B_{12} deficiency. It seems likely that the adjustments in oxygen transport occurring with thyroid dysfunction are more dependent on other components in the oxygen transport system than on hemoglobin concentration per se. In thyrotoxicosis, an increase in cardiac output (72) and a decrease in hemoglobin affinity for oxygen (45) mediated by an increased 2,3-diphosphoglycerate content of the red cell (67) would appear to be more than enough to compensate for the increased tissue oxygen requirements. No studies have yet been carried out in myxedema to evaluate the composite adjustments in oxygen transport.

Increased *estrogen* levels may play a role in the 1 to 3 g. reduction in hemoglobin concentration observed in pregnancy (34). In the rat, estrogen administration results in a hematocrit fall, an effect not seen with progesterone (46). In low doses, estradiol has been reported as decreasing the marrow response to erythropoietin (25), an effect antagonized by the simultaneous administration of 17α-OH progesterone or of testosterone propionate. *Prolactin* has been shown to stimulate erythropoiesis in normal, polycythemic, and orchiectomized rodents, presumably by increasing erythropoietin production (35), although no clear effect on erythropoiesis in man has been defined.

Other unspecified *pituitary* factors have been suspected of having additional effects on the erythron, since pituitary failure is associated with a more marked anemia (hemoglobin 6 to 12 g. per 100 ml.) than is seen with the hypofunction of individual target organs (14). This may well be due to a summation of the effects of individual target gland hypofunction, although another "pituitary effect" as well is not excluded (35, 70). While somatotropin administered to intact rats and given to pituitary dwarfs increases erythropoietin production (13, 36, 54), the direct effect of this hormone on erythropoietin production must be separated from its secondary effects on growth and blood volume.

The various normocytic normochromic anemias resulting from endocrine dysfunction are associated with a normal red cell maturation and life span and, therefore, depend on changes in the rate of red cell production. The mechanism by which these hormones influence erythropoiesis appears largely mediated by erythropoietin. Initially it was suggested that the primary effect of the circulating hormones was on tissue metabolism and that changes in erythropoietin output resulted from changes in tissue oxygen requirements (38). However, changes in tissue oxygen requirements are met principally by an adjustment in cardiac output (17).

Effects of Hormones on Blood Volume

In addition to the changes in erythropoiesis already discussed, hormones also affect plasma volume, which in turn modifies total blood volume and red cell mass (Table 21–3). For example, patients with myxedema or hypopituitarism have a decreased blood volume and, consequently, a decrease in red cell mass greater than that suggested by the hematocrit change (47). In hyperthyroidism, the blood volume is enlarged, with proportionate increases in plasma and red cells. It seems likely that these volume changes, which are rapidly reversed by treatment, have to do with the level of body metabolism and oxygen requirements, and that changes in plasma volume per se do not alter hemoglobin concentration if sufficient time has passed for equilibrium to be reached.

In Cushing's disease, the blood volume is often reduced, with a disproportionate decrease in plasma volume, similar to changes described in so-called "stress polycythemia." The reason for the reduction in plasma volume with excess glucocorticoids is unclear but may be related in part to protein depletion. In the untreated patient with Addison's disease, the plasma volume is diminished because of saline depletion. If this occurs acutely, hemoglobin concentration rises above normal, and the presence of any red cell deficit will be apparent only after saline balance is regained. High dose androgen administration may produce an increased plasma volume through sodium retention. Increased catecholamine output produces hypovolemia which, if acute, is associated with increased hemoglobin concentration but, if chronic, may result in a symmetrical decrease in plasma volume and red cell mass (11). In pregnancy, a mean blood volume increase of about 50 per cent is associated with a somewhat smaller increase in red cell mass (43). The volume increase undoubtedly has several explanations, including increases in body metabolism, size of the vascular bed, and body sodium. Sodium retention appears to be due to the effect of placental lactogen. Hyperaldosteronism, while producing a modest increase in extracellular fluid, has little effect on blood volume or hemoglobin concentration.

The clinical significance of these various volume changes lies in the reduced ability of individuals with hormone-induced hypovolemia to compensate further for volume change. Patients with hypopituitarism, hypoadrenalism, and Cushing's disease tolerate hemorrhage poorly and are unduly susceptible to shock from various causes; they are likewise unusually susceptible to volume overload. Those hypervolemic states associated with increased extracellular fluid volume, such as pregnancy, are unduly susceptible to pulmonary edema.

LEUKOCYTES

Primary Hormonal Regulation

The granulocyte system is known to be regulated by one or more humoral substances, although the chemical nature of and point of origin of the regulator(s) within the body are unknown. A humoral substance capable of increasing the number of granulocytes within a millipore chamber (61) or the number of granulocyte colony-forming units *in*

TABLE 21–3. BLOOD VOLUME

Increase	Decrease
Thyrotoxicosis	Hypothyroidism
Androgens (variable)	Hypopituitarism
Placental lactogen	Cushing's disease
	Addison's disease
	Epinephrine

vitro (57, 64) has been shown to appear after induction of granulocytopenia or exposure to endotoxin. A leukocytosis-inducing factor present in the plasma and capable of releasing neutrophils from the marrow has also been demonstrated (10, 23). Plasma from leukopenic subjects has been shown to produce a granulocyte response in other humans (44).

Measurements of granulocyte kinetics based on blood sampling have been difficult and have had limited application to the study of hormonal regulation of granulopoiesis. Most adult granulocytes are held in marrow storage, and circulating granulocytes comprise a very small fraction of the total mass. The rapid turnover of granulocytes and their variable distribution between the circulating and marginal pool lead to rapid fluctuations in the blood granulocyte count which bear little relationship to actual rates of production and destruction.

Little is known of the regulation of lymphocytes. It has been reported that lymphopenia induced by antilymphocytic serum results in the appearance of a lymphocytosis-producing factor within the plasma (58). However, the number of circulating lymphocytes probably has little quantitative relationship to the activity of the immunocyte systems; cellular proliferation within lymph nodes and increased circulating immunoglobulins may be more meaningful criteria. Antigenic stimulation appears to be the main factor inducing proliferation and increased function of lymphoid tissue, and other specific hormonal regulation is not well defined.

General Effects of Hormones

The granulocyte and lymphocyte systems, although their specific functions differ, both participate in host resistance to infection and in the inflammatory reaction. Central to this response is the adrenal cortex which, through its output of glucocorticoids, either mediates the leukocyte response to inflammation or at least permits this response to occur. With either bacterial infection or glucocorticoid administration, there is an increase in circulating granulocytes and, at the same time, a decrease in eosinophils and lymphocytes (7). Although the subject with Addison's disease displays near-normal blood values at rest (Table 21–4), he shows no change when exposed to stress or bacterial infection (8). Kinetic studies of granulocyte turnover after glucocorticoid administration show an increased movement of granulocytes from marrow to blood and a decrease in margination of circulating granulocytes (9). The increase in circulating granulocytes in response to a dose of glucocorticoids has been used as a means of evaluating marrow granulocyte reserve. There is some evidence that egress of granulocytes into tissues may be interfered with, particularly by some glucocorticoid compounds (55). However, the total circulating granulocyte pool is increased, and an overall effect may be the reduction of purposeless granulocyte penetration into unaffected areas and the focus of the extravascular migration more specifically on that portion of the vascular bed affected by inflammation. The lysosome-stabilizing effect of glucocorticoids is held largely responsible for their anti-inflammatory properties (74).

Quantitative enumeration of circulating eosinophils has been employed to evaluate adrenal function (7). For example, a normal eosinophil count in a patient under stress is suggestive of adrenal insufficiency. Similarly, Cushing's disease is also associated with eosinopenia; thus, a normal eosinophil count militates against this diagnosis. However, the basal level of eosinophils may be greatly increased by allergy; therefore it has been difficult to interpret a single eosinophil count without knowledge of the individual's previous values.

Glucocorticoids also affect the immune system. With decreased hormone levels, there is an increase in the bulk of lymph nodes and thymus. With increased glucocorticoid levels, the germinal centers of the thymus and lymph nodes are reduced in size (12), and the afferent limb of the immunologic response (antigen recognition and processing) is impaired by the suppression of cellular migration and phagocytosis at the inflammatory site. Glucocorticoids are particularly effective in the treatment of lymphocytic malignancies. In lymphocytic lymphoma or chronic lymphocytic leukemia, glucocorticoids may destroy large numbers of abnormal circulating cells and reduce tissue masses. A unique and poorly understood action of glucocorticoids is their effect in acute lymphocytic leukemia of childhood, in which the administration of pharmacologic amounts of the hormone may result in the disappearance of malignant cells and the reinstitution of normal marrow function. It has been suggested that this action is the result of effects of glucocorticoids on nucleic acid synthesis within the lymphoblasts, leading to the production of protein lethal to the neoplastic cell.

Placental hormones increase circulating granulocytes without significantly affecting lymphocytes or eosinophils (59). Thyroid hormone does not appear to have a significant effect on circulating leukocytes, although occasional patients with hyperthyroidism show leukopenia, granulocytopenia, and slight eosinophilia; more prominent are increases in tissue lymphocytes manifested by lymphadenopathy and occasional splenomegaly. *Etiocholanolone,* when injected intramuscularly, produces local inflammation and fever

TABLE 21–4. ENDOCRINE EFFECTS ON CIRCULATING LEUKOCYTE COUNTS*

	Granulocytes	Eosinophils	Lymphocytes
Normal	4200	150	2100
Cushing's Disease	9200	20	1500
Addison's Disease	4200	250	2900
Pregnancy (3–9 mo.)	8000	145	2200

*Mean levels (per mm.³) in circulating blood.

and granulocyte changes secondary to this (71). This granulocyte response appears to result from inflammation at the injection site rather than from a direct hormonal effect, since it is not seen following intravenous injection.

THROMBOCYTES

Primary Hormonal Regulation

The megakaryocyte-thrombocyte system has been shown to respond to thrombocytopenia and thrombocytosis by respectively increasing and decreasing platelet production (15, 30, 49). These responses have been shown to be humorally mediated (31, 66). While almost nothing is known of the nature of this circulating substance, called thrombopoietin, it is known to affect both the number of megakaryocytes found within the marrow and their proliferative behavior (30). With stimulation, there is an increase in the rate of maturation of the megakaryocyte, an increase in megakaryocyte size resulting from an increase in the number of mitoses within the individual cells, and possibly an increase in the size of platelets appearing in circulation. With suppression, megakaryocytes are smaller and contain a decreased number of nuclei. These changes affect the number of platelets produced per megakaryocyte. An inverse relationship is also normally found between the number of platelets in circulation and the size of megakaryocytes within the marrow (32). In the thrombocytosis accompanying inflammatory states and iron deficiency, however, there is dissociation between increased megakaryocyte number and the number of platelets produced per megakaryocyte. At the present time it is impossible to say whether megakaryocyte stimulation is mediated by one or more stimulating factors.

General Effects of Hormones on Platelets

There do not appear to be any significant effects of the hormones on the megakaryocyte-thrombocyte system; when changes in the number of circulating platelets are observed in endocrinopathies, other causes should be sought. While estrogens administered in large doses have been shown to cause thrombocytopenia in animals (69), there is little evidence for this in man, and the thrombocytopenia occasionally occurring at or before the time of menses is not known to be hormonally mediated. Glucocorticoids have no effect on normal thrombopoiesis but are often effective in decreasing the immune destruction of platelets and occasionally help to interrupt the increased platelet consumption seen with small vessel vasculitis.

REFERENCES

1. Adamson, J. W.: *Blood 32*:597, 1968.
2. Adamson, J. W., Alexanian, R., et al.: *Blood 28*:354, 1966.
3. Adamson, J. W., Eschbach, J. W., et al.: *Amer. J. Med. 44*:725, 1968.
4. Alexanian, R.: *Blood 33*:564, 1969.
5. Alexanian, R., Nadell, J., et al.: *Blood 40*:353, 1972.
6. Allen, D. M., and Diamond, L. K.: *Amer. J. Dis. Child. 102*:416, 1961.
7. Archer, R. K.: *The Eosinophil Leucocytes.* Philadelphia, F. A. Davis Co., 1963.
8. Báez-Villaseñor, J., Rath, C. E., et al.: *Blood 3*:769, 1948.
9. Bishop, C. R., Athens, J. W., et al.: *J. Clin. Invest. 47*:249, 1968.
10. Boggs, D. R., Marsh, J. C., et al.: *Proc. Soc. Exp. Biol. Med. 127*:689, 1968.
11. Brunjes, S., Johns, V. J., Jr., et al.: *New Eng. J. Med. 262*:393, 1960.
12. Claman, H. N.: *New Eng. J. Med. 287*:388, 1972.
13. Crafts, R. C., and Meineke, H. A.: *Ann. N. Y. Acad. Sci. 77*:501, 1959.
14. Daughaday, W. H., Williams, R. H., et al.: *Blood 3*:1342, 1948.
15. Evatt, B. L., and Levin, J.: *J. Clin. Invest. 48*:1615, 1969.
16. Finch, C. A., Deubelbeiss, K., et al.: *Medicine 49*:17, 1970.
17. Finch, C. A., and Lenfant, C.: *New Eng. J. Med. 286*:407, 1972.
18. Finkel, H. E., Kimber, R. J., et al.: *Amer. J. Med. 43*:771, 1967.
19. Frenkel, E. P., Douglass, C. C., et al.: *Arch. Intern. Med.* (Chicago) *125*:1050, 1970.
20. Fried, W., Marver, D., et al.: *J. Lab. Clin. Med. 68*:947, 1966.
21. Goldwasser, E., and Kung, C. K.: *Proc. Nat. Acad. Sci. USA 68*:697, 1971.
22. Gordon, A. S., Cooper, G. W., et al.: *Seminars Hemat. 4*:337, 1967.
23. Gordon, A. S., Handler, E. S., et al.: *Ann. N. Y. Acad. Sci. 113*:766, 1964.
24. Gordon, A. S., Kadow, P. C., et al.: *Amer. J. Med. Sci. 212*:385, 1946.
25. Gordon, A. S., Zanjani, E. D., et al.: *Proc. Soc. Exp. Biol. Med. 129*:871, 1968.
26. Gordon, A. S., Zanjani, E. D., et al.: *Blood 35*:151, 1970.
27. Granick, S., and Kappas, A.: *J. Biol. Chem. 242*:4587, 1967.
28. Gross, M., and Goldwasser, E.: *Biochemistry 8*:1795, 1969.
29. Gross, M., and Goldwasser, E.: *J. Biol. Chem. 246*:2480, 1971.
30. Harker, L. A.: *J. Clin. Invest. 47*:458, 1968.
31. Harker, L. A.: *Amer. J. Physiol. 218*:1376, 1970.
32. Harker, L. A., and Finch, C. A.: *J. Clin. Invest. 48*:963, 1969.
33. Hillman, R. S.: *J. Clin. Invest. 48*:443, 1969.
34. Jepson, J. H.: *Canad. Med. Ass. J. 98*:844, 1968.
35. Jepson, J. H., and Lowenstein, L.: *Acta Haemat.* (Basel) *38*:292, 1967.
36. Jepson, J. H., and McGarry, E. E.: *Ann. Intern. Med. 68*:1169, 1968.
37. Krantz, S. B., and Goldwasser, E.: *Biochim. Biophys. Acta 108*:455, 1965.
38. Krantz, S. B., and Jacobson, L. O.: *Erythropoietin and the Regulation of Erythropoiesis.* Chicago, University of Chicago Press, 1970.
39. Krantz, S. B., and Kao, V.: *Blood 34*:1, 1969.
40. Lange, R. D., McDonald, T. P., et al.: *J. Lab. Clin. Med. 73*:78, 1969.
41. Larsson, S. O.: *Acta Med. Scand. 157*:349, 1957.
42. Lipsett, M. B., Odell, W. D., et al.: *Ann. Intern. Med. 61*:733, 1964.
43. Low, J. A., Johnston, E. E., et al.: *Amer. J. Obstet. Gynec. 91*:356, 1965.
44. Marsh, J. C., and Levitt, M.: *Blood 37*:647, 1971.
45. Miller, W. W., Delivoria-Papadopoulos, M., et al.: *J.A.M.A. 211*:1824, 1970.
46. Mirand, E. A., and Gordon, A. S.: *Endocrinology 78*:325, 1966.
47. Muldowney, F. P., Crooks, J., et al.: *Clin. Sci. 16*:309, 1957.
48. Necheles, T. F., and Rai, U. S.: *Blood 34*:380, 1969.
49. Odell, T. T., Jackson, C. W., et al.: *Acta Haemat.* (Basel) *38*:34, 1967.
50. Papayannopoulou, T., and Finch, C. A.: *J. Clin. Invest. 51*:1179, 1972.
51. Parker, J. P., Beirne, G. J., et al.: *New Eng. J. Med. 287*:381, 1972.
52. Perrotta, A. L., and Finch, C. A.: *Amer. J. Clin. Path. 57*:471, 1972.
53. Peschle, C., and Condorelli, M.: *Blood 38*:828, 1971.
54. Peschle, C., Rappaport, I. A., et al.: *Endocrinology 91*:511, 1972.

55. Peters, W. P., Holland, J. F., et al.: *New Eng. J. Med. 286*:342, 1972.
56. Plotz, C. M., Knowlton, A. I., et al.: *Amer. J. Med. 13*:597, 1952.
57. Quesenberry, P., Morley, A., et al.: *New Eng. J. Med. 286*:227, 1972.
58. Rakowitz, F., Schultz, E. F., et al.: *J. Lab. Clin. Med. 78*:363, 1971.
59. Rath, C. E., Caton, W., et al.: *Surg. Gynec. Obstet. 90*:320, 1950.
60. Rosse, W. F., and Waldmann, T. A.: *Blood 24*:739, 1964.
61. Rothstein, G., Hügl, E. H., et al.: *J. Clin. Invest. 50*:2004, 1971.
62. Sánchez-Medal, L., Gomez-Leal, A., et al.: *Blood 34*:283, 1969.
63. Schooley, J. C.: *Proc. Soc. Exp. Biol. Med. 122*:402, 1966.
64. Shadduck, R. K., and Nagabhushanam, N. G.: *Blood 38*:559, 1971.
65. Shaldon, S., Koch, K. M., et al.: *Brit. Med. J. 3*:212, 1971.
66. Shreiner, D. P., and Levin, J.: *J. Clin. Invest. 49*:1709, 1970.
67. Snyder, L. M., and Reddy, W. J.: *Science 169*:879, 1970.
68. Tudhope, G. R., and Wilson, G. M.: *Quart. J. Med. 29*:513, 1960.
69. Tyslowitz, R., and Dingemanse, E.: *Endocrinology 29*:817, 1941.
70. Van Dyke, D. C., Contopoulos, A. N., et al.: *Acta Haemat.* (Basel) *11*:203, 1954.
71. Vogel, J. M., Kimball, H. R., et al.: *Ann. Intern. Med. 67*:1226, 1967.
72. Wade, O. L., and Bishop, J. M.: *Cardiac Output and Regional Blood Flow.* Oxford, Blackwell Scientific Publications, 1962.
73. Ward, H. P., Kurnick, J. E., et al.: *J. Clin. Invest. 50*:332, 1971.
74. Weissmann, G., and Thomas, L.: *Recent Progr. Hormone Res. 20*:215, 1964.

CHAPTER 22

Allergy, Immunology, and Hormones

By Paul P. VanArsdel, Jr.

The disciplines of endocrinology and immunology interact, in one way or another, in practically all the organ systems of the body. This chapter will cover only the highlights of this interaction, giving priority to that material not likely to be emphasized elsewhere in this book.

NATURE OF THE IMMUNE RESPONSE

Immunologically uncommitted stem cells are produced in large numbers by the bone marrow. There are two major pathways for development of these cells into immunologically competent lymphocytes. One pathway involves obligatory processing by the thymus gland. Most cells develop into short-lived lymphocytes (thymocytes), which have no known immunologic function. A few, under the influence of antigen, become long-lived, immunologically competent lymphocytes (T cells) which are responsible for cell-mediated immunity (CMI).

The other pathway involves the development of lymphocytes capable of responding to antigen with the production of humoral antibodies. In fowl, the bursa of Fabricius is the organ responsible for programming lymphocytes for antibody production. No homologous organ exists in mammals; functionally, a bursal equivalent almost certainly exists, and the processed lymphocytes — precursors of plasma cells in lymphoid germinal centers — are called B cells. To complicate matters, optimal response of B lymphocytes to some antigens also requires the participation of T lymphocytes, the so-called "helper" cells. The reader should refer to recent review articles (5, 20) for further information on this very complex subject.

Immunodeficiency States

Much of the knowledge concerning the immune response in man has come from the study of patients in whom the potential for such a response is deficient. Immunodeficiencies fall into three general categories: (1) low immunoglobulin levels and no antibody response to antigen stimulation (B-cell defect); (2) absence of cell-mediated immunity (T-cell defect); and (3) severe combined immunodeficiency (possible stem-cell defect). In the second category is a condition of special interest to the endocrinologist, congenital thymic aplasia (DiGeorge syndrome). Infants with this condition soon succumb to overwhelming bacterial, viral, or fungal infections despite normal antibody responses. The defect is caused by failure of development of the entodermal derivatives of the third and fourth pharyngeal pouches from which the parathyroid glands also develop. Thus hypoparathyroidism is part of the syndrome, and neonatal tetany is the first diagnostic clue (18).

Endocrine Function of the Thymus

It has been known for over two decades that cell-free thymus extracts produce lymphocytopoiesis when injected into animals of the same or different species. The immunologic capacity of thymectomized animals has been found to be partially restored by thymus grafts enclosed in an implanted millipore chamber, suggesting that a secreted humoral factor was responsible (24). Efforts to purify such a factor are not yet complete, but a partially purified protein named "thymosin" (11) apparently stimulates the development of immunologically competent lymphocytes. This should not be confused with thymin, another hormonelike substance which affects neuromuscular transmission (12).

Thymosin differs substantially from the thymic humoral factor studied by Trainin and Small (35), which contains nucleic acid and has a molecular weight of 1,000 or less and yet has an action similar to thymosin. By rigid criteria, these substances should be identified in the blood before they can qualify as hormones.

Influence of Conventional Hormones on the Immune Response

It is likely that any endocrine system which influences cell growth and metabolism will exert a modest, nonspecific effect on the cell proliferation and protein synthesis involved in CMI and antibody production. Thus, only the more specific and better-known effects will be presented here.

Growth hormone is required for the normal development of the thymus-dependent immune system in lower mammals. That this represents a specific thymotropic effect is supported by several observations summarized by Pierpaoli et al. (27). Of particular interest is their observation that the pituitaries of neonatally thymectomized mice have enlarged, degranulated acidophilic cells, suggesting a specific interrelationship. Growth hormone also stimulates thymocytes *in vitro* (25). Other studies indicate a possible alteration of immune reactions by hypo- or hyperthyroidism but were not designed to rule out alterations in tissue reaction to the immune response rather than in the response itself.

There is no known human counterpart of the above observations. Specifically, pituitary or thyroid deficiencies are not associated with any significant deficiency in the immune response.

Mention should also be made of the effect of androgen, specifically 19-nortestosterone, on the developing chick embryo. This hormone prevents the development of the bursa of Fabricius and, thus, humoral immunity; the thymus is unaffected (33). This is a well-known model for the study of humoral immunity, but there is no evidence for a comparable androgenic effect in humans.

Glucocorticosteroids have received by far the greatest amount of attention, clinically and experimentally. Very little of this attention has been devoted to the influence of normal adrenocortical activity on the immune response, although there is some evidence that the development of the lymphoid system is impaired by the absence of the adrenal cortex. On the other hand, an extensive and confusing literature exists regarding the inhibitory effect of pharmacologic doses of glucosteroids on lymphocytes and the immune response. The confusion is due partly to marked species differences in sensitivity to glucosteroids and partly to the difference in glucosteroid sensitivity of the several stages of lymphocyte development. In sensitive species, such as the mouse, rat, and rabbit, glucosteroids produce marked lysis of the short-lived cells of the thymic cortex and of those B lymphocytes which have not yet been activated by antigen. Humoral antibody response can be inhibited by glucosteroid administration in these species. Once either the T or B cells have been activated by antigen, however, they become steroid-resistant. In other species, including man, glucosteroids have essentially no effect on the immune response at any step. Even though they can produce peripheral lymphopenia in humans and reduction in thymus size in infants, this effect is immunologically insignificant. One must look to the inflammatory and other host responses to hypersensitivity reactions in man to identify significant glucosteroid effects (3).

MEDIATORS OF IMMUNOLOGIC TISSUE INJURY

When a sensitized individual is exposed to antigen, the resulting reaction develops in one of several characteristic patterns which differ in their immunologic mechanisms. These patterns have been classified by Coombs and Gell (4) into four general types:

Type I: anaphylactic and atopic reactions. These are initiated by antigen reacting with antibody that has a strong affinity for basophils and tissue mast cells and that generally is of the immunoglobulin E (IgE) class.

Type II: cytotoxic reactions. These occur when antibody reacts with antigen which is part of, or closely associated with, cells or other tissue elements.

Type III: arthus-type or immune complex reactions. In these, antigen reacts with antibody (usually IgG) in the fluid phase; the deposition of these complexes leads to tissue injury.

Type IV: tuberculin-type or cell-mediated reactions.

Although this classification has certain imperfections, it is convenient, widely used, and sufficient for this discussion. The activity of vasoactive mediators is of paramount importance in the development of type I reactions, in which the antigen-antibody reaction triggers mediator release from mast cells and basophils; this amplification step permits very minute amounts of antigen and antibody to initiate what may be major clinical reactions. The two mediators important in man are histamine and slow-reacting substance of anaphylaxis (SRS-A).*

---

*Serotonin, a mediator in certain lower animals, has no such function in man.

Histamine

Histamine, the best known and most extensively studied of the autacoids or local hormones (8), is formed by the enzymatic decarboxylation of histidine in mast cells and basophils and is stored within their granules, where it is biologically inert. When antigen and antibody react on the cell surface, a series of two or more enzymatic steps are activated, leading to the active release of histamine by exocytosis. The released histamine is then metabolized rapidly by oxidative deamination and conjugation and excreted in the urine (36, 22). The cells are not damaged by the process and proceed to resynthesize their histamine stores. Of course, if damaged by other means, they would also release histamine.

In the short time between release and destruction, histamine causes an increase in vascular permeability associated with constriction of postcapillary venules, vasodilatation, contraction of bronchial and visceral smooth muscle, and stimulation of mucus glands. It can produce the characteristic clinical features of atopic diseases in man, such as urticaria, bronchospasm, rhinitis, and anaphylaxis.

Slow-Reacting Substance of Anaphylaxis (SRS-A)

The other mediator, SRS-A, is an acidic lipid of as yet undetermined chemical structure which is released following antigen challenge from the lungs of several animal species including man. It is a potent stimulator of bronchial smooth muscle contraction and may have some effect on vascular permeability as well. The response of smooth muscle to this mediator is slower than that to histamine, hence the name. It is not a prostaglandin (22). The lack of any significant response in most asthmatic patients to antihistaminic drugs lends further support for the concept that SRS-A is the major mediator in asthma. Parenthetically, prostaglandins also are found in the lungs of several species, and $PGF_{2\alpha}$ is a potent bronchoconstrictor (14). However no evidence exists that these interesting lipids are involved in antigen-induced reactions.

Eosinophil Chemotactic Factor of Anaphylaxis

This mediator was recently identified under conditions similar to those for release of histamine and SRS-A. With a molecular weight of less than 1,000, it has a specific chemotactic effect on eosinophils but no other known action (16).

Kinins

An extensive literature has accumulated regarding the so-called "kinin hormones." These are specific basic peptides produced by the action of glandular or plasma enzymes (kallikreins) on certain alpha globulins (kininogens). The major plasma kinin is bradykinin, a nonapeptide with potent physiologic effects: smooth muscle stimulation, vasodilatation, increase in vascular permeability, and pain production [see Table XXI, Rocha e Silva, 1970 (29)]. Such effects indicate that the kinins may be important mediators of hypersensitivity reactions; in fact, kinin activation does occur with certain antigen-antibody reactions in experimental animals and, in a few instances, in man. However, kinin activation can be produced nonspecifically with any tissue injury, and it is not yet known if kinins act as primary mediators in type I or type III reactions (22).

Other Mediators

A variety of other substances mediate tissue injury in type III reactions. These macromolecular substances include leukocyte lysosomal enzymes and split products of the third and fifth components of complement. In the presence of antigen, lymphocytes produce several substances called *lymphokines* which mediate tissue injury in type IV reactions (2, 7). Only time will tell if the macromolecular mediators and lymphokines will be classified as hormones.

INFLUENCE OF THE ENDOCRINE SYSTEM ON THE EXPRESSION OF ALLERGIC AND IMMUNOLOGIC REACTIONS

Epinephrine

The autonomic nervous system has a major regulator role in enhancing or antagonizing physiologic changes in the skin, mucous membranes, and bronchi which are characteristic of type I reactions. For example, acetylcholine can aggravate bronchospasm through psychogenic or nonspecific reflex pathways. However, it is not a specific mediator of antigen-antibody reactions and thus was not included in the discussion of mediators in the previous section nor will it be discussed further, despite its obvious physiologic importance. Epinephrine might suffer a similar fate were it not for its pharmacologic importance in type I reactions. It is a pharmacologic, or nonspecific, antagonist of histamine and other mediators. By its alpha adrenergic action, it is a vasoconstrictor, and by its beta adrenergic action, it is a bronchodilator. Not so well known is the inhibition by epinephrine of antigen-induced release of histamine and SRS-A from sensitized tissues (23). This inhibition is shared by all agents known to increase the intracellular concentration of cyclic adenosine monophosphate and is blocked by the beta adrenergic antagonist, propranolol. This may be an important part of the therapeutic action of epinephrine in treating reactions such as anaphylaxis. The eosinopenia produced by epinephrine also appears to be a beta adrenergic effect, since it also is blocked by propranolol (17). Whether some patients with asthma and eosinophilia suffer from a relative resistance to endogenous epinephrine ("intrinsic β-adrenergic blockade") is a matter of active investigation [see review by Szentivanyi (34)].

Adrenal Glucosteroids

In contrast to the lack of substantial effect on antibody production or antigen-antibody interaction, the glucosteroids in pharmacologic doses can reduce substantially the physiologic abnormalities and other signs of tissue injury which are the consequences of hypersensitivity reactions. Extensive clinical observations have established the efficacy of steroids in such widely divergent conditions as asthma, serum sickness, and transplant rejection. Fundamental knowledge regarding the mechanisms involved, however, has lagged far behind the accumulation of empirical clinical observations.

The response of type I reactions to steroid treatment is least well understood. In animals given glucosteroids, the tissue histamine content is diminished, and mast cell synthesis of new histamine following histamine release is inhibited. However, this is not a significant effect in man. During glucosteroid therapy, the typical wheal-and-flare response to an antigen skin test is not altered, indicating in addition that histamine release is not inhibited. The vasoconstriction and vascular permeability inhibition produced by glucosteroids may play a role, but this is speculative. Steroids do inhibit the enzymatic production of kinins from their substrate, but as yet the role of kinins in type I reactions is not established [see review by David et al. (6)]. Since blood and tissue eosinophilia is so characteristic of type I hypersensitivity, one might expect some explanation from the eosinopenic effect of glucosteroids. However, even this effect is not completely understood. It seems to involve decreased marrow release and increased sequestration in some unknown compartment (13), but such information does not help to explain the therapeutic action of glucosteroids.

More is known about the action of glucosteroids on other types of hypersensitivity. Stabilization of leukocytic lysosomal membranes retards the release of one class of macromolecular mediators (lysosomal enzymes) thought to be important in type III reactions. Less specific effects include reduction in accumulation of macrophages and polymorphonuclear leukocytes in sites of inflammation. As in type I reactions, inhibition of kinin production also may play a role (6).

The inhibitory effect of glucosteroids on type IV reactions probably involves the several nonspecific anti-inflammatory actions mentioned above. In addition, lymphocyte metabolism is suppressed. This action has been particularly well demonstrated in respect to the response of lymphocytes in tissue culture to mitogenic stimulation by substances such as phytohemagglutinin. Either prior glucosteroid treatment of the cell donor or addition of any glucosteroid to the culture medium markedly inhibits RNA and DNA synthesis, amino acid incorporation, and, of course, cell replication. The production of one or more lymphocyte mediators of inflammation may also be suppressed. How important this action is in the glucosteroid suppression of the many cell-mediated phenomena in man, ranging from the tuberculin skin reaction to allograft rejection, remains to be determined (3, 6).

ALLERGIC AND IMMUNOLOGIC REACTIONS INVOLVING ENDOCRINE HORMONES

Hormone Administration

All the polypeptide hormones can, of themselves, induce an antibody response, and this effect is utilized widely for the preparation of reagents for immunoassay (see below). However, protein contaminants are responsible for most allergic reactions, which are usually type I, characterized by urticaria and, rarely, anaphylactic shock following hormone injection or by allergic rhinitis and asthma following inhalation of posterior pituitary powder for treatment of diabetes insipidus. Occasionally, sensitivity to posterior pituitary snuff has been manifested by a form of infiltrative lung disease similar to Farmer's lung associated with precipitating antibodies and thus presumably a type III reaction (26). The risk of allergic reactions makes prior skin testing advisable before injecting a hormone such as bovine ACTH. Synthetic corticotropin (Cosyntropin), on the other hand, rarely if ever produces allergic reactions and is now the agent of choice for diagnostic testing. Similarly, synthetic lysine vasopressin has largely supplanted posterior pituitary powder for nasal administration and has produced very few allergic reactions.

The situation with insulin is considerably more complex. Probably all persons given insulin respond with the production of an insulin-binding antibody, usually of the IgG class. A small proportion of diabetics produce sufficient antibody to be markedly insulin resistant; as the insulin dose is increased, the antibody titer is likely to rise even further (28). In some instances, antibodies to insulin lack species specificity, reacting not only with bovine insulin but also with all other insulins, including desalinated pork and even human insulin, rendering management extremely difficult. Tissue injury, such as vasculitis or glomerulitis, produced by circulating antibody-insulin complexes is surprisingly rare. Faulk et al. (9) have described one insulin-resistant patient with hepatosplenomegaly and a Coombs' test-positive hemolytic anemia due to insulin-antibody complexes, but other stigmata of vasculitis or serum sickness were lacking.

Insulin allergy has little if any relationship to insulin resistance. Except for local erythema and induration, allergy is extremely rare in patients maintained on continuous insulin treatment. Reactions are most likely to occur after a lapse in treatment and are characterized usually by urticaria, occasionally by anaphylactic shock. As expected in type I reactions, the antibody is of the IgE class. Reactions are most common to protein contaminants, but the insulin molecule itself, even synthetic human insulin, can induce positive skin tests in sensitive patients (19). Fortunately, desensitization is usually successful. Cell-mediated (type IV) sensitivity may play a role in some reactions, characterized by the delayed appearance of erythema and induration (10).

Allergic reactions to nonpolypeptide hormones seldom, if ever, occur. Steroids, for example, are nonimmunogenic unless chemically coupled to carrier protein by reactions which do not occur *in vivo*. Rare reports of steroid allergy are anecdotal and have not been confirmed. The same can be said of the so-called "endogenous steroid allergy" proposed as a cause of cyclical urticaria and other skin reactions in women in scattered reports over half a century.

Disorders of Endocrine Function

In contrast to the scanty evidence for hormone autoimmunity, a vast amount of clinical and experimental information has accumulated on immunologically mediated tissue injury involving endocrine glands, particularly the thyroid and adrenal. Evidence for a similar pathogenesis for diabetes and hypoparathyroidism is not yet conclusive enough to warrant discussion here.

The Thyroid.   The thyroid gland is most susceptible to autoimmune tissue injury, possibly because it is rich in organ-specific antigens, particularly thyroglobulin which normally is isolated from lymphocyte surveillance and thus is recognized as "foreign" when it escapes from the gland or is injected elsewhere. Thyroiditis can be induced quite easily in a number of species by immunization with thyroglobulin and is characterized by the appearance of circulating antibodies and cell-mediated immunity. Passive transfer of lymphocytes from sensitized animals to normal animals produces thyroiditis in the recipients, indicating the importance of cell-mediated immunity. Under special circumstances, however, thyroiditis can also be induced by transfer of cytotoxic antibody (30).

The human counterpart, Hashimoto's thyroiditis, is discussed in Chapter 4. Briefly, it is characterized by varying degrees of thyroid gland enlargement and inflammation leading eventually to atrophy and hypothyroidism. Histologically, the gland becomes depleted of colloid and shows infiltrates of round cells that may be organized into lymphoid follicles with germinal centers. Most patients have circulating thyroglobulin antibodies of the IgG class, usually detected by the agglutination of thyroglobulin-coated tanned red cells. The presence of such antibodies is useful diagnosti-

cally, particularly when they are present in high titer. It should be noted, however, that antibodies in low titer may be present in as many as 20 per cent of normal subjects and in a higher percentage of those with other thyroid diseases.

Another antibody found in the sera of most patients with Hashimoto's disease reacts with the microsomes of thyroid epithelial cells and can be detected by immunofluorescence or by complement fixation. This may be the same antibody that is cytotoxic to thyroid cells in tissue culture. Another antibody, about which much less is known, reacts with some antigen in colloid (not thyroglobulin). Antinuclear antibodies, which are not organ-specific, may also be present (32).

Comparable antibody studies in myxedema and Graves' disease have led to substantial recent changes in concepts of their pathogenesis, which may have the same immunologic common denominator as Hashimoto's disease. A majority of patients with idiopathic primary myxedema have thyroglobulin antibodies. This suggests that myxedema is the end stage of asymptomatic or unrecognized thyroiditis.

Graves' disease is more complex immunologically. Lymphocytic infiltration in the thyroid, lymphadenopathy, and even thymic enlargement have been recognized for several decades. Most patients have both thyroglobulin and microsomal antibodies in their serum. Werner et al. (37) have recently identified by immunofluorescence specific deposition of IgG, IgM, and two components of complement (C1q and C3) both in stroma and in follicular basement membranes of thyroid glands from patients with Graves' disease. This is not too surprising, but they also found deposits of IgE, suggesting the contribution of a type I reaction, which fit with no known clinical features of the disease. Graves' disease and Hashimoto's disease also tend to be associated in family studies, and further circumstantial evidence is provided by the fate of patients with Graves' disease after surgery or radioiodine therapy, in which the risk of eventual myxedema is associated with the presence and amount of antibody. Yet Graves' disease is entirely unique in one respect at least. The serum of many patients contains a substance that stimulates radioiodine release from the thyroid for as long as 24 hours, much longer than the response to TSH. This long-acting thyroid stimulator (LATS) is an immunoglobulin (IgG). Thus LATS possibly is a stimulatory antibody (not unknown experimentally) contributing to the clinical activity of the disease (1). Yet the ultimate significance of LATS has yet to be determined. If it is an antibody, the specific thyroid antigen remains unknown.

The Adrenal.   Circulating serum antibodies to adrenal tissue have been found in a large proportion of patients with idiopathic Addison's disease but only rarely in that secondary to tuberculosis. The antibody is IgG, which reacts with the cytoplasm of secretory cells, particularly with the microsomal fraction. The concept that this represents an autoimmune disease is supported by the experimental production of adrenalitis in animals and the occurrence of lymphocytic infiltration in the adrenal cortex of patients with the disease. As in Hashimoto's disease, associated cell-mediated sensitivity may be necessary for tissue injury, but this matter has not been settled (15).

Immunologic Cross-Reactivity. Antithyroid antibodies are often found in other apparent autoimmune diseases, such as systemic lupus erythematosus. Conversely, other tissue- and organ-specific antibodies have been found in the thyroid diseases. The association with pernicious anemia (gastric parietal cell antibodies) is particularly impressive. Patients with idiopathic Addison's disease frequently have antithyroid, antigastric, antigonadal, and antiparathyroid antibodies; this is particularly significant in view of the common association of this uncommon disease with pernicious anemia, hypothyroidism, and hypoparathyroidism. The development of more than one autoantibody in a single person suggests that the immunologic abnormality is a general one, possibly representing a loss of competence for self-recognition.

The Gonads. There is little evidence that the endocrine function of testes or ovaries can be impaired experimentally or clinically by autoimmune mechanisms. In numerous experiments involving immunization with testicular tissue, the most consistent result has been aspermatogenesis, with little inflammation and no evidence of Leydig cell destruction. Accordingly, the main thrust of clinical studies has been in the investigation of male infertility, which has been correlated with the presence of sperm agglutinating autoantibodies, but the role of these antibodies clinically has yet to be determined. Similarly, the presence of sperm agglutinating antibodies in women may contribute to female infertility (31).

ANTIBODIES AS HORMONE ASSAY REAGENTS

The development and application of immunoassay for the measurement of hormones in biologic fluids has expanded rapidly over the last decade and is becoming a specialty in itself, quite distinct conceptually from the role of immune mechanisms in disease with which this chapter is primarily concerned. Most of the human peptide hormones will produce specific antibody without special preparation when injected into lower animals. The larger their molecular weight, the greater the antibody response; generally, peptides with a molecular weight less than 5,000 are weak immunogens and may need to be conjugated to a carrier protein to produce a satisfactory antibody response. There are exceptions; satisfactory antisera can be produced to unconjugated vasopressin and gastrin if these are injected with complete adjuvant.

To be immunogenic, all nonpeptide hormones, as well as certain small molecular weight peptides, must be conjugated to an appropriate carrier protein (such as human albumin) and thus act as hap-

tens. Effective conjugation involves the formation of a strong covalent bond. Such a reaction between hormones and protein does not occur naturally.* Conjugation requires synthetic manipulations involving the use of activating chemicals. Agents such as the carbodiimides activate carboxyl groups to form a CO-NH bond. Others, such as the diisocyanates, link two amino groups.

Optimal conditions for antibody production vary widely from one hormone to another relative to species used, mode of administration, and duration of immunization. Within a species, some animals are better antibody producers than others, and a dozen or more may need to be immunized to ensure at least one source of high-titered, high-affinity antibody.

Because of the low concentration and small molecular weight of the hormones, conventional methods of measuring antigen-antibody reactions, such as precipitation in agar, cannot be used for hormone assay. Of numerous methods tried, radioimmunoassay is the most sensitive and can be adapted to assays of all hormones that are available in chemically pure form and that can be labeled with a radioisotope. Standard amounts of antibody and labeled hormone are mixed with the material to be tested. The more unlabeled hormone in the test material, the less labeled hormone is bound to the antibody. This method, then, is a special application of competitive protein-binding assays in which the sensitivity can be very high, because the affinity of specific antibody for a hormone is usually much higher than the affinity of natural hormone-binding serum proteins. A critical step in the procedure is the separation of the radiolabeled hormone bound to antibody from free radiolabeled hormone. In many applications, free hormone can be separated by solid adsorbents such as dextran-treated charcoal. Separation can also be achieved by electrophoresis, by affixing antibody to solids such as agarose beads or the surface of plastic tubes, or by precipitating antigen-antibody complexes with an appropriate anti-immunoglobulin serum (the "double antibody" method).

The lower the concentration of antibody and labeled hormone that can be used in the assay, the greater the sensitivity of the method. Thus the specific activity of the radioisotope label and the binding affinity of the antibody should be as high as possible. Sufficient sensitivity can now be achieved with good reagents to reliably measure hormone concentrations of only a few picograms per milliliter. For detailed information regarding the problems in developing, standardizing, and validating assays for specific hormones, the reader should refer to Odell and Daughaday (21).

Most of the hormones that can now be measured by immunoassay are listed in Table 22–1. A few assays (particularly that for thyroxine) probably will not have any clinical application, but several,

---

*As mentioned earlier, this fact makes the whole concept of autoimmunity to such hormones as the steroids very tenuous.

TABLE 22–1. HORMONES MEASURED BY RADIOIMMUNOASSAY

Peptides		Nonpeptides
Insulin	Vasopressin	Aldosterone
Glucagon	Oxytocin	Testosterone
GH	Parathyroid hormone	Estrone
ACTH	Calcitonin	Estradiol
TSH	Bradykinin	Progesterone
FH	Angiotensin	Prostaglandins
LH	Gastrin	Triiodothyronine
MSH	Secretin	Thyroxin
HCG		

such as those for insulin and the pituitary hormones, have proven the best, or even the only, assay methods available; their use is discussed in appropriate sections elsewhere in this book.

REFERENCES

1. Beall, G. N., and Solomon, D. H.: Hashimoto's disease and Graves' disease, In *Immunological Diseases.* 2nd ed. Samter, M. (ed.), Boston, Little, Brown and Co., 1971, Ch. 73.
2. Bloom, B. R.: *In vitro* approaches to the mechanism of cell-mediated immune reactions, In *Advances in Immunology.* Vol. 13. Dixon, F. J., Jr., and Kunkel, H. G. (eds.), New York, Academic Press, 1971, pp. 101–208.
3. Claman, H. N.: Corticosteroids and lymphoid cells. *New Eng. J. Med.* 287:388, 1972.
4. Coombs, R. R. A., and Gell, P. G. H.: Classification of allergic reactions responsible for clinical hypersensitivity and disease, In *Clinical Aspects of Immunology.* 2nd ed. Gell, P. G. H., and Coombs, R. R. A. (eds.), Philadelphia, F. A. Davis Co., 1968, Ch. 20.
5. Craddock, C. G., Longmire, R., et al.: Lymphocytes and the immune response. *New Eng. J. Med.* 285:324, 378, 1971.
6. David, D. S., Grieco, M. H., et al.: Adrenal glucocorticoids after twenty years: A review of their clinically relevant consequences. *J. Chronic Dis.* 22:637, 1970.
7. David, J. R.: Lymphocytic factors in cellular hypersensitivity, In *Immunobiology.* Good, R. A., and Fisher, D. W. (eds.), Stamford, Sinauer, 1971, Ch. 7.
8. Douglas, W. W.: Autacoids, In *The Pharmacological Basis of Therapeutics.* 4th ed. Goodman, L. S., and Gilman, A. (eds.), New York, Macmillan, 1970, p. 620.
9. Faulk, W. P., Tomsovic, E. J., et al.: Insulin resistance in juvenile diabetes mellitus. *Amer. J. Med.* 49:133, 1970.
10. Federlin, K.: *Immunopathology of Insulin.* New York, Springer-Verlag, 1971.
11. Goldstein, A. L., and Slater, F. D., et al.: Preparation, assay and partial purification of a thymic lymphocytopoietic factor (thymosin). *Proc. Nat. Acad. Sci. USA* 56:1010, 1966.
12. Goldstein, G., and Mackay, I. R.: *The Human Thymus.* London, Heinemann, 1969, p. 61.
13. Honsinger, R. W., Jr., and Silverstein, D., et al.: The eosinophil and allergy: Why? *J. Allerg. Clin. Immun.* 49:142, 1972.
14. Horton, E. W.: *Prostaglandins.* New York, Springer-Verlag, 1972, Ch. XIV.
15. Irvine, W. J.: Adrenalitis, hypoparathyroidism, and associated diseases, In *Immunological Diseases.* 2nd ed.

Samter, M. (ed.), Boston, Little, Brown and Co., 1971, Chapter 74.
16. Kay, A. B., and Austen, K. F.: The IgE-mediated release of an eosinophil leukocyte chemotactic factor from human lung. *J. Immun.* 107:899, 1971.
17. Koch-Weser, J.: Beta-adrenergic blockade and circulating eosinophiles. *Arch. Intern. Med.* (Chicago) 121:255, 1968.
18. Kretschmer, R., Say, B., et al.: Congenital aplasia of the thymus gland (DiGeorge's syndrome). *New Eng. J. Med.* 279:1295, 1968.
19. Lieberman, P., Patterson, R., et al.: Allergic reactions to insulin. *J.A.M.A.* 215:1106, 1971.
20. Mills, J. A., and Cooperband, S. R.: Lymphocyte physiology. *Ann. Rev. Med.* 22:185, 1971.
21. Odell, W. D., and Daughaday, W. H.: *Principles of Competitive Protein-Binding Assays.* Philadelphia, Lippincott, 1971.
22. Orange, R. P., and Austen, K. F.: Chemical mediators of immediate hypersensitivity, In *Immunobiology.* Good, R. A., and Fisher, D. W. (eds.), Stamford, Sinauer, 1971, Ch. 12.
23. Orange, R. P., Austen, W. G., et al.: Immunological release of histamine and slow-reacting substance of anaphylaxis from human lung. I. Modulation by agents influencing cellular levels of cyclic 3′,5′-adenosine monophosphate. *J. Exp. Med.* 134:136s, 1971.
24. Osoba, D., and Miller, J. F. A. P.: The lymphoid tissues and immune responses of neonatally thymectomized mice bearing thymus tissue in millipore diffusion chambers. *J. Exp. Med.* 119:117, 1964.
25. Pandian, M. R., and Talwar, G. P.: Effect of growth hormone on the metabolism of thymus and on the immune response against sheep erythrocytes. *J. Exp. Med.* 134:1095, 1971.
26. Pepys, J.: *Hypersensitivity Diseases of the Lungs Due to Fungi and Organic Dusts.* Basel, S. Karger, 1969, p. 112.
27. Pierpaoli, W., Fabris, N., et al.: Developmental hormones and immunological maturation, In *Hormones and the Immune Response.* Wolstenholme, G. E. W., and Knight, J. (eds.), London, J. & A. Churchill, 1970, p. 126.
28. Pope, C. G.: The immunology of insulin, In *Advances in Immunology.* Vol. 5. Dixon, F. J., Jr., and Humphrey, J. H. (eds.), New York, Academic Press, 1966, p. 209.
29. Rocha e Silva, M.: *Kinin Hormones.* Springfield, Illinois, Charles C Thomas, 1970.
30. Rose, N. R., and Witebsky, E.: Experimental thyroiditis, In *Immunological Diseases.* 2nd ed. Samter, M. (ed.), Boston, Little, Brown and Co., 1971, Chapter 72.
31. Shulman, S.: Antigenicity and autoimmunity in sexual reproduction: A review. *Clin. Exp. Immun.* 9:267, 1971.
32. Shulman, S.: Thyroid antigens and autoimmunity, In *Advances in Immunology.* Vol. 14. Dixon, F. J., and Kunkel, H. G. (eds.), New York, Academic Press, 1971, pp. 85–185.
33. Szenberg, A.: Influence of testosterone on the primary lymphoid organs of the chicken, In *Hormones and the Immune Response.* Wolstenholme, G. E. W., and Knight, J. (eds.), London, Churchill, 1970, p. 42.
34. Szentivanyi, A.: The beta adrenergic theory of the atopic abnormality in bronchial asthma. *J. Allerg.* 42:203, 1968.
35. Trainin, N., and Small, M.: Studies on some physicochemical properties of a thymus humoral factor conferring immunocompetence on lymphoid cells. *J. Exp. Med.* 132:885, 1970.
36. VanArsdel, P. P., Jr., and Beall, G. N.: The metabolism and functions of histamine. *Arch. Intern. Med.* (Chicago) 106:714, 1960.
37. Werner, S. C., Wegelius, O., et al.: Immunoglobulins (E, M, G) and complement in the connective tissues of the thyroid in Graves's disease. *New Eng. J. Med.* 287:421, 1972.

CHAPTER 23

Skin and Hormones

By Frank Parker

The skin is unusually heterogeneous in its cellular composition, comprising, as it does, rapidly proliferating keratinizing epidermal and hair follicle cells, lipid-synthesizing sebaceous glands, pigment-producing melanocytes, and dermal connective tissue cells responsible for the production of fibrous tissue and ground substances. Each cell type has its own unique metabolic pattern, and therefore the integument is capable of a wide variety of biochemical activities.

Many of these metabolic activities are under hormonal regulation. The control of cutaneous pigmentation by melanocyte-stimulating hormone is well known, as are the stimulatory effects of androgens on sebaceous glands and certain hair follicles. The regulatory effects of insulin on cutaneous carbohydrate and lipid metabolism are now receiving much attention, and there is a growing awareness that the skin, the largest organ of the body, plays an important role in the total body metabolism of several hormones.

The variety of hormonal effects upon various cellular elements in the skin will be reviewed in this chapter and, when possible, this information will be related to cutaneous clinical findings. In many instances, metabolic aberrations occurring in the skin have helped to explain clinical cutaneous alterations which accompany endocrine diseases.

HORMONES AND THE EPIDERMIS AND DERMIS

Glucose and Lipid Metabolism

Qualitatively the skin—in particular, the epidermis—is capable of metabolizing carbohydrate by the same pathways as other tissues to provide both energy (ATP) for the synthetic, energy-requiring processes and various intermediate substances for other metabolic pathways utilized by epidermal cells. Biochemical studies on human and experimental animal epidermis have verified the presence of the anaerobic glycolytic pathway, as well as the oxidative phosphorylative hexose monophosphate shunt and tricarboxylic acid cycle (Fig. 23–1).

Studies on the relative importance of these major pathways in skin have revealed some differences from other tissues of the body. Glycolysis produces ATP at a maximal rate of about 0.1 μM/hr./mg. wet weight epidermis, while the respiratory pathways generate the majority of the energy (80 per cent of epidermal ATP) at a rate of

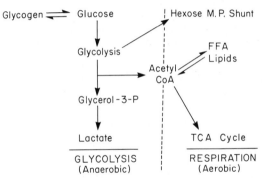

Figure 23–1. A brief résumé of the major pathways of glucose and lipid metabolism demonstrated in the skin.

977

about 0.5 μM ATP/hr. Estimates of respiratory activity of human epidermis indicate a CO_2 value of 5.0, higher than the value for smooth muscle or lung tissue. An unusual feature of epidermal metabolism is that most of the glucose assimilated is converted by glycolysis to pyruvate and, particularly, lactic acid (70 per cent) without further degradation to CO_2 by glycolytic or oxidative pathways. Moreover, only 2 per cent of the glucose finds its way through the direct oxidative (hexose monophosphate shunt) pathway, in contrast to glucose metabolism in such organs as liver and muscle. Therefore, although considerable amounts of glucose are assimilated by human epidermis, most of this is not oxidized to CO_2 for energy production through the oxidative pathways. Rather, the primary substrate for epidermal respiration is apparently lipid. This conclusion is supported by the fact that the respiratory quotient (RQ, the ratio of CO_2 formed to oxygen consumed) of epidermis is less than 1.0, a value that results from fatty acid oxidation. β-Oxidation of fatty acids generates two-carbon units (acetyl CoA) and reduces nucleotides which in turn form approximately 5 moles of ATP for each mole of acetyl CoA produced (Fig. 23–1).

The epidermis is also an active site of sterol, fatty acid, and polar lipid synthesis, utilizing pyruvate, some amino acids, acetate, and glucose as substrates. Glucose, however, seems to be the major precursor of lipogenesis, being the only compound that stimulates this process *in vitro*. Glucose also appears to regulate lipogenesis *in vivo*, since glucose feeding accelerates cutaneous lipid synthesis, while fasting produces the opposite effect. The level of L-glycerol 3-phosphate in the skin fluctuates parallel to lipogenic activity, and the addition of this substance *in vitro* stimulates lipogenesis, suggesting that this intermediate in the glycolytic pathway (Fig. 23–1) may play a regulatory role in the lipid synthetic processes. Although the hexose monophosphate shunt plays a relatively minor role in epidermal respiration, it does function significantly in lipogenesis, as it supplies about one-half the necessary NADPH for these synthetic reactions.

Cutaneous sterol synthesis proceeds by way of two alternate routes, the Kandutsch-Russell and the Block pathways, which differ in the intermediary steps between lanosterol and cholesterol. One of the Kandutsch-Russell intermediates is 7-dehydrocholesterol, which can be converted by sunlight to vitamin D, providing a teleological basis for the explanation of the operation of this pathway in skin.

Several examples can be cited to demonstrate how hormones may affect cutaneous glucose and lipid metabolism, although it is still difficult to relate these metabolic alterations directly to clinical changes in the skin. Hormones have been shown to alter epidermal metabolism in diabetes mellitus. Glucose uptake and utilization and cutaneous lipogenesis are severely impaired in both human and experimental animal diabetics. Insulin reverses these alterations *in vivo* and even *in vitro* in skin in contrast to the reported unresponsiveness to insulin of diabetic leukocytes and adipose tissue *in vitro*. Insulin even stimulates glucose uptake and lipogenesis (via its effect on the hexose monophosphate shunt) in normal skin. How these disturbances in epidermal metabolism contribute, alone or in concert with a variety of other systemic alterations, to the cutaneous complications of diabetics, such as the propensity to bacterial, yeast, and fungal infection, is not yet clear.

A second example of hormonal effects on cutaneous metabolism may be found in the case of thyroxine. Thyrotoxicosis in animals has been shown to stimulate cutaneous respiration as well as to augment glucose assimilation and aerobic metabolism. Whether these changes are brought about directly by the action of thyroxine on the skin or indirectly by altered vascular blood flow or hormone interactions cannot be stated. Nevertheless, the presence of changes in cutaneous metabolism in experimental thyrotoxicosis suggests that these alterations may accompany and underlie clinical abnormalities of the skin in states of thyroid dysfunction.

A final example of hormonal effects on epidermal metabolism is seen in the relationship of cutaneous sterol metabolism to sex hormones. Testosterone and progesterone significantly accelerate sterol ester synthesis via the Kandutsch-Russell pathway. Estrogens inhibit steroidogenesis and concomitantly cause thinning of the epidermis. This decrease in epidermal thickness in relation to alterations in sterol metabolism emphasizes the critical role sterols and their esterification play in the process of epidermal maturation and keratinization. Several drugs, such as nicotinic acid and triparanol, that inhibit cutaneous sterol synthesis induce scaly lesions in the skin reminiscent of ichthyosis. In addition, deficiencies of essential fatty acids which are normally esterified to sterols also lead to abnormal keratinization and scaliness.

Cutaneous Metabolism of Hormones

Sex hormones have long been known to play an important role in the development of secondary sexual characteristics by influencing hair growth and sebaceous gland activity (see below), but recently the skin has also been noted to participate actively in the metabolism of several hormones including testosterone, progesterone, estrogens, and cortisol. In view of the fact that the skin constitutes 15 per cent of the total body weight, its role in overall body hormone homeostasis and metabolism may be more important than has been assumed.

An unusual feature of normal cutaneous steroid metabolism is that the metabolites of the steroids studied to date all have the 5α configuration in contrast to those of other organs, such as the liver, in which both 5α and 5β isomers are produced. This cutaneous stereospecific reduction at C-5, under the influence of 5α reductase enzymatic activity, operates upon C-21 steroids (cortisol and progesterone) and C-19 steroids (androgens and estrogens). There is evidence that these steroids compete for the same reductase enzyme, which suggests a complex interplay between the metabolism of one steroid hormone and that of another. For example, progesterone inhibits the 5α reduction of testosterone to the more potent androgen, 5α-dihydrotestosterone. No known direct effect on the skin can at present be attributed to the 5α-pregnane derivatives formed from progesterone, but if these metabolites actively inhibit the reduction of testosterone, they could regulate the formation of potent androgenic substances by the skin. Another comparable situation of steroid competition for the same enzymatic site is seen in the oxidation of the 17β-OL in estradiol and in testosterone by microsomal preparations of human skin. In this instance, an androgen and an estrogen seem to share the same dehydrogenase, which might represent one mechanism by which antagonism between these steroids occurs.

The skin is capable of both activation and inactivation of steroid hormones (Fig. 23–2). Several pairs of steroids are known to be reversibly transformed in the skin, including cortisol and cortisone, testosterone and androstenedione, and estradiol and estrone. The equilibrium of these reversible reactions appears to favor oxidative formation of ketones which are less active hormones, i.e., cortisone has less anti-inflammatory activity than cortisol, androstenedione is less androgenic than testosterone, and estrone is less estrogenic than estradiol. In some instances, however, the reverse reductive reactions occur in the skin or mucous membranes, transforming the steroids into more active products. This has been shown, for example, in human vaginal mucosa, where the main product of the interconversion of estrone and estradiol favors the stronger estrogenic substance, estradiol, but not in human abdominal skin and foreskin, which produce primarily estrone. Another such example is found in the ability of both male and female skin to form testosterone from the relatively weak androgen, dehydroepiandrosterone, and to further reduce testosterone to the even more potent androgen, 5α-dihydrotestosterone. It would appear that dihydrotestosterone is the most important androgenic metabolite in human skin, and, as in the case of the prostate gland, it may be the active form of androgenic hormone at the tissue receptor site. Those areas of skin that demonstrate the most active conversion rates of testosterone to dihydrotestosterone in both men and women arise from a common anlage in the urogenital ridge (prepuce, clitoris, scrotum, and labium majus), and each of these tissues develops in response to androgenic stimulae. It seems likely that these areas of skin can be likened to accessory sex target organs, and hence steroid metabolism in these specific sites might be particularly sensitive to pathologic aberrations in this metabolic realm.

This point is dramatically demonstrated clinically in the testicular feminization syndrome, in which a basic biochemical defect characteristic of this disorder has been demonstrated in the skin. These patients have a normal male chromosomal pattern, sclerotic but functioning testes, and normal plasma testosterone levels, but they display a phenotypic female physiognomy. Such individuals appear to be suffering from an inherited defect in the target organ response to testosterone, since skin samples are unable to convert testosterone to 5α-dihydrotestosterone. Although it has been suggested that these patients lack the 5α-reductase enzyme in the skin, they do not respond to dihydrotestosterone therapy either, which implies there is a more basic defect in androgen retention or binding by the target tissues.

Dermal Connective Tissue, Cells, and Hormones

The great bulk of skin is connective tissue stroma consisting of cells (fibroblasts, mast cells,

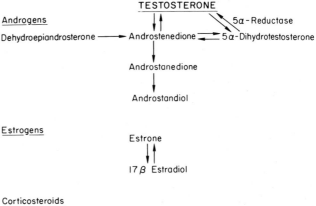

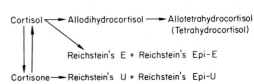

Figure 23–2. The metabolites and interconversions of androgens, estrogens, and corticosteroids by human skin as determined by *in vitro* studies. The formation of allodihydrocortisol and allotetrahydrocortisol is confirmed only in foreskin. Oxidation of 11-β-OH and reduction of 20-one are common to all anatomical sites studied.

histiocytes), fibrils (collagen and elastic fibers), and interfibrillar amorphous ground substances (glycosaminoglycans). The extracellular components are synthesized by fibroblasts, which are suspended in a three dimensional network of dense collagen fibers embedded in the nonfibrous, semi-fluid ground substances.

Glycosaminoglycans are single chain linear macromolecular polymers of disaccharides, whose configuration in solution and moist environs of the dermis assumes random coils which play an important role, along with collagen, in determining the skin's resilience and resistance to compression. Of the half dozen glycosaminoglycans characterized to date, two occur predominantly in the dermis: hyaluronic acid (repeating units of glucuronic acid and N-acetyl glucosamine) and dermatan sulfate (chondroitin sulfate B, consisting of iduronic acid and N-acetyl galactosamine).

Both the fibrillar and ground substance constituents undergo continuous turnover, and their synthesis and catabolism appear in certain instances to be under hormonal influence. Abnormalities in this balance between the catabolism and anabolism of various dermal components may therefore occur in association with endocrinopathies in the form of changes in cutaneous thickness, compliability, and texture.

Alterations in skin thickness may indicate changes in the dermal collagen content, and several endocrinologic conditions affect decreases or increases in the collagen composition of the dermis. Corticosteroid hormones accelerate the catabolism of collagen and reduce the amount of collagen synthesized by fibroblasts. Thus patients with Cushing's syndrome, from either overproduction of endogenous glucosteroids or from exogenous administration of these hormones in unphysiologic doses, have atrophic, tissue paper–thin skin. The clinical impression of atrophic skin in Cushing's syndrome has been verified by direct measurements. This loss of collagen accounts for the increased transparency of the skin, which allows the dermal and subcutaneous vasculature to become apparent, as manifested by plethoric facies and purple striae over the upper arms, abdomen, and thighs. Identical atrophic striae can be produced by applying corticosteroids under occlusive material to the skin for many weeks. Minor trauma readily produces ecchymosis, presumably because the blood vessels have less support secondary to the decrease in dermal collagen. Since glucosteroids have been shown experimentally to inhibit wound healing, it is not surprising that patients with Cushing's syndrome also suffer from this problem. In contrast to corticosteroids, increased circulating levels of growth hormone, as occur in acromegaly, cause fibroblastic proliferation and increased quantities of dermal collagen deposition recognizable clinically as thickening, coarseness, and a leathery consistency to the skin. Over the face, neck, and scalp the excessive mass of dermis causes the skin surface to buckle into folds and furrows, imparting a corrugated appearance resembling gyri of the cerebral cortex (cutis verticis gyrata). The cutaneous thickening in these patients has been verified by direct radiologic measurements on the forearm and heel, although the degree of thickening does not correlate closely with the severity of the acromegaly.

Thyrotropin and thyroid and sex hormones appear to affect the metabolism of dermal glycosaminoglycans rather than collagen. As is the case for connective tissue in other organs of the body (e.g., gastrointestinal tract, pericardium, larynx), there is an accumulation of glycosaminoglycans in the dermis of patients with hypothyroidism. Specifically, hyaluronic acid collects throughout the dermal collagenous network. It would seem that thyroxine is primarily concerned with the catabolism of dermal hyaluronic acid, its absence leading to a slowing of these degradative processes and the accumulation of ground substance within the skin, while thyrotropin acts directly on connective tissue to stimulate the formation of glycosaminoglycans (increased sulfate-S^{35} incorporation into mucopolysaccharides). This may explain why the accumulation of hyaluronic acid is so marked in patients with primary myxedema, in whom thyroxine is deficient and thyrotropin levels are increased, when compared with secondary myxedematous patients, whose thyrotropin levels are decreased and whose skin amasses much smaller quantities of hyaluronic acid. The large amounts of hydrophilic hyaluronic acid are responsible for the puffy, doughy, nonpitting edematous features of the skin in hypothyroid patients. There is also dryness of the skin surface with roughness and scaling, particularly over the extensor surfaces of the limbs. In long-standing cases, this becomes so marked as to mimic "tree bark" in appearance and texture. Replacement therapy with thyroid hormones mobilizes the dermal glycosaminoglycans with increases in urinary hexosamines.

A similar accumulation of hyaluronic acid occurring in localized form on the anterolateral aspects of the legs in patients with Graves' disease is called pretibial myxedema. It may appear while the patient is hypermetabolic, but more often it follows surgical or radioiodine therapy. Hence the skin alterations cannot be directly related to known thyroid function. The skin lesions appear as pink or violaceous infiltrated plaques and nodules with prominent, dilated, follicular orifices in the overlying skin (peau d'orange). In extreme cases, the entire lower leg may be involved, with thickened skin thrown into folds overhanging the ankles. Pretibial myxedema frequently occurs concomitantly with exophthalmos and occasionally with clubbing and osteoarthropathy of the digits (acropachy). Exophthalmos results from the accumulation of hyaluronic acid and fluid interposed between the bony socket and the eyeball. The etiology of pretibial myxedema is unknown, but its occurrence is correlated best with the presence in the blood of long-acting thyroid stimulating substance (LATS), being found in high concentrations in 90 per cent of patients with this dermopathy. Whether LATS, an IgG antibody, is directly responsible for initiating the skin lesions is undetermined. Some investigators postulate that this antibody fixes to the skin and elicits a localized antigen-antibody reaction which secondarily stimulates the accumulation of hyaluronic acid. Other workers, however, have failed to demonstrate the presence of LATS in the skin lesions, and several cases have had normal levels of circulating LATS. The cutaneous lesions respond impressively to topically applied fluorinated steroids under occlusive thin plastic wraps.

Sex hormones also influence dermal glycosaminoglycans, although their importance in the human can only be inferred at the present time from observations in animals. The rhythmic swelling in the sex skin of female monkeys in relation to the rising levels of estrogens appears to be due to enormous localized accumulations of hyaluronic acid and water which readily binds to this hydrophilic substance. It could be that the generally recognized phenomenon in women of increased water-binding and retention in connective tissues before and during the menstrual periods and concomitant with pregnancy is analogous to this event in nonhuman Primates.

In addition to the effects hormones have on fibroblasts and the fibrous and amorphous substances they synthesize, the dermal histiocyte also occasionally plays a role in the clinical aberrations of certain endocrine diseases. Patients with diabetes and myxedema and those receiving estrogenic hormones may develop an abnormality in lipoprotein metabolism, leading to large elevations both in beta and pre-beta lipoproteins and in chylomicrons. These blood lipids infiltrate through dermal capillaries, preferentially in areas subject to stress and pressure, where dermal histiocytes phagocytize the lipids to evolve into foam cells and form xanthomas. Eruptive (small, yellow papules on the extensor surfaces) and tuberous (large, reddish nodules on the elbows and knees) xanthomas are the most common clinical forms found in these patients. The xanthomas resolve concomitant with the decrease in circulating lipoproteins when insulin or thyroid replacement is given for the specific underlying endocrinologic problem.

Dermal Vasculature and Hormones

Certain cutaneous features of endocrine diseases are related to physiologic or anatomic alterations in the dermal vascular bed. For example, the vasodilatation and increase in cutaneous blood flow in thyrotoxicosis (3–4 times normal) may account for the soft, smooth, warm characteristics of the skin. Patients with pheochromocytomas suffer from paroxysms of blanching and sweating in response to the intermittent release of vasoconstrictive catecholamines, while episodes of cutaneous flushing are characteristic of patients with carcinoid tumors. The cyanotic or bright red flushes over the face and upper trunk of patients with carcinoid tumors of ileal origin are mediated by kinins formed in response to the release of kallikreins synthesized by the tumor. Gastric carcinoid tumors producing large quantities of histamine cause

flushes which are patchy with sharply delineated serpentine borders over the face, trunk, and extremities, while tumors of bronchial origin, synthesizing large amounts of 5-hydroxytryptophan, induce flushes of long duration (several days) accompanied by dramatic facial edema.

Patients with increased quantities of circulating estrogens form numerous spider angiomas over the face, trunk, and upper extremities as well as palmar erythema. These situations obtain in pregnancy and in patients on estrogen therapy or with cirrhosis of the liver.

Certain skin alterations associated with diabetes mellitus owe their pathogenesis to alterations in the vasculature. It is likely that abnormalities in lipid, glycolipid, and glycoprotein metabolism, prevalent in diabetics, are responsible for the pathologic changes occurring in the vascular walls of vessels of all sizes, including large muscular and elastic arteries, arterioles, and capillaries. Premature peripheral large vessel insufficiency secondary to arteriosclerotic changes is a frequent occurrence in diabetics, leading initially to loss of hair, shininess, atrophy, and coolness of the skin over the toes and lower legs, with subsequent ulceration and gangrene. Multiple, sharply demarcated, gangrenous ulcerations may occur over the lower extremities in the presence of adequate flow through the large peripheral arteries when arterioles (arteriolosclerosis) and capillaries (microangiopathy) are the major site of vascular damage.

Several unique cutaneous lesions are seen in diabetics with endarteritic obliterative small vessel disease (intimal proliferation and basement membrane thickening), including necrobiosis lipoidica diabeticorum (NLD), shin spots (pigmented pretibial patches), and bullae (bullosis diabeticorum). Although these lesions can occur in individuals without diabetes, they are found with sufficient frequency in association with the microangiopathy of this disease that their presence should alert the physician to search for the presence of diabetes. It should also be stressed that little is known of how these small-vessel pathologic alterations initiate the clinical features of each of these skin changes.

Necrobiosis lipoidica diabeticorum (NLD) appears as asymptomatic, sharply circumscribed, shiny, atrophic plaques with an erythematous border and a yellowish central region through which telangiectatic vessels course. Ulceration commonly occurs and may require skin grafting. The plaques, which vary in size and number, usually occur over the pretibial areas, although they have been found on the trunk, arms, and head. In about 15 per cent of patients, the NLD may precede the onset of chemical evidence of diabetes (prediabetes) by about two years (range of one-half to 14 years). In 25 per cent of cases, NLD and diabetes (latent, chemical, and overt diabetes) appear concomitantly, while in the remainder, the skin lesions are present after the diabetic condition is diagnosed. Spontaneous resolution of small NLD plaques occurs in 13–19 per cent of cases, but the resolution or progression does not appear to be related to the severity of, the activity of, or the adequacy of control of the diabetes.

Shin spots, the second cutaneous sign of diabetes, begin as asymptomatic red-brown papules that evolve into sharply circumscribed, atrophic, depressed, hyperpigmented patches over the shins and less frequently on the arms. Identical skin lesions are observed in 2 per cent of normal individuals and in 20 per cent of patients with a variety of endocrinopathies whose glucose tolerance is normal. The age and sex distributions of the occurrence of diabetic shin spots are different from those of NLD. Shin spots occur in 10–30 per cent of female diabetics and 60–65 per cent of male diabetics past the age of 30, while NLD occurs in far fewer diabetics and usually in female diabetics between the second and fourth decades. The incidence of shin spots rises with the increasing duration of the presence of the diabetic state.

The third cutaneous lesion attributed to microangiopathic changes observed in diabetes is recurrent crops of bacteriologically sterile, tense bullae without a surrounding inflammatory reaction over the toes, fingers, and forearms. These asymptomatic bullae, varying in size from several millimeters to several centimeters in diameter, usually occur in patients with recognized diabetes (3 to 20 years' duration), although occasionally they may be the presenting feature leading to the diagnosis of diabetes. The lesions usually heal without scarring, but several cases have been reported in which the bullae evolve into circumscribed atrophic patches.

HORMONES, MELANOCYTES, AND PIGMENTATION

Melanin, the major product of the melanocyte, is largely responsible for the coloring of skin. Melanocytes originate in the embryonic neural crest, from which they migrate to form a horizontal network of cells with many cytoplasmic processes or dendrites that intermesh between the basal cells of the epidermis. Melanin is a complex of insoluble, polyquinone, brown or red pigment and protein, formed by the oxidation of tyrosine and 3,4-dihydroxyphenylalanine (DOPA) in the presence of the oxidative enzyme, tyrosinase. Tyrosinase is found within distinctive ultrastructural organelles of the melanocytes, called melanosomes, which are membrane-bound ovoid structures enclosing regularly packed and coiled lamellae upon which melanin is synthesized and deposited. Eventually when the melanosomes are filled with melanin pigment, all enzymatic activity ceases. They are then referred to as melanin granules, and the granules move out along the melanocytic dendritic processes, where they are transferred to the surrounding epidermal cells (cytocrine activity). Human skin pigmentation, therefore, depends upon not only the amount of melanin synthesized by melanocytes but also the number and dispersion of melanin granules in the adjacent basal cells.

Hormones profoundly influence the melanin pigmentation of man as well as other mammals and amphibia. The precise action of hormones at the cellular level is obscure, although certain parallels exist with a comparable phenomenon in frogs, whereby a number of hormones *in vitro* and *in vivo* rapidly produce hyperpigmentation or lightening of pigmentation by causing dispersion or aggregation of melanin granules throughout the melanocyte's cytoplasm and dendritic processes. This movement of granules in response to hormones can be observed by light microscopy. Table 23–1 lists the effects of certain hormones on both frog and human skin. Note that, in most instances where hormones cause dispersion of melanin granules and thus darkening of amphibian skin, these same hormones cause increased pigmentation in humans, whereas hormones aggregating the granules and thus lightening frog skin have no clinical effect on human pigmentation. Cyclic AMP has been shown to cause pigment dispersion in frog melanocytes, so that the dispersive effect of MSH and other darkening hormones may be mediated by cyclic AMP. It further appears that microfilaments within the melanocyte's cytoplasm are the transducer between cyclic AMP and pigment granule dispersion. In humans, the increase or decrease in pigmentation initiated by the presence of too much of or the absence of certain hormones, such

TABLE 23–1. COMPARATIVE EFFECTS OF VARIOUS HORMONES ON SKIN PIGMENTATION IN FROGS AND MAN

Hormone	Frog Skin		Human Skin	
	Dispersion of Melanin Granules (Darkening Effect)	*Aggregation of Melanin Granules (Lightening Effect)*	*Increased Pigmentation*	*Decreased Pigmentation*
ACTH	+		+ (in large doses)	
α MSH	+		+	
β MSH	+		+	
Estrogens	+		+	
Progesterone	+		+	
Thyroxine		+	+	
Epinephrine		+	No effect	No effect
Norepinephrine		+	No effect	No effect
Hydrocortisone		+	No effect	No effect

TABLE 23–2. HORMONE-INDUCED AND ENDOCRINE-RELATED CHANGES IN CUTANEOUS PIGMENTATION

Increased Pigmentation		Decreased Pigmentation	
Generalized	*Localized*	*Generalized*	*Localized*
Adrenal insufficiency	Pregnancy and anovulatory drugs	Panhypopituitarism	Vitiligo associated with thyroid diseases, adrenal insufficiency, or diabetes
Ectopic ACTH- & MSH-producing neoplasms	Acanthosis nigricans associated with endocrinopathies		
Thyrotoxicosis	Polyostotic fibrous dysplasia (Albright's syndrome)		
	Neurofibromatosis and pheochromocytoma		

as ACTH, MSH, estrogen, and progesterone, may partially be due to the movement of melanin granules via the same system as in amphibian skin, but it is more likely such changes in pigmentation are the result of alterations in the rate of melanin synthesis and melanin transfer to epidermal cells. MSH increases cyclic AMP in experimental melanomas, and it is possible that this nucleotide is responsible for initiating tyrosinase synthesis and melanin production in human melanocytes. The administration of α MSH to humans results in hyperpigmentation in several days, characterized histologically by increased numbers of melanin granules in the dendrites of melanocytes as well as in epidermal cells.

Marked regional variation exists in the sensitivity of certain melanocytes to specific hormones. For example, during pregnancy estrogens and progesterones stimulate melanogenesis in melanocytes of the areolae and nipples and to a lesser extent in those on the face, midline of the anterior abdominal wall, and genitals.

Table 23–2 summarizes the hormonal imbalances and endocrinologic conditions associated with either hyperpigmentation or hypopigmentation. These changes in pigmentation can be further subdivided, depending upon whether the pigmentary alteration is generalized in nature or localized.

Hyperpigmentation and Endocrinopathies

Generalized Hyperpigmentation

Three pituitary hormones, ACTH, α MSH, and β MSH, are capable of causing generalized hyperpigmentation in man. A 13 amino-acid polypeptide, α MSH has the same sequence as the first 13 amino acids of ACTH, while human β MSH consists of 22 amino acids whose arrangement is almost identical to the first one-third of the ACTH polypeptide. Humans given injections of MSH begin to darken in 24 hours, and continued daily doses increase the general darkening until the hormone is discontin-

ued, following which normal color returns in 3–5 weeks. The pigmentation in these subjects is most pronounced over the face and mucous membranes and within nevi. Similar pigmentation occurs following ACTH administration, but massive doses (2,400 units/day) must be used.

Normal human pituitary glands contain α MSH and β MSH as identified and quantitated by radioimmunoassay. β MSH accounts for 98 per cent of the MSH activity, while α MSH contributes 2 per cent. In view of the predominance of β MSH in the human pituitary and the somewhat unphysiologic amounts of ACTH required to cause hyperpigmentation, it is generally accepted that β MSH plays the major role in maintaining human pigmentation.

Patients with adrenal cortical insufficiency develop diffuse darkening of the exposed parts, such as face, neck, arms, and dorsum of the hands as well as the axillae, palmar creases, anogenital region, and buccal mucosa. Nevi darken, new ones may appear, and occasionally darkening of nevi occur several years before any other pigmentary changes. Scars that develop after the onset of adrenal insufficiency become hyperpigmented as well. The pigmentary changes are brought on by increased levels of MSH and ACTH in the plasma. Diminution of plasma levels of cortisol provokes a compensatory increased release of pituitary MSH and ACTH, probably mediated through activation of the respective hypothalamic releasing factor(s).

Generalized hyperpigmentation like that seen in Addison's disease also occurs in some patients with Cushing's disease who undergo bilateral adrenalectomy (with subsequent recognition of enlarging pituitary tumors) and in the ectopic ACTH syndrome caused by various neoplasms, such as carcinomas of the lung, liver, pancreas, and thymus. In each of these instances, plasma ACTH, α MSH, and β MSH have been characteristically elevated. The pigmentary changes are due to β MSH, because the quantity of ACTH and α MSH is too small to account for the amount of melanocyte-stimulating activity. Radioimmunoassays of tumors taken from hyperpigmented patients with the ectopic ACTH syndrome show large concentrations of β MSH, suggesting these nonpituitary neoplasms are capable of synthesizing this hormone. Such observations clearly account for the raised plasma levels of this polypeptide and the associated cutaneous pigmentation. In some patients, surgical removal of the tumor has resulted in reversal of cutaneous pigmentation.

The close biologic relationship among α MSH, β MSH, and ACTH can be appreciated from consideration of the fact that all these hormones are found to accompany each other not only in pituitary tissue but also in tumors associated with the ectopic ACTH syndrome, even though the tumors themselves arise from a variety of tissues. One could speculate, therefore, that the synthesis and secretion of these three polypeptides may be controlled by some common mechanism.

Chronic hyperthyroidism can be complicated by generalized hyperpigmentation similar to that seen in Addison's disease. This pigmentation is caused by increased MSH secretion by the pituitary.

Localized Hyperpigmentation

Melasma is a common disorder of large, pale, or sometimes dark brown, irregularly shaped macules over the forehead, upper lips, cheeks, chin, and neck seen in pregnant females. It occurs in association with the hyperpigmentation of the nipples, genitalia, and linea alba universally seen during pregnancy. Existing nevi also darken during pregnancy. Melasma clears several months after delivery, but it is likely to recur with subsequent pregnancies. During pregnancy, increased amounts of MSH and the high levels of estrogens and progesterone augment the pigmentary changes, particularly those over the face.

Melasma is also seen in 23–25 per cent of patients on oral contraceptives. Exposure to ultraviolet light accentuates this facial pigmentation. Unfortunately, in most patients, cessation of the anovulatory pills rarely results in complete resolution of the pigmentation.

Similar facial pigmentation may occur in association with ovarian tumors, diethylstilbestrol treatment of prostatic carcinoma in men, and conjugated estrogens for menopausal women.

Acanthosis nigricans, chiefly recognized for its ominous identification with upper gastrointestinal tract adenocarcinoma in adults, is more commonly seen in a benign setting in children and young adults with several metabolic and endocrinologic diseases. Acanthosis nigricans appears as hyperpigmented, soft, verrucous lesions found symmetrically distributed in the body folds and flexural areas (axillae, neck, groin, and antecubital and popliteal fossae). The lesions can occasionally involve the face, breasts, and inner aspects of the thighs. Perhaps most important in making the diagnosis is the soft, velvety texture imparted to the involved skin, which can be appreciated by gently stroking the skin. Acanthosis is most commonly seen in association with obesity, and if sufficient weight reduction is achieved, the lesions

improve. In some instances of acanthosis nigricans, the obesity is related to hypothalamic derangements, as seen in several case reports in children who sustained cranial trauma with concomitant hypothalamic obesity. In other instances, the obesity and acanthosis may be seen in patients with Stein-Leventhal syndrome. Brown et al. demonstrated additional links between acanthosis and endocrine disease in a series of 72 patients with these cutaneous lesions, including diabetes mellitus, lipodystrophic diabetes, adrenal insufficiency, hyperthyroidism, myxedema, and testicular carcinoma. In addition, these authors reported upon seven individuals without obesity who had pituitary tumors associated with acromegaly, gigantism, and Cushing's disease, all of whom had marked acanthosis nigricans. The acanthosis improved in only a few patients after their various endocrine disorders were successfully treated. The association of acanthosis with this seemingly large number of unrelated diseases is perplexing and as yet unexplained in the absence of any common denominator in these endocrine diseases which might serve as a pathogenetic mechanism. It is known, however, that diethylstilbestrol and corticosteroids can induce acanthosis in some individuals, so alterations in the levels of circulating hormones may play a direct role.

Two other well recognized but poorly understood diseases have localized pigmentary changes on the skin and may also be associated with endocrinologic disorders. The first, polyostotic fibrous dysplasia (Albright's syndrome), consists of disseminated osteitis fibrosa bone lesions, often in a segmental distribution; large, circumscribed, irregularly-shaped, dark brown, melanotic macules arranged in a linear or segmental pattern on one side of the midline of the body and generally overlying the hyperostotic and hypo-ostotic bone lesions; and precocious puberty in females but not males. The coincidence of the cutaneous and bony lesions involving similar segments of the body suggests that a neurologic or embryonic relationship underlies the pathogenesis of this syndrome, but it does not readily explain the association with precocious puberty in the female. The second disease associated with localized cutaneous pigmentation is neurofibromatosis (von Recklinghausen's disease), a dominantly inherited disorder in which a variety of neurogenic tumors are found in conjunction with localized melanin pigmentary macules or so-called café-au-lait spots. The neurogenic tumors involve the cutaneous nerves (neurofibromas), cranial nerves (optic and acoustic neuromas), and even the autonomic nervous system (pheochromocytoma). Approximately 10–15 per cent of patients with neurofibromatosis have pheochromocytomas and associated hypertension. The café-au-lait spots are light brown macules which are usually smaller, more numerous, have less irregular borders, and are more generally distributed over the body than the pigmented macules in Albright's disease. One other useful clinical feature in diagnosing neurofibromatosis is the presence of small, pigmented macules in the axillae (axillary freckling) in a very high percentage of patients. Neural cells and melanocytes both arise from the embryonic neural crest. It appears that proliferation of these neural crest derivatives, including melanocytes, accounts for the clinical findings of neurofibromatsis, suggesting an embryonic defect of neural crest origin.

Hypopigmentation and Endocrinopathies

Generalized Hypopigmentation

Loss of pituitary function results in a decrease in ACTH and MSH, with a resulting generalized hypopigmentation and pallor. Such patients have a decreased ability to tan.

Localized Hypopigmentation

Vitiligo is most commonly seen in patients without endocrine abnormalities, but in some vitiligo patients there appears to be a significant association of such disorders as Addison's disease, thyroid disease, and diabetes. Vitiligo presents as multiple, depigmented, oval or irregularly shaped macules, often symmetrically distributed over the extremities and around the body orifices.

Vitiligo is seen superimposed upon the generalized hyperpigmentation of Addison's disease in 15 per cent of patients. Successful therapy of the adrenal insufficiency not only causes the hyperpigmentation to regress but also may cause the vitiliginous areas to undergo repigmentation.

Vitiligo also appears more frequently in patients with thyroid disease (myxedema, thyroiditis, and thyrotoxicosis) than would occur by chance alone. Among patients with Graves' disease, 7 per cent have been reported to have vitiligo, but in these instances the clinical pattern of depigmentation is unusual in that it is confined primarily to the extremities, particularly the palms and soles. In some instances, the vitiligo precedes the onset of thyroid dysfunction by several years.

Recently seven patients with vitiligo have been reported in whom several endocrine diseases were found in each individual, including diabetes, hypothyroidism, and pernicious anemia (another disease in which vitiligo is more frequently found). In these patients, the vitiligo often preceded the development of the multiple diseases by many years; therefore, vitiligo may be an important external manifestation of impending or occult endocrine abnormalities.

The cause for this apparent increased frequency of vitiliginous lesions found in association with endocrine disease is unknown, but some studies suggest autoimmune processes might play a role since patients with vitiligo with or without endocrinopathies have various antithyroid, antiadrenal, and antiparietal cell antibodies in their circulation. It has been recognized that melanocytes are absent in vitiliginous skin, and, in like manner, in some patients with diabetes, myxedema, adrenal insufficiency, and pernicious anemia there is a loss of pancreatic islet cells, thyroid acinar cells, adrenal cortical cells, and gastric parietal cells, respectively. There is, of course, no direct evidence that the presence of antibodies directed toward these glands results in this cellular loss, but the analogy of cellular destruction in these endocrine diseases and vitiligo is apparent.

HORMONES AND CUTANEOUS APPENDAGES

Sebaceous Glands

Sebaceous glands on the face, upper back, and chest are dependent upon androgenic stimulation for their development and secretory activity. The glands' holocrine secretion (sebum) is composed of disintegrating sebaceous cells containing large amounts of triglycerides, squalene, and wax esters. The formation of sebum, oiliness of the skin, and occurrence of papulopustular acne result from cellular proliferations and lipid synthesis within the sebaceous glands. Androgens promote cellular turnover and increase the size of the sebaceous gland cells.

The amount of sebum production can be quantitated by collecting and measuring the amount of sebum delivered to a given area of facial skin per unit of time. Sebum production and the histologic size of facial sebaceous glands at various ages reflect the amounts of androgenic hormones produced by the testes, ovaries, and adrenal glands (Fig. 23–3). Before puberty the glands are small, and little sebum is secreted. Early in puberty, the glands enlarge, sebum production increases severalfold, and acne may develop in response to the increased production of testicular and ovarian androgens. The administration of low doses of androgen (5 mg. methyltestosterone daily) to prepubertal subjects stimulates sebaceous gland size and sebum production within 1–3 weeks. Sebaceous glands, therefore, are exquisitely sensitive to small amounts of androgens in the circulation. Testicular androgens play the predominant role in regulating sebaceous gland activity in the adult male, while androgens synthesized in the ovaries are of prime importance in the female. When testicular or ovarian androgenic stimulation is lost, as occurs after orchiectomy in men being treated for prostatic carcinoma or following menopause in females, there is a diminution in sebum production, but some sebaceous activity is retained in response to the remaining adrenal androgens (mainly dehydroepiandrosterone).

Estrogens administered in large doses to either men or women inhibit sebum production by decreasing the turnover time of the sebaceous cells. This may explain the therapeutic benefits of estrogens and anovulatory drugs in acne patients. It requires large pharmacologic doses of estrogens,

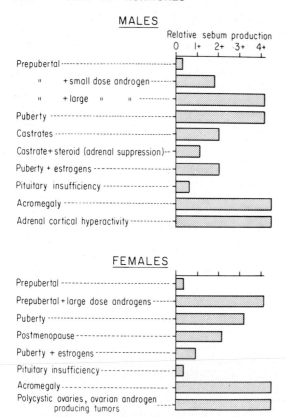

MALES

Relative sebum production
0   1+   2+   3+   4+

Prepubertal
"   + small dose androgen
"   + large   "   "
Puberty
Castrates
Castrate + steroid (adrenal suppression)
Puberty + estrogens
Pituitary insufficiency
Acromegaly
Adrenal cortical hyperactivity

FEMALES

Prepubertal
Prepubertal + large dose androgens
Puberty
Postmenopause
Puberty + estrogens
Pituitary insufficiency
Acromegaly
Polycystic ovaries, ovarian androgen
        producing tumors

Figure 23–3.   Relative amounts of sebum produced in normal males and females in relation to certain endocrinologic disorders.

however, to overcome the effects of physiologic amounts of androgens.

The apparent central role of androgens in regulating sebaceous gland activity has led to investigations of the metabolism of androgens *in vitro* by sebaceous glands. These studies reveal that the major metabolite of testosterone produced by the glands is dihydrotestosterone. It has, in turn, been suggested that dihydrotestosterone, a very potent androgen, is the primary androgenic stimulus for sebaceous gland activity. Acne-bearing skin produces 2–20 times more dihydrotestosterone than does normal skin, and normal facial skin converts more testosterone to dihydrotestosterone than normal skin from the back. These kinds of studies suggest that there are differences in sebaceous gland androgen metabolism and thus "end-organ" sensitivity to androgens in different regions of the body surface. These regional differences account in part for the distribution of acne, mediated by differential rates of conversion of testosterone to dihydrotestosterone. The individual rates of conversion may also explain the variability in severity of acne seen from patient to patient and the presence of severe acne in some women who have relatively low levels of plasma testosterone as compared to men.

Various endocrinologic disorders are accompanied by changes in sebum production and sometimes

acne (Fig. 23–3). Pituitary insufficiency causes decreased sebum production probably indirectly through its effects on other endocrine glands. Administration of gonadotropin to hypopituitary males results in a rise in sebum secretion. Increased sebum production in patients with acromegaly accounts for their greasy skin. Pituitary ablation decreases sebum excretion, and this decrease is greater in patients with a good therapeutic response to ablation than in those who obtain a poor result. Sebum excretion is said to be a more sensitive indicator of clinical activity in treated acromegaly patients than measurements of serum growth hormone.

Patients with masculinizing androgenic conditions, such as Cushing's disease, adrenal tumors, and adrenogenital syndrome, have significantly elevated rates of sebum production and often concomitant acne. Total or subtotal adrenalectomy in patients with Cushing's disease decreases sebaceous gland activity to normal.

Increased sebum secretion and acne also appear in those ovarian diseases characterized by increased androgen production, such as in certain tumors and polycystic ovaries. When clomiphene is given or wedge resection is performed in patients with polycystic ovaries, the acne disappears.

One additional form of hormonally induced acne should be mentioned—that caused by glucosteroids. Steroid acne is actually a follicular hyperkeratinization, or folliculitis, rather than a stimulation of sebaceous glands. Steroid acne differs from androgen-mediated acne in that the acneform eruption due to steroids consists of numerous small pustules and red papules all in the same stage of development, and no comedones are present. Steroid acne is found mainly on the trunk, shoulders, and upper arms with less involvement of the face, and it may appear as early as 2 weeks after large doses (i.e., greater than 60 mg. of prednisone) of steroids are begun.

Hair Growth

Abnormalities in hair growth must be regarded as affecting both hair growth cycle and pattern of distribution of hair types. Hormonal imbalances can alter each of these two aspects of hair growth to cause either increases or decreases in body hair. In assessing clinical problems of hair growth as they may relate to endocrine diseases, it is often of practical value to distinguish between hair pattern abnormalities and growth cycle changes.

Hair Pattern Defined.   Hair pattern is determined by the distinctive distribution of two kinds of hair over the body: (1) vellus hairs, which are fine textured and unpigmented and impart a nonhairy appearance to the integument, and (2) terminal hairs, which are coarse, thick, and heavily pigmented and give the impression of hairiness. The proportionate distribution of these two types of hair in various areas of the body is referred to as an individual's hair pattern. Normal hair pattern is determined by the patient's hereditary background as well as hormones, which collectively determine the formation of terminal or vellus hairs in various portions of the skin. An example of this is seen in male pattern baldness, which is genetically determined but requires the presence of androgenic hormones to initiate the transformation of terminal hairs to vellus hairs over the vertex of the scalp in some 60 per cent of Caucasian males by the age of 50 and to a lesser degree in 15 per cent of women past menopause.

Hair Pattern and Hormonal Control

There appear to be three general groupings of hairs, the patterns of which are distinguished by their response to physiologic hormone changes at the time of puberty. These three groups of hair are noted in Table 23–3. They are as follows:

1. Nonsexual hair, which does not depend on hormone stimulation. These hairs are generally of the same type in both pre- and postpubertal individuals (e.g., eyebrows, eyelashes, and hair on forearms and lower legs).

2. Ambosexual hair, which generally changes from vellus to terminal type at puberty in both males and females. These hairs, such as in the axilla and lower pubic triangle, depend upon low levels of circulating androgens from the adrenals and ovaries, as is found in normal females. Ambosexual hair is also found along the frontal hairline, and at puberty these terminal hairs are replaced by vellus hairs with a reshaping and some recession of the facial outline in 80 per cent of girls and nearly 100 per cent of males.

3. Male sexual hairs, such as those found in the beard areas, ears, tip of nose, presternal region, upper pubic triangle, and over certain areas of the temples and vertex of the scalp, occur in follicles which require high levels of circulating androgens for their stimulation. These follicles evolve into terminal hairs in places like the beard area and

into vellus hairs over the vertex of the scalp (male baldness) only in the presence of the large amounts of androgens produced in the male.

The pituitary plays a role in determining normal hair patterns to the extent that it controls androgen production by the ovary, testis, and adrenal. It is likely, however, that pituitary hormones also directly influence hair growth, as in the case of growth hormone, which causes a gradual increase in hair shaft diameter over the limbs and scalp from birth to puberty.

Hormone-Induced Abnormalities in Hair Pattern (Table 23–4). Clinically it is important to determine if hypertrichosis or alopecia is confined to any one or more of these three groups of hair follicles. If changes occur in nonsexual hair follicles, underlying causative endocrine disturbances are unlikely, whereas cases in which ambosexual or male sexual hair follicles exclusively are affected are usually associated with endocrine disease.

Ambosexual hair is lost in post-pubertal females who develop Addison's disease, and these hairs never grow in females who develop adrenal insufficiency prior to the onset of puberty. On the other hand, Addison's disease in the adult male is not accompanied by hair loss since the loss of adrenal androgens is overshadowed by the presence of large quantities of testicular androgens. In patients with ovarian agenesis, ambosexual hair is sparse, emphasizing the important role ovarian androgens play in maintaining growth of hair in these follicles. Patients with polycystic ovaries, whose abnormal ovaries synthesize increased amounts of androgens, often have mild to modest amounts of hirsutism of the face, breasts, and upper pubic triangle. Androgen-producing tumors of the ovaries or adrenals cause male sexual hair growth and male pattern baldness in association with other manifestations of masculinization, such as amenorrhea, clitoromegaly, deep voice, and acne. A similar series of events occurs in some pa-

TABLE 23–3. HORMONAL CLASSIFICATION OF HAIR PATTERN

| Type of Hair Follicle | Hair Regions | Types of Hair Produced | | Hormone | |
		Prepubertal	Postpubertal	Dependent	Source
Nonsexual hair	Eyebrows and lashes	Terminal	Terminal	Growth hormone	Pituitary
	Forearms and lower legs	Vellus	Terminal		
	Lower parts of scalp	Terminal	Terminal		
Ambosexual hair	Axilla	Vellus	Terminal	Androgen in low concentrations	Adrenal, ovary (females)
	Lower pubic triangle	Vellus	Terminal		
	Temporal and vertical parts of scalp	Terminal	Vellus		Adrenal (males)
Male sexual hair	Beard	Vellus	Terminal	Androgen in high concentrations	Testis
	Ears, nasal tip	Vellus	Terminal		
	Trunk (sternal)	Vellus	Terminal		
	Upper pubic triangle	Vellus	Terminal		
	Temporal and vertical parts of scalp	Terminal	Vellus		

TABLE 23-4. ABNORMALITIES OF HAIR PATTERN*
IN PATIENTS WITH ENDOCRINE DISEASES

Disease	Hair Change		
	Ambosexual Dec.	Male Sexual Inc.	Male Sexual Dec.
Addison's disease	+		
Ovarian agenesis	+		
Polycystic ovaries		+	
Androgen-secreting tumor of ovary or adrenal		+	
Cushing's syndrome		+	
Congenital adrenal hyperplasia		+	
Klinefelter's syndrome			+
Male Turner's syndrome			+
Eunuchism			+
Panhypopituitarism	+	+	
Acromegaly			+
Hypothyroidism	+	+	

*See Table 23-3 for listing of hair types.

tients with Cushing's syndrome and congenital adrenal hyperplasia. In women with virilizing syndromes, the extent of sexual hair growth is influenced in part by the genetic constitution and age of the patient.

Endocrine abnormalities of the testes also affect hair patterns, as exemplified by patients with Klinefelter's syndrome and male Turner's syndrome, in which the hypoandrogenemia accounts for the sparse beard and the axillary and suprapubic male sexual hair. Male eunuchs or males castrated before puberty have similar derangements in male sexual hair patterns, and these patients do not display male pattern baldness unless exogenous testosterone therapy is instituted.

Diseases of the pituitary gland also affect hair growth patterns. Acromegaly with high plasma levels of growth hormone causes an increase in hair shaft diameter, giving the hair over the extremities and scalp a coarse, thick texture. Hypopituitary dwarfs may be totally hairless, and panhypopituitarism in adults results in loss of axillary and pubic hair.

Although diseases of the thyroid gland do not specifically alter ambosexual or male sexual hair, they are associated with changes in hair texture that alter hair pattern. Hyperthyroidism induces a fine, silky textured hair, occasionally associated with diffuse scalp hair loss, while the lack of thyroxine in hypothyroidism causes the hair to be coarse, dry, and brittle. There may also be diffuse and occasionally marked loss of scalp hair as well as loss of hair from the lateral half of the eyebrows. A curious local alteration in hair growth is seen in the pretibial myxedematous plaques of patients with Graves' disease. In these plaques, the hair is coarse and pigmented and grows at an accelerated rate.

Hair Cycle and Hormonal Control

From the completion of its development in the last month of fetal life, every hair follicle undergoes recurring cycles of active growth, regression and rest. These stages are known as (1) anagen, the phase of active growth when a new hair shaft is formed by the follicle; (2) catagen, the phase of regression when the hair shaft stops growing and the hair root moves upward within the follicle and becomes club-shaped; and (3) telogen, the resting phase which heralds the ultimate loss of hair from the follicle after a new anagen hair forms in the underlying follicle. When hairs are pulled from the integument, they can be clinically identified. Anagen hairs have elongate roots surrounded by a conspicuous translucent sheath, while catagen and telogen hairs have short, club-shaped roots without a surrounding sheath. If clinical disorders of hair cycle are suspected, it is often useful to examine the roots of a number of hairs under the microscope after forcibly plucking them to determine the relative ratio of anagen to telogen hairs (A/T ratio) in the sampling.

The relative ratio of the number of anagen to telogen hairs in any given region of the body helps to determine the hairiness of that body surface. Regions such as the scalp with large numbers of follicles in anagen phase for long periods of time relative to telogen normally have a high A/T ratio and appear hairy, whereas the generally sparse-appearing general body hair has a low A/T ratio.

Hormone-Induced Abnormalities in Hair Cycle. Hormones influence the hair cycle by either (1) shortening telogen by initiating or prolonging anagen or both in more hair follicles (increase in A/T ratio and increased hairiness), or (2) prolonging telogen while inhibiting the initiation of anagen (decrease in A/T ratio and loss of hair).

Estrogens and probably progesterones stimulate hair growth by initiating anagen. Pregnant females or those on anovulatory drugs may note increasing hairiness over the face, breasts, and extremities. After the estrogenic stimulus is withdrawn, many hairs go into telogen and a telogen effluvium is observed, often involving the scalp with diffuse loss of hair. This occurs 2-3 months after the estrogenic stimulus is withdrawn. Patients concerned about this often impressive loss of scalp hair can be reassured since it is transient and will be replaced in several months. Inexplicably some women note diffuse balding while on anovulatory drugs. Hair growth commences when the medications are stopped.

Thyroxine stimulates hair growth by initiating anagen, although this does not cause clinical hirsutism in hyperthyroid patients. On the other hand, the diffuse alopecia of the scalp, eyebrow, and other body hair seen in hypothyroidism is partly explained by this loss of anagen stimulus, with a resulting increase in the number of telogen hairs and consequently a decrease in the A/T ratio. Normal anagen-telogen hair relationships are re-

TABLE 23–5. GENERAL SUMMARY OF SOME HORMONAL EFFECTS OF VARIOUS COMPONENTS OF THE INTEGUMENT

	Glucose Metabolism	Lipogenesis and Steroidogenesis	Epidermal Hormone Metabolism	Connective Tissue	Vasculature	Melanocytes	Sebaceous Glands	Hair
Insulin	X				X			
Testosterone		X	X				X	X
Estrogens		X	X		X	X	X	X
Progesterone		X	X					
Corticosteroids			X	X				
ACTH						X		
MSH						X		
Growth hormone				X			X	
Thyroxine	X			X	X	X		X
TSH				X				

Insulin controls glucose uptake and utilization as well as epidermal lipogenesis. Its relative absence in diabetes is thought to play a role in large and small vessel insufficiency, which leads to gangrene, necrobiosis lipoidica, shin spots, and bullosis diabeticorum.

Testosterone has been shown to accelerate sterol ester synthesis. It is actively metabolized by the epidermis as well as by the sebaceous glands and hair follicles. Indeed, its conversion to dihydrotestosterone correlates with acceleration of sebum production and hair growth, suggesting it is a tissue-active hormone.

Estrogens inhibit sterol metabolism and cause thinning of the epidermis. These hormones are actively metabolized by the epidermis, sebaceous glands, and hair. They suppress sebum production and stimulate hair growth. Excessive amounts cause cutaneous "spiders" and increase pigmentation over the face and nipples.

Progesterone inhibits steroidogenesis in human epidermis and is metabolized by human epidermis.

Corticosteroids are also metabolized by human epidermis. These hormones decrease dermal collagen synthesis, accounting for the thin skin, striae, easy bruising, and poor wound healing seen in Cushing's syndrome.

ACTH in large doses may cause generalized hyperpigmentation.

MSH, particularly β MSH, is the most important hormone in regard to hyperpigmentation. Lack of MSH, as in panhypopituitarism, causes decreased pigmentation.

Growth hormone induces fibroblastic proliferation with increased dermal collagen synthesis, causing thickening of the skin in patients with acromegaly. It also initiates thickening and coarsening of the hair and increased sebum production in patients with acromegaly.

Thyroxine stimulates cutaneous respiration and glucose assimilation in epidermis. It also controls the catabolism of dermal hyaluronic acid, so that in myxedema the catabolism is decreased and hyaluronic acid accumulates in the dermis. High levels of thyroxine, as occur in thyrotoxicosis, increase cutaneous blood flow, giving a soft, smooth texture to the skin. Diffuse pigmentation occasionally occurs in thyrotoxicosis, and thyroxine also stimulates hair growth.

TSH appears to directly stimulate the synthesis of glycosaminoglycans in the dermis.

stored during replacement therapy with thyroid hormone.

Idiopathic Hirsutism

Most cases of hirsutism occur in women with no demonstrable endocrinologic disease. Some of these cases are merely the expression of a wide variation in hairiness dependent upon hereditary factors. In general, dark haired, pigmented Caucasians of either sex, such as persons of Mediterranean stock, tend to be more hirsute, while Orientals and American Indians have scanty hair. McKnight reported on 400 consecutive observations of normal women students attending a general medical clinic; 84 per cent had terminal hair on the lower arms and legs, 26 per cent had such hair on the face and upper lip, 17 per cent had hair on the chest, and in 35 per cent, abdominal hair extending up the linea alba was noted.

It is obvious that endocrine disease is more likely to account for the hirsutism if features of defeminization or masculinization are present. It is of help to the clinician in analyzing such cases if he finds either (1) coarse ear hair or (2) a "disperse" pattern of pubic hair in females, since these kinds of hair growth are considered to be truly masculine and suggest altered androgen metabolism.

Although the cause of idiopathic hirsutism is unknown, several lines of evidence suggest that it may be a manifestation of subtle hypersecretion of adrenocortical androgens. Some patients have increases in total or fractional 17-ketosteroid excretion, and Perloff et al. showed that daily prednisone treatment reduced this increased secretion. The adrenal glands of some patients with idiopathic hirsutism may be more sensitive to ACTH stimulation than those of nonhirsute females. Plasma and urinary testosterone levels show a tendency toward elevated levels, but there is considerable overlap with normal values. Bardin and Lipsett, however, found increased production rates of adrenal testosterone in these women, often associated with increased androgen metabolic clearance rates, explaining why absolute plasma testosterone concentrations were often normal.

Hair Follicle Metabolism

Studies on isolated hair follicles have provided information on the metabolic effects hormones have on the follicle cells responsible for hair growth and have further suggested that individual variations in hair growth may reflect differences in hair follicle end-organ response to hormones.

Growing hairs from human integument reveal net shifts in glucose metabolic pathways during the transformation of the resting into the growing anagen stage, which can be summarized as follows: compared with that in resting follicles, glucose utilization in growing follicles increases 200 per cent, glycolysis 200 per cent, activity of the pentose

cycle 800 per cent, and metabolism by other pathways 150 per cent. The most remarkable metabolic change in the transition from telogen to anagen hair, then, is the activation of one of the respiratory pathways, the hexose monophosphate shunt, which also produces large amounts of NADPH. NADPH is apparently important in the metabolism of testosterone by hair follicles. Hair follicles metabolize testosterone to either dihydrotestosterone or androstenedione, but the 5α reductase pathway to dihydrotestosterone is dependent upon NADPH. Thus the growing hair follicles, which generate more NADPH, convert larger amounts of testosterone to dihydrotestosterone than resting hairs. Dihydrotestosterone (but not testosterone or androstenedione) in turn has been shown to inhibit adenyl cyclase and reduce intracellular cyclic AMP in scalp hair follicles, while estrone has an opposite effect, increasing follicular cells' cyclic AMP. Therefore, there is a close relationship between growing hairs and follicles which convert more dihydrotestosterone from testosterone in the presence of decreased cyclic AMP, and in an opposite manner those follicles converting more estradiol to estrone are in a resting phase with increased intracellular follicular cyclic AMP.

These alterations in steroid metabolism and cyclic AMP content probably have diverse effects on various pathways of energy metabolism, which in turn inhibit or increase hair growth by affecting the energy supply for keratin synthesis. Further studies on the metabolism of various hormones by isolated hair follicles will continue to identify the means by which hormones influence hair patterns and hair growth cycles in normal individuals and in those with endocrine diseases.

CONCLUSION

The wide variety of effects hormones have on the integument clearly marks the skin as an important endocrine end organ (Table 23–5). Although some of the effects can now be directly related to certain clinical cutaneous alterations seen in endocrinologic diseases, for the most part this is not possible, as the hormonal influences on the skin are just now beginning to receive investigative attention. Even so, the cutaneous changes in endocrine disease compel the clinician to examine the skin carefully.

REFERENCES

Hormones and the Epidermis and Dermis

GLUCOSE AND LIPID METABOLISM

Bloch, K.: Biogenesis and transformations of squalene, In *Biosynthesis of Terdenes and Sterols.* Wolstenholme, G. E. W., and O'Connor, M. (eds.), Boston, Little, Brown and Co., 1959.

Crounse, R. G., and Rothberg, S.: Evaluation of the enzymes of the Krebs-Henseleit cycle in human epidermis. *J. Invest. Derm. 36:*287, 1961.

Decker, R. H.: Nature and regulation of energy metabolism in the epidermis. *J. Invest. Derm.* 57:351, 1971.

Freinkel, R. K.: Effect of thyroxine administration on the metabolism of guinea pig skin. *J. Invest. Derm.* 38:31, 1962.

Freinkel, R. K.: Metabolism of glucose-C-14 by human skin *in vitro. J. Invest. Derm.* 34:37, 1960.

Gilbert, D.: Demonstration of a respiratory control mechanism in human skin *in vitro. J. Invest. Derm.* 43:45, 1964.

Halprin, K. M., and Ohkawara, A.: Glucose and glycogen metabolism in the human epidermis. *J. Invest. Derm.* 46:43, 1966.

Horlick, L.: Effect of diethylstilbestrol on skin sterols of the male rat. *J. Lipid Res.* 9:773, 1968.

Hsia, S. L.: Potentials in exploring the biochemistry of human skin, In *Essays in Biochemistry.* Vol. 7. Academic Press, 1971.

Hsia, S. L., Dreize, M. A., et al.: Lipid metabolism in human skin. II. A study of lipogenesis in skin of diabetic patients. *J. Invest. Derm.* 47:443, 1966.

Hsia, S. L., Fulton, J. E., et al.: Lipid synthesis from acetate-1-¹⁴C by suction blister epidermis and other skin components. *Proc. Soc. Exp. Biol. Med.* 135:285, 1970.

Kalenberg, A., and Kalant, N.: The effect of insulin and diabetes on glucose metabolism in human skin. *Canad. J. Biochem.* 44:801, 1966.

Kandutsch, A. A., and Russell, A. E.: Preputial gland tumor steroids. III. A metabolic pathway from lanosterol to cholesterol. *J. Biol. Chem.* 235:2256, 1960.

Liebsohn, E., Appel, B., et al.: Respiration of human skin: normal values, pathologic changes and effect of certain agents on oxygen uptake. *J. Invest. Derm.* 30:1, 1958.

Menton, D. N.: The effects of essential fatty acid deficiency on the skin of the mouse. *Amer. J. Anat.* 122:337, 1968.

Mier, P. D.: The carbohydrate metabolism of skin. *Brit. J. Derm.* 81 (Suppl. 2):14, 1969.

Nicolaides, N., Reiss, O. K., et al.: Studies of the *in vitro* lipid metabolism of the human skin. I. Biosynthesis in scalp skin. *J. Amer. Chem. Soc.* 77:1535, 1955.

Pomerantz, S. H.: Citric acid cycle in young rat skin. *J. Biol. Chem.* 236:2863, 1961.

Pomerantz, S. H., and Asbornsen, M. T.: Glucose metabolism in young rat skin. *Arch. Biochem. Biophys.* 93:147, 1961.

Srere, P. A., Chaikoff, J. L., et al.: The extrahepatic synthesis of cholesterol. *J. Biol. Chem.* 182:629, 1950.

Vroman, H. E., Nemecek, R. A., et al.: Synthesis of lipids from acetate by human preputial and abdominal skin *in vitro. J. Lipid Res.* 10:507, 1969.

Wheatley, V. R., Hodgins, L. T., et al.: Cutaneous lipogenesis: precursors utilized by guinea pig skin for lipid synthesis. *J. Lipid Res.* 12:347, 1971.

Wilson, J. D.: Studies on the regulation of cholesterol synthesis in the skin and preputial gland of the rat, In *Advances in Biology of Skin.* Vol. IV. *The Sebaceous Glands.* Montagna, W., Ellis, R. A., et al. (eds.), New York, Pergamon Press, 1963.

Yardley, H. J.: Sterol and keratinization. *Brit. J. Derm.* 81 (Suppl. 2):29, 1969.

Yardley, H. J., and Godfrey, G.: Direct evidence for the hexose monophosphate pathway of glucose metabolism in skin. *Biochem. J.* 86:101, 1963.

Yardley, H. J., and Godfrey, G.: Metabolism of phosphate esters and phospholipids in skin maintained *in vitro. J. Invest. Derm.* 43:51, 1964.

Ziboh, V. A., and Hsia, S. L.: Lipogenesis in rat skin: a possible regulatory role of glycerol 3-phosphate. *Arch. Biochem. Biophys.* 131:153, 1969.

Ziboh, V. A., Dreize, M. A., et al.: Inhibition of lipid synthesis and glucose-6-phosphate dehydrogenase in rat skin by dehydroepiandrosterone. *J. Lipid Res.* 11:346, 1970.

CUTANEOUS METABOLISM OF HORMONES

Cameron, E. H. D., Baillie, A. H., et al.: Transformation *in vitro* of (7α-³H) dehydroepiandrosterone to (³H) testosterone by skin from men. *J. Endocr.* 35:XIX, 1966.

Frost, P., Gomez, E. C., et al.: Metabolism of progesterone-4-¹⁴C in human skin and vaginal mucosa. *Biochemistry, Easton* 8:948, 1969.

Gomez, E. C., and Hsia, S. L.: Studies on cutaneous metabolism of testosterone-4-¹⁴C and Δ⁴-androstene-3,17-dione-4-¹⁴C in human skin. *Biochemistry, Easton* 7:24, 1968.

Grant, J. K.: The metabolism of steroids by skin in man. *Brit. J. Derm.* 81 (Suppl. 2):1969.

Hsia, S. L., and Hao, Y. L.: Metabolic transformations of cortisol-4-¹⁴C in human skin. *Biochemistry, Easton* 5:1469, 1966.

Hsia, S. L., and Hao, Y. L.: Transformation of cortisone to cortisol in human skin. *Steroids* 10:489, 1967.

Kelch, R. P., Lindholm, U. B., et al.: Testosterone metabolism in target tissues. 2. Human fetal and adult reproductive tissues, perianal skin and skeletal muscle. *J. Clin. Endocr.* 32:449, 1971.

Kim, M. H., and Herrmann, W. L.: *In vitro* metabolism of dehydroepiandrosterone sulfate in foreskin, abdominal skin and vaginal mucosa. *J. Clin. Endocr.* 28:187, 1968.

Mauvis-Jarvis, P., Bercovici, J. P., et al.: *In vitro* studies on testosterone metabolism by skin of normal males and patients with the syndrome of testicular feminization. *J. Clin. Endocr.* 29:417, 1969.

Mauvis-Jarvis, P., Crepy, O., et al.: Further studies on the pathophysiology of testicular feminization syndrome. *J. Clin. Endocr.* 32:568, 1971.

Northcut, R. C., Island, D., et al.: An explanation for target organ unresponsiveness to testosterone in the testicular feminization syndrome. *J. Clin. Endocr.* 29:422, 1969.

Rogone, E. L.: Testosterone metabolism by human male mammary skin. *Steroids* 7:489, 1966.

Rosenfeld, R. L., Lawrence, A. M., et al.: Androgens and androgen responsiveness in the feminizing testicular syndrome. *J. Clin. Endocr.* 32:625, 1971.

Stickland, A. L., and French, F. S.: Absence of response to dihydrotestosterone in the syndrome of testicular feminization. *J. Clin. Endocr.* 29:1284, 1969.

Strauss, J. S., and Pochi, P. E.: Recent advances in androgen metabolism and their relation to the skin. *Arch. Derm.* 100:621, 1969.

Voigt, W., Fernandez, E. P., et al.: Transformation of testosterone into 17β-hydroxy-5α-androstan-3-one by microsomal preparations of human skin. *J. Biol. Chem.* 245:5594, 1970.

Weinstein, G. D., Frost, P., et al.: *In vitro* interconversion of estrone and 17β-estradiol in human skin and vaginal mucosa. *J. Invest. Derm.* 51:4, 1968.

Wilson, J. D., and Walker, J. D.: The conversion of testosterone to 5-α-androstan-17β-ol-3-one (dihydrotestosterone) by skin of man. *J. Clin. Invest.* 48:371, 1969.

Wotiz, H. H., Mescon, H., et al.: The *in vitro* metabolism of testosterone by human skin. *J. Invest. Derm.* 26:113, 1956.

DERMAL CONNECTIVE TISSUE AND HORMONES

Asboe-Hansen, G.: Hormonal effects on connective tissue. *Physiol. Rev.* 38:446, 1958.

Asboe-Hansen, G. (ed.): *Hormones and Connective Tissue.* Baltimore, Williams and Wilkins Co., 1966.

Kriss, J. P., Pleshakov, V., et al.: Isolation and identification of the long-acting thyroid stimulator and its relation to hyperthyroidism and circumscribed pretibial myxedema. *J. Clin. Endocr.* 24:1005, 1964.

Kriss, J. P., Pleshakov, V., et al.: Therapy with occlusive dressings of pretibial myxedema with fluocinolone acetonide. *J. Clin. Endocr.* 27:595, 1967.

Parker, F., and Short, J. M.: Xanthomatosis associated with hyperlipoproteinemia. *J. Invest. Derm.* 55:71, 1970.

Schermer, D. R., Roenigk, H. H., et al.: Relationship of long-acting thyroid stimulator to pretibial myxedema. *Arch. Derm.* 102:62, 1970.

Sheppard, R. H., and Meema, H. E.: Skin thickness in endocrine disease. *Ann. Intern. Med.* 66:531, 1967.

Sisson, J. C.: Hyaluronic acid in localized myxedema. *J. Clin. Endocr.* 28:433, 1968.

Szirmai, J. A.: The organization of the dermis, In *Advances in Biology of Skin.* Vol. X. *The Dermis.* Montagna, W., Bentley, J. P., et al. (eds.), New York, Meredith Corp., 1968.

DERMAL VASCULATURE AND HORMONES

Allen, G. E.: Diabetes mellitus and the skin. *Practitioner* 203:189, 1969.

Allen, G. E., and Hadden, D. R.: Bullous lesions of the skin in diabetes (bullosis diabeticorum). *Brit. J. Derm.* 82:216, 1970.

Braverman, I. M.: *Skin Signs of Systemic Disease.* Philadelphia, W. B. Saunders Co., 1970.

Danowski, T. S., Sabeh, G., et al.: Shin spots and diabetes mellitus. *Amer. J. Med. Sci.* 251:570, 1966.

Fox, R. H., Goldsmith, R., et al.: Bradykinin as a vasodilator in man. *J. Physiol.* 157:589, 1961.

Jelinek, J. E.: Oral contraceptives and the skin. *Amer. Fam. Physician* 4:68, 1971.

Kontos, H. A., Shapiro, W., et al.: Mechanism of certain abnormalities of the circulation to the limbs in thyrotoxicosis. *J. Clin. Invest.* 44:947, 1965.

Kurwa, A., Roberts, P., et al.: Concurrence of bullous and atrophic skin lesions in diabetes mellitus. *Arch. Derm.* 103:670, 1971.

Levine, R. J., and Sjoersdma, A.: Pressor amines and the carcinoid flush. *Ann. Intern. Med.* 58:818, 1963.

Mason, D. T., and Melmon, K. L.: Abnormal forearm vascular responses in the carcinoid syndrome: the role of kinins and kinin generating system. *J. Clin. Invest.* 45:1685, 1966.

Melin, H.: An atrophic circumscribed skin lesion in the lower extremities of diabetics. *Acta Med. Scand.* 176(Suppl. 423):1, 1964.

Melmon, K. K., Sjoersdma, A., et al.: Distinctive clinical and therapeutic aspects of the syndrome associated with bronchial carcinoid tumors. *Amer. J. Med.* 39:568, 1965.

Muller, S. A., and Winkelmann, R. K.: Necrobiosis lipoidica diabeticorum. *Arch. Derm.* 93:272, 1966.

Oates, J. A., and Melmon, K. L.: Biochemical and physiologic studies of the kinins in carcinoid syndrome, In *Symposium on Hypotensive Peptides.* Erdos, E. G., Back, N., et al. (eds.), Berlin, Springer Verlag, 1966.

Oates, J. A., and Sjoersdma, A.: A unique syndrome associated with secretion of 5-hydroxytryptophan by metastatic gastric carcinoids. *Amer. J. Med.* 32:333, 1962.

Hormones, Melanocytes, and Pigmentation

Abe, K., Island, D. P., et al.: Radioimmunologic evidence for α-MSH (melanocyte stimulating hormone) in human pituitary and tumor tissues. *J. Clin. Endocr.* 27:46, 1967.

Abe, K., Nicholson, W. E., et al.: Radioimmunoassay of β-MSH in human plasma and tissues. *J. Clin. Invest.* 46:1609, 1967.

Benedict, P. H., Szabo, G., et al.: Melanotic macules in Albright's syndrome and in neurofibromatosis. *J.A.M.A.* 205:618, 1968.

Bloom, R. E., and Rothman, S.: Juvenile acanthosis nigricans. *Arch. Derm.* 71:413, 1955.

Brostoff, J., Bor, S., et al.: Autoantibodies in patients with vitiligo. *Lancet* 2:177, 1969.

Brown, J., and Winkelmann, R. K.: Acanthosis nigricans. A study of 90 cases. *Medicine* 47:33, 1968.

Brown, J., Winkelmann, R. K., et al.: Acanthosis nigricans and pituitary tumors. *J.A.M.A.* 198:619, 1966.

Crowe, F. W.: Axillary freckling as a diagnostic aid in neurofibromatosis. *Ann. Intern. Med.* 61:1142, 1964.

Cunliffe, W. J., Hall, R., et al.: Vitiligo, thyroid disease and autoimmunity. *Brit. J. Derm.* 80:135, 1968.

Fitzpatrick, T. B., and Mihm, M. C.: Abnormalities of the melanin pigmentary system. In *Dermatology in General Medicine.* Fitzpatrick, T. B., Arndt, K. A., et al. (eds.), New York, McGraw-Hill, 1971.

Katzenellenbogen, I.: Dermatoendocrinological syndrome due to diethylstilbestrol. *J.A.M.A.* 161:1695, 1956.

Kawamura, T., Fitzpatrick, T. B., et al.: *Biology of Normal and Abnormal Melanocytes.* Tokyo, University of Tokyo Press, 1971.

Lee, T. H., and Lee, M. S.: Measurement and electrophoretic study of MSH-like substances in human pregnancy urine. *J. Clin. Endocr.* 29:660, 1969.

Lerner, A. B.: Hormones and skin color. *Sci. Amer.* 205:99, 1961.

Lerner, A. B., and McGuire, J. S.: Melanocyte-stimulating hormone and adrenocorticotrophic hormone. *New Eng. J. Med.* 270:539, 1964.

Lerner, A. B., Shizume, K., et al.: The mechanism of endocrine control of melanin pigmentation. *J. Clin. Endocr.* 14:1463, 1954.

McGregor, B. C., Katz, H. I., et al.: Vitiligo and multiple glandular insufficiencies. *J.A.M.A.* 219:724, 1972.

McGuire, J., Moellmann, G., et al.: Cytochalasin B and pigment granule translocation. *J. Cell Biol.* 52:754, 1972.

Nelson, D. H., Meakin, J. W., et al.: ACTH-producing tumor of the pituitary gland. *New Eng. J. Med.* 259:161, 1958.

Ochi, Y., and DeGroot, L. J.: Vitiligo in Graves' disease. *Ann. Intern. Med.* 71:935, 1969.

Quevedo, W. C., Szabo, G., et al.: Biology of the melanin pigmentary system, In *Dermatology in General Medicine.* Fitzpatrick, T. B., Arndt, K. A., et al. (eds.), New York, McGraw-Hill, 1971.

Resnik, C. S.: Melasma induced by oral contraceptive drugs. *J.A.M.A.* 199:601, 1967.

Snell, R. S.: Hormonal control of pigmentation in man and other mammals, In *The Pigmentary System.* Vol. 8. *Advances in Biology of Skin.* Montagna, W., and Hu, F. (eds.), New York, Pergamon Press, 1967.

Snell, R. S., and Bischitz, P. G.: The melanocytes and melanin in human abdominal wall skin: a survey made at different ages in both sexes and during pregnancy. *J. Anat.* 97:361, 1963.

Taleisnik, S., and Orias, R.: A melanocyte-stimulating hormone releasing factor in hypothalamic extracts. *Amer. J. Physiol.* 208:293, 1965.

Taleisnik, S., and Tomatis, M. E.: Melanocyte-stimulating hormone—releasing and inhibiting factors in two hypothalamic extracts. *Endocrinology* 81:819, 1967.

Tucker, W. R., Klink, D., et al.: Insulin resistance and acanthosis nigricans. *Diabetes* 13:395, 1964.

Hormones and Cutaneous Appendages

SEBACEOUS GLANDS

Burton, J. L., Libman, L. J., et al.: Sebum excretion in acromegaly. *Brit. Med. J.* 139:406, 1972.

Milne, J. A.: The metabolism of androgens by sebaceous glands. *Brit. J. Derm.* 81(Suppl. 2):23, 1969.

Montagna, W., Ellis, R. A., et al.: The sebaceous glands, In *Advances in Biology of Skin IV.* New York, Macmillan Co., 1963.

Pochi, P. E., and Strauss, J. S.: Effect of cyclic administration of conjugated equine estrogens on sebum production in women. *J. Invest. Derm.* 47:582, 1966.

Pochi, P. E., and Strauss, J. S.: Effect of prednisone on sebaceous gland secretion. *J. Invest. Derm.* 49:456, 1967.

Pochi, P. E., and Strauss, J. S.: Effect of sequential mestranol-chlormadinone on sebum production. *Arch. Derm.* 95:47, 1967.

Pochi, P. E., and Strauss, J. S.: Sebaceous gland response in man to the administration of testosterone, Δ⁴-androstenedione, and dehydroisoandrosterone. *J. Invest. Derm.* 52:32, 1969.

Pochi, P. E., Strauss, J. S., et al.: Plasma testosterone and estrogen levels, urine testosterone excretion, and sebum production in males with acne vulgaris. *J. Clin. Endocr.* 25:1660, 1965.

Sansone, G., and Reisner, R. M.: Differential rates of conversion of testosterone to dihydrotestosterone in acne and in normal human skin—a possible pathogenic factor in acne. *J. Invest. Derm.* 56:366, 1971.

Strauss, J. S.: Diseases of sebaceous glands, In *Dermatology in General Medicine.* Fitzpatrick, T. B., Arndt, K. A., et al. (eds.), New York, McGraw-Hill, 1971.

Strauss, J. S., and Pochi, P. E.: The hormonal control of human sebaceous glands: observations in certain endocrine disorders. *Clin. Endocr.* 2:798, 1968.

Strauss, J. S., and Pochi, P. E.: The human sebaceous gland: its regulation by steroidal hormones and its use as an end organ for assaying androgenicity *in vivo. Recent Progr. Hormone Res.* 19:385, 1963.

Summerly, R., and Woodbury, S.: The *in vitro* incorporation of ¹⁴C-acetate into the isolated sebaceous glands and appendage-freed epidermis of human skin. *Brit. J. Derm.* 85:424, 1971.

Sweeney, T. M., Szarnicki, R. J., et al.: The effect of estrogen and androgen on the sebaceous gland turnover time. *J. Invest. Derm.* 53:8, 1969.

HAIR GROWTH

Adachi, K., and Kano, M.: Adenyl cyclase in human hair follicles: its inhibition by dihydrotestosterone. *Biochem. Biophys. Res. Commun.* 41:884, 1970.

Adachi, K., Takayasu, S., et al.: Human hair follicles: metabolism and control mechanisms. *J. Soc. Cosmet. Chem.* 21:901, 1970.

Baker, L., Kaye, R., et al.: Diazoxide treatment of idiopathic hypoglycemia of infancy. *J. Pediat.* 71:494, 1967.

Bardin, C. W., and Lipsett, M. B.: Testosterone and androstenedione blood production rates in normal women and women with idiopathic hirsutism or polycystic ovaries. *J. Clin. Invest.* 46:891, 1967.

Brooksbank, B. W. L.: Endocrinological aspects of hirsutism. *Physiol. Rev.* 41:623, 1961.

Forbes, A. P.: Hirsutism, In *Dermatology in General Medicine.* Fitzpatrick, T. B., Arndt, K. A., et al. (eds.), New York, McGraw-Hill, 1971.

Freinkel, R. K., and Freinkel, N.: Hair growth and alopecia in hypothyroidism. *Arch. Derm. 106*:349, 1972.

Garn, S. M.: Types and distribution of the hair in man. *Ann. N.Y. Acad. Sci. 53*:498, 1951.

Liddle, G. W.: Cushing's syndrome and problems of hirsutism, In *The Hirsute Female.* Greenblatt, R. B. (ed.), Springfield, Illinois, Charles C Thomas, 1963.

Livingston, S., Petersen, D., et al.: Hypertrichosis occurring in association with dilantin therapy. *J. Pediat. 47*:351, 1955.

Lloyd, C. W., Moses, A. M., et al.: Studies of adrenocortical function of women with idiopathic hirsutism: response to 25 units of ACTH. *J. Clin. Endocr. 23*:413, 1963.

Lynfield, Y. L.: Effect of pregnancy on the human hair cycle. *J. Invest. Derm. 35*:323, 1960.

McKnight, E.: The prevalence of "hirsutism" in young women. *Lancet 1*:410, 1964.

Muller, S. A.: Hirsutism. *Amer. J. Med. 46*:803, 1969.

Munroe, D. D.: Disorders of hair, In *Dermatology in General Medicine.* Fitzpatrick, T. B., Arndt, K. A., et al. (eds.), New York, McGraw-Hill, 1971.

Perloff, W. H., Channick, B. T., et al.: Clinical management of idiopathic hirsutism (adrenal virilism). *J.A.M.A. 167*:2041, 1958.

Plager, J. E., Cushman, P., et al.: The plasma cortisol response to ACTH in "idiopathic hirsutism." *J. Clin. Invest. 40*:1315, 1961.

Rampini, E., Davis, B. P., et al.: Cyclic changes in the metabolism of estradiol by rat skin during the hair cycle. *J. Invest. Derm. 57*:75, 1971.

Rook, A.: Endocrine influences on hair growth. *Brit. Med. J. 1*:609, 1965.

Strauss, J. S., and Pochi, P. E.: Recent advances in androgen metabolism and their relation to the skin. *Arch. Derm. 100*:621, 1969.

Wieland, R. G., Vorys, N., et al.: Studies of female hirsutism. *Amer. J. Med. 41*:927, 1966.

CHAPTER 24

Muscle and Hormones

By Carl M. Pearson

The general concept that disorders of metabolism, especially those mediated by endocrine glands, may induce disorders of the neuromuscular system has long been recognized. On the other hand, it is not always clear whether the effects of hyper- or hyposecretion of one of the endocrine glands is directed primarily at the muscle fiber or its motor end plate or at the peripheral nerve or the anterior horn cell supplying muscle. It is likely that the effect may be exerted to a variable extent at each of those levels. Aside from the use of very special diagnostic techniques such as electron microscopy, nerve conduction measurements, or special histochemical procedures directed at delineating the nature of the neuromuscular junction (motor end plate), for assessment of nerve or motor end plate dysfunction, it is not possible to be certain that these structures are in some fashion involved in the abnormal metabolic or endocrinologic disorder. Thus descriptions of the various "myop-

athies," as defined in the following sections, have as an added implication the possible involvement of the neural apparatus at one or more levels in addition to involvement of a myopathic component.

Since the peripheral action of the hormones is so complex, involving such widespread chemical responders as cyclic AMP (Butcher et al.), it is possible that the hormonal effects may be multiple. Furthermore, in such states as diabetes and periodic paralysis, either the accumulation of glycogen (or depletion thereof) or alterations in the permeability of muscle cell membranes may be at fault.

The detection of myopathy or neuropathy by clinical methods alone presents significant difficulties. For instance, weakness and wasting, which are the most obvious clinical signs of disease of muscle and its peripheral nerve, may not be due specifically to the endocrinopathy alone but may be secondary to musculoskeletal pain which develops in some pathologic conditions. Furthermore, if muscular weakness occurs in conjunction with a mild endocrinopathy in an elderly patient, it is most difficult to differentiate the somewhat subtle effect of over- or undersecretion of one of the endocrine glands in comparison with the natural aging processes that may be occurring at the same time.

It is probable that most if not all of the endocrine glands have some effect upon muscle fiber metabolism. Such effects may alter energy metabolism within muscle, thereby leading to weakness from depletion of energy stores, membrane alterations, or insufficient replacement of contractile or other protein constituents of the muscle fiber itself. Furthermore, muscle carbohydrate metabolism is clearly regulated by insulin and glucagon and very likely by growth hormones (as in acromegalic myopathy). Intrafiber electrolyte imbalances may occur from malfunction of the adrenal glands, of the parathyroid glands, and possibly of the thyroid gland in certain susceptible persons.

The ultimate in clinical detection of a myopathic state is demonstrable muscle weakness, muscular wasting, or both. Skill in detecting such weakness and careful assessment of the degree of muscle involvement are required before concluding that such a situation exists. Even though muscle weakness is clinically demonstrable in some of the endocrine myopathies or neuromyopathies, upon histologic examination little pathologic change can be found in muscle tissue. Thus a number of the subtle changes of "endocrine myopathy" may reside in the metabolic state of muscle and its capacity to perform its primary function, contraction, without any significant morphologic counterpart that can be demonstrated by the techniques currently available to the pathologist, the histochemist, or the electron microscopist.

THYROID DYSFUNCTION

Of all the myopathies associated with endocrine disease, those associated with alterations of thyroid function are the most clearly defined. The myopathies associated with thyroid hormone dysfunction have been subclassified into several categories by Millikan and Haines.

Thyrotoxic Myopathy

Since Basedow and Graves described hyperthyroidism, muscular weakness and atrophy have been known as common features of this disorder. An actual myopathy, however, was considered to be a relatively rare disorder until the studies by Hed et al. Much of this work was done in the early 1960's and was primarily the result of careful electromyographic studies which delineated that, in a consecutive series of patients with thyrotoxicosis, about 80 per cent of them had physical evidence of muscle weakness or electromyographic signs of myopathy or both.

It should be noted that, at the end of the last century, Bathurst was the first to publish a case of thyrotoxicosis that was accompanied by profound muscular weakness and atrophy. In more recent years, Satoyoshi and his associates have done a great deal to delineate not only the electrical but also the histologic aspects of the myopathy that appears in thyrotoxicosis. From their study of 240 hospitalized patients in Japan, where this condition appears to occur more frequently than elsewhere in the world, these authors have demonstrated that, regardless of sex, almost 62 per cent of thyrotoxic patients demonstrated weakness or atrophy or both of the muscles of the shoulder and pelvic girdle. The proportion of persons with muscle atrophy or weakness or both of moderate or marked severity seemed to increase with age. These features in their very severe form were encountered in nearly 30 per cent of persons with a history of unrecognized hyperthyroidism of over three years in duration. Regardless of the initial severity, it was possible to observe almost complete return to normal muscle bulk and strength following adequate treatment of the hyperthyroidism. There were many suggestions in these studies that

a definite myopathy frequently resulted from prolonged but unrecognized hyperthyroidism.

In chronic thyrotoxic myopathy, which appears to occur more often in the older thyrotoxic patients, the muscle lesion may be the presenting complaint. In most patients, however, the onset of muscle symptoms is usually concurrent with those of the hyperthyroid state itself. Involvement of bulbar musculature with weakness of speech and dysphagia and normal or even hyperactive tendon reflexes may suggest the diagnosis of a motor neuron disease, a differential diagnosis of which is also justified by the clinical occurrence of fasciculations, which may be found in more than 50 per cent of cases (Shy).

Histopathologic studies of muscle biopsy specimens in thyrotoxic myopathy have produced varied and often inconclusive results. In many patients, even though there is significant weakness present, the findings on routine histology may be almost negligible. Occasionally one does find spotty, atrophic muscle fibers as well as rare degeneration of isolated muscle fibers, minimal connective tissue proliferation or fatty infiltration, and occasional increases in sarcolemmal nuclei. About the most frequent but not necessarily most characteristic histologic feature of thyrotoxic myopathy is the presence of lymphorrhages (Thorn and Eder). In concert with the histology of muscle in thyrotoxicosis, the histologic changes in thyrotoxic myopathy are also rarely striking. They correlate very poorly with the often striking clinical weakness. It has therefore been suggested by several authors (Satoyoshi, Harvard) that thyrotoxic myopathy is not a morphologic disease but rather a biochemical or a metabolic disorder with no significant or specific anatomical correlate.

Chemical analysis of muscle tissue and serum from patients with thyrotoxic myopathy has led to variable and somewhat uncertain results. In most patients, creatinuria and an elevated level of serum and urine creatine or a diminished creatine tolerance are well-recognized features of hyperthyroidism. These findings could be the results of an increased rate of metabolism of creatine phosphate in muscle in patients with the hypermetabolic state. In one study (Satoyoshi et al., 1963a), the mean creatine content in muscle biopsy specimens from 20 patients with thyrotoxicosis was found to be 28.8 per cent lower (per wet weight of tissue) than in control subjects. Moreover, these authors found that creatine phosphate and ATP in muscle, which are naturally essential substances in energy production and muscle contraction, showed a significant decrease in their content of 44 per cent and 26 per cent, respectively.

In further studies by Satoyoshi and his associates, the quantities of water and of electrolytes in muscle were measured, and each of these substances was found to be diminished by an average of about 12 per cent when compared with normal muscle on a solid-tissue basis. The intracellular potassium content was found to be decreased by nearly 21 per cent, whereas the intracellular content of sodium was reciprocally increased in thyrotoxic muscle.

Whether these biochemical abnormalities in muscle tissue were the cause or the result of the myopathic weakness is not clear. It is possible, however, that the loss of water and potassium from muscles may be attributable to increased membrane permeability, which in turn may be due to an excess of thyroid hormone, as shown by Green and Matty (1964).

More elaborate studies have been carried out recently by Peter, who focused upon the function, intactness, and qualitative and quantitative aspects of skeletal muscle mitochondria and sarcotubular vesicles, since these structures not only are involved in oxidative metabolism in hyperthyroidism but also are responsible for the rapidity of contraction and relaxation of muscle. Employing improved techniques for isolation of skeletal muscle mitochondria, Peter demonstrated that the mitochondria possessed *normal* respiratory control and oxidative phosphorylation in seven patients with severe hyperthyroidism and muscle weakness. On the other hand, he found that there was a significant increase in the *number* of mitochondria isolated from the muscles of these patients. Such an increase in yield of mitochondria could account at least in part for the hypermetabolism of long-standing hyperthyroidism in humans. Furthermore, Peter demonstrated an increased number of sarcotubular vesicles in thyrotoxic muscles, which, he concludes, may help to explain the rapid contraction and relaxation of muscle that occurs in this disease. Vesicles from thyrotoxic human muscles showed no increase, however, in their rate of calcium transport or in their maximal capacity for calcium accumulation under the conditions employed. Thus the biochemical abnormalities that are responsible for the muscular weakness in thyrotoxicosis as yet have not been fully clarified.

The possibility remains that the effect of thyroxine in producing muscular weakness does not reside precisely within the muscle fibers but rather in the central nervous system or in the spinal motor neurons. Obviously tremor or hyperirritability or both are common features in thyrotoxicosis, and brisk tendon reflexes as well as coarse fibrillations or fasciculations of muscle are frequently observed. Only minimal studies have been made on the neurogenic aspects of thyrotoxic myopathy. Magladery et al. studied thyrotoxic patients and normal controls with reference to electrical stimuli of peripheral motor nerves as attained by two shocks at varying intervals from 30–400 msec. to the peroneal nerve. Following this, the recovery rate for nerve impulses was determined. Such studies were further elaborated upon by Satoyoshi and Kinoshita using similar techniques. Here it was found that the nerve fiber recovery curves in normal individuals were similar to those described by Magladery et al., although those in thyrotoxic patients showed marked shortening of the maximal recovery period with a steep upward curve.

The latter was similar to the type of curve seen in patients with upper motor neuron disease. Although it is not clear from these studies how much influence abnormal spinal motor neuron excitability has on muscle function, it probably contributes to the muscular weakness in thyrotoxic myopathy.

It may therefore be deduced that there are as yet unclear biochemical or metabolic disorders or both of muscle fibers, as well as an indeterminate component of CNS or spinal motor neuron effects, both of which contribute to the weakness and other features characteristic of thyrotoxic myopathy.

Thyrotoxicosis and Myasthenia Gravis

Thyrotoxicosis occurs in about 5 per cent of patients with myasthenia gravis. The incidence of some other thyroid disorders (such as thyroiditis) is even higher in myasthenia (Simpson). Myasthenia gravis is rarely found as a complication of thyroid disease, however. Some observers have mentioned a "see-saw" relationship between thyrotoxicosis and myasthenic symptoms, the myasthenia waning with hyperthyroidism and waxing with the treatment of hyperthyroidism, though others have not clearly observed this effect.

Further evidence for the increase in frequency of hyperthyroidism in myasthenia gravis comes from some interesting observations. If one accepts that the usual incidence of myasthenia gravis is about 3/100,000 population, occurrence calculations show that the incidence of myasthenia gravis in patients affected with thyrotoxicosis is 10–100 times higher than would be expected by chance alone (Bartels and Kingsley, Osserman et al.).

The ultimate reason for this interrelationship between myasthenia gravis and hyperthyroidism is not certain. There is more than suggestive evidence that myasthenia gravis is an autoimmune disease or is at least associated with autoimmunity (Simpson). Furthermore, LATS (long-acting thyroid stimulating hormone) has antibody characteristics which suggest that some forms of hyperthyroidism are immunologically motivated (Burke). Although hyperthyroidism is certainly not the cause of myasthenia gravis, some clinical as well as experimental evidence seems to imply that an excess of thyroid hormone may alter the function of the motor end plates. This observation is fortified by the fact that, occasionally in hyperthyroidism, an unfavorable effect on the motor end plate may also be found.

Nonetheless, an anatomical alteration of the motor end plate is the least acceptable hypothesis of an interrelationship between the two conditions. A functional alteration, however, is not excluded. Possibilities for research are still open in this field, especially with regard to the influence of thyroxine on (a) electrolyte metabolism in muscle, (b) acetylcholine, and (c) cholinesterases *in situ,* all of which may be involved in the myasthenic syndrome. The possibility that autoimmune phenomena may sometimes provide the link between myasthenia gravis and thyrotoxicosis is intriguing.

Thyrotoxicosis and Periodic Paralysis

Hypokalemic periodic paralysis may occur in conjunction with hyperthyroidism. The occurrence of this disorder is very uncommon in Caucasians but quite common in Orientals, especially in Japanese, as reported by Satoyoshi and his associates. This combined condition usually occurs in young adults in whom there is no prior family history of episodic paralysis. The periodic paralysis is clinically typical, characterized by rapid onset of generalized flaccid muscular weakness that occurs in sporadic attacks, usually succeeding a heavy carbohydrate meal and exercise followed by a period of rest. Furthermore, the attacks are chemically typical, since the serum potassium may fall to very low levels (K^+ of 1.8–2.2 mEq./liter) during the early stages of an attack, just as in familial hypokalemic periodic paralysis (Pearson and Kalyanaraman). It appears that the attacks of periodic paralysis always completely disappear when these patients are restored to the euthyroid state and that, rather surprisingly, once the patient achieves a euthyroid state, further attacks *cannot* be provoked by any possible means that have so far been tried.

Exophthalmic Ophthalmoplegia and Hyperthyroidism

Weakness of the extraocular muscles occurs during the course of thyrotoxicosis in a significant number of persons. Clinically there appears to be a special predilection for the inferior rectus muscles, and it is extremely rare for total ophthalmoplegia to occur. There is an inconstant relationship between the degree of exophthalmos and the severity of the ocular paresis. In a few cases, bilateral ophthalmoplegia may be the only manifestation of thyrotoxicosis, especially during the early phases of that disease (Kissel et al.).

Electromyographic examination of the extraocular muscles seems to imply that the disorder is a primary disease of the muscle, a myopathy, with occasional electrical evidences of neurogenic disease also being found (Hed et al., Petersen et al.). Pathologic examination of the ocular muscles confirms the electromyographic findings indicating that this is a disease of muscle. There are fatty infiltration, increase in interstitial connective tissue, proliferation of lymphocytes and of other inflammatory elements, as well as degenerative changes of the muscle fibers themselves, the latter occurring to varying degrees in different reports (Dobyns).

Theories concerning the pathogenesis of exophthalmic ophthalmoplegia in thyrotoxicosis have undergone a substantial revision during the past decade. It was initially thought that the exophthalmos was linked to an increased secretion of thyrotropin (TSH) which was unaffected by the corresponding increases of circulating thyroxine and triiodothyronine. The discovery, however, in 1957 by Adams and Purves, and by McKenzie, of a factor that was called long-acting thyroid stimulator (LATS) which is endowed with antibody-like activity as well as stimulating activity on the thyroid, placed the entire status of "exophthalmic ophthalmopathy" under reinvestigation. It now appears that the exophthalmos, and in some cases the ophthalmoplegia, might be due to the direct action of LATS or to the toxic effects of the antigen-antibody complex (thyroid antigen–LATS) on the extraocular muscles. Such an explanation could account for a number of the histologic changes that occur in the extraocular muscles in this disease, including the inflammatory reaction, the degeneration of muscle fibers, and to a smaller extent the fatty infiltration.

Myopathy in Hypothyroidism or Myxedematous Myopathy

Neuromuscular and neurologic symptoms are common in myxedema. The majority of these consist of paresthesias and other sensory features which suggest that the central and the peripheral nervous systems are affected in hypothyroidism.

It is also well known, however, that there is an altered speed of contractility of muscle in hypothyroidism, with a slow ankle jerk, especially during the relaxation phase. Less commonly recognized is the fact that in hypothyroidism a myopathy with proximal limb muscle weakness may occur and may respond satisfactorily to thyroid medication (Salick et al.).

In addition to the clinical evidence of hypothyroidism, slowness of movement and delayed relaxation of tendon jerks, myoedema to percussion of a muscle is also a frequent finding in myxedematous myopathy (Salick et al.). Furthermore, nerve conduction times are slowed, especially motor conduction velocities.

Histologic examination of affected muscles has presented variable results. With the usual hematoxylin-eosin staining, the muscle fibers appear to be essentially normal (Salick et al.), or there may be a slight increase in the number of sarcolemmal nuclei and occasionally a peculiar accumulation of a bluish mucoid substance within the muscle fibers. In other instances of hypothyroid myopathy, however, muscle biopsies have been reported to be completely within the normal range.

For some inexplicable reason, probably enhanced membrane permeability, the serum level of creatine phosphokinase (CPK) is often elevated two- to eightfold in patients with severe myxedema, with or without myopathy. Those with myopathy frequently show the highest levels and, like the clinical state, the enzymes return to the normal level as the patient is brought back to the euthyroid state with appropriate therapy. It should also be noted that CPK levels are *not* elevated in any of the other myopathies associated with thyroid dysfunction, except possibly transitorily in hypokalemic periodic paralysis, in which the elevated CPK level probably results from membrane leakage from muscle; this is associated with hypokalemia.

CUSHING'S SYNDROME, MUSCULAR WEAKNESS, AND CORTICOSTEROID-INDUCED MYOPATHIES

Endogenous Cushing's Syndrome

Muscular weakness and fatigue are common symptoms in Cushing's syndrome, as first described by Cushing in 1932. In the 33 patients studied in 1952 by Plotz and co-workers, these symptoms occurred in 83 per cent. Muscular weakness may also be associated with muscular wasting (Fig. 24–1), especially if the hormonal disease has been present for several months or more. In the myopathy or neuromyopathy in Cushing's syndrome as described by Müller and Kugelberg in six patients, five had major weakness of the muscles of the thighs, especially the quadriceps, and of the pelvic girdle muscles. Electromyographic studies revealed what were interpreted as "myopathic changes" in all these patients. In muscle biopsies from these patients, evidence of isolated fiber destruction may be present; however, the histologic changes were fewer than may have been expected from the fairly significant clinical weakness and electromyographic alterations. No vacuolar changes were mentioned in muscle fibers in this study. After treatment of Cushing's syndrome, moderate to significant improvement in muscular strength, which takes place over a matter of months, has been noted.

Corticosteroid-Induced Myopathy

Muscular weakness and wasting involving the limb girdle muscles may result from long-term treatment with corticosteroids, and this "steroid myopathy" is often reversible upon reduction in dosage or withdrawal of the steroids or even through changing from a daily to a 48-hour dosage schedule.

Since a number of patients who require steroid

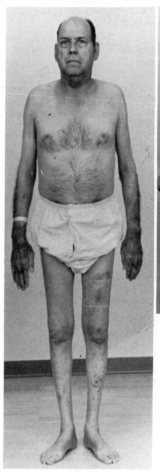
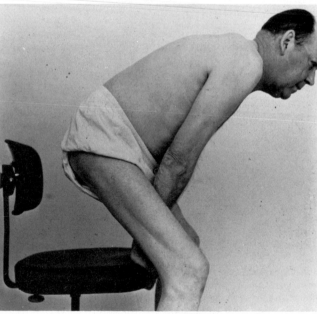

Figure 24–1. Photographs of a man aged 55 with a functioning adrenal adenoma and symptoms and signs of severe muscular weakness. Diffuse proximal and distal atrophy of muscles and other features of Cushing's disease are apparent.

treatment have diseases such as polymyositis, rheumatoid arthritis, or systemic lupus erythematosus (SLE) which themselves may be associated with muscular weakness, it is often difficult to differentiate a so-called steroid myopathy from the effects of the underlying disease. One differential feature, however, is that the electromyograph shows only very minimal alterations in steroid myopathy, whereas it shows very significant changes in diseases such as myositis. To date there is also little evidence that steroid myopathy per se causes an elevation of the serum creatine phosphokinase and other enzymes that are indicative of muscle necrosis. These distinctive points may be used in some instances to differentiate from one another disorders that cause weakness in man.

The interval between starting corticosteroid treatment and the development of weakness is extremely variable. The weakness is usually dose-related; the patients on heavy dosage may show weakness within a matter of a month or two. On the other hand, in those individuals on modest doses of prednisone, 15–20 mg./day, weakness (if it appears at all) may not develop for six months to a year. This weakness is usually associated with easy fatigability or inability to climb stairs or to hold the arms up for prolonged periods. There may be an increase in weight associated with fluid and electrolyte retention, which may appear to intensify the weakness somewhat. It has been said that the halogenated corticosteroids have a greater propensity than other corticosteroids for producing myopathy. They also cause other side effects with greater frequency. The halogenated steroids include triamcinolone and dexamethasone.

The limited studies that have been achieved so far in humans on steroid-induced myopathy have demonstrated minimal electromyographic findings, although it is reasonably certain that there is atrophy of the type II fibers with relative preservation of the type I fibers (W. K. Engel).

Studies on Experimentally Induced Corticosteroid Myopathy

Since the corticosteroids do have the capacity to induce significant myopathic changes in a number of experimental animals, this type of experimental study has been applied to animals with interesting results, which are not always compatible with those that are found in human muscle. In the experimental situation, studies comparing the effects of various steroids have shown that many steroid compounds produce decreases in total body and individual muscle weight in dogs, mice, rats, and rabbits (Sheahan and Vignos).

The most extensive histologic and ultrastructural study on induced steroid myopathy was that of Afifi and Bergman, in which they followed sequentially the necrotic changes that occurred within a matter of a few hours after rabbits were given a large daily dose (10 mg./kg. IM) of cortisone acetate. In their animals, necrosis and other significant alterations, including glycogen depletion, began within 24 hours and continued throughout the administration of steroids. The rabbits became extremely weak, and by the twelfth day of treatment they became almost immobile. The sequential histologic changes that occurred in these animals were followed by and reported in detail by these authors.

Other workers have performed similar experiments. Surprisingly, in the rabbit and other animals, a rapid degree of muscle regeneration occurs along with recovery of muscle capacity once the injurious agent (corticosteroid) is discontinued. Furthermore, histochemical studies have demonstrated significant atrophy of the type II fibers (which usually contain more glycogen) in these animals; as W. K. Engel has described, these type II fibers may be affected first, followed later by the red fibers.

The precise reason for all these muscle fiber changes (either endogenous or exogenous) following steroid administration in animals or, to a much smaller extent, in the Cushingoid patient is at the present time not completely clear. Peter and his associates found that isolated mitochondria and sarcotubular vesicles *were not* the sites of a steroid-induced defect in muscle biochemistry in the rats they studied following the administration of triamcinolone. Others have suggested that the cause is a depletion of glycogen, increased vacuolization of muscle fibers, and so on, but none has been fully confirmed. Since W. K. Engel has observed that there is clear type II fiber atrophy, the corticosteroids may have their predominant effect on the central nervous system or on selected anterior horn cells that dictate this histochemical type fiber rather than on the muscle metabolism. In summary, it is likely that the effects of steroids are multiple both on the nervous system and on muscle metabolism.

THE PANCREAS AND NEUROMYOPATHIES

Diabetes Mellitus and Neuromyopathy and Amyotrophy

The neuropathies and presumably also the myopathies that are associated with diabetes mellitus are polyneuropathy, mononeuropathy, and diabetic amyotrophy. The frequency of occurrence of these neuropathies in patients with diabetes varies considerably according to the criteria applied in the definition of neuropathy. If the term is restricted to patients who have significant symptoms and therefore are forced to seek medical advice (Gilliatt), a neuropathy may be found in more than 40 per cent of most series, while considerably lower figures appear when only objective clinical signs are accepted as criteria of a neuropathy.

Diabetic polyneuropathy is a syndrome of pain, symmetric-distal sensory loss, tendon areflexia, distal weakness or paralysis, and disturbances of autonomic function, usually presenting insidiously (Thage). Isolated nerve palsies usually occur in untreated or uncontrolled diabetics in the middle or older age groups, and these mononeuropathies rarely regress completely. Most commonly affected are the third and sixth cranial nerves and the femoral nerves; pain is a prominent feature before or during the onset of the paresis, and sensory changes are rarely found.

The symptomatology of diabetic polyneuropathy is chiefly related to the duration of the diabetes. The cause of the multitude of neuropathic conditions found in diabetes mellitus may be the carbohydrate metabolism disorder alone, while intraneural microangiopathy may explain why diabetic neuropathy of long standing is not greatly influenced by the control of the glycosuria.

So-called *diabetic amyotrophy* has been accepted as a separate entity since Garland in 1955, in a follow-up of five cases of "diabetic myelopathy," added seven patients of his own, all of whom had uncontrolled diabetes and a clinical picture that presented as an asymmetrical weakness and wasting of the pelvic girdle and thigh muscles with associated loss of reflexes and diffuse pain. Although arguments have continued to be raised, the question as to whether this condition is truly a myopathy or merely a manifestation of proximally localized multiple mononeuropathy has not been completely settled. The reports by Bischoff and Esslen and by Locke et al. described a histologic pattern of single muscle fiber atrophy in the biopsied muscles in these cases, which is somewhat different from the usual pattern of clustered neuroatrophy. So far as is known, the muscle enzymes are not elevated in the serum in these cases, and histochemical studies on muscle biopsies have not been done to a degree that would allow one to draw differential conclusions between myopathy and neuropathy.

There are two reports in the literature (Gårde and Kugelberg, Swash et al.) that seem to have clearly described a diabetic myopathy. The former authors mentioned 12 patients with proximal weakness. All the patients had electromyographic signs of a myopathy, and six had histologic evidence of "a myogenic lesion." None of the latter, however, had good clinical evidence for a myopathy. In the series described by Swash and his associates, a late onset of proximal myopathy occurred in conjunction with diabetes mellitus in four sisters. These patients were found in a family of six. All had a slowly progressive myopathy of late onset, all affected were female members of the family, and there was further association of cataracts and bilateral Dupuytren's contractures. Enzyme histochemistry, tissue analysis, and ischemic exercise studies were all normal. Muscle biopsies showed prominent central migration of sarcolemma nuclei and an occasional single fiber degeneration and regeneration. It was unclear even to the authors whether the diabetes mellitus in this family had any direct association with the prox-imal myopathy, which could have been a very slowly evolving type of myopathic disease, such as a completely separate and unrelated adult-onset form of muscular dystrophy.

PITUITARY (GROWTH HORMONE) MYOPATHY IN ACROMEGALY

On a number of occasions, references have been made in the literature to enlarged muscles with moderate weakness that occur in patients with acromegaly. This finding could be consistent with a high amount of continuous circulating growth hormone secretion in man, which apparently produces hypertrophy of many tissues with some associated functional impairment.

Despite these observations, there has been almost no comment concerning the presence of myopathy or neuropathy in acromegaly except for two studies. The most thorough study, done by Mastaglia and his associates in 1970, encompasses 11 patients with acromegaly, all of whom had had their disease for more than three years. Most were under adequate replacement therapy with corticosteroids and thyroxine, and none had obvious diabetes. Therefore, it appears that the effects, as observed in their muscles, were due to the excess quantity of circulating growth hormone, although this could not be stated with certainty. Of the 11 patients, 3 complained of mild generalized weakness and 3 of tiring easily during the course of the day. By quantitative measurement, there was mild weakness of the proximal limb muscles in 6 of the patients. All had enlarged muscles, and there was considerable discrepancy between the size of the muscles and their apparent decrease in strength.

A number of detailed studies were done in these patients. Several had elevated serum creatine phosphokinase levels, suggestive of or indicative of a myopathy, and a number had electromyographic alterations that revealed a significant increase in motor-unit action potential duration, indicating a progressive fallout of muscle fibers from motor units or the failure of certain fibers to contribute to the electrical changes. These findings were, however, nonspecific and relatively mild in degree.

Muscle biopsies in this series were obtained in all patients from proximal muscles, and there were some histologic abnormalities to be found in five of the biopsy specimens. These changes comprised segmental necrosis of isolated muscle fibers in three cases, increased numbers of internal sarcolemmal nuclei in five cases, and a small number of ringed fibers in one specimen. Detailed histochemical stains showed a relatively high glycogen content in muscle fibers in 6 of the 11 biopsies, but there was no significant abnormality in either oxidative or glycolytic metabolism. The relative numbers of and arrangement of type I and type II fibers were normal, but the average mean diameter of both type I and type II fibers was increased by about 15 per cent above the average when compared with similar measurements on age-matched normal control subjects.

Another series (Lundberg et al.) was composed of eight patients: four women and four men between the ages of 25 and 60 years. All eight patients had clinically well-established acromegaly, and most were also under treatment. A variety of studies undertaken by these authors failed to reveal significant electromyographic or histologic changes in muscle, despite the fact that the muscles themselves were moderately large. The authors did find a significant number of entrapment neuropathies in this group of patients, but since the carpal-tunnel syndrome and other types of compression neuropathies are common in acromegaly, this is not surprising. Lundberg's laboratory studies were generally quite inconclusive; the histologic and histochemical details were not as complete as one might have desired.

From the detailed studies of Mastaglia et al., it appears that the relatively mild nature of the pathologic changes in the muscle biopsy specimens, as well as the mild clinical muscle weakness, suggests that the myopathic process is a mild and protracted one with a very gradual loss of muscle fibers. Alternatively, as may occur in thyrotoxic and other endocrine myopathies, the reduction in motor-unit action potential duration could have been due to a *functional failure* of the muscle fibers, most of which were morphologically normal. This view would be consistent with the observation made previously in animals (Bigland and Jehring) that muscular hypertrophy induced by growth hormone is functionally inefficient, in that the contractile strength of the hypertrophied muscles is paradoxically reduced rather than increased.

In conclusion, it appears from clinical, serum enzyme, histologic, histochemical, and muscle strength studies that all findings indicate there is a mild form of myopathy that occurs in acromegaly, which is probably due to a direct effect on muscle of continuously circulating growth hormone. The mechanisms whereby this occurs have not been clarified. These findings indicate that the proximal muscles of patients with acromegaly are commonly the sites of a mild and patchy myopathic process.

EFFECTS OF TESTOSTERONE ON MUSCLE

Although there are no definitive reports of androgenic hormones in human muscle, it is common experience in the athletic community to use androgenic hormones plus exercise to improve muscular strength and bulk. Experiments in rats (Pellegrino) have shown an effect of testosterone on muscle (the levator ani), even within a few hours after its administration. Pellegrino has shown that in this study testosterone causes a rapid increase in (a) sugar penetration into muscle, (b) hexose phosphorylation, and (c) glycogen synthesis, possibly in part due to induction of glycogen synthetase.

THE PARATHYROID GLAND AND MYOPATHY

Hyperparathyroid Myopathy

It has been apparent for several years that a type of mild myopathy occurs in association with hyperparathyroidism or functioning tumors of the parathyroid gland or both. This myopathy is characterized by muscular weakness and fatigability, atrophy of muscles, intact deep tendon reflexes, and pressure tenderness of bones (Richet et al., Vicale). The myopathy has been reported in both primary and secondary hyperparathyroidism and seems mainly to affect the proximal limb muscles. The pathogenesis of this muscle disorder is unknown, and there is some doubt as to its direct relationship with hyperparathyroidism. In one study (Frame et al.) there appeared to be no direct correlation between the level of the total serum calcium and the degree of the myopathy or other electrolyte disorders that were found in hyperparathyroidism.

In most of the reported series, light-microscopic studies of the muscle have revealed only minimal changes, which frequently have been interpreted as myositis or as simple atrophy of muscles (Bischoff and Esslen). In one study (Hudson et al.) of two sisters, each of whom had an adenoma of the parathyroid and muscle weakness of 3–5 years' duration, evaluations were carried out in considerable detail. Each patient, one aged 40 and one aged 29, described difficulties in climbing stairs and fatigue after walking even short distances. Examination revealed outward bowing of the femora, wasting and marked weakness of the quadriceps bilaterally, and other features indicative of a myopathic process. Each had generalized skeletal pain and tenderness, as is common in this syndrome.

Muscle biopsy specimens were obtained from the quadriceps muscle of each patient and were studied by light microscopy as well as by histochemistry and electron microscopy. Sections revealed normal distributions of both type I and type II fibers, but with an increased vacuolization within the muscle fibers themselves. This vacuolization was never very marked. The majority of the muscle fibers were normal by light microscopy, but these normal fibers were interspersed with bundles of atrophic fibers, and there was some increase in sarcolemmal nuclei. The smallest arterioles were thickened, particularly in the 40-year-old woman.

The authors chose to presume that the changes in muscle were secondary to thickening of the arterioles and the basement membranes of the endomesial capillaries. They felt that this vascular factor was primarily responsible for the muscular weakness and other changes. They speculated that the changes in muscle, for example, could have been due to the direct action of parathyroid hormone on muscle cell metabolism. It is possible that there was a compensatory increase in calcitonin that directly affected cells. Another explanation could be that the changes were due to alterations in concentration of divalent ions in the tissues (muscle fibers), particularly to an increase in calcium. At any rate, a clear-cut myopathy was not demonstrated in hyperparathyroidism. Serum enzymes were normal, and even though the patients were weak and had atrophy, the precise role of the excessive parathyroid hormone, its interrelationship with calcitonin, or both, require a good deal of further study before elucidation of the cause of the "myopathic" changes in hyperparathyroidism is fully possible.

Creatine Phosphokinase (CPK) Activity in Hypoparathyroidism

Although a myopathy has not been described in hypoparathyroidism, there are one or two references in the literature to elevated serum enzymes in conjunction with this condition. The reasons for the elevated CPK have not so far been clarified but could possibly be due to a variation in membrane permeability of the sarcolemmal membrane. Electromyographic recordings in these cases have been normal, and deltoid muscle biopsy in one patient (Hower et al.) was apparently normal. Strikingly, the elevated serum CPK was as much as ten times normal in two females with idiopathic hypoparathyroidism (Hower et al.). These authors report that in one patient, after institution of vitamin D_3 therapy in doses adequate enough to maintain serum calcium levels within the normal range, the elevated enzyme levels declined to half their previous levels, but they never did return to normal values during the subsequent eight weeks. In the other patient, the CPK levels were threefold above normal, and the patient was admitted to the hospital with tetany (which could have explained some of the elevated CPK levels). After adequate therapy with vitamin D_3 as well as maintenance of the serum calcium levels with intravenous serum calcium administration, the elevated serum CPK levels returned completely to normal.

REFERENCES

Adams, D. D., and Purves, H. D.: Abnormal response in the assay of thyrotropin. *Metabolism* 6:26, 1957.

Afifi, A. K., and Bergman, R. A.: Steroid myopathy: A study of the evolution of muscle lesions in rabbits. *Johns Hopkins Med. J.* 124:66, 1969.

Afifi, A. K., Bergman, R. A., et al.: Steroid myopathy: Clinical, histologic, and cytologic observations. *Johns Hopkins Med. J.* 123:158, 1968.

Astrom, K. E., Kugelberg, E., et al.: Hypothyroid myopathy. *Arch. Neurol.* 5:472, 1961.

Bartels, E. C., and Kingsley, J. W., Jr.: Hyperthyroidism associated with myasthenia gravis. *Lahey Clin. Bull.* 6:101, 1949.

Bathurst, L. W.: A case of Graves' disease associated with idiopathic muscular atrophy. *Lancet* 2:529, 1895.

Bigland, H., and Jehring, B. J.: Muscle performance in rats, normal and treated with growth hormone. *J. Physiol.* (London) 116:129, 1952.

Bischoff, A., and Esslen, E.: Myopathy with primary hyperparathyroidism. *Neurology* 15:64, 1965.

Burke, G.: The long-acting thyroid stimulator of Graves' disease. *Amer. J. Med.* 45:435, 1968.

Butcher, R. W., Robison, G., et al.: *Cyclic AMP.* New York, Academic Press, 1971.

Cushing, H.: The basophile adenomas of the pituitary body and their clinical manifestations. *Bull. Johns Hopkins Hosp.* 50:137, 1932.

Dobyns, B. M.: Present concept of the pathologic physiology of exophthalmos. *J. Clin. Endocr.* 10:1202, 1950.

Engel, A. G.: Electron microscopic observations in thyrotoxic and corticosteroid-induced myopathies. *Mayo Clin. Proc.* 47:97, 1966.

Engel, W. K.: Muscle biopsy, type II fiber atrophy in humans. *Clin. Orthop.* 39:80, 1965.

Faludi, G., Gotlief, J., et al.: Factors influencing the development of steroid-induced myopathies. *Ann. N.Y. Acad. Sci.* 138:62, 1966.

Frame, B., Heinz, E. G., et al.: Myopathy in generalized hyperparathyroidism: Observation in three patients. *Ann. Intern. Med.* 68:1022, 1968.

Gårde, A., and Kugelberg, E.: Myopatier vid diabetes. (Abstr.). *Nord. Med.* 70:1252, 1963.

Garland, H.: Diabetic amyotrophy. *Brit. Med. J.* 2:1287, 1955.

Gilliatt, R. W.: Clinical aspects of diabetic neuropathy, In *Biochemical Aspects of Neurological Disorders.* 2nd series. Cummings, J. J., and Kremer, M. (eds.), Oxford, Blackwell, 1965, p. 117.

Golding, D. H., Murray, S. M., et al.: Corticosteroids and myopathy. *Ann. Phys. Med.* 6:171, 1961.

Green, K., and Matty, A. J.: Action of thyroxin on active transport in isolated membranes of *Bufo bufo. Gen. Comp. Endocr.* 3:244, 1963.

Green, K., and Matty, A. J.: The effect of thyroid hormones on water permeability of the isolated bladder of the toad *Bufo bufo. J. Endocr.* 28:205, 1964.

Harman, J. B.: Muscular wasting in corticosteroid therapy. *Lancet* 1:887, 1959.

Harvard, C. W. H., Campbell, E. D. R., et al.: Electromyographic and histological findings in the muscles of patients with thyrotoxicosis. *Quart. J. Med.* 32:145, 1963.

Hed, R., Kirstin, L., et al.: Thyrotoxic myopathy. *J. Neurol. Neurosurg. Psychiat.* 21:270, 1958.

Hower, J., Struck, H., et al.: CPK activity in hypoparathyroidism. (Letter to the editor.) *New Eng. J. Med.* 287:1096, 1972.

Hudson, A. J., Cholod, E. J., et al.: Familial hyperthyroid myopathy, In *Muscle Diseases.* Walton, J. N., Canal, N., et al. (eds.) (Excerpta Medica Int. Congr. Ser., no. 199) Amsterdam, Excerpta Medica Foundation, 1970, p. 526.

Kissel, P., Gartemann, P., et al.: *Les Syndromes des Myothyridiens.* Paris, Masson et Cie, 1965, p. 24.

Locke, S., Lawrence, D. G., et al.: Diabetic amyotrophy. *Amer. J. Med.* 34:775, 1963.

Lundberg, P. O., Osterman, P. O., et al.: Neuromuscular signs and symptoms in acromegaly, In *Muscle Diseases.* Walton, J. N., Canal, N., et al. (eds.) (Excerpta Medica Int. Congr. Ser., no. 199), Amsterdam, Excerpta Medica Foundation, 1970, p. 531.

McKenzie, J. M.: Studies on the thyroid activator of hyperthyroidism. *J. Clin. Endocr.* 21:635, 1961.

Magladery, J. W., Teasdall, R. D., et al.: Electrophysiological studies of reflex activity in patients with lesions of the nervous system. A comparison of spinal motor-neurone excitability following afferent nerve valleys in normal persons and patients with upper motor-neurone lesions. *Bull. Johns Hopkins Hosp.* 91:219, 1952.

Mastaglia, F. L., Barwick, D. D., et al.: Myopathy in acromegaly. *Lancet* 2:907, 1970.

Millikan, C., and Haines, S. S.: Thyroid gland in relation to neuromuscular disease. *Res. Publ. Ass. Nerv. Ment. Dis.* 32:87, 1953.

Müller, R., and Kugelberg, E.: Myopathy in Cushing's syndrome. *J. Neurol. Neurosurg. Psychiat.* 22:314, 1959.

Osserman, E., Tsairis, P., et al.: Myasthenia gravis and thyroid disease: Clinical and immunologic correlations. *J. Mount Sinai Hosp.* 34:469, 1967.

Pearson, C. M., and Kalyanaraman, K.: The periodic paralyses, In *The Metabolic Basis of Inherited Disease.* Stanbury, J. B., Wyngaarden, J. B., et al. (eds.), New York, McGraw-Hill, 1972, p. 1180.

Pellegrino, C.: The effects of testosterone on the ultrastructure and glycogen synthesis in the levator ani muscle of the rat, In *Muscle Diseases.* Walton, J. N., Canal, N., et al. (eds.) (Excerpta Medica Int. Congr. Ser., no. 199), Amsterdam, Excerpta Medica Foundation, 1970, p. 704.

Perkoff, G. T., Silber, R., et al.: Myopathy due to administration of therapeutic amounts of 17-hydroxycorticosteroids. *Amer. J. Med.* 26:891, 1959.

Peter, J. B.: Studies of human skeletal muscle mitochondria. *Biochem. Med. 2*:179, 1968.

Peter, J. B.: Hyperthyroidism. *Ann. Intern. Med. 69*:1016, 1968.

Petersen, I., Tengroth, B., et al.: Electromyographic study of the eye muscle in endocrine exophthalmos. *Acta Opthalmol.* (Kbh.) *39*:171, 1961.

Plotz, C. M., Knowlton, A. I., et al.: The natural history of Cushing's syndrome. *Amer. J. Med. 13*:597, 1952.

Ramsey, I. D.: Electromyography and thyrotoxicosis. *Quart. J. Med. 34*:255, 1965.

Ramsey, I. D.: Muscle dysfunction in hyperthyroidism. *Lancet 2*:931, 1966.

Richet, C., Sourdel, M., et al.: Syndromes parathyroïdomusculaires: Myopathies scléreuses liées à des troubles parathyroïdiens. *J. Med. Franc. 26*:377, 1937.

Rowland, L. P., Aranow, H., et al.: Endocrine aspects of myasthenia gravis. In *Progressive Muskeldystrophil-Myotenie-Myasthenie.* Vol. I. Kuhn, E. (ed.), Berlin, Springer-Verlag, 1966, p. 416.

Salick, A. E., Colachis, S. C., et al.: Myxedema myopathy: Clinical, electrodiagnostic and pathologic findings in an advanced case. *Arch. Phys. Med. Rehabil. 49*:230, 1968.

Satoyoshi, E., and Kinoshita, M.: Some aspects of thyrotoxic and steroid myopathy, In *Muscle Diseases.* Walton, J. N., Canal, N., et al. (eds.), (Excerpta Medica Int. Congr. Ser., no. 199), Amsterdam, Excerpta Medica Foundation, 1970, p. 455.

Satoyoshi, E., Murakama, K., et al.: Myopathy and thyrotoxicosis, with special emphasis on an effect of potassium ingestion on serum and urinary creatine. *Neurology 13*:645, 1963a.

Satoyoshi, E., Murakama, K., et al.: Periodic paralysis in hyperthyroidism. *Neurology 13*:746, 1963b.

Sheahan, M. G., and Vignos, P. J.: Experimental corticosteroid myopathy. *Arthritis Rheum. 12*:491, 1969.

Shy, G. M.: Neuromuscular disorders: Diseases of muscle, In *Textbook of Medicine.* Beeson, P. B., and McDermott, W. (eds.), Philadelphia, W. B. Saunders Co., 1967, p. 1659.

Simpson, J. A.: The correlations between myasthenia gravis and disorders of the thyroid gland. Proc. 4th Symp., *Research in Muscular Dystrophy.* Milhorat, A. D. (ed.), London, Pitman, 1968, p. 31.

Swash, M., van den Noort, S., et al.: Late-onset proximal myopathy with diabetes mellitus in four sisters. *Neurology 20*:694, 1970.

Thage, O.: Metabolic neuropathies and myopathies in adults: Clinical aspects. *Acta Neurol. Scand. 46*(Suppl. 43):120, 1970.

Thorn, G. W., and Eder, H. A.: Studies on chronic thyrotoxic myopathy. *Amer. J. Med. 1*:583, 1946.

Vicale, C. T.: The diagnostic features of the muscular syndrome resulting from hyperparathyroidism, osteomalacia owing to renal tubular acidosis, and perhaps to related disorders of calcium metabolism. *Trans. Amer. Neurol. Ass. 74*:143, 1949.

CHAPTER 25

Genetics and Endocrinology

By Joseph L. Goldstein and
Arno G. Motulsky

GENERAL PRINCIPLES OF
HEREDITARY DISEASES

As with disease affecting other body systems, genetic factors play a significant role in the pathogenesis of many endocrine and metabolic diseases. In many instances the genetic effects are clearly discernible and easy to analyze. Not infrequently, however, the role of hereditary factors is hard to prove, and the mechanisms involved remain obscure.

In general, "classic" genetic or hereditary diseases transmitted by single-factor inheritance are believed to result from mutations affecting specific parts of the desoxyribonucleic acid (DNA), which carries the genetic information possessed by each cell. These mutations may be of several types, ranging from the substitution of one nucleotide base for another to the addition or deletion of large segments of DNA. Visible chromosomal aberrations are not found in this type of disease. The principal manifestations of single gene mutations are usually mediated through alterations in the synthesis or structure of proteins. If the mutation affects *structural genes* — genes which control the amino acid sequences of specific proteins — abnormal proteins may be made, or the synthesis of the proteins may be prevented. On the other hand, mutations involving *regulatory genes* possibly exist and may result in the synthesis of abnormal amounts of protein by disturbances in the metabolic and temporal control of their synthesis. At present, the concepts of structural gene mutations have been admirably documented in man, especially for the various abnormal hemoglobins, haptoglobins, and glucose-6-phosphate dehydrogenases (1). However, understanding of regulatory gene mutations is, so far, based mainly on work carried out in microorganisms. Although it is reasonable and probable that many concepts derived from unicellular organisms, which differ genetically in many important regards from mammals, will prove applicable to man, more direct evidence of the action of regulatory genes in man is required.

In some hereditary diseases it is possible to demonstrate directly a genetically determined abnormality or absence of a specific protein or enzyme (1). In many or even most genetic disorders, only the distal physiologic effects of the mutation are recognizable, and the underlying, or primary, defect is unknown. Nevertheless, it generally seems reasonable to assume that a single primary defect exists whenever a disease is transmitted by a single gene mechanism and that the various manifestations of the disease can all be related to the mutational event by a more or less complicated "pedigree of causes." Whenever the identification of a primary defect is claimed for a disease, it becomes necessary that all clinical and biochemical observations be satisfactorily explained, and that transmission of the proposed defect conforms with the observed mode of inheritance.

Recent work in genetic diseases has resulted in the almost constant finding that an entity that appears clinically uniform may represent the end result of different gene mutations (genetic heterogeneity) (2). Considering the complex enzymatic control of metabolism, it is not surprising that interference with different metabolic steps necessary for a given function may lead to a similar end result. In order to demonstrate that a given disease is the result of different mutations, one must ultimately demonstrate biochemical differences between the various forms of the disease. However, such heterogeneity can be strongly suspected if different modes of inheritance (i.e., autosomal recessive or X-linked recessive) are detected in different families with a similar disease. This approach, with careful correlation of detailed genetic, clinical, and biochemical data, has been extremely helpful in the definition of disease entities and for an understanding of the pathophysiology of diseases.

Mechanisms of Genetic Disease

Autosomal Dominant Diseases

Mendelian patterns of inheritance can be divided into autosomal dominant, autosomal recessive, and X chromosome–linked traits. The distinction between "dominant" and "recessive" must be understood as one of convenience in pedigree analysis rather than as necessarily implying a fundamental difference in genetic mechanisms (3). The term *dominant* implies that a mutation will be clinically manifest when an individual has a single dose of this mutation (or is heterozygous for it), while *recessive* implies that the double dose (or homozygosity) is required for clinical detection. Genes themselves are never dominant or recessive; their effects, however, are reflected by dominant or

recessive inheritance. Individuals who are heterozygous for "recessive" genes often have demonstrable biochemical abnormalities, while those who are homozygous for "dominant" genes may be more severely affected than the heterozygotes.

Autosomal dominant diseases often exhibit considerable clinical variability, both in their penetrance (whether or not they manifest at all) and in their expressivity (the degree to which they manifest). Penetrance is a relative concept, since its assessment varies with the technique used for detection of the trait. In many diseases, penetrance may be rather low if one relies only on history and physical examination but becomes significantly higher when specific laboratory tests are used. Penetrance of less than 100 per cent may be caused by various genetic or environmental modifiers. The genetic modifiers may be genes located on other chromosomes. Not infrequently, the partner gene or allele on the nonmutant homologous chromosome may itself affect clinical expression of the mutant gene. It has been suggested that such modification may be caused by the presence of a series of multiple "normal" allelic forms (isoalleles) that function with different degrees of efficiency (4). If the normal isoallele works at high capacity, the effect of a mutation might be relatively mild and age of onset delayed. A less efficient isoallele might not produce enough functional gene product, and in that case the mutant allele on the other chromosome would cause more severe disease with an earlier age of onset.

Not infrequently a patient with a dominant disorder is found to have unaffected parents, and a mutation is suspected. A mutation is most likely when the disease under study is highly deleterious and unlikely to lead to reproduction. In less severe disorders, a smaller proportion of cases will be caused by fresh mutations. In general, the frequency of new mutations observed clinically correlates directly with the genetic lethality of the disease. The more lethal the disease, the more common will be cases due to new mutations. For example, some of the rare nonfamilial disorders of sexual development, such as congenital anorchism and congenital absence of the vagina and uterus (Rokitansky-Küstner syndrome), may be the result of a new dominant mutation. Since individuals with these disorders cannot reproduce, the mutation is not transmitted, and the disorder, therefore, appears sporadically. For practical purposes, the presence of several affected sibs rules out mutation since cluster mutations in a gonadal sector are extremely rare (5). Often when the parents are unaffected, the gene may be carried by one parent in whom the disease was nonpenetrant or of low expressivity. Extramarital paternity is another source of difficulty in interpretation since it is found in about 3 per cent of randomly studied children in the United States and Western Europe.

Autosomal Recessive Diseases

The clinical picture of autosomal recessive diseases tends to be more uniform than that of dominant diseases, and the age of onset is often early. As a general rule, recessive diseases are more commonly seen in children, while dominant diseases are more frequently encountered in adults. Since with recessive inheritance only one of four children is expected to be affected, multiple cases in a family may not occur, and many isolated or sporadic cases will be found. It can be shown that, in a population in which families with two, three, and four children exist in equal proportions, over 50 per cent of all cases of a disease due to recessive inheritance will be sporadic, and the genetic etiology will not be apparent from the family history. The presence of autosomal recessive inheritance implies that each clinically normal parent has contributed a single mutant gene to the patient. In the parents, the gene product of the normal allele is sufficient for normal function. With rare recessive diseases, the frequency of consanguineous marriages among the parents is often elevated; the rarer the gene, the higher the proportion of parental consanguinity.

X-linked Diseases

Mutant genes carried on the X chromosome are characterized by full expression in males (hemizygotes) and variability of expression and penetrance in females (heterozygotes) depending on the particular mutation and on the individual carrying it. X-linked inheritance can be distinguished from male sex-limited autosomal dominant inheritance by pedigree analysis. Demonstration of genetic linkage to other X-linked traits (such as glucose-6-phosphate dehydrogenase variants, color vision defects, or the blood group Xg^a is also of great assistance, as is the observation of cellular mosaicism (see below). X-linked inheritance of rare traits is ruled out by the demonstration of father to son transmission. In common X-linked traits, the mother may be a carrier without clinical manifestation, and spurious father to son transmission may be mimicked.

The understanding of the mechanisms of gene expression for X-linked genes has been greatly advanced by the Lyon hypothesis (6). According to this hypothesis, only one of the two X chromosomes functions genetically in female cells. Female cells would, therefore, be equivalent in terms of X-chromosome activity to male cells. The nonfunctional X chromosome is heteropyknotic (very condensed in appearance), replicates late in the mitotic cycle ("late-labeling" with tritiated thymidine), and gives rise to the sex chromatin or Barr body (7). In abnormal states with more than two X chromosomes such as XXX, all but one of the X chromosomes appear to be inactivated. The process of X chromosome inactivation takes place early in embryonic development and is thought to be random, with inactivation of either the paternally or maternally derived X chromosome in each cell occurring with equal probability. Once inactivation has occurred, the inactivated X chromosome remains nonfunctional, and all progeny of the initial cell will have the same X chromosome inactivated.

As a result of the inactivation process, mosaicism of cells in females who are heterozygous for an X-linked mutation will be particularly apparent. One group of cells in a given tissue will be normal; the other will manifest the mutant genotype. Because of the statistically random nature of the inactivation process, about half the cells will, on the average, have the normal X chromosome, while the other half will have the mutant X chromosome. However, chance or selection of one or the other sets of clones of cells may disturb these proportions in any given individual. Depending on the nature of the biochemical defect and on the proportions of mutant and normal X chromosomes in an individual, a genetically heterozygous female may be either virtually undetectable or may be mildly or severely manifested in the heterozygous state.

Although the Lyon hypothesis assumes complete inactivation of one X chromosome, the phenotype of human sex chromosome abnormalities and other evidence suggests that this may not be completely true (7). For example, XO individuals should be identical to XX females and XXY individuals identical to XY males. The existence of considerable differences in these phenotypes suggests that either irreparable damage has been done before the time of inactivation, or that complete inactivation does not occur. Moreover, the common X-linked blood group locus Xg does not undergo inactivation (8).

Chromosomal Disorders

Still another category of genetic disease results from chromosomal abnormalities. Chromosomal abnormalities may consist of an increase or a decrease in chromosome number, deletion or inversion of portions of chromosomes, or translocation of bits of chromosomes from one to another. If the sex chromosomes are affected, abnormalities in sexual differentiation may result (e.g., Klinefelter's and Turner's syndromes). Abnormalities of autosomal chromosomes may cause congenital malformations as in Down's syndrome (mongolism). Diseases due to chromosomal aberrations are not usually hereditary or familial but are most frequently caused by an abnormal division of germ cells before fertilization or by mitotic errors in the early cell divisions after fertilization. However, certain chromosome anomalies such as translocations may rarely be carried in a "balanced" state by phenotypically normal carriers and may thus be both hereditary and familial. Since the detection of chromosomal errors is carried out by conventional light microscopy, aberrations involving small chromosomal segments are beyond the resolving power of present methods. A class of genetic diseases with complex malformations which are caused by minute chromosomal defects affecting more than one gene may exist.

Polygenic Disorders

The genetic element in most common disorders is rarely based on either single gene (mendelian) or chromosomal abnormalities. Instead, multiple genes interact with each other as well as with environmental factors to produce the familial aggregation that is observed in common diseases. The common thyroid diseases, such as thyrotoxicosis, primary hypothyroidism, chronic lymphocytic thyroiditis, and nonendemic goiter, fit into this category, as do, probably, certain forms of diabetes mellitus and coronary heart disease. In polygenic disorders there is an underlying genetically determined and continuously distributed predisposition, often with a threshold beyond which individuals are at risk to the development of disease (9, 10). In general, both the first-degree relatives (i.e., parents, sibs, children) and second-degree relatives (i.e., uncles, aunts, nieces, nephews, grandchildren) of a proband with a polygenic disorder will have an increased absolute risk for the development of the disorder, first-degree relatives being more frequently affected than second-degree relatives. Polygenic disorders rarely affect more than 5 to 10 per cent of first-degree relatives. The hypothesis of polygenic inheritance has been made more plausible in recent years by the demonstration of polymorphisms at many gene loci. Thus, at as many as one-third of all gene loci, different forms of a gene (alleles) are present with frequencies that cannot be explained by mutation (11). Such a large degree of variation in normal genes undoubtedly exerts an important influence on the phenotypic expression of various traits and disease states in man and provides the "genetic background" against which a given gene or genes act.

GENE ACTION IN ENDOCRINE GLANDS

The identification of a gene affecting a specific endocrine function is usually inferred from genetic analysis of family pedigrees showing mendelian inheritance of an endocrine abnormality. The existence of a normal gene can only be demonstrated by the presence and expression of its mutant allele. Since at least 50 phenotypically distinct and simply inherited disorders of the endocrine glands are currently recognized (comprising about 5 per cent of all mendelian disorders presently known to exist in man) (12), at least 50 genes exist which affect endocrine function in a major way. Mutation of these genes causes endocrine dysfunction, which is manifested at different physiologic levels, including glandular differentiation and neoplasia; hormone synthesis, secretion, and transport; and hormone action at the target cell level. In most cases, the elucidation of the biochemical nature of these 50 genes (i.e., the isolation and characterization of the normal and abnormal proteins specified by the normal and mutant alleles for each gene) has not been achieved.

As more of these endocrine gene products become identified, more "markers" will become available for linkage studies to map the human chromosomes. Genetic linkage needs to be distinguished from association of two traits (13, 14). Genetic linkage refers to the demonstrable presence of one or several genes on a given chromosome. X-chromosomal linkage of recessive genes is easy to infer because of the typical pedigree patterns with "criss-cross" inheritance and affected maternal relatives. Autosomal linkage between two genes is much more difficult to demonstrate and has been proved for about 30 genes [including the ABO blood group genes and the nail-patella syndrome, the Rh gene(s) and one type of hereditary elliptocytosis, and the loci for secretor blood group, Lutheran blood group, and myotonic dystrophy (15)]. In a population, specific alleles of linked genes do not necessarily occur more frequently in association. Thus hemophiliacs have no increased frequency of color blindness, and there is no association between a given ABO blood group and the nail-patella syndrome. Conversely, association of two inherited traits in an individual does not imply location on the same chromosome. It is sometimes stated that different manifestations in a given hereditary syndrome are due to the presence of closely linked mutant genes. Such a hypothesis would imply that mutations occurred simultaneously at different linked loci. It is highly unlikely that mutations occur in this manner. In most cases, the association of apparently unrelated signs and symptoms in a patient is caused by the common action of a single mutant gene on multiple organ systems.

Several generalizations can be made regarding the relationship between molecular pathophysiology and mechanism of inheritance in endocrine disorders. The endocrine neoplasia syndromes, such as multiple endocrine adenomatosis, familial hyperparathyroidism without other endocrine gland involvement, and the medullary thyroid carcinoma-pheochromocytoma syndromes, are each inherited as autosomal dominant traits, as is frequently the case for other heritable tumors (16). As for most enzyme deficiency states in man, the disorders affecting hormone biosynthesis (such as the adrenogenital syndromes and the familial goiters) show an autosomal recessive pattern of inheritance. Finally, it is noteworthy that the best documented examples of hormone resistance in man—e.g., Albright's hereditary osteodystrophy, vitamin D-resistant rickets, nephrogenic diabetes insipidus, and the testicular feminization syndrome (complete type)—result from mutations involving different genes on the X chromosome.

Single gene-determined endocrine disorders have provided superb investigative models for unraveling the complexities of endocrine physiology and biochemistry. Most impressive has been the use of the various adrenogenital syndromes and of the familial goiters in the delineation of the biosynthesis of adrenocortical hormones and thyroxine respectively. Since at least 15 mendelian disorders of sexual development are now recognized, it is predictable that the elucidation of the basic defect in each of them will similarly provide the biochemical information necessary to define the basis of sexual differentiation in man.

Many family studies of endocrinologic disease have been published because the operation of genetic factors is striking. Unfortunately, apart from extremely rare disorders, such studies usually are of little value in assessing the total role of heredity in the disease under study. In some published reports, genetic factors may be inferred from the data in the family history, but detailed studies on affected family members have not been performed. To obtain full appreciation of the role of genetic factors in endocrinology, it is imperative that complete individual and family studies be made on nonselected consecutive patients and their family members, using identical criteria in every subject investigated. Although time consuming and expensive, such studies will be of great help in affording an understanding of the pathophysiology and natural history of these diseases.

Table 25–1 lists those endocrine disorders in which genetic factors have generally been demonstrated to play a significant role. In most of these cases, familial occurrence is frequent enough to warrant a family study. On the other hand, there are a number of endocrine diseases which rarely if ever show familial aggregation (Table 25–2). Al-

TABLE 25–1. ENDOCRINE DISORDERS INFLUENCED BY GENETIC FACTORS

Pituitary disorders
  Diabetes insipidus
  Pituitary dwarfism
  Pituitary hypogonadism

Parathyroid disorders
  Hypoparathyroidism
  Albright's hereditary osteodystrophy
  Hyperparathyroidism
  Vitamin D-resistant rickets

Thyroid disorders
  Goiter
  Cretinism
  Myxedema
  Chronic lymphocytic thyroiditis
  Thyrotoxicosis

Pancreatic disorders
  Diabetes mellitus
  Hypoglycemia

Adrenal disorders
  Adrenogenital syndromes
  Adrenal insufficiency
  Bartter's syndrome

Disorders of sexual development
  XX gonadal dysgenesis   XY gonadal dysgenesis
  True hermaphroditism   Testicular feminization
  Reifenstein's syndrome
  Primary male hypogonadism   Pseudovaginal perineoscrotal
  Sertoli-cell-only syndrome   hypospadias
  Stein-Leventhal syndrome   Precocious puberty

Endocrine tumor syndromes
  Multiple endocrine adenomatosis
  Medullary thyroid carcinoma-pheochromocytoma syndromes

Others
  Baldness
  Hirsutism
  Myotonic dystrophy
  Werner's syndrome
  Laurence-Moon-Bardet-Biedl syndrome
  Congenital lipodystrophy

TABLE 25–2. ENDOCRINE DISORDERS WHICH RARELY OCCUR IN FAMILIAL FORM

Pituitary disorders
  Acromegaly
  Amenorrhea-galactorrhea syndrome
  Hypopituitarism of adult onset
  Inappropriate secretion of ADH
  Anorexia nervosa

Parathyroid disorders
  DiGeorge syndrome

Adrenal disorders
  Cushing's syndrome
  Primary hyperaldosteronism
  Hypoaldosteronism of adult onset

Disorders of sexual development
  Turner's syndrome
  Klinefelter's syndrome
  XYY syndrome
  Mixed gonadal dysgenesis
  Sex-reversed 46/XX male syndrome
  Persistent müllerian duct syndrome (hernia uteri inguinale)
  Congenital anorchia
  Congenital absence of the vagina and uterus (Rokitansky-
    Küstner syndrome)

Others
  Polyostotic fibrous dysplasia (Albright-McCune-
    Sternberg syndrome)
  Ectopic hormone-producing tumors

though one or two isolated case reports have appeared suggesting familial occurrence of acromegaly, the galactorrhea-amenorrhea syndrome, and primary aldosteronism, most of the available evidence suggests a nongenetic etiology for these as well as the other disorders listed in Table 25–2.

The ectopic polypeptide hormone-producing tumors, although not strictly genetic in the sense that the tumors are heritable, are nevertheless of great genetic interest. Their biologic importance lies not only in that ectopic hormone production can serve as a clue to early diagnosis of cancer, but also in that it provides a model system for the study of the mechanism of genetic derepression of cellular function (17). These ectopic hormone syndromes are discussed in Chapter 30.

GENETIC COUNSELING IN ENDOCRINOLOGY

When advising parents or potential parents about the risk to subsequent children of having a disorder that has already affected someone in the family, the first step is to be sure of the diagnosis — in particular, to make certain that the problem in question is really of genetic origin. This is especially important in endocrine disorders with genetic and nongenetic etiologies, such as diabetes insipidus, panhypopituitarism, hypoglycemia, and hyperparathyroidism. Second, if the disease has a hereditary element, there is the problem of genetic heterogeneity (2). Clinically similar genetic disorders may show different patterns of inheritance. For example, there are two types of familial isolated growth hormone deficiency that resemble each other quite closely, but one shows autosomal recessive and the other autosomal dominant inheritance (18).

Estimates of recurrence risk are derived in a variety of ways (19). These will take into account what is known of the genetic mechanism which determines the relevant disorder. When more than one genetic mechanism or when environmental or secondary factors can determine clinically indistinguishable traits, then the *relative* probabilities of the different mechanisms operating in the particular family are considered. For conditions determined by simple mendelian inheritance, there is no particular difficulty in predicting the probability of an offspring being affected, provided that the genotypes of the parents can be recognized. These are, of course, complications associated with failure of penetrance, variability in expression, and new mutations, but in general mendelian principles apply. When advising families about disorders of polygenic causation or disorders in which the inheritance pattern is not clear-cut, such as diabetes mellitus (see p. 1023), the counselor must resort to empirical risk estimates which are derived from retrospectively assembled data.

The genetic prognosis is usually presented in terms of probability that the couple will produce another affected child. It is important that the counselor makes sure that the couple understands the meaning of such absolute risk figures. Although different families initially react in different ways to the same risk (and not always in the way one expects), most couples who ask for genetic advice can be expected to take a responsible course of action on the basis of the information quoted. For genetic diseases in general, when the recurrence risk is high—that is, equal to or greater than 1 in 10—most parents [66 per cent in Carter's genetic clinic (20)] are deterred from planning further children. When the risks are low—that is, less than 1 in 10—few (25 per cent) are deterred.

Nearly 50 inherited disorders can now be diagnosed prenatally by amniocentesis (21). The 21-hydroxylase variety of the adrenogenital syndrome is the only endocrine disorder that has been successfully detected by this technique (22 to 24). Elevated levels of pregnanetriol have been found in the amniotic fluid during the *last* trimester of several pregnancies in which the fetus was subsequently proved to be affected with this disorder. Attempts at diagnosis *in utero* earlier in gestation have not been successful (25). Prenatal knowledge of diagnosis may be life-saving in the management of male infants known to be at risk for this disease. Affected males often have no genital abnormalities at birth and are thus frequently discharged from the newborn nursery only to return subsequently in adrenal crisis.

Certain inherited endocrine disorders in which expression of the mutant gene is limited to only one sex can be avoided by determining the sex of the fetus and selectively aborting fetuses of the appropriate sex. In the diseases listed in Table 25–3,

TABLE 25–3. INHERITED ENDOCRINE DISORDERS PREVENTABLE BY SELECTIVE ABORTION

Disorder	Method of Prevention
Diabetes insipidus, vasopressin-resistant type	Selective abortion of XY fetuses
Familial true hermaphroditism	Selective abortion of XX fetuses
Familial XX gonadal dysgenesis	Selective abortion of XX fetuses
Familial XY gonadal dysgenesis	Selective abortion of XY fetuses
Testicular feminization	Selective abortion of XY fetuses
Reifenstein's syndrome	Selective abortion of XY fetuses
Familial pseudovaginal perineoscrotal hypospadias	Selective abortion of XY fetuses

selective abortion is a feasible means of prevention because the disorder is X-linked recessive and affects only males (e.g., diabetes insipidus, vasopressin-resistant type) or because the disorder involves sexual development and is expressed in only one sex (e.g., testicular feminization). In any mendelian disorder for which selective abortion is carried out on the basis of sex alone, one-half of the aborted fetuses will be normal and one-half will be affected. However, many parents prefer abortion on these grounds to prevent the birth of a sick child, particularly if amniocentesis can guarantee a nonaffected infant in a future pregnancy. A more rational approach ultimately will be to make the specific prenatal diagnosis so that only affected fetuses are aborted.

Table 25–4 lists those inherited endocrine disorders in which asymptomatic relatives at risk can be diagnosed by simple laboratory tests and then successfully treated by either hormone replacement, prophylactic surgery, or by other indicated means. In order that therapy be successful, it must be initiated within the first few months of life for certain of these disorders (e.g., diabetes insipidus, vasopressin-resistant type; vitamin D-resistant rickets; athyrotic cretinism; the adrenogenital syndromes; and familial leucine-sensitive hypoglycemia). In those forms of pituitary dwarfism which respond to treatment (e.g., familial hypopituitarism and isolated growth hormone deficiency), administration of growth hormone must be started in childhood to ensure normal growth. Moreover, in those individuals identified as asymptomatic gene carriers of the familial medullary thyroid carcinoma syndrome, a prophylactic thyroidectomy carried out in adolescence or early adulthood may be lifesaving. Family study to detect and treat affected relatives who are unaware of this disease is, therefore, mandatory in this disorder.

GENETIC DISORDERS OF THE PITUITARY

Diabetes Insipidus

Two hereditary forms of diabetes insipidus are recognized: (1) vasopressin-sensitive diabetes insipidus and (2) vasopressin-resistant, or nephrogenic, diabetes insipidus. Together these two

TABLE 25–4. TREATABLE OR PREVENTABLE INHERITED ENDOCRINE DISORDERS FOR WHICH SEARCH IN FAMILY MEMBERS OF AFFECTED PATIENTS IS MANDATORY

Disorder	Mode of Inheritance	Age of Onset	Method of Diagnosis	Treatment	Advantages of Early Diagnosis and Treatment
Diabetes insipidus, vasopressin-resistant type	X-linked recessive	Infancy	Urine concentration tests	Adequate hydration; chlorothiazide	Prevent mental retardation
Familial panhypopituitarism	Autosomal recessive; X-linked recessive	Infancy	Measurement of pituitary, adrenal, gonadal, and thyroid hormones	Replace deficient hormones	Prevent dwarfism, cretinism, adrenal insufficiency, gonadal failure
Isolated growth hormone deficiency	Autosomal recessive; autosomal dominant	Childhood	Measurement of growth hormone responses	Growth hormone	Prevent dwarfism
Pituitary hypogonadism	X-linked recessive; autosomal recessive	Adolescence	Plasma FSH, LH, testosterone	Testosterone	Prevent eunuchoidism
Primary male hypogonadism	X-linked recessive	Adolescence	Plasma FSH, LH, testosterone	Testosterone	Prevent eunuchoidism
Hypoparathyroidism	X-linked recessive; autosomal recessive	Infancy; adolescence	Serum calcium, phosphorus, parathyroid hormone	Calcium lactate; vitamin D	Prevent cataracts and tetany
Hyperparathyroidism	Autosomal dominant	Adulthood	Serum calcium, phosphorus, parathyroid hormone	Parathyroidectomy	Prevent renal damage and other complications of hypercalcemia
Vitamin D-resistant rickets	X-linked dominant	Infancy	Serum calcium, phosphorus, aklaline phosphatase; measurement of urine TRP	Vitamin D (high doses); oral phosphate	Prevent rickets
Familial goiters	Autosomal recessive	Infancy; childhood	PBI; perchlorate test; measurement of iodotyrosines in urine; audiogram	Thyroxine	Prevent cretinism
Hereditary form of athyrotic cretinism	Autosomal recessive	Infancy	PBI	Thyroxine	Prevent cretinism
Adrenogenital syndromes	Autosomal recessive	Infancy	Urinary 17-ketosteroids, pregnanetriol; buccal smear; serum electrolytes	Cortisone acetate	Prevent adrenal crisis and avoid sex identification problems
Adrenal insufficiency	Autosomal recessive; autosomal dominant; X-linked recessive	Infancy; adolescence; adulthood	Serum cortisol, ACTH	Cortisone acetate; DOC	Prevent adrenal crisis
Aldosterone deficiency	Autosomal recessive	Infancy; childhood	Serum electrolytes; measurement of aldosterone secretion	DOC	Prevent hyperkalemia and dehydration
Leucine-sensitive hypoglycemia	Autosomal recessive	Infancy	Blood sugar; measurement of plasma insulin responses	Low protein diet; diazoxide	Prevent convulsions
Multiple endocrine adenomatosis	Autosomal dominant	Adulthood	Serum calcium, phosphorus, blood sugar; gastrointestinal series	Parathyroidectomy; pancreatectomy; ulcer surgery	Prevent complications of hyperparathyroidism, hypoglycemia, peptic ulcer, metastatic cancer
Medullary thyroid carcinoma-pheochromocytoma syndromes	Autosomal dominant	Adulthood	Plasma calcitonin; measurement of blood pressure	Prophylactic thyroidectomy; removal of pheochromocytoma	Prevent thyroid carcinoma and complications of hypertension

hereditary disorders comprised about one-third of all types of diabetes insipidus seen on the Children's Service of the Massachusetts General Hospital (26). In this particular series, the familial form of nephrogenic diabetes insipidus was at least 6.5 times more frequent than the familial vasopressin-sensitive type (26). The most common cause of diabetes insipidus in all series is a nonfamilial form of the vasopressin-sensitive disorder due to brain tumor, such as craniopharyngioma in children (26) and metastatic carcinoma in adults (27, 28).

Vasopressin-Sensitive Diabetes Insipidus

Hereditary vasopressin-sensitive diabetes insipidus is due to a quantitative reduction in the number of nerve cells in the supraoptico-hypophysial system (29), resulting in a deficiency of circulating plasma vasopressin (30). A number of families have been reported in which the disease showed the pedigree characteristics of autosomal dominant inheritance. The age of onset is often delayed until adolescence and early adulthood, and there is a wide variability in symptoms in both males and females. Females may be particularly symptomatic during pregnancy with improvement after menopause (31). In contrast to nephrogenic diabetes insipidus, hypocaloric dwarfism and mental retardation infrequently occur (26, 31).

X-linked inheritance of vasopressin-sensitive diabetes insipidus has also been documented in several kindreds (32). In such families, the males are moderately to severely affected, but female carriers show only mild defects in urine concentration or polyuria, particularly during the last trimester of pregnancy. Such mild effects in heterozygous females are readily understandable on the basis of a partial reduction in hormone secreting cells, as predicted from the X-inactivation hypothesis. Neither clinical nor laboratory examinations can differentiate between the autosomal and the X-linked varieties of vasopressin-sensitive diabetes insipidus.

Nephrogenic Diabetes Insipidus

In vasopressin-resistant or nephrogenic diabetes insipidus, the renal tubule is completely insensitive to the action of antidiuretic hormone (33). The biochemical basis for the end-organ unresponsiveness may be related to a deficiency in the renal cyclic AMP receptor system mediated by vasopressin (34). Almost all cases of nephrogenic diabetes insipidus beginning in childhood are familial, and the genetic pattern is compatible with X-linked recessive inheritance. All males thus far reported exhibit severe clinical signs, while most but not all carrier females manifest a mild form of the disorder, i.e., an abnormal urinary concentration test (35, 36). One severely affected girl was found to have a deletion of one X chromosome (37). Bode and Crawford have traced a large number of families to a group of Ulster Scots who settled in Nova Scotia in 1761 and have, therefore, suggested that most North American Caucasian patients with the disorder descended from these original settlers (37). At least three Negro families have been reported with X-linked nephrogenic diabetes insipidus (38, 40). No close linkage exists between the gene for diabetes insipidus and the Xg^a blood group (41).

Pituitary Dwarfism

Pituitary dwarfism refers to a heterogeneous group of disorders in which shortness of stature results from a deficiency of growth hormone (HGH). At least eight genetically distinct forms of familial dwarfism and HGH deficiency have been identified (Table 25–5 and below) (42). Sporadic cases and those forms secondary to tumors and congenital abnormalities are also recognized. In Norway, the prevalence of pituitary dwarfism is estimated at 1 case per 100,000 population, with 25 per cent of all cases being hereditary, 60 per cent sporadic, and 15 per cent secondary (43).

Two of the genetic forms of pituitary dwarfism, congenital absence of the pituitary (44) and abnormal sella turcica syndrome (Ferrier-Stone syndrome) (45), have each been reported in only one family. Both disorders occurred in sibs of both sexes and are, therefore, presumed to be transmitted as autosomal recessive traits.

Familial Panhypopituitarism

Familial panhypopituitarism (asexual ateliotic dwarfism) is associated with a deficiency of growth

TABLE 25–5. GENETIC FORMS OF PITUITARY DWARFISM*

Disorder	Inheritance
Congenital absence of pituitary	Autosomal recessive
Familial panhypopituitarism	
Type I	Autosomal recessive
Type II	X-linked recessive
Isolated growth hormone deficiency	
Type I	Autosomal recessive
Type II	Autosomal dominant
Laron-type dwarfism	Autosomal recessive
Pygmies	Probably polygenic
	(*not* autosomal dominant)
Abnormal sella turcica	Autosomal recessive

*Modified from Rimoin, D. L., and Schimke, R. N.: *Genetic Disorders of the Endocrine Glands*. St. Louis, C. V. Mosby Co., 1971, with permission.

hormone *and* of one or more other pituitary hormones as well. Although many cases are nongenetic, a number of inbred kindreds reported from Switzerland (46), Yugoslavia (47), and the Hutterite community of Western Canada (48) provide evidence that the most common familial form of panhypopituitary dwarfism is inherited as an autosomal recessive trait (42). Two recent reports have appeared suggesting that panhypopituitarism may occasionally occur as an X-linked trait. One of these reports described four male cases in three related sibships connected through females of normal height (49), and the other one showed panhypopituitarism in two half-brothers with the same mother (50). The primary defects causing autosomal recessive and X-linked recessive panhypopituitary dwarfism are unknown.

Isolated Growth Hormone Deficiency

Analysis of the clinical, genetic, and metabolic features of normally proportioned dwarfs with normal sexual function (midgets or sexual ateliotics) indicates at least two genetically distinct types of isolated HGH deficiency (48). Type I HGH deficiency, the more common type, is associated with insulin deficiency, prolonged hypoglycemia following insulin administration, HGH responsiveness, wrinkled skin, and autosomal recessive inheritance. Type II HGH deficiency, characterized by hyperinsulinemia, poor response to administered growth hormone, and normal skin, usually occurs as a sporadic disorder, but when it is genetic, it is transmitted as an autosomal dominant trait.

Although puberty is frequently delayed to between 16 and 19 years, sexual development, once it occurs, is normal (48). Caesarean section is required in pregnant affected females since their offspring will be of normal birth weight and length, regardless of whether the child is normal or ateliotic (42). Pregnancy in these women is followed by normal lactation, suggesting that HGH is not essential for normal postpartum lactation (51).

Laron-Type Dwarfism

Although clinically indistinguishable from Type I HGH deficiency, this form of familial pituitary dwarfism is distinct metabolically in that it is associated with high fasting levels of immunoreactive growth hormone, low somatomedin (sulfation factor) activity, and metabolic resistance to the action of administered HGH (42). The basic defect is not known with certainty. A primary lack of somatomedin would not readily explain the observed manifold metabolic changes except for dwarfism (52). Laron has suggested that the primary defect may result from a mutation in the structural gene for growth hormone, resulting in an immunologically active but functionally inactive molecule that blocks growth hormone receptor sites in peripheral tissues (53). This hypothesis of competitive receptor saturation is supported experimentally by the finding that newborns and a patient with acromegaly were resistant to the influence of exogenous HGH while the concentration of plasma HGH was high but showed a normal response when HGH levels were decreased (52). Although originally reported in inbred families of Oriental Jewish origin, the Laron-type dwarfism has since been described in non-Jewish families from Western Europe and the United States (42).

Laron has documented diminished size of penis and testicles in five out of six patients with this disorder, suggesting that HGH may play a primary role in development of the external genitalia and gonads (54).

Pygmies

The African Pygmies vaguely resemble pituitary dwarfs in their size and skeletal proportions but differ in their lack of truncal obesity and wrinkled skin (42). Metabolically, the Pygmies show the unique combination of peripheral unresponsiveness to HGH administration in the presence of normal levels of immunoreactive plasma HGH and normal serum somatomedin activity (42). Since Pygmy-Bantu hybrids have a normal metabolic response to HGH administration, dominant inheritance of the HGH unresponsiveness seems unlikely (55). Further studies in Pygmy-Bantu hybrids may help define the genetic mechanism.

Pituitary Hypogonadism

Pituitary hypogonadism, resulting from an isolated lack of either one or both of the gonadotropic hormones, FSH and LH, occurs as an accompaniment of organic pituitary impairment and malnutrition and as a primary genetic disorder. Although the heterogeneity of the genetic forms of pituitary hypogonadism has not been well delineated, at least two genetically distinct disorders exist: hyopgonadotropic hypogonadism with anosmia (Kallman's syndrome), inherited as an X-linked trait, and familial isolated gonadotropin deficiency, inherited as an autosomal recessive trait.

Hypogonadotropic Hypogonadism with Anosmia (Kallman's Syndrome)

The most frequent from of familial hypogonadotropic hypogonadism occurs in males in association with anosmia or hyposmia and is known as Kallman's syndrome (56). It appears to be inherited as an X-linked recessive (or as a male-limited autosomal dominant), the trait being transmitted through females who either are normal or show partial or complete anosmia. Since the anosmia is secondary to an absence of the olfactory lobes of the brain, and since hypoplasia of the hypothalamus has been reported in several autopsied cases (57), the gonadotropin deficiency may be caused by a developmental anomaly of the brain. The presence of any one of a number of abnormalities, such as cleft lip and palate, unilateral renal agenesis, ichthyosis, epilepsy, and short metacarpals, has been reported in some families with Kallman's syndrome (58 to 60), but their genetic relationship to the endocrine defect is not well defined. Rarely, hypogonadotropic hypogonadism with anosmia and midline facial anomalies occurs as an autosomal recessive disorder (61).

Familial Isolated Gonadotropin Deficiency

An isolated deficiency of gonadotropin involving both LH and FSH without anosmia or somatic anomalies has been described as a cause of familial hypogonadism in both males and females in at least four kindreds (62). Autosomal recessive inheritance is suggested by involvement of siblings only and the presence of first-cousin parental consanguinity in one of the families.

Isolated deficiency of LH with normal serum FSH is reported to be the cause of the fertile eunuch syndrome, a disorder of males in which androgen deficiency is seen in combination with near-normal spermatogenesis (63). This disorder is almost always sporadic, though one sibship with two affected brothers has been reported (64).

GENETIC DISORDERS OF THE PARATHYROIDS

Hypoparathyroidism

The hereditary forms of hypoparathyroidism are rare disorders and probably comprise no more than one-fourth of all cases of idiopathic hypoparathyroidism (65, 66). At least three genetically distinct disorders are recognized: (1) familial neonatal hypoparathyroidism, (2) familial hypoparathyroidism without Addison's disease and moniliasis, and (3) familial hypoparathyroidism with Addison's disease and moniliasis.

Familial Neonatal Hypoparathyroidism

Hypoparathyroidism developing in the first weeks of life and manifesting as neonatal tetany is due either to congenital absence of the thymus and parathyroid glands (DiGeorge syndrome), which occurs as a sporadic disorder in both males and females, or to familial neonatal hypoparathyroidism, which is inherited as an X-linked recessive and affects only males (67, 68). Rarely, unrecognized maternal hyperparathyroidism may lead to suppression of parathyroid function of the newborn causing a clinical picture that transiently resembles neonatal hypoparathyroidism (69).

Familial Hypoparathyroidism With and Without Addison's Disease and Moniliasis

Idiopathic hypoparathyroidism *without* Addison's disease and moniliasis usually appears after the first six months of life and before age 20 years. The distributions of the age of onset do not differ in the familial and nonfamilial cases (65). Genetic analysis in 13 families suggests autosomal recessive inheritance (65). Consanguinity has been recorded in several instances (70).

Hypoparathyroidism developing between the ages of six months and 20 years has also been associated with idiopathic Addison's disease and mucocutaneous moniliasis (75). Most of these cases have been familial, and the inheritance is autosomal recessive (65). Moniliasis is usually the first manifestation of the disorder, and hypoparathyroidism generally reveals itself before the adrenal insufficiency. In addition, affected siblings may occasionally manifest any combination of pernicious anemia, thyroiditis, ovarian failure, or juvenile cirrhosis. Furthermore, since high titers of antiendocrine-organ antibodies are found in the sera of affected individuals, an inherited autoimmune basis for the disorder has been postulated (71).

Albright's Hereditary Osteodystrophy

Albright's hereditary osteodystrophy (AHO) is an inherited disorder in which affected family members manifest either pseudohypoparathyroidism (PHP) or pseudopseudohypoparathyroidism (PPHP). The population frequency of the disorder is not known, but at least 227 cases had been reported as of 1966 (72). Patients with PHP seek aid at an average age of eight years with all the clinical and biochemical findings of true idiopathic hypoparathyroidism but do not respond to the administration of parathyroid hormone (73). In addition, they manifest a variety of skeletal and developmental defects, including shortness of stature, subcutaneous calcifications, ectopic bone formation, shortened metacarpals, roundness of the face, and mental retardation. Not all features are present in all cases, and patients with the skeletal but not the biochemical abnormalities of hypocalcemia and hyperphosphatemia have been designated as having PPHP. It is now generally concluded that PHP and PPHP are part of the same genetic syndrome, since single patients have had both conditions at different ages and many families have been reported in which members with both PHP and PPHP were present (72).

Aurbach has suggested that the basic defect in AHO may involve a deficient parathyroid hormone receptor-adenyl cyclase system in kidney, bone, and other tissue (74). Experimental data in support of this hypothesis are based on the observation that little or no cyclic AMP appears in the urine after the administration of parathyroid hormone to subjects with PHP, whereas there is a ten- to twentyfold increase in normal subjects, in patients with true idiopathic hypoparathyroidism, and in patients with a variety of unusual skeletal and developmental defects that resemble AHO, including the basal cell nevus syndrome, familial calcification of the cerebral basal ganglia, Gardner's syndrome, vitamin D-resistant rickets, and Turner's syndrome (74, 75). The specific component of the parathyroid hormone-sensitive adenyl cyclase receptor system that is deficient is not known, but studies *in vitro* of renal tissue from one patient with PHP showed normal membrane-bound adenyl cyclase activity (76). This result suggests that the primary defect may lie at a site in the action of parathyroid hormone more distal than membrane-bound adenyl cyclase.

On the basis of genetic analysis showing lack of evidence of male to male transmission in families and an affected female:affected male ratio of 2:1, it has been inferred that an X-linked dominant mode of inheritance is operating (77). On the other hand, the finding that hemizygous males are not more severely affected than are heterozygous females is contrary to what is observed in other X-linked traits. Moreover, the observation that at least 13 unaffected daughters have been born to affected males with AHO (72) is not in keeping with current concepts of X-chromosome inheritance. Finally, while the female to male ratio of all probands with AHO reported as of 1966 is 2.2:1 (72), the sex ratio of their affected sibs is 1.2:1, a value which approaches unity. Taken together, these data suggest either that AHO is in fact inherited as a sex-influenced autosomal dominant rather than an X-linked dominant or that AHO is genetically heterogeneous, comprising both X-linked and autosomal forms.

Hyperparathyroidism

Primary hyperparathyroidism is a common endocrine disorder occurring with a population frequency of 1 in 800 (78). In adults, hereditary forms of primary hyperparathyroidism account for about 20 per cent of all cases and thus occur at a frequency of about 1 in 4,000 (78). Three genetic forms are currently recognized, one affecting neonates and two affecting adults. Familial neonatal primary hyperparathyroidism is extremely rare; it affects young infants in the neonatal period and is inherited as an autosomal recessive trait (79).

Hyperparathyroidism in adults may occur in families in whom there is no other endocrine involvement, or it may be a component of multiple endocrine adenomatosis. Both disorders appear to be inherited as autosomal dominant traits and are probably genetically distinct, but this remains to be clarified. Within the same family, both hyperplasia and adenomas of the parathyroid glands have been seen, suggesting that both histologic types are manifestations of the same pathologic process (78).

Jackson has pointed out that male patients with hyperparathyroidism are three times more likely to have a familial disorder than are females. This is because the disorder in general has a male to female ratio of 1:3, while the ratio in hereditary hyperparathyroidism is 1:1. Therefore, if one in five patients with hyperparathyroidism has the hereditary type, then two of every five male patients and two of every 15 female patients should have affected relatives (78).

Vitamin D-Resistant Rickets with Hypophosphatemia

Familial vitamin D-resistant rickets with hypophosphatemia is a disorder characterized by the development of rickets or osteomalacia, metabolic unresponsiveness to physiologic amounts of vitamin D, and the presence of hypophosphatemia due to diminished renal tubular reabsorption of phosphate (80). Although an abnormality in the metabolism of vitamin D—a decrease in the hepatic conversion of the vitamin to one of its biologically active products, 25-hydroxycholecalciferol—has been demonstrated in several patients with the disorder (81), it is not yet known whether this deficient conversion reflects a primary or secondary manifestation of the genetic defect (80).

When hypophosphatemia alone is used to identify the presence of the trait, all available genetic data, including sex ratios and segregation analyses, are consistent with a pattern of X-linked dominant inheritance with complete penetrance. Males usually have more severe skeletal disease than do females, as expected from the X-inactivation hypothesis (80). Not all cases of vitamin D-resistant rickets are clearly inherited. Of 24 index cases studied by Burnett and Dent, eight (three males, five females) were found to be the only affected member of their respective kindreds (82). Such sporadic cases could be due to phenocopy, an autosomal recessive trait, illegitimacy, or to a new mutation. At least two instances of new mutations in this disorder have been identified (82).

GENETIC DISORDERS OF THE THYROID

Familial Goiter Resulting from Defects in Thyroxine Biosynthesis

This group of diseases is an excellent example of a genetically heterogeneous disorder. Pathophysio-

TABLE 25–6. DEFECTS IN THYROXINE BIOSYNTHESIS CAUSING FAMILIAL GOITER*

Failure to transport iodide
Failure to form organic iodine
    Complete peroxidase deficiency (85)
    Altered binding of hemin to peroxidase (86)
Pendred's syndrome (goiter with deaf-mutism)
Failure of coupling of iodotyrosines
Failure of iodotyrosine deiodinase activity
Diminished or altered thyroglobulin synthesis
Abnormal iodinated polypeptides in serum

*Modified from J. B. Stanbury (83).

logic and biochemical studies have elucidated at least eight different biochemical defects in thyroxine biosynthesis that have the common end result of defective thyroid hormone secretion, hypothyroidism, and goiter formation (Table 25–6) (83). In general, patients affected with the complete defect in these disorders have retarded mental and skeletal development and, if untreated, show the outward appearance of thyroid hormone deficiency. Goiter may be present at birth but more commonly becomes noticeable during childhood. Although these disorders are the only types of thyroid disease in which a marked preponderance of affected females does not occur, females tend to be more severely involved (84). Most of these defects appear to be inherited as autosomal recessive traits, and, with the exception of the Pendred syndrome, homozygotes are extremely rare, probably occurring no more frequently than one in 100,000 for each disorder.

The importance of these rare disorders, however, is out of all proportion to their frequency and relates to the light they throw on the modes of gene action in the causation of thyroid disease in general (84). In all these defects, heterozygotes, who can be expected to be quite common, show a propensity to goiter formation much in excess of the normal population (83). Thus, it is likely that the heterozygous states of these disorders contribute to the causation of milder and more common thyroid diseases such as nontoxic goiter (see below).

Pendred's Syndrome (Familial Goiter with Deaf-Mutism)

Pendred's syndrome, characterized by the unique association of goiter and nerve deafness, is the most frequent of the inherited defects in thyroxine biosynthesis. It comprises 7.5 per cent of all individuals with congenital deafness. Moreover, the incidence of the disorder in the general population is estimated at 1 in 50,000 (87, 88). Family studies clearly indicate autosomal recessive inheritance.

Studies with I^{131} have shown that the administration of perchlorate to these patients characteristically causes the thyroid to discharge iodine only partially, a finding which suggests that the basic defect may involve an incomplete failure of organification of iodine (83). Since direct measurements and characterization of peroxidase activity in

TABLE 25-7. FORMS OF ADRENOGENITAL SYNDROME*

Deficiency	Virilization	Dominant Steroid Secreted	Urinary 17-Ketosteroids	Salt Loss	Miscellaneous
Desmolase	0	Cholesterol	Low	Usually	Rare; males have female external genitalia
3β-Hydroxysteroid dehydrogenase	+	Δ⁵-3β-OH compounds	Elevated	Usually	Rare; males have female external genitalia
11-Hydroxylase	+++++	S and DOC	Elevated	No	Usually hypertensive
17-Hydroxylase	0	B and DOC	Low	No	No sex hormones; males have ambiguous genitalia, no second-degree sex development; hypertensive
21-Hydroxylase	+++++	17-HP	Elevated	Often	Most common type

*From Bongiovanni, A. M., In *The Metabolic Basis of Inherited Disease.* 3rd ed. Stanbury, J. B., Wyngaarden, J. B., et al. (eds.), New York, McGraw-Hill Book Co., 1972, with permission.

thyroid homogenates from patients with Pendred's syndrome have not yet been carried out, its precise biochemical relationship to the several other recognized organification defects listed in Table 25-7 is not known.

In addition to their nerve deafness, patients with Pendred's syndrome can also be distinguished from most other patients with familial goiter by their smaller goiters and euthyroid status. Nerve deafness has been reported, albeit infrequently, in other forms of familial goiter. A single case of cochlear deafness with a partial defect in coupling of iodotyrosines has been reported (88). Moreover, two brothers with deafness, one of whom was goitrous and had a defect in the coupling of iodotyrosines, have been described (89). The combination of familial goiter and deaf-mutism has also been reported in a brother and sister who, in addition, had "stippled" epiphyses and end-organ refractoriness to thyroid hormone as determined by elevated plasma thyroxine-bound iodine levels in the presence of euthyroidism. Since the parents of these two siblings were consanguineous, autosomal recessive inheritance is likely (97).

Nontoxic Goiter

Probably the most frequent cause of simple nontoxic goiter is iodine deficiency, the pathologic changes in the thyroid being due to attempts to compensate for the interference with normal hormone production. The fact that not every person in a hyperendemic area develops goiter, as well as the occasional familial occurrence of simple goiter in nonendemic areas, suggests that genetic factors affect susceptibility to goiter formation (91). The higher proportion of nontasters of phenylthiocarbamide [PTC tasting is a dominantly inherited genetic polymorphism in which tasters are of the genotypes TT and Tt, while nontasters are tt (92)] among patients in some populations with goiter, and the possibility of genetically determined, thyroid autoimmunity in goitrous patients (see below) may explain some of this genetic susceptibility. Moreover, there is further evidence that the

mild or incomplete defects in thyroid hormone biosynthesis present in heterozygotes for the various types of familial goiter may sometimes express as euthyroid goiter (discussed above). Fraser has estimated that approximately 8 per cent of the general population is heterozygous for one of the genes causing familial goiter (84). However, heterozygosis of this type alone is clearly not sufficient to cause goiter, since if it were, the family history in cases of nontoxic goiter would be more striking than it is.

Thus it is likely that nontoxic goiter is due to an interaction of the various genetic factors with secondary modifying factors, of which female sex, dietary deficiency of iodine, and dietary excess of goitrogens are the major etiologic factors thus far identified. In this sense, the inheritance of most nontoxic goiters is likely to be polygenic and multifactorial.

At least one form of euthyroid nontoxic goiter is determined by a single gene. Murray and associates described a Scottish family in which 13 members of 5 generations had nontoxic goiters which appeared in childhood and were characterized by marked intrathyroidal calcification demonstrable roentgenologically. None of the known defects in thyroxine biosynthesis could be implicated. The pedigree was consistent with an autosomal dominant mode of inheritance (93).

Athyrotic Cretinism

This disorder results from a failure of thyroid development and is probably twice as common a cause of childhood hypothyroidism as are the familial goiters (94). Most cases are sporadic and occur in females, but a number of families with affected sibs of both sexes have been described, consanguinity having been present in at least three instances (95).

It is likely that athyrotic cretinism is as heterogeneous as are the familial goiters. One possible mendelian variant of this group is the very rare Kocher-Debre-Semelaigne syndrome, which is characterized by agoitrous cretinism in association with muscular hypertrophy. Cross and associates have identified two affected sibs in an inbred Amish family, thus making autosomal recessive inheritance likely (96).

Thyroiditis and Adult Hypothyroidism

Thyroid autoantibodies are frequently found in adult patients with both chronic lymphocytic thyroiditis and primary hypothyroidism. Furthermore, a number of family studies have demonstrated an increased occurrence of thyroid autoantibodies in apparently normal relatives of patients with these disorders (97). Although fathers as well as mothers can transmit the tendency to thyroid autoantibody formation (98), no firm statement regarding the mode of inheritance can be made yet (97). In addition to familial clustering of autoantibodies, the familial occurrence of various types of thyroid diseases, including nontoxic goiter and thyrotoxicosis, has been noted among relatives of patients with thyroiditis and primary hypothyroidism (97). It has been estimated that about one-third of all adult patients with thyroid disease have family members affected with the same or a closely related thyroid disorder (99).

Thyrotoxicosis

Genetic factors that influence susceptibility to hyperthyroidism have been demonstrated directly in families with thyrotoxicosis. Twin studies strongly suggest the operation of genetic factors, since 47 per cent of identical twins and only 3.1 per cent of nonidentical twins were concordant for thyrotoxicosis (100).

Several family studies have shown a significant excess of thyrotoxicosis in relatives of those with the disease (84). Both dominant and recessive modes of inheritance, with relative limitation to women and low penetrance of the gene, have been claimed. Various investigators have found that the incidence of thyroid autoantibodies, as well as of nontoxic goiter, thyroiditis, and primary hypothyroidism, is higher in relatives of thyrotoxic patients than in controls. These findings, coupled with data demonstrating a higher frequency of thyrotoxicosis among relatives of patients with both chronic lymphocytic thyroiditis and thyroid autoantibodies alone, suggest that thyroid autoimmunity may be the most important genetic factor supplying the common etiologic link among thyrotoxicosis, primary hypothyroidism, and thyroiditis. It is not yet clear, however, whether this genetic factor is primarily related to an inherited tendency to form autoantibodies or whether the autoimmune phenomena are secondary to a more fundamental basic lesion. An individual patient with chronic lymphocytic thyroiditis may be clinically hyperthyroid, euthyroid, or hypothyroid at different stages of his disease, thus providing an explanation for the finding of both myxedema and nontoxic goiter in relatives of patients with thyro-

toxicosis. Further evidence that a common genetic factor or factors can produce different clinical forms of thyroid disease comes from studies in monozygotic twins, in whom either hypothyroidism with lymphocytic thyroiditis (101) or congenital athyrotic hypothyroidism (102) has been found in one twin and hyperthyroidism in the other.

That thyroid autoimmunity may not be the only genetic factor in thyrotoxicosis is suggested by the demonstration by Ingbar et al. of increased thyroxine turnover and increased uptake by the thyroid of I^{131} in euthyroid relatives of thyrotoxic patients (103). These workers postulated the existence of a familial metabolic abnormality predisposing to the development of diffuse toxic goiter.

Variants of Serum Thyroxine-binding Globulin

Several plasma proteins, including prealbumin and thyroxine-binding globulin (TBG), bind thyroxine. Elevation and depression of TBG is associated with high and low protein-bound iodine values, respectively, and occurs as a familial condition in euthyroid individuals (104, 105). Family studies indicate that both TBG deficiency and TBG elevation are inherited as X-linked dominant traits (105, 106), and both conditions affect the same protein (TBG) with at least two different mutations. The discovery of an XO female with absent TBG is in accord with these genetic data (107). No linkage of the locus for elevated TBG to the Xg blood group locus could be demonstrated in one family study (108). Neither condition appears to produce any clinical difficulties, but both must be remembered as causes of falsely low or high PBI values.

GENETIC DISORDERS OF THE ADRENAL

Adrenogenital Syndromes

The disorders of adrenocortical steroid biosynthesis leading to the adrenogenital syndromes and congenital adrenal hyperplasia have been resolved into at least five different specific genetic disorders, each presumably due to a different enzymatic defect (109). The clinical manifestations vary in each disorder and are dependent on the specific actions of the particular intermediate steroid compound that accumulates (Table 25–7).

All these disorders appear to be inherited as autosomal recessive traits. Most are rare, except for the 21-hydroxylase deficiency, which accounts for more than 90 per cent of all cases currently recognized (109). The gene frequency for the latter disorder varies among different populations. In the United States, determined in Maryland, the homozygous state is reported at 1 in 67,000 (110), giving a heterozygote frequency of 1 in 125. Figures for Switzerland are 1 in 5,000 and 1 in 35, respectively (111). Southwestern Alaskan Eskimos have the highest frequencies yet reported: 1 in 490 for homozygosity and 1 in 11 for heterozygosity (112). The reason for these striking population differences in gene frequency is not completely known, but they probably reflect differences in inbreeding in these different areas. While gene frequencies are not affected by inbreeding, a higher frequency of affected homozygotes would be found with high inbreeding levels. If such estimates of homozygote frequency are used for calculations of gene and heterozygote frequencies, as is usually done, misleadingly high gene frequency estimates are obtained.

Money and Lewis have reported that among 70 patients with the adrenogenital syndrome, 60 per cent rather than the expected 25 per cent had an IQ of 110 or higher. These data were interpreted to indicate that the higher intelligence in homozygotes is a result of a positive effect of elevated fetal androgen on intellectual development (113).

Biochemical studies in the rare patients with the desmolase, 3β-hydroxysteroid dehydrogenase, and 17-hydroxylase deficiencies are of particular genetic interest because they indicate that the synthesis of each of these enzymes in both adrenal gland and gonad is under the control of the same gene, since the enzyme deficiency is found in both organs (109).

Familial Adrenocortical Insufficiency

The familial forms of adrenocortical insufficiency consist of a number of different genetic disorders, each of which is relatively rare. The age of onset of symptoms may provide an initial clue to differential diagnosis. Congenital adrenal hypoplasia, Wolman's disease, and the adrenogenital syndromes (discussed above) become clinically evident in the newborn period; hereditary unresponsiveness to ACTH, uncomplicated Addison's disease, Addison's disease with diffuse cerebral sclerosis, and Addison's disease with hypoparathyroidism and moniliasis usually appear in early childhood, while adrenal insufficiency associated with Schmidt's syndrome develops in late childhood or early adulthood (see below).

Congenital Adrenal Hypoplasia

On the basis of both histologic and genetic evidence, there are at least two heritable forms of this disorder: (1) an X-linked recessive form involving males and characterized by the persistence of large fetal cells in the adrenal cortex, and (2) an autosomal recessive form involving both sexes in which the histologic abnormality does not appear (114). The X-linked form has been reported more often than the autosomal recessive form. Both disorders are fatal if not immediately treated with steroids.

Wolman's Disease

This is an abnormality of lipid storage causing adrenal insufficiency, hepatosplenomegaly, and steatorrhea (115). It is invariably fatal by the age of six months despite treatment with steroids. In a newborn with failure to thrive, the presence of bilateral calcification of the adrenals on the abdominal x-ray is highly suggestive of this disorder. Over 20 patients have been reported, and the inheritance is consistent with that of an autosomal recessive mode. The significant biochemical feature is the accumulation of both cholesterol esters and triglycerides in many organs, presumably because of a total deficiency of one form of acid lipase activity (116).

Hereditary Unresponsiveness to ACTH

At least 11 sibships with adrenocortical dysfunction, characterized by deficient hydrocortisone production but normal aldosterone production, have been described (119). Careful clinical studies have demonstrated ACTH unresponsiveness. Hypoglycemic convulsions and hyperpigmentation have been the two prominent features of this syndrome. Genetic analysis by Franks and Nance revealed an excess of males and a deficiency of consanguineous matings, suggesting the occurrence of both autosomal recessive and X-linked recessive forms of the disorder (118). ACTH levels in these patients as determined by both immunoassay and bioassay are elevated, thus excluding the possibility of a biologically inactive ACTH molecule (118). The basic lesion(s) most likely involves a cellular interaction between ACTH and the cortisol biosynthetic system.

Addison's Disease

Idiopathic Addison's disease unassociated with other disorders is frequently familial, especially when it occurs in males below 10 years of age. Spinner et al. found affected relatives in the families of about one-third of all cases of uncomplicated Addison's disease seen at the Endocrine Clinic at Johns Hopkins Hospital (65). The presence of normal sexual differentiation and the absence of autoantibodies and associated endocrinopathies in these patients separate this entity from other forms of familial adrenal insufficiency (discussed below). Most cases are inherited as a recessive trait, either autosomal or X-linked. The preponderance of males suggests the latter (65, 119), but no unequivocal X-linked pedigree has yet been reported.

The unique combination of idiopathic Addison's disease and diffuse cerebral sclerosis (Schilder's disease) has been reported in at least 13 families. All fully documented cases have been limited to males, and the pedigrees are characteristic of X-linked recessive inheritance (120). Close linkage to the Xg^a blood group has been excluded (121). Clinically, the patients usually first develop adrenal insufficiency during childhood, followed several years later by the onset of spastic paraplegia and mental deterioration. The basic defect is not known, but presumably it involves a process common to brain and adrenal cortex.

Addison's disease with hypoparathyroidism and moniliasis is discussed on p. 1013.

The occurrence of Addison's disease of adult onset in association with thyroiditis is called Schmidt's syndrome (122). An increased incidence of diabetes mellitus, vitiligo, and pernicious anemia, as well as the presence of circulating antiendocrine tissue antibodies, is also characteristic of this disorder. Patients with Schmidt's syndrome usually have family members who manifest other types of autoimmune diseases. Rarely, the disorder itself has been reported in sibs of both sexes (123). The mechanism of inheritance remains unclear. If the disorder is due to a single gene, then autosomal recessive inheritance is likely (65). However, a polygenic mechanism with an inherited liability to develop pluriglandular endocrine failure and autoantibody formation has not been excluded.

Familial Aldosterone Deficiency

Familial aldosterone deficiency results from an abnormality in the conversion of progesterone to aldosterone. Two forms are recognized: one due to a deficiency of 18-hydroxylase (124) and the other due to a deficiency of 18-hydroxydehydrogenase (134). Both disorders appear to be inherited as autosomal recessive traits. The affected members of one inbred family reported with the 18-hydroxylase defect were severely ill with hyperkalemia, sodium depletion, and intermittent fever. On the other hand, the several families reported with the 18-hydroxydehydrogenase defect manifested only subtle signs, such as mild growth retardation and transient electrolyte disturbances.

Bartter's Syndrome

Bartter's syndrome is a unique disorder in which juxtaglomerular hyperplasia and hyperaldosteronism are associated with severe hypokalemic alkalosis in the absence of hypertension (126). Onset is usually in childhood. Dwarfism and chronic renal disease are often present. A disturbance in sodium transport unrelated to elevated levels of aldosterone or renin has been demonstrated *in vitro* in the red blood cells of affected patients, and this may relate to the primary defect of the disorder (127). Autosomal recessive inheritance seems likely since of 26 cases reported, about half either occurred in sibs, including one pair of monozygotic twins, or resulted from a consanguineous or incestuous mating (128). More than half of the cases described have occurred in Blacks, suggesting a high frequency of the mutant gene in this race (128).

Variants of Corticosteroid-Binding Globulin

As in the case of thyroxine-binding globulin, inherited variation in the level of serum corticosteroid-binding globulin (CBG) is also known. Both decreases (139) and increases (130) in CBG occur, neither of which has been associated with clinical abnormalities, though both cause abnormalities in the serum cortisol level. The mode of inheritance for CBG decrease appears to be dominant, either autosomal or X-linked, while that of CBG increase presumably involves the same genetic locus, although critical studies are lacking.

DISORDERS OF SEXUAL DEVELOPMENT

Abnormalities in sexual development usually result either from nonfamilial aberrations in sex chromosomes or from inherited single-gene mutations. However, several rare disorders of sexual development have been described in which neither a chromosomal error nor familial aggregation of the disease can be demonstrated, such as the sex reversed 46/XX male syndrome (131), the persistent müllerian duct syndrome in the male (hernia uteri inguinale) (132), congenital anorchia (133), and congenital absence of the vagina and uterus (Rokitansky-Küstner syndrome) (134). It is possible that each of these abnormalities is due to a new dominant single-gene mutation that cannot be transmitted because affected individuals are always sterile. Such cases, therefore, appear as "sporadic" disorders. These "sporadic" abnormalities and the chromosomal errors of sexual development (e.g., Turner's syndrome, Klinefelter's syndrome, and mixed gonadal dysgenesis) are discussed in detail in Chapter 8.

At least ten different inherited mendelian disorders affecting a variety of steps in sexual development (other than those described for the adrenogenital syndromes) are recognized, and their genetics are discussed in this section. The importance of such rare disorders lies in the fact that the elucidation of the specific biochemical nature of each of these mutations can be expected ultimately to provide the basis of a methodology for carrying out genetic analyses of sexual differentiation in man. These disorders are classified in terms of the presumed site of action of the mutation (Table 25-8).

Familial XX and XY Gonadal Dysgenesis

Pure gonadal dysgenesis refers to the occurrence of streak gonads in phenotypic females who lack the somatic anomalies and short stature present in Turner's syndrome. Such women usually have either a 46/XX karyotype (XX gonadal dysgenesis) or a 46/XY karyotype (XY gonadal dysgenesis) (135, 136). Familial gonadal dysgenesis should not

TABLE 25-8. MENDELIAN DISORDERS OF
SEXUAL DEVELOPMENT

Abnormalities involving gonadal differentiation in the embyro
Familial XX gonadal dysgenesis
Familial XY gonadal dysgenesis
Familial true hermaphroditism

Abnormalities involving androgen production or action
in the embryo
Adrenogenital syndromes
Testicular feminization syndrome (complete type)
Partial testicular feminization
Reifenstein's syndrome
Familial pseudovaginal perineoscrotal hypospadias

Abnormalities involving gonadal function in the adult
Familial male hypogonadism
Sertoli-cell-only syndrome
Stein-Leventhal syndrome

---

be confused with Noonan's syndrome, a disorder in which both males and females affected manifest the Turner phenotype but without gonadal abnormalities (137).

At least 61 individuals with normal female chromosomal complements (46/XX) and histologically proven streak gonads have been reported (136). Nerve deafness has been particularly frequent in this group (incidence of 25 per cent). Although deafness may occur in patients with 45/XO Turner's syndrome, it is usually not due to nerve damage but rather is secondary to middle ear infections (138).

The occurrence of 16 of these cases in seven sibships is highly suggestive of autosomal recessive inheritance. Moreover, in three of these seven families, and in another family in which a sporadic case appeared, the parents were consanguineous (139 to 142). Male sibs in these families appeared to be normal. The autosomal nature of the inheritance of this disorder suggests that genes other than on the X chromosome may be necessary for normal female gonadal development and differentiation.

Of the 62 individuals reported with 46/XY pure gonadal dysgenesis, all have had female phenotypes, and 17 were familial cases (136). Unlike familial XX gonadal dysgenesis which is inherited as an autosomal recessive trait, familial XY gonadal dysgenesis is not associated with increased parental consanguinity, and affected relatives are not limited to sibs but may also include cousins and aunts. Thus either X-linked recessive or autosomal dominant inheritance with expression only in chromosomal males is the most likely hereditary pattern in this disorder (136, 142).

Although no family has yet been reported in which pure gonadal dysgenesis was found in both a genetic male and a genetic female, one sibship has been described in which XY gonadal dysgenesis and male pseudohermaphroditism with partial masculinization occurred in two sisters (144). Patients with XY gonadal dysgenesis, but not XX gonadal dysgenesis, are especially prone to the development of tumors in their streak gonads (136). It is not known whether the abnormal gene

product in this disorder directly suppresses testis-determining loci on the Y chromosome and autosomes or whether it blocks some early stage of testicular morphogenesis.

Familial True Hermaphroditism

True hermaphroditism, defined by the presence of gonadal tissue of both sexes in one individual, is a heterogeneous entity. Sex chromosomal mosaicism, although infrequently demonstrated, is believed to account for the majority of cases (135). Several examples of true XY/XX hermaphroditism in association with genetic chimeras resulting from the double fertilization of an egg by two sperm have also been reported (135). Furthermore, a familial form of true hermaphroditism inherited as an autosomal recessive trait represents another mechanism by which this disorder can be produced (144 to 146). In the sibship reported by Clayton et al., all three affected "brothers" had a 46/XX karyotype, hypospadias, and gynecomastia, in addition to both ovarian and testicular tissues (144).

The presence of testicular tissue in the absence of a Y chromosome in the single-gene-determined form of 46/XX true hermaphroditism seems to contradict the generally accepted notion that a Y chromosome is necessary for testicular development. Additional evidence in favor of autosomal genes contributing to testicular differentiation comes from the recent discovery of an autosomal dominant mutation in mice which causes true sex reversal in 46/XX females (147).

Since the familial form of true hermaphroditism in man appears to be inherited as an autosomal recessive, it is possible that many of the sporadic cases of hermaphroditism in which karyotypes fail to show sex-chromosomal mosaicism are, in fact, examples of the inherited form. It is unknown whether homozygosity for this gene, which causes true hermaphroditism in genetic females, has any aberrant effects on the sexual development of genetic males.

Testicular Feminization Syndrome

In contrast to the true hermaphrodite who is usually a genetic female with gonadal tissue of both sexes, the male pseudohermaphrodite is a genetic male who has unequivocal male gonadal differentiation (i.e., only testes are present) but has some of the genital appearance of females (135). In other words, the male pseudohermaphrodite is a genetic and gonadal male who fails to virilize. Based on degree of deficiency in masculinization, which presumably reflects different biochemical errors in testosterone action or production during embryonic sexual differentiation, at least four different inherited forms of male pseudohermaphroditism can be distinguished: testicular feminization syndrome (complete type), partial testicular feminization, the Reifenstein syndrome, and pseudovaginal perineoscrotal hypospadias.

Complete Testicular Feminization

The testicular feminization syndrome (complete type) represents the extreme form of male pseudohermaphroditism due to complete failure of virilization. Affected individuals are unmistakably feminine in phenotype (i.e., they develop breasts and a typical female body build, with female external genitalia, despite the presence of intra-abdominal testes and the absence of internal female structures such as ovaries, uterus, and fallopian tubes). As a result of the clinical observation that topical and parenteral administration of high doses of methyltestosterone caused no growth of sexual hair in patients with testicular feminization, Wilkins was the first to propose that this disorder was due to end-organ unresponsiveness to this male sex hormone (148). Experimental proof of this hypothesis of androgen resistance is based on evidence obtained both in man and in mice with testicular feminization. First, in affected adult patients, despite normal blood levels of testosterone and normal rates of androgen production by the intra-abdominal testes, there is no detectable metabolic response to endogenous or administered testosterone or dihydrotestosterone (149, 150). Second, in mouse embryos affected with testicular feminization, recent studies have directly demonstrated that the failure of male sexual differentiation is a result of a primary resistance to the action of androgen during embryogenesis (151). Although a number of human investigations have been carried out to explore the biochemical basis of androgen resistance in this disorder, the results have been difficult to interpret because, in all studies, mature target tissues were used in place of fetal tissue with its critical androgen-sensitive cell line. However, studies of testicular feminization in fetal tissues of mice indicate that neither the reduction of testosterone to dihydrotestosterone by 5α-reductase nor the binding of dihydrotestosterone to its cytoplasmic receptor is deficient. Rather, the underlying defect may involve an inability to transfer the dihydrotestosterone-receptor complex from the cell cytoplasm to the nucleus (152).

The testicular feminization syndrome (complete type) is the most common form of hereditary male pseudohermaphroditism, the estimated frequency being 1 in 20,000 men in Switzerland (153) and 1 in 62,000 men in Great Britain (154). Approximately 1 to 2 per cent of females with inguinal hernias prove to have this disorder (155). Genetic analysis of published pedigree data on this condition is compatible with either X-limited recessive inheritance or with autosomal dominant inheritance limited to the male sex. Female carriers can often be recognized by the sparseness of their pubic and axillary hair. Linkage studies in man using the X-linked markers—Xg^a blood group, color blindness, and hemophilia—have failed to show measurable linkage between these genes and that for the testicular feminization syndrome (156 to 158). Probably the best evidence to date that the gene in man may be X-linked is the finding of a homologous mutation in the mouse which is unequivocally X-linked (159).

Partial Testicular Feminization

Partial testicular feminization resembles the complete form of the syndrome in respect to female phenotype, bilateral intra-abdominal testes, and 46/XY karyotype but differs in that ambiguous genitalia are present at birth, and some degree of virilization occurs at puberty. The unique clinical feature of the partial syndrome is the finding of breast development and ambiguous genitalia in a phenotypic female (160). Although the genitalia are primarily female, with clitoromegaly and partially fused labia, the degree of masculinization of the genitalia can be quite variable in different families, suggesting that this disorder is not genetically homogeneous (160 to 164). Furthermore, metabolic studies performed in several of these patients indicate heterogeneity in that some patients show a partial peripheral response to the action of testosterone (161), while others have a partial deficiency in testicular 17-ketosteroid reductase without manifesting androgen resistance (163).

Although the pathogenesis of this group of disorders is not known, its close phenotypic resemblance to the complete form of testicular feminization suggests that the basic defect(s) may involve a variety of different biochemical steps, each of which is normally necessary for male sexual differentiation (136). In almost all of the familial cases of partial testicular feminization, affected male sibs have been related through unaffected females, suggesting a pattern of inheritance similar to that of the complete form of testicular feminization.

Reifenstein's Syndrome

Reifenstein's syndrome is clinically distinct from the partial forms of testicular feminization in that the affected individuals are usually raised as males and develop a male phenotype (165). Hypospadias is a cardinal manifestation of the syndrome and is often associated with incomplete fusion of the scrotal folds, a normal-sized penis, cryptorchidism, and gynecomastia, the last developing at puberty. The development of severe psychological problems has been a prominent feature in all affected males of one large family (166). Whether this is simply a result of the psychological stress of sexual ambiguity or reflects a primary effect of the mutation on behavior is not known. Although the pathogenesis of this disorder has not been worked out, it is likely to involve either deficient androgen production or resistance to androgen action during embryonic sexual differentiation. The inheritance is that of either X-linked recessive or male-limited autosomal dominant.

Familial Pseudovaginal Perineoscrotal Hypospadias

This disorder is characterized by a congenital anomaly of the external genitalia in an otherwise normal male and may represent the most localized form of inherited male pseudohermaphroditism. Affected individuals are nearly always raised as females because the genitalia have a severe hypospadias with a perineal urethral opening, cleft scrotum, testes in labioscrotal folds, and a phallus which is mistaken for an enlarged clitoris. At the time of puberty, complete masculinization occurs (167). Unlike the other forms of male pseudohermaphroditism, there is no breast development. The pathogenesis is not known but may involve a partial form of embryonic androgen resistance localized to the genital tubercle and urogenital sinus without involvement of the wolffian ducts or the mammary buds. The description of at least eight families with multiple affected sibs and the finding of parental consanguinity in several of these families suggests that this disorder is inherited as an autosomal recessive trait (167) and is thus genetically distinct from all other forms of male pseudohermaphroditism.

Familial Male Hypogonadism

A number of families have been described in which hypogonadism unassociated with hermaphroditism, pseudohermaphroditism, and pituitary gonadotropin deficiency occurred in multiple male relatives (168). Pathogenesis is presumably related to defective androgen production in the testes, though it is unknown whether the mutation(s) involves a biosynthetic enzyme(s) or causes a failure of Leydig cell differentiation. As in most inherited disorders of male sexual development, pedigree analysis cannot distinguish between X-linked recessive and sex-limited autosomal dominant inheritance. This disorder should be distinguished from familial gynecomastia, in which gonadal function is normal and the breast enlargement is thought to be the result of familial sensitivity of the breast to normal circulating levels of androgen and estrogens. Since affected males with familial gynecomastia can reproduce, pedigree analysis can be informative, and it indicates that this trait is transmitted as an autosomal dominant trait limited to males (169).

Sertoli-Cell-Only Syndrome

In the Sertoli-cell-only syndrome, the seminiferous tubules and germ cells of the testis fail to develop, despite normal Leydig cell development and function (170). The patients are normally virilized and their only complaint is infertility. The testes are smaller than normal but larger than those of patients with Klinefelter's syndrome. Single-gene inheritance is indicated by the occurrence of two or more affected brothers in several families (170, 171). The mode of inheritance could either be X-linked or autosomal recessive. The nature of the defect is unknown but may involve a critical step in germ cell differentiation that occurs after formation of the testes from the indifferent gonad.

Stein-Leventhal Syndrome

This disorder is characterized by infertility, secondary amenorrhea, menstrual abnormalities, and hirsutism in women who have enlarged polycystic ovaries. The pathogenesis is not known, though it may involve altered steroid metabolism in the ovary. Detailed genetic analysis in 18 families by Cooper et al. has demonstrated an increased frequency of oligomenorrhea, elevated levels of androgen metabolites in urine and blood, and an increased frequency of polycystic ovaries among the mothers and sisters of index patients. Male relatives were noted to be abnormally hairy. From these data, the inheritance appears to be dominant, probably autosomal (172).

FAMILIAL PRECOCIOUS PUBERTY

Most cases of isosexual precocious puberty are nonfamilial and are either idiopathic or associated with a central nervous system lesion, a gonadal or adrenal tumor, or polyostotic fibrous dysplasia. These nonfamilial cases occur more often in females than in males (173). Among the idiopathic forms of precocious puberty, there is a familial variety which predominantly affects males (174, 175). Since the condition can be transmitted by unaffected females, as well as by affected males, to their sons, X-linked inheritance is excluded, and an autosomal dominant mode of inheritance with male limitation is indicated. Carrier females may either appear normal (176, 177) or show signs of virilization, such as frontal baldness and hirsutism (175). Certain of the adrenogenital syndromes also cause familial isosexual precocious puberty in males. Familial forms of precocious puberty in females are extremely rare (173) and need to be distinguished from the early onset of sexual development and menarche which may represent the extreme of the normal distribution curve. Since the time of onset of menarche in mothers and daughters, as well as between sisters, shows a significant correlation (r = 0.4), it is likely that multiple genes control this physiologic process (178).

HIRSUTISM AND BALDNESS

Hair growth patterns show marked variation both qualitatively and quantitatively. That such variation is particularly pronounced when certain racial groups are compared suggests the operation of multiple genetic factors. For example, in African Blacks and Orientals, chest and beard growth is greatly diminished (179).

Probably the best evidence that hair growth is polygenically determined comes from Lorenzo's detailed family studies of American women with all types of hirsutism (adrenal, ovarian, and idiopathic) (180). For each type of hirsutism, the pattern of hair distribution in female relatives ranged from the normal female distribution to the abnormally hirsute. Correlation coefficients for hair distribution between propositi and their mothers averaged 0.50. No evidence for a major gene effect on hirsutism could be demonstrated in these data.

Pattern baldness, on the other hand, may be controlled by a major gene, whose expression is influenced by both age and hormones (181, 182). This form of baldness results in the progressive transformation of large stout terminal hairs to short thin vellus hairs and ultimately leads to a reduction in the number of hair follicles of the scalp. Castration before puberty prevents male pattern baldness (183), while masculinizing tumors will produce pattern baldness in women with bald male relatives (179, 181).

The action of the presumed gene(s) for baldness at the molecular level has not been defined, but its product(s) may interact directly with dihydrotestosterone, the active androgen in male target organs (184). Based on experimental data demonstrating that dihydrotestosterone, but not testosterone or estradiol, inhibits adenyl cyclase and lowers cyclic AMP levels in scalp hair follicles, it has been suggested that the sequence of events in balding consists of (1) conversion of testosterone to dihydrotestosterone, (2) lowering of cyclic AMP by dihydrotestosterone's inhibition of adenyl cyclase, (3) diminution in protein synthesis, and (4) ultimately, premature termination of the growing stage of the hair follicle (185).

FAMILIAL ENDOCRINE TUMOR SYNDROMES

Most endocrine tumors are not heritable, but there are several types of endocrine neoplasia which are determined by a single-gene mechanism. These genetic endocrine tumor syndromes include multiple endocrine adenomatosis and the medullary thyroid carcinoma-pheochromocytoma syndromes. Since the action of the genes causing these tumors has not been identified, very little is known about the pathogenesis of these disorders.

Multiple Endocrine Adenomatosis

Thirty-six families have been described in which members have had hyperplasia or tumors (adenomas and, less often, carcinomas) involving one or more of the following endocrine organs: parathyroids, pituitary, pancreatic islets, thyroid, and adrenal cortex (186 to 190). The parathyroid and islet-cell tumors are frequently multicentric, and all four parathyroids may be involved. In addition, multiple lipomas of the skin, bronchial adenomas, and intestinal carcinoids may occur. Many of the tumors are functional, and clinical hyperparathyroidism is frequently found. The islet-cell tumors may be either insulin- or gastrin-secreting, giving rise, respectively, to hypoglycemia or the Zollinger-Ellison syndrome of gastric hypersecretion and fulminating peptic ulcerations (191). In a series of 25 patients with the Zollinger-Ellison syndrome, about 50 per cent had familial multiple

endocrine tumors (191). It is now generally accepted that multiple endocrine adenomatosis and the Zollinger-Ellison syndrome are phenotypic variants of the same mutant gene (187). Likewise, over half of the families with hereditary hyperparathyroidism actually have multiple endocrine adenomatosis (78).

The disorder is inherited as an autosomal dominant trait with high penetrance. When 27 asymptomatic adult relatives of five index patients with multiple endocrine tumors were examined, 14 showed evidence of either hypercalcemia, lipomas, or peptic ulcers (189). Similar to other dominant traits, there is a great deal of phenotypic variability. In the studies of Johnson et al., the frequency of involvement rose from zero in relatives studied during the first decade of life to more than 50 per cent of those examined during the fifth and sixth decades (192).

Familial Medullary Thyroid Carcinoma-Pheochromocytoma Syndromes

Schimke has defined a spectrum of six familial syndromes involving medullary thyroid carcinoma and pheochromocytoma (193) (Table 25–9). Medullary thyroid carcinoma comprises less than 10 per cent of all thyroid carcinomas (194) and is characterized histologically by the deposition of amyloid.

Family studies of patients with medullary thyroid carcinoma indicate that the disorder is inherited in an autosomal dominant pattern (193). While some families show only medullary thyroid carcinoma, others have shown the combination of this tumor with bilateral pheochromocytomas and parathyroid adenomas. The parathyroid tumors are believed to represent a reactive hyperplasia secondary to hypocalcemia that results from excess thyrocalcitonin produced by the medullary thyroid tumor (195). Studies by Melvin and Miller indicate that the first manifestation of this disorder in asymptomatic heterozygotes is an elevated plasma level of thyrocalcitonin determined by radioimmunoassay. This assay, therefore, can be used to predict which relatives in an affected family should undergo prophylactic thyroidectomy in order to prevent the onset of thyroid carcinoma (196).

TABLE 25–9. SPECTRUM OF FAMILIAL SYNDROMES INVOLVING MEDULLARY THYROID CARCINOMA AND PHEOCHROMOCYTOMA*

Medullary thyroid carcinoma alone
Medullary thyroid carcinoma with pheochromocytoma and parathyroid adenoma
Medullary thyroid carcinoma, pheochromocytoma, mucosal neuromas and neurofibromas
Pheochromocytoma alone
Pheochromocytoma with neurofibromatosis (von Recklinghausen's disease)
Pheochromocytoma with hemangioblastoma of the retina and cerebellum (Lindau-von Hippel syndrome)

*From Schimke, R. N., In *The Clinical Delineation of Birth Defects. X. The Endocrine System.* Baltimore, Williams and Wilkins Co., 1971, with permission.

Patients with medullary thyroid carcinoma and pheochromocytoma may also manifest mucosal neuromas of the tongue, buccal mucosa, and eyelids. These patients also have a characteristic appearance: patulous lips, prognathic jaw, and Marfan-like body habitus (193). Most cases of this disorder have been sporadic, but several instances of autosomal dominant transmission have been recorded (193).

In addition to its association with the above syndromes, pheochromocytoma may occur as a familial disorder unassociated with other diseases. As many as 5 per cent of all pheochromocytomas are familial (198). These familial tumors are often bilateral and multifocal and may be extra-adrenal in location, while the sporadic lesion is usually single. Pheochromocytomas are also rarely seen in association with two mendelian disorders: von Recklinghausen's neurofibromatosis and Lindau-von Hippel disease (193).

All these various syndromes involving medullary thyroid carcinoma and pheochromocytoma appear to be inherited in an autosomal dominant pattern. Whether they are the result of different gene mutations at the same locus (allelic) or at different loci (nonallelic) or merely reflect variable expression of a single-gene mutation is not known.

DIABETES MELLITUS

While diabetes mellitus has long been considered a hereditary disease and certainly the most common inherited endocrinologic disorder, the mode of inheritance has been the subject of much debate. Rimoin has extensively reviewed the nature of the controversy concerning the genetics of diabetes mellitus (199 to 201).

Many studies have demonstrated a higher frequency of diabetes mellitus among relatives of patients than in control populations (202, 203). Furthermore, studies of twins indicate a higher concordance rate for diabetes between both members of a pair of monozygotic twins compared with dizygotic twins [for example, 48 per cent and 3 per cent (205), 96.6 per cent and 9.1 per cent (206), and 73.0 per cent and 32 per cent (207), respectively]. However, when the precise analysis of the genetic basis of diabetes mellitus has been attempted, the subject has become "in many respects a geneticist's nightmare . . . (which) . . . presents almost every impediment to a proper genetic study" (208). Neel has summarized the difficulties involved: (1) frequency of the disease is age-dependent, (2) environmental factors including nutrition influence expression, (3) the nature of the basic defect is unknown, (4) genetic heterogeneity is likely, and (5) precise diagnostic criteria and genetic markers are lacking (209).

Despite these difficulties, often with investigations in which sources of bias were not or could not be controlled and in which methods of ascertainment and diagnosis were not ideal, many genetic mechanisms have been proposed (199, 201, 205). Chief among them are autosomal recessive (simple) inheritance and polygenic (complex) inheritance. The most convincing evidence in favor of single-gene inheritance is the demonstration of clear-cut bimodality in the glucose tolerance distributions of adult Pima Indians (210). This contrasts with the unimodal distributions described in the general United States population. Steinberg feels that this difference in glucose distributions is attributable to the lower prevalence of diabetes in the United States [5 per cent as compared to the 50 per cent prevalence in adult Pimas over age 35 (211)] which would obscure the identification of bimodality even if it existed. The mode of inheritance in the Pimas has not yet been determined.

Against the autosomal recessive or single-gene hypothesis for the general American population is the failure to find diabetes in 100 per cent of the children of conjugal diabetics. Even if decreased penetrance is invoked, one still finds no more than 50 per cent of the offspring of two diabetic parents affected, regardless of the criteria used (i.e., clinical diabetes, abnormal oral glucose tolerance, abnormal intravenous glucose tolerance, abnormal cortisone-glucose tolerance, or thickening of muscle capillary basement membranes) (201). More and better data are obviously required. It is quite possible that a satisfactory genetic analysis will not be possible until the basic defect(s) is known.

In mice (Mus musculus), inappropriate hyperglycemia may result from not one but at least six distinct mutations, some of which are transmitted as autosomal dominant and others as autosomal recessive traits. Polygenic forms of hyperglycemia have also been described (212). If these observations in mice are applicable to the genetics of diabetes in man, then it is quite likely that human diabetes is genetically heterogeneous, and its genetic complexity may, in part, be due to the occurrence in different individuals of various combinations of "diabetes genes," some having a major action and others having minor effects. In support of the idea of genetic heterogeneity in human diabetes is the finding of abnormal carbohydrate tolerance in at least 30 distinct genetic disorders (211). The hyperglycemia found in association with many of these genetic syndromes, such as that found in isolated growth hormone deficiency and myotonic dystrophy, occurs in the absence of capillary basement membrane thickening (213, 214) and is, therefore, probably a different disorder from "garden-variety" diabetes mellitus, the hallmark of which is microangiopathy (215).

The relationship between insulin-sensitive (juvenile) and insulin-resistant (adult) diabetes is still undecided. Although cases of both types have appeared in the same family, many populations are known in which there is a high prevalence of adult diabetes alone (211, 216, 222). Current evidence does not support the proposal that patients with juvenile diabetes are homozygous for the "diabetes gene," while adult onset cases are heterozygous.

Whatever the exact mode of inheritance, the high frequency of this disease [at least 2 per cent clinically affected in the United States (212)] is of great genetic interest. Since diabetes was commonly a lethal disease until 50 years ago, one would have expected gradual elimination of the gene or genes leading to diabetes. On the contrary, diabetes is a frequently found disease. Since there is no reason to believe that mutations of the genes causing diabetes are more common than other mutations, and since it has not been proved that carriers of the gene(s) for diabetes have an increased number of offspring, a yet undetected advantage of the diabetic gene or genes unrelated to the disease itself must be seriously considered. Neel speculated that the ability to mobilize glucose readily may have been of great survival value during times in human evolution in which difficulty in obtaining food was common (the "thrifty genotype" hypothesis) (223).

Genetic Counseling

Since the mode of inheritance and nature of the genetic mechanisms causing diabetes mellitus are not known, precise genetic counseling on risks to relatives is nearly impossible. However, guidelines for the counselor of diabetic families are available and are based on empirical risk figures derived from averages from the literature for a series of common counseling situations (202 to 204). The risk figures presented in Table 25–10 represent our assessment of this literature. These figures may need to be modified as more extensive empiric data become available. The major weakness in all previously published empiric data on the familial occurrence of diabetes is that the true lifetime risk to the development of diabetes in normoglycemic relatives cannot be determined by current diagnostic tests. Nonetheless, as indicated by the risk figures in Table 25–10, the observed absolute risks to relatives of diabetics are not as large as the mendelian autosomal recessive genetic risks of 25 per cent and 100 per cent that are often quoted to sibs of diabetics and to children of conjugal diabetics, respectively. In general, the risks outlined in Table 25–10 will be slightly increased (perhaps $1\frac{1}{2}$ times) if the diabetes in the index case was of early onset and severe and if diabetes mellitus is present in both maternal and paternal second-degree relatives (aunts, uncles, nieces, and nephews). Although only about 5 per cent of the children of juvenile diabetics married to nondiabetics actually develop clinical diabetes mellitus during childhood and adolescence, their relative risk is 22 times that of the general population (203). This low observed frequency for development of diabetes despite high relative risk occurs because juvenile diabetes is a very uncommon disorder in the population at large. Thus, *in quoting risk figures to the relative at risk, the counselor should emphasize the absolute risk figures.*

It frequently happens that young couples want to know the risk of having diabetic children when one member of the couple has clinical diabetes and the other is not diabetic by glucose tolerance testing but has a first-degree relative (parent or sib) with known diabetes. Based on the empiric data in Table 25–10, the absolute risk to the child would probably be greater than 5 per cent (1 parent diabetic) and less than 10 to 15 per cent (both parents diabetic).

A newer and more quantitative approach to the genetic counseling of families with diabetes mellitus involves the use of computer programs to estimate recurrence risks. Smith has recently reported one such program which uses parameters on population prevalence, heritability of liability of the condition, and details of the family history (224).

A recent controversy on whether or not two diabetics should be allowed to marry one another and have children has arisen as a result of the advice of the World Health Organization, which feels "that conjugal diabetics may increase the number of diabetic offspring and perhaps determine the appearance of diabetes at earlier ages" (225). This view has been challenged by Edwards, who argues that the marriage of two diabetics would probably not result in an increase in the number of subsequent diabetics but would merely influence their allocation (226). In other words, if diabetics marry each other, there will only be half as many marriages involving diabetics. Furthermore, Edwards points out that the impaired fertility of double diabetic matings will tend to prevent any increase in the population of diabetics. In actual practice, it has been found that *clinical* diabetes is found in no more than 10 to 15 per cent of the offspring of conjugal diabetics, though several studies have re-

TABLE 25–10. ESTIMATED ABSOLUTE RISKS FOR CLINICAL DIABETES*

Relative at Risk	Diabetic Status of Near Relatives				Absolute Risk
	One Parent Diabetic	Both Parents Diabetic	One Sib Diabetic	> One Sib Diabetic	
Child	+	−	−	−	~5%
Child	−	+	−	−	~10–15%
Child	+	−	+	−	~10%
Sib	−	−	+	−	~5%
Sib	+	−	+	−	~10%
Sib	−	+	+	−	~20%
Sib	−	−	−	+	~10%

*These risk figures represent our assessment of the published empirical data on common counseling situations in diabetes mellitus (202, 203, 204, 224) and are meant to serve as approximate guidelines.

ported as many as 37.5 per cent affected (199). When more sensitive criteria are used to diagnose the diabetic state, such as an oral glucose tolerance test (227) and capillary basement membrane thickening (215), as many as 50 per cent of the offspring of two diabetic parents are found to be affected.

In addition to quoting risk figures to diabetic families, the genetic counselor should also indicate the alleged relationship between clinical diabetes or chemical diabetes in the mother and congenital defects in her offspring. The most extensive study found that 44 of 853 infants of diabetic mothers (5.2 per cent) had *major* defects as compared to a 1.2 per cent frequency in control infants of non-diabetic mothers (228). The most characteristic diabetic embryopathy is the caudal regression syndrome, which consists of agenesis of the sacrum and coccyx, hypoplasia of both femurs, and urogenital abnormalities (229). Finally, it should be emphasized that, although gestation in the diabetic female is associated with an increased incidence of toxemia and polyhydramnios, the great majority of such pregnancies can be successfully managed with good obstetric care.

FAMILIAL HYPOGLYCEMIAS

The most common form of familial hypoglycemia not associated with other disease affects infants in the first six months of life and is characterized by excessive insulin release due to leucine sensitivity. Several families showing autosomal dominant inheritance of this disorder have been reported (230, 231). Symptoms, including convulsions, may abate with age. Affected family members are often detected only after a challenge with leucine.

Familial hypoglycemia may also be associated with a number of different mendelian disorders including galactosemia, hereditary fructose intolerance, maple syrup urine disease, familial adrenal insufficiency, leprechaunism, various forms of pituitary dwarfism, glycogen storage disease (types I, III, V, and VI), fructose-1-6-diphosphatase deficiency, and multiple endocrine adenomatosis (232). The hypoglycemias are discussed in detail in Chapter 10.

OBESITY

In man, obesity has been found in association with several rare mendelian disorders, including the Laurence-Moon-Bardet-Biedl syndrome (233) and the Alström syndrome (234). However, the genetic aspects of the common forms of obesity are less well understood. An association of obesity with both diabetes mellitus (235) and hypertriglyceridemia (236) is unquestioned, and it is possible that a clarification of the genetics of these latter two disorders will provide insight into the genetics of the more common forms of obesity.

Studies of human families show striking aggregation of obesity, and segregation analyses of mating types (stout × stout, stout × normal, nor-

mal × normal) suggest a significant genetic contribution (237). However, because of the problem of assortative matings (i.e., stouts marry stouts and thins marry thins), and because family groups share common eating habits, the genetic significance of these investigations is difficult to interpret. Although studies of twins have been criticized for similar reason, they do suggest that identical twins are more closely related in weight than are fraternal twins or sibs taken at the same age.

In view of man's variable genetic background, familial obesity is more likely to be polygenic rather than due to a single factor. Thus the weights of sibs of obese index cases are unimodally distributed with a higher modal weight than the control population, as would be expected with polygenic inheritance (238). A variety of physiologic mechanisms leading to obesity, such as the control of the number and size of adipose tissue cells, could be influenced by heredity.

OTHER HEREDITARY SYNDROMES WITH MAJOR ENDOCRINOLOGIC COMPONENTS

Myotonic Dystrophy

The characteristic clinical findings in myotonic dystrophy include myotonia, progressive muscular atrophy, frontal baldness, cataracts, and endocrine symptoms (239 to 241). Over 50 per cent of affected males develop testicular atrophy with age, which causes impotence and loss of libido but *not* gynecomastia or loss of male secondary sex characteristics. The frontal baldness does not appear to be directly related to the degree of hypogonadism. Affected females have normal menarche, but about 20 per cent of them have menstrual irregularities, infertility, abortions, or early menopause. A low basal metabolism rate is common, while thyroid function, as assessed by specific tests, is usually normal. Although glucose intolerance and hyperinsulinemia are frequently present (241), the microangiopathy of "garden-variety" diabetes mellitus does not occur (214).

The disorder is inherited as an autosomal dominant, usually with delayed onset and marked clinical variability. About 25 per cent of index cases are the result of a new mutation (242). The most useful clinical methods for identifying subclinical cases in families at risk listed in order of diagnostic success are slit-lamp examination (for lens changes), followed by electromyography (for myotonic discharges), followed by measurement of immunoglobulins (for low IgG) (242). Since the genetic locus for myotonic dystrophy is closely linked to the locus determining the secretor blood group, application of such genetic linkage offers an additional technique for the diagnosis and counseling of family members at risk (243). The most valuable information can be offered in a family where the affected parent is a secretor married to a nonsecretor, and the coupling phase is known from study of other relatives. If, in such an affected parent, the gene for myotonic dystrophy is on the same chromosome as the gene for secretor, and if the clinically normal offspring is secretor-negative, the probability of normality for that offspring is 92 per cent, even when allowance is made for genetic recombination (243). Since the secretor status can be assessed by amniotic fluid assay, intrauterine diagnosis of myotonic dystrophy and selective abortion may occasionally be possible.

Werner's Syndrome

Werner's syndrome is a condition characterized by autosomal recessive inheritance which simulates premature aging. It is characterized by shortness of stature, a peculiar habitus with thin extremities, cataracts, early graying and loss of hair, a high-pitched voice, atrophy of the skin (especially below the knees), severe vascular disease, and intractable ulcerations of the feet and ankles. Although many endocrinologic defects have been claimed, the only two that are consistently found are a severe testicular atrophy in most males and a mild, relatively insulin-resistant diabetes mellitus affecting about half of all patients (244). Although patients of both sexes have had children, fertility is markedly reduced. Females often have irregular menses, early menopause, and poor breast development, and the male external genitalia are usually small.

Laurence-Moon-Bardet-Biedl Syndrome

The Laurence-Moon-Bardet-Biedl syndrome is characterized by retinitis pigmentosa, obesity, mental deficiency, polydactylia, and hypogonadotropic hypogonadism (233, 245, 246). Many other congenital anomalies, such as congenital heart disease, dwarfism, ataxia, nystagmus, and structural defects of the kidney and urogenital tract, have also been reported. There is a high rate of consanguinity among parents (25 per cent), and autosomal recessive inheritance is likely.

In Switzerland, homozygotes occur at a frequency of 1 in 160,000 (246). The syndrome is often seen in an incomplete form, and the basic defect and the reason for the marked clinical variability are not understood. One disorder which superficially resembles the Laurence-Moon-Bardet-Biedl syndrome, but which is probably a separate entity, is the Alström syndrome, an autosomal recessive condition characterized by profound childhood blindness due to retinal degeneration, severe nerve deafness, infantile obesity, chronic nephropathy associated with aminoaciduria and vasopressin-resistant diabetes insipidus, and carbohydrate intolerance. A variety of other metabolic and endocrine abnormalities are present, including baldness, primary hypogonadism in males, hypertriglyceridemia, hyperuricemia, and acanthosis nigricans (234, 247). The absence of both mental retardation and polydactylylia in the

Alström syndrome also serves to distinguish this disorder from the Laurence-Moon-Bardet-Biedl syndrome.

Congenital Total Lipodystrophy

Congenital generalized lipodystrophy (Seip-Laurence syndrome) is inherited as an autosomal recessive. It is to be distinguished from noninherited forms of lipodystrophy (partial and total) which usually have an adult onset (248). Congenital total lipodystrophy has been reported in association with many endocrine and metabolic abnormalities, including hypertriglyceridemia; insulin-resistant, nonketotic diabetes mellitus; elevation in basal metabolic rate without other evidence of hyperthyroidism; polycystic ovaries; and acanthosis nigricans. Mental retardation, hepatomegaly, systemic cystic angiomatosis, and acromegaloid facial and acral features have also been described in these patients (249). The basic defect is not known, and it is also unclear as to whether congenital lipodystrophy is genetically heterogeneous.

REFERENCES

1. Stanbury, J. B., Wyngaarden, J. B., et al., *The Metabolic Basis of Inherited Disease.* 3rd ed. New York, McGraw-Hill Book Co., 1972.
2. Childs, B., and DerKaloustian, V. M.: *New Eng. J. Med.* 279:1205–1212, 1267–1274, 1968.
3. Allison, A. C., and Blumberg, B. S.: *Amer. J. Med.* 25:933, 1958.
4. Sutton, H. E. (ed.), *Genetics, Genetic Information, and the Control of Protein Structure and Function.* Transactions of the First Conference. New York, Josiah Macy, Jr., Foundation, 1960.
5. Reed, T. E., and Falls, H. F.: *Amer. J. Hum. Genet.* 7:28, 1959.
6. Lyon, M. F.: *Ann. Rev. Genet.* 2:31, 1968.
7. Epstein, C. J.: *New Eng. J. Med.* 296:318, 1972.
8. Fialkow, P. J.: *Amer. J. Hum. Genet.* 22:460, 1970.
9. Cavalli-Sforza, L. L., and Bodmer, W. F.: *The Genetics of Human Populations.* San Francisco, W. H. Freeman and Co., 1971, pp. 508–633.
10. Carter, C. O.: *Brit. Med. Bull.* 25:52, 1969.
11. Harris, H.: *Brit. Med. Bull.* 25:5, 1969.
12. McKusick, V. A.: *Mendelian Inheritance in Man.* 3rd ed. Baltimore, Johns Hopkins University Press, 1971.
13. Roberts, J. A. F.: *An Introduction to Medical Genetics.* 5th ed. London, Oxford University Press, 1970, pp. 136–153.
14. McConnell, R. B.: *Amer. J. Med.* 34:692, 1963.
15. Renwick, J. H.: *Ann. Rev. Genet.* 5:81, 1971.
16. Rimoin, D. L., and Schimke, R. N., In *The Clinical Delineation of Birth Defects. X. The Endocrine System.* Baltimore, Williams and Wilkins Co., 1971, pp. 5–11.
17. Omenn, G. S.: *Ann. Intern. Med.* 72:136, 1970.
18. Merimee, T. J., Hall, J. G., et al.: *Lancet* 1:963, 1969.
19. Stevenson, A. C., and Davison, B. C. C.: *Genetic Counseling.* Philadelphia, J. B. Lippincott Co., 1970.
20. Carter, C. O., Roberts, J. A. F., et al.: *Lancet* 1:281, 1971.
21. Milunsky, A., Littlefield, J. W., et al.: *New Eng. J. Med.* 283:1370–1381, 1441–1447, 1470–1504, 1970.
22. Jeffcoate, T. N. A., Fliegner, J. R. H., et al.: *Lancet* 2:533, 1965.
23. Nichols, J.: *Lancet* 1:1151, 1969.
24. Nichols, J.: *Lancet* 1:83, 1970.
25. Merkatz, I. R., New, M. I., et al.: *J. Pediat.* 75:977, 1969.

26. Crawford, J. D., and Bode, H. H., In *Endocrine and Genetic Diseases of Childhood.* Gardner, L. I. (ed.), Philadelphia, W. B. Saunders Co., 1969, pp. 126–141.
27. Blotner, H.: *Metabolism* 7:191, 1958.
28. Thomas, W. C.: *J. Clin. Endocr.* 17:565, 1957.
29. Braverman, L. E., Mancini, J. R., et al.: *Ann. Intern. Med.* 63:503, 1965.
30. Robertson, G. L., Klein, L. A., et al.: *Proc. Natl. Acad. Sci. USA* 66:1298, 1970.
31. Martin, F. I. R.: *Quart. J. Med.* 28:573, 1959.
32. Forssman, H.: *Amer. J. Hum. Genet.* 7:21, 1955.
33. Orloff, J., and Burg, M., In *The Metabolic Basis of Inherited Disease.* 3rd ed. Stanbury, J. B., Wyngaarden, J. B., and Fredrickson, D. S. (eds.), New York, McGraw-Hill Book Co., 1972, pp. 1567–1580.
34. Fichman, M. P., and Brooker, C.: *Clin. Res.* 20:217, 1972.
35. Carter, C., and Simpkiss, M.: *Lancet* 2:1069, 1956.
36. Childs, B., and Sidbury, J. B.: *Pediatrics* 20:177, 1957.
37. Bode, H., and Crawford, J. D.: *New Eng. J. Med.* 280:750, 1969.
38. Kaplan, S. A.: *Amer. J. Dis. Child.* 97:308, 1957.
39. Feigin, R. D., Rimoin, D. L., et al.: *Amer. J. Dis. Child.* 120:64, 1970.
40. Bianchine, J. W., Stambler, A. A., et al., In *The Clinical Delineation of Birth Defects. X. The Endocrine System.* Baltimore, Williams and Wilkins Co., 1971, pp. 280–281.
41. Bode, H. E., and Miettinen, O. S.: *Amer. J. Hum. Genet.* 22:221, 1970.
42. Rimoin, D. L., and Schimke, R. N.: *Genetic Disorders of the Endocrine Glands.* St. Louis, C. V. Mosby Co., 1971, pp. 29–42.
43. Seip, M., Trygstad, O., et al., In *The Clinical Delineation of Birth Defects. X. The Endocrine System.* Baltimore, Williams and Wilkins Co., 1971, p. 33.
44. Steiner, M. M., and Boggs, J. D.: *J. Clin. Endocr.* 25:1591, 1965.
45. Ferrier, P. E., and Stone, E. F.: *Pediatrics* 43:858, 1969.
46. Hanhart, E.: *Arch. Klaus Stift. Vererbungsforsch.* 1:181, 1925.
47. Zergollern, L., In *The Clinical Delineation of Birth Defects. X. The Endocrine System.* Baltimore, Williams and Wilkins Co., 1971, pp. 28–32.
48. Rimoin, D. L., Merimee, T. J., et al.: *Recent Prog. Hormone Res.* 24:365, 1968.
49. Phelan, P. D., Connelly, J., et al., In *The Clinical Delineation of Birth Defects. X. The Endocrine System.* Baltimore, Williams and Wilkins Co., 1971, pp. 24–27.
50. Schimke, R. N., Spaulding, J. J., et al., In *The Clinical Delineation of Birth Defects. X. The Endocrine System.* Baltimore, Williams and Wilkins Co., 1971, pp. 21–23.
51. Rimoin, D. L., Holzman, G. B., et al. *J. Clin. Endocr.* 28:1183, 1968.
52. Laron, Z., Pertzelan, A., et al.: *J. Clin. Endocr.* 33:332, 1971.
53. Laron, Z., Pertzelan, A., et al.: *Israel J. Med. Sci.* 2:152, 1966.
54. Laron, Z., and Sarel, R.: *Acta Endocr.* (Kobenhavn) 63:625, 1970.
55. Merimee, T. J., Rimoin, D. L., et al.: *J. Clin. Invest.* 51:395, 1972.
56. Federman, D. D.: *Abnormal Sexual Development: A Genetic and Endocrine Approach to Differential Diagnosis.* Philadelphia, W. B. Saunders Co., 1967, p. 166.
57. Gauthier, S.: *Acta Neuroveg.* (Wien) 21:345, 1960.
58. Sparkes, R. S., Simpson, R. W., et al.: *Arch. Intern. Med.* (Chicago) 121:534–538, 1968.
59. Barden, C. W., In *The Clinical Delineation of Birth Defects. X. The Endocrine System.* Baltimore, Williams and Wilkins Co., 1971, pp. 175–178.
60. Christian, J. C., Bixler, D., et al., In *The Clinical Delineation of Birth Defects. X. The Endocrine System.* Baltimore, Williams and Wilkins Co., 1971, pp. 166–171.
61. Rosen, S. W.: *Proc. 47th Meeting Endocrine Society,* 1965.
62. Ewer, R. W.: *J. Clin. Endocr.* 28:783, 1968.
63. Faiman, C., Hoffman, D. L., et al.: *Mayo Clin. Proc.* 43:661, 1968.
64. McCullagh, E. P., Beck, J. C., et al.: *J. Clin. Endocr.* 13:489, 1953.
65. Spinner, M. W., Blizzard, R. M., et al.: *J. Clin. Endocr.* 28:795, 1968.
66. Aurbach, G. D., In *The Clinical Delineation of Birth Defects. X. The Endocrine System.* Baltimore, Williams and Wilkins Co., 1971, pp. 48–54.
67. Peden, V. H.: *Amer. J. Hum. Genet.* 12:323, 1960.
68. Bronsky, D., Kiamko, R. T., et al.: *J. Clin. Endocr.* 28:61, 1968.
69. Hutchin, P., and Kessner, D. M.: *Ann. Intern. Med.* 61:1109, 1964.
70. Rimoin, D. L., and Schimke, R. N.: *Genetic Disorders of the Endocrine Glands.* Saint Louis, C. V. Mosby Co., 1971, p. 83.
71. Wuepper, K. D., and Fudenberg, H. H.: *Clin. Exp. Immun.* 2:71, 1967.
72. Spranger, J. W., In *The Clinical Delineation of Birth Defects. IV. Skeletal Dysplasias.* Baltimore, Williams and Wilkins Co., 1969, pp. 122–128.
73. Potts, J. T., Jr., In *The Metabolic Basis of Inherited Disease.* 3rd ed. Stanbury, J. B., Wyngaarden, J. B., and Fredrickson, D. S. (eds.), New York, McGraw-Hill Book Co., 1972, pp. 1305–1319.
74. Chase, L. R., Nelson, G. L., et al.: *J. Clin. Invest.* 48:1832, 1969.
75. Aurbach, G. D., Marcus, R., et al.: *Metabolism* 19:799, 1970.
76. Marcus, R., Wieber, J. F., et al.: *J. Clin. Endocr.* 33:537, 1971.
77. Mann, J. B., Alkerman, S., et al.: *Ann. Intern. Med.* 56:315, 1962.
78. Jackson, C. E., and Frame, B., In *The Clinical Delineation of Birth Defects. X. The Endocrine System.* Baltimore, Williams and Wilkins Co., 1971, pp. 66–68.
79. Hillman, D. A., Scriver, C. R., et al.: *New Eng. J. Med.* 270:483, 1964.
80. Williams, T. F., and Winters, R. W., In *The Metabolic Basis of Inherited Disease.* 3rd ed. Stanbury, J. B., Wyngaarden, J. B., and Fredrickson, D. S. (eds.), New York, McGraw-Hill Book Co., 1972, pp. 1465–1481.
81. Avioli, L. V., Williams, R. F., et al.: *J. Clin. Invest.* 46:1907, 1967.
82. Burnett, C. H., Dent, C. E., et al.: *Amer. J. Med.* 36:222, 1964.
83. Stanbury, J. B., In *The Metabolic Basis of Inherited Disease.* 3rd ed. Stanbury, J. B., Wyngaarden, J. B., et al. (eds.), New York, McGraw-Hill Book Co., 1972, pp. 223–265.
84. Fraser, G. R., In *Progress in Medical Genetics.* Vol. VI. Steinberg, A. G., and Bearn, A. G. (eds.), New York, Grune and Stratton, 1969, pp. 89–116.
85. Valenta, L., Bode, H. H., et al.: *J. Clin. Invest.* 50:94a, 1971.
86. Hagen, G. A., Niepomniszcze, H., et al.: *New Eng. J. Med.* 285:1394, 1971.
87. Nilsson, L. R., Borgfors, N., et al.: *Acta Pediat.* 53:117, 1964.
88. Hollander, C. S., Prout, T. E., et al.: *Amer. J. Med.* 37:630, 1964.
89. Fontan, A., Rubiana, M., et al.: *Arch. Franc. Pediat.* 22:897, 1965.
90. Refetoff, S., DeWind, L. T., et al.: *J. Clin. Endocr.* 27:279, 1967.
91. Malmos, B., Koutras, D. A., et al.: *J. Clin. Endocr.* 26:688, 1966.
92. Harris, H., Kalmus, H., et al.: *Lancet* 2:1038, 1949.
93. Murray, I. P., Thomson, J. A., et al.: *J. Clin. Endocr.* 26:1039, 1966.
94. Fraser, G. R.: *J. Genet. Hum.* 18:169, 1970.
95. Rimoin, D. L., and Schimke, R. N.: *Genetic Disorders of the Endocrine Glands.* Saint Louis, C. V. Mosby Co., 1971, pp. 116–117.
96. Cross, H. E., Hollander, C. S., et al.: *Pediatrics* 41:413, 1968.
97. Fialkow, P. J., In *Progress in Medical Genetics.* Vol. VI. Steinberg, A. G., and Bearn, A. G. (eds.), New York, Grune and Stratton, 1969, pp. 117–167.
98. Beierwalters, W. H., In *The Thyroid.* Hazard, J. B., and Smith, D. E. (eds.), Baltimore, Williams and Wilkins Co., 1964, pp. 58–75.
99. Klein, E.: *Deutsch. Med. Wschr.* 85:314, 1960.
100. Von Verschuer, O.: *Verh. Deutsch. Ges. Inn. Med.* 64:262, 1959.
101. Jayson, M. I. V., Doniach, D., et al.: *Lancet* 2:15, 1967.
102. Townes, P. L., and Bradford, W. L.: *J. Med. Genet.* 8:471, 1971.
103. Ingbar, S. H., Freinkel, N., et al.: *J. Clin. Invest.* 35:714, 1956.

104. Beierwalters, W. H., and Robbins, J.: *J. Clin. Invest.* 38:1683, 1959.
105. Marshall, J. S., Levy, R. P., et al.: *New Eng. J. Med.* 274:469, 1966.
106. Nusynowitz, M. L., Clark, R. F., et al.: *Amer. J. Med.* 50:458, 1971.
107. Refetoff, S., and Selenkow, H.: *New Eng. J. Med.* 278:1081, 1968.
108. Fialkow, P. J., Giblett, E. R., et al.: *J. Clin. Endocr.* 30:66, 1970.
109. Bongiovanni, A. M., In *The Metabolic Basis of Inherited Disease.* 3rd ed. Stanbury, J. B., Wyngaarden, J. B., et al. (eds.), New York, McGraw-Hill Book Co., 1972, pp. 857–885.
110. Childs, B. Grumbach, M. M., et al.: *J. Clin. Invest.* 35:213, 1956.
111. Prader, A.: *Helv. Paediat. Acta* 13:426, 1958.
112. Hirschfeld, A. J., and Fleshman, J. K.: *J. Pediat.* 75:492, 1969.
113. Money, J., and Lewis, V.: *Bull. Johns Hopkins Hosp.* 118:365, 1966.
114. Wein, L., and Mellinger, R. C.: *J. Med. Genet.* 7:27, 1970.
115. Sloan, H. R., and Fredrickson, D. S., In *The Metabolic Basis of Inherited Disease.* 3rd ed. Stanbury, J. B., Wyngaarden, J. B., and Fredrickson, D. S. (eds.), New York, McGraw-Hill Book Co., 1972, pp. 808–832.
116. Lake, B. D., and Patrick, A. D.: *J. Pediat.* 76:262, 1970.
117. Kelch, R. P., Daniels, G., et al.: *Clin. Res.* 19:202, 1971.
118. Franks, R. C., and Nance, W. E.: *Pediatrics* 45:43, 1970.
119. Martin, M. M., In *The Clinical Delineation of Birth Defects. X. The Endocrine System.* Baltimore, Williams and Wilkins Co., 1971, pp. 98–100.
120. Forsyth, C. C., Forbes, M., et al.: *Arch. Dis. Child.* 46:273, 1971.
121. Spira, T. J., Adam, A., et al.: *Lancet* 2:820, 1971.
122. Carpenter, C. C. J., Solomon, N., et al.: *Medicine* 43:153, 1964.
123. Phair, J. P., Bondy, P. K., et al.: *J. Clin. Endocr.* 25:260, 1965.
124. Visser, H. K. A., and Cost, W. S.: *Acta Endocr.* (Kobenhavn) 47:589, 1964.
125. David, R., Golan, S., et al.: *Pediatrics.* 41:403, 1968.
126. Bartter, F. C., Pronove, P., et al.: *Amer. J. Med.* 33:811, 1962.
127. Gardner, J., Lapey, A., et al.: *J. Clin. Invest.* 49:32a, 1970.
128. Sutherland, L. E., Hartroft, P., et al.: *Acta Pediat. Scand.* (Suppl) 201:1, 1970.
129. Doe, R. P., Lohrenz, R. N., et al.: *Metabolism* 14:940, 1965.
130. Lohrenz, F., Doe, R. P., et al.: *J. Clin. Endocr.* 18:1073, 1968.
131. de la Chapelle, A.: *Amer. J. Hum. Genet.* 24:71, 1972.
132. Morillo-Cucci, G., and German, J., In *The Clinical Delineation of Birth Defects. X. The Endocrine System.* Baltimore, Williams and Wilkins Co., 1971, pp. 229–231.
133. Simpson, J. L., Horwith, M., et al., In *The Clinical Delineation of Birth Defects. X. The Endocrine System.* Baltimore, Williams and Wilkins Co., 1971, pp. 196–200.
134. Leduc, B., Van Campenhout, J., et al.: *Amer. J. Obstet. Gynec.* 100:512, 1968.
135. Federman, D. D.: *Abnormal Sexual Development: A Genetic and Endocrine Approach to Differential Diagnosis.* Philadelphia, W. B. Saunders Co., 1967, p. 54.
136. Simpson, J. L., Christakos, A. C., et al., In *The Clinical Delineation of Birth Defects. X. The Endocrine System.* Baltimore, Williams and Wilkins Co., 1971, pp. 215–228.
137. Noonan, J. A.: *Amer. J. Dis. Child.* 116:373, 1968.
138. Szpunar, J., and Rybak, M.: *Arch. Otolaryng.* (Chicago) 87:34, 1968.
139. Simpson, J. L., and Christakos, A. C.: *Obstet. Gynec. Survey* 24:580, 1969.
140. Perrault, M., Klotz, B., et al.: *Bull. Soc. Med. Paris* 67:79, 1951.
141. Guisti, G., Borghi, A., et al.: *Acta Genet. Med. Gemellol.* (Roma) 15:51, 1966.
142. Sternberg, W. H., Barclay, D. L., et al.: *New Eng. J. Med.* 278:695, 1968.
143. Barr, M. L., Carr, D. H., et al.: *Amer. J. Obstet. Gynec.* 99:1047, 1967.
144. Clayton, G. W., Smith, J. D., et al.: *J. Clin. Endocr.* 18:1349, 1958.
145. Milner, W. A., Garlick, W. B., et al.: *J. Urol.* 79:1003, 1958.

146. Rosenberg, H. S., Clayton, W., et al.: *J. Clin. Endocr.* 10:121, 1963.
147. Cattanach, B. M., Pollard, C. E., et al.: *Cytogenetics* 10:318, 1971.
148. Wilkins, L. M.: *The Diagnosis and Treatment of Endocrine Disorders in Childhood and Adolescence.* 2nd ed. Springfield, Illinois, Charles C Thomas, 1957.
149. French, F. S., Van Wyk, J. J., et al.: *J. Clin. Endocr.* 26:493, 1966.
150. Strickland, A. L., and French, F. S.: *J. Clin. Endocr.* 29:1284, 1969.
151. Goldstein, J. L., and Wilson, J. D.: *J. Clin. Invest.* 51:1647, 1972.
152. Wilson, J. D., and Goldstein, J. L.: *J. Biol. Chem.* 247: 7342, 1972.
153. Hauser, G. A., In *Intersexuality.* Overdizer, C. (ed.), London, Academic Press, 1963, p. 255.
154. Jagiello, G., and Atwell, J. D.: *Lancet* 1:329, 1962.
155. Kaplan, S. A., Synder, W. H., et al.: *Amer. J. Dis. Child.* 117:243, 1969.
156. Sanger, R., Tippett, P., et al.: *J. Med. Genet.* 6:26, 1969.
157. Stewart, J. S. S.: *Lancet* 2:592, 1959.
158. Nillson, I. M., Bergman, S., et al.: *Lancet* 2:264, 1959.
159. Lyon, M. F., and Hawkes, S. G.: *Nature* (London) 225:1217, 1970.
160. Park, J. I., and Jones, H. W., Jr.: *Amer. J. Obstet. Gynec.* 108:1197, 1970.
161. Rosenfeld, R. L., Laurence, A. M., et al.: *J. Clin. Endocr.* 32:625, 1971.
162. Saez, J. M., Peretili, E. de, et al.: *J. Clin. Endocr.* 32:604, 1971.
163. Lubs, H. A., Jr., Vilpar, O., et al.: *J. Clin. Endocr.* 19:1110, 1959.
164. Gilbert-Dreyfus, S., Sebaoun, C. A., et al.: *Ann. Endocr.* (Paris) 18:93, 1957.
165. Bowen, P., Lee, C. S. N., et al.: *Ann. Intern. Med.* 62:252, 1965.
166. Wilson, J. D.: Personal communication, 1972.
167. Simpson, J. L., New, M., et al., In *The Clinical Delineation of Birth Defects. X. The Endocrine System.* Baltimore, Williams and Wilkins Co., 1971, pp. 140–144.
168. Nowakowski, H., and Lenz, W.: *Recent Prog. Hormone Res.* 17:53, 1961.
169. Wallach, E. F., and Garcia, S. R.: *J. Clin. Endocr.* 22:1201, 1962.
170. Howard, R. P., Sniffer, R. C., et al.: *J. Clin. Endocr.* 10:121, 1950.
171. Weyeneth, R.: *Praxis* 45:21, 1956.
172. Cooper, H. E., Spellacy, W. N., et al.: *Amer. J. Obstet. Gynec.* 100:371, 1968.
173. Federman, D. D.: *Abnormal Sexual Development: A Genetic and Endocrine Approach to Differential Diagnosis.* Philadelphia, W. B. Saunders Co., 1967, pp. 159–160, 174–176.
174. Rimoin, D. L., and Schimke, R. N.: *Genetic Disorders of the Endocrine Glands.* Saint Louis, C. V. Mosby Co., 1971, pp. 338–340.
175. Beas, F., Zurbrugg, R. P., et al.: *J. Clin. Endocr.* 22:1095, 1962.
176. Jacobson, A. W., and Macklin, M. T.: *Pediatrics* 9:682, 1952.
177. Jungck, E. C., Brown, N. H., et al.: *Amer. J. Dis. Child.* 91:138, 1956.
178. Zacharias, L., and Wurtman, R. J.: *New Eng. J. Med.* 280:868, 1969.
179. Munro, D. D., In *Dermatology in General Medicine.* Fitzpatrick, T. B., Arndt, K. A., et al. (eds.), New York, McGraw-Hill Book Co., 1971, pp. 297–330.
180. Lorenzo, E. M.: *J. Clin. Endocr.* 31:556, 1970.
181. Rook, A.: *Brit. Med. J.* 1:609, 1965.
182. Synder, L. H., and Yingling, H. C.: *Hum. Biol.* 7:608, 1935.
183. Hamilton, J. B.: *Amer. J. Anat.* 71:451, 1942.
184. Bruchovksy, N., and Wilson, J. D.: *J. Biol. Chem.* 243:2012, 1968.
185. Adachi, K., and Kano, M.: *Biochem. Biophys. Res. Commun.* 41:884, 1970.
186. Wermer, P.: *Amer. J. Med.* 35:205, 1963.
187. Ballard, H. S., Frame, B., et al.: *Medicine* 43:481, 1964.
188. Karback, H. E., and Golindo, D. L.: *Texas Med.* 66:54, 1970.
189. Synder, N., Scurry, M. T., et al.: *Ann. Intern. Med.* 76:53, 1972.
190. Zollinger, R. M., and Craig, T. V.: *Amer. J. Med.* 29:29, 1960.

191. Huizenga, K. A., Goodrick, W. I. M., et al.: *Amer. J. Med.* *37*:564, 1964.
192. Johnson, G. J., Summerskill, W. H. J., et al.: *New Eng. J. Med.* 1379, 1967.
193. Schimke, R. N., In *The Clinical Delineation of Birth Defects. X. The Endocrine System.* Baltimore, Williams and Wilkins Co., 1971, pp. 55–65.
194. Williams, E. D.: *J. Clin. Path. 18*:288, 1965.
195. Melvin, K. E. W., and Tashijian, A. H.: *Proc. Nat. Acad. Sci. USA 59*:1216, 1968.
196. Melvin, K. E. W., Miller, H. H., et al.: *New Eng. J. Med. 285*:1115, 1971.
197. Williams, E. D., and Pollack, D. J.: *J. Path. Bact. 91*:71, 1966.
198. Herman, H., and Mornex, R.: *Human Tumors Secreting Catecholamines.* New York, MacMillan Co., 1964.
199. Rimoin, D. L.: *Med. Clin. N. Amer. 55*:807, 1971.
200. Rimoin, D. L.: *Diabetes 16*:346, 1967.
201. Rimoin, D. L., and Schimke, R. N.: *Genetic Disorders of the Endocrine Glands.* Saint Louis, C. V. Mosby Co., 1971, pp. 150–216.
202. College of General Practitioners: *Brit. Med. J. 1*:960, 1965.
203. Simpson, N. E.: *Canad. Med. Ass. J. 98*:427, 1968.
204. Stevenson, A. C., Davison, B. C. C., et al.: *Genetic Counseling.* Philadelphia, J. B. Lippincott Co., 1970, pp. 258–259.
205. White, P.: *Med. Clin. N. Amer. 49*:857, 1965.
206. Steiner, F.: *Deutsch. Arch. Klin. Med. 178*:497, 1936.
207. Harvald, B., and Hauge, M.: *Acta Med. Scand. 173*:459, 1963.
208. Neel, J. V., Fajans, S. S., et al., In *Genetics and the Epidemiology of Chronic Diseases.* Neel, J. V., Shaw, M. W., and Schull, W. J. (eds.), Public Health Service Publication No. 1163, 1965.
209. Neel, J. V., In *Early Diabetes.* Camerini-Davalos, R., and Cole, H. S. (eds.), New York, Academic Press, 1970, pp. 3–10.
210. Rushforth, N. B., Bennett, P. H., et al.: *Diabetes 20*:756, 1971.
211. Bennett, P. H., Burch, T. A., et al.: *Lancet 2*:125, 1971.
212. Renold, A. E., Stauffacher, W., et al.: In *The Metabolic Basis of Inherited Disease.* 3rd ed. Stanbury, J. B., Wyngaarden, J. B., and Fredrickson, D. S. (eds.), New York, McGraw-Hill Book Co., 1972, pp. 83–118.
213. Merimee, T. J., Siperstein, M. D., et al.: *J. Clin. Invest. 49*:2161, 1970.
214. Danowski, T. S., Khurana, R. C., et al.: *Amer. J. Med. 51*:757, 1971.
215. Siperstein, M. D., Unger, R. H., et al.: *J. Clin. Invest. 47*:1973, 1968.
216. Stein, J. H., West, K. M., et al.: *Arch. Intern. Med.* (Chicago) *116*:842, 1965.
217. Blackard, W. G., Omori, Y., et al.: *J. Chronic Dis. 18*:415, 1965.
218. Khachadurian, A. K., and Somerville, I.: *J. Chronic Dis. 18*:1309, 1965.
219. Drevets, C. C.: *J. Okla. Med. Ass. 58*:322, 1965.
220. Harris, H.: *Ann. Eugen.* (London) *14*:293, 1949.
221. Steinberg, A. G.: *Eugen. Quart. 2*:26, 1955.
222. Grunnet, J.: *Op. Domo Biol. Hered. Hum. Univ. Hafniensis.* Vol. 39. Copenhagen, Munksgaard, 1957.
223. Neel, J. V.: *Amer. J. Hum. Genet. 14*:353, 1964.
224. Smith, C.: *Brit. Med. J. 1*:495, 1972.
225. World Health Organization: *Who Techn. Rep. Ser.* No. 310, 1965.
226. Edwards, J. H.: *Lancet 1*:1045, 1969.
227. Kahn, C. B., Soeldner, J. S., et al.: *New Eng. J. Med. 281*:343, 1969.
228. Miller, H. C.: *Advances Pediat. 8*:137, 1956.
229. Fields, G. A., Schwarz, R. H., et al.: *Obstet. Gynec. 32*:778, 1968.
230. Ebbin, A. J., Huntley, C., et al.: *Metabolism 16*:926, 1967.
231. Snyder, R. D., and Robinson, A.: *Amer. J. Dis. Child. 113*:566, 1967.
232. Rimoin, D. L., and Schimke, R. N.: *Genetic Disorders of the Endocrine Glands.* St. Louis, C. V. Mosby Co., 1971, pp. 194–200.
233. Blumel, J., and Kniker, W. R.: *Texas Rep. Biol. Med. 17*:391, 1959.
234. Goldstein, J. L., and Fialkow, P. J.: *Medicine 52*:53, 1973.
235. Oakley, W. G., Pyke, D. A., et al.: *Clinical Diabetes and Its Biochemical Basis.* Oxford, Blackwell Scientific Publications Ltd., 1968.
236. Badgade, J. D., Bierman, E. L., et al.: *Diabetes 20*:664, 1971.
237. Mayer, J.: *Bull. N. Y. Acad. Med. 36*:323, 1960.
238. Lenz, W.: *Medizinische Genetik.* 2nd ed. Stuttgart, Georg Thieme Verlag, 1970, pp. 234–238.
239. Caughey, E., and Myrianthopoulos, N. C.: *Dystrophia Myotonia and Related Disorders.* Springfield, Ill., Charles C Thomas, 1963.
240. Drucker, W. D., Rowland, L. P., et al.: *Amer. J. Med. 31*:941, 1961.
241. Huff, T. A., and Lebovitz, H. E.: *J. Clin. Endocr. 28*:992, 1968.
242. Bundey, S., Carter, C. O., et al.: *J. Neurol. Neurosurg. Psychiat. 33*:279, 1970.
243. Renwick, J. H., Bundey, S. E., et al.: *J. Med. Genet. 8*:407, 1971.
244. Epstein, C. J., Martin, G. M., et al.: *Medicine 45*:177, 1966.
245. Cockayne, E. A., Drestin, D., et al.: *Quart. J. Med. 4*:93, 1935.
246. Ammann, F.: *J. Genet. Hum.* (Suppl.) *18*:1, 1970.
247. Alström, C. H., Hallgren, B., et al.: *Acta Psychiat. Neurol. Scand.* (Suppl. 129) *34*:1, 1959.
248. Seip, M., and Trygstad, O.: *Arch. Dis. Child. 38*:447, 1963.
249. Brunzell, J. D., Schankle, S. S., et al.: *Ann. Intern. Med. 69*:501, 1968.

CHAPTER 26

The Influence of the Endocrine Glands Upon Growth and Development

By Jo Anne Brasel and
Robert M. Blizzard

MULTIFACTORIAL NATURE OF CONTROL OF GROWTH (137, 141)

Childhood and adolescence are periods during which the endocrinologist has an excellent opportunity to study certain effects of various hormones. In adults hormonal dysfunctions are manifested largely by metabolic and physiologic disturbances. During embryonic life and childhood, however, these same hormonal dysfunctions may alter the growth and differentiation of tissue, causing marked deviations from the usual patterns of somatic or sexual growth and development. Cognizance of these structural changes aids greatly in the diagnosis of some endocrinopathies. On the other hand, the fact that endocrine disturbances in childhood are frequently accompanied by gross abnormalities of body structure has led erroneously to overemphasizing their importance and to attributing many observed abnormalities to hormonal deficiencies. This has resulted in mistakes of diagnosis and irrational trials of therapy. The clinician must not forget or minimize the many other factors which regulate growth.

The growth, differentiation, and development of the body structures depend both upon intrinsic regulators within the individual and upon extrinsic influences. Failure to thrive in the infant and poor linear growth or short stature in the child are nonspecific signs of disease, since any serious or significant disease process will alter the growth rate. Indeed, most patients with poor growth have major organ system disease and not an endocrine or metabolic disorder. Therefore, it is important to exclude evidence that points to disease in the central nervous system and in the cardiovascular, gastrointestinal, pulmonary, and renal organ systems before progressing to more erudite considerations and often complicated diagnostic evaluations. To discuss such a differential diagnosis, therefore, means writing a textbook of pediatrics, which is not the purpose of this chapter.

During fetal life, external influences and maternal disease, such as rubella, syphilis, toxoplasmosis, cytomegalic inclusion disease, vitamin deprivation or excess, protein malnutrition, toxemia, and drug ingestion, to name a few, may alter growth and development. It may be impossible to differentiate between an anomaly or mutation which is genetically determined and a phenocopy due to prenatal environmental or maternal factors. The term "congenital anomaly" should include both. Alterations in fetal growth may or may not persist to influence postnatal growth patterns.

Even more dramatic and mysterious are the intrinsic regulators which govern the orderly pattern of growth and cellular differentiation from the time of formation of the zygote to the time of full adult maturity. The pattern of genes or genotype determines the plan for the future growth, development, and biologic constitution of the individual. It is only late in the fetal period that certain tissues become specialized as endocrine glands and begin to secrete hormones which have specific metabolic activities or which control the development of different parts of the body. Genetic influences may also give rise to constitutional variations in the pattern of the hypothalamic-endocrine system, which may account for differences in the time and pattern of puberty. Tendencies to thyrotoxicosis, autoimmune disease of the endocrine glands, and other endocrine disorders may also be influenced by genetic factors. It is now apparent that some endocrine disorders, such as congenital virilizing adrenal hyperplasia and familial goitrous cretinism, result from genetically transmitted defects of the enzyme systems necessary for the biosynthesis of the normal hormones of the adrenal and thyroid glands, respectively.

Obviously from what has been said, when one encounters patients showing significant deviations from the norms of growth and development, it is important (1) to exclude nutritional or metabolic factors or major organ system diseases, (2) to determine whether the variations depend solely upon genetic factors or prenatal injuries, (3) to determine if variations are caused by minor and often temporary constitutional differences in the endocrine pattern, or (4) to ascertain if growth deviations are due to specific disorders of the endocrine glands or brainstem. Most major organ system disease is apparent if one takes a thorough history and does a complete physical examination; renal disease is the one frequent exception to this generalization. However, since the type of renal disease associated with growth failure in an almost asymp-

tomatic patient is that characterized by inability to concentrate urine and loss of fixed base, other symptoms, such as nocturia, polyuria, or polydypsia, can often be gleaned from the history. A routine urinalysis should reveal a low specific gravity and, usually, an alkaline pH. When a child or adolescent is suspected of having an endocrine disorder, the evaluation involves assessment of the level and the pattern of somatic and sexual growth and development and application of tests for the measurement of specific hormonal functions. The differential diagnosis of short stature as well as evaluation techniques will be discussed later in this chapter.

INFLUENCE OF HORMONES ON DEVELOPMENTAL CHANGES DURING GROWTH

During childhood, there are bodily changes not only in terms of increases in height and size but also in terms of the skeletal proportions and the contours of the face and head, progressive ossification of the epiphysial cartilages, the shape of the metaphyses, and finally fusion of the epiphyses with cessation of growth. Dental development consists of both the formation of the tooth buds and the eruption of teeth. At puberty, maturation of the gonads occurs, the genital organs grow, and the secondary sexual characteristics develop, together with an adolescent spurt of growth and muscular development. Mental development is most rapid during the earliest years but continues throughout childhood, with further emotional and psychic maturation in adolescence. Obviously, many of these maturational changes are hormone-dependent, and these interrelationships are briefly outlined below. Since it is often desirable to compare the rate of development of a number of parameters with one another, a few simple indices of development which are helpful will be discussed.

Height and Weight (137, 141)

Various tables of height and weight have been published, showing the wide range of variations in "normal" children of the same age and sex. The deviations from the mean or average height are generally expressed as percentiles, and the fiftieth percentile on most developmental curves indicates the mean height or weight at a particular age. In order to compare growth with various developmental indices such as osseous or mental development, it is helpful to express height in terms of "height age." Thus, if a child is said to have a height age of 3 years, it is meant that he has the mean height of 3-year-old children of the same sex. The height age can then be compared with bone age, as determined by roentgenograms of the epiphysial development, or with mental age. The rates of growth and development can be recorded on simple charts as shown in Figure 26–1. Weight can be expressed and compared similarly as

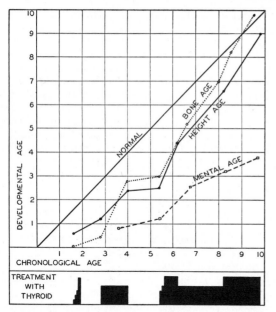

Figure 26-1. Chart illustrates method of following and comparing growth and development in multiple parameters. Chronologic age is plotted horizontally and developmental age vertically. The patient's "height age" indicates that he has the height of an average child of the same sex of the age specified. For example, at 4 years of age the bone age was 2.8 years, the height age about 2.4 years, and the mental age nearly 1 year.

In this cretin, thyroid medication was omitted during two periods because of failure of the parents to cooperate. The resulting retardation in growth and development is shown. By this method of charting, inadequate treatment sometimes is detected by a lag in growth and development before other signs of deficiency are obvious. (From Wilkins, L.: *The Diagnosis and Treatment of Endocrine Disorders in Childhood and Adolescence.* 3rd ed. Springfield, Ill., Charles C Thomas, 1965.)

"weight age." Tanner et al. (132) have recently published data for the calculation of percentile growth from 2 to 9 years of age based on midparent height. Such charts increase the precision in determining the expected growth pattern for any one child and make the differential diagnosis of genetic short stature or tall stature considerably more straightforward.

Somatic growth and development are accelerated by at least four groups of hormones: pituitary growth hormone, thyroxine or triiodothyronine, androgens derived from either the adrenal or the testes, and estrogens. All of these have been shown to stimulate protein anabolism to varying extents and to increase retention of nitrogen, potassium, phosphorus, and calcium needed for building protein and bony tissues. Much remains to be learned about the details of their action both in accelerating growth and in bringing it to an end through fusion of the epiphyses. It is probable that each of these hormones manifests its effect at a somewhat different period of life and in a different way.

The ultimate height attained by an individual depends not only upon the rate of growth but also upon the duration of growth as determined by the time of epiphysial fusions. The cause of the fusion and the relative role of the various hormones are not totally understood (121, 142). When rapid growth is induced by the administration of growth hormone, the epiphysial plates become wider. Testosterone accelerates both epiphysial ossification and fusion. The importance of estrogen in somatic growth and epiphysial fusion remains unclear. Studies of the use of estrogen in tall but otherwise normal girls are felt to support a role for estrogen in growth and bone fusion (138–140). The interpretation of data is difficult, however, because in most instances of increased estrogen secretion or administration there are concomitant changes in the secretion of adrenal androgens. In both sexes, there is a remarkable acceleration of growth and muscular development during adolescence. Since it has been shown that this can be produced by the administration of testosterone, even in patients with true pituitary dwarfism, it seems probable that the adolescent growth spurt, at least in males, is related to testicular and adrenal androgens. Estrogens have the least effect of all the anabolic hormones upon nitrogen retention and in large doses may even inhibit it. Therefore, it seems probable that the adolescent growth spurt of females is due to adrenal androgens rather than to estrogens.

Thyroxine or triiodothyronine or both are essential for normal growth and development throughout the growing period. A deficiency is manifested most spectacularly during the early years of life, when growth and development normally progress most rapidly. The exact nature of the relationship between thyroxine or triiodothyronine and growth hormone is not completely understood. Hypothyroidism in man reduces or delays the expected peak elevation in plasma growth hormone following insulin-induced hypoglycemia, however (119). In addition, the pituitary content of growth hormone in hypothyroid rats is greatly reduced (22, 71, 89, 124). Both of these abnormalities can be restored to normal with thyroid hormone replacement.

The glucocorticosteroids (cortisol and cortisone) of the adrenal, when present in greater than physiologic amounts, either as a result of Cushing's syndrome or when administered therapeutically, inhibit growth. This is in part attributable to their catabolic or antianabolic action, by which the amino acids of the metabolic pool are diverted from the formation of protoplasm toward carbohydrate and fat synthesis. In addition, the growth hormone production rate is blunted in patients receiving corticosteroids (45, 56, 129). The fact that administering glucocorticoid to rats increases the pituitary content of growth hormone (78, 89) suggests that the defect may be due to diminished release rather than to decreased synthesis. Furthermore, an inhibitory effect on the peripheral growth-promoting action of human growth hormone has been demonstrated (127, 128).

Skeletal Proportions (141, 142)

Because the upper/lower ratio varies with age and is hormonally determined in part, this physical measurement must be understood by the physician. The lower segment of the measurement is the

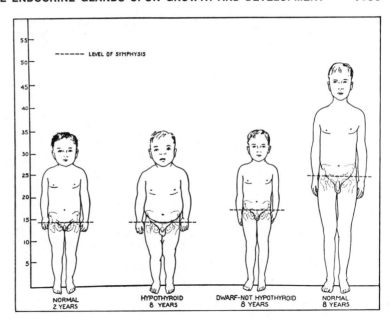

Figure 26–2. The figures of normal boys 2 and 8 years respectively illustrate the change in the ratio of upper and lower skeletal segments measured from the symphysis pubis. At birth the ratio is 1.7/1 and at 10 years, 1/1.

The hypothyroid dwarf having the height of a 2-year-old retains the infantile proportions of 2 years. Dwarfs of pituitary or primordial types, however, attain the more mature proportions of their chronological age. (From Wilkins, L.: *The Diagnosis and Treatment of Endocrine Disorders in Childhood and Adolescence.* 3rd. ed. Springfield, Ill., Charles C Thomas, 1965.)

distance, while the child is standing, from the top of the symphysis pubis to the floor. The upper segment is obtained by subtracting the lower from the total height. At birth, the upper/lower ratio is approximately 1.7:1. The legs grow more rapidly than the trunk; consequently, by the age of 10 years, the segments are normally of equal length and remain approximately equal thereafter. As shown in Figure 26–2, hypothyroid dwarfs frequently retain very infantile skeletal proportions which correspond to their actual heights. A similar infantile upper/lower ratio is seen with most chondrodystrophies. In other types of dwarfs, the skeletal proportions become more mature and are commensurate with the chronological age. In eunuchoidism, the lower segment becomes relatively long because of delayed epiphysial fusion.

Maturation of the Features (137)

During the early months and years of infancy, the facial features undergo marked changes, largely as a result of growth of the bridge of the nose. At adolescence, there is further maturation of the features because of lengthening of the nose and jaw. There are no simple measurements of these changes, but clinical observations make one familiar with them. The infantile cretinoid facies results from the lack of maturation. The features of pituitary dwarfs remain juvenile, whereas some primordial dwarfs and patients with gonadal dysgenesis develop more mature features (Figs. 26–3 to 26–8).

Osseous Development (52, 58, 87, 104, 121, 135, 141, 142)

This is an objective index of maturation which can be measured by studying x-ray films of the epiphysial centers. A number of tables have been

compiled for estimating the bone age on the basis of the time of ossification of various cartilages. Since considerable variation in the bone age in different epiphysial centers frequently occurs, it is preferable to obtain roentgenograms of all the centers rather than to make an evaluation from a single area such as the hand and wrist. This procedure is valuable, for example, when the bone age determination of the hand and wrist alone does not agree with the clinical impression. Mellits et al. (86) have demonstrated a better correlation between "bone age," which was determined on the hand using the Gruelich and Pyle atlas as opposed to the hemiskeleton method using multiple centers, and "biologic age," which was determined by using appropriate equations involving parameters of cell growth and body composition.

Pituitary growth hormone and thyroid hormone deficiencies result in delayed osseous maturation. Androgens, especially when present in excess, advance bone development at a rate greater than the increase in linear growth. Therefore, characteristically bone age is more advanced than height age in androgen-induced overgrowth. This aspect of the biologic activity negates the therapeutic effectiveness of androgens in the treatment of growth failure. Glucocorticoids in excess may cause not only osteoporosis but also mild to moderate delay in bone maturation. Whether this results from a primary action on bone or is mediated by corticoid inhibition of growth hormone release or its peripheral action or both is incompletely known. However, the failure of skeletal maturation to advance significantly in hypopituitary patients receiving growth hormone and pharmacologic doses of cortisol suggests the latter.

Dental Development (83, 114–117, 137)

Abnormalities in the formation of the tooth buds, as revealed by roentgenography, are proba-
(*Text continued on page 1037*)

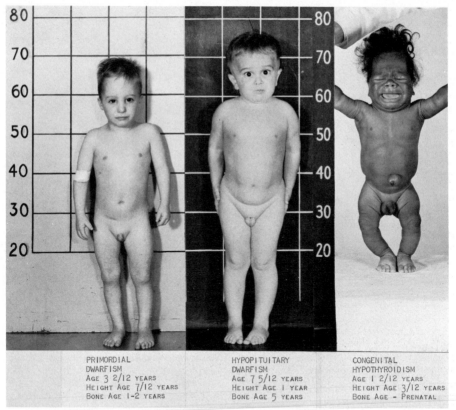

Figure 26–3

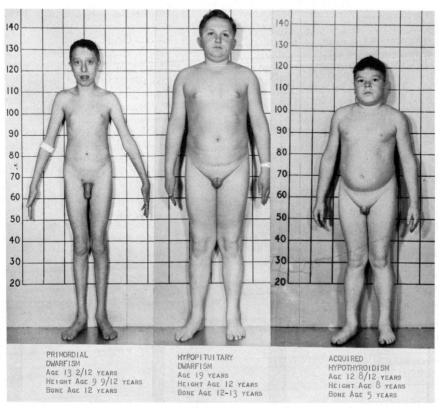

Figure 26–4

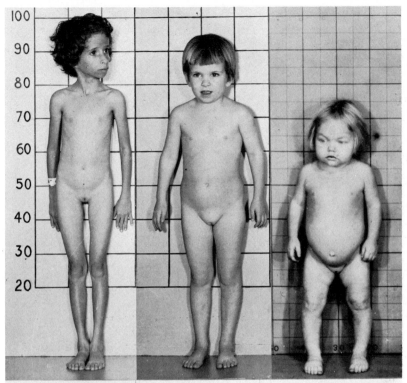

PRIMORDIAL
DWARFISM
Age 9 3/12 years
Height Age 3 9/12 years
Bone Age 9 6/12 years

HYPOPITUITARY
DWARFISM
Age 9 years
Height Age 3 years
Bone Age 6 years

CONGENITAL
HYPOTHYROIDISM
Age 5 9/12 years
Height Age 1 3/12 years
Bone Age 5/12 years

Figure 26–5

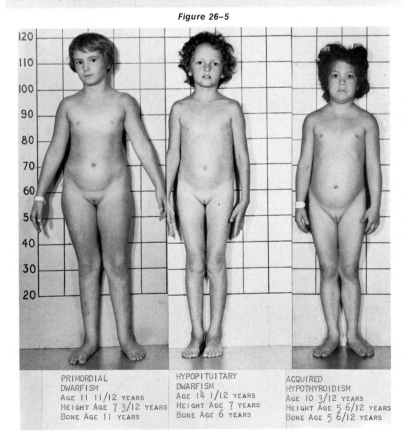

PRIMORDIAL
DWARFISM
Age 11 11/12 years
Height Age 7 3/12 years
Bone Age 11 years

HYPOPITUITARY
DWARFISM
Age 14 1/12 years
Height Age 7 years
Bone Age 6 years

ACQUIRED
HYPOTHYROIDISM
Age 10 3/12 years
Height Age 5 6/12 years
Bone Age 5 6/12 years

Figure 26–6

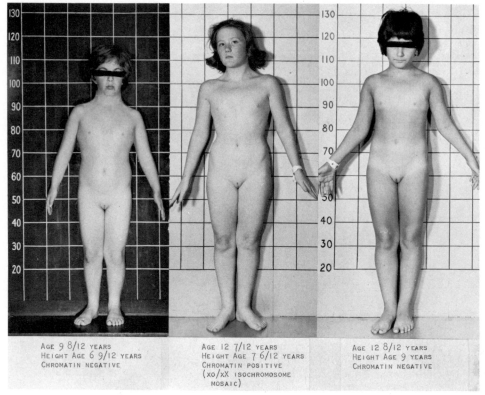

AGE 9 8/12 YEARS
HEIGHT AGE 6 9/12 YEARS
CHROMATIN NEGATIVE

AGE 12 7/12 YEARS
HEIGHT AGE 7 6/12 YEARS
CHROMATIN POSITIVE
(XO/XX ISOCHROMOSOME
MOSAIC)

AGE 12 8/12 YEARS
HEIGHT AGE 9 YEARS
CHROMATIN NEGATIVE

Figure 26–7

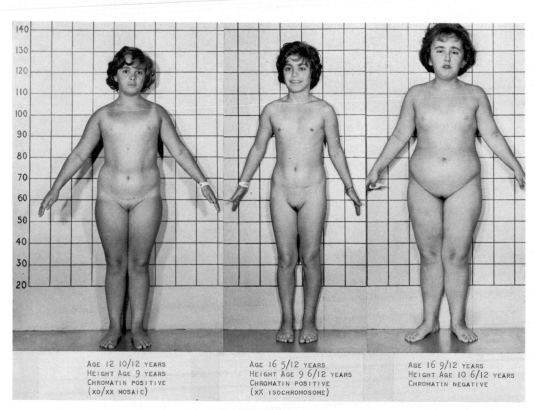

AGE 12 10/12 YEARS
HEIGHT AGE 9 YEARS
CHROMATIN POSITIVE
(XO/XX MOSAIC)

AGE 16 5/12 YEARS
HEIGHT AGE 9 6/12 YEARS
CHROMATIN POSITIVE
(XX ISOCHROMOSOME)

AGE 16 9/12 YEARS
HEIGHT AGE 10 6/12 YEARS
CHROMATIN NEGATIVE

Figure 26–8

bly more significant than is the time of eruption of the teeth, as the latter may depend upon growth of the alveolar processes. Delayed dental eruption is characteristic of hypothyroidism and hypopituitarism, however, and some delay may occur in constitutional slow growth. In primordial dwarfism and in gonadal dysgenesis, the dentition and eruption are usually within normal limits.

Mental Development (137)

This is evaluated by psychometric tests, such as the Wechsler (Adults' and Children's Scale), the Stanford-Binet (children over 2 years), and the Cattell (infants), and can be expressed as an IQ or as a mental age which then can be compared with the chronological age, height age, and bone age. Certain hormones, particularly the thyroid hormones, are essential for normal central nervous system development during fetal and infantile life. An excellent review of intelligence and personality evaluation in hypopituitarism, gonadal dysgenesis, achondroplasia, and psychosocial dwarfism can be found in the paper by Drash, Greenberg, et al. (30).

Sexual Development (80, 81, 141)

Adolescent sexual development is preceded by beginning maturation of the gonads. One obtains some information by measuring the testes, but testicular biopsies or examination of the seminal ejaculate is necessary to determine the state of spermatogenesis. Changes in areolae, extent of glandular breast development, and the degree of epithelial cornification observed in the vaginal smear provide an index of sexual development in the premenarchial girl. Ovulation can be assessed by basal temperature records or serial vaginal smears. Data have been compiled showing the time and order of development of various secondary sexual changes in both boys and girls (80, 81). Data on the developmental patterns of gonadotropin secretion appear later in this chapter.

Sexual development is primarily related to gonadotropin secretion, followed by the secretion of the sex hormones by the gonads. Growth hormone or thyroid hormone deficiency may alter the onset of puberty, however. Hypopituitary patients without gonadotropin deficiency often enter adolescence somewhat later than average. Primary hypothyroidism has been associated with both adolescent delay (141) and precocious puberty (65), both of which return toward normal patterns with thyroid hormone replacement.

INFLUENCE OF HORMONES ON CELLULAR GROWTH

The role of hormones in protein synthesis is presented in Chapter 17. These effects are, of course, basic to their mode of action in cell growth,

but there is another aspect to their action to be presented in this section, i.e., their more global effects on cell hyperplasia or hypertrophy or both in hormone-sensitive tissues. Such information depends in part upon methodology for the measurement of cell number and the assessment of cell mass at various ages.

The constancy of deoxyribonucleic acid (DNA) content of the diploid nucleus in a given vertebrate species was first proposed by Boivin, Vendrely, et al. in 1948 (11) and confirmed by Mirsky and Ris in 1949 (92). This information had fundamental implications for the study and documentation of patterns of cellular growth. Davidson and Leslie (26) ably reviewed the rationale, the usefulness, and the pitfalls of monitoring DNA content in tissues as an index of cell multiplication or as a reference unit for comparing compositional changes in the cell during growth.

Although the measurement of total DNA and protein content and calculation of the number of diploid nuclei and protein/DNA or weight/DNA ratios may not provide actual or precisely accurate values for cell number or cell size, it is valid to assume that increases in total DNA content represent one aspect of growth, that due primarily to DNA replication and cell division (hyperplasia). Increases in weight or total protein content out of proportion to increases in DNA represent another aspect of growth, that due to cell enlargement (hypertrophy). In cases of ploidy or multinucleated cells, interpretation of data must be altered. In liver, protoplasmic mass has been shown to increase commensurately with the increase in DNA (34), so that protein/DNA ratios remain valid indices. In skeletal or cardiac muscle, one can think in terms of nuclear number and of the average mass or territory presided over by one nucleus within the larger muscle cell.

Enesco and Leblond (32) published one of the first studies reporting changes in weight and in DNA content or nuclear number in the major organs and tissues of a mammalian species from before birth to adulthood. On the basis of their findings in the rat, they defined two populations of different cell growth characteristics: (1) expanding cell populations, in which moderate cell enlargement accounts for a considerable portion of the growth in mass of the total organ or tissue; and (2) renewing cell populations, in which cell enlargement is small or absent and growth in mass is achieved predominantly by increases in cell number. They further concluded that cell growth can be divided into three periods: (1) cellular proliferation with little or no change in cell size; (2) continued, but reduced, proliferation with the associated onset of increases in cell size; and (3) cessation of proliferation with continued increases in cell size. Even though data on growth of specific cell types are not delineated by these techniques, the measurement of DNA and protein provides important information regarding growth at a cellular level not available from mass measurements alone.

Studies of the rat have documented rather precisely the temporal patterns of the phases of cell growth for various tissues during normal growth. For example, brain and lung complete DNA synthesis by 22 days of age (144), muscle nuclear number continues to increase through adolescence (18), and DNA synthesis persists in liver, forming tetraploid and octaploid parenchymal cells well into "middle age" (57). Far fewer data are available for human tissues. It is known, however, that DNA synthesis ceases in human brain between 12 and 18 months of age (147), and that muscle nuclear number increases at least into adolescence in males (17). Histochemical studies at autopsy also suggest continued increases in the number of polyploid cells into the sixth decade (57, 77). Lymphoid tissue in both species grows by an increase in cell number, with little or no increment of the average cell mass during maturation. The nonregenerating tissues in all cases studied continue to grow in mass and protein content and therefore in cell size after the cessation of DNA synthesis or growth in cell number. With such data on cell growth as a background, it is then possible to study the effect of hormones on these parameters.

Growth Hormone

In the case of pituitary dwarfism, we are particularly fortunate to have an ideal animal model. Panhypopituitarism occurs as a simple recessive trait in the Snell Smith strain of mice. A group of these mice was studied by Winick and Grant (143), and the body weight curves are shown in Figure 26–9. Before 10–12 days of age, the dwarf cannot be identified as different from littermate normals. Soon thereafter, however, he stops gaining weight and growth essentially ceases. When one examines the tissues, the most striking changes are in DNA content, as shown in Figure 26–10. Similar reductions in DNA were noted in other tissues, includ-

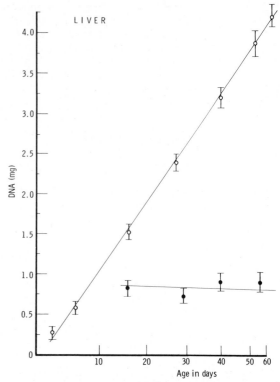

Figure 26–10.   Liver content of DNA in Snell Smith dwarf mice. The dwarf mice fail to demonstrate the normal increase in DNA with increasing age so that values fall further and further behind control levels with time. (Compiled from the data of Winick, M., and Grant, P.: *Endocrinology 83*:544, 1968.)

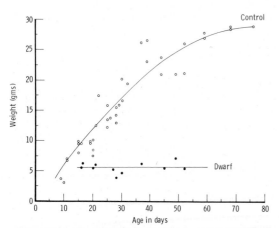

Figure 26–9.   Growth of Snell Smith dwarf mice. In comparison to normal littermates, the dwarf mice demonstrate considerable growth retardation first noted at 10 to 12 days of age. Prior to that time, body weight measurements reveal no differences from control values. (Compiled from the data of Winick, M., and Grant, P.: *Endocrinology 83*:544, 1968.)

ing muscle. These reductions in total tissue DNA content corroborate the earlier findings of Helweg-Larson (57) and others (15, 29, 48, 77) of diminished to absent liver ploidy in these animals. Moreover, mitotic activity in liver and in gut mucosa has been shown to be less than normal in the absence of growth hormone (74). Using radiothymidine, Winick and Grant (143) have shown that DNA synthesis not only is occurring at a slower rate than normal but also may cease prematurely in the dwarf mouse. Cheek et al. (20) have reported a decrease in DNA content in both liver and muscle of hypopituitary mice and rats and an increase toward normal with growth hormone therapy. In general, these same studies reveal a commensurate reduction in protein content, so that protein/DNA ratios are those expected for the size of the animal. Daughaday and Reeder (25) have demonstrated that thymidine uptake in cartilage can be returned toward normal by growth hormone treatment in the hypophysectomized rat. Epstein et al. (35) have shown that growth hormone treatment will elevate thymidine kinase activity, an enzyme involved in the synthesis of one of the DNA precursors, in adipose tissue of hypophysectomized rats. Recent studies (64) have investigated the levels of DNA polymerase activity in hypophysectomized rats before and after growth hormone therapy. The very low values in the deficient rats' livers were markedly increased by the replacement

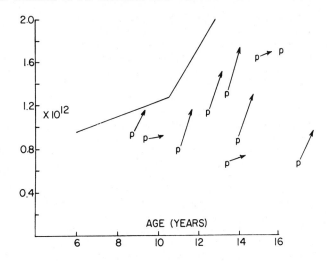

Figure 26–11. Muscle nuclear number in hypopituitary dwarfs. Muscle nuclear number in males with idiopathic hypopituitary dwarfism is plotted against age. In comparison to normal male children, as shown by the unbroken line, the dwarfs show considerable reduction in nuclear number prior to therapy with human growth hormone. Following eight months of treatment, there is an accelerated rate of increase in the nuclear number, shown by the slope of the line from the initial point (p) to the tip of the arrow. However, these increases are no greater in slope than is seen for normal males during the adolescent growth spurt which begins at $10\frac{1}{2}$ years of age. The three patients who did not show an increase in nuclear number could not be separated from the rest of the group on the basis of age, other tropic hormone deficiencies, or their linear growth response to therapy; their lack of response is unexplained. (Modified from Cheek, D. B.: *Human Growth.* Philadelphia, Lea & Febiger, 1968.)

therapy. Thus the animal data point to DNA replication or synthesis, i.e., growth by cell number, as an important site of action of growth hormone in young animals.

Very little data are available in humans. Cheek (16), however, using creatinine to calculate muscle mass and measuring the DNA concentration in a biopsy sample of gluteal muscle, was able to calculate muscle nuclear number in preadolescent male hypopituitary dwarfs before and after eight months of growth hormone therapy. In comparison with age-matched controls, the dwarfs showed a marked reduction in total muscle DNA, which was corrected toward normal at an accelerated rate by growth hormone (Fig. 26–11). Therefore, the limited human data support the animal studies in pointing to DNA biosynthesis as one site of the action of growth hormone on cellular growth.

Thyroid Hormone

The majority of studies on the effects of thyroid hormone on growth have focused on RNA and protein metabolism (Ch. 17). Some data are available, however, on its effects on DNA synthesis in the young, growing animal and in tissues with continued mitotic activity throughout life. One study of protein, RNA, and DNA content in young rats that were made hypothyroid during the second week of life revealed nearly proportionate reductions of all three constituents in the tissues (12). Furthermore, the tissues most sensitive to the hormone deficiency were those in the most active state of cell division at the time of the insult. For example, spleen was markedly affected, whereas brain and lung were only mildly altered. The deficient animals, therefore, at 25 days of age had disproportionately large brains and small spleens. Muscle nuclear number and total liver DNA were markedly reduced in rats two, five, and seven weeks after I^{131} administration at one week of age (20). In both of these studies, cell size, i.e., the protein/DNA ratio, was much less severely affected

than was cell number, i.e., DNA content. Other methods of study have also suggested a role for thyroid hormone in DNA biosynthesis. Thyroid deficiency decreases mitotic activity in gut epithelium (74) and retards the rate of appearance of polyploid nuclei in liver (15, 48, 130); hormone replacement returns these abnormalities towards normal. Triiodothyronine-induced metamorphosis in the tadpole is associated with increased thymidine uptake into DNA in the liver (14). Triiodothyronine administration to thyroidectomized rats enhances the mitotic index and thymidine uptake into DNA in liver (75); these changes are inhibited by actinomycin D and cycloheximide. Finally, mean doubling time of human kidney epithelial cells in tissue culture can be reduced by 25 per cent after exposure to exogenous thyroxine (120).

An area of intensive investigation has been the study of thyroid hormone and brain development. The reader is referred to the collection of papers in *Hormones in Development* (55) for a particularly comprehensive review of work in this area. Of particular interest in the present context are the papers by Balazs et al. and Hamburgh et al. In young male rats, hypothyroidism or hyperthyroidism was produced just before or after birth and brain growth and development assessed. The findings based on DNA and protein measurements and radioautography after thymidine injection showed that the growth of the cerebrum under these circumstances is little affected, but the cerebellum, on the other hand, is significantly affected. Hormone deficiency retards the rate of DNA synthesis and prolongs the usual period of synthesis, so that eventually the DNA content reaches normal adult values. Exogenous hormone administration accelerates the rate of DNA synthesis and brings it to a premature cessation, so that the final result is a cerebellum with a significant reduction in DNA content. The changes in DNA content are accompanied by persistence of the fetal external granular zone in the cerebellar cortex of the hypothyroid rats and prolongation of mitosis in and delayed migration of these cells to their final destination. The authors suggest that thyroid hormone may push cells into the "differentiation" phase of growth by pulling them out of the proliferative phase. Excessive hormone may cause premature cessation of this latter phase, while inadequate amounts of hormone may prolong this phase and delay differentiation. Errors in timing in either direction could then lead to permanent or transitory abnormalities in brain development.

In summary, thyroid hormone at any age or stage of development has profound effects on RNA and protein synthesis which alter the cellular content of these constituents. In addition, the hormone exerts significant effects on DNA biosynthesis during proliferative cell growth which are apt to produce permanent alterations in total DNA content or subsequent differentiation and development or both. The alterations in DNA synthesis may well be secondary to the hormone's effects on RNA and protein synthesis, since some investigations have shown them to be sensitive to actinomycin D and cycloheximide. At any rate, such studies emphasize the particular vulnerability of tissues in proliferative growth to growth-affecting stimuli and point out the necessity of employing young animals in any comprehensive study of the effects of hormones on cell growth.

Insulin

Similar to growth hormone and thyroid hormone, insulin has significant effects on RNA and protein synthesis and on amino acid transport across cell membranes. It has even been proposed that insulin may exert its primary effects on cell size (19, 50). The nature of its action may well be more complicated, however, as suggested by other studies. The fetal overgrowth accompanying maternal diabetes is associated with an increase in fetal DNA content in the rat (101). Placentas of the human diabetic contain increased amounts of DNA (146). Microscopic analysis also suggests a true hyperplastic response (93). Moreover, the studies previously cited (19, 50), demonstrating little insulin effect on DNA content, were performed either in the absence of growth hormone or in older animals. In either instance, the experimental design was not such as to provide favorable circumstances for demonstrating any alterations in DNA synthesis. Additionally, Younger et al. (149) have shown a 70 per cent increase in total liver DNA and in elevations of DNA polymerase activity and thymidine incorporation within 72 hours of insulin administration to diabetic rats. Growth hormone is not an absolute requirement for this insulin-mediated response, but in its absence, the response is curtailed. Therefore, the majority of the data would suggest that under the appropriate conditions insulin will affect the synthesis of DNA as well as that of RNA and protein.

In the preceding discussions of the effects of the major somatic growth-promoting hormones, several recurring features are to be noted. The growth failure or growth stimulation pursuant to alterations in their production may well vary with the age of the organism at the time of the alterations. During the proliferative growth phase, DNA synthesis or growth in cell number will be affected with or without effects on cell size. Once this growth phase is past, the major effects are upon cell size. Thus the developmental stage of the animal or tissue would appear to be the critical factor in determining the cell growth effects. The mechanisms by which these changes occur are not entirely understood. Determinations of DNA polymerase activity have already been cited (14, 64, 149) which suggest that levels of this enzyme, at least, reflect the state of proliferative cell growth and that, at most, the enzyme may even represent one site of hormone action on cell growth. Whether or not alterations in polymerase activity are secondary to changes in *de novo* RNA and protein synthesis in all instances is as yet unknown. It is also important to point out that it is nearly impossible to isolate experimentally the action of one of these hormones from the others and from changes secondary to differences in dietary intake. For example, hypophysectomy decreases both thyroid hormone and insulin secretion as well as growth hormone. Hypothyroidism alters the pituitary content of growth hormone and probably its secretion as well. Fluctuations in blood glucose consequent to insulin deficiency or excess probably affect growth hormone secretion. Finally, dietary intake is almost always altered by these hormone deficiencies or excesses, and altered nutrition per se will affect cell growth (145). This is not to suggest that it is impossible to separate the actions of specific hormones and nutritional influences from one another. They produce distinctly different clinical and biochemical pictures. Replacement of one hormone will not correct the deficits of another, and pair-feeding does not produce the same picture as does the hormone deficiency. It is certain, however, that considerable additional information is needed to provide an overall understanding of their complex interrelationships.

INTERRELATIONSHIPS, ONTOGENY, AND CONTROL OF HORMONES CONCERNED WITH SOMATIC GROWTH AND DEVELOPMENT

Interrelations of the Endocrine System (See Also Chs. 1 and 2)

The relationship of the hypothalamus and the endocrine glands principally concerned with growth and development is a complex one. There are releasing factors (hormones) for growth hormone, prolactin, thyrotropin, adrenocorticotropin, and gonadotropin (47, 72). The thyrotropin releasing factor (TRF) also acts as a prolactin releasing factor when given in large doses (42). Two factors inhibit the release of pituitary hormones, i.e., prolactin releasing inhibiting factor and growth hormone releasing inhibiting factor. The releasing factors are made in the hypothalamus and are subsequently transported from the area of the median eminence by the pituitary portal vascular system to the anterior pituitary. The tropic hormones are then released to act upon the peripheral glands or tissues against which they are directed. The negative feedback control exerted by the hormones or tissue metabolites is at the hypothalamic level and is directed against the release or synthesis or both of releasing factors. The exception to this feedback principle relates to TRF and TSH, as thyroxine exerts its negative feedback at the pituitary by interfering with the action of TRF on TSH release. The releasing factors also are under central nervous system control, possibly via the limbic system. Therefore, clinical manifestations of a deficiency of thyroxine, cortisol, estrogen, or testosterone can result from a defect at one of at least three levels: the hypothalamus, the pituitary, or in the peripheral gland or tissue (109). In addition to defects at the hypothalamic and pituitary levels, apparent growth hormone deficiency can be attributable to an inability to generate somatomedin (sulfation factor) or to an inability of the tissues to respond to somatomedin. Somatomedin is a circulating, growth-promoting hormone which is deficient in growth hormone-deficient humans and which rises to normal levels with the injection of growth hormone, but is not the hormone itself. Further discussion concerning the various types of growth hormone deficiency is presented on pages 1045–1047.

Ontogeny of Pituitary Growth Hormone

In the fetus, this hormone apparently plays little role in the growth of any of the tissues (9). Growth hormone-deficient fetuses who are born to growth hormone-deficient mothers are of normal birth weight and length. The possibility that placental lactogen, which has the same effect as growth hormone (GH) on carbohydrate and lipid metabolism, crosses the placenta in adequate amounts to substitute for absent pituitary growth hormone has not been excluded. Regardless, the fetal production of pituitary growth hormone is not essential to fetal growth. Immediately or shortly after birth, it becomes essential, since at least 30 per cent of growth hormone-deficient children exhibit growth retardation in the first year of life (13).

The neonate has a somewhat different regulatory apparatus for releasing immunoreactive growth hormone (IGH) than have older children. The levels are in the acromegalic range for the first few hours of life. Franchimont et al. (44) found a progressive decrease in premature infants from a value of 48 ± 18.1 ng./ml. on day 1 to 14 ± 8.2 ng./ml. on day 4. These infants when infused with insulin had a rise in plasma growth hormone concentrations, but not as significant a rise as had older children. Hyperglycemia did not have the same inhibitory effect on GH release in the neonatal period as it did subsequently. In addition, the peak release of growth hormone, which occurs with

stage 4 of sleep in adults, does not develop in children until approximately 4–5 years of age.

The comparable production rates of growth hormone at various ages and the comparable somatomedin levels are not known. Theoretically, production rates should be greatest when growth is maximal. Determination of production rates by the usual means, i.e., the urinary and blood production methods, is unsatisfactory. A satisfactory technique for determining production rates or even a mean 24-hour concentration of IGH only recently has become available. The limited data available (134) indicate that male children over the age of 8 years make 4–5 times the amount of GH, regardless of the stage of sexual development, as do men between 30 and 50 years of age. Younger children and female children have not been evaluated. That the adolescent growth spurt may be in part due to increased growth hormone concentrations is suggested by Finkelstein et al. (39), who reported that peaks of GH release were more frequent in children during adolescence than in younger children. Regardless of the IGH levels, until somatomedin levels are determined for various ages, the data pertaining to IGH must be interpreted with caution; for example, estrogen increases IGH concentrations, but such levels are not associated with increased growth.

Ontogeny of Thyrotropin, Thyroxine, and Triiodothyronine (79)

These hormones act significantly in the fetus only on the growth and development of the central nervous system. TSH and free thyroxine are at term concentrations by 16 weeks gestation (51). Since the placental transfer of thyroid hormones is very limited (107), the infant with deficient thyroxine because of a primary thyroid defect often has mental retardation and neurologic sequelae. Immediate adequate hormonal replacement in the newborn period offers the opportunity for increased cerebral and cerebellar maturation in addition to normal physical growth. Apparently, fetuses with deficient TSH production maintain adequate autonomous thyroid function, so that such infants do not suffer significant cerebral dysfunction.

If thyroxine and triiodothyronine deficiencies occur between 0 and 18 months of age, growth and development, both cerebral and physical, are affected (141). If the deficiency occurs after 18 months of age, only physical growth is affected, although mental sluggishness, which is temporary and reversible, is often seen.

Ontogeny of Gonadotropins (5, 10, 66) (See Also Variations in Adolescent Development)

The gonadotropins increase in both boys and girls at approximately 9–10 years of age, and early secondary sexual characteristics become visible shortly thereafter. Serum LH concentrations reach adult levels at the mean age of 14 years in females and 17 years in males (10). These data are in accord with the attainment of full sexual maturation in a majority of girls prior to that in a majority of boys. Ninety per cent of normal girls develop breast enlargement with pouting of the nipples before sexual hair appears. This may reflect that ovarian maturation precedes adrenal maturation by several months, but there is no documentation that this is fact. The adrenal is probably responsible for the majority of androgens that produce growth of sexual hair in adolescent females.

Testosterone acts to stimulate the growth of sexual hair, thickening of the vocal cords, and penile and prostatic growth. Estrogen acts on the mammary tissue to stimulate duct proliferation and on the uterus to increase the thickness of the myometrium and to produce duct proliferation in the endometrium.

CAUSES OF SHORT STATURE (141)

The differential diagnosis of short stature, once major organ system disease has been excluded, is outlined in Table 26–1. The relative frequency of the types of short stature presenting to our pediatric endocrine clinic is reported in Table 26–2.

Familial Short Stature

Familial short stature occurs with a variable degree of stunting, depending upon the particular

TABLE 26–1. DIFFERENTIAL DIAGNOSIS OF SHORT STATURE

Familial Short Stature

Constitutional Slow Growth with Delayed Adolescence

Chromosomal Disorders
  Trisomy syndromes
  Gonadal dysgenesis

Metabolic Disorders
  Inborn errors of metabolism
  Renal tubular defects

Skeletal Disorders
  Chondrodystrophies
  Epiphysial dysplasias
  Metaphysial dysplasias
  Diseases of the spine
  Pseudo- & pseudopseudohypoparathyroidism

Primordial Dwarfism (Intrauterine Dwarfism)
  Dwarfism without congenital anomalies
  Dwarfism with congenital anomalies
  Dwarfism with intrauterine infection

Endocrine Disorders
  Primary hypothyroidism
  Anterior pituitary insufficiency
    Organic hypopituitarism
    Idiopathic hypopituitarism
    Familial hypopituitarism
    Psychosocial dwarfism
  Excessive androgen or estrogen production with early
    epiphysial fusion
  Glucocorticoid excess
  Insulin deficiency

TABLE 26–2. PATIENTS WITH SHORT STATURE: INCIDENCE BY TYPES AND SEX (1965–1972)

	Male		Female		Total	
	No.	*%*	*No.*	*%*	*No.*	*%*
Constitutional delay	173	35	15	6	188	25
Familial short stature	43	9	38	15	81	11
Familial short stature + constitutional delay	32	6	—	—	32	4
Idiopathic hypopituitarism						
Multiple tropic hormones	40	8	10	4	50	7
Isolated growth hormone	8	2	—	—	8	1
Organic hypopituitarism	14	3	6	2	20	3
Gonadal dysgenesis	—	—	50	20	50	7
Psychosocial dwarfism	26	5	17	7	43	6
Chondrodystrophy	18	4	5	2	23	3
Primary hypothyroidism	7	1	11	4	18	2
Intrauterine growth retardation	15	3	16	6	31	4
Crohn's disease (+ steroids)	8	2	1	0.4	9	1
Crohn's disease (− steroids)	2	0.4	1	0.4	3	0.4
Steroid-induced short stature without Crohn's disease	4	0.8	—	—	4	0.5
Cushing's syndrome	1	0.2	2	0.8	3	0.4
Prader-Willi syndrome	3	0.6	—	—	3	0.4
Diabetes insipidus	4	0.8	—	—	4	0.5
Diabetes mellitus	1	0.2	6	2.4	7	0.8
Other	94	19	77	30	171	23
Total:	493	100	255	100	748	100

family's growth pattern. Characteristically the rate of growth, osseous and dental development, and sexual maturation are normal. No endocrine abnormalities are present.

Constitutional Slow Growth with Delayed Adolescence

The largest proportion of children who are brought to physicians because of their small size have no true endocrine disorder or other medical abnormality. A majority of the males in this category have constitutional slow growth with delayed adolescence. Throughout childhood their growth may lag consistently 2–4 years behind the average for their age. Frequently, x-ray studies reveal a comparable retardation in the epiphysial development. When such a pattern is found and the growth parallels that of the average boy, it is safe to predict that the onset of puberty and the adolescent spurt of growth will be correspondingly delayed. Such patients become more conspicuous at the time their age-mates are maturing sexually, growing rapidly, developing muscularly, and maturing emotionally. If they remain untreated, they eventually mature sexually and, because of delayed epiphysial fusion, continue to grow for a longer than average period. Eventually, they attain normal adult height. This condition should be regarded as a constitutional variant of the normal pattern of growth and development. Often there is a strong familial history of parents or other relatives who have followed this same pattern, though this is not invariably the case. Perhaps there are inborn constitutional differences in the activities or rates of maturation of the hypothalamic-pituitary-gonadal axis. During childhood it is often difficult to differentiate on clinical grounds patients with marked slow growth and development from those with true pituitary deficiency. The growth hormone levels following insulin or arginine stimulation in the relatively small number of these patients who have been studied are within the normal range (68), however, as are other studies of an endocrine nature. The gonadotropin and sex hormone levels are consistent with the clinical stage of development rather than the chronological age (10).

Chromosomal Disorders

Trisomy of the autosomes in man has been reported for the 13–15 group of chromosomes, the 16–18 group, and the twenty-first chromosome (63, 108). The last is seen in mongolism. In addition, translocation of parts of chromosomes leading to an effective trisomic condition with a normal chromosomal number has been noted. In addition to growth failure, often prenatal in onset, a characteristic set of congenital anomalies is seen with each of the trisomic syndromes, which often allows recognition of the chromosome involved prior to karyotypic analysis. Except in the 21-trisomy syndrome, the congenital defects are usually too severe to be compatible with prolonged survival.

Patients who are phenotypic females with the syndrome of gonadal dysgenesis and stunted growth are often easily recognizable because of their appearance (Ch. 8). Twenty per cent of 255 girls reporting to our clinic with short stature had this diagnosis. The short stature is believed to depend upon factors other than endocrine dysfunction. Recent studies by Peake et al. (100) of hormonal and metabolic responses, however, suggest that patients with gonadal dysgenesis may have a selective inability to retain nitrogen following human growth hormone administration, which reflects an end-organ unresponsiveness to the protein anabolic effects of the hormone. Although fasting growth hormone levels were greater than control values, the integrated secretion following arginine infusion was within normal limits. Moreover, the calciuria and sulfation factor levels before and after hormone administration were comparable to controls. Almqvist et al. (3), on the other hand, reported elevated levels of sulfation factor activity.

About 80 per cent of these patients have a chromatin-negative nuclear pattern in their buccal smears and have a single X chromosome when the karyotype is determined rather than the two X chromosomes of normal females. The other 20 per cent have a chromatin-positive pattern and either are mosaics for the X chromosome or have an isochromosome "X." The gonads are undeveloped and exist in the majority only as fibrous streaks in the broad ligament. The external and internal genitalia otherwise are of normal female structure. At the usual age of puberty, these patients show no breast or vaginal development or other estrogenic manifestations. Unlike the hypopituitary dwarfs, however, they usually develop some pubic and axillary hair at adolescence. During childhood, these patients usually are brought to attention because of their small stature. Epiphysial development and fusion are only slightly delayed, if at all. More than 50 per cent of the patients have other somatic anomalies (33, 53, 76), such as webbed neck, coarctation of the aorta, lymphedema of the extremities, renal anomalies, and intestinal telangiectasia. Hypertension unrelated to renal or vascular anomalies is relatively common.

Even in early childhood, the diagnosis may be established in 80 per cent of the cases by the finding of a chromatin-negative nuclear pattern in the buccal smear. After puberty, the finding of elevated or even normal levels of urinary gonadotropins in the absence of secondary sexual characteristics distinguishes these patients from females with hypopituitary dwarfism. Since a number of these patients may not demonstrate the characteristic phenotype, and since 20 per cent of the group as a whole are not chromatin-negative, the diagnosis may not be readily apparent without karyotypic analysis of the patient's chromosomes. The wide variation in phenotypes is shown in Figures 26–7 and 26–8.

Metabolic Disorders (62, 85, 95, 99)

Such disorders, as exemplified by the mucopolysaccharidoses, may cause growth failure by a variety of mechanisms, though many share either a deficiency or an excess of a substance or substances which interfere with the normal metabolic pathways at a cytoplasmic level. Many have characteristic physical or chemical abnormalities which lead to the correct diagnosis. Patients also may give off characteristic odors. Mental retardation is a common feature of the inborn errors of amino acid metabolism, especially if the treatment is delayed. As with other inborn errors, the family history may be positive for similarly affected relatives. In some, treatment can be directed toward the primary disorder, and in others, the cytoplasmic environment can be improved through diet or by other means to partially correct the biochemical abnormality or to bypass it altogether. Disorders of the renal tubules are of particular interest, and their diagnosis can be missed, unless studies of urine specific gravity and pH or serum electrolytes are made to exclude these etiologies.

Skeletal Disorders (112)

Skeletal disorders are usually easily recognized because of typical physical characteristics or radiologic findings. In those which affect primarily the growth of long bones, the upper to lower segment ratios will show retardation when compared with those of the same chronological age, since the trunk will be of normal length and the legs shorter than normal. In those which affect primarily the spine, the reverse is true, and the skeletal proportions may become eunuchoid, even though dwarfing is present. Pseudo- and pseudopseudohypoparathyroidism are listed as skeletal defects, since there are bone abnormalities in these disorders and because there is no reason to implicate parathyroid dysfunction as the cause of the short stature.

Primordial Dwarfism
(4, 8, 21, 27, 59, 94, 113, 118, 122)

Primordial dwarfism (Figs. 26–3 to 26–6) is at best a poor term, which implies that there are unknown factors causing poor growth. Because the infants in this category are often small for their gestational age, the term "intrauterine dwarfism" has also been used to designate those who have growth retardation at birth. Characteristically, growth is slow from earliest infancy, although epiphysial maturation and sexual development occur normally or at an only slightly retarded rate. Growth hormone levels are usually normal. Usually, studies to determine endocrine function are also normal. Intellect may be affected. This pattern of growth is seen sporadically, without other congenital anomalies in some and in association with a number of characteristic anomalies in others. Progeria "bird-headed" dwarfism, with peculiar craniofacial anomalies, and hemiatrophy or hemihypertrophy with dwarfism are but a few of the latter type that have been described. Until more is known regarding pathogenesis and the basic defects involved, little is gained from trying to segregate each patient into a particular diagnostic category. Severe congenital defects of the central nervous system of unknown etiology may be associated with growth failure. Placental insufficiency may be associated with variable degrees of growth retardation, which may persist postnatally. In addition, growth failure and multiple congenital anomalies can be seen following intrauterine infection, as in congenital rubella, syphilis, toxoplasmosis, or cytomegalic inclusion disease.

Endocrine Disorders Causing Stunted Growth (141)

Primary Hypothyroidism

Hypothyroidism, if untreated during the growing period, always leads to marked impairment of growth. It is the most characteristic and readily diagnosable of any of the endocrine disorders of childhood. The clinical picture (Figs. 26–3 to 26–6), however, varies according to the age at which the deficiency begins and the span of life during which it remains untreated. The most conspicuous signs of developmental retardation are found in those cases in which the deficiency is congenital or begins in the earliest years of life when growth and development progress most rapidly. As indicated in Table 26–3, thyroid deficiency is accompanied by abnormal physiologic signs, such as sluggishness, circulatory impairment, coolness of the

TABLE 26–3.   DIAGNOSIS OF HYPOTHYROIDISM

Physiologic Signs
Torpor
    Physical and mental
    Anorexia
Circulatory impairment
    Grayish pallor of lips
    Cool, mottled extremities
    Slow pulse, small pulse pressure
Hypotonia
    Poor skeletal muscle tone
    Constipation
    Abdominal distention and umbilical hernia
Myxedema
    "Puffy" appearance
    Thick tongue
    Hoarse cry

Retarded Growth and Development
Stunted growth
Immature facies
Infantile skeletal proportions
Delayed dentition
Delayed epiphysial ossification
Epiphysial dysgenesis (diagnostic when present)

Laboratory Data
PBI, thyroxine, and/or free thyroxine low
I^{131} uptake absent or low in athyrotic types, normal or high
    with most enzymatic defects
Serum TSH elevated
Cholesterol frequently elevated
Serum carotene frequently elevated

skin, and constipation. Myxedema is a late sign and may not be present in milder cases.

Impairment of growth is invariably accompanied by marked retardation of all the developmental changes that normally occur in the skeleton, such as the proportions of the upper and lower skeletal segments, maturation of the naso-orbital configuration, ossification of the epiphyses, and dental development. Such delays, including retardation of epiphysial development, however, are not in themselves diagnostic of hypothyroidism as they may occur in other conditions. Of much greater diagnostic significance is the finding of the characteristic epiphysial dysgenesis which is frequently present when thyroid deficiency has existed in the early months of life. X-rays of multiple sites will often be of assistance.

After 18 months of age, the serum cholesterol is often high (over 300 mg./100 ml.), but not invariably so. Serum carotene values may also be elevated. The study of the radioiodine (I^{131}) uptake is of value principally to differentiate between the athyrotic type of cretinism or acquired hypothyroidism and that due to enzymatic defects of biosynthesis (Ch. 4). In the majority of patients with primary hypothyroidism, the PBI, thyroxine, and free thyroxine will be decreased. In a few patients with certain types of enzymatic defects or lymphocytic thyroiditis, however, the PBI may be within the normal range because of circulating iodoproteins which are not calorigenically active. In these instances, the PBI-thyroxine discrepancy will be abnormally elevated to greater than 2 μg./100 ml., and thyroxine or free thyroxine determinations will more accurately represent the thyroid status of the patient. Serum TSH levels are markedly elevated in primary hypothyroidism in children as in adults.

Anterior Pituitary Insufficiency

This is one of the least common causes of dwarfism and the one most difficult to diagnose during childhood. It must be distinguished from constitutional delays of growth and adolescence on the one hand and from various "primordial" types of dwarfism and from the syndrome of gonadal dysgenesis on the other (Table 26–4). Hypopituitary dwarfs often but not always remain sexually undeveloped; individuals with constitutional delay of growth and development have a late but otherwise normal adolescence; primordial dwarfs mature sexually at about the average time, and patients with gonadal dysgenesis have elevated serum and urinary gonadotropins but no secondary characteristics except scanty sexual hair.

Organic hypopituitarism (13) in children occurs most commonly in association with craniopharyngiomas but is also seen with destructive diseases in the brainstem which affect the synthesis or release or both of the pituitary releasing hormones and with an unusual and rare congenital anomaly in which there is absence of the septum pellucidum, very small optic discs, nystagmus, and sometimes diabetes insipidus (49).

Organic hypopituitarism is the only type in which posterior pituitary deficiency is also seen. Most commonly, patients manifest neurologic abnormalities, especially of vision, but on occasion growth failure may be the chief complaint. For-

tunately, the differential diagnosis between organic and idiopathic pituitary failure is not difficult, since x-rays of the skull and sella turcica are usually abnormal in the former, and the neurologic examination is normal in the latter. Rarely, however, air studies may be necessary to document a suspected brainstem lesion.

The majority of cases have *idiopathic hypopituitarism* (13, 49, 68), in which localized central nervous system signs cannot be detected. As a cause of short stature, it is still a relatively rare condition, accounting for only 8 per cent of the short stature cases reporting to the Pediatric Endocrine Clinic at the Johns Hopkins Hospital in the last eight years. These patients are usually of normal size at birth but may not grow and develop normally during the following two or three years. In one series of such patients (13), one-third of the group demonstrated significant growth failure by one year of age, and one-half were abnormally small by two years. Growth and bone development proceed at a slow rate, lagging farther below the average as the years pass. There are no distinguishing characteristics in their habitus or facies (Figs. 26–3 to 26–6). They appear like normal children, except for juvenile features which make them seem much younger than their age-mates. In these respects, they cannot be distinguished during childhood from patients with the constitutional type of slow growth and development. Males are usually affected 2–4 times more often than females.

By definition, hypopituitary dwarfs have decreased growth hormone production or release or both with or without other tropic hormone deficiencies. The rare cases of presumed growth hormone resistance will be covered later in this

TABLE 26–4. DIAGNOSIS OF DWARFISM*

	Idiopathic Hypopituitarism	Constitutional Delay	Familial Short Stature	Primordial Dwarfism	Gonadal Dysgenesis
History					
Family history	±	±	+	−	−
Birth weight	Usually normal	Normal	Usually normal	Decreased	Often decreased
Hypoglycemic symptoms	Not uncommon	Absent	Absent	Absent	Absent
Physical Examination					
Facial features	Immature but normal	Normal	Normal	Often characteristic	Often characteristic
Dentition	Retarded	Minimally retarded	Normal	Normal	Normal
Dwarfing	Usually marked	Minimal to marked	Minimal to moderate	Usually marked	Usually marked
Sexual development	Infantile	Delayed	Normal	Normal	Infantile except for sparse sexual hair
Laboratory Studies					
Bone age	Retarded	Minimally to markedly retarded	Normal	Normal	Normal or minimally retarded
Metyrapone†	Usually abnormal	Normal	Normal	Normal	Normal
Insulin sensitivity†	Usually present	Absent	Absent	Absent	Absent
PBI, T$_4$, or free T$_4$	Often decreased	Normal	Normal	Normal	Normal
RAI	Often decreased	Normal	Normal	Normal	Normal
HGH levels	Decreased	Normal	Normal	Normal	Normal

*Modified from Blizzard, R. M., and Brasel, J. A.: Dwarfism, In *Current Therapy*. Conn, H. F. (ed.). Philadelphia, W. B. Saunders Co., 1966.

†For details of testing procedures and interpretation see Brasel, J. A., Wright, J. C., et al.: *Amer. J. Med.* 38:484, 1965.

chapter. Numerous stimuli have been used to cause growth hormone release. These include insulin-induced hypoglycemia, arginine infusion, L-dopa, glucagon, and exercise. A negative response to at least two stimuli must be obtained before a diagnosis of growth hormone deficiency can be accepted (Ch. 2).

In addition to growth hormone deficiency, many patients have deficient secretion of other pituitary tropic hormones as well. Gonadotropin deficiency is the next most common hormone deficiency (13), but unfortunately its evaluation is of limited diagnostic use during childhood. ACTH deficiency can be demonstrated in a majority of patients by measuring the basal excretion of 17-hydroxycorticosteroids and the response to metyrapone (SU-4885). In a significant number of patients, only the metyrapone response is abnormal, as the baseline 17-hydroxycorticosteroids are normal. In some patients, TSH deficiency is suggested by low or low-normal thyroxine levels and radioactive iodine uptake values, both of which will increase with TSH administration. Overt myxedematous features and epiphysial dysgenesis are not usually seen in this type of secondary hypothyroidism.

Other findings may include elevation of the serum urea nitrogen, elevation of the cholesterol unrelated to the thyroid status, and hypoglycemia. The hypoglycemia rarely causes spontaneous symptoms but is often demonstrated during some tests. Abnormalities of carbohydrate metabolism are common and consist of fasting hypoglycemia, reactive hypoglycemia, failure to return to fasting glucose levels 4–5 hours after a glucose load, and insulin sensitivity – all manifestations of hypoglycemic unresponsiveness. Curiously, a significant percentage of patients also demonstrate hyperglycemic unresponsiveness after a glucose load, showing abnormally high blood sugar peaks or a delayed fall in blood sugar. This latter phenomenon may be related to the insulinopenia these patients demonstrate (88). The occurrence of these carbohydrate abnormalities does not correlate with ACTH or TSH status, and they return to normal solely by the administration of growth hormone (23, 148).

Familial hypopituitarism (109, 111) is not as rare as it was once thought. The first type is *familial isolated growth hormone deficiency.* On the basis of the 24 patients studied at Johns Hopkins Hospital by Rimoin et al. (111) and a review of the literature, this form of hypopituitarism usually appears to occur as a result of autosomal recessive inheritance. The observations of multiple affected siblings, a high consanguinity frequency, the occurrence of only affected siblings in a conjugal mating, and concordance among monozygotic twins support the hypothesis that this is recessive. In Rimoin's series, there were two families in which two affected parents gave birth to normal children, who are, therefore, exceptions from the recessive inheritance concept. They suggest that isolated growth hormone deficiency may occasionally occur in families as a dominant trait or, as an alternative, that one of the parents may have had isolated growth hormone deficiency of a nonhereditary na-

ture. Only further study of additional families will determine which of these possibilities is the more likely. Nonetheless, it is fair to state that the majority of cases of familial isolated growth hormone deficiency occur as the result of the expression of an autosomal recessive trait.

Familial panhypopituitarism has also been reported. Although the majority of patients with multiple tropic hormone deficiencies have a negative family history for a similar disorder, at least 15 kindreds with multiple affected members have been reported with panhypopituitarism. Again the recessive inheritance is suggested by the presence of affected siblings of both sexes and a high incidence of consanguinity. Rimoin et al. (111) have studied extensively a large inbred Hutterite kindred from Canada and have documented panhypopituitarism by the appropriate laboratory procedures.

The genetics of *familial dwarfism with high growth hormone levels* has been discussed by Laron's group (73), who reported cases of dwarfism in which familial occurrence or parental consanguinity or both were seen in association with normal or high levels of plasma growth hormone. Many of these patients were derived from families of Oriental Jewish origin rather than European origin, which again suggests an autosomal recessive inheritance. These patients have the clinical signs and symptoms of isolated growth hormone deficiency, including insulinopenia. It was postulated that these patients represent a CRM*-positive mutant, resulting in the production of an immunologically active but biologically inactive growth hormone molecule. Certain patients have subsequently been found, however, who demonstrate no sulfation factor (somatomedin) in their serum following HGH administration (24). This finding suggests that the error is in the production of somatomedin. The liver or kidney or both may play an important role in this conversion (136), but further work is needed to determine the nature of the biochemical reaction before the defect in dwarfs can be approached in the laboratory.

The African Pygmies are felt to have a hereditary *resistance to growth hormone at the tissue level* (110). They are a particularly interesting group, as they have the metabolic abnormalities of growth hormone deficiency but lack many of the physical characteristics, such as the baby face, wrinkled skin, and infantile body fat distribution. Their growth hormone responses to insulin and arginine are comparable to those of normal controls; yet they demonstrate insulin sensitivity and insulinopenia. Furthermore, exogenous HGH administration does not result in the expected changes in serum urea nitrogen or free fatty acids or in correction of the insulinopenia as occurs in hypopituitarism.

In summary, we can state that most of the patients with hypopituitarism are sporadic, nonfamilial, nonhereditary cases. However, a significant

---

*Cross-reactive material.

number of families, usually coming from highly inbred populations, have been reported and the familial occurrence of hypopituitarism documented. Cases of isolated growth hormone deficiency, panhypopituitarism, and dwarfism with normal or high growth hormone levels have all been reported. In these instances, the mode of inheritance appears to be autosomal recessive.

In both the sporadic and familial forms of the disease, the basic defect often is of hypothalamic rather than pituitary origin (1, 82). The administration of thyrotropin releasing factor in patients with growth hormone and TSH deficiency produced TSH release in 10 to 13 such patients (42). Therefore, TRF can be used to differentiate between the hypothalamic and the pituitary types of hypopituitarism.

Children with severe growth failure who come from disturbed homes in which there is a history of emotional deprivation and abnormal parent-child relationships were placed in a category of functional hypopituitarism by Talbot (131) some years ago. The syndrome has more recently been termed *psychosocial dwarfism*. It has been shown that many of these patients do have transient pituitary insufficiency (103). Growth hormone and ACTH deficiencies are the most common abnormalities detectable. They characteristically manifest with bizarre polyphagia and polydipsia and immature speech and behavior (102). The growth failure, endocrine abnormalities, and behavior problems largely disappear without any drug therapy upon the child's removal from the home. Figures 26–12 to 26–14 illustrate the clinical picture and the remarkable "catch-up" growth and maturation which occur at rapid pace once the child is removed from the adverse environmental circumstances. Although many patients show total recovery with respect to growth deficits if they are diagnosed early and are maintained in a psychologically satisfactory environment, the psychic scars and apparent mental retardation may not be entirely reparable. Only prolonged follow-up will answer this important question. The nature of the pituitary defect is not clear. It is assumed, however, that the abnormality probably involves a disturbance in hypothalamic releasing hormones rather than a primary defect of the anterior pituitary.

Excessive Androgen or Estrogen Production (31, 37, 141)

Sexual precocity, which may be due to various causes, leads to marked acceleration of both growth and epiphysial development. This is probably due to the effects of increased androgen. Accordingly, the patients are overgrown and have markedly advanced bone ages during childhood, but early epiphysial fusion brings growth to an end, often before normal adult height is attained. The earlier sexual precocity begins, the greater the stunting. Sexual precocity is, of course, readily recognized; diagnosis is concerned largely with the determination of its etiology.

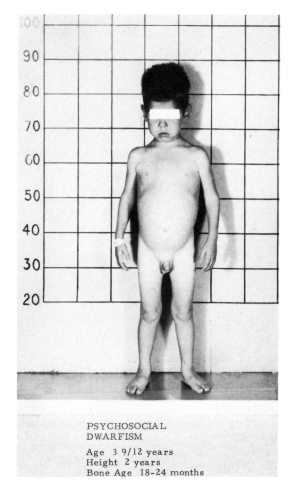

PSYCHOSOCIAL
DWARFISM

Age 3 9/12 years
Height 2 years
Bone Age 18-24 months

Figure 26–12. Child with classical psychosocial dwarfism, who had no growth hormone release with arginine or insulin and an abnormal SU-4885 test. He was removed from the adverse environment and grew 10.0 cm. in the first year.

The terms "precocious puberty" and "sexual precocity" should be applied only to those patients in whom sexual development begins before the age of 9 years, which is the lower range of constitutional variation in the onset of puberty. In at least 90 per cent of females and in approximately 50 per cent of males, precocious puberty is idiopathic in origin. That is, it seems to be initiated by a normal pituitary-gonadal mechanism which, for some unknown reason, has been activated at an unusually early age. Accordingly, the pituitary secretes gonadotropins which in turn stimulate the ovaries or the testes to develop and mature. Ovulation and regular menstrual cycles may develop in females and spermatogenesis in males. Although sexual development may occur at any time during childhood, it sometimes begins at a surprisingly early age (84). The menarche, followed by regular menstrual cycles, has occurred within the first few weeks of life, and male secondary sexual development may be evident during the early months.

Before the early activation of the pituitary-gonadal mechanism is labeled "idiopathic," the possibility that it might be initiated by some in-

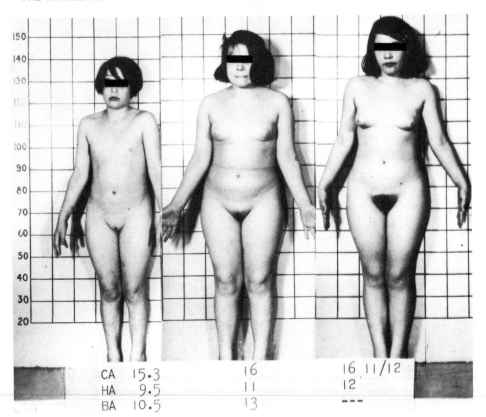

CA	15.3	16	16 11/12
HA	9.5	11	12
BA	10.5	13	---

Figure 26–13.   Girl of adolescent age who came from disruptive home environment. By history, the behavior pattern was classical at 6 to 8 years of age. The laboratory findings were those of idiopathic hypopituitarism (abnormal arginine-insulin tolerance test, SU-4885, and serum gonadotropins). After six weeks away from the adverse environment, breast enlargement was occurring, and linear growth increased 2.5 cm. Subsequent spontaneous maturation was as depicted.

tracranial lesion acting through the hypothalamus must be considered. Brain tumors usually give some intracranial, neurologic, or ophthalmologic signs or symptoms. Occasionally, hamartomas of the tuber cinereum occur which are too small to give any diagnostic signs. Encephalitic lesions and perhaps congenital defects of the hypothalamus may give rise to sexual precocity. Albright's syndrome of sexual precocity, skin pigmentation, and polyostotic fibrous dysplasia also may act through the hypothalamus.

In contrast to sexual precocity of the idiopathic or the hypothalamic type are cases due to tumors of the ovary, testes, or adrenal and cases of virilizing hyperplasia in males. In these cases, the sex hormones of gonadal or adrenal origin usually inhibit the pituitary secretion of gonadotropins. Accordingly, ovulation or spermatogenesis usually does not occur.

The granulosa cell tumor is the usual ovarian neoplasm which causes sexual precocity, although a few cases have been due to luteomas and chorioepitheliomas. At the time that sexual precocity is evident, the granulosa cell tumor is almost always sufficiently large to be readily palpable by rectal-abdominal examination. One would expect to be able to distinguish between sexual precocity induced by estrogen-secreting tumors and idiopathic or hypothalamic sexual precocity on the basis of laboratory measurements of estrogen and gonado-

tropins, estrogens presumably being high and gonadotropins absent in cases of tumor, and estrogens and gonadotropins being at normal adult levels in early activation of the pituitary. Unfortunately, this is not always so. In some cases of granulosa cell tumor, estrogens are not above the normal adult level, and in cases of the idiopathic or hypothalamic type, urinary gonadotropins are not always measurable. The sensitive radioimmunoassay of serum gonadotropins, however, should make laboratory differentiation possible in the majority of cases (10, 66, 70).

Occasionally, a tumor of the adrenal will produce only estrogen or primarily estrogen. In all children reported with sexual precocity secondary to this etiology, the 17-ketosteroids have been elevated beyond that which would be expected in constitutional sexual precocity. A Decadron suppression test should be done in all cases of sexual precocity, male or female, when the 17-ketosteroids are elevated. A normal suppression test usually eliminates serious consideration of a tumor.

In males, precocious secondary sexual development occurs with about equal frequency because of the idiopathic or hypothalamic type or because of the adrenogenital syndrome. The urinary 17-ketosteroids are considerably elevated with the adrenogenital syndrome in contrast to the other types of precocity; the testes are usually small

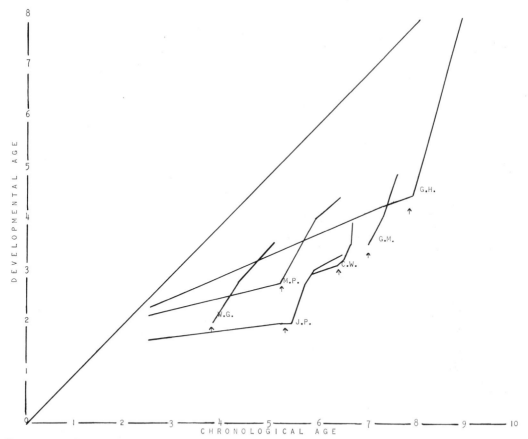

Figure 26–14. Growth rates of psychosocial dwarfs are presented before and after removal from the adverse environment.

and show no Leydig cells or spermatogenesis on biopsy, but this is not invariably the case. With early activation of the pituitary, the testes undergo adult maturation. Leydig cell tumors of the testes are exceedingly rare and are generally palpable. In cases reported, the urinary 17-ketosteroids have ranged from 3–64 mg./day.

Glucocorticoid Excess

When glucocorticoids are present in amounts greater than physiologic requirements demand, whether of endogenous or exogenous origin, poor linear growth is a common occurrence. The relationship of the glucocorticoids to growth has been covered earlier in this chapter. Ordinarily the characteristic features of Cushing's syndrome permit diagnosis of the primary entity, and there should be no confusion with the other causes of short stature (Ch. 5). It is worthwhile emphasizing that, in childhood, obesity alone without short stature or growth failure is *inconsistent* with the diagnosis of Cushing's syndrome.

Insulin Deficiency

Poorly controlled diabetes as a cause of poor growth and short stature should present no diagnostic difficulties.

HORMONAL TREATMENT OF SHORT STATURE (SEE TABLE 26–5)

Androgens

Testosterone is the most potent of all androgens. Because of its maturing effect on the skeletal system, the advancement of skeletal maturation usually is more rapid than the acceleration of linear growth (141). This disproportionate effect is particularly noticeable when the bone age is less than 11–12 years. Therefore, there is *no* reason for prescribing testosterone in any dosage whatsoever before the chronological age of 14 years. Because sexual infantilism is an added problem to that of short stature in boys with constitutional delayed growth and adolescence or hypopituitarism, testosterone treatment may be indicated in boys aged 14 or older. However, these boys should be given a choice of growing for a while longer to a greater ultimate height and remaining sexually infantile, or developing sexually and growing for a limited period of time to a lesser ultimate height.

In *constitutional delay of sexual development,* methyltestosterone, 30 mg./day, can be given orally, or testosterone enanthate, 200–300 mg. every 3–4 weeks, can be given intramuscularly. After six months, some evidence of sexual maturation occurs, along with growth of 2–3 inches and a

TABLE 26-5. HORMONAL TREATMENT OF SHORT STATURE

Hormone	Comments on Use
Human growth hormone	Of documented effectiveness only in cases of demonstrated pituitary deficiency and certain types of intrauterine dwarfism. Demand still greatly exceeds supply.
Thyroid hormone	Useful in primary hypothyroidism and in hypopituitarism, especially on an organic basis when TSH deficiency is present. Care must be taken not to provoke cortisol deficiency by the administration of thyroid hormone alone if both ACTH and TSH are deficient. No evidence of efficacy in other types of growth failure.
Androgens	Growth spurt produced is almost always counteracted by more rapid advancement in skeletal maturation. Therapeutic usefulness in short stature is, therefore, limited to selected cases of constitutional delayed growth and adolescence in boys over 14 years of age and to prepubertal girls with gonadal dysgenesis (see text). Careful monitoring of growth versus bone age advancement is obligatory during treatment.
Estrogens	Female sex hormones are not growth-promoting agents; indeed, like androgens, they may hasten epiphysial fusion and result in ultimate shortening. In gonadotropin-deficient hypopituitary dwarfs and in patients with gonadal dysgenesis, estrogens are useful in bringing about adolescent development when the age of expected puberty is reached.
Glucocorticoids and mineralocorticoids	The specific and judicious use of these agents in congenital virilizing hyperplasia and adrenal insufficiency will permit normal growth and epiphysial fusion. Patients with ACTH deficiency, especially of an organic nature, may also require glucocorticoid but not mineralocorticoid replacement therapy. Care must be taken not to inhibit the effectiveness of growth hormone therapy when the two agents are used jointly.

weight gain of 10–20 pounds; this restores self-confidence to the otherwise normally adjusted boy, and treatment is usually stopped for at least six months. Occasionally, a second course is administered after a gap of 6–8 months, but normal sexual development is usually progressing by this time and no further therapy is required.

Human chorionic gonadotropin, 1000–2000 I.U. 3 times a week, can be used alternatively. The advantage is that testicular enlargement occurs, and the disadvantage is the significant expense.

Males with *hypogonadotropism* plus growth hormone deficiency virilize when given the same regimens. Usually, this therapy is reserved until the patient reaches five feet in height or, for psychological reasons, until the boy needs to develop sexually, even if he does not reach that height. Females with hypopituitarism are given methyltestosterone, 10 mg./day, when the need for sexual development becomes apparent.

In patients with *gonadal dysgenesis,* some of the "protein anabolic–weaker androgenic" synthetic steroids are used to accelerate growth with the hope of increasing ultimate height. Johanson et al. (67) reported that giving 6-fluoxymesterone, 2.5 mg./day, to patients 12–18 years of age significantly increased their growth rate and ultimate height. The maximum effect was observed in the first 12–24 months of administration, with marked diminution in effect thereafter. Consequently, this agent or oxandrolone, 0.1–0.15 mg./kg. body weight, now are administered for 12 months, beginning at age 10, if the diagnosis is made this early. It is then discontinued for 12 months. Side effects are minimal with this dosage.

The only other justifiable use of androgens is for younger patients with severe growth retardation secondary to *hypopituitarism,* and then only if human growth hormone is not available. Oxandro-

lone, 0.1 mg./kg. body weight, increases growth significantly in many such patients. Skeletal maturation must be observed at 6-month intervals to ascertain that it does not exceed that expected for the increase in linear growth. Occasionally, children with *severe constitutional delay of growth* who are less than 14 years of age do require small doses to advance their growth. Oxandrolone, because of its weak androgenicity, is used instead of testosterone because sexual maturation has not yet become a problem; the same cautions apply for these patients as in patients with hypopituitarism. Before any compounds of this nature are administered, a proper diagnosis must be made.

Estrogens

Estrogens are used therapeutically in the treatment of short stature only for girls with *sexual infantilism* of whatever cause. Either Premarin, 1.25–2.5 mg./day, or ethynylestradiol, 0.05–0.1 mg./day, is administered for a 3-week period. This period is followed by one week without medication, during which time menstruation usually occurs, but menstruation may not occur until several cycles have been pursued. Progesterone compounds can be given during the third week of the 3-week cycle simultaneously with estrogen therapy to promote breast development. Because of the epiphysial fusion induced by the estrogen, the girls should be 14 years of age or older and should elect to have sexual development, even if it means sacrificing some ultimate height. In patients with *gonadal dysgenesis,* we usually use estrogen only after androgen has produced epiphysial fusion, but it is used earlier when the patient sincerely feels she needs sexual maturation more than additional height.

Growth Hormone (105, 106, 128, 133, 148)

Human growth hormone is effective in the treatment of *hypopituitarism* when given in dosages of approximately 1 I.U./day. Patients of early adolescent age may require a somewhat larger dose. Unfortunately, the limitation of available hormone, which must be prepared only from human pituitaries, prevents its use for many patients in whom it could be of benefit. Because the action of growth hormone occurs via generation of somatomedin, which has a longer half-life than does growth hormone, the daily total dose can be administered on an every-other-day basis. In approximately 5 per cent of hypopituitary patients receiving human growth hormone, antibodies of a type and titer that inhibit further growth develop. The parents and patient must be made aware of this possibility. Antibodies do develop in approximately 50 per cent of patients receiving growth hormone, but there is no diminution in response because of these antibodies. There is no way of predicting which patient will develop resistance. When using growth hormone for hypopituitary patients, the use of glucocorticoids should be minimal. Cortisol and cortisone markedly inhibit the action of growth hormone peripherally, as mentioned previously. Cortisol or cortisone is preferable to prednisone in the treatment of such patients because the increments administered can be smaller. No more than 10 mg./M.^{2} of oral cortisone should be used in patients receiving growth hormone.

Human growth hormone is also beneficial in some patients with *intrauterine growth retardation* (43). Approximately 50 per cent of such patients who have received extended courses of growth hormone have responded with significant increase in their growth rates. The patients who have responded have been primarily those with intrauterine dwarfism with unexplained delayed skeletal maturation. Patients with normal birth weights and lengths but subsequent growth retardation of unexplained origin (primordial dwarfs) have not responded favorably in the limited studies conducted to date (133, 148). In Figure 26–15, one such patient with intrauterine growth retardation is presented. The accompanying Figure 26–16 shows the growth rates during growth hormone therapy and when it is omitted.

Since growth hormone is a complex polypeptide which will be difficult to synthesize in large quantities, the eventual identification and synthesis of growth hormone releasing factor may make therapy more readily available to patients with hypopituitarism, intrauterine growth retardation, and other causes of short stature which may respond to growth hormone.

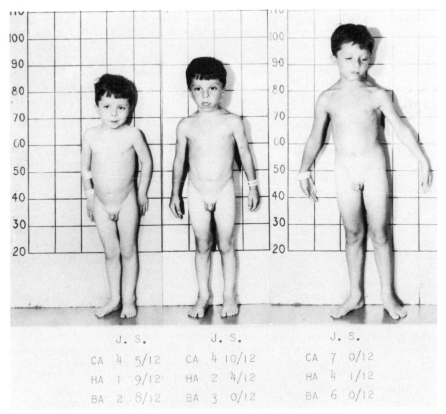

Figure 26–15. This patient with intrauterine growth retardation had a birth length of 17.0 inches and weighed 3 pounds 8 ounces at 40 weeks gestation. Growth hormone treatment (see Fig. 26–16) was associated with marked acceleration of growth over an extended period.

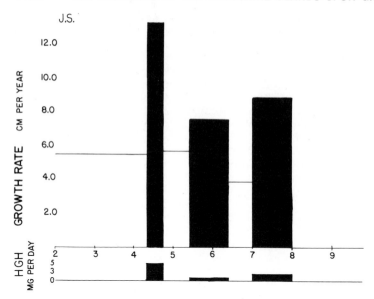

Figure 26–16. The growth rate of J. S. (Fig. 26–15) before and after growth hormone administration. Growth rates during growth hormone therapy are represented by the solid black bars in the top of the figure. Growth rates without therapy are recorded by horizontal black lines.

Thyroxine and Triiodothyronine (141)

Thyroxine is used to accelerate growth only in patients with either *primary or secondary thyroid hormone deficiency*. U.S.P. desiccated thyroid, 65 mg./day, is recommended for infants between 1 month and 18 months of age. The dosage increases to 100 mg. between 18 months and 6 years of age, and to 100–130 mg. between 6 and 12 years of age. Subsequently, 130–195 mg. are adequate for total replacement. A dose of 65 mg. (1 grain) of U.S.P. desiccated thyroid is the equivalent of 0.1 mg. thyroxine. Triiodothyronine is not necessary as a replacement drug, although it forms 50 per cent of the active hormone synthesized daily in the normal individual. The newer combination preparations which contain both thyroxine and triiodothyronine are as satisfactory as desiccated thyroid but more expensive. If thyroid hormone is given to patients with organic hypopituitarism, cortisol or cortisone should be given simultaneously, 10–20 mg./M.² /day, in divided doses. Acute cortisone deficiency is thus prevented when thyroxine is administered. This may otherwise occur since, in the euthyroid state, cortisol is metabolized more rapidly, and the patient who could previously tolerate cortisol insufficiency can no longer do so when made euthyroid.

Occasionally, reports are published concerning the use of thyroid hormone in normal but short children to increase growth. To date, all such reports require confirmation, and this type of treatment should be reserved for a few investigators who can adequately evaluate the data generated.

Glucocorticoids

The production rate of cortisol is 13.0 mg./M.²/day, and when oral cortisone or cortisol is administered, the replacement dose is twice the production rate (90). If intramuscular maintenance cortisone is used, the dosage is the same as the production rate, but the total 3-day production (37.5 mg./M.²) can be given in one injection every three days. Cortisol is used in the treatment of short stature either in patients with hypopituitarism or in patients with congenital virilizing adrenal hyperplasia. The caution required in the use of cortisol in hypopituitarism is mentioned in a previous paragraph. With appropriate use of cortisol to suppress the hyperactive adrenals in virilizing hyperplasia, growth rate decelerates and epiphysial maturation is delayed. Greater ultimate growth is therefore attained.

CAUSES OF OVERGROWTH

Many of the fundamental factors which control growth are entirely unknown. Most instances of overgrowth probably represent an unexplained constitutional variant from the normal pattern of growth and development opposite to that seen in "constitutional slow growth." Endocrine evaluation and studies of carbohydrate metabolism reveal no abnormalities suggestive of hyperpituitarism in these cases.

Familial Tall Stature

Unusually tall girls or boys often have one or both parents taller than average. Bayley's tables (6, 7) offer an approximate prediction of eventual height according to whether the bone age is normal or above or below the chronological age. Those with advanced osseous development may stop growing before they become unusually tall. Excessive height in girls, because of its social handicap, is a cause of great anxiety to both the girls and their parents, who plead for some hormonal treatment to stop further growth. Some workers have claimed that estrogenic therapy will do this by hastening epiphysial fusion (138–140). Treatment may have to be continued for a number of years before epiphysial fusion occurs. This will cause endometrial hyperplasia with menorrhagia unless artificial menstruation is produced by administering the estrogen cyclically. In spite of the physiologic rationale behind such hormonal intervention, it has yet to be proved conclusively that ultimate restriction of height is consistently accomplished. Further follow-up studies are needed. Data suggest that the earlier treatment is begun, the more likely it is to be successful. Little effect on growth is seen in the already pubertal girl. In any event, no assurances regarding final height should be given to the patient or her family, and such treatment should probably not even be considered for any girl predicted to become less than 6 feet in height. If it is used, the estrogen compound should be given in large doses (e.g., 10 mg. of Premarin daily) and continuously. Every fourth week, a progestational compound is administered; with cessation of this drug, menstruation occurs.

Pituitary or Hypothalamic Gigantism

The rare cases of hyperpituitary gigantism due to eosinophilic adenoma of the pituitary developing in childhood present a very different picture from the constitutionally overgrown children. A boy of $9\frac{1}{4}$ years with a pituitary tumor who had a height age of 14 years was compared with three constitutionally overgrown boys of similar age and height (28). The latter had advanced epiphysial development, whereas the bone age was normal in the hyperpituitary patient. It also was most striking that the boy with the pituitary tumor, even at this early age, showed cortical thickening of the bones with tufting of the terminal phalanges, overgrowth of soft tissues, and coarsening of features of an acromegalic type.

In rare cases, hypothalamic disease may also result in excess height that probably is caused by alterations in the synthesis or release or both of releasing hormones. A number of hypothalamic tumors associated with normal or accelerated linear growth, markedly excessive weight gain, severe polyphagia, absent immunoreactive growth hormone, and normal or increased somatomedin levels have been reported (40, 41, 46, 60, 69). It is interesting that in several instances this constellation of signs and symptoms does not appear until after surgical removal of the tumor.

Cerebral Gigantism (2, 61, 98, 126)

Some infants are of very large size at birth, weighing 10–13 pounds, after a gestation of normal duration. Postnatally, some of these continue to grow rapidly and may attain the average height of 5 or 6 years by the time they are 2 or 3 years of age. The osseous development is usually accelerated, but not to the same degree as the height.

Such children are frequently mentally retarded. In some instances, this may have resulted from anoxia at birth or some other birth trauma, often due to labor problems associated with a large head. In the majority of cases, the pathogenesis of cerebral gigantism is unknown. A normal sella turcica, a large skull, and slightly dilated ventricles are common. The extremities have none of the changes seen in acromegaly. Laboratory findings are inconsistent. On occasion, some evidence of a disturbed hypothalamic axis has been noted. The growth hormone studies reported are normal.

Infants of Diabetic Mothers
(36, 54, 91, 96, 97)

The macrosomia of infants whose mothers were prediabetic or overtly diabetic has been appreciated for years. Body composition studies reveal an increase in lean body mass as well as in adipose tissue mass. Animal studies (101, 146) and evaluation of human placentas suggest this excess growth is, at least in part if not totally, a hyperplastic phenomenon. The overgrowth is self-limited and presents no practical problem. The difficulties in management lie in the treatment of the often severe neonatal hypoglycemia which occurs as a result of the pancreatic hyperplasia and excessive insulin production.

Beckwith-Wiedemann Syndrome (38, 125)

A third group of infants with neonatal gigantism has been described which can be separated from the above two categories despite some similar characteristics. Congenital macrosomia, organomegaly including the characteristic macroglossia, and congenital umbilical anomalies are the hallmarks of this syndrome. Other usually minor congenital anomalies are frequent. The overgrowth persists after birth for several years and is often associated with some advancement in bone age. Neonatal hypoglycemia is common and is associated with pancreatic hyperplasia and presumed hyperinsulinism. Adrenal cortical cytomegaly is also seen. No studies of cortisol production have been reported. Mental development is usually normal unless the hypoglycemia has been severe. A positive family history has been reported in a few cases.

Miscellaneous Causes of Overgrowth

Other causes of overgrowth to be considered in the differential diagnosis of tall stature include neurofibromatosis, lipodystrophy, Marfan's syndrome, homocystinuria, and thyrotoxicosis. In most cases, the characteristics peculiar to these disorders allow ready recognition of the primary disease. Sexual precocity, as noted earlier, is associated with rapid growth during childhood, but early epiphysial fusion brings growth to an end, often before normal adult height is achieved.

VARIATIONS IN ADOLESCENT DEVELOPMENT (141)

Endocrine Factors Concerned with Adolescent Sexual Development

The development of secondary sexual characteristics depends upon the secretion by the anterior pituitary of gonadotropins, which are not liberated in easily measurable amounts during earlier childhood. The factors responsible for activating these functions of the pituitary are not known. Normal maturation of the ovary with the establishment of menstrual cycles and ovulation depends on the secretion of follicle stimulating hormone (FSH) and luteinizing hormone (LH). These must be secreted cyclically in varying amounts. The development of breasts, labia minora, vagina, uterus, and fallopian tubes is brought about by estrogens secreted by the graafian follicle under the influence of FSH. The secretory changes of the endometrium and acinar budding of the breasts are caused by progesterone secreted by the corpus luteum under the control of LH and LTH. In females, androgens which are primarily secreted by the adrenal cortex are necessary for the growth of sexual hair. It is not known what causes the adrenals to begin secreting androgens (11-deoxy-19-carbon steroids) shortly before the onset of puberty, whereas previously they formed mainly glucocorticoids (21-carbon steroids). Maturation of the testes with spermatogenesis depends upon the secretion of both LH and FSH. Secondary sexual development, such as deepening of the voice, changes in the scrotal skin, development of the penis, prostate, and seminal vesicles, and development of sexual hair and beard, is caused by androgen secreted by the Leydig cells under the influence of LH. Spermatogenesis is dependent upon stimulation of the seminiferous tubules by FSH.

Puberty (10) is a time of great transition in the functions of the endocrine system during which the main activities of the hypothalamic-pituitary centers change from those governing somatic growth and development to those regulating secretion of the sex hormones. The normal maturation of secondary sexual characteristics depends upon the orderly development and functioning of the pituitary-gonadal-adrenal mechanism. It is not surprising that there are differences in the time of onset of these pituitary activities or temporary imbalances in the amounts of the numerous hormones secreted during this period of transition. It is also natural that there be individual differences in the responsiveness of the sexual end-organs to the various hormones.

The age ranges of onset of specific aspects of sexual development for white British children were published by Marshall and Tanner (80, 81). Genital development in 95 per cent of boys began between 9½ and 13½ years, with a mean of 11.6 years; full adult genital development was reached on an average of three years after its onset. Peak height velocity occurred at the mean age of 14.1 years. In girls, the first signs of puberty were noted in 95 per cent between 8½ and 13 years. Mean menarchial age was 13.47 years and was preceded in all cases by the peak height velocity, which occurred at a mean of 12.14 years. Thus peak adolescent growth rate in girls precedes that in boys by nearly two years.

Constitutional Variations in Time of Onset and Pattern of Sexual Development (141)

Delayed Adolescence (141)

Just as the rate of somatic growth and the final height that a normal individual attains may depend upon inborn constitutional traits, there are also wide variations in the time of onset of sexual development and the rate at which it progresses. Extensive studies have shown that in entirely normal males and females the first signs of puberty may appear at any time between the ages of 9 and 17 years. Children who are slow in somatic growth and osseous development are more apt to have a delayed adolescence. At times, however, children of normal height may have a late onset of puberty. These individuals are perfectly normal except for the eunuchoid proportions which usually result. Treatment was discussed in the previous section.

Gynecomastia in Adolescent Boys (141)

This condition should be distinguished from the fat padding which frequently simulates breasts in obese individuals. A slight degree of hyperplasia of the mammary ducts occurs in a large percentage of boys during adolescence. More marked breast development is not uncommon and may be bilateral or unilateral. It is usually transient, disappearing after a year or two, but sometimes it persists for years. The cause is not clearly understood. It should not be considered evidence of "femininity"; in fact, it is usually seen in boys who are virilizing rapidly. It should be distinguished from the gynecomastia that may occur in Klinefelter's syndrome or testicular dysgenesis. Patients with the latter disorder have small testes, aspermia or oligospermia, elevated urinary gonadotropins, and usually a chromatin-positive nuclear pattern of the buccal smear. Hormonal therapy, such as testosterone or chorionic gonadotropins, should not be given, as these make the condition worse. Mastectomy is indicated only when the hyperplasia is very marked and persistent or causes severe psychologic problems, and then it should be done only by an experienced surgeon.

Premature Development of Breasts in Girls ("Premature Thelarche") (37, 66, 70, 123, 141)

The isolated development of the breasts without signs of sexual maturation is not uncommon at any time during infancy and childhood and is usually not related to the neonatal breast hyperplasia. The

TABLE 26-6. TYPES OF EARLY SEXUAL DEVELOPMENT IN FEMALES

	Premature Thelarche	Premature Pubarche	Sexual Precocity
Areolar changes	None usually	None	Present
Glandular breast tissue	Present	None	Present
Vaginal smear	Minimal or no estrogen effect	No estrogen effect	Definite estrogen effect
Sexual hair	None	Present	Often present
Somatic growth	Normal	Normal or slightly advanced	Advanced
Osseous development	Normal	Normal or slightly advanced	Advanced
17-ketosteroid excretion	Normal	Normal or slightly increased	Variable
Serum gonadotropins	Normal for age	Normal for age	Commensurate with stage of puberty

enlargement is usually bilateral but sometimes is unilateral. Frequently the condition is transient, but it may persist for a number of years. It can be distinguished usually from true sexual precocity by the fact that the labia minora, vagina, and uterus do not develop and the vaginal smear has no or minimal estrogenization. The condition is benign, and no treatment is needed (see Table 26-6).

✓ bone age.

Premature Development of Sexual Hair ("Premature Pubarche") (66, 70, 141)

Occasionally pubic and axillary hair appear early, especially in girls, without the development of any other secondary sexual characteristics. The absence of breast, labial, or vaginal development distinguishes the condition from true sexual precocity in girls (see Table 26-6). It can be differentiated from the adrenogenital syndrome by the fact that the clitoris is not enlarged, there is no progressive virilization, and the 17-ketosteroid excretion is only slightly elevated above the normal for the age. The condition is entirely harmless, and no treatment is needed. For unknown reasons, this condition is more common in patients with cerebral dysfunction. The patients go into normal puberty at about the average time.

Menstrual Irregularities

The occurrence of regular ovulatory menstrual cycles depends upon the full maturation of the complicated pituitary-ovarian mechanism responsible for the cyclic secretion of both pituitary and ovarian hormones in varying amounts. During the first few years after the menarche, it is not surprising that there are frequent irregularities of menstruation and anovulatory cycles because of temporary imbalances. When irregular anovulatory menses persist, hormonal therapy may be indicated. This should be undertaken, however, only

after careful gynecologic examination by someone thoroughly familiar with gynecologic endocrine problems.

REFERENCES

1. Aarskog, D., Blizzard, R. M., et al.: The response to methapyrapone (SU-4885) and pyrogen test in idiopathic hypopituitarism. *J. Clin. Endocr.* 25:439, 1965.
2. Abraham, J. M., and Snodgrass, G. J.: Soto's syndrome of cerebral gigantism. *Arch. Dis. Child.* 44:203, 1969.
3. Almqvist, S., Lindsten, J., et al.: Linear growth, sulfation factor activity and chromosome constitution in 22 subjects with Turner's syndrome. *Acta Endocr.* 42:168, 1963.
4. Andrews, B. F.: The small-for-date infant. *Pediat. Clin. N. Amer.* 17:1, 1970.
5. August, G. P., Grumbach, M. M., et al.: Hormonal changes in puberty. III. Correlation of plasma testosterone, LH, FSH, testicular size, and bone age with male pubertal development. *J. Clin. Endocr.* 34:319, 1972.
6. Bayer, L. M., and Bayley, N.: *Growth Diagnosis.* Chicago, University of Chicago Press, 1959.
7. Bayley, N., and Pinneau, S. R.: Tables for predicting adult height from skeletal age: revised for use with the Greulich-Pyle hand standards. *J. Pediat.* 40:423, 1952.
8. Black, J.: Low birth weight dwarfism. *Arch. Dis. Child.* 36:633, 1961.
9. Blizzard, R. M.: Differentiation, morphogenesis, and growth with emphasis on the role of pituitary growth hormone, In *Human Growth.* Cheek, D. B. (ed.), Philadelphia, Lea & Febiger, 1968.
10. Blizzard, R. M., Penny, R., et al.: Pituitary gonadal interrelationship in relation to puberty, In *Gonadotropins. An International Symposium.* Saxena, B. B., Beling, C. G., et al. (eds.), New York, Wiley-Interscience, 1972.
11. Bovin, A., Vendrely, R., et al.: L'Acide désoxyribonucléique du noyau cellulaire, dépositaire des caratères héréditaires; arguments d'ordre analytique. *C. R. Acad. Sci.* (Paris) 226:1061, 1948.
12. Brasel, J. A., and Winick, M.: Differential cellular growth in the organs of hypothyroid rats. *Growth* 34:197, 1970.
13. Brasel, J. A., Wright, J. C., et al.: An evaluation of seventy-five patients with hypopituitarism beginning in childhood. *Amer. J. Med.* 38:484, 1965.
14. Campbell, A. M., and Keir, H. M.: The effect of triiodothyronine on the biosynthesis of deoxyribonucleic acid in *Rana catesbeiana* tadpoles. *Biochem. J.* 114:38, 1969.
15. Carriere, R.: Influence of growth hormone and thyroxine on nuclear size in rat liver. *Anat. Rec.* 121:273, 1955.
16. Cheek, D. B.: Muscle cell growth in abnormal children, In *Human Growth.* Cheek, D. B. (ed.), Philadelphia, Lea & Febiger, 1968.
17. Cheek, D. B.: Muscle cell growth in normal children, In *Human Growth.* Cheek, D. B. (ed.), Philadelphia, Lea & Febiger, 1968.
18. Cheek, D. B., Brasel, J. A., et al.: Muscle cell growth in rodents: Sex difference and the role of hormones, In *Human Growth.* Cheek, D. B. (ed.), Philadelphia, Lea & Febiger, 1968.
19. Cheek, D. B., and Graystone, J. E.: The action of insulin, growth hormone, and epinephrine on cell growth in liver, muscle and brain of the hypophysectomized rat. *Pediat. Res.* 3:77, 1969.
20. Cheek, D. B., Powell, G. K., et al.: Growth of muscle cells (size and number) and liver DNA in rats and Snell Smith mice with insufficient pituitary, thyroid or testicular function. *Bull. Johns Hopkins Hosp.* 117:306, 1965.
21. Cockayne, E. A.: Dwarfism with retinal atrophy and deafness. *Arch. Dis. Child.* 21:52, 1946.
22. Contopoulos, A. N., Simpson, M. E., et al.: Pituitary function in the thyroidectomized rat. *Endocr.* 63:642, 1958.
23. Costin, G., Kogut, M. D., et al.: Effect of low-dose human growth hormone on carbohydrate metabolism in children with hypopituitarism. *J. Pediat.* 80:796, 1972.
24. Daughaday, W. H., Laron, Z., et al.: Defective sulfation factor generation: A possible etiological link in dwarfism. *Trans. Ass. Amer. Physicians* 82:129, 1969.

25. Daughaday, W. H., and Reeder, C.: Synchronous activation of DNA synthesis in hypophysectomized rat cartilage by growth hormone. *J. Lab. Clin. Med.* 68:357, 1966.

26. Davidson, J. N., and Leslie, I.: Nucleic acids in relation to tissue growth: A review. *Cancer Res.* 10:587, 1950.

27. DeBusk, F. L.: The Hutchinson-Gilford progeria syndrome. *J. Pediat.* 80:697, 1972.

28. deMajo, S. F., and Onativia, A.: Acromegaly and gigantism in a boy: comparison with 3 overgrown non-acromegalic children. *J. Pediat.* 57:382, 1960.

29. DiStefano, H. S., and Diermeier, H. F.: Effects of hypophysectomy and growth hormone on ploidy distribution and mitotic activity of rat liver. *Proc. Soc. Exp. Biol. Med.* 92:590, 1956.

30. Drash, P. W., Greenberg, N. E., et al: Intelligence and personality in four syndromes of dwarfism, In *Human Growth.* Cheek, D. B., (ed.), Philadelphia, Lea & Febiger, 1968.

31. Eberlein, W. R., Bongiovanni, A. M., et al: Ovarian tumors and cysts associated with sexual precocity. Report of three cases and review of literature. *J. Pediat.* 57:484, 1960.

32. Enesco, M., and Leblond, C. P.: Increase in cell number as a factor in the growth of the organs of the young male rat. *J. Embryol. Exp. Morphol.* 10:530, 1962.

33. Engel, E., and Forbes, A. P.: Cytogenetic and clinical findings in 48 patients with congenitally defective or absent ovaries. *Medicine* 44:135, 1965.

34. Epstein, C. J.: Cell size, nuclear content, and the development of polyploidy in the mammalian liver. *Proc. Nat. Acad. Sci. (USA)* 57:327, 1967.

35. Epstein, S., Esanu, C., et al: The effect of growth hormone and cortisone on thymidine kinase activity in rat adipose tissue. *Biochim. Biophys. Acta* 186:280, 1969.

36. Fee, B. A., and Weil, W. B., Jr.: Body composition of infants of diabetic mothers by direct analysis. *Ann. N.Y. Acad. Sci.* 110:869, 1963.

37. Ferrier, P., Shepard, T. H., et al.: Growth disturbances and values for hormone excretion in various forms of precocious sexual development. *Pediatrics* 28:258, 1961.

38. Filippi, G., and McKusick, V. A.: Beckwith-Wiedemann syndrome: Exomphalos-macroglossia-gigantism syndrome. Report of two cases and review of the literature. *Medicine* 49:279, 1970.

39. Finkelstein, J. W., Boyar, R. M., et al.: Age-related change in the 24-hour spontaneous secretion of growth hormone. *J. Clin. Endocr.* 35:665, 1972.

40. Finkelstein, J. W., Kream, J., et al.: Sulfation factor (Somatomedin): An explanation for continued growth in the absence of immunoassayable growth hormone in patients with hypothalamic tumors. *J. Clin. Endocr.* 35:13, 1972.

41. Fishman, M. A., and Peake, G. T.: Paradoxical growth in a patient with the diencephalic syndrome. *Pediatrics* 45:973, 1970.

42. Foley, T. P., Jr., Jacobs, L. S., et al.: Human prolactin and thyrotropin concentrations in the serums of normal and hypopituitary children before and after the administration of synthetic thyrotropin-releasing hormone. *J. Clin. Invest.* 51:2143, 1972.

43. Foley, T. P., Jr., Shaw, M., et al.: Growth hormone as a therapeutic agent in patients with intrauterine growth retardation. (In preparation).

44. Franchimont, P., Legros, J. J., et al.: Anterior pituitary function in human fetal life. *Sympos. Deutsch. Ges. Endocr.* 16:47, 1970.

45. Frantz, A. G., and Rabkin, M. T.: Human growth hormone. Clinical measurement, response to hypoglycemia and suppression by corticosteroids. *New Eng. J. Med.* 27:1375, 1964.

46. Frasier, S. D., and Smith, F. G.: Return of normal growth following removal of a craniopharyngioma. *Amer. J. Dis. Child.* 116:311, 1968.

47. Frohman, L. A.: Clinical pharmacology of hypothalamic releasing factors. *New Eng. J. Med.* 286:1391, 1972.

48. Geschwind, I. I., Alfert, M., et al.: The effects of thyroxin and growth hormone on liver polyploidy. *Biol. Bull.* 118:66, 1960.

49. Goodman, H. G., Grumbach, M. M., et al.: Growth and growth hormone. II. Comparison of isolated growth-hormone deficiency and multiple pituitary hormone defi-

50. Graystone, J. E., and Cheek, D. B.: The effects of reduced caloric intake and increased insulin-induced caloric intake on the cell growth of muscle, liver, and cerebrum and on skeletal collagen in the postweanling rat. *Pediat. Res.* 3:66, 1969.

51. Greenberg, A. H., Czernichow, P., et al.: Observations on the maturation of thyroid function in early fetal life. *J. Clin. Invest.* 49:1790, 1970.

52. Greulich, W. W., and Pyle, S. I.: *Radiographic Atlas of Skeletal Development of the Hand and Wrist.* 2nd ed. Stanford, Calif., Stanford University Press, 1959.

53. Haddad, H. M., and Wilkins, L.: Congenital anomalies associated with gonadal aplasia. *Pediatrics* 23:885, 1959.

54. Hagbard, L.: Pregnancy and diabetes mellitus. *Acta Obstet. Gynec. Scand.* 35 (Suppl. 1.):138, 1956.

55. Hamburgh, M., and Barrington, E. J. W. (eds.), *Hormones in Development.* New York, Appleton-Century-Crofts, 1971.

56. Hartog, M., Gaafar, M. A., et al.: Effect of corticosteroids on serum growth hormone. *Lancet* 2:376, 1964.

57. Helweg-Larson, H. F.: Nuclear series; studies on frequency distribution of nuclear sizes and quantitative significance of formation of nuclear class series for growth of organs in mice with special reference to influence of pituitary growth hormone. *Acta Path. Microbiol. Scand.* (Kbn.), *Suppl.* 92, 1952, p. 3.

58. Hoerr, N. L., Pyle, S. I., et al.: *Radiographic Atlas of Skeletal Development of the Foot and Ankle.* Springfield, Ill., Charles C Thomas, 1962.

59. Holden, J. D.: Russell-Sliver's dwarf. *Dev. Med. Child. Neurol.* 9:457, 1967.

60. Holmes, L. B., Frantz, A. G., et al.: Normal growth with subnormal growth hormone levels. *New Eng. J. Med.* 279:559, 1968.

61. Hook, E. B., and Reynolds, J. W.: Cerebral gigantism: Endocrinologic and clinical observations of six patients including a congenital giant, concordant monozygotic twins and a child who achieved adult gigantic size. *J. Pediat.* 70:900, 1967.

62. Howell, R. R.: Diagnostic procedures for genetic metabolic defects, In *Genetics in Medical Practice.* Bartalos, M. (ed.), Philadelphia, J. B. Lippincott Co., 1968.

63. Jacobson, C. B.: Cytogenetic techniques and their clinical uses, In *Genetics in Medical Practice.* Bartalos, M. (ed.), Philadelphia, J. B. Lippincott Co., 1968.

64. Jasper, H. G., and Brasel, J. A.: The effects of growth hormone on DNA polymerase activity in the liver of normal and hypophysectomized rats. *J. Clin. Endocr.* 92:194, 1973.

65. Jenkins, M. E.: Precocious menstruation in hypothyroidism. *Amer. J. Dis. Child.* 109:252, 1965.

66. Jenner, M. R., Kelch, R. P., et al.: Hormonal changes in puberty. IV. Plasma estradiol, LH, and FSH in prepubertal children, pubertal females, and in precocious puberty, premature thelarche, hypogonadism, and in a child with a feminizing ovarian tumor. *J. Clin. Endocr.* 34:521, 1972.

67. Johanson, A. J., Brasel, J. A., et al.: Growth in patients with gonadal dysgenesis receiving fluoxymesterone. *J. Pediat.* 75:1015, 1969.

68. Kaplan, S. L., Abrams, C. A. L., et al.: Growth and growth hormone. I. Changes in serum level of growth hormone following hypoglycemia in 134 children with growth retardation. *Pediat. Res.* 2:43, 1968.

69. Kenny, F. M., Iturzaeta, N. F., et al.: Iatrogenic hypopituitarism in craniopharyngioma: Unexplained catch-up growth in three children. *J. Pediat.* 72:766, 1968.

70. Kenny, F. M., Midgley, A. R., et al.: Radioimmunoassayable serum LH and FSH in girls with sexual precocity, premature thelarche and adrenarche. *J. Clin. Endocr.* 29:1272, 1969.

71. Knigge, K. M.: Cytology and growth hormone content of rat's pituitary gland following thyroidectomy and stress. *Anat. Rec.* 130:543, 1958.

72. Krieger, D. T.: The hypothalamus and neuroendocrine pathology. *Hosp. Pract.* Nov., 1971, p. 127.

73. Laron, Z., Pertzelan, A., et al.: Pituitary dwarfism with high serum levels of growth hormone. *Israel J. Med. Sci.* 4:883, 1968.

ciencies in 35 patients with idiopathic hypopituitary dwarfism. *New Eng. J. Med.* 278:57, 1968.

74. Leblond, C. P., and Carriere, R.: The effect of growth hormone and thyroxine on the mitotic rate of the intestinal mucosa of the rat. *Endocrinology* 56:261, 1955.

75. Lee, K. L., Sun, S. C., et al.: Stimulation of incorporation by triiodothyronine of thymidine-methyl-³H into hepatic DNA of the rat. *Arch. Biochem. Biophys.* 125:751, 1968.

76. Lemli, L., and Smith, D. W.: The XO syndrome: Study of the differential phenotype in 25 patients. *J. Pediat.* 63:577, 1963.

77. Leuchtenberger, C., Helweg-Larson, H. F., et al.: Relationship between hereditary pituitary dwarfism and the formation of multiple desoxyribose nucleic acid (DNA) classes in mice. *Lab. Invest.* 3:245, 1954.

78. Lewis U. J., Cheever, E. V., et al.: Alteration of the proteins of the pituitary gland of the rat by estradiol and cortisol. *Endocrinology* 76:362, 1965.

79. Liu, N.: Some aspects of endocrinology in the fetus and newborn. *Pediat. Clin. N. Amer.* 13:1047, 1966.

80. Marshall, W. A., and Tanner, J. M.: Variations in pattern of pubertal changes in girls. *Arch. Dis. Child.* 44:291, 1969.

81. Marshall, W. A., and Tanner, J. M.: Variations in the pattern of pubertal changes in boys. *Arch. Dis. Child.* 45:13, 1970.

82. Martin, L. G., Martul, P., et al.: Hypothalamic origin of idiopathic hypopituitarism. *Metabolism* 21:1472, 1972.

83. Massler, M., Schour, I., et al.: Developmental pattern of the child as reflected in the calcification pattern of the teeth. *Amer. J. Dis. Child.* 62:33, 1941.

84. McGeorge, M., and Connor, D. V.: A case of precocious puberty in a female. *Arch. Dis. Child.* 36:439, 1961.

85. McKusick, V. A.: Some principles of medical genetics, In *Genetics in Medical Practice.* Bartalos, M., (ed.), Philadelphia, J. B. Lippincott Co., 1968.

86. Mellits, E. D., Dorst, J. P., et al.: Bone age: Its contribution to the prediction of maturational or biological age. *Amer. J. Phys. Anthrop.* 35:381, 1971.

87. Mellman, W. J., Bongiovanni, A. M., et al.: The diagnostic usefulness of skeletal maturation in an endocrine clinic. *Pediatrics* 23:530, 1959.

88. Merimee, T. J., Rabinowitz, D., et al.: Isolated human growth hormone deficiency. III. Insulin secretion in sexual atelitotic dwarfism. *Metabolism* 17:1005, 1968.

89. Meyer, Y. N., and Evans, E. S.: Acidophil regranulation and increased growth hormone concentration in the pituitary of thyroidectomized rats after cortisol administration. *Endocrinology* 74:784, 1964.

90. Migeon, C. J., Green, O. C., et al.: Study of adrenocortical function in obesity. *Metabolism* 12:718, 1963.

91. Miller, H. C.: Offspring of diabetic and prediabetic mothers. *Advances Pediat.* 8:137, 1956.

92. Mirsky, A. E., and Ris, H.: Variable and constant components of chromosomes. *Nature* 163:666, 1949.

93. Naeye, R. L.: Infants of diabetic mothers: A quantitative, morphologic study. *Pediatrics* 35:980, 1965.

94. Neill, C. A., and Dingwall, M. A.: A syndrome resembling progeria: a review of two cases. *Arch. Dis. Child.* 25:213, 1950.

95. Nyhan, W. L. (ed.), *Amino Acid Metabolism and Genetic Variation.* New York, McGraw-Hill, 1967.

96. Osler, M.: Body water of newborn infants of diabetic mothers. *Acta Endocr.* 34:261, 1960.

97. Osler, M.: Body fat of newborn infants of diabetic mothers. *Acta Endocr.* 34:277, 1960.

98. Ott, J. E., and Robinson, A.: Cerebral gigantism. *Amer. J. Dis. Child.* 117:357, 1969.

99. Paine, R. S.: Diagnosis of inherited metabolic diseases, In *Genetics in Medical Practice.* Bartalos, M. (ed.), Philadelphia, J. B. Lippincott Co., 1968.

100. Peake, G. T., Rimoin, D., et al.: Hormonal and metabolic response to human growth hormone (HGH) in 45XO patients. *Clin. Res.* 20:436, 1972.

101. Pitkin, R. M., Plank, C. J., et al.: Fetal and placental composition in experimental maternal diabetes. *Proc. Soc. Exp. Biol. Med.* 138:163, 1971.

102. Powell, G. F., Brasel, J. A., et al.: Emotional deprivation and growth retardation simulating idiopathic hypopituitarism. I. Clinical evaluation of the syndrome. *New Eng. J. Med.* 276:1271, 1967.

103. Powell, G. F., Brasel, J. A., et al.: Emotional deprivation and growth retardation simulating idiopathic hypopitui-

104. Pyle, S. I., and Hoerr, N. L.: *Radiographic Atlas of Skeletal Development of the Knee.* Springfield, Ill., Charles C Thomas, 1955.

105. Raben, M. S., Matsuzaki, F., et al.: Growth promoting and metabolic effects of growth hormone. *Metabolism* 13:1102, 1964.

106. Raiti, S., and Blizzard, R. M.: Human growth hormone: Current role in normal and abnormal metabolic states. *Advances Pediat.* 17:99, 1970.

107. Raiti, S., Holzman, G. B., et al.: The passage of triiodothyronine across the human placenta in the last trimester and at term. *New Eng. J. Med.* 277:456, 1967.

108. Reisman, L. E.: Chromosomal abnormalities and intrauterine growth retardation. *Pediat. Clin. N. Amer.* 17:101, 1970.

109. Rimoin, D. L.: Genetic defects of growth hormone. *Hosp. Pract.* Feb., 1971, p. 113.

110. Rimoin, D. L., Merimee, T. J., et al.: Peripheral subresponsiveness to human growth hormone in the African pygmies. *New Eng. J. Med.* 281:1383, 1969.

111. Rimoin, D. L., Merimee, T. J., et al.: Genetic aspects of clinical endocrinology. *Recent Progr. Hormone Res.* 24:365, 1968.

112. Rubin, P.: *Dynamic Classification of Bone Dysplasias.* Chicago, Year Book Medical Publishers, 1964.

113. Russell, A.: A syndrome of "intra-uterine" dwarfism recognizable at birth with craniofacial dysostosis, disproportionately short arms, and other anomalies (5 examples). *Proc. Roy. Soc. Med.* 47:1040, 1954.

114. Schour, I., and Massler, M.: Endocrines and dentistry. *J.A.D.A.* 30:595, 1943.

115. Schour, I., and Massler, M.: Endocrines and dentistry. Part II. *J.A.D.A.* 30:763, 1943.

116. Schour, I., and Massler, M.: Endocrines and dentistry. Part III. *J.A.D.A.* 30:943, 1943.

117. Schour, I., and Massler, M.: Studies in tooth development: the growth pattern of human teeth. *J.A.D.A.* 27:1778, 1940.

118. Seckel, H. P. G.: *Bird-Headed Dwarfs: Studies in Developmental Anthropology Including Human Proportions.* Basel, S. Karger, 1960.

119. Sheikholislam, B. M., Lebovitz, H. E., et al.: Growth hormone secretion in hypothyroidism. Forty-eighth Annual Meeting, Endocrine Society, Chicago, June 21, 1966.

120. Siegel, E., and Tobias, C. A.: Actions of thyroid hormones on cultured human cells. *Nature* 212:1318, 1966.

121. Simpson, M. E., Arling, C. W., et al.: Some endocrine influences on skeletal growth and differentiation. *Yale J. Biol. Med.* 23:1, 1950.

122. Silver, H. K.: Asymmetry, short stature and variations in sexual development: Syndrome of congenital malformations. *Amer. J. Dis. Child.* 107:495, 1964.

123. Silver, H. K., and Sami, D.: Premature thelarche. Precocious development of breast. *Pediatrics* 34:1067, 1964.

124. Solomon, J., and Greep, R. O.: The effect of alterations in thyroid function on the pituitary growth hormone content and acidophil cytology. *Endocrinology* 65:158, 1959.

125. Sotelo-Avila, C., and Singer, D. B.: Syndrome of hyperplastic fetal visceromegaly and neonatal hypoglycemia (Beckwith's syndrome): Report of seven cases. *Pediatrics* 46:240, 1970.

126. Sotos, J. F., Dodge, P. R., et al.: Cerebral gigantism in childhood. A syndrome of excessively rapid growth with acromegalic features and a nonprogressive neurologic disorder. *New Eng. J. Med.* 271:109, 1964.

127. Soyka, L. F., and Crawford, J. D.: Antagonism by cortisone of the linear growth induced in hypopituitary patients and hypophysectomized rats by human growth hormone. *J. Clin. Endocr.* 25:469, 1965.

128. Soyka, L. F., Ziskind, A., et al.: Treatment of short stature in children and adolescents with human pituitary growth hormone (Raben). Experience with thirty-five cases. *New Eng. J. Med.* 271:754, 1964.

129. Stempfel, R. S., Jr., Sheikholislam, B. M., et al.: Pituitary growth hormone suppression with low-dosage, long-acting corticoid administration. *J. Pediat.* 73:767, 1968.

130. Swartz, F. J., and Ford, J. D., Jr.: Effect of thyroidectomy on

development of polyploid nuclei in rat liver. *Proc. Soc. Exp. Biol. Med. 104*:756, 1960.

131. Talbot, N. B., Sobel, E. H., et al.: Dwarfism in healthy children: Its possible relation to emotional, nutritional and endocrine disturbances. *New Eng. J. Med. 236*:783, 1947.

132. Tanner, J. M., Goldstein, H., et al.: Standards for children's height at ages 2–9 years allowing for height of parents. *Arch. Dis. Child. 45*:755, 1970.

133. Tanner, J. M., Whitehouse, R. H., et al.: Effect of human growth hormone treatment for 1 to 7 years on growth of 100 children, with growth hormone deficiency, low birthweight, inherited smallness, Turner's syndrome and other complaints. *Arch. Dis. Child. 46*:745, 1971.

134. Thompson, R. G., Rodrigues, A., et al.: Integrated concentrations of growth hormone correlated with plasma testosterone and bone age in preadolescent and adolescent males. *J. Clin. Endocr. 35*:334, 1972.

135. Todd, T. W.: *Atlas of Skeletal Maturation.* St. Louis, C. V. Mosby Co., 1937.

136. Wallace, A. L. C., Thorburn, G. D., et al.: Role of the kidneys and liver in the degradation and excretion of injected growth hormone. *Aust. J. Exp. Biol. Med. Sci. 47*:35, 1969.

137. Watson, E. H., and Lowrey, G. H.: *Growth and Development of Children.* 5th ed. Chicago, Year Book Medical Publishers, 1967.

138. Wettenhall, H. N. B., and Roche, A. F.: Tall girls. Assessment and management. *Aust. Paediat. J. 1*:210, 1965.

139. Whitelaw, M. J., and Foster, T. N.: Treatment of excessive height in girls. *J. Pediat. 61*:566, 1962.

140. Whitelaw, M. J., Foster, T. N., et al.: Estradiol valerate: Its effects on anabolism and skeletal age in the prepubertal girl. *J. Clin. Endocr. 23*:1125, 1963.

141. Wilkins, L.: *The Diagnosis and Treatment of Endocrine Disorders in Childhood and Adolescence.* 3rd ed. Springfield, Ill., Charles C Thomas, 1965.

142. Wilkins, L.: Hormonal influence on skeletal growth. *Ann. N.Y. Acad. Sci. 60*:763, 1955.

143. Winick, M., and Grant, P.: Cellular growth in the organs of the hypopituitary dwarf mouse. *Endocrinology 83*:544, 1968.

144. Winick, M., and Noble, A.: Quantitative changes in DNA, RNA, and protein during prenatal and postnatal growth in the rat. *Develop. Biol. 12*:451, 1965.

145. Winick, M., and Noble, A.: Cellular response in rats during malnutrition at various ages. *J. Nutr. 89*:300, 1966.

146. Winick, M., and Noble, A.: Cellular growth in human placenta. II. Diabetes mellitus. *J. Pediat. 71*:216, 1967.

147. Winick, M., Rosso, P., et al.: Cellular growth of cerebrum, cerebellum, and brain stem in normal and marasmic children. *Exp. Neurol. 26*:393, 1970.

148. Wright, J. C., Brasel, J. A., et al.: Studies with human growth hormone (HGH). An attempt to correlate metabolic response during short-term administration with linear growth during prolonged therapy. *Amer. J. Med. 38*:499, 1965.

149. Younger, L. R., King, J., et al.: Hepatic proliferative response to insulin in severe alloxan diabetes. *Cancer Res. 26*:1408, 1966.

CHAPTER 27

Aging and Hormones

By Robert I. Gregerman and
     Edwin L. Bierman

In past years, aging has been thought by some scientists to be the direct result of deficiency states resulting from age-related failure of the endocrine glands to secrete their hormones. Such thinking now seems naive as the complexities of the processes of aging have become more apparent. Moreover, an overt hormone deficiency state, such as that which occurs at the menopause with ovarian failure and subsequent estrogen lack, is the exception rather than the rule for age-related endocrine changes. In contrast with other hormones, either no deficiency exists in the classical sense, or else the age-related alteration of hormone physiol-

ogy is subtle. Nonetheless, although mastery of the organs of internal secretion can no longer be viewed as the key to longevity, normal aging does produce a variety of effects on hormone production, secretion, and action. For these reasons, an understanding of age-related changes in endocrine function can make a significant contribution to our concepts of what constitutes "disease," as opposed to time-related physiologic alteration, and to our understanding of the processes of aging.

The practical need for such age-based information has become obvious, and it is now clear that standards of normality in clinical tests of endocrine function must take into account the effects of aging that occur throughout the population. For example, over a number of years, failure to appreciate this phenomenon in connection with age-related changes of glucose tolerance led to probable overestimation of the incidence of diabetes in the adult population and to the frequent initiation of unnecessary therapeutic measures. At the present time, age-related data from normal subjects are beginning to appear earlier and with greater regularity in the evolution of new testing procedures, but the issue of age-based standards from normal subjects for the clinical interpretation of endocrine tests will continue to arise as new tests are developed.

It should be emphasized that useful physiologic and biochemical clinical tests may fail completely to reveal significant age-related events. An unaltered concentration of a hormone in blood, for example, does not mean that age has necessarily been unaccompanied by physiologic changes. The blood level of a hormone is the balance of a number of processes, each of which can be age-influenced. The concentration in blood of a hormone with a relatively constant rate of production results not only from the rate of secretion but also from the concentration in plasma of specific carrier binding proteins, which in turn determine the "free" or metabolically active hormone in plasma and the rate of metabolic destruction or disposal of the hormone, an event which need bear no direct relation to its biologic action. For those hormones whose secretion is episodic or cyclic, the amplitude of the secretory cycles and their frequency are additional age-related variables bearing on the integrated hormonal effect. In addition, concentration in blood is frequently determined by feedback control mechanisms, often in the hypothalamus, the sensitivity of which may be affected by age. Beyond consideration of blood hormone concentration, however, age affects the sensitivity of target tissue responsiveness through effects on hormone receptors, intracellular binding proteins, and other steps related to the expression of hormonal effects. Examples of these age-related phenomena will be pointed out, insofar as they are known, in the discussions of specific hormones, but it should be obvious already that the determination of plasma hormone concentration at a given moment or even of the secretion rate of a hormone may give a very incomplete picture of age-related events.

Our attempts to understand endocrine-aging interrelationships in man are, of course, dependent on animal model systems, but the use of animal models is complicated by the fact that it is frequently inappropriate to extrapolate observations made in animals to the situation in man. There are so many qualitative and quantitative differences in the endocrinology of experimental animals and that of the human that such extrapolations, although frequently and sweepingly made, are dangerously deceptive, especially so in connection with age-related events. In our discussion we shall attempt to point out where major differences occur between animals and man and shall mention some occurrences which so far have no counterpart in man, but our major emphasis shall be on what is known about the effects of aging on endocrine gland activity and the metabolism of hormones in the human. A number of reviews are available which cover general aspects of the biology of aging and the endocrine system, including much experimental work dealing with hormonal effects on the processes of growth, development, and alteration of life span (Bellamy, Comfort, Gusseck), as well as experimental work dealing with age-related autoimmune phenomena and their relationships to the endocrines (Blumenthal).

ANTERIOR PITUITARY: HORMONE CONTENT AND MORPHOLOGY

A review of the many reports dealing with the weight, histologic appearance, and tropic hormone content of the anterior pituitary during growth and senescence in man and animals can be found elsewhere (Verzár). Only a summary will be given here. The human data are extremely difficult to interpret, because the gland is of necessity obtained mainly at autopsy, at which time it has usually suffered the effects of one or more disease states, a problem which has been best described in relation to thyroid stimulating hormone (TSH) (Bakke et al.). With all reservations in mind, it appears that in advanced age the size of the human pituitary decreases not more than 20 per cent. It is not certain whether there is a decrease in ACTH and growth hormone (GH) content in old age (Verzár), but there appears to be no gross decrease in GH (Gershberg). Thyrotropin (TSH) content seems not to be altered (Bakke et al.). There is a considerable increase in follicle stimulating hormone (FSH) in the pituitary of the postmenopausal female, which is in keeping with the increased secretion of FSH that occurs as the result of failure of ovarian estrogen secretion at menopause. Comparative data from elderly males are few and inconclusive but show no gross increases such as are seen in the female.

Functionally or physiologically it matters little whether the amount of a pituitary hormone changes with age. The important considerations relate to the release of the hormone in response to appropriate stimuli, which in turn relates to such parameters as age-determined changes in releasing factor secretion, pituitary sensitivity to the releasing factors, and hypothalamic threshold to feedback inhibition, to mention a few. In several instances, limited data that indicate age-related changes are available and are discussed below.

RELEASING HORMONES: HYPOTHALAMUS

Information on the hypothalamic regulatory hormones is rapidly accumulating, and the subject has been recently reviewed (Schally et al.). Although there are as yet only a few reports, age has already been shown to affect the physiology of these hormones both during postnatal development and in senescence. Responsiveness of the rat pituitary to luteinizing hormone releasing hormone (LHRH) reaches a peak during the first weeks of life and then falls off as the animal reaches maturity (Debeljuk et al.). A more extreme change of pituitary sensitivity to a releasing hormone is seen in the senescent rat, the pituitary of which responds only minimally to hypothalamic extracts which have potent GH releasing activity in young animals (Pecile et al.). Moreover, GHRH appears to be absent from the hypothalamus of the senescent rat. The latter observations may have their counterpart in man and, if so, could form the basis of the decreased growth hormone responses seen in elderly persons after such stimuli as hypoglycemia and arginine infusion. The impaired response of the pituitary of elderly men to thyrotropin releasing hormone (TRH) should also be recalled in this connection (see TSH and TRH).

It has been suggested that the age changes observed in human plasma GH result from a raising of the threshold to feedback inhibition of GH secretion. Other age-related changes of hypothalamic sensitivity have also been proposed (Dilman). These observations as applied to man are open to criticism on numerous grounds, and at this time the conclusions derived from them can only be considered as speculative. Nonetheless, there is some evidence that human hypothalamic reactivity is altered during senescence (see Sympathetic Nervous System: Catecholamines). Moreover, recent studies in the rat indicate an extremely complex pattern of age-related alterations of hypothalamic function. Evidence has been presented, on the one hand, for increased sensitivity during senescence to direct stimulation by catecholamines and acetylcholine and, on the other, for decreased responses of the hypothalamico-neurohypophyseal system when complex neural pathways are involved (Frolkis and Bezrukov, 1972).

GROWTH HORMONE (GH)

Regardless of age, overnight fasting at rest results in basal plasma GH levels which are low or not detectable by ordinary immunoassay techniques. Even in old people, however, mean basal levels of growth hormone are higher in females than in males, as is the case in young people. Following stimulation of GH secretion by insulin-induced hypoglycemia, plasma GH levels rise in young and old alike. The mean increase in elderly men and women is considerably diminished, however (Laron et al.). Among the elderly, 20 per cent have such grossly decreased responses that, were they younger subjects, a diagnosis of inadequate GH reserve or GH deficiency would be made. The available data suggest that such diminished responses are seen only in persons over age 65. Further evidence for age-related impairment of GH release has been reported. The surges of GH secretion which have been regularly observed during deep sleep in younger adults were entirely absent in a significant proportion of older persons studied (Carlson et al.). Moreover, GH release in response to stimulation by arginine is diminished in the elderly (Dudl and Ensinck). With regard to growth hormone effects in old age, the limited evidence available indicates that certain metabolic responses are blunted in elderly subjects (Root and Oski).

THYROTROPIN (TSH) AND THYROTROPIN RELEASING HORMONE (TRH)

Although plasma TSH concentration does not change with age, a striking decrease has recently been demonstrated in the responsiveness of the pituitary of elderly subjects to stimulation by exogenous TRH. Elderly subjects (60–80 years) show a maximal mean increment of plasma TSH following TRH infusion which is only about 40 per cent of that of young adults (Snyder and Utiger). Since the amount of TSH in the pituitary does not appear to decrease with age, the decreased responsiveness to TRH probably represents an age-related impairment of the mechanism of TSH release. This age effect in man recalls the impaired responsiveness of the pituitary of aged rats to GHRH (see Hypothalamus). The two sets of observations taken together raise the issue of whether impaired responsiveness of the pituitary to hypothalamic releasing hormones may be a widespread phenomenon.

POSTERIOR PITUITARY: ANTIDIURETIC HORMONE (ADH)

Conclusions drawn from a number of extensive studies are that, in the aged rat, neurohypophyseal function and ADH secretion are impaired, and that the senescent animal has a modified form of diabetes insipidus (Friedman et al.; see also Dunihue, Frolkis, 1972). With administration of ADH, a variety of age-related alterations (impaired ability to concentrate urine, increased size of organs, increased muscle sodium, impaired muscle function) are all reversed toward those of the young animal, and life span has been claimed to have been extended. These results have been extrapolated from the rat to account for certain age-related changes in man, but the extrapolation is not justified. The aged human does not exhibit evidence of diabetes insipidus. It is true that the maximum achievable urine osmolality following water deprivation decreases with increasing age, but the defect is apparently a renal one, since the ability of the kidney to respond to exogenous ADH is also decreased. The decrease of maximum urine concentrating ability is in turn related to the decreased glomerular filtration rate that occurs with age rather than to decreased sensitivity to ADH (Lindeman et al.).

A disturbance of the mechanism for ADH release has been postulated to account for a syndrome of inappropriate ADH activity in certain elderly diabetics treated with chlorpropamide (Diabinese) (Weissman et al.). Since this drug appears to potentiate ADH rather than to cause its release, it has been theorized that the syndrome reflects an inability of certain individuals to reduce their output of ADH in response to the stimulus of volume expansion and hypo-osmolality. To date the phenomenon has been seen only in elderly diabetics, suggesting an age-related alteration of hypothalamic-posterior pituitary regulation of ADH secretion. It should be noted in this connection that in man two important ADH-secreting sites, the supraoptic and paraventricular nuclei, both show striking age-specific cytologic changes without evidence of cell destruction (Buttlar-Brentano, Andrew).

THYROID

Attention was drawn many years ago to the influence of age on the thyroid by observations that basal metabolic rate (BMR) decreases with increasing age. Since thyroid hormone (TH) is a major determinant of metabolic rate, a direct relationship between age, TH secretion, and the BMR was suspected. It is now clear that, while BMR and TH secretion rate decrease with age, the two events are not causally related. The decrease of BMR is best explained by an age-related decrease

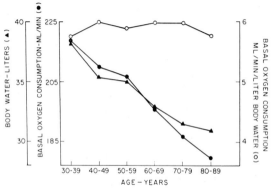

Figure 27–1. Basal oxygen consumption (BMR) and age in male subjects. Note decrease of oxygen consumption with age (●—●). Metabolic mass, in this study estimated from total body water (▲—▲), also decreases with age. Oxygen consumption calculated per unit metabolic mass (○—○), however, shows no such decrease. Thus the age-related decrease of BMR is considered to be a function of altered body composition with age rather than a result of diminished thyroid function. Similar age-related decreases of metabolic mass (lean tissue, cell mass) can also be shown with measurements of intracellular water or of body potassium. All of these estimates (see also Fig. 27–2) decrease with age. (From Gregerman, R. I., In *Endocrines and Aging.* Chapter 8. Gitman, L. (ed.), Springfield, Illinois, Charles C Thomas, 1967.)

of metabolic mass; oxygen consumption per unit of metabolic mass does not decrease with age (Fig. 27–1). The decrease of TH secretion, on the other hand, is currently viewed as a homeostatic adjustment to slowed metabolic disposal of thyroid hormone. These considerations have been reviewed in greater detail elsewhere, together with functional changes related to the neonatal period and age-related data from animal studies (Gregerman, 1971).

Thyroid Anatomy

With advancing age, the thyroid undergoes fibrosis, cellular infiltrations, and follicular alterations. Microscopic and clinically palpable nodularity also increase with age. There is controversy about whether the overall size of the gland is increased or decreased, but from a functional point of view, the significance of these anatomic changes is minimal, since the thyroid of even very elderly persons appears to function adequately and maintains its reserve capacity.

Thyroid Function Studies

Radioiodide Uptake

While the technical and conceptual limitations of the use of conventional thyroid "function tests" to assess age-related physiologic changes have been reviewed elsewhere (Gregerman, 1971), the effect of age on the results of the more commonly used tests deserves some mention here. Decreases of radioiodide uptake have been described in el-

derly subjects, but the magnitude of such changes is small and the statistical variance so large that it serves no useful purpose to establish age-related normal clinical ranges. A partial explanation for the small magnitude of the age-related decrease of uptake is the decrease of renal function in the elderly, which results in alteration of handling of tracer iodide by the thyroid.

Plasma Thyroid Hormones and Binding Protein Concentrations

In normal healthy elderly adults, plasma thyroxine (T_4), as measured by protein-bound iodine (PBI) or directly as T_4, shows no change with age; the free or non–protein-bound T_4 also shows no change. Triiodothyronine (T_3) concentration decreases by 25–40 per cent in subjects over the age of 50–60 years (Snyder and Utiger, Brunelle and Bohuon). Thyroxine-binding globulin (TBG) rises slightly and thyroxine-binding prealbumin (TBPA) falls, but the latter is a carrier of relatively minor importance. Acute and chronic illnesses can affect the plasma T_4, the concentration of both TBG and TBPA, and the free T_4 (Lutz et al.). Since such illnesses are, of course, frequent in the elderly, changes of these parameters are not attributable to age alone (Jefferys et al.).

Thyroxine Disposal and Secretion Rate

A number of studies in man have shown a progressive decrease of the rate of thyroxine (T_4) disposal with advancing age (Gregerman et al., Gregerman, 1971). The magnitude of the change is a loss of about 50 per cent over the entire adult age span. This is attributed largely to a progressive slowing of the rate of cellular degradation of the hormone. Since the total plasma T_4 is unchanged, and since in the steady state disposal equals secretion, the decrease in the secretion rate of the thyroid is viewed as being homeostatic.

Functional State of the Thyroid

For several reasons, the decrease with age of thyroidal secretion of T_4 should not be viewed as gland "failure." First, the thyroid of the elderly person has good reserve, as judged by an unaltered response to stimulation by exogenous TSH. Second, the plasma T_4 does not fall as is the case when decreased output of hormone is a primary event. Third, the mechanism for activating hormone secretion at a greatly accelerated rate is maintained even in old age, as evidenced by gross acceleration of T_4 turnover during infectious illness in both old and young subjects (Gregerman, 1967). Finally, plasma TSH, a sensitive indicator of primary hypothyroidism, is not elevated in elderly individuals and shows an age-related decreased response to TRH stimulation rather than the increase that is seen in hypothyroidism (Snyder and Utiger).

T_4 Versus T_3: Physiologic Considerations

Recent studies have somewhat obscured this simple view of the functional state of the thyroid in old age. The plasma concentration of T_3, unlike that of T_4, does decrease in elderly individuals. Moreover, at the present time, it is not clear whether T_4 is merely a prohormone or not, or to what extent it contributes directly to metabolic effects relative to T_3. Thus the exact significance of the age-related decrease of plasma T_3 remains to be determined. If peripheral metabolic effects are exerted primarily by T_3, then in the elderly there is a decrease of peripherally effective hormone of up to 40 per cent. This implies that the negative-feedback control of TSH release is grossly affected at advanced age, since plasma TSH does not increase. Decreased plasma T_3 may be due to an age-related change of peripheral T_4 metabolism as well, since much of the circulating T_3 appears to originate from circulating T_4 rather than from thyroidal secretion.

Mechanism of Altered Metabolic Rate of T_4 and T_3

The mechanism of the age-related slowing of T_4 disposal is not established, but it may relate in part to altered physical activity, since strenuous exercise appears to accelerate the rate of T_4 metabolism in both animals and man. In the available studies of the relationship of age to T_4 disposal rate, the possible importance of exercise was not appreciated and was not controlled. It remains to be shown, however, whether exercise is an important determinant of T_4 disposal rate within the range of normal activities or whether decreased activity such as that seen in the elderly results in decreased disposal rate. The slowed disposal of T_4 with age does provide an explanation for the clinical impression that elderly hypothyroid subjects appear to require less replacement hormone than do young persons to maintain a euthyroid status. These observations are also in keeping with increased sensitivity of the senescent rat to T_4 (Grad).

In normal man, the rate of metabolism of T_4 and T_3 in the liver is undoubtedly the major determinant of overall TH disposal rate. In animals, disposal is clearly linked to the metabolic pathway for certain drugs and other chemical agents (Oppenheimer et al.) and can be considered as an adaptive mechanism; the same is probably true in the human. The age-related slowing of T_4 disposal in normal man and the acceleration of T_4 and T_3 disposal during certain acute illnesses, even in the elderly, would appear to be best explained at present in terms of an alteration in this adaptive regulatory mechanism which is clearly influenced by a variety of physiologic and pathophysiologic factors.

ADRENALS

Age-related changes in adrenal structure and function are highly species-specific. Unique and perhaps the most dramatic are the massive hypertrophy and hyperactivity of the adrenal of the spawning (senescent) Pacific salmon. In other species, however, involutional changes are the rule. Microscopically, one sees accumulation of pigment, connective tissue proliferation, and loss of steroid-containing lipid. Vascular dilation and small hemorrhages are common. Cytologically, the most striking and perhaps functionally most important alteration is the fragmentation and gross alteration of the mitochondrial structure (Bourne). Size changes in the adrenal may also be seen. In the fowl, for example, the adrenals show an overall decrease in size with age, while in the rat, the zona glomerulosa is selectively and grossly atrophied, with the remainder of the gland relatively little affected. Loss of the zona glomerulosa correlates with decreased juxtaglomerular cell granularity in the kidney and with diminished neurosecretory material in the neurohypophysis. These changes are interpreted as showing diminished activity of the renin-angiotensin-aldosterone system in the aging rat (Dunihue). Alterations of neurohypophyseal function in the rat are discussed elsewhere (see Antidiuretic Hormone).

The human adrenal shows no major anatomic changes, such as those of decreased gland size or loss of zona glomerulosa, but the microscopic alterations described above are seen, and cortical nodule formation is frequent. Moreover, a variety of age-related alterations of adrenal secretory activity have been extensively studied and will be discussed below.

Glucocorticoids

For the most important glucocorticoid of man, cortisol, the age-related alterations resemble those of T_4. Plasma cortisol concentration remains unaltered, even at very advanced age, but secretion rate decreases about 30 per cent over the entire adult age span. This is a consequence of slowed metabolic disposal and undoubtedly the result of an age-related alteration of the enzymatic activities involved in hepatic steroid metabolism (West et al., Gherondache et al., Romanoff et al.). The reduced secretion rate is closely paralleled by a corresponding age-related decrease of urinary excretion of the 17-hydroxy steroid metabolites of cortisol. In several species other than man (cattle, goat, rat) (Riegle and Nellor, Riegle et al., Hess and Riegle), plasma glucocorticoid concentrations do not decrease with advancing age.

Many investigators have attributed significance to the observation that the excretion of glucocorticoid metabolites and the secretion rate of cortisol, when expressed per unit of creatinine excretion, do not decrease with age (Pincus, Gherondache et al.). The observation is true, but the physiologic significance of this calculation is nil, since it is total muscle mass that determines creatinine excretion, while the liver, not muscle, is the major site of adrenal steroid metabolism (Moncloa et al.). Thus there is no good basis for directly relating steroid production to muscle mass or to creatinine excretion. To express glucocorticoid excretion or secretion in terms of any other unrelated measurement that shows an age-correlated decrease would also "abolish" or "correct" the age-related glucocorticoid change and would be equally meaningless.

Adrenal Androgens

The progressive decrease in men and women of the urinary excretion of 17-ketosteroids with age to mean levels in the elderly that are about one-half those in young adults is a reflection of the decreasing production of the so-called adrenal androgens, secreted chiefly as the sulfate conjugates of dehydroepiandrosterone (DHA) and androsterone. The plasma levels of these specific steroids are closely age-related (Vihko) and in some individuals practically disappear from the plasma at advanced age (Migeon et al.). Decrease of urinary excretion of DHA is considerably greater than that of total 17-ketosteroids (Gherondache et al.).

The biologic significance of these adrenal secretory products is not known. In the past, attempts have been made to attribute "anabolic" function to the adrenal androgens and to relate them to a "balance" with "catabolic" glucocorticoids and in turn to age-related phenomena, such as osteoporosis and even neoplasia; to date, however, no definite concepts have been established. Unfortunately, the adrenal androgens have not received the study they deserve. Certainly, roles for these steroids in such functions as the maintenance of muscle or of bone have not been excluded (Pincus). In terms of quantities produced, the adrenal androgens equal or even exceed those of all the other adrenal steroids combined. It would be most remarkable, considering merely the amounts secreted, if they were proved to be devoid of physiologic effects, but until such time as a functional role is demonstrated, we shall remain ignorant of the significance of one of the most striking age-related alterations of hormone secretion.

Aldosterone

Age-related measurements of plasma aldosterone in man have not yet been reported, but isotopic studies have indicated a decreased metabolic clearance rate, a decreased secretory rate, and a decreased calculated plasma concentration in elderly subjects to levels about one-half those in young adults (Flood et al.). The urinary excretion of aldosterone also decreases progressively with age. When sodium intake is unrestricted, the decrease is approximately 50 per cent. Although older persons do increase aldosterone excretion with sodium restriction, those over age 60 show increases which are only 30–40 per cent of those seen in young adults (Crane and Harris). In terms of control mechanisms for aldosterone, the secretion of renin shows an age-related decrease which parallels that of aldosterone. In one-third of females over age 70, however, plasma renin levels not only are low but also fail to show the characteristic rise which is usually seen in young subjects during sodium restriction or postural change. These striking age-related alterations of aldosterone and renin secretion have obvious importance for interpreting data from hypertensive populations and, in this context, stress the need for age-related standards.

ACTH and Tests of Adrenocortical Reserve

Adrenal Responses to ACTH

The effect of age on the response of the human adrenal to stimulation by ACTH is controversial. In terms of glucocorticoids, several investigators have reported decreased urinary 17-hydroxysteroid excretion by elderly subjects after ACTH administration, while others have observed no effect of age on urinary excretion or on plasma glucocorticoid response (Gherondache et al., Moncloa et al.). In regard to the excretion of adrenal androgens after ACTH administration, there is also some disagreement, but definitely decreased responses have been reported (Moncloa et al.). In some species (cow, goat), a striking age effect is seen. Despite the fact that basal levels of plasma corticosteroids are unchanged with age, the old animals show little or no response to ACTH stimulation as measured by plasma concentration of cortisol and corticosterone (Riegle and Nellor, Riegle et al.). Response to ACTH appears to be grossly intact in the senescent rat, although the steroid output of the old animals is somewhat less after stimulation (Hess and Riegle). Recent studies have indicated that a longer time is required for initiation of ACTH action in the old animals (Rotenberg and Adelman).

Secretion of dehydroepiandrosterone (DHA) in elderly people has been studied by measurements of plasma DHA following ACTH administration. Basal DHA concentrations were very much lower in the elderly than in the young (see Adrenal Androgens). Although plasma levels increased after ACTH in both groups, responses in the elderly ranged from minimal to delayed, and in no instance did they approach the levels seen in younger subjects (Yamaji and Ibayashi). This and other observations clearly indicate that age has a greater effect on adrenal androgen production than on the glucocorticoids, and thus age has a highly selective effect on specific pathways of synthesis in the adrenal. The mechanism of this age effect is not known, but recent evidence suggests that adrenal androgen production is regulated by gonadal hormones (Barmach de Niepomniszsze et al.). Since both estrogen and testosterone secretion decrease with age (see Gonads), at least part of the age-related decrease of adrenal androgen secretion may be a consequence of altered gonadal function during aging.

ACTH Reserve: Metyrapone Test

A simple interpretation of the effect of age on the most commonly used test of ACTH reserve is not possible. When metyrapone is given orally, the response, as measured by the excretion of 17-ketogenic steroids, of some elderly subjects is diminished. However, when large doses of the inhibitor are given intravenously and the response is measured in terms of increased plasma compound S (deoxycortisol), the values in the elderly are identical to those in young persons (Jensen and Blichert-Toft). The explanation for this discrepancy could lie in either the dosage or route of administration of the drug or both, but it is more likely that it is related to the measured end point of the response. In view of the slowed rate of steroid disposal in the elderly, it could be expected that a moderately diminished adrenal response, due either to impaired ACTH release or diminished adrenal responsiveness, would be masked when plasma steroid level rather than urine excretion is used as the index of the response. Thus the only available evidence fails to indicate any gross impairment in the elderly of the negative feedback mechanism for the release of ACTH, but some degree of impairment is not excluded.

PANCREATIC HORMONES

Insulin

The gradual decline of glucose tolerance with age has been well documented (Ch. 9) and the mechanisms extensively investigated. Some of the earlier attempts to explain the effect of age on glucose utilization in terms of impaired insulin secretion, as indicated by plasma insulin concentration, supported such an explanation, but other studies were contradictory (Andres, Chlouverakis et al., Crockford et al., Danowski et al., Hales et al., Joffe et al., O'Sullivan et al.). Although the reasons for them are not clear, the discrepant results are probably due partly to the characteristics of the populations sampled. The problem of subject selection is complicated by the increased prevalence in older subjects of at least one factor, adiposity, known to affect glucose tolerance. Since adiposity is known to result in increased insulin secretion, obese subjects can simply be excluded from study. However, age is also associated with the development of relative adiposity. Age-related changes in body composition, as characterized by loss of muscle and increase of fat (Fryer; Novak), are shown (Fig. 27–2). Probably it is because of these factors that insulin levels following glucose loading were unchanged or even elevated with age, although other data seemed clearly to indicate a

BODY COMPOSITION AND AGE

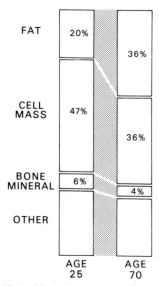

Figure 27–2. Idealized representation of the age-related change of body composition of male subjects. (Young females [age 25] have nearly twice as much body fat as do males but show a smaller increase of fat [and loss of cell mass] with age than do males.) Since adiposity (increased total body fat) has a major effect on glucose tolerance and insulin secretion (see text), this age-related change of body composition (relative adiposity) may account for some of the effect of age on glucose and insulin metabolism.

decrease. Most reports have indicated that basal insulin levels are not affected by age, and in only one study was basal insulin elevated. Further complicating the interpretation of plasma insulin changes during glucose tolerance studies is the question of what constitutes an appropriate plasma insulin level for a given level of blood glucose.

Taking the latter factor into account, Andres, Tobin, and their collaborators have reported experiments in non-obese elderly male subjects in whom blood sugar was controlled to the same elevated level in young and old (Andres; Sherwin et al.). Both the early and late phases of insulin secretion were clearly less in the old subjects than in the young. Since early insulin release is an important determinant of glucose tolerance (Ch. 9), it is as yet impossible to distinguish by this measurement alone the age-related decrease of glucose tolerance from the appearance in the elderly of glucose intolerance resulting from a genetic diabetic trait.

The influence of age on other parameters of insulin physiology has also been recently studied. Neither the sensitivity of peripheral tissues to insulin, the metabolic clearance rate of the hormone, nor the basal delivery (secretory) rate is affected by age (Sherwin et al.). In regard to the nature of the immunologically measured insulin of plasma, in older subjects following glucose administration a larger portion of immunologically reactive hormone is actually proinsulin (Duckworth and Kitabchi). Since proinsulin is metabolically less effective than insulin, this age-related alteration of secretory pattern contributes to an explanation of the observed decline of glucose tolerance. Heretofore reported plasma insulin values, determined by immunoassay, have been based on the assumption that all of the measured material is metabolically active, when in fact in older subjects, less than the total amount of the hormone is effective.

Glucagon

Preliminary observations indicate that neither basal levels of plasma glucagon (immunoassay) nor the glucagon response to arginine stimulation is impaired in older individuals. It is unlikely, therefore, that altered glucagon secretion contributes to the decline of glucose tolerance with age. It is of interest in this connection, that, in contrast to glucagon, plasma insulin response to arginine stimulation, like that to glucose, is reduced in elderly people (Dudl and Ensinck).

GONADS

Testosterone

Although wide individual variation exists, sexual interest, drive, and vigor in the adult male declines with advancing age. This event cannot, however, be attributed to decreasing testosterone secretion in persons below age 50, although it may be true of some older individuals (see below). Sexual behavior in both elderly men and women appears to be closely related to habits formed during earlier adult life (Pfeiffer and Davis), and, on the basis of present knowledge, age-changes in sexual function would probably be better related to this fact than to changes of endocrine function. No studies are as yet available, however, that relate sexual functioning, age, and testosterone levels in specific individuals.

The first reports of the quantitation of plasma testosterone in males suggested that no decrease of hormone occurred, even in the very elderly. More recent studies provide extensive data that appear to account for the earlier failure to appreciate an age change. From adolescence to early adulthood, plasma testosterone increases greatly, but thereafter no decrease is seen until beyond age 50, after which mean values decrease considerably. The mean for subjects at age 80–90 is about 40 per cent of that in the group under age 50. The variability is very great, however. Some subjects in their 80's or even 90's have levels that exceed those in normal young men in their 20's, while in other elderly men the values are as low as those found in normal females (Vermeulen et al., 1972). This extreme variation, together with the relatively small numbers of subjects, especially those of very advanced age, appears to account for failure of the first reports to appreciate the decrease with age of plasma testosterone.

An additional change with age of plasma testosterone exists beyond the decrease of total hormone concentration. Some 98 per cent of the testosterone in plasma is normally associated with a specific testosterone-binding globulin. With advancing age, the concentration of the binding globulin increases, with the consequence that there is an increase of that fraction of hormone that is bound to protein. The two events are additive and the concentration of free or physiologically active hormone thus decreases by about one-third more than does the total testosterone of plasma (Vermeulen et al., 1971; 1972).

Kinetic studies have directly demonstrated that decreased plasma testosterone is due to a decreased rate of hormone production. An age-related decrease of the amount and alteration of the pattern of excretion of testosterone metabolites (androstanediols) has also been seen (Vermeulen et al., 1972). Although plasma testosterone is much lower in females than in males, the available data indicate that no decrease of testosterone occurs during senescence in the female.

Estrogens and Progesterone

As an invariable accompaniment to aging in the human female, diminished estrogen production is to be contrasted to the far less predictable decrease of testosterone in the male. Decreased estrogen excretion is known to occur after age forty at a time close to the menopause, although the available data are cross-sectional rather than longitudinal and do not establish the exact time sequence or the rate of decrease in specific individuals (Pincus et al.). Mean values for estrogen excretion decline further between ages 50 and 60, but thereafter no additional change is evident. In the elderly female, the ovary ceases completely to secrete either estradiol or estrone. Estradiol blood levels decline by over 90 per cent and those of estrone by about 70 per cent (Longcope). Nonetheless, the urinary excretion of biologically active estrogen is still about one-fifth of that before the menopause. What estrogen remains is produced from the peripheral conversion of steroid precursors, and, in the case of estrone, continued production originates from androstenedione of adrenal origin.

Recent kinetic studies have indicated that metabolic clearance rates of both estradiol and estrone decrease by about 25 per cent, a change similar in magnitude to that for testosterone and aldosterone. The recent estimates of decreased production rates of estradiol and estrone are in good agreement with older information obtained from bioassays of urinary estrogens (Pincus et al.).

Estrogen production in the male, although always much less than in the female, decreases progressively with age, about 30 per cent less total estrogen being excreted at age 70 as compared with that at age 30. However, the biologically more active hormones, estradiol and estrone, together decrease by over 50 per cent, while estriol is relatively unchanged until late in life, when it decreases slightly by about 15 per cent (Pincus). Estrogen in the male arises from both the adrenals and the testes, but the relative contribution of each source to the age-related decrease of estrogen production is not established. The male also produces significant quantities of progesterone, again with both the adrenals and the testes contributing. The production rate in elderly males falls to 40 per cent of that in young subjects. Excretion of urinary pregnanediol, the major metabolite of progesterone, decreases at advanced age to 25 per cent of that seen in young adults (Gherondache et al.).

PARATHYROID HORMONE (PTH)– ESTROGEN INTERRELATIONSHIPS

The progressive decrease of bone density that accompanies aging in both men and women is one of the almost invariable accompaniments of senescence. A clear distinction between this process and that of "osteoporosis" is not possible (Newton-John and Morgan), but osteoporosis is said to be present when the demineralization is severe and symptomatic and there are fractures, or when the age at onset is unusually early. Diminished gonadal hormone secretion in senescence, and especially postmenopausal loss of the protective effect of estrogen in preventing the action of PTH on bone, was postulated many years ago as a factor in the pathogenesis of this process. Experimentally, estrogen appears to decrease the sensitivity of bone to PTH (Orimo et al.). Moreover, postmenopausal evidences of increased bone resorption, slightly elevated levels of serum calcium, and increased calcium excretion are significantly diminished by treatment with physiologic amounts of estrogen (Gallagher and Nordin, Riggs et al.).

There is recent preliminary evidence that PTH levels in blood decrease slightly with age. In overtly osteoporotic subjects, however, the normal age decrement of PTH is not seen, and blood levels are significantly higher than in normal subjects of corresponding age (Fujita et al.). Thus both increased sensitivity to PTH and increased blood levels may contribute to the bone resorption in osteoporosis. Interestingly, plasma PTH rises after estrogen administration, apparently secondary to a small decrease of plasma calcium (Riggs et al.).

While the exact role of PTH and its interrelationship with estrogen remains to be determined, two lines of evidence strongly indicate that the pathogenesis of osteoporosis involves more than a loss of estrogen effect. In the first place, data exist which show that demineralization begins years before the menopause, the time when estrogen secretion presumably first diminishes. Secondly, with estrogen replacement given at menopause, bone density when measured after 5–10 years was clearly greater than when replacement was not given (Davis et al.). Thereafter, the difference between those receiving estrogen and those without became progressively less, although a significant difference was still seen after 10–15 years of therapy. By the end of 15–20 years, a significant difference was no longer demonstrable. While this study seems clearly to establish a delay in demineralization lasting at least 10–15 years, even those given estrogen show progressive demineralization.

Recent studies of estrogen treatment of patients with overt osteoporosis have shown that, while bone resorption decreased after both short-term and, to a lesser extent, long-term treatment, bone formation, initially unaffected, ultimately decreased (Riggs et al.). Thus, over the longer period (2–3 years), the beneficial effect of estrogen was partially negated. Taken together, the available data indicate that estrogen therapy is worthwhile for arresting or slowing the progressive bone loss of osteoporosis, but the age-related demineralization process clearly involves other contributing factors. It is of interest to note here, in connection with the progressive loss of adrenal androgens with age (see Adrenal Androgens), that a synthetic anabolic steroid has short-term and long-term effects similar to those of estrogen (Riggs et al.).

Heightened sensitivity to PTH in the estrogen-lacking postmenopausal woman has been postulated to account for the high incidence of hyperparathyroidism at this age, the hypersecretion of PTH by previously undetected adenomas being thought to become apparent only after the restraining effect of estrogen is removed. Treatment with a physiologic amount of estrogen is, indeed, effective in some such cases, with a reduction of hypercalcemia and hypercalciuria and a beneficial effect on bone resorption (Gallagher and Nordin).

THYROCALCITONIN (TCT)

The effectiveness of TCT is greatly decreased during maturation in the rat. When one-year-old adult rats are compared with young ones, markedly diminished hypocalcemic and hypophosphatemic effects are seen, even with large doses of hormone (Hirsch and Munson). Data are not yet available for senescent rats (2 or more years old). The aged human does respond to exogenous TCT, although no comparison between the responses of old and young has been reported. Experiments with rats and sheep indicate that TCT secretion following the stimulus of hypercalcemia is decreased during maturation, but comparable measurements are not as yet available in the human.

Since TCT decreases bone resorption, its potential usefulness in the therapy of age-related demineralization and osteoporosis has been explored. Several preliminary studies have shown beneficial results, but the most recent data are not so encouraging, and truly long-term results are not yet at hand (Jowsey et al.).

SYMPATHETIC NERVOUS SYSTEM: CATECHOLAMINES

Urinary excretion of epinephrine, reflecting basal function of the adrenal medulla, does not change with advancing age in adult man, nor does the excretion of norepinephrine (Kärki). Nonetheless, elderly subjects differ from young in having diminished adrenal medullary and sympathetico-adrenal responses to certain pharmacologic and psychophysiologic stresses (insulin hypoglycemia, vasomotor conditioning). The response to hypoglycemia is mediated by the hypothalamus, and the effect of age could well be exerted here rather than in the adrenal. Reduced hypothalamic reactivity in the aged has, in fact, been inferred from impaired vascular responses to certain drugs (Cohen and Shmavonian) (see also Hypothalamus and Anti-diuretic Hormone).

Progress in this area has been limited by methodologic problems related to the difficulties of measuring catecholamines in plasma and the necessity of relying on urinary catecholamine excretion. The available observations, however, are in keeping with the clinical impression that elderly diabetics with insulin-induced hypoglycemia are less likely to show the obvious sympathetic symptoms seen in young diabetics, although autonomic dysfunction related to diabetes rather than to age may be responsible.

That alterations of other catecholamine-mediated events in the central nervous system will eventually become apparent is suggested by the recent finding of decreased levels of norepinephrine and increased monoamine oxidase in human brain with aging (Robinson et al.). In addition to the age-related changes of the complex sympathetic functions already described, however, considerable information suggests impaired tissue responsiveness to catecholamines. Examples of such changes include diminished arterial contractile response to norepinephrine in the senescent rat (Tuttle), and the decreased lipolytic effect of catecholamines during maturation and senescence in both rat and man (see Adenyl Cyclase).

HORMONE-MEDIATED ENZYME INDUCTION

Although the mechanisms of specific enzyme adaptation or induction are complex, hormonal stimuli trigger this phenomenon in many instances. Recent work in the rat has led to an emerging concept that aging results in a progressive increase in the time required for certain hormone-mediated adaptive enzyme responses. Examples to date of this age-related time lag include the inductions of hepatic glucokinase by glucose via insulin and of tyrosine aminotransferase by glucocorticoids via ACTH release (Adelman). In the former, diminished insulin release in response to glucose appears to be the mechanism, while in the latter response the aged rat adrenal requires increased time for the expression of ACTH action (Rotenberg and Adelman). Induction of the drug-metabolizing enzyme, NADPH–cytochrome c reductase, by phenobarbital also requires greater time in old animals, suggesting that delayed hormonal responses may be part of a more general age-related change. However, direct inductions of enzymes, such as hepatic tyrosine aminotransferase and tryptophan pyrrolase by cortisol (Gregerman, 1959; Adelman) and hepatic α-glycerophosphate dehydrogenase by thyroxine (Bulos et al.), are not impaired during senescence in the rat, so the time-lag phenomenon is certainly not universal. Nonetheless, some observations indicate that dose-response effects may be important in demon-strating an effect of age on the rate of enzyme induction (Frolkis, 1970) and emphasize the complexity of this area. No comparable data are as yet available for enzyme inductions in man.

ADENYL CYCLASE SYSTEM

Alterations of membrane structure and function have been thought by many to be of critical importance during aging. Although little definitive information regarding age-related changes of membrane function is available, some changes have been described in relation to adenyl cyclase (Ch. 16). In the rat, adenyl cyclase activity of heart, lung, liver, and skeletal muscle decreases during maturation. Similar decreases in the related enzyme, guanyl cyclase, as well as in the phosphodiesterases that metabolize both cyclic nucleotides have been reported (Williams and Thompson). Catecholamine-induced lipolysis, which decreases progressively with aging both in the rat (Jelínková et al.) and in man (Berger et al.), is a cAMP-mediated process. A decrease with age of cyclase activation in rat fat cells by catecholamines has been recently reported. In this instance, an age-related alteration of phosphodiesterase appears to augment the altered hormonal response, since phosphodiesterase activity increases as adenyl cyclase decreases (Forn et al.). Age-related loss of cyclase responsiveness is selective for specific hormones within a given tissue and varies from one tissue to another. During maturation in the rat, there is a greater decrease in activation of fat-cell adenyl cyclase by glucagon than by epinephrine or ACTH (Manganiello and Vaughan), while the loss of epinephrine responsiveness by hepatic adenyl cyclase is greater than that of glucagon (Bitensky et al.). These reports barely begin to describe this area, but they already clearly indicate that endocrine-related membrane function, i.e., the adenyl cyclase system, is involved in the aging process, and they provide an important clue to the explanation of age-related alterations of hormone sensitivity.

CONCLUSIONS

Aging affects many aspects of endocrine regulation but does not affect all the endocrine glands or all the different hormones secreted by the same gland to the same extent. Although our present knowledge in this area is limited, examples are known of age-related alterations of hormone secretion rates, patterns of secretion, and altered secretory responses to physiologic or pharmacologic stimulation (Fig. 27–3). Diminished secretion is sometimes a primary phenomenon, but age-related decreases of the rate of metabolic disposal of some hormones also lead to decreased hormone secretion rates as secondary or homeostatic mechanisms. Age not only can affect the concentration of a specific plasma protein involved in hormone transport but also can influence the concentration of the free or metabolically active portion of that hormone in blood. Target-tissue sensitivity to hormonal effects

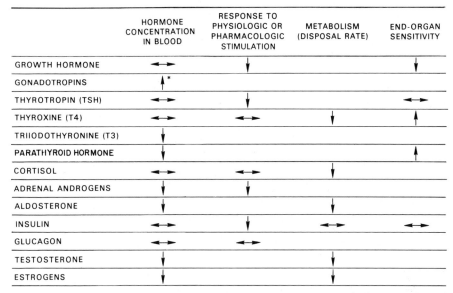

	HORMONE CONCENTRATION IN BLOOD	RESPONSE TO PHYSIOLOGIC OR PHARMACOLOGIC STIMULATION	METABOLISM (DISPOSAL RATE)	END-ORGAN SENSITIVITY
GROWTH HORMONE	⟷	↓		↓
GONADOTROPINS	↑ *			
THYROTROPIN (TSH)	⟷	↓		⟷
THYROXINE (T4)	⟷	⟷	↓	↑
TRIIODOTHYRONINE (T3)	↓			
PARATHYROID HORMONE	↓			↑
CORTISOL	⟷	⟷	↓	
ADRENAL ANDROGENS	↓	↓		
ALDOSTERONE	↓		↓	
INSULIN	⟷	↓	⟷	⟷
GLUCAGON	⟷	⟷		
TESTOSTERONE	↓		↓	
ESTROGENS	↓		↓	

Figure 27–3. Changes of plasma hormones during aging in man. Symbols: ↑, increase; ↓, decrease; ⟷, no change; *, postmenopausal. Blank spaces indicate that no data are presently available.

is sometimes age-related and in certain instances appears to involve hormone receptor mechanisms via alterations of adenyl cyclase responses. From a practical clinical viewpoint, aside from these physiologic considerations, age is a variable which must be considered in evaluating normal endocrine function by laboratory methods and in interpreting diagnostic tests.

REFERENCES

Adelman, R. C.: Age-dependent control of enzyme adaptation. *Adv. Gerontol. Res. 4*:1, 1972.

Andres, R.: Aging and diabetes. *Med. Clin. N. Amer. 55*:835, 1971.

Andrew, W.: Structural alterations with aging in the nervous system. *J. Chronic Dis. 3*:575, 1956.

Bakke, J. L., Lawrence, N., et al.: A correlative study of the content of thyroid stimulating hormone (TSH) and cell morphology of the human adenohypophysis. *Amer. J. Clin. Path. 41*:576, 1964.

Barmach de Niepomniszsze, A. J., Rosenfield, R. L., et al.: Adrenal androgen production: dependence on ACTH and gonadal function. Program 55th Annual Meeting Endocrine Society, A-194 (abstract 292), 1973.

Bellamy, D.: Hormonal effects in relation to ageing in mammals. *Symp. Soc. Exp. Biol. 21*:427, 1967.

Berger, M., Preiss, H., et al.: Altersabhängigkeit der Fettzellgrösse und der lipolytischen Aktivität im menschlichen Fettgewebe. *Gerontologia 17*:312, 1971.

Bitensky, M. W., Russell, V., et al.: Independent variation of glucagon and epinephrine responsive components of hepatic adenyl cyclase as a function of age, sex and steroid hormones. *Endocrinology 86*:154, 1970.

Blumenthal, H. T.: Age-related autoimmune phenomena of the endocrine glands, In *Endocrines and Aging.* Gitman, L. (ed.), Springfield, Illinois, Charles C Thomas, Publisher, 1967.

Bourne, G. H.: Aging changes in the endocrines, In *Endocrines and Aging.* Gitman, L. (ed.), Springfield, Illinois, Charles C Thomas, Publisher, 1967.

Brunelle, P., and Bohuon, C.: Baisse de la triiodothyronine serique avec l'age. *Clin. Chim. Acta 42*:201, 1972.

Bulos, B., Shukla, S., et al.: The rate of induction of the mitochondrial α-glycerophosphate dehydrogenase by thyroid hormone in adult and senescent rats. *Mech. Age. Dev. 1*:227, 1972.

Buttlar-Brentano, K. von: Zur Lebensgeschichte des nucleus basalis, tuberomammillaris, supraopticus und paraventricularis unter normalen und pathogenen Bedingungen. *J. Hirnforsch. 1*:337, 1954.

Carlson, H. E., Gillin, J. C., et al.: Absence of sleep-related growth hormone peaks in aged normal subjects and in acromegaly. *J. Clin. Endocr. 34*:1102, 1972.

Chlouverakis, C., Jarrett, R. J., et al.: Glucose tolerance, age, and circulating insulin. *Lancet 1*:806, 1967.

Cohen, S. I., and Shmavonian, B. M.: Catecholamines, vasomotor conditioning and aging, In *Endocrines and Aging.* Gitman, L. (ed.), Springfield, Illinois, Charles C Thomas, Publisher, 1967.

Comfort, A.: The prevention of ageing in cells. *Lancet 2*:806, 1967.

Crane, M. G., and Harris, J. J.: Effect of aging on renin activity and urinary aldosterone levels. Program 55th Annual Meeting Endocrine Society, A-74 (abstract 51), 1973.

Crockford, P. M., Harbeck, R. J., et al.: Influence of age on intravenous glucose tolerance and serum immunoreactive insulin. *Lancet 1*:465, 1966.

Danowski, T. S., Tsai, C. T., et al.: Serum growth hormone and insulin in females without glucose intolerance. *Metabolism 18*:811, 1969.

Davis, M. E., Lanzl, L. H., et al.: Estrogens and the aging process. The detection, prevention, and retardation of osteoporosis. *J.A.M.A. 196*:219, 1966.

Debeljuk, L., Arimura, A., et al.: Pituitary responsiveness to LH-releasing hormone in intact female rats of different ages. *Endocrinology 90*:1499, 1972.

Dilman, V. M.: Age-associated elevation of hypothalamic threshold to feedback control, and its role in development, aging, and disease. *Lancet 1*:1211, 1971.

Duckworth, W. C., and Kitabchi, A. E.: Direct measurement of plasma pro-insulin in normal and diabetic subjects. *Amer. J. Med. 53*:418, 1972.

Dudl, R. J., and Ensinck, J. W.: The role of insulin, glucagon, and growth hormone in carbohydrate homeostasis during aging. *Diabetes 21*:357, 1972.

Dunihue, F. W.: Reduced juxtaglomerular cell granularity, pituitary neurosecretory material, and width of the zona glomerulosa in aging rats. *Endocrinology 77*:948, 1965.

Flood, C., Gherondache, C., et al.: The metabolism and secretion of aldosterone in elderly subjects. *J. Clin. Invest. 46*:961, 1967.

Forn, J., Schonhofer, P. S., et al.: The effect of aging on adenyl cyclase and phosphodiesterase activity of isolated fat cells of the rat. *Biochim. Biophys. Acta 208*:304, 1970.

Friedman, S. M., Friedman, C. L., et al.: Adrenal-neurohypophyseal regulation of electrolytes and work performance. Age-related changes in the rat, In *Endocrines and Aging.* Gitman, L. (ed.), Springfield, Illinois, Charles C Thomas, Publisher, 1967.

Frolkis, V. V.: On the regulatory mechanism of molecular-genetic alterations during aging. *Exp. Gerontol. 5*:37, 1970.

Frolkis, V. V., and Bezrukov, V. V.: The hypothalamus in aging. *Exp. Gerontol. 7*:169, 1972.

Fryer, J. H.: Studies of body composition in men aged 60 and over, In *Biological Aspects of Aging*. Shock, N. W. (ed.), New York, Columbia University Press, 1962, p. 59.

Fujita, T., Orimo, H., et al.: Age and parathyroid hormone in plasma. Ninth International Congress Gerontology 3:317, 1972.

Gallagher, J. C., and Nordin, B. E. C.: Treatment with estrogens of primary hyperparathyroidism in postmenopausal women. *Lancet* 1:503, 1972.

Gershberg, H.: Growth hormone content and metabolic actions of human pituitary glands. *Endocrinology* 61:160, 1957.

Gherondache, C. N., Romanoff, L. P., et al.: Steroid hormones in aging men, In *Endocrines and Aging*. Gitman, L. (ed.), Springfield, Illinois, Charles C Thomas, Publisher, 1967.

Grad, B.: The metabolic responsiveness of young and old female rats to thyroxine. *J. Gerontol.* 24:5, 1969.

Gregerman, R. I.: Adaptive enzyme responses in the senescent rat: tryptophan peroxidase and tyrosine transaminase. *Amer. J. Physiol.* 197:63, 1959.

Gregerman, R. I.: The age-related alteration of thyroid hormone function and thyroid hormone metabolism in man, In *Endocrines and Aging*. Gitman, L. (ed.), Springfield, Illinois, Charles C Thomas, Publisher, 1967.

Gregerman, R. I.: Effects on thyroid hormone economy: Intrinsic physiologic variables and nonthyroidal illness; environmental effects, In *The Thyroid*. Werner, S. C., and Ingbar, S. H. (eds.), New York, Harper and Row, 1971.

Gregerman, R. I., and Solomon, N.: Acceleration of thyroxine and triiodothyronine turnover during infections and fever: Implications for the functional state of the thyroid during stress and in senescence. *J. Clin. Endocr.* 27:93, 1967.

Gregerman, R. I., Gaffney, G. W., et al.: Thyroxine turnover in euthyroid man with special reference to changes with age. *J. Clin. Invest.* 41:2065, 1962.

Gusseck, D. J.: Endocrine mechanisms and aging. *Adv. Gerontol. Res.* 4:105, 1972.

Hales, C. N., Greenwood, F. C., et al.: Blood-glucose, plasma-insulin and growth hormone concentrations of individuals with minor abnormalities of glucose tolerance. *Diabetologia* 4:73, 1968.

Hess, G. D., and Riegle, G. D.: Effects of chronic ACTH stimulation on adrenocortical function in young and aged rats. *Amer. J. Physiol.* 222:1458, 1972.

Hirsch, P. F., and Munson, P. L.: Thyrocalcitonin. *Physiol. Rev.* 49:548, 1969.

Jefferys, P. M., Hoffenberg, R., et al.: Thyroid-function tests in the elderly. *Lancet* 1:924, 1972.

Jelinková, M., Stuchlíková, E., et al.: Hormone-sensitive lipolytic activity of the aorta of different age groups of rats. *Exp. Gerontol.* 7:263, 1972.

Jensen, H. K., and Blichert-Toft, M.: Pituitary-adrenal function in old age evaluated by the intravenous metyrapone test. *Acta Endocr.* 64:431, 1970.

Joffe, B. I., Vinik, A. I., et al.: Insulin reserve in elderly subjects. *Lancet* 1:1292, 1969.

Jowsey, J., Riggs, B. L., et al.: Effects of prolonged administration of porcine calcitonin in postmenopausal osteoporosis. *J. Clin. Endocr.* 33:752, 1971.

Kärki, N. T.: The urinary excretion of noradrenaline and adrenaline in different age groups, its diurnal variation and the effect of muscular work on it. *Acta Physiol. Scand.* 39 (Suppl. 132):7, 1956.

Laron, Z., Doron, M., et al.: Plasma growth hormone in men and women over 70 years of age, In *Medicine and Sport*. Vol. 4. Brunner, D., and Jokl, E. (eds.), White Plains, New York, Phiebig, 1969.

Lindeman, R. D., Lee, T. D., Jr., et al.: Influence of age, renal disease, hypertension, diuretics, and calcium on the antidiuretic responses to suboptimal infusions of vasopressin. *J. Lab. Clin. Med.* 68:206, 1966.

Longcope, C.: Metabolic clearance and blood production rates of estrogens in postmenopausal women. *Amer. J. Obstet. Gynec.* 111:778, 1971.

Lutz, J. H., Gregerman, R. I., et al.: Thyroxine binding proteins, free thyroxine and thyroxine turnover interrelationships during acute infectious illness in man. *J. Clin. Endocr.* 35:230, 1972.

Manganiello, V., and Vaughan, M.: Selective loss of adipose cell responsiveness to glucagon with growth in the rat. *J. Lipid Res.* 13:12, 1972.

Migeon, C. J., Keiler, A. R., et al.: Dehydroepiandrosterone and androsterone levels in human plasma. *J. Clin. Endocr.* 17:1051, 1957.

Moncloa, F., Gómez, R., et al.: Response to corticotrophin and correlation between excretion of creatinine and urinary steroids and between the clearance of creatinine and urinary steroids in ageing. *Steroids* 1:437, 1963.

Newton-John, H. F., and Morgan, D. B.: Osteoporosis: Disease or senescence? *Lancet* 1:232, 1968.

Novak, L. P.: Aging, total body potassium, fat-free mass, and cell mass in males and females between ages 18 and 85 years. *J. Gerontol.* 27:438, 1972.

Oppenheimer, J. H., Bernstein, G., et al.: Increased thyroxine turnover and thyroidal function after stimulation of hepatocellular binding of thyroxine by phenobarbital. *J. Clin. Invest.* 47:1399, 1968.

Orimo, H., Fujita, T., et al.: Increased sensitivity of bone to parathyroid hormone in ovariectomized rats. *Endocrinology* 90:760, 1972.

O'Sullivan, J. B., Mahan, C. M., et al.: Effect of age on carbohydrate metabolism. *J. Clin. Endocr.* 33:619, 1971.

Pecile, A., Müller, E., et al.: Growth hormone-releasing activity of hypothalamic extracts at different ages. *Endocrinology* 77:241, 1965.

Pfeiffer, E., and Davis, G. C.: Determinants of sexual behavior in middle and old age. *J. Amer. Geriatr. Soc.* 20:151, 1972.

'incus, G.: Steroid hormones and aging in man, In *Growth in Living Systems*. Zarrow, M. X. (ed.), New York, Basic Books, 1961.

Pincus, G., Romanoff, L. P., et al.: The excretion of urinary steroids by men and women of various ages. *J. Gerontol.* 9:113, 1954.

Riegle, G. D., and Nellor, J. E.: Changes in adrenocortical function during aging in cattle. *J. Gerontol.* 22:83, 1967.

Riegle, G. D., Przekop, F., et al.: Changes in adrenocortical responsiveness to ACTH infusion in aging goats. *J. Gerontol.* 23:187, 1968.

Riggs, B. L., Jowsey, J., et al.: Short- and long-term effects of estrogen and synthetic anabolic hormone in postmenopausal osteoporosis. *J. Clin. Invest.* 51:1659, 1972.

Robinson, D. S., Nies, A., et al.: Ageing, monoamines, and monoamine-oxidase levels. *Lancet* 1:290, 1972.

Romanoff, L. P., Morris, C. W., et al.: The metabolism of cortisol-4-C^{14} in young and elderly men. *J. Clin. Endocr.* 21:1413, 1961.

Root, A. W., and Oski, F. A.: Effects of human growth hormone in elderly males. *J. Gerontol.* 24:97, 1969.

Rotenberg, S., and Adelman, R. C.: Age-dependent adaptive regulation of adrenocortical function. *Gerontologist* 12:34, 1972.

Schally, A. V., Arimura, A., et al.: Hypothalamic regulatory hormones. *Science* 179:341, 1973.

Sherwin, R. S., Insel, P. A., et al.: Computer modeling: An aid to understanding insulin action. *Diabetes* 21 (Suppl. 1):347, 1972.

Snyder, P. J., and Utiger, R. D.: Response to thyrotropin releasing hormone (TRH) in normal man. *J. Clin. Endocr.* 34:380, 1972.

Tobin, J. D., Andres, R., et al.: Sensitivity of beta cells to programmed hyperglycemia in man: effect of age. *Diabetes* 18:332, 1969.

Tuttle, R. S.: Age-related changes in the sensitivity of rat aortic strips to norepinephrine and associated chemical and structural alterations. *J. Gerontol.* 21:510, 1966.

Vermeulen, A., Stöica, T., et al.: The apparent free testosterone concentration, an index of androgenicity. *J. Clin. Endocr.* 33:759, 1971.

Vermeulen, A., Rubens, R., et al.: Testosterone secretion and metabolism in male senescence. *J. Clin. Endocr.* 34:730, 1972.

Verzár, F.: Anterior pituitary function in age, In *The Pituitary Gland*. Vol. 2. Donovan, B. T., and Harris, G. W. (eds.), Berkeley, University of California Press, 1966.

Vihko, R.: Gas chromatographic-mass spectrometric studies on solvolyzable steroids in human peripheral plasma. *Acta Endocr.* (Kbh.) 52(Suppl. 109):1, 1966.

Weissman, P. N., Shenkman, L., et al.: Chlorpropamide hyponatremia: Drug-induced inappropriate antidiuretic-hormone activity. *New Eng. J. Med.* 284:65, 1971.

West, C. D., Brown, H., et al.: Adrenocortical function and cortisol metabolism in old age. *J. Clin. Endocr.* 21:1197, 1961.

Williams, R. H., and Thompson, W. J.: Effect of age upon guanyl cyclase, adenyl cyclase, cyclic nucleotide phosphodiesterases in rats. *Proc. Soc. Biol. Med.* 143:382, 1973.

Yamaji, T., and Ibayashi, H.: Plasma dehydroepiandrosterone sulfate in normal and pathological conditions. *J. Clin. Endocr.* 29:273, 1969.

CHAPTER 28

Endocrine Responsive Cancers of Man

By Mortimer B. Lipsett

INTRODUCTION

The current resurgence of interest in the hormone-sensitive cancers derives from increased knowledge of the mechanism of action of hormones. However, the concept underlying many endocrine therapies is essentially simple, namely that some tumors remain dependent on the hormones that are necessary for growth and maintenance of function of the normal tissue from which the tumor originated. This concept was presaged by the remarkable clinical experiment of Beatson (1) in 1896, who achieved regression of metastatic breast cancer by oophorectomy. Lacassagne (2) suggested that hormones might be involved in the development of cancer, since he was able to induce mammary carcinoma by estrone in mice with low natural incidences of cancer. Huggins et al. (3) demonstrated that carcinoma of the human prostate regressed after orchiectomy and thereby initiated the modern era of endocrine therapy of cancer. This study was based on his earlier observations that androgen was necessary for function of the prostate, and he then surmised that this dependence survived the process of neoplastic transformation.

In this chapter breast cancer is discussed in depth, first because the principles of endocrine therapy derived from the study of this disease are applicable generally, and second because the large volume of research in experimental and clinical mammary cancer illuminates the direction of research and therapy to a greater extent than that in other cancers. We shall also discuss endocrine therapy of carcinoma of the prostate, uterine endometrium, and kidney, with emphasis on the basic endocrinology underlying therapy.

BREAST CANCER

Endocrinology

Estrogen Receptors

The modern studies of the mechanism of steroid hormone action are directly relevant to human breast cancer. As discussed in Chapter 7, when a steroid hormone acts at its target tissue, it is bound by a biologically specific, high affinity, receptor protein in the cytoplasm. The estrogen receptor (estrophile) is present in some experimental and human mammary cancers. When mammary cancer is induced in the rat by dimethylbenzanthracene (DMBA), oophorectomy causes regression in 90% of the cancers. Estradiol receptors were noted to be present in the responsive tumors and absent in the autonomous tumor (4). Using a different rat mammary cancer that does not regress after ovariectomy, estradiol receptors were identified but only at very low concentration (5). The correlation of abundant, high affinity, estradiol receptors with hormone-dependent mammary cancer was affirmed in the mouse (6) and rat (7). However, low concentrations of receptors are not the only defects in hormone-independent tumors, since in one such tumor, receptor was apparently present, but the receptor-hormone complex did not accumulate in the nucleus (8) as it does in estrogen-responsive tissues. From these and data in human breast cancer (see later section), it seems probable that an important correlate of endocrine-insensitive tumors is loss of specific receptors.

To anticipate subsequent sections, it has been

recognized that human breast cancer may respond to removal of estrogens. It was thus logical to attempt to correlate estradiol receptors in breast cancer with response to therapy. Following the demonstration of the presence of receptors in some human breast cancer (9), Jensen reported that the absence of estrophile predicted that there would be no response to adrenalectomy. However, when receptors were present, about a 50% response rate was noted (10). This finding has been affirmed in other studies (11).

It has been noted that estradiol receptors are present in as many as two-thirds of primary breast cancers (12, 13) and did not appear to be correlated with the histologic grade of the tumor. This latter observation is in accord with older data showing that response to removal of estrogen by ablative surgery could not be predicted from the grade of the cancer.

These findings raise a series of questions about the responsiveness of metastatic breast cancer to therapy. For example, if two-thirds of primary breast cancers contain the estradiol receptor, why is the response to oophorectomy in patients with metastatic disease only 30%? A facile answer is that the population of cancer cells in a tumor is mixed and that the response to therapy will depend on which clone metastasizes. Such a hypothesis can account for the resumption of growth after a remission has been achieved by removal of estrogen, i.e., the cells lacking the estrophile are those that resume growth. These problems demand exploration in order to establish a rational procedure for therapy.

Prolactin

Prominent among the other endocrine factors affecting the growth and function of mammary tissue is prolactin. It has been shown that administration of estrogen induces the release of prolactin and that in the absence of estrogen prolactin release is inhibited (Chapter 7). Increased release of prolactin achieved by an appropriate hypothalamic lesion stimulates the growth of DMBA-induced mammary cancer (14). Conversely, administration of a prolactin anti-serum stops the growth of this tumor (15). The interrelations between estrogen and prolactin acting on the cancer cell have not been clarified. Ovariectomy did induce regression of the rat mammary cancer when prolactin secretion was increased by hypothalamic lesions (16). When ovaries were grafted into these rats, tumor growth resumed although prolactin levels were unchanged. Thus the effect of ovariectomy in the DMBA-induced rat mammary tumor cannot be assumed to be solely the result of changes in prolactin secretion.

In man, data are fragmentary. There is as yet no evidence that differences in prolactin concentration can be associated with differences in incidence or growth rate of cancer or with the response to hypophysectomy. The lability of the plasma prolactin concentration makes single determinations of little value in assessing the tissue exposure to prolactin. A recent report (17) suggests that prolactin improved the growth and function of some human mammary cancer cells *in vitro*. If prolactin were a significant factor for the growth rate of human breast cancer, then hypophysectomy should give better results than adrenalectomy. This has been confirmed in single reports (18, 19) and denied in a large combined series of experiences (20).

Epidemiologic Considerations

The distribution of breast cancer among the population with respect to variables such as sex, age, race, country, reproductive history, and other indices can give valuable direction to biochemical research. The fact that breast cancer occurs 100 times as frequently in women than in men suggests that the hormonal milieu is significant. This may be, but the mass of epithelial tissue in the breast from which clinical carcinoma arises is 100 times as great in women, so that the carcinogenic event would be expected to occur more frequently on a random basis.

A significant epidemiologic finding is the striking variation in rates of breast cancer among various areas of the world. At age 50, the incidence of breast cancer is about six times higher in the United States or Scandinavia than in Japan or Taiwan (21). This initially was interpreted as genetic in origin, but the descendants of the Chinese living in Hawaii for several generations have the same rate of breast cancer as do the Caucasians, and first and second generation Japanese in Hawaii have rates higher than do those in Japan (22). Therefore, environmental factors must be considered.

The rates with age also have interesting and differential characteristics (Fig. 28–1). In countries with a high incidence of breast cancer, there is a continued increase with age. But in "low-risk" countries, the rate of development of breast cancer decreases after the menopause (Fig. 28–1). De-Waard (23) has suggested that these data are derived from two different etiologic types of breast cancer. Superimposed on the curve for breast cancer incidence in Japan or China is an additional type of cancer associated with increased food consumption and consequent obesity (23). Support for this hypothesis comes from studies of estrogen metabolism. Obese postmenopausal women were shown to have a greater frequency of estrogen effect in their vaginal smear (24), and the rate of conversion of the adrenal steroid, androstenedione, to estrone is higher in obese than in thin women (25). Although these data scarcely constitute proof, they connect seemingly remote environmental effects with estrogen metabolism.

Reproductive experience is an obvious factor that has often been considered in the epidemiology of breast cancer. It is now the consensus that lactation does not lower breast cancer risk (26, 27), although it may have this effect in countries with

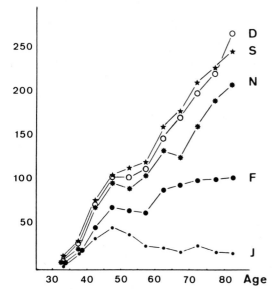

Figure 28-1.   Incidence of breast cancer with age in countries with high and low cancer rates. D = Denmark; S = Sweden; N = Norway; F = France; J = Japan. (From DeWaard, F.: *Int. J. Cancer* 4:577, 1969.)

low breast cancer rates (28). An intriguing finding is that breast cancer risk increases with age at first birth (29). Women whose first pregnancy occurs after age 35 have three times the risk of development of breast cancer as do those who are first parous before age 18. This remarkable finding has not been explained, but data from studies of carcinogenesis are pertinent. In the rat, pregnancy before administration of DMBA decreases the incidence of mammary cancer (30, 31). Similarly, prolactin decreases the yield of tumors induced by DMBA (16). A hypothesis consistent with the findings is that earlier differentiation and function renders the tissue less susceptible to carcinogenesis.

Genetic factors should be mentioned briefly. Familial aggregation of breast cancer has been documented (32), and a close relative of a woman with breast cancer has a risk of breast cancer two to three times greater than the population. The association of "soft" and "hard" ear wax with populations of high and low risk for breast cancer, respectively, supports the genetic component (32). Genetic effects can, of course, be appreciated through a variety of mechanisms not yet susceptible to study in man.

Carcinogenesis

The epidemiologic studies are one avenue into carcinogenesis. Since it is probable that carcinogenesis in man may require 10–20 years, events preceding the development of clinical breast cancer must be examined. The difficulties of correlating these events with hormonal alteration are formidable, and the task of defining susceptibility to the development of breast cancer will require exten-

sive measurements of several hormones in a population large enough so that follow-up can be adequate during twenty years, and so that sufficient cases of breast cancer can be expected.

The hormones may be considered as cocarcinogens or promoters of carcinogenesis. The administration of prolactin or estrogen increases the susceptibility to cancer produced by the Bittner virus in the mouse (34). Similarly, ovariectomy reduces the incidence of DMBA-induced tumors in the rat (35). In dogs, a species susceptible to mammary cancer, early oophorectomy markedly reduces the rate of development of cancer (36). In women, early menopause or surgical castration has a marked protective effect that is greater the earlier the age of oophorectomy (37). The data, therefore, are in accord with the fact that some aspect of ovarian function (most probably estrogen secretion, in man at least) appreciably increases the risk of developing breast cancer. Similar inferences about prolactin are not possible, since the history of the duration of lactation is relatively unimportant (see above).

Since the evidence is good that reduction of estrogenic load in young women reduces breast cancer risk, the question of whether increased estrogen load increases cancer risk is important. There is no evidence for this at present. Using combined data from several small studies, it was concluded that increased use of estrogen did not increase cancer risk (38). In a case control study, no evidence of a higher incidence of breast cancer patients was noted with use of oral contraceptives (39). Since the patient-years of exposure in both studies are small, judgment must still be withheld. It seems fair to conclude, however, that exogenous estrogens, in man, do not produce a large increase in the incidence of breast cancer.

The Hormonal Milieu

It has long been supposed that the hormonal environment may influence the risk of development of breast cancer and the rate of progression of established cancer. This concept had experimental support from studies of induction of mammary cancer in mice, in which the cocarcinogen or promoter role of estrogens could be demonstrated clearly. Investigations of this area in man have been slow for many reasons. Among these were inadequate methods of measurement; rapid fluctuations in the plasma concentrations of some hormones; a variety of characteristics of patients, such as thyroid status, nutrition, age, and liver function, that affect steroid metabolism; and, possibly most importantly, the real probability that measurement at the time of development of clinical disease has little relevance to the hormonal milieu present during the initial stage of carcinogenesis.

In 1960, Bulbrook and his colleagues (40) derived a discriminant function for predicting the success of adrenalectomy and hypophysectomy in the treatment of metastatic breast cancer. To do this, they measured several urinary steroids and

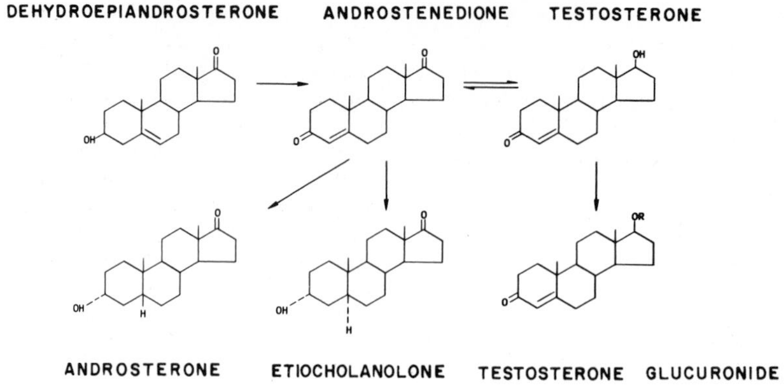

DEHYDROEPIANDROSTERONE   ANDROSTENEDIONE   TESTOSTERONE

ANDROSTERONE   ETIOCHOLANOLONE   TESTOSTERONE GLUCURONIDE

Figure 28–2. Adrenal steroid precursors of urinary 17-ketosteroids.

found that a formula using the excretion of etiocholanolone (Fig. 28–2) and 17-hydroxycorticosteroids gave the best separation between responders and nonresponders. In subsequent work by Bulbrook's group (41) and others, it became apparent that a favorable prognosis was correlated with a higher excretion of either of the urinary 11-deoxy-17-ketosteroids, androsterone and etiocholanolone. Since these ketosteroids (KS) are predominantly metabolites of the adrenal secretory product, dehydroepiandrosterone (Fig. 28–2), it was assumed that subtle alterations in adrenal function were correlated with the responsivity to ablative endocrine procedures. The success of these measurements as a discriminant has been variably confirmed (42) and denied (43–45).

These data have been interpreted somewhat differently by Zumoff et al. (46), who studied the metabolism of 17-KS precursors and found that severe illness lowered the rate of conversion to the 11-deoxy-17-KS. This implied that the discriminant distinguished between sicker and healthier patients, and that this was the important prognostic factor. Discrimination between response and nonresponse can be improved if the free interval (the period between onset and recurrence of disease) is taken into account (47). This may reflect the biologic nature of the cancer, i.e., slower growing cancers respond better. Although the theoretical basis for the discriminant may still be obscure, the data suggest that neither adrenalectomy nor hypophysectomy should be performed when the discriminant predicts failure.

Bulbrook (48) has presented one important datum supporting the importance of the endocrine milieu at the inception of breast cancer. They collected urine samples from 5000 apparently healthy women and froze them. When breast cancer developed, the urine of that woman and those of matched controls were analyzed. In 27 patients who developed breast cancer 6 months to 5 years after urine collection, etiocholanolone excretion was significantly lower than that of matched controls. It seems doubtful that the rate of metabolism of dehydroepiandrosterone to the 17-KS was abnormal when the breast cancer was subclinical. Thus an abnormality either of C-19 steroid secre-

tion or metabolism with breast cancer has been suggested.

Since the relationship of breast cancer to estrogens seems obvious, the measurement of urinary estrogens has been undertaken by several groups; there were, however, no differences between women with breast cancer and those in the normal population. These studies also suffer from the criticism that estrogens should have been measured during the stage of carcinogenesis rather than at some stage of clinical disease. Further, the large fluctuations of estrogens during the menstrual cycle and the alterations in route of metabolism with disease or with drugs make interpretation difficult.

The problem of estrogens and breast cancer has been approached by another route. Estriol, a metabolite of estradiol, is a weak estrogen which can antagonize the effects of estradiol (49). It was proposed, therefore, that women with a high excretion of estriol were relatively protected against the cancer-promoting effects of estradiol (50), and a few data were offered to support the hypothesis. Because of the lower incidence of breast cancer in Japan, this hypothesis was tested by measuring estrogen excretion in Japanese women and in Australian women. Estriol excretion was increased in the Japanese women, thereby supporting the hypothesis (51). The physiologic significance of these data are obscure, however, since estriol exists in the urine as the glucuronide conjugate and is derived mostly from plasma estradiol and estrone. The observation, however, may have empirical significance, or it may be an epiphenomenon having little relevance to breast cancer. It should be noted that a careful study of urinary estriol excretion and formation from estradiol in a limited number of women with breast cancer did not support the above hypothesis (52).

Most of the data regarding the hormonal milieu relate to hormones present in plasma. However, in 1968, Adams and Wong (53–55) reported that human breast cancer tissue could metabolize dehydroepiandrosterone to androstenedione and possibly to estriol. Cholesterol was converted to C-19 steroids. Dao et al. (56) found that breast cancer tissue could aromatize ring A and isolated estrone and estradiol after incubation with C-19 steroids. Thus the breast cancer cell may create its own microenvironment and thereby defeat efforts to lower estradiol levels in the surrounding medium. Some breast cancers have the capacity to sulfurylate various steroids, and it has been noted that the absence of the sulfokinase was correlated with a lack of response to adrenalectomy (56). When the tumor was able to sulfurylate dehydroepiandrosterone more efficiently than estradiol, 9 of 10 patients responded to adrenalectomy. How this biochemical parameter correlates with the presence of the estrogen receptor is not known, but if these characteristics are independent, then the predictive potential of the two tests should be very high.

Comment: There is little general agreement about the role of hormones in genesis and growth of breast cancer. There is, however, some certainty on two points. Some breast cancers have cytoplasmic estrogen receptors, and estrogen in several species, including man, "prepares the soil" for the carcinogenic event(s).

Therapy

Introduction

Before discussing the therapy of patients with metastatic breast cancer, it is necessary to consider some general principles of management. In contrast to chemotherapy, there is no evidence that concurrent use of two modalities of endocrine therapy is beneficial. Thus any method should be employed singly and continued until there is either evidence of failure or a resumption of growth after a remission.

Even casual perusal of the literature makes it clear that remission is defined variously by many groups, thereby accounting for the variations in the response rate. The rigid criteria employed by the Cooperative Breast Cancer Group (57) ensures that their remission rates will be lowest. They require evidence of a measurable decrease in the size of a metastasis and do not accept biochemical evidence for remission. Thus a patient with hypercalcemia who becomes normocalcemic after therapy is not classified as being a remission unless there is x-ray evidence of bone healing. The rigid criteria may be important in comparing modalities of therapy, since subjective components are of limited value, but important clinical aspects of response are overlooked. It is common clinical experience, when following the response to treatment of a patient with progressive disease, to observe either no progression or a greatly slowed rate of progression. Since alterations in tumor growth rate can occur spontaneously, it is difficult to quantify this type of response. Nevertheless, "arrest" of disease is common with therapy and is a significant benefit accruing to such therapy.

Breast cancer is a chronic disease, and the time from mastectomy to metastatic disease may be many years. Against this setting, one must evaluate the 9- to 12-month remissions produced by endocrine therapy. Data have been presented showing that life is prolonged in patients who respond to androgen, estrogen, adrenalectomy, or hypophysectomy. More than that, though, is the return to normal life that often accompanies such a remission. It is, therefore, fair to state that these remissions are important to the patient and, as a corollary, that it is necessary to improve predictive capacity to avoid unnecessary and potentially dangerous treatment.

Oophorectomy

If there is one area of general agreement about therapy, it is that women with metastatic breast cancer who have functioning ovaries should have oophorectomy. Using rigid criteria, the regression rate is 25–30% (58–60), and the median duration of remission is 9 months. In general, surgery is the method of choice, since radiation may require several weeks to be effective, and incomplete destruction of the follicles has been reported.

It is important to be able to evaluate ovarian status accurately. As noted in Chapter 7, a high plasma FSH is a reliable indication of loss of follicles and consequent cessation of estradiol secretion. The low plasma estradiol (< 20 pg./ml.) is also characteristic of cessation of ovarian function, but whether concentrations this low can also occur in patients with secondary amenorrhea needs further study. The vaginal smear is unreliable for distinguishing between a low secretion rate of estradiol and cessation of ovarian function. In perimenopausal and postmenopausal patients, the regression rate from oophorectomy is well below that of women with ovarian function (61).

It is probable that the presence of an estrogen receptor in tumor tissue will predict response to ovariectomy. This assumption needs to be tested in ongoing studies. However, tissue for these studies will often not be available, so that the empirical use of oophorectomy will continue.

Although the ovary secretes many steroids, indirect evidence has been presented that it is the decrease in estrogen secretion following ovariectomy that causes tumor regression. The process of osteolysis by metastatic cancer, characterized by hypercalciuria and hypercalcemia, has been halted by oophorectomy and accelerated by estrogen (62). In no other situation does estrogen cause hypercalciuria. Thus, in women whose tumors regress with oophorectomy, estrogen stimulates that function of the tumor involved with osteolysis. This has been equated with tumor growth. In fact, patients whose urine calcium excretion becomes normal following ovariectomy or other ablative procedures generally have remission of disease.

It is appropriate to discuss the question of early and late oophorectomy. Early oophorectomy has been called "prophylactic" in several writings; however, this is a misnomer, since if cancer is not present there is no prophylaxis, and if it is present oophorectomy is therapeutic. Early oophorectomy implies that metastases are not evident. It was hoped that early oophorectomy would prolong survival. This has not been the case, although the period before the development of clinical metastatic disease is apparently increased (63). There is a disadvantage to early oophorectomy. Since the response to oophorectomy defines an endocrine-responsive tumor (59, 64), the failure to respond suggests strongly that other endocrine modalities of therapy are likely to be unsuccessful and that chemotherapy would be the treatment of choice. Conversely, if metastases regress after castration, other ablative measures have an increased likelihood of success. Thus so-called prophylactic oophorectomy is not warranted.

Adrenalectomy and Hypophysectomy

Estrogens persist in blood and urine after ovariectomy. The adrenal cortex secretes estrone (65), but the main source of estrone after castration is the transformation of androstenedione, secreted by the adrenal cortex, to estrone in peripheral tissues (25). It has been difficult to prove, except inferentially, that the low concentrations of estradiol and estrone characteristic of the menopause are sufficient to support the growth of endocrine-sensitive tumors. However, the demonstration that the absence of an estrogen receptor in tumor tissue predicts that adrenalectomy will fail to be beneficial (10) is additional evidence for this concept.

The criteria for selection of patients for adrenalectomy or hypophysectomy are several. First, if an estrogen receptor can be identified in metastatic tissue, then the chance of response is about 50% (10). If the patient has responded to castration, then the likelihood of subsequent response to ablative surgery is also 50%. Whether these two criteria identify the same patients is not known, but it is likely. The role of measurement of the discriminant has been discussed, and it is also likely that the longer the free interval, the higher is the remission rate (47).

The rate of response to adrenalectomy or hypophysectomy has been variously estimated as equal (20) or somewhat in favor of hypophysectomy (18, 19). The mean duration of remission was also longer after hypophysectomy (15 months versus 8 months) (19). Although these data suggest that hypophysectomy may offer some advantages, the choice of operation must usually be made from more pragmatic considerations, such as the surgical skills available, the sites of metastases, and the age of patient. The problems of management of adrenal and pituitary insufficiency have been discussed elsewhere in this book. It is only necessary to state that the patient can be treated adequately in either case and, when a remission occurs, can often resume full activity.

The timing of these operative procedures is still debated. There is no reason to recommend them for the premenopausal woman, since the benefits are less than those obtainable by sequential oophorectomy and a major ablative procedure. When a

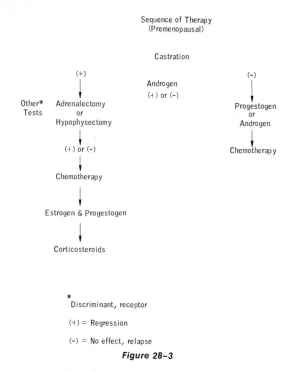

Figure 28–3.

woman has had a clear-cut regression following ovariectomy, then it is wise to consider surgery at the time of relapse (Fig. 28–3). In the postmenopausal patient, adrenalectomy or hypophysectomy may be postponed until after therapy with hormonal steroids (Figs. 28–4 and 28–5), since success or failure with one of the steroid regimens does not prejudice the probability of response to major ablative surgery (66). It is curious that in the period one year after the menopause most endocrine procedures are less effective than later. It is not clear whether such patients should initially be treated by chemotherapy or by adrenalectomy or hypophysectomy.

The suggestion has been made that the favorable effects of the major ablative procedures are due

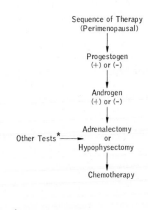

*
Discriminant, receptor

Figure 28–4.

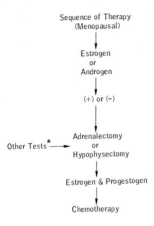

Sequence of Therapy
(Menopausal)

↓

Estrogen
or
Androgen

↓

(+) or (−)

↓

Other Tests* ⟶ Adrenalectomy
or
Hypophysectomy

↓

Estrogen & Progestogen

↓

Chemotherapy

*
Discriminant, receptor

Figure 28–5

solely to the administration of cortisone. In one randomized trial, adrenalectomy produced results clearly superior to those obtained with cortisone treatment (67).

Androgen Therapy

Lacassagne, who was the first to show that estrogens promoted development of mammary tumors in mice, found that the growth of these tumors could be inhibited by testosterone propionate (68). Androgen therapy of women with metastatic cancer was initiated 30 years ago. The Cooperative Breast Cancer Group surveyed the response of 521 patients treated with testosterone propionate and reported a remission rate of 21% (57). The response depended on menopausal status and on sites of metastases. Within one year of the menopause, the remission rate was less than 10% and was highest 5 years after the menopause. Soft tissue metastases responded most favorably and visceral metastases least (Table 28–1). The median period of remission was 8 months. Given the long clinical course of breast cancer, it is fair to ask whether remissions of this length actually prolong survival. The Cooperative Breast Cancer Group

TABLE 28–1. RESPONSE TO TESTOSTERONE THERAPY*

	Number of Cases	Remission (%)
Postmenopausal (<1 yr.)	92	9
Postmenopausal (1–5 yr.)	100	17
Postmenopausal (5–10 yr.)	82	26
Postmenopausal (>10 yr.)	247	27
Site of soft tissue	127	32
Bone metastasis	189	19
Visceral metastasis	205	18

*From Cooperative Breast Cancer Group: *J.A.M.A. 188*:106, 1964.

found that patients who responded to androgen therapy survived twice as long as did the nonresponders. Similar conclusions have been reached for responders to other modes of endocrine therapy.

It is clear from the data of Table 28–1 that androgens are used advantageously after the menopause. They should not be used either before or after oophorectomy in the premenopausal patient. Testosterone is converted to estrogen (25), but, more importantly, the concurrent use of two modalities will not permit the physician to assess the response to oophorectomy. If the patient has responded to oophorectomy, androgen may be used with good results following relapse. However, the response rate in castration failures is low (57), and, as noted above, chemotherapy then is the treatment of choice. The dose and type of androgen need not be discussed in detail. Any androgen, given in large amounts, produces about the same rate of regression. Usual doses are testosterone propionate, 50 mg. IM three times a week, or fluoxymesterone, 40 mg. daily. Long-acting preparations should be avoided, since it is then impossible to stop therapy should the disease accelerate, e.g., the sudden development of severe hypercalcemia. The results of trials with many androgens have been summarized (69).

Attempts have been made to find steroids less androgenic than testosterone, since it may produce virilization that is severe and often distressing. This quest has been generally unsuccessful. A synthetic steroid, Δ'-testololactone, has essentially no androgenic activity and has been reported to produce a few regressions (70). Although the incidence of remissions was low, their occurrence is evidence that antitumor effect can be independent of androgenicity.

One other point should be noted. In patients who respond to androgen, eventual relapse demands cessation of androgen therapy. Before attempting other therapies, the patient should be observed, since about 10% of such patients will experience remission again with androgen withdrawal (71). It may be suggested that relapse in this situation is due to growth of a partially androgen-dependent clone of cells.

Estrogens

The observation that some patients with breast cancer can respond to estrogen therapy was not predictable nor was it based on data from animal models. Following the initial observations, however, remission rates of 30–37% were reported in two large series (72, 73) when estrogen was used as initial therapy. In a randomized trial of steroid therapy, estrogen produced a 29% remission rate and androgen a 10% remission rate (74). The duration of response to estrogen has been longer than that to androgen in most series. Estrogen responsiveness increases with years after the menopause. As with androgen and the ablative procedures, the longer the free interval, the higher is the probability of response to estrogen.

When estrogens are used in patients who have relapsed from other therapy, remission rates are low, the chances of response being less than 10%. Estrogen is generally ineffective following hypophysectomy or adrenalectomy, although some success has been recorded with the combined use of estradiol and progesterone (24). Since estrogen in small doses may exacerbate breast cancer in the premenopausal woman after oophorectomy, its use in this period is hazardous. Very large doses of estrogen, however, have caused regressions (76).

The toxicity from estrogens even at high doses is small. Endometrial hyperplasia and breakthrough bleeding are not uncommon and can usually be managed by giving a progestogen, followed by a short period of cessation of hormone therapy to permit sloughing of the endometrium. Salt and water retention, particularly in the elderly, may occur with any estrogen. Of greatest consequence, however, is hypercalcemia. This can occur abruptly in any patient but is rare in patients 10 or more years after the menopause. Hypercalcemia is managed by withdrawal of estrogen and hydration. Often, on reinstitution of therapy, a regression will be obtained without recurrence of hypercalcemia.

The phenomenon of a response following withdrawal of estrogen has been recorded (71). Thus, as with androgens, new attempts at therapy should generally not be started until at least 2 months after stopping estrogens. Rapidly advancing disease will, of course, constitute an exception to this suggestion.

Progestogens

A variety of progestogens both of the C-21-17α-hydroxysteroids, such as medroxyprogesterone, and of the C-19 steroids, such as norethisterone, have been used in patients with breast cancer. In general, remission rates have clustered about 20% (77, 78), the same as that noted with androgens. The response to progestogens was not influenced by previous response to castration, estrogen, or androgen. Thus progestogens may be given a trial in patients failing to respond to other therapeutic modalities. In general, these agents are without important side effects. Regression appears to be more common with soft tissue metastases and unusual with bone metastases.

Glucocorticoids

There is little doubt that large doses of any glucocorticoid (equivalent to 200–300 mg. of cortisol daily) can induce regression of disease at any site. These are short-lived, but the rapid effect of the glucocorticoids makes them useful in rapidly advancing disease. A response to glucocorticoids is not predictive of response to other endocrine modalities.

The finding that androgens, estrogens, progestogens, and glucocorticoids can induce regression of some human breast cancers makes it difficult to construct a unifying mechanism. It is known that the rate of growth of a tumor is due to the fraction of cells that enter the proliferative pool (leave the "resting" state) and to the rate of cell loss of dividing cells. Since specific hormones, such as estradiol and prolactin, stimulate growth and function of mammary cells, it is reasonable to assume that they increase the proliferative pool and, conversely, that removal of estrogen will thereby decrease growth rate in estrogen-sensitive tumors. Since the cell cycle is apparently independent of hormones, the hormones in pharmacologic doses must act in ways other than on cell division. It has been proposed (79) that the steroid hormones increase the rate of cell loss following division and thereby slow the growth rate.

ENDOMETRIAL CANCER

Endocrinology

The uterine endometrium is a classic example of a hormone-dependent tissue, its growth and morphology changing cyclically in response to varying concentrations of the ovarian hormones, estradiol and progesterone. Specific uterine cytosol receptors for estradiol were first identified in 1960 (80) and have been studied extensively since then (Ch. 7). Progesterone receptors were shown to be present in the guinea pig uterus in 1968 (81) and subsequently in human endometrium (82). About one-third of endometrial cancers have estrophile (83), and its presence has been correlated positively with the degree of differentiation of the tumor (84). Progesterone receptors are present in endometrial cancer (85), but their presence could not be correlated with degree of differentiation.

The modern biochemical evidence for endocrine relationships with endometrial cancer was preceded by many suggestive clinical data and by some therapeutic successes. Gusberg (86) defined adenomatous hyperplasia as a precursor of endometrial carcinoma. Since adenomatous hyperplasia is preceded by endometrial hyperplasia (87) and this can be caused by estrogen (86), the path from estrogen effect to endometrial cancer can be traced. Experimentally high doses of estrogens have produced endometrial hyperplasia and cancer in rabbits (88, 89).

Since an endometrial carcinoma is manifested predominantly during the menopause, the emphasis on estrogen may seem misplaced. However, the events favoring carcinogenesis must have happened at least 5–10 years earlier, because of the long latent period between carcinogenesis and clinical cancer. Secondly, excess estrogen secretion is probably not the important consideration in carcinogenesis. Larson (90), reviewing the data, concluded that estrogens are not involved in the etiology of endometrial carcinoma but noted their high association with several types of ovarian disorder. The association of the estrogen-producing granulosa–theca cell tumor and endometrial carcinoma is convincing (91). In the Stein-Leventhal syndrome, the incidence of endometrial carcinoma is increased (92). This is true also for several other ovarian abnormalities, such as cortical stromal hyperplasia (93) and persistent stromal thecal cells (94). In each case, there is reason to believe that estrogen secretion is not excessive. It is continuous, however, since there are no ovulatory cycles with progesterone secretion and consequent endometrial sloughing. The recent report of endometrial cancer in women with Turner's syndrome who were treated with estrogens only (95) is further evidence for this concept. The causal role of continued, unopposed, estrogenic stimulus is supported by the high incidence of irregular menses in women with endometrial cancer (96, 97). The resumption of cyclic ovarian function in response to ovarian wedge resection in the Stein-Leventhal syndrome (98) results in regression of endometrial hyperplasia.

A cause for increased estrogen secretion in the menopause has been suggested. The origin of estrogens in the postmenopausal woman has been shown to be predominantly from androstenedione (25, 99). Since the rate of conversion of androstenedione to estrone increases with age and is high enough to cause endometrial hyperplasia in some women (25), this mechanism acting after the menopause may be of significance.

The literature on gynecology is replete with suggestions that the constellation of abnormal estrogen stimulation, disordered anterior pituitary function, diabetes mellitus, obesity, and infertility occur with high frequency in women with endometrial cancer. Using matched groups, the factors associated with the cancer were obesity and infertility (100). Nevertheless, there is, in fact, some support for the existence of other factors. Abnormal glucose tolerance tests have been documented in cases of cancer, and abnormalities of growth hormone secretion were noted in women with breast cancer (101) and, more recently, in women with endometrial cancer (102). Whether these abnormalities are cause or effect is unknown. The increased frequency of breast cancer in women with endometrial cancer (103) also suggests common etiologic factors. The abnormalities of estrogen secretion have been discussed. In biochemical-epidemiologic studies, it was shown that the ratio of estriol to etiocholanolone differed between patients with endometrial cancer and normal controls (104). A similar study of individual 17-KS and corticoid excretion by patients with endometrial cancer revealed differences between them and several types of matched controls, permitting the construction of a discriminant function (105). The findings in these last reports do not, of course, distinguish between abnormalities of secretion or of metabolism. However, the excretion of the three classic estrogens — estrone, estradiol, and estriol — was the same in patients with cancer as in an age-matched normal population (106). The data cited above suggest that the hormonal milieu is an important determinant in the pathogenesis of endometrial cancer.

Therapy

In 1961 Kelley and Baker reported that progestogens could cause regression in about one-third of patients with metastatic endometrial cancer (107). This has been confirmed in a large series of patients treated at many centers (108). The response to therapy did not depend on age of patient, site of metastasis, or previous or concurrent therapy. However, women with slowly growing or more differentiated tumors responded better than did those with aggressive cancers. Duration of life after initiation of therapy was 27 months in those who responded and only 7 months in those who did not. These combined data have been duplicated in other reports (109, 110). It has not mattered which progestogen was used, neither was the dose important (110), except that large doses seemed to be necessary.

It is the consensus that progestogens should be used in any patient with metastatic disease. It is claimed that the response of pulmonary metastases is better than that of bone metastases, but responses have been noted in all groups. To cite a personal experience, a woman with extensive lytic disease of the pelvis has remained in remission for 12 years, with calcification and remodeling of pelvic bones, on a dose of 100 mg. of medroxyprogesterone daily. The remissions seen with progestogens are unique, since they are accomplished with essentially no toxicity.

The mechanism behind the effects of progestogen is still only speculation. In the normal estrogen-primed uterus, progesterone causes specific maturational changes, followed by atrophy when a progestogen is continued for long periods. Following administration of progestogens to women with endometrial cancer, mitotic activity ceases, there is increased glandular differentiation, and an increase in cytoplasm:nucleus ratio is seen (109, 111). Atrophy is also noted (112). Thus these changes duplicate those of the normal endometrium during progesterone therapy.

CANCER OF THE PROSTATE

Endocrinology

Although the influence of the testis on prostatic function had been suspected in the nineteenth century, the pioneering work of Huggins (113, 114) established its role and gave rise to the concept of androgen dependence. The subsequent demonstration that castration caused regression of prostatic cancer in man (3, 115) initiated the era of hormonal management of cancer of the prostate.

In broad outlines, the mechanism of androgen action resembles that of estrogen, i.e., the androgen is bound to a cytosol receptor and transported to the nucleus where it interacts with chromatin (116). It is almost certain that, in man and many other species, the active intracellular androgen is dihydrotestosterone, a metabolite of testosterone (117). It has been suggested from studies of prostate in organ culture that a metabolite of dihydrotestosterone, 5α-androstane-3α, 17β-diol, specifically stimulates secretion, whereas dihydrotestosterone induces growth (118). Although both testosterone and androstenedione are precursors of intracellular dihydrotestosterone, apparently high plasma concentrations of testosterone are necessary, since prostate weight is not maintained following castration. Stimulation of the adrenal cortex in the castrate rat will cause growth of the prostate (119), probably via the mechanism of increasing androstenedione secretion. In the only modern study of testosterone production, Isurugi (120) found that testosterone production rates were the same in men with prostatic cancer as in normal controls.

There are studies of rodents that delineate a role for prolactin in prostatic growth. Hypophysectomy causes a more profound atrophy of the rat prostate than does castration (121), and endogenous prolactin has been shown to synergize with testosterone in maintaining the male mouse sexual accessory glands (122). Injection of a prolactin antiserum inhibits prostate growth in rabbits (123). How prolactin effects growth is unknown, but there is some evidence that prolactin increases the uptake of testosterone by the prostate (124, 125). It should be noted, however, that in rodents prolactin may have biochemical effects not seen in other species. Thus it has marked effects on corpus luteum function and spermatogenesis in the rat but is inactive at these sites in other species. Nevertheless, the data are intriguing and offer some rationale for the use of hypophysectomy in patients with metastatic disease.

Therapy

The incidence of cancer of the prostate is second only to that of bronchogenic carcinoma in men in the United States (126). Over 60% of the cases occur in men over 70 years of age. From histologic criteria, it has been estimated that at age 100, the prevalence of prostatic carcinoma is close to 100%, although in many it is not clinically apparent.

Although the principles of therapy are simple, there remains some controversy about tactics. If, as proposed by Huggins and those who followed him, it is necessary to decrease plasma androgens to a low level, then orchiectomy should suffice. However, estrogen can inhibit the effect of androgen in prostatic secretion in the absence of the pituitary gland (127), implying a direct effect of estrogen in addition to its suppression of LH. Thus reasons can be cited for the simultaneous use of orchiectomy and estrogen.

In large, collected series of patients with metastatic disease (128–130), 3- and 5-year survival rates of treated patients were always better than those of untreated patients. The differences among regimens of castration, estrogen therapy, or combined treatment were not significant at 3 and 5 years. In a more recent study using randomized assignments to therapeutic regimens, no difference was found among the three regimens (131); however, estrogen therapy was associated with increased mortality from cardiovascular disease (131), and these data have been confirmed recently in a study of treatment of patients with coronary artery disease. Since estrogen carries increased risks as well as the side effects of fluid retention and gynecomastia, it seems wise to use orchiectomy only. Estrogen, given prophylactically to men with prostatic cancer apparently free of metastases, did not significantly decrease cancer deaths but did increase mortality from cardiovascular disease (131).

Remission of disease has usually been defined as a significant lowering of acid phosphatase and relief of pain. Since bone metastases are usually osteoblastic, sufficient remodeling to permit diagnosis of remission may take several years. Nevertheless, regression rates from either orchiectomy or estrogen have been 50–80%, varying with grade and stage of disease (132). The average duration of remission has been 15 months, although remissions lasting over 5 years have been noted.

There is no evidence that any estrogen has superiority over another, although individual patients may have lesser gastrointestinal reaction to one or the other. Since there are no adequate studies of dosage versus response, a large enough dose of estrogen must be used to ensure suppression of LH, such as stilbestrol, 15 mg. daily, or ethinylestradiol, 1.5 mg. daily. When patients have responded to either orchiectomy or estrogen, the alternative mode of therapy may be tried after relapse. Remissions are rare, however.

It has been claimed (133) that in some patients 17-KS excretion rises following orchiectomy, and that this may be associated with reactivation of disease. This idea has persisted without further adequate studies. Recently, it was shown that androstenedione and testosterone plasma concentrations are higher in some patients with prostatic cancer after orchiectomy than has been found generally (134). Suppression of the adrenal cortex reduced these levels. It seems quite possible that some men, like some postmenopausal women with endometrial hyperplasia (25), produce higher amounts of androstenedione than does the general population, and that possibly adrenal suppression would be beneficial in this group. Trials of cortisone have been inconclusive, however, although some improvement has been recorded (135). There is no correlation between clinical relapse and increasing testosterone levels after orchiectomy (136).

Progestational agents have been used in treatment. As discussed previously, these agents suppress LH and, in addition, can act as antiandrogens, competing directly with testosterone for the prostate androgen receptors. In three studies (137–139), remissions were reported in response to cyproterone acetate, an effective antiandrogen. The agent was given before castration or estrogen therapy and has been ineffective following castration. The latter finding indicates that resumption of tumor growth following remission from orchiectomy is not androgen-dependent.

Because of residual androgen production by the adrenal cortex and the possible role of prolactin in maintaining prostate growth, adrenalectomy and hypophysectomy have been performed in patients who have relapsed after primary therapy with estrogen or orchiectomy. In general, responses to adrenalectomy have been less satisfactory than to hypophysectomy (140). In three series, the remission rate for hypophysectomy varied between 40% and 63% (140–142). The survival of patients classified as having remission was considerably longer than that of the nonresponders (140). However, in the absence of objective evidence of regression of disease, this criterion cannot be used to judge the success of the procedure, for those patients with less advanced disease may more easily have claimed benefit. Although the acid phosphatase was reported to decrease in responders to hypophysectomy (140), the data are not convincing. It is thus still premature to recommend any of these procedures routinely in the patient after relapse.

Testosterone has been given to patients in relapse following orchiectomy. Not all patients show evidence of acceleration of disease, and some have responded symptomatically with relief of pain and increased sense of well-being (143). There was no objective evidence of regression of disease.

CANCER OF THE KIDNEY

Endocrinology

The kidney is not usually considered an endocrine-responsive tissue, although in the rat, androgen administration causes hypertrophy of the kidney (144), and an androgen receptor has been identified in mouse kidney (145). Experimental models of adenocarcinoma of the kidney are rare, the only one being the estrogen-induced renal cell adenoma and adenocarcinoma of the hamster (146). The histologic pattern of the cancer closely resembles that of the human adenocarcinoma (147). These tumors can be transplanted to male hamsters only after pretreatment with estrogen (148). They cannot be induced in females except after ovariectomy, suggesting that ovarian progesterone inhibits induction. The growth of the tumors can be suppressed by cortisone and medroxyprogesterone given concurrently but not by either agent alone (149). An estrogen antagonist decreases the growth rate of a transplantable tumor (150).

Evidence that studies of this unique system are relevant to the treatment of human kidney cancer is sparse and depends chiefly on the observation that hormonal therapy, particularly with progestogens, occasionally causes regression of disease. Renal cell cancer occurs twice as commonly in men as in women (151), thereby minimizing a role for estrogens in tumor induction.

Therapy

The group of patients treated longest with hormonal therapy has been summarized by Bloom (152). Of the 80 patients with metastatic disease, 55% underwent remissions (mean duration of 11.5 months). All were treated initially with high doses of medroxyprogesterone and a few secondarily with testosterone. Remissions were rare in the women. The results reported in this series are much better than those given in other reports (153–156). The sex difference among responses recorded by Bloom has not been confirmed because of the limited number of responses noted. An occasional good response to testosterone has also been recorded.

The use of medroxyprogesterone acetate is associated with few side effects. Although this steroid in high doses has a low glucocorticoid potency, neither adrenal atrophy nor Cushing's syndrome has been reported in adults on long-term therapy. The agent causes loss of libido in men via its suppressive effect on LH (157).

REFERENCES

1. Beatson, G. T.: *Lancet* 2:104, 162, 1896.
2. Lacassagne, A.: *C. R. Soc. Biol.* (Paris) 195:630, 1932.
3. Huggins, C., Stevens, R. E., et al.: *Arch. Surg.* 43:209, 1941.
4. Mobbs, B. G.: *J. Endocr.* 36:409, 1966.
5. McGuire, W. L., Julian, J. A.: *Endocrinology* 89:969, 1971.
6. Terenius, L.: *Europ. J. Cancer* 8:55, 1972.
7. McGuire, W. L., and Julian, J. A.: *Cancer Res.* 31:1440, 1971.
8. Shyamala, G.: *Biochem. Biophys. Res. Commun.* 46:1623, 1972.
9. Korenman, S. G., and Dukes, B. A.: *J. Clin. Endocr.* 30:639, 1970.
10. Jensen, E. V., In *Cancer Medicine.* Holland, J. F., and Frei, E. M. (eds.), Philadelphia, Lea and Febiger, 1972.
11. Maass, H., Engel, B., et al.: *Amer. J. Obstet. Gynec.* 113:377, 1972.
12. Feherty, P., Farber-Brown, G., et al.: *Brit. J. Cancer* 26:697, 1971.
13. Wittliff, J. L., Hilf, R., et al.: *Cancer Res.* 32:1983, 1971.
14. Clemens, J. A., Welsch, C. W., et al.: *Proc. Soc. Exp. Biol. Med.* 127:969, 1968.
15. Butler, T. P., and Pearson, O. H.: *Cancer Res.* 31:817, 1971.
16. Sinha, D., Cooper, D., et al.: *Cancer Res.* 33:411, 1973.
17. Salih, H., Brander, W., et al.: *Lancet* 2:1103, 1972.
18. Hayward, J. L., Atkins, H. J. B., et al., In *The Clinical Management of Advanced Breast Cancer.* Second Tenovus Workshop. Joslin, C. A. F., and Gleave, E. N. (eds.), Cardiff, Livingstone, 1970, p. 50.
19. Pearson, O. H., and Ray, B. S., In *Cancer (Hormone Therapy).* Vol. 6. Chapter 12. Raven, R. W. (ed.), London, Butterworth & Co., 1959.
20. Joint Committee on Endocrine Ablative Procedures in Disseminated Mammary Carcinoma. *J.A.M.A.* 175:787, 1961.
21. Doll, R., Muir, C., et al.: *Cancer Incidence in Five Continents.* Vol. 2. Berlin, Springer-Verlag, 1966.
22. Haenszel, W., and Kurihara, M.: *J. Nat. Cancer Inst.* 40:43, 1968.
23. DeWaard, F.: *Intern. J. Cancer* 4:577, 1969.
24. DeWaard, F., Pot, H., et al.: *Acta Cytol.* 16:273, 1972.
25. Grodin, J. M., Siiteri, P. K., et al.: *J. Clin. Endocr.* 36:207, 1973.
26. Wynder, E. L., Bross, I. J., et al.: *Cancer* 13:559, 1960.
27. MacMahon, B., Cole, P., et al.: *Bull. WHO* 43:185, 1970.
28. Kamoi, M.: *Tohoku J. Exp. Med.* 72:59, 1960.
29. MacMahon, B., Cole, P., et al.: *Bull. WHO* 43:209, 1970.
30. Dao, T. L.: *Progr. Exp. Tumor Res.* 14:59, 1971.

31. Moon, R. C.: *Intern. J. Cancer 43*:312, 1969.
32. Lilienfeld, A. M.: *Cancer Res. 23*:1503, 1963.
33. Petrakis, N. L.: *Science 173*:347, 1971.
34. Furth, J., In *Prolactin and Carcinogenesis*. Fourth Tenovus Workshop. Boyns, A. R., and Griffiths, K. (eds.), Cardiff, Livingstone, 1972.
35. Dao, T. L.: *Progr. Exp. Tumor Res. 5*:157, 1964.
36. Schneider, R., Dorn, C. R., et al.: *J. Nat. Cancer Inst. 43*:1249, 1969.
37. Feinleib, M.: *J. Nat. Cancer Inst. 41*:315, 1968.
38. Arthes, F. G., Sartwell, P., et al.: *Cancer 28*:1391, 1971.
39. Vessey, M. P., Doll, R., et al.: *Brit. Med. J. 3*:719, 1972.
40. Bulbrook, R. D., Greenwood, F. C., et al.: *Lancet 1*:1154, 1960.
41. Atkins, H., Bulbrook, R. D., et al.: *Lancet 2*:1263, 1968.
42. Kumaoka, S., Sakauchi, N., et al.: *J. Clin. Endocr. 28*:667, 1968.
43. Sarfaty, G., and Tallis, M.: *Lancet 2*:685, 1970.
44. Wade, A. P., Tweedie, M. C. K., et al.: *Lancet 1*:853, 1969.
45. Ahlquist, K. A., Jackson, A. W., et al.: *Brit. Med. J. 1*:217, 1968.
46. Zumoff, B., Bradlow, H. L., et al.: *J. Clin. Endocr. 32*:824, 1971.
47. Wilson, R. E., and Moore, F. D., In *Prognostic Factors in Breast Cancer*. Forrest, A. P. M., and Kunkler, P. B. (eds.), Edinburgh, Livingstone Press, 1968.
48. Bulbrook, R. D., Hayward, J. L., et al.: *Lancet 2*:395, 1971.
49. Huggins, C., and Jensen, E. V.: *J. Exp. Med. 102*:335, 1955.
50. Lemon, H. M., Wotiz, H. H., et al.: *J.A.M.A. 196*:1128, 1966.
51. MacMahon, B., Cole, P., et al.: *Lancet 2*:900, 1971.
52. Hellman, L., Zumoff, B., et al.: *J. Clin. Endocr. 33*:138, 1971.
53. Adams, J. B., and Wong, M. S. F.: *J. Endocr. 41*:41, 1968.
54. Adams, J. B., and Wong, M. S. F.: *J. Endocr. 44*:69, 1968.
55. Adams, J. B., and Wong, M. S. F.: *Steroids 11*:313, 1968.
56. Dao, T. L., Varela, R., et al., In *Estrogen Target Tissues and Neoplasia*. Dao, T. L. (ed.), Chicago, University of Chicago Press, 1972.
57. Cooperative Breast Cancer Group: *J.A.M.A. 188*:106, 1964.
58. Taylor, S. G.: *Surg. Gynec. Obstet. 115*:443, 1962.
59. Hall, T. C., Dederich, M. M., et al.: *Cancer Chemother. Rep. 31*:47, 1963.
60. Lewison, E. F.: *Cancer 18*:558, 1965.
61. Fracchia, A. A., Farrow, J. N., et al.: *Surg. Gynec. Obstet. 128*:1221, 1969.
62. Pearson, O. H., West, C. D., et al.: *J.A.M.A. 95*:357, 1955.
63. Kennedy, B. J., Meilke, P. W., et al.: *Surg. Gynec. Obstet. 118*:524, 1964.
64. Stewart, H. J., In *The Clinical Management of Advanced Breast Cancer*. Second Tenovus Workshop. Joslin, C. A. F., and Gleave, A. N. (eds.), Cardiff, Livingstone, 1970.
65. Saez, J. M., Morera, A. M., et al.: *J. Endocr. 55*:41, 1972.
66. Hayward, J. L., In *The Clinical Management of Advanced Breast Cancer*. Second Tenovus Workshop. Joslin, C. A. F., and Gleave, A. N. (eds.), Cardiff, Livingstone, 1970.
67. Dao, T. L., Tan, E., et al.: *Cancer 14*:1259, 1961.
68. Lacassagne, A.: *C. R. Soc. Biol.* (Paris) *126*:385, 1936.
69. Cooperative Breast Cancer Group: *Cancer Chemother. Rep. 11*:109, 1961.
70. Goldenberg, J. S.: *Cancer 23*:109, 1969.
71. Kaufman, R. J., and Escher, G. C.: *Surg. Gynec. Obstet. 113*:635, 1961.
72. Kennedy, B. J.: *Cancer 24*:1345, 1969.
73. Stoll, B. A.: *Med. J. Aust. 1*:980, 1964.
74. Kennedy, B. J.: *Surg. Gynec. Obstet. 120*:1246, 1965.
75. Landau, R. L., Ehrlich, E. N., et al.: *J.A.M.A. 182*:632, 1962.
76. Kennedy, B. J.: *Cancer 15*:641, 1962.
77. Stoll, B. A.: *Brit. Med. J. 2*:338, 1967.
78. Briggs, M. H., Caldwell, A. D. S., et al.: *Hosp. Med. 2*:63, 1967.
79. Lipsett, M. B.: *Cancer Res. 29*:2408, 1969.
80. Jensen, E. V., and Jacobson, H. I.: *Recent Progr. Hormone Res. 18*:387, 1962.
81. Milgrom, E., and Baulieu, E. E.: *C. R. Soc. Biol.* (Paris) *267*:2005, 1968.
82. Wiest, W. G., and Rao, B. R.: *Advances Biosci. 7*:251, 1971.
83. Rubin, B. L., Gusberg, S. B., et al.: *Amer. J. Obstet. Gynec. 114*:660, 1972.
84. Terenius, L., Lindell, A., et al.: *Cancer Res. 31*:1895, 1971.
85. Haukkamaa, M., Karjalainen, O., et al.: *Amer. J. Obstet. Gynec. 11*:205, 1971.

86. Gusberg, S. B.: *Amer. J. Obstet. Gynec. 54*:905, 1947.
87. Novak, E., and Yui, E.: *Amer. J. Obstet. Gynec. 32*:674, 1936.
88. Burrows, H., and Horning, E. S.: *Oestrogens and Neoplasia*. Springfield, Illinois, Charles C Thomas, 1952.
89. Meissner, W. A., Sommers, S. C., et al.: *Cancer 10*:500, 1957.
90. Larson, J. A.: *Obstet. Gynec. 3*:551, 1954.
91. Gusberg, S. B.: *Obstet. Gynec. 30*:287, 1967.
92. Jackson, R. L., and Dockerty, M. B.: *Amer. J. Obstet. Gynec. 73*:161, 1957.
93. Sommers, S. C., and Meissner, W. A.: *Cancer 10*:516, 1957.
94. Fienberg, R.: *Cancer 24*:32, 1969.
95. Cutler, B. S., Forks, A. P., et al.: *New Eng. J. Med. 287*:628, 1972.
96. Peterson, E. P.: *Obstet. Gynec. 31*:702, 1968.
97. Sherman, A. I., and Woolf, R. B.: *Amer. J. Obstet. Gynec. 77*:233, 1959.
98. Kaufman, R. H., Abbott, W. P., et al.: *Amer. J. Obstet. Gynec. 77*:1271, 1959.
99. Longcope, C.: *Amer. J. Obstet. Gynec. 111*:778, 1971.
100. Dunn, L. J., and Bradbury, J. T.: *Amer. J. Obstet. Gynec. 97*:465, 1967.
101. Pearson, O. H., Llerena, O., et al.: In *Prognostic Factors in Breast Cancer*. First Tenovus Symposium. Forrest, A. P. M., and Kunkler, P. B. (eds.), Cardiff, Livingstone, 1967.
102. Benjamin, F., Casper, D. J., et al.: *New Eng. J. Med. 281*:1448, 1969.
103. MacMahon, B.: *Cancer 23*:275, 1969.
104. DeWaard, F., Thyssen, J. H. N., et al.: *Cancer 22*:988, 1968.
105. Sall, S., and Calanog, A.: *Amer. J. Obstet. Gynec. 114*:153, 1972.
106. Hausknecht, R. V., and Gusberg, S. B.: *Amer. J. Obstet. Gynec. 105*:1161, 1969.
107. Kelley, R. M., and Baker, W. H.: *New Eng. J. Med. 264*:216, 1961.
108. Reifinstein, E. C., Jr.: *Cancer 27*:485, 1971.
109. Sherman, I.: *Obstet. Gynec. 28*:309, 1966.
110. Malkasian, G. D., Jr., Decker, D. G., et al.: *Amer. J. Obstet. Gynec. 110*:15, 1971.
111. John, A. H., Cornes, J. C., et al.: *Proceedings St. Thomas' Hosp. Med. School Symposium*. London, 1971.
112. Bonte, J.: *Proceedings St. Thomas' Hosp. Med. School Symposium*. London, 1971.
113. Huggins, C., and Clark, P. J.: *J. Exp. Med. 72*:547, 1940.
114. Huggins, C., Masina, M. H., et al.: *J. Exp. Med. 70*:543, 1939.
115. Huggins, C., and Hodges, C. V.: *Cancer Res. 1*:293, 1941.
116. Liao, S., and Fang, S.: *Vitam. Horm. 27*:17, 1969.
117. Wilson, J. D.: *New Eng. J. Med. 287*:1284, 1972.
118. Baulieu, E. E., Lasnitzki, I., et al.: *Nature* (London) *219*:1155, 1968.
119. Tullner, W. W.: *Nat. Cancer Inst. Monographs 12*:211, 1963.
120. Isurugi, K.: *J. Urol. 97*:903, 1967.
121. Grayhack, J. T.: *Nat. Cancer Inst. Monographs 12*:189, 1963.
122. Peyre, A., Ravault, J. P., et al.: *C. R. Soc. Biol.* (Paris) *162*:1592, 1968.
123. Asano, M., Karizaki, S., et al.: *J. Urol. 106*:248, 1971.
124. Lawrence, A. M., and Landau, R. L.: *Endocrinology 77*:1119, 1965.
125. Farnsworth, W. E., In *Some Aspects of the Activity and Biochemistry of Prostatic Cancer*. Third Tenovus Workshop. Griffiths, K., and Pierrepoint, C. G. (eds.). Cardiff, Livingstone, 1970.
126. *Vital Statistics of the United States*. Vol. II, Part A, 1966, p. 1.
127. Goodwin, D. A., Rasmussen-Tasdal, D. S., et al.: *J. Urol. 69*:152, 1961.
128. Nesbit, R. M., and Baum, W. C.: *J.A.M.A. 143*:1317, 1950.
129. Emmett, O. L., Greene, L. F., et al.: *Brit. J. Urol. 83*:471, 1960.
130. Nesbit, R. M., and Plumb, R. T.: *J. Urol. 89*:236, 1963.
131. Veterans Administration Cooperative Urological Research Group: *Surg. Gynec. Obstet. 124*:1011, 1967.
132. Schirmer, H. K. A., Murphy, G. P., et al.: *Urol. Digest 4*:15, 1965.
133. Scott, W. W., and Vermeulen, C.: *J. Clin. Endocr. 2*:450, 1942.
134. Sciarra, F., Sorcini, G., et al.: *Clin. Endocr. 2*:101, 1973.
135. Mellinger, G. T.: *Surg. Clin. N. Amer. 45*:1413, 1965.

136. Young, H. H., II, and Kent, J. R.: *J. Urol. 99*:788, 1968.
137. Brendler, H., and Prout, G.: *Cancer Chemother. Rep. 16*:323, 1962.
138. Scott, W. W., and Schirmer, H. K. A.: *Trans. Amer. Ass. Genitourin. Surg. 58*:54, 1966.
139. Giller, J., Fruchtman, B., et al.: *Cancer Chemother. Rep. 51*:51, 1967.
140. Murphy, P., Reynoso, G., et al.: *J. Urol. 105*:817, 1971.
141. Scott, W. W., and Schirmer, H. K. A., In *On Cancer and Hormones: Essays in Experimental Biology.* Boyland, E., et al. (eds.), Chicago, University of Chicago Press, 1962, p. 175.
142. Maddy, J. A., Winterinitz, W. W., et al.: *Cancer 28*:322, 1971.
143. Prout, G. R., and Brewer, W. R.: *Cancer 20*:1871, 1967.
144. Korenchevsky, V., and Ross, M. A.: *Brit. Med. J. 1*:645, 1940.
145. Bullock, L. P., Bardin, C. W., et al.: *Biochem. Biophys. Res. Commun. 44*:1537, 1971.
146. Kirkman, H.: *Nat. Cancer Inst. Monographs,* No. 1, Washington, D.C., U. S. Government Printing Office, 1959.
147. Horning, E. S., and Whittick, J. W.: *Brit. J. Cancer 8*:451, 1954.
148. Horning, E. S.: *Brit. J. Cancer 10*:678, 1956.
149. Bloom, H. J. G., Dukes, C. E., et al.: *Brit. J. Cancer 17*:611, 1963.
150. Bloom, H. J. G., Roe, F. J. C., et al.: *Cancer 20*:2118, 1967.
151. Wagle, D. G., and Scal, D.: *J. Surg. Oncol. 2*:23, 1970.
152. Bloom, H. J. G.: *Brit. J. Cancer 25*:250, 1971.
153. Samuels, M. L., Sullivan, P., et al.: *Cancer 22*:525, 1968.
154. Talley, R. W., Moorhead, E. L., et al.: *J.A.M.A. 207*:322, 1969.
155. Paine, C. H., Wright, F. W., et al.: *Brit. J. Cancer 24*:277, 1970.
156. Wagle, D. G., and Murphy, G. P.: *Cancer 28*:318, 1971.
157. Gordon, G. G., Southren, S. L., et al.: *J. Clin. Endocr. 30*:449, 1970.

CHAPTER 29

The Endocrinologic Manifestations of the Carcinoid Tumor

By Kenneth L. Melmon

INTRODUCTION

Carcinoid tumors long have been known to be composed of enterochromaffin cells. These cells, which contain granules and often have an affinity for silver salts (argentaffin cells), normally are found throughout the gastrointestinal tract, bronchus, gallbladder, and ducts of the pancreas. They are called Kulchitsky cells. Although their physiologic role is poorly understood, they are innervated cells that contain several biologically active substances (19). Wherever Kulchitsky cells are found, a high concentration of serotonin (5-hydroxytryptamine) is often detected. The cells are identified in various tissues by a specific formaldehyde-induced fluorescence test (157) and appear to give rise to all of the carcinoid tumors in a variety of locations (203). Although widely scattered throughout the body, the cells apparently have a common embryologic origin. Because of this common cellular origin, Williams and Sandler have classified carcinoid tumors on the basis of the original location of the cell of the primary tumor (203). The ileal carcinoid tumor (most frequent of the group) is derived from midgut cells and contains a high concentration of 5-hydroxytryptamine. The tumor is associated with the classical carcinoid syndrome. On the other hand, carcinoid tumors arising from the hindgut, especially the rectum, have different staining characteristics from their midgut relatives, only very rarely contain serotonin, and have not been associated with a syndrome related to hormone release (144). Carcinoid tumors derived from cells of the foregut (bronchial, pancreatic, duodenal, and gallbladder areas) are particularly interesting. Cells from this area contain only small amounts of serotonin; since there is often high urinary excretion of 5-HIAA (5-hydroxyindole acetic acid) in patients with the tumor, however, a rapid release of synthesized amine is indicated. The tumors are able to make a variety of hormones and are frequently associated with atypical carcinoid syndromes (Table 29–1).

The endocrine potential of carcinoid tumors was not recognized until 1953, when Lembeck discovered that they contained large amounts of serotonin (5-hydroxytryptamine) (105). Almost simultaneously, three independent investigating teams defined a syndrome associated with the presence of malignant carcinoid tumors of the ileum. The most prominent features included flushes, bronchial constriction, lesions of the valves of the heart, and diarrhea, not all of which could be due to serotonin (190). It is now known that these tumors can produce histamine, catecholamines, prostaglandins, vasoactive peptides, and more complex pep-

*The original studies reported here were supported in part by USPHS Grants HL–09964, GM–01791, GM–16496, and a special fellowship 1-FO-HL-50,244-01.

TABLE 29–1. CHARACTERISTICS OF CARCINOID TUMORS DERIVED FROM DIFFERENT EMBRYONIC DIVISIONS OF THE GUT

	Foregut	Midgut	Hindgut
Histologic structure	Tendency to be trabecular; may differ widely from classical pattern	Characteristic	Tendency to be trabecular
Argentaffin and diazo reactions	Usually negative	Positive	Often negative
Association with the carcinoid syndrome	Frequent	Frequent	None
Tumor 5-HT content	Low	High	Not detected
Urinary 5-HIAA	High	High	Normal
5-HTP secretion	Frequent	Rare	Not detected
Metastases into bone (usually osteoblastic) and skin	Common	Unusual	Common
Association with other endocrine secretion	Frequent	Not described	Not described

5-HT, 5-hydroxytryptamine; 5-HIAA, 5-hydroxyindole acetic acid; 5-HTP, 5-hydroxytryptophan.

tides similar to, if not identical with, adrenocorticotropic hormone, melanocyte stimulating hormone, calcitonin, and insulin.

The spectrum of pharmacologically active substances produced by the tumor can be related to the pathogenesis of different manifestations of the syndrome (178). It is known that 5-hydroxytryptamine is not the only agent which produces manifestations of the carcinoid syndrome and that the syndrome in any patient at any given time is the sum of effects of the active substances being elaborated by the tumor. In addition, tumors that arise in primary sites other than the small intestine may produce characteristic syndromes distinct from the classic carcinoid syndrome.

CLASSIC CARCINOID SYNDROME

Morbid Anatomy

The primary tumor is usually derived from the enterochromaffin cells of the midgut and is located most frequently in the terminal ileum (Fig. 29–1). The tumor can be as small as a few millimeters in diameter and rarely is large enough to produce symptoms of intestinal obstruction (Fig. 29–2). The tumor is usually yellow and firm and consists of regularly dispersed epithelial cells with little evidence of mitosis, surrounded by well-defined fibrous borders (Fig. 29–3). The epithelial cells frequently contain intracellular granules that stain with silver salts. The average period of time before a primary tumor metastasizes is unknown, but it has been estimated that 38 per cent of extra-appendicular tumors, or approximately 1–6 per cent of all carcinoid tumors, spread (117, 138, 167). Metastatic lesions first involve the mesenteric lymph nodes and then the liver (Fig. 29–4). The right lobe of the liver, which receives most of the venous drainage of the ileum, enlarges more frequently than does the left lobe. With only a single possible exception (66, 71), the carcinoid syndrome does not appear until after metastases

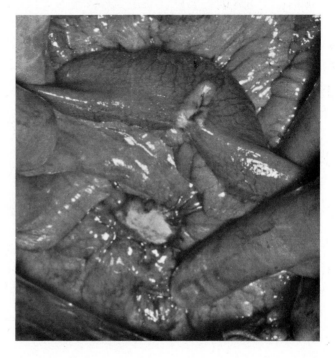

Figure 29–1. A primary ileal carcinoid tumor that has already metastasized to a regional mesenteric lymph node.

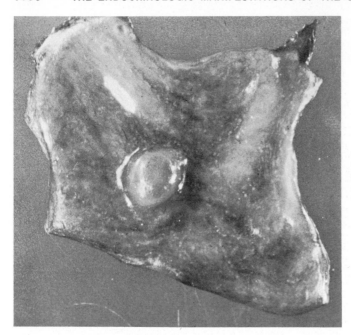

Figure 29–2. A typical primary ileal lesion that was only 3 mm. in diameter and was not located until the bowel was examined carefully during autopsy. Although the tumor was quite small, it had metastasized extensively to the peritoneum and liver (Figs. 29–3 and 29–4).

have occurred in the liver and biochemical substances produced by the tumor can bypass the portal circulation. The metastatic lesions are confined most commonly to the abdominal cavity.

Cutaneous lesions associated with the carcinoid syndrome include *telangiectasia of the skin* over the cheeks and the bridge of the nose. Mast cells sometimes infiltrate the area of telangiectasia (184). However, since human mast cells contain no serotonin, the substance cannot be incriminated in a pathogenetic relationship between the mast cells and the telangiectasia.

The *lesions of the heart* are confined to the endocardial surface and are highly specific (163).

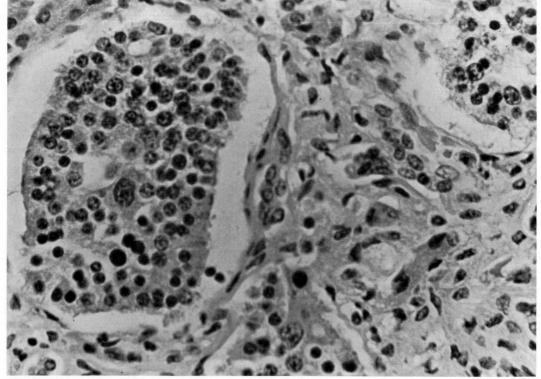

Figure 29–3. Carcinoid tumor illustrated in Figure 29–2. Nests of evenly dispersed epithelial cells are surrounded by bands of fibrous tissue. This tumor was argentaffin-negative but produced and contained large amounts of serotonin. (Hematoxylin and eosin stain, original magnification × 340.)

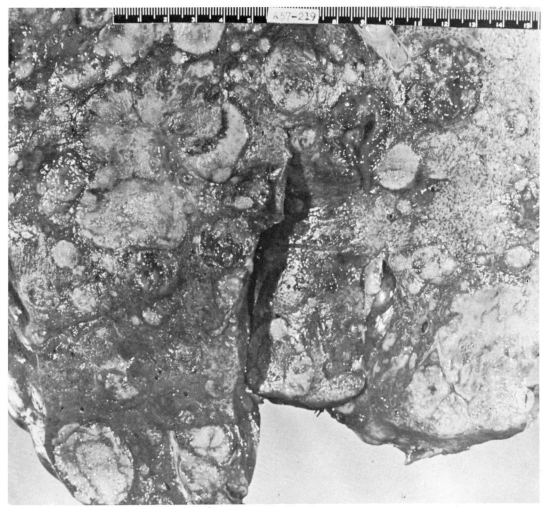

Figure 29-4. A carcinoid tumor which has metastasized from the ileal primary tumor (shown in Fig. 29–2) to the liver. Despite massive replacement of liver parenchyma, hepatic function was normal by usual parameters.

Collagenous deposits are most prominent in the chambers of the right side and often extend to the intima of the great veins and arteries. The deposits may involve the valve leaflets and chordae tendineae and may produce valvular stenosis or insufficiency. While the tricuspid and pulmonic lesions are most prominent, the subendocardium of the chambers on the left side can be affected and may become clinically important when an atrial septal defect with right-to-left shunting is present (79, 163). The myocardium is separated from the fibrotic process by the intact internal elastic membrane, the limiting feature which makes the lesion quite specific (Fig. 29–5). Severe fibrotic lesions in other areas of the body have been reported with the carcinoid tumor. Lesions involving the *peritoneum and mesentery of the small bowel* resulting in extensive matting and fibrous adhesions may occur spontaneously (79) but usually follow abdominal surgery. These adhesions may be responsible for obstruction of the intestine. Because they so characteristically follow any abdominal incisions, a surgeon must have especially good reasons for performing a laparotomy. Thirty-three of 49 small bowel obstructions were caused by fibrosis around the bowel after a surgical procedure which usually did not involve the bowel itself (138).

The location of the endocardial lesions suggests a circulating humoral substance as a mediator of the fibrosis. Administration of indole precursors of serotonin or serotonin alone (188) has not produced similar pathologic changes in rats. However, prolonged serotonin administration to tryptophan-deficient guinea pigs whose livers were damaged by a hepatotoxin was associated with proliferative fibroplasia of the endocardium (183). The conditions simulated the major biochemical abnormalities seen in patients with carcinoid tumors (i.e., excessive utilization of tryptophan for the production of serotonin by metastatic hepatic lesions). The pathogenetic role of other substances manufactured by the tumor which can produce fibrosis (histamine, prostaglandins, and bradykinin) has not been evaluated.

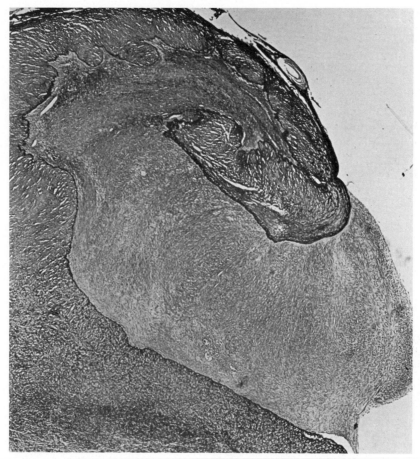

Figure 29–5. The collagenous deposit on the pulmonary valve of a patient with carcinoid syndrome is separated from the muscular tissue by the intact internal elastic membrane. (Hematoxylin and eosin stain, original magnification × 100.)

Clinical Features

Most symptoms of the syndrome are a result of the pharmacologic or endocrinologic effects of the tumor, not its size or its replacement of normal tissues. While there is a distinct complex of symptoms which constitutes the complete syndrome, most patients have few or only one of these symptoms as an indication of the presence of tumor. Because the symptoms appear and disappear, and because the course of the disease is so long, the physician may care for a patient with "bizarre complaints" for several years before the true diagnosis is made.

The unique *vasomotor phenomena* are the most dramatic features of the carcinoid syndrome. They may develop gradually, and the only hint of disease may be slow development (over a year or two) of telangiectases associated with a chronic cyanotic hue over the blush area. Most patients, however, experience several cyanotic, tricolored, or bright red *flushes* over the face and upper chest. These may be caused by stimuli which activate the autonomic nervous system; i.e., anger, tension, severe exercise, sudden position change, or the Valsalva maneuver may predictably provoke a flush.

Indeed, administration of exogenous catecholamines (see Diagnosis) also may provoke flushes in these patients, as will ingestion of food and alcohol. Catecholamines and alcohol provoke flushes by indirect effects. Their actions are delayed for several seconds or minutes after injection or ingestion, respectively. The flush-provoking activity of the drugs is inhibited by alpha-adrenergic blocking agents (2, 3). Both the catecholamines and the alcohol work in part by the release of an enzyme (kallikrein) from the tumor which produces bradykinin from plasma substrates. The flushes may occur 20–30 times a day, last for minutes, and may be associated with a feeling of warmth, with perspiration, and on occasion with increased lacrimation and salivation. They may also be associated with remarkable hypotension, tachycardia, bronchial constriction, increased respiratory rate, increased gastrointestinal motility (borborygmus), and occasionally diarrhea. If flushes are prolonged, periorbital and facial edema as well as oliguria may occur.

The *pulmonary manifestations* of the syndrome are less frequently observed than early published work suggested (71). Hyperventilation may occur during the flush. Evidence of asthma may be present between flushes and exacerbated during them. Most frequently, however, patients do not have symptoms referable to the chest, and evidence of bronchial constriction is found only during flushing attacks. It is not at all unusual to find patients with no signs or symptoms of pulmonary disease. If bronchoconstriction does become a threatening symptom, therapeutic measures must be carefully considered. Intravenous catecholamines will usually exacerbate both the flush and the bronchoconstriction. Aerosol sprays of isoproterenol may be sparingly employed to distribute the drug to the affected area in reasonable concentrations. By such a route, the amount reaching the peripheral circulation is minimized and usually insufficient to continue the old flush or initiate a new one.

Cardiac manifestations of the syndrome may be of two varieties. The most prominent kind are associated with stenosis or insufficiency of the pulmonary or tricuspid valves. These lesions can lead to intractable right-sided congestive heart failure. The presence of collagen deposits immediately beneath other areas of the endocardium usually is not apparent clinically. If there is evidence of mitral or aortic valve disease, the possibility of an atrial septal defect with right-to-left shunting of blood, a bronchial carcinoid with direct venous drainage to the left side of the heart, or acquired or congenital valvular defects unrelated to the carcinoid tumor should be considered (163). In addition to the anatomical abnormalities of the heart, a high cardiac output at rest has been recorded in patients with flushing. This functional abnormality does not seem to be related to an excess of serotonin but has been attributed to the release of a vasodilator substance (perhaps bradykinin) by the tumor (171).

The *gastrointestinal symptoms* may represent the most debilitating aspect of the carcinoid syndrome. Probably the most common initial complaint is abdominal discomfort and frequent diarrheal stools. There is considerable evidence that serotonin is the mediator of the diarrhea and intestinal hypermotility. Serotonin is found mainly in two areas of the body, the gastrointestinal tract and the brain. (It is also present in high concentration in the lungs and platelets.) In the gut and brain, the amine is synthesized and stored in nerve endings (27, 193). When the preganglionic myenteric nerves are stimulated, the serotonin is released as a neurotransmitter (27, 36, 40). That specific serotoninergic nerves also exist in the brain has recently been established (193). The nerves are not part of the adrenergic system, and they specifically take up and release serotonin (63, 97, 98). Any degenerative lesion of the nerves (either physical or chemical [e.g., by a drug, 6-hydroxytryptamine, which works by being specifically transported into serotoninergic nerves and selectively destroying them (14, 15)]) results in a major depletion of the stores of serotonin. In the gut, serotonin seems to have a role in peristalsis and perhaps absorption of fats.

Serotonin is released into the venous effluent of the normal intestine when the serosal surface is scratched, when acetylcholine is administered intra-arterially, or when intraluminal pressure is increased (30). Evidence that the amine reaches specific receptors in various tissues is developing (6, 7, 102, 152, 187), but there are few data regarding its second messenger. In the gut, serotonin may reduce the threshold of excitation of mucosal sensory nerve endings, so that a lower than usual increase in intraluminal pressure will be sufficient to elicit a peristaltic reflex (28, 85, 153). The amine also directly stimulates an increase in the tone and motility of the small intestine (82, 145) and inhibits the motility of the stomach and colon (17, 57, 83). The pattern of diarrhea in patients with the carcinoid syndrome is quite consistent with the effects of serotonin (136). It would be important to know whether the stores of serotonin in the specific serotoninergic neurons of the gut are expanded in patients with the carcinoid syndrome. If they are, normal stimulation of the nerves would result in exaggerated release and effects of serotonin. Thus the amine could produce effects on the gut whether or not it was released from the tumor into blood. An analogy with the pheochromocytoma seems appropriate: the pheochromocytoma slowly releases catecholamines into the blood. The amines are taken up into usable stores of the adrenergic nerve endings as one process of biologic inactivation. The stores in the nerve thus are expanded, and more catecholamines can be released following normal or pharmacologic (e.g., tyramine or glucagon) stimulation of the nerves. Stores of serotonin are expanded in platelets in patients with the carcinoid syndrome. It would be logical to assume that stores are also expanded in other sites (43) wherever active transport mechanisms for the indolamines are found.

Indirect pharmacologic data also implicate serotonin in the mediation of diarrhea and perhaps the malabsorption found in a number of patients (50, 100, 132, 146). Agents which retard inactivation of serotonin (e.g., monoamine oxidase inhibitors) will increase diarrhea (93), while drugs which are pharmacologic antagonists of serotonin (e.g., methysergide) usually ameliorate the abdominal cramps, diarrhea, or malabsorption (132). In addition, parachlorophenylalanine, an effective inhibitor of the synthesis of serotonin, alleviates the diarrhea in patients with the carcinoid syndrome (52). The antagonists and inhibitors of the synthesis of serotonin do not decrease the other symptoms and signs of carcinoid syndrome—the flush, heart lesions, or asthma. During an acute flushing episode accompanied by hyperperistalsis, however, serotonin is released infrequently into the blood (164). Both bradykinin and prostaglandins (recently isolated from carcinoid tumors) are found in high concentration in the circulation during a flush (168). Both have direct pharmacologic effects on the gut and could contribute to changes in intestinal motility during acute flushes. Their role in intestinal motility of the carcinoid patient is not known.

There are two additional abdominal symptoms in patients with carcinoid syndrome:

1. The *acute abdominal "crisis"* (abdominal pain, fever, leukocytosis, and thrombocytosis) is

usually associated with necrosis of metastatic lesions in the liver. The pathogenesis of the necrosis is thought to be due to the tumor's outgrowing its blood supply. Indeed, the crisis can be precipitated by ligation of the hepatic artery, which has been done in some patients following hepatic artery perfusion with antitumor agents (143). The symptoms may be due to liberation of pharmacologically active substances by the metastasis and distention of the liver capsule by hemorrhage. The crisis may end with marked pulmonary complications (pleural effusions and pneumonia) secondary to immobilization and irritation of the diaphragm overlying the liver. These crises are often difficult to distinguish from true small bowel obstruction, which does not occur often unless there has been preceding abdominal surgery and sufficient time for development of fibrous adhesions. Spontaneous fibrosis also may produce small bowel obstruction or even retroperitoneal fibrosis (33, 78, 140). The peptic ulcer occurs with high incidence when the primary tumor is in the stomach (151).

2. *Deficiency syndromes* may develop in patients with the carcinoid syndrome. Normally, hydroxylation of tryptophan accounts for about 1 per cent of the dietary intake of the amino acid. If the tumors are sufficiently large, more than half the dietary tryptophan can be converted to serotonin, thereby diverting this amino acid from niacin and protein formation. Thus patients may have hypoalbuminemia and pellagra. Recently, questions have been raised as to whether diversion of 50 per cent of tryptophan into unusual pathways would be sufficient to cause pellagra (39, 128) and whether the only abnormality of tryptophan metabolism was represented by the increased synthesis of 5-hydroxytryptophan, serotonin, and their metabolites. Some 5,6-hydroxylated products of tryptophan and tryptamine have been found in normal animal tissues. They could conceivably produce biologic effects, but they have not been sought in normal man or patients with the carcinoid syndrome (106). Williams et al. have demonstrated, in 3 of 11 patients with biopsy-proven carcinoid tumor and some symptoms of the syndrome, that nonhydroxylated products of tryptophan can be abnormally elevated and could participate in both the shunt of tryptophan away from protein synthesis and its keinuremic pathway, and perhaps in the symptoms of the disease (204). These studies, still preliminary, indicated that when the three patients with unusual patterns of indole acid excretion were given tryptophan loads, the biochemical abnormality became pronounced, and during the loading, unusual psychological features, such as anxiety, depression, amnesia, and in one patient visual hallucinations, occurred. These psychological features were not seen in the other eight patients with classical increased 5-hydroxylated products but did mimic some of the spontaneous symptoms the three patients had previously described. A major function of this chapter is to present the multipotential qualities of the carcinoid tumor and the scientific and clinical drawbacks of concentrating on one obvious abnormality (e.g., excess serotonin production) and concluding

that it is responsible for all symptoms (69, 71, 72, 147). The data discussed above simply serve as an example of one of the many lessons in biochemistry, pharmacology, and endocrinology that the carcinoid tumor is likely to teach us.

Evidence of *hepatic insufficiency* is relatively rare in the carcinoid syndrome until extensive metastases have developed. Then hyperbilirubinemia, bleeding, hypoalbuminemia, and hepatic coma may occur. Like others suffering from neoplastic disease, patients with carcinoid tumors may become cachectic before death.

Perhaps abnormalities in *glucose tolerance and metabolism* were to be expected in the presence of the carcinoid tumor. The metastatic tumor grows to massive sizes. Some tumors of foregut origin (bronchial and pancreatic carcinoid tumors) have been suspected of producing ACTH and growth hormone and have recently been proven to contain and release insulin (1). Even an ileal tumor can make and inappropriately release enough insulin to cause symptomatic hypoglycemia. All the above factors could contribute to abnormal handling of glucose. Symptoms of hypoglycemia, unusual patterns of hunger and eating, or osmotic diuresis related to high blood glucose levels should be sought and objectively documented in patients with the carcinoid syndrome. During medical evaluation in three patients (two with ileal carcinoids and one with bronchial carcinoid) with symptoms of hypoglycemia and a craving for foods with high sugar content, we were surprised to find normal glucose tolerance and rates of glucose utilization. Further evaluation did little more to define the pathogenesis of the symptoms other than to reveal that the three patients had normal to low basal circulating levels of immunoreactive insulin (16). When challenged with an oral or intravenous glucose load, the K values of glucose disappearance were normal, *but* release of immunoreactive insulin was minimal or absent. Response of growth hormone was appropriate. Only a beginning of our understanding of these phenomena can be derived from available information. Serotonin may inhibit glucose-induced release of insulin (107) and perhaps contribute, in ill-defined ways, to maintenance of normal glucose concentrations in plasma (176). Whether these activities of serotonin are operating in these patients is as yet unknown. Even more puzzling is the possibility that the tumor may be making an unidentified noninsulin substance capable of promoting transport of glucose into tissues. Again, the carcinoid syndrome provides us with the challenge of understanding fundamental facts related to endocrinology.

Abnormal Chemistry and Pathogenesis

Serotonin Synthesis and Metabolism (Fig. 29-6)

Although carcinoid tumors differ widely in their ability to produce or store serotonin, the excessive production of 5-hydroxytryptamine (serotonin) remains their most characteristic chemical abnor-

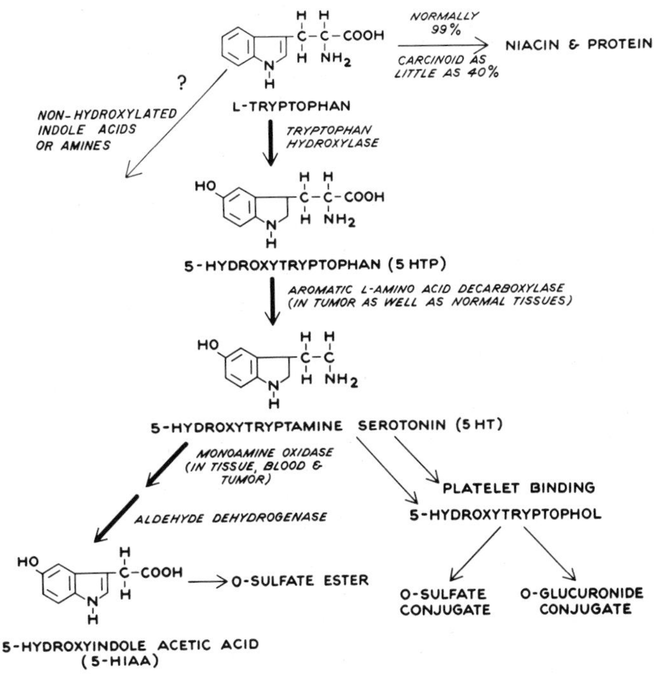

Figure 29-6. Metabolism of tryptophan in a patient with carcinoid syndrome. Heavy arrows indicate the shunting of tryptophan away from its usual metabolic pathway to form niacin and protein. Heavy arrows leading from serotonin show the major metabolites of serotonin excreted in the urine. Several gastric and some bronchial tumors lack aromatic-L-amino acid decarboxylase and release large amounts of 5-hydroxytryptophan into the blood. Metabolites in the urine then include 5-hydroxytryptophan, 5-hydroxytryptamine, and less 5-hydroxyindole acetic acid than is expected.

mality. The production of serotonin depends upon hydroxylation of the amino acid tryptophan to form 5-hydroxytryptophan. Tryptophan hydroxylase has only recently been isolated from tumors and normal animal tissues, including the brain stem, pineal gland, and liver of the rat, dog, cow, and mouse, and the mouse mast-cell tumor (113, 114, 115). The enzyme was difficult to isolate as it was sometimes confused with phenylalanine hydroxylase, but it has been well characterized (115). It appears to originate from either the cell cytoplasm or the mitochondria and has an absolute requirement for oxygen, a reduced pteridine, and ferrous iron. In most preparations, the K_m for the substrate is reasonably low (3×10^{-4} to 4×10^{-5}), but it has been characterized as responsible for the rate-limiting step in the synthesis of serotonin and melatonin. The enzymatic production of 5-hydroxytryptophan can be accelerated by increasing substrate availability (55) and inhibited by either norepinephrine or phenylalanine (115).

There is no feedback inhibition of tryptophan hydroxylase by serotonin as there is of tyrosine hydroxylase by norepinephrine (111). There is a complex relationship between the turnover rates of serotonin and norepinephrine, however (10, 54, 173, 211). Generally speaking, it is inverse: when catecholamine synthesis decreases or stores of catecholamines are depleted, the synthesis rate of serotonin increases and the amine accumulates. Since the rate of serotonin synthesis is dependent on tryptophan availability, diet and the state of liver function may substantially influence serotonin synthesis (56, 191). The unusual mental symptoms in some patients with carcinoid tumors perhaps may be explained by their diets or by the relative availability in the brain of substrate for tryptophan hydroxylase. Perhaps the functional states of the circulation or the liver can alter distribution of an amino acid to various parts of the central nervous system so as to alter significantly the synthesis of serotonin.

The fact that phenylalanine inhibits tryptophan hydroxylase in the majority of tissues in which the enzyme is found is clinically important (115). In fact, the reason for the low rates of synthesis of 5-hydroxytryptophan in liver preparations apparently is that the liver enzyme is phenylalanine hydroxylase and not tryptophan hydroxylase. Derivatives of phenylalanine have been synthesized, and not surprisingly they inhibit tryptophan hydroxylase. The inhibition is noncompetitive and involves inactivation of the enzyme. It also is associated with decreased levels of serotonin in brain and decreased rates of synthesis. One derivative has been used clinically to inhibit serotonin synthesis (41, 52, 169, 177). Although it decreases the diarrhea in patients with the carcinoid syndrome, it also induces psychiatric effects, implying that serotonin deficiency in the brain may in part be responsible for some affective illnesses. The drug also inhibits phenylalanine hydroxylase in vivo, resulting in substantial rises in concentrations of serum phenylalanine (186). Whether the phenylalanine itself contributes to any of the effects of parachlorophenylalanine is not known.

Besides diet, liver function, and general availability of tryptophan to the enzyme, other factors participate in regulation of serotonin synthesis. Psychological stress increases the rate of both synthesis and metabolism of serotonin in the brain (200); the serotonin-associated physiologic events that accompany stress seem dependent on a small portion of the total pool, predominantly the portion most recently synthesized (67, 70, 73). It is likely that stress or midbrain stimulation induces synthesis of tryptophan hydroxylase, accounting for the rapid synthesis rates (49). Serotonin synthesis in the pineal gland has a circadian rhythm that is dependent on the amount of light that the animal can visually appreciate (11, 182) (Ch. 13). The serotonin thus synthesized has important relationships to a number of endocrine functions, including secretion of luteinizing hormone (210) and the circadian rhythm of 17-hydroxycorticoids (103).

Effects of Drugs

A number of drugs also affect the synthesis, action, or metabolism of serotonin. Reserpine depletes serotonin from a variety of tissue stores in the same manner as it affects stores of norepinephrine and dopamine (see Ch. 5, Part II) (189). Monoamine oxidase inhibitors promote retention of amine and expansion of amine stores in a variety of tissues. Lithium can either increase or decrease the turnover rate of serotonin in various areas of the brain (86); morphine also seems to affect serotonin synthesis and metabolism. Tolerance to morphine may be related to its effects on serotonin synthesis (120, 174, 207). Chlorpromazine, which has a profound effect on transport and synthesis of catecholamines, appears to block the peripheral effects of serotonin [i.e., it may prevent serotonin action in the same way that adrenergic blocking agents inhibit the effects of catecholamines on effector organs (68)].

Central Nervous System and Serotonin

During studies in animals of the drugs that altered the production, stores, and metabolism of serotonin, many pharmacologic effects observed began to be linked to serotonin (142). We now realize that the physiologic functions of serotonin go far beyond its activity on blood vessels, inflammatory processes, the lung, and the heart (26, 75, 153, 199). Serotonin deprival states were induced in laboratory animals with parachlorophenylalanine; they were associated with affective disorders, retardation of passive-avoidance learning, suppression of rapid eye movements during sleep, and increases in sexual activity (46, 177, 185). In man, serotonin is strongly indicated as an influence in the central nervous system on a variety of behavioral patterns including sleep, perception of pain, arousal, emotionality, and social behavior (20, 29, 92, 112, 126).

Although serotonin does not cross the blood-brain barrier, factors in the periphery may influence the brain. If, for example, tryptophan is shunted from normal pathways in the periphery, less amino acid than usual will reach the brain; this may occur in patients with the carcinoid tumor. Since synthesis is so dependent on availability of substrate, a relative depletion of serotonin in the brain may result. Parachlorophenyl-

alanine treatment could yield the same effect, parachlorophenylalanine reduces serotonin synthesis in both the brain and periphery. Chlorpromazine may block the central as well as the peripheral effects of serotonin. No doubt more attention should be directed to the mental symptoms in patients with the carcinoid syndrome. If necessary, drugs might be designed to selectively alter specific organ function by altering local serotonin turnover.

Metabolism of Serotonin

The 5-hydroxytryptophan produced by tryptophan hydroxylase is stereospecific and has a high affinity (K_m 2×10^{-5}) for aromatic-L-amino acid decarboxylase (74). This enzyme converts 5-hydroxytryptophan to 5-hydroxytryptamine. Of the indoles produced by the tumor, serotonin seems to be the most pharmacologically active. It may be metabolized by the enzyme, monoamine oxidase, in the tumor (in which case it produces little pharmacologic effect) or in the blood after release from the tumor. Serotonin is oxidized to 5-hydroxyindole acetaldehyde, which is converted to 5-hydroxyindole acetic acid by aldehyde dehydrogenase. Small amounts of circulating serotonin are inactivated by ATP-dependent binding to platelets or by conversion to the alcohol, 5-hydroxytryptophol, or its conjugates, 5-hydroxytryptophol-O-sulfate and 5-hydroxytryptophol-O-glucuronide. Most of the 5-hydroxyindole acetic acid is excreted in the urine as the free acid, although small amounts may be conjugated to the O-sulfate ester before excretion. Patients with the syndrome usually have an expanded pool of serotonin (179), a twofold to tenfold increase in blood and platelet concentrations of serotonin, and elevations of 5-hydroxyindole acetic acid in the urine.

It is important to note that some patients with the "carcinoid syndrome" do not have elevations of urinary 5-hydroxyindole acetic acid (108). In contrast, patients with carcinoid tumors but without the syndrome may have marked urinary elevations of the acid (197). The absence of symptoms during excessive 5-hydroxyindole acetic acid excretion may indicate that the metabolism of serotonin is occurring within the tumor substance and that only biologically inactive metabolites are being released from the tumor. Conversely, it is possible that a tumor could rapidly produce and release critical amounts of amine only at the times symptoms are caused. If the tumor sporadically releases serotonin but does not metabolize or release oxidation products of serotonin, the total urinary 5-hydroxyindole acetic acid over a day should be minimally elevated or even normal. An analogous situation was discussed in Chapter 5, Part II. Even very small pheochromocytomas may produce symptoms without elevating urinary excretion of the metabolites of catecholamines. In such an instance, the turnover of catecholamines is rapid, little amine is bound or metabolized in the tumor, and sufficient amine is released from the tumor to create symptoms. The only abnormality associated with the symptoms is an elevated concentration of amines but not their metabolites, either in blood or urine.

Urinary serotonin is not routinely measured in patients with carcinoid syndrome. We do not know whether symptoms in patients with normal urinary 5-HIAA are associated with changes in urinary serotonin. When serotonin is released from the tumor into the blood, the severity of the gastrointestinal aspects of the syndrome frequently correlates with the quantity of the amine produced.

Other Amines and the Carcinoid Tumor

Other amines have been found in the urine of carcinoid patients. Histamine excretion is frequently and consistently elevated in patients with gastric carcinoid tumors and inconsistently elevated in patients with ileal tumors. Available evidence in these patients indicates that the amine is not made in mast cells and is most often seen in tumors which lack aromatic-L-amino acid decarboxylase, i.e., gastric and bronchial carcinoids (147, 151). Urinary catecholamines and their metabolites also have been elevated in some patients with the carcinoid syndrome (194). This abnormality is unusual and has not been correlated with specific symptoms or tumor locations.

Mediators of the Flush and Bradykinin

Evidence indicates that serotonin is not the only biologically active substance mediating the flush in the carcinoid syndrome: (1) Intravenous injection of 5-hydroxytryptamine does not reproduce the typical spontaneous attacks of flushing in carcinoid patients (109, 147, 154, 164). (2) There is little correlation between free plasma 5-hydroxytryptamine levels and flushing episodes (108). (3) Although the infusion of epinephrine or norepinephrine provokes typical flushing attacks, it is not often accompanied by elevation of 5-hydroxytryptamine in the blood from either the hepatic vein or the brachial artery (155, 164). (4) The carcinoid syndrome with flushing is not always accompanied by elevations of 5-hydroxyindole acetic acid excretion (44). (5) Metastatic carcinoid tumors can be present without the syndrome, even though

elevations of 5-hydroxyindole acetic acid excretion occur (197).

Recent data implicate a group of vasodilator peptides among the mediators of the flush in some patients with carcinoid syndrome (148, 209). Kinins (lysyl-bradykinin and bradykinin) are produced by the action of the enzyme kallikrein on an α_2-globulin substrate kininogen (Fig. 29–7) (134, 161, 162). Kallikrein is normally found as an inactive enzyme in plasma and in many tissues including the gut (38, 62, 205). The kallikrein in plasma is chemically distinct from kallikreins derived from other tissues. Activation of plasma kallikrein usually depends on activation of either a component of the clotting system or critical components of complement, or upon some unusual functions of the granulocyte (38, 94, 124, 205). Plasma kallikrein probably has nothing to do with production of kinin in patients with the carcinoid syndrome.

In tissues such as the submaxillary gland, kallikrein appears to be stored in granules (62). In the same granules, or at least in similar cells, renin-like activity has also been found. The activation of glandular kallikrein is not well understood. Since it exists in granules, it is likely that a secretory process is involved, but whether this depends on exocytosis is not known. The enzyme can be released by hormones such as catecholamines. It has recently been implicated in dissimilar dysfunctions such as hypertension (118), the dumping syndrome (58), reactions to antilymphocytic globulin (22), and after gastric surgery (42).

The peptides produced by kallikrein are potent vasodilators, they may release catecholamines from nerve endings and they have been implicated by many studies as mediators of various aspects of the inflammatory process (135, 166, 175). They normally are present in plasma in concentrations of less than 2.5 ng./ml. and have a half-life of only seconds (127). Because kallikrein is present normally in gut tissue which gives rise to the carcinoid tumor, and because it may be released by catecholamines which also may provoke a flush, the role of kinins in the carcinoid flush was investigated. When synthetic bradykinin was infused rapidly into patients with the carcinoid syndrome, the resultant flush closely mimicked spontaneous flushes (59, 149). Bradykinin was elevated in the hepatic venous blood of some patients during spontaneous and epinephrine-induced flushes (150). Tumors from patients with the carcinoid syndrome

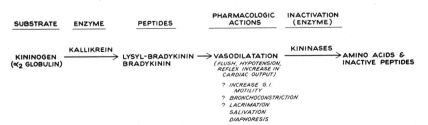

Figure 29–7. Kinin production and destruction in the human. The pharmacologic actions listed have been produced by kinins in man and other species. The role of the kinins in the carcinoid syndrome is related to vasodilatation in some patients. Their role in other symptoms of the syndrome is pharmacologically possible but as yet is unproven.

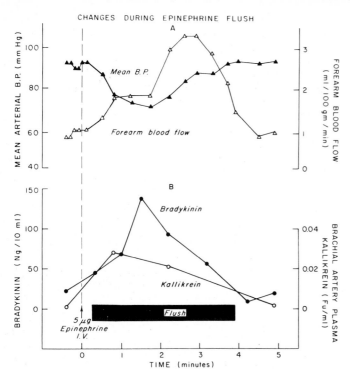

Figure 29-8. Serial determination of mean arterial pressure (B.P.) (solid triangles) and forearm blood flow (open triangles), top panel (*A*), and of bradykinin (closed circles) and kallikrein (open circles), bottom panel (*B*), before and after injection of epinephrine into a patient with carcinoid syndrome. The subnormal control values for forearm blood flow are compatible with the fact that the patient was in congestive heart failure. (From Mason, D. T., and Melmon, K. L.: *J. Clin. Invest.* *45*:1691, 1966.)

and prominent flushing have been extracted, and most contained a type of tissue kallikrein (130). These results have been broadly confirmed (2, 61, 121, 181). In addition, kallikrein has been located in a carcinoid tumor by immunofluorescent techniques (12). Finally, in several patients who flush, the release of kallikrein has correlated with production of the flush, increase in forearm blood flow, and decrease in systemic arterial pressure (Fig. 29-8) (2, 121, 122, 181).

It is now believed that the flush in any given patient with the carcinoid syndrome is caused by a variety of biologically active substances (159), among which are lysyl-bradykinin and bradykinin. From available data, it would appear that the flush-provoking stimuli, such as epinephrine, sympathetic discharge, and alcohol ingestion, liberate kallikrein from the tumor (Fig. 29-9). The mechanisms causing the liberation are not known. Once in the blood, kallikrein splits lysyl-bradykinin from kininogen. The lysyl-bradykinin is rapidly converted to bradykinin by a plasma aminopeptidase. Both lysyl-bradykinin and bradykinin are capable of producing profound vasodilatation, systemic hypotension, edema, and tachycardia and an increase in salivation, lacrimation, and cardiac output.

In addition, in some species the kinins are bronchial constrictors and, as mediators of inflammation, may participate in fibrosis. It is conceivable that they may be contributing to the asthma and increased fibrosis that occur in patients with the carcinoid syndrome.

Just as serotonin is not likely to be the only mediator of the flush, there is evidence that bradykinin is not either. The most convincing evidence

is from three separate laboratories including our own: abnormally high concentrations of bradykinin cannot be detected in the venous blood of every patient who has a carcinoid flush. In addition, substances such as histamine and prostaglandin can be released from some tumors and certainly are capable of influencing a carcinoid flush. Possibly not all the vasoactive agents in a given flush come from the actual tumor; excesses of one

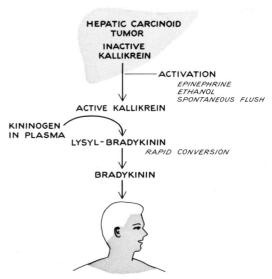

Figure 29-9. Summary of present concepts by which kallikrein and kinins may contribute to the carcinoid flush. The flush mechanism, however, is complex; in some patients, kinin levels are normal. (From *Physiol. Pharmacol. Physicians, 1*:6, 1966.)

substance may act to release other hormones from normal tissues. Thus prostaglandin can be released from kidney by the direct action of bradykinin (125). Knowing the particular chemical abnormality responsible for a flush in any given patient may be critical in designing effective therapy.

Additional Biologically Active Compounds Produced by or Associated with the Tumor

There is more than suggestive evidence that carcinoid tumors may be ectopic sites of ACTH production (23, 25, 95, 170). Such tumors produce a syndrome similar to Cushing's syndrome and are usually in sites other than the ileum. To date, the only tumors actually found to contain the ACTH substance [by bioassay (80) and immunofluorescence studies (90)] were carcinoids unassociated with a syndrome. The carcinoid tumor can produce and release insulin, and the syndrome may appear concomitantly with other tumors of the pancreas that release a substance with insulin-like activity (48, 180). The carcinoid tumor also may be associated with pluriglandular adenomatosis, type I (parathyroid adenomas, pancreatic nonbeta islet-cell tumors, and pituitary adenomas) (202), and may be seen with acromegaly or with melanocyte-stimulating hormone production (80). Since these observations are relatively recent, it seems reasonable to assume, by analogy with other polypeptide hormone–producing neoplasms, that substances such as antidiuretic hormone, parathyroid hormone, erythrocyte-stimulating factor, or other vasodilatory peptides may also be produced by these tumors but have simply remained undetected to date. The precedent for the manufacture of some of these biologically active substances by other tumors, such as oat-cell carcinomas, cerebellar hemangioblastomas, and pheochromocytomas, has already been established (21).

The hormones produced at various ectopic sites are similar if not identical to the natural hormones made by normal tissues (21, 110) (Ch. 30). Hormone production appears to be a highly organized and biochemically economical function of tumor tissue. The question arises as to whether elements of normal endocrine glands have infiltrated or been mixed with the tumor tissues producing the ectopic hormones. Such an elaborate explanation depending upon mixing of cell types in order to produce unusual hormones in carcinoid tissue is equivocal and debatable (84).

The differentiation of cells is ultimately an expression of their genetic instructional material (76, 77). Any cells capable of division may theoretically develop any form or function within the range and competence of their genetic information. The inappropriate biochemical properties of carcinoid tumors may suggest that a large amount of genetic knowledge is retained in neoplastic cells and is derepressed in the process of autonomous control of growth, and that reactivation of latent information is relatively common in a variety of malignant tissues (201). The most direct evidence to support such an explanation comes from experiments in which normally nucleated intestinal epithelial cells of an adult frog were transplanted into enucleated eggs of *Xenopus laevis*. Normal adult frogs resulted. In addition, nearly normal tail-bud tadpoles can be produced by transplanting nuclei from renal adenocarcinoma cells to enucleated eggs of *Rana esculenta* (76, 77). Some argue that nuclei of differentiated somatic cells do not generally undergo restrictive changes that affect the genetic material itself (76, 77).

A variety of tumors, including carcinoma of the pancreas, nonbeta islet-cell carcinoma of the pancreas, oat-cell carcinoma of the lung, ovarian neoplasms, carcinoma of the gallbladder, and anaplastic carcinomas of unknown origin, may produce clinical syndromes resembling the carcinoid syndrome (64, 137). Most of these tumors produce typical flushes, and many patients have experienced diarrhea and bronchial constriction. At least two oat-cell carcinomas have been associated with the fibrous subendocardial lesions typical of carcinoid tumor (13). While these tumors frequently are associated with an increased production of 5-hydroxyindole acetic acid, few have demonstrated evidence of abnormal indole metabolism. Kallikrein activity has been found in at least one patient with oat-cell carcinoma of the bronchus (47). The discovery of additional biologically active substances that might be elaborated by these tumors is the object of current research. A number of the noncarcinoid, endocrine-active tumors have been examined by electronmicroscopy. Beusch and co-workers postulated the finding of Kulchitsky cells at least in the bronchial tumors (18). They concluded that, in the case of oat-cell carcinoma, some hormonal production could be under the control of "ectopically" placed Kulchitsky cells, and even went so far as to suggest that the bronchial carcinoid tumor is a more benign form of the oat-cell carcinoma.

There is no need to accept the pluripotential cell theory over the ectopic cell theory of unnatural hormone production. A reasonable and rational compromise has been proposed by Weichert (198). He suggests that the enterochromaffin cell system is derived from cells of the neuroectoderm, which probably migrate into the primitive alimentary tract during embryonic development. These neuroectodermal "stem" cells may migrate with endocrine glands developing from the embryonic foregut—the anterior pituitary, thyroid, parathyroid, and pancreatic islets. These cells may also form the chromaffin cell system of the adrenals and paraganglia, autonomic ganglia, and cells in the hypothalamus which produce the posterior pituitary hormones. Weichert suggests that ectopic hormone-producing tumors and tumors in the syndrome of multiple endocrine adenomatosis arise from cells with a common neuroectodermal embryonic precursor. Their capacity to synthesize a variety of peptide and amine hormones may be revealed as their genetic material is derepressed during tumor formation.

The precise role of each of the biologically active

substances produced by the carcinoid tumor in each instance is not well defined, but certainly serotonin is not the exclusive mediator of the symptoms of the carcinoid syndrome.

VARIANTS OF THE CLASSIC CARCINOID SYNDROME

Deviations from the classic syndrome include (1) unusual syndromes associated with a carcinoid tumor in a location other than the small bowel (Table 29–2), and (2) syndromes resembling the classic carcinoid syndrome but caused by a heterogeneous group of neoplasms that have no histologic relation to carcinoid tumor (described above). Variant forms of the carcinoid syndrome may sometimes be managed with specific medical therapy.

The Gastric Carcinoid Tumor (151)

The gastric carcinoid syndrome is distinguished from the classic syndrome by the pattern of flushes. They are patchy and extend over the face and neck to the arms, trunk, and legs. The flush has a geographic distribution with sharply delineated serpentine borders (Fig. 29–10). The patches of discoloration will become confluent if the attacks last long enough. Characteristic production of large amounts of histamine may contribute to the geographic pattern of the flushes. The excessive histamine may also be responsible for the increased production of gastric acid and hence peptic ulcers in these patients. Other gastrointestinal symptoms are less common in these patients, whose primary tumor is in the stomach, than in patients with the classic lesion.

In addition to fairly consistent increases in urinary histamine, the pattern of excretion of indoles can be distinct for the patient with gastric carcinoid syndrome. The tumor usually lacks aromatic-L-amino acid decarboxylase and consequently releases unconverted 5-hydroxytryptophan rather than serotonin into the blood, thus causing normal platelet serotonin values and increased urinary 5-hydroxytryptophan. A portion of the 5-hydroxytryptophan is decarboxylated in the kidney, resulting in elevated urinary serotonin and a concomitant decrease in the fraction of indoles (to less than 90 per cent of total urinary indoles) excreted as 5-hydroxyindole acetic acid since serotonin is not available for oxidation.

Oates and Sjoerdsma state that patients with gastric carcinoid are less likely to have cardiac lesions than are those with ileal tumors (151). Perhaps the decreased serotonin production is responsible for the absence of both prominent cardiac lesions and gastrointestinal symptoms. The decarboxylase inhibitor (alpha-methyldopa) can be therapeutically used to substantially diminish serotonin production in other parts of the body and is accompanied by less severe flushing episodes. This clinical response to alpha-methyldopa is unusual in patients with the classic carcinoid syndrome.

TABLE 29–2. COMPARATIVE FEATURES OF THE SYNDROME ASSOCIATED WITH PRIMARY CARCINOID TUMORS IN VARIOUS SITES

Features	Tumor Site		
	Ileal	*Gastric*	*Bronchial*
Flush	Brief, multiple, occurs over head and neck areas	Generalized, bright red, geographic distribution	Prolonged, severe, may include anxiety, tremulousness, periorbital and facial edema, lacrimation, salivation, diaphoresis, fever, and oliguria
Heart lesions	Right sided	May be rare	Frequently left-sided, with pulmonary edema during flushing
Metastases	Rarely beyond abdominal cavity	Rarely beyond abdominal cavity	Widespread metastases with osteoblastic bone lesions
Chemistry	Urinary 5-HIAA accounts for more than 90% indole products; elevation histamine inconstant	Tumor often lacks decarboxylase enzyme. Therefore, 5-HIAA may account for less than 90% of indoles and 5-HT and 5-HTP are frequently elevated. Urinary histamine is often continuously elevated	Often has large amounts of 5-HTP as well as 5-HIAA in urine
Association with other disorders	Rare	High frequency of peptic ulceration	High incidence of other endocrine disorders
Treatment	Determined by symptoms and specific chemical abnormalities	Aromatic-L-amino acid decarboxylase inhibitors may be helpful	Corticosteroids may have unique and dramatic effects on symptoms
Prognosis	Fair: 10–15 year survival not unusual	Fair	Very poor

5-HIAA, 5-hydroxyindole acetic acid; 5-HT, 5-hydroxytryptamine; 5-HTP, 5-hydroxytryptophan.

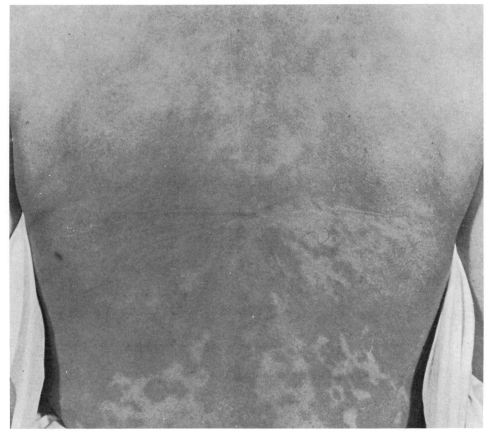

Figure 29–10. A generalized flush with geographic distribution and sharply delineated serpentine borders as seen in a patient with a gastric carcinoid tumor.

The Bronchial Carcinoid Tumor

The bronchial tumors produce the most striking clinical variants of the carcinoid spectrum and serve as the best example of the carcinoid tumor's multiple endocrine functions (131).

By far the most important clinical features that separate the bronchial syndrome from the ileal are the acute episodes of flushing. The flushes may be severe and prolonged, lasting as long as three or four days. They are often preceded by disorientation, anxiety, and tremulousness of the hands. They are associated with periorbital and facial edema and striking increases in lacrimation (Fig. 29–11, *A* and *B*), salivation, sweating, temperature, and heart rate. Nausea, vomiting, explosive diarrhea, dyspnea, and wheezing common to the flush period are usually totally absent between flushes. The flushes may be associated with profound hypotension, oliguria, and, if left-sided cardiac lesions are present, pulmonary edema. The attacks of pulmonary edema may be fatal. Other unusual and prominent features of the syndrome are the prevalence of mitral rather than pulmonic and tricuspid valve lesions and associated, seemingly unrelated disorders. For example, the increased incidence of Cushing's syndrome, pluriglandular adenomatosis, and acromegaly may be due to tropic proteins elaborated by the tumor itself or to the coexistence of other endocrine-producing tumors (see section on chemistry). The tumors may produce large amounts of 5-hydroxytryptophan as well as serotonin. The association of 5-hydroxyindole acetic acid excretion with an *asymptomatic* pulmonary "coin" lesion, discovered during routine roentgenologic examinations, has encouraged Warner et al. to suggest the use of 5-hydroxyindole acetic acid screening tests in these individuals (197).

Patients with bronchial carcinoids seem to have a poorer prognosis than do those with the usual carcinoid tumor. Widespread metastases are more common and include osteoblastic bone lesions and involvement of lymph nodes, heart, lungs, kidneys, gallbladder, pancreas, and adrenal and thyroid glands. However, these patients may respond dramatically to treatment with corticosteroids. Such treatment has permitted patients with regular and life-threatening flushes to remain asymptomatic for as long as two years. One patient first examined because of increased salivation and lacrimation, and later for severe flushes, was given a therapeutic trial of 15 mg. of prednisone a day. Because of her dramatic response to corticosteroids, the patient was suspected of having a bronchial carcinoid tumor, and a previously overlooked pulmonary

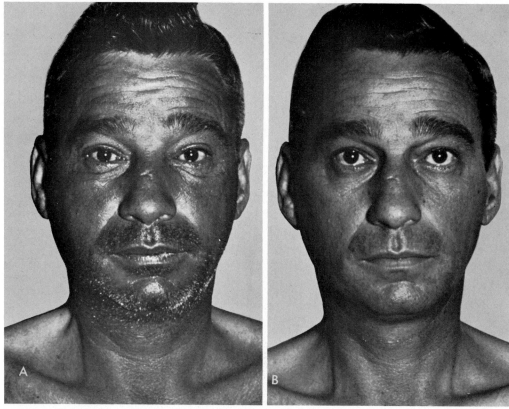

Figure 29-11. *A*, Appearance of patient during a severe and prolonged flush associated with a bronchial carcinoid tumor. Note the periorbital and facial edema, glistening of the eyes due to lacrimation, and parotid swelling. *B*, After recovery, patient appears normal and asymptomatic. (From Melmon, K. L., Sjoerdsma, A., et al.: *Amer. J. Med. 39*:568, 1965.)

density was then observed in chest roentgenograms. Several months later the patient died; an autopsy revealed the bronchial carcinoid tumor.

The reason for the dramatic response of patients with bronchial carcinoids to steroid therapy is not understood. For those patients who produce primarily the kinin peptides, preliminary but controversial evidence suggests that steroids may affect the kinin-generating system by either preventing kallikrein activation or kinin generation after activation (37). Perhaps the corticosteroids also affect prostaglandin release or activity.

DIAGNOSIS

General

When a patient has the fully developed clinical syndrome, the diagnosis may be easy. However, a patient seldom has all the features of the carcinoid syndrome, and the disease should be suspected in patients with unexplained intermittent diarrhea, development of telangiectasia over the face, episodes of flushing, bronchial constriction, or psychosis appearing late in life. A physical examination may disclose no more than isolated hepatomegaly or bronchoconstriction as a clue to the underlying pathologic changes. If the primary tumor can be removed before metastases occur, the patient can be cured. Female patients with suggestive symptoms and signs should be accorded special attention because an ovarian carcinoid or teratoma may give rise to symptoms before it has metastasized (87). Similarly, an early discovery of a bronchial lesion may permit a complete cure.

Routine clinical laboratory tests are seldom helpful. Thrombocytosis and leukocytosis during abdominal crisis may be seen, however. Liver function tests may show elevated alkaline phosphatase without hyperbilirubinemia — signs consistent with neoplastic involvement of this organ. Hypoalbuminemia and excessive sulfobromophthalein retention may be seen in the later course of the disease. The ^{131}I sodium *o*-iodohippurate (Hippuran) "liver scan" is a helpful but not completely reliable test for detection of early hepatic involvement. Liver biopsy can aid in the proper diagnosis in a patient with or without evidence of hepatomegaly or chemical evidence of abnormalities of liver function. In three patients without other evidence of metastatic spread, the biopsy revealed positive involvement of the liver with typical carcinoid tumor.

Determination of serum levels of cholesterol, carotene, and vitamin A and the results of xylose tolerance tests as well as quantitation of stool fat while the patient is on controlled fat intake may expose occult malabsorption or steatorrhea, even in the absence of diarrhea (132).

Roentgenographic studies may be helpful in detecting the presence of a bronchial carcinoid tumor or metastasis, peptic ulcer, a primary gastric neoplasm, or rapid transit of a barium meal through the small bowel in patients with the carcinoid syndrome (88). The gastrointestinal examination rarely reveals the primary ileal tumor. Sigmoidoscopy may detect a rectal carcinoid, but since these tumors so rarely produce a syndrome, they are usually discovered during examinations done for reasons other than a search for a carcinoid tumor.

Special Studies

The excessive excretion of *5-hydroxyindole acetic acid* continues to be the most useful means for discovering the carcinoid tumor. The qualitative test is positive if the 5-hydroxyindole acetic acid excretion exceeds 25–30 mg./day. Since some carcinoid tumors will not produce enough serotonin to elevate 5-hydroxyindole acetic acid above 15 mg./day, it is worthwhile to perform a quantitative determination of this indole metabolite when the diagnosis is strongly suspected. Elevations in the range of 9–25 mg./day can be seen with either carcinoid syndrome or nontropical sprue (101). The acid may be deceptively low when the patient has a gastric carcinoid tumor. In such a patient, 5-hydroxytryptamine and 5-hydroxytryptophan should be sought by paper chromatography of the urine. Low excretion of 5-hydroxyindole acetic acid can occur during either diet-induced or spontaneous pyridoxal phosphate deficiencies (34, 60). Then the decarboxylation of tryptophan and other amino acids may be inhibited by lack of the essential cofactor. Some have advocated, but generally on relatively weak grounds, that diets deficient in vitamin B_6 and containing inhibitors of pyridoxal phosphate might be tried in patients with the carcinoid syndrome. Falsely negative results may occur in patients with carcinoid tumors that do not excrete excessive 5-hydroxyindole acetic acid. Patients with intestinal obstruction (5) or small intestinal resection also may have unusually low excretions of 5-hydroxyindole acetic acid. Falsely negative results also may occur when patients are taking phenothiazine drugs. Eating bananas (8, 195), walnuts (96), or other foods containing serotonin may elevate 5-hydroxyindole acetic acid excretion in the absence of a tumor. Some proprietary cough medications containing glyceryl guaiacolates may produce falsely positive results. Therefore, urine specimens should be collected after the patient has stopped taking drugs for three or four days. Levels of urinary histamine, of catecholamines, and of metabolites may be elevated, but elevation is not specifically related to carcinoid tumors (119).

Determination of the 5-hydroxytryptamine content of whole blood, plasma, or platelets may help to confirm the diagnosis. Measurements of kinins or the tumor-kallikrein released into the peripheral circulation are feasible, but the methods are specialized and laborious.

Provocation of a flush by the intravenous administration of subpharmacologic doses of epinephrine or a few ounces of orally administered ethyl alcohol (2) may help in detecting a carcinoid tumor in patients complaining of flushes (109, 156). A flush similar in quality to those that the patient experiences spontaneously, as well as conjunctival suffusion and increased lacrimation and respiratory rate, may be seen 1–2 minutes after the administration of 1–5 μg. of epinephrine. The epinephrine test also may be positive in patients who have not experienced or been aware of flushes in the past (108). The incidence of falsely positive and falsely negative results has not been determined, but in general this test has been a useful adjunct to the chemical screening tests.

Treatment and Prognosis

Surgical removal of an isolated primary tumor is the best treatment. However, the diagnosis is seldom made before metastasis has occurred. After metastasis has occurred, surgical removal of the primary tumor is only justified if the tumor is large or is causing mechanical obstruction. In rare instances, resection of large, isolated, hepatic lesions has substantially but only temporarily eased the patient's symptoms (71, 141, 208). Such procedures also have considerable morbidity and mortality associated with them (208). If metastases are extensive, the treatment should be tailored to the patient's symptoms, the defined chemical abnormalities, and the location of the primary tumor. Even after metastasis of the tumor, supportive and symptomatic treatment is extremely important; some patients, particularly those with ileal carcinoid tumor, have lived as long as 23 years, and others may live 10 or more years after the syndrome appears. The clinician should not necessarily be discouraged by excretion of large quantities of 5-hydroxyindole acetic acid in the urine. There is no correlation between indole acid excretion and prognosis.

There are some reports that antitumor agents, e.g., 5-fluorouracil or cyclophosphamide, diminish liver size, particularly when infused into the hepatic artery (71, 133, 143, 147, 160). This treatment must be studied further and probably should be used only when other forms of medication have failed or when the major clinical problem results from the enlarged liver. At present there is no evidence that these toxic agents significantly alter the long-term prognosis.

When directed at specific chemical abnormalities, specific pharmacologic therapy may be very helpful. Thus, if 5-hydroxyindole acetic acid excretion is elevated and gastrointestinal symptoms are the major complaint of the patient, antiserotonin agents (either competitive inhibitors, e.g., methysergide, or inhibitors of synthesis of serotonin, e.g., parachlorophenylalanine) may diminish abdominal cramps and diarrhea and may even reverse steatorrhea (132). The effect of antiserotonin agents on flushes is inconsistent. These drugs appear to have no controlling effect on growth of the tumor, development of heart lesions, or bronchial manifestations of the syndrome. Agents such as methysergide and cyproheptadine will antagonize the peripheral effects of serotonin without altering its synthesis or metabolism. Because methysergide may produce retroperitoneal fibrosis, prolonged use must be carefully supervised or avoided (32, 65). Decarboxylase inhibitors such as alpha-methyldopa may be helpful in ameliorating the symptoms of some patients with gastric carcinoid tumors but are not generally useful therapeutic agents. When the patient's prime symptoms are flushes, antiserotonin agents rarely help. Phenothiazine drugs, which are effective alpha adrenergic blocking agents as well as antikinin agents, may be beneficial in the treatment of flushes (165). Phenoxybenzamine, an alpha adrenergic blocking drug, but not propranolol, a beta adrenergic blocking drug, appears to be useful in control of the flushes in some patients (71). In the bronchial carcinoid patient, corticosteroids may be of immense help (see Bronchial Carcinoid Tumor).

Hypotension may be a difficult problem to manage during surgical procedures. In such a situation it is important to avoid the use of pressor agents which are catecholamines (e.g., norepinephrine or epinephrine) or which primarily act by release of endogenous catecholamines (e.g., metaraminol). These agents quite likely will produce further hypotension by activation of tumor-kallikrein or by release of other as yet unidentified vasodilator substances. Methoxamine or angiotensin, whose major action is direct constriction of arterioles, will increase peripheral vascular resistance and effectively raise blood pressure in carcinoid patients.

Supportive therapy must include good nutrition and vitamin supplements (particularly niacin when there is evidence of pellagra or when 5-hydroxyindole acetic acid excretion exceeds 200–300 mg./day). Deodorized tincture of opium may be used alone or in conjunction with antiserotonin agents in the management of severe diarrhea. When therapy is rationally administered, it is often quite effective. We hope that, as we learn more about the endocrine potential of these tumors, therapy will become more specific and successful.

MASTOCYTOSIS

Comparisons with the Carcinoid Syndrome

Recurrent severe diarrhea, occasionally associated with intestinal malabsorption, flushing in association with tachycardia and hypotension, telangiectatic lesions of the skin, hepatomegaly, and bone lesions are common to both the carcinoid syndrome and systemic mastocytosis. Waldenström was first to point out the analogy between the diseases (196). This analogy has been supported by the finding of mast cell infiltration beneath the telangiectatic lesions of patients with carcinoid syndrome and the presence of large numbers of mast cells in some carcinoid tumors (51). Despite the similarity of signs and symptoms, however, the two diseases are distinct entities, differing in etiology and pathogenesis (Table 29–3).

Mastocytosis may occur during childhood as a benign, self-limited disease or commonly in adulthood as a systemic disease (Table 29–4). Occasionally, solitary tumors in the lungs may resemble plasmacytomas (35, 123). In the child, the most common clinical manifestation is an accumulation of mast cells in the skin, either in the form of a single fairly well circumscribed nodule, 2–3 cm. in diameter, or as multiple smaller, diffuse infiltrates which blister and urticate after minor trauma. This form of mast-cell proliferation usually regresses spontaneously before or shortly after puberty. In systemic mastocytosis, the proliferating mast cells invade multiple organs of the reticuloendothelial system (skin, lymph nodes, liver, spleen, bone marrow), where they produce and release certain biologically active substances in sufficient quantity to cause dermatographism, pruritus, bronchial spasm, and peptic ulceration of the pylorus and stomach in addition to the symptoms already described. Despite the extensive mast cell infiltration required to produce these abnormalities, prognosis is usually good, and the disease progresses to a malignant or "pseudoleukemic" phase in only a small number of patients. Since mast cells multiply and produce symptoms by release of their hormones, they, like enterochromaffin cells, have become the subject of intensive biochemical research.

Biochemistry of the Mast Cell

Mast cells from different species have different biochemical capabilities (172). The mast cells of all species are relatively large and contain cytoplasmic granules which stain metachromatically with thiazine dyes such as toluidine blue. Cells from several species synthesize heparin, 5-hydroxytryptamine (serotonin), and histamine (158), are able to take up and store dopamine and other catecholamines (51), and contain proteolytic enzymes, as well as tryptophan, phenylalanine hydroxylase, and carbonic anhydrase (99, 104, 116). Human mast cells, however, synthesize and store only heparin and histamine. Serotonin may be present in low concentrations but is not synthesized in the cell (53). Despite the low concentration or complete absence of serotonin in the cells, trauma to the skin of patients with urticaria pigmentosa may result in increased urinary excretion of 5-hydroxyindole acetic acid (45). An enzyme from malignant mast cells from the mouse has esterolytic properties [hydrolyzes paratoluenesulfonyl-L-arginine methyl ester (TAME)] and may be able to form small quantities of kinin from human α_2-globulin (129). Whether the human mast cell contains a kallikrein or releases kinin as a mediator of the flush and hypotension of systemic mastocytosis remains to be determined. Recent data, however, indicate that intravenous injection of epinephrine

TABLE 29-3. COMPARISON OF SYSTEMIC MASTOCYTOSIS AND CARCINOID TUMORS

	Mastocytosis	Carcinoid Tumor
Pathogenesis	Increased infiltration of "normal" mast cells; rarely malignant	Malignant enterochromaffin cell tumor
Symptoms		
Skin		
Pruritus	Prominent	
Cardiovascular		
Flush	Childhood	Any age
Tachycardia and hypotension	Common	Common
Gastrointestinal		
Diarrhea	Common	Common
Steatorrhea	Rare	Rare
Ulcers	Common	High incidence, especially with primary gastric tumors
Pulmonary		
Wheezing	Infrequent	Infrequent
Signs		
Skin		
Telangiectasia	Generalized	Localized
Dermatographism	Common	Rare
Pellagra		Rare
Lymph node enlargement	Common	
Cardiovascular		
Valvular lesions		Common
Abdominal		
Liver enlargement	Common (mast cell infiltration)	Common (metastasis)
Spleen enlargement	Common	
Skeletal		
Osteoblastic lesions	Diffuse osteosclerosis or isolated osteoblastic lesions	Common, especially with primary bronchial tumors
Other	Osteoporosis and isolated osteoclastic lesions	
Chemical Mediators		
Known		
Histamine	+	+
Serotonin	±	+
Kinins	?	+
Catecholamines	−	+
Heparin	+	−
Prostaglandins	?	+
Other, suspected	+	+

into patients with mastocytosis does not result in flushes (192). Presumably, neither kallikrein nor bradykinin causes the spontaneous flushes.

In patients with mastocytosis, the occurrence of urticaria and flushes is related to the release of histamine from the mast cell (31, 45). Heparin probably is released also (31), judging from the prolonged clotting time of venous blood obtained directly from a lesion; apparently, however, it is not released in sufficient quantities to cause systemic blood-clotting abnormalities. When gross bleeding does occur in patients with mastocytosis, it can usually be attributed to thrombocytopenia associated with cellular infiltration of the bone marrow.

Oxygen, glucose, compounds with disulfide linkage, magnesium, and a critical concentration of SH groups are requisites for histamine release (139,

158). Degranulation of normal cells can occur during antigen-antibody reactions, during heterophile anaphylaxis, and after exposure to certain pharmacologic agents. Perhaps analogous situations occur in patients with mastocytosis whose gastrointestinal symptoms resemble celiac disease but apparently depend on degranulation of the mast cells (24). In addition, Janoff et al. (89) have characterized a cationic nonpyrogenic protein (molecular weight greater than 10,000) obtained from leukocytes. The protein induces leukotaxis, increases vascular permeability, and by destroying mast cells liberates their biologically active substances. Whether any of these mechanisms are involved in the release of histamine in mastocytosis is not known. Perhaps once histamine is released, other vasoactive substances (e.g., serotonin, kinins) may be liberated from normal tissues and

TABLE 29–4.   CLASSIFICATION OF MASTOCYTOSIS

Classification	Age at Time of Onset	Comment
Benign		
Solitary lesions (mastocytoma)	Birth or shortly after; rarely in adult	
Multiple lesions (urticaria pigmentosa)	Infancy or early childhood	
Multiple lesions	Late childhood, adolescence, or adulthood	Approximately 20% of cases progress to systemic mastocytosis
Malignant		
Systemic mastocytosis	Adulthood	May be associated with amyloidosis, Hodgkin's disease, or intestinal carcinoma

thesis (histidine decarboxylase), while not yet available for clinical use, may have a role in the management of systemic mastocytosis in the future. Protamine is of little value in therapy, since the amount of heparin released is usually not sufficient to cause bleeding. Standard therapy of ulcers may be required. Splenectomy is indicated if hypersplenism offers a threat to life.

No treatment yet known has altered the prognosis of systemic mastocytosis. Although radiation therapy may ameliorate pain in sites of local bone or soft tissue invasion, neither radiation nor antitumor agents have produced objective long-term benefits; in addition, such measures may result in massive release of histamine and the patient's death.

contribute to the symptoms. As with the carcinoid syndrome, it cannot be assumed that all the biochemical mediators of the symptoms in mastocytosis have been identified.

Diagnosis and Treatment

The disease should be suspected in any patient with flushing, tachycardia, gastrointestinal complaints, and headaches. The demonstration of excessive amounts of histamine or its metabolite, 1,4-methylimidazole acetic acid, in the urine will help to confirm the diagnosis. A definitive diagnosis, however, must be based on histologic examination of a biopsy specimen of the red-brown macules or slightly raised papules. Repeated biopsies may be required to detect the characteristic extensive concentrations of mast cells in the upper corium. When the disease is widespread (systemic mastocytosis), the cells will be found in a variety of organs of the reticuloendothelial system. If bone is involved, either discrete isolated radiolucent or radiopaque lesions or generalized osteoporosis or osteosclerosis may be present. Such bone involvement is associated at times with bone pain, anemia secondary to hypoplasia of cellular elements, or bleeding secondary to thrombocytopenia.

Since the disease is usually self-limiting, symptomatic treatment is often sufficient. Antihistamines may be helpful during acute exacerbations of the disease. Other anti-inflammatory drugs which can inhibit certain types of mast cell degranulation have not been evaluated in patients with the disease (206). Intriguing data related to restriction of magnesium and gluten from the diet have been presented recently by Broitman et al. (24). Perhaps their experience will prove to be unusual, but certainly these maneuvers have appeared to reverse the severe malabsorption in one patient. The positive effects of hypomagnesemia may be related to an inability of the mast cells to regranulate once their contents are released (24).

Drugs that can release histamine, such as morphine (4) or similar alkaloids and cortisone, should be avoided. Effective inhibitors of histamine syn-

REFERENCES

1. Adamson, A. R., Grahame-Smith, D. G., et al.: *Brit. Med. J.* 3:93, 1971.
2. Adamson, A. R., Grahame-Smith, D. G., et al.: *Amer. Heart J.* 81:141, 1971.
3. Adamson, A. R., Grahame-Smith, D. G., et al.: *Lancet* 2:293, 1969.
4. Akcasu, A., and Unna, K. R.: *Europ. J. Pharmacol.* 13:103, 1970.
5. Alfthan, O., Lempinen, M., et al.: *Ann. Med. Exp. Biol. Fenn.* 47:285, 1969.
6. Alivisatos, S. G. A., Papaphilis, A. D., et al.: *Nature* 226:455, 1970.
7. Alivisatos, S. G. A., Ungar, F., et al.: *Science* 171:809, 1971.
8. Anderson, J. A., Zeigler, M. R., et al.: *Science* 127:236, 1958.
9. Aronsen, K. F., Steiner, H., et al.: *Acta Chir. Scand.* 135:177, 1969.
10. Axelrod, J., In *Mechanisms of Release of Biogenic Amines.* Proc. Int. Wenner-Gren Sympos., Stockholm, Oxford, Pergamon Press, 1966, p. 189.
11. Axelrod, J., and Wurtman, R. J.: *Advances Pharmacol.* 6:157, 1968, p. 157.
12. Back, N., In *Symposium on Hypotensive Peptides.* Erdos, E. G., Back, N., et al. (eds.), Berlin, Springer-Verlag, 1966.
13. Bates, H. R., Jr.: *Lancet* 1:1111, 1967.
14. Baumgarten, H. G., Bjoerklund, A., et al.: *Acta Physiol. Scand.* 84(Suppl. 373):1971.
15. Baumgarten, H. G., Evetts, K. D., et al.: *J. Neurochem.* 19: 1587, 1972.
16. Becker, N., Burrill, K., et al.: *Clin. Res.* 19:186, 1971.
17. Bennett, A., and Whitney, B.: *Gut* 7:307, 1966.
18. Beusch, K. G., Corrin, B., et al.: *Cancer* 22:1163, 1968.
19. Beusch, K. G., Gordon, G. B., et al.: *J. Ultrastruct. Res.* 12:668, 1965.
20. Boelkins, C.: Unpublished manuscript. Stanford University School of Medicine, Stanford, California, 1971.
21. Bower, B. F., and Gordon, G. S.: *Ann. Rev. Med.* 16:83, 1965.
22. Bradley, J., Mason, K., et al.: *Lancet* 2:578, 1971.
23. Branson, J., Oleesky, S., et al.: *Postgrad. Med. J.* 42:518, 1966.
24. Broitman, S. A., McCray, R. S., et al.: *Amer. J. Med.* 48:382, 1970.
25. Brown, H., and Lane, M.: *Arch. Intern. Med.* 115:490, 1965.
26. Buccino, R. A., Covell, J. W., et al.: *Amer. J. Physiol.* 213:483, 1967.
27. Bulbring, E., and Gershon, M. D.: *Advances Pharmacol.* 6A:323, 1968.
28. Bulbring, E., and Lin, R. C. Y.: *J. Physiol.* 140:381, 1958.
29. Bunney, W. E., Jr., Murphy, D. L., et al.: *Lancet* 1:1022, 1970.
30. Burks, T. F., and Long, J. P.: *Amer. J. Physiol.* 211:619, 1966.
31. Caplan, R. M.: *J.A.M.A.* 194:1077, 1965.
32. Carr, R. J., and Biswas, B. K.: *Brit. Med. J.* 2:1116, 1966.
33. Cater, D. B., and Taylor, C. R.: *Brit. J. Cancer* 20:517, 1966.

34. Chabner, B. A., DeVita, V. T., et al.: *New Eng. J. Med.* 282:838, 1970.
35. Charrette, E. E., Mariano, A. V., et al.: *118*:358, 1966.
36. Chase, T. N., Katz, R. I., et al.: *J. Neurochem.* 16:607, 1969.
37. Cline, M. J., and Melmon, K. L.: *Science* 153:1135, 1966.
38. Cochrane, C. G., and Wuepper, K. D.: *J. Exp. Med.* 134:986, 1971.
39. Cohen, R. M.: *Calif. Med.* 114:1, 1971.
40. Cottrell, G. A.: *Nature* 225:1060, 1970.
41. Cremata, V. Y., and Koe, B. K.: *Clin. Pharmacol. Ther.* 7:768, 1966.
42. Cuschieri, A., and Onabanjo, O. A.: *Brit. Med. J.* 3:565, 1971.
43. DaPrada, M., and Pletscher, A.: *Life Sci.* 8:65, 1969.
44. Davis, R. B., and Rosenberg, J. C.: *Amer. J. Med.* 30:167, 1961.
45. Demis, D. J.: *Ann. Intern. Med.* 59:194, 1963.
46. DiChiara, G., Camba, R., et al.: *Nature* 233:272, 1971.
47. DiMattei, P.: *Biochem. Pharmacol.* 16:909, 1967.
48. Dollinger, M. R., Ratner, L. H., et al.: *Arch. Intern. Med.* 120:575, 1967.
49. Eccleston, D., Ritchie, I. M., et al.: *226*:84, 1970.
50. Egan, T. J.: *Isreal J. Med. Sci.* 3:587, 1970.
51. Enerbäck, L.: *Acta Path. Microbiol. Scand.* 64:491, 1965.
52. Engelman, K., Lovenberg, W., et al.: *New Eng. J. Med.* 277:1103, 1967.
53. Erspamer, V.: *Progr. Drug Res.* 3:151, 1961.
54. Feer, H., and Wirz-Justice, A.: *Experientia* 27:885, 1971.
55. Fernstrom, J. D., and Wurtman, R. J.: *Science* 173:149, 1971.
56. Fernstrom, J. D., and Wurtman, R. J.: *Nature (New Biol.)* 234:62, 1971.
57. Fishlock, D. J., and Parks, A. G.: *Brit. J. Pharmacol.* 28:164, 1966.
58. *Canad. Med. Ass. J.* 96:1282, 1967.
59. Fox, R. H., Goldsmith, R., et al.: *J. Physiol.* 157:589, 1961.
60. Gailani, S., Roque, A. L., et al.: *Ann. Intern. Med.* 65:1044, 1966.
61. Gardner, B., Dollinger, M., et al.: *Surgery* 61:846, 1967.
62. Geipert, F., and Erdös, E. G.: *Experientia* 27:912, 1971.
63. Gershon, M. D., and Altman, R. F.: *J. Pharmacol. Exp. Ther.* 179:29, 1971.
64. Gowenlock, A. H., Platt, D. S., et al.: *Lancet* 1:304, 1964.
65. Graham, J. R., Suby, H. I., et al.: *New Eng. J. Med.* 274:359, 1966.
66. Grahame-Smith, D. G., and Ferriman, D. G.: *Proc. Roy. Soc. Med.* 68:701, 1965.
67. Grahame-Smith, D. G.: Unpublished report. St. Mary's Hospital Medical School, London, 1971.
68. Grahame-Smith, D. G.: *Brit. J. Pharmacol.* 43:856, 1971.
69. Grahame-Smith, D. G. *Gut* 11:189, 1970.
70. Grahame-Smith, D. G.: *J. Neurochem.* 18:1053, 1971.
71. Grahame-Smith, D. G.: *Hosp. Med.* 4:556, 1968.
72. Grahame-Smith, D. G.: *Amer. J. Cardiol.* 21:376, 1968.
73. Grahame-Smith, D. G.: Unpublished report. St. Mary's Hospital Medical School, London, 1971.
74. Grahame-Smith, D. G.: *Biochim. Biophys. Acta* 86:175, 1964.
75. Grimson, B. S., Robinson, S. C., et al.: *Amer. J. Physiol.* 216:50, 1969.
76. Gurdon, J. B.: *Quart. Rev. Biol.* 38:54, 1963.
77. Gurdon, J. B., In *Advances in Morphogenesis.* Abercrombie, M., and Bracket, J. (eds.), New York, Academic Press, 1964, p. 1.
78. Hale, J. F., and Lane-Mitchell, W.: *Cent. Afr. J. Med.* 10:162, 1964.
79. Hallen, A.: *Lancet* 1:746, 1964.
80. Hallwright, G. P., North, A. K., et al.: *J. Clin. Endocr.* 24:496, 1964.
81. Harvey, J. A., and Yunger, L. M.: Unpublished report. Univ. of Iowa, Iowa City, Iowa, 1972.
82. Haverback, B. J., and Davidson, J. D.: *Gastroenterology* 35:570, 1958.
83. Hendrix, T. R., Atkinson, M., et al.: *Amer. J. Med.* 23:886, 1957.
84. Hernandez, F. J., and Reid, J. D.: *Arch. Path.* 88:489, 1969.
85. Hiatt, R. B., Goodman, I., et al.: *Amer. J. Surg.* 119:527, 1970.
86. Ho, A. K. A., Loh, H. H., et al.: *Europ. J. Pharmacol.* 10:72, 1970.
87. Hoch, Z., Lichtig, C., et al.: *Amer. J. Obstet. Gynec.* 110:1141, 1971.

88. Hudson, H. L., and Margulis, A. R.: *Amer. J. Roentgen.* 91:833, 1964.
89. Janoff, A., Schaefer, S., et al.: *J. Exp. Med.* 122:841, 1965.
90. Jarrett, L., Lacy, P. E., et al.: *J. Clin. Endocr.* 24:543, 1964.
91. Jones, J. E., Shane, S. R., et al.: *J. Clin. Endocr.* 29:1, 1969.
92. Jouvet, M.: *Science 163*:32, 1969.
93. Kabakow, B., Weinstein, J. B., et al.: *Fed. Proc.* 17:382, 1958.
94. Kaplan, A. P., Kay, A. B., et al.: *J. Exp. Med.* 135:81, 1972.
95. Kinloch, J. D., Webb, J. N., et al.: *Brit. Med. J.* 1:1533, 1965.
96. Kirberger, E.: *Deutsch. Med. Wschr.* 87:929, 1962.
97. Klingman, G. I.: *Biochem. Pharmacol.* 18:2061, 1969.
98. Klingman, G. I., and Klingman, J. D.: *Biochem. Pharmacol.* 18:2069, 1969.
99. Korhonen, L. K., and Korhonen, E.: *Experientia* 21:628, 1965.
100. Kowlessar, O. D., Law, D. H., et al.: *Amer. J. Med.* 27:673, 1959.
101. Kowlessar, O. D., Williams, R. C., et al.: *New Eng. J. Med.* 259:340, 1958.
102. Krasner, J., and McMenamy, R. H.: *J. Biol. Chem.* 241:4186, 1966.
103. Krieger, D. T., and Rizzo, F.: *Amer. J. Physiol.* 217:1703, 1969.
104. Lagunoff, D., and Benditt, E. P.: *Ann. N.Y. Acad. Sci.* 103:185, 1962.
105. Lembeck, F.: *Nature 172*:910, 1953.
106. Lemberger, L., Axelrod, J., et al.: *J. Pharmacol. Exp. Ther.* 177:169, 1971.
107. Lernmark, A.: *Horm. Metab. Res.* 3:305, 1971.
108. Levine, R. J., Elsas, L. J., et al.: *J.A.M.A.* 186:905, 1963.
109. Levine, R. J., and Sjoerdsma, A.: *Ann. Intern. Med.* 58:818, 1963.
110. Liddle, G. W., Nicholson, W. E., et al.: *Recent Progr. Hormone Res.* 25:283, 1969.
111. Lin, R. C., Neff, N. H., et al.: *Life Sci.* 8:1077, 1969.
112. Lipton, M. A.: In *Neurobiological Aspects of Psychopathology.* Grune & Stratton, New York, 1969, pp. 310–330.
113. Lovenberg, W., Bensinger, R. E., et al.: *Anal. Biochem.* 43:269, 1971.
114. Lovenberg, W., and Engelman, K.: *Methods Biochem. Anal.* 19:1, 1971.
115. Lovenberg, W., Jequier, E., et al.: *Advances Pharmacol.* 6:21, 1968.
116. Lovenberg, W., Levine, R. J., et al.: *Biochem. Pharmacol.* 14:887, 1965.
117. MacDonald, R. A.: *Amer. J. Med.* 21:867, 1956.
118. Margolius, H. S., Geller, R., et al.: *Lancet* 2:1063, 1971.
119. Marshall, P. B.: *J. Pharm. Pharmacol.* 18:764, 1966.
120. Maruyama, Y., Hayashi, G., et al.: *J. Pharmacol. Exp. Ther.* 178:20, 1971.
121. Mashford, M. L., and Zacest, R.: *Aust. Ann. Med.* 16:326, 1967.
122. Mason, D. T., and Melmon, K. L.: *J. Clin. Invest.* 45:1685, 1966.
123. McBride, T. I., McDonald, G. A., et al.: *Postgrad. Med. J.* 43:176, 1967.
124. McConnell, D. J., and Mason, B.: *Brit. J. Pharmacol.* 38:490, 1970.
125. McGiff, J. C., Terrango, N. A., et al.: *Circ. Res.* 31:36, 1972.
126. McGinty, D. J., Fairbanks, M. K., et al., In *Serotonin Behavior.* Barchus, J., and Usdin, E. (eds.), New York, Academic Press, 1973 (in press).
127. Melmon, K. L.: *Physiol. Pharmacol. Physicians* 1:1, 1966.
128. Melmon, K. L.: *Calif. Med.* 114:33, 1971.
129. Melmon, K. L., and Cline, M. J., In *International Symposium on Vasoactive Peptides, Bradykinin and Related Kinins.* Rocha é Silva, M., and Rothschild, H. A. (eds.), Sao Paulo, Brazil, Livraria Editora Flamboyant Ltda., 1967, p. 223.
130. Melmon, K. L., Lovenberg, W., et al.: *Clin. Chim. Acta* 12:292, 1965.
131. Melmon, K. L., Sjoerdsma, A., et al.: *Amer. J. Med.* 39:568, 1965.
132. Melmon, K. L., Sjoerdsma, A., et al.: *Gastroenterology* 48:18, 1965.
133. Mengel, C. E.: *Ann. Intern. Med.* 62:587, 1965.
134. Miller, R. L., and Melmon, K. L., In *Clinical Pharmacology: Basic Principles in Therapeutics.* Melmon, K. L., and Morrelli, H. F. (eds.), New York, MacMillan Co., 1972, p. 382.

135. Miller, R. L., Reichgott, M. J., et al.: *J. Infect. Dis.*, 1973 (in press).
136. Misiewicz, J. J., Waller, S. L., et al.: *Gut 7*:208, 1966.
137. Moertel, C. G., Beahrs, O. H., et al.: *New Eng. J. Med. 273*:244, 1965.
138. Moertel, C. G., Sauer, W. G., et al.: *Cancer 14*:901, 1961.
139. Mongar, J. L., and Perera, B. A. V.: *Immunology 8*:511, 1965.
140. Morin, L. J., and Zuerner, R. T.: *J.A.M.A. 216*:1647, 1971.
141. Mosenthal, W. T.: *Surg. Clin. N. Amer. 45*:1253, 1963.
142. Mouret, J., Bobillier, P., et al.: *Europ. J. Pharmacol. 5*:17, 1968.
143. Murray-Lyon, I. M., Parsons, V. A., et al.: *Lancet 2*:172, 1970.
144. Murray-Lyon, I. M., Sandler, M., et al.: *Gut 13*:385, 1972.
145. Murrell, T. G. C., Wangel, A. G., et al.: *Gastroenterology 51*:656, 1966.
146. Nash, D. T., and Borin, M.: *New York J. Med. 64*:1128, 1964.
147. Oates, J. A.: *Advances Pharmacol. 5*:109, 1967.
148. Oates, J. A., and Melmon, K. L., In *Symposium on Hypotensive Peptides.* Erdos, E. G., Back, N., et al. (eds.), Berlin, Springer-Verlag, 1966.
149. Oates, J. A., Melmon, K. L., et al.: *Lancet 1*:514, 1964.
150. Oates, J. A., Pettinger, W. A., et al.: *J. Clin. Invest. 45*:173, 1966.
151. Oates, J. A., and Sjoerdsma, A.: *Amer. J. Med. 32*:333, 1962.
152. Offermeier, J., and Ariens, E. J.: *Arch. Int. Pharmacodyn. 164*:192, 1966.
153. Page, I. H.: *Serotonin.* Chicago, Year Book Medical Publishers, 1968.
154. Page, I. H., and McCubbin, J. W.: *Amer. J. Physiol. 184*:265, 1956.
155. Peart, W. S., Andrews, T. M., et al.: *Lancet 1*:577, 1961.
156. Peart, W. S., Robertson, J. I. S., et al.: *Lancet 2*:715, 1959.
157. Pentilla, A., and Lempinen, M.: *Gastroenterology 54*:375, 1968.
158. Perera, B. A. V., and Mongar, J. L.: *Immunology 8*:519, 1965.
159. *Lancet 1*:404, 1968.
160. Reed, M. L., Kuipers, F. M., et al.: *New Eng. J. Med. 269*:1005, 1963.
161. Reichgott, M. J., and Melmon, K. L.: *Circulation 42*:563, 1970.
162. Reichgott, M. J., and Melmon, K. L., In *Methods in Investigative and Diagnostic Endocrinology.* Berson, S. A., and Yalow, R. S. (eds.), Amsterdam, North-Holland Publishing Co., 1973 (in press).
163. Roberts, W. C., and Sjoerdsma, A.: *Amer. J. Med. 36*:5, 1964.
164. Robertson, J. I. S., Peart, W. S., et al.: *Quart. J. Med. 31*:103, 1962.
165. Rocha é Silva, M., and Garcia Lerne, J.: *Med. Exp. 8*:287, 1963.
166. Rothschild, A. M.: *Brit. J. Pharmacol. 42*:631, 1971.
167. Sander, R. J., and Axtell, H. K.: *Surg. Gynec. Obstet. 199*:369, 1964.
168. Sandler, M., Karim, S. M. M., et al.: *Lancet 2*:1053, 1968.
169. Satterlee, W. G., Serpick, A., et al.: *Ann. Intern. Med. 72*:919, 1970.
170. Sayle, B. A., Lang, P. A., et al.: *Ann. Intern. Med. 63*:58, 1965.
171. Schwaber, J. R., and Lukas, D. S.: *Amer. J. Med. 32*:846, 1962.
172. Selye, H.: *The Mast Cells.* New York, Appleton-Century-Crofts, 1965, p. 320.
173. Shaskan, E. G., and Snyder, S. H.: *J. Pharmacol. Exp. Ther. 175*:404, 1970.
174. Shen, Fu-Hsiung, Loh, H. H., et al.: *J. Pharmacol. Exp. Ther. 175*:427, 1970.
175. Shionoya, S., Nakata, Y., et al.: *Angiology 22*:456, 1971.
176. Sirek, A., Geerling, E., et al.: *Amer. J. Physiol. 211*:1018, 1966.
177. Sjoerdsma, A., Lovenberg, W., et al.: *Ann. Intern. Med. 73*:607, 1970.
178. Sjoerdsma, A., and Melmon, K. L.: *Gastroenterology 47*:104, 1964.
179. Sjoerdsma, A., Weissback, H., et al.: *Amer. J. Med. 23*:5, 1957.
180. Sluys, V. J., Chonfoer, J. C., et al.: *Lancet 1*:1416, 1964.
181. Smith, A. N., and Zeitlin, I. J.: *Brit. J. Surg. 53*:867, 1966.
182. Snyder, S. H., Axelrod, J., et al.: *J. Pharmacol. Exp. Ther. 158*:206, 1967.
183. Spatz, M.: *Lab. Invest. 13*:288, 1964.
184. Steiner, K.: *Arch. Derm. 84*:477, 1961.
185. Stevens, D. A., and Fechter, L. D.: *Life Sci. 8*:379, 1969.
186. Szeinberg, A., Shani, M., et al.: *Israel J. Med. Sci. 6*:475, 1970.
187. Takagi, K., and Takayanagi, I.: *Europ. J. Pharmacol. 4*:96, 1968.
188. Tammes, A. R.: *Arch. Pathol. 79*:626, 1965.
189. Thompson, J. H., and Campbell, L. B.: *Experientia 23*:826, 1967.
190. Thorson, A., Biork, G., et al.: *Amer. Heart J. 47*:795, 1954.
191. Tyce, G. M., Flock, E. V., et al.: *Biochem. Pharmacol. 16*:979, 1967.
192. Vaidya, A. B., Wustrack, K. O., et al.: *Ann. Intern. Med. 74*:711, 1971.
193. van Praag, H. M.: *Psychiatr., Neurol. Neurochir.* (Amst.) *73*:9, 1970.
194. von Studnitz, W.: *Scand. J. Clin. Lab. Invest. 11*:309, 1959.
195. Waalkes, T. P., Sjoerdsma, A., et al.: *Science 127*:648, 1958.
196. Waldenström, J.: *Acta Endocr. 17*:432, 1954.
197. Warner, R. R. P., Kirschner, P. A., et al.: *J.A.M.A. 178*:1175, 1961.
198. Weichert, R. F.: *Amer. J. Med. 49*:232, 1970.
199. Weiner, R., and Altura, B. M.: *Proc. Soc. Exp. Biol. Med. 124*:494, 1967.
200. Welch, A. S., and Welch, B. L.: *Biochem. Pharmacol. 17*:699, 1968.
201. Williams, E. D.: *Lancet, 2*:1108, 1969.
202. Williams, E. D., and Celestin, L. R.: *Thorax 17*:120, 1962.
203. Williams, E. D., and Sandler, M.: *Lancet 1*:238, 1963.
204. Williams, H. E., Wilson, K. M., et al.: *Clin. Res. 18*:541, 1970.
205. Wuepper, K. D., and Cochrane, C. G.: *J. Exp. Med. 135*:1, 1972.
206. Yamasaki, H., and Saeki, K.: *Arch. Int. Pharmacodyn. 168*:166, 1967.
207. Yarbrough, G. G., Buxbaum, D. M., et al.: *Life Sci. 10*:977, 1971.
208. Zeegen, R., Rothwell-Jackson, R., et al.: *Gut 10*:617, 1969.
209. Zeitlin, I. J., In *Symposium on Hypotensive Peptides.* Erdos, E. G., Back, N., et al. (eds.), Berlin, Springer-Verlag, 1966.
210. Zenker, N., Hanker, J. S., et al.: *Science 159*:1104, 1968.
211. Zweig, M., and Axelrod, J.: *J. Neurobiol. 1*:87, 1969.

CHAPTER 30

Humoral Manifestations of Nonendocrine Neoplasms—Ectopic Hormone Production*

By William D. Odell

INTRODUCTION

A great variety of endocrine syndromes are manifestations of hormone production by neoplasms (benign or malignant) not usually considered to be derived from endocrine tissues. Since physicians have become more generally aware of the existence of such syndromes and assay techniques have become more widely available in the past ten years, the number of such patients and the variety of such syndromes have increased enormously (Table 30–1). These syndromes are of great interest to the physician for both practical and theoretical reasons. First, the physician *must* be aware of these syndromes in order to correctly diagnose the presence of a neoplasm and to avoid erroneous treatment directed to other causes. Detectable hormone production by the neoplasm may precede any other evidence of the neoplasm by months or years, and diagnosis in some instances thus may be possible when the neoplasm is easily resectable or treata-

ble. At times, a positive diagnosis of a hormone-producing neoplasm can be made when increased production of the particular hormone is the only manifestation. Second, these tumors that elaborate hormones are of great interest to the oncologist, since the hormone produced serves as a label or tag of the neoplastic cell. Changes in production rates of this substance may be utilized not only to localize the tumor (in some instances) but also to follow the response to chemotherapeutic, surgical, or radiation treatment. Third, such tumor modification of hormonal substances is of great theoretical interest.

All cells of an organism contain genetic material coded with the same information. Presumably, much of this information is repressed as differentiation proceeds and special cell functions are derived. It is possible that during neoplasia formation, derepression occurs and results in polypeptide hormone elaboration. It is of great significance that all ectopic hormone syndromes are manifestations of *polypeptide* hormone production; steroids

TABLE 30–1. EXAMPLES OF HUMORAL SYNDROMES ASSOCIATED WITH NEOPLASMS

1. Ectopic hormone production (the subject of this chapter)
2. Carcinoembryonic antigen
3. Hepatoma antigen (alpha fetal globulin)
4. Alkaline phosphatase
5. Central nervous system degenerative conditions
6. Myopathies
7. Myasthenic syndromes
8. Dermatologic diseases (i.e., dermatomyositis, acanthosis nigricans, pachydermia)
9. Digital clubbing and arthropathies
10. Hematologic diseases (i.e., aplastic anemias, gamma globulin abnormalities, thrombophlebitis)
11. Cardiovascular syndromes (i.e., nonbacterial endocarditis)
12. Fever

---

*This term was introduced by Dr. Grant Liddle in 1962.

or thyronines have not been produced. This is believed to be true because synthesis of steroids and thyronines requires an *orderly sequence* of several enzymatic steps, and ectopic tissue presumably does not have the types and amounts of chemicals for this kind of synthesis. On the other hand, synthesis of a polypeptide presumably requires only a single alteration in cellular genetic material.

Recently it has been shown that four hormones (LH, FSH, TSH, and chorionic gonadotropin) are composed of two polypeptide chains, α and β (10, 28–30). The α chains of each of these hormones are very similar in structure; the β chain of each is different and confers biologic and immunologic specificity. Neither chain alone has biologic potency. Furthermore, when an α chain from any of the four hormones is mixed in vitro with a β chain from one of the other three, a two-chain polypeptide molecule is produced with the biologic activity determined only by the particular β chain. It is not known whether the α and β chains are produced by cleavage of a single, very large molecule, as are the α and β chains of insulin, or whether each is synthesized separately and assembly takes place afterwards. If the latter is true, it appears possible for some neoplasms to elaborate only α or β chains of these molecules; since no biologic activity would result, however, humoral syndromes would not be produced.* Nevertheless, such polypeptide elaboration by neoplasms could be detected and quantified by immunologic means. Alternatively, it is also possible that aberrant polypeptide or protein synthesis is a common or universal property of neoplasms. In this chapter we discuss only those we *recognize*, that is, those tumors that produce polypeptides with biologic activity. It appears likely that the ectopic hormone syndrome represents only a small fraction of a more common phenomenon of abnormal protein synthesis by neoplasms. If this is true, and if means of detecting and quantifying such production are available, specific diagnosis and intelligent follow-up of response to therapy should be possible for *any* malignancy. Thus such syndromes are of great theoretical interest to the experimental oncologist.

Recent experience with neoplastic elaboration of nonhormonal polypeptides, carcinoembryonic antigen (CEA), and α fetal globulin adds further support to these postulates. CEA is a protein or polypeptide originally extracted and partially purified from carcinomas of the colon. Immunoassays have been developed, and evidence accumulating at the time of the writing of this chapter indicates that the vast majority of carcinomas of the thorax and abdomen elaborate this material. CEA also is present in large amounts in fetal tissue and appears to

---

*Indeed, this may explain why production of *pituitary* TSH, LH, and FSH by neoplasms is so rare relative to other ectopic hormone production. The gonadotropin produced by neoplasms is usually similar to chorionic gonadotropin and different from pituitary LH and FSH. Ectopic production of pituitary TSH-like material has not been reported, though substances with thyroid-stimulating ability similar to *placental* thyrotropin have been described.

TABLE 30–2. HORMONES REPORTED TO BE PRODUCED BY NONENDOCRINE NEOPLASMS*

1. ACTH
2. α and β MSH
3. Gonadotropin
4. Vasopressin
5. Parathyroid hormone
6. Hypoglycemic producing factor
7. Erythropoietin
8. Gastrin
9. Thyroid stimulating factor
10. Hypophosphatemia producing factor
11. Corticotropin releasing hormone
12. Prolactin
13. Growth hormone
14. Kinins
15. Prostaglandins
16. Secretin
17. Glucagon

*The order is approximately in relation to the numbers of patients reported with these syndromes.

be a protein elaborated by rapidly dividing tissues. Alpha fetal globulin was originally described in sera of human fetuses. This protein is present in large amounts in most patients with hepatomas and in many with other types of neoplasms. Its function, if any, is unknown.

I emphasize, then, that the humoral syndromes discussed in this chapter in all probability are only in small part responsible for the circumstances under which neoplasms elaborate polypeptides. Furthermore, I am of the opinion that the majority of neoplasms or possibly all neoplasms elaborate polypeptides in increased amounts. Table 30–2 lists some of the known examples of *hormonal* or *nonhormonal* compounds produced by neoplasms.

Before discussing the specific syndrome, the following case history is presented to illustrate how the diagnosis of neoplasms can be based upon hormonal production and the difficulty which at times can be encountered in locating the neoplasm (34).

A 22-year-old man reported to his physician with mild breast soreness. The physician detected minimal gynecomastia on physical examination; the rest of the examination was entirely normal. All laboratory determinations including x-rays were normal, except that serum immunoassayable gonadotropin in the LH assay was 5,000 mI.U./ml. This LH value was higher than is ever observed under physiologic conditions, even in castrate men, and a certain diagnosis of a gonadotropin-producing neoplasm was made. In spite of an extensive search over eight months' time, however, no neoplasm was found. The search included all routine x-rays, plus arteriograms of abdominal vasculature, tomograms of the mediastinum, catheterization, gonadotropin measurement at 2- to 3-inch intervals throughout the truncal venous and arterial tree, surgical exploration of the testes with testicular vein gonadotropin measurements, and surgical exploration of the mediastinum. Finally, metabolic turnover studies of the tumor gonadotropin showed the degradation time was very long, thus production rates were low. Therefore, in spite of the 5,000 mI.U./ml. concentration, detection of the differences between tumor venous and peripheral venous blood would have been unlikely. One year after the onset of gynecomastia, pulmonary metastases suddenly appeared, and serum LH increased to over 300,000 mI.U./ml. He expired with widespread disease in a few weeks. At postmortem examination, it was decided that the likely primary source was a 4 mm. testicular teratocarcinoma.

This case report illustrates the following important four facts:

1. The only indication that a neoplasm is present may be the ectopic hormone production.

2. Given a precise assay system and a knowledge of normal endocrine physiology, a syndrome caused by a neoplasm can be differentiated from an alteration in normal endocrine gland function. For this patient, a hypogonadal state or any other manipulation of the hypothalamic-pituitary-testicular axis could not result in 5,000 mI.U./ml. of LH or its equivalent; this could be caused only by ectopic hormone production.

3. Knowledge of the production and degradation rates of hormones may be of more than theoretical interest. In this instance, catheterization studies were unlikely to succeed, because the half-time of degradation of the gonadotropin was so long that only a low production rate was required to produce these blood concentrations of gonadotropin. Localization attempts based on definite increases in blood hormone concentration proximate to a neoplasm are much more likely to be successful if the degradation rate of a hormone is relatively rapid ($T_{1/2}$ less than one hour). Fortunately, this is true for most hormones, and this approach of localizing a neoplasm is usually likely to succeed.

4. Given knowledge of all three principles above, knowledge of the nature of tumors producing given hormones and their age distributions may be helpful in planning diagnostic procedures.

It appears likely that, for the patient presented, unilateral castration followed by quantification of gonadotropin concentrations to ascertain response might have resulted in a cure during the stable period of this disease. If the testicle harboring the neoplasm had been removed, blood gonadotropin would have fallen to normal. If it did not, the remaining testicle could have been removed. This approach is suggested (a) because the most likely location of gonadotropin-producing tumors in a 22-year-old man is a teratoma of the testes; (b) because after such a thorough search, gonadotropin-producing neoplasms other than testicular were unlikely; and (c) because cure of other gonadotropin-producing neoplasms is infrequent. Rosen et al. (32) have presented a similar patient.

HYPERADRENOCORTICISM (ECTOPIC ACTH PRODUCTION)

Cushing's syndrome* (excess glucocorticoid effects) is one of the most common manifestations of

*Cushing's *syndrome* may be defined as the symptomatology and physical findings associated with *any cause* of excess glucocorticoid action; Cushing's *disease* may be defined as bilateral adrenal hyperplasia caused by a derangement in hypothalamic-pituitary control of ACTH secretion.

TABLE 30-3. NEOPLASMS ASSOCIATED WITH ECTOPIC ACTH PRODUCTION

Tumor Type	Approximate Percentage of Cases
Carcinoma of lung	50
Thymic carcinoma	10
Pancreatic carcinoma (including islet cell and carcinoid)	10
Neoplasms from neural crest tissue (pheochromocytoma, neuroblastoma, paraganglioma, ganglioma)	5
Bronchial adenoma (including carcinoid)	2
Medullary carcinoma of the thyroid	5
Miscellaneous*	each <2

*Carcinoma of ovary, prostate, breast, thyroid, kidney, salivary glands, testes, stomach, colon, gallbladder, esophagus, appendix, etc.

†These interesting neoplasms also elaborate thyrocalcitonin and are associated, frequently in the same patient, with pheochromocytomas, hyperparathyroidism, Marfan's habitus, increased frequency of peptic ulcers, intestinal diverticulosis, and humor-caused diarrhea. According to our definition, calcitonin elaboration by medullary carcinoma is not an example of *ectopic* hormone production.

ectopic ACTH production. Several hundred patients with this syndrome have been reported; Liddle et al. (21) alone have studied over 88 patients with this syndrome. The neoplasms associated with this syndrome are shown in Table 30-3. Among such patients, 70 per cent have harbored carcinomas of the lung, thymic carcinomas, or pancreatic carcinomas; carcinoma of the lung alone accounts for about 50 per cent. The types of neoplasms causing this syndrome in childhood (or at any selected age) are different. Omenn (27) reviewed 11 patients under age 16; five had neural crest neoplasms, three had thymic carcinoma or anaplastic carcinoma of the lung, one had pancreatic islet cell carcinoma, one adrenal carcinoma, and one carcinoma of the "liver." It is noteworthy that in adults some of the other common neoplasms, such as carcinoma of the breast, colon, stomach, and cervix, are only infrequently associated with this syndrome. Liddle (21) assayed 78 nonselected visceral carcinomas for ACTH content and found six to contain increased concentrations. This suggests that the syndrome may be much more common (8 per cent of visceral neoplasms) than recognized.

Clinical Manifestations

The Cushing's syndrome associated with ectopic ACTH production may occur coincidentally with other manifestations of the tumor or, rarely, as long as 1-4 years prior to the diagnosis of the neoplasm. Although the blood ACTH concentrations are extremely high, clinical signs and symptoms of Cushing's syndrome are often subtle. It is uncommon for patients with ectopic ACTH syndrome to manifest classic symptoms and findings of hyperadrenocorticism. This is explained by the

TABLE 30–4. SOME LABORATORY FEATURES OF ASSISTANCE IN DIAGNOSIS OF ECTOPIC ACTH SYNDROMES

	Plasma ACTH	Hypokalemia, Alkalosis	24-Hour Urinary 17-Ketosteroid Excretion (Times Normal)	Suppression by Dexamethasone (0.5 mg. q. 6 hr.)	Suppression by Dexamethasone (2 mg. q. 6 hr.)
Cushing's disease	Slightly increased	Rare	1–2	No	Yes
Primary adrenal cortical tumor	Low	Common	1–10	No	No
Ectopic ACTH	High	Common	1–10	No	No*
Pituitary adenoma secreting ACTH	High	Rare	1–2	No	No

*Except bronchial adenoma or neoplasm that elaborates ACTH or corticotropin-releasing hormone or both.

fact that usually several years of excess cortisol production are required to produce such symptoms, whereas in ectopic ACTH syndrome, the duration of disease is usually short. Because of this, diagnosis is often difficult. Any patient with a neoplasm and hypokalemia, abnormal glucose tolerance, marked weakness, or increased pigmentation should be examined for this syndrome (Table 30–4).

The cortisol production in ectopic ACTH syndrome is usually much greater than in bilateral adrenal hyperplasia or in adrenal neoplasms. Cortisol in large amounts causes hypokalemic alkalosis, and this is much more common in ectopic ACTH syndrome than in Cushing's disease (bilateral adrenal hyperplasia). This difference is so great that any patient with manifestations of Cushing's syndrome *and hypokalemia* should be suspected of having ectopic ACTH syndrome rather than Cushing's disease. In addition, whereas excretion of 17-ketosteroids is usually normal or only slightly increased in Cushing's disease, excretion of large amounts is common with ectopic ACTH syndrome. Additional assistance may be obtained by use of the dexamethasone suppression test. Whereas secretion of ACTH and cortisol is diminished by *large* doses of dexamethasone in patients with Cushing's disease, this is *usually* not true in patients with ectopic ACTH syndrome and in patients with adrenal cortical adenomas or carcinomas. An exception exists to the statement that in patients with ectopic ACTH syndrome, ACTH is not suppressible by

glucosteroids; when this syndrome is caused by bronchial carcinoids, dexamethasone treatment *usually* results in suppression of cortisol production. A possible explanation for this unexpected finding is given by the studies in two patient with oatcell carcinoma of the lung and two with pancreatic carcinomas reported by Upton and Amatruda (41). All four patients showed suppression of cortisol secretion with dexamethasone. These neoplasms elaborated both ACTH and a peptide with ability to stimulate ACTH secretion by the pituitary (corticotropin releasing hormone = CRH). If in a given patient, tumor secretion of CRH were principally responsible for excess ACTH secretion, then suppression with dexamethasone might be expected.

Figure 30–1 schematically illustrates the pathophysiology involved in the various disease states resulting in excess glucocorticoid production. In the normal state, ACTH is influenced by three factors: (1) time of day (diurnal variation of ACTH); (2) stress; and (3) a delicate feedback by cortisol. Cushing's *disease* is associated with a change in this feedback. The feedback of cortisol on ACTH secretion is still present, as evidenced by the ability of large doses of glucocorticoids to suppress ACTH and cortisol secretion. In the presence of adrenal neoplasms elaborating cortisol, CRH and ACTH secretion are suppressed. With an autonomous pituitary tumor secreting ACTH, the pathophysiology is uncertain; conceivably CRH may be involved in tumor production and maintenance. In the usual ectopic ACTH syndrome, pituitary

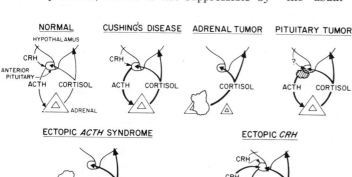

Figure 30–1. Schematic representation of the hypothalamic-pituitary-adrenal interrelationships in normal subjects and in those with various causes of excess ACTH secretion.

ACTH secretion is low, and presumably CRH secretion is low. In ectopic CRH production, however, it is presumed that hyperstimulation of *pituitary* ACTH occurs but may be suppressed by cortisol action directly on the pituitary. Direct proof of this hypothesis does not exist.

Bailey (3) has reported the interesting phenomenon of periodicity in ACTH elaboration by a malignant carcinoid. In this patient, regular cyclic variation in 17-hydroxycorticoid excretion occurred with periodicity of approximately 18 days. During such cycles, excretion of 17-hydroxycorticoids ranged from normal (<10 mg./day) to as high as 150 mg./day. This has not been previously reported. No explanation is available, and whether cyclic variation in hormone production is a common phenomenon in patients with ectopic hormone production is unknown.

The ACTH produced by neoplasms appears to be identical to pituitary ACTH when tested by a variety of immunologic and physiochemical means. Behavior of the two has been identical when tested in several chemical systems, in several radioimmunoassays with different immunologic specificities, and by inactivation through chemical and enzymatic means.*

Treatment of patients with ectopic ACTH syndrome follows well-defined guidelines. As we have tried to emphasize, *recognition* of the syndrome is the most difficult aspect. This is exemplified by a patient described by Vingerhoeds et al. (43). The man had Cushing's syndrome associated with failure of 8 mg. of dexamethasone per day to suppress cortisol production. Bilateral adrenal hyperplasia was found at surgery, and adrenalectomy was performed. Careful search of the abdomen at surgery and of the thorax by x-ray procedures failed to reveal a neoplasm. Eighteen months later a malignant bronchial carcinoid was identified in the thorax and was removed surgically. Although, as I have indicated, dexamethasone suppression and the presence of highly elevated 17-ketosteroid production and hypokalemia are common associates of the ectopic ACTH syndromes, these findings are not infallible. Unfortunately, failure of glucosteroid to suppress ACTH secretion has been reported in Cushing's disease, and the patient of Vingerhoeds et al. was not reported to have hypokalemia (electrolyte levels were not given in the

case report). Excretion of 17-ketosteroids was increased to 37 mg./day.

The main emphasis of treatment is obviously to remove or treat the neoplasm effectively. If this is not possible and the effects of excess cortisol are producing the majority of symptoms, bilateral adrenalectomy or treatment with sufficient doses of the 11-hydroxylase inhibitor, metyrapone, to reduce cortisol production to normal is indicated. The doses of metyrapone required are frequently extremely large—several gram quantities per day. Caution is required in interpreting response to treatment, as some common methods of quantifying cortisol in blood and urine also show reaction to 11-deoxycortisol, the product found in response to metyrapone treatment.

ECTOPIC MELANOCYTE STIMULATING HORMONE PRODUCTION

In mammals, it appears likely that beta melanocyte stimulating hormone (β MSH) is secreted in parallel with ACTH. In 1972 Phifer et al. (31), using specific antisera for identification of cell types, showed that β MSH and ACTH are secreted by the same cells in the normal pituitary. In addition, the pigmentation of patients with Addison's disease and of patients with ACTH-producing pituitary tumors is not solely attributable to the pigmentary effects of ACTH. In 1967 Abe et al. (1) showed that, although some α MSH also was present, the biologic MSH activity in ectopic tumors was predominantly due to β MSH. Several patients with marked hyperpigmentation have been reported, and, when studied, the degree of hyperpigmentation has been correlated with the elevation in circulating β MSH. The frequency of this syndrome is unknown, but it may be as common as the ectopic ACTH syndrome, if ACTH and MSH secretion are usually coexistent. Assays for β MSH and α MSH have not been widely available, but recently Phifer et al. (31) showed that all tumors from four patients with ectopic ACTH syndrome also had increased MSH activity by radioimmunoassay. Isolated MSH production by neoplasms has not been reported, and the frequency of occurrence and types of neoplasms involved must await further study.

ECTOPIC GONADOTROPIN PRODUCTION

Production of polypeptides with gonadotropic activity by *nonpituitary* tissues is rare in nature. In primates, the trophoblastic cells produced during normal gestation produce chorionic gonadotropin, but as far as is known, such a phenomenon does not occur in any other mammals or in lower vertebrates.* Neoplasms derived from trophoblastic cells or from teratomas containing trophoblastic

---

*Since preparation of this chapter, additional data are available. Ratcliffe et al. (*Clin. Endocr. 1:27*, 1972) showed that the ratio of the amino end of ACTH to the carboxyl end as determined by immunoassay was about 10 in the ectopic—considerably higher than in normal pituitary tissue. This could result from unequal degradation of the two ends of ACTH or disproportionate production. Gewertz and Yalow (*Proceedings Endocr. Soc.*, 1973, p. A-53) found that a large amount of ACTH was present in bronchial carcinomas. This ACTH was present in all such carcinomas, whether or not ectopic ACTH syndrome was present, although the content was higher in the tumors associated with the syndrome. Schneider et al. (*Proceeding Endocr. Soc.*, 1973, p. A-52) found that big ACTH had no biologic activity in an *in vitro* assay. Treatment with trypsin produced a biologically potent ACTH indistinguishable from pituitary ACTH. These studies help support the belief that peptide elaboration by neoplasms is common and that immunologically active, biologically inactive material may be produced.

---

*Two nonprimate species possess an extrapituitary gonadotropin: (1) the pregnant mare produces a gonadotropin (pregnant mare's serum gonadotropin) which is elaborated by endometrial cups; (2) the pregnant elephant has also been reported to excrete a pregnancy gonadotropin in urine. Its source is not known.

TABLE 30–5. NEOPLASMS ASSOCIATED WITH GONADOTROPIN PRODUCTION

	Approximate Frequency
Gestational trophoblastic neoplasms (choriocarcinoma, chorioadenoma destruens, hydatidiform mole, etc.)	90%
Carcinoma of the lung	9%
Teratomas (testes, ovary, pineal, mediastinum)	1%
Miscellaneous (hepatoblastoma, malignant melanoma, bladder papillomas, etc.)	Rare*

*Only a few case reports.

cells secrete a gonadotropin similar to chorionic gonadotropin. Other neoplasms not containing trophoblastic cells, such as carcinoma of the lung and hepatoblastomas, also may produce gonadotropin, but the chemical nature of this gonadotropin has not been well studied. Table 30–5 lists the neoplasms that secrete gonadotropins and the approximate relative frequency of their occurrence. Secretion of FSH by neoplasms is extremely rare. Only one patient has been reported for whom such a claim has been made (11). In this tumor, arterial-venous differences were shown for both LH and FSH, using specific radioimmunoassays.

Interestingly, hepatoblastomas which produced precocious puberty by secreting a gonadotropin have been reported only in boys. Precocious puberty also has been caused by pinealomas, ectopic pinealomas, or teratomas of the pineal. While in some patients these tumors have been said to produce precocious puberty by anatomically interfering with the normal process of puberty, those studied by my colleagues and me did so by secreting excess gonadotropin. Few such neoplasms have been routinely studied using sensitive gonadotropin assays, and it is likely that many pinealomas produce precocious puberty by gonadotropin production.

The symptoms of ectopic gonadotropin production are few; thus, this syndrome is probably not detected in many of the patients who have it. If excess gonadotropin production occurs in prepubertal children, precocious sexual maturation occurs, and the neoplasm is generally recognized as being responsible. If excess gonadotropin is produced in adult men, however, the *only* symptom likely to occur is minimal gynecomastia. This minor but very significant finding is frequently missed by the examining physician. In women, amenorrhea or menometrorrhagia may occur.

As was indicated in the introduction to this chapter, however, detection of gonadotropin-producing neoplasms can be extremely important. Unfortunately, screening or following the response to treatment is frequently (but erroneously) performed by physicians using standard pregnancy tests. Urinary pregnancy tests are designed to respond to more than 500–1,000 I.U. of chorionic

gonadotropin per liter. Thus, for a 24-hour urine volume of 2,000 ml., such a test would be positive when 1,000–2,000 I.U./24 hrs. was excreted. The excretion of LH or its equivalent in the urine of normal men and women usually ranges between 1 and 20 I.U./24 hrs. Thus a great range of *abnormal* gonadotropin excretion could exist and not be detected by standard pregnancy tests. Such tests are unlikely to give a false *positive* reaction with normally pregnant women, since gonadotropin production is then very great. However, about 20 per cent of women with nonmetastatic gestational neoplasms studied at the National Institutes of Health by my co-workers and me had negative pregnancy tests, but all produced increased amounts of tumor gonadotropin when studied by adequate assays (33). In men, carcinomas of the lung seldom produce sufficient gonadotropin to give a "positive" pregnancy test. It thus follows that *pregnancy tests should not be used to diagnose or follow response of treatment of gonadotropin-producing neoplasms.* When studied by sufficiently sensitive means, it may be found that gonadotropin production by carcinomas of the lung is more common than realized. Rosen (32) studied nonselected patients with carcinoma of the lung and found about 10 per cent had excess gonadotropin production.

As was stated earlier, the LH, FSH, chorionic gonadotropin, and TSH molecules are composed of two peptide chains. Biologic activity requires that both chains be present. These hormones also contain considerable carbohydrate. The content of sialic acid in chorionic gonadotropin is directly related to the half-time of disappearance of the hormone and to the hormone's biologic properties in some bioassays. Desialated human chorionic gonadotropin has a very short half-life and also possesses very little biologic activity, but it does possess full immunologic activity (42). Table 30–6 presents these data. It is conceivable that some neoplasms elaborate the peptides of chorionic gonadotropin without carbohydrate and the activity is missed by screening such patients with bioassays.

ECTOPIC VASOPRESSIN PRODUCTION

Another syndrome associated with neoplasms is characterized by hyponatremia, persistently hy-

TABLE 30–6. CHANGES IN POTENCIES AS DETERMINED BY BIOASSAY AND RADIOIMMUNOASSAY OF DESIALATED HUMAN CHORIONIC GONADOTROPIN

Per Cent Sialic Acid Removed	Per Cent Biologic Activity Remaining	Per Cent Immunologic Activity Remaining
0	100	100
47	2 to 10*	136†
70	<1	100
100	<1	100

*Bioassay activity was greater using the ventral prostate weight assay than the ovarian ascorbic acid depletion bioassay.

†Immunologic activity was significantly greater than in starting materials.

perosmotic urine, and difficulty with sodium conservation. This syndrome is attributed to the elaboration of vasopressin-like peptides by certain neoplasms. The first description of this syndrome and its explanation was that of Schwartz et al. (35), and since then large numbers of patients have been reported. Amatruda et al. (2), using bioassays, demonstrated the presence of large amounts of antidiuretic substance in an extract of an oatcell carcinoma. Bower and Mason (6) demonstrated a similar material in a primary neoplasm and in its metastasis. That this material was not elicited by excess elaboration of vasopressin from the posterior pituitary was evident because, in the patient of Bower and Mason, the posterior pituitary was replaced by metastatic neoplasm. In 1967 Bartter and Schwartz (4) reported 12 patients with this syndrome and showed that the vasopressin-like material reacted in immunoassay for arginine vasopressin. Vorherr et al. (44) in 1968 also reported a series of such patients in whom the vasopressin reacted identically to arginine vasopressin in radioimmunoassay.

Almost all the patients with this syndrome suffer from bronchogenic carcinoma, but a few isolated reports of other tumor types exist. Treatment of patients with this syndrome should again be directed against the tumor itself. If such treatment is ineffective, then the following temporary alleviations are indicated. Sustained hypersecretion of vasopressin is *not* associated with any symptoms *unless* access to water is permitted; thus restriction of water intake to less than insensible losses will be associated with increase in serum sodium and reversal of symptoms produced by profound water retention and hypo-osmolality.

HYPERCALCEMIA AND CANCERS

Hypercalcemia has been found in association with a great number of neoplasms. In many patients, metastases have been present in bone, and rapid dissolution of bone matrix may exceed the capacity of body control systems to excrete or deposit calcium, thus producing hypercalcemia. Probably many patients with hypercalcemia and metastases in bone also have tumor elaboration of humoral substances which increase blood calcium as well as increased osteoclasia via direct metastases. For example, Table 30-7 lists tumors associated with hypercalcemia and ectopic hormone production. Such lists have not included carcinoma of the breast because patients with metastatic carcinoma of the breast invariably have bone metastases. However, hypercalcemia is very commonly encountered in patients with breast carcinoma and is usually attributed to bone dissolution. Mavligit et al. (23) reported a patient with breast carcinoma, widespread bone metastases, and increased parathyroid hormone content in the neoplasm. In 12 other patients with carcinoma of the breast and *normal* serum calcium, no parathyroid hormone activity was found in tumor extracts. A list of tumors producing hypercalcemia *without* bone metastases may

TABLE 30-7. NEOPLASMS ASSOCIATED WITH ECTOPIC PARATHYROID HORMONE PRODUCTION

Tissue of Origin	Approximate Frequency (Per Cent)
Carcinoma of lung	35
Carcinoma of kidney	24
Carcinoma of ovary	8
Miscellaneous*	each <3

*Carcinoma of breast, uterus, pancreas, urinary bladder, colon, prostate, penis, esophagus, parotid gland, testis (a child), hepatoblastoma (a child), hemangiosarcoma.

falsely indicate that these are the most common neoplasms associated with ectopic parathyroid hormone production. Such may not be the case. However, the causal relationship in such cases is more likely to be correct, especially if tumor treatment results in return of calcium to normal. The majority of patients who have hypercalcemia associated with tumor parathyroid hormone production also have low or low-normal serum phosphorus, as do patients with classic hyperparathyroidism. In contrast, many of the patients with bone metastases and hypercalcemia have hyperphosphatemia. Successful tumor treatment of more than 20 patients, with return of serum calcium to normal, has been reported.

In the majority of patients, when examination has been possible and renal failure was not present, the parathyroid glands have been normal. This indicates that neither primary hyperparathyroidism nor a substance stimulating the parathyroid gland was present. Munson et al. (24) reported immunologic quantification (hemagglutination inhibition) of parathyroid hormone in tumor extracts. Sherwood et al. (36) studied a number of tumor extracts from patients with hypercalcemia; a substance identical to parathyroid hormone by chemical, physical, and immunologic properties was present. Buckle et al. (8) studied a patient with renal adenocarcinoma and hypercalcemia with great care. Tumor extracts gave a dose-response curve identical to bovine parathyroid hormone, and the tumor contained 2,200 ng./ml. parathyroid hormone. Extracts of normal kidney contained none. The parathyroid hormone concentration in renal artery and vein blood from the kidney containing the tumor was 0.62 and 2.55 ng./ml., respectively, illustrating an arteriovenous difference of 1.93 ng./ml. Postoperatively, plasma parathyroid hormone fell to normal.

Recognition of the symptoms of hypercalcemia is important. Patients with polyuria, anorexia, constipation, lethargy, or fatigue, or any patient who is comatose should be suspected of having hypercalcemia. Any patient with a neoplasm should have periodic measurement of serum calcium. Often these neoplasms cause death from hypercalcemia, and intelligent recognition and treatment is of major importance. For example, a patient may be able to maintain a normal or near normal calcium level when up and active. After surgery for any cause and during postoperative inactivity with bed rest, serum calcium may rapidly increase to dangerous levels. Marked inactivity tends to result in mobilization of bone calcium. This mobilization in a patient with ectopic parathyroid hormone production may be the important modifying factor. Treatment of hypercalcemia follows several well-established lines. The simplest form of treatment consists of increasing renal solute load with NaCl infusions. For others, treatment with sodium sulfate infusions, 1–3 liters given continuously over 24 hours, may be required. Treatment with chelating agents (EDTA) (18) or hemodialysis using a calcium-free medium may be required if the first two forms of treatment are inadequate. Obviously, primary treatment of the neoplasm will remove the source of ectopic parathyroid hormone, but frequently this is not rapidly effective if chemotherapy is used, or not possible if the neoplasm is widely metastatic.

There is one other possible etiology of hypercalcemia in patients with carcinoma of the breast. Gordan et al. (13) reported the presence of large amounts of vitamin D–like steroids, stigmasterol acetate, and 17–hydroxysitosterol acetate in the plasma and breast tissue of some patients. Breast tissue from subjects without breast cancer did not contain these potent hypercalcemic agents. This finding was of particular interest, since these are plant steroids not previously reported to be present in human tissues. This report has not been confirmed by other investigators to date.

HYPOGLYCEMIA AND CANCERS

Another interesting syndrome is hypoglycemia caused by nonpancreatic neoplasms. Table 30–8 lists the neoplasms reported to cause hypoglycemia and their estimated frequency. It is noteworthy that about two-thirds of these patients suffer from the relatively rare mesenchymal tumors typified by the fibrosarcoma. Fifty of these mesenchymal tumors causing hypoglycemia were distributed as follows: 12 retroperitoneally, 20 peritoneally (including pelvis), and 18 intrathoracically. No predilection for retroperitoneal areas is thus evident, although these tumors are commonly attributed to retroperitoneal fibromas. All the tumors have been

large, ranging in weight from 800–10,000 g. Many such tumors are benign, and symptoms are completely alleviated by their removal.

The nature of the humoral agent producing hypoglycemia remains unknown. Although these are often called "insulin"-producing tumors, there is no solid evidence to convince one that insulin is being elaborated. Ten extracts of 25 tumors producing hypoglycemia contained an *insulin-like* material by bioassay; that is, using the rat diaphragm or rat epididymal fat pad bioassay (22), this substance *in vitro* stimulated uptake and utilization of glucose. Bushell et al. (9) reported that this substance could increase conversion of glucose to carbon dioxide, also a property shared by insulin. In addition, these workers reported that this activity could be neutralized by excess anti-insulin antiserum. However, in no published account did this material react in insulin immunoassays. It is important to note that neutralization of biologic activity by excess antiserum is not a sensitive test of immunologic similarity or identity; reaction in an immunoassay with production of identical dose-response curves to natural insulin is a more sensitive test. *Failure to react in an insulin immunoassay is powerful evidence that this material is different from insulin.* Field et al. (12) studied in detail extracts of four tumors producing this syndrome. Two had no insulin activity by either bioassay or radioimmunoassay. More importantly, however, two extracts that had insulin-like activity by bioassay failed to react at all in the radioimmunoassay. This study also indicated that these extracts had a biologically active material which was different from human insulin or insulin from many other animal species.*

Although it has often been said that hypoglycemia is caused by excess glucose utilization by the neoplasm itself, there is little evidence to support this. When measured, differences in arterial and venous blood glucose concentrations across the neoplasm have not been great. Furthermore, in an animal neoplasm that produces hypoglycemia, C^{14}-glucose studies failed to reveal excessive glucose utilization by the neoplasm. Silverstein et al. (37) investigated this animal neoplasm. It was capable of producing hypoglycemia in alloxan diabetic mice. Furthermore, three extraction techniques for the neoplasm were studied: saline, acetone, and a standard insulin extraction. Only the acetone extract (not insulin extraction techniques) produced hypoglycemia when injected into other mice; the material from 1 g. of tumor lowered blood sugar by an average of 27 per cent.

Lastly, it has been stated that the hypoglycemia produced by hepatomas may be explained by inadequate glucose output by the liver. Evidence to support this statement is meager. Large amounts of normal liver tissue are often found at autopsy, and liver function studies are often only slightly

TABLE 30–8. TYPES OF NEOPLASMS CAUSING HYPOGLYCEMIA

Tumor Types	Approximate Percentage of Cases
Mesenchymal*	64
Hepatic	21
Adrenal carcinomas	6
Miscellaneous (anaplastic carcinomas, adenocarcinomas, pseudomyxomas, cholangiomas)	9

*Included in this category are fibrosarcomas, mesotheliomas, neurofibromas, neurofibrosarcomas, spindle cell sarcomas, rhabdomyosarcomas, and leiomyosarcomas.

---

*It has recently been shown that somatomedin, a peptide, is probably the same substance previously called "nonsuppressible insulin-like activity" (see Ch. 9). One might postulate that such neoplasms elaborate somatomedin. No data exist to substantiate this hypothesis.

deranged. Hepatic glucose output is a primitive hepatic function and is only inadequate with specific hormonal deficiency states (cortisol and perhaps growth hormone and glucagon deficiency in children), or with terminal hepatic failure when evidence of hepatic dysfunction is clinically *overt*. Hypoglycemia attacks often occur months *before* the presence of a hepatoma is known.

Treatment of hypoglycemia related to these neoplasms is difficult. Obviously, surgical removal of the tumor will completely alleviate symptoms. If this is not possible, drug therapy is sometimes useful. Continuous intravenous administration of 10 or 20 per cent glucose will alleviate symptoms over periods of days. Sometimes, but not commonly, treatment with high doses of glucocorticoids is of assistance. Zinc glucagon (long-acting) and streptozotocin constitute additional and generally more effective measures of preventing hypoglycemia in the presence of inoperable neoplasms.

ECTOPIC ERYTHROPOIETIN PRODUCTION

Erythremia or erythrocytosis has been found in association with a number of neoplasms, and well over 200 patients have been described with this syndrome (22). Table 30–9 lists the types and estimated frequency of these neoplasms. These neoplasms are often not readily apparent, and specific studies directed toward disclosing the presence of a tumor are required. Patients with polycythemia vera often have enlarged spleen, leukocytosis, and thrombocytosis, whereas patients having tumor-caused erythrocytosis usually have only erythremia. Polycythemia has been noted to occur in 1.3–4.5 per cent of patients with renal tumors and in 9–20 per cent of patients with cerebellar hemangioblastomas. The kidney is known to be the normal source of erythropoietin, the hormone that controls the rate of red cell production. Thus, strictly speaking, the renal neoplasm–polycythemia syndrome is not an ectopic hormone syndrome. However, the erythremia associated with cerebellar hemangioblastomas and with pheochromocytomas is observed in the same patient in Lindau-von Hippel syndrome.

This syndrome appears to be caused by elaboration of an erythropoietin-like material by the neoplasm. In over 70 patients, the polycythemia has been reversed following surgical removal of the neoplasm. Erythropoietin has not yet been purified to a high degree, and radioimmunoassays have not yet been developed. Thus, only bioassay data may be reviewed at the time of this writing. Several groups have performed bioassays of tumor extracts or cyst fluid of patients with this syndrome and have found high concentrations of erythropoietin-like activity. The technique of radiation inactivation of biologic activity, a technique that does not require purification, has been used to estimate molecular weight of tumor erythropoietin (22). The molecular weight of tumor and "normal" erythropoietin was identical as determined by the technique. Furthermore, the erythropoietin-like activity associated with neoplasms, in common with true erythropoietin, was inactivated by trypsin or by removal of sialic acid and migrated identically in zone electrophoresis. Interestingly, however, with a single exception, extracts of hepatomas, uterine fibromas, virilizing adrenal cortical tumors, and ovarian tumors have not been shown to possess erythropoietin. Thus the etiology of polycythemia associated with these neoplasms may be different from that associated with cerebellar hemangioblastoma and renal tumors.

HYPERTHYROIDISM AND CANCERS

Fewer than 25 patients who had neoplasms containing trophoblastic cells and a peculiar form of hyperthyroidism have been described (17, 25, 26). Almost all these patients were women with hydatid moles or choriocarcinoma; two men with testicular teratocarcinomas have been reported with this syndrome. All patients reported also excreted huge amounts (over 100,000 I.U. HCG/24 hr.) of gonadotropin. Characteristically, these patients have had few clinical symptoms suggestive of hyperthyroidism. Furthermore, there were few physical findings suggesting thyrotoxicosis. Table 30–10 lists the frequency of physical findings in these patients. Nevertheless, laboratory studies disclosed markedly abnormal increases in thyroidal func-

TABLE 30–9. NEOPLASMS ASSOCIATED WITH POLYCYTHEMIA

Neoplasm	Approximate Percentage of Cases
Renal carcinomas	46
Cerebellar hemangioblastomas	21
Benign renal lesions*	16
Uterine fibromas	6
Adrenal cortical carcinoma or hyperplasia	3
Ovarian neoplasms	3
Hepatomas	3
Pheochromocytomas	1

*Such as hydronephrosis, cysts, and adenomas.

TABLE 30–10. PHYSICAL FINDINGS IN PATIENTS WITH HYPERTHYROIDISM ASSOCIATED WITH TROPHOBLASTIC NEOPLASMS

Finding	Approximate Percentage of Cases*
Tachycardia	100
Skin changes	55
Widened pulse pressure	55
Tremor	20
Goiter	20
Eye signs	10

*Based upon 15 patients.

TABLE 30–11. LABORATORY DATA IN PATIENTS WITH NEOPLASMS AND HYPERTHYROIDISM

	24-hour Urinary Gonadotropin Excretion* (Mouse Units)	Protein-Bound Iodine* (μg./100 ml.)	24-hour Thyroid I^{131} Uptake* (Per Cent)	Plasma TSH Bioassay** (μU./ml.)‡	Plasma TSH RIA† (μU./ml.)‡	LATS (Long-Acting Thyroid Stimulator)†	Tumor TSH Bioassay† (mU./100 g.)‡
	$2–10 \times 10^6$	9.2–18.0	46–82	15–33	4.5	None detected	40 and 300
Normal	200	4–8	15–45	1.0–6.0	0.8–10.0	None	None

*Eight patients.
**Four patients; day-old chick assay using discharge of thyroidal radioiodine.
†Two patients.
‡In terms of Human International Reference Preparation A.

tion. Table 30–11 summarizes the available data. In my laboratory (25) we found that the tumor TSH reacted in TSH bioassays but had little reaction in human pituitary TSH radioimmunoassay. Later Hennen and Pierce (14) and Hershman (16) isolated and partially purified a substance with TSH activity from normal placenta and termed it human placental thyrotropin (HCT). HCT also reacted poorly in human TSH immunoassays but showed significant bioassay activity and, most interestingly, reacted with antisera produced against bovine TSH. Presumably HCT is similar to the TSH substance produced by trophoblastic neoplasms. However, Hershman (15) has recently reported that HCT and tumor TSH are similar but not entirely identical.

MISCELLANEOUS ECTOPIC HORMONE SYNDROMES

A number of other hormonal syndromes exist which will be discussed as a group. These syndromes include gastrin, secretin, kinin, prostaglandin, and growth hormone production. The best known and studied is the Zollinger-Ellison syndrome, which is associated with single or multiple non–beta cell adenomas of the pancreas, single or multiple ulcers in the stomach, commonly in the esophagus and second to fourth portions of the duodenum, and refractoriness to usual medical or surgical treatment. These tumors elaborate a peptide, gastrin, which is normally secreted by the antrum of the stomach and acts to control acid secretion hormonally. Diagnosis may be confirmed by serum gastrin measurements, which are constantly elevated, generally outside the physiologic range. Recently, Yalow and Berson (45) have shown that gastrin activity is associated with molecules of two sizes, a large and a small, perhaps similar to insulin and proinsulin. Serum from one patient studied with the Zollinger-Ellison syndrome contained 80 per cent large gastrin. Further studies are required to determine whether this syndrome is commonly or always associated with an increased fraction of circulating large gastrin. In some instances, pancreatic adenomas are associated with severe diarrhea, and occasionally diarrhea and excess gastrin production occur in the

same patient (7, 40). The etiology of the diarrhea is probably kinin or prostaglandin production, but the evidence is circumstantial. It also appears likely that some of the manifestation of the carcinoid syndromes may stem from kinin production. These syndromes are discussed in a separate chapter.

Ectopic growth hormone production has been only rarely reported. Steiner et al. (39) reported a patient with bronchial carcinoma and osteoarthropathy who had ectopic growth hormone production. Beck and Burger have reported increased growth hormone content in 18 bronchogenic and 8 stomach adenocarcinomas (5a). However, increased growth hormone secretion existing for a few months in adults produces few symptoms, and these few patients may again represent examples of a more widespread, but not commonly recognized abnormality.

About 30 patients have been reported with profound hypophosphatemia associated with neoplasms.* Table 30–12 lists the approximate distribution of these neoplasms; interestingly, many of the neoplasms have been considered incidental or difficult to detect. We have recently seen a patient with this syndrome who had profound hypophosphatemia and osteopenia for 12 years prior to the knowledge that he had a neoplasm. Removal of the neoplasm was associated with reversal of symptoms. The etiology of this syndrome remains obscure. Parathormone was undetectable in one patient when the tumor was present, and was

*For an excellent review see Stanbury, S. W.: Tumour-associated hypophosphatemic osteomalacia and rickets, In *Clinics in Endocrinology & Metabolism.* London, W. B. Saunders Co. Ltd., Vol. 1, March, 1972, p. 256.

TABLE 30–12. NEOPLASMS ASSOCIATED WITH HYPOPHOSPHATEMIA

Neoplasm	Approximate Percentage of Cases
Mesenchymomas, pleomorphic sarcomas, or neurofibromas	60
Sclerosing or cavernous hemangiomas	30
Miscellaneous (e.g., giant cell tumor of rib)	10

present in normal concentrations after tumor removal (34a). All patients studied have profound phosphaturia. This syndrome is often termed "idiopathic acquired hypophosphatemic osteomalacia," and it is possible that both a tumor-caused and a true idiopathic form exist. However, careful and continued search for the presence of a neoplasm is indicated in all patients with this syndrome. Differentiation from "normocalcemic" hyperparathyroidism, familial vitamin D–resistant rickets, and hypophosphatemia caused by excess phosphate-binding antacid ingestion is necessary. The first is unusual in the United States, where vitamin D intake is relatively high.

ECTOPIC PRODUCTION OF MULTIPLE HORMONES BY A SINGLE NEOPLASM

As was mentioned, it appears likely that all neoplasms secreting ectopic ACTH also elaborate peptide fragments with MSH activity. Several patients have been reported with neoplasms that secreted two or more hormones. For example, Law et al. (20) described a 35-year-old woman with non–beta cell carcinoma of the pancreatic islets of Langerhans that produced ACTH, MSH, and gastrin. Becker et al. (5) reported a patient with hepatoma that caused hypercalcemia, erythremia, and hypoglycemia. It is likely that multiple ectopic hormone syndromes will be more commonly described as more widespread availability of bioassay, immunoassay, and receptor assay techniques are available.

REFERENCES

1. Abe, K., Nicholson, W. E., et al.: Radioimmunoassay of βMSH in human plasma and tissues. *J. Clin. Invest.* 46:1609, 1967.
2. Amatruda, T. T., Jr., Mulrow, P. J., et al.: Carcinoma of the lung with inappropriate antidiuresis. *New Eng. J. Med.* 269:544, 1963.
3. Bailey, R. E.: Periodic "hormonogenesis"—a new phenomenon. *J. Clin. Endocr.* 32:317, 1971.
4. Bartter, F. C., and Schwartz, W. B.: The syndrome of inappropriate secretion of antidiuretic hormone. *Amer. J. Med.* 42:790, 1967.
5. Becker, D. J., Sternberg, M. S., et al.: Hepatoma associated with hypoglycemia, polycythemia and hypercalcemia. *J.A.M.A.* 186:1018, 1963.
5a. Beck, C., and Burger, H. G.: Evidence for the presence of immunoreactive growth hormone in cancers of the lung and stomach. *Cancer* 30:75, 1972.
6. Bower, B. F., and Mason, D. M.: Measurement of antidiuretic activity in plasma and tumor in carcinoma of the lung with inappropriate antidiuresis. *Clin. Res.* 12:121, 1964.
7. Brunt, P. W., and Small, W. P.: Secretory tumours of the pancreas: Pancreatic tumour associated with life-threatening diarrhoea. *J. R. Coll. Surg. Edinb.* 15:200, 1970.
8. Buckle, R. M., McMillan, M., et al.: Ectopic secretion of parathyroid hormone by a renal adenocarcinoma in a patient with hypercalcaemia. *Brit. Med. J.* 4:724, 1970.
9. Bushell, B. R., Kirschenfeld, J. J., et al.: Extrapancreatic insulin-secreting tumor. *New Eng. J. Med.* 270:338, 1964.
10. Canfield, R. E., Morgan, F. J., et al.: Studies of human chorionic gonadotropin. *Recent Progr. Hormone Res.* 27:121, 1971.
11. Faiman, C., Colwell, J. A., et al.: Gonadotropin secretion from

12. Field, J. B., Keen, H., et al.: Insulin-like activity of nonpancreatic tumors associated with hypoglycemia. *J. Clin. Endocr.* 23:1229, 1963.
13. Gordan, G. S., Cantino, T., et al.: Osteolytic sterol in human breast cancer. *Science* 151:1226, 1966.
14. Hennen, G., and Pierce, J. G.: Further characterization of the human chorionic thyroid-stimulating factor (HCTSF), In *Protein and Polypeptide Hormones.* Part 2. Margoulies, M. (ed.), Amsterdam, Excerpta Medica Foundation, 1968, p. 511.
15. Hershman, J. M., Higgins, H. P., et al.: Differences between thyroid stimulator in hydatidiform mole and human chorionic thyrotropin. *Metabolism* 19:735, 1970.
16. Hershman, J. M., and Starnes, W. R.: Extraction and characterization of a thyrotropic material from the human placenta. *J. Clin. Invest* 48:923, 1969.
17. Hershman, J. M., and Higgins, H. P.: Hydatidiform mole—a cause of clinical hyperthyroidism. Report of two cases with evidence that the molar tissue secreted a thyroid stimulator. *New Eng. J. Med.* 284:573, 1971.
18. Holland, J. F., Danielson, E., et al.: Use of ethylenediamine tetraacetic acid in hypercalcemic patients. *Proc. Soc. Exp. Biol. Med.* 84:359, 1953.
19. Jones, J. E., Shane, S. R., et al.: Cushing's syndrome induced by the ectopic production of ACTH by a bronchial carcinoid. *J. Clin. Endocr.* 29:1, 1969.
20. Law, D. H., Liddle, G. W., et al.: Ectopic production of multiple hormones (ACTH, MSH and gastrin) by a single malignant tumor. *New Eng. J. Med.* 273:292, 1965.
21. Liddle, G. W., Nicholson, W. E., et al.: Clinical and laboratory studies of ectopic humoral syndromes. *Recent Progr. Hormone Res.* 25:283, 1969.
22. Lipsett, M. B., Odell, W. D., et al.: Humoral syndromes associated with non-endocrine tumors. *Ann. Intern. Med.* 61:733, 1964.
23. Mavligit, G. M., Cohen, J. L., et al.: Ectopic production of parathyroid hormone by carcinoma of the breast. *New Eng. J. Med.* 285:154, 1971.
24. Munson, P. L., Tashjian, A. H., Jr., et al.: Evidence for parathyroid hormone in nonparathyroid tumors associated with hypercalcemia. *Cancer Res.* 25:1062, 1965.
25. Odell, W. D., Bates, R. W., et al.: Increased thyroid function without clinical hyperthyroidism in patients with choriocarcinoma. *J. Clin. Endocr.* 23:658, 1963.
26. Odell, W. D., Hertz, R., et al.: Endocrine aspects of trophoblastic neoplasms. *Clin. Obstet. Gynec.* 10:290, 1967.
27. Omenn, G. S.: Ectopic hormone syndromes associated with tumors in childhood. *Pediatrics* 47:613, 1971.
28. Papkoff, H., and Ekblad, M.: Ovine follicle stimulating hormone: preparation and characterization of its subunits. *Biochem. Biophys. Res. Commun.* 40:614, 1970.
29. Papkoff, H., and Samy, T. S. A.: Isolation and partial characterization of the polypeptide chains of ovine interstitial cell-stimulating hormone. *Biochim. Biophys. Acta* 147:175, 1967.
30. Pierce, J. G., Liao, T. H., et al.: Studies on the structure of thyrotropin: its relationship to luteinizing hormone. *Recent Progr. Hormone Res.* 27:165, 1971.
31. Phifer, R. F., Orth, D. N., et al.: Immunohistologic evidence that β–melanocyte stimulating hormone (βMSH) and adrenocorticotropin (ACTH) are produced by the same human hypophyseal cells. Fourth Int. Cong. Endocrinology, Abstract 573, Washington, D.C., 1972.
32. Rosen, S. W., Becker, C. E., et al.: Ectopic gonadotropin production before clinical recognition of bronchogenic carcinoma. *New Eng. J. Med.* 279:640, 1968.
33. Ross, G. T., Hammond, C. B., et al.: Chemotherapy of metastatic and non-metastatic gestational trophoblastic neoplasms. *Tex. Rep. Biol. Med.* 24:326, 1966.
34. Rudnick, P., and Odell, W. D.: In search of a cancer. *New Eng. J. Med.* 284:405, 1971.
34a. Salassa, R. M., Jowsey, J., et al.: Hypophosphatemic osteomalacia associated with "nonendocrine" tumors. *New Eng. J. Med.* 283:65, 1970.
35. Schwartz, W. B., Bennett, W., et al.: A syndrome of renal sodium loss and hyponatremia probably resulting from inappropriate secretion of antidiuretic hormone. *Amer. J. Med.* 23:529, 1957.

a bronchogenic carcinoma. Demonstration by radioimmunoassay. *New Eng. J. Med.* 277:1395, 1967.

36. Sherwood, L. M., O'Riordan, J. L. H., et al.: Production of parathyroid hormone by non-parathyroid tumors. *J. Clin. Endocr.* 27:140, 1967.

37. Silverstein, M. N., Wakim, K. G., et al.: A hypoglycemic factor in leukemic tumors. *Proc. Soc. Exp. Biol. Med. 103:* 824, 1960.

38. Steigbigel, N. H., Oppenheim, J. J., et al.: Metastatic embryonal carcinoma of the testis associated with elevated plasma TSH-like activity and hyperthyroidism. *New Eng. J. Med. 271:*345, 1964.

39. Steiner, H., Dahlbäck, O., et al.: Ectopic growth hormone production and osteoarthropathy in carcinoma of the bronchus. *Lancet 1:*783, 1968.

40. Tompkins, R. K., Kraft, A. R., et al.: Secretin-like choleresis produced by a diarrheogenic non-beta islet cell tumor of the pancreas. *Surgery 66:*131, 1969.

41. Upton, G. V., Amatruda, T. T.: Evidence for the presence of tumor peptides with corticotropin releasing factor–like activity in the ectopic ACTH syndrome. *New Eng. J. Med. 285:*419, 1971.

42. Van Hall, E. V., Vaitukaitis, J. L., et al.: Immunological and biological activity of HCG following progressive desialylation. *Endocrinology 88:*456, 1971.

43. Vingerhoeds, A. C., der Kinderen, P. J., et al.: Detection of an ACTH secreting bronchial carcinoid tumour, eighteen months after adrenalectomy for Cushing's syndrome. *Acta Endocr. 67:*625, 1971.

44. Vorherr, H., Massry, S. G., et al.: Antidiuretic principle in malignant tumor extracts from patients with inappropriate ADH syndrome. *J. Clin. Endocr. 28:*162, 1968.

45. Yalow, R. S., and Berson, S. A.: Problems of validation of radioimmunoassays, In *Principles of Competitive Protein Binding Assays.* Odell, W. D., and Daughaday, W. H. (eds.), Philadelphia, J. B. Lippincott Co., 1971, p. 374.

INDEX

Note: Page numbers in *italics* refer to illustrations. Page numbers followed by the letter *t* refer to tables.